Vasculitis

Vasculitis

SECOND EDITION

Edited by

Gene V. Ball, MD

The Jane Knight Lowe Professor of Medicine Emeritus
Division of Clinical Immunology and Rheumatology
The University of Alabama at Birmingham
Birmingham, Alabama, USA

and

S. Louis Bridges, Jr., MD, PhD

Professor
Departments of Medicine and Microbiology
Division of Clinical Immunology and Rheumatology
The University of Alabama at Birmingham
Birmingham, Alabama, USA

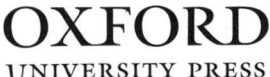
OXFORD
UNIVERSITY PRESS

OXFORD

UNIVERSITY PRESS

Great Clarendon Street, Oxford OX2 6DP

Oxford University Press is a department of the University of Oxford.
It furthers the University's objective of excellence in research, scholarship,
and education by publishing worldwide in

Oxford New York

Auckland Cape Town Dar es Salaam Hong Kong Karachi
Kuala Lumpur Madrid Melbourne Mexico City Nairobi
New Delhi Shanghai Taipei Toronto

With offices in

Argentina Austria Brazil Chile Czech Republic France Greece
Guatemala Hungary Italy Japan Poland Portugal Singapore
South Korea Switzerland Thailand Turkey Ukraine Vietnam

Oxford is a registered trade mark of Oxford University Press
in the UK and in certain other countries

Published in the United States
by Oxford University Press Inc., New York

British Library Cataloguing in Publication Data

Data available

Library of Congress Cataloging-in-Publication Data

ISBN 978–0–19–857019–6

10 9 8 7 6 5 4 3 2 1

Typeset in Minion
by Cepha Imaging Private Ltd., Bangalore, India
Printed in Great Britain
on acid-free paper by
Antony Rowe Ltd., Chippenham

Whilst every effort has been made to ensure that the contents of this book are as complete,
accurate and up-to-date as possible at the date of writing, Oxford University Press is not
able to give any guarantee or assurance that such is the case. Readers are urged to take
appropriately qualified medical advice in all cases. The information in this book is
intended to be useful to the general reader, but should not be used as a means of
self-diagnosis or for the prescription of medication.

This book is dedicated to our families: Sara Jane Ball; Rebecca
Anne and Doug Campagna; Hilary Ball, Julius Ball-Heldman, and
Sam Heldman; and to Ginny, Mary Katherine, and Jack Bridges,
and to the memory of Jeanne LeBlanc Bridges.

Preface

This, the second edition of *Vasculitis*, has been compiled to revise and update all chapters, while adding others, to reflect the major recent advances in the science of immunology as they apply to diagnostic and pathogenetic aspects of vasculitic syndromes and their treatment.

The improvement in treatment is exemplified by the stunning performance in the 2006 Winter Olympics of Irina Slutskaya, a figure skater, whose vasculitis was noted by a television commentator. Prior to 2003, she had won 18 gold medals at various international ice skating competitions, but in that summer she became ill with 'pneumonia, asthmatic bronchitis, pericarditis' and what was finally diagnosed as 'vasculitis'. She was treated with 'strong medication' and improved slowly, returning to international competitions in 2004 and more gold and silver medals. In an interview at the Olympics, she stated that she remained on medication for her vasculitic symptoms and that she hoped to inspire people 'to have faith that you can find your way out of anything'.

Although most vasculitic syndromes are present world-wide, their incidence may vary markedly among different regions of the globe. The geographical distribution of these syndromes has again influenced our choice of authors: vasculitis is uncommon, and experience of dealing with it is acquired slowly. The authors were identified through our knowledge of their clinical or research accomplishments, and their national or international reputations. Our goal was to have chapters written by authors with the greatest expertise, without geographic constraints. For this reason, half of the contributors are from the USA and half from Europe, Asia, and the Middle East. Chapters dealing specifically with pathology, complement, autoantibodies, animal models, PET scanning, and gastrointestinal and cardiopulmonary manifestations have been added. Many of the authors are rheumatologists, but radiologists, immunologists, dermatologists, nephrologists, ophthalmologists, and others contributed substantially. We are grateful to these persons who are busily engaged in patient care and research, and who have given their time and expertise to make the text authoritative. Immunology is one of the areas of biomedical science displaying marked vitality and expansion, and discoveries relevant to the pathogenesis and physiology of inflammation and autoimmunity proceed at an accelerating rate. There are now enough solid data to propose a reasonable explanation for many of the phenomena of vasculitis, and to blend this with clinical observations. Vasculitis causes symptoms primarily through ischemia, which results in a degree of uniformity in some of the syndromes. They all differ in some respects, but their similarities lead inevitably to some repetition in the clinical descriptions as well as in those of diagnostic tools, and treatment. A few chapters in this text deal only with concepts of generic vasculitis. Most, though, describe the pathogenesis of individual syndromes integrated with clinical descriptions and treatment strategies. Elucidations of mechanisms pertaining to the immune response and inflammation are accruing constantly; however, the clinical descriptions in this book are less likely to change with time.

Non-invasive diagnostic tools have been refined considerably in the last decade, and the chapters on diagnosis by imaging studies, particularly non-invasive, are a reflection of their increasing importance in determining the extent of disease, and its management. The discussions of these diagnostic modalities should be useful to clinicians whose circumstances may not allow them first hand experience with these techniques.

Prompt recognition of the various types of inflammatory disorders affecting the vascular system is necessary for distinguishing between those syndromes that are less serious, and those that are threatening to life or limb. Some are trivial and resolve without treatment, while others require the 'desperate appliances' of Hamlet. We are confident this text will guide physicians of varied disciplines to better patient care, the goal of any clinical text.

Acknowledgements

The editors gratefully acknowledge the secretarial assistance of Paula Kiley, the editorial assistance of Helen Liepman and Anna Winstanley of Oxford University Press, and the support of research in clinical immunology and rheumatology at UAB provided by Marguerite Jones Harbert.

Contents

Contributors

Adil Al-Nahhas, MSc, FRCP Consultant and Chief of Service, Department of Nuclear Medicine, Hammersmith Hospital, London, England, UK.

T. Prescott Atkinson, MD, PhD Associate Professor of Pediatrics, Division of Developmental and Clinical Immunology, University of Alabama at Birmingham, Birmingham, Alabama, USA.

Gülsevim Azizlerli, MD Professor of Dermatology, Istanbul University Faculty of Medicine, Istanbul, Turkey.

Paul A. Bacon, MD, FRCP Rheumatology Department, University of Birmingham, Edgbaston, Birmingham, England, UK.

Gene V. Ball, MD Jane Knight Lowe Professor Emeritus, Division of Clinical Immunology and Rheumatology, University of Alabama at Birmingham, Birmingham, Alabama, USA.

Holly Bastian, MD, MSPH Assistant Professor of Medicine, Division of Clinical Immunology and Rheumatology, University of Alabama at Birmingham, Birmingham, Alabama, USA.

S. Louis Bridges, Jr, MD, PhD Professor of Medicine and Microbiology, Division of Clinical Immunology and Rheumatology, University of Alabama at Birmingham, Birmingham, Alabama, USA.

Daniel E. Bullard, PhD Associate Professor, Department of Genetics, University of Alabama at Birmingham, Birmingham, Alabama, USA.

Leonard H. Calabrese, DO Professor of Medicine, Cleveland Clinic Lerner College of Medicine of Case Western Reserve University, Vice Chairman, Department of Rheumatic and Immunologic Diseases, R. J. Fasenmyer Chair of Clinical Immunology, The Cleveland Clinic Foundation, Cleveland, Ohio, USA.

Sumapa Chaiamnuay, MD Fellow, Division of Clinical Immunology and Rheumatology, University of Alabama at Birmingham, Birmingham, Alabama, USA.

W. Winn Chatham, MD Professor of Medicine, Division of Clinical Immunology and Rheumatology, University of Alabama at Birmingham, Birmingham, Alabama, USA.

Sharon A. Chung, MD Clinical Fellow, Division of Rheumatology, University of California at San Francisco, San Francisco, California, USA.

Andrew Churg, MD Department of Pathology, University of British Columbia, Vancouver, BC, Canada.

Professor Jan W. Cohen Tervaert, MD, PhD Department of Clinical Immunology, University Hospital Maastricht, Maastricht, The Netherlands.

Elena Csernok, PhD Associate Professor, Medical University at Lübeck, Lübeck, Germany.

David P. D'Cruz, MD FRCP The Lupus Research Unit, The Rayne Institute, St Thomas' Hospital, London, England, UK.

Amy E. DeVore, MD Resident, Department of Dermatology, Wake Forest University School of Medicine, Winston-Salem, North Carolina, USA.

George F. Duna, MD, FACP Associate Professor of Medicine, Baylor College of Medicine, Chief of Rheumatology, St. Luke's Episcopal Hospital, Houston, Texas, USA.

Barri J. Fessler, MD Assistant Professor of Medicine, Director, Multidisciplinary Vasculitis Clinic, Division of Clinical Immunology and Rheumatology, University of Alabama at Birmingham, Birmingham, Alabama, USA.

C. Stephen Foster, MD, FACS Clinical Professor of Ophthalmology, Harvard Medical School, Boston, Massachusetts, USA.

Stephen K. Frankel, MD Assistant Professor of Medicine, Division of Pulmonary Sciences and Critical Care Medicine, University of Colorado at Denver and Health Sciences Center, Denver, Colorado, USA.

Izzet Fresko, MD Associate Professor, Division of Rheumatology, Cerrahpaşa Medical Faculty, University of Istanbul, Istanbul, Turkey.

Massimo Galli, MD, PhD Associate Professor, Institute of Infectious Diseases, University of Milan, Milan, Italy.

Carlos Garcia-Porrúa, MD, PhD Rheumatology Staff, Hospital Xeral-Calde, Lugo, Spain.

Miguel A. Gónzalez-Gay, MD, PhD Rheumatology Staff, Hospital Xeral-Calde, Lugo, Spain.

Wolfgang L. Gross, MD Professor of Internal Medicine and Rheumatology, Director, Department of Rheumatology, University Hospital of Schleswig-Holstein, Campus Lübeck and Rheumaklinik Bad Bramstedt, Lübeck, Germany.

Loïc Guillevin, MD Professor of Medicine, Department of Internal Medicine, Hôpital Cochin, University of Paris 5 René-Descartes, Assistance Publique–Hôpitaux de Paris, Paris, France.

Bernhard Hellmich, MD, PhD Department of Rheumatology, University Hospital of Schleswig-Holstein, Campus Luebeck, and Rheumaklinik Bad Bramstedt, Lübeck, Germany.

Konstanze Holl-Ulrich, MD Department of Pathology, University of Lübeck, Lübeck, Germany.

Larry Horesh, MD Memorial Health University Physicians, Savannah Vascular Institute, Provident Professorial Building, Savannah, Georgia, USA.

Graham R.V. Hughes, MD Consultant Rheumatologist, The Louise Coote Lupus Unit, St. Thomas Hospital, London, England, UK.

Laura B. Hughes, MD, MSPH Assistant Professor of Medicine, Division of Clinical Immunology and Rheumatology, University of Alabama at Birmingham, Birmingham, Alabama, USA.

K. Kwasind Huston, MD Fellow, Division of Rheumatology, Johns Hopkins University School of Medicine, Baltimore, Maryland, USA.

Fulvio Invernizzi, MD, PhD St. Paul Hospital, University of Milan, Milan, Italy.

Joseph L. Jorizzo, MD Department of Dermatology, Wake Forest University School of Medicine, Winston-Salem, North Carolina, USA.

Cees G. M. Kallenberg, MD, PhD Department of Clinical Immunology, University Hospital Groningen, Groningen, The Netherlands.

Saravanan Kasthuri, MD Interventional Radiologist, Pacific Medical Imaging, Wenatchee, Washington, USA.

Hirohisa Kato, MD, PhD, FACC Professor Emeritus, Department of Pediatrics, Honorary Director, The Cardiovascular Research Institute, Kurume University, Kurume, Japan

Munther A. Khamashta, MD Consultant Physician, The Louise Coote Lupus Unit, St. Thomas Hospital, London, England, UK.

Yasushi Kobayashi, MD, PhD Section of Immunobiology, Yale University School of Medicine, New Haven, Connecticut, USA.

Alisa Erika Koch, MD Frederick G. L. Huetwell and William D. Robinson, MD Professor of Rheumatology, Division of Rheumatology, Department of Internal Medicine, University of Michigan Medical School, Ann Arbor, Michigan, USA.

Emire Kural-Seyahi, MD Division of Rheumatology, Department of Medicine, Cerrahpaşa Medical Faculty, University of Istanbul, Istanbul, Turkey.

Professor Peter Lamprecht Department of Rheumatology, University Hospital of Schleswig-Holstein, Campus Lübeck, and Rheumaklinik Bad Bramstedt, Lübeck, Germany.

Robert Leonardo, MD Interventional Radiologist, Department of Radiology, The Long Island College Hospital, Brooklyn, New York, USA.

Raashid A. Luqmani, DM, FRCP (E) Rheumatology Department, University of Edinburgh, Edinburgh, Scotland, UK.

Melike Melikoglu, MD Fellow in Rheumatology, Cerrahpaşa Medical Faculty, University of Istanbul, Istanbul, Turkey.

Giuseppe Monti, MD Chief, Medicine Department, Saronno Hospital, Saronno, Italy.

Gideon Nesher, MD Clinical Associate Professor of Medicine, The Hebrew University Medical School, Chairman of Department of Internal Medicine and the Rheumatology Service, Shaare-Zedek Medical Center, Jerusalem, Israel.

Ronit Nesher, MD Lecturer in Ophthalmology, Tel-Aviv University Sackler School of Medicine, Department of Ophthalmology, Meir Medical Center, Kfar-Saba, Israel.

Shin J. Oh, MD Professor of Neurology, Department of Neurology, University of Alabama at Birmingham, Birmingham VA Medical Center, Birmingham, Alabama, USA.

Sumru Onal, MD Fellow, Massachusetts Eye Research and Surgery Institute, Cambridge, Massachusetts, USA. Instructor, Department of Ophthalmology, Marmara University, School of Medicine, Istanbul, Turkey.

Christian Pagnoux Department of Internal Medicine, Hôpital Cochin, University of Paris 5 René-Descartes, Assistance Publique–Hôpitaux de Paris, Paris France.

Ross E. Petty, MD, PhD Professor of Pediatrics, University of British Columbia, and Head, Division of Rheumatology, Department of Pediatrics, British Columbia Children's Hospital, Vancouver, British Columbia, Canada.

Gaafar M. Ragab, MD Rheumatology and Immunology, Faculty of Medicine, Cairo University, Cairo, Egypt.

Brad K. Rodu, DDS Professor of Medicine, University of Louisville School of Medicine, Louisville, Kentucky, USA.

Enrique A. Sabater, MD Senior Associate Consultant, Department of Diagnostic Radiology, Mayo Clinic, Rochester, Minnesota, USA.

Kenneth E. Sack, MD Professor of Clinical Medicine, University of California at San Francisco, San Francisco, California, USA.

Souheil Saddekni, MD Professor of Radiology, Director of Vascular and Interventional Radiology, University of Alabama at Birmingham, Birmingham, Alabama, USA.

Trenton R. Schoeb, DVM, PhD Professor of Genetics, University of Alabama at Birmingham, Birmingham, Alabama, USA.

Marvin I. Schwarz, MD James C. Campbell Professor of Pulmonary Medicine, Division of Pulmonary Sciences and Critical Care Medicine, University of Colorado at Denver and Health Sciences Center, Denver, Colorado, USA.

David G. I. Scott, MD, FRCP Honorary Professor, School of Health, University of East Anglia, Norwich, England, UK.

Philip Seo, MD, MHS Assistant Professor of Medicine, Division of Rheumatology, Department of Medicine, John Hopkins University School of Medicine, Baltimore, Maryland, USA.

Ulrich Specks, MD Professor of Medicine, Mayo Clinic College of Medicine, Division of Pulmonary and Critical Care Medicine, Mayo Clinic, Rochester, Minnesota, USA.

Anthony W. Stanson, MD Professor of Radiology, Department of Diagnostic Radiology, Mayo Clinic, Rochester, Minnesota, USA.

John H. Stone, MD, MPH Associate Professor of Medicine, Director, Johns Hopkins Vasculitis Center, Johns Hopkins University School of Medicine, Baltimore, Maryland, USA.

Zoltán Szekanecz, MD, PhD, DSc Associate Professor of Medicine, Immunology and Rheumatology, 3rd Department of Medicine, University of Debrecen Medical Center, Debrecen, Hungary.

Kei Takahashi, MD, PhD Associate Professor of Pathology, Toho University, Tokyo, Japan

Luis Teixeira Department of Internal Medicine, Hôpital Cochin, University of Paris 5 René-Descartes, Assistance Publique–Hôpitaux de Paris, Paris, France.

Gim Gee Teng, MD Fellow, Division of Clinical Immunology and Rheumatology, University of Alabama at Birmingham, Birmingham, Alabama, USA.

Kitti Totemchokchyakarn, MD Assistant Professor of Medicine, Division of Allergy, Immunology, and Rheumatology, Department of Medicine, Ramathibodi Hospital, Mahidol University, Bangkok, Thailand.

Nadarajah Vigneswaran, BSS, DMD Associate Professor, Department of Stomatology, The University of Texas – Houston Health Science Center, Houston, Texas, USA.

John E. Volanakis, MD Professor Emeritus, Department of Medicine, University of Alabama at Birmingham, Birmingham, Alabama, USA.

Richard A. Watts, DM, FRCP Honorary Consultant Rheumatologist, Norfolk and Norwich Hospital, Honorary Senior Lecturer, University of East Anglia, Norwich, England, UK.

Myles Webb, FRACP Department of Nuclear Medicine, The Prince Charles Hospital, Brisbane, Australia.

Fredrick M. Wigley, MD Professor of Medicine, Associate Director, Division of Rheumatology, Director, Johns Hopkins Scleroderma Center, Johns Hopkins University School of Medicine, Baltimore, Maryland, USA.

Allan S. Wiik, MD, D.Sci (Med) Department of Autoimmunology, Statens Serum Institut, Copenhagen, Denmark.

Hasan Yazici, MD Professor and Chief, Division of Rheumatology, Department of Medicine, Cerrahpaşa Medical Faculty, University of Istanbul, Istanbul, Turkey.

Abbreviations

ACE	angiotensin-converting enzyme	GMB	glomerular basement membrane
ACR	American College of Rheumatology	GCA	giant cell arteritis
ADCC	antibody-dependent cellular toxicity	G-CSF	granulocyte-colony stimulating factor
AECA	antiendothelial cell antibodies	GSE	gluten-sensitive enteropathy
AGBMA	antiglomerular basement membrane antibodies	HBV	hepatitis B virus
ANCA	antineutrophil cytoplasmic antibody	HCL	hairy cell leukemia
BRVO	branch retinal vein occlusion	HCV	hepatitis C virus
BS	Behçet's syndrome	HeAU	herpetiform aphthous ulcers
BUN	blood urea nitrogen	HIV	human immunodeficiency virus
BVAS	Birmingham Vasculitis Activity Score	HRCT	high-resolution computed tomography
CBC	complete blood count	HSP	Henoch–Schönlein purpura
CD	Crohn's disease	HSV	herpes simplex virus
CHCC	Chapel Hill Consensus Conference	HUV	hypocomplementemic urticarial vasculitis
CMV	cytomegalovirus	HUVEC	human umbilical vein endothelial cell
CNS	central nervous system	ICAM-1	intercellular adhesion molecule-1
CPN	classis periarteritis nodosa	IFN	interferon
CRP	C-reactive protein	ISKDC	International Study for Kidney Disease in Children
CRVO	central retinal vein occlusion		
CSS	Churg–Strauss syndrome	IVIG	intravenous immunoglobulin
CSVV	cutaneous small-vessel vasculitis	JDM	juvenile dermatomyositis
CT	computed tomography	JRA	juvenile rheumatoid arthritis
CTA	computed tomography angiography	KD	Kawasaki's disease
CUS	chronic ulcerative stomatitis	LFA-1	lymphocyte function-associated antigen-1
CYC	cyclophosphamide	LMV	lupus mesenteric vasculitis
DAH	diffuse alveolar hemorrhage	MAbs	monoclonal antibodies
DEI	disease extent index	MALT	mucosa-associated lymphoid tissue
DMARD	disease modifying antirheumatic drug	M-CSF	macrophage-colony stimulating factor
DSA	digital subtraction angiography	MDS	melodysplastic syndromes
EBV	Epstein–Barr virus	MHC	major histocompatibility complex
EC	endothelial cells	MiAU	minor aphthous ulcers
ECP	eosinophil cationic protein	MjAU	major aphthous ulcers
EED	erythema elevatum diutinum	MPA	microscopic polyangiitis
ELAM-1	endothelial–leukocyte adhesion molecule-1	MPO	myeloperoxidase
ELISA	enzyme-linked immunoabsorbent assay	MRA	magnetic resonance angiography
EM	erythema multiforme	MRI	magnetic resonance imaging
EMC	essential mixed cryoglubulinemia	MTX	methotrexate
ESR	erythrocyte sedimentation rate	NIH	National Institutes of Health
fMLP	formyl-methionine leucine phenylalanine	NK	natural killer cell
FUO	fever of unknown origin	PAN	polyarteritis nodosa
GACNS	granulomatous angiitis of the central nervous system	PACNS	primary angiitis of the central nervous system
		PCR	polymerase chain reaction

PET	positron emission tomography	TA	Takayasu's arteritis
PMN	polymorphonuclear neutrophil	TAO	thromboangiitis obliterans
PPD	purified protein derivative	TNF	tumor necrosis factor
PTA	percutaneous balloon angioplasty	TSST	toxic shock syndrome toxin
RA	rheumatoid arthritis	UC	ulcerative colitis
RAS	recurrent aphthous stomatitis	US	ultrasonography
RBC	red blood cell	VCAM	vascular cell adhesion molecule
RMSF	Rocky Mountain spotted fever	VGEF	vascular endothelial growth factor
SLE	systemic lupus erythematosus	VZV	varicella zoster virus
SPECT	single photon emission computed tomography	WBC	white blood cell
		WG	Wegener's granulomatosis

PART 1

Introductory chapters

CHAPTER 1

Classification of vasculitic syndromes

Gene V. Ball and S. Louis Bridges, Jr

Much has been written about the inadequacies of present schemes for classifying and diagnosing vasculitis, and the misapplication of classification schemes to the diagnosis of an individual's illness. The most frequently cited classification in the recent past was devised by a committee of the American College of Rheumatology (ACR) for the purpose of facilitating research (Bloch *et al.* 1990; Fries *et al.* 1990; Hunder *et al.* 1990a). The authors of this scheme for classifying seven distinct vasculitic syndromes (Arend *et al.* 1990; Calabrese *et al.* 1990; Hunder *et al.* 1990b; Leavitt *et al.* 1990; Lightfoot *et al.* 1990; Masi *et al.* 1990; Mills *et al.* 1990) stated explicitly that the criteria were not meant for diagnostic purposes in an individual patient. They have, however, have been useful in differentiating one vasculitis syndrome from another. Recognizing the widespread use of the criteria for diagnosis, Rao, Allen, and Pincus (1998) evaluated their effectiveness in diagnosing Wegener's granulomatosis (WG), giant cell arteritis (GCA), polyarteritis nodosa (PAN), and hypersensitivity vasculitis in 198 patients referred to medical centers with diagnoses of possible vasculitis. They concluded that when the criteria were applied to these patients, their positive predictive values for WG, GCA, PAN, and hypersensitivity vasculitis ranged from only 17% to 29%. Thus, there is empirical evidence that the ACR criteria should not be used for diagnosis of specific syndromes in patients without confirmed diagnosis of vasculitis. This is in accordance with the intent of the committee: that the criteria not be used to distinguish vasculitis from other diseases, and that the criteria were established to insure uniformity in epidemiologic and other research studies (Hunder *et al.* 1990a). The ACR and later definitional criteria require that vasculitis be established as a prerequisite for defining a specific vasculitic syndrome. For most syndromes, a histologic diagnosis of vasculitis, whose classical features are endothelial swelling, inflammatory infiltrates, and fibrinoid necrosis, is required or recommended strongly but the biopsy findings must be correlated with clinical and laboratory data, and with the understanding that the histologic features of vascular lesions may change with time (see Chapter 9).

The concept of surrogate markers of vasculitis such as antineutrophil cytoplasmic antibodies (ANCA) and imaging studies, which are not features of the ACR classification criteria, recognizes that histologic diagnosis is not always possible. Although the ACR classification criteria have been useful for establishing uniform criteria for inclusion of patients in research studies, they were promulgated before widespread availability of reliable assays for ANCA. They did not differentiate PAN and microscopic polyangiitis (MPA); however, the specificity for WG and Churg–Strauss syndrome (CSS) appear to be 92% and 99.7%, respectively.

Because of confusion concerning classification *vis-à-vis* diagnosis, one might consider the dictionary definitions of these two words. The Oxford English Dictionary defines classification as arranging in classes according to common characteristics or affinities. Diagnosis is defined as identification of a disease by careful investigation of its symptoms and history, or distinctive characterization in precise terms. The definition of diagnosis stresses the identification of the nature and cause of a disease through evaluation of all clinical and laboratory data. Jennette *et al.* (1994), in their influential proposal on the nomenclature of systemic vasculitides, observed that "it is advantageous for everyone to use the same name for the same disease, and to do this, there must be clear agreement on the definition of the name and therefore of the disease." This seems straightforward; however, while acknowledging that a diagnosis is, in essence, the name of a disease, they disavowed determination of clinical criteria required to classify or diagnose individual patients. Diagnostic criteria would require analysis of large numbers of patients with unequivocal defining features. Jennette *et al.* (1994) tabulated the names and definitions of 10 of the more common vasculitides (see Table 26.2 in Chapter 26). These definitions are expanded in the chapters of this text dealing with individual diseases. Discussion of criteria for the classification/diagnosis of childhood vasculitis can be found in Chapter 22.

The ambiguities of clinical presentations, limited diagnostic laboratory tests, and difficulty in obtaining appropriate tissue for histologic examination (which may not provide categorical information) may impede precise diagnosis/ classification at any time. Furthermore, a diagnosis that is perfectly tenable at a given time, may later be inappropriate for a patient whose disease has evolved over time. This is particularly true of cutaneous leukocytoclastic angiitis, probably the most common of the vasculitides, which may be the sole manifestation of a vasculitis that later blossoms into a systemic disease. This concept of a changing clinical condition, requiring the rethinking of a diagnosis, applies to many non-vasculitic diseases as well.

One of the first descriptions of a specific systemic vasculitis was that of polyarteritis (periarteritis) nodosa (PAN) by Kussmaul and

Maier in 1866. Despite their detailed and careful description of the gross and microscopic anatomy of a disease defined by anatomical characteristics, the term was used thereafter in a generic sense to encompass all types of vasculitis. Other distinctive vasculitic syndromes were recognized as WG in 1936, and CSS in 1951, and in 1952, Zeek proposed a classification of vasculitis, from which most, if not all, others have descended. Her "necrotizing angiitis" differentiated hypersensitivity angiitis; allergic granulomatous angiitis; rheumatic arteritis; periarteritis nodosa; and temporal arteritis.

Disease characteristics that have been used for diagnosis/classification have included: size, type, and distribution of involved vessels; histologic appearance of the vessels and extravascular lesions; clinical and laboratory features; and associations with other disorders. The size of diseased vessels has been the major criterion for classifying these disorders in most schemes, and size is the major determinant of the clinical symptoms. Large size signifies the aorta and its branches; medium signifies vessels that, while smaller than the major branches of the aorta, contain an internal elastic membrane as well as muscular media and adventitia. Small size denotes capillaries, and post capillary venules and arterioles. The value of this diagnostic classification is limited by the difficulty in acquiring tissue from visceral organs, as well as the variation within major syndromes in regards to the predominant size of affected vessels. For example, although GCA is predominantly a disease of large arteries, smaller vessels are sometimes involved. Another example, using GCA again: this disease, described by Hutchinson in 1890, may differ significantly in its clinical features from Takayasu's arteritis, which was described in 1909, yet both affect large arteries primarily, as do other, albeit, rare syndromes. The distinctions between these two syndromes are based in large part on age of onset, the former after 50 years, and the latter before age 50. Any valid classification that will be used for diagnostic purposes must be based on other features as well. These include: the organ distribution of lesions; the presence or absence of granulomatous inflammation; the presence of certain infections; autoantibodies such as ANCA; and the age of the patient.

The Chapel Hill Consensus Conference (CHCC) on the Nomenclature of Systemic Vasculitides definition of PAN makes it accord more closely to the classic description by Kussmaul and Maier (1866) of a medium or small-sized arteritis, without disease in arterioles, venules, and capillaries, and with sparing of pulmonary arteries (Jennette *et al.* 1994) (see Table 26.4 in Chapter 26). The CHCC nomenclature purges PAN of small-vessel disease, assigning this and glomerulonephritis to the syndrome of MPA, which was probably first described (as microscopic periarteritis nodosa) in 1923 by Friedrich Wohlwill (Wohlwill 1923). Cupps and Fauci, in their textbook *The Vasculitides* (1981), referred to a group of patients with clinical and pathologic characteristics of both classic PAN and allergic angiitis, but who did not fit precisely into either category. Lesions of muscular arteries, arterioles, and venules typified the syndrome, which they referred to as an "overlap". This is probably the group now referred to as ANCA-associated vasculitis which differs from classic PAN, not only in size of affected vessels, but in the relative absence of immune complex deposits, the frequent presence of ANCA, and involvement of lungs and glomeruli, which are characteristic of MPA, CSS, and WG. ANCA are found in about 75% of these three disorders.

In general, about 75% of patients with WG are cANCA positive; about 40–75% of CSS patients are positive for either cANCA or pANCA, and pANCA is found in about 50–75% of MPA. Either type of ANCA can be found in any of these three disorders, and are absent in 5 to 30%. The important role of ANCA in the diagnosis of various forms of vasculitis was recognized in the Chapel Hill Consensus Conference on nomenclature, which led to promulgation of definitions for 10 vasculitic syndromes.

The classification scheme given here (Table 1.1) embodies features of both ACR and CHCC criteria and the vasculitides *per se*, some of which are secondary to other defined diseases such as sarcoidosis. Vasculitis embraces complex syndromes, the clinical and laboratory features of which are to be found in individual chapters in this text. The clinician caring for a patient with presumed vasculitis must integrate all the data obtained by direct observation and by clinical laboratory testing. Although there is much emphasis placed in these chapters on the need for microscopic examination of material obtained by biopsy, it is increasingly clear that imaging studies can often be satisfactory surrogates for invasive biopsies. An object of the clinician's assessment is to determine the presence or absence of lesions in vital organs, their activity, and their functional consequences. Assessment is not usually a one-time thing: the clinician should view vasculitis as not necessarily static. The application of classification criteria to diagnosis requires careful integration of all available data.

Table 1.1 Classification of vasculitis emphasizing the predominant size of involved vessels

Large vessel	
More common	*Less common*
Giant cell (temporal) arteritis	Sarcoidosis (may be large, medium, or small)
Takayasu's arteritis	Cogan's syndrome (may be large or medium)
Wiskott–Aldrich syndrome (may be large or small)	
Medium vessel	
Polyarteritis nodosa	
Hepatitis B virus-related	
Familial Mediterranean fever	
Cutaneous polyarteritis nodosa	
Kawasaki's disease	
Medium to small vessel	
More common	*Less common*
Wegener's granulomatosis	Primary angiitis of the CNS
Churg–Strauss syndrome	Thromboangiitis obliterans
Microscopic polyangiitis (polyarteritis)	
Vasculitis of connective tissue diseases	
Behçet's syndrome (may be large)	
Small vessel	
More common	*Less common*
Cutaneous leukocytoclastic angiitis	Paraneoplastic
Henoch–Schönlein purpura	Degos' disease
Cryoglobulinemic vasculitis	Urticarial vasculitis
	Myelodysplastic syndromes
	Erythema elevatum diutinum
	Hyperimmunoglobulin D

References

Arend, W. P., Michel, B. A., Bloch, D. A., Hunder, G. G., Calabrese, L. H., Edworthy, S. M., Fauci, A. S., Leavitt, R. Y., Lie, J. T. and Lightfoot, R. W. Jr. (1990). The American College of Rheumatology 1990 criteria for the classification of Takayasu arteritis. *Arthritis and Rheumatism*, **33,** 1129–34.

Bloch, D. A., Michel, B. A., Hunder, G. G., McShane, D. J., Arend, W. P., Calabrese, L. H., Edworthy, S. M., Fauci, A. S., Fries, J. F. and Leavitt, R. Y. (1990). The American College of Rheumatology 1990 criteria for the classification of vasculitis. Patients and methods. *Arthritis and Rheumatism*, **33,** 1068–73.

Calabrese, L. H., Michel, B. A., Bloch, D. A., Arend, W. P., Edworthy, S. M., Fauci, A. S., Fries, J. F., Hunder, G. G., Leavitt, R. Y. and Lie, J. T. (1990). The American College of Rheumatology 1990 criteria for the classification of hyper-sensitivity vasculitis. *Arthritis and Rheumatism*, **33,** 1108–13.

Cupps, T. R. and Fauci, A. S. (1981). *The vasculitides: major problems in internal medicine*, vol. 21. W. B. Saunders, Philadelpia.

Fries, J. F., Hunder, G. G., Bloch, D. A., Michel, B. A., Arend, W. P., Calabrese, L. H., Fauci, A. S., Leavitt, R. Y., Lie, J. T. and Lightfoot, R. W. Jr. (1990). The American College of Rheumatology 1990 criteria for the classification of vasculitis. Summary. *Arthritis and Rheumatism*, **33,**1135–6.

Hunder, G. G., Arend, W. P., Bloch, D. A., Calabrese, L. H., Fauci, A. S., Fries, J. F., Leavitt, R. Y., Lie, J. T., Lightfoot, R. W. Jr. and Masi, A. T. (1990a). The American College of Rheumatology 1990 criteria for the classification of vasculitis. Introduction. *Arthritis and Rheumatism*, **33,**1065–7.

Hunder, G. G., Bloch, D. A., Michel, B. A., Stevens, M. B., Arend, W. P., Calabrese, L. H., Edworthy, S. M., Fauci, A. S., Leavitt, R. Y. and Lie, J. T. (1990b). The American College of Rheumatology 1990 criteria for the classification of giant cell arteritis. *Arthritis and Rheumatism*, **33,** 1122–8.

Jennette, J. C., Falk, R. J., Andrassy, K., Bacon, P. A., Churg, J., Gross, W. L., Hagen, E. C., Hoffman, G. S., Hunder, G. G. and Kallenberg, C. G. (1994). Nomenclature of systemic vasculitides. Proposal of an international consensus conference. *Arthritis and Rheumatism*, **37,** 187–92.

Kussmaul, A. and Maier, R. (1866). On a previously undescribed peculiar arterial disease (periarteritis nodosa), accompanied by Bright's disease and rapidly progressive general muscle weakness. *Deutsches Archiv fur klinische Medicin*, **1,** 484. (Translated by E. Matteson.)

Leavitt, R. Y., Fauci, A. S., Bloch, D. A., Michel, B. A., Hunder, G. G., Arend, W. P., Calabrese, L. H., Fries, J. F., Lie, J. T. and Lightfoot, R. W. Jr. (1990). The American College of Rheumatology 1990 criteria for the classification of Wegener's granulomatosis. *Arthritis and Rheumatism*, **33,** 1101–107.

Lightfoot, R. W. Jr., Michel, B. A., Bloch, D. A., Hunder, G. G., Zvaifler, N. J., McShane, D. J., Arend, W. P., Calabrese,L. H., Leavitt, R. Y. and Lie, J. T. (1990). The American College of Rheumatology 1990 criteria for the classification of polyarteritis nodosa. *Arthritis and Rheumatism*, **33,** 1088–93.

Masi, A. T., Hunder, G. G., Lie, J. T., Michel, B. A., Bloch, D. A., Arend, W. P., Calabrese, L. H., Edworthy, S. M., Fauci, A. S. and Leavitt, R. Y. (1990). The American College of Rhematology 1990 criteria for the classification of Churg–Strauss syndrome (allergic granulomatosis and angiitis). *Arthritis and Rheumatism*, **33,** 1094–100.

Mills, J. A., Michel, B. A., Bloch, D. A., Calabrese, L. H., Hunder, G. G., Arend, W. P., Edworthy, S. M., Fauci, A. S., Leavitt, R. Y. and Lie, J. T. (1990). The American College of Rheumatology 1990 criteria for the classification of Henoch–Schönlein purpura. *Arthritis and Rheumatism*, **33,** 1114–21.

Rao, J. K., Allen, N. B. and Pincus, T. (1998). Limitations of the 1990 American College of Rheumatology classification criteria in the diagnosis of vasculitis. *Annals of Internal Medicine*, **129,** 345–52.

Wohlwill, F, (1923). Über die nur mikroskopisch erkennbare Form der Periarteritis nodosa. *Virchows Arch Pathol Anat Physiol*, **246,** 377–411.

CHAPTER 2

Epidemiology of vasculitis

Richard A. Watts and David G. I. Scott

Introduction

The vasculitis syndromes are a group of relatively uncommon conditions whose etiology is still poorly understood, thus impeding accurate epidemiological studies. They affect individuals of all ages but are predominately diseases of the extremes of age (Figure 2.1). Over the past few years prospective, population-based registers have been established and results from these are now becoming available.

The classification of the vasculitides is based on the size of the predominant vessels involved (Table 2.1). Until the 1990s there was a lack of consensus in evidence based classification of individual patients with vasculitic syndromes. This was addressed by the American College of Rheumatology (ACR) in 1990, which proposed criteria for the classification of seven different vasculitides with sensitivities varying from 71.0% to 95.3% and specificities of 78.7 to 99.7% (Fries *et al.* 1990). The most sensitive and specific criteria were found in Churg–Strauss syndrome (CSS), giant cell arteritis (GCA), and Takayasu's arteritis (TA); hypersensitivity (leukocytoclastic) vasculitis was the least well-defined condition. This development was important because it allowed epidemiological studies to be performed using established criteria. The ACR criteria are not perfect; the main criticism is that they do not include microscopic polyangiitis (MPA) or consider antineutrophil cytoplasmic antibodies (ANCA). Furthermore, they were established by comparing patients with different types of vasculitis, but not patients prior to the diagnosis of vasculitis, or with other systemic diseases or other connective tissue diseases. The reliability of these criteria when used in patients in whom vasculitis is suspected but not yet diagnosed is poor (Rao *et al.* 1998) (Chapter 21).

Table 2.1 Classification of systemic vasculitis

Dominant vessel involved	Primary	Secondary
Large arteries	Giant cell arteritis Takayasu's arteritis	Aortitis associated with RA Infection (e.g. syphilis, tuberculosis)
Medium arteries	Classical PAN Kawasaki disease	Hepatitis B associated PAN
Small vessels and medium arteries	Wegener's granulomatosis[1] Churg–Strauss syndrome[1] Microscopic polyangiitis[1]	Vasculitis secondary to RA, SLE, Sjögren's syndrome Drugs Infection (e.g. HIV)
Small vessels (leukocytoclastic)	Henoch–Schönlein purpura Cryoglobulinemia Cutaneous leukocytoclastic angiitis	Drugs[2] Hepatitis C associated Infection

RA, rheumatoid arthritis; PAN, polyarteritis nodosa; SLE, systemic lupus erythematosus.

[1] Diseases most commonly associated with ANCA (antimyeloperoxidase and antiproteinase 3 antibodies), with a significant risk of renal involvement and which are most responsive to immunosuppression with cyclophosphamide.

[2] For example sulfonamides, penicillins, thiazide diuretics, and many others.

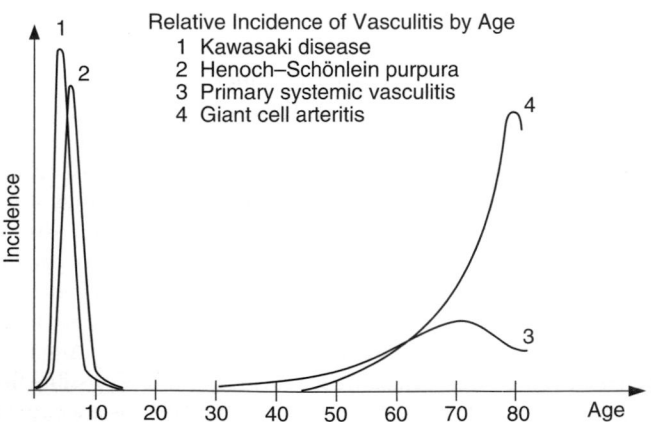

Relative Incidence of Vasculitis by Age
1 Kawasaki disease
2 Henoch–Schönlein purpura
3 Primary systemic vasculitis
4 Giant cell arteritis

Figure 2.1 Relative incidence of vasculitis by age.

In 1994, the Chapel Hill Consensus Conference (CHCC) produced definitions for vasculitis (Jennette *et al.* 1994). They included for the first time MPA, but were not intended as classification or diagnostic criteria. They also recognized that histologic data would not be available for all patients, especially when the clinical condition of the patient might preclude obtaining appropriate biopsies or the sample might not be representative and miss salient histologic features. This is particularly a problem for focal lesions such as granulomata. The concept of surrogate markers of vasculitis was therefore introduced. In addition, the potential importance of ANCA in diagnosis was recognized, but not included in the definitions.

The ACR criteria and CHCC definitions are widely used for epidemiological studies. Comparative epidemiology requires the use of well-validated and generally accepted classification criteria. For some types of vasculitis, for example GCA, TA, WG, and CSS, this condition is satisfied, however for others such as MPA and PAN there is no consensus (see below). This lack of consensus on case definition and distinction between the different types of vasculitis has hindered progress. While differences in incidence between geographic areas may reflect a genuine difference due to environmental or ethnic factors, there remains the possibility that a systematic difference in the application of the criteria/definitions may be responsible for at least some of the variation. There is therefore an urgent need to develop a better classification system for the vasculitides.

The etiology of vasculitis is unknown but is clearly multifactorial; among the influences on disease expression are ethnicity, genes (HLA and others), gender, and environment (UV light, infections, toxins, drugs, smoking, and surgery). There are sufficient differences, even with the limited epidemiological data available, to suggest that not all these factors work in the same direction in the various vasculitic syndromes described. In this chapter, we will review the available evidence and attempt to identify the key epidemiological factors involved in the major vasculitis syndromes. We have structured this around a classification system based on the size of vessels predominately involved (Table 2.1), and considered vasculitis in children separately.

Large-vessel vasculitis

Giant cell arteritis

Giant cell arteritis is a vasculitic disease in which the characteristic feature is the presence of giant cells in a biopsy of a large artery. Although the ACR criteria for GCA (Hunder *et al.* 1990a) do not require histological evidence of arteritis, many studies only report biopsy-positive cases. Clearly the biopsy rate and intensity of histological search for evidence of vasculitis have influenced the reported incidence. Furthermore, many of the studies have been hospital based and retrospective. GCA is closely related to polymyalgia rheumatica (PMR); population-based studies of PMR have shown that 16–21% of patients have biopsy-proven GCA (Salvarani *et al.* 1995a; Franzen *et al.* 1992). Conversely, 40–60% of GCA patients have PMR symptoms (Salvarani *et al.* 1995b). Many studies include patients with PMR and do not clearly distinguish those with pure GCA.

Prospective studies from Scandinavia have reported annual incidence figures for biopsy-proven GCA of 15–35 per 100,000 individuals aged over 50 years and a similar rate has been reported from Olmsted County (Minnesota, USA) (Table 2.2). There is an increasing incidence with age, peaking in persons aged 80 years or greater; very few cases occur in those aged less than 50 years. Most series report a greater incidence in women, with a female to male ratio of around 2:1; however, an occasional series describes an excess in men (female: male 1:1.4) (González-Gay *et al.* 1997). The reasons for this discrepancy are not clear.

Time trends

Several studies have suggested an increase in the incidence of GCA with time. In Olmsted County between 1950–54 and 1980–84 there was an increase from 6.7/100,000 to 28.5/100,000 in persons aged >50 years. The rate then stabilized and has not risen further (Salvarani *et al.* 2004). A similar increase in incidence has been documented in Göteborg, Sweden between 1976 and 1995 from 16.8/100,000 to 30.1/ 100,000 persons aged >50 years (Petursdottir *et al.* 1999). The estimated rate of increase was 10.9% per year. González-Gay and colleagues in northwest Spain reported an increasing incidence of GCA between 1981 and 1998, but noted that the frequency of classic manifestations decreased (González-Gay *et al.* 1997) and that the increase was more marked in women (González-Gay and García-Porrúa 1999). This increase is independent of changing population structures in which there is an increase in the elderly and very elderly (aged >80 years) population (Salvarani *et al.* 2004; Nordborg *et al.* 2003).

Geographical factors

The majority of studies have come from Scandinavia or from populations with a similar ethnic background (Olmsted County, Minnesota, USA includes a significant population of Scandinavian ancestry). Studies from southern Europe (Italy and Spain) and France have consistently reported lower incidence rates than those from Scandinavia. Jews from Jerusalem also seem to have a very low incidence. In the USA, there is only one study from a population other than Olmsted County: this study is from Tennessee and reports a lower incidence in the southern USA Caucasian population (Smith *et al.* 1983). The prevalence of GCA in Japan was reported in a nationwide survey to be 1.47/100,000 in persons aged >50 years, considerably lower than in Europe (Kobayashi *et al.* 2003). There are no epidemiological studies and only scattered cases reports from Africa, Latin America, the Indian subcontinent, and Asia including China.

Ethnic differences

GCA is uncommon in non-Caucasians, although there are few substantive epidemiological data. The Tennessee study reported a low incidence in African-Americans (Smith *et al.* 1983). A retrospective review from the Texas Gulf Coast reported that 13/27 patients were black women, but that the disease was rare in Hispanics (González *et al.* 1989). No incidence figures are available from that study. Liu and colleagues reported, from Southern California, a retrospective study from an ophthalmology unit (1986–98) of 121 patients undergoing temporal artery biopsy (Liu *et al.* 2001). Nineteen of 66 (29%) Caucasian patients had a positive biopsy compared to 1/9 Asian patients (11.0%), 0/40 Hispanic, and 0/6 African-American patients. Few clinical details were provided and it is possible that referral bias might account for their results. There is a low prevalence in Japan compared with Europe (Kobayashi *et al.* 2003). The paucity of reports from non-Caucasian populations could

Table 2.2 Annual incidence of giant cell arteritis

Year(s)	Place	Incidence (per 100,000)[1]	Case definition	Study type	Reference
1964–77	Lothian, Scotland	4.2	Biopsy	Retrospective	Jonasson *et al.* 1979
1969–89	Tampere, Finland	7.2	Biopsy	Retrospective	Rajala *et al.* 1993
1970–79	Loire, France	9.4	Biopsy/clinical	Retrospective	Barrier *et al.* 1982
1973–75	Goteborg, Sweden	16.8	Biopsy	Retrospective	Bengtsson and Malmvall 1981
1977–86	Goteborg, Sweden	18.3	Biopsy	Retrospective	Nordborg and Bengtsson 1990
1980–88	Reggio Emilia, Italy	6.9	Biopsy	Retrospective	Salvarani *et al.* 1991
1981–98	Lugo, NW Spain	10.3	Biopsy	Retrospective	González-Gay *et al.* 2001
1982	Ribe, Denmark	23.3	Biopsy	Prospective	Boesen and Sorensen 1987
1982–94	Denmark	20.4	Biopsy	Prospective (since 1984)	Elling *et al.* 1996
1984–90	Iceland	27.0	ACR[2]	Retrospective	Baldursson *et al.* 1994
1984–87	W Nyland, Finland	17.4	Biopsy/clinical	Retrospective	Franzen *et al.* 1992
1987–88	W Nyland, Finland	26.2	Biopsy/clinical	Prospective	Franzen *et al.* 1992
1986	S Sweden	33.6	Biopsy/clinical	Prospective, population	Noltrop and Svensson 1991
1986–88	Frederiksborg, Denmark	17.6	Biopsy/clinical	Retrospective	Fledelius and Nissen 1992
1987–94	Aust Agder, Norway	29.0	Biopsy/clinical	Retrospective, hospital	Gran and Myklebust 1997
1992–96	Bodø, Norway	27.5	Biopsy/ACR	Retrospective, hospital	Haugeberg *et al.* 2003
1992–96	Ålesund, Norway	36.7	Biopsy/ACR	Retrospective, hospital	Haugeberg *et al.* 2003
1992–96	Kristiansand, S. Norway	32.8	Biopsy/ACR	Retrospective, hospital	Haugeberg *et al.* 2003
1976–95	Goteborg, Sweden	22.2	Biopsy, clinical	Retrospective	Nordborg *et al.* 2003
1998–2002	Schleswig Holstein, Germany	3.2	CHCC	Prospective, population	Reinhold-Keller *et al.* 2005
1990–99	Vilnius, Lithuania	0.72	ACR	Prospective, hospital	Dadoniene *et al.* 2005
1960–78	Israel	0.5	Biopsy	Retrospective	Friedman *et al.* 1982
1980–91	Jerusalem, Israel	10.2	Biopsy	Retrospective	Sonnenblick *et al.* 1986
1950–99	Olmsted County, Minnesota, USA	18.8	ACR[2]	Retrospective (to 1985), population	Salvarani *et al.* 1995; 2004
1971–80	Shelby, Tennessee, USA	1.6	Biopsy/clinical	Retrospective	Smith *et al.* 1983

[1] Population aged over 50 years.

[2] ACR (1990) criteria.

Studies grouped by continental location and chronologically.

reflect non-recognition or a true ethnic difference with non-white individuals protected from the disease.

Cardiovascular risk factors

In the Olmsted county population, smoking was associated with a statistically significant, two-fold increase in biopsy-proven GCA (Machado *et al.* 1989). In a prospective case–control study from France, past or present smoking in women, but not men, was associated with biopsy-positive or biopsy-negative GCA with an odds ratio of 6, and heavy smoking (defined as greater than 10 pack-years), with an odds ratio of 16. Previous atheromatous disease was associated with a 4.5-fold increase in women with GCA (Duhaut *et al.* 1998). This was an independent effect. For men, no significant cardiovascular risk factors for GCA were identified. The same group of investigators also reported that previous pregnancy was not an additional risk factor for GCA, and might even be protective (Duhaut *et al.* 1999a). The reason for this is unclear but may

be related to the protective effect of pregnancy on cardiovascular disease.

Environmental factors

The incidence of GCA shows a marked variation with latitude. Multiple regression analysis correcting for the effect of increasing incidence with time suggests that there is a significant trend to increasing incidence with more northerly (higher) latitude (Watts *et al.* 2000). This geographical trend is similar to that seen in multiple sclerosis and rheumatoid arthritis in both hemispheres. Exposure to ultraviolet (UV) light has been proposed as an etiological factor for autoimmunity: the amount of UV radiation (UVR) reaching the earth's surface varies inversely with latitude, UVR down-regulates cellular immunity, and low levels of UVR are associated with low vitamin D synthesis (Staples *et al.* 2003). Hence UVR might have a protective effect on the development of GCA. Further studies are required to investigate the role of UVR and vitamin D in the development of GCA. An alternative explanation is that there might be an infectious agent which is either more common or operates more effectively at higher latitudes.

The Olmsted County study identified peaks in incidence occurring every 7 years, a finding that would be consistent with an infectious etiology (Salvarani *et al.* 1995a). In Denmark, peak incidences were correlated with the occurrence of epidemics of *Mycoplasma pneumoniae* infection (Elling *et al.* 1996). Using a matched case–control method, Russo *et al.* (1995) showed a correlation between infection and onset of GCA but could not identify a specific infection. In addition to cyclic peaks, occasional clusters have been reported; in Jerusalem, Sonnenblick and colleagues observed five cases in a 7-week period when the expected background rate was one case per year (Sonnenblick *et al.* 1986). Temporal clusters have been reported from general practice in the UK, with six cases occurring among a population of 4400 in a 7-month period (McCreay 1986). Several cases of GCA occurring in families or in close temporal relation have been reported and used to adduce an infectious or genetic etiology; both sibling and spouse pairs have been reported (Faerk 1992). In contrast, neither the Swedish nor Spanish groups observed any cyclical fluctuations (Petursdottir *et al.* 1999; Gonzalez-Gay *et al.* 2001). In Germany, GCA was observed to be more prevalent in urban environments compared with rural areas, with a 2.25 relative risk (Reinhold-Keller *et al.* 2000).

A seasonal pattern of onset has been identified by several studies but the precise season of maximum occurrence has not been consistent. In addition, some studies have failed to document a seasonal effect. Kinmont and McCallum (1965) initially described a peak in summer, while Mowat and Hazleman (1974) also noted a peak in winter. Duhaut and colleagues reported a winter peak for biopsy-positive GCA and a spring–summer peak for biopsy-negative GCA (Duhaut *et al.* 1999a). Petursdottir noted peaks in autumn and late winter (Petursdottir *et al.* 1999).

The factors described above point towards an infectious etiology; however, despite intensive searches no specific infectious agent has been identified. The striking feature of the epidemiology of GCA is the age distribution. As the immune system ages it becomes more vulnerable to infections (Butcher *et al.* 2000). Viral infections have been considered causative, and a small number of serological studies have looked for a variety of viruses. Those include hepatitis B; herpes zoster; Epstein–Barr virus (EBV); herpes simplex virus (HSV 1 and 2); respiratory syncytial virus; and adenovirus. A large case–control study suggested that reinfection with human parainfluenza virus (HPIV), a virus known to induce human multinucleated giant cells, was associated with the onset of GCA (Duhaut *et al.* 1999b). No association was seen with other viruses that induce multinucleated giant cells, such as measles virus, HSV, EBV, and respiratory syncytial virus, nor was there an association with temporal artery biopsy-negative patients with PMR. The presence of parvovirus B19 and *Chlamydia pneumoniae* in temporal artery biopsy specimens from GCA patients has not been consistently observed.

In summary, despite all the available epidemiological data on GCA/PMR, including large studies looking at infectious causes, which have been far more extensive than for most other vasculitides, no unifying hypothesis has emerged.

Takayasu's arteritis

Takayasu's arteritis (TA) was first described in Japan in 1908. Since then it has generally been considered to be more common in Asia

Table 2.3 Annual incidence of Takayasu's arteritis

Year	Place	Incidence/million	Reference:
1982–84	Japan	1–2	Koide 1992
1971–83	Olmsted County, Minnesota, USA	2.6	Hall *et al.* 1985
1969–75	Sweden	0.8	Waern *et al.* 1983
1989–94	Kuwait	3.3	El-Reshaid *et al.* 1995
1998–02	Schleswig-Holstein, Germany	04–1.0	Reinhold-Keller *et al.* 2005
1990–99	Vilnius, Lithuania	1.3	Dadoniene *et al.* 2005

although it has been described world-wide. The annual incidence in most populations is 1–3/million (Table 2.3). The peak age of disease onset is in the third decade and the disease is more common in women. There are too few studies to reliably assess time trends, but the available data suggest no major change (Table 2.3). TA has been described in most ethnic groups including African, for which quite large series have been published (Vanoli *et al.* 2005; Mwipatayi *et al.* 2005). Many series suggest that the condition is most common in Asians compared with Caucasians or black Africans; however, at present there are no epidemiological studies from Asian countries to support this assertion. The clinical phenotype appears to be different in some populations with a different pattern of aortic involvement. In South African patients, lower abdominal aorta involvement with leg ischemia is more common than in Japan. Aneurysmal disease is much more common in Africa compared with Japan (Mwipatayi *et al.* 2005).

The etiopathogenesis of TA is unknown; possible environmental factors to be considered include tuberculosis (TB) because of the granulomatous nature of the disease and its more frequent occurrence in areas endemic for TB, but no clear causal relationship has been established.

Medium and small-vessel vasculitis

The classification of the medium/small-vessel primary systemic vasculitides (PSV) poses a particular difficulty to the epidemiologist

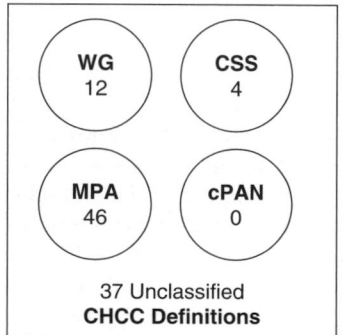
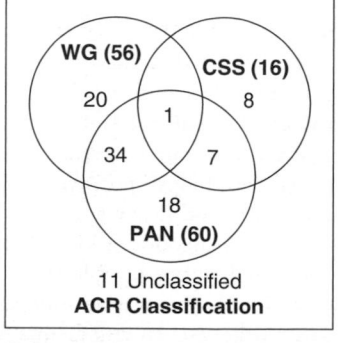

(a)   (b)

Figure 2.2 Results of the application of (a) the CHCC definitions and (b) the ACR (1990) criteria for WG, CSS, and PAN to a cohort of 99 patients. Data from Lane *et al.* 2005a.

Table 2.4 Annual incidence of polyarteritis nodosa

Diagnosis	Years	Place	Incidence (million)	Reference
PAN	1972–80	Bristol/Bath, UK	4.6	Scott *et al.* 1982
PAN	1951–67	Olmsted County MN, USA	7.0	Kurland *et al.* 1969
PAN	1957–71	Michigan, USA	2.0	Sack *et al.* 1975
PAN[1]	1974–85	Alaska	77.0	McMahon *et al.* 1989
PAN	1976–79	Olmsted County MN, USA	9.0	Kurland *et al.* 1984
ACR	1992–96	Kristiansand, Norway	6.6	Haugeberg *et al.* 1998
ACR	1990–99	Vilnius, Lithuania	7.7	Dadoniene *et al.* 2005
ACR	1988–97	Norwich, UK	8.0	Watts *et al.* 2000
CHCC	1993–96	Kuwait	16.0	El-Reshaid *et al.* 1997
ACR	1988–97	Lugo, Spain	6.6	González-Gay and García-Porrúa 1999
CHCC	1988–01	Lugo, Spain	0.9	González-Gay *et al.* 2003
ACR + CHCC	1990–01	Lund, Sweden	1.4	Selga *et al.* 2006
CHCC	1998–2002	Schleswig-Holstein, Germany	04–2.0	Reinhold-Keller *et al.* 2005

[1] Hepatitis B positive

as there is no uniform agreement on the application of the ACR (1990) criteria and CHCC definitions. Use of the two systems in parallel has resulted in considerable conflict. We have applied in parallel the ACR criteria (WG, CSS, PAN) and CHCC (WG, CSS, classical PAN and MPA) definitions to a cohort of 99 patients from a well-defined population. From an application of the ACR (1990) criteria, there was significant overlap between diagnoses (34 patients could be classified as both WG and PAN, seven as both CSS and PAN, and one as CS, WG, and PAN) and 11 patients were unclassifiable (Figure 2.2b). Applying the CHCC definitions without surrogate markers/ANCA resulted in no overlapping diagnoses but 37 patients could not be classified (Figure 2.2a). Figure 2.2 demonstrates that patients classified as MPA by the CHCC definitions are classified as either WG or PAN using the ACR criteria (Lane *et al.* 2005b). To address this issue, a consensus approach to the use of the ACR (1990) and CHCC definitions has been developed and validated by a group of European physicians interested in the epidemiology of the vasculitides. This uses an algorithm to sort patients into a single category with only a minimum of unclassifiable patients (Watts *et al.* 2007).

The majority of the data on the incidence and prevalence of the PSV has come from Europe with studies from the UK, Spain, France, Norway, Sweden, and Germany (Tables 2.4, 2.5, 2.6, 2.7). There is a broad consensus that: (i) the overall annual incidence is approximately 10–20/million; (ii) the peak age of onset is in those aged 65–74 years (Figure 2.1); (iii) these disease are slightly more common in men; and (iv) they are very rare in childhood (Gardner-Medwin 2002). We have recently completed a 15-year prospective study of the incidence of PSV in a well-defined population in Norfolk (UK). The overall annual incidence of the PSV was stable between 1989 and 2003 at 19.6/million (Watts *et al.* 2005). The PSV are under-reported from India, Africa, Asia, and Latin

Table 2.5 Annual incidence of microscopic polyangiitis

Diagnosis	Year	Place	Incidence (per million)	Reference
MPA[1,2]	1971–93	Lund, Sweden	2.5	Westman *et al.* 1998
MPA	1980–86	Leicester, UK	0.5	Andrews *et al.* 1990
MPA	1987–89	Leicester, UK	3.0	Andrews *et al.* 1990
MPA[1]	1984–89	Heidelberg, Germany	1.5	Andrassy *et al.* 1991
MPA[2]	1988–97	Norwich, UK	8.0	Watts *et al.* 2000
MPA[2]	1988–01	Lugo, Spain	7.9	González-Gay *et al.* 2003
MPA[1,2]	1993–96	Kuwait	24.0	El-Reshaid *et al.* 1997
MPA	1998–2002	Schleswig-Holstein, Germany	3	Reinhold-Keller *et al.* 2005
MPA[3]	2000–04	Miyazaki, Japan	14.8	Fujimoto *et al.* 2006
MPA	1990–99	Vilnius, Lithuania	3.0	Dadoniene *et al.* 2005
MPA	1993–2004	Western Montana, USA	2.9	Zeft *et al.* 2005

[1] Renal involvement only.

[2] Chapel Hill Consensus definition.

[3] Includes renal limited vasculitis

Table 2.6 Annual incidence of Wegener's granulomatosis

Year	Place	Criteria	Incidence (per million)	Reference
1971–93	Lund, Sweden	ACR[1]	2.1	Westman et al. 1998
1980–86	Leicester, UK	Fauci[2]	0.7	Andrews et al. 1990
1987–89	Leicester, UK	Fauci	2.8	Andrews et al. 1990
1988–97	Norwich, UK	ACR[1]	9.7	Watts et al. 2000
1988–97	Lugo, Spain	ACR[1]	4.8	González-Gay and García-Porrúa, 1999
1992–96	Kristiansand, Norway	ACR[1]	6.6	Haugeberg et al. 1998
1998–2002	Schleswig-Holstein, Germany	CHCC	6–12	Reinhold-Keller et al. 2005
1990–99	Vilnius, Lithuania	ACR	2.1	Dadionne et al. 2005
1984–98	Tromsø, Norway	ACR	8.0	Koldingsnes and Nossent 2000
	Lugo, Spain	CHCC	2.95	Gonzalez-Gay et al. 2003
1990–99	Olmsted County, USA	ACR	11.0	Ng et al. 2003
1993–2004	Western Montana, USA		8.6	Zeft et al. 2005

[1] ACR (1990) criteria.

[2] Fauci et al. 1983.

Table 2.7 Prevalence of Wegener's granulomatosis

Year	Classification	Place	Prevalence (million)	Reference
1994	CHCC	Germany (North)	58	Reinhold-Keller et al. 2000
1994	CHCC	Germany (South)	42	Reinhold-Keller et al. 2000
1986–90	ACR	New York, USA	32.0	Cotch et al. 1996
1986–90	ACR	USA	26.0	Cotch et al. 1996
1988–97	ACR/CHCC	Norwich, UK	106.4	Watts et al. 2000
1997[1]	ACR/CHCC	Norwich, UK	62.9	Watts et al. 2000
1992–96	ACR	Norway	53.0	Haugeberg et al. 1998
1999–2003	ACR	Canterbury, New Zealand	131	Gibson et al. 2006
2000	ACR	Paris, France	23.7	Mahr et al. 2004
2003[2]	ACR	Canterbury, New Zealand	93.5	Gibson et al. 2006
2004	ACR	Western Montana, USA	90	Zeft et al. 2005

[1] Point prevalence on 31 December, 1997.

[2] Point prevalence on 31 December, 2003.

America; while this could reflect genuine differences in incidence, failure of recognition and diagnosis is very likely. A confounding factor is the very different age demography in these populations, which are younger compared with Western Europe and the USA. As PSV is most common in the older age groups this could influence the apparent frequency with which these conditions are seen.

Polyarteritis nodosa and microscopic polyangiitis

The original description of periarteritis nodosa by Kussmaul and Maier (1866) was of a patient with inflammation and necrosis of medium-sized arteries leading to aneurysm formation and organ infarction. Davson et al. (1948) described patients with segmental necrotizing glomerulonephritis who also had features of polyarteritis nodosa (PAN) with extrarenal small and medium artery involvement. The term microscopic polyarteritis (MPA) was used to describe these patients in whom the dominant feature was rapidly progressive renal failure. The dominant feature of PAN is organ infarction (gut, nerve) due to involvement of medium-sized arteries. This illness is now termed classical PAN. The literature on the epidemiology of PAN and MPA has to be carefully interpreted, because many older studies used the term polyarteritis nodosa as a generic term for any form of necrotizing vasculitis. WG, CSS, and MPA are associated with antineutrophil cytoplasmic antibodies (ANCA) and are sometimes considered as ANCA-associated vasculitis, whereas classical PAN is typically ANCA-negative.

Time trends

In Europe and the USA the estimated annual incidence of PAN ranges from 2.0 to 9.0/million (Table 2.4). Re-analysis of the data from the Bath/Bristol study in the 1970s suggests that their polyarteritis group included patients who would now be considered to have MPA or CSS (Scott et al. 1982; Scott, unpublished data). Overall, the European and American studies of PAN do not suggest a change over time (Table 2.4), nor does our Norwich study over 15 years, but differences in classification make direct comparison difficult. Application of the ACR (1990) criteria and CHCC definitions to the same cohort of patients results in very different number of patients with PAN (Figure 2.2). Use of the CHCC definitions makes classical PAN appear to be a much rarer disease; this has been observed in a number of studies (Table 2.4), the exception being one from Kuwait. A prevalence study from France suggests that improved public health control of HBV infection by vaccination is producing a fall in the prevalence of PAN (Mahr et al. 2004). In Leicester (UK) the annual incidence of MPA between 1980 and 1986 was 0.5/million and between 1987 and 1989 it was 3.3/million (Andrews et al. 1990) (Table 2.5). This increase followed introduction of testing for ANCA and was possibly ascribed to increased physician awareness. A recent study from Norwich UK reported an incidence of 8.0/million (Watts et al. 2005). A renal biopsy study in Stockholm reported a doubling of the annual incidence of pauci-immune necrotizing and crescentic glomerulonephritis from 6.0 to 12.0/million between 1986 and 1992 (Pettersson et al. 1995). More recent studies suggest that the incidence was greater during the 1990s than the 1980s (González-Gay and Garcia-Porrua 1999). In our prospective Norwich study, there was no significant change in incidence during the period 1988–2004 (Watts et al. 2005). Tidman et al. (1998) also did not observe an increase in incidence during 1986–1995. During this period they noted a periodic fluctuation with peaks every 3–4 years. It is possible that MPA is becoming more common but the number of series is small and the reported increases could represent increasing physician awareness and changing ideas of diagnosis and classification.

Geographical factors

In Europe there appears to be a North–South gradient in incidence, with MPA being more common in Southern Europe (Lugo, Spain latitude 43°N) compared with Tromsø in Northern Norway (latitude 70°N) (Watts *et al.* 2001). Care was taken in this study to eliminate variations in classification. The period prevalence in New Zealand in 2000–2003, which has a similar latitude south (40–44°S) to Paris in the north (49°N), is 58/million and appears to be similar to that observed in Paris (Gibson *et al.* 2006; Mahr *et al.* 2004).

Two geographical regions with an apparently high incidence of MPA and PAN are Japan and Kuwait. In the Kuwaiti national population, the incidence of MPA, PAN, and patients with angiographic findings compatible with PAN was 45/million (El-Reshaid *et al.* 1997). The incidence of classical PAN was 16/million and MPA 24/million. In Japan, the incidence of MPA was 14.8/million, higher than any European figure (Fujimoto *et al.* 2006).

Ethnic differences

Clues are beginning to emerge that PAN may have an ethnic variation, with a higher incidence in non-Caucasian ethnic groups. The highest incidence of PAN recorded was 77/million in Alaskan Indians (McMahon *et al.* 1989). The population was, however, small (14,000) and all the cases were positive for hepatitis B surface and e antigen at diagnosis. Detailed hepatitis serology is not available in most other studies. Whether these data reflect geographical and ethnic differences or the high infection rate with hepatitis B virus is unclear as no other comparable study has been reported. A study from Paris reported a prevalence of classical PAN of 30.7/million (Mahr *et al.* 2004), higher than in Germany (2–9/million) (Reinhold-Keller *et al.* 2000) or Scandinavia (3.3/million using the ACR criteria) (Haugeberg *et al.* 1998). Of the French PAN patients, 30% were HBV positive.

In the Kuwait study the incidence figures were only calculated for Kuwaitis but MPA and PAN also occurred in other non-white groups. In the Miyazaki prefecture, Japan, the incidence of MPA is higher than in European Caucasian populations (Fujimoto *et al.* 2006), and MPO-ANCA associated disease is seen more frequently than PR3-ANCA associated disease. Whether this reflects ascertainment bias or a genuine difference in response to the (as yet unknown) triggering factor(s) remains to be determined.

Most of the populations studied in Europe have been predominantly white Caucasians. In Paris, France, a study from a multiethnic urban area reported that the prevalence of PSV was twice as high in individuals of European descent (104.7/million) as in non-Europeans (52.5/million) (Mahr *et al.* 2004). WG was relatively less frequent than MPA in non-Europeans, and none of the WG patients came from Africa. The non-European population was derived from the Maghreb, sub-Saharan Africa, Asia, and the Caribbean, and comprised 28% of the study population (1.09 million).

Environmental factors

The PSV have been associated with a number of environmental factors including silica, hydrocarbons, drugs, and infections. Many of these studies discuss MPA and WG together and these data are presented below.

Drugs

Drug exposure has been predominately associated with MPO-ANCA positive vasculitis (see Chapter 7). The most commonly reported are propylthiouracil and hydralazine although penicillamine, minocycline, methimazole, carbimazole, thiamazole, sulfasalazine, phenytoin, and allopurinol have also been implicated (Holder *et al.* 2002). There has been a growing number of reports of vasculitis in hyperthyroid patients treated with propylthiouracil; of these, pANCA with specificity for MPO is most common (Choi *et al.* 2000). Choi *et al.* reviewed 250 MPO-positive systemic vasculitis patients and detected hydralazine, propylthiouracil, allopurinol, penicillamine, or sulfasalazine use in 18 cases within 9 months prior to the onset of disease (Choi *et al.* 2000). Positivity for MPO-ANCA, IgM anticardiolipin antibodies, and antihistone antibodies is characteristic of drug-induced vasculitis syndromes. Skin vasculitis and arthralgias are more common than in idiopathic vasculitis, with renal lesions being less common. The condition is milder than idiopathic vasculitis and may remit on withdrawal of the precipitating drug.

Infection

The major environmental factor associated with PAN has been hepatitis B virus infection (HBV); one of the highest rates for PAN yet reported comes from an area endemic for HBV infection. Many studies do not report HBV infection rates and only two of 13 patients with PAN in Spain were positive for HBV (González-Gay and Garcia-Porrua 1999). In France, as HBV infection rates have fallen due to vaccination, the prevalence of PAN has also decreased (Mahr *et al.* 2004).

Wegener's granulomatosis

Wegener, in 1936, first described a disease characterized by necrotizing granulomata of the upper and lower respiratory tract, focal glomerulonephritis, and necrotizing systemic vasculitis (Godman and Churg 1954). The ACR (1990) criteria for WG have high sensitivity and specificity (Leavitt *et al.* 1990).

Time trends

The incidence of WG may have increased from the 1980s to 1990s. Andrews and colleagues (1990) in Leicester (UK) reported an increase in the annual incidence of WG from 0.7/million (1980–1986) to 2.8/million (1987–1989) (Table 2.5). This was partially attributed to heightened diagnostic awareness following the introduction of assays for ANCA in 1987, as occurred for MPA. Studies conducted during the late 1990s and early 2000s suggest a relatively stable incidence. We did not observe any significant change during the 15-year period of our Norwich study (Watts *et al.* 2005). Different diagnostic criteria have been used to define patients with WG. For example, the Leicester study used the criteria described by Fauci in 1983 (Fauci *et al.* 1983) whereas more recent studies used the ACR (1990) criteria or CHCC definitions.

Geographical factors

The annual incidence of WG since 1986 in Europe is in the range of 2 to 10/million (Table 2.5). The prevalence of WG has been reported by several groups from the Europe and the USA (Table 2.6). The estimated prevalence of WG in the USA was estimated to be 26.0/million in 1986–1990 (Cotch *et al.* 1996). In 1994, the prevalence of WG in north Germany was reported to be 58/million and

42/million (Reinhold- Keller *et al.* 2000). A retrospective study from Norway in 1996 reported a prevalence of 53/million (Haugeberg *et al.* 1998). In Norwich, the point prevalence on 31 December 1997 was 63.8/million with a 10-year period prevalence of 106/million. The higher prevalence in Norwich could represent either better case capture or a genuine geographical variation.

There are little data on the incidence or prevalence of WG outside North America or Europe. In Japan, WG and PR3-ANCA associated vasculitis are relatively rare compared with MPA and MPO-associated vasculitis (Fujimoto *et al.* 2006). Case series from India suggest that WG is being recognized more frequently (Malaviya *et al.* 1990). Reviews of patients attending rheumatology clinics in both urban and rural Africa do not substantiate an occurrence of WG. Other forms of autoimmune disease are seen, possibly implying that WG is rare in Africa. In areas where TB is common, patients presenting with pulmonary vasculitis are liable to be misdiagnosed with tuberculosis.

A recent study of the prevalence of WG in New Zealand reported a 5-year prevalence of 131 cases/million and a point prevalence of 37/million on 31 December 2003 (Gibson *et al.* 2006). Using the ACR criteria, these prevalence rates are similar to Northern Norway; the patients in this study were all Caucasian of European ancestry.

Ethnic factors

Most reports have dealt with Caucasian populations. The French prevalence study suggested that WG is less common in persons of non-European ancestry than MPA (Mahr *et al.* 2004). In Japan WG is also less common than MPA, and cANCA-associated disease is less frequent than pANCA-associated disease.

Environmental factors

Raynauld and colleagues in 1993 reported a higher rate of onset in winter (29.8%) compared with summer (14.3%). In Norwich, the onset was most common in the winter, with 43% of patients first developing symptoms in December through February (Carruthers *et al.* 1996). This trend was also supported by a study of ANCA-associated glomerulonephritis and systemic vasculitis, which showed a higher onset in winter (Falk *et al.* 1990). The USA prevalence study did not, however, support the notion of seasonality (Cotch *et al.* 1996), nor did a study of environmental exposure (Duna *et al.* 1998). Tidman *et al.* (1998) noted winter onset of symptoms in a group of patients with ANCA-positive disease, but when those who fulfilled the classification criteria for WG were analyzed, there was no obvious seasonality.

The occurrence of ENT and pulmonary disease in WG has led to the notion that dust exposure might be important in the pathogenesis. Some counties in New York state have a higher prevalence than others but this does not appear to be linked to rural/urban differences (Cotch *et al.* 1996). Similarly, there was no urban/rural difference in Germany (Reinhold-Keller *et al.* 2000). Duna and colleagues (1998) studied self-reported exposure to heat, fumes, and particulates. There was a higher incidence of exposure in WG patients compared with normal control subjects, but no difference between WG patients and patients with other types of lung disease. Paradoxically, smoking appears to be protective for ANCA-associated small-vessel vasculitis (Haubitz *et al.* 2005).

The possible role of infection both in triggering *de novo* disease and its relapse has been extensively investigated for many years. No clear associations have been demonstrated except for *Staphylococcus*

aureus infection. *Staphylococcus aureus* is the organism most commonly isolated in cultures from the upper airways of WG patients and nasal carriage of *S. aureus* has been associated with increased risk of relapse in WG (Stegeman *et al.* 1996).

Clusters of WG occurring in families have been described (Nowack *et al.* 1999). In most clusters, no more than two people have been affected, usually one parent and a child or two siblings. Distant family members are rarely involved. The occurrence of clusters in first degree relatives and not in more distant family members suggests that environmental triggers play an important role in the etiology, as parents and children or siblings share environment as well as genetic background.

Systemic vasculitis has been associated with exposure to particulate silica, for example quartz, granite, sandstone, and grain dust. Case reports have described systemic vasculitis in association with pulmonary silicosis and in individuals exposed to high levels of silica, for example miners and quarrymen (Cohen-Tervaert *et al.* 1998). Clinical cases of MPA, limited WG, and MPO-ANCA-positive disease have been reported. A study of individuals exposed to silica found a significantly higher number positive for MPO-ANCA compared to healthy individuals but not disease controls (systemic lupus erythematosus and systemic sclerosis). A causal association was suggested between the high levels of silica dust experienced after the 1995 great earthquake in Kobe, Japan and the subsequent increase in MPO-ANCA-associated vasculitis (Yashiro *et al.* 2000). Five case–control studies have found significant associations between systemic vasculitis and silica. Hogan *et al.* (2001) found an odds ratio of 4.6 (95% CI 1.8–12.1) for reported silica exposure in ANCA-positive patients (36 MPA, 21 WG, 8 necrotizing glomerulonephritis) compared to renal controls and Gregorini *et al.* (1993) reported that ANCA-positive patients with rapidly progressive glomerulonephritis were 14 times more likely to have been exposed to silica dust than controls. Nuyts *et al.* (1995) found an odds ratio of 5 (95% CI 1.4–11.6) for silica exposure in 16 cases of WG compared to community controls. In a recent case–control study from Norfolk (UK), we reported ORs of 3.0 (95% CI 1.0–8.4) in 75 cases of PSV (47 WG, 12 MPA, 16 CSS) and 5.0 (95% CI 1.3–23.5) in CSS. There was no significant association between MPA or WG and occupational silica exposure (Lane *et al.* 2003). Stratta *et al.* reported an odds ratio of 2.4 (p = 0.04) for silica exposure in 31 cases of biopsy-proven vasculitis compared to controls but no other significant risk factors including hydrocarbons, metals, and asbestos (Stratta *et al.* 2001).

Inhaled fumes, particulates and hydrocarbons

A case–control study carried out at the National Institutes of Health (NIH) reported an association of inhaled fumes and particulates and pesticides with WG compared to healthy and rheumatic disease controls, but not respiratory disease controls (Duna *et al.* 1998). Metal fumes have been associated with pulmonary vasculitis in Russian brass bronze smelters, and Nuyts *et al.* reported significantly raised ORs for exposure to various metals and welding fumes (OR 2.0, 95% CI 1.1–4.6) in a group of renal patients with WG and glomerulonephritis (Nuyts *et al.* 1995). Our case–control study failed to find an association with occupational metal exposure and primary systemic vasculitis (Lane *et al.* 2003).

There has been conflicting evidence regarding a link between occupational exposure to hydrocarbons, for example paints and glues, and systemic vasculitis. Pai *et al.* reported significantly higher hydrocarbon exposure in male MPA and WG patients compared to matched blood donors and non-significantly greater exposures in female patients with pulmonary hemorrhage (Pai *et al.*1998). We found odd ratios of 4.8 (95% CI 1.2–19.8) for exposure to occupational solvents compared to matched controls for PSV overall (Lane *et al.* 2003). Heavy metals (mercury, lead) have been linked to WG (Albert *et al.* 2004).

Farming

We recently conducted a case–control study in Norfolk (UK) and observed an association between farming and the development of PSV. Farming in the year prior to the onset of vasculitis was associated with primary systemic vasculitis with an odds ratio of 2.3 (WG 2.7 and MPA 6.3). It was not possible to distinguish between exposures to crops, livestock, or animal species, as most individuals were exposed to more than one type, but the association appeared stronger in livestock than crops (Lane *et al.* 2003). The earlier NIH study failed to find a significant association between WG and farming (Duna *et al.* 1998).

Churg–Strauss syndrome

In 1951, Churg and Strauss described the post-mortem features of 13 patients who died following an illness characterized by asthma, eosinophilia, fever, and granulomatous necrotizing vasculitis (Churg and Strauss, 1951). The annual incidence of CSS appears to be broadly similar in all populations studied (Table 2.8), and it is much less common than WG or MPA. The data are too limited to draw conclusions about changes in incidence with time. Prevalence data confirm that CSS is much rarer than WG or MPA in New Zealand and France (Gibson *et al.* 2006; Mahr *et al.* 2004).

Environmental factors

The majority of cases of CSS are idiopathic; inhaled antigens, vaccination, and desensitization have been reported as triggering factors (Guillevin *et al.* 1999). Drugs, including sulfonamides, penicillin, anticonvulsants, and thiazides have also been allied to the syndrome as have leukotriene inhibitors including zafirlukast, montelukast, and pranlukast (Gross 2002). There has been some debate as to whether the introduction of a leukotriene inhibitor in a steroid-resistant asthmatic permits a reduction in corticosteroid dose and unmasking of CSS. The incidence of CSS in asthma drug users in general is higher (34.6/million person years)

than in the general population but is not especially high in those taking leukotriene antagonists (Harrold *et al.* 2005).

Small-vessel vasculitis

Henoch–Schönlein purpura and leukocytoclastic vasculitis

Schönlein (1837) first described a childhood illness characterized by acute purpura and arthritis. Henoch (1874) described the additional features of colicky abdominal pain and nephritis. Vasculitis due to allergic or hypersensitivity mechanisms has been considered a distinct entity since the 1940s and was included by Zeek in her original classification (Zeek 1952). The ACR (1990) considered Henoch–Schönlein purpura (HSP) and leukocytoclastic vasculitis (LCV) (hypersensitivity vasculitis) to be separate conditions. The criteria for LCV were the least sensitive (71.0%) and specific (78.5%) (Fries *et al.* 1990). There is considerable overlap between the ACR and CHCC criteria (Watts *et al.* 1998). The CHCC definition for HSP makes a much better distinction between HSP and cutaneous leukocytoclastic angiitis (their preferred term for cutaneous vasculitis; they did not consider hypersensitivity vasculitis), because they included the presence of IgA deposits in the definition (Jeanette *et al.* 1994).

HSP occurs predominately in children (see below). The incidence in adults is approximately 10-fold less than in children (Table 2.9) at around 3–10/million. In Norfolk, from 1990 to 1994, the annual incidence of LCV using the ACR (1990) criteria was 17.8/million with an increased frequency in females (Watts *et al.* 1998). In northwest Spain the incidence rate for biopsy-proven LCV was 30/million with an increased frequency in males (38/million) compared with 22/million in women (García-Porrúa and González-Gay 1999).

Table 2.8 Annual incidence of Churg–Strauss syndrome

Year	Place	Criteria	Incidence (per million)	Reference
1976–79	Olmsted County, Minnesota		4.0	Kurland *et al.* 1984
1988–97	Norwich, UK	ACR[1]	2.8	Watts *et al.* 2000
1988–97	Lugo, Spain	ACR[1]	1.1	González-Gay and García-Porrúa 1999
1998–2002	Schleswig-Holstein, Germany	CHCC	1	Reinhold-Keller *et al.* 2005
1990–99	Vilnius, Lithuania	ACR	1.3	Dadionne *et al.* 2005
1988–2001	Lugo, Spain	CHCC and ACR	1.3	Gonzalez-Gay *et al.* 2003

[1] ACR (1990) criteria.

Table 2.9 Annual incidence of Henoch–Schönlein purpura

Year	Place	Criteria	Incidence	Reference
Aged <17 years			**/ 100,000**	
1997–99	Czech Republic		10.2	Dolezalova *et al.* 2004
1999–2002	Taiwan	ACR	12.9	Yang *et al.* 2005
	Lugo, Spain	ACR[1]	10.5[3]	González-Gay and García-Porrúa, 1999
	Birmingham, UK		20.4	Gardner-Medwin *et al.* 2002
			13.5	Stewart *et al.* 1988
Adults			**/million**	
1998–2002	Schleswig-Holstein, Germany	CHCC	3–10[2]	Reinhold-Keller *et al.* 2005
	Norfolk, UK	ACR	13.0	Watts *et al.* 1998
	Norfolk, UK	CHCC	3.4	Watts *et al.* 1998
1990–99	Vilnius, Lithuania	ACR	3.0	Dadoniene *et al.* 2005
1988–1997	Lugo, Spain	Biopsy positive	14.0	García-Porrúa and González-Gay 1999

[1] ACR (1990) criteria.

[2] Includes adults and children.

[3] Aged <14 years.

There is insufficient data to determine any time-related, geographical, or ethnic factors. In Vilnius, hypersensitivity vasculitis had an incidence of 26/million (Dadoniene *et al.* 2005).

Environmental factors

In the Spanish study a history of drug use (antibiotics, especially beta-lactams, analgesics, or NSAIDs), or upper respiratory tract infections shortly before development of vasculitis, was more common in patients with LCV than in those with HSP (García-Porrúa and González-Gay, 1999). All patients in this study who had drug-induced vasculitis met ACR (1990) criteria for LCV or HSP, and none fulfilled criteria for PAN or WG.

Cutaneous leukocytoclastic vasculitis (angiitis)

Cutaneous vasculitis can occur either as part of a generalized systemic vasculitis or in isolation. The CHCC considered isolated cutaneous vasculitis (cutaneous leukocytoclastic vasculitis) to be a distinct entity (Jennette *et al.* 1998) based essentially on histopathological criteria. Many of these patients fulfill ACR (1990) criteria for hypersensitivity vasculitis (Watts *et al.* 1998). In Norwich during 1990–1994, the annual incidence of biopsy-proven cutaneous leukocytoclastic vasculitis was 15.4/million with a higher incidence in females (Watts *et al.* 1998). These figures are an underestimate as many mild or classical cases would not have been undergone biopsy. The German study reported that the incidence of CHCC-defined cutaneous leukocytoclastic angiitis was 4–9/million between 1998 and 2002 (Reinhold-Keller *et al.* 2005).

Vasculitis in childhood

The spectrum of vasculitis seen in children is very different from that seen in adult. In children the predominant diseases are Kawasaki disease and HSP (Figure 2.1). No validated classification criteria exist for childhood vasculitis but recent proposals have been based on the adult ACR (1990) criteria and CHCC definitions (Ozen *et al.* 2005). The large-vessel vasculitides are rare in both adults and children. Takayasu's arteritis occurs rarely in children and GCA does not occur. The medium/small-size vasculitides associated with ANCA are all very rare in children, with incidence figures of probably <1/million aged <15 years (Gardner-Medwin *et al.* 2003). A recent series of WG presenting in childhood observed that the mean age of onset was 14.5 years; unlike adult WG, there was a 1:4 male to female ratio (Akikusa *et al.* 2005).

Kawasaki's disease

Kawasaki's disease (mucocutaneous lymph node syndrome) (KD) is an acute vasculitis. The striking feature of the epidemiology of KD is the predominance of infants and young children. The condition was first recognized in Japan in 1967 (Kawasaki 1967). KD occurs in both epidemic and endemic forms world-wide. The occurrence of epidemic KD has led to speculation that the condition is caused by an infectious agent. In most populations the incidence rates are increasing.

Geographical factors

Early studies on the epidemiology of KD came from Japan, where nationwide epidemiological surveys carried out between 1970 and 1992 found a total of 116,848 cases. The annual incidence of KD in 1991–1992 in Japan was 900/million in children aged less than 5 years (Yanagawa *et al.* 1995). Because KD is rare in children over

5 years of age, most incidence figures are quoted as age-specific, making the incidence seem high compared with other diseases. The peak incidence is at age 1 year.

Because of the relative frequency of KD there are now a large number of epidemiological studies showing quite a variation in incidence (Table 2.10). KD is relatively infrequent in the UK and Northern Europe.

Ethnic factors

KD has been reported in all ethnic groups, but there are marked variations. Within the USA and UK populations the highest incidence is in individuals from southeast Asia. In Birmingham, UK, the incidence

Table 2.10 Annual incidence of Kawasaki's disease

Year	Place	Criteria	Incidence /100,000 children aged <5 years	Reference
1997–1998	Japan	Japanese	108	Yanagawa *et al.* 2001
1995	Beijing, China	Japanese	18.2	Du *et al.* 2002
1996			27.8	
1993	Shaanxi, China	Japanese	2.4	Jiao *et al.* 2001
1997			2.4	
2000–02	Korea		86.4	Park *et al.* 2005
1997–00	Hong Kong		39	Ng *et al.* 2005
1996–02	Taiwan	ICD	66	Chang *et al.* 2004
1997	USA		17.6	Holman *et al.* 2003
2000			17.1	
1995–99	California, USA	ICD-9	15.3	Chang 2002b
1996–01	Hawaii		45.2	Holman *et al.* 2005
1997–98	Georgia	CDC	9.8	Gibbons *et al.* 2002
1991–92	UK	ICD-9	4.0	Harnden *et al.* 2002
1999–00		ICD-10	8.1	
1996–99	UK	AHA	5.5	Gardner-Medwin *et al.* 2002
	Sweden		6.2	Schiller *et al.* 1995
1996–00	Ireland	ICD-9	15.2	Lynch *et al.* 2003
1998–02	Schleswig-Holstein, Germany	CHC	0–1[1]	Reinhold-Keller *et al.* 2005
1997–99	Czech Republic		1.6	Dolezalova *et al.* 2004
1995–00	Guadelope, West Indies	AHA	25.4	Tourneux *et al.* 2005
1993–95	Australia		3.7	Royle *et al.* 1998

ICD = International classification of disease

CDC = Centers for disease control

AHA = American Heart Association

[1] /million population

in Asians (from the Indian subcontinent) was 14.6/100,000, Black Afro-Caribbeans 5.9/100,000, and Caucasians 4.6/100,000 (Gardner-Medwin *et al.* 2002). In Washington State (USA), the annual incidence was greatest in Asian Americans aged less than 5 years (33.3/100,000) compared with African-Americans (23.4/100,000) and Caucasians (12.7/100,000) (Davis *et al.* 1995). Furthermore, the incidence of KD in Japanese Americans in Hawaii (197.7/100,000 aged <5 years) is higher than the rates reported in Japanese residents of Japan (Holman *et al.* 2005). The incidence in Asian and Pacific Islander children was 70.9/100,000 and in white children 35.3/100,000. These differences between ethnic groups in the same environment, and presumably therefore exposed to the same infections, suggest that genetic factors are key in determining susceptibility.

Environmental factors

There is indirect evidence to support an infectious etiology. KD rarely occurs before the age of 6 months or after the age of 5 years, suggesting that early in life the infant is protected by passively acquired maternal immunity, or that the immature immune system is unable to mount a response to induce KD. The low frequency after 5 years of age suggests early exposure to a common pathogen against which most children mount an appropriate and protective immune response.

A seasonal variation in KD has long been observed but the season of highest incidence varies. In Japan there is a bimodal distribution with peak incidence in January and June/July and a nadir in October. This pattern is consistent throughout the Japanese archipelago (Burns *et al.* 2005). Spring and summer predominate in China (Du *et al.* 2002), and summer in Korea (Park *et al.* 2005). In the UK, USA, and Australia, KD is most common in spring (Harnden 2002; Royle *et al.* 1998; Chang *et al.* 2002a,b).

There has been an extensive, and so far fruitless, search for a single causative organism; numerous organisms have been proposed but not proven (Burgner and Harnden 2005). Other proposed risk factors include a history of shampooing household rugs, proximity to water, mercury, and house dust mites. The failure to identify a single organism suggests either that KD can occur as a final common pathway response to many different organisms or that a novel infectious agent is involved.

KD, among all the vasculitides, has the strongest evidence for the importance of both genetic and environmental factors in its pathogenesis.

Henoch–Schönlein purpura

The annual incidence of HSP in children is 10–20/100,000 (Table 2.9). The peak age of onset in most studies is 5–6 years (Yang *et al.* 2005) with a peak onset in autumn and winter.

Ethnic factors

In Birmingham (UK), HSP was more common in Asians from the Indian subcontinent (24.0/100,000) compared with white Caucasians (17.8/100,000), and blacks (predominantly Afro-Caribbean) (6.2/100,000). The Chinese population in Taiwan has an annual incidence of 12.9/100,000 children aged <17 years (Yang *et al.* 2005).

Secondary vasculitis

Vasculitis occurring in the presence of a connective tissue disease or infection is usually considered to be secondary (Table 2.1). This most typically occurs in patients with rheumatoid arthritis (RA),

systemic lupus erythematosus (SLE), or Sjögren's syndrome. There are no recognized criteria for the definition of vasculitis occurring in association with SLE or Sjögren's syndrome and hence no data on the epidemiology of these conditions.

Systemic rheumatoid vasculitis

Vasculitis as a complication of RA was first described in 1898 in a patient with histological evidence of vascular inflammation of the vasa nervorum. The early clinical descriptions in the 1940s and 1950s were of the classical features of peripheral gangrene and mononeuritis multiplex (Bywaters and Scott 1963). Since then a wider spectrum of disease has been recognized to include carditis, scleritis, nodules, and systemic disease (Scott *et al.* 1981). All sizes of vessel may be involved, from aorta to capillaries. Small-vessel vasculitis can occur in isolation as small nail edge or nail fold lesions which are considered benign but which may herald or coexist with major arterial disease (Watts *et al.* 1995). Systemic rheumatoid vasculitis usually occurs in patients with long-standing, rheumatoid factor-positive, erosive RA. Males with RA are at greater risk than females.

Time trends

Systemic rheumatoid vasculitis first became widely recognized and reported during the 1960s, a period when glucocorticoids were widely used for the management of RA. This has led to the notion that vasculitis could be caused by the inappropriate use of (by current standards) high doses of glucocorticoids, although this is conjectural. It has also been suggested that RA is becoming less severe and that therefore the frequency of rheumatoid vasculitis should also be declining.

In Spain, the annual incidence of biopsy-proven rheumatoid vasculitis during 1988–1997 was 6.4/million (González-Gay and García-Porrúa 1999). In our population in Norfolk, UK, between 1988 and 2002 the overall annual incidence was 7.9/million (males 7.7/million; females 8.1/million) (Watts *et al.* 2004). From 1988 to 1992 the incidence was 11.6/million and this fell to 3.6/million during 1998–2002. A similar pattern was seen for males and females. There was no difference in age or disease duration at onset during the study. This decline could be due to better disease control (increased use of immunosuppressive agents such as methotrexate) or changes in smoking habits.

These results are consistent with a study in California (USA) which showed the rates of hospital admissions for vasculitis in the context of RA was one-third lower in 1998–2001 compared with 1983–1987 (Ward 2004). Other evidence of severe RA, such as splenectomy for Felty syndrome and surgery for cervical spine instability, also diminished. A retrospective review of 609 cases from Rochester, Minnesota (USA) diagnosed from 1955 to 1994 suggested that the incidence of extra-articular disease, including rheumatoid vasculitis, had not changed significantly over the decades (Turesson *et al.* 2004).

Conclusions

The vasculitides continue to present a challenge to the epidemiologist. There is increasing interest in these rare diseases and improvements in classification mean that the picture is gradually unfolding. There is clearly age tropism, suggesting that the causes of vasculitis in childhood are likely to be very different from those triggering vasculitis in the elderly. Ethnic differences are beginning to emerge;

this has been most clearly described in KD, but there are clues that GCA, WG, and MPA may occur with different frequencies in different ethnic groups. Slow progress is being made in understanding the causative factors, with environmental agents such as silica being important in WG and MPA. Search for an infectious cause continues to be fruitless.

References

Akikusa, J., Silverman, E. D., Laxer, R. M., Schneider, R. (2005). Clinical features and outcome of paediatric Wegener's granulomatosis. *Arthritis and Rheumatism*, **52**, S534.

Albert, D., Clarkin, C., Komoroski, J., *et al.* (2004). Wegener's granulomatosis: possible role of environmental agents in its pathogenesis. *Arthritis and Rheumatism*, **51**, 656–64.

Andrassy, K., Küster, S., Waldherr, R., *et al.* (1991). Rapidly progressive glomerulonephritis: analysis of prevalence and clinical course. *Nephron*, **59**, 206–12.

Andrews, M., Edmunds, M., Campbell, A., *et al.* (1990). Systemic vasculitis in the 1980's – is there an increasing incidence of Wegener's granulomatosis and microscopic polyarteritis? *Journal Royal College of Physicians*, **24**, 284–8.

Baldursson, O., Steinsson, K., Bornsson, L., *et al.* (1994). Giant cell arteritis in Iceland. An epidemiologic and histopathologic analysis. *Arthritis and Rheumatism*, **37**, 1007–12.

Barrier, J. H., Pion, P., Massari, R., *et al.* (1982). Approche epidemiologique de la maladie de Horton dans le departement de Loire-Atlantique – 110 cas en 10 ans (1970–9). *Revue Medicine Interne*, **1**, 13–20.

Bengtsson, B-Å. and Malmvall, B. E. (1981). The epidemiology of giant cell arteritis including temporal arteritis and polymyalgia rheumatica: incidences of different clinical presentations and eye complications. *Arthritis and Rheumatism*, **24**, 899–904.

Boesen, P. and Sorensen, S. F. (1987). Giant cell arteritis, temporal arteritis and polymyalgia rheumatica in a Danish county. *Arthritis and Rheumatism*, **30**, 294–9.

Bonaci-Nikolic, B., Nikolic, M. M., Andrejivic, S., *et al.* (2005). Antineutrophil cytoplasmic antibody asoociated autoimmune diseases induced by thyroid drugs: comparison with idiopathic ANCA vasculitides. *Arthritis Research Therapy*, **7**, R1072–81.

Burgner, D. and Harnden, A. (2005). Kawasaki disease: what is the epidemiology telling us about the aetiology? *International Journal of Infectious Disease*, **9**, 185–94.

Burns, J. C., Cayan, D. R., Tong, G., *et al.* (2005). Seasonality and temporal clustering of Kawasaki syndrome. *Epidemiology*, **16**, 220–5.

Butcher, S., Chahel, H. and Lord, J. M. (2000). Ageing and the neutrophil: no appetite for killing. *Immunology*, **100**, 411–6.

Bywaters, E. G.L. and Scott, J. T. (1963). The natural history of vascular lesions in rheumatoid arthritis. *Journal of Chronic Disease*, **16**, 905–14.

Carruthers, D. C., Watts, R. A., Symmons, D. P.M., *et al.* (1996). Wegener's granulomatosis – Increased incidence or increased recognition? *British Journal of Rheumatology*, **35**, 142–5.

Chang, L. Y., Chang, I. S., Lu, C. Y., *et al.* (2004). Epidemiologic features of Kawasaki disease in Taiwan, 1996–2002. *Pediatrics*, **114**, e678–82.

Chang, R-K. (2002a). Hospitalizations for Kawasaki disease among children in the United States, 1988–97. *Pediatrics,* **109**, e87.

Chang, R-K. (2002b). Epidemiologic characteristics of children hospitalized for Kawasaki disease in California. *Pediatric Infectious Diseases*, **21**,1150–5.

Choi, H. K., Merkel, P. A., Walker, A. M. and Niles, J. L. (2000). Drug induced antineutrophil cytoplasmic antibody positive vasculitis -prevalence among patients with high titres of myeloperoxidase antibodies. *Arthritis Rheumatism*, **43**, 405–413.

Churg, J. and Strauss, L. (1951). Allergic granulomatosis, allergic angiitis and periarteritis nodosa. *American Journal of Pathology*, **27**, 277–301.

Cohen Tervaert, J. W., Stegeman, C. A. and Kallenberg, C. G.M. (1998). Silicon exposure and vasculitis. *Current Opinion in Rheumatology*, **10**, 12–7.

Cotch, M. F., Hoffman, G. S., Yerg, D. E., *et al.* (1996). The epidemiology of Wegener's granulomatosis: estimates of the five year period prevalence, annual mortality and geographic disease distribution from population based data sources. *Arthritis and Rheumatism*, **39**, 87–92.

Dadoniene. J., Kirdaite. G., Mackiewicz, Z., Rimkevicus, A. and Haugeber, G. (2005). Incidence of primary systemic vasculitis in Vilnius: a university hospital population based study. *Annals of the Rheumatic Diseases*, **64**, 335–6.

Davis, R. L., Waller, P. L., Mueller, B. A., *et al.* (1995). Kawasaki syndrome in Washington State. Race specific incidence rates and residential proximity to water. *Archives of Pediatric and Adolescent Medicine*, **149**, 66–9.

Davson, J., Ball, J. and Platt, R. (1948). The kidney in periarteritis nodosa. *Quarterly Journal of Medicine*, **17**, 175–202.

Dhillon, R., Newton, L., Rudd, P. T., *et al.* (1993). Management of Kawasaki disease in the British Isles. *Archives of Diseases of Children*, **69**, 631–8.

Dolezalova, P., Telekesova, P., Nemcova, D. and Hoza, J. (2004). Incidence of vasculitis in children in the Czech Republic: 2-year prospective epidemiology survey. *Journal of Rheumatology*, **31**, 2295–9.

Du, Z. D., Zhang, T., Liang, L., *et al.* (2002). Epidemiologic picture of Kawasaki disease in Beijing from 1995 through 1999. *Pediatric Infectious Disease Journal*, **21**, s103–7.

Duhaut, P., Pinede, L., Demolombe-Rague, S., *et al.* (1998). Giant cell arteritis and cardiovascular risk factors. A multi-centre, prospective case-control study. *Arthritis and Rheumatism*, **41**, 1960–5.

Duhaut, P., Pinede, L., Demolombe-Rague, S., *et al.* (1999a). Giant cell arteritis and polymyalgia rheumatica: are pregnancies a protective factor? A multicentre, prospective case-control study. *Rheumatology*, **38**, 118–23.

Duhaut, P., Bosshard, S., Calvet, A., *et al.* (1999b). Giant cell arteritis, polymyalgia rheumatica, and viral hypothesis: A multicenter, prospective case-control study. *Journal of Rheumatology*, **26**, 361–9.

Duna, G. F., Cotch, M. F., Galperin, C., *et al.* (1998). Wegener's granulomatosis: role of environmental exposures. *Clinical and Experimental Rheumatology*, **16**, 669–74.

Elling, P., Olsson, A. T., and Elling, H. (1996). Synchronous variations of the incidence of temporal arteritis and polymyalgia rheumatica in different regions of Denmark, association with epidemics of *Mycoplasma pneumoniae* infection. *Journal of Rheumatology*, **23**, 112–9.

El-Reshaid, K., Varro, J., Al-Duwairi, Q., *et al.* (1995). Takayasu arteritis in Kuwait. *Journal of Tropical Medicine and Hygiene*, **98**, 299–305.

El-Reshaid, K., Kapoor, M., El-Reshaid, W., *et al.* (1997). The spectrum of renal disease associated with microscopic polyangiitis and classical polyarteritis nodosa in Kuwait. *Nephrology Dialysis and Transplant*, **12**, 1874–82.

Faerk, K. K. (1992). Simultaneous occurrence of polymyalgia rheumatica in a married couple. *Journal of Internal Medicine*, **231**, 621–2.

Falk, R., Hogan, S., Carey, T., *et al.* (1990). Clinical course of anti-neutrophil cytoplasmic antibody associated glomerulonephritis and systemic vasculitis. *Annals of Internal Medicine*, **113**, 656–63.

Fauci, A. S., Haynes, B. F., Katz, P., *et al.* (1983). Wegener's granulomatosis: prospective clinical and therapeutic experience with 85 patients for 21 years. *Annals of Internal Medicine*, **98**, 76–85.

Fledelius, H. C. and Nissen, K. R. (1992). Giant cell arteritis and visual loss. *Acta Ophthalmologica*, **70**, 801–5.

Franzen, P., Sutinen, S. and Von Knorring, J. (1992). Giant cell arteritis and polymyalgia rheumatica in region of Finland: an epidemiologic, clinical and pathologic study, 1984–1988. *Journal of Rheumatology*, **19**, 273–80.

Friedman, G., Friedman, B. and Benbassat, J. (1982). Epidemiology of temporal arteritis in Israel. *Israel Journal of Medical Science*, **18**, 241–4.

Fries, J. F., Hunder, G. G., Bloch, D. A., *et al.* (1990). The American College of Rheumatology 1990 criteria for the classification of vasculitis: summary. *Arthritis and Rheumatism*, **33**, 1135–6.

Fujimoto, S., Uezono, S., Hisanaga, S., *et al.* (2006). Incidence of ANCA-Associated Primary Renal Vasculitis in the Miyazaki Prefecture: The First Population-Based, Retrospective, Epidemiologic Survey in Japan. *Clin J Am Soc Nephrol,* **1,** 1016–22.

García-Porrúa, C. and González-Gay, M. A. (1999). Comparative clinical and epidemiological study of hyper- sensitivity vasculitis versus Henoch Schönlein purpura in adults. *Seminars in Arthritis and Rheumatism,* **28,** 404–12.

Gardner-Medwin, J. M., Dolezalova, P., Cummins, C. and Southwood, T. R. (2002). Incidence of Henoch Schönlein purpura, Kawasaki disease, and rare vasculitides in children of different ethnic origins. *Lancet,* **360,** 1197–1202.

Gibbons, R. V., Parashar, U. D., Holman, R. C., *et al.* (2002). An evaluation of hospitalizations for Kawasaki syndrome in Georgia. *Archives of Pediatric Adolescent Medicine,* **156,** 492–6.

Gibson, A., Stamp, L. K., Chapman, P. T. and O'Donnell, J. L. (2006). The epidemiology of Wegner's granulomatosis and microscopic polyangiitis in a southern hemisphere region. *Rheumatology,* (Oxford) **45,** 624–8.

Godman, G. C. and Churg, J. (1954). Wegener's granulomatosis: pathology and review of the literature. *Archives of Pathology,* **58,** 533–53.

González, E. B., Varner, W. T., Lisse, J. R., *et al.* (1989). Giant cell arteritis in the Southern United States. *Archives of Internal Medicine,* **149,** 1561–5.

González-Gay, M. A., Blanco, R., Sánchez-Andrade, A., *et al.* (1997). Giant cell arteritis in Lugo, Spain: A more frequent disease with fewer classic features. *Journal of Rheumatology,* **24,** 2166–70.

González-Gay, M. A. and García-Porrúa, C. (1999). Systemic vasculitis in adults in North Western Spain 1988–97. Clinical and epidemiological aspects. *Medicine,* **78,** 292–308.

Gonzalez-Gay, M., García-Porrúa, C., Rivas, M. J., Rodriguez-Ledo, P., Llorca, J. (2001). Epidemiology of biopsy proven giant cell arteritis in northwestern Spain: trend over an 18 year period. *Annals of the Rheumatic Diseases,* **60,** 367–71.

Gonzalez-Gay, M., García-Porrúa, C., Guerrero, J., Rodriguez-Ledo, P., Llorca, J. (2003). The epidemiology of the primary systemic vasculitides in northwest Spain: implications of the Chapel Hill Consensus Conference definitions. *Arthritis Rheumatism,* **49,** 388–93.

Gran, J. T. and Myklebust, G. (1997). The incidence of polymyalgia rheumatica and temporal arteritis in the County of Aust Agder, South Norway: A prospective study 1987–94. *Journal of Rheumatology,* **24,** 1739–43.

Gregorini, G., Ferioli, A., Donato, F., *et al.* (1993). Association between silica exposure and necrotizing crescentic glomerulonephritis with p-ANCA and anti-MPO antibodies: a hospital-based case control study. *Advances in Experimental Medicine and Biology,* **336,** 435–40.

Gross, W. L. (2002). Churg-Strauss syndrome: update on recent developments. *Current Opinion in Rheumatology,* **14,** 11–4.

Guillevin, L. (1999). Virus-associated vasculitides. *Rheumatology,* **38,** 588–90.

Guillevin, L., Cohen, P., Gayraud, M., *et al.* (1999). Churg Strauss Syndrome: clinical study and long term follow up of 96 patients. *Medicine,* **78,** 26–37.

Hall, S., Barr, W., Lie, J. T., *et al.* (1985). Takayasu arteritis: a study of 32 North American patients. *Medicine,* **64,** 89–99.

Harnden, A., Alves, B. and Sheikh, A. (2002). Rising incidence of Kawasaki disease in England: analysis of hospital admission data. *British Medical Journal,* **324,** 1424–5.

Harrold, L. R., Andrade, S. E. and Go, A. S., *et al.* (2005). Incidence of Churg Strauss syndrome in asthma drug users: a population based perspective. *Joournal of Rheumatology,* **32,** 1076–80.

Haubitz, M., Waywadt, A., De Groot, K., *et al.* (2005). Smoking habits in patients diagnosed with ANCA associated small vessel vasculitis. *Annals of Rheumatic Disease,* **64,** 1500–02.

Haugeberg, G., Bie, R., Bendvold, A., *et al.* (1998). Primary vasculitis in a Norwegian community hospital: a retrospective study. *Clinical Rheumatology,* **17,** 364–8.

Haugeberg, G., Irgens K. A. and Thomsen, R. S. (2003). No major differences in incidence of temporal arteritis in northern and western Norway compared with reports from southern Norway. *Scandinavian Journal of Rheumatology,* **32,** 318–9.

Henoch, E. H. (1874). Uber ein eigenthumlioche Form von Purpura. *Berliner Klinika Wochenschrift,* **11,** 641–3.

Hoffman, G. S., Kerr, G. S., Leavitt, R. Y., *et al.* (1992). Wegener's granulomatosis: an analysis of 158 patients. *Annals of Internal Medicine,* **116,** 488–98.

Hogan, S. L., Satterly, K. K., Dooley, M. A., Nachman, P. H., Jennette, J. C. and Falk, R. J. (2001). Silica exposure in antineutrophil cytoplasmic antibody-associated glomerulonephritis and lupus nephritis. *Journal American Society of Nephrology,* **12,** 134–42.

Holder, S. M., Joy, M. S. and Falk, R. J. (2002). Cutaneous and systemic manifestations of drug-induced vasculitis; *Annals of Pharmacotherapy,* **36,** 130–47.

Holman, R. C., Curns, A. T., Belay, E. D., Steiner, C. A. and Schonberger, L. B. (2003). Kawasaki syndrome hospitalizations in the United States, 1997 and 2000. *Pediatrics,* **112,** 495–501.

Holman, R. C., Curns, A. T., Belay, E. D., *et al.* (2005). Kawasaki syndrome in Hawaii. *Pediatric Infectious Disease Journal,* **24,** 429–33.

Hunder, G. G., Arend, W. P., Bloch, D., *et al.* (1990b). The American College of Rheumatology 1990 criteria for the classification of vasculitis: introduction. *Arthritis and Rheumatism,* **33,** 1065–7.

Hunder, G. G., Bloch, D. A., Michel, B. A., *et al.* (1990a). The American College of Rheumatology 1990 criteria for the classification of giant cell arteritis. *Arthritis and Rheumatism,* **33,** 1122–8.

Jennette, J. C., Falk, R. J., Andrassy, K., *et al.* (1994). Nomenclature of systemic vasculitides. Proposal of an international consensus conference. *Arthritis and Rheumatism,* **37,** 187–92.

Jiao, F., Yang, L., Li, Y., *et al.* (2001). Epidemiologic and clinical characteristics of Kawasaki disease in Shaanxi province, China, 1993–1997. *Journal of Tropical Pediatrics* **47,** 54–6.

Jonasson, F., Cullen, J. F. and Elton, R. A. (1979). Temporal arteritis: a 14 year epidemiological, clinical and prognostic study. *Scottish Medical Journal,* **24,** 111–7.

Kawasaki, T. (1967). Acute febrile mucocutaneous syndrome with lymphoid involvement with specific desquamation of the fingers and toes in children: clinical observations in 50 cases. *Japanese Journal of Allergology,* **16,** 178–222.

Kinmont, P. C. and McCallum, D. I. (1965). The etiology, pathology and course of giant cell arteritis the possible role of light sensitivity. *British Journal of Dermatology,* **77,** 193.

Kobayashi, S., Yano, T., Matsumoto, Y., *et al.* (2003). Clinical and epidemiological analysis of giant cell arteritis from a nationwide survey in 1998 in Japan: The first government supported nationwide survey. *Arthritis Rheumatism (Arthritis Care Research),* **49,** 594–8.

Koide, K. (1992). Takayasu arteritis in Japan. *Heart Vessels,* **7,** 48–52.

Koldingsnes, W. and Nossent, J. C. (2000). Epidemiology of Wegener's granulomatosis in northern Norway. *Arthritis Rheumatism,* **43,** 2481–7.

Kurland, L. T., Hauser, W. A., Ferguson, R. H., *et al.* (1969). Epidemiologic features of diffuse connective tissue disorders in Rochester, Minn., 1951 through 1967, with special reference to systemic lupus erythematosus. *Mayo Clinic Proceedings,* **44,** 649–63.

Kurland, L. T., Chuang, T. Y. and Hunder, G. G. (1984). The epidemiology of systemic arteritis. In *The epidemiology of the rheumatic diseases* (eds. R. C. Lawrence and L. E. Shulman), pp. 196–205. Gower Publishing, New York.

Kussmaul, A. and Maier, R. (1866). Uber eine bisher nicht beschriebene eigenthümliche Arterienerkrankung (Periarteritis nodosa), die mit Morbus Brightü und rapid fortschreitender allgemeiner Muskellähmung einhergeht. *Deutsche Archive Klinical Medizine,* **1,** 484–514.

Lane, S. E., Scott, D. G.I., Watts, R. A., *et al.* (2000). Primary renal vasculitis in Norfolk – Increasing incidence or increasing recognition? *Nephrology Dialysis and Transplantation,* **15,** 23–27.

Lane, S. E., Watts, R. A., Bentham, G., Innes, N. J. and Scott, D. G. (2003). Are environmental factors important in primary systemic vasculitis? A case control study. *Arthritis and Rheumatism,* **48,** 124–32.

Lane, S. E., Watts, R. A. and Scott, D. G.I. (2005a). Primary systemic vasculitis: clinical features and mortality. *Quarterly Journal of Medicine,* **98,** 97–112.

Lane, S. E., Watts, R. A., Scott DGI on behalf EMEA vasculitis group. (2005b). Towards a practical classification of classification for vasculitis for epidemiological studies. *Arthritis Rheumatism,* **52** (suppl.), S224 (abstract).

Leavitt, R. Y., Fauci, A. S., Bloch, D. A., *et al.* (1990). The American College of Rheumatology criteria for the classification of Wegener's Granulomatosis. *Arthritis Rheumatism,* **33,** 1101–7.

Liu, N. H., LaBree, L. D., Feldon, S. E. and Rao, N. A. (2001). The epidemiology of giant cell arteritis: a 12 year retrospective study. *Ophthalmology,* **108,** 1145–9.

Lynch, M., Holman, R. C., Mulligan, A., Belay, E. D., Schonberger, L. B. (2003). Kawasaki syndrome hospitalizations in Ireland, 1996 through 2000. *Pediatric Infectious Disease Journal,* **22,** 959–63.

Machado, E. B., Gabriel, S. E., Beard,C. M., *et al.* (1989). A population based case-control study of temporal arteritis: evidence for an association between temporal arteritis and degenerative vascular disease? *International Journal of Epidemiology,* **18,** 836–41.

Mahr, A., Guillevin, L., Poissonnet, M., Ayme, S. (2004). Prevalences of Polyarteritis nodosa, microscopic polyangiitis, Wegener's granulomatosis, and Churg Strauss syndrome in a French Urban mulit ethnic population in 2000: a capture-recapture estimate. *Arthritis and Rheumatism,* **51,** 92–9.

Malaviya, A. N., Kumar, A., Singh, Y. N., *et al.* (1990). Wegener's granulomatosis in India: not so rare. *British Journal of Rheumatology,* **29,** 499–500.

McCreay, R. D. (1986). 'Epidemic' of polymyalgia and temporal arteritis. *Journal of Royal College of General Practitioners,* **36,** 523–4.

McMahon, B. J., Heyward, W. L., Templin, D. W., *et al.* (1989). Hepatitis B associated polyarteritis nodosa in Alaskan eskimos: clinical and epidemiological features and long term follow up. *Hepatology,* **9,** 97–101.

Mowat, A. G. and Hazleman, B. L. (1974). Polymyalgia rheumatica: a clinical study with particular reference to arterial disease. *Journal of Rheumatology,* **1,** 190–202.

Mwipatayi, B. P., Jeffrey, P. C., Beningfield. S. J., *et al.* (2005). Takayasu arteritis: clinical features and management: repport of 272 cases. *Australian New Zealand Journal of Surgery,* **75,** 1107.

Ng, B., Specks, U., Offord, K. P., Matteson, E. L. (2003). Epidemiology of Wegener Granulomatosis Since the Introduction of ANCA Testing in Olmsted County, MN, 1990–1999. *Journal of Clinical Rheumatology,* **9,** 387–8.

Ng, Y. M., Sung, R. Y., So, L. Y., *et al.* (2005). Kawasaki disease in Hong Kong. *Hong Kong Medical Journal,* **11,** 331–5.

Noltrop, S. and Svensson, B. (1991). High incidence of polymyalgia rheumatica and giant cell arteritis in a Swedish community. *Clinical and Experimental Rheumatology,* **9,** 351–5.

Nordborg, E. and Bengtsson, B-Å. (1990). Epidemiology of biopsy-proven giant cell arteritis (GCA). *Journal of Internal Medicine,* **227,** 233–6.

Nordberg, C., Johanssen, H., Petursdottir, V., Nordberg, E. (2003). The epidemiology of giant cell arteritis: special reference to changes in the age of the population. *Rheumatology,* **42,** 549–52.

Nowack, R., Lehamnn, H., Flores-Suarez, L. F., *et al.* (1999). Familial occurrence of systemic vasculitis and rapidly progressive glomerulonephritis. *American Journal of Kidney Disease,* **34,** 364–73.

Nuyts, G. D., van Vlem, E., de Vos, A., *et al.* (1995). Wegener's granulomatosis is associated with exposure to silicon compounds: a case control study. *Nephrology Dialysis and Transplantation,* **10,** 1162–5.

Ozen, S., Ruperto N., Dillon, M., *et al.* (2006). EULAR/PRES endorsed consensus criteria for the classification of childhood vasculitides. *Annals of the Rheumatic Diseases,* **65,** 936–41.

Pai, P., Bone, J. M. and Bell, G. M. (1998). Hydrocarbon exposure and glomerulonephritis due to systemic vasculitis. *Nephrology Dialysis Transplantation,* **13,** 1321–3.

Park, Y. W., Han, J. W., Park, I. S., *et al.* (2005). Epidemiologic picture of Kawasaki disease in Korea, 2000–2002. *Pediatrics International,* **47,** 382–7.

Pettersson, E. E., Sundelin, B. and Heigl, Z. (1995). Incidence and outcome of pauci-immune necrotising glomerulonephritis in adults. *Clinical Nephrology,* **43,** 141–9.

Petursdottir, V., Johannsson, H., Nordborg, C. and Nordborg, E. (1999). The epidemiology of biopsy-positive giant cell arteritis: special reference to cyclic fluctuations. *Rheumatology.* **38,** 1208–12.

Rajala, S. A., Ahvenainen, J. E., Mattila, K. J., *et al.* (1993). Incidence and survival rate in cases of biopsy-proven temporal arteritis. *Scandinavian Journal of Rheumatology,* **22,** 89–91.

Rao, J. K., Allen, N. B. and Pincus, T. (1998). Limitations of the 1990 American College of Rheumatology Classification Criteria in the diagnosis of vasculitis. *Annals of Internal Medicine,* **129,** 345–52.

Raynauld, J-P., Bloch, D. A. and Fries, J. F. (1993). Seasonal variation in the onset of Wegener's granulomatosis, polyarteritis nodosa and giant cell arteritis. *Journal of Rheumatology,* **20,** 1524–6.

Reinhold-Keller, E., Zeidler, A., Gutfleisch, J., *et al.* (2000). Giant cell arteritis is more prevalent in urban than rural populations: results of an epidemiological study of primary systemic vasculitides in Germany. *Rheumatology,* **39,** 1396–402.

Reinhold-Keller, E., Herlyn, K., Wagner-Bastmeyer, R. and Gross, W. L. (2005). Stable incidence of primary systemic vasculitides over five years: results from the German vasculitis register. *Arthritis Rheumatism,* **53,** 93–9.

Royle, J. A., Williams, K., Elliott, E., *et al.* (1998). Kawasaki disease in Australia, 1993–95. *Archives of Diseases of Childhood,* **78,** 33–39.

Russo, M. G., Waxman, J., Abdoh, A. A., *et al.* (1995). Correlation between infection and the onset of the giant cell arteritis (temporal) arteritis syndrome. *Arthritis and Rheumatism,* **38,** 374–80.

Sack, M., Cassidy, J. T. and Bole, G. G. (1975). Prognostic factors in polyarteritis. *Journal of Rheumatology,* **2,** 411–20.

Salo, E. (1993). Kawasaki disease in Finland 1982–1992. *Scandinavian Journal of Infectious Diseases,* **25,** 497–502.

Salvarani, C., Macchioni, P., Zizzi, F., *et al.* (1991). Epidemiologic and immunogenetic aspects of polymyalgia rheumatica and giant cell arteritis in northern Italy. *Arthritis and Rheumatism,* **34,** 351–6.

Salvarani, C., Gabriel, S. E., O'Fallon, W. M., *et al.* (1995a). The incidence of giant cell arteritis in Olmstead County, Minnesota: apparent fluctuations in a cyclic pattern. *Annals of Internal Medicine,* **123,** 192–4.

Salvarani, C., Gabriel, S. E., O'Fallon, W. M., *et al.* (1995b). Epidemiology of polymyalgia rheumatica in Olmsted County, Minnesota, 1970–91. *Arthritis and Rheumatism,* **38,** 369–73.

Salvarani, C., Crowson, C. S., O'Fallon, W. M., Hunder, G. G. and Gabriel, S. E. (2004). Reappraisal of the epidemiology of giant cell arteritis in Olmsted County, Minnesota, over a 50 year period. *Arthritis Rheumatism (Arthritis Care Research),* **51,** 264–8.

Schiller, B., Fasth, A., Bjorkheim, G., *et al.* (1995). Kawasaki disease in Sweden: incidence and clinical features. *Acta Paediatrica,* **84,** 769–74.

Schönlein, H. (1837). *Allgemeine und Specielle Pathologie und Therapie,* Vol 2, 3rd edn. Wurzburg, Herisau.

Scott, D. G.I., Bacon, P. A. and Tribe, C. R. (1981). Systemic rheumatoid vasculitis: a clinical and laboratory study of 50 cases. *Medicine,* **60,** 288–97.

Scott, D. G.I., Bacon, P. A., Elliott, P. J., *et al.* (1982). Systemic vasculitis in a district general hospital 1972–80: clinical and laboratory features, classification and prognosis of 80 cases. *Quarterly Journal of Medicine*, **203,** 292–311.

Selga D, Mohammad A, Sturfelt G, Segelmark M. (2006). Polyarteritis nodosa when applying the Chapel Hill nomenclature–a descriptive study on ten patients. *Rheumatology* (Oxford), **45,** 1276–81.

Smith, C. A., Fidler, W. J. and Pinals, R. S. (1983). The epidemiology of giant cell arteritis. Report of a ten year study in Shelby County, Tennessee. *Arthritis and Rheumatism*, **26,** 1214–9.

Sonnenblick, M., Nesher, G., Friedlande, Y., *et al.* (1986). Giant cell arteritis in Jerusalem: A 12 year epidemiological study. *British Journal of Rheumatology*, **33,** 938–41.

Staples, J. A., Ponsonby, A-L., Lim, L.L-Y. and McMichael, A. M. (2003). Ecologic analysis of some immune related disorders, including type I diabetes, in Australia: Latitude, regional ultraviolet radiation, and disease prevalence. *Environmental Health Perspective,* **111,** 518–23.

Stegeman, C. A., Cohen Tervaert, J. W., de Jong, P. E., *et al.* (1996). Trimethoprim-ulphamethoxazole (co-trimoxazole) for the prevention of relapses in Wegener's granulomatosis. *New England Journal of Medicine*, **335,** 16–20.

Stewart, M., Savage, J. M., Bell, B., *et al.* (1988). Long term renal prognosis of Henoch Schönlein purpura in an unselected childhood population. *European Journal of Paediatrics*, **147,** 113–5.

Stratta, P., Messuerotti, A., Canavese, C., Coen, M. and Luccoli, L. (2001). The role of metals in autoimmune vasculitis: epidemiological and pathogenic study. *Science Total Environment*, **270,** 179–90.

Tidman, M., Olander, R., Svalander, C., *et al.* (1998). Patients hospitalised because of small vessel vasculitides with renal involvement in the period 1975–95: organ involvement, anti-neutrophil cytoplasmic antibodies patterns, seasonal attack rates and fluctuation of annual frequencies. *Journal of Internal Medicine*, **244,** 133–41.

Tourneux, P., Dufillot, D., Belloy, M., *et al.* (2005). Kawasaki disease in Guadeloupe. *Presse Med*, **15,** 25–8.

Turesson, C., McClelland, R. L., Christianson, T. J.H. and Matteson, E. L. (2004). No decrease over time in the incidence of vasculitis or other extra-articular manifestations in rheumatoid arthritis: results from a community base study. *Arthritis Rheumatism*, **50,** 3729–32.

Vanoli, M., Daina, E., Salvarani, C., *et al.* (2005). Takayasu arteritis: a study of 107 Italian patients. *Arthritis Rheumatism,* **53,** 100–7.

Waern, A. U., Andersson, P. and Hemmingsson, A. (1983). Takayasu's arteritis: a hospital-region based study on occurrence, treatment and prognosis. *Angiology*, **34,** 311–20.

Ward, M. M. (2004). Decreases in rates of hospitalizations for manifestations of severe rheumatoid arthritis, 1983–2001. *Arthritis Rheumatism*, **50,** 1122–31.

Watts, R. A., Carruthers, D. M., and Scott, D. G. (1995). Isolated nail fold vasculitis in rheumatoid arthritis. *Annals of the Rheumatic Diseases*, **54,** 927–9.

Watts, R. A., Gonzalez-Gay, M., Garcia-Porrua, C., Lane, S., Bentham, G. and Scott, D. G.I. (2001). Geoepidemiology of systemic vasculitis. *Annals of the Rheumatic Disease*, **60,** 170–72.

Watts, R. A., Jolliffe, V. A., Grattan, C. E.H., *et al.* (1998). Cutaneous vasculitis in a defined population – clinical and epidemiological associations. *Journal of Rheumatology*, **25,** 920–4.

Watts, R. A., Lane, S. E., Bentham, G., *et al.* (2000). Epidemiology of systemic vasculitis – a ten year study in the United Kingdom. *Arthritis and Rheumatism*, **43,** 414–19.

Watts, R. A., Lane, S., Bentham, G. and Scott, D. G.I. (2000). Is giant cell arteritis more common in the north of Europe. *Clinical Experimental Immunology*, **120** (suppl. 1), 63.

Watts, R. A., Lane, S. E., Mooney, J. and Scott, D. G.I. (2005). Primary systemic vasculitis – unchanged incidence over 15 years. *Rheumatology*, **44** (suppl.), i22.

Watts, R. A., Mooney, J., Lane, S. E. and Scott, D. G.I. (2004). Rheumatoid vasculitis – becoming extinct? *Rheumatology*, **43,** 920–3.

Watts R., Lane S., Hanslik T., *et al.* (2007). Development and validation of a consensus methodology for the classification of the ANCA-associated vasculitides and polyarteritis nodosa for epidemiological studies. *Ann Rheum Dis*, **66,** 222–7.

Wechsler, M. E., Garpestad, E., Flier, S. R., *et al.* (1998). Pulmonary infiltrates, eosinophilia, and cardiomyopathy following corticosteroid withdrawal in patients with asthma receiving Zafirlukast. *Journal of the American Medical Association*, **279,** 455–7.

Westman, K. W.A., Bygren, P. G., Olsson, H., *et al.* (1998). Relapse rate, renal survival, and cancer morbidity in patients with Wegener's granulomatosis or microscopic polyangiitis and renal involvement. *Journal of American Society for Nephrology*, **9,** 842–52.

Yanagawa, H., Yashiro, M., Nakamura, Y., *et al.* (1995). Epidemiologic pictures of Kawasaki disease in Japan from the nationwide incidence survey in 1991 and 1992. *Paediatrics*, **95,** 475–9.

Yanagawa, H., Nakamura, Y., Yashiro, M., *et al.* (2001). Incidence survey of Kawasaki disease in 1997 and 1998 in Japan. *Pediatrics*, **107,** E33.

Yang, Y. H., Hung, C. F., Hsu, C. R., *et al.* (2005). A nationwide survey on epidemiological characteristics of childhood Henoch Schonlein purpura in Taiwan. *Rheumatology,* **44,** 618–22.

Yashiro, M., Muso, E., Itoh-Ihara, T., *et al.* (2000). Significantly high regional morbidity of MPO-ANCA related angiitis and/or nephritis with respiratory tract involvement after the 1995 great earthquake in Kobe (Japan). *American Journal of Kidney Disease*, **35,** 889–95.

Zeek, P. M. (1952). Periarteritis nodosa – a critical review. *American Journal of Clinical Pathology*, **22,** 777–90.

Zeft, A., Schlesinger, M., Weiss, N. and Emery, H. (2005). Case control study of ANCA associated vasculitis in Western Montana. *Arthritis and Rheumatism*, **52,** S648 (abstract).

PART 2

Basic science

CHAPTER 3

Hypersensitivity

T. Prescott Atkinson

Introduction

The study of hypersensitivity reactions, in which tissue damage occurring as a result of an immunologic response, is inextricably entwined in the roots of the science of immunology in the late nineteenth and early twentieth centuries. Many of the giants of the early days of immunology made indelible marks in science through their studies of hypersensitivity phenomena. The impetus for discovery in the preantibiotic era was the inadequate medical treatment of infections in patients for whom little could be done outside immunologic modulation. At the dawn of the twenty-first century, it is ironic that scientific interest in immunomodulation using vaccines and other biologic agents as prevention and cure for infectious and inflammatory diseases is renewed with the realization that microbial resistance to antibiotics is inexorably increasing. This chapter is an attempt to review the history of the various hypersensitivity phenomena, the framework for differentiating them, and recent advances in our understanding of the complex mechanisms at work within the context of vasculitis diseases and syndromes.

The history of the discovery of hypersensitivity reactions is punctuated by many famous names. As in any area of science, few of these researchers could claim that their work was not built upon an edifice of knowledge constructed by a multitude of predecessors and contemporaries whose names are much less well known today. It is noteworthy that in 1798, long before the development of the science of immunology, Edward Jenner published the first example of delayed hypersensitivity in a controlled setting with his description of a local cutaneous "reaction of immunity" which developed over 24–48 hours in subjects reinoculated with vaccinia virus (Movat 1979). Robert Koch rediscovered the phenomenon in 1890 with his description of a similar reaction in tuberculous patients injected intradermally with tuberculin. The phenomenon of anaphylaxis described by Paul Portier and Charles Richet in 1902 (Portier and Richet 1902), for which work Richet received the Nobel prize in 1913, provided evidence of the existence of explosive hypersensitivity reactions which obviously differed fundamentally from the delayed reactions described by Koch and Jenner.

The term "allergy," meaning "other reactivity" (as opposed to "normergy," the normal host response) was first suggested in 1906 by Clemens P. von Pirquet, who believed that immunity and hypersensitivity, host protection and tissue damage, were opposite ends of the spectrum of the immune response, a concept which is arguably still acceptable today. Together with Bela Schick 1 year earlier, von Pirquet had described serum sickness, a peculiar illness which developed in individuals who had been given horse serum as treatment for diphtheria (Pirquet and Schick 1905). Maurice Arthus at about the same time described the reaction that bears his name, a necrotizing, hemorrhagic local skin reaction which developed in rabbits repeatedly injected with horse serum subcutaneously at 6-day intervals (Arthus 1903). Thus, within a 15-year period in the early twentieth century, hypersensitivity reactions later recognized as involving IgE-mast cell activation, antibody-complement-Fc receptor interactions, and T cell activation had been identified. All primarily depend upon the adaptive portion of the immune system. It would be decades before even the most basic molecular details of the mechanisms at work in these reactions became clear, and it would be fair to say that none are completely understood at present.

To these classical immunologic hypersensitivity reactions should be added at least one more, which involves the innate arm of the immune response. Gregory Shwartzman first described the "phenomenon of local tissue reactivity" in the late 1930s (Shwartzman 1937). In his systematic exploration of this remarkable hypersensitivity reaction Shwartzman demonstrated that a preparatory intradermal injection of culture filtrate from a variety of Gram-negative bacteria followed by an intravenous injection of filtrate about 24 hours later resulted in a thrombohemorrhagic reaction at the site of the original injection. The phenomenon did not seem to involve classical immunologic reactivity as it occurred too rapidly and was not transferable by serum; however, it could be blocked by pretreatment with antiserum to the specific bacterial agent used.

A generalized form of the Shwartzman reaction, resembling disseminated intravascular coagulation (DIC), was probably observed prior to Schwartzman's work by Sanarelli (Sanarelli 1924) and later by Apitz (Apitz 1934). This systemic thrombohemorrhagic reaction characterized by coagulopathy, microthrombi, reduced platelets and leukocytes, and often bilateral renal cortical hemorrhage, could be reliably induced by the intravenous injection of live Gram-negative bacteria or culture supernatant 24 hours apart.

Later workers who explored the pathogenesis of the generalized reaction included such famous researchers as Lewis Thomas and Robert A. Good (Thomas and Good 1952). Insight (albeit as yet incomplete) into the pathogenesis of the Shwartzman reaction would have to wait until the close of the twentieth century with the explosion of knowledge regarding inflammatory cytokines and the cellular elements of the immune system that generate them. The generalized Shwartzman reaction has been shown to depend upon the action of IFN-γ, TNF-α, and IL-12 (Ozmen *et al.* 1994). Lipopolysaccharide (LPS)-induced IL-12 and IL-15 from macrophages appear to induce IFN-γ production which then sensitizes macrophages to the second exposure 18–24 hours later (Fehniger *et al.* 2000). The primary subsets of cells which generate the key inflammatory cytokine IFN-γ, at least in mice, appear to be CD3+ natural killer T (NKT) cells when low doses of LPS are used and orthodox natural killer (NK) cells at higher doses of endotoxin (Kim *et al.* 2000; Dieli *et al.* 2000). A storm of inflammatory cytokines following the second injection results in DIC and life-threatening shock.

The best known classification scheme for hypersensitivity reactions involving the adaptive immune system was published by P.G.H. Gell and R.R.A. Coombs in 1963 (Table 3.1) (Coombs and Gell 1963), and it is still a useful framework for thinking about them today. Although the different forms of antigen-specific hypersensitivity disorders will be discussed within this setting, it should be kept in mind that they offer only a general reference point for understanding the initiation of the complex processes of inflammation which ensue. As knowledge increases with regard to certain elements of the immune system, for example NK cells, NKT cells, or γδ T cells, our ability to distinguish specific hypersensitivity disorders related to those elements may improve.

Table 3.1 Gell and Coombs classification of hypersensitivity reactions

Type I: Anaphylactic
Allergic rhinoconjunctivitis
Acute urticaria
Allergic asthma
Atopic dermatitis
Anaphylaxis

Type II: Cytolytic or cytotoxic
Drug-induced immune cytopenias
Infection-induced (e.g. Goodpasture's syndrome)
Transfusion reactions
Hyperacute graft rejection
Hemolytic disease of the newborn (Rh incompatibility)

Type III: Immune complex/Arthus reaction
Drug-induced immune complex disease ('serum-sickness like')
Infection-induced (e.g. acute rheumatic fever)
Arthus reactions (e.g. to immunizations)
Hypersensitivity pneumonitis
Serum sickness

Type IV: Cell-mediated
Drug reactions
Delayed-type hypersensitivity (e.g. insect bites, vaccines)
Contact hypersensitivity (e.g. Rhus dermatitis)
Hypersensitivity pneumonitis
Foreign body reaction
Chronic graft rejection

Type I hypersensitivity

Disorders such as "summer catarrh" or "hay fever" (allergic rhinoconjunctivitis) had been described beginning in the early 1800s but the pathogenic mechanism was unclear (Bostock 1828). In 1923 Coca and Cooke first proposed the term "atopy" (from the Greek meaning "without place") to describe a heterogeneous group of hypersensitivity disorders including hay fever, allergic asthma, and atopic dermatitis (or "flexural neurodermatitis" as it was then known) which had hitherto been difficult to categorize (Coca and Cooke 1923). The existence of a transferable serum factor in systemic anaphylaxis had been demonstrated in animals by Charles Richet and a similar factor was shown to exist in humans with local cutaneous anaphylaxis by Prausnitz and Kustner in 1921 (Prausnitz and Küstner 1921). The nature of this transferable "reaginic" hypersensitivity remained undefined for another 50 years until the discovery of IgE by Kimishige Ishizaka and colleagues in 1966 (Ishizaka *et al.* 1966).

The genetic basis for atopy is the subject of intensive ongoing study. A number of chromosomal regions have been associated with allergic disease, including most prominently 11q13 (containing the high affinity IgE receptor (FcεRI) beta subunit), 5q31–33 (containing the cytokine gene cluster of interleukin-3,4,5,9,13, and granulocyte-macrophage colony-stimulating factor), and 12q (containing IFN-γ, KIT ligand (stem cell factor), insulin-like growth factor-1 (IGF-1), and the constitutive form of nitric oxide synthetase (NOS1)) (Manian 1997). Specific polymorphisms have been identified in a number of candidate genes which appear to confer susceptibility to atopy and/or allergic asthma (Barnes 1999; Blumenthal 2000; Borish 1999; Rosenwasser 1999). These include the IL-4 receptor alpha chain (Hershey *et al.* 1997; Kruse *et al.* 1999; Ober *et al.* 2000; Oisoet al. 2000; Rosa-Rosa *et al.* 1999), the promoter region of the IL-4 gene (Burchard *et al.* 1999; Song *et al.* 1996), the β$_2$ adrenergic receptor (Green *et al.* 1993; Reihsaus *et al.* 1993), the 5′ flanking region of the CD14 gene (Baldini *et al.* 1999), and acidic mammalian chitinase (Zhu *et al.* 2004; Bierbaum *et al.* 2005). A recent review of hundreds of genetic association studies revealed that eight genes had been linked with asthma/atopy in at least five studies each: interleukin-4 (IL4), interleukin-13 (IL13), β$_2$ adrenergic receptor (ADRB2), human leukocyte antigen DRB1 (HLA-DRB1), TNF-α (TNF), lymphotoxin-alpha (LTA), FcεRI beta subunit (FCER1B), and IL-4 receptor alpha subunit (IL4RA) (Hoffjan *et al.* 2003). With convincing evidence for contributions from such a wide variety of genes, atopy is most likely the product of contributions from multiple genes as well as the environment.

The aptly named hygiene hypothesis postulates that it is the low level of infection and parasitism in Western society that has fostered the rise in Type I Hypersensitivity disorders (Schaub *et al.* 2006; Liu and Leung 2006). Under this line of reasoning, individuals with a polygenic predisposition for atopy have a lower threshold for specific IgE formation, a trait which may be adaptive in regions where helminth infections are endemic but are detrimental in developed nations where such parasites are less common. In atopic individuals, the IgE system is thus more likely to respond inappropriately to environmental antigens from pollen and foods, producing symptoms in the absence of high levels of parasite-specific IgE. This predisposition to exuberant IgE responses is exacerbated in environmental conditions lacking in Th1-stimulating infections and microbial compounds such as LPS.

Mast cells are of fundamental importance in Type I hypersensitivity. Particularly abundant along mucosal and epithelial surfaces and in perivascular locations, mast cells are well suited to early amplification of local inflammatory responses and appear to act as sentinels for local injury. IgE binds to the multimeric high affinity IgE receptor, FcεRI, primarily on mast cells and basophils, where it may remain on the cell surface for weeks or months. Atopic individuals respond to antigenic stimulation, particularly at low levels over mucosal borders, with Th2 type cytokine production which results in specific IgE production (Biedermann and Rocken 1999). Dosing of antigen-mediated receptor aggregation on mast cells has revealed that the EC50 for IL-4 production is among the lowest of all the cytokines produced by mast cells (Gonzales-Espinosa et al. 2003), occurring even below the threshold for histamine release, and this may be at least part of the explanation for the tendency for Th2 responses to occur at low-level antigen stimulation.

Experimental activation of mucosal mast cells through the high affinity IgE receptor with allergen challenge results in two distinct phases of inflammation in many subjects: an acute phase marked by angioedema, pruritus, and vasodilatation and a delayed phase some 6–12 hours later which is characterized by a cellular infiltrate, principally with neutrophils, eosinophils, and basophils (Charlesworth et al. 1989; White 1999). With intracellular amounts at approximately 10 pg/cell, histamine can reach millimolar concentrations locally around the mast cell when released. The bioactivity of histamine accounts for virtually all the acute phase effects of mast cell activation while TNF-α accounts for a major portion of delayed phase effects (Wershil et al. 1991).

A bewildering array of cytokines is synthesized by mast cells including IL-1, IL-2, IL-3, IL-4, IL-5, IL-6, IL-8, IL-13, IL-16, GM-CSF, TNF-α, TGF-β, bFGF, FGF-2, PDGF, NGF, VPF/VEGF, and several C-C chemokines (Wedemeyer and Galli 2000). In at least some mast cell populations in humans and rodents TNF-α and IL-4 can be stored preformed in granules, potentially reducing the time required for initial release following cellular activation (Bradding et al. 1993; Bradding et al. 1995; MacLeod et al. 1997; Wedemeyer and Galli 2000). Early activation of mast cells in mice appears to be essential for protection from fast moving infections in the peritoneal cavity; mice genetically deficient in mast cells succumb to experimental peritonitis induced by cecal ligation and puncture (Echtenacher et al. 1996; Malaviya et al. 1996). IL-4 is essential for the production of IgE and the induction of Th2 responses (Brown and Hural 1997; Kuhn et al. 1991).

Mast cell activation also results in rapid de novo synthesis of lipid-derived mediators including leukotrienes C4 and D4 (LTC4 and LTD4), which act primarily to increase vascular permeability at the site of mediator release, and prostaglandin D2 (PGD2), which acts to increase smooth muscle tone, to increase blood flow locally, and to stimulate mucus (Henderson 1994; Kay 1983; Ramos et al. 1992; Boyce 2005). Platelet-activating factor (PAF), another lipid-derived mediator probably also produced by mast cell activation, increases smooth muscle tone, produces increased microvascular permeability, and activates local endothelial cells promoting expression of adhesion molecules (Stafforini et al. 2003).

Mast cell granules contain a variety of enzymes, particularly neutral proteases (Lutzelschwab et al. 1997), as well as a proteoglycan matrix which is responsible for their distinctive metachromatic staining property in histological sections. At least five different chymases and two different tryptases are associated with mast cell granules. The functions of mast cell-derived tryptases appear to include a kallikrein-like activity catalyzing the formation of bradykinin, which enhances increased vascular permeability produced by histamine (Imamura et al. 2004; Fiorucci and Ascoli 2004). Activation of diverse cellular responses to mast cell-derived chymases and tryptases occurs partly through the activation of G-protein-coupled proteinase-activated receptors (PAR), with chymases selectively activating PAR_1 and tryptases PAR_2 (Reed and Kita 2004).

Mast cells are capable of responding to a variety of other stimuli including complement fragments C5a and C3a, and physical stimuli such as heat, cold, and hyperosmolarity. Polyamines such as Compound 48/80, spermine, and a variety of basic polypeptides such as Substance P elicit rapid exocytosis from rodent mast cells as well as human skin mast cells (Ansel et al. 1993; Mousli et al. 1994; Yano et al. 1989). Plant lectins such as Concanavalin A aggregate cell surface glycoproteins on the cell including the IgE receptor and produce robust mast cell activation. Finally, a number of cytokines, particularly stem cell factor, have been found to induce degranulation in mast cells (Alam et al. 1994; Galli and Costa 1995; Lukacs et al. 1996; Tsai, Tam, and Galli 1993). The ability of mast cells to respond to such a wide array of stimuli highlights their importance in the early phase of the inflammatory response.

The late-phase inflammatory response, which follows extensive mast cell degranulation, is marked by a cellular influx rich in neutrophils and eosinophils, but basophils have also been recognized to play a role in allergic inflammation. Like mast cells, basophils also express the high affinity IgE receptor at relatively high surface densities, enabling their response to allergens in the area, and they also release stored histamine as well as newly synthesized eicosanoids and cytokines, particularly IL-4 and IL-13, in response to IgE receptor aggregation by allergen (Guo et al. 1994; Iliopoulos et al. 1992; Lichtenstein and Bochner 1991; Marone et al. 1997; Redrup et al. 1998). Mast cell elaboration of cytokines such as IL-5, IL-8, and TNFα with concomitant activation of local endothelium is likely the major factor controlling the influx of these granulocytic cell types (Bradding et al. 1993; Moller et al. 1993; Tanimoto, Takahashi, and Kimura 1992; Zhang et al. 1995). Finally, mast cells may induce the influx of T lymphocytes both by direct production of IL-16 and by histamine-induced IL-16 production in some tissues (Laberge et al. 1999; Mashikian et al. 1998; Rumsaeng et al. 1997). The immigrant cell populations called in by initial mast cell activation are thus able to potentiate the regional inflammatory response with their own mediators.

Type II hypersensitivity

Despite extensive experimental work over the course of the entire twentieth century, many of the details of the Type II and Type III hypersensitivity reactions remain to be deciphered. The distinction between the two is probably somewhat artificial, but there is some merit in discriminating between antibody reactions directed against surfaces (cells or structural elements of the extracellular matrix) (Type II) and those which occur in liquid phase (Type III). The production of cellular damage from binding of antibody to the surfaces of cells or tissue structures followed by activation of complement and Fc receptor bearing cells such as neutrophils and macrophages is the traditional model used to explain tissue injury in Type II hypersensitivity. Since the reaction occurs against components of tissues, not surprisingly many examples involve autoimmunity. The involvement of autoantibodies against endothelial cell antigens at present is a plausible but unproven cause of vasculitis (Youinou *et al.* 2005), which will be discussed elsewhere in this volume.

The development of animal models that accurately reflect human autoimmune diseases is an important step in understanding the pathogenesis of these disorders and in the production of novel therapies (Table 3.2) (Cohen and Miller 1994; Bigazzi 1998). The roles and relative importance of complement and Fc receptors have proven particularly difficult to understand. In animal models of antibody-mediated autoimmune disease, such as glomerulonephritis induced by heterologous antibody to renal tissues or specific glomerular components, the involvement of phagocytes is generally essential to full expression of the disease (Cochrane *et al.* 1965; Schrijver *et al.* 1990; Suzuki *et al.* 1998). In certain cases, however, such as Heymann nephritis, which is induced by immunization of rats with brush border antigens, particularly megalin, the resultant nephritis appears to be also dependent on the assembly of terminal complement components into the membrane attack (Farquhar *et al.* 1995).

Fcγ receptors on phagocytes have recently assumed an increasingly important role in understanding Type II and Type III hypersensitivity disorders. Using mice homozygous for a targeted deletion of the Fc receptor common gamma chain, Clynes and Ravetch (1995) have shown that even prototypical Type II disorders, such as immune hemolytic anemia and thrombocytopenia in mice, do not develop in the absence of functional Fc receptors. Importantly, mutational deletion of a specific Fc receptor, FcγRIIB, which downregulates the activation of other Fc receptors, renders the animals more susceptible to tissue damage by cytotoxic antibodies (Nakamura *et al.* 2000; Suzuki *et al.* 1998).

The production of antibodies to cell surface molecules may also result in modulation of cellular functions when the surface molecule is a receptor, a transmembrane channel, or other molecule with a signaling function. Cell bound antibody may either block normal receptor function, as in myasthenia gravis, or stimulate abnormal receptor activity, as in Graves' disease. Recent evidence indicates that chronic urticaria, formerly thought to be a form of Type I hypersensitivity is caused in about 50% of cases by autoantibodies against

Table 3.2 Animal models in Type II hypersensitivity

Animal Model	Reference
Heymann nephritis	Farquhar *et al.* 1995
Anti-Thy-1 antibody-induced glomerulonephritis	Eppel *et al.* 2000
Autoimmune glomerular basement membrane disease	Nakamura *et al.* 2000; Tang *et al.* 2000
Experimental autoimmune myasthenia gravis	Vincent 1994
Experimental Graves' disease	Ludgate 2000
Collagen-induced arthritis	Myers *et al.* 1997
Experimental bullous pemphigoid	Liu *et al.* 1993; Liu *et al.* 1995
Experimental autoimmune hemolytic anemia	Cox and Howles 1981; Nisitani *et al.* 1997; Sharon and Naor 1992

the alpha chain of the high affinity IgE receptor, which triggers mast cell degranulation and the typical pruritic rash (Greaves 2000).

Type III hypersensitivity

Tissue damage produced by soluble immune complexes (IC) has been studied extensively over the past century. IC probably form routinely during the clearance of antigens derived from infectious agents and under normal circumstances are cleared without sequelae. Under certain conditions, however, IC may occasionally produce devastating tissue damage. As with Type II reactions, IC disease may also be due to autoimmunity when the antigen involved is self-derived, but the source of the offending complexes in this disorder is frequently related to infection or drug therapy. Much of the morbidity and mortality in the prototypical autoimmune disease systemic lupus erythematosus is mediated by immune complexes. In contrast to the situation in Type II disorders, IC disease is clearly implicated in at least one form of vasculitis, often designated hypersensitivity vasculitis, discussed in detail elsewhere in this volume (Chapter 39) (Russell and Gibson 2006).

Immune complex injury to tissues may be induced by reaction of antigen and antibody to form IC (a) within the vessel lumen where they subsequently move into the vessel and tissues (serum sickness reaction) or (b) within the vessel wall and outside the vessel within the tissues (Arthus reaction). Different forms of the Arthus reaction have been produced, and, although usually elicited in the skin, the reaction may be produced in any vascular tissue (Ranadive and Movat 1979). The active or direct reaction occurs when antigen is injected intradermally in a hyperimmune animal. In this situation, IgG antibody within the extravascular space reacts with the injected antigen locally. Passive reactions are produced when antibody and antigen are both injected in a naïve animal, the reverse passive reaction occurs when antibody is injected intradermally and antigen is given intravenously.

Perhaps not surprisingly, experimental evidence demonstrates that the most severe vascular injury results when the reaction occurs within the vessel wall as in the reverse passive Arthus reaction, as opposed to administration of both antibody and antigen either intravenously or intradermally (Cochrane and Weigle 1958). Mast cells appear to be important in the evolution of the direct response because extravasation of Evan's blue dye from the vasculature is seen within 3–5 minutes after injection, and this increased permeability is suppressible by antihistamines (Hayashi *et al.* 1964). This immediate increase in local vascular permeability is largely absent in the passive Arthus reaction.

The mechanisms involved in immune complex disease have been the focus of intensive study. It has been known for decades that neutrophils are required for the development of Arthus lesions (Cochrane *et al.* 1959). Phagocytosis and clearance of IC within vessel walls begins within minutes of initiation (Hopken *et al.* 1997). More recent studies using mice in which the Fc receptor common gamma chain has been eliminated by targeted genetic deletion demonstrate that, as with cytotoxic antibodies in Type II reactions, Type III reactions require the presence of functional Fc receptors (Clynes *et al.* 1999; Clynes *et al.* 1998). At least a part of this requirement appears to relate to a necessary function for FcγRIII on mast cells in the direct Arthus reaction (Sylvestre and Ravetch 1996). Finally, as in Type II hypersensitivity reactions, deletion of the down-regulatory FcγRIIB receptor in mice potentiates IC-mediated tissue damage (Clynes *et al.* 1999). The interaction of Fc receptors on phagocytes and mast cells with IC thus forms an essential step in both the clearance of IC and the production of the severe inflammatory lesion. Our understanding of the complexity of interactions between the complement system and Fc-phagocyte compartment was increased by the recent discovery that the anaphylatoxin C5a may regulate the levels of activating and inhibitory Fc receptors on phagocytes (Shushakova *et al.* 2002).

The importance of Fc receptors in human immune complex diseases is underscored by two recently recognized pairs of polymorphisms in FcγRIIA and FcγRIIIA which correlate with disease phenotype in the prototypical autoimmune immune complex disorder, systemic lupus erythematosus (SLE). Two common polymorphisms in the extracellular domain of human FcγRIIA produce different binding affinities for IgG2 (Salmon *et al.* 1996); one, the H131 allele, is significantly under-represented among African Americans with SLE. Similarly, a pair of common polymorphisms in FcγRIIIA produces a difference in affinities for IgG1 and IgG3 (Wu *et al.* 1997). The allele with the lower affinity is significantly associated with SLE, especially with renal involvement. One possible interpretation of these observations is that Fcγ alleles with low affinities for IgG subclasses are associated with impaired IC clearance, predisposing affected individuals to chronic inflammation and subsequent autoimmune disease.

The involvement of complement in the pathogenesis of Arthus lesions is complex and may be more important in some species and tissues than others. Decomplementation of animals with cobra venom factor generally does not abrogate immune complex-mediated inflammatory reactions, although the resulting tissue damage may be diminished (Ranadive and Movat 1979). Activation of complement and release of anaphylatoxins C3a and C5a have been regarded as important in the activation of local mast cells (in the direct reaction), basophils and platelets within the vasculature, and in directing the neutrophilic influx. In support of this suggestion, deletion of the receptor for C5a in mice eliminates IC-mediated pulmonary inflammation and significantly reduces, but does not eliminate, the inflammatory response to the reverse passive Arthus reaction (Hopken *et al.* 1997).

A somewhat different mechanism of tissue injury occurs when massive quantities of immune complexes arise within the circulation during the development of serum sickness. The condition can be readily produced in rabbits by intravenous injection of 10 ml of xenogeneic serum or 0.25 g of purified foreign protein (e.g. albumin) per kg of weight (Ranadive and Movat 1979). Early studies determined that antigen (bovine serum albumin) elimination in rabbits occurs in three phases: the first 2 days being that of equilibration in the extravascular and intravascular compartments, the second consisting of relatively slow catabolism over the next 8 days, and a final rapid phase of elimination over 2–3 days as immune complex formation progresses. The size of the complexes increases with increasing antibody concentration until antibody excess occurs, and the development of vasculitis and glomerulonephritis is accompanied by a significant fall in the serum hemolytic complement (Cochrane and Hawkins 1968; Dixon *et al.* 1958). Vascular and glomerular lesions in rabbits correlate almost entirely with the appearance of large circulating IC (greater than 19S). IC decline in serum and free antibody appears by day 13, approximately 2–3 days prior to resolution of vasculitis. In the course of a reaction to a single injection, segmental vasculitic lesions are produced which are typically within the heart, joints, and glomeruli. There is usually a transmural neutrophilic infiltrate but little necrosis or hemorrhage.

Deposition of immunoglobulin and complement in vessel walls, on the surface of the synovium, and in glomeruli is readily demonstrated in fresh lesions in serum sickness. Severe glomerulonephritis in experimental animals usually develops only with chronic antigenemia induced by repeated injections. The mild glomerular injury in acute serum sickness is ablated neither by decomplementation nor by induced leukopenia, but the arteritis is significantly decreased by either manipulation. Interestingly, vasoactive amines potentiate the development of vascular lesions. Passive anaphylaxis or injection of anaphylatoxins in experimental animals worsens inflammatory lesions, and their appearance in response to these agents is blocked by antihistamines (Ranadive and Movat 1979). In human patients with circulating immune complexes, injection of histamine into uninvolved areas of skin can elicit necrotizing cutaneous vasculitis (Chossegros *et al.* 1987; Gower *et al.* 1977; Jorizzo *et al.* 1983; Wolff *et al.* 1978). On the basis of these studies, the activation of basophils and platelets with release of vasoactive amines in individuals with circulating IC is likely to worsen the vascular injury during a serum sickness reaction.

Abnormal complement clearance of soluble IC as well as those which have become deposited in vessel walls and other tissues is believed to explain the pronounced tendency for individuals with genetic deficiencies in early classical pathway components (C1, C2, C4) to develop SLE. Genetic deficiency of C1 has a nearly 100% association with SLE, the strongest risk factor yet identified (Walport *et al.* 1998). In addition, autoantibodies to C1q, particularly of the IgG$_2$ subclass, are strongly associated with lupus nephritis, especially in combination with the FcγRIIB R131 allele, which binds IgG$_2$ poorly (Haseley *et al.* 1997). In aggregate, these observations, both in animals and in humans, suggest that complement generally plays an augmentative but not an essential role in IC-mediated inflammation. On the other hand, deposition of complement in immune complexes is important in targeting complexes for clearance by phagocytes; persistence of complexes in tissues produced either by deficiencies in early classical pathway complement components or in the phagocyte receptors for complement appears to set the stage for chronic inflammation and eventual autoimmunity.

Type IV hypersensitivity

As noted in the introduction, cellular hypersensitivity as a clinical phenomenon was noted by Jenner and Koch. It had been observed that delayed-type hypersensitivity (DTH) was most often seen in subjects suffering from infections, particularly chronic infections, with mycobacteria, fungi, or viruses (Pappenheimer and Freund 1959). The diagnostic use of DTH reactions to intradermal antigens derived from the organisms causing tuberculosis, histoplasmosis, brucellosis, leptospirosis, and a variety of other infections has been extensively employed in the clinic. However, immunization of control subjects or animals with purified microbial products from the same organisms or other foreign proteins elicited antibody formation but usually little DTH unless the antigens were injected intradermally (Lipton and Freund 1953; Mote and Jones 1936; Salvin 1958). The addition of microbial products, particularly from mycobacteria, as adjuvants greatly increased the DTH response elicited with routes of administration other than intradermal (Pappenheimer and Freund 1959). One of the earliest and most efficient methods discovered involved the injection of protein antigens directly into tuberculous foci such as lymph nodes (Hay 1979). The separate nature of DTH reactions from those involving antibody was convincingly demonstrated by the ready elicitation of DTH in patients with Bruton's agammaglobulinemia (Good *et al.* 1957; Porter 1957).

Extensive experimental work was carried out to explore the clinical observation of DTH. Landsteiner and colleagues did much to shed light on the underlying mechanisms (Landsteiner and Jacobs 1935). The dependence of DTH reactions upon cells rather than humoral factors was first demonstrated convincingly in work by Landsteiner, Chase, and Lawrence in the 1940s (Landsteiner and Chase 1940; Chase 1945; Chase 1946; Lawrence 1949). With the identification of thymus-derived lymphocytes as a distinct lineage of lymphoid cells, it quickly became apparent that it was this fraction of circulating leukocytes that transferred the DTH reaction (Cooper 1972; Jaffer *et al.* 1973; Youdim *et al.* 1973). Following the discovery of the Th1/Th2 T cell paradigm in mice by Mosmann and colleagues (Mosmann *et al.* 1986; Mosmann 1992), most cellular hypersensitivity reactions, including those involved in experimental animal models of organ-specific autoimmunity (Table 3.3) were subsequently found to depend upon cells with a Th1 phenotype (Cher and Mosmann 1987; De Carli *et al.* 1994; Ohta *et al.* 1997). Although the dichotomy of functional T cell subsets has not proven to be as well-defined in humans, the general patterns of cytokine production remain a useful conceptual framework in the analysis of immune responses leading to DTH.

DTH reactions differ from antibody-mediated reactions in their slow development, generally peaking after 1–2 days rather than minutes (Type I reactions) or hours (Types II–III reactions) (Hay 1979). A variety of somewhat different reactions can be elicited depending on the tissue and antigen used. These include contact hypersensitivity, tuberculin-type hypersensitivity, hypersensitivity pneumonitis, granulomatous hypersensitivity, and allograft rejection. The classic reaction is that seen following the intradermal injection of tuberculin in an individual who has been previously infected with *M. tuberculosis*. Within several hours, erythema appears around the injection site which represents increased blood flow, often several-fold higher than the baseline flow rates in surrounding skin (Hay *et al.* 1975). Increased vascular permeability can simultaneously be demonstrated experimentally using Evan's blue and is not affected by antihistamines, indicating that mast cell-derived mediators play a minimal role in the evolving response (Phair *et al.* 1970). Although neutrophils may appear in variable numbers within hours of challenge, the most characteristic cellular infiltrate is composed of lymphocytes and monocytes, typically in prominent perivenular cuffs. The increased blood flow, vascular permeability, and the cellular infiltrate create induration in the tissues which is useful as a measure of the intensity of the reaction in experimental animals. This can be semiquantified, for example by measuring changes in footpad or ear thickness.

IL-12 produced by dendritic cells and macrophages during the initial stages of inflammation is a key cytokine involved in driving Th1 development (Trinchieri 1996). The Th1 subset of T lymphocytes elaborates an arsenal of inflammatory cytokines which function in amplifying the activation of phagocytes in the defense against intracellular pathogens such as viruses, atypical bacteria, and fungal pathogens. Among these, IFNγ is perhaps the most crucial in further activating tissue macrophages and in suppression of Th2 differentiation (Mosmann *et al.* 1995). IFNγ produced by Th1 cells forms part of a positive feedback loop with IL-12 produced by phagocytes, each driving the other higher (Trinchieri 1996). This feedback loop is opposed by Th2 cytokines, particularly IL-10.

Some of the clearest evidence for the importance of the Th1 response in resistance to intracellular infections has come from experimental infection of mice with *Leishmania major*. This infection results in a Th1 pattern of T cell activation which, when opposed by the injection of anti-IFNγ antibody, is converted to a Th2 cytokine pattern with a lethal outcome (Belosevic *et al.* 1989). The importance of the IL-12–IFNγ amplification loop in protection from intracellular pathogens is further illustrated by the propensity of human patients deficient in the receptor for IFNγ, IL-12, or the IL-12 receptor (or essential downstream signaling components, e.g. STAT 1) to develop recurrent infections with *Listeria monocytogenes* and atypical mycobacteria (Rosenzweig and Holland 2005). Well-formed granulomas are not seen in the tissues of such patients despite abundant mycobacteria, indicating that cellular activation by this cytokine pathway is an essential step in containing the pathogen.

Conclusion

Hypersensitivity reactions are exaggerated normal immune responses of various arms of the immune system to antigenic stimulation which have become so exuberant that they damage the host which they evolved to protect. In living animals they rarely occur in isolation, but are combined with each other during the evolution of an inflammatory response. Natural infections frequently induce both cellular and humoral immunity, and the relative balance of these two arms of the specific immune response is critical in the defense against pathogens which vary from obligate intracellular pathogens such as viruses to complex extracellular parasites such as helminths. The study of these phenomena has provided the science of immunology with windows into the intricate workings of immunity.

Table 3.3 Animal models in Type IV hypersensitivity

Animal Model	Reference
Antigen-dependent	
Murine hypersensitivity pneumonitis	Fink *et al.* 2005
Infection-induced	
Murine Leishmaniasis	Belosevic *et al.* 1989
Murine Listeriosis	Mielke *et al.* 1997; North *et al.* 1997
Autoimmunity	
Experimental autoimmune uveitis	Merryman *et al.* 1987; Tarrant *et al.* 1998; Xu *et al.* 1997
Experimental autoimmune encephalomyelitis	Smeltz and Swanborg 1998
Experimental autoimmune thyroiditis	Braley-Mullen *et al.* 1985; Okayasu 1985
Experimental autoimmune neuritis	Zhu *et al.* 1998
Experimental autoimmune myocarditis	Smith and Allen 1993
Experimental autoimmune sialoadenitis	Greiner *et al.* 1991

References

Alam, R., Kumar, D., Anderson-Walters, D. and Forsythe, P. A. (1994). Macrophage inflammatory protein-1 alpha and monocyte chemoattractant peptide-1 elicit immediate and late cutaneous reactions and activate murine mast cells in vivo. *Journal of Immunology*, **152**, 1298–303.

Ansel, J. C., Brown, J. R., Payan, D. G. and Brown, M. A. (1993). Substance P selectively activates TNF-alpha gene expression in murine mast cells. *Journal of Immunology*, **150**, 4478–85.

Apitz, K. (1934). Die Wirkung bakterieller Kulturfiltrate nach Umstimmung des gesamten Endothels beim Kaninchen. *Virchows Archiv*, **293**, 1–33.

Arthus, M. (1903). Injections répétées de sérum de cheval chez le lapin. *Comptes Rendus de la Societé de Biologie*, **55**, 817–20.

Baldini, M., Lohman, I. C., Halonen, M., Erickson, R. P., Holt, P. G. and Martinez, F. D. (1999). A Polymorphism in the 5'flanking region of the CD14 gene is associated with circulating soluble CD14 levels and with total serum immunoglobulin E. *American Journal of Respiratory Cell and Molecular Biology*, **20**, 976–83.

Barnes, K. C. (1999). Gene-environment and gene-gene interaction studies in the molecular genetic analysis of asthma and atopy. *Clinical and Experimental Allergy*, **29** (Suppl. 4), 47–51.

Belosevic, M., Finbloom, D. S., Van Der Meide, P. H., Slayter, M. V. and Nacy, C. A. (1989). Administration of monoclonal anti-IFNγ antibodies in vivo abrogates natural resistance of C3H/HeN mice to infection with Leishmania major. *Journal of Immunology*, **143**, 266–74.

Biedermann, T. and Rocken, M. (1999). Th1/Th2 balance in atopy. *Springer Seminars in Immunopathology*, **21**, 295–316.

Bierbaum, S., Nickel, R., Coch, A., Lau, S., Deichmann, K. A., Wahn, U., Superti-Furga, A. and Heinzmann, A. (2005). Polymorphisms and haplotypes of acid mammalian chitinase are associated with bronchial asthma. *American Journal of Respiratory and Critical Care Medicine*, **172**, 1505–9.

Bigazzi, P. E. (1998). Animal models of autoimmunity: spontaneous and induced. In *The Autoimmune Diseases*, 3rd edn, (eds N. R. Rose and I. R. Mackay), pp. 211–44. Academic Press.

Blumenthal, M. N. (2000). Genetics of asthma and allergy. *Allergy and Asthma Proceedings*, **21**, 55–9.

Borish, L. (1999). Genetics of allergy and asthma. *Annals of Allergy, Asthma, and Immunology*, **82**, 413–24.

Bostock, J. (1828). On the catarrhus aestivus or summer catarrh. *Medico-Chirurgical Transactions* (London), **XIV**, 437–46.

Boyce, J. A. (2005). Eicosanoid mediators of mast cells: receptors, regulation of synthesis, and pathobiologic implications. *Chemical Immunology and Allergy*, **87**, 59–79.

Bradding, P., Feather, I. H., Wilson, S., Bardin, P. G., Heusser, C. H., Holgate, S. T. and Howarth, P. H. (1993). Immunolocalization of cytokines in the nasal mucosa of normal and perennial rhinitic subjects. The mast cell as a source of IL-4, IL-5, and IL-6 in human allergic mucosal inflammation. *Journal of Immunology*, **151**, 3853–65.

Bradding, P., Okayama, Y., Howarth, P. H., Church, M. K. and Holgate, S. T. (1995). Heterogeneity of human mast cells based on cytokine content. *Journal of Immunology*, **155**, 297–307.

Braley-Mullen, H., Johnson, M., Sharp, G. C. and Kyriakos, M. (1985). Induction of experimental autoimmune thyroiditis in mice with in vitro activated splenic T cells. *Cellular Immunology*, **93**, 132–43.

Brown, M. A. and Hural, J. (1997). Functions of IL-4 and control of its expression. *Critical Reviews in Immunology*, **17**, 1–32.

Burchard, E. G., Silverman, E. K., Rosenwasser, L. J., Borish, L., Yandava, C., Pillari, A., Weiss, S. T., Hasday, J., Lilly, C. M., Ford, J. G. and Drazen, J. M. (1999). Association between a sequence variant in the IL-4 gene promoter and FEV(1) in asthma. *American Journal of Respiratory and Critical Care Medicine*, **160**, 919–22.

Charlesworth, E. N., Iliopoulos, O., MacDonald, S. M., Kagey-Sobotka, A. and Lichtenstein, L. M. (1989). Cells and secretagogues involved in the human late-phase response. *International Archives of Allergy and Applied Immunology*, **88**, 50–3.

Chase, M. W. (1945). The cellular transfer of cutaneous hypersensitivity to tuberculin. *Proceedings of the Society for Experimental Biology and Medicine*, **59**, 134–5.

Chase, M. W. (1946). The cellular transfer of cutaneous hypersensitivity. *Journal of Bacteriology*, **51**, 643.

Cher, D. J. and Mosmann, T. R. (1987). Two types of murine helper T cell clone. II. Delayed-type hypersensitivity is mediated by TH1 clones. *Journal of Immunology*, **138**, 3688–94.

Chossegros, P., Wu, R., Hermier, C., Doutre, M. S., Brette, R. and Trepo, C. (1987). [Satellite vasculitis of B or non-A non-B hepatitis. Diagnostic value of a provocation test by intradermal injection of histamine]. *Annales de Medecine Interne*, **138**, 193–8.

Clynes, R., Dumitru, C. and Ravetch, J. V. (1998). Uncoupling of immune complex formation and kidney damage in autoimmune glomerulonephritis. *Science*, **279**, 1052–4.

Clynes, R., Maizes, J. S., Guinamard, R., Ono, M., Takai, T. and Ravetch, J. V. (1999). Modulation of immune complex-induced inflammation in vivo by the coordinate expression of activation and inhibitory Fc receptors. *Journal of Experimental Medicine*, **189**, 179–85.

Clynes, R. and Ravetch, J. V. (1995). Cytotoxic antibodies trigger inflammation through Fc receptors. *Immunity*, **3**, 21–6.

Coca, A. F. and Cooke, R. A. (1923). On the classification of the phenomena of hypersensitiveness. *Journal of Immunology*, **8**, 163–75.

Cochrane, C. G. and Hawkins, D. (1968). Studies on circulating immune complexes III. Factors governing the ability of circulating complexes to localize in blood vessels. *Journal of Experimental Medicine*, **127**, 137–54.

Cochrane, C. G., Unanue, E. R. and Dixon, F. J. (1965). A role of polymorphonuclear leukocytes and complement in nephrotoxic nephritis. *Journal of Experimental Medicine*, **122**, 99–119.

Cochrane, C. G. and Weigle, W. O. (1958). The cutaneous reaction to soluble antigen-antibody complexes. A comparison with the Arthus reaction. *Journal of Experimental Medicine*, **108**, 591–604.

Cochrane, C. G., Weigle, W. O. and Dixon, F. J. (1959). The role of polymorphonuclear leukocytes in the initiation and cessation of the Arthus vasculitis. *Journal of Experimental Medicine*, **110**, 481–94.

Cohen, I. R. and Miller, A. (eds) (1994). *Autoimmune disease models*. Academic Press, Inc., New York.

Coombs, R. R.A. and Gell, P. G.H. (1968). Classification of allergic reactions responsible for clinical hypersensitivity and disease. In *Clinical aspects of immunology*, 2nd edn, (eds R. R.A. Coombs and P. G.H. Gell), pp. 575–96. Alden Press, Oxford.

Cooper, M. G. (1972). Delayed-type hypersensitivity in the mouse. II. Transfer by thymus-derived (T) cells. *Scandinavian Journal of Immunology*, **1**, 237–45.

Cox, K. O. and Howles, A. (1981). Induction and regulation of autoimmune hemolytic anemia in mice. *Immunological Reviews*, **55**, 31–53.

De Carli, M., D'Elios, M. M., Zancuoghi, G., Romagnani, S., Del and Prete, G. (1994). Human Th1 and Th2 cells: functional properties, regulation of development and role in autoimmunity. *Autoimmunity*, **18**, 301–8.

Dieli, F., Sireci, G., Russo, D., Taniguchi, M., Ivanyi, J., Fernandez, C., Troye-Blomberg, M., De Leo, G. and Salerno, A. (2000). Resistance of natural killer T cell-deficient mice to systemic Shwartzman reaction. *Journal of Experimental Medicine*, **192**, 1645–51.

Dixon, F. J., Vazquez, J. J., Weigle, W. O. and Cochrane, C. G. (1958). Pathogenesis of serum sickness. A. M.A. *Archives of Pathology*, **65**, 18–28.

Echtenacher, B., Mannel, D. N. and Hultner, L. (1996). Critical protective role of mast cells in a model of acute septic peritonitis. *Nature*, **381**, 75–7.

Eppel, G. A., Takazoe, K., Nikolic-Paterson, D. J., Lan, H. Y., Atkins, R. C. and Comper, W. D. (2000). Characteristics of albumin processing during renal passage in anti-Thy1 and anti-glomerular basement membrane glomerulonephritis. *American Journal of Kidney Diseases*, **35**, 418–26.

Farquhar, M. G., Saito, A., Kerjaschki, D. and Orlando, R. A. (1995). The Heymann nephritis antigenic complex: megalin (gp330) and RAP. *Journal of the American Society of Nephrology*, **6**, 35–47.

Fehniger, T. A., Yu, H., Cooper, M. A., Suzuki, K., Shah, M. H. and Caligiuri, M. A. (2000). Cutting Edge: IL-15 costimulates the generalized Shwartzman reaction and innate immune IFN-γ production in vivo. *Journal of Immunology*, **164**, 1643–7.

Fink, J. N., Ortega, H. G., Reynolds, H. Y., Cormier, Y. F., Fan, L. L., Franks, T. J., Kreiss, K., Kunkel, S., Lynch, D., Quirce, S., Rose, C., Schleimer, R. P., Schuyler, M. R., Selman, M., Trout, D. and Yoshizawa, Y. (2005). Needs and opportunities for research in hypersensitivity pneumonitis. *American Journal of Respiratory and Critical Care Medicine*, **171**, 792–8.

Fiorucci, L. and Ascoi, F. (2004). Mast cell tryptase, a still enigmatic enzyme. *Cellular and Molecular Life Sciences*, **61**, 1278–95.

Galli, S. J. and Costa, J. J. (1995). Mast-cell-leukocyte cytokine cascades in allergic inflammation. *Allergy*, **50**, 851–62.

Gonzales-Espinosa, C., Odom, S., Olivera, A., Hobson, J. P., Martinez, M. E.C., Oliveira-dos-Santos, A., Barra, L., Spiegel, S., Penninger, J. M. and Rivera, J. (2003). Preferential signaling and induction of allergy-promoting lymphokines upon weak stimulation of the high affinity IgE receptor on mast cells. *Journal of Experimental Medicine*, **197**, 1453–65.

Good, R. A., Zak, S. J., Jensen, D. R. and Pappenheimer, A. M. (1957). Delayed allergy and agammaglobulinemia. *Journal of Clinical Investigation*, **36**, 894.

Gower, R. G., Sams, W. M., Jr., Thorne, E. G., Kohler, P. F. and Claman, H. N. (1977). Leukocytoclastic vasculitis: sequential appearance of immunoreactants and cellular changes in serial biopsies. *Journal of Investigative Dermatology*, **69**, 477–84.

Greaves, M. (2000). Chronic urticaria. *Journal of Allergy and Clinical Immunology*, **105**, 664–72.

Green, S. A., Cole, G., Jacinto, M., Innis, M. and Liggett, S. B. (1993). A polymorphism of the human beta 2-adrenergic receptor within the fourth transmembrane domain alters ligand binding and functional properties of the receptor. *Journal of Biological Chemistry*, **268**, 23116–21.

Greiner, D. L., Angelillo, M., Wayne, A. L., Fitzgerald, K. M., Rozenski, D. and Cutler, L. S. (1991). Experimental autoallergic sialadenitis in the LEW rat. III. Role of CD4+ T cells in EAS induction. *Cellular Immunology*, **135**, 354–9.

Guo, C. B., Liu, M. C., Galli, S. J., Bochner, B. S., Kagey-Sobotka, A. and Lichtenstein, L. M. (1994). Identification of IgE-bearing cells in the late-phase response to antigen in the lung as basophils. *American Journal of Respiratory Cell and Molecular Biology*, **10**, 384–90.

Haseley, L. A., Wisnieski, J. J., Denburg, M. R., Michael-Grossman, A. R., Ginzler, E. M., Gourley, M. F., Hoffman, J. H., Kimberly, R. P. and Salmon, J. E. (1997). Antibodies to C1q in systemic lupus erythematosus: characteristics and relation to Fc gamma RIIA alleles. *Kidney International*, **52**, 1375–80.

Hay, J. B. (1979). Delayed (cellular) hypersensitivity. In *Inflammation, immunity, and hypersensitivity*, 2nd edn, (ed. H. Z. Movat), pp. 271–318. Harper and Row, New York.

Hay, J. B., Johnston, M. G., Hobbs, B. B. and Movat, H. Z. (1975). The use of radioactive microspheres to quantitate hyperemia in dermal inflammatory sites. *Proceedings of the Society for Experimental Biology and Medicine*, **150**, 641–4.

Hayashi, H., Yoshinaga, M., Koono, M., Miyoshi, H. and Matsumura, M. (1964). Endogenous permeability factors and their inhibitors affecting vascular permeability in cutaneous Arthus reactions and thermal injury. *British Journal of Experimental Pathology*, **45**, 419–35.

Hershey, G. K., Friedrich, M. F., Esswein, L. A., Thomas, M. L. and Chatila, T. A. (1997). The association of atopy with a gain-of-function mutation in the alpha subunit of the interleukin-4 receptor. *New England Journal of Medicine*, **337**, 1720–5.

Hoffjan, S., Nicolae, D. and Ober, C. (2003). Association studies for asthma and atopic diseases: a comprehensive review of the literature. *Respiratory Research*, **4**, 14–25.

Hopken, U. E., Lu, B., Gerard, N. P. and Gerard, C. (1997). Impaired inflammatory responses in the reverse Arthus reaction through genetic deletion of the C5a receptor. *Journal of Experimental Medicine*, **186**, 749–56.

Iliopoulos, O., Baroody, F. M., Naclerio, R. M., Bochner, B. S., Kagey-Sobotka, A. and Lichtenstein, L. M. (1992). Histamine-containing cells obtained from the nose hours after antigen challenge have functional and phenotypic characteristics of basophils. *Journal of Immunology*, **148**, 2223–8.

Imamura, T., Potempa, J. and Travis, J. (2004). Activation of the kallikrein-kinin system and release of new kinins through alternative cleavage of kininogens by microbial and human cell proteinases. *Biological Chemistry*, **385**, 989–96.

Ishizaka, K., Ishizaka, T. and Hornbrook, M. M. (1966). Physicochemical properties of human reaginic antibody. IV. Presence of a unique immunoglobulin as a carrier of reaginic activity. *Journal of Immunology*, **97**, 75–85.

Jaffer, A. M., Jones, G., Kasdon, E. J. and Schlossman, S. F. (1973). Local transfer of delayed hypersensitivity by T lymphocytes. *Journal of Immunology*, **111**, 1268–9.

Jorizzo, J. L., Daniels, J. C., Apisarnthanarax, P., Gonzalez, E. B. and Cavallo, T. (1983). Histamine-triggered localized vasculitis in patients with seropositive rheumatoid arthritis. *Journal of the American Academy of Dermatology*, **9**, 845–51.

Kim, S., Iizuka, K., Aguila, H. L., Weissman, I. L. and Yokoyama, W. M. (2000). In vivo natural killer cell activities revealed by natural killer cell-deficient mice. *Proceedings of the National Academy of Sciences (USA)*, **97**, 2731–6.

Kruse, S., Japha, T., Tedner, M., Sparholt, S. H., Forster, J., Kuehr, J., and Deichmann, K. A. (1999). The polymorphisms S503P and Q576R in the interleukin-4 receptor alpha gene are associated with atopy and influence the signal transduction. *Immunology*, **96**, 365–71.

Kuhn, R., Rajewsky, K. and Muller, W. (1991). Generation and analysis of interleukin-4 deficient mice. *Science*, **254**, 707–10.

Laberge, S., Pinsonneault, S., Ernst, P., Olivenstein, R., Ghaffar, O., Center, D. M. and Hamid, Q. (1999). Phenotype of IL-16-producing cells in bronchial mucosa: evidence for the human eosinophil and mast cell as cellular sources of IL-16 in asthma. *International Archives of Allergy and Immunology*, **119**, 120–5.

Landsteiner, K. and Chase, M. W. (1940). Studies on the sensitization of animals with simple compounds. VII. Skin sensitization by intraperitoneal injections. *Journal of Experimental Medicine*, **71**, 237–45.

Landsteiner, K. and Jacobs, J. (1935). Studies on the sensitization of animals with simple chemical compounds. *Journal of Experimental Medicine*, **61**, 643–56.

Lawrence, H. S. (1949). The cellular transfer of cutaneous hypersensitivity to tuberculin in man. *Proceedings of the Society for Experimental Biology and Medicine*, **71**, 516–22.

Lichtenstein, L. M. and Bochner, B. S. (1991). The role of basophils in asthma. *Annals of the New York Academy of Sciences*, **629**, 48–61.

Lipton, M. M. and Freund, J. (1953). Allergic encephalomyelitis in the rat induced by the intracutaneous injection of central nervous tissue and adjuvants. *Journal of Immunology*, **71**, 98.

Liu, A. H. and Leung, D. Y.M. (2006). Renaissance of the hygiene hypothesis. *Journal of Allergy and Clinical Immunology*, **117**, 163–6.

Liu, Z., Diaz, L. A., Troy, J. L., Taylor, A. F., Emery, D. J., Fairley, J. A. and Giudice, G. J. (1993). A passive transfer model of the organ-specific autoimmune disease, bullous pemphigoid, using antibodies generated against the hemidesmosomal antigen, BP180. *Journal of Clinical Investigation*, **92**, 2480–8.

Liu, Z., Giudice, G. J., Swartz, S. J., Fairley, J. A., Till, G. O., Troy, J. L. and Diaz, L. A. (1995). The role of complement in experimental bullous pemphigoid. *Journal of Clinical Investigation*, **95**, 1539–44.

Ludgate, M. (2000). Animal models of Graves' disease. *European Journal of Endocrinology*, **142**, 1–8.

Lukacs, N. W., Kunkel, S. L., Strieter, R. M., Evanoff, H. L., Kunkel, R. G., Key, M. L. and Taub, D. D. (1996). The role of stem cell factor (c-kit ligand) and inflammatory cytokines in pulmonary mast cell activation. *Blood*, **87**, 2262–8.

Lutzelschwab, C., Pejler, G., Aveskogh, M. and Hellman, L. (1997). Secretory granule proteases in rat mast cells. Cloning of 10 different serine proteases and a carboxypeptidase A from various rat mast cell populations. *Journal of Experimental Medicine*, **185**, 13–29.

MacLeod, J. D., Anderson, D. F., Baddeley, S. M., Holgate, S. T., McGill, J. I. and Roche, W. R. (1997). Immunolocalization of cytokines to mast cells in normal and allergic conjunctiva. *Clinical and Experimental Allergy*, **27**, 1328–34.

Malaviya, R., Ikeda, T., Ross, E. and Abraham, S. N. (1996). Mast cell modulation of neutrophil influx and bacterial clearance at sites of infection through TNF-alpha. *Nature*, **381**, 77–80.

Manian, P. (1997). Genetics of asthma: a review. *Chest*, **112**, 1397–408.

Marone, G., Casolaro, V., Patella, V., Florio, G. and Triggiani, M. (1997). Molecular and cellular biology of mast cells and basophils. *International Archives of Allergy and Immunology*, **114**, 207–17.

Mashikian, M. V., Tarpy, R. E., Saukkonen, J. J., Lim, K. G., Fine, G. D., Cruikshank, W. W. and Center, D. M. (1998). Identification of IL-16 as the lymphocyte chemotactic activity in the bronchoalveolar lavage fluid of histamine-challenged asthmatic patients. *Journal of Allergy and Clinical Immunology*, **101**, 786–92.

Merryman, C. F., Donoso, L. A., Sery, T. W., Sciutto, E., Bauer, A. and Shinohara, T. (1987). S-antigen. Adoptive transfer of experimental autoimmune uveitis following immunization with a small synthetic peptide. *Archives of Ophthalmology*, **105**, 841–3.

Mielke, M. E., Peters, C. and Hahn, H. (1997). Cytokines in the induction and expression of T-cell-mediated granuloma formation and protection in the murine model of listeriosis. *Immunological Reviews*, **158**, 79–93.

Moller, A., Lippert, U., Lessmann, D., Kolde, G., Hamann, K., Welker, P., Schadendorf, D., Rosenbach, T., Luger, T. and Czarnetzki, B. M. (1993). Human mast cells produce IL-8. *Journal of Immunology*, **151**, 3261–6.

Mosmann, T. R. (1992). T lymphocyte subsets, cytokines, and effector functions. *Annals of the New York Academy of Sciences*, **664**, 89–92.

Mosmann, T. R., Cherwinski, H., Bond, M. W., Giedlin, M. A., and Coffman, R. L. (1986). Two types of murine helper T cell clone. I. Definition according to profiles of lymphokine activities and secreted proteins. *Journal of Immunology*, **136**, 2348–57.

Mosmann, T. R., Sad, S., Krishnan, L., Wegmann, T. G., Guilbert, L. J. and Belosevic, M. (1995). Differentiation of subsets of CD4+ and CD8+ T cells. *Ciba Foundation Symposium*, **195**, 42–54.

Mote, J. R. and Jones, T. D. (1936). The development of foreign protein sensitization in human beings. *Journal of Immunology*, **30**, 149–167.

Mousli, M., Hugli, T. E., Landry, Y. and Bronner, C. (1994). Peptidergic pathway in human skin and rat peritoneal mast cell activation. *Immunopharmacology*, **27**, 1–11.

Movat, H. Z. (1979). The acute inflammatory reaction. In *Inflammation, immunity, and hypersensitivity*, 2nd edn, (ed. H. Z. Movat), pp. 1–161. Harper and Row.

Myers, L. K., Rosloniec, E. F., Cremer, M. A. and Kang, A. H. (1997). Collagen-induced arthritis, an animal model of autoimmunity. *Life Sciences*, **61**, 1861–78.

Nakamura, A., Yuasa, T., Ujike, A., Ono, M., Nukiwa, T., Ravetch, J. V. and Takai, T. (2000). Fcgamma receptor IIB-deficient mice develop Goodpasture's syndrome upon immunization with type IV collagen: a novel murine model for autoimmune glomerular basement membrane disease. *Journal of Experimental Medicine*, **191**, 899–906.

Nisitani, S., Murakami, M. and Honjo, T. (1997). Anti-red blood cell immunoglobulin transgenic mice. An experimental model of autoimmune hemolytic anemia. *Annals of the New York Academy of Sciences*, **815**, 246–52.

North, R. J., Dunn, P. L. and Conlan, J. W. (1997). Murine listeriosis as a model of antimicrobial defense. *Immunological Reviews*, **158**, 27–36.

Ober, C., Leavitt, S. A., Tsalenko, A., Howard, T. D., Hoki, D. M., Daniel, R., Newman, DL, Wu, X., Parry, R., Lester, L. A., Solway, J., Blumenthal, M., King, R. A., Xu, J., Meyers, D. A., Bleecker, E. R. and Cox, N. J. (2000). Variation in the interleukin 4-receptor alpha gene confers susceptibility to asthma and atopy in ethnically diverse populations. *American Journal of Human Genetics*, **66**, 517–26.

Ohta, A., Sato, N., Yahata, T., Ohmi, Y., Santa, K., Sato, T., Tashiro, H., Habu, S. and Nishimura, T. (1997). Manipulation of Th1/Th2 balance in vivo by adoptive transfer of antigen-specific Th1 or Th2 cells. *Journal of Immunological Methods*, **209**, 85–92.

Oiso, N., Fukai, K. and Ishii, M. (2000). Interleukin 4 receptor alpha chain polymorphism Gln551Arg is associated with adult atopic dermatitis in Japan. *British Journal of Dermatology*, **142**, 1003–6.

Okayasu, I. (1985). Transfer of experimental autoimmune thyroiditis to normal syngeneic mice by injection of mouse thyroglobulin-sensitized T lymphocytes after activation with concanavalin A. *Clinical Immunology and Immunopathology*, **36**, 101–9.

Ozmen, L., Pericin, M., Hakimi, J., Chizzonite, R. A., Wysocka, M., Trinchieri, G., Gately, M. and Garotta, G. (1994). Interleukin 12, interferon, and tumor necrosis factor α are the key cytokines of the generalized Shwartzman reaction. *Journal of Experimental Medicine*, **180**, 907–15.

Pappenheimer, A. M. and Freund, J. (1959). Induction of delayed hypersensitivity to protein antigens. In *Cellular and humoral aspects of the hypersensitive states*, (ed. H. S. Lawrence), pp. 67–88. P. B. Hoeber.

Phair, J. P., Eisenfeld, A. J., Levine, R. J. and Kantor, F. S. (1970). Effects of pharmacological inhibition of histamine synthesis upon immunological reactions in guinea-pigs. *Immunology*, **18**, 611–9.

Pirquet, C. V. and Schick, B. (1905). *Die Serumkrankheit*. Franz Deuticke, Leipzig. (English translation by B. Schick, 1951, Williams and Wilkins.)

Porter, H. M. (1957). Demonstration of delayed type reactivity in congenital agammaglobulinemia. 2nd Tissue Homotransplantation Conference. *Annals of the New York Academy of Sciences*, **64**, 932.

Portier, P. and Richet, C. (1902). De l'action anaphylactique de certains venins. *Comptes Rendus de la Societé de Biologie*, **54**, 170–2.

Prausnitz, C. and Küstner, H. (1921). Studien über die Ueberempfindlichkeit. *Zentrabl Bakteriol*, **86**, 160–9.

Ranadive, N. S. and Movat, H. Z. (1979). Tissue injury and inflammation induced by immune complexes. In *Inflammation, immunity and hypersensitivity*, 2nd edn, (ed. H. Z. Movat), pp. 409–43. Harper and Row.

Redrup, A. C., Howard, B. P., MacGlashan, D. W., Jr., Kagey-Sobotka, A., Lichtenstein, L. M. and Schroeder, J. T. (1998). Differential regulation of IL-4 and IL-13 secretion by human basophils: their relationship to histamine release in mixed leukocyte cultures. *Journal of Immunology*, **160**, 1957–64.

Reed, C. E. and Kita, H. (2004). The role of protease activation of inflammation in allergic respiratory diseases. *Journal of Allergy and Clinical Immunology*, **114**, 997–1008.

Reihsaus, E., Innis, M., MacIntyre, N. and Liggett, S. B. (1993). Mutations in the gene encoding for the beta 2-adrenergic receptor in normal and asthmatic subjects. *American Journal of Respiratory Cell and Molecular Biology*, **8**, 334–339.

Rosa-Rosa, L., Zimmermann, N., Bernstein, J. A., Rothenberg, M. E., and Khurana Hershey, G. K. (1999). The R576 IL-4 receptor alpha allele correlates with asthma severity. *Journal of Allergy and Clinical Immunology*, **104**, 1008–14.

Rosenwasser, L. J. (1999). Promoter polymorphism in the candidate genes, IL-4, IL-9, TGF-beta1, for atopy and asthma. *International Archives of Allergy and Immunology*, **118**, 268–70.

Rosenzweig, S. D. and Holland, S. M. (2005). Defects in the interferon- and interleukin-12 pathways. *Immunological Reviews*, **203**, 38–47.

Rumsaeng, V., Cruikshank, W. W., Foster, B., Prussin, C., Kirshenbaum, A. S., Davis, T. A., Kornfeld, H., Center, D. M. and Metcalfe, D. D. (1997). Human mast cells produce the CD4+ T lymphocyte chemoattractant factor, IL-16. *Journal of Immunology*, **159**, 2904–10.

Russell, J. P. and Gibson, L. E. (2006). Primary cutaneous small vessel vasculitis: approach to diagnosis and treatment. *International Journal of Dermatology*, **45**, 3–13.

Salmon, J. E., Millard, S., Schachter, L. A., Arnett, F. C., Ginzler, E. M., Gourley, M. F., Ramsey-Goldman, R., Peterson, M. G. and Kimberly, R. P. (1996). Fc gamma RIIA alleles are heritable risk factors for lupus nephritis in African Americans. *Journal of Clinical Investigation*, **97**, 1348–54.

Salvin, S. B. (1958). Occurrence of delayed hypersensitivity during the development of Arthus type hypersensitivity. *Journal of Experimental Medicine*, **107**, 109–24.

Sanarelli, G. (1924). De la pathogenie du cholera (neuvieme memoire). Le Cholera Experimentale. *Annales de l'Institut Pasteur*, **38**, 11–72.

Schaub, B., Lauener, R. and von Mutius, E. (2006). The many faces of the hygiene hypothesis. *Journal of Allergy and Clinical Immunology*, **117**, 969–77.

Schrijver, G., Bogman, M. J., Assmann, K. J., *et al.* (1990). Anti-GBM nephritis in the mouse: role of granulocytes in the heterologous phase. *Kidney International*, **38**, 86–95.

Sharon, R. and Naor, D. (1992). Experimental model of autoimmune hemolytic anemia induced in mice with levodopa by intraperitoneal injection or oral feeding. *International Journal of Immunopharmacology*, **14**, 1241–7.

Shushakova, N., Skokowa, J., Schulman, J., Bauman, U., Zwirner, J., Schmidt, R. E. and Gessner, J. E. (2002). C5a anaphylatoxin is a major regulator of activating versus inhibitory Fc_Rs in immune complex-induced lung disease. *Journal of Clinical Investigation*, **110**, 1823–30.

Shwartzman, G. (1937). *Phenomenon of local tissue reactivity*. Paul B. Hoeber, Inc., New York.

Smeltz, R. B. and Swanborg, R. H. (1998). Concordance and contradiction concerning cytokines and chemokines in experimental demyelinating disease. *Journal of Neuroscience Research*, **51**, 147–53.

Smith, S. C. and Allen, P. M. (1993). The role of T cells in myosin-induced autoimmune myocarditis. *Clinical Immunology and Immunopathology*, **68**, 100–6.

Song, Z., Casolaro, V., Chen, R., Georas, S. N., Monos, D. and Ono, S. J. (1996). Polymorphic nucleotides within the human IL-4 promoter that mediate overexpression of the gene. *Journal of Immunology*, **156**, 424–9.

Stafforini, D. M., McIntyre, T. M., Zimmerman, G. A. and Prescott, S. M. (2003). Platelet-activating factor, a pleiotrophic mediator of physiological and pathological processes. *Critical Reviews in Clinical Laboratory Sciences*, **40**, 643–72.

Suzuki, Y., Shirato, I., Okumura, K., Ravetch, J. V., Takai, T., Tomino, Y. and Ra, C. (1998). Distinct contribution of Fc receptors and angiotensin II-dependent pathways in anti-GBM glomerulonephritis. *Kidney International*, **54**, 1166–74.

Sylvestre, D. L. and Ravetch, J. V. (1996). A dominant role for mast cell Fc receptors in the Arthus reaction. *Immunity*, **5**, 387–90.

Tang, W. W., Feng, L., Loskutoff, D. J. and Wilson, C. B. (2000). Glomerular extracellular matrix accumulation in experimental anti-GBM Ab glomerulonephritis. *Nephron*, **84**, 40–8.

Tanimoto, Y., Takahashi, K. and Kimura, I. (1992). Effects of cytokines on human basophil chemotaxis. *Clinical and Experimental Allergy*, **22**, 1020–5.

Tarrant, T. K., Silver, P. B., Chan, C. C., Wiggert, B. and Caspi, R. R. (1998). Endogenous IL-12 is required for induction and expression of experimental autoimmune uveitis. *Journal of Immunology*, **161**, 122–7.

Thomas, L. and Good, R. A. (1952). Studies on the generalized Shwartzman reaction: I. General observations concerning the phenomenon. *Journal of Experimental Medicine*, **96**, 605–25.

Trinchieri, G. (1996). Role of interleukin-12 in human Th1 response. *Chemical Immunology*, **63**, 14–29.

Tsai, M., Tam, S. Y. and Galli, S. J. (1993). Distinct patterns of early response gene expression and proliferation in mouse mast cells stimulated by Stem Cell Factor, Interleukin-3, or IgE and antigen. *European Journal of Immunology*, **23**, 867–72.

Vincent, A. (1994). Experimental autoimmune myasthenia gravis. In *Autoimmune disease models*, (eds I. R. Cohen and A. Miller), pp. 83–106. Academic Press.

Walport, M. J., Davies, K. A. and Botto, M. (1998). C1q and systemic lupus erythematosus. *Immunobiology*, **199**, 265–85.

Wedemeyer, J. and Galli, S. J. (2000). Mast cells and basophils in acquired immunity. *British Medical Bulletin*, **56**, 936–55.

Wershil, B. K., Wang, Z. S., Gordon, J. R. and Galli, S. J. (1991). Recruitment of neutrophils during IgE-dependent cutaneous late phase reactions in the mouse is mast cell-dependent. Partial inhibition of the reaction with antiserum against tumor necrosis factor-alpha. *Journal of Clinical Investigation*, **87**, 446–53.

White, M. (1999). Mediators of inflammation and the inflammatory process. *Journal of Allergy and Clinical Immunology*, **103**, S378–81.

Wolff, H. H., Maciejewski, W., Scherer, R. and Braun-Falco, O. (1978). Immunoelectronmicroscopic examination of early lesions in histamine induced immune complex vasculitis in man. *British Journal of Dermatology*, **99**, 13–24.

Wu, J., Edberg, J. C., Redecha, P. B., Bansal, V., Guyre, P. M., Coleman, K., Salmon, J. E. and Kimberly, R. P. (1997). A novel polymorphism of FcgammaRIIIa (CD16) alters receptor function and predisposes to autoimmune disease. *Journal of Clinical Investigation*, **100**, 1059–70.

Xu, H., Rizzo, L. V., Silver, P. B. and Caspi, R. R. (1997). Uveitogenicity is associated with a Th1-like lymphokine profile: cytokine-dependent modulation of early and committed effector T cells in experimental autoimmune uveitis. *Cellular Immunology*, **178**, 69–78.

Yano, H., Wershil, B. K., Arizono, N. and Galli, S. J. (1989). Substance P-induced augmentation of cutaneous vascular permeability and granulocyte infiltration in mice is mast cell dependent. *Journal of Clinical Investigation*, **84**, 1276–86.

Youdim, S., Stuntman, O. and Good, R. A. (1973). Thymus dependency of cells involved in transfer of delayed hypersensitivity to Listeria monocytogenes in mice. *Cellular Immunology*, **8**, 395–402.

Youinou, P., le Dantec, C., Bendaoud, B., Renaudineau, Y., Pers, J. O. and Jamin, C. (2005). Endothelium, a target for immune-mediated assault in connective tissue disease. *Autoimmunity Reviews*, **5**, 222–8.

Zhang, Y., Ramos, B. F., Jakschik, B., Baganoff, M. P., Deppeler, C. L., Meyer, D. M., Widomski, D. L., Fretland, D. J. and Bolanowski, M. A. (1995). Interleukin 8 and mast cell-generated tumor necrosis factor-alpha in neutrophil recruitment. *Inflammation*, **19**, 119–32.

Zhu, J., Mix, E. and Link, H. (1998). Cytokine production and the pathogenesis of experimental autoimmune neuritis and Guillain-Barre syndrome. *Journal of Neuroimmunology*, **84**, 40–52.

Zhu, Z., Zheng, T., Homer, R. J., Kim, Y. K., Chen, N. Y., Cohn, L., Hamid, Q. and Elias, J. A. (2004). Acidic mammalian chitinase in asthmatic Th2 inflammation ad IL-13 pathway activation. *Science*, **304**, 1678–82.

CHAPTER 4

Biology of endothelial cells

Zoltán Szekanecz and Alisa E. Koch

Introduction

Endothelial cells (ECs) line the lumina of blood vessels and thus separate and connect the blood and the extravascular interstitial matrix. In inflammatory processes, such as vasculitis, ECs interact with multiple cell types, such as leukocytes, fibroblasts, smooth muscle cells, and others, and adhere to components of the extracellular matrix (ECM). ECs secrete numerous soluble inflammatory mediators and proteolytic enzymes, express cellular adhesion molecules (CAMs) on their surface, and thus regulate inflammation in the surrounding tissue. ECs also respond to inflammatory mediators produced by leukocytes (Pober and Cotran 1990; Cotran 1993; Szekanecz and Koch, 2004, 2005).

Through the distinct processes of stimulation and activation, ECs are involved in the inflammatory process of vasculitis. EC stimulation by vasoactive substances, such as serotonin or histamine, is a rapid process (occurring within minutes) and is independent of new protein synthesis. These rapid EC responses are accompanied by cell contraction and the redistribution of certain CAMs, such as P-selectin (Pober and Cotran 1990; Cotran 1993). In contrast, EC activation occurs after several hours or days. Activation is associated with new protein synthesis and involves the action of proinflammatory cytokines, predominantly tumor necrosis factor-α (TNF-α), interleukin-1 (IL-1), or interferon-γ (IFN-γ). EC activation may also involve increased expression of CAMs, particularly E-selectin. EC activation is also indicated by up-regulation of major histocompatibility complex (MHC) class II antigen on these cells (Pober *et al.* 1983; Bevilacqua *et al.* 1987; Cotran 1993; Szekanecz and Koch 2004, 2005).

In this chapter, we briefly review those mechanisms which are most relevant for the pathogenesis of vascular inflammation. Some aspects of EC morphology, leukocyte–EC adhesion, transendothelial inflammatory cell migration, and angiogenesis will be discussed in more detail. All these important processes are involved in the onset of vasculitis and the progression of inflammation. Although we will describe these mechanisms as distinct entities, there is certainly significant overlap between them and the outcome of vascular inflammation is highly dependent on this complex inflammatory network (Leibovich *et al.* 1987; Szekanecz *et al.* 1998a, 1999, 2005; Szekanecz and Koch 2004, 2005).

Endothelial morphology and function in vascular inflammation

During vasculitis, the vascular endothelium may undergo morphological changes, including vasodilatation and increased permeability (leakage) (Cotran 1993; Szekanecz and Koch 2004). Vasodilatation itself may indirectly enhance vascular leakage. The latter can result from several processes, including EC contraction and retraction as well as leukocyte- or anti-EC antibody (AECA)-mediated vascular injury and regeneration (Table 4.1) (Cotran 1993; Szekanecz and Koch 2004, 2005).

Vasodilatory mediators may originate from plasma, blood cells, or the ECs themselves. ECs produce prostacyclin (PGI$_2$), nitric oxide (NO), and platelet-activating factor (PAF) (Brenner *et al.* 1989; Cotran 1993). Thrombin, histamine, and leukotriene C$_4$ enhance the synthesis of these EC-derived vasodilators (Jaffe *et al.* 1987).

A number of crucial mechanisms may be involved in increased vascular permeability. Factors triggering EC leakage include: histamine, serotonin, C3a, C5a, bradykinin, leukotrienes, PAF, and AECA (Joris *et al.* 1987; Brenner *et al.* 1989; Cotran 1993; Szekanecz and Koch 2005). The morphological basis for vascular leakage is EC retraction and contraction. These result in the formation and widening of intercellular gaps between ECs (Cotran 1993). The gaps form as a result of EC contraction mediated by vasoactive agents, primarily histamine (Cotran 1993). EC retraction, associated with cytoskeletal reorganization, occurs in EC monolayers exposed to proinflammatory cytokines, such as IL-1, TNF-α, or IFN-γ. Treatment of EC cultures with these cytokines for 4–6 hours results in cytoskeletal reorganization and EC retraction, leading to increased vascular permeability lasting for a day or more (Brett *et al.* 1989; Szekanecz and Koch 2004). Thus, the mechanism of EC retraction, which is long-term and is influenced by cytokines, is different from that of EC contraction, which occurs more rapidly and is histamine dependent. Moreover, EC retraction is a good example of EC stimulation, while EC contraction is a manifestation of EC activation (Cotran 1993; Joris *et al.* 1987; Brett *et al.* 1989; Szekanecz and Koch 2004, 2005).

Leukocyte–EC interactions may themselves cause EC injury and thus increased vascular leakage. The molecular mechanisms of leukocyte–EC adhesion will be discussed in detail below.

Table 4.1 Morphological changes of blood vessels in inflammation

Vasodilatation
Increased vascular permeability (vascular leakage)
Endothelial contraction ("histamine-mediated injury")
Endothelial retraction ("cytokine-mediated injury")
Leukocyte-mediated endothelial injury
Antiendothelial antibody-mediated injury
Endothelial regeneration

The key mediators in this process are reactive oxygen intermediates (ROI) and matrix metalloproteinase (MMP) enzymes primarily produced by inflammatory leukocytes (Varani *et al.* 1989; Szekanecz and Koch 2004). The outcome of leukocyte-mediated vascular injury depends highly on activated leukocytes. Non-activated neutrophils extravasate without affecting endothelial permeability. In contrast, the transendothelial migration of activated leukocytes results in vascular leakage (Hurley 1972). Inhibition of neutrophil adhesion or inhibition of production of ROIs in animal models of inflammation suppresses vascular leakage and edema formation (Mulligan *et al.* 1991).

AECAs have been detected in several autoimmune and inflammatory diseases, including RA and rheumatoid vasculitis, systemic sclerosis (SSc), systemic lupus erythematosus (SLE), and mixed connective tissue disease (MCTD) (Editorial 1991; Van der Zee *et al.* 1991; Westphal *et al.* 1994; Bodolay *et al.* 2004). AECA has been implicated in vascular injury underlying SLE and MCTD. In addition, AECA production has been correlated with some markers of clinical activity in these disorders (Baguley and Hughes 1988; Westphal *et al.* 1994; Bodolay *et al.* 2004). Circulating AECAs may be markers of vascular damage. AECAs have been found more frequently in the sera of patients with rheumatoid vaculitis compared to RA patients without vasculitis (Van der Zee *et al.* 1991; Westphal *et al.* 1994). AECA of the IgG isotype has also been described in other forms of vasculitis (Baguley and Hughes 1988). Thus, AECAs may be involved in the evolution of vasculitis-associated endothelial injury.

Vascular regeneration occurring after injury or during angiogenesis may also be associated with leakage. Open intercellular junctions and the incomplete basement membranes are observed in differentiating ECs (Schoefl 1963; Szekanecz *et al.* 1999, 2005; Szekanecz and Koch 2005). Endothelial regeneration may also occur without the formation of new blood vessels. In this situation, regeneration is accompanied by increased capillary permeability. These processes may occur in the vicinity of necrotic tissues, as is seen near areas of infarction (Joris *et al.* 1990).

Leukocyte–endothelial adhesion and transendothelial cell migration in inflammation

Adhesion of peripheral blood leukocytes to ECs is a key event in leukocyte ingress into inflammatory sites (Albelda and Buck 1990; Springer 1990; Szekanecz and Szegedi 1992; Carlos and Harlan 1994; Haskard 1995; Szekanecz *et al.* 1996; Szekanecz and Koch 1999). The process of leukocyte extravasation occurs via venules

resembling specialized high-endothelial venules (HEV), naturally found in lymphoid organs which play a role in lymphocyte homing (Haskard 1995; Szekanecz *et al.* 1996). HEV-like structures are seen in certain inflammatory tissues, such as in inflamed synovium (van Dinther-Janssen *et al.* 1990; Szekanecz *et al.* 1996). Thus, leukocyte migration through these HEV-like vessels in inflammation may be considered a form of pathological homing (Haskard 1995; Szekanecz *et al.* 1996; Szekanecz and Koch 2004, 2005). The adhesion of ECs to the surrounding ECM is also important for EC activation, contraction, retraction, proliferation, migration, and neovascularization (Albelda and Buck 1990; Springer 1990; Szekanecz and Szegedi 1992; Haskard 1995; Szekanecz *et al.* 1996; Szekanecz and Koch 1999).

EC adhesion to leukocytes or to ECM components is mediated by adhesion receptors. CAMs have been classified into a number of distinct superfamilies including integrins, selectins, and those of the immunoglobulin superfamily (Albelda and Buck 1990; Springer 1990; Szekanecz and Szegedi 1992; Carlos and Harlan 1994; Szekanecz *et al.* 1996; Szekanecz and Koch 1999) (Table 4.2). Although there are exceptions, integrins are mainly involved in EC adhesion to the ECM, while selectins and members of the immunoglobulin superfamily are involved in EC adhesion to other cell types (Albelda and Buck 1990; Springer 1990; Szekanecz and Szegedi 1992; Carlos and Harlan 1994; Szekanecz *et al.* 1996; Szekanecz and Koch 1999).

The selectin superfamily includes E-, P-, and L-selectin. All selectins contain an extracellular N-terminal domain related to lectins, an epidermal growth factor (EGF)-like motif, and moieties related to complement regulatory proteins. E- and P-selectin are expressed by ECs, while L-selectin is mostly expressed by leukocytes (Albelda and Buck 1990; Springer 1990; Szekanecz and Szegedi 1992; Carlos and Harlan 1994).

E-selectin is not expressed on resting cultured ECs, however, upon stimulation with IL-1 or TNF-α, for even less than 1 hour, ECs will express E-selectin on their surface. Maximal E-selectin expression is observed after 4 to 6 hours of cytokine exposure

Table 4.2 Relevant endothelial adhesion molecules in inflammation

Adhesion molecule superfamily	Receptor on endothelium	Ligand(s)
Integrins	β_1 integrins	ECM components (laminin, fibronectin, collagen, vitronectin, etc.)
	$\alpha_4\beta_1$ integrin	VCAM-1, fibronectin
	$\alpha_V\beta_3$ integrin	ECM components (fibronectin, fibrinogen, thrombospondin)
Immunoglobulins	ICAM-1, (ICAM-3?) VCAM-1 LFA-3 PECAM-1 (CD31)	β_2 integrins: LFA-1, Mac-1 A4β1 and α4β7 CD2 Homophilic, $\alpha v\beta 3$
Selectins	E-selectin P-selectin	ESL-1, PSGL-1, CLA PSGL-1
Cadherins	VE-cadherin	Homophilic
Others	CD44 Endoglin VAP-1, VAP-2	Hyaluronic acid TGF-β ?

(Bevilacqua *et al.* 1987). Thus, as described above, E-selectin expression is a good marker of cytokine-dependent EC activation (Pober *et al.* 1983; Bevilacqua *et al.* 1987; Cotran 1993). Furthermore, cytokine-activated ECs shed this CAM, thus releasing soluble E-selectin to the surface of ECs (Koch *et al.* 1993a; Haskard 1995; Szekanecz *et al.* 1996). E-selectin mediates the adhesion of neutrophils and some eosinophils, monocytes, and memory T cells to ECs (Bochner *et al.* 1991). Ligands for E-selectin, such as E-selectin ligand-1 (ESL-1), P-selectin ligand-1 (PSGL-1), and cutaneous leukocyte antigen (CLA), contain sialylated glycan motifs, such as sialyl Lewis-X (sLX) (Asa *et al.* 1995; Borges *et al.* 1997).

There is substantial evidence that E-selectin plays an important role in mediating leukocyte–EC adhesion in inflammation *in vivo.* Abundant endothelial expression of E-selectin is observed in lymphocyte-rich areas in inflammatory sites (Ishikawa *et al.* 1993; Szekanecz *et al.* 1996). E-selectin has been associated with animal models of inflammation (Mulligan *et al.* 1991; Carlos and Harlan 1994; Kavanaugh 1996; Borges *et al.* 1997). Regarding humans, abundant expression of E-selectin has been detected in synovial tissues of patients with rheumatoid arthritis (RA) (Koch *et al.* 1991). In addition, elevated serum and synovial fluid concentrations of soluble E-selectin are detected in RA (Koch *et al.* 1991, 1993a; Szekanecz *et al.* 1996).

P-selectin is constitutively present on the membrane of EC Weibel–Palade bodies. Its expression on the plasma membrane of endothelial cells is rapidly up-regulated by histamine or thrombin (McEver *et al.* 1989). P-selectin is involved in neutrophil and monocyte adhesion to endothelium *in vitro* (Geng *et al.* 1990). PSGL-1 is a known ligand for P-selectin (Asa *et al.* 1995; Borges *et al.* 1997). In contrast to E-selectin, the induction of P-selectin on ECs is an example of endothelial stimulation rather than activation. The up-regulation of P-selectin expression occurs within seconds. Thus, this CAM is thought to be involved in the very early phases of adhesion (Lawrence and Springer 1991). As described above, P-selectin plays a role in rapid EC responses, such as in histamine-dependent EC stimulation (Pober and Cotran 1990; Cotran 1993). P-selectin may also shed from the cell surface and appear in a soluble form in the sera and synovial fluids (Hosaka *et al.* 1996). P-selectin acts in concert with PAF to induce the expression of β_2 integrins on neutrophils leading to maximal neutrophil adherence in inflammation (Lorant *et al.* 1991). Stimulation of neutrophil PSGL-1 expression also enhances β_2 integrin-dependent leukocyte adhesion (Blanks *et al.* 1998). In a model of neutrophil-dependent acute lung injury, a rapid up-regulation of P-selectin expression was observed after the induction of inflammation. Furthermore, an antibody to P-selectin had a protective effect against vascular injury in this model (Mulligan *et al.* 1992). An anti-PSGL-1 antibody blocked the migration of T cells into skin inflammatory sites (Borges *et al.* 1997). P-selectin is expressed on synovial ECs in RA (Johnson *et al.* 1993; Szekanecz *et al.* 1996). Moreover, abundant soluble P-selectin has been detected in RA synovial fluids (Hosaka *et al.* 1996).

L-selectin is absent from ECs but present on most types of leukocytes, including lymphocytes and neutrophils. L-selectin mediates physiological lymphocyte homing by binding to its ligands, which include CD34, MadCAM-1, and GlyCAM-1 expressed by HEVs (Albelda and Buck 1990; Springer 1990). There is an increasing body of evidence that L-selectin may also be involved in neutrophil–EC interactions or, as termed above, pathological homing underlying inflammatory situations (Albelda and Buck 1990; Springer 1990;

Von Andrian *et al.* 1991; Carlos and Harlan 1994; Szekanecz *et al.* 1996; Szekanecz and Koch 1999). In experimental cases of E- and P-selectin deficiency, L-selectin was solely able to mediate leukocyte rolling (Ley *et al.* 1993). Nevertheless, L-selectin expression on leukocytes is down-regulated upon cytokine activation (Ichikawa *et al.* 1992). Therefore, the exact role of L-selectin in inflammation remains to be fully elucidated.

Integrins are $\alpha\beta$ heterodimers and are classified into subfamilies with respect to their common β subunits. Each of the common β chains is associated with one or more α subunits (Albelda and Buck 1990; Springer 1990; Szekanecz and Szegedi 1992; Carlos and Harlan 1994; Szekanecz and Koch 1999). β_1 and β_3 integrins are expressed on ECs. Integrins, such as $\alpha_1\beta_1$ to $\alpha_9\beta_1$, and $\alpha_V\beta_3$, mediate EC adhesion to ECM components including various types of collagen, laminin, fibronectin, fibrinogen, tenascin, vitronectin, thrombospondin, and von Willebrand factor (Albelda and Buck 1990; Springer 1990; Szekanecz and Szegedi 1992; Carlos and Harlan 1994). The $\alpha_1\beta_1$ and $\alpha_2\beta_1$ heterodimers mediate EC adhesion to various types of collagen, as well as to laminin (Albelda and Buck 1990; Springer 1990; Szekanecz and Szegedi 1992). Laminin is also recognized by the $\alpha_6\beta_1$ integrin. There are two important receptors for fibronectin: $\alpha_5\beta_1$ recognizes the RGD (arginyl-glycyl-aspartyl) motif in fibronectin, while $\alpha_4\beta_1$ binds to an RGD-independent site (Albelda and Buck 1990; Springer 1990; Szekanecz and Szegedi 1992; Szekanecz and Koch 1999). Both fibronectin receptor integrins as well as another fibronectin, laminin, and collagen receptor ($\alpha_3\beta_1$) have been detected on ECs (Albelda 1991; Szekanecz and Koch 1999). Integrins containing the β_3 subunit play a role in EC adhesion to fibronectin, vitronectin, thrombospondin, von Willebrand factor, and fibrinogen (Albelda and Buck 1990; Springer 1990; Albelda 1991; Szekanecz and Szegedi 1992). Microvascular and macrovascular ECs may exert different integrin profiles suggesting that ECs, under certain conditions, may alter their CAM expression pattern during angiogenesis (Albelda 1991; Szekanecz *et al.* 1996, 2005; Szekanecz and Koch 2005). Most β_1 integrins, as well as $\alpha_V\beta_3$, are highly involved in EC migration on various substrata, and angiogenesis (see later), and are required for the survival and maturation of new blood vessels (Brooks *et al.* 1994; Szekanecz *et al.* 1998a, 2005; Szekanecz and Koch 2004).

Integrins are not only involved in EC adhesion to ECM, but they are also able to mediate cell-to-cell contacts. In the latter situation, integrins bind to CAMs belonging to the immunoglobulin superfamily. The two most relevant receptor–counterreceptor pairs are $\alpha_4\beta_1$ integrin recognizing vascular cell adhesion molecule-1 (VCAM-1) and β_2 integrins binding to intercellular adhesion molecule-1 (ICAM-1) (Albelda and Buck 1990; Springer 1990). These integrin-mediated adhesive pathways have been implicated in leukocyte–EC interactions during inflammatory processes. For example, β_1 and β_2 integrins have been implicated in animal models of arthritis (Jasin *et al.* 1992; Barbadillo *et al.* 1995; Szekanecz *et al.* 1996; Szekanecz and Koch 1999). Anti-$\alpha_4\beta_1$ integrin antibodies suppress leukocyte accumulation in animal models of colitis, peritonitis, and experimental allergic encephalomyelitis (Carlos and Harlan 1994; Kavanaugh 1996). In humans, abundant expression of EC integrins was described in synovial inflammation (El Gabalawy and Wilkins 1993; Johnson *et al.* 1993; Haskard 1995; Szekanecz *et al.* 1996; Szekanecz and Koch 1999).

As described above, VCAM-1 is a member of the immunoglobulin superfamily of CAMs. VCAM-1 is a ligand for the integrins

$\alpha_4\beta_1$ and $\alpha_4\beta_7$. VCAM-1 is constitutively expressed on resting ECs and its expression is strongly up-regulated by proinflammatory cytokines (Thornhill and Haskard 1990; Szekanecz et al. 1996). Antibodies to VCAM-1 inhibit leukocyte adhesion to ECs (Cotran 1993) and attenuate experimental colitis (Sans et al. 1999) and leukocyte infiltration associated with murine cardiac allograft rejection (Orosz et al. 1993). Abundant in situ VCAM-1 expression has been associated with synovitis, scleroderma, and various other types of inflammation (Koch et al. 1991; Wilkinson et al. 1993; Koch et al. 1993b; Szekanecz et al. 1996). There is a high concentration of soluble VCAM-1 in RA sera and synovial fluid of RA patients (Wellicome et al. 1993). ICAM-1 is a ligand for the β_2 integrins LFA-1 ($\alpha_L\beta_2$), Mac-1 ($\alpha_M\beta_2$), and p150,95 ($\alpha_X\beta_2$) (Albelda and Buck 1990; Springer 1990; Szekanecz and Szegedi 1992; Szekanecz et al. 1994, 1996).

The expression of ICAM-1 on ECs can be induced by IL-1, TNF-α, and IFN-γ (Pober et al. 1986). The maximal expression of ICAM-1 on ECs is observed later (>24 hours) than that of E-selectin or VCAM-1 (Pober et al. 1986; Pober and Cotran 1990). The ICAM-1/β_2 integrin-dependent adhesion pathway is crucial in inflammation, as patients with leukocyte-adhesion deficiency (LAD) syndrome, in which there are mutations in the gene encoding the β_2 integrin subunit, show marked suppression of the inflammatory response (Anderson and Springer 1978). ICAM-1 is highly expressed on ECs in inflammatory sites (Koch et al. 1991; Szekanecz et al. 1996). Anti-ICAM-1 antibody inhibits experimental arthritis, allergic encephalomyelitis, and glomerulonephritis in animal models (Iigo et al. 1991; Carlos and Harlan 1994; Kavanaugh 1996). High levels of soluble ICAM-1 are detected in the synovia of RA patients (Cush et al. 1993; Koch et al. 1994).

Other CAMs mediating EC adhesion to other cells in inflammation include LFA-3, platelet-endothelial cell adhesion molecule-1 (PECAM-1; CD31), CD44, vascular adhesion proteins (VAP-1 and VAP-2), endoglin, VE-cadherin, junctional adhesion molecules (JAMs), CD99, and possibly ICAM-3 (Hale et al. 1989; Albelda and Buck 1990; Springer 1990; Szekanecz and Szegedi 1992; Salmi et al. 1993; Szekanecz et al. 1994, 1995a, 1996; Szekanecz and Koch 1999, 2004, 2005; Cunningham et al. 2000; Arrate et al. 2001; Schenkel et al. 2002). LFA-3 and its counterreceptor, CD2, are members of the immunoglobulin superfamily. LFA-3 is present on ECs and the CD2/LFA-3 adhesion pathway is involved in T cell adhesion to ECs in various inflammatory responses (Hale et al. 1989; Szekanecz et al. 1996). PECAM-1, another CAM in the immunoglobulin superfamily, mediates homotypic adhesion by binding to PECAM-1, as well as heterotypic adhesion by recognizing the $\alpha_V\beta_3$ integrin (Albelda and Buck 1990; Springer 1990; Piali et al. 1995; Szekanecz et al. 1996). PECAM-1 is a marker of activated EC and it is abundantly expressed in inflamed synovium (Johnson et al. 1993; Szekanecz et al. 1995b). CD44 is a receptor for hyaluronate (Albelda and Buck 1990; Szekanecz and Szegedi 1992). CD44 is present on activated ECs in inflammatory sites (Haynes et al. 1991; Johnson et al. 1993; Szekanecz et al. 1996).

VAP-1 was originally isolated from synovial ECs. The expression of VAP-1 is increased in synovial inflamation (Salmi et al. 1993). Furthermore, VAP-1 is an important inflammation-associated EC marker used for endothelial characterization (Holmen et al. 2005). Endoglin is a receptor for transforming growth factor-β (TGF-β). Endoglin is involved in EC adhesion and is highly expressed in inflammation, such as in RA (Szekanecz et al. 1995a). VE-cadherin mediates homophilic binding between endothelial cells. It shows colocalization with many other CAMs including PECAM-1 and endoglin. VE-cadherin is involved in endothelial migration and polarization (Dejana 1996). JAMs (JAM1, JAM2, and JAM3), as well as CD99 have also been implicated in leukocyte migration through endothelial junctions (Cunningham et al. 2000; Arrate et al. 2001; Schenkel et al. 2002). ICAM-3, a leukocyte CAM, is a known ligand for LFA-1. It is absent from most types of ECs, but it is present on a portion of RA synovial ECs, suggesting a role for endothelial ICAM-3 in inflammation (Szekanecz et al. 1994; Szekanecz and Koch 1997).

Leukocyte adhesion to ECs occurs in several steps. An early, weak adhesion termed rolling, occurring within the first 1–2 hours, is mediated mostly by selectins and their ligands. Leukocyte activation occurs next due to the interactions between chemokine receptors on leukocytes and proteoglycans on ECs. PECAM-1 is involved in this step. Activation-dependent, firm adhesion involves mostly $\alpha_4\beta_1$ integrin/VCAM-1, LFA-1/ICAM-1, and JAM/integrin interactions. This step is accompanied by the secretion of multiple chemokines. Transendothelial migration or diapedesis, mostly involving integrins, occurs when secreted chemokines bind to endothelial heparan sulfate. Chemokines preferentially attract EC-bound leukocytes (Butcher 1991; Carlos and Harlan 1994; Imhof and Aurrand-Lions 2004).

The regulation of leukocyte–EC interactions is dependent on a number of factors (Table 4.3). Physical factors, such as altered shear stress, stimulate the rolling and adhesion of neutrophils to endothelium (Lawrence and Springer 1991). The state of leukocyte activation is also important. For example, resting neutrophils readily adhere to E-selectin and VCAM-1 but not to ICAM-1. In contrast, activated neutrophils adhere to ICAM-1 (Jutila et al. 1989). As described above, exogenous proinflammatory cytokines may up-regulate endothelial CAM expression and stimulate leukocyte–EC adhesion (Pober et al. 1986; Thornhill and Haskard 1990; Szekanecz et al. 1996). ECs themselves also produce a number of inflammatory mediators including IL-1; IL-6; IL-8; granulocyte-colony stimulating factor (G-CSF); granulocyte/monocyte-colony stimulating factor (GM-CSF); monocyte chemoattractant protein-1 (MCP-1); and the groα chemokine (Table 4.4). Other soluble mediators may also regulate CAM expression and intercellular adhesion. For example, PAF is involved in P-selectin-dependent rolling (Lorant et al. 1991), while chemokines play a role in integrin-dependent firm adhesion (Butcher 1991). Certain CAMs can also crosstalk with each other, resulting in strengthened intercellular adhesion. For example, E-selectin and P-selectin stimulate the adhesive activity of β_2 integrins on neutrophils (Lo et al. 1991; Lorant et al. 1991). The crosstalk between selectins and integrins is crucial for the transition from rolling to firm adhesion. Finally, intercellular contact itself may result in increased cytokine release

Table 4.3 Regulatory factors of leukocyte–endothelial adhesion

Physical factors
State of activation of neutrophils
Exogenous cytokines
Endogenous endothelial mediators
Cross talk between adhesion molecules

Table 4.4 Endothelial-derived inflammatory mediators

Cytokines

    Interleukin-1 (IL-1)

    Interleukin-6 (IL-6)

Chemokines

    Interleukin-8 (IL-8)

    Monocyte chemoattractant protein-1 (MCP-1)

    Growth-regulated oncogene-α (groα)

Growth factors

    Endothelial cell-derived growth factor (ECGF)

    Transforming growth factor-β (TGF-β)

Colony-stimulating factors

    Granulocyte colony-stimulating factor (G-CSF)

    Granulocyte-macrophage colony-stimulating factor (GM-CSF)

Others

    Platelet-activating factor (PAF)

    Nitric oxide (NO)

    Prostacyclin (PGI$_2$)

and CAM expression (Bombara *et al.* 1993). These mechanisms may synchronize the sequence of steps and events described above and they may be important in the regulation of leukocyte extravasation and the inflammatory process.

The endothelium in angiogenesis

Angiogenesis or neovascularization is a physiologically important process in reproduction, development, and tissue repair. The formation of new blood vessels is enhanced in numerous disease states, such as inflammatory diseases and malignancies. Inflammation is associated with an increased turnover of capillaries. Several cytokines, growth factors, chemokines, ECM components, CAMs, and other mediators can stimulate neovascularization. The suppression of neovascularization by blocking the action of angiogenic mediators, or by the administration of angiostatic compounds, may be useful to control inflammation (Folkman and Klagsbrun 1987; Auerbach and Auerbach 1994; Diaz-Flores *et al.* 1994; Schweigerer 1995; Koch 1998; Szekanecz *et al.* 1998a, 1999, 2005; Szekanecz and Koch 2004).

Angiogenesis is a program of several distinct steps. New capillaries develop from existing blood vessels (Koch 1998; Szekanecz and Koch 2004) and there are preferential endothelial precursor stem cells carrying receptors for vascular endothelial growth factor (VEGF) among circulating CD34$^+$ cells (Peichev *et al.* 2000). First, angiogenic mediators (described below) activate ECs. This is associated with the production of MMPs. These enzymes degrade the basement membrane and the interstitium, thus enabling endothelial outgrowth. Among these enzymes, collagenase (MMP-1) and gelatinases (MMP-2 and MMP-9) seem to be the most relevant for angiogenesis. In addition to MMPs, other enzymes, termed serine proteases, including tissue-plasminogen activator (tPA) and urokinase-type plasminogen activator (uPA), are also involved in neovascularization. The migration of loose ECs results in the formation of capillary sprouts. ECs in the midsection of the sprout

undergo mitosis while others at the tip of the sprout migrate but do not proliferate. This is followed by lumen formation within the sprout. Two sprouts then link with each other, thus forming capillary loops and new basement membrane is then synthesized. The continuous emigration of ECs results in the development of second and later generations of new vessels (Folkman and Klagsbrun 1987; Colville-Nash and Scott 1992; Szekanecz *et al.* 1999; Szekanecz and Koch 2004).

As mentioned above, preferential CD34$^+$ EC precursors carrying receptors for VEGF exist within the population of blood stem cells. These precursors, under certain circumstances, may develop into ECs. They are important in blood vessel growth and they also have relevance for future therapies for vascular disorders (Peichev *et al.* 2000; Gehling *et al.* 2000; Freedman and Isner 2001). Endothelial progenitor cell dysfunction and impaired angiogenic function have been described in vasculitis such as Wegener's granulomatosis (Holmen *et al.* 2005).

Some angiogenic factors (Table 4.5) directly effect EC proliferation and migration by interacting with their cognate receptors expression on ECs. In contrast, other mediators act indirectly by stimulating the production of other angiogenic factors (Folkman and Klagsbrun 1987; Koch 1998; Szekanecz *et al.* 1998a, 1998b, 1999; Szekanecz and Koch 1999, 2004). Only naturally produced angiogenic and angiostatic factors which may be involved in inflammatory reactions such as vaculitis will be discussed here.

Among growth factors, VEGF is probably the best known angiogenic factor associated with chronic inflammation (Fava *et al.* 1994; Koch 1998; Szekanecz *et al.* 1998a, 1999, 2005; Manley *et al.* 2002; Shibuya 2003). There have been several attempts to therapeutically interrupt VEGF-dependent angiogenesis using inhibitors of VEGF and VEGF receptors (Manley *et al.* 2002; Shibuya 2003). VEGF, as well as basic (bFGF) and acidic fibroblast growth factors (aFGF), and hepatocyte growth factor (HGF)/scatter factor, are bound to heparin and heparan sulfate in the ECM. These growth factors are mobilized by heparanase and plasmin during neovascularization (Folkman and Klagsbrun 1987; Koch 1998; Szekanecz *et al.* 1998a, 1999, 2005). Hypoxia, which may be a feature of inflamed tissue, stimulates the production of VEGF (Etherington *et al.* 2002). In addition, hypoxia-inducible factors (HIF-1α and HIF-2α) that regulate VEGF gene transcription have also been implicated in angiogenesis (Giatromanolaki *et al.* 2003). Some growth factors that do not bind to heparin may also stimulate new vessel formation. These include platelet-derived growth factor (PDGF),

Table 4.5 Some mediators of angiogenesis in inflammation

VEGF and other growth factors
Cytokines (TNF-α, IL-1, IL-6, IL-15, IL-18, etc.)
ELR+ C-X-C chemokines (IL-8, ENA-78, gro, CTAP-III)
Fractalkine
Extracellular matrix components
Adhesion molecules (some integrins, E-selectin, VEGF, etc.)
Angiogenin
Angiopoietin-1
Prostaglandin E$_2$
Platelet-activating factor

platelet-derived endothelial cell growth factor (PD-ECGF)/
gliostatin, epidermal growth factor (EGF), insulin-like growth
factor-I (IGF-I), and TGF-β (Folkman and Klagsbrun 1987;
Szekanecz et al. 1998a; Koch 1998). Among these growth factors,
TGF-β may exert dose-dependent stimulatory or inhibitory effects
on angiogenesis as well as other inflammatory processes (Wiseman
et al. 1988).

Among proinflammatory cytokines, TNF-α, IL-1, IL-6, IL-8,
IL-15, IL-18, G-CSF, GM-CSF, and oncostatin M are involved in
angiogenesis. The effects of IL-1 on angiogenesis are similar to
those of TGF-β. These cytokines are abundantly produced in the
sera and synovia of RA patients (Folkman and Klagsbrun 1987;
Leibovich et al. 1987; Sachs 1991; Auerbach and Auerbach 1994;
Angiolillo et al. 1997; Wijelath et al. 1997; Koch 1998; Szekanecz
et al. 1998a, 1999, 2005; Park et al. 2001; Voronov et al. 2003).

C-X-C chemokines containing the ELR (glutamyl-leucyl-arginyl)
amino acid motif stimulate angiogenesis. These chemokines include
IL-8 (CXCL8); epithelial neutrophil activating protein-78
(ENA-78; CXCL5); growth-related oncogene α (groα; CXCL1);
and connective tissue activating protein-III (CTAP-III; CXCL6).
In contrast, other C-X-C chemokines lacking the ELR sequence
suppress neovascularization (Strieter et al. 1996; Walz et al. 1996;
Koch et al. 1996; Szekanecz et al. 1998a, 1998b, 1999). Stromal cell-
derived factor-1 (SDF-1; CXCL12) is a C-X-C chemokine that
lacks the ELR motif but is still angiogenic (Strieter et al. 1995, 1996;
Szekanecz and Koch 2001). Fractalkine (CX3CL1) is a C-X3-C chemokine promoting neovascularization (Szekanecz and Koch 2001).
These chemokines are also involved in leukocyte recruitment into
inflammatory sites, such as the arthritic synovium (Szekanecz and
Koch 2001). Among chemokine receptors, CXCR2 may be the most
important receptor (on ECs) for ELR-containing angiogenic
C-X-C chemokines. CXCR2 is a major receptor for IL-8, ENA-78,
and groα (Addison et al. 2000).

Several ECM components, including type I collagen, fibronectin,
laminin, vitronectin, tenascin, thrombospondin, proteoglycans,
and others, play a role in EC adhesion and migration during neovascularization (Madri and Williams 1983; Folkman and Klagsbrun
1987; Montesano et al. 1991; Colville-Nash and Scott 1992; Nicosia
et al. 1993; Canfield and Schor 1995; Szekanecz et al. 1999, 2005;
Szekanecz and Koch 1999). The role of ECM-degrading enzymes in
angiogenesis is discussed above.

CAMs also play a crucial role in inflammation-associated angiogenesis. Among CAMs expressed on ECs, the following mediate cellular adhesion during angiogenesis: β$_1$ and β$_3$ integrins; E-selectin;
the L-selectin ligand CD34; selectin-related glycoconjugates including Lewis^y/H and MUC18; VCAM-1; PECAM-1; and endoglin
(Albelda 1991; Nguyen et al. 1993; Brooks et al. 1994; Koch et al.
1995; Dejana 1996; Maier et al. 1997; Szekanecz et al. 1998a, 1999;
Szekanecz and Koch 1999, 2004; Szekanecz et al. 2005).

Other angiogenic mediators include members of the cyclooxygenase
(COX)/prostaglandin system including prostaglandin E$_2$, as well as
angiogenin, angiotropin, angiopoietin-1, pleiotrophin, PAF, histamine, substance P, erythropoietin, adenosine, fibrinogen, and thrombin (Folkman and Klagsbrun 1987; Colville-Nash and Scott 1992;
Diaz-Flores et al. 1994; Camussi et al. 1995; Koch 1998; Szekanecz
et al. 1998a, 1999, 2005; Pufe et al. 2003; Woods et al. 2003).

Angiostatic factors (Table 4.6) may directly suppress neovascularization or may indirectly interfere with the action of the angiogenic mediators discussed above. Among cytokines, IFN-α, IFN-γ,

Table 4.6 Some inhibitors of angiogenesis in inflammation

Anti-inflammatory agents
Anti-TNF biologicals
ELR- C-X-C chemokines (PF4, IP-10, MIG)
VEGF inhibitors
MMP inhibitors
Adhesion blocking
Angiostatin, endostatin
Angiopoietin-2
Thrombospondin-1
TNP-470 (fumagillin) and other derivatives of antibiotics

IL-4, IL-12, and leukemia inhibitory factor (LIF), indirectly suppress neovascularization by blocking the secretion of angiogenic
cytokines and chemokines (Folkman and Klagsbrun 1976; Waring
et al. 1993; Auerbach and Auerbach 1994; Szekanecz et al. 1998a,
1999, 2005).

As described above, C-X-C chemokines lacking the ELR motif
may be angiostatic. Among these chemokines, platelet factor-4
(PF4, CXCL4); monokine induced by interferon-g (MIG, CXCL9);
and IFN-g-inducible protein (IP-10; CXCL10) inhibit neovascularization. As IP-10 and MIG bind to CXCR3, this chemokine receptor
may be involved in chemokine-mediated angiostasis (Koch et al.
1996; Strieter et al. 1996, Szekanecz et al. 1998a, 1998b; Szekanecz
and Koch 2001).

Protease inhibitors, such as tissue inhibitors of MMPs (TIMPs)
and plasminogen activator inhibitors (PAIs) antagonize the effects
of ECM-degrading enzymes during angiogenesis (Dameron et al.
1994; Auerbach and Auerbach 1994; Koch et al. 1998; Szekanecz
et al. 1999; Szekanecz and Koch 2001; Apparailly et al. 2002). Gene
transfer of urokinase PAI inhibits angiogenesis (Apparailly et al.
2002). Heparin-binding factors, such as thrombospondin-1 and the
PF4 chemokine, block growth factor binding to heparin (Dameron
et al. 1994; Auerbach and Auerbach 1994; Koch et al. 1998;
Szekanecz et al. 1999; Szekanecz and Koch 2001).

A number of anti-inflammatory and antirheumatic agents currently used for the treatment of rheumatic diseases suppress EC
migration and neovascularization. These compounds include, among
others, dexamethasone, chloroquine, sulfasalazine, methotrexate,
azathioprine, cyclophosphamide, leflunomide, thalidomide, minocycline, anti-TNF agents, and possibly cyclosporine A (Auerbach
and Auerbach 1994; Koch 1998; Szekanecz et al. 1998a, 2005).

Some antibiotics and their derivatives may suppress angiogenesis
via the inhibition of VEGF or MMP action. Apart from minocycline mentioned above, TNP-470, an angiostatic analogue of fuma-
gillin, a naturally occurring product of Aspergillus fumigatus,
decreases serum levels of VEGF and inhibits angiogenesis.
Deoxyspergualin and clarithromycin may also inhibit neovascularization (Auerbach and Auerbach 1994; Koch 1998; Szekanecz et al.
1998a, 2005).

Other angiogenesis inhibitors include the following: taxol, osteo-
nectin, opioids, angiopoietin-2, angiostatin, endostatin, retinoids,
troponin I, chondromodulin-1, Secreted Protein Acidic and Rich in
Cysteine (SPARC), and others (Folkman and Klagsbrun 1987;
Colville-Nash and Scott 1992; Auerbach and Auerbach 1994;

Schweigerer 1995; Koch 1998; Szekanecz *et al.* 1998a, 2005; Setoguchi *et al.* 2004). Some of these agents, particularly angiostatin and endostatin, gave promising results in cancer therapy trials and preclinical arthritis studies (Kim *et al.* 2002; Matsuno *et al.* 2002; Szekanecz *et al.* 2005).

The outcome of angiogenesis, and thus leukocyte recruitment into inflammatory sites through newly formed vessels, depends on the imbalance between angiogenic mediators and inhibitors of neovascularization. A regulatory network consisting of numerous interactive mechanisms and feedback loops exists in inflamed tissues. For example, soluble and cell surface-bound angiogenic factors may interact with each other: VEGF, in part, acts via integrin-dependent pathways (Senger *et al.* 1997). Other regulatory mechanisms include: the balance between specific antagonistic pairs, such as MMPs and TIMPs; the stimulation of angiostatic factors by angiogenic mediators (negative feedback); suppression of angiogenic mediator production by antagonists; and interactions between angiostatic molecules. The use of synthetic compounds in order to inhibit neovascularization is also a method of regulation which is relevant for antiangiogenic therapy (Colville-Nash and Scott 1992; Sato *et al.* 1993; Rathanaswami *et al.* 1993; Martel-Pelletier *et al.* 1994; Schweigerer 1995; Strieter *et al.* 1996; Szekanecz *et al.* 1998a, 1998b, 1999; Szekanecz and Koch 1999).

Endothelial activation, adhesion, and angiogenesis in vasculitis

Most of the complex mechanisms described above are involved in the pathogenesis of vascular injury underlying autoimmune vasculitis (Table 4.7). It has been speculated that circulating AECAs may play a central role in immune injury to endothelium (Cotran and Pober 1990). Circulating IgG antibodies against human umbilical vein ECs can be found in 70% of patients with SLE, 30% of those with scleroderma, and 28% of those with RA (Heurkens *et al.* 1989). Circulating cytotoxic antibodies that reacted with ECs have been described in a variety of vasculitides, such as in Kawasaki disease (Brasile *et al.* 1989; Grunebaum *et al.* 2002).

It has been shown that CAMs play a role in leukocyte–EC interactions underlying vasculitides associated with other autoimmune syndromes. Increased expression of $\alpha_4\beta_1$ and LFA-1 integrins is found on peripheral blood lymphocytes derived from SLE patients with vasculitis. In contrast, only LFA-1 but not $\alpha_4\beta_1$ integrin is up-regulated in SLE patients without vasculitis. Functional studies confirm that the adhesion of lymphocytes to cytokine-activated human umbilical vein ECs, as well as to the CS-1 motif of fibronectin, the ligand for $\alpha_4\beta_1$, is increased in SLE patients with vasculitis (Takeuchi *et al.* 1993). ANCA may play an important role in the regulation of CAM expression as it can induce β_2 integrin

Table 4.7 Key mechanisms in vasculitis

Antiendothelial cell antibodies (AECA)
Cell adhesion molecules (CAM)
Tissue expression
Production of soluble CAMs
ANCA may trigger CAM expression
Altered angiogenesis

expression on neutrophils leading to the perpetuation of neutrophil influx in vasculitis (Calderwood *et al.* 2005). ICAM-1 and VCAM-1 have been associated with the development of vasculitis in Sjögren's syndrome (Turkcapar *et al.* 2005). VCAM-1 is involved in the pathogenesis of hepatitis C-induced mixed cryoglobulinemic vasculitis (Kaplanski *et al.* 2005). There is an altered CAM expression profile on coronary artery aneurysm ECs in acute Kawasaki disease (Miura *et al.* 2004). There is increased production of circulating, soluble ICAM and E-selectin in ANCA-associated vasculitis (Di Lorenzo *et al.* 2004). In rheumatoid vasculitis, increased concentrations of serum soluble ICAM-1 and ICAM-3 are found in comparison to RA patients without vasculitis. Furthermore, soluble ICAM-3 levels are significantly higher in active versus inactive disease (Voskuyl *et al.* 1995). Increased production of soluble ICAM-1 has been associated with more intensive vascular changes in rheumatoid vasculitis, as assessed by nailfold capillaroscopy (Witkowska *et al.* 2003). These data suggest that CAM expression and soluble CAM production may be useful markers of vascular inflammation in patients with vasculitis.

Impaired angiogenesis based on endothelial progenitor cell dysfunction has been reported in various types of vasculitis with kidney involvement. Patients with active disease had decreased numbers of progenitor cell colony forming units linked to high expression of VAP-1 on kidney ECs. As described above, VAP-1 is a marker of inflammatory ECs. Thus, endothelial progenitor cell dysfunction is highly dependent on activated, inflammatory EC-mediated vascular damage (Holmen *et al.* 2005).

Summary

ECs are involved in a number of mechanisms underlying vascular inflammation. These cells are able to produce vasodilatory mediators including prostacyclin, NO, or PAF. Several factors lead to increased vascular permeability, including endothelial contraction caused by histamine, endothelial stimulation and endothelial retraction triggered by cytokines, and endothelial activation. In addition, increased permeability results from vascular injury mediated by leukocytes and AECAs, as well as from endothelial regeneration.

ECs play a central role in leukocyte extravasation, a key feature of inflammation including vasculitis. A number of CAMs termed integrins, selectins, immunoglobulins, and others act in concert and regulate the sequence of distinct steps. The most important adhesive pathways are determined by receptor-ligand pairs, including endothelial E- and P-selectin and their respective ligands, VCAM-1 and $\alpha_4\beta_1$ or $\alpha_4\beta_7$ integrin, ICAM-1 and LFA-1, or Mac-1 integrin. These CAMs interact with soluble inflammatory mediators, such as chemokines or PAF. The presence of various CAM pairs and the existence of distinct steps of rolling, activation, adhesion, and migration account for the diversity and specificity of leukocyte-endothelial interactions.

ECs are active participants in new vessel formation which is initiated by a number of soluble and cell-bound factors. Angiogenic mediators form a complex interactive network that regulates the perpetuation of this process. Naturally produced angiogenesis inhibitors down-regulate the effects of angiogenic factors. Changes in the morphology and function of ECs play a crucial role in the pathogenesis of vasculitis and other inflammatory conditions. Specific targeting of these mechanisms may be useful for the future management of vascular inflammatory diseases.

References

Addison, C. L., Daniel, T. O., Burdick, M. D., Liu, H., Ehlert, J. E., Xue, Y. Y., Buechi, L., Walz, A., Richmond, A. and Strieter, R. M. (2000). The CXC chemokine receptor 2, CXCR2, is the putative receptor for ELR+ CXC chemokine-induced angiogenic activity. *Journal of Immunology*, **65**, 5269–77.

Albelda, S. M. (1991). Differential expression of integrin cell-substratum adhesion receptors on endothelium. *EXS*, **59**, 188–92.

Albelda, S. M. and Buck, C. A. (1990). Integrins and other cell adhesion molecules. *FASEB Journal*, **4**, 2868–80.

Anderson, R. and Springer, T. A. (1978). Leukocyte adhesion deficiency. *Annual Review of Medicine*, **38**, 175–90.

Angiolillo, A. L., Kanegane, H., Sgadari, C., Reaman, G. H. and Tosato, G. (1997). Interleukin-15 promotes angiogenesis in vivo. *Biochemical and Biophysical Research Communication*, **233**, 231–7.

Apparailly, F., Bouquert, C., Millet, V., Noel, D., Jacquet, C., Opolon, P., Perricaudet, M., Sany, J., Yeh, P. and Jorgensen, C. (2002). Adenovirus-mediated gene transfer of urokinase plasminogen inhibitor inhibits angiogenesis in experimental arthritis. *Gene Therapy*, **9**, 192–200.

Arrate, M. P., Rodriguez, J. M., Tran, T. M., Brock, T. A. and Cunningham, S. A. (2001). Cloning of human junctional adhesion molecule 3 (JAM3) and its identification as the JAM2 counter-receptor. *Journal of Biological Chemistry*, **276**, 45826–32.

Asa, D., Raycroft, L., Ma, L., Aeed, P. A., Kaytes, P. S., Elhammer, A. P. and Geng, J. G. (1995). The P-selectin glycoprotein ligand functions as a common human leukocyte ligand for P- and E-selectins. *Journal of Biological Chemistry*, **270**, 11662–70.

Auerbach, W. and Auerbach, R. (1994). Angiogenesis inhibition: a review. *Pharmacotherapy*, **63**, 265–311.

Baguley, E. and Hughes, G. R. (1988). Lytic IgG anti-endothelial cell antibodies in vasculitis. *Lancet*, **2**, 907.

Barbadillo, C., Arroyo, A., Salas, C., Mulero, J., Sanchez-Madrid, F. and Andreu, J. L. (1995). Anti-integrin immunotherapy in rheumatoid arthritis: protective effect of anti-alpha 4 antibody in adjuvant arthritis. *Springer Seminars in Immunopathology*, **16**, 427–36.

Bevilacqua, M. P., Pober, J. S., Mendrick, D. L., Cotran, R. S. and Gimbrone, M. A. Jr. (1987). Identification of an inducible endothelial-leukocyte adhesion molecule. *Proceedings of the National Academy of Sciences of the USA*, **84**, 9238–42.

Blanks, J. E., Moll, T., Eytner, R. and Vestweber, D. (1998). Stimulation of P-selectin glycoprotein ligand-1 on mouse neutrophils activates beta 2-integrin mediated cell attachment to ICAM-1. *European Journal of Immunology*, **28**, 433–43.

Bochner, B. S., Luscinskas, F. W., Gimbrone, M. A. Jr, Newman, W., Sterbinsky, S. A., Derse-Anthony, C. P., Klunk, D. and Schleimer, R. P. (1991). Adhesion of human basophils, eosinophils, and neutrophils to interleukin 1-activated human vascular endothelial cells: contributions of endothelial cell adhesion molecules. *Journal of Experimental Medicine*, **173**, 1553–7.

Bodolay, E., Csipo, I., Gal, I., Sipka, S., Gyimesi, E., Szekanecz, Z. and Szegedi, G. (2004). Anti-endothelial cell antibodies in mixed connective tissue disease: frequency and association with clinical symptoms. *Clinical and Experimental Rheumatology*, **22**, 419–15.

Bombara, M. P., Webb, D. L., Conrad, P., Marlor, C. W., Sarr, T., Ranges, G. E., Aune, T. M., Greve, J. M. and Blue, M. L. (1993). Cell contact between T cells and synovial fibroblasts causes induction of adhesion molecules and cytokines. *Journal of Leukocyte Biology*, **54**, 399–406.

Borges, E., Tietz, W., Steegmaier, M., Moll, T., Hallmann, R., Hamann, A. and Vestweber, D. (1997). P-selectin glycoprotein ligand-1 (PSGL-1) on T helper 1 but not on T helper 2 cells binds to P-selectin and supports migration into inflamed skin. *Journal of Experimental Medicine*, **185**, 573–8.

Brasile, L., Kremer, J. M., Clarke, J. L. and Cerilli, J. (1989). Identification of an autoantibody to vascular endothelial cell-specific antigens in systemic vasculitis. *American Journal of Medicine*, **87**, 74–9.

Brenner, B. M., Troy, J. L. and Ballermann, B. J. (1989). Endothelium-dependent vascular responses. Mediators and mechanisms. *Journal of Clinical Investigation*, **84**, 1373–8.

Brett, J., Gerlach, H., Nawroth, P., Steinberg, S., Godman, G. and Stern, D. (1989). Tumor necrosis factor/cachectin increases permeability of endothelial cell monolayers by a mechanism involving regulatory G proteins. *Journal of Experimental Medicine*, **169**, 1977–91.

Brooks, P. C., Clark, R. A. and Cheresh, D. A. (1994). Requirement of vascular integrin alpha v beta 3 for angiogenesis. *Science*, **264**, 569–71.

Butcher, E. C. (1991). Leukocyte-endothelial cell recognition: three (or more) steps to specificity and diversity. *Cell*, **67**, 1033–6.

Calderwood, J. W., Williams, J. M., Morgan, M. D., Nash, G. B. and Savage, C. O. (2005). ANCA induces beta2 integrin and CXC chemokine-dependent neutrophil-endothelial cell interactions that mimic those of highly cytokine-activated endothelium. *Journal of Leukocyte Biology*, **77**, 33–43.

Camussi, G., Montrucchio, G., Lupia, E., De Martino, A., Perona, L., Arese, M., Vercellone, A., Toniolo, A. and Bussolino, F. (1995). Platelet-activating factor directly stimulates in vitro migration of endothelial cells and promotes in vivo angiogenesis by a heparin-dependent mechanism. *Journal of Immunology*, **154**, 6492–501.

Canfield, A. E. and Schor, A. M. (1995). Evidence that tenascin and thrombospondin-1 modulate sprouting of endothelial cells. *Journal of Cell Science*, **108**, 797–809.

Carlos, T. M. and Harlan, J. M. (1994). Leukocyte-endothelial adhesion molecules. *Blood*, **84**, 2068–101.

Colville-Nash, P. R. and Scott, D. L. (1992). Angiogenesis in rheumatoid arthritis: pathogenic and therapeutic implications. *Annals of the Rheumatic Diseases*, **51**, 919–25.

Cotran, R. S. (1993). Endothelial cells. In *Textbook of Rheumatology*, 4th edn, (eds W. N. Kelley, E. D. Harris, S. Ruddy and C. Sledge), pp. 327–36. W. B. Saunders Co., Philadelphia.

Cotran, R. S. and Pober, J. S. (1990). Cytokine-endothelial interactions in inflammation, immunity and vascular injury. *Journal of the American Society of Nephrology*, **1**, 225–35.

Cunningham, S. A., Arrate, M. P., Rodriguez, J. M., Bjercke, R. J., Vanderslice, P., Morris, A. P., Brock, T. A. (2000). A novel protein with homology to the junctional adhesion molecule. Characterization of leukocyte interactions. *Journal of Biological Chemistry*, **275**, 34750–6.

Cush, J. J., Rothlein, R., Lindsley, H. B., Mainolfi, E. A. and Lipsky, P. E. (1993). Increased levels of circulating intercellular adhesion molecule 1 in the sera of patients with rheumatoid arthritis. *Arthritis and Rheumatism*, **36**, 1098–102.

Dameron, K. M., Volpert, O. V., Tainsky, M. A. and Bouck, N. (1994). Control of angiogenesis in fibroblasts by p53 regulation of thrombospondin-1. *Science*, **265**, 1582–4.

Dejana, E. (1996). Endothelial adherens junctions: implications in the control of vascular permeability and angiogenesis. *Journal of Clinical Investigation*, **98**, 1949–53.

Diaz-Flores, L., Gutierrez, R. and Varela, H. (1994). Angiogenesis: an update. *Histology Histopathology*, **9**, 807–43.

Di Lorenzo, G., Pacor, M. L., Mansueto, P., Lo Bianco, C., Di Natale, E., Rapisarda, F., Pellitteri, M. E., Ditta, V., Gioe, A., Giammarresi, G., Rini, G. B. and Li Vecchi, M. (2004). Circulating levels of soluble adhesion molecules in patients with ANCA-associated vasculitis. *Journal of Nephrology*, **17**, 800–7.

Editorial (1991). Antibodies to endothelial cells. *Lancet*, **337**, 649–50.

El Gabalawy, H. and Wilkins, J. (1993). Beta 1 (CD29) integrin expression in rheumatoid synovial membranes. *Journal of Rheumatology*, **20**, 231–7.

Etherington, P. J., Winlove, P., Taylor, P., Paleolog, E. and Miotla, J. M. (2002). VEGF release is associated with reduced oxygen tensions in experimental inflammatory arthritis. *Clinical and Experimental Rheumatology*, **20**, 799–805.

Fava, R. A., Olsen, N. J. and Spencer-Green, G. (1994). Vascular permeability factor/endothelial growth factor (VPF/VEGF): accumulation and expression in human synovial fluids and rheumatoid synovial tissue. *Journal of Experimental Medicine*, **180**, 341–6.

Folkman, J. and Klagsbrun, M. (1987). Angiogenic factors. *Science*, **235**, 442–7.

Freedman, S. B. and Isner, J. M. (2001). Therapeutic angiogenesis for ischemic cardiovascular disease. *Journal of Molecular and Cellular Cardiology*, **33**, 379–93.

Gehling, U. M., Ergun, S., Schumacher, U., Wagener, C., Pantel, K., Otte, M., Schuch, G., Schafhausen, P., Mende, T., Kilic, N., Kluge, K., Schafer, B., Hossfeld, D. K., Fiedler, W. (2000). In vitro differentiation of endothelial cells from AC133-positive progenitor cells. *Blood*, **95**, 3106–12.

Geng, J. G., Bevilacqua, M. P., Moore, K. L., McIntyre, T. M., Prescott, S. M., Kim, J. M., Bliss, G. A., Zimmerman, G. A. and McEver, R. P. (1990). Rapid neutrophil adhesion to activated endothelium mediated by GMP-140. *Nature*, **343**, 757–60.

Giatromanolaki, A., Sivridis, E., Maltezos, E., Athanassou, N., Papazoglou, D., Gatter, K. C., Harris, A. L. and Koukourakis, M. I. (2003). Upregulated hypoxia inducible factor-1α and -2α pathway in rheumatoid arthritis and osteoarthritis. *Arthritis Research and Therapy*, **5**, R193–8.

Grunebaum, E., Blank, M., Cohen, S., Afek, A., Kopolovic, J., Meroni, P. L., Youinou, P. and Shoenfeld, Y. (2002). The role of anti-endothelial cell antibodies in Kawasaki disease – in vitro and in vivo studies. *Clinical and Experimental Immunology*, **130**, 233–40.

Hale, L. P., Martin, M. E., McCollum, D. E., Nunley, J. A., Springer, T. A., Singer, K. H. and Haynes, B. F. (1989). Immunohistologic analysis of the distribution of cell adhesion molecules within the inflammatory synovial microenvironment. *Arthritis and Rheumatism*, **32**, 22–30.

Haskard, D. O. (1995). Cell adhesion molecules in rheumatoid arthritis. *Current Opinion in Rheumatology*, **7**, 229–34.

Haynes, B. F., Hale, L. P., Patton, K. L., Martin, M. E. and McCallum, R. M. (1991). Measurement of an adhesion molecule as an indicator of inflammatory disease activity. Up-regulation of the receptor for hyaluronate (CD44) in rheumatoid arthritis. *Arthritis and Rheumatism*, **34**, 1434–43.

Heurkens, A. H.M., Hiemstra, P. S., Lafebvre, G. J.M., Daha, M. R. and Breedveld, F. C. (1989). Anti-endothelial cell antibodies in patients with rheumatoid arthritis complicated by vasculitis. *Clinical and Experimental Immunology*, **78**, 7–12.

Holmen, C., Elsheikh, E., Stenvinkel, P., Qureshi, A. R., Pettersson, E., Jalkanen, S. and Sumitran-Holgersson, S. (2005). Circulating inflammatory endothelial cells contribute to endothelial progenitor cell dysfunction in patients with vasculitis and kidney involvement. *Journal of the American Society of Nephrology*, **16**, 3110–20.

Hosaka, S., Shah, M. R., Pope, R. M. and Koch, A. E. (1996). Soluble forms of P-selectin and intercellular adhesion molecule-3 in synovial fluids. *Clinical Immunology and Immunopathology*, **78**, 276–82.

Hurley, J. V. (1972). *Acute inflammation*. Williams and Wilkins, Baltimore.

Ichikawa, Y., Shimizu, H., Yoshida, M., Takaya, M. and Arimori, S. (1992). Accessory molecules expressed on the peripheral blood or synovial fluid T lymphocytes from patients with Sjogren's syndrome or rheumatoid arthritis. *Clinical and Experimental Rheumatology*, **10**, 447–54.

Iigo, Y., Takashi, T., Tamatani, T., Miyasaka, M., Higashida, T., Yagita, H., Okumura, K. and Tsukada, W. (1991). ICAM-1-dependent pathway is critically involved in the pathogenesis of adjuvant arthritis in rats. *Journal of Immunology*, **147**, 4167–71.

Imhof, B. A. and Aurrand-Lions, M. (2004). Adhesion mechanisms regulating the migration of monocytes. *Nature Reviews in Immunology*, **4**, 432–44.

Ishikawa, H., Nishibayashi, Y., Kita, K., Ohno, O., Imura, S. and Hirata, S. (1993). Adhesion molecules in the lymphoid cell distribution in rheumatoid synovial membrane. *Bulletin of the Hospital of Joint Diseases*, **53**, 23–8.

Jaffe, E. A., Grulich, J., Weksler, B. B., Hampel, G. and Watanabe, K. (1987). Correlation between thrombin-induced prostacyclin production and inositol trisphosphate and cytosolic free calcium levels in cultured human endothelial cells. *Journal of Biological Chemistry*, **262**, 8557–65.

Jasin, H. E., Lightfoot, E., Davis, L. S., Rothlein, R., Faanes, R. B. and Lipsky, P. E. (1992). Amelioration of antigen-induced arthritis in rabbits treated with monoclonal antibodies to leukocyte adhesion molecules. *Arthritis and Rheumatism*, **35**, 541–9.

Johnson, B., Haines, G. K., Harlow, L. A. and Koch, A. E. (1993). Adhesion molecule expression in human synovial tissues. *Arthritis and Rheumatism*, **36**, 137–46.

Joris, I., Majno, G., Corey, E. J. and Lewis, R. A. (1987). The mechanism of vascular leakage induced by leukotriene E4. Endothelial contraction. *American Journal of Pathology*, **126**, 19–24.

Joris, I., Cuenoud, H. F., Doern, G. V., Underwood, J. M. and Majno, G. (1990). Capillary leakage in inflammation. A study by vascular labeling. *American Journal of Pathology*, **137**, 1353–63.

Jutila, M. A., Berg, E. L., Kishimoto, T. K., Picker, L. J., Bargatze, R. F., Bishop, D. K., Orosz, C. G., Wu, N. W. and Butcher, E. C. (1989). Inflammation-induced endothelial cell adhesion to lymphocytes, neutrophils and monocytes. Role of homing receptors and other adhesion molecules. *Transplantation*, **48**, 727–31.

Kaplanski, G., Maisonobe, T., Marin, V., Gres, S., Robitail, S., Farnarier, C., Harle, J. R., Piette, J. C. and Cacoub, P. (2005). Vascular cell adhesion molecule-1 (VCAM-1) plays a central role in the pathogenesis of severe forms of vasculitis due to hepatitis C-associated mixed cryoglobulinemia. *Journal of Hepatology*, **42**, 334–40.

Kavanaugh, A. (1996). Adhesion molecules as therapeutic targets in the treatment of allergic and immunologically mediated diseases. *Clinical Immunology and Immunopathology*, **80**, S15–22.

Kim, J. M., Ho, S. H., Park, E. J., Hahn, W., Cho, H., Jeong, J. G., Lee, Y. W., Kim, J. (2002). Angiostatin gene transfer as an effective treatment strategy in murine collagen-induced arthritis. *Arthritis and Rheumatism*, **46**, 793–801.

Koch, A. E. (1998). Angiogenesis: implications for rheumatoid arthritis. *Arthritis and Rheumatism*, **41**, 951–62.

Koch, A. E., Burrows, J. C., Haines, G. K., Carlos, T. M., Harlan, J. and Leibovich, S. J. (1991). Immunolocalization of leukocyte and endothelial adhesion molecules in human rheumatoid and osteoarthritic synovial tissue. *Laboratory Investigation*, **64**, 313–20.

Koch, A. E., Turkiewicz, W., Harlow, L. A. and Pope, R. M. (1993a). Soluble E-selectin in arthritis. *Clinical Immunology and Immunopathology*, **69**, 29–35.

Koch, A. E., Kronfeld-Harrington, L. B., Szekanecz, Z., Cho, M. M., Haines, G. K., Harlow, L. A., Strieter, R. M., Kunkel, S. L., Massa, M. C., Barr, W. G. and Jimenez, S. A. (1993b). In situ expression of cytokines and cellular adhesion molecules in the skin of patients with systemic sclerosis. *Pathobiology*, **61**, 239–46.

Koch, A. E., Shah, M. R., Harlow, L. A., Lovis, R. M. and Pope, R. M. (1994). Soluble intercellular adhesion molecule-1 in arthritis. *Clinical Immunology and Immunopathology*, **71**, 208–15.

Koch, A. E., Halloran, M. M., Haskell, C. J., Shah, M. R. and Polverini, P. J. (1995). Angiogenesis mediated by soluble forms of E-selectin and vascular cell adhesion molecule-1. *Nature*, **376**, 517–9.

Koch, A. E., Kunkel, S. L. and Strieter, R. M. (1996). Chemokines in arthritis. In *Chemokines in disease*, (ed. A. E. Koch and R. M. Strieter), pp. 103–16. RG Landes Company, Austin.

Koch, A. E., Szekanecz, Z., Friedman, J., Haines, G. K., Langman, C. B. and Bouck, N. P. (1998). Effects of thrombospondin-1 on disease course and angiogenesis in rat adjuvant-induced arthritis. *Clinical Immunology and Immunopathology*, **86**, 199–208.

Lawrence, M. B. and Springer, T. A. (1991). Leukocytes roll on a selectin at physiologic flow rates: distinction from and prerequisite for adhesion through integrins. *Cell*, **65**, 859–73.

Leibovich, S. J., Polverini, P. J., Shepard, H. M., Wiseman, D. M., Shively, V. and Nuseir, N. (1987). Macrophage-induced angiogenesis is mediated by tumour necrosis factor-α. *Nature*, **329**, 630–2.

Ley, K., Tedder, T. F. and Kansas, G. S. (1993). L-selectin can mediate leukocyte rolling in untreated mesenteric venules in vivo independent of E- or P-selectin. *Blood*, **82**, 1632–8.

Lo, S. K., Lee, S., Ramos, R. A., Lobb, R., Rosa, M., Chi-Rosso, G. and Wright, S. D. (1991). Endothelial-leukocyte adhesion molecule 1 stimulates the adhesive activity of leukocyte integrin CR3 (CD11b/CD18, Mac-1) on human neutrophils. *Journal of Experimental Medicine*, **173**, 1493–500.

Lorant, D. E., Patel, K. D., McIntyre, T. M., McEver, R. P., Prescott, S. M. and Zimmerman, G. A. (1991). Coexpression of GMP-140 and PAF by endothelium stimulated by histamine or thrombin: a juxtacrine system for adhesion and activation of neutrophils. *Journal of Cell Biology*, **115**, 223–34.

Madri, J. A. and Williams, K. S. (1983). Capillary endothelial cell cultures: phenotypic modulation by matrix components. *Journal of Cell Biology*, **97**, 153–65.

Maier, J. A., Delia, D., Thorpe, P. E. and Gasparini, G. (1997). In vitro inhibition of endothelial cell growth by the antiangiogenic drug AGM-1470 (TNP-470) and the anti-endoglin antiody TEC-11. *Anticancer Drugs*, **8**, 238–44.

Manley, P. W., Martiny-Baron, G., Schlaeppi, J. M. and Woods, J.M (2002). Therapies directed at vascular endothelial growth factor. *Expert Opinion on Investigational Drugs*, **11**, 1715–36.

Martel-Pelletier, J., McCollum, R., Fujimoto, N., Obata, K., Cloutier, J. M. and Pelletier, J. P. (1994). Excess of metalloproteases over tissue inhibitor of metalloprotease may contribute to cartilage degradation in osteoarthritis and rheumatoid arthritis. *Laboratory Investigation*, **70**, 807–15.

Matsuno, H,. Yudoh, K., Uzuki, M., Nakazawa, F., Sawai, T., Yamaguchi, N., Olsen, B. R. and Kimura, T. (2002). Treatment with the angiogenesis inhibitor endostatin: a novel therapy in rheumatoid arthritis. *Journal of Rheumatology*, **29**, 890–5.

McEver, R. P., Beckstead, J. H., Moore, K. L., Marshall-Carlson, L. and Bainton, D. F. (1989). GMP-140, a platelet alpha-granule membrane protein, is also synthesized by vascular endothelial cells and is localized in Weibel-Palade bodies. *Journal of Clinical Investigation*, **84**, 92–9.

Miura, M., Garcia, F. L., Crawford, S. E. and Rowley, A. H. (2004). Cell adhesion molecule expression in coronary artery aneurysms in acute Kawasaki disease. *Pediatric Infectious Diseases Journal*, **23**, 931–6.

Montesano, R., Pepper, M. S., Vassalli, J.-D. and Orci, L. (1991). Modulation of angiogenesis in vitro. *EXS*, **59**, 129–36.

Mulligan, M. S., Varani, J., Dame, M. K., Lane, C. L., Smith, C. W., Anderson, D. C. and Ward, P. A. (1991). Role of endothelial-leukocyte adhesion molecule 1 (ELAM-1) in neutrophil-mediated lung injury in rats. *Journal of Clinical Investigation*, **88**, 1396–406.

Mulligan, M. S., Polley, M. J., Bayer, R. J., Nunn, M. F., Paulson, J. C. and Ward, P. A. (1992). Neutrophil-dependent acute lung injury. Requirement for P-selectin (GMP-140) *Journal of Clinical Investigation*, **90**, 1600–7.

Nguyen, M., Strubel, N. A. and Bischoff, J. (1993). A role for sialyl Lewis-X/A glycoconjugates in capillary morphogenesis. *Nature*, **365**, 267–9.

Nicosia, R. F., Bonanno, E. and Smith, M. (1993). Fibronectin promotes the elongation of microvessels during angiogenesis in vitro. *Journal of Cellular Physiology*, **154**, 654–61.

Orosz, C. G., Ohye, R. G., Pelletier, R. P., Van Buskirk, A. M., Huang, E., Morgan, C., Kincade, P. W. and Ferguson, R. M. (1993). Treatment with anti-vascular cell adhesion molecule 1 monoclonal antibody induces long-term murine cardiac allograft acceptance. *Transplantation*, **56**, 453–60.

Park, C. C., Morel, J. C., Amin, M. A., Connors, M. A., Harlow, L. A. and Koch, A.E (2001). Evidence of IL-18 as a novel angiogenic mediator. *Journal of Immunology*, **167**, 1644–53.

Peichev, M., Naiyer, A. J., Pereira, D., Zhu, Z., Lane, W. J., Williams, M., Oz, M. C., Hicklin, D. J., Witte, L., Moore, M. A. and Rafii, S. (2000). Expression of VEGFR-2 and AC133 by circulating human CD34(+) cells identifies a population of functional endothelial precursors. *Blood*, **95**, 952–8.

Piali, L., Hammel, P., Uherek, C., Bachmann, F., Gisler, R. H., Dunon, D. and Imhof, B. A. (1995). CD31/PECAM-1 is a ligand for alpha v beta 3 integrin involved in adhesion of leukocytes to endothelium. *Journal of Cell Biology*, **130**, 451–60.

Pober, J. S. and Cotran, R. S. (1990). Cytokines and endothelial cell biology. *Physiology Reviews*, **70**, 427–34.

Pober, J. S., Gimbrone, M. A. Jr., Cotran, R. S., Reiss, L. S. and Burakoff, S. J. (1983). Ia expression by vascular endothelium is inducible by activated T cells and by human gamma interferon. *Journal of Experimental Medicine*, **157**, 1339–45.

Pober, J. S., Gimbrone, M. A. Jr., Lapierre, L. A., Mendrick, D. L., Fiers, W., Rothlein, R. and Springer, T. A. (1986). Overlapping patterns of activation of human endothelial cells by interleukin 1, tumor necrosis factor, and immune interferon. *Journal of Immunology*, **137**, 1893–6.

Pufe, T., Bartscher, M., Petersen, W., Tillmann, B. and Mentlein, R. (2003). Expression of pleiotrophin an embryonic growth and differentiation factor, in rheumatoid arthritis. *Arthritis and Rheumatism*, **48**, 660–7.

Rathanaswami, P., Hachicha, M., Wong, W. L., Schall, T. J. and McColl, S. R. (1993). Synergistic effect of interleukin-1 beta and tumor necrosis factor alpha on interleukin-8 gene expression in synovial fibroblasts. Evidence that interleukin-8 is the major neutrophil-activating chemokine released in response to monokine activation. *Arthritis and Rheumatism*, **36**, 1295–304.

Sachs, L. (1991). Angiogenesis – cytokines as part of a network. *EXS*, **59**, 20–2.

Salmi, M., Kalimo, K. and Jalkanen, S. (1993). Induction and function of vascular adhesion protein-1 at sites of inflammation. *Journal of Experimental Medicine*, **178**, 2255–60.

Sans, M., Panes, J., Ardite, E., Elizalde, J. I., Arce, Y., Elena, M., Palacin, A., Fernandez-Checa, J. C., Anderson, D. C., Lobb, R. and Pique, J. M. (1999). VCAM-1 and ICAM-1 mediate leukocyte-endothelial cell adhesion in rat experimental colitis. *Gastroenterology*, **116**, 874–83.

Sato, N., Beitz, J. G., Kato, J., Yamamoto, M., Clark, J. W., Calabresi, P. and Frackelton, A. R. (1993). Platelet-derived growth factor indirectly stimulates angiogenesis in vitro. *American Journal of Pathology*, **142**, 1119–30.

Schenkel, A. R., Mamdouh, Z., Chen, X., Liebman, R. M. and Muller, W. A. (2002). CD99 plays a major role in the migration of monocytes through endothelial junctions. *Nature Immunology*, **3**, 153–50.

Schoefl, G. (1963). Studies on inflammation. III. Growing capillaries. *Virchows Archiv*, **A337**, 97–100.

Schweigerer, L. (1995). Antiangiogenesis as a novel therapeutic concept in pediatric oncology. *Journal of Molecular Medicine*, **73**, 497–508.

Senger, D. R., Claffey, K. P., Benes, J. E., Perruzzi, C. A., Sergiou, A. P. and Detmar, M. (1997). Angiogenesis promoted by vascular endothelial growth factor: regulation through α1β1 and α2β1 integrins. *Proceedings of the National Academy of Sciences USA*, **94**, 13612–7.

Setoguchi, K., Misaki, Y., Kawahata, K., Shimada, K., Juji, T., Tanaka, S., Go, H., Shukunami, C., Nishizaki, Y; Hiraki, Y. and Yamamoto, K. (2004). Suppression of T cell responses by chondromodulin 1, a cartilage-derived angiogenesis inhibitory factor: therapeutic potential in rheumatoid arthritis. *Arthritis and Rheumatism*, **50**, 828–39.

Shibuya, M. (2003). VEGF-receptor inhibitors for anti-angiogenesis. *Nippon Yakurigaku Zasshi*, **122**, 498–503.

Springer, T. A. (1990). Adhesion receptors of the immune system. *Nature*, **346**, 425–33.

Strieter, R. M., Polverini, P. J., Kunkel, S. L., Arenberg, D. A., Burdick, M. D., Kasper, J., Dzuiba, J., Van-Damme, J., Walz, A. and Marriott, D. (1995). The functional role of the ELR motif in CXC chemokine-mediated angiogenesis. *Journal of Biological Chemistry*, **270**, 27348–57.

Strieter, R. M., Kunkel, S. L., Shanafelt, A. M., Arenberg, D. A., Koch, A. E. and Polverini, P. J. (1996). The role of C-X-C chemokines in regulation of angiogenesis. In *Chemokines in disease*, (eds A. E. Koch and R. M. Strieter), pp. 195–209. R. G. Landes Company, Austin.

Szekanecz, Z. and Koch, A. E. (1997). Intercellular adhesion molecule (ICAM)-3 expression on endothelial cells. *American Journal of Pathology*, **151**, 313–4.

Szekanecz, Z. and Koch, A. E. (1999). Adhesion molecules: potent inducers of endothelial cell chemotaxis. In *Tissue engineering of prosthetic vascular grafts* (eds P. P. Zilla and H. P. Greisler), pp. 271–7. R. G. Landes, Austin.

Szekanecz, Z. and Koch, A. E. (2001). Chemokines and angiogenesis. *Current Opinion in Rheumatology*, **13**, 202–8.

Szekanecz, Z. and Koch, A. E. (2004). Vascular endothelium and immune responses: implications for inflammation and angiogenesis. *Rheumatology Disease Clinics of North America*, **30**, 97–114.

Szekanecz, Z. and Koch, A. E. (2005). Endothelial cells in inflammation and angiogenesis. *Current Drug Targets in Inflammation and Allergy*, **4**, 319–23.

Szekanecz, Z. and Szegedi, G. (1992). Cell surface adhesion molecules: structure, function, clinical importance. *Orvosi Hetilap*, **133**, 135–42.

Szekanecz, Z., Haines, G. K., Lin, T. R., Harlow, L. A., Goerdt, S., Rayan, G. and Koch, A. E. (1994). Differential distribution of ICAM-1, ICAM-2 and ICAM-3, and the MS-1 antigen in normal and diseased human synovia. *Arthritis and Rheumatism*, **37**, 221–31.

Szekanecz, Z., Haines, G. K., Harlow, L. A., Shah, M. R., Fong, T. W., Fu, R., Lin, S. J-W., Rayan, G. and Koch, A. E. (1995a). Increased synovial expression of transforming growth factor (TGF)-β receptor endoglin and TGF-β1 in rheumatoid arthritis: possible interactions in the pathogenesis of the disease. *Clinical Immunology and Immunopathology*, **76**, 187–94.

Szekanecz, Z., Haines, G. K., Harlow, L. A., Shah, M. R., Fong, T. W., Fu, R., Lin, S. J-W. and Koch, A. E. (1995b). Increased synovial expression of the adhesion molecules CD66a, CD66b and CD31 in rheumatoid and osteoarthritis. *Clinical Immunology and Immunopathology*, **76**, 180–6.

Szekanecz, Z., Szegedi, G. and Koch, A. E. (1996). Cellular adhesion molecules in rheumatoid arthritis. Regulation by cytokines and possible clinical importance. *Journal of Investigative Medicine*, **44**, 124–35.

Szekanecz, Z., Szegedi, G. and Koch, A. E. (1998a). Angiogenesis in rheumatoid arthritis: pathogenic and clinical significance. *Journal of Investigative Medicine*, **46**, 27–41.

Szekanecz, Z., Kunkel, S. L., Strieter, R. M. and Koch, A. E. (1998b). Chemokines in rheumatoid arthritis. *Springer Seminars in Immunopathology*, **20**, 115–32.

Szekanecz, Z., Halloran, M. M., Haskell, C. J., Shah, M. R., Polverini, P. J. and Koch, A. E. (1999). Mediators of angiogenesis: the role of cellular adhesion molecules. *Trends in Glycoscience and Glycotechnology*, **11**, 73–93.

Szekanecz, Z., Gaspar, L. and Koch, A. E. (2005). Angiogenesis in rheumatoid arthritis. *Frontiers in Bioscience*, **10**, 1739–53.

Takeuchi, T., Amano, K., Sekine, H., Koide, J. and Abe, T. (1993). Upregulated expression and function of integrin adhesive receptors in systemic lupus erythematosus patients with vasculitis. *Journal of Clinical Investigation*, **92**, 3008–16.

Thornhill, M. H. and Haskard, D. O. (1990). IL-4 regulates endothelial cell activation by IL-1, tumor necrosis factor, or IFN-gamma. *Journal of Immunology*, **145**, 865–72.

Turkcapar, N., Sak, S. D., Saatci, M., Duman, M. and Olmez, U. (2005). Vasculitis and expression of vascular cell adhesion molecule-1, intercellular adhesion molecule-1, and E-selectin in salivary glands of patients with Sjogren's syndrome. *Journal of Rheumatology*, **32**, 1063–70.

Van der Zee, J. M., Heurkens, A. H.M., van der Voort, E. A.M., Daha, M. R. and Breedveld, F. C. (1991). Characterization of anti-endothelial antibodies in patients with rheumatoid arthritis complicated with vasculitis. *Clinical and Experimental Immunology*, **9**, 589–94.

van Dinther-Janssen, A. C.H. M., Pals, S. T., Scheper, R., Breedveld, F. and Meijer, C. J. (1990). Dendritic cells and high endothelial venules in the rheumatoid synovial membrane. *Journal of Rheumatology*, **17**, 11–7.

Varani, J., Ginsburg, I., Schuger, L., Gibbs, D. F., Bromberg, J., Johnson, K. J., Ryan, U. S. and Ward, P. A. (1989). Endothelial cell killing by neutrophils. Synergistic interaction of oxygen products and proteases. *American Journal of Pathology*, **135**, 435–8.

Von Andrian, U. H., Chambers, J. D., McEvoy, L. M., Bargatze, R. F., Arfors, K. E. and Butcher, E. C. (1991). Two-step model of leukocyte-endothelial cell interaction in inflammation: distinct roles for LECAM-1 and the leukocyte beta 2 integrins in vivo. *Proceedings of the National Academy of Sciences of the USA*, **88**, 7538–42.

Voronov, E., Shouval, D. S., Krelin, Y., Cagnano, E., Benharroch, D., Iwakuchi, Y., Dinarello, C. A. and Apte, R. N. (2003). IL-1 is required for tumor invasiveness and angiogenesis. *Proceedings of the National Academy of Sciences USA*, **100**, 2645–50.

Voskuyl, A. E., Martin, S., Melchers, I., Zwinderman, A. H., Weichselbraun, I. and Breedveld, F. (1995). Levels of circulating intercellular adhesion molecule-1 and -3 but not circulating endothelial leukocyte adhesion molecule are increased in patients with rheumatoid vasculitis. *British Journal of Rheumatology*, **34**, 311–5.

Walz, A., Kunkel, S. L. and Strieter, R. M. (1996). C-X-C chemokines – an overview. In *Chemokines in disease* (eds A. E. Koch and R. M. Strieter), pp. 1–25. R. G. Landes Company, Austin.

Waring, P. M., Carroll, G. J., Kandiah, D. A., Buirski, G. and Metcalf, D. (1993). Increased levels of leukemia inhibitory factor in synovial fluid from patients with rheumatoid arthritis and other inflammatory arthritides. *Arthritis and Rheumatism*, **36**, 911–5.

Wellicome, S. M., Kapahi, P., Mason, J. C., Lebranchu, Y., Yarwood, H. and Haskard, D. O. (1993). Detection of a circulating form of vascular cell adhesion molecule-1: raised levels in rheumatoid arthritis and systemic lupus erythematosus. *Clinical and Experimental Immunology*, **92**, 412–8.

Westphal, J. R., Boerbooms, A. M.Th., Schalkwijk, C. J.M., Kwast, H., De Weijert, M., Jacobs,. C., Vierwinden, G., Ruiter, D. J., Van de Putte, L. B.A. and De Waal, R. M.W. (1994). Anti-endothelial cell antibodies in sera of patients with autoimmune diseases: comparison between ELISA and FACS analysis. *Clinical and Experimental Immunology*, **96**, 444–9.

Wijelath, E. S., Carlsen, B., Cole, T., Chen, J., Kothari, S. and Hammond, W. P. (1997). Oncostatin M induces basic fibroblast growth factor expression in endothelial cells and promotes endothelial cell proliferation, migration and spindle morphology. *Journal of Cell Science*, **110**, 871–9.

Wilkinson, L. S., Edwards, J. C., Poston, R. N. and Haskard, D. O. (1993). Expression of vascular cell adhesion molecule-1 in normal and inflamed synovium. *Laboratory Investigation*, **68**, 82–8.

Wiseman, D. M., Polverini, P. J., Kamp, D. W. and Leibovich, S. J. (1988). Transforming growth factor-beta (TGFβ) is chemotactic for human monocytes and induces their expression of angiogenic activity. *Biochemical and Biophysical Research Communications*, **157**, 793–800.

Witkowska, A. M., Kuryliszyn-Moskal, A., Borawska, M. H., Hukalowicz, K. and Markiewicz, R. (2003). A study on soluble intercellular adhesion molecule-1 and selenium in patients with rheumatoid arthritis complicated by vasculitis. *Clinical Rheumatology*, **22**, 414–9.

Woods, J. M., Mogollon, A., Amin, M. A., Martinez, R. J. and Koch, A. E. (2003). The role of COX-2 in angiogenesis and rheumatoid arthritis. *Experimental and Molecular Pathology*, **74**, 282–90.

CHAPTER 5

Complement in vasculitis

John E. Volanakis

Complement and complement activation

The human complement system consists of more than 35 plasma and membrane-bound proteins, including recognition molecules, proteases, cellular receptors, and regulatory proteins. Together they constitute a major recognition and effector system in host defense and act in a self-controlled fashion (Volanakis 1998; Walport 2001) The system aims at eliminating invading pathogens from blood and tissues and also participates in regulation of adaptive immune responses. Activation of complement is necessary for expression of biologic function and is initiated through three independent recognition mechanisms, the classical, the lectin, and the alternative pathways. The three pathways merge at C3 cleavage, which is catalyzed by two distinct but structurally similar and catalytically identical proteases, termed C3 convertases. Although complement activation is necessary for optimal host defense against pathogens, complement-mediated inflammatory responses can lead to tissue damage under conditions of excessive or inappropriate activation (Volanakis 2005).

The three complement activation pathways recognize a wide range of pathogens and necrotic or apoptotic cells of the host and initiate the assembly of the complement convertases by using different proteins and different mechanisms; however, all three pathways result in the production of the same biological activities. In the classical pathway, recognition of activators is through the C1q component of the C1 complex. C1 is a large protein complex comprising one molecule of C1q and a Ca^{2+}-dependent tetramer C1s-C1r-C1r-C1s, consisting of two serine proteases in their zymogen form (Gaboriaud et al. 2004). C1q recognizes antigen-bound antibodies, ligand-bound CRP, and certain bacteria and apoptotic cells. Binding of C1q to a target cell or molecule elicits a signal that triggers self-activation of C1r, which in turn activates C1s. Activated C1s then cleaves sequentially C4 and C2 to form the C4b2a complex, which is a C3 convertase (Figure 5.1). In the lectin pathway, recognition of pathogens is carried out by mannan-binding lectin (MBL) and the serum ficolins L and H (Holmskov 2003; Matsushita and Fujita 2001). All three proteins are pattern recognition lectins, composed of collagen and globular lectin domains. They are oligomers of homotrimeric subunits in which the collagen regions form a triple helix. In MBL the recognition domain is a C-type lectin, while in the ficolins, it is a fibrinogen domain. MBL has binding specificity for mannose, glucose, fucose, N-acetylmannosamine,

and N-acetylglucosamine. The ficolins have specificity for N-acetylglucosamine. Their lectin specificity endows these proteins with the ability to bind to a wide variety of Gram-positive and Gram-negative bacteria. In blood all three proteins circulate as complexes with homodimers of MBL-associated serine protease (MASP)-1, -2, or –3. Binding of the lectin to a bacterial cell surface leads to activation of MASP, through a currently unknown mechanism. Activated MASP-2 can then activate sequentially C4 and C2 to form the C4b2a, C3 convertase. The function of MASP-1 and -3 is currently unknown.

The alternative pathway is activated by a variety of cellular surfaces, including those of certain bacteria, viruses, fungi, and parasites (Fearon and Austen 1980; Pangburn and Müller-Eberhard 1984). Antibodies, particularly in the form of large, insoluble complexes with antigen, can also activate this pathway. Assembly of the C3 convertase is initiated by the covalent attachment of freshly generated, metastable C3b to the activator surface. A supply of metastable C3b is always available in the blood through a mechanism termed C3 tick-over. The chemical nature of the activator surface allows factor B to form a complex with C3b. Factor B bound to C3b is then cleaved by factor D into two fragments, the largest of which, Bb, remains attached to C3b. The resulting C3bBb complex is the C3 convertase of the alternative pathway. This complex has a short half-life, but it is stabilized by the binding of properdin (P)

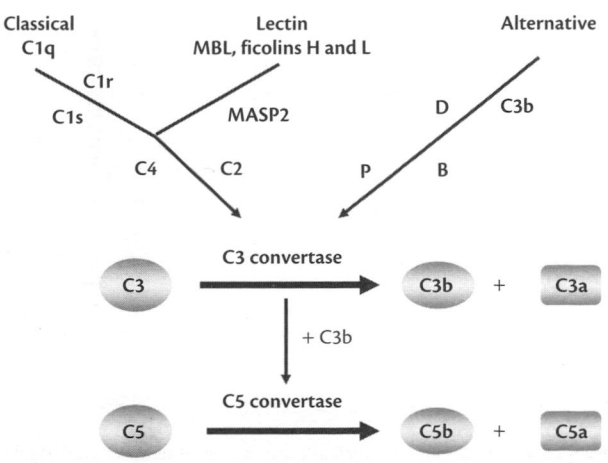

Figure 5.1 Complement activation pathways.

and is usually termed the amplification C3 convertase because it generates many C3b fragments and, thus, additional C3 convertase complexes.

Biologically-active complement activation products

A C3 convertase assembled on the surface of a complement activator can catalyze the cleavage of numerous C3 molecules into the small peptide C3a and the large fragment C3b. A portion of the resulting metastable C3b binds covalently to the surface of the activator around the C3-convertase site. Such C3b molecules have multiple functions. They can initiate the assembly of additional C3-convertase, they can be recognized by complement receptor 1 (CR1; CD35), or can serve as precursors for smaller C3 fragments (iC3b, C3dg), produced by factor I cleavage and recognized by complement receptors 2 (CR2; CD21) or 3 (CR3; CD11b/CD18). Binding of C3b or its fragments to these complement receptors triggers important biologic functions. For example, binding of immune complex-bound C3b to CR1 on red blood cells provides the main mechanism for removal of immune complexes from the circulation (Davies and Walport 1998); binding of iC3b fragments to CR3 enhances phagocytosis of bacteria and other particles; binding of C3dg to CR2 on B cells contributes to B cell activation and maturation (Fearon and Locksey 1996; Carroll 2004).

Metastable C3b, generated by the action of a C3 convertase, can also bind to the non-catalytic subunit, C4b or C3b, of the convertase, giving rise to a trimolecular complex, C4b2a3b or (C3b)$_2$Bb, respectively (Takata *et al.* 1987; Kinoshita *et al.* 1988). Both of these complexes express C5 convertase proteolytic activity, restricted to the cleavage of C5. Cleavage of C5 by a C5 convertase generates two fragments: C5a, a small peptide, and C5b, a large two-polypeptide chain fragment. C5b can initiate the assembly of a large protein–protein complex, termed membrane attack complex (MAC), by interacting sequentially with single molecules of C6, C7, and C8, and with 6 to 18 molecules of C9 (Podack and Tschopp 1984; Esser 1994). During these sequential interactions, hydrophobic regions of the participating proteins become exposed on the surface of the complex. Assembly of the MAC on the surface of a biologic membrane favors interactions of these hydrophobic regions with the fatty acid chains of phospholipids (Figure 5.2) The complex becomes gradually

inserted into the lipid bilayer and eventually forms a transmembrane channel, which can elicit cellular functions (Rus *et al.* 2001) or lead to apoptosis or killing of susceptible cells.

The acute inflammatory response is the principal means of host defense against infection by pyogenic bacteria. Complement can elicit all aspects of acute inflammation and frequently is activated not only during infections but also in inflammatory diseases of autoimmune etiology. Three products of complement activation, C3a, C5a, and the MAC, elicit vascular changes characteristic of inflammation. The two small peptides, C3a and C5a, termed anaphylatoxins, interact with their respective receptors, C3aR (Ames *et al.* 1996) and C5aR (Gerard and Gerard 1991) on mast cells and tissue basophils, causing the release of vasoactive amines such as histamine. Both receptors have a structure typical of seven transmembrane domain, G-protein coupled, rhodopsin family receptors and they are expressed on various cells, including myelomonocytic cells. Engagement of these receptors by anaphylatoxins triggers additional aspects of the inflammatory response, including activation and chemotactic responses of phagocytic cells.

Complement regulation

Several mechanisms ensure that the self-destructing potential of complement activation products is normally kept under control (Liszewski *et al.* 1996). Complement convertases have a short half life; therefore production of active products is limited and proportional to the magnitude and persistence of the activating insult. In addition, three serum proteins, C4b-binding protein (C4bp) and factors H and I regulate the convertases. C4bp dissociates the classical and lectin pathway convertase and inhibits its assembly. It also serves as cofactor for cleavage/inactivation of C4b by factor I, a serine protease. Factor H has a similar function in the alternative pathway, dissociating the C3bBb convertase, inhibiting its formation, and serving as factor I cofactor in cleavage of C3b. As mentioned above, cleavage of C3b by factor I produces fragments (iC3b, C3dg) with distinct biological activities, which however, unlike C3b, cannot form a C3 convertase. At the level of the initiating enzymes of the classical and lectin pathways, control is exercised by C1 inhibitor (C1 INH), a serpin that inhibits activated C1r, C1s, and MASPs. The action of anaphylatoxins is regulated by anaphylatoxin inactivator, a serum carboxypeptidase N (Plummer and

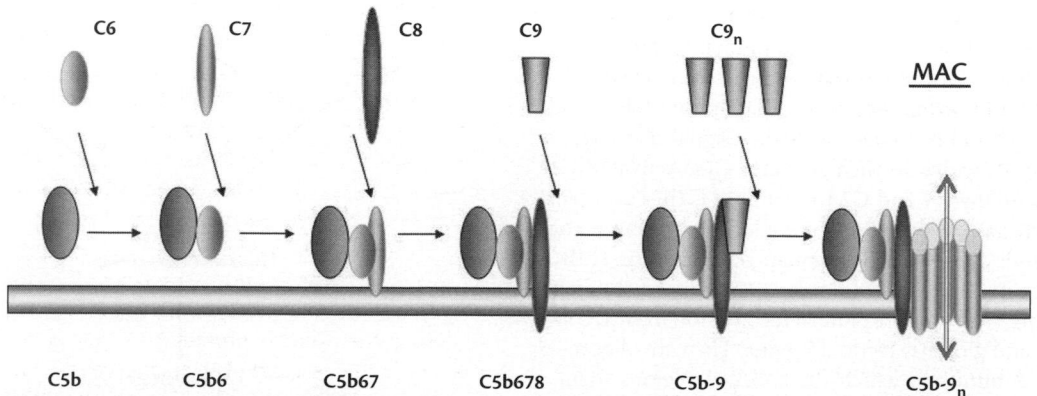

Figure 5.2 Sequential non-enzymatic protein–protein interactions among the terminal complement proteins initiated by C5b and leading to the formation of the membrane attack complex (MAC).

Hurwitz 1978), and the serum proteins vitronectin (S-protein) and clusterin inhibit the formation of the MAC, thereby precluding its insertion into lipid bilayers (Morgan 1999).

Four cell-associated proteins, decay-accelerating factor (DAF, CD55) (Lukacik *et al.* 2004), membrane-cofactor protein (MCP, CD46) (Liszewski *et al.* 2005), CR1 (Weisman *et al.* 1990), and CD59 (Huang *et al.* 2005) play a major role in protecting host tissues from the damaging potential of complement activation. DAF, MCP, and CD59 are widely distributed in human tissues, while the distribution of CR1 is limited mainly to blood cells, follicular dendritic cells, and glomerular podocytes. DAF inhibits formation and dissociates both assembled C3 convertases, MCP serves as factor I cofactor for C4b and C3b cleavage, while CR1 expresses all four of these functions. CD59 inhibits incorporation of C9 into the MAC and prevents C9 polymerization. DAF and CD59 are glycan phosphatidylinositol (GPI)-linked membrane proteins. GPI serves as a membrane anchor for many additional cell surface proteins and its biosynthesis is initiated by an enzyme complex called GPI-*N*-acetylglucosaminyltransferase. DAF, MCP, and CD59 exhibit species-specificity, effectively protecting tissues from self complement activation, but not from complement of other species (Atkinson *et al.* 1991). Such "homologous restriction" is not, however, absolute and considerable overlap exists among different species (Morgan *et al.* 2005).

The importance of the regulatory proteins in protecting self tissues from complement activation is demonstrated by the clinical syndromes associated with mutations of their genes. Heterozygous C1 INH deficiency is associated with hereditary angioneurotic edema (Davis 3rd 2005) and factor I deficiency with susceptibility to infection, vasculitis, and glomerulonephritis (Genel *et al.* 2005). Mutations of the factor H, MCP, or factor I genes predispose to membranoproliferative glomerulonephritis and also to atypical hemolytic uremic syndrome, a thrombotic microangiopathy characterized by hemolytic anemia, thrombocytopenia, and acute renal failure (Dragon-Durey and Fremeaux-Bacchi 2005). Finally, somatic mutation and subsequent clonal expansion of the pig-A gene, a component of the GPI-*N*-acetylglucosaminyltransferase, results in absence from cell membranes of DAF and CD59, as well as all other GPI-linked proteins. The defect is associated with paroxysmal nocturnal hemoglobinuria, characterized by hemolysis, venous thrombosis, and cytopenia (Takeda *et al.* 1993).

While the combined action of the regulatory proteins adequately protects host tissues from bystander complement activation damage, they are unable to protect tissues that become targets of complement activation either as a result of attachment of tissue-specific autoantibodies or as a result of deposition of immune complexes, or because of changes of the surface characteristics of the tissue. It is not surprising that the vascular endothelium, which is in constant contact with complement in the blood, is particularly susceptible to complement attack.

Complement-induced endothelial damage

Activation of complement directed against the vascular endothelium leads to profound changes in its structure and function. Endothelial damage is mediated mainly by the action of C5a and the MAC (Figure 5.3). C5a has both direct and indirect effects, the latter mediated mainly by neutrophils. Neutrophils activated by C5a produce reactive oxygen species and release elastase and

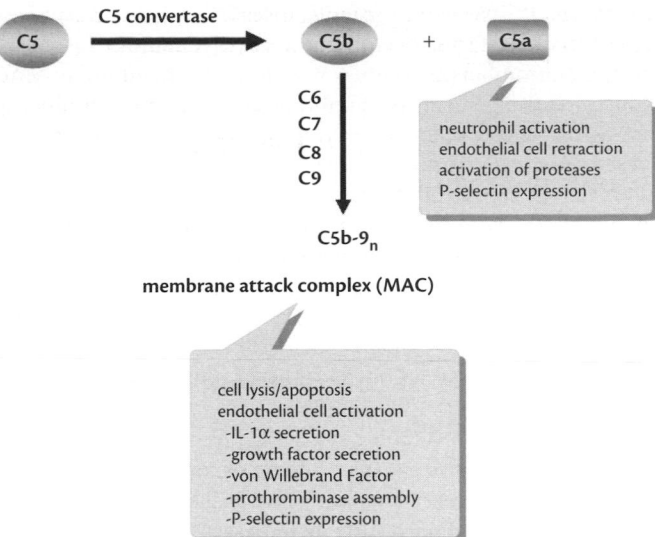

Figure 5.3 Biological activities of C5a and MAC that play a role in the pathogenesis of endothelial injury.

cathepsin G, which may disrupt the intercellular junctions and impair the barrier function of the endothelium (Owen *et al.* 1995). Elastase cleaves proteoglycan on the endothelial surface, causing the release of heparin sulfate and leading to loss of the anticoagulant, anti-inflammatory, and barrier function (Key *et al.* 1992). Direct effects of C5a are mediated through its receptor, which is expressed on endothelial cells (Haviland *et al.* 1995). Engagement of C5aR by its ligand leads to multiple effects, including a sustained pertussis toxin-sensitive cytoskeletal response, resulting in cell retraction and increased paracellular permeability (Albrecht *et al.* 2004). It also leads to transient expression of P-selectin by fusion of Weibel–Palade bodies containing P-selectin, as well as von Willebrand factor and coagulation factor V (Foreman *et al.* 1994). C5a also causes activation of serine and cysteine proteases secreted by endothelial cells (Ihrcke and Platt 1996). P-selectin causes adhesion of neutrophils and facilitates their infiltration into tissues (Geng *et al.* 1990), while activated proteases cleave core proteoglycan, resulting in the release of heparin sulfate. *In vitro* stimulation of endothelial cells with C5a results in induction of a number of genes encoding cell adhesion molecules, including E-selectin, ICAM-1, and V-CAM, and of cytokines and their receptors, such as IL-6 and IL-18R (Albrecht *et al.* 2004).

Insertion of sublytic numbers of the MAC into the endothelial cell membrane also has multiple effects (Acosta *et al.* 2004). One of the most significant structural effects is the disruption of intercellular junctions, leading to formation of gaps and disruption of the barrier function of the endothelium (Saadi and Platt 1995). Another important consequence of MAC insertion is the induction of the IL-1α gene and the secretion of this cytokine, which acts in an autocrine fashion to mediate expression of E-selectin, plasminogen activator inhibitor-1, and tissue factor (Saadi *et al.* 1995; Acosta *et al.* 1996). Additional cytokines and growth factors, including monocyte chemotactic protein-1 (Acosta *et al.* 2004), basic fibroblast growth factor, and platelet-derived growth factor (Benzaquen *et al.* 1994) are secreted following insertion of sublytic MAC. The formation of MAC in endothelial cell membranes also initiates secretion of the endothelial storage pool of von Willebrand factor

(Hattori *et al.* 1989) and promotes release of plasma membrane vesicles that bind factor Va and expose a catalytic surface for assembly of prothrombinase (Hamilton *et al.* 1990). In addition, MAC induces rearrangement of membrane phospholipids, leading to increased presence in the outer leaflet of the bilayer of phosphatidyl serine, which may promote plasma clotting by increasing tissue factor activity (Sims and Wiedmer 1995).

Combined, the pleiotropic effects of complement activation products lead to structural damage of the vascular endothelium associated with inflammatory, proliferative, and thrombotic reactions, commonly seen in vasculitis.

Animal models of complement-induced vascular damage

The study of the *in vivo* damaging effects of complement activation on the vasculature has been made possible by the use of animal models. The oldest such model is the Arthus reaction (Arthus 1903), in which antibodies in blood encounter their intradermally injected cognitive antigen at the level of the vascular wall. Antibodies are in large excess, so large, insoluble immune complexes are formed with consequent activation of complement and neutrophils. A violent, acute inflammatory reaction ensues, with destruction of the vascular wall followed by edema, hemorrhage, and necrosis. The Arthus reaction is relevant to immune complex vasculitis, as exemplified by leukocytoclastic (hypersensitivity) vasculitis and perhaps also by the vasculitis of SLE. Participation of complement in the pathogenesis of the Arthus reaction was questioned recently on the basis of experiments demonstrating development of the lesion in mice deficient in C3 or C4, whereas grossly diminished reactions were observed in animals deficient in IgG receptors (FcγR) (Sylvestre *et al.* 1996). Subsequent experiments, however, indicated that complement was indeed necessary for development of the Arthus reactions. Specifically, it was shown that animals deficient in C5aR failed to develop the reaction (Hopken *et al.* 1997; Baumann *et al.* 2001). These divergent results were reconciled by the observation that C5a is a major inducer of the genes of activating, but not inhibitory, FcγRs (Shushakova *et al.* 2002). Thus, it appears that both complement and FcγRs are necessary for a fully developed Arthus reaction.

Xenotransplantation has also been used extensively to study complement participation in acute vascular injury. An organ transplanted into a recipient of another species is subject to hyperacute rejection, a severe reaction that destroys the xenograft within minutes to a few hours and is characterized by local ischemia, endothelial swelling, interstitial hemorrhage, edema, and intravascular coagulation (Platt 2000). Because of the possibility that it may represent a broader set of vascular diseases, there has been intense interest in understanding how hyperacute rejection arises (Saadi *et al.* 2004). There is considerable evidence that the rejection is initiated by natural IgM antibodies against endothelial cells that activate the classical complement pathway. In primates, the main xenoreactive antibodies against endothelial cells of a xenograft are directed against Galα1–3Gal, a disaccharide expressed by lower mammals but not primates (Lin *et al.* 1997). Hyperacute rejection also occurs in allotransplantation when the recipient is presensitized to donor MHC antigens. The dominant role of complement in the development of the reaction has been studied extensively by several methods, including depleting the recipient's complement using cobra venom factor (Leventhal *et al.* 1993), using

complement inhibitors such as soluble CR1 (Pruitt *et al.* 1994), or using animals genetically deficient in complement proteins (Brauer *et al.* 1995). Attempts at transplanting pig organs into primates emphasized the role of the cell-membrane-associated regulatory proteins in protecting endothelial cells from complement damage. The pig xenografts were subject to hyperacute rejection in part because of incompatibility between pig DAF, MCP, and CD59 with primate complement (Dalmasso *et al.* 1991) or alternatively because of inadequate numbers of these molecules on pig endothelium (Morgan *et al.* 2005). To overcome this problem, pigs transgenic for human DAF and/or CD59 were generated (Pascher *et al.* 1997; Storck *et al.* 1997; Byrne *et al.* 1997). Organs from these transgenic pigs transplanted into non-human primates survive much longer than organs from non-transgenic animals.

In recent years, animal models of ischemia/reperfusion (I/R) injury have been used extensively to investigate the role of complement in the vascular injury associated with this syndrome. I/R injury is an acute inflammatory response at the level of the vascular endothelium occurring after an ischemic event and subsequent restoration of blood flow. I/R injury is a major participant in many clinical conditions, including myocardial infarction, stroke, intestinal ischemia, cardiovascular surgery, and trauma (Hart *et al.* 2004). Evidence derived mainly from experimental animal models has indicated that complement activation plays a major role in the pathogenesis of I/R injury of the myocardial, skeletal, cerebral, renal, and intestinal tissues (Weisman *et al.* 1990; Weiser *et al.* 1996; Zhao *et al.* 2002). Activation of the classical pathway is initiated by natural antibodies reacting with endothelial cells altered by oxidative stress (Weiser *et al.* 1996; Zhang *et al.* 2004). Studies using animals deficient in complement proteins have demonstrated that the lectin pathway also plays a dominant role in complement activation in I/R injury (Walsh *et al.* 2005; Hart *et al.* 2005), while the alternative pathway is necessary for full development of the injury (Stahl *et al.* 2003).

Complement in clinical vasculitis

Complement has been implicated in the pathogenesis of many vasculitic syndromes, although supporting evidence has not always been convincing. It is, however, generally accepted that complement plays a significant role in the pathogenesis of the vasculitis associated with cryoglobulinemia (Sansonno and Dammacco 2005), Henoch–Schönlein purpura (Kawana *et al.* 1990), diabetes (Acosta *et al.* 2000), rheumatoid arthritis (Danning *et al.* 1998), and leukocytoclastic (hypersensitivity) vasculitis (Claudy 2003).

References

Acosta, J., Hetinga, J., Fluckiger, R., *et al.* (2000). Molecular basis for a link between complement and the vascular complications of diabetes. *Proceedings of the National Academy of Sciences USA*, **97**, 5450–5.

Acosta, J. A., Benzaquen, L. R., Goldstein, D. J., Tosteson, M. T. and Halperin, J. A. (1996). The transient pore formed by homologous terminal complement complexes functions as a bidirectional route for the transport of autocrine and paracrine signals across human cell membranes. *Molecular Medicine*, **2**, 755–65.

Acosta, J., Qin, X. and Halperin, J. (2004). Complement and complement regulatory proteins as potencial molecular targets for vascular diseases. *Current Pharmaceutical Design*, **10**, 203–11.

Albrecht, E. A., Chinnaiyan, A. M., Varambally, S., *et al.* (2004). C5a-induced gene expression in human umbilical vein endothelial cells. *American Journal of Pathology*, **164**, 849–59.

Ames, R. S., Li, Y., Sarau, H. M., *et al.* (1996). Molecular cloning and characterization of the human anaphylatoxin C3a receptor. *Journal of Biological Chemistry*, **271**, 20231–4.

Arthus, M. (1903). Injections repetees de serum de cheval chez le lapin. *Comptes Rendus des Seances de la Societe de Biologie et de ses Filiales*, **55**, 817–25.

Atkinson, J. P., Oglesby, T. J., White, D., Adams, E. A., Liszewski and M. K. (1991). Separation of self from non-self in the complement system: a role for membrane cofactor protein and decay accelerating factor. *Clinical Experimental Immunology*, **86** (Suppl. 1), 27–30.

Baumann, U., Chouchakova, N., Gewecke, B., *et al.* (2001). Distinct tissue site-specific requirements of mast cells and complement components C3/C5a receptor in IgG immune complex-induced injury of skin and lung. *Journal of Immunology*, **167**, 1022–7.

Benzaquen, L. R., Nicholson-Weller, A. and Halperin, J. A. (1994). Terminal complement proteins C5b-9 release basic fibroblast growth factor and platelet-derived growth factor from endothelial cells. *Journal of Experimental Medicine*, **179**, 985–92.

Brauer, R. B., Baldwin, W. M. 3rd, Ibrahim, S. and Sanfilipo, F. (1995). The contribution of terminal complement components to acute and hyperacute allograft rejection in the rat. *Transplantation* **59**, 288–93.

Byrne, G. W., McCurry, K. R., Martin, M. J., McClellan, S. M., Platt, J. L. and Logan, J. S. (1997). Transgenic pigs expressing human CD59 and decay-accelerating factor produce an intrinsic barrier to complement-mediated damage. *Transplantation*, **63**, 149–53.

Carroll, M. C. (2004). The complement system in regulation of adaptive immunity. *Nature Immunology*, **5**, 981–6.

Claudy, A. (1998). Pathogenesis of leukocytoclastic vasculitis. *European Journal of Dermatology*, **2**, 75–9.

Dalmasso, A. P., Vercellotti, G. M., Platt, J. L. and Bach, F. H. (1991). Inhibition of complement-mediated endothelial cell cytotoxicity by decay accelerating factor: potential for prevention of xenograft hyperacute rejection. *Transplantation*, **52**, 530–3.

Danning, C. L., Illei, G. G. and Boumpas, D. T. (1998). Vasculitis associated with primary rheumatologic diseases. *Current Opinion in Rheumatology*, **10**, 58–65.

Davies, K. A. and Walport, M. J. (1998). Processing and clearance of immune complexes by complement and the role of complement in immune complex diseases. In *The Human Complement System in Health and Disease*, (eds J. E. Volanakis and M. M. Frank), pp. 423–53. Marcel Dekker, New York.

Davis, A. E., 3rd (2005). The pathophysiology of hereditary angioedema. *Clinical Immunology*, **114**, 3–9.

Dragon-Durey, M.-A. and Fremeaux-Bacchi, V. (2005). Atypical haemolytic uraemic syndrome and mutations in complement regulator genes. *Springer Seminars in Immunopathology*, **27**, 359–74.

Esser, A. F. (1994). The membrane attack complex of complement. Assembly, structure, and cytotoxic activity. *Toxicology*, **87**, 229–47.

Fearon, D. T. and Austen, K. F. (1980). The alternative pathway of complement: a system for host defense of microbial infection. *New England Journal of Medicine*, **303**, 259–63.

Fearon, D. T. and Locksley, R. M. (1996). The instructive role of innate immunity in the acquired immune response. *Science*, **272**, 50–4.

Foreman, K. E., Vaporciyan, A. A., Bonish, B. K., *et al.* (1994). C5a-induced expression of P-selectin in endothelial cells. *Journal of Clinical Investigation*, **94**, 1147–55.

Gaboriaud, C., Thielens, N. M., Gregory, L. A., Rossi, V., Fontecilla-Camps, J. C. and Arlaud, G. J. (2004). Structure and activation of the C1 complex of complement: unraveling the puzzle. *Trends in Immunology*, **25**, 368–73.

Genel, F., Sjoholm, A. G., Skattum, L. and Truedsson, L. (2005). Complement factor I deficieny associated with recurrent infections, vasculitis and immune complex glomerulonephritis. *Scandinavian Journal of Infectious Diseases*, **37**, 615–18.

Geng, J. G., Bevilacqua, M. P., Moore, K. L., *et al.* (1990). Rapid neutrophil adhesion to activated endothelium mediated by GMP-140. *Nature*, **343**, 757–60.

Gerard, N. P. and Gerard, C. (1991). The chemotactic receptor for human C5a anaphylatoxin. *Nature*, **349**, 614–17.

Hamilton, K. K., Hattori, R., Esmon, C. T. and Sims, P. J. (1990). Complement proteins C5b-9 induce vesiculation of the endothelial plasma membrane and expose catalytic surface for assembly of the prothrombinase enzyme complex. *Journal of Biological Chemistry*, **265**, 3809–14.

Hart, M. L., Walsh, M. C. and Stahl, G. L. (2004). Initiation of complement activation following oxidative stress. In vitro and in vivo observations. *Molecular Immunology*, **41**, 165–71.

Hart, M. L., Ceonzo, K. A., Shaffer, L. A., *et al.* (2005). Gastrointestinal ischemia-reperfusion injury is lectin complement pathway dependent without involving C1q. *Journal of Immunology*, **174**, 6373–80.

Hattori, R., Hamilton, K. K., McEver, R. P. and Sims, P. J. (1989). Complement proteins C5b-9 induce secretion of high molecular weight multimers of endothelial von Willebrand factor and translocation of granule membrane protein GMP-140 to the cell surface. *Journal of Biological Chemistry*, **264**, 9053–60.

Haviland, D. L., McCoy, R. L., Whitehead, W. T., *et al.* (1995). Cellular expression of the C5a anaphylatoxin receptor (C5aR): demonstration of C5aR on nonmyeloid cells of the liver and lung. *Journal of Immunology*, **154**, 1861–69.

Holmskov, U., Thiel, S. and Jensenius, J. C. (2003). Collectins and Ficolins: Humoral lectins of the innate immune system. *Annual Review of Immunology*, **21**, 547–78.

Hopken, U. E., Lu, B., Gerard, N. P. and Gerard, C. (1997). Impaired inflammatory responses in the reverse Arthus reaction through genetic deletion of the C5a receptor. *Journal of Experimental Medicine*, **186**, 749–56.

Huang, Y., Smith, C. A., Song, H., Morgan, B. P., Abagyan, R. and Tomlinson, S. (2005). Insights into human CD59 complement binding interface toward engineering new therapeutics. *Journal of Biological Chemistry*, **280**, 34073–79.

Ihrcke, N. S. and Platt, J. L. (1996). Shedding of heparin sulfate proteoglycan by stimulated endotheliasl cells: evidence for proteolysis of cell surface molecules. *Journal of Cell Physiology*, **168**, 625–37.

Kawana, S., Shen, G. H., Kobayashi, Y. and Nishiyama, S. (1990). Membrane attack complex of complement in Henoch-Schoenlein purpura skin and nephritis. *Archives of Dermatological Research*, **282**, 183–7.

Key, N. S., Platt, J. L. and Vercellotti, G. M. (1992). Vascular endothelial cell proteoglycans are susceptible to cleavage by neutrophils. *Arteriosclerosis and Thrombosis*, **12**, 836–42.

Kinoshita, T., Takata, Y., Kozono, H., Takeda, J., Hong, K. S. and Inoue, K. (1988). C5 convertase of the alternative complement pathway: covalent linkage between two C3b molecules within the trimolecular complex enzyme. *Journal of Immunology*, **141**, 3895–901.

Leventhal, J. R., Dalmasso, A. P., Cromwell, J. W., *et al.* (1993). Prolongation of cardiac xenograft survival by depletion of complement. *Transplantation*, **55**, 857–66.

Lin, S. S., Kooyman, D. L., Daniels, L. J., *et al.* (1997). The role of natural anti-Gal alpha 1–3Gal antibodies in hyperacute rejection of pig-to-baboon cardiac xenotransplants. *Transplant Immunology*, **5**, 212–18.

Liszewski, M., Farries, T., Lublin, D., Rooney, I. and Atkinson, J. (1996). Control of the complement system. *Advances in Immunology*, **61**, 201–83.

Liszewski, M. K., Kemper, C., Price, J. D. and Atkinson, J. P. (2005). Emerging roles and new functions of CD46. *Springer Seminars in Immunopathology*, **27**, 345–58.

Lukacik, P., Roversi, P., White, J., *et al.* (2004). Complement regulation at the molecular level: The structure of decay-accelerating factor. *Proceedings of the National Academy of Sciences, USA*, **101**, 1279–84.

Matsushita, M. and Fujita, T. (2001). Ficolins and the lectin complement pathway. *Immunological Reviews*, **180**, 78–85.

Morgan, B. P. (1999). Regulation of the complement membrane attack pathway. *Critical Reviews in Immunology*, **19**, 173–98.

Morgan, B. P., van den Berg, C. W. and Harris, C. L. (2005). "Homologous restriction" in complement lysis: roles of membrane complement regulators. *Xenotransplantation*, **12**, 258–65.

Owen, C. A., Campbell, M. A., Sannes, P. L., Boukedes, S. S. and Campbell, E. J. (1995). Cell surface bound elastase and cathepsin G on human neutrophils: a novel non-oxidative mechanism by which neutrophils focus and preserve catalytic activity of serine proteinases. *Journal of Cell Biology*, **131**, 775–89.

Pangburn, M. K. and Müller-Eberhard, H. J. (1984). The alternative pathway of complement. *Springer Seminars in Immunopathology*, **7**, 163–92.

Pascher, A., Poehlein, C., Storck, M., *et al.* (1997). Immunological observations after xenogeneic liver perfusions using donor pigs transgenic for human decay-accelerating factor. *Transplantation*, **64**, 384–91.

Platt, J. L. (2000). Immunobiology of xenotransplantation. *Transplant International*, **13** Suppl 1:S7–10.

Plummer, T. H., Jr. and Hurwitz, N. Y. (1978). Human plasma carboxypeptidase N. *Journal of Biological Chemistry*, **253**, 3907–12.

Podack, E. R. and Tschopp, J. (1984). Membrane attack by complement. *Molecular Immunology*, **21**, 589–603.

Pruitt, S. K., Kirk, A. D., Bolinger, R. R., *et al.* (1994). The effect of soluble complement receptor type 1 on hyperacute rejection of porcine xenografts. *Transplantation*, **57**, 363–70.

Rus, H. G., Niculescu, F. I. and Shin, M. L. (2001). Role of the C5b-9 complement complex in cell cycle and apoptosis. *Immunological Reviews*, **180**, 49–55.

Saadi, S. and Platt, J. L. (1995). Transient perturbation of endothelial integrity induced by antibodies and complement. *Journal of Experimental Medicine*, **181**, 21–31.

Saadi, S., Holzkhecht, R. A., Patte, C. P., Stern, D. M. and Platt, J. L. (1995). Complement-mediated regulation of tissue factor activity in endothelium. *Journal of Experimental Medicine*, **182**, 1807–14.

Saadi, S., Takahashi, T., Holzknecht, R. A. and Platt, J. L. (2004). Pathways to acute humoral rejection. *American Journal of Pathology*, **164**, 1073–80.

Sansonno, D. and Dammacco, F. (2005). Hepatitis C virus, cryoglobulinaemia, and vasculitis: immune complex relations. *Lancet Infectious Diseases*, **5**, 227–36.

Shushakova, N., Skokowa, J., Schulman, J., *et al.* (2002). C5a anaphylatoxin is a major regulator of activating versus inhibitory FcγRs in immune complex-induced lung disease. *Journal of Clinical Investigation*, **110**, 1823–30.

Sims, P. J. and Wiedmer, T. (1995). Induction of cellular procoagulant activity by the membrane attack complex of complement. *Seminars in Cell Biology*, **6**, 275–82.

Stahl, G. L., Xu, Y., Hao, L., *et al.* (2003). Role for the alternative complement pathway in ischemia/reperfusion injury. *American Journal of Pathology*, **162**, 449–55.

Storck, M., Abendroth, D., Prestel, R., *et al.* (1997). Morphology of hDAF (CD55) transgenic pig kidneys following ex-vivo hemoperfusion with human blood. *Transplantation*, **63**, 304–10.

Sylvestre, D., Clynes, R., Ma, M., Warren, H., Carroll, M. and Ravetch, J. (1996). Immunoglobulin G-mediated inflammatory responses develop normally in complement-deficient mice. *Journal of Experimental Medicine*, **184**, 2385–92.

Takata, Y., Kinoshita, T., Kozono, H., *et al.* (1987). Covalent association of C3b with C4b within C5 convertase of the classical complement pathway. *Journal of Experimental Medicine*, **165**, 1494–507.

Takeda, J., Miyata, T., Kawagoe, K., *et al.* (1993). Deficiency of the GPI anchor caused by a somatic mutation of the PIG-A gene in paroxysmal nocturnal hemoglobinuria. *Cell*, **73**, 703–11.

Volanakis, J. E. (1998). Overview of the Complement System. In *The Human Complement System in Health and Disease*, (eds J. E. Volanakis and M. M. Frank), pp. 9–32. Marcel Dekker, New York.

Volanakis, J. E. (2005). The molecular biology of the complement system. In *Arthritis & Allied Conditions – A Textbook of Rheumatology*, 15th edn, (eds W. J. Koopman and L. W. Moreland), pp. 490–503. Williams and Wilkins Co., Maryland.

Walport, M. J. (2001). Complement. *New England Journal of Medicine*, **344**, 1058–66, 1140–4.

Walsh, M. C., Bourcier, T., Takahashi, T., *et al.* (2005). Mannose-binding lectin is a regulator of inflammation that accompanies myocardial ischemia and reperfusion injury. *Journal of Immunology*, **175**, 541–6.

Weiser, M. R., Williams, J. P., Moore, Jr F. D., Kobzik, I., Ma, M., Hechtman, H. B. and Carroll, M. C. (1996). Reperfusion injury of ischemic skeletal muscle is mediated by natural antibody and complement. *Journal of Experimental Medicine*, **183**, 2343–8.

Weisman, H. F., Bartow, T., Leppo, M. K., *et al.* (1990). Soluble human complement receptor type 1: In vivo inhibitor of complement suppressing post-ischemic myocardial inflammation and necrosis. *Science*, **249**, 146–51.

Zhang, M., Austen, Jr. W. G., Chiu, I., *et al.* (2004). Identification of a specific self-reactive IgM antibody that initiates intestinal ischemia/reperfusion injury. *Proceedings of the National Academy of Sciences USA*, **101**, 3886–91.

Zhao, H., Montalto, M. C., Pfeiffer, K. J., Hao, L. and Stahl, G. L. (2002). Murine model of gastrointestinal ischemia associated with complement-dependent injury. *Journal of Applied Physiology*, **93**, 338–45.

CHAPTER 6

Autoantibodies in vasculitis

Allan S. Wiik

Introduction

In many chronic inflammatory diseases characterized by localized or widespread inflammation investigators have been searching for autoantibodies that might reflect pathogenetic disease mechanisms, tissue damage, or clues to etiology. This has certainly also been the case in the area of vasculitic conditions without a known cause, the so-called primary vasculitides (Jennette *et al.* 1994).

The first searches for autoantibodies focused on antibodies to the endothelial cells of blood vessels. Indeed, early studies detected antiendothelial antibodies (AECA) in both small and large-vessel vasculitis (reviewed by Meroni *et al.* 1999). Obstacles to their accurate characterizations have been: uncertainties about the type of substrate to use; doubts about use of fixatives; and issues pertaining to cytokine stimulation of endothelial cells, etc. Even with standard methodology, it has been difficult to secure reasonable reproducibility of results from different institutions. The common occurrence of AECA (or AECA-like activity) in a large variety of inflammatory conditions has diminished the value of positive findings for differential diagnosis.

It seemed logical to examine other cellular and tissue elements involved in chronic inflammatory processes of vasculitis as autoantigens that can give rise to autoantibody production, at least in phases of pronounced disease activity. Investigators who have used this approach have found autoantibodies to a large variety of constituents of inflammatory cells, endothelial cells, vascular basement membranes, and the adjacent extracellular matrix compartment, as illustrated in Table 6.1. In addition to these, some patients with primary small-vessel vasculitis produce autoantibodies to circulating antigens such as complement proteins (immunoconglutinins) that have not been shown to be of value for clinical use in this regard.

Since antineutrophil cytoplasm antibodies (ANCA) have been shown to be closely associated with systemic small-vessel vasculitis (SVV), and are likely to be instrumental in pathogenesis, and relate to the clinical phenotype of these conditions, ANCA is the main topic of this chapter. As other autoantibodies may become interesting for subdividing the classical ANCA-positive vasculitides into subgroups with different manifestations and prognosis, other SVV-related antibodies are also discussed. The ANCA-associated SVV are Wegener's granulomatosis (WG), microscopic polyangiitis (MPA),

Table 6.1 Autoantibodies that may reflect pathogenetic events occurring in primary small-vessel vasculitides (SVV)

Antiendothelial cell antibodies (AECA)[1]
Antineutrophil cytoplasm antibodies (ANCA)[1]
Antiglomerular basement membrane (collagen type IV) antibodies (Anti-GBM)[1]
Antientactin antibodies
Antilaminin antibodies
Anti-α-enolase antibodies[1]
Antiphospholipid (β_2-glycoprotein I antibodies)

[1] These antibodies have been found to fluctuate with disease activity, higher levels being found in phases of active disease.

Churg–Strauss syndrome (CSS), and limited forms of these vasculitides, for example renal-limited necrotizing glomerulonephritis (Jennette *et al.* 1994; Jennette and Falk 1994).

Terminology used for neutrophil-specific autoantibodies

Neutrophil-specific autoantibodies (NSA) were initially detected in the 1960s by an indirect immunofluorescence technique (IIF) using peripheral blood cells as the substrate for studying antibodies to cells in patients with leukopenia (Calabresi *et al.* 1959). NSA were found later in patients with ulcerative colitis (Calabresi *et al.* 1961). They were first termed leukocyte-specific autoantibodies and, later, granulocyte-specific antinuclear antibodies due to their predominant reactivity with nuclei of neutrophils and monocytes (Wiik 1980). When antibodies to cytoplasmic granules of neutrophils were found in SVV patient sera in the 1980s they were named anticytoplasmic antibodies, but this inclusive term was altered to antineutrophil cytoplasm antibodies (ANCA) in 1989 (Wiik and van der Woude 1990).

At the same time it was agreed to call the cytoplasmic granular ANCA "cANCA" and the perinuclear ANCA that decorate the area around and sometimes over the whole neutrophil nuclei "pANCA" (Figure 6.1a and b). Some groups use the term atypical ANCA for staining patterns that do not fit these descriptions

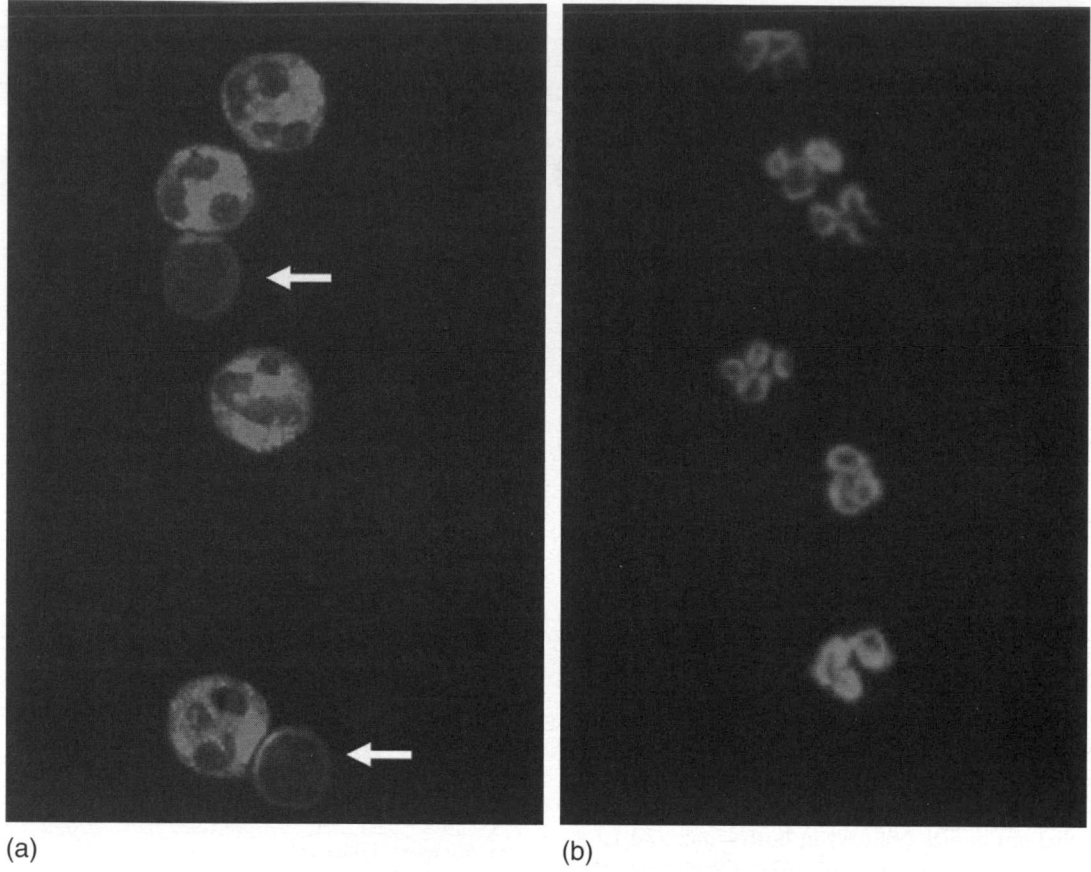

(a)   (b)

Figure 6.1 Patterns of ANCA staining. (a) Typical staining pattern of buffy coat cells with cANCA/PR3-ANCA positive serum using an IgG-specific fluorescent conjugate. Note positive neutrophils and negative lymphocytes (arrows). (b) Staining pattern of buffy coat cells with pANCA/MPO-ANCA positive serum using an IgG specific fluorescent conjugate.

(Figures 6.1c and d). This designation is less important if the specificity of a positive IIF reaction is always sought by testing for reactivity to the main ANCA antigens involved in all positive cases (Hagen et al. 1998; Savige et al.1999, Vassilopoulos et al. 2003). Atypical patterns of reactivity are especially common in non-vasculitic conditions and mostly fall into the suggested category of unspecified NSA (Wiik 2002). Numerous studies from many groups have shown that such NSA are commonly produced in many forms of chronic inflammation dominated by neutrophil granulocyte infiltration, such as ulcerative colitis, primary sclerosing cholangitis, chronic active hepatitis, RA, Felty's syndrome, Sweet's syndrome, and certain chronic infections (Lesavre et al. 1993; Bang la Cour et al. 1995; Zhao et al. 1996; Wiik et al. 1999; Wiik 2002a, 1980, 2001).

Today, we still know little about the actual autoantigens recognized by NSA in non-vasculitic conditions, and the finding of a positive NSA as shown by IIF, without determination of a precise neutrophil target antigen, seems to have little influence on diagnoses or prognoses of these diseases, as exemplified by chronic inflammatory bowel diseases (Hertervig *et al.* 1995; Roozendaal *et al.* 1999). Autoantibodies to neutrophils in patients with ulcerative colitis can target a 50 kD myeloid-cell-specific nuclear-envelope protein (Terjung *et al.* 2000), histone H1 (Eggena *et al.* 2000), and the non-histone chromosomal proteins HMG1 and HMG2

(Sobajima *et al.* 1997) as well as lactoferrin (Peen *et al.* 1993). Demonstration of NSA in early RA patients has been found to predict an erosive disease course (Mustila *et al.* 2000).

In contrast, the subgroup of NSA called ANCA, because of their reactivity with myeloid cell azurophilic and primary granule components, augment clinical diagnosis of necrotizing SVV and rational decision-making in the clinic (Jennette and Falk 1990; Guillevin *et al.* 1996; Franssen *et al.* 1998; Hagen *et al.* 1998; Guillevin *et al.* 1999; Segelmark *et al.* 2000; Wiik 2001; Falk and Jennette 2004). These conditions are now referred to as ANCA-associated SVV, and histopathologically characterized as pauci-immune SVV due to the absence of immunoglobulin deposits in active vasculitic lesions such as those in glomeruli (Jennette and Falk 1990; Jennette and Falk 2004; Ferrario and Rastaldi 2005).

A current definition of vasculitis-associated ANCA thus involves demonstration of positive IgG class IIF ANCA as well as demonstration of IgG antibodies to a neutrophil granule antigen target, for example proteinase 3 (PR3), myeloperoxidase (MPO), elastase (EL), or bacterial permeability-increasing protein (BPI) (Hagen *et al.* 1998; Savige *et al.* 1999; Choi *et al.* 2001; Savige *et al.* 2003; Vassilopoulos *et al.* 2003). To avoid unintended misuse of a positive IIF NSA in the absence of a defined antigen target as support for a diagnosis of SVV, it has been proposed to term the latter antibodies NSA and not ANCA until further research

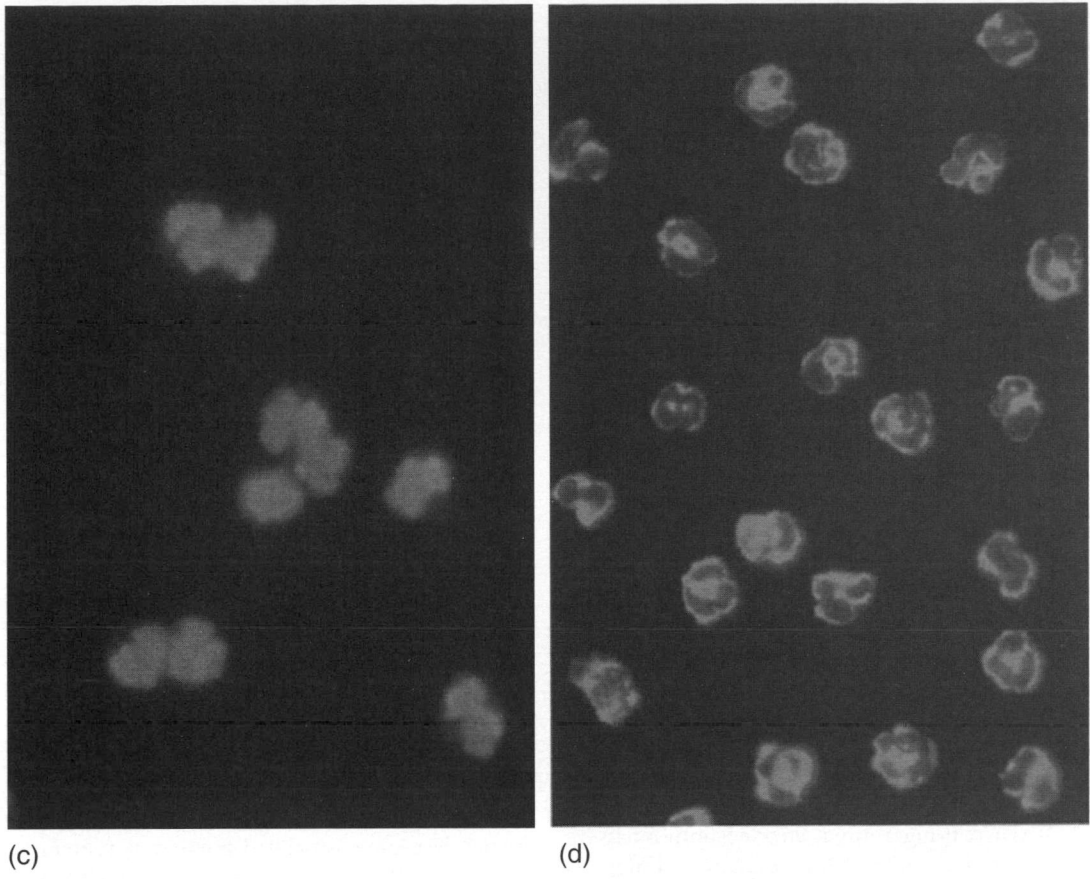

(c)   (d)

Figure 6.1 (c) Cauliflower-like staining pattern of buffy coat cells with NSA-positive serum from a patient with rheumatoid arthritis. Note that many such sera contain autoantibodies to neutrophil and monocyte nuclear constituents. (d) Distinctly narrow peripheral staining pattern of buffy coat cells with NSA-positive serum from a patient with ulcerative colitis. Note that such patients may have antibodies to nuclear membrane and heterochromatin constituents.

can clarify their specificity and relevance for clinical medicine (Wiik 2002).

ANCA targets in small-vessel vasculitides

The first published studies on necrotizing SVV describing antibodies binding to cytoplasmic granules of neutrophils in serum of patients with focal necrotizing glomerulonephritis were done in Australia (Davies *et al.* 1982). Apparently similar antibodies were described in two independent studies on WG patients in 1985, and both studies concluded that these antibodies were especially expressed in active phases of the disease (Rasmussen and Wiik 1985; van der Woude *et al.* 1985).

Proteinase 3 (PR3)

In the First International Workshop on ANCA, in Copenhagen in 1988, the main antigen targeted by WG-associated ANCA was defined as a 29–30kD serine protease in azurophilic granules isolated from the alpha-fraction of neutrophils, and from supernatants of degranulated neutrophils (Lüdemann *et al.* 1988; Goldschmeding *et al.* 1989a). These ANCA were soon after found to react with the proteolytic enzyme proteinase 3 (PR3) of azurophilic granules (Niles *et al.*1989; Goldschmeding *et al.* 1989b; Jenne *et al.* 1990).

The antibody reactivity depends on the native conformation of the PR3 molecule (Bini *et al.* 1992; Specks *et al.* 1996), and most PR3-ANCA react with the enzymatically active PR3 after cleavage of its N-terminal activation dipeptide (Sun *et al.* 1998a). PR3-ANCA directed to the pro-form of PR3 have been found in some patients with WG and MPA, particularly during phases of disease activity (Russell *et al.* 2001).

PR3 is a linear polypeptide containing 228 amino acids. The crystal structure of PR3 was reported in 1996 (Fujinaga *et al.* 1996). Interestingly, it was suggested that the linear epitopes shown to react with PR3-ANCA in WG (Williams *et al.* 1994) occurred in regions of the three-dimensional structure that could implicate the inactive pro-form of the enzyme in the pathogenesis of the disease (Fujinaga *et al.* 1996). Cloning of cDNA for proteinase 3 was accomplished in 1990 (Campanelli *et al.* 1990a).The gene encoding PR3 is located on chromosome 19 (Sturrock *et al.* 1992) close to the EL and azurocidin gene sites (Jenne 1994). The PR3 gene is mainly expressed during the early myelocyte maturation stage of bone marrow development (Sturrock *et al.* 1992; Müller-Bérat *et al.* 1994).

Several groups have shown that PR3-ANCA can inhibit the enzyme activity of PR3, especially during active disease (Daouk *et al.* 1995), but there is no clear consensus on this finding. The PR3 enzyme can degrade a large variety of proteins, among them

IgG molecules and PR3-ANCA molecules themselves (Dolman *et al.* 1995). Most human PR3-ANCA seem to target epitopes close to the catalytic site where four out of five linear epitopes are found (Griffith *et al.* 2001). The fact that PR3 can degrade its bound ANCA would suggest that this type of inhibition is not likely to have lasting biological relevance. Characterization of epitopes using mouse monoclonal antibodies indicated the presence of at least four different epitopes (van der Geld *et al.* 1999). Some of these monoclonal antibodies have been shown to inhibit binding of human PR3-ANCA (Sommarin *et al.* 1995).

Myeloperoxidase (MPO)

In the late 1980s several authors described the presence of ANCA directed to MPO in sera from SVV. Falk and Jennette published their first study on MPO-ANCA in sera from patients with necrotizing glomerulonephritis in 1988 (Falk and Jennette 1988), and Goldschmeding reported the presence of MPO-ANCA and EL-ANCA in patients with SVV (Goldschmeding *et al.* 1989a). Later studies have confirmed the presence of MPO-ANCA in patients with necrotizing SVV, especially when the disease is manifest in the kidneys and lungs (Jennette and Falk 1990; Roberts *et al.* 1991; Saxena *et al.* 1995; Niles *et al.* 1996; Westman *et al.* 1997; Franssen *et al.*1998; Choi *et al.* 2001). The antibody reactivity has been shown to depend on the native conformation of the 140 kD heterodimeric MPO molecule (Falk *et al.* 1992). The MPO-encoding gene has been localized to chromosome 17 (Chang *et al.* 1987). Recombinant MPO seems to function just as well as native MPO as antigen for detection of MPO-ANCA using a direct enzyme-immunoassays (EIA) technique (Short *et al.* 1995). When capture technique is used for MPO-ANCA detection, results are superior with the recombinant MPO molecule (Boomsma *et al.* 2001).

The MPO molecule is quite unstable due to cleavage at a light-sensitive site located to the Met[409] position of the heavy chain (Taylor *et al.* 1992), and this property has great importance for preservation of the molecule as an antigen for MPO-ANCA detection (Hagen *et al.* 1996). The number of epitopes recognized by human MPO-ANCA has been difficult to estimate, partly due to the instability of MPO, but it appears to be restricted (Short and Lockwood 1997). Interestingly, human monoclonal MPO-ANCA has similar restricted epitope reactivity (Ehrenstein *et al.* 1992). For unknown reasons some MPO-ANCA produce a cANCA pattern by IIF technique (Segelmark *et al.* 1994).

Elastase (EL)

ANCA directed to the other main azurophilic granule serine protease, EL, have been found in patients with primary SVV (Apenberg *et al.* 1996) although they may be rare (Cohen Tervaert *et al.* 1993). In patients with drug-induced vasculitis they are more common (Dolman *et al.* 1993; Choi *et al.* 2000; Herlin *et al.* 2002). They can occur together with ANCA directed to PR3, MPO, or lactoferrin.

Lactoferrin

Lactoferrin-ANCA are found rarely in primary SVV but more commonly in systemic lupus erythematosus (Sinico *et al.* 1993), in Felty's syndrome, and RA with vasculitis (Coremans *et al.* 1992).

Bacterial/permeability-increasing protein (BPI)

Some patients with SVV who are ANCA-positive by IIF but negative for PR3-ANCA and MPO-ANCA may harbor BPI-ANCA (Zhao *et al.* 1995). BPI-ANCA typically give rise to a finely granular and often weak cytoplasmic staining pattern on neutrophils, most likely because the molecule is anchored to the inside of azurophilic granules. If a patient with vasculitis is found to harbor ANCA directed to BPI, one should suspect that the underlying cause could be an infection or a condition that gives rise to leakage of bacterial components to the blood stream and hence the systemic immune system (Zhao *et al.* 1996; Stoffel *et al.* 1996; Kobayashi *et al.* 1998; Sediva *et al.* 2003).

Azurocidin

ANCA directed to the cationic antimicrobial and monocyte attractant protein azurocidin (Pereira *et al.* 1990), a homologue to EL and PR3 without enzyme activity (Campanelli *et al.* 1990), are rare in patients with SVV and not more frequent than antiazurocidin ANCA found in other glomerular diseases (Yang *et al.* 1996). They produce a pANCA pattern on ethanol-fixed neutrophils.

Lysozyme

Lysozyme may be a target autoantigen in many different inflammatory conditions, for example RA, systemic lupus erythematosus, inflammatory bowel disease, and WG, but no particular clinical features seem to be associated with this antibody (Schmitt *et al.* 1993).

Human lysome-associated membrane protein (H-lamp-2)

In active phases of necrotizing SVV, ANCA can be directed to a human lysosome-associated membrane protein named h-lamp-2 (Kain *et al.* 1995). These antibodies target glycoproteins gp170 and 80–110 of human neutrophils.

Technical aspects of IIF NSA detection

The main reason for assembling people with an interest in SVV in the First International Workshop on ANCA in Copenhagen was the emergence of various methods to detect these antibodies, leading to discrepant results and attenuation of their value.

The use of one method for IIF demonstration of NSA, including ANCA, was agreed upon (Wiik 1989). This method employed washed, isolated buffy coat cells free of platelets, and smeared or cytocentrifuged onto glass slides, followed by ethanol fixation, serum and conjugate incubation, and evaluation with an incident light-illuminated fluorescence microscope (Wiik 1989, 2002b). Slides can be kept at 4°C in the dark for up to a month after ethanol fixation. The use of whole buffy coat cells as substrate for ANCA detection allows discrimination between NSA and non-organ-specific antibodies such as antinuclear antibodies (ANA). This method has been detailed in many recent publications and is available at www.vasculitis.org. Unfortunately, no commercial vendors of slides for IIF detection of NSA have followed this recommendation, so lymphocytes are generally missing in commercially available leukocyte slides.

The designations cANCA and pANCA (Figure 6.1a and b) are based on the reactivity patterns seen on ethanol- or acetone-fixed leukocytes as cellular substrate. The pANCA pattern is the result of reactivity of antibodies with cationically charged hydrophilic constituents, for example MPO, EL, lysozyme, azurocidin, and cathepsin G, that have redistributed to oppositely charged structures in and around nuclei of neutrophils, monocytes, and sometimes closely adjacent lymphocytes (Wiik 2002b). If neutrophils are pre-fixed with the cross-linking agent formalin, the pANCA pattern caused by MPO-ANCA turns into a cANCA pattern (Falk and Jennette 1988). This fixation has been shown to be less reproducible and it is infrequently used in expert laboratories, and is unnecessary when a positive IIF reaction is followed by specificity testing (Savige et al. 1999; Savage et al. 2003). Securing the presence of all peripheral blood cells in the cell substrate (buffy coat cells) allows easy distinction between pANCA and homogeneous/peripheral antinuclear antibodies (ANA), as the latter stain all lymphocytes as well.

Semiquantification of ANCA levels is usually accomplished by titration of IIF-positive samples. A novel image analysis approach for the quantification of ANCA levels in WG patient sera was recently described (Boomsma et al. 2003). No clear differences were shown between conventional ANCA titration and image analysis based quantification, whereas capture-PR3 ANCA EIA was superior (see below).

Relationship between IIF ANCA staining patterns and antigenic targets

Though it is generally true that cANCA are directed to PR3 or BPI, the pattern does not give definite clues to the antigenic target recognized. Thus, some sera showing a cANCA pattern have been found to exclusively target MPO (Segelmark et al. 1994). Similarly, sera harboring pANCA (or atypical ANCA) can sometimes be found to contain PR3-ANCA or BPI-ANCA. Thorough studies have not been done to eliminate the possibility that a pANCA pattern has been caused by simultaneous presence of ANCA directed to other lysosomal components, such as lysozyme or azurocidin, that redistribute to the nuclei upon ethanol fixation (Yang et al. 1996). To ascertain relationships between a particular ANCA staining pattern and antigen specificity it is necessary to do absorption studies with single antigens and look for disappearance of the IIF pattern (Segelmark et al. 1994).

An atypical NSA staining pattern is likely caused by antibodies directed to several neutrophil constituents, each antibody resulting in a particular reaction pattern which becomes superimposed on others (Savige et al. 1999, 2003). A particular staining pattern stands out as rather characteristic for RA (Figure 6.1c) and another for ulcerative colitis (Figure 6.1d) but no dominant antigen has been found to cause these IIF staining patterns (Wiik 2001, 2002a).

Methods used to determine ANCA specificity

The first EIA used to detect PR3-ANCA were described in the First International Workshop on ANCA by Lüdeman, who used 30 kD protein isolated from neutrophil degranulation supernatant as substrate, and by Goldschmeding who used the antigen captured by a mouse monoclonal antibody coated to the microplates (Lüdemann et al. 1988; Goldschmeding et al. 1989b). These assays gave somewhat different results on identical sera, and it was concluded that a multicenter study on the use of PR3 isolated by different methods from neutrophils or from human sputum as substrate needed to be done. In the following years studies were done in many centers in Europe. These studies concluded that different methods could be used to isolate well-preserved PR3 for EIA to detect and quantify PR3-ANCA (Hagen et al. 1996). Each purified antigen was sent to the study participants with a precise description of how to coat the PR3, the optimal buffers and conjugates to be used, etc. The overall concordance of positive results was ~20% between participating centers with varying levels of experience and expertise. The final proof of the usability of preserved PR3 for clinical diagnosis was established by studies on sera both from newly and formerly diagnosed patients with systemic SVV, for example WG, MPA, CSS, and renal-limited rapidly progressive glomerulonephritis, as well as from inflammatory disease controls and healthy donors (Hagen et al. 1998). It was concluded that all of the PR3 preparations could be used for direct EIA.

EIA for demonstrating and quantifying MPO-ANCA had also obtained discrepant results with identical SVV sera. Therefore one commercially available MPO preparation was used by investigating centers to test the same sera as those used for the PR3-ANCA standardization studies (Hagen et al. 1996, 1998). It was shown that MPO that had been sent by mail could not be used, as it gave different results in different centers, most probably due to instability of the MPO during transfer and subsequent handling. As a consequence, MPO was coated onto microplates in one center and then distributed to all participating laboratories with a precise description from one expert center on how to keep the plates intact for use, and how to handle them identically during performance of the assay. After this, reproducible results were attained between the different centers. This assay was again critically tested on the SVV and disease control materials mentioned above, and was found to be suitable for clinical differential diagnosis (Hagen et al. 1998).

If sera from healthy donors are used as controls, a positive cut-off is usually chosen as the mean value plus 2–3 standard deviations. The resulting cut-off will categorize a number of non-vasculitic patient sera as ANCA positive, that is the diagnostic specificity is low. In the multicenter study, we found that low positive values of MPO-ANCA were common in inflammatory disease controls, and thus a high cut-off value had to be chosen to attain useful differential diagnostic properties of the EIA (Hagen et al. 1998).

Use of the EIA format is practical for high-throughput, low-cost autoantibody testing, and the laboratory equipment needed is available in most centers. Nevertheless, little has been done to critically grade the performance of various EIA ANCA assays with regard to nosographic sensitivity and diagnostic specificity, values that are indispensable for predicting the clinical value of a test, expressed as positive or negative predictive values (Hagen et al. 1998). Evaluation of commercial EIAs for ANCA testing using sera from patients with WG and MPA has been done using the preset conditions for testing recommended by the different manufacturers (Holle et al. 2005), but a direct comparison of these kits with regard to differential diagnostic utility has not been done.

Experiences from other areas of autoimmune serology indicate that the use of a single batch of EIA kits can give very different results in the hands of experienced technicians compared to those with little experience, and a minimal performance target of correlation values for EIA should be established (Fritzler et al. 2003).

Today the commercial industry has introduced several other methods for detection of PR3-ANCA and MPO-ANCA using new types of technical platforms, for example addressable laser bead immunoassays (ALBIA), line immunoassays (LIA), and multiple antigen arrays in a number of formats (Fritzler et al. 2003; Wiik et al. 2004), but little has been done to standardize these methods.

The postmarketing surveillance and quality assurance of their utility for differential diagnostics has been less than satisfactory, since this effort requires close collaboration between the industry, experienced clinicians, and patients who are willing to donate their serum for such purposes.

Capture techniques for quantification of PR3-ANCA and MPO-ANCA have been used in certain expert centers and a slightly better correlation between IIF cANCA titer and capture EIA level has been shown for capture PR3-ANCA than those attained with direct EIA (Westman *et al.* 1998; Sun *et al.* 1998b; Segelmark *et al.* 2003; Boomsma *et al.* 2003). The capture EIA technique for determination of MPO-ANCA may have an advantage over direct EIA by distinguishing better between positive and negative results (Boomsma *et al.* 2001). The advantages of the capture EIA principle for monitoring ANCA levels during follow-up will be described below.

A new solid phase assay for detecting and quantifying PR3-ANCA and MPO-ANCA in SVV patients has been introduced. Initial publications using inflammatory disease controls indicate that the performance characteristics are similar to that of direct EIA, although the capture EIA for PR3-ANCA quantification may be superior (Villalta *et al.* 2004; Sinico *et al.* 2005a). Interestingly, IIF ANCA testing was still more sensitive than the other methods studied, but as expected was less specific. Further studies along the lines of these two studies are warranted.

Use of ANCA results for diagnosis and prognosis

The main indication for ordering ANCA testing is a tentative or definite diagnosis of a primary SVV condition (Bizzaro and Wiik 2003). The simple, non-overlapping nomenclature with useful practical definition of each condition proposed by the Chapel Hill Consensus Conference in 1992 (Jennette *et al.* 1994; Falk and Jennette 2004) is used in this chapter. The article describing this terminology made it clear that ANCA are predominantly found in WG, MPA, CSS, and several more limited forms of these conditions, for example necrotizing glomerulonephritis and subglottic stenosis, which usually is one type of limited WG. ANCA are rarely found in other small and intermediate size vessel vasculitides. Recent publications from France have clearly indicated that ANCA are not present in classical polyarteritis nodosa, and presence of ANCA in a patient suspected of having this type of vasculitis should prompt a search for small vessel involvement, a shift in diagnosis, and commonly a change in therapeutic strategy (Guillevin *et al.* 1996).

Frequencies of PR3-ANCA in the published literature from Europe and the United States vary from 60 to 95% for PR3-ANCA in WG, 30 to 40% in MPA, and 9 to 30 % in CSS (Table 6.2), probably due to differences in patient cohorts chosen for study, differences in disease activity, and extent of active involvement at time of serum sampling. The geographic area from which a study appears should also be considered. A recent study indicated that Chinese patients with WG predominantly produce MPO-ANCA (around 60%) while PR3-ANCA was found in less than 40% (Chen *et al.* 2005). An interesting finding is the negative ANCA on repeated testing of serum from some WG patients with CNS vasculitis (Reinhold-Keller *et al.* 2001).

It should be emphasized that not all patients whose sera exhibit PR3-ANCA suffer from WG. PR3-ANCA have been detected in

Table 6.2 Reported frequencies of PR3-ANCA and MPO-ANCA in different forms of ANCA-associated small-vessel vasculitis

Disease	PR3C-ANCA (%)	MPO-ANCA (%)
Wegener's granulomatosis	40[1]–95	5–60[1]
Microscopic polyangiitis	25–30	50–70
Churg–Strauss syndrome	9–30	30–40
Renal limited vasculitis	25–30	50–70
Drug induced vasculitis	10–15[2]	80–90[2]

[1] These percentages come from studies of Chinese WG patients (Chen *et al.* 2005).

[2] Values estimated from rather limited patient populations in the published literature.

Values are dependent on populations studied, disease activity and disease extent at time of sampling, cut-off values chosen for positivity, and other factors.

patients with subacute bacterial endocarditis (Choi *et al.* 2000) and certain other infections, such as tuberculosis (Flores-Suarez *et al.* 2003), but there is not general agreement about this finding (Teixera *et al.* 2005).

Differences in prevalence of ANCA reported in CSS may in part be due to uncertainty of the diagnosis in some studies, since differentiation of CSS from non-vasculitic eosinophilic syndromes is not always possible (Sinico *et al.* 2005b; Sable-Fortassou *et al.* 2005).

Differences in methodology and in cut-off values chosen for grading a result as positive are important causes of the different frequencies reported for PR3-ANCA. Similar considerations also apply to frequencies of MPO-ANCA in literature published from Europe and the United States which shows ranges from 5 to 20% in WG, 50 to 70% in MPA, and 30 to 40% in CSS (Table 6.2). As mentioned above, the majority of Chinese WG patients were found to produce MPO-ANCA (Chen *et al.* 2005). MPO-ANCA positive WG patients in Europe as well as China commonly exhibit pronounced impairment of renal function.

Monitoring ANCA levels in follow-up of patients

A strongly debated topic in clinics treating patients with SVV is the use of serial measurements of ANCA levels for monitoring disease activity. Early investigations indicated that IIF ANCA titers fluctuated with disease activity, especially in cases having cANCA, high values being characteristic of active disease (Cohen Tervaert *et al.* 1989; Egner and Chapel 1990). This was partly confirmed by Jayne *et al.* (1995), who found that the majority of their SVV patients showed a rise in ANCA levels before or during a disease relapse. More recent studies have found that cANCA/PR3-ANCA levels increased preceding disease flares in 92% of patients (Boomsma *et al.* 2000). This may indicate that thoroughly validated and standardized methods for ANCA determination may be useful for monitoring patients. A recent study with the new enzyme fluoroimmunoassay (EliA[TM]) assay platform indicates that this automated system may be useful for following disease activity (Sinico *et al.* 2005a).

A recent review summarizing the value of serial measurements for monitoring disease activity concluded that studies have been different with regard to the methodology chosen, the patient material studied, and lack of a prospective design (Birck *et al.* 2006). Furthermore, no comparison was made between the index test and reference tests. Thus, much better validation and standardization is needed to ensure comparisons of prospectively studied patients, and new serum standards for alignment of results between different laboratories are needed. Such standards will soon be a reality following multicenter collaborative work in the IUIS/WHO/AF/CDC International Autoantibody Standardization Committee; these will be made available through the CDC in Atlanta.

Several studies have indicated that the use of a capture EIA technique for measuring PR3-ANCA is superior to direct EIA for predicting disease flares (Westman *et al.* 1998; Sun *et al.* 1998b; Arranz *et al.* 2001; Segelmark *et al.* 2003; Sinico *et al.* 2005a). Long-term studies using this sensitive technology for follow-up of PR3-ANCA positive, non-vasculitic disease patients (such as the renal disease control patients studied in Sweden) are warranted in order to reveal its potential for predicting later development of SVV (Westman *et al.* 1998).

When should ANCA testing be ordered in the clinic?

The impetus for ordering ANCA testing needs to rest on characteristic as well as non-specific clinical symptoms and manifestations (Wiik 2001). For example, testing should be ordered for a patient in the clinic with one or two early symptoms known to be common in primary SVV, and with constitutional symptoms such as fatigue, weight loss, myalgias, and arthralgias. A clearly positive ANCA at this early stage will influence plans for evaluation of organ involvement and lesions which can be biopsied. Histological verification of necrotizing SVV is still necessary for unequivocal diagnosis. The most rational approach to diagnostic evaluation is to establish a multidisciplinary team of vasculitis experts who can help estimate the extent and type of disease, and make use of a laboratory that can distinguish vasculitis-associated ANCA from other types of NSA. Because a positive NSA without specificity can be misinterpreted by clinicians as presence of ANCA, this term should only be used when both the IIF test and EIA results are clearly positive, and these results should preferably not be reported to the clinic until both results are ready (Savige *et al.* 1999).

ANCA in drug-induced vasculitic syndromes

For the purposes of differential diagnosis, one needs to note the common presence of ANCA directed to more than one granule constituent in serum of patients with drug-induced syndromes (Dolman *et al.* 1993; Choi *et al.* 2000; Wiik 2001; Herlin *et al.* 2002). Presence of more than one specific ANCA in a patient is uncommon in primary SVV (Hagen *et al.* 1998). Thus, presence of MPO-ANCA together with PR3-ANCA, EL-ANCA, lactoferrin-ANCA, etc., should prompt consideration of drug-induced vasculitis.

Drug-induced vasculitis mainly localizes to the skin and rarely to the kidneys. Arthralgias are prominent, and tests for antinuclear antibodies (ANA) often become positive with specificity for histones (Bonaci-Nikolic *et al.* 2005), especially the nucleosome subunit (H2A-H2B)-DNA (Burlingame and Rubin 1996). AECA and antiphospholipid antibodies often accompany this syndrome, in which complement consumption may also be present. The rare combination of ANCA and anticardiolipin antibodies can be caused by thiazides (Larsson *et al.* 1993), indicating that drug-induced lupus-like syndromes caused by drugs other than antithyroid agents can induce this same autoimmune response.

There may be a common pathway of metabolic transformation of lupus-inducing drugs to cytotoxic products caused by activated neutrophils and the enzymatic action of myeloperoxidase (Jiang *et al.* 1994). Discontinuation of the offending drug usually leads to complete resolution of the condition (Rubin 2005; Choi *et al.* 2000). The presence of antiphospholipid antibodies may indicate that antithrombotic therapy should be used, at least for a period of time, as in other secondary antiphospholipid syndrome patients (Bertolaccini *et al.* 2005).

Autoantibody specificity may reflect the complex nature of pathogenesis

As indicated in the introduction, other autoantibodies are commonly found in sera of SVV patients (Table 6.1). These different autoantibodies likely reflect essential inflammatory processes operating in the affected vascular tissues. A breakdown of self-tolerance to certain molecules that are turned into autoantigens by the inflammation, as is assumed for other autoantigens, cause autoantibody production (Utz and Anderson 1998). A short review of contemporary hypotheses concerning pathogenetic events in necrotizing SVV hopefully can clarify this view.

ANCA

It is assumed that both PR3-ANCA and MPO-ANCA play a role in the pathogenesis of ANCA-associated SVV (Savage *et al.* 1992; Kallenberg *et al.* 1995; Harper and Savage 2000; Falk and Jennette 2002). This hypothesis is supported by experiments showing that antibodies to mouse MPO give rise to systemic necrotizing SVV similar to the human disease (Xiao *et al.* 2002).

It has been known for many years that human ANCA directed to PR3 or MPO can activate neutrophils *in vitro* to release toxic oxygen radicals and lytic enzymes (Falk *et al.* 1990; Savage *et al.* 1992). Hyperactivation by IgG ANCA causes neutrophils to firmly adhere to endothelial cells where they degranulate and undergo apoptosis (Harper *et al.* 2001). When exposed to IgG fractions of WG sera, neutrophils upregulate adhesion molecules and secrete several cytokines and chemokines (Harper and Savage 2000; Radford *et al.* 2000). Patients with SVV were recently shown to have hypogalactosylated IgG molecules in their serum which can activate the complement cascade through the mannan-binding lectin pathway (Holland *et al.* 2002), a finding which is in accordance with the early recognition of complement-fixing properties in WG-associated ANCA (Rasmussen and Wiik 1985).

PR3 and EL released from neutrophils can bind directly to the endothelial cell surface, cause internalization of PR3 and MPO (Yang *et al.* 2001), and subsequently lead to endothelial cell apoptosis. After entering into endothelial cells, both enzymes degrade important intracellular molecules such as NFκB and cause proapoptotic changes in JNK, ERK, and p38 MAPK signalling pathways (Preston *et al.* 2002). Neutrophils are assumed to be instrumental in the development of necrotizing SVV (Cockwell and Savage 2000; Xiao *et al.* 2005), but monocytes are also likely to have a role (Casselman *et al.* 1995; Ralston *et al.* 1997; Weidner *et al.* 2001). Experiments indicate that both PR3-ANCA and MPO-ANCA can also stimulate endothelial cells directly in the absence of neutrophils, resulting in increased adherence of unstimulated neutrophils to the cells with ensuing cytotoxicity (Harper and Savage 2000).

WG is a disease with putative complex genetic influences (Jagiello *et al.* 2005a). Disease-related genetic markers in the MHC region contain the extended haplotype DPB1*0401/RXRB03 (Jagiello *et al.* 2004). The PTPN22 620W allele that predisposes to several forms of autoimmune diseases may also play a role in the development of WG (Jagiello *et al.* 2005b). It is not known which of these genes are associated with particular autoantibodies.

AECA

AECA have been found in many types of vasculitis, their presence and titers increasing with active disease (Meroni *et al.* 1999; Yu *et al.* 2005). AECA are assumed to be pathogenic to small vessels independent of ANCA (Del Papa *et al.* 1996; Damianovich *et al.* 1996). When AECA are present in SVV patient sera, some authors have found increased levels of endothelial cell damage markers (Carvalho *et al.* 1999; Meroni *et al.* 1999). A rise in AECA levels has been observed in patients with ANCA negative WG, and AECA positive/ANCA negative patients are at risk of relapses of disease without ANCA production (Meroni *et al.* 1999). Longitudinal studies have shown that AECA and ANCA levels fluctuate independently and do not cross-react (Chan *et al.* 1993).

The precise nature of the surface-exposed endothelial antigens recognized by AECA in WG is not known, though a 125 kD protein on unprimed endothelial cells was selectively targeted in some WG patients (Meroni *et al.* 1999). AECA detected in patients with MPA target several different endothelial cell antigens compared to patients with other types of SVV (Chanseaud *et al.* 2003). AECA levels were generally found to be much higher in SVV patients than in those with large and intermediate size vessel disease (Salojin *et al.* 1996). Interestingly, non-cytotoxic AECA from patients with WG have been shown to react especially well with unprimed endothelial cells from the nose, lung, and kidney, which perhaps relates to the most common distribution of lesions in these patients (Holmen *et al.* 2004). Priming with IFN-γ or TNFα resulted in total loss of endothelial cell binding.

AECA found in Kawasaki's disease (KD) are predominately of the IgM isotype. They have complement-fixing properties and are cytotoxic towards cytokine-stimulated endothelial cells (Meroni *et al.* 1999; Grunebaum *et al.* 2002). Multiple antigens appear to be recognized as targets by AECA in KD but tropomyosin and T plastin seem to be the main targets (Kaneko *et al.* 2004). IgG ANCA are usually not found in KD.

AECA from patients with Henoch–Schönlein purpura seem to especially stimulate IL-8 production in endothelial cells, which corresponds with an increased level of IL-8 in serum of active disease patients (Yang *et al.* 2004).

Studies aimed at standardizing AECA determination are necessary to solve the question of whether AECA determination should be done more frequently in the evaluation of vasculitis.

Antiglomerular basement membrane (GBM) antibodies

Antibodies to the α3 non-collagenous domain of type IV collagen are present in nearly all patients with anti-GBM disease in the lungs and kidneys (formerly called Goodpasture syndrome) (Gunnarsson *et al.* 2000). This type of vasculitis is also classified as a primary SVV and has been added to the array of SVV in Chapel Hill consensus classification terminology. In older individuals with SVV it is not uncommon to find anti-GBM antibodies co-occurring with

ANCA, which are primarily directed to MPO (Bygren *et al.*1992; Rutgers *et al.* 2003). The syndrome of lung hemorrhage and nephritis is most commonly seen in the presence of ANCA (Saxena *et al.* 1995; Niles *et al.* 1996; Rutgers *et al.* 2003). It should be emphasized that both anti-GBM and ANCA should be looked for in renopulmonary syndromes (Westman *et al.* 1997). Patients who harbor ANCA as well as anti-GBM have symptoms similar to those of MPO-ANCA associated SVV and relapses are common (Bygren *et al.* 1992; Rutgers *et al.* 2003). The co-occurrence of anti-GBM and ANCA may influence the disease outcome, with a worse survival and end-stage kidney disease (Levy *et al.* 2004). Determination of anti-GBM antibodies should be done using the isolated epitope coated on a solid support, for example EIA. The epitope in type IV collagen in anti-GBM/ANCA positive disease is the same as the one targeted in anti-GBM disease alone (Hellmark *et al.* 1997). There are suggestions that presence of more than one vasculitis-associated autoantibody, for example ANCA plus anti-GBM antibody, can aggravate vasculitic disease in animal models (Heeringa *et al.* 1996) suggesting that these autoantibodies also have synergistic pathogenic effects in humans.

Antilaminin and antientactin antibodies

Antibodies to the basement membrane component laminin have been found in ~20% of patients with ANCA-associated vasculitis (Vecchi *et al.* 2000). Further studies are needed to judge the clinical importance of this antibody. Antibodies to the GBM component entactin have been detected in patients with isolated glomerulonephritis, but they are probably less important for diagnosing SVV (Saxena *et al.* 1991).

Anti-α-enolase antibodies

α-Enolase is a cytosol constituent of many different cell types, among them macrophages and endothelial cells. α-Enolase is surface expressed on endothelial cells and macrophages and is a plasminogen receptor on these cells (Moscato *et al.* 2000). Production of autoantibodies to this molecule most likely reflects pathogenetic events in the affected tissues. α-Enolase antibodies have been found in ANCA-associated SVV (Moodie *et al.* 1993) and many other inflammatory diseases. In Behçet's disease the antibodies mainly belong to the IgM isotype and react with endothelial cell α-enolase (Lee *et al.* 2003).

Antiphospholipid antibodies

Autoantibodies directed to phospholipid binding proteins, such as β_2-glycoprotein 1 or thrombin, are hallmarks in the diagnosis of primary and secondary antiphospholipid syndromes (Roubey 1994; Wilson *et al.*1999) (Chapter 44) and are detected by many different assays. The commonly used anticardiolipin assay detects β_2-glycoprotein 1 protein in an EIA where cardiolipin forms the bottom layer and human or bovine β_2-glycoprotein 1 is the attached antigen (Bertolaccini *et al.* 2005). Autoantibodies demonstrated by this EIA technique recognize either the complex or the attached β_2-glycoprotein 1 in a new conformational state with exposed cryptic epitopes (Kasahara *et al.* 2005). Antibodies to β_2-glycoprotein 1 or thrombin are also detected by the lupus inhibitor (lupus anticoagulant) assay.

Anti-β_2-glycoprotein 1 antibodies may mimic AECA if the antibodies attach to endothelial cell-adherent β_2-glycoprotein 1, and *in vitro* studies have shown that this binding induces endothelial cell activation (Del Papa *et al.* 1997). Antiphospholipid antibodies are rarely found in classical primary SVV patient sera (Rees *et al.* 2006), but case reports suggest that organ lesions become more extensive, possible reflecting synergy between autoantibodies. Antiphospholipid antibodies of the IgM isotype are frequently found in sera from patients with vasculitis induced by antithyroid drugs (Bonaci-Nikolic *et al.* 2005). The presence of antiphospholipid antibodies and ANCA to one or more ANCA targets thus indicates probable drug-induced vasculitis. From a therapeutic standpoint, use of an antithrombotic agent in patients with drug-induced lupus should be considered to avoid thrombosis and organ damage.

Conclusions

Autoantibodies to cellular and structural elements involved in the pathology of primary SVV are frequent and diverse. Until further methodological and molecular biological advances have been made, ANCA will remain the most important specific autoantibodies for clinical use.

Some data discussed in this chapter imply that the occurrence of a particular profile of antibodies in a patient can be regarded as an "immunological read-out" of a pathophysiologic process characteristic of a defined type of SVV condition, and can lead to insights into etiology, pathology, and therapeutic options. Alternatively, as suggested by many investigators, the different autoantibodies may be direct contributors to inflammation and a particular pathology. AECA directed at nose, lung, and kidney endothelium in ANCA-positive WG may determine the characteristic distribution of the lesions in this disease, while anti-GBM against type IV collagen expressed in lung and glomerular basement membranes can act directly or synergize with ANCA in inciting inflammation in these organs. Similarly, antiphospholipid antibodies together with ANCA and antichromatin antibodies may give rise to lupus-like drug-induced syndromes. Thus, future studies of autoantibody profiles in individual patients are desirable, and will likely lead to better differentiation between different forms of SVV and facilitate use of tailored therapies.

References

Apenberg, S., Andrassy, K., Wörner, I., *et al.* (1996). Antibodies to neutrophil elastase: a study in patients with vasculitis. *American Journal of Kidney Diseases*, **28**, 178–85.

Arranz, O., Ara, J., Rodriguez, R., *et al.* (2001). Comparison of anti-PR3 capture and anti-PR3 direct ELISA for detection of antineutrophil cytoplasmic antibodies (ANCA) in long-term clinical follow-up of PR3-ANCA-associated vasculitis patients. *Clinical Nephrology*, **56**, 295–301.

Bang la Cour, B., Wiik, A., Høier-Madsen, M. and Baslund, B. (1995). Clinical correlates and substrate specificities of antibodies exhibiting neutrophil nuclear reactivity – a methodological study. *Journal of Immunological Methods*, **187**, 287–95.

Bertolaccini, M. L., Gomez, S., Pareja, J. F., *et al.* (2005). Antiphospholipid antibody tests: spreading the net. *Annals of the Rheumatic Diseases*, **64**, 1639–43.

Bini, P., Gabay, J. E., Teitel, A., *et al.* (1992). Antineutrophil cytoplasmic autoantibodies in Wegener's granulomatosis recognize conformational epitope(s) on proteinase 3. *Journal of Immunology,* **149**, 1409–15.

Birck, R., Schmidt, W. H., Kaelsch, I. A. and van der Woude, F. J. (2006). Serial ANCA determinations for monitoring disease activity in patients with ANCA-associated vasculitis: systematic review. *American Journey of Kidney Diseases*, **47**, 15–23.

Bizzaro, N. and Wiik, A. (2003). Appropriateness in antinuclear antibody testing: from clinical request to strategic laboratory practice. *Clinical and Experimental Rheumatology*, **22**, 349–55.

Bonaci-Nikolic, B., Nikolic, M. M., Andrejevic, S., Zoric, S. and Bukilica, M. (2005). Antineutrophil cytoplasmic antibody (ANCA)-associated autoimmune diseases induced by antithyroid drugs: comparison with idiopathic ANCA vasculitides. *Arthritis Research and Therapy*, **7**, R1072–81.

Boomsma, M. M., Damoiseaux, J. G., Stegeman, C. A., *et al.* (2003). Image analysis: a novel approach for the quantification of antineutrophil cytoplasmic antibody levels in patient s with Wegener's granulomatosis. *Journal of Immunological Methods*, **274**, 27–35.

Boomsma, M. M., Stegeman, C. A. and van der Leij, M. J., *et al.* (2000). Prediction of relapses in Wegener's granulomatosis by measurement of antineutrophil cytoplasmic antibody levels: a prospective study. *Arthritis and Rheumatism*, **43**, 2025–33.

Boomsma, M. M., Stegeman, C. A., Oost-Kort, W. W., *et al.* (2001). Native and recombinant proteins to analyze auto-antibodies to myeloperoxidase in pauci-immune glomerulonephritis. *Journal of Immunological Methods*, **254**, 47–58.

Burlingame, R. W. and Rubin, R. L. (1996). Autoantibody to the nucleosome subunit (H2A-H2B)-DNA is an early and ubiquitous feature of lupus-like conditions. *Molecular Biology Reports*, **20**, 159–66.

Bygren, P., Rasmussen, N., Isaksson, B. and Wieslander, J. (1992). Antineutrophil cytoplasmic antibodies, anti-GBM antibodies and anti-dsDNA antibodies in glomerulonephritis. *European Journal of Clinical Investigation*, **22**, 783–92.

Calabresi, P., Edwards, E. A. and Schilling, R. F. (1959). Fluorescent anti-globulin studies in leukopenic and related disorders. *Journal of Clinical Investigation*, **38**, 2091–2100.

Calabresi, P., Thayer, W. R. and Spiro, H. M. (1961). Demonstration of circulating antinuclear globulins in ulcerative colitis. *Journal of Clinical Investigation*, **40**, 2126–33.

Campanelli, D., Detmers, P. A., Nathan, C. F. and Gabay, J. E. (1990b). Azurocidin and a homologous serin protease from neutrophils. Differential antimicrobial and proteolytic properties. *Journal of Clinical Investigation*, **85**, 904–15.

Campanelli, D., Melchior, M., Fu, Y., *et al.* (1990a). Cloning of cDNA for proteinase 3: a serine protease, antibiotic, and autoantigen from human neutrophils. *Journal of Experimental Medicine*, **172**, 1709–15.

Carlsson, M., Eriksson, L., Erwander, I., Wieslander, J. and Segelmark, M. (2003). Pseudomonas-induced lung damage in cystic fibrosis correlates to bactericidal-permeability-increasing protein (BPI)-autoantibodies. *Clinical and Experimental Rheumatology*, **21** (Suppl. 32), S95–100.

Carvalho, D., Savage, C. O., Isenberg, D. and Pearson, J. D. (1999). IgG anti-endothelial cell autoantibodies from patients with systemic lupus erythematosus or systemic vasculitis stimulate the release of two endothelial cell-derived mediators, which enhance adhesion molecule expression and leukocyte adhesion in an autocrine manner. *Arthritis and Rheumatism*, **42**, 631–40.

Casselman, B. L., Kilgore, K., Miller, B. F. and Warren, J. S. (1995). Antibodies to neutrophil cytoplasmic antigens induce monocyte chemoattractant protein-1 secretion from human monocytes. *Journal of Clinical Laboratory Medicine*, **126**, 495–502.

Chan, T. M., Frampton, G., Jayne, D. R.W., Perry, G. J., Lockwood, C. M. and Cameron, J. S. (1993). Clinical significance of anti-endothelial cell antibodies in systemic vasculitis: a longitudinal study comparing anti-endothelial cell antibodies and anti-neutrophil cytoplasm antibodies. *American Journal of Kidney Diseases*, **22**, 387–92.

Chang, K. S., Schroeder, W., Siciliano, M. J., *et al.* (1987). The localization of the human myeloperoxidase gene is in close proximity to the translocation breakpoint in acute promyelocytic leukaemia. *Leukaemia*, **1**, 458–62.

Chanseaud, Y., Pena-Lefebvre, P. G., Guilpain, P., *et al.* (2003). IgM and IgG autoantibodies from microscopic polyangiitis patients but not those with other small- and medium-sized vessel vasculitides recognize multiple endothelial cell antigens. *Clinical Immunology,* **109,** 165–78.

Chen, M. M., Feng, Y., Zhang, Y., Zou, W.-Z., Zhao, M.-H. and Wang, H.-Y. (2005). Characteristics of Chinese patients with Wegener's granulomatosis with anti-myeloperoxidase autoantibodies. *Kidney International,* **68,** 2225–29.

Choi, H. K., Merkel, P. A., Walker, A. M., *et al.* (2000). Drug-associated antineutrophil cytoplasmic antibody-positive vasculitis: prevalence among patients with high titers of antimyeloperoxidase antibodies. *Arthritis and Rheumatism,* **43,** 405–13.

Choi, H. K., Liu, S., Merkel, P. A., Colditz, G. A. and Niles, J. L. (2001). Diagnostic performance of antineutrophil cytoplasmic antibody tests for idiopathic vasculitides: metananlysis with a focus on antimyeloperoxidase antibodies. *Journal of Rheumatology,* **28,** 1584–90.

Cockwell, P. and Savage, C. O. (2000). Role of leukocytes in the immunopathogenesis of ANCA-associated glomerulonephritis. *Nephron,* **85,** 287–306.

Cohen Tervaert, J. W., van der Woude, F. J., Fauci, A. S., *et al.* (1989). Association between active Wegener's granulomatosis and anticytoplasmic antibodies. *Archives of Internal Medicine,* **149,** 2461–65.

Cohen Tervaert, J. W., Mulder, L., Stegeman, C., *et al.* (1993). Occurrence of autoantibodies to human leucocyte elastase in Wegener's granulomatosis and other inflammatory disorders. *Annals of the Rheumatic Diseases,* **52,** 155–20.

Coremans, I. E. M., Hagen, E. C., Daha, M. R., *et al.* (1992). Antilactoferrin antibodies in patients with rheumatoid arthritis are associated with vasculitis. *Arthritis and Rheumatism,* **53,** 1466–75.

Damianovich, M., Gilburd, B., George, J., *et al.* (1996). Pathogenic role of anti-endothelial cell antibodies in vasculitis. *Journal of Immunology,* **156,** 4946–51.

Daouk, G. H., Palsson, R. and Arnaout, M. A. (1995). Inhibition of proteinase 3 by ANCA and its correlation with disease activity. *Kidney International,* **47,** 1528–36.

Davies, D., Moran, M. E., Niall, J. F. and Ryan, G. B. (1982). Segmental glomerulonephritis with antineutrophil antibody: possible arbovirus aetiology. *British Journal of Medicine,* **285,** 606.

Del Papa, N., Guidali. L., Sironi, M., *et al.* (1996). Anti-endothelial cell IgG antibodies from patients with Wegener's granulomatosis bind to human endothelial cells in vitro and induce adhesion molecule expression and cytokine secretion. *Arthritis and Rheumatism,* **39,** 758–66.

Del Papa, N., Guidali, N., Tincani, A., Balestrieri, G., Ishikawa, I. and Koike, T. (1997). Endothelial cells as targets for antiphospholipid antibodies: human polyclonal and monoclonal anti-ß2 glycoprotein I react in vitro with endothelial cells through adherent ß2 glycoprotein I and induce endothelial cell activation. *Arthritis and Rheumatism,* **40,** 551–61.

Dolman, K. M., Gans, R. O. B., Vervaadt, Th. J., *et al.* (1993). Vasculitis and anti-neutrophil cytoplasmic autoantibodies with propylthiouracil therapy. *Lancet,* **342,** 651–2.

Dolman, K. M., Jager, A., Sonnenberg, A., *et al.* (1995). Proteolysis of classical anti-neutrophil cytoplasmic autoantibodies (C-ANCA) by neutrophil proteinase 3. *Clinical and Experimental Immunology,* **101,** 8–12.

Eggena, M., Cohavy, O., Parsegian, M. H., *et al.* (2000). Identification of histone H1 as a cognate antigen of the ulcerative colitis-associated marker pANCA. *Journal of Autoimmunity,* **14,** 83–97.

Egner, W. and Chapel, H. M. (1990). Titration of antibodies against neutrophil cytoplasmic antigens is useful in monitoring disease activity in systemic vasculitides. *Clinical and Experimental Immunology,* **82,** 244–9.

Ehrenstein, M. R., Leaker, B., Isenberg, D. and Cambridge, G. (1992). Production of human monoclonal antibodies to myeloperoxidase. *Immunology,* **76,** 617–20.

Falk, R. J., Becker, R., Terrell, R. and Jennette, C. J. (1992). Anti-myeloperoxidase autoantibodies react with native but not denatured myeloperoxidase. *Clinical and Experimental Immunology,* **89,** 274–78.

Falk, R. J. and Jennette, J. C. (1988). Anti-neutrophil cytoplasmic autoantibodies with specificity for myeloperoxidase in patients with systemic vasculitis and idiopathic necrotizing and crescentic glomerulonephritis. *New England Journal of Medicine,* **318,** 1651–7.

Falk, R. J. and Jennette, J. C. (2002). ANCA are pathogenic – oh yes they are! *Journal of Nephrology,* **13,** 1977–9.

Falk, R. J. and Jennette, J. C. (2004). Thoughts about the classification of small vessel vasculitis. *Journal of Nephrology,* **17** (Suppl. 8), S3–9.

Ferrario, F. and Rastaldi, M. P. (2005). Histopathological atlas of renal diseases: ANCA-associated vasculitis (second part). *Journal of Nephrology,* **18,** 217–20.

Flores-Suarez, L. F.,Cabiedes, J., Villa, A. R., van der Woude, F. J. and Alcocer-Varela, J. (2003). Prevalence of antineutrophil cytoplasmic antibodies in patients with tuberculosis. *Rheumatology,* **42,** 223–9.

Franssen, C., Gans, R., Kallenberg, C. G. M., Hageluken, C. and Hoorntje, S. (1998). Disease spectrum of patients with antineutrophil cytoplasmic autoantibodies of defined specificity: distinct differences between patients with anti-proteinase 3 and anti-myeloperoxidase autoantibodies. *Journal of Internal Medicine,* **244,** 209–16.

Fritzler, M. J., Wiik, A., Fritzler, M. L. and Barr, S. G. (2003). The use and abuse of commercial kits used to detect autoantibodies. *Arthritis Research and Therapy,* **5,** 192–201.

Fujinaga, M., Cgernaia, M., Halenbeck, R., *et al.* (1996). The crystal structure of PR **3,** a neutrophil serine proteinase antigen of Wegener's granulomatosis antibodies. *Journal of Molecular Biology,* **261,** 267–78.

Goldschmeding, R., Cohen Tervaert, J. W., van der Schoot, C. E., *et al.* (1989a). ANCA, anti-myeloperoxidase, and anti-elastase: three members of a novel class of autoantibodies against myeloid lysosomal enzymes. *Acta Pathologica et Microbiologica Scandinavica,* **97,** (Suppl. 6), 48–9.

Goldschmeding, R., van der Schoot, C. E., Ten Bokkel Huininck, D., *et al.* (1989b). Wegener's granulomatosis autoantibodies identify a novel diiso-fluorophosphate-binding protein in the lysosomes of normal human neutrophils. *Journal of Clinical Investigations,* **84,** 1577–87.

Griffith, M. E., Coulthart, S., Pemberton, A., *et al.* (2001). Anti-neutrophil cytoplasmic antibodies (ANCA) from patients with systemic vasculitis recognize restricted epitopes of proteinase 3 involving the catalytic site. *Clinical and Experimental Immunology,* **123,** 170–7.

Grunebaum, E., Blank, M., Cohen, S., *et al.* (2002). The role of anti-endothelial cell antibodies in Kawasaki disease – in vitro and in vivo studies. *Clinical and Experimental Immunology,* **130,** 233–40.

Guillevin, L., Durand-Gasselin, B., Cevallos, R., *et al.* (1999). Microscopic polyangiitis: clinical and laboratory findings in eighty-five patients. *Arthritis and Rheumatism,* **42,** 421–30.

Guillevin, L., Lhote, F., Amouroux, J., Gherardi, R., Callard, P. and Cassasus, P. (1996). Antineutrophil cytoplasmic antibodies, abnormal angiograms and pathological findings in polyarteritis nodosa and Churg-Strauss syndrome: indications for the classification of vasculitides of the polyarteritis nodosa group. *British Journal of Rheumatology,* **35,** 958–64.

Gunnarsson, A., Hellmark, T. and Wieslander, J. (2000). Molecular properties of the Goodpasture epitope. *Journal of Biological Chemistry,* **275,** 30844–8.

Hagen, E. C., Andrassy, K., Csernok, E., *et al.* (1996). Development and standardization of solid phase assays for the detection of anti-neutrophil cytoplasmic antibodies (ANCA). A report on the second phase of an international cooperative study on the standardization of ANCA assays. *Journal of Immunological Methods,* **196,** 1–15.

Hagen, E. C., Daha, M., Hermans, J., *et al.* (1998). The diagnostic value of standardized assays for anti-neutrophil cytoplasmic antibodies (ANCA) in idiopathic systemic vasculitis. *Kidney International,* **53,** 743–53.

Harper, L. and Savage, C. O. (2000). Pathogenesis of ANCA-associated systemic vasculitis. *Journal of Pathology*, **190**, 349–59.

Harper, L. and Savage, C. O. (2001). Leucocyte-endothelial interactions in anti-neutrophil cytoplasmic antibody-associated vasculitis. *Rheumatic Disease Clinics of North America*, **27**, 887–903.

Heeringa, P., Brouwer E., Klok, P. A., *et al.* (1996). Autoantibodies to myeloperoxidase aggravate mild anti-glomerular basement membrane-mediated glomerular injury in the rat. *American Journal of Pathology*, **149**, 1695–706.

Hellmark, T., Niles, J. L., Collins, A. B., McCluskey, R. T. and Brunmark, C. (1997). Comparison of anti-GBM antibodies in sera with and without ANCA. *Journal of the American Society for Nephrology*, **8**, 376–85.

Herlin, T., Birkebaek, N. H., Wolthers, O. D., Heegaard, N. H. and Wiik, A. (2002). Anti-neutrophil cytoplasmic autoantibody (ANCA) prophiles in propylthiouracil-induced lupus-like manifestations in monozygotic triplets with hyperthyroidism. *Scandinavian Journal of Rheumatology*, **31**, 46–9.

Hertervig, E., Wieslander, J., Johansson, C., Wiik, A. and Nilsson, A. A. (1995). Anti-neutrophil cytoplasmic antibodies in chronic inflammatory bowel disease. Prevalence and diagnostic role. *Scandinavian Journal of Gastroenterology*, **30**, 693–8.

Holland, M., Takada, K., Okumoto, T., *et al.* (2002). Hypogalactosylation of serum IgG in patients with ANCA-associated systemic vasculitis. *Clinical and Experimental Immunology,* **129**, 183–90.

Holle, J. U., Hellmich, B., Backes, M., Gross, W. L. and Csernok, E. (2005). Variations in the performance characteristics of commercial enzyme immunoassay kits for detection of antineutrophil cytoplasmic antibodies: what is the optimal cut-off? *Annals of the Rheumatic Diseases*, **64**, 1773–9.

Holmen, C., Christensson, M., Pettersson, E., *et al.* (2004). Wegener's granulomatosis is associated with organ-specific antiendothelial cell antibodies. *Kidney International*, **66**, 1049–60.

Jagiello, P., Gencik, M., Arning, L., *et al.* (2004). New genomic region for Wegener's granulomatosis as revealed by an extended association screen with 202 apoptosis-related genes. *Human Genetics*, **114**, 468–77.

Jagiello, P., Aries, P., Arning, L., *et al.* (2005b). The PTPN22 620W allele is a risk factor for Wegener's granulomatosis. *Arthritis and Rheumatism*, **52**, 4039–43.

Jagiello, P., Gross, W. L. and Epplen, J. T. (2005a). Complex genetics of Wegener's granulomatosis. *Autoimmunity Reviews*, **4**, 42–7.

Jayne, D. R.W., Gaskin, G., Pusey, C. D. and Lockwood, C. M. (1995). ANCA and predicting relapse in systemic vasculitis. *Quarterly Journal of Medicine*, **88**, 127–33.

Jenne, D. E., Tshopp, J., Lüdemann, J., Utecht, B. and Gross, W. L. (1990). Wegener's autoantigen decoded. *Nature*, **346**, 520.

Jenne, D. E. (1994). Structure of azurocidin, proteinase 3, and neutrophil elastase genes. Implications for inflammation and vasculitis. *American Journal of Respiratory and Critical Care Medicine,* **150**, S147–54.

Jennette, J. C. and Falk, R. N. (1990). Antineutrophil cytoplasmic autoantibodies and associated diseases: a review. *American Journal of Kidney Diseases*, **15**, 517–29.

Jennette, J. C. and Falk, R. J. (1994). The pathology of vasculitis involving the kidney. *American Journal of Kidney Diseases*, **24**, 130–41.

Jennette, J. C., Falk, R. J., Andrassy, K., *et al.* (1994). Nomenclature of systemic vasculitides: proposal of an international consensus conference. *Arthritis and Rheumatism*, **37**, 187–92.

Jiang, X., Khursigara, G. and Rubin, R. L. (1994). Transformation of lupus-inducing drugs to cytotxic products by activated neutrophils. *Science*, **266**, 810–3.

Kain, R., Matsui, K., Exner, M., *et al.* (1995). A novel class of autoantigens of anti-neutrophil cytoplasmic antibodies in necrotizing and crescentic glomerulonephritis: the lysosomal membrane glycoprotein h-lamp-2 in neutrophil granulocytes and a related membrane protein in glomerular endothelial cells. *Journal of Experimental Medicine*, **181**, 585–97.

Kallenberg, C. G. M., Brouwer, E., Mulder, A. H.L., Stegeman, C. A., Weening, J. J. and Cohen Tervaert, J. W. (1995). ANCA – pathophysiology revisited. *Clinical and Experimental Immunology*, **100**, 1–3.

Kaneko, M., Ono, T., Matsubara, T., *et al.* (2004). Serological identification of endothelial antigens predominantly recognized in Kawasaki disease patients by expression cloning. *Microbiology and Immunology*, **48**, 703–11.

Kasahara, H., Matsuura, E., Kaihara, K., *et al.* (2005). Antigenic structures recognized by anti-beta2-glycoprotein I autoantibodies. *International Immunology*, **17**, 1533–42.

Kobayashi, O. (1998). Clinical role of autoantibody against bactericidal/permeability-increasing protein in chronic airway infection. *Journal of Infection and Chemotherapy,* **4**, 83–93.

Larssson, G. B., Langer, L. and Nässberger, L. (1993). *Journal of Internal Medicine*, **233**, 493–4.

Lee, K. H., Chung, H. S., Kim, H. S., *et al.* (2003). Human alpha-enolase from endothelial cells as a target antigen of anti-endothelial cell antibody in Behçet's disease. *Arthritis and Rheumatism*, **48**, 2025–35.

Lesavre, P., Noël, L. H., Gayno, P., *et al.*(1993). Atypical autoantigen targets of perinuclear antineutrophil cytoplasm antibodies (P-ANCA): specificity and clinical associations. *Journal of Autoimmunity*, **6**, 185–95.

Levy, J. B., Hammad, T., Coulthart, A., Dougan, T. and Pusey, C. D. (2004). Clinical features and outcome of patients with both ANCA and anti-GBM antibodies. *Kidney International*, **66**, 1535–40.

Lucena-Fernandes, F., Dalpé, G., Dagenais, P., *et al.* (1995). Detection of anti-neutrophil cytoplasmic antibodies by immunoprecipitation. *Clinical Investigative Medicine*, **18**, 1995.

Lüdemann, J., Utecht, B. and Gross, W. L. (1988). Detection and quantitation of anti-neutrophil cytoplasmic antibodies in Wegener's granulomatosis by ELISA using affinity-purified antigen. *Journal of Immunological Methods*, **114**, 167–74.

Meroni, P. L., Del Papa, N., Raschi, E., Tincani, A., Balestrieri, G. and Youinou, P. (1999). Antiendothelial cell antibodies (AECA): from laboratory curiosity to another useful autoantibody. In *The Decade of Autoimmunity* (ed. Y. Shoenfeld), pp. 285–94. Elsevier Science, Amsterdam.

Moodie, F. D., Leaker, B., Cambridge, G., Totty, N. F. and Sega, A. W. (1993). Alpha-enolase: a novel cytosolic autoantigen in ANCA positive vasculitis. *Kidney International*, **43**, 675–81.

Moscato, S., Pratesi, F., Sabbatini, A., *et al.* (2000). Surface expression of a glycolytic enzyme, a-enolase, recognized by autoantibodies in connective tissue disorders. *European Journal of Immunology*, **30**, 3575–84.

Mustila, A., Paimela, L., Leirisalo-Repo, M., Huhtala, H. and Miettinen, A. (2000). Antineutrophil cytoplasmic antibodies in patients with early rheumatoid arthritis: an early marker of progressive erosive disease. *Arthritis and Rheumatism,* **43**, 1371–77.

Müller-Bérat, N., Minowada, J., Tsuji-Takayama, K., *et al.* (1994). The phylogeny of proteinase 3/myeloblastin, the autoantigen in Wegeren's granulomatosis, and myeloperoxidase as shown by immunohistochemical studies on human leukemic cell lines. *Clinical Immunology and Immunopathology*, **70**, 51–9.

Niles, J. L., McCluskey, R. T., Ahmad, M. E. and Arnaout, M. A. (1989). Wegener's granulomatosis autoantigen is a novel neutrophil serine proteinase. *Blood*, **74**, 1888–93.

Niles, J. L., Böttinger, E. P., Saurina, G. R., *et al.* (1996). The syndrome of lung hemorrhage and nephritis is usually an ANCA-associated condition. *Archives of Internal Medicine,* **156**, 440–5.

Peen, E., Almer, S., Bodemar, G., *et al.* (1993). Anti-lactoferrin antibodies and other types of ANCA in ulcerative colitis, primary sclerosing cholangitis, and Crohn's disease. *Gut*, **34**, 56–62.

Pereira, H. A., Shafer, W. M., Pohl, J., Martin, L. E. and Spitznagel, J. K. (1990). CAP37, a human neutrophil-derived chemotactic factor with monocyte specific activity. *Journal of Clinical Investigation*, **85**, 1468–76.

Preston, G. A., Zarella, C. S., Pendergraft, W. F., *et al.* (2002). Novel effects of neutriophil-derived proteinase 3 and elastase on the vascular endothelium involve *in vivo* cleavage of NF-kappa B and proapoptotic changes in JNK. ERK, and MAPK signalling pathways. *Journal of the American Society for Nephrology*, **13**, 2840–9.

Radford, D. J., Savage, C. O. S. and Nash, G. B. (2000). Treatment of rolling neutrophils with antineutrophil cytoplasmic antibodies causes conversion to firm integrin-mediated adhesion. *Arthritis and Rheumatism*, **43**, 1337–45.

Ralston, D. R., Marsh, C. B., Lowe, M. P. and Wewers, M. D. (1997). Antineutrophil cytoplasmic antibodies induce monocyte IL-8 release. *Journal of Clinical Investigation,* **100**, 1416–24.

Rasmussen, N. and Wiik, A. (1985). Autoimmunity in Wegener's granulomatosis. In *Immunology, Autoimmunity and Transplantation in Otolaryngology: Proceedings for the First International Conference in Immunology and Immunopathology as applied to Otology and Rhinology* (eds J. E. Veldman, J. E. McCabe, E. H. Huizing and N. Mygind), pp. 231–6. Kugler, Utrecht.

Rees, J. D., Lanca, S., Marques, P. V., *et al.* (2006). Prevalence of the antiphospholipid syndrome in primary systemic vasculitis. *Annals of the Rheumatic Diseases*, **65**, 109–11.

Reinhold-Keller, E., de Groot, K., Holl-Ulrich, K., *et al.* (2001). Severe CNS manifestations as the clinical hallmark in generalized Wegener's granulomatosis consistently negative for antineutrophil cytoplasmic antibodies (ANCA). A report of 3 cases and a review of the literature. *Clinical and Experimental Rheumatology*, **19**, 541–9.

Roberts, D. E., Peebles, C., Curd, J. G., Tan, E. M. and Rubin, R. L. (1991). Autoantibodies to native myeloperoxidase in patients with pulmonary hemorrhage and acuterenal failure. *Journal of Clinical Immunology*, **11**, 389–97.

Roozendaal, C., Pogany, K., Horst, G., *et al.* (1999). Does analysis of the antigenic specificities of anti-neutrophil cytoplasmic antibodies contribute to their clinical significance in the inflammatory bowel diseases? *Scandinavian Journal of Gastroenterology*, **34**, 1123–31.

Roubey, R. A. S. (1994). Autoantibodies to the phospholipid-binding plasma proteins: a new view of the lupus anticoagulants and other "antiphospholipid" autoantibodies. *Blood*, **84**, 2854–67.

Rubin, R. L. (2005). Drug-induced lupus. *Toxicology*, **15**, 135–47.

Russell, K. A., Fass, D. N. and Specks, U. (2001). Antineutrophil cytoplasmic antibodies reacting with the pro form of proteinase 3 and disease activity in patients with Wegener's granulomatosis and microscopic polyangiitis. *Arthritis and Rheumatism*, **44**, 463–8.

Rutgers, A., Heeringa, P., Damoiseaux, J. G. and Cohen Tervaert, J. W. (2003). ANCA and anti-GBM antibodies in diagnosis and follow-up of vasculitic disease. *European Journal of Internal Medicine*, **14**, 287–95.

Sable-Fortassou, R., Cohen, P., Mahr, A., *et al.* (2005). Antineutrophil cytoplasmic antibodies and the Churg-Strauss syndrome. *Annals of Internal Medicine*, **143**, 632–8.

Salojin, K. V., Le Tonqueze, M., Nassonov, E. L., *et al.* (1996). Anti-endothelial cell antibodies in patients with various forms of vasculitis. *Clinical and Experimental Rheumatology*, **14**, 163–9.

Savage, C. O. S., Pottinger, B. E., Gaskin, G., Pusey, C. D. and Pearson, J. D. (1992). Autoantibodies developing to myeloperoxidase and proteinase 3 in systemic vasculitis stimulate neutrophil cytotoxicity toward cultured endothelial cells. *American Journal of Pathology*, **141**, 335–42.

Savige, J., Gillis, D., Benson, E., *et al.* (1999). International consensus statement on testing and reporting of antindutrophil cytoplasmic antibodies (ANCA). *American Journal of Clinical Pathology*, **111**, 507–13.

Savige, J., Dimech, W., Frotzler, M., *et al.* (2003). Addendum to the international consensus statement on testing and reporting of antineutrophil cytoplasmic antibodies. Quality control guidelines, comments, and recommendations for testing in other autoimmune diseases. *American Journal of Clinical Pathology*, **120**, 312–8.

Saxena, R., Bygren, P., Arvastson, B. and Wieslander, J. (1995). Circulating autoantibodies as serological marker in the differential diagnosis of pulmonary-renal syndrome. *Journal of Internal Medicine*, **238**, 143–52.

Saxena, R., Bygren, P., Rasmussen, N. and Wieslander, J. (1991). Circulating autoantibodies in patients with extracapillary glomerulonephritis. *Nephrology Dialysis Transplantation*, **6**, 389–97.

Schmitt, W. H., Csernok, E., Flesch, B. K., Hauschild, S. and Gross, W. L. (1993). Autoantibodies directed against lysozyme: a new target antigen for anti-neutrophil cytoplasmic antibodies (ANCA). In *ANCA-associated Vasculitides: Immunological and Clinical Aspects* (ed. W. L. Gross), pp. 267–71. Plenum Press, New York.

Sediva, A., Bartunkova, J., Bartosova, J., Jennette, C., Falk, R. J. and Jethwa, H. S. (2003). Antineutrophil cytoplasmic antibodies directed against bactericidal/permeability-increasing protein detected in children with cystic fibrosis inhibit neutrophil-mediated killing of Pseudomonas aeruginosa. *Microbes and Infections*, **5**, 27–30.

Segelmark, M., Baslund, B., Wieslander, J., *et al.* (1994). Some patients with anti-myeloperoxidase autoantibodies have a C-ANCA pattern. *Clinical and Experimental Immunology*, **96**, 458–65.

Segelmark, M., Phillips, B. D., Hogan, S. L., Falk, R. J. and Jennette, J. C. (2003). Monitoring proteinase 3 antineutrophil cytoplasmic antibodies for detection of relapses in small vessel vasculitis. *Clinical and Diagnostic Laboratory Immunology*, **10**, 769–74.

Segelmark, M., Westman, K. and Wieslander, J. (2000). How and why should we detect ANCA? *Clinical and Experimental Rheumatology*, **18**, 629–35.

Short, A. K., Lockwood, C. M., Bollen, A. and Moguilevsky, N. (1995). Neutrophil native and recombinant myeloperoxidase as antigens in ANCA positive systemic vasculitis. *Clinical and Experimental Immunology*, **102**, 106–11.

Short, A. K. and Lockwood, C. M. (1997). Studies of epitope restriction on myeloperoxidase (MPO), an important antigen in systemic vasculitis. *Clinical and Experimental Immunology*, **110**, 270–6.

Sinico, R. A., Pozzi, C., Radice, A., *et al.* (1993). Clinical significance of antineutrophil cytoplasmic autoantibodies with specificity for lactoferrin in renal diseases. *American Journal of Kidney Diseases*, **22**, 253–60.

Sinico, R. A., DiToma, L., Maggiore, U., *et al.* (2005b). Prevalence and clinical significance of antineutrophil cytoplasmic antibodies in Churg-Strauss syndrome. *Arthritis and Rheumatism*, **52**, 2589–93.

Sinico, R. A., Radice, A., Corace, C., DiToma, L. and Sabadini, E. (2005a) Value of new automated fluorescence immunoassay (ELiA) for PR3 and MPO-ANCA in monitoring disease activity in ANCA-associated systemic vasculitis. *Annals of the New York Academy of Sciences*, **1050**, 185–92.

Sobajima, J., Ozaki, S., Osakada, F., *et al.* (2000). Novel autoantigens of perinuclear anti-neutrophil cytoplasmic antibodies (P-ANCA) in ulcerative colitis: non-histone chromosomal proteins, HMG1 and HMG2. *Clinical and Experimental Immunology*, **107**, 135–40.

Sommarin, Y., Rasmussen, N. and Wieslander, J. (1995). Characterization of monoclonal antibodies to proteinase-3 and application in the study of epitopes for classical anti-neutrophil cytoplasm antibodies. *Experimental Nephrology*, **3**, 249–56.

Specks, U., Fass, D. N., Fautsch, M. P., Hummel, A. M. and Viss, M. A. (1996). Recombinant human proteinase 3, the Wegener's autoantigen, expressed in HMC-1 cells is enzymatically active and recognized by C-ANCA. *Federation of European Biochemical Societies Letters*, **390**, 265–70.

Spickett, G. P. and Broomhead, V. (1995). Formalin fixation and patterns of antineutrophil cytoplasmic antibodies. *Journal of Clinical Pathology*, **48**, 89–90.

Stoffel, M. P., Csernok, E., Herzberg, C., Johnston, T., Caroll, S. F. and Gross, W. L. (1996). Anti-neutrophil cytoplasmic antibodies (ANCA) directed against bactericidal permeability increasing protein (BPI): a new seromarker for inflammatory bowel disease and associated disorders. *Clinical and Experimental Immunology*, **104**, 54–9.

Sturrock, A. B., Franklin, K. F., Rao, G., *et al.* (1992). Structure, chromosomal assignment, and expression of the gene for proteinase 3, the Wegener's granulomatosis autoantigen. *Journal of Biological Chemistry,* **267,** 21193–9.

Sun, J., Fass, D. N., Hudson, J. A., *et al.* (1998b). Capture ELISA based on recombinant PR3 is sensitive for PR3-ANCA testing and allows detection of PR3-ANCA/PR3 immune complexes. *Journal of Immunological Methods,* **211,** 111–23.

Sun, J., Fass, D. N., Viss, M. A., *et al.* (1998a). A proportion of proteinase 3 (PR3)-specific anti-neutrophil cytoplasmic antibodies (ANCA) only react with PR3 after cleavage of its N-terminal activation dipeptide. *Clinical and Experimental Immunology,* **114,** 320–6.

Taylor, K., Pohl, J. and Kinkade, J. M. (1992). Unique autolytic cleavage of human myeloperoxidase. *Journal of Biological Chemistry,* **267,** 25282–8.

Teixera, L., Mahr, A., Jaurguy, F., *et al.* (2005). Low prevalence and poor specificity of antineutrophil cytoplasmic antibodies in tuberculosis. *Rheumatology,* **44,** 247–50.

Terjung, B., Spengler, U., Sauerbruch, T. and Worman, H. J. (2000). "Atypical p-ANCA" in IBD and hepatobiliary disorders react with a 50-kilodalton nuclear envelope protein of neutrophils and myeloid cell lines. *Gastroenterology,* **119,** 310–22.

Utz, P. and Anderson, P. (1998). Posttranslational protein modifications, apoptosis and the bypass of tolerance to autoantigens. *Arthritis and Rheumatism,* **41,** 1152–60.

van der Geld, Y. M., Limburg, P. C. and Kallenberg, C. G. M. (1999). Characterization of monoclonal antibodies to proteinase 3 (PR3) as candidate tools for epitope mapping of human anti-PR3 autoantibodies. *Clinical and Experimental Immunology,* **118,** 487–96.

van der Woude, F. J., Rasmussen, N., Lobatto, S., Wiik, A., Permin, H. and van Es, L. A. (1985). Autoantibodies against neutrophils and monocytes: tool for diagnosis and marker of disease activity in Wegener's granulomatosis. *Lancet,* **i,** 425–9.

Vassilopoulos, D., Niles, JL., Villa-Forte, A., *et al.* (2003). Prevalence of antineutrophil cytoplasmic antibodies in patients with various pulmonary diseases or multiorgan dysfunction. *Arthritis and Rheumatism (Arthritis Care and Research),* **49,** 151–5.

Vecchi, M. L., Radice, A., Renda, F., Mule, G. and Sinico, R. A. (2000). Anti-laminin autoantibodies in ANCA-associated vasculitis. *Nephrology Dialysis Transplantation,* **15,** 1600–3.

Villalta, D., Tonutti, E., Tampoia, M., *et al.* (2004). Analytical and diagnostic accuracy of the ELiA automated enzyme fluoroimmunoassay for antineutrophil cytoplasmic autoantibody detection. *Clinical Chemical Laboratory Medicine,* **42,** 1161–7.

Weidner, S., Neupert, W., Goppelt-Struebe, M. and Rupprecht, H. D. (2001). Antineutrophil cytoplasmic antibodies induce human monocytes to produce oxygen radicals in vitro. *Arthritis and Rheumatism,* **44,** 1698–706.

Westman, K. W., Bygren, P. G., Eilert, I., Wiik, A. and Wieslander, J. (1997). Rapid screening assay for anti-GBM antibody and ANCAs: an important tool for the differential diagnosis of pulmonary-renal syndromes. *Nephrology Dialysis Transplantation,* **12,** 1863–8.

Westman, K. W. A., Selga, D., Bygren, P., *et al.* (1998). Clinical evaluation of a capture ELISA for detection of proteinase-3 antineutrophil cytoplasmic antibody. *Kidney International,* **53,** 1230–6.

Wiik, A. (1980). Granulocyte-specific antinuclear antibodies. Possible significance for the pathogenesis, clinical features and diagnosis of rheumatoid arthritis. *Allergy,* **35,** 263–89.

Wiik, A. (1989). Delineation of a standard procedure for indirect immunofluorescence detection of ANCA. *Acta Pathologica et Microbiologica Scandinavica,* **97** (Suppl. 6), 12–3.

Wiik, A. (2001) Clinical use of serological tests for ANCA: what do the studies say? *Rheumatic Disease Clinics of North America,* **27,** 799–813.

Wiik, A. (2002a). Neutrophil-specific autoantibodies in chronic inflammatory bowel diseases. *Autoimmunity Reviews,* **1,** 67–72.

Wiik, A. (2002b). Antineutrophil cytoplasmic antibodies (ANCAs) and ANCA testing. In *Manual of Clinical Laboratory Immunology,* 6th edn (eds N. R. Rose, R. G. Hamilton, B. Detrick), pp. 981–6. ASM Press, Washington D. C.

Wiik, A., Brimnes, J. and Heegaard, N. H. H. (1999). Distinct differences in autoantigen specificity of anti-neutrophil cytoplasm antibodies in systemic vasculitides and other inflammatory diseases. *Israel Medical Association Journal,* **1,** 4–7.

Wiik, A. and van der Woude, F. J. (1990). The new ACPA/ANCA nomenclature. *Netherland Journal of Medicine,* **36,** 107–9.

Wiik, A., Gordon, T. P., Kavanaugh, A., *et al.* (2004). Cutting edge diagnostics in rheumatology: the role of patients, clinicians, and laboratory scientists in optimising the use of autoimmune serology. *Arthritis and Rheumatism (Arthritis Care and Research),* **51,** 291–8.

Williams, R. C., Staud, R., Malone, C. C., *et al.* (1994). Epitopes on proteinase-3 recognized by antibodies from patients with Wegener's granulomatosis. *Journal of Immunology,* **152,** 4722–37.

Wilson, W. A., Gharavi, A. E. and Koike, T., *et al.* (1999). International consensus statement on preliminary classification criteria for definite antiphospholipid syndrome: report of an international workshop. *Arthritis and Rheumatism,* **42,** 1309–11.

Xiao, H., Heeringa, P., Hu, P., *et al.* (2002). Antineutrophil cytoplasmic autoantibodies specific for myeloperoxidase cause glomerulonephritis and vasculitis in mice. *Journal of Clinical Investigation,* **110,** 955–63.

Xiao, H., Heeringa, P., Liu, Z., *et al.* (2005). The role of neutrophils in the induction of glomerulonephritis by anti-myeloperoxidase antibodies. *American Journal of Pathology,* **167,** 39–45.

Yang, J. J., Tuttle, R., Falk, R. J. and Jennette, J. C. (1996). Frequency of anti-bactericidal/permeability-increasing protein (BPI) and anti-azurocidin in in patients with renal disease. *Clinical and Experimental Immunology,* **104,** 125–31.

Yang, J. J., Preston, G. A., Pendergraft, W. F., *et al.* (2001). Internalization of proteinase 3 is concomitant with endothelial cell apoptosis and internalization of myeloperoxidase with generation of intracellular oxidants. *American Journal of Pathology,* **158,** 581–92.

Yang, Y. H., Lai, H. J., Huang, C. M., Wang, L. C., Lin, Y. T. and Chiang, B. L. (2004). Sera from children with active Henoch-Schonlein purpura can enhance the production of interleukin 8 by human umbilical venous endothelial cells. *Annals of the Rheumatic Diseases,* **63,** 1511–3.

Yu, F., Zhao, M. H., Zhang, Y. and Wang, H. Y. (2005). Anti-endothelial cell antibodies (AECA) in patients with propylthiouracil (PTU)-induced ANCA positive vasculitis are associated with disease activity. *Clinical and Experimental Immunology,* **139,** 569–74.

Zhao, C., Zhao, M.-H., Xin, G. and Hai-yan, W. (2005). Characteristics and prognosis of Chinese patients with anti-glomerular basement membrane disease. *Nephron Clincal Practice,* **99,** c49–c55.

Zhao, M. H., Jayne, D. R. W., Ardiles, L. G., Culley, F., Hodson, M. E. and Lockwood, C. M. (1996). Autoantibodies against bactericidal/permeability-increasing protein in patients with cystic fibrosis. *Quarterly Journal of Medicine,* **89,** 259–65.

Zhao, M. H., Jones, S. J. and Lockwood, C. M. (1995). Bactericidal/permeability-increasing protein (BPI) is an important antigen for anti-neutrophil cytoplasmic antibodies (ANCA) in vasculitis. *Clinical and Experimental Immunology,* **99,** 49–56.

CHAPTER 7

Pathogenesis of vasculitis

Gene V. Ball and S. Louis Bridges, Jr

The pathogenesis of vasculitis is complex, and our understanding of it is an evolving process, as is true of almost every human disease. Major participants in the pathogenetic mechanisms of vasculitic diseases and syndromes are listed in Table 7.1. Gross and microscopic pathologic findings in various forms of vasculitis, which provide the basis for many of the current hypotheses on the causes and mechanisms of vasculitis, are discussed in Chapter 9. Pathologic findings and clinical responses of patients with vasculitis to anti-inflammatory and immunosuppressive therapy support the concept that immunologic mechanisms play an active role in the pathogenesis of vasculitic diseases. Proposed mechanisms include: (1) pathogenic immune complex formation and deposition in vessel walls; (2) autoantibodies such as antineutrophil cytoplasmic antibodies (ANCA) and antiendothelial cell antibodies (AECA); (3) cellular and molecular immune responses involving cytokines and adhesion molecules; (4) granuloma formation; and (5) damaged or altered endothelial cell function due to infectious organisms, tumors, or toxins. Immune complexes appear to initiate the inflammation of cutaneous small-vessel (leukocytoclastic) vasculitis related to infections and medications, of Henoch–Schönlein purpura (HSP), polyarteritis nodosa (PAN), and of some cryoglobulinemias. ANCAs are probably major participants in the pathogenesis of so-called pauci-immune vasculitis, and pathologic responses of T cells may be involved in others. Rapid expansion of our knowledge of the molecules that regulate interactions among circulating and infiltrating cells of the immune system and endothelial cells promises greater insight into the pathogenesis of vessel damage, and potential sites for drug intervention. The underpinnings of applied clinical research on vasculitis are described in detail in separate chapters focused on hypersensitivity (Chapter 3); the biology of endothelial cells (Chapter 4); complement (Chapter 5); and autoantibodies, including ANCA (Chapter 6). Animal models pertinent to vasculitis are discussed in Chapter 8.

In this chapter we focus on general pathogenetic mechanisms as they apply to the vasculitides. The discussion is organized as follows: (1) immune complexes and complement in vasculitis; (2) ANCA; (3) cytokines, growth factors, and chemokines; (4) AECA; (5) drug-induced vasculitis; (6) infectious agents; (7) tumor cell-mediated vascular damage; and (8) cell-mediated immune responses and granuloma formation. Chapters dealing with specific vasculitis diseases and syndromes, which include discussions germane to

pathogenetic aspects, are: giant cell arteritis (GCA); Takayasu's arteritis (TA); PAN and microscopic polyangiitis (MPA); Kawasaki's disease (KD); Wegener's granulomatosis (WG); Churg–Strauss syndrome (CSS); vasculitis of primary connective tissue diseases; Behçet's syndrome (BS); CNS vasculitis; thromboangiitis obliterans (TAO); cutaneous small-vessel vasculitis (CSVV); and cryoglobulinemic vasculitis.

Immune complexes and complement in vasculitis

Deposition of immune complexes in blood vessels has long been implicated as an instigating mechanism of vascular inflammation. Animal models of serum sickness and the Arthus reaction provide most of the support for this role of immune complexes. In the acute serum sickness model, the single injection of a large amount of a heterologous serum protein is followed in 10–14 days by arteritis, glomerulonephritis, and endocarditis. The vasculitic lesions, which appear when circulating antigen–antibody complexes are formed in slight antigen excess, contain antigen, immunoglobulin, and complement (Dixon et al. 1958). After immune complexes deposit, the vasculitis of acute serum sickness resembles PAN histologically with segmental infiltration of arterial walls by neutrophils and mononuclear cells, intimal proliferation, and fibrinoid necrosis. Antigen has not been detected by fluorescent antibody techniques in glomeruli, arteries, or the endocardium prior to immune complex deposition, suggesting that in situ formation is not the mechanism involved, as it is in the Arthus reaction (Dixon et al. 1958).

Vasculitis is absent from animal models of chronic serum sickness. There is a variable host response to intravenous injections of foreign protein given daily for several weeks. The majority of animals rapidly clear antigen, others acquire immunologic tolerance, and 10–20% form immune complexes that are slowly removed from the circulation, resulting in chronic glomerulonephritis (Christian and Sergent 1976). An explanation of the difference between acute and chronic serum sickness with respect to the development of arteritis has not been forthcoming.

A likely explanation is that other factors contributing to the quantity and quality of the host immune response account for the inconsistent expression of vasculitis in animal and human immune complex disease. Cytokines and adhesion molecules expressed by

Table 7.1 Participants in the pathogenesis of vasculitis

Cells

   T lymphocytes

   B lymphocytes

   Monocytes/ macrophages

   Platelets

   NK cells

   Eosinophils

   Neutrophils

   Endothelial cells

Growth factors

   Vascular endothelial growth factor

   Platelet-derived growth factor

   Granulocyte-colony stimulating factor

   Macrophage-colony stimulating factor

Autoantibodies

   Antineutrophil cytoplasmic antibodies

   Antiendothelial cell antibodies

Complement components (see Chapter 5)

Cytokines and chemokines

   Cytokines

   Tumor necrosis factor (TNF)

   Interferon-gamma (IFN-γ)

   Interleukin (IL)-1, IL-1Ra

   IL-2

   IL-4

   IL-6

   IL-10

   IL-12

   IL-15

   IL-18

   Chemokines

   IL-8

   RANTES

Adhesion molecules/ cellular receptors

   β_2-integrin

   E-selectin

   ICAM-1

   VCAM-1

   Fcγ receptors

Drugs (see Chapter 39)

Infectious agents (see Chapters 37, 40, 42, and 45)

neutrophils and endothelial cells are undoubtedly necessary for generation of the inflammatory response in immune vasculitis. The role of antibodies in specific pathologic processes is uncertain. The mere presence of circulating immune complexes is not sufficient to produce vasculitis, as indicated by the paucity of vasculitis

in animals injected with preformed immune complexes (McCluskey and Fienberg 1983). Cochrane and colleagues demonstrated that the release of vasoactive amines from platelets is necessary for the tissue deposition of immune complexes in experimental acute serum sickness (Cochrane 1971). Pretreatment with antihistamines or depletion of platelets clearly suppressed the deposition of immune complexes and prevented vasculitis. Physical properties of the immune complexes are also important as only those with a sedimentation coefficient greater than 19S are deposited in vessel walls (Cochrane 1971). Other specific factors that influence their proinflammatory nature include the ability of the immune complex to activate complement, the antigen–antibody combining ratio, and structural and hemodynamic differences between various blood vessels (Haynes 1992). The tendency for immune complexes to deposit at vessel branching sites, heart valves, and dependent areas is partly explained by hydrostatic forces.

Detection of immunoglobulin and complement in human vasculitic lesions by immunofluorescent or immunochemical techniques provides circumstantial evidence of immune complex mediation of disease. These proteins are most readily detected in cutaneous vasculitis, but inconsistently in systemic vasculitis. Definitive support for a pathogenetic role for immune complexes requires the detection of a relevant antigen and specific antibody simultaneously in the circulation and in sites of vascular injury. This has been a fruitless pursuit in most cases of vasculitis because the inciting antigen is seldom known, and it is not usually possible to elute sufficient material from vasculitic lesions to isolate and quantify specific antibodies (McCluskey and Fienberg 1983). Failure to detect immunoglobulin in vasculitic lesions argues against their pathogenic role only when early lesions are examined since neutrophils have been shown to degrade immune complexes within 24–48 hours after their deposition (Cochrane *et al.* 1959).

After treatment of bone marrow failure with horse antithymocyte globulin, serum sickness appeared, coincident with increased circulating immune complexes, decreased serum complement, and the localization of immunoglobulin and complement in affected small cutaneous blood vessels (Lawley *et al.* 1984). Prospective evaluation of human serum sickness has confirmed the immunologic observations made in experimental animals. Current evidence also implicates immune complex deposition as the primary pathogenic mechanism in some forms of vasculitis such as HSP and vasculitis associated with hepatitis B, hepatitis C, and cryoglobulinemia, which primarily affects small- or medium-sized vessels (Hoffman 1997).

In the 1970s, persistent hepatitis B infection was linked to some cases of PAN and cryoglobulinemic vasculitis (Gocke *et al.* 1970; Levo *et al.* 1977). Several vasculitic syndromes, cutaneous and systemic, have been associated with hepatitis B infection. Hepatitis B surface antigen (HBsAg)-antibody complexes have been found in the circulation (Gocke *et al.* 1970; Trepo *et al.* 1974), and deposits of HBsAg, immunoglobulin, and complement have been found in lesions of muscular arteries (Gocke *et al.* 1970; Michalak 1978), dermal vessels (Gower *et al.* 1978), glomeruli (Combes *et al.* 1971), and vasa nervorum (Tsukada *et al.* 1983). Hypocomplementemia may accompany vasculitis associated with hepatitis B infection, and cryoglobulins have been shown to contain HBsAg and particles resembling the virus (Levo *et al.* 1977). Several investigators were able to elute all of the HBsAg and part of the immunoglobulin from vascular deposits by treatment with buffers known to dissociate antigen–antibody bonds but not with phosphate buffered saline, arguing against non-specific binding to pre-existing lesions (Michalak 1978). Substantial evidence therefore correlates the immunopathologic events of hepatitis B-associated vasculitis with experimental serum sickness. In addition, the causative relationship between hepatitis C and cryoglobulinemic vasculitis is well-established (Agnello *et al.* 1992, Cacoub *et al.* 2002) (see Chapter 41).

For years, the presumed pathogenesis of leukocytoclastic vasculitis (also referred to as cutaneous small-vessel vasculitis, see Chapter 39) has been that circulating immune complexes are deposited in the small blood vessels of the skin, with inflammation occurring after complement activation. The ability of immune complexes to trigger polymorphonuclear cells and induce production of tumor necrosis factor-alpha (TNF-α), perforin, and Fas ligand has been shown *ex vivo* (Nishimura *et al.* 2004). Activated neutrophils release collagenase and elastase which, in conjunction with free oxygen radicals, result in necrosis of vessels (Sindrilaru *et al.* 2006). Cytokines from T cells and endothelial cells are involved, and various antibodies such as those reacting with endothelial cells may contribute to the complex phenomena of inflammation (Claudy 1998). Immunoglobulins and complement are seen on direct immunofluorescence of vasculitic skin lesions. Circulating immune complexes may be detected but serum complement levels are not usually decreased (Kammer *et al.* 1980; Sunderkotter *et al.* 2001).

Intradermal injection of histamine and epinephrine into uninvolved skin of patients with cutaneous vasculitis reproduces the histopathologic findings of spontaneous lesions. Although deposition of immunoreactants can be demonstrated in normal-appearing skin of patients with leukocytoclastic vasculitis, increased deposition of immunoglobulin and complement follows the injection of histamine in a few hours, but neither is detected after 24 hours (Braverman and Yen 1975; Gower *et al.* 1977). Using direct immunofluorescence, Grunwald and colleagues were able to demonstrate immunoreactants in skin biopsies of vasculitis of various causes and of early, mature, and healing stages. Biopsies from 92% of patients were positive, in increasing concentration, for fibrinogen, albumin, IgG, IgM, IgA, and C4 (Grunwald *et al.* 1997). Gower and colleagues also demonstrated that the deposition of immune complexes and complement precedes the inflammatory infiltrate (Gower *et al.* 1977).

IgA plays a primary role in Henoch–Schönlein purpura (see Chapter 40). IgA deposits have been found in vasculitic lesions obtained simultaneously from skin, kidney, and small intestine (Stevenson *et al.* 1982). IgA, C3, and fibrin have been found together in affected skin and glomeruli (Giangiacomo and Tsai 1977). There are increased numbers of IgA-producing lymphocytes in HSP (Kondo *et al.* 1992; Kuno-Sakai *et al.* 1979), and high levels of circulating IgA-containing immune complexes (Kauffmann *et al.* 1980). Sera from children with active HSP contain IgA antibodies which bind with endothelial cells and enhance production of IL-8 via the MEK/ERK signaling pathway (Yang *et al.* 2006). The data are consistent with the concept of impaired clearance of IgA immune complexes by complement and the reticuloendothelial system. IgA immune complexes do not activate the classical complement pathway and are ineffective in fixing C3 (Schifferli *et al.* 1986). Indeed, there has been little evidence of classical pathway activation in HSP, as C1q, C3 and C4 are usually not depressed

(Garcia-Fuentes *et al.* 1978). Waxman and colleagues have also shown that IgA complexes bind poorly to erythrocytes, are inefficiently cleared by the liver, and become deposited in the kidney and lungs (Waxman *et al.* 1986). The membrane-attack complex, C5b-9, is a component of IgA and C3 deposits in vessel walls of the skin, in capillary walls and in mesangium of glomeruli of patients with HSP nephritis (Kawana and Nishiyama 1992). C5b-9 appears to damage dermal vascular endothelial cells in the absence of polymorphonuclear cells.

The frequent conjunction of genetic deficiencies of complement and immune complex diseases implies an important pathogenetic interaction between the two (Genel *et al.* 2005) (see Chapter 5). Activation of the classical and alternative complement pathways results in the adherence of C3b to immune complexes, facilitating their clearance by the reticuloendothelial system and modifying their structure and biologic activity. An intact classical complement pathway is required for this binding of C3b, which inhibits precipitation of the complexes. Activation of the alternative pathway may solubilize precipitated immune complexes (Miller and Nussenzweig 1975; Schifferli *et al.* 1986). This conceivably allows for diffusion of antigen–antibody complexes from the site of their formation and minimizes the local inflammatory response (Schifferli *et al.* 1986).

The C3b component of immune complexes binds to a specific receptor, complement receptor type 1 (CR1). This binding prevents immune complex interaction with other structures such as vascular endothelium. As much as 90–95% of the CR1 in humans is located on the surface of erythrocytes (Schifferli *et al.* 1986), but it is also found on polymorphonuclear leukocytes, macrophages, B lymphocytes, some T lymphocytes, dendritic cells in germinal centers, and glomerular podocytes. Immune complexes bound to CR1 on red blood cells are then removed from the circulation by spleen and liver macrophages (Cornacoff *et al.* 1983). CR1 is also a potent inhibitor of the complement cascade, serving as a cofactor for the enzyme (Factor 1) that inactivates C3b by cleavage (Fearon 1984; Medof *et al.* 1982).

Thus, experimental evidence corroborates the critical role of complement in processing immune complexes so that they remain soluble and can be transported to tissue macrophages for elimination. There are several plausible reasons for failure of the normal processes for eliminating immune complexes that could lead to the development of vasculitis and other manifestations of immune complex disease: (1) depletion or deficiency of complement components; (2) failure of various antibody classes within immune complexes to bind complement; (3) depletion or blockade of CR1; and (4) impairment of tissue macrophage function (Haynes 1992). There is a complex interaction between complement components and activation products, and endothelial cells which stimulates their proinflammatory status (Fischetti and Tedesco 2006). Acosta *et al.* (2004) have reviewed complement and complement regulatory proteins focusing on blood vessels and vasculitis diseases. Ghebrehiwet *et al.* (2006) have proposed a model of inflammation in which factors such as immune complexes, viruses, and bacteria convert the vascular endothelium into a procoagulant and proinflammatory surface and enhance expression of cell surface molecules including gC1qR, a component of the receptor for the globular heads of C1q. This might lead to high affinity C1q binding and cell production of proinflammatory factors and generation of bradykinin and possibly coagulation.

Antineutrophil cytoplasmic antibodies (ANCA)

There is a wealth of emerging literature on the role of ANCA in systemic vasculitis. Jennette and Falk, who first described pANCA in patients with necrotizing glomerulonephritis and microscopic polyangiitis, and who identified the antigen as myeloperoxidase (MPO), have summarized their views of the role of ANCA in pathogenesis, as well as the evidence supporting their pathogenicity (Jennette and Falk 1998). A partial listing of the clinical evidence they adduce includes: (1) the frequent occurrence of ANCA in the sera of patients with vasculitis and necrotizing crescentic glomerulonephritis; (2) the response of these diseases to immunosuppressive drugs; (3) their pauci-immune nature; and (4) the induction of ANCA and vasculitis by medications such as propylthiouracil and hydralazine which may disappear after cessation of the offending medication. Thus, there is considerable evidence supporting a role for ANCA in pathogenesis of vasculitis diseases. Current recommendations for ANCA testing, methodologies, and clinical utility in patients with suspected or known vasculitic syndromes are discussed in detail in Chapter 6.

Antigenic specificity and diagnostic utility

ANCA have been thought to be specific for cytoplasmic antigens located in primary granules of neutrophils and lysosomes of monocytes; however, Witko-Sarsat and colleagues identified proteinase 3 (PR3), a major target antigen, in plasma membrane secretory vesicles (Witko-Sarsat *et al.* 1999). By indirect immunofluorescence (IIF), ANCA are identified as cytoplasmic (cANCA), with coarse granular staining of cytoplasm; perinuclear (pANCA), with staining of the nucleus and perinuclear area; and atypical ANCA. The antigens responsible for cytoplasmic IIF are usually PR3 and those detected as perinuclear are often MPO. Antibodies to other neutrophil constituents such as elastase, cathepsin G, lysozyme, and lactoferrin produce pANCA (or atypical pattern); but the ANCA of diagnostic significance for vasculitis are those directed against PR3 and MPO. The antigen epitopes of ANCA have recently been analyzed by Erdbrugger *et al.* (2006). These investigators have found that MPO-ANCA do not target a single epitope, but rather a small number of regions of MPO, primarily in the carboxy-terminus of the heavy chain.

It is important to keep in mind that positive tests for ANCA are found in disorders other than vasculitis. ANCA directed against bactericidal/permeability-increasing protein have been described in patients with inflammatory bowel disease, cystic fibrosis, and rheumatic diseases, and ANCA reacting with azurocidin have been found in 18–25% of sera from patients with WG, cystic fibrosis, and chronic active hepatitis (Cooper *et al.* 2000). pANCA was detected, using a commercial antibody panel, in 70% of 54 children and young adults with ulcerative colitis and in 18% of 81 children and young adults with Crohn's disease (Zholudev *et al.* 2004). A study from India detected ANCA in 30% of 70 patients with tuberculosis; in 7% of 30 with interstitial lung disease; and in 4% of 100 normal controls (Pradhan *et al.* 2004). By ELISA analysis, 47.6% of the ANCAs were anti-MPO; 28.6% were anti-PR3; and 19.1% were antilactoferrin. It should be noted that in this study, the prevalence of antinuclear antibodies and antihistone antibodies was unusually high (24.3% and 21.4% respectively), suggesting possible drug induction of these antibodies and ANCA. Similarly, a study from Mexico showed that 44% of 45 patients with tuberculosis were ANCA positive; 40% were PR3-ANCA positive by ELISA testing (Flores-Suarez *et al.* 2003). The ANCA results were not related to stage of disease, comorbidities, or known ANCA-inducing pharmacotherapy.

Pathogenicity of ANCA

There is compelling clinical and experimental evidence that MPO-ANCA are pathogenic in vasculitis, and laboratory evidence that PR3-ANCA can amplify locally produced inflammation. The clinical evidence is represented by transplacental transfer of MPO-ANCA from a mother to a 33-week gestational age neonate whose cord blood contained IgG MPO levels identical to that of the mother's serum, and which resulted in neonatal pulmonary hemorrhage and renal disease. The neonate was treated with high dose glucocorticoids and exchange transfusion, and became asymptomatic (Bansal and Tobin 2004).

The first definitive, controlled demonstration that MPO-ANCA can cause vasculitis and glomerulonephritis was reported in 2002 by Xiao and colleagues. MPO knockout mice were immunized with mouse MPO. Splenocytes from these mice were injected into Rag2 knockout (Rag2$^{-/-}$) mice lacking B and T lymphocytes. The recipient mice developed necrotizing glomerulonephritis and systemic necrotizing vasculitis. Furthermore, purified anti-MPO IgG injected into Rag2$^{-/-}$ mice and wild type mice caused necrotizing glomerulonephritis (Xiao *et al.* 2002).

Another murine model for anti-MPO mediated glomerulonephritis and vasculitis which documents the pathogenic potential of ANCA has been described by Schreiber *et al.* (2006). This study used MPO knockout mice (Mpo$^{-/-}$) to show that bone marrow-derived cells are sufficient targets to cause anti-MPO disease in the absence of MPO in other cell types. Chimeric Mpo$^{-/-}$ mice with circulating MPO-positive neutrophils developed pauci-immune necrotizing and crescentic glomerulonephritis whereas chimeric Mpo$^{+/+}$ mice with circulating MPO-negative neutrophils did not. Thus, bone marrow-derived cells are not only sufficient but also necessary for induction of anti-MPO disease. Experimental evidence for pathogenicity of PR3-ANCA in vasculitis has not been obtained, primarily because ANCA epitopes on human PR3 are not shared by the murine homolog (Wiesner *et al.* 2005). Pfister *et al.* made ANCAs against recombinant murine PR3 in PR3/neutrophil elastase-deficient mice. These ANCAs, which recognized the mouse PR3 antigen on the surface of neutrophils, were then analyzed in a model of local inflammation. They found that intradermal injection of TNF-α produced a stronger subcutaneous panniculitis in the presence of passively transferred systemic PR3-ANCA than in the presence of control immune serum. Liposaccharide (LPS)-primed wild type mice that were treated with PR3 ANCA did not develop more vigorous inflammation of the lungs or kidneys than mice treated with control immune serum (Pfister *et al.* 2004).

In contrast to the other systemic vasculitides, there is little, if any, direct evidence for a direct pathogenic role of ANCA in CSS (Hellmich *et al.* 2005). Pagnoux *et al.* (2007) have suggested that ANCA are probably more important in the vasculitic manifestations of CSS, for example glomerulonephritis, while eosinophil tissue infiltration and associated cytotoxicity are responsible for non-vasculitis manifestations, such as cardiomyopathy.

The mechanisms by which ANCA-expressing B lymphocytes are generated are poorly understood. It is possible that there are aberrant pathways in which B cell selection occurs, resulting in proliferation of autoantibody-producing B cells and plasma cells. In WG, as in rheumatoid arthritis (Zhang and Bridges 2001), auto-immune thyroid disease (Weyand *et al.* 2001), and other autoimmune inflammatory conditions, there are germinal center-like structures in the inflamed non-lymphoid tissue. In WG, these structures form within granulomas, suggesting antigen-driven B cell maturation; the PR3 autoantigen, the target for autoreactive B and T cells, is also expressed in granulomas. The expressed immunoglobulin gene repertoire from WG lesions indicates a predominance of V_H3+ B cells with affinity to PR3 as well as to the *S. aureus* B cell superantigen SPA (Voswinkel *et al.* 2005). Hence, *S. aureus* SPA or another antigen might drive the maturation of PR3-specific B cells within the WG lesion, suggesting that granulomatous tissue could function similar to lymphoid tissue.

As reviewed by Jennette *et al.* (2006), experimental studies from many laboratories have shown that both PR3-ANCA and MPO-ANCA activate neutrophils to release mediators of acute inflammation. Figure 7.1 illustrates a hypothetical sequence of pathogenic events that could result in ANCA-mediated vascular inflammation. We will use this model to discuss the following aspects of the role

of ANCAs in the pathogenesis of vasculitis: (1) cytokines and other priming factors that induce neutrophils to express ANCA antigens on the cell surface; (2) activation of neutrophils by binding of ANCA antigens to ANCAs; (3) interaction of ANCA-activated neutrophils with endothelial cells; and (4) release of toxic factors that cause apoptosis and necrosis.

Cytokines and other factors that induce neutrophils to express ANCA antigens on the cell surface

Several studies have analyzed expression of membrane PR3 in neutrophils and monocytes. Van Rossum *et al.* (2003) have shown that PR3 expression on resting neutrophils and the percentage of neutrophils expressing membrane PR3 (mPR3) is stable over time for a given individual, suggesting a genetic determinant. They have also shown that patients with ANCA-positive vasculitis have increased constitutive expression of mPR3 on resting neutrophils compared to healthy controls. High levels of mPR3 on resting neutrophils are a potential risk factor for relapse in persons with PR3-ANCA-positive vasculitis, possibly through increasing the susceptibility of neutrophils to binding of ANCA, leading to activation. Ohlsson *et al.* (2005) found that circulating monocytes from patients with

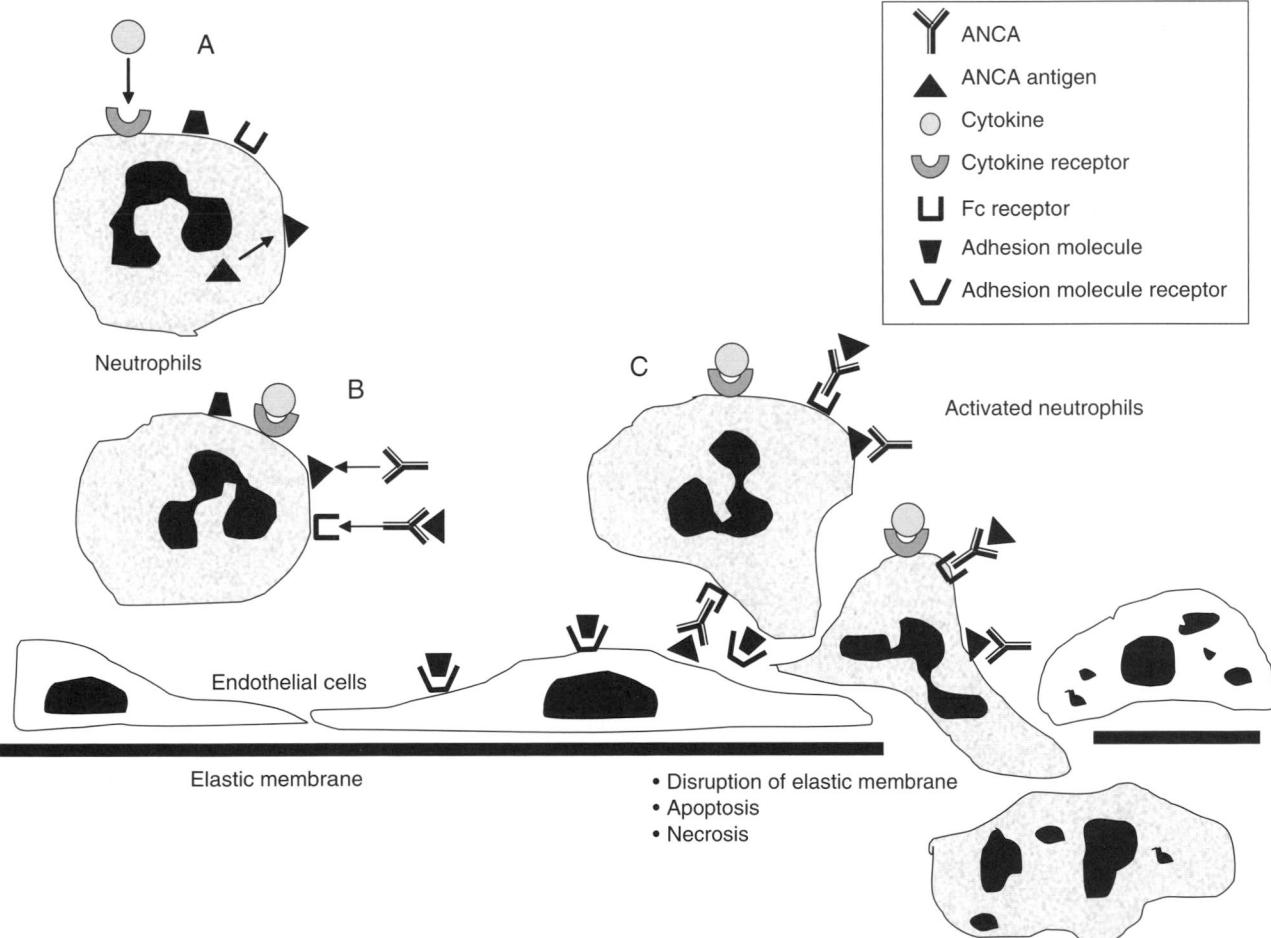

Figure 7.1 Events in the pathogenesis of ANCA small-vessel vasculitis that have been observed *in vitro*. (A) Cytokines or other priming factors induce neutrophils to express more ANCA antigens at the cell surface, where they are available for binding to ANCA. (B) ANCA binds to ANCA antigens, which activates neutrophils by both Fc receptor engagement and direct Fab'2 ligation. (C) Neutrophils that have been activated by ANCA interact with endothelial cells via adhesion molecules and release toxic factors that cause apoptosis and necrosis. From Jennette *et al.* (2006) with permission.

systemic vasculitis display increased PR3 transcription compared to healthy controls and patients with SLE. Schreiber *et al.* (2004) reported a bimodal distribution of cells expressing membrane PR3, and that cells expressing low amounts of membrane PR3 can be distinguished from cells with high expression. PR3-high neutrophils showed more superoxide generation, more degranulation, and more PI$_3$-K/Akt activation compared to mPR3-low neutrophils. There were no differences in β_2-integrin, FcγRIIa, and FcγRIII expression with respect to the PR3 subtype, and no differences in immobilization of PR3-containing granules or migration through fibronectin.

Muller Kobold *et al.* (1998) have found increased expression of PR3 on neutrophils from patients with active WG but not from those with quiescent disease or healthy controls. The expression correlated with disease activity. They concluded that the availability of PR3, and the interaction of ANCA and PR3 are central to WG. The same investigators reported that markers of monocyte activation, including neopterin, IL-6, and CD11b, were increased with active disease (Muller Kobold *et al.* 1999b). Activated monocytes release significant amounts of the neutrophil chemoattractant IL-8, when exposed to ANCA (Ralston *et al.* 1997).

Treatment with tumor necrosis factor (TNF) can cause neutrophils to express both MPO and PR3 on their cell surface where they may interact with ANCA. This interaction stimulates a respiratory burst and degranulation in the primed neutrophils (Charles *et al.* 1991; Falk *et al.* 1990). It has also been shown that granulocyte-macrophage colony-stimulating factor (GM-CSF), but not granulocyte colony-stimulating factor (G-CSF), increases PR3 membrane expression on intact neutrophils as well as those primed with TNF (Hellmich *et al.* 2000). In addition, the increased deposition of IL-18 in renal biopsies from ANCA-positive vasculitis led Hewins *et al.* (2006) to analyze the role of IL-18. They found that superoxide production by ANCA activated polymorphonuclear leukocytes (PMN) primed with IL-18 comparably to TNF. IL-18 primed, ANCA-induced superoxide production was unaffected by anti-TNF antibody (which abrogated TNF priming), implicating an independent role for IL-18 priming.

Cytokine priming of neutrophils, as might occur with infection, may not be necessary for translocation of primary granules to their surface. This translocation occurs as well during neutrophil apoptosis, and experiments have shown that ANCA-positive sera will react with the apoptotic neutrophils (Gilligan *et al.* 1996; Yang *et al.* 2000). For ANCA-activated neutrophils to cause vasculitis, they must adhere to and injure endothelial cells, as has been shown to occur *in vitro* using cultured human umbilical vein endothelial cells (HUVEC) (Ewert *et al.* 1992; Savage *et al.* 1992). There is evidence that ANCA can directly activate neutrophils to become adherent to vessel walls (Radford *et al.* 2000). Incubation of endothelial cells with anti-PR3 antibodies leads to an increase in VCAM-1 expression, and increased adhesion of T lymphocytes to the cells. Thus, ANCA can contribute to regulation of T lymphocyte migration (Mayet *et al.* 1996).

In this regard, it is of interest that the Chapel Hill group did not find transcripts for PR3 or MPO in human endothelial cells from umbilical vein or artery, or from lung microvasculature. They concluded that endothelial cell presentation of these antigens was not involved in the pathogenesis of ANCA-associated vasculitis (Pendergraft *et al.* 2000). Schwarting *et al.* found PR3 mRNA and PR3 protein in distal tubular epithelial cells and glomerular epithelial cells in normal kidney tissue and in crescentic glomerulonephritis. There was restriction of strong glomerular PR3 mRNA expression to the site of cellular crescents in patients with WG, and they concluded that the glomerular expression of PR3 is associated with crescent formation in WG (Schwarting *et al.* 2000).

Rarok *et al.* (2002) tested the hypothesis that the presence of PR3 on the surface of non-stimulated neutrophils enables interaction with PR3-ANCA and influences clinical manifestations of the disease. They compared mPR3 expression on neutrophils of 89 WG patients in complete remission to that in 72 healthy controls. There was an increased percentage of mPR3-positive neutrophils and an elevated level of mPR3 expression in WG patients compared to healthy individuals. Furthermore, within WG patients, an elevated level of mPR3 expression was significantly associated with an increased risk for relapse, supporting the hypothesis that PR3 expression on membrane of neutrophils plays a role in the pathophysiology of PR3-ANCA-associated vasculitis.

There is evidence that circulating ANCA and antiendothelial cell antibodies (AECA) might directly activate endothelial cells to express E-selectin and IL-6. Immunoglobulin preparations from 28 patients with WG or MPA (17 of whom were anti-PR3-positive) were incubated with HUVEC. One sample up-regulated E-selectin expression and four induced both IL-6 production and E-selectin up-regulation (Muller Kobold *et al.* 1999a).

Drugs may play a role in inducing ANCA and vasculitis (see below). It is theoretically possible that these drugs prime cellular expression of ANCA antigens, although there are no data to currently support this hypothesis.

Activation of neutrophils by binding of ANCA antigens to ANCA

In refutation of Abdel-Salam *et al.* (2004), van Rossum *et al.* (2005) presented evidence that human PR3-ANCA specifically bind to PMN that express PR3 on their membrane. Binding of IgG was concentration dependent as shown by dilution of plasma and serum. Double staining for PR3 and IgG demonstrated that IgG in plasma or serum from PR3-ANCA-positive patients only bound to those PMN that expressed PR3 and not to PMN that lacked PR3 membrane expression. Two recent reviews have focused on the mechanisms of neutrophil activation by ANCA (Rarok *et al.* 2003; Reumaux *et al.* 2004). An obligatory role for neutrophils in the pathogenesis of murine anti-MPO antibody-induced glomerulonephritis was demonstrated by Xiao *et al.* (2005). Mice were injected with antibodies specific for mouse MPO, which caused necrotizing glomerulonephritis with neutrophil infiltration at the sites of glomerular necrosis and crescent formation. Depletion of circulating neutrophils with rat monoclonal antibodies abrogated anti-MPO IgG induced lesions. Van Rossum *et al.* (2005) have shown PR3-ANCA in undiluted serum or plasma from PR3-ANCA-positive WG patients bind to TNF-primed and PMA-stimulated PMN that express PR3 on their membrane.

ANCA activation of neutrophils requires ligation of FcγRIIa receptor, and ANCA also bind to FcγRIIIb. Pretreatment of TNF-primed neutrophils with antibodies against FcγRII and FcγRIII inhibited MPO-ANCA and PR3-ANCA induced superoxide generation, confirming that FcγR ligation is involved in ANCA-mediated neutrophil activation. However, although stimulation of TNF-primed neutrophils by conventional FcγR ligation, either using antibody mediated cross linking of FcγR or aggregated IgG, induced phospholipase D activation, ANCA stimulation did not. In addition, the kinetics of activation of protein kinase B differs between conventional FcγR ligation and ANCA stimulation of neutrophils. These results demonstrate that though ligation of FcγRIIa and FcγRIIIb may be necessary, it is likely that ANCAs require other membrane cofactors for neutrophil activation (Ben-Smith *et al.* 2001).

The cell signaling pathways involved in activation of neutrophils by ANCA binding have recently been explored. Schreiber *et al.* (2004) found that PR3-high neutrophils showed more PI$_3$-K/Akt activation than mPR3-low neutrophils. Hewins *et al.* (2004) reported that ANCA-IgG induces phosphorylation of the tyrosine kinase Syk in human neutrophils via Fcγ receptors and CD18. Given the central role of tyrosine kinase Syk in both the Fcγ receptor and β$_2$-integrin-mediated respiratory burst, the authors speculate that Syk represents a central component of the signaling pathways recruited by ANCA that lead to inappropriate neutrophil activation. Furthermore, the authors conclude, coligation of antigens and receptors by ANCA may form novel heteromers and confer different characteristics on Syk recruitment compared with conventional Fcγ receptor cross-linking.

Tse *et al.* (2005) have proposed a novel mechanism by which ANCA may contribute to tissue damage through activation of neutrophils and which might explain the predilection for small vessels in ANCA-associated vasculitis. They tested the hypothesis that ANCA, by inducing actin polymerization, increases rigidity of neutrophils and contributes to their sequestration in capillaries. IgG-ANCA was found to significantly increase dose-dependent actin polymerization and distortions in the shape of neutrophils. Actin polymerization required engagement of FcγRIIa receptor, tyrosine phosphorylation, and calcium fluxes.

Interaction of ANCA-activated neutrophils with endothelial cells

Chapter 4 contains a full discussion of endothelial activation, and adhesion and transmigration of neutrophils in vasculitis. Cohen Tervaert and colleagues have recently argued that ANCA are a primary pathogenic factor in renal vasculitis, mainly through their action in augmenting leukocyte-endothelial interactions (Heeringa *et al.* 2005; van Paassen *et al.* 2006). Using isolated human neutrophils, Radford *et al.* (2001) found that ANCA treatment promoted the transmigration of neutrophils through the endothelium. Little *et al.* (2005) used a rat model of ANCA-associated experimental autoimmune vasculitis, induced by immunization with human MPO, to directly analyze the effect of ANCAs on leukocyte-venular wall interactions *in vivo* by intravital microscopy. These rats developed anti-MPO antibodies directed against rat leukocytes, showed pathologic evidence of small-vessel vasculitis, and had enhanced leukocyte adhesion and transmigration in response to the chemokine Gro-alpha (CXCL1 [CXC ligand 1]). This was thought to provide a mechanism by which ANCAs could exert pathogenic effects in systemic vasculitis.

Wikman *et al.* studied eight patients with PR3-ANCA-positive acute vasculitis, looking at PMN expression of adhesion molecules, Fc receptors and ANCA-antigen PR3 at inclusion of patients and at 1, 3, 6, and 9 months (Wikman *et al.* 2005). Additional markers of inflammation and endothelial activation (IL-8 and soluble VCAM-1) were analyzed at the same times. The main finding was an activated neutrophil adhesion phenotype at diagnosis and after

1 month, with normalized expression of adhesion molecules at 3–9 months. This may be germane to endothelial damage seen in vasculitis.

Release of toxic factors that cause apoptosis and necrosis

How neutrophils damage vessels in vasculitis mediated by immune complexes is incompletely understood. *In vitro* studies have demonstrated that ANCA IgG augment several neutrophil functions, inducing degranulation (Falk *et al.* 1990), and the release of superoxide (Radford *et al.* 1999). Cytokines released after ANCA activation of neutrophils include IL-1β (Brooks *et al.* 1996) and IL-8 (Cockwell *et al.* 1999). In addition, ANCA induce neutrophils to firmly adhere to endothelial cells, leading to increased migration across the endothelial barrier (Radford *et al.* 2001).

von Willebrand factor (vWF), a glycoprotein involved in arterial thrombus formation, is secreted into the circulation by endothelial cells (Vischer 2006). Lu *et al.* (2006) have recently reported an analysis of the factors that control the neutrophil respiratory burst and endothelial release of vWF during neutrophil–endothelial cell interactions. Paradoxically, endothelial cells were shown to inhibit superoxide generation by ANCA-activated neutrophils. The release of vWF was sensitive to serine protease, but not NADPH oxidase inhibition, suggesting that serine proteases play a more important role than reactive oxygen species in mediating endothelial injury during ANCA-associated systemic vasculitis.

It is uncertain what factors prevent degradative enzymes and oxygen radicals released from neutrophils adherent to the luminal side of the vessel from being washed away or neutralized by serum protease inhibitors. Work by Sindralaru *et al.* (2006) suggests that immune complexes induce tight interactions between the neutrophils and endothelial cells which shield the cytotoxic products from the blood stream.

Reactive oxygen species resulting from degranulation and respiratory burst from neutrophils are important in triggering apoptosis (Jacobson *et al.* 1996) involving the CD95 (Fas/APO-1) pathway (Kasahara *et al.* 1997). Apoptosis of endothelial cells can be induced by the neutrophil serine proteases proteinase 3 and elastase (Yang *et al.* 1996). Harper *et al.* (2001) reported that PMN from patients with active vasculitis became apoptotic at a greater rate than those of controls and that opsonization of apoptotic PMN with ANCA enhanced recognition and phagocytosis by macrophages, leading to increased secretion of IL-1 and IL-8, thus possibly contributing to chronic inflammation.

IFN-activated neutrophils are able to release TNF-related apoptosis-inducing ligand (TRAIL/APO2 ligand), a molecule involved in apoptosis of tumor cells and virus-infected cells, as well as immunoregulatory functions on activated T lymphocytes. The majority of the newly synthesized TRAIL is retained intracellularly, can be rapidly mobilized to the cell surface, and secreted following exposure to a variety of proinflammatory mediators such as TNF, LPS, formyl-methionyl-leucyl-phenylalanine (fMLP), CXC chemokine ligand 8/IL-8, insoluble immune complexes, and heat shock protein Gp96 (Cassatella *et al.* 2006). This represents a novel mechanism by which neutrophils may be involved in immunomodulation relevant to ANCA-associated vasculitis.

Although apoptosis is an important process in ANCA-associated vasculitis, proliferation is a prominent lesion in the glomerulonephritis of the necrotizing small-vessel vasculitides. Kettritz *et al.* (2006) examined apoptosis, apoptosis-regulating proteins, and proliferation in skin biopsies from patients with leukocytoclastic vasculitis and renal biopsies from patients with ANCA-associated vasculitis, ANCA-negative crescentic glomerulonephritis, and a variety of other renal lesions. There was a relatively low rate of apoptosis and a relatively high rate of proliferation (assessed by Ki-67 expression) in renal biopsy tissue of patients with ANCA-positive necrotizing crescentic glomerulonephritis.

Cytokines, growth factors, and chemokines

Cytokines

As discussed above, cytokines are key players in ANCA-associated vasculitis. A Th1 cytokine profile has been reported in WG (see Chapter 30). Ludviksson *et al.* (1998) showed that PBMC from clinically active WG patients exhibited increased proliferation and increased secretion of IFN-γ and TNF-α, but not of IL-4, IL-5, or IL-10. Monocytes from both inactive and active WG patients produced increased amounts of IL-12, while *in vitro* IFN-γ production was inhibited by exogenous IL-10 in a dose-dependent manner. Gross and colleagues (Csernok *et al.* 1999) analyzed T cell clones and cell lines, and polyclonal CD4+ and CD8+ T cells derived from biopsied nasal mucosal tissue, bronchoalveolar lavage fluid, and peripheral blood of patients with WG. IFN-γ, but not IL-4, was frequently expressed at the sites of tissue injury. These data support a predominantly Th1-type response in the pathogenesis of WG. Ben Ahmed *et al.* (2004) found a similar Th1-type response in BS. A somewhat similar study concluded that Th1-associated cytokines (particularly IFN-γ and IL-12) may play a critical role in the development of skin and intestinal lesions in patients with BS, and implicated Txk, a member of the Tec family of tyrosine kinases which acts as a Th1 cell-specific transcription factor (Suzuki *et al.* 2006). In TA, there also appears to be an inflammatory cytokine signature with key roles for TNF-α, IL-4, IL-6, IL-8, IL-10, and IL-12 in pathological processes of the disease (Tripathy *et al.* 2004; Chauhan *et al.* 2006).

In contrast to other primary systemic vasculitides, there seems to be a prominent role for both Th1 and Th2-type cytokines in CSS. PBMCs secrete large amounts of Th1-type cytokines, particularly IFN-γ, and Th2-type 2 cytokines such as IL-4 and IL-13. PBMCs from patients with CSS cultured with T-cell specific stimuli secrete significant amounts of IL-5, the most potent stimulator of eosinophil production and activation of mature eosinophils, suggesting that it contributes significantly to eosinophilia in CSS (Hellmich *et al.* 2005).

Additional data supporting a role of TNF-α are the findings of Huugen *et al.* (2005), who used a mouse model of anti-MPO IgG-induced glomerulonephritis using bacterial LPS as the pro-inflammatory stimulus. Systemic administration of LPS was found to increase glomerular crescent formation and glomerular necrosis induced by anti-MPO. A transient induction of circulating TNF levels was observed after administration of LPS, and anti-MPO IgG induced an *in vitro* respiratory burst in murine neutrophils only after priming with TNF. Finally, anti-TNF treatment attenuated, but did not prevent, the LPS-mediated aggravation of anti-MPO IgG-induced glomerulonephritis.

There is circumstantial evidence that IL-1 and its endogenous antagonist, interleukin 1 receptor antagonist (IL-1Ra), may play a role in vasculitis. Mice that are homozygous for a null mutation in the gene encoding the anti-inflammatory molecule *IL-1Ra*, develop

lethal arterial inflammation (Nicklin *et al.* 2000). In these animals, there is massive transmural infiltration of neutrophils, macrophages, and CD4+ T cells, and they die from vessel wall collapse, stenosis, and organ infarction or from hemorrhage from ruptured aneurysms. Heterozygous individuals do not die from arteritis within a year of birth but do develop small lesions, suggesting that a reduced level of IL-1Ra is insufficient to fully control inflammation in arteries. These results suggest a significant role of IL-1Ra in vasculitis and that recombinant IL-1Ra may be an efficacious treatment.

IL-6 is one of the most extensively studied cytokines in vasculitis. It has been suggested that in GCA patients, IL-6 levels are a more sensitive marker of disease activity than the erythrocyte sedimentation rate (Weyand *et al.* 2000). Among 25 patients with GCA, plasma IL-6 levels were abnormal in 92% of untreated patients. The ESR was elevated during 58% of disease flares, but plasma IL-6 levels were increased in 89% of disease recurrences. Similarly, IL-6 appears to reflect disease activity in TA (Noris *et al.* 1999). Among 18 patients with TA, all had an increased serum concentration of IL-6 (compared with healthy control subjects) during the active phase of the disease, and reflected disease activity. In contrast, serum concentrations of IL-1 were not detectable in either healthy subjects or patients with TA.

IL-15 appears to also contribute to the pathogenesis of vasculitis, particularly BS. Hamzaoui *et al.* (2006) measured IL-15 in the serum and CSF of 40 patients with BS, 20 of whom had active disease. Those with active BS had higher serum IL-15 levels (median 10.4 pg/ml) than those with inactive BS (6.1 pg/ml) and controls (4.7 pg/ml). The presence of cerebral vascular BS lesions was associated with high CSF/serum IL-15 ratios.

Cytokines purported to play a pathogenetic role in KD include IL-1β, IL-2, IL-6, IL-8, IL-10, interferon-gamma (IFN-γ), and TNF (Yoshioka *et al.* 1999). TNF may be particularly important in the pathogenesis of coronary artery lesions in KD, as shown by correlation of TNF production with the presence of inflammatory infiltrates and aneurysms in a murine model, along with relative resistance to induction of TNF-induced lesions after treatment with the TNF inhibitor etanercept (Hui-Yuen *et al.* 2006).

IL-18, as mentioned above, may play a role in ANCA-associated vasculitis by priming PMNs to produce superoxide after ANCA binding (Hewins *et al.* 2006). Serum IL-18 and IL-6 levels are elevated in patients with TA, especially those with active disease (Park *et al.* 2006).

Growth factors

A role for vascular endothelial growth factor (VEGF), a regulator of angiogenesis and blood vessel permeability, has been invoked in KD (Terai *et al.* 1999) and leukocytoclastic vasculitis (Viac *et al.* 1999). In 30 patients with acute KD, peak plasma levels of VEGF were significantly elevated compared with controls. The plasma levels of VEGF highly correlated with those of TGF-β1 but not of TNF, leading to the conclusion that the up-regulated production of VEGF may be influenced by TGF-β1. Mitsuyama *et al.* (2006) found that serum VEGF levels were significantly higher in CSS patients than in patients with asthma or acute bronchitis. Serum VEGF levels decreased significantly after therapy, and infiltrating eosinophils in CSS lesions showed immunohistochemical staining for VEGF, suggesting that VEGF might be involved in the pathogenesis of CSS.

Angiogenic cytokines and growth factors have also been studied in GCA. Temporal arteries from patients with GCA were compared with controls (Kaiser *et al.* 1999). In normal arteries, vasa vasorum were found only in the adventitia, but in affected arteries, capillaries were noted in the media and the intima. Neovascularization correlated with significant intimal proliferation, fragmentation of the internal elastic lamina, and the presence of multinucleated giant cells. VEGF, supplied by giant cells and CD68-positive macrophages at the media-intima junction, and IFN-γ appeared to mediate neovascularization.

A small study (10 patients) suggested a role of granulocyte-colony stimulating factor (G-CSF) and macrophage-colony stimulating factor (M-CSF) in KD (Igarashi *et al.* 1999). Levels of serum M-CSF (and to a lesser extent G-CSF and IL-6) were higher in the acute phase than in the convalescent phase. Of note, patients with ANCA-positive vasculitis had disease flares after administration of rhuG-CSF, given to improve collection of stem cells prior to autologous stem cell transplantation, implicating this growth factor in the pathogenesis of ANCA-associated vasculitis (Iking-Konert *et al.* 2004).

Chemokines

Chemokines, which serve to recruit leukocytes to sites of inflammation, are also likely to have an important role in vasculitis. For example, serum concentrations of RANTES (*r*egulated upon *a*ctivation, *n*ormal *T*-cell *e*xpressed and *s*ecreted) have been reported to be elevated in active TA (Noris *et al.* 1999). Serum levels tended to normalize in remission, but values remained higher than those of control subjects. Anti-PR3 antibodies purified from sera of patients with active WG induce *in vitro* expression of another chemokine, IL-8, in endothelial cells (Mayet *et al.* 1999). NF-κB plays a crucial role in anti-PR-3 antibody induced endothelial IL-8 production. Chung *et al.* (2004) compared production of three chemokines: IFN-γ-inducible protein-10 (IP-10); monocyte chemoattractant protein-1 (MCP-1); and growth related onco-gene-alpha (gro-α) in KD, HSP, and acute febrile illnesses. Plasma levels of IP-10 and MCP-1 were elevated in KD and acute febrile illnesses compared with HSP. Gro-alpha levels were elevated only in acute febrile illnesses. Ben Ahmed *et al.* (2004) found elevated expression of MCP-1, as well as IL-8, in mucocutaneous lesions of patients with BS. Recently, a role for soluble fractalkine (Fkn; CX$_3$CL1), a chemokine for monocytes, NK cells, and T lymphocytes that is produced by endothelial cells, has been analyzed in rheumatoid vasculitis (Matsunawa *et al.* 2006). Serum soluble Fkn levels were significantly higher in RA patients with rheumatoid vasculitis than in those without vasculitis; they correlated with disease activity, and decreased significantly following clinical improvement.

Role of antiendothelial cell antibodies

A role for AECA in the pathogenesis of vasculitis has been inferred from their presence in WG, MPA, and KD, as well as in vasculitis associated with SLE and RA. Despite the data presented below, it still remains unclear whether AECA are contributors to the pathogenesis of vasculitis or are a result of vasculitis-associated inflammation (Eichhorn *et al.* 1996; Belizna *et al.* 2006; Cid *et al.* 2004). One finding that can potentially repudiate the importance of AECA in vasculitis is their presence in disease states not thought to be primarily inflammatory in nature. For example,

Papadopoulos *et al.* (2006) found that healthy subjects with blood pressure in the high end of normal have significantly higher levels of both IgG and IgM AECA than healthy subjects with normal blood pressure.

High titers of these antibodies have been found in the sera of 18 of 19 patients with Takayasu's arteritis (Eichhorn *et al.* 1996). Salojin and colleagues have also found increased levels of AECA in patients with vasculitis of large- and medium-sized arteries (Salojin *et al.* 1996). Park *et al.* (2006) found that IgM AECA and IgG AECA were more prevalent in patients with TA than in controls and that IgM AECA titers correlated well with the disease activity of TA, corroborating the findings of Brasile *et al.* who detected AECA in 86% of 21 patients with systemic necrotizing vasculitis and found that they correlated with disease activity (Brasile *et al.* 1989). Other investigators have reported AECA in 19% of 27 patients with WG and in 2% of 43 patients with microscopic polyangiitis (Varagunam *et al.* 1993). Holmen *et al.* (2004) reported that Wegener's granulomatosis is significantly associated with non-cytotoxic AECA that selectively bind surface antigens on unstimulated nasal, kidney, and lung endothelial cells.

The identity of the antigens inducing AECAs remains unknown, but they may be important in the initiation of WG. Brasile *et al.* (1989) reported preferential binding of the AECA to splenic and inferior mesenteric endothelium in comparison with aortic endothelium, findings that are compatible with visceral arterial involvement in vasculitis. Yu *et al.* (2005) analyzed sera from 11 patients with PTU-induced ANCA positive vasculitis during active and quiescent phases, sera from 10 patients with PTU-induced ANCA but no evidence of vasculitis, and sera from 30 healthy controls. Soluble proteins from HUVECs were used as antigens in an immunoblotting assay to determine the presence of AECA. Ten of the 11 patients with active PTU-induced ANCA vasculitis were serum IgG-AECA positive and six protein bands of endothelial antigens could be detected. In the quiescent phase, seven of the 10 positive sera were negative. None of the other subjects tested were AECA positive. Chauhan *et al.* (2006) recently sought to delineate the precise role of antigenic targets of AECA and the pathogenic mechanism of antibodies directed against aortic AECAs in TA. After isolating aortic AECAs using a cellular ELISA, their antigenic targets were detected by immunoblotting. Aortic AECAs were detected in 86% of patients with TA and in 9% of controls. Sera obtained from aortic AECA-positive TA patients recognized a total of nine antigens ranging in size from 18 kD to 200 kD. The most common antigen was a 60–65-kD triplet. The precise molecular composition of the antigens binding to AECA remains to be determined.

AECA can induce endothelial cell injury and lysis via complement-mediated cytotoxicity or antibody-dependent cellular cytotoxicity (ADCC). Using sera from patients with KD and systemic vasculitis, AECA have been shown to participate in complement-mediated cytotoxicity of cultured human umbilical vein endothelial cells (HUVEC) (Brasile *et al.* 1989; Leung *et al.* 1986a, 1986b), an observation not confirmed by all investigators (Savage *et al.* 1991). ADCC is a process by which specific antibody binds to a target cell and engages a natural killer cell via its Fc receptor, resulting in lysis of the cell. Its role in systemic vasculitis is unclear, but ADCC has been demonstrated *in vitro* against endothelial cells (Del Papa *et al.* 1992). These activities of AECA may account for observed elevations of vWF and factor VIII-related antigen in the serum of patients with vasculitis. Holmen *et al.* (2004) found that

IFN-γ and TNF were cytotoxic to nasal and lung endothelial cells; that cell lysis was increased by the addition of serum from patients with systemic vasculitis; and that WG serum caused agglutination of cytokine-stimulated nasal endothelial cells.

Another mechanism by which AECA may contribute to the pathogenesis of systemic vasculitis is through increasing leukocyte adhesion to endothelial cells. Purified IgG from each of three AECA-positive systemic vasculitis patients was found to up-regulate the expression of adhesion molecules (ICAM-l, VCAM-l, E-selectin) *in vitro*. In contrast, AECA-negative samples had no effect (Carvalho *et al.* 1999). AECA-mediated leukocyte adhesion to endothelium is thought to be mediated, in part, by increasing the release of endothelium-derived IL-l. The analysis of a panel of monoclonal AECA generated from a patient with TA by Blank *et al.* supports the concept that AECA directly stimulate EC. Again, there was evidence of adhesion of monocytes and upregulation of adhesion molecule expression, perhaps mediated by NF-κB activation (Blank *et al.* 1999). Finally, sera from aortic AECA-positive patients with TA induces expression of E-selectin, and VCAM1, suggesting that AECAs may cause vascular dysfunction through a variety of mechanisms (Chauhan *et al.* 2006).

Drug-induced vasculitis

The causes of most vasculitis are unknown; however, there has been clear evidence for many years that they can be caused by drugs. While drug-induced vasculitis is most often cutaneous, it can be systemic and life-threatening. Among the earliest reported cases of serious drug induced vasculitis (DIV) were those due to methamphetamine abuse, with visceral and intracranial lesions, and a histologic picture indistinguishable at times from classic PAN (Weiss *et al.* 1970; Margolis and Newton 1971). Drug-related vascular inflammation can result from pharmacological or immunological mechanisms. Pharmacological toxicity can be predicted in animal toxicology studies and thus usually avoided but animal studies have not predicted immunologically-mediated DIV in humans (Kerns *et al.* 2005). Drug-related hypersensitivity reactions have been explained by the hapten concept in which a small antigen covalently modifies an endogenous protein. More recent studies have shown that non-covalent drug presentation can lead to the activation of drug-specific T cells. In some instances, a drug-induced hypersensitivity may occur within hours of even first exposure to the drug, suggesting the reaction may be mediated by existing, preactivated T cells that display cross-reactivity for the drug. This implies that drugs may bypass the checkpoints for immune activation by the classical antigen processing mechanisms. Gerber and Pichler (2006) propose this to explain the idiosyncratic nature of some drug hypersensitivity reactions. Choi *et al.* looked at 30 patients with vasculitis and the highest titers of anti-MPO found in their laboratory over a 5-year period. Ten of the 30 had taken hydralazine and three had taken propythiouracil. Others of the 30 patients had been exposed to penicillamine, allopurinol, and sulfasalazine. The investigators recommended that clinicians should examine the histories of patients with MPO-positive vasculitis for exposure to these drugs (Choi *et al.* 2000b).

The differentiation of idiopathic and drug induced vasculitis may be difficult, with few clues other than those from a careful chronologic history of drug intake. A study of 16 patients with DIV and 47 with idiopathic vasculitis, however, found a significant difference in the mean eosinophil counts obtained on histopathologic examination of biopsied tissue (mean eosinophil ratio of 5.20 in the former versus 1.05), suggesting that tissue eosinophilia can be a relative indicator of drug-induced disease (Bahrami *et al.* 2006). The importance of recognizing DIV was underscored by the clinical evidence of systemic vasculitis in 13% of the drug-induced group.

Recognition of an offending drug and its withdrawal usually leads to recovery; however, a literature review in 2002 reported that death was the result in 10% of all published cases, predominantly in patients with multiple organ involvement. Furthermore, the interval between first exposure and appearance of symptoms was highly variable, from hours to years, sometimes confounding recognition of the condition as drug-induced. The drugs most frequently incriminated were propylthiouracil, hydralazine, colony-stimulating factors, allopurinol, cefaclor, minocycline, D-penicillamine, phenytoin, isotretinoin, and methotrexate (Ten Holder *et al.* 2002). Another recent review listed 100 drugs associated with vasculitis, with the caveat that the level of evidence for each causing vasculitis varied greatly, and the authors advised the readers to investigate agents individually when making clinical decisions. The drugs were subdivided into the following categories (Merkel 2001):

- antimicrobials
- vaccines
- interferons
- antithyroid agents
- anticonvulsants/antiarrhythmics
- diuretics
- other cardiovascular agents
- anticoagulants/thrombolytics
- antineoplastic/antimetabolites
- hematopoietic growth factors
- NSAIDs
- leukotriene inhibitors
- psychoactive agents
- sympathomimetics
- miscellaneous.

Postmarketing surveillance of drugs will often uncover adverse reactions not evident in premarketing controlled studies, as has happened with some of the newer drugs used to treat rheumatic disorders. Paradoxically, leflunomide, infliximab, etanercept, adalimumab, and rituximab, which affect immunological mediators of inflammation, can themselves cause vasculitis (MacDonald *et al.* 2004; Mohan *et al.* 2004; Srivastava *et al.* 2005; Haraoui and Keystone 2006; Duffy *et al.* 2006; Orpin *et al.* 2006). The risk is slight, and the vasculitis has most often been cutaneous although there are rare reports of systemic disease. Bosentan, which is used in some patients with scleroderma, has also been reported to cause leukocytoclastic vasculitis (Gasser *et al.* 2004).

A contentious association is that between asthma drugs and CSS. Independent of its treatment, asthma has been recognized as a significant risk factor for CSS since the latter's identification as a distinctive entity. Since 1998 there have been numerous anecdotal reports of CSS appearing after the introduction of leukotriene receptor antagonists (LTA) into the asthma treatment regimen. It has been postulated that with improvement of asthma following the administration of LTA, CSS is unmasked as glucocorticoids are decreased or withdrawn (Wechsler *et al.* 1999; Keogh and Specks 2003). There are contrasting reports of the appearance of CSS in patients who have been treated with LTA and low-dose or no glucocorticoids (Kobayashi *et al.* 2003; Oberndorfer *et al.* 2004; Conen *et al.* 2004; DuMouchel *et al.* 2004). Thus, whether treatment of asthma with LTAs can induce CSS or not remains an unanswered question. The rarity of CSS, both before and after introduction of LTAs, precludes using epidemiologic data to provide a definite answer; however, clinicians using these drugs should be mindful of the irresolution and its implications.

The association of antithyroid drugs (carbimazole, methimazole, propylthiouracil) and vasculitis, although uncommon, has been accepted since its recognition in 1950 (McCormick 1950), and in 1993 Dolman *et al.* reported an association of antineutrophil cytoplasmic autoantibodies and propylthiouracil (PTU) related vasculitis (Dolman *et al.* 1993). In a subsequent study of 56 patients with Graves' disease who were given PTU, antimyeloperoxidase antibodies (MPO-ANCA) appeared in 21; of these, 12 had no symptoms, but nine complained of myalgia or arthralgia. The proportion of patients positive for MPO-ANCA increased with prolongation of PTU treatment (Sera *et al.* 2000). Several studies have noted the appearance of MPO-ANCA following PTU treatment without development of vasculitis (Noh *et al.* 2001; Wada *et al.* 2002). Bonaci-Nikolic and colleagues compared the clinical and laboratory characteristics of 56 patients with idiopathic systemic vasculitis (ISV) and 16 who became ANCA-positive during treatment with PTU or methimazole (Bonaci-Nikolic *et al.* 2005). Kidney disease was present in 75% of the former and 18% of the antithyroid drug treated patients; skin lesions were noted in 62.5% of those taking the drugs, and 25% of ISV patients. MPO-ANCA, ANA, anticardiolipin antibodies, cryoglobulins, and low serum C4 were more common in the patients treated with antithyroid drugs. Four of these 16 had drug-induced ANCA vasculitis and 12 had lupus-like illness. A similar investigation in China examined sera from 216 patients with hyperthyroidism and found ANCA in 22.6 % of PTU treated patients versus 2.9% of untreated patients. Of the 216 samples, 33 were positive for ANCA and antineutrophil antibodies by indirect immunofluorescence. By ELISA testing of 22 ANCA positive sera, antibodies were found against lactoferrin, elastase, MPO, and three against PR3 (Gao *et al.* 2004). It thus appears that PTU-induced ANCA may be due to polyclonal activation of B cells.

Vanek and Samuels (2005) found reports of 42 cases of antithyroid drug related ANCA positive vasculitis since 1992, noting that kidneys, skin, and the musculoskeletal systems were most often involved, that the mean duration of treatment was 35 months "prior to presentation," and they described a patient with central nervous system vasculitis with resolution of symptoms after withdrawal of PTU. ANCA have also been found in children with Graves' disease who were treated with PTU: MPO-ANCA was present in 6.7% prior to and in 64% after treatment, but no child had vasculitis (Sato *et al.* 2000).

There are rare reports of ANCA-positive DIV in patients taking other drugs such as hydralazine; allopurinol; penicillamine; sulfasalazine; minocycline (one of whom had cutaneous polyarteritis); proton pump inhibitors; and cephotaxime (Pelletier *et al.* 2003; Jacobs-Kosmin *et al.* 2006; Feriozzi *et al.* 2000). Positivity for MPO-ANCA, IgM anticardiolipin antibodies, and antihistone antibodies is characteristic of some DIV.

It is obvious that almost any drug might cause vasculitis. Illicit drugs, preservatives (Moneret-Vautrin *et al.* 1986), and drug additives (Lowry *et al.* 1994) may also cause vasculitis syndromes. Thus, a meticulous history of drug consumption should be an important part of the evaluation of any patient with vasculitis, either cutaneous or systemic although there are many pitfalls in definitively determining that a particular drug is the etiologic agent in vasculitis.

Genetic influences

The frequent conjunction of genetic deficiencies of complement components and immune complex diseases implies an important pathogenetic interaction (see Chapter 5). Furthermore, as the molecular pathways important in the pathogenesis of vasculitis are unraveled, genetic variants in the proteins and other molecules involved will be sought. Such studies have grown dramatically since the completion of the Human Genome Project and the rapidly expanding databases of single nucleotide polymorphisms (SNPs), including those that tag particular haplotypes. For example, Oztas *et al.* (2005) reported that serum IL-18 (and TNF) levels are increased in BS. Lee *et al.* (2006) subsequently sought an association between susceptibility to the BS and polymorphisms in the promoter region of the IL-18 gene. A full review of reports of associations between vasculitides and polymorphisms in candidate genes is beyond the scope of this text, but selected examples are discussed below.

Because of the physiological role of Fc receptors in processing immune complexes, the genes encoding these proteins have been extensively analyzed for polymorphisms important in the pathogenesis of vasculitis. It has been postulated that FcγR alleles are a genetic risk factor for disease expression in WG (Tse *et al.* 2000), and these investigators explored the importance of FcγRIIIb polymorphism as a risk factor for development of ANCA-associated systemic vasculitis/nephritis. Receptor genotyping was determined by allele-specific polymerase chain reaction on 101 patients with ANCA-positive vasculitis, of whom 84 had nephritis, and 100 matched controls. ANCA from 71 of the patients were PR3 positive; 30 were specific for MPO. There was no overall significant difference in genotype distribution or allele frequencies between patients and controls, or between patients with nephritis and controls. There was a trend towards increased homozygosity for the NA1 allele in patients with vasculitis, and this was significant in patients who were MPO-ANCA-positive. The investigators concluded that FcγRIIIb receptor polymorphism is not a major factor predisposing to development of ANCA-positive vasculitis or nephritis (Tse *et al.* 2000).

Another polymorphism that has been studied in this regard is the SNP at amino acid residue 131 of FcγRIIa that encodes arginine (the R131 allele) or hisitidine (the H131 allele). These alleles differ in their ability to bind human IgG$_2$ and IgG$_3$. Neutrophils from individuals homozygous for the FcγRIIa-H131 allele bind more efficiently to IgG3 than do those from individuals with the FcγRIIa-R131 allele and are the only human FcγR that bind IgG$_2$. There is a similar variant at amino acid reside 158 of FcγRIIIa that encodes either valine (V158 allele) or phenylalanine (F158 allele). In a study of 91 patients with WG and 154 controls, patients homozygous for both the R131 allele of FcγRIIa and the F158 allele of FcγRIIIa were more susceptible to disease relapse (Dijstelbloem *et al.* 1999).

Tse and colleagues (1999) performed genotyping of 107 Caucasian patients with ANCA+ vasculitis (of whom 89 had renal disease) and 100 ethnically matched controls. Of the patients with ANCA-positive systemic vasculitis, 75 had ANCA with specificity for proteinase 3 and 32 with specificity for myeloperoxidase. As was the case with FcγRIIIb (Tse *et al.* 2000), there was no skewing in FcγRIIa allotypes in patients versus controls. No significant increase of the FcγRIIa-H131 allotype was found among patients, regardless of ANCA specificity, and no association between the FcγRIIa genotype and nephritis was found. Other investigators have found no association between FcγRIIa genotypes and susceptibility to leukocytoclastic vasculitis (Groger *et al.* 1999).

Another gene relevant to vasculitis is that encoding the protease inhibitor (Pi) alpha-1-antitrypsin (α1-AT), which is considered to be the major physiological inhibitor of PR3 and elastase through its large circulating excess (Esnault *et al.* 1997). The serum concentration of α1-AT is genetically determined by the polymorphic Pi genes (Brandrup and Ostergaard 1978). A 2-year-old child with α1-AT deficiency of the PiZZ type and cutaneous vasculitis was described in 1978 (Brandrup and Ostergaard 1978). Subsequently, several studies have addressed a possible pathogenetic relationship between α1-AT deficiency and anti-PR3-positive systemic vasculitis (Esnault *et al.* 1997.) Patients with ANCA-positive systemic vasculitis may have a genetically determined protease/antiprotease imbalance (in the case of patients with genotypes associated with α1-AT deficiency) or an acquired decrease in formation of PR3/α1-AT complexes by anti-PR3 ANCA.

Mazodier *et al.* reported eight patients with systemic necrotizing vasculitis (six with microscopic polyangiitis, one with WG, and one with HSP) and severe α1-AT deficiency and reviewed six previously reported cases (Mazodier *et al.* 1996). In a study of the potential association between ANCA-positive vasculitis and α1-AT alleles in 198 ANCA-positive vasculitis patients and 2310 controls, cANCA patients showed an increased frequency of the Z allele (0.055 versus 0.018 in controls), conferring a relative risk of about 3 (Griffith *et al.* 1996). In an analysis of 18 PiZ-positive and 81 PiZ-negative PR3-ANCA patients, PiZ-positive patients had more disseminated disease and a slightly higher mortality rate (Segelmark *et al.* 1995). α1-AT may play a role in the pathogenesis of retinal vasculitis (Wakefield *et al.* 1985).

Audrain *et al.* (2001) tested 191 persons with homozygous (PiZZ) alpha1-antitrypsin-deficient persons for ANCA activity and compared them to 272 PiMM matched control subjects. The incidence of antibodies directed against PMN alpha granules and human leukocyte elastase, but not PR3, MPO, lactoferrin, or bactericidal/permeability increasing protein, was increased in the PiZZ compared to the PiMM group. The authors concluded that ANCA not directed against MPO and PR3 may be found in PiZZ patients, who do not develop systemic vasculitis. Thus, these authors hypothesize that alpha 1 antitrypsin deficiency is not sufficient to induce ANCA positive vasculitis, but may act as a second hit to amplifying the immune response.

Physicians should consider α1-AT deficiency in patients with systemic vasculitis and emphysema or cirrhosis. Concomitant α1-AT deficiency and vasculitis may have treatment ramifications.

For example, a 49-year-old man with α1-AT deficiency and refractory cutaneous vasculitis responded to treatment with alpha 1-protease inhibitor (Dowd *et al.* 1995). In addition, treatments decreasing plasma α1-AT (such as plasmapheresis without plasma replacement) may be deleterious in systemic vasculitis.

Finally, a SNP in the gene encoding an intracellular tyrosine phosphatase (*PTPN22*) has been found to be important in susceptibility to rheumatoid arthritis (Begovich *et al.* 2004) and subsequently in other diseases, including type 1 diabetes, systemic lupus erythematosus, and Hashimoto's thyroiditis. Jagiello *et al.* (2005) examined this *PTPN22* SNP in 199 patients with WG and in 399 healthy individuals. They found that the *PTPN22* 620W allele frequency was significantly increased in ANCA-positive WG patients compared with healthy controls, particularly in those with generalized WG. The 620W allele appears to influence thresholds for T cell receptor signaling (Gregersen *et al.* 2006), invoking a variety of potential disease models involving central and peripheral T lymphocyte tolerance. The precise mechanisms for these associations, however, remain unclear.

Infectious agents as triggers of vasculitis

It is conceivable that any infectious agent or foreign antigen that induces an immune response might result in vasculitis, but some infectious agents probably cause vasculitis through nonimmunologic mechanisms. Evidence to support a pathogenetic role for infectious organisms in vasculitis includes case reports of concominant vasculitis and infection. Indirect support for a potential role for an infectious agent in ANCA-associated vasculitis is the finding that a peptide translated from the antisense DNA strand of PR3 and homologous to several microbial peptides may be involved in induction of PR3 ANCA (Pendergraft *et al.* 2004). In equine viral arteritis, evidence supports viral infection of the vascular endothelium (Estes and Cheville 1970). A more convincing example of an arteritis without immunologic mediation has come from experimental central nervous system arteritis in turkeys infected with *Mycoplasma gallisepticum* (Thomas *et al.* 1966). Inoculation of a large dose of organisms resulted in arteritic lesions within 24 hours, implicating a direct toxic effect of mycoplasma, or their products, on vascular endothelium. Numerous exotic parasites and microbes also cause animal, and less often human, vasculitis.

In humans, invasion by infectious organisms resulting in direct vascular injury is seen with bacteria, mycobacteria, spirochetes, and rickettsia. Varicella zoster virus, herpes simplex virus (HSV), and cytomegalovirus appear to cause human vasculitis (see Chapter 42). Viral inclusion bodies have been detected within and closely adjacent to vessel walls in several patients (Doyle *et al.* 1983; Linnemann and Alvira 1980; Reyes *et al.* 1976). HSV-1 infection of human endothelial cells results in expression of C3b and Fc receptors on the cell surface (Cines *et al.* 1982). There is conflicting evidence on the presence of HSV DNA within tissues affected by vasculitis. Powers *et al.* (2005) detected HSV DNA in 21 of 24 histologically-positive temporal artery biopsies from patients with GCA and in eight of 15 histologically-negative specimens, compared to none of 10 renal artery samples from age matched controls. On the other hand, no viral genomes of HSV-1, CMV, or EBV were found in 35 biopsy specimens of histologically-positive temporal arteries by Cankovic *et al.* (2006). A similar study found no evidence of herpesvirus DNA in GCA (Rodriguez-Pla *et al.* 2004).

The human retrovirus HTLV-1 has been shown to infect human endothelial cells *in vitro*, which may explain the cutaneous vasculitis associated with HTLV-1 induced T cell leukemia (Haynes 1992). Human immunodeficiency virus (HIV) appears to directly cause vasculitis; however, other causes of vasculitis, such as medications and opportunistic infections, may be identified in persons with AIDS (Gisselbrecht 1999). Other infectious agents that have been implicated in vasculitis syndromes are discussed elsewhere (see Chapter 42) and include *Mycobacterium tuberculosis* (Allins *et al.* 1999; Blanco Garcia *et al.* 1999); hepatitis C virus; dengue fever (Ishikawa *et al.* 1999); brucellosis (Nagore *et al.* 1999; Perez *et al.* 1999); and Salmonella (Soravia-Dunand *et al.* 1999).

Parvovirus B19 has been implicated in GCA (Gabriel *et al.* 1999; Alvarez-Lafuente *et al.* 2005) and HSP (Watanabe and Oda 2000), but a causative relationship has not been established with either disease. Although a case report of a 9-month-old boy with prolonged febrile illness thought to be KD was noted to have increased serum levels of IgG and IgM antibodies to antihuman herpesvirus (HHV)-6, and HHV-6 DNA in serum, blood mononuclear cells and lymph nodes (Toyabe *et al.* 2001), Alvarez-Lafuente *et al.* (2005) found no evidence of HHV-6 in GCA.

The role of bacterial superantigens (SAg) in vasculitis, most notably KD, has been a focus of recent investigation (Cohen Tervaert *et al.* 1999). SAg may activate autoreactive T cells that participate in vessel damage, or B cells that produce autoantibodies such as ANCA or AECA. In support of a role of superantigens is the finding that the acute phase of KD is associated with the polyclonal expansion of T cells (primarily CD4+) expressing the Vβ2 and Vβ8.1 gene segments (Abe *et al.* 1993). In another study, toxin-producing bacteria were isolated in cultures from 13 of 16 KD patients but from only one of 15 controls (Leung *et al.* 1993). *Staphylococcus aureus* secreting toxic shock syndrome toxin (TSST) was isolated from 11 of the 13 toxin-positive cultures, and streptococcal pyogenic exotoxin B and C were found in the remaining two cultures. Because TSST preferentially stimulates Vβ2-bearing T cells, this finding has been used to further support a role for bacterial superantigens in KD. Serologic evidence in at least one study, however, does not support a significant contribution of superantigens in KD (Morita *et al.* 1997) and their importance in its pathogenesis is not universally accepted (Uchiyama and Kato 1999).

Cases of vasculitis have been associated with a plethora of parasitic diseases, including toxoplasmosis, trichinosis, strongyliasis, ascardiosis, sarcocystosis, amebiasis, leishmaniosis, and toxocarosis. Unusual parasitic infections have been anecdotally reported in conjunction with vasculitis. For example, a 50-year-old Chilean man had systemic vasculitis, and was found to have *Fasciola hepatica* infection. He was treated with triclabendazole and all symptoms and systemic manifestations resolved within weeks (Llanos *et al.* 2006).

Tumor cell-mediated vascular damage

Cancers primarily associated with vasculitis are lymphomatoid and myeloproliferative malignancies (see Chapter 42 for detailed discussion). The pathogenesis of malignancy-associated vasculitis is unclear and likely multifactorial. As mentioned in Chapter 42, potential mechanisms include: (1) direct effects of tumor cells

(such as hairy cells in hairy cell leukemia) on vascular walls (Klima and Waddell 1984; Gabriel and Scott 1986); (2) tumor release or tumor-induced release of cytokines that promote destruction of vascular structures; and (3) formation of immune complexes of tumor associated antigen/antibodies (Sanchez-Guerrero and Alarcon-Segovia 1990; Kurzrock and Cohen 1993). Because of its rarity, there is a paucity of data on the pathogenesis of vasculitis in the setting of malignancy. It is assumed that a tumor antigen activates cellular immunity, or participates in immune complex formation. The vasculitis of hairy cell leukemia is the best studied of these. Of 42 persons with this disease, 17 had polyarteritis, 21 had leukocytoclastic vasculitis, and four had vessel wall infiltration by hairy cells. Immune complexes were found in three of four patients tested. Three patients, of 12 tested, were HBsAg positive. Vasculitis most often occurred after splenectomy (Hasler *et al.* 1995; Klima and Waddell 1984; Krol *et al.* 1983). Unidentified viral infections may also play a role through either immune complex disease or direct infection of endothelial cells. Direct invasion of vascular walls has also been documented in hairy cell leukemia (Klima and Waddell 1984), mycosis fungoides, HTLV-1-associated T cell leukemia, and in the premalignant syndrome of lymphomatoid granulomatosis (Haynes 1992). Peripheral vasculitis complicated by gangrene of the fingers has been reported in a patient with the eosinophilic variant of chronic myeloid leukemia (Gotlib *et al.* 2003).

Cell-mediated immune responses and granuloma formation in vasculitis

The occurrence of granulomas in WG and CSS is indicative of activation of lymphocytes and macrophages. It has been hypothesized that CD4+ T cells are triggered by antigens in the circulation or within vascular walls. Despite the involvement of T cells in vasculitis, there is no consistent evidence of association between genes in the major histocompatibility complex and vasculitic syndromes, with the exception of Behçet's syndrome (see Chapter 30). After stimulation, T cells release cytokines chemotactic for monocytes. Monocytes transformed into macrophages are then capable of releasing lysosomal enzymes that damage endothelial cells (Fauci *et al.* 1978). Experimental evidence for this comes from mice that were injected with syngeneic T cells sensitized *in vitro* to cultured vascular smooth muscle cells (Hart *et al.* 1985). Twenty percent of the mice developed granulomatous vasculitis of the pulmonary arterioles.

In human vasculitis, cell-mediated immunity has been studied primarily in WG. Activated T cells, particularly the CD4+ and CD8+ subtypes, have been found in biopsies from the upper and lower respiratory tracts and kidneys (Gephardt *et al.* 1983; Rasmussen *et al.* 1988; ten Berge *et al.* 1985). The expanded populations show high expression of activation markers HLADR and CD25, independent of activity of disease and there are high levels of intracellular and secreted IFN- and IL-2 (Giscombe *et al.* 1998). Patients with active WG had higher percentages of CD38-positive (activated) B cells than did those in remission, or control subjects; however, activated T cells persisted during remission of the vasculitis (Popa *et al.* 1999). Earlier studies found significant elevations of soluble IL-2 receptor (sIL-2R) levels in active generalized WG (Schmitt *et al.* 1992). Peripheral blood mononuclear cells (PBMC) from patients with WG proliferate *in vitro* on exposure to PR3, suggesting the presence of antigen-primed memory T cells

(Kallenberg *et al.* 1991). A sustained response to monoclonal anti-bodies directed against CD4+ T cells (Campath 1-H and anti-CD4) has also been observed in four patients with life-threatening systemic vasculitis that had been unresponsive to conventional immunosuppressive agents (Lockwood *et al.* 1993)

In addition to T cells, macrophages play an important role in vasculitis and Weyand and colleagues have studied mechanisms of the contribution of these cells. They used differential display poly-merase chain reaction to identify genes differentially expressed in inflamed and unaffected temporal artery specimens (Rittner *et al.* 1999). Multinucleated giant cells and CD68+ macrophages charac-teristic of those that aggregate in the media-intima junction had increased expression of mitochondrial products and were able to synthesize metalloproteinase 2. Products of lipid peroxidation were found on nearby smooth muscle cells suggesting the action of reactive oxygen species.

References

Abdel-Salam, B., Iking-Konert, C., Schneider, M., Andrassy, K. and Hansch, G. M. (2004). Autoantibodies to neutrophil cytoplasmic antigens (ANCA) do not bind to polymorphonuclear neutrophils in blood. *Kidney International*, **66**, 1009–17.

Abe, J., Kotzin, B. L., Meissner, C., Melish, M. E., Takahashi, M., Fulton, D., Romagne, F., Malissen, B. and Leung, D. Y. (1993). Characterization of T cell repertoire changes in acute Kawasaki disease. *Journal of Experimental Medicine*, **177**, 791–6.

Acosta, J., Qin, X. and Halperin, J. (2004). Complement and complement regulatory proteins as potential molecular targets for vascular diseases. *Current Pharmaceutical Design*, **10**, 203–11.

Agnello, V., Chung, R. T. and Kaplan, L. M. (1992). A role for hepatitis C virus infection in type II cryoglobulinemia. *New England Journal of Medicine*, **327**,1490–5.

Allins, A. D., Wagner, W. H., Cossman, D. V., Gold, R. N. and Hiatt, J. R. (1999). Tuberculous infection of the descending thoracic and abdominal aorta: case report and literature review. *Annals of Vascular Surgery*, **13**, 439–44.

Alvarez-Lafuente, R., Fernandez-Gutierrez, B., Jover, J. A., Judez, E., Loza, E., Clemente, D., Garcia-Asenjo, J. A. and Lamas, J. R. (2005). Human parvovirus B19, varicella zoster virus, and human herpes virus 6 in temporal artery biopsy specimens of patients with giant cell arteritis: analysis with quantitative real time polymerase chain reaction. *Annals of the Rheumatic Diseases*, **64**, 7890–2.

Argenbright, L. W. and Barton, R. W. (1992). Interactions of leukocyte integrins with intercellular adhesion molecule l in the production of inflammatory vascular injury *in vivo*. The Shwartzman reaction revisited. *Journal of Clinical Investigation*, **89**, 259–72.

Audrain, M. A., Sesboue, R., Baranger, T. A., Elliott, J., Testa, A., Martin, J. P., Lockwood, C. M. and Esnault, V. L. (2001). Analysis of anti-neutrophil cytoplasmic antibodies (ANCA): frequency and specificity in a sample of 191 homozygous (PiZZ) alpha1-antitrypsin-deficient subjects. *Nephrology, Dialysis, Transplantation*, **16**, 39–44.

Bahrami, S., Malone, J. C., Webb, K. G. and Callen, J. P. (2006). Tissue eosinophilia as an indicator of drug-induced cutaneous small-vessel vasculitis. *Archives of Dermatology*, **142**, 155–61.

Bansal, P. J. and Tobin, M. C. (2004). Neonatal microscopic polyangiitis secondary to transfer of maternal myeloperoxidase-antineutrophil cytoplasmic antibody resulting in neonatal pulmonary hemorrhage and renal involvement. *Annals of Allergy Asthma and Immunology*, **93**, 398–401.

Barak, A., Morse, L. S. and Schwab, I. R. (2000). Atypical retinal vasculitis associated with ticlopidine hydrochloridine use. *American Journal of Ophthalmology*, **129**, 684–5.

Barbano, G., Ginevri, F., Ghiggeri, G. M. and Gusmano, R. (1999). Disseminated autoimmune disease during levamisole treatment of nephrotic syndrome. *Pediatric Nephrology*, **13**, 602–603.

Begovich, A. B., Carlton, V. E., Honigberg, L. A., Schrodi, S. J., Chokkalingam, A. P., Alexander, H. C., *et al.* (2004). A missense single-nucleotide polymorphism in a gene encoding a protein tyrosine phosphatase (PTPN22) is associated with rheumatoid arthritis. *American Journal of Human Genetics*, **75**, 330–7.

Belizna, C., Duijvestijn, A., Hamidou, M., and Cohen Tervaert, J. W. (2006). Antiendothelial cell antibodies in vasculitis and connective tissue disease. *Annals of the Rheumatic Diseases*, **65**, 1545–50.

Ben Ahmed, M., Houman, H., Miled, M., Dellagi, K. and Louzir, H. (2004). Involvement of chemokines and Th1 cytokines in the pathogenesis of mucocutaneous lesions of Behcet's disease. *Arthritis and Rheumatism*, **50**, 2291–5.

Ben-Smith, A., Dove, S. K., Martin, A., Wakelam, M. J. and Savage, C. O. (2001). Antineutrophil cytoplasm autoantibodies from patients with systemic vasculitis activate neutrophils through distinct signaling cascades: comparison with conventional Fcgamma receptor ligation. *Blood*, **98**, 1448–55).

Blanco Garcia, F. J., Sanchez, B. M. and Freire, G. M. (1999). Histopathologic features of cerebral vasculitis associated with mycobacterium tuberculosis. *Arthritis and Rheumatism*, **42**, 383.

Blank, M., Krause, I., Goldkorn, T., Praprotnik, S., Livneh, A., Langevitz, P., Kaganovsky, E., Morgenstern, S., Cohen, S., Barak, V., Eldor, A., Weksler, B. and Shoenfeld, Y. (1999). Monoclonal anti-endothelial cell antibodies from a patient with Takayasu arteritis activate endothelial cells from large vessels. *Arthritis and Rheumatism*, **42**, 1421–32.

Bonaci-Nikolic, B., Nikolic, M. M., Andrejevic, S., Zoric, S. and Bukilica, M. (2005). Antineutrophil ctoplasmic antibody (ANCA)-associated immune diseases induced by antithyroid drugs: comparison with idiopathic ANCA vasculitides. *Arthritis Research and Therapy*, **7**, R72–81.

Brandrup, F. and Ostergaard, P. A. (1978). Alphal-antitrypsin deficiency associated with persistent cutaneous vasculitis. Occurrence in a child with liver disease. *Archives of Dermatology*, **114**, 921–4.

Brasile, L., Kremer, J. M., Clarke, J. L and Cerilli, J. (1989). Identification of an autoantibody to vascular endothelial cell-specific antigens in patients with systemic vasculitis. *American Journal of Medicine*, **87**, 74–80.

Braverman, I. M. and Yen, A. (1975). Demonstration of immune complexes in spontaneous and histamine-induced lesions and in normal skin of patients with leukocytoclastic angiitis. *Journal of Investigative Dermatology*, **64**, 105–12.

Brooks, C. J., King, W. J., Radford, D. J., Adu, D., McGrath, M. and Savage, C. O. (1996). IL-1beta production by human polymorphonuclear leucocytes stimulated by anti-neutrophil cytoplasmic autoantibodies: relevance to systemic vasculitis. *Clinical and Experimental Immunology*, **106**, 273–9.

Cacoub, P., Costedoat-Chalumeau, N., Lidove, O. and Alric, L. (2002). Cryoglobulinemia vasculitis. *Current Opinion in Rheumatology*, **14**, 29–35.

Cambridge, G., Rampton, D. S., Stevens, T. R., McCarthy, D. A., Kamm, M. and Leaker, B. (1992). Anti-neutrophil antibodies in inflammatory bowel disease: prevalence and diagnostic role. *Gut*, **33**, 668–74.

Cankovic, M. and Zarbo, R. J. (2006). Failure to detect human herpes simplex virus, cytomegalovirus and EB virus viral genomes in giant cell arteritis biopsy specimens by real time quantitative polymerase chain reaction. *Cardiovascular Pathology*, **15**, 280–6.

Carrasco, M. D., Riera, C., Clotet, B., Grifol, M. and Foz, M. (1987). Cutaneous vasculitis associated with propylthiouracil therapy. *Archives of Internal Medicine*, **147**, 1677.

Carvalho, D., Savage, C. O., Isenberg, D. and Pearson, J. D. (1999). IgG anti-endothelial cell autoantibodies from patients with systemic lupus erythematosus or systemic vasculitis stimulate the release of two endothelial cell-derived mediators, which enhance adhesion molecule expression and leukocyte adhesion in an autocrine manner. *Arthritis and Rheumatism*, **42**, 631–40.

Cassatella, M. A., Huber, V., Calzetti, F., Margotto, D., Tamassia, N., Peri, G., Mantovani, A., Rivoltini, L. and Tecchio, C. (2006). Interferon-activated neutrophils store a TNF-related apoptosis-inducing ligand (TRAIL/Apo-2 ligand) intracellular pool that is readily mobilizable following exposure to proinflammatory mediators. *Journal of Leukocyte Biology*, **79**, 123–32.

Charles, L. A., Caldas, M. L., Falk, R. J., Terrell, R. S. and Jennette, J. C. (1991) Antibodies against granule proteins activate neutrophils *in vitro*. *Journal of Leukocyte Biology*, **50**, 539–46.

Chauhan, S. K., Tripathy, N. K. and Nityanand, S. (2006). Antigenic targets and pathogenicity of anti-aortic endothelial cell antibodies in Takayasu arteritis. *Arthritis and Rheumatism*, **54**, 2326–33.

Choi, H. K., Merkel, P. A. and Niles, J. L. (1998). ANCA-positive vasculitis associated with allopurinol therapy. *Clinical and Experimental Rheumatology*, **16**, 743–4.

Choi, H. K., Merkel, P. A., Tervaert, J. W., Black, R. M., McCluskey R. T. and Niles, J. L. (1999). Alternating antineutrophil cytoplasmic antibody specificity: drug-induced vasculitis in a patient with Wegener's granulomatosis. *Arthritis and Rheumatism*, **42**, 384–8.

Choi, H. K., Lamprecht, P., Niles, J. L., Gross, W. L. and Merkel, P. A. (2000a). Subacute bacterial endocarditis with positive cytoplasmic antineutrophil cytoplasmic antibodies and anti-proteinase 3 antibodies. *Arthritis and Rheumatism*, **43**, 226–31.

Chung, H. S., Kim, H. Y., Kim, H. S., Lee, H. J., Yuh, J. H., Lee, E. S., Choi, K. H. and Lee, Y. H. (2004). Production of chemokines in Kawasaki disease, Henoch-Schönlein purpura and acute febrile illness. *Journal of Korean Medical Science*, **19**, 800–4.

Choi, H. K., Merkel, P. A., Walker, A. M. and Niles, J. L. (2000b). Drug-associated antineutrophil cytoplasmic antibody-positive vasculitis: prevalence among patients with high titers of antimyeloperoxidase antibodies. *Arthritis and Rheumatism*, **43**, 405–413.

Christian, C. L. and Sergent, J. S. (1976). Vasculitis syndromes: clinical and experimental models. *American Journal of Medicine*, **61**, 385–92.

Cid, M. C., Segarra, M., Garcia-Martinez, A. and Hernandez-Rodriguez, J. (2004). Endothelial cells, antineutrophil cytoplasmic antibodies, and cytokines in the pathogenesis of systemic vasculitis. *Current Rheumatology Reports*, **6**, 184–94.

Cines, D. B., Lyss, A. P., Bina, M., Corkey, R. Kefalides, N. A. and Friedman, H. M. (1982). Fc and C3 receptors induced by herpes simplex virus on cultured human endothelial cells. *Journal of Clinical Investigation*, **69**, 123–8.

Claudy, A. (1998). Pathogenesis of leukocytoclastic vasculitis. *European Journal of Dermatology*, **8**, 75–9.

Cochrane, C. G. (1971). Mechanisms involved in the deposition of immune complexes in tissues. *Journal of Experimental Medicine*, **134** (Suppl.), 89s.

Cochrane, C. G., Weigle, W. O. and Dixon, F. J. (1959). The role of polymorphonuclear leukocytes in the initiation and cessation of the Arthrus vasculitis. *Journal of Experimental Medicine*, **110**, 481–94.

Cockwell, P., Brooks, C. J., Adu, D. and Savage, C. O. (1999). Interleukin-8: a pathogenic role in antineutrophil cytoplasmic autoantibody (ANCA)-associated glomerulonephritis. *Kidney International*, **55**, 852–63.

Cohen Tervaert, J. W., Popa, E. R. and Bos, N. A. (1999). The role of superantigens in vasculitis. *Current Opinion in Rheumatology*, **11**, 24–33.

Combes, B., Shorey, J., Barrera, A., Stastny, P., Eigenbrodt, E. H., Hull, A. R. and Carter, N. W. (1971). Glomerulonephritis with deposition of Australia antigen-antibody complexes in glomerular basement membrane. *Lancet*, **2** (7718), 234–7.

Conen, D., Leuppi, J., Budendorf, L. *et al.* (2004). Montelukast and Churg-Strauss syndrome. *Swiss Medical Weekly* **134**, 377–80.

Cooper, T., Savige, J., Nassis, L., Paspaliaris, B., Neeson, P., Neil, J., Knight, K. R., Daskarakis, M. and Doery, J. C. (2000). Clinical associations and characterisation of antineutrophil cytoplasmic antibodies directed against bactericidal/permeability-increasing protein and azurocidin. *Rheumatology International*, **19**, 129–36.

Cornacoff, J. B., Hebert, L. A., Smead, W. L., VanAman, M. E., Birmingham, D. J. and Waxman, F. J. (1983). Primate erythrocyte-immune complex-clearing mechanism. *Journal of Clinical Investigation*, **71**, 236–47.

Csernok, E., Trabandt, A., Muller, A., Wang, G. C., Moosig, F., Paulsen, J., Schnabel, A. and Goss, W. L. (1999). Cytokine profiles in Wegener's granulomatosis: predominance of type 1 (Th1). in the granulomatous inflammation. *Arthritis and Rheumatism*, **42**, 742–50.

D'Cruz, D., Chesser, A. M., Lightowler, C., Coiner, M., Hurst, M. J., Baker, L. R. and Raine, A. E. (1995). Antineutrophil cytoplasmic antibody-positive crescentic glomerulonephritis associated with anti-thyroid drug treatment. *British Journal of Rheumatology*, **34**, 1090–1.

Dal Canto, A. J. and Virgin, H. W., IV (1999). Animal models of infection-mediated vasculitis. *Current Opinion in Rheumatology*, **11**, 17–23.

de Bandt, M., Meyer, O., Haim, T. and Kahn, M. F. (1996). Antineutrophil cytoplasmic antibodies in rheumatoid arthritis patients. *British Journal of Rheumatology*, **35**, 38–43.

Del Papa, N., Meroni, P. L., Barcellini, W., Sinico, A., Radice, A., Tincani, A., D'Cruz, D., Nicoletti, F., Borghi, M. O. and Khamashta, M. A. (1992). Antibodies to endothelial cells in primary vasculitides mediate *in vitro* endothelial cytotoxicity in the presence of normal peripheral blood mononuclear cells. *Clinical Immunology and Immunopathology*, **63**, 267–74.

Dijstelbloem, H. M., Scheepers, R. H., Oost, W. W., Stegeman, C. A., van der Pol, W. L., Sluiter, W. J., Kallenberg, C. G., van de Winkel, J. G. and Tervaert, J. W. (1999). Fcgamma receptor polymorphisms in Wegener's granulomatosis: risk factors for disease relapses. *Arthritis and Rheumatism*, **42**, 1823–27.

Dixon, F. J., Vazquez, J. J., Weigle, W. O. and Cochrane, C. G. (1958). Pathogenesis of serum sickness. *Archives of Pathology*, **65**, 18–28.

Dolman, K. M., Gans, R. O., Vervaat, T. J., Zevenbergen, G., Maingay, D., Nikkels, R. E., Donker, A. J., dem Borne, A. E. and Goldschmeding, R. (1993). Vasculitis and antineutrophil cytoplasmic autoantibodies associated with propylthiouracil therapy. *Lancet*, **342** (8872), 651–2.

Dowd, S. K., Rodgers, G. C. and Callen, J. P. (1995). Effective treatment with alpha 1-protease inhibitor of chronic cutaneous vasculitis associated with alpha 1-antitrypsin deficiency. *Journal of the American Academy of Dermatology*, **33**, 913–6.

Doyle, P. W., Gibson, G. and Dolman, C. L. (1983). Herpes zoster ophthalmicus with contralateral hemiplegia: identification of cause. *Annals of Neurology*, **14**, 84–5.

Duffy, T. N., Genta, M., Moll, S., Martin, P. Y. and Gabay, C. (2006). Henoch Schonlein purpura following etanercept treatment of rheumatoid arthritis. *Clinical and Experimental Rheumatology*, **24**, S106.

DuMouchel, W., Smith, E. T., Beasley, R., Nelson, H., Yang, X., Fram, D. and Almenoff, J. S. (2004). Association of asthma therapy and Churg-Strauss syndrome: an analysis of postmarketing surveillance data. *Clinical Therapeutics*, **26**, 1092–104.

Eichhorn, J., Sima, D., Thiele, B., Lindschau, C., Turowski, A., Schmidt, H., Schneider, W., Haller, H. and Luft, F. C. (1996). Anti-endothelial cell antibodies in Takayasu arteritis. *Circulation*, **94**, 2396–401.

Elkayam, O., Yaron, M. and Caspi, D. (1999). Minocycline-induced autoimmune syndromes: an overview. *Seminars in Arthritis and Rheumatism*, **28**, 392–7.

Enat, R., Katz, R., Munichor, M. and Pollack, S. (1988). Hypersensitivity vasculitis induced by terbutaline sulfate. *Annals of Allergy*, **61**, 275–6.

Erdbrugger, U., Hellmark, T., Bunch, D. O., Alcorta, D. A., Jennette, J. C., Falk, R. J., Nachman, P. H. (2006). Mapping of myeloperoxidase epitopes recognized by MPO-ANCA using human-mouse MPO chimers. *Kidney International*, **69**, 1799–805.

Escudero, A., Lucas, E., Vidal, J. B., Sanchez-Guerrero, I., Martinez, A., Illan, F. and Ramos, J. (1996). Drug-related Henoch-Schönlein Purpura. *Allergologia et Immunopathologia*, **24**, 22–4.

Esnault, V. L., Audrain, M. A., and Sesboue, R. (1997). Alpha-1-antitrypsin phenotyping in ANCA-associated diseases: one of several arguments for protease/antiprotease imbalance in systemic vasculitis. *Experimental and Clinical Immunogenetics*, **14**, 206–13.

Estes, P. C. and Cheville, N. F. (1970). The ultrastructure of vascular lesions in equine viral arteritis. *American Journal of Pathology*, **58**, 235–53.

Ewert, B. H., Jennette, J. C. and Falk, R. J. (1992). Anti-myeloperoxidase antibodies stimulate neutrophils to damage human endothelial cells. *Kidney International*, **41**, 375–83.

Falk, R. J., Terrell, R. S., Charles, L. A. and Jennette, J. C. (1990). Anti-neutrophil cytoplasmic autoantibodies induce neutrophils to degranulate and produce oxygen radicals *in vitro*. *Proceedings of the National Academy of Sciences of the United States of America*, **87**, 4115–9.

Fauci, A. S., Haynes, B. and Katz, P. (1978). The spectrum of vasculitis: clinical, pathologic, immunologic and therapeutic considerations. *Annals of Internal Medicine*, **89**, 660–76.

Fearon, D. T. (1984). Cellular receptors for fragments of the third component of complement. *Immunology Today*, **5**, 105–10.

Feriozzi, S., Muda, A. O., Gomes, V., Montanaro, M., Faraggiana, T. and Ancarani, E. (2000). Cephotaxime-associated allergic interstitial nephritis and MPO-ANCA positive vasculitis. *Renal Failure*, **22**, 245–51.

Fischetti, F. and Tedesco, F. (2006). Cross-talk between the complement system and endothelial cells in physiologic conditions and in vascular diseases. *Autoimmunity*, **39**, 417–28.

Flores-Suarez, L. F., Cabiedes, J., Villa, A. R., van der Woude F. J. and Alcocer-Varela, J. (2003). Prevalence of antineutrophil cytoplasmic autoantibodies in patients with tuberculosis. *Rheumatology*, **42**, 223–9.

Franssen, C., Gans, R., Kallenberg, C., Hageluken, C. and Hoorntje, S. (1998). Disease spectrum of patients with anti-neutrophil cytoplasmic autoantibodies of defined specificity: distinct differences between patients with anti-proteinase 3 and anti-myeloperoxidase autoantibodies. *Journal of Internal Medicine*, **244**, 209–16.

Fredericks, R. K., Leflcowitz, D. S., Challa, V. R. and Troost, B. T. (1991). Cerebral vasculitis associated with cocaine abuse. *Stroke*, **22**, 1437–9.

Gabriel, S. E., Espy, M., Erdman, D. D., Bjornsson, J., Smith, T. F. and Hunder, G. G. (1999). The role of parvovirus B19 in the pathogenesis of giant cell arteritis: a preliminary evaluation. *Arthritis and Rheumatism*, **42**, 1225–8.

Gaffey, C. M., Chun, B., Harvey, J. C. and Manz, H. J. (1986). Phenytoin-induced systemic granulomatous vasculitis. *Archives of Pathology and Laboratory Medicine*, **110**, 131–5.

Galaria, N. A., Werth, V. P. and Schumacher, H. R. (2000). Leukocytoclsatic vasculitis due to etanercept. *Journal of Rheumatology*, **27**, 2041–4.

Gammeltoft, M. and Kristensen, J. K. (1982). Propylthiouracil-induced cutaneous vasculitis. *Acta Dermato-Venereologica*, **62**, 171–3.

Gao, Y., Zhao, M. H., Guo, X. H., Xin, G., Gao, Y. and Wang, H. Y. (2004). The prevalence and target antigens of antithyroid drugs induced antineutrophil cytoplasmic antibodies (ANCA) in Chinese patients with hyperthyroidism. *Endocrine Research*, **30**, 205–13.

Garcia-Fuentes, M., Martin, A., Chantler, C. and Williams, D. G. (1978). Serum complement components in Henoch-Schönlein purpura. *Archives of Disease in Childhood*, **53**, 417–9.

García-Porrua, C., González-Gay, M. A. and Lopez-Lazaro, L. (1999). Drug associated cutaneous vasculitis in adults in northwestern Spain. *Journal of Rheumatology*, **26**, 1942–4.

Gasser, S., Kuhn, M. and Speich, R. (2004). Severe necrotising leucocytoclastic vasculitis in a patient taking bosentan. *British Medical Journal*, **329**, 430.

Gavura, S. R. and Nusinowitz, S. (1998). Leukocytoclastic vasculitis associated with clarithromycin. *Annals of Pharmacotherapy*, **32**, 543–5.

Geffriaud-Ricouard, C., Noel, L. H., Chauveau, D., Houhou, S., Grunfeld, J. P. and Lesavre, P. (1993). Clinical spectrum associated with ANCA of defined antigen specificities in 98 selected patients. *Clinical Nephrology*, **39**, 125–36.

Genel, F., Sjoholm, A. G., Skattum, L. and Truedsson, L. (2005). Complement factor I deficiency associated with recurrent infections, vasculitis and immune complex glomerulonephritis. *Scandinavian Journal of Infectious Diseases*, **37**, 615–18.

Gephardt, G. N., Ahmad, M. and Tubbs, R. R. (1983). Pulmonary vasculitis (Wegener's granulomatosis) Immunohistochemical study of T and B cell markers. *American Journal of Medicine*, **74**, 700–704.

Gerber, B. O. and Pichler, W. J. (2006). Noncovalent interactions of drugs with immune receptors may mediate drug-induced hypersensitivity reactions. *The AAPS Journal*, **8**, E160–5.

Ghebrehiwet, B., CebadaMora, C., Tantral, L., Jesty, J. and Peerschke, E. I. (2006). gC1qR/p33 serves as a molecular bridge between the complement and contact activation systems and is an important catalyst in inflammation. *Advances in Experimental Medicine and Biology*, **586**, 95–105.

Giangiacomo, J. and Tsai, C. C. (1977). Dermal and glomerular deposition of IgA in anaphylactoid purpura. *Journal of Diseases of Children*, **131**, 981–3.

Gilligan, H. M., Bredy, B., Brady, H. R. *et al.* (1996). Antineutrophil cytoplasmic autoantibodies interact with primary granule constituents on the surface of apoptotic neutrophils in the absence of neutrophil priming. *Journal of Experimental Medicine*, **184**, 2231–41.

Giscombe, R., Nityanand, S., Lewin, N., Grunewald, J. and Lefvert, A. K. (1998). Expanded T cell populations in patients with Wegener's granulomatosis: characteristics and correlates with disease activity. *Journal of Clinical Immunology*, **18**, 404–13.

Gisselbrecht, M. (1999). Vasculitis during human acquired immunodeficiency virus infection. [French] *Pathologie Biologie*, **47**, 245–7.

Glick, R., Hoying, J., Cerullo, L. and Perlman, S. (1987). Phenylpropanolamine: an over-the-counter drug causing central nervous system vasculitis and intracerebral hemorrhage. Case report and review, *Neurosurgery*, **20**, 969–74.

Gocke, D. J., Hsu, K., Morgan, C., Bombardieri, S., Lockshin, M. and Christian, C. L. (1970). Association between polyarteritis and Australia antigen. *Lancet*, **2** (7684), 1149–53.

Goldberg, E. I., Shoji, T. and Sapadin, A. N. (1999). Henoch-Schönlein purpura induced by clarithromycin. *International Journal of Dermatology*, **38**, 706–8.

Gotlib, V., Darji, J., Bloomfield, K., Chadburn, A., Patel, A. and Braunschweig, I. (2003). Eosinophilic variant of chronic myeloid leukemia with vascular complications. *Leukemia and Lymphoma*, **44**, 1609–13.

Gower, R. G., Sams, W. M., Jr., Thorne, E. G., Kohler, P. F. and Claman, H. N. (1977). Leukocytoclastic vasculitis: sequential appearance of immunoreactants and cellular changes in serial biopsies. *Journal of Investigative Dermatology*, **69**, 477–84.

Gower, R. G., Sausker, W. F., Kohler, P. F., Thorne, G. E. and McIntosh, R. M. (1978). Small vessel vasculitis caused by hepatitis B virus immune complexes. Small vessel vasculitis and HBsAG. *Journal of Allergy and Clinical Immunology*, **62**, 222–8.

Gregersen, P. K., Lee, H. S., Batliwalla, F. and Begovich, A. B. (2006). PTPN22: setting thresholds for autoimmunity. *Seminars in Immunology*, **18**, 214–23.

Grennan, D. M., Jolly, J., Holloway, L. J. and Palmer, D. G. (1979). Vasculitis in a patient receiving naproxen. *New Zealand Medical Journal*, **89**, 48–9.

Griffith, M. E., Lovegrove, J. U., Gaskin, G., Whitehouse, D. B. and Pusey, C. D. (1996). C-antineutrophil cytoplasmic antibody positivity in vasculitis patients is associated with the Z allele of alpha-1-antitrypsin, and P-antineutrophil cytoplasmic antibody positivity with the S allele. *Nephrology, Dialysis, Transplantation*, **11**, 438–43.

Groger, M., Fischer, G. F., Wolff, K. and Petzelbauer, P. (1999). Immune complexes from vasculitis patients bind to endothelial Fc receptors independent of the allelic polymorphism of FcgammaRIIa. *Journal of Investigative Dermatology*, **113**, 56–60.

Grunwald, M. H., Halevy, S. and Livni, E. (1989). Allergic vasculitis induced by hydrochiorothiazide: confirmation by mast cell degranulation test. *Israel Journal of Medical Sciences*, **25**, 572–4.

Grunwald, M. H., Avinoach, I., Amichai, B. and Halevy, S. (1997). Leukocytoclastic vasculitis-correlation between different histologic stages and direct immunofluorescence results. *International Journal of Dermatology*, **36**, 349–52.

Gupta, M. N., Sturrock, R. D. and Gupta, G. (2000). Cutaneous leucocytoclastic vasculitis caused by cyclosporin A (Sandimmun). *Annals of the Rheumatic Diseases*, **59**, 319.

Hamzaoui, K., Hamzaoui, A., Ghorbel, I., Khanfir, M. and Houman, H. (2006). Levels of IL-15 in serum and cerebrospinal fluid of patients with Behçet's disease. *Scandinavian Journal of Immunology*, **64**, 655–60.

Haraoui, B. and Keystone, E. (2006). Musculoskeletal manifestations and autoimmune diseases related to new biologic agents. *Current Opinion in Rheumatology*, **18**, 96–100.

Harper, L., Cockwell, P., Adu, D. and Savage, C. O. (2001). Neutrophil priming and apoptosis in anti-neutrophil cytoplasmic autoantibody-associated vasculitis. *Kidney International*, **59**, 1729–38.

Harris, A., Chang, G., Vadas, M. and Gillis, D. (1999). ELISA is the superior method for detecting antineutrophil cytoplasmic antibodies in the diagnosis of systemic necrotising vasculitis. *Journal of Clinical Pathology*, **52**, 670–6.

Hart, M. N., Tassell, S. K., Sadewasser, K. L., Schelper, R. L. and Moore, S. A. (1985). Autoimmune vasculitis resulting from *in vitro* immunization of lymphocytes to smooth muscle. *American Journal of Pathology*, **119**, 448–55.

Hasler, P., Kistler, H. and Gerber, H. (1995). Vasculitides in hairy cell leukemia. *Seminars in Arthritis and Rheumatism*, **25**, 134–42.

Haynes, B. F. (1992). Vasculitis: pathogenic mechanisms of vessel damage. In: *Inflammation: basic principles and clinical correlates*, 2nd edn (eds J. I. Gallin and I. M.S. R. Goldstein), pp. 921–41. Raven Press, New York.

Heeringa, P., Huugen, D. and Tervaert, J. W. (2005). Anti-neutrophil cytoplasmic autoantibodies and leukocyte-endothelial interactions: a sticky connection? *Trends in Immunology*, **26**, 561–4.

Hellmich, B., Csernok, E., Trabandt, A., Gross, W. L. and Ernst, M. (2000). Granulocyte-macrophage colony-stimulating factor (GM-CSF) but not granulocyte colony-stimulating factor (G-CSF) induces plasma membrane expression of proteinase 3 (PR3). on neutrophils *in vitro*. *Clinical and Experimental Immunology*, **120**, 392–8.

Hellmich, B., Csernok, E. and Gross, W. L. (2005). Proinflammatory cytokines and autoimmunity in Churg-Strauss syndrome. *Annals of the New York Academy of Science*, **1051**, 121–31.

Hewins, P., Williams, J. M., Wakelam, M. J. and Savage, C. O. (2004). Activation of Syk in neutrophils by antineutrophil cytoplasm antibodies occurs via Fcgamma receptors and CD18. *Journal of the American Society for Nephrology*, **15**, 796–808.

Hewins, P., Morgan, M. D., Holden, N., Neil, D., Williams, J. M., Savage, C. O. and Harper, L. (2006). IL-18 is upregulated in the kidney and primes neutrophil responsiveness in ANCA-associated vasculitis. *Kidney International*, **69**, 605–15.

Hoffman, G. S. (1997). Vasculitic syndromes. *Current Opinion in Rheumatology*, **9**, 1–2.

Holmen, C., Christensson, M., Pettersson, E., Bratt, J., Stjarne, P., Karrar, A. and Sumitran-Holgersson, S. (2004). Wegener's granulomatosis is associated with organ-specific antiendothelial cell antibodies. *Kidney International*, **66**, 1049–60.

Holt, P. (1999). Systemic vasculitis associated with long-term phenytoin therapy. *New Zealand Medical Journal*, **112**, 100.

Hui-Yuen, J. S., Duong, T. T. and Yeung, R. S. (2006). TNF-alpha is necessary for induction of coronary artery inflammation and aneurysm formation in an animal model of Kawasaki disease. *Journal of Immunology*, **176**, 6294–301.

Huugen, D., Xiao, H., van Esch, A., Falk, R. J., Peutz-Kootstra, C. J., Buurman, W. A., Tervaert, J. W., Jennette, J. C. and Heeringa, P. (2005). Aggravation of anti-myeloperoxidase antibody-induced glomerulonephritis by bacterial lipopolysaccharide: role of tumor necrosis factor-alpha. *American Journal of Pathology*, **167**, 47–58.

Igarashi, H., Hatake, K., Tomizuka, H., Yamada, M., Gunji, Y. and Momoi, M. Y. (1999). High serum levels of M-CSF and G-CSF in Kawasaki disease. *British Journal of Haematology*, **105**, 613–15.

Iking-Konert, C., Ostendorf, B., Foede, M., Fischer-Betz, R., Jung, G., Haensch, M. G. and Schneider, M. (2004). Granulocyte colony-stimulating factor induces disease flare in patients with ANCA associated vasculitis. *Journal of Rheumatology*, **31**, 1655–8.

Imai, H., Nakamoto, Y., Hirokawa, M., Akihama, T. and Miura, A. B. (1989). Carbamazepine-induced granulomatous necrotizing angiitis with acute renal failure. *Nephron*, **51**, 405–408.

Iredale, J. P., Sankaran, R. and Wathen, C. G. (1989). Cutaneous vasculitis associated with rifampin therapy. *Chest*, **96**, 215–16.

Ishikawa, H., Okada, S., Katayama, I., Mazaki, H., Nagatake, T., Hasebe, F. and Igarashi, A. (1999). A Japanese case of dengue fever with lymphocytic vasculitis: diagnosis by polymerase chain reaction. *Journal of Dermatology*, **26**, 29–32.

Jacobs-Kosmin, D., Derk, C. T. and Sandorfi, N. (2006). Pantoprazole and perinuclear antineutrophil cytoplasmic antibody-associated vasculitis. *Journal of Rheumatology*, **33**, 629–32).

Jacobson, M. (1996). Reactive oxygen species and programmed cell death. *Trends in Biological Sciences*, **21**, 83–7.

Jagiello, P., Aries, P., Arning, L., Wagenleiter, S. E., Csernok, E., Hellmich, B., Gross, W. L. and Epplen, J. T. (2005). The PTPN22 620W allele is a risk factor for Wegener's granulomatosis. *Arthritis and Rheumatism*, **52**, 4039–43.

Jahangiri, M., Jayatunga, A. P., Bradley, J. W. and Goodwin, T. J. (1992). Naproxen-associated vasculitis. *Postgraduate Medical Journal*, **68**, 766–7.

Jennette, J. C. and Falk, R. J. (1998). Pathogenesis of the vascular glomerular damage in ANCA-positive vasculitis. *Nephrology, Dialysis, Transplantation*, **13** (Suppl. 1), 16–20.

Jennette, J. C., Xiao, H. and Falk, R. J. Pathogenesis of vascular inflammation by anti-neutrophil cytoplasmic antibodies (2006). *Journal of the American Society for Nephrology* **5**, 1235–42.

Kaiser, M., Younge, B., Bjornsson, J., Goronzy, J. J. and Weyand, C. M. (1999). Formation of new vasa vasorum in vasculitis. Production of angiogenic cytokines by multinucleated giant cells. *American Journal of Pathology*, **155**, 765–74.

Kallenberg, C. G., Cohen Tervaert, J. W., van der Woude, F. J., Goldschmeding, R., dem Borne, A. E. and Weening, J. J. (1991). Autoimmunity to lysosomal enzymes: new clues to vasculitis and glomerulonephritis? *Immunology Today*, **12**, 61–4.

Kammer, G. M., Soter, N. A. and Schur, P. H. (1980). Circulating immune complexes in patients with necrotizing vasculitis. *Clinical Immunology and Immunopathology*, **15**, 658–72.

Kasahara, Y., Iwai, K., Yachie, A. *et al.* (1997). Involvement of reactive oxygen intermediaries in spontaneous and CD95 (Fas/APO-1)-mediated apoptosis of neutrophils. *Blood*, **89**, 1748–53.

Kauffmann, R. H., Herrmann, Meyer, C. J., Daha, M. R. and Van Es, L. A. (1980). Circulating IgA-immune complexes in Henoch-Schonlein purpura. A longitudinal study of their relationship to disease activity and vascular deposition of IgA. *American Journal of Medicine,* **69,** 859–66.

Kawana, S. and Nishiyama, S. (1992). Serum SC5b-9 (terminal complement complex) level, a sensitive indicator of disease activity in patients with Henoch-Schonlein purpura. *Dermatology,* **184,** 171–6.

Keogh, K. A. and Specks, U. (2003). Churg-Strauss syndrome: clinical presentation, antineutrophil cytoplasmic antibodies, and leukotriene receptor antagonists. *American Journal Medicine,* **115,** 284–90.

Kerns, W., Schwartz, L., Blanchard, K., Burchiel, S., Essayan, D., Fung, E., *et al.*; Expert Working Group on Drug-Induced Vascular Injury. (2005). Drug-induced vascular injury-a quest for biomarkers. *Toxicology and Applied Pharmacology,* **203,** 62–87.

Kettritz, R., Wilke, S., von Vietinghoff, S., Luft, F. and Schneider, W. (2006). Apoptosis, proliferation and inflammatory infiltration in ANCA-positive glomerulonephritis. *Clinical Nephrology,* **65,** 309–16.

Kitahara, T., Hiromura, K., Maezawa, A., Ono, K., Narabara, N., Yano, S., Naruse, T., Takenouchi, K., and Yasumoto, Y. (1997). Case of propylthiouracil-induced vasculitis associated with anti-neutrophil cytoplasmic antibody (ANCA); review of literature. *Clinical Nephrology,* **47,** 336–40.

Klima, M. and Waddell, C. C. (1984). Hairy cell leukemia associated with focal vascular damage. *Human Pathology,* **15,** 657–9.

Knox, J. P., Welykyj, S. E., Gradini, R. and Massa, M. C. (1988). Procainamide-induced urticarial vasculitis. *Cutis,* **42,** 469–72.

Kobayashi, S., Ishizuka, S., Tamura, N., Takaya, M., Kaneda, K. and Hashimoto, H. (2003). Churg-Strauss syndrome (CSS) in a patient receiving pranlukast. *Clinical Rheumatology,* **22,** 491–2.

Kondo, N., Kasahara, K., Shinoda, S. and Orii, T. (1992). Accelerated expression of secreted alpha-chain gene in ana-phylactoid purpura. *Journal of Clinical Immunology,* **12,** 193–6.

Krol, T., Robinson, J., Bekeris, L. and Messmore, H. (1983). Hairy cell leukemia and a fatal periarteritis nodosa-like syndrome. *Archives of Pathology and Laboratory Medicine,* **107,** 583–5.

Kuno-Sakai, H., Sakai, H., Nomoto, Y., Takakura, I. and Kimura, M. (1979). Increase of IgA-bearing peripheral blood lymphocytes in children with Henoch-Schoenlein purpura. *Pediatrics,* **64,** 918–22.

Lambert, W. C., Kolber, L. R. and Proper, S. A. (1982). Leukocytoclastic angiitis induced by clindamycin. *Cutis,* **30,** 615–9.

Lawley, T. J., Bielory, L., Gascon, P., Yancey, K. B., Young, N. S. and Frank, M. M. (1984). A prospective clinical and immunologic analysis of patients with serum sickness. *New England Journal of Medicine,* **311,** 1407–13.

Lee, A. Y. (1999). A case of leukocytoclastic vasculitis associated with haloperidol [letter]. *Clinical and Experimental Dermatology,* **24,** 430.

Lee, S. and Lawton, J. W. (2000). Heterogeneity of anti-PR3 associated disease in Hong Kong. *Postgraduate Medical Journal,* **76,** 287–8.

Lee, Y. J., Kang, S. W., Park, J. J., Bae, Y. D., Lee, E. Y., Lee, E. B. and Song, Y. W. (2006). Interleukin-18 promoter polymorphisms in patients with Behcet's disease. *Human Immunology,* **67,** 812–8.

Leung, D. Y., Meissner, H. C., Fulton, D. R., Murray, D. L., Kotzin, B. L. and Schlievert, P. M. (1993). Toxic shock syndrome toxin-secreting *Staphylococcus aureus* in Kawasaki syndrome. *Lancet,* **342** (8884), 1385–8.

Leung, D. Y. M., Geha, R. S., Newburger, J. W., *et al.* (1986a). Two monokines, interleukin-l and tumor necrosis factor, render cultured vascular endothelial cells susceptible to lysis by antibodies circulating during Kawasaki syndrome. *Journal of Experimental Medicine,* **164,** 1958–72.

Leung, K. Y. M., Collins, T., Lapierre, L. A., Geha, R. S. and Pober, J. S. (1986b). Immunoglobulin M antibodies present in the acute phase of Kawasaki syndrome lyse cultured vascular endothelial cells stimulated by gamma interferon. *Journal of Clinical Investigation,* **77,** 1428–35.

Levo, Y., Gorevic, P. D., Kassab, H. J., Zucker-Franklin, D. and Franklin, E. C. (1977). Association between hepatitis B virus and essential mixed cryoglobulinemia. *New England Journal of Medicine,* **296,** 1501–504.

Lie, J. T. and Dixit, R. K. (1996). Nonsteroidal antiinflammatory drug induced hypersensitivity vasculitis clinically mimicking temporal arteritis. *Journal of Rheumatology,* **23,** 183–5.

Linnemann, C. C. and Alvira, M. M. (1980). Pathogenesis of varicella-zoster angitis in the CNS. *Archives of Neurology,* **37,** 239–40.

Little, M. A., Smyth, C. L., Yadav, R., Ambrose, L., Cook, H. T., Nourshargh, S. and Pusey, C. D. (2005). Antineutrophil cytoplasm antibodies directed against myeloperoxidase augment leukocyte-microvascular interactions *in vivo. Blood,* **196,** 2050–8.

Llanos, C., Soto, L., Sabugo, F., Gallegos, I., Valenzuela, O., Verdaguer, J. and Cuchacovich, M. (2006). Systemic vasculitis associated with Fasciola hepatica infection. *Scandinavian Journal of Rheumatology,* **35,** 143–6.

Lockwood, C. M., Thiru, S., Isaacs, J. D., Hale, G. and Waldmann, H. (1993). Long-term remission of intractable systemic vasculitis with monoclonal antibody therapy. *Lancet,* **341,** 1620–2.

Lowry, M. D., Hudson, C. F. and Callen, J. P. (1994). Leukocytoclastic vasculitis caused by drug additives. *Journal of the American Academy of Dermatology,* **30,** 854–5.

Lu, X., Garfield, A., Rainger, G. E., Savage, C. O. and Nash, G. B. (2006). Mediation of endothelial cell damage by serine proteases, but not superoxide, released from antineutrophil cytoplasmic antibody-stimulated neutrophils. *Arthritis and Rheumatism,* **54,** 1619–28.

Ludviksson, B. R., Sneller, M. C., Chua, K. S., Talar-Williams, C., Langford, C. A., Ehrhardt, R. O., Fauci, A. S. and Strober, W. (1998). Active Wegener's granulomatosis is associated with HLA–DR + CD4 + T cells exhibiting an unbalanced Th1-type T cell cytokine pattern: reversal with IL-10. *Journal of Immunology,* **160,** 3602–609.

MacDonald, J., Zhong, T., Lazarescu, A., Gan, B. S. and Harth, M. (2004). Vasculitis associated with the use of leflunomide. *Journal Rheumatology,* **31,** 2076–8.

McCluskey, R. T. and Fienberg, R. (1983). Vasculitis in primary vasculitides, granulomatoses, and connective tissue diseases. *Human Pathology,* **14,** 305–15.

Margolis, M. T. and Newton, T. H. (1971). Methamphetamine ("Speed"). *Arteritis Neuroradiology,* **2,** 179–182.

Martinez-Taboada, V. M., Blanco, R., Garcia-Fuentes, M. and Rodriguez-Valverde, V. (1997). Clinical features and outcome of 95 patients with hypersensitivity vasculitis. *American Journal of Medicine,* **102,** 186–91.

Matsunawa, M., Isozaki, T., Odai, T., Yajima, N., Takeuchi, H. T., Negishi, M., Ide, H., Adachi, M. and Kasama, T. (2006). Increased serum levels of soluble fractalkine (CX3CL1). correlate with disease activity in rheumatoid vasculitis. *Arthritis and Rheumatism,* **54,** 3408–16.

Mayet, W. J., Schwarting, A., Orth, T., Duchmann, R., Meyer, Z. and Buschenfelde, K. H. (1996). Antibodies to proteinase 3 mediate expression of vascular cell adhesion molecule-1 (VCAM-1). *Clinical and Experimental Immunology,* **103,** 259–67.

Mayet, W., Schwarting, A., Barreiros, A. P., Schlaak, J. and Neurath, M. (1999). Anti-PR-3 antibodies induce endothelial IL-8 release. *European Journal of Clinical Investigation,* **29,** 973–9.

Mazodier, P., Elzouki, A. N., Segelmark, M. and Eriksson, S. (1996). Systemic necrotizing vasculitides in severe alpha1-antitrypsin deficiency. *Quarterly Journal of Medicine,* **89,** 599–611.

McCormick, R. V. (1950). Periarteritis occurring during propylthiouracil therapy. *Journal of the American Medical Association,* **144,** 1453–4.

Medof, M. E., Iida, K., Mold, C. and Nussenzweig, V. (1982). Unique role of the complement receptor CR1 in the degradation of C3b associated with immune complexes. *Journal of Experimental Medicine,* **156,** 1739–54.

Merkel, P. A. (2001). Drug-induced vasculitis. *Rheumatic Disease Clinics of North America,* **27,** 849–62.

Mesec, A., Rot, U., Perkovic, T., Lunder, T. and Sibanc, B. (1999). Carbamazepine hypersensitivity syndrome presenting as vasculitis of the CNS [letter]. *Journal of Neurology, Neurosurgery and Psychiatry*, **66**, 249–50.

Michalak, T. (1978). Immune complexes of hepatitis B surface antigen in the pathogenesis of periarteritis nodosa. A study of seven necropsy cases. *American Journal of Pathology*, **90**, 619–32.

Miller, G. W. and Nussenzweig, V. (1975). A new complement function: solubilization of antigen-antibody aggregates. *Proceedings of the National Academy of Sciences of the United States of America*, **72**, 418–22.

Miller, R. M., Savige, J., Nassis, L. and Cominos, B. I. (1998). Antineutrophil cytoplasmic antibody (ANCA)-positive cutaneous leucocytoclastic vasculitis associated with antithyroid therapy in Graves' disease. *Australian Journal of Dermatology*, **39**, 96–9.

Mitchell, G. G., Magnusson, A. R. and Weiler, J. M. (1983). Cimetidine-induced cutaneous vasculitis. *American Journal of Medicine*, **75**, 875–6.

Mitsuyama, H., Matsuyama, W., Iwakawa, J., Higashimoto, I., Watanabe, M., Osame, M. and Arimura, K. (2006). Increased serum vascular endothelial growth factor level in Churg-Strauss syndrome. *Chest*, **129**, 407–11.

Mockel, M., Kampf, D., Lobeck, H. and Frei, U. (1999). Severe panarteritis associated with drug abuse. *Intensive Care Medicine*, **25**, 113–7.

Mohan, N., Edwards, E. T., Cupps, T. R., Slifman, N., Lee, J. H., Siegel, J. N. and Braun, M. M. (2004). Leucocytoclastic vasculitis associated with tumor necrosis factor-alpha blocking agents. *Journal of Rheumatology*, **31**, 1955–8.

Moneret-Vautrin, D. A., Faure, G. and Bene, M. C. (1986). Chewing-gum preservative induced toxidermic vasculitis. *Allergy*, **41**, 546–8.

Morita, A., Imada, Y., Igarashi, H. and Yutsudo, T. (1997). Serologic evidence that streptococcal superantigens are not involved in the pathogenesis of Kawasaki disease. *Microbiology and Immunology*, **41**, 895–900.

Morrow, P. L. and McQuillen, J. B. (1993). Cerebral vasculitis associated with cocaine abuse. *Journal of Forensic Sciences*, **38**, 732–8.

Muller Kobold, A. C., Kallenberg, C. G. and Tervaert, J. W. (1998). Leucocyte membrane expression of proteinase 3 correlates with disease activity in patients with Wegener's granulomatosis. *British Journal of Rheumatology*, **37**, 901–7.

Muller Kobold, A. C., van Wijk, R. T., Franssen, C. F., Molema, G., Kallenberg, C. G. and Tervaert, J. W. (1999a). *in vitro* up-regulation of E-selectin and induction of inter-leukin-6 in endothelial cells by autoantibodies in Wegener's granulomatosis and microscopic polyangiitis. *Clinical and Experimental Rheumatology*, **17**, 433–40.

Muller Kobold, A. C., Kallenberg, C. G. and Tervaert, J. W. (1999b). Monocyte activation in patients with Wegener's granulomatosis. *Annals of the Rheumatic Diseases*, **58**, 237–45.

Nagore, E., Sanchez-Motilla, J. M., Navarro, V., Febrer, M. I. and Aliaga, A. (1999). Leukocytoclastic vasculitis as a cutaneous manifestation of systemic infection caused by *Brucella melitensis*. *Cutis*, **63**, 25–7.

Nicklin, M. J., Hughes, D.E., Barton, J. L., Ure, J. M. and Duff, G. W. (2000). Arterial inflammation in mice lacking the interleukin 1 receptor antagonist gene. *Journal of Experimental Medicine*, **191**, 303–12.

Niehaus, L. and Meyer, B. U. (1998). Bilateral borderzone brain infarctions in association with heroin abuse. *Journal of the Neurological Sciences*, **160**, 180–2.

Nishimura, M., Ishikawa, Y. and Satake, M. (2004). Activation of polymorphonuclear neutrophils by immune complex: possible involvement in development of transfusion-related acute lung injury. *Transfusion Medicine*, **14**, 359–67.

Noh, J. Y., Asari, T., Hamada, N. *et al.* (2001). Frequency of appearance of myeloperoxidase-antineutrophil cytoplasmic antibody (MPO-ANCA) in Graves' disease patients treated with propylthiouracil and the relationship between MPO-ANCA and clinical manifestations. *Clinical Endocrinology (Oxford)*, **54**, 651–4.

Noris, M., Daina, E., Gamba, S., Bonazzola, S. and Remuzzi, G. (1999). Interleukin-6 and RANTES in Takayasu arteritis: a guide for therapeutic decisions? *Circulation*, **100**, 55–60.

Oberndorfer, S., Beate, U., Sabine, U., Peter, H., Heinz, L., Barabra, H. and Wolfgang, G. (2004). Churg-Strauss syndrome during treatment of bronchial asthma with a leucotriene receptor antagonist presenting with polyneuropathy. *Neurologia*, **19**, 134–8.

Ohlsson, S., Hellmark, T., Pieters, K., Sturfelt, G., Wieslander, J. and Segelmark, M. (2005). Increased monocyte transcription of the roteinase 3 gene in small vessel vasculitis. *Clinical and Experimental Immunology*, **141**, 175–82.

Orpin, S. D., Majmudar, V. B., Soon, C., Azam, N. A. and Salim, A. (2006). Adalimumab causing vasculitis. *British Journal of Dermatology*, **154**, 998–9.

Oztas, M. O., Onder, M., Gurer, M. A., Bukan, N. and Sancak, B. (2005). Serum interleukin 18 and tumour necrosis factor-alpha levels are increased in Behcet's disease. *Clinical and Experimental Dermatology*, **30**, 61–3.

Pagnoux, C., Guilpain, P. and Guillevin, L. (2007). Churg-Strauss syndrome. *Current Opinion in Rheumatology*, **19**, 25–32.

Papadopoulos, D. P., Makris, T. K., Krespi, P., Papazachou, U., Stavroulakis, G., Hatzizacharias, A. and Votteas, V. (2006). Antiendothelial cell antibody levels in healthy normotensives with high normal blood pressure. *Clinical and Experimental Hypertension*, **28**, 663–7.

Park, M. C., Park, Y. B., Jung, S. Y., Lee, K. H. and Lee, S. K. (2006). Anti-endothelial cell antibodies and antiphospholipid antibodies in Takayasu's arteritis: correlations of their titers and isotype distributions with disease activity. *Clinical and Experimental Rheumatology*, **24** (2 Suppl. 41), S10–6.

Park, M. C., Lee, S. W., Park, Y. B. and Lee, S. K. (2006). Serum cytokine profiles and their correlations with disease activity in Takayasu's arteritis. *Rheumatology* (Oxford), **45**, 545–8.

Pelletier, F., Puzenate, E. *et al.* (2003). Minocycline-induced cutaneous polyarteritis nodosa with antineutrophil cytoplasmic antibodies. *European Journal of Dermatology*, **13**, 396–8.

Pendergraft, W. F., Alcorta, D. A., Segelmark, M., Yang, J. J., Tuttle, R., Jennette, J. C., Falk, R. J. and Preston, G. A. (2000). ANCA antigens, proteinase 3 and myeloperoxidase, are not expressed in endothelial cells. *Kidney International*, **57**, 1981–90.

Pendergraft, W. F., Preston, G. A., Shah, R. R., Tropsha, A., Jennette, J. C. and Falk, R. J. (2004). cPR3105–206, a protein complementary to the autoantigen proteinase 3, triggers autoimmunity. *Nature Medicine*, **10**, 72–9.

Perez, C., Hernandez, R., Murie, M., Vives, R. and Guarch, R. (1999). Relapsing leucocytoclastic vasculitis as the initial manifestation of acute brucellosis [letter]. *British Journal of Dermatology*, **140**, 1177–8.

Pfister, H., Ollert, M., Frohlich, L. F., Quintanilla-Martinex, L., Colby, T. V., Specks, U. and Jenne, D. E. (2004). Antineutrophil cytoplasmic autoantibodies against the murine homolog of proteinase 3 (Wegener autoantigen) are pathogenic in vivo. *Blood*, **104**, 1411–8.

Popa, E. R., Stegeman, C. A., Bos, N. A., Kallenberg, C. G. and Tervaert, J. W. (1999). Differential B- and T-cell activation in Wegener's granulomatosis. *Journal of Allergy and Clinical Immunology*, **103**, 885–94.

Powers, J. F., Bedri, S., Hussein, S., Salomon, R. N. and Tischler, A. S. (2005). High prevalence of herpes simplex virus DNA in temporal arteritis biopsy specimens. *American Journal of Clinical Pathology*, **123**, 261–4.

Pradhan, V. D., Badakere, S. S., Ghosh, K. and Pawar, A. R.(2004). Spectrum of anti-neutrophil cytoplasmic antibodies in patients with pulmonary tuberculosis overlaps with that of Wegener's granulomatosis. *Indian Journal of Medical Science*, **58**, 283–8.

Radford, D. J., Lord, J. M. and Savage, C. O. (1999). The activation of the neutrophil respiratory burst by anti-neutrophil cytoplasm antibody (ANCA) from patients with systemic vasculitis requires tyrosine kinases and protein kinase C activation. *Clinical and Experimental Immunology*, **118**, 171–9.

Radford, D. J., Savage, C. O. and Nash, G. B. (2000). Treatment of rolling neutrophils with antineutrophil cytoplasmic antibodies causes conversion to firm integrin-mediated adhesion. *Arthritis and Rheumatism*, **43**, 1337–45.

Radford, D. J., Luu, N. T., Hewins, P., Nash, G. B. and Savage, C. O. (2001). Antineutrophil cytoplasmic antibodies stabilize adhesion and promote migration of flowing neutrophils on endothelial cells. *Arthritis and Rheumatism*, **44**, 2851–61.

Ralston, D. R., Marsh, C. B., Lowe, M. P. and Wewers, M. D. (1997). Antineutrophil cytoplasmic antibodies induce monocyte IL-8 release. Role of surface proteinase-3, alphal-antitrypsin, and Fcgamma receptors. *Journal of Clinical Investigation*, **100**, 1416–24.

Rarok, A. A., Stegeman, C. A., Limburg, P. C. and Kallenberg, C. G. (2002). Neutrophil membrane expression of proteinase 3 (PR3). is related to relapse in PR3-ANCA-associated vasculitis. *Journal of the American Society for Nephrology*, **13**, 2232–8.

Rarok, A. A., Limburg, P. C. and Kallenberg, C. G. (2003). Neutrophil-activating potential of antineutrophil cytoplasm autoantibodies. *Journal Leukocyte Biology*, **74**, 3–15.

Rasmussen, N., Petersen, J., Ralfkiaer, E., Avnstom, S. and Wiik, A. (1988). Spontaneous and induced immunoglobulin synthesis and anti-neutrophil cytoplasm antibodies in Wegener's granulomatosis: relation to leukocyte subpopulations in blood and active lesions. *Rheumatology International*, **8**, 153–8.

Reumaux, D., Duthilleul, P. and Roos, D. (2004). Pathogenesis of diseases associated with antineutrophil cytoplasm autoantibodies. *Human Immunology*, **65**, 1–12.

Reyes, M. G., Fresco, R., Chokroverty, S. and Salud, E. Q. (1976). Viruslike particles in granulomatous angiitis of the central nervous system. *Neurology*, **26**, 797–9.

Rittner, H. L., Kaiser, M., Brack, A., Szweda, L. I., Goronzy, J. J. and Weyand, C. M. (1999). Tissue-destructive macrophages in giant cell arteritis. *Circulation Research*, **84**, 1050–8.

Rodriguez-Pla, A., Bosch-Gil, J. A., Echevarria-Mayko, J. E., Rossello-Urgell, J., Solans-Laque, R., Huguet-Redecilla, P., Stone, J. H. and Vilardell-Tarres, M. (2004). No dection of parvovirus B19 or herpesvirus DNA in giant cell arteritis. *Journal of Clinical Virology*, **31**, 11–5.

Rosenberg, J. L., Edlow, D. and Sneider, R. (1978). Liver disease and vasculitis in a patient taking cromolyn. *Archives of Internal Medicine*, **138**, 989–91.

Rote, W. E., Dempsey, E., Maki, S., Vlasuk, G. P. and Moyle, M. (1996). The role of CD11/CD18 integrins in the reverse passive Arthus reaction in rat dermal tissue. *Journal of Leukocyte Biology*, **59**, 254–61.

Rothwell, P. M. and Grant, R. (1996). Cerebral vasculitis following allopurinol treatment. *Postgraduate Medical Journal*, **72**, 119–20.

Salojin, K. V., Le Tonqueze, M., Nassovov, E. L., Blouch, M. T., Baranov, A. A., Sarau A., Guillevin, L., Fiessinger, J. N., Piette, J. C. and Youinou, P. (1996). Anti-endothelial cell antibodies in patients with various forms of vasculitis. *Clinical and Experimental Rheumatology*, **14**, 163–9.

Santos, L. L., Huang, X. R., Berndt, M. C. and Holdsworth, S. R. (1998). P-selectin requirement for neutrophil accumulation and injury in the direct passive Arthus reaction. *Clinical and Experimental Immunology*, **112**, 281–6.

Sato, H., Hattori, M., Fujieda, M. *et al.* (2000). High prevalence of antineutrophil cytoplasmic antibody positivity in childhood onset Graves' disease treated with propylthiiouracil. *Journal of Clinical Endocrinology and Metabolism*, **85**, 4270–3.

Savage, C. O., Pottinger, B. E., Gaskin, G., Lockwood, C. M., Pusey, C. D. and Pearson, (1991). Vascular damage in Wegener's granulomatosis and microscopic polyarteritis: presence of anti-endothelial cell antibodies and their relation to anti-neutrophil cytoplasm antibodies. *Clinical and Experimental Immunology*, **85**, 14–19.

Savage, C. O., Pottinger, B. E., Gaskin, G., Pusey, C. D. and Pearson, J. D. (1992). Autoantibodies developing to myeloperoxidase and proteinase 3 in systemic vasculitis stimulate neutrophil cytotoxicity toward cultured endothelial cells. *American Journal of Pathology*, **141**, 335–42.

Savage, J., Gillis, D. and Benson, E. *et al.* (1999). International consensus statment on testing and reporting of antineutrophil cytoplasmic antibodies. *American Journal of Clinical Pathology*, **111**, 507–13.

Schifferli, J. A., Ng, Y. C. and Peters, D. K. (1986). The role of complement and its receptor in the elimination of immune complexes. *New England Journal of Medicine*, **315**, 488–95.

Schreiber, A., Xiao, H., Falk, R. J. and Jennette, J. C. (2006). Bone marrow-derived cells are sufficient and necessary targets to mediate glomerulonephritis and vasculitis induced by anti-myeloperoxidase antibodies. *Journal of the American Society for Nephrology*, **17**, 3355–64.

Schreiber, A., Luft, F. C. and Kettritz, R. (2004). Membrane proteinase 3 expression and ANCA-induced neutrophil activation. *Kidney International*, **65**, 2172–83.

Schmitt, W. H., Heesen, C., Csernok, E., Rautmann, A. and Gross, W. L. (1992). Elevated serum levels of soluble inter-leukin-2 receptor in patients with Wegener's granulomatosis. Association with disease activity. *Arthritis and Rheumatism*, **35**, 1088–96.

Schrodt, B. J., Kulp-Shorten, C. L. and Callen, J. P. (1999). Necrotizing vasculitis of the skin and uterine cervix associated with minocycline therapy for acne vulgaris. *Southern Medical Journal*, **92**, 502–4.

Schwarting, A., Hagen, D., Odenthal, M., Brockmann, H., Dienes, H. P., Wandel, E., Rumpelt, H. J., Zum Buschenfeld, K. H., Galle, P. R. and Mayet, W. (2000). Proteinase-3 mRNA expressed by glomerular epithelial cells correlates with crescent formation in Wegener's granulomatosis. *Kidney International*, **57**, 2412–22.

Segelmark, M., Elzouki, A. N., Wieslander, J. and Eriksson, S. (1995). The PiZ gene of alpha l-antitrypsin as a determinant of outcome in PR3-ANCA-positive vasculitis. *Kidney International*, **48**, 844–50.

Seibold, F., Brandwein, S., Simpson, S., Terhorst, C. and Elson, C. O. (1998). pANCA represents a cross-reactivity to enteric bacterial antigens. *Journal of Clinical Immunology*, **18**, 153–60.

Sera, N., Ashizawa, K., Ando, T. *et al.* (2000). Treatment with propythiouracil is associated with appearance of antineutrophil cytoplasmic antibodies in some patients with Graves' disease. *Thyroid*, **10**, 595–9.

Sheehan-Dare, R. A. and Goodfield, M. J. (1988). Widespread cutaneous vasculitis associated with diltiazem. *Postgraduate Medical Journal*, **64**, 467–8.

Sindrilaru, A., Seeliger, S., Ehrchen, J. M., Peters, T., Roth, J., Scharffetter-Kochanek, K. and Sunderkotter, C. H. (2007). Site of Blood Vessel Damage and Relevance of CD18 in a Murine Model of Immune Complex-Mediated Vasculitis. *Journal of Investigative Dermatology*, **127**, 447–54.

Smith, R. J., Chosay, J. G., Dunn, C. J., Manning, A. M. and Justen, J. M. (1996). ICAM-l mediates leukocyteendothelium adhesive interactions in the reversed passive Arthus reaction. *Journal of Leukocyte Biology*, **59**, 333–40.

Soravia-Dunand, V. A., Loo, V. G. and Salit, I. E. (1999). Aortitis due to Salmonella: report of 10 cases and comprehensive review of the literature. *Clinical Infectious Diseases*, **29**, 862–8.

Srivastava, M. D., Alexander, F. and Tuthill, R. J. (2005). Immunology of cutaneous vasculitis associated with both etanercept and infliximab. *Scandinavian Journalof Immunology*, **61**, 329–36.

Stevenson, J. A., Leong, L. A., Cohen, A. H. and Border, W. A. (1982). Henoch-Schönlein purpura: simultaneous demonstration of IgA deposits in involved skin, intestine, and kidney. *Archives of Pathology and Laboratory Medicine*, **106**, 192–5.

Subra, J. F., Michelet, C., Laporte, J., Carrere, F., Reboul, P., Cartier, F., Saint-Andre, J. P. and Chevailler, A. (1998). The presence of cytoplasmic antineutrophil cytoplasmic antibodies (C-2 ANCA) in the course of subacute bacterial endocarditis with glomerular involvement, coincidence or association? *Clinical Nephrology*, **49**, 15–18.

Sunderkotter, C., Seeliger, S., Schonlau, F., Roth, J., Hallmann, R., Luger, T. A., Sorg, C. and Kolde, G. (2001). Different pathways leading to cutaneous leukocytoclastic vasculitis in mice. *Experimental Dermatology*, **10**, 391–404.

Suzuki, N., Nara, K. and Suzuki, T. (2006). Skewed Th1 responses caused by excessive expression of Txk, a member of the Tec family of tyrosine kinases, in patients with Behcet's disease. *Clinical Medicine and Research*, **4**, 147–51.

ten Berge, I. J. M., Wilmink, J. M., Meyer C. J.L. M. *et al.* (1985). Clinical and immunological follow-up of patients with severe renal disease in Wegener's granulomatosis. *American Journal of Nephrology*, **5**, 2l–9.

Ten Holder, S. M., Joy, M. S. and Falk, R. J. (2002). Cutaneous and systemic manifestations of drug-induced vasculitis. *Annals of Pharmacotherapy*, **36**, 130–47.

Terai, M., Yasukawa, K., Narumoto, S., Tateno, S., Oana, S. and Kohno, Y. (1999). Vascular endothelial growth factor in acute Kawasaki disease. *American Journal of Cardiology*, **83**, 337–9.

Thomas, L., Davidson, M. and McCluskey, R. T. (1966). Studies of PPLO infection. I. The production of cerebral polyarteritis by *Mycoplasma gallisepticum* in turkeys; the neurotoxic property of the *Mycoplasma*. *Journal of Experimental Medicine*, **123**, 897–912.

Toyabe, S., Harada, W., Suzuki, H., Hirokawa, T. and Uchiyama, M. (2001). Large vessel arteritis associated with human herpesvirus 6 infections. *Clinical Rheumatology*, **21**, 528–32.

Torres, R. A., Lin, R. Y., Lee, M. and Barr, M. R. (1992). Zidovudine-induced leukocytoclastic vasculitis. *Archives of Internal Medicine*, **152**, 850–1.

Trepo, C. G., Zucherman, A. J., Bird, R. C. and Prince, A. M. (1974). The role of circulating hepatitis B antigen/antibody immune complexes in the pathogenesis of vascular and hepatic manifestations in polyarteritis nodosa. *Journal of Clinical Pathology*, **27**, 863–8.

Tripathy, N. K., Chauhan, S. K. and Nityanand, S. (2004). Cytokine mRNA repertoire of peripheral blood mononuclear cells in Takayasu's arteritis. *Clinical and Experimental Immunology*, **138**, 369–74.

Tse, W. Y., Abadeh, S., McTiernan, A., Jefferis, R., Savage, C. O. and Adu, D. (1999). No association between neutrophil FcgammaRIIa allelic polymorphism and anti-neutrophil cytoplasmic antibody (ANCA)-positive systemic vasculitis. *Clinical and Experimental Immunology*, **117**, 198–205.

Tse, W. Y., Abadeh, S., Jefferis, R., Savage, C. O. and Adu, D. (2000). Neutrophil FcgammaRJllb allelic polymorphism in anti-neutrophil cytoplasmic antibody (ANCA)-positive systemic vasculitis. *Clinical and Experimental Immunology*, **119**, 574–7.

Tse, W. Y., Nash, G. B., Hewins, P., Savage, C. O. and Adu, D. (2005). ANCA-induced neutrophil F-actin polymerization: implications for microvascular inflammation. *Kidney International*, **67**, 130–9.

Tsukada, N., Koh, C. S., Owa, M. and Yanagisawa, N. (1983). Chronic neuropathy associated with immune complexes of hepatitis B virus. *Journal of the Neurological Sciences*, **61**, 193–210.

Uchiyama, T. and Kato, H. (1999). The pathogenesis of Kawasaki disease and superantigens. *Japanese Journal of Infectious Diseases*, **52**, 141–5.

Vanek, C. and Samuels, M. H. (2005). Central nervous system vasculitis caused by propylthiouracil therapy: a case report and literature review. *Thyroid*, **15**, 80–4.

van Paassen, P., Cohen Tervaert, J. W. and Heeringa, P. (2006). Mechanisms of vasculitis: how pauci-immune is ANCA-associated renal vasculitis? *Nephron. Experimental Nephrology*, e10–16.

van Pesch, V., Jadoul, M., Lefebvre, C., Lauwerys, B. R., Tomasi, J. P., Devogelaer, J. P. and Houssiau, F. A. (1999). Clinical significance of antiproteinase 3 antibody positivity in cANCA-positive patients. *Clinical Rheumatology*, **18**, 279–82.

Van Rossum, A. P., van der Geld, Y. M., Limburg, P. C. and Kallenberg, C. G. (2005). Human anti-neutrophil cytoplasm autoantibodies to proetinase 3 (PR3-ANCA) bind to neutrophils. *Kidney International*, **68**, 537–41.

Van Rossum, A. P., Limburg, P. C. and Kallenberg, C. G. (2003). Membrane proteinase 3 expression on resting neutrophils as a pathogenic factor in PR3-ANCA-associated vasculitis. *Clinical and Experimental Rheumatology*, **21**, S64–8.

Varagunam, M., Nwosu, Z., Adu, D., Garner, C., Taylor, C. M., Michael, J. and Thompson, R. A. (1993). Little evidence for anti-endothelial cell antibodies in microscopic polyarteritis and Wegener's granulomatosis. *Nephrology Dialysis, Transplantation*, **8**, 113–7.

Vasconcelos, C., Magina, S., Quirino, P., Barros, M. A. and Mesquita-Guimaraes, J. (1998). Cutaneous drug reactions to piroxicam. *Contact Dermatitis*, **39**, 145.

Vasily, D. B. and Tyler, W. B. (1980). Propylthiouracil-induced cutaneous vasculitis. Case presentation and review of the literature. *Journal of the American Medical Association*, **243**, 458–61.

Viac, J., Pernet, I., Schmitt, D. and Claudy, A. (1999). Overexpression of circulating vascular endothelial growth factor (VEGF) in leukocytoclastic vasculitis. *Archives of Dermatological Research*, **291**, 622–3.

Vischer, U. M. (2006). von Willebrand factor, endothelial dysfunction, and cardiovascular disease. *Journal of Thrombosis and Haemostasis*, **4**, 1186–93.

Vittecoq, O., Joen-Beades, F., Krzanowska, K., Bichon-Tauvel, I., Menard, J. F., Daraagon, A., Gilbert, D., Tron, F. and Le Loet, X. (2000). Prospective evaluation of the frequency and clinical significance of antineutrophil cytoplasmic and anti-cardiolipin antibodies in community cases of patients with rheumatoid arthritis. *Rheumatology (Oxford)*, **39**, 481–9.

Voswinkel, J., Muller, A. and Lamprecht, P. (2005). Is PR3-ANCA formation initiated in Wegener's granulomatosis lesions? Granulomas as potential lymphoid tissue maintaining autoantibody production. *Annals of the New York Academy of Science*, **1051**, 12–9.

Wada, N., Mukai, M., Kohno, M., Notoya, A., Ito, T. and Yoshioka, N. (2002). Prevalence of serum anti-myeloperoxidase antineutrophil cytoplasmic antibodies (MPO-ANCA) in patients with Graves' disease treated with propylthiouracil and thiamazole. *Endocrinology Journal*, **49**, 329–34.

Wakefield, D., Easter, J., Breit, S. N., Clark, P. and Penny, R. (1985). Alpha 1 antitrypsin serum levels and phenotypes in patients with retinal vasculitis. *British Journal of Ophthalmology*, **69**, 497–9.

Watanabe, T. and Oda, Y. (2000). Henoch-Schönlein purpura nephritis associated with human parvovirus B19 infection. *Pediatrics International*, **42**, 94–6.

Waxman, F. J., Hebert, L. A., Cosio, F. G., Smead, W. L., VanAman, M. E., Taguiam, J. M. and Birmingham, D. J. (1986). Differential binding of immunoglobulin A and immunoglobulin G1 immune complexes to primate erythrocytes in vivo. Immunoglobulin A immune complexes bind less well to erythrocytes and are preferentially deposited in glomeruli. *Journal of Clinical Investigation*, **77**, 82–9.

Wechsler, M. E., Finn, D., Gunawardena, D., Westlake, R., Barker, A., Haranath, S. P., Pauwels, R. A., Kips, J. C. and Drazen, J. M. (2000). Churg-Strauss syndrome in patients receiving montelukast as treatment for asthma. *Chest*, **117**, 708–13.

Wechsler, M. E., Garpestad, E., Flier, S. R., Kocher, O., Weiland, D. A., Polito, A. J., Klinek, M. M., Bigby, T. D., Wong, G. A., Helmers, R. A. and Drazen, J. M. (1998). Pulmonary infiltrates, eosinophilia, and cardiomyopathy following corticosteroid withdrawal in patients with asthma receiving zafirlukast. *Journal of the American Medical Association*, **279**, 455–7.

Wechsler, M. E., Pauwels, R. and Drazen, J. M. (1999). Leukotriene modifiers and Churg-Strauss syndrome: adverse effect or response to corticosteroid withdrawal? *Drug Safety*, **21**, 241–51.

Weiss, S. R., Raskind, R., Morganstern, N. L., Pytlyk, P. J. and Baiz, T. C. (1970). Intracerebral and subarachnoid hemorrhage following use of methamphetamine "speed". *International Surgery*, **53**, 123–127.

Weyand, C. M., Kurtin, P. J. and Goronzy, J. J. (2001). Ectopic lymphoid organogenesis: a fast track for autoimmunity. *American Journal of Pathology*, **159**, 787–93.

Wikman, A., Lundahl, J. and Jacobson, S. H. (2005). Neutrophil activation in anti-proteinase 3 positive vasculitis–a prospective study. *Scandinavian Journal of Immunology*, **62**, 539–45.

Weyand, C. M., Fulbright, J. W., Hunder, G. G., Evans, J. M. and Goronzy, J. J. (2000). Treatment of giant cell arteritis: interleukin-6 as a biologic marker of disease activity. *Arthritis and Rheumatism*, **43**, 1041–8.

Wiesner, O., Litwiller, R. D., Hummel, A. M., Viss, M. A., McDonald, C. J., Jenne, D. E., Fass, D. N. and Specks, U. (2005). Differences between human proteinase 3 and neutrophil elastase and their murine homologues are relevant for murine model experiments. *FEBS Letters*, **579**, 5305–12.

Witko-Sarsat, V., Cramer, E. M., Hieblot, C., Guichard, J., Nusbaum, P., Lopez, S., Lesavre, P. and Halbwachs-Mecarelli, L. (1999). Presence of proteinase 3 in secretory vesicles: evidence of a novel, highly mobilizable intracellular pool distinct from azurophil granules. *Blood*, **94**, 2487–96.

Wolf, R., Ophir, J., Elman, M. and Krakowski, A. (1989). Atenolol-induced cutaneous vasculitis. *Cutis*, **43**, 231–3.

Xiao, H., Heeringa, P., Hu, P., Liu, Z., Xhao, M., Aratani, Y., Maeda, N., Falk, R. J. and Jennette, J. C. (2002). Antineutrophil cytoplasmic autoantibodies specific for myeloperoxidase cause glomerulonephritis and vasculitis in mice. *Journal of Clinical Investigation*, **110**, 955–63.

Xiao, H., Heeringa, P., Liu, Z., Huugen, D., Hu, P., Maeda, N., Falk, R. J. and Jennette, J. C. (2005). The role of neutrophils in the induction of glomerulonephritis by anti-myeloperoxidase antibodies. *American Journal of Pathology*, **167**, 39–45.

Yang, J. J., Kettritz, R., Falk, R. J., Jennette, J. C. and Gaido, M. L. (1996). Apoptosis of endothelial cells induced by the neutrophil serine proteases proteinase 3 and elastase. *American Journal of Pathology*, **149**, 1617–26.

Yang, J. J., Tuttle, R. H., Hogan, S. L., Taylor, J. G., Phillips, B. D., Falk, R. J. and Jennette, J. C. (2000). Target antigens for anti-neutrophil cytoplasmic autoantibodies (ANCA) are on the surface of primed and apoptotic but not unstimulated neutrophils. *Clinical and Experimental Immunology*, **121**, 165–72.

Yang, Y. H., Huang, Y. H., Lin, Y. L., Wang, L. C., Chuang, Y. H., Yu, H. H., Lin, Y. T. and Chiang, B. L. (2006). Circulating IgA from acute stage of childhood Henoch-Schönlein purpura can enhance endothelial interleukin (IL)-8 production through MEK/ERK signalling pathway. *Clinical and Experimental Immunology*, **144**, 247–53.

Yarman, S., Sandalci, O., Tanakol, R., Azizlerli, H., Oguz, H. and Alagol, F. (1997). Propylthiouracil-induced cutaneous vasculitis. *International Journal of Clinical Pharmacology and Therapeutics*, **35**, 282–6.

Yoshioka, T., Matsutani, T., Iwagami, S., Toyosaki-Maeda, T., Yutsudo, T., Tsuruta, Y., Suzuki, H., Uemura, S., Takeuchi, T., Koike, M. and Suzuki, R. (1999). Polyclonal expansion of TCRBV2-and TCRBV6-bearing T cells in patients with Kawasaki disease. *Immunology*, **96**, 465–72.

Yu, F., Zhao, M. H., Zhang, Y. K., Zhang, Y. and Wang, H. Y. (2005). Anti-endothelial cell antibodies (AECA) in patients with propylthiouracil (PTU)-induced ANCA positive vasculitis are associated with disease activity. *Clinical and Experimental Immunology*, **139**, 569–74.

Zhang, Z. and Bridges, S. L. Jr. (2001). Pathogenesis of rheumatoid arthritis. Role of B lymphocytes. *Rheumatic Disease Clinics of North America*, **27**, 335–53.

Zholudev, A., Zurakowski, D., Young, W., Leichtner, A. and Bousvaros, A. (2004). Serologic testing with ANCA, ASCA, and anti-OmpC in children and young adults with Crohn's disease and ulcerative colitis: diagnostic value and correlation with disease phenotype. *American Journal of Gastroenterology*, **99**, 2235–41.

CHAPTER 8

Animal models of vasculitis

Daniel E. Bullard and Trenton R. Schoeb

Introduction

As described in other chapters in this book, vasculitis can occur as a primary or secondary feature of a wide variety of disorders of inflammation, including drug hypersensitivities and response to infection. Many such conditions are of complex etiology and pathogenesis in which genetic or environmental factors or both are likely to be important. Identifying etiologic and genetic susceptibility factors and elucidating pathogenetic pathways are thus the fundamental challenges in vasculitis research. Many different animal models in mice and other species have been described, both spontaneously occurring and induced by experimental treatment, but space limitations preclude a comprehensive review. In this chapter, we present an overview of models that are well recognized or that offer the greatest potential for productive research, and do not discuss most models for which few publications exist. Data from animal models relevant to Wegener's granulomatosis (WG) are also discussed in Chapter 30.

Mouse models with spontaneously occurring vasculitis

Spontaneously occurring vasculitis has been described in several different inbred and F_1 hybrid mouse strains. Many of these have been characterized as models for systemic lupus erythematosus (SLE), as they develop systemic autoimmunity with loss of immune tolerance, autoantibody formation, and immune complex-mediated glomerulonephritis. In general, the incidence and prevalence of vasculitis, types of vessels affected, organ distribution, and age of onset is highly variable among the different strains. One of the best-characterized and most frequently used animal models of vasculitis is the MRL/MpJ-Fas^{lpr} ($Tnfrsf6^{lpr}$) mouse strain (Theofilopoulos and Dixon, 1985). Necrotizing vasculitis occurs in these mice in many organs, including lung, liver, kidney, skin, salivary gland, testis, and others (Alexander et al. 1985; Moyer et al. 1987; Berden et al. 1983). Vasculitis most commonly affects small and medium-sized arteries and veins and arterioles and venules. The etiology and pathogenesis are not fully understood, but important factors are thought to include immune complex deposition, antineutrophil cytoplasmic antibodies (ANCA), antiendothelial cell antibodies (AECA), TNF-α, and IL-1β (Theofilopoulos and

Dixon 1985; McHale et al. 1999; Dimitriu-Bona et al. 1995; Harper et al. 1998; Hewicker and Trautwein 1987).

Most publications concerning vasculitis in MRL/MpJ-Fas^{lpr} mice have focused on lesion development in relatively young mice, in which three distinct patterns are evident: (a) perivascular or adventitial accumulation of lymphoid and other mononuclear cells without evidence of injury to the vessel wall, such as necrosis, fibrin deposition, or edema; (b) lymphocyte infiltration of the vessel wall, which can be, but is not necessarily, accompanied by vessel wall injury; and (c) classic "leukocytoclastic" necrotizing vasculitis, which is characterized by necrosis, often with fibrin deposition, of any or all layers of the vessel wall but most prominently in the medial smooth muscle, and which typically is accompanied by infiltration of neutrophils, some or many of which have undergone nuclear fragmentation ("leukocytoclasis") (Alexander et al. 1985; Moyer et al. 1987; Berden et al. 1983). Some investigators have concluded, from results of in vitro studies and because the lymphocytic lesions tend to appear in mice younger than those developing neutrophilic vasculitis, that mechanisms involving delayed type hypersensitivity initiate vascular inflammation in MRL/MpJ-Fas^{lpr} mice (Moyer and Reinisch 1984). Our observations to date of older MRL/MpJ-Fas^{lpr} mice that died or were sacrificed due to advanced disease are similar, in that necrotizing vasculitis (Figure 8.1) is much more common than lymphocytic vasculitis. Such lesions vary considerably in cellularity, and any size vessel can be affected, including large elastic arteries (Figures 8.2 and 8.3). In some organs, such as the lung, perivascular accumulation of lymphocytes without vasculitis is common (Figure 8.4). We think the different types of lesions observed probably reflect the complexity of the pathogenesis of vasculitis in these mice and in immune-mediated vasculitis in general, in which different mechanisms may predominate in different vessels or at different times.

Several other mouse vasculitis models originating from crosses of MRL/MpJ-Fas^{lpr} and other inbred strains of mice have been described. One of these models, termed spontaneous crescentic glomerulonephritis/Kinjoh or SCG/Kj mice, develop necrotizing vasculitis that primarily affects small arteries and arterioles in multiple organs, including the ovary, uterus, spleen, heart, and stomach (Kinjoh et al. 1993). Development of vasculitis and glomerulonephritis in this model has been linked with high circulating levels of myeloperoxidase-specific ANCA (MPO-ANCA)

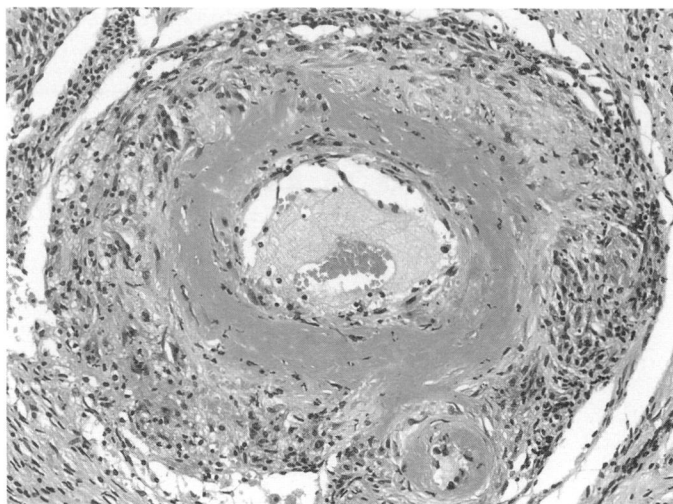

Figure 8.1 Severe necrotizing arteritis of a muscular artery in the uterus of an MRL/MpJ-*Fas^lpr* mouse. H & E stain. Original magnification 20×. (See Color Plate 1.)

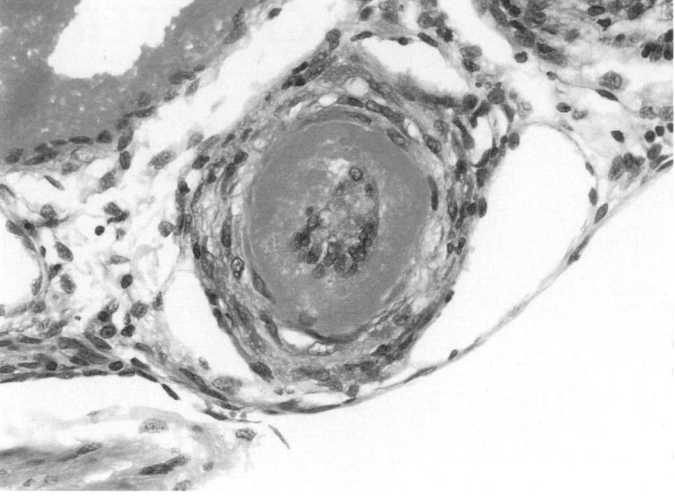

Figure 8.3 Medial necrosis in a muscular artery of the uterus of an MRL/MpJ-*Fas^lpr* mouse. H & E stain. Original magnification 40×. (See Color Plate 3.)

(Ishida-Okawara *et al*. 2004; Neumann *et al*. 2003), and thus may represent a model for ANCA-associated vasculitides.

The MRL/MpJ-*Fas^lpr* and Kinjoh models have also been used in genetic screens to identify chromosomal regions that contain loci (alleles) that contribute to the development of vasculitis in this strain. Similar approaches have been used in other mouse inflammatory disease models to identify specific loci or genetic pathways that may be involved in the development of the human counterpart. These studies have generally performed linkage analyses on intercross (F$_2$) or backcross mice (N$_2$) generated by breeding MRL/MpJ-*Fas^lpr* or SCG/Kj mice to vasculitis-resistant strains. At least six different chromosomal regions have been identified that contain loci involved in the development of vasculitis (Wang *et al*. 1997; Nose *et al*. 1998; Nose *et al*. 2000; Yamada *et al*. 2003; Qu *et al*. 2000; Hamano *et al*. 2006; Zhang *et al*. 2006). Further studies are necessary to identify the specific alleles that show altered expression

or function in these regions, and their potential roles in the development of human vasculitides.

Palmerston North mice

Palmerston North (PN) mice also develop a systemic autoimmune disease with similarities to human SLE, including glomerulonephritis and vasculitis (Walker *et al*. 1978). R.D. Wigley reported polyarteritis nodosa (PAN)-like disease in outbred PN mice in 1966 (Wigley and Couchman 1966). These mice were subsequently inbred through brother–sister matings, and the incidence and distribution of the lesions were further characterized. Female PN mice show a more rapid and severe form of glomerulonephritis and vasculitis than males (Walker *et al*. 1978). Venulitis with an associated mononuclear cell infiltrate was observed in the kidney and liver as early as 3 months of age in female PN mice (Luzina *et al*. 1999). Arteritis was only observed in older mice, with lesions appearing in

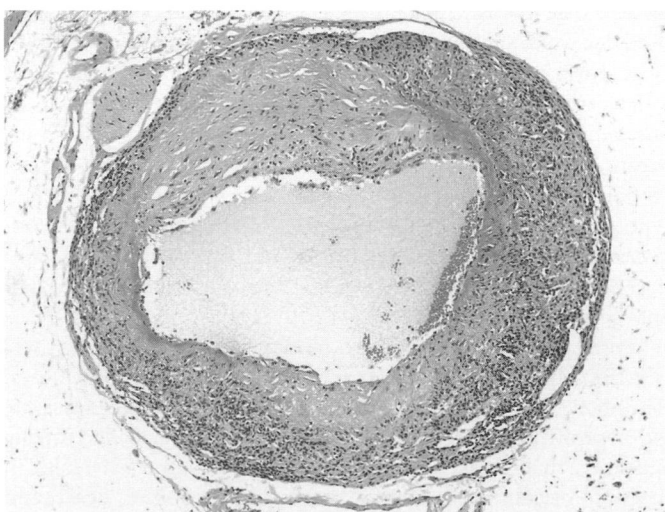

Figure 8.2 Severe chronic active arteritis of an external carotid artery (a large, elastic artery) of an MRL/MpJ-*Fas^lpr* mouse. H & E stain. Original magnification 10×. (See Color Plate 2.)

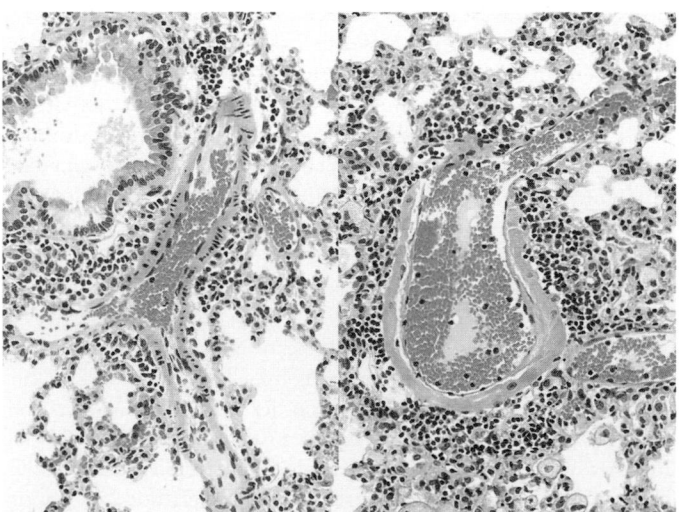

Figure 8.4 Perivascular lymphocyte accumulation without vasculitis of a pulmonary artery (left) and pulmonary vein (right) of an MRL/MpJ-*Fas^lpr* mouse. H & E stain. Original magnification 20×. (See Color Plate 4.)

the thymus, spleen, ovary, skeletal muscle, kidney, and other tissues, starting around 9 months of age (Luzina *et al.* 1999; Walker *et al.* 1978; Wigley *et al.* 1975). Development of vasculitis in PN mice also was found to be incompletely penetrant, with only about 60% of older mice having vasculitis at the time of death (Walker *et al.* 1978).

Interleukin-1 receptor antagonist mutant mice

IL-1 receptor antagonist (IL-1ra) is a structural homolog of IL-1 and acts as an anti-inflammatory cytokine through antagonizing IL-1α and IL-1β binding to the IL-1 receptor (Arend *et al.* 1998). Certain strains of mice containing a gene targeted or knockout mutation of the IL-1ra gene (*Il1rn*) develop chronic arthropathy, psoriasiform dermatitis, and vasculitis affecting the elastic arteries, primarily the aorta and its branches (Horai *et al.* 2000; Shepherd *et al.* 2004; Nicklin *et al.* 2000). Lesions are characterized by infiltrating monocyte/macrophages and CD4[+] T cells, many of which express IFN-γ (Shepherd and Nicklin 2005). Thus, these mice may be considered a model for Takayasu's arteritis and giant cell arteritis (Shepherd and Nicklin 2005). *Il1rn* mutant BALB/c mice show a high incidence of vasculitis, starting as early as 4 weeks of age, whereas C57BL/6 mice having the same mutation are resistant, indicating that loci other than *Il1rn* have important roles (Matsuki *et al.* 2005).

NZB × NZW F1 mice

NZB × NZW F$_1$ or B/W mice derived from breeding the inbred strains New Zealand Black (NZB) and New Zealand White (NZW) together are a well-studied model of SLE (Theofilopoulos and Dixon 1985). Glomerulonephritis occurs consistently in these mice, but fewer reports describe vasculitis in the kidneys or other organs (Burnet and Holmes 1965; Hicks 1966; Staszak and Harbeck 1985). In a 1966 paper, Hicks (Hicks 1966) reported that 20% of B/W and 10% of NZB mice showed necrotizing arteritis in the kidneys. Wigley *et al.* (Wigley *et al.* 1970) reported a similar frequency of renal arteritis, but also observed a high incidence of spleen and lymph node arteriolitis. Pulmonary vasculitis, affecting primarily the arterioles, veins, and venules, has also been described in B/W mice (Staszak and Harbeck 1985). In this study, pulmonary vasculitis was not observed in mice 4 months of age but was seen in 50% of 8-month-old mice. At 12 months of age, all of the mice had severe multifocal lesions. In the last 20 years, B/W mice, or strains of mice derived from them, have not been used extensively as models of vasculitis, probably due to the low penetrance and slow development of vasculitis.

NZW × BXSB F$_1$ Mice

BXSB mice, similar to MRL/MpJ-*Fas^lpr* and NZB × NZW F$_1$ strains, develop a severe lupus-like syndrome with glomerulonephritis but not vasculitis (Dixon *et al.* 1978; Berden *et al.* 1983). However, F$_1$ hybrids of BXSB and NZW mice (W/BF$_1$) can develop arteritis in various organs (Mizutani *et al.* 1995; Kono *et al.* 2003). Mizutani *et al.* (Mizutani *et al.* 1995) analyzed W/BF$_1$ mice at different ages for vasculitis in the GI tract and observed vasculitis in small arteries and arterioles in 20% of 8 to 12-week-old mice and 61% of 12 to 18-week-old mice. The duodenum, jejunum, and ileum were most often affected, with almost half of the mice also having pancreatic vasculitis.

Naturally occurring vasculitis in non-murine species

Spontaneous vasculitis has been reported in many other species, including rats, mink, pigs, dogs, sheep, and horses (Wigley 1970; Bishop 1989; Mathieson *et al.* 1993, Burns *et al.* 1991). In some cases, such as Aleutian mink disease and porcine reproductive and respiratory syndrome, vasculitis was later found to be associated with a specific viral infection (Thibault *et al.* 1998; Rossow *et al.* 1995; Bishop 1989). Canine juvenile polyarteritis syndrome or canine pain syndrome is an interesting, potential model for mucocutaneous lymph node syndrome or Kawasaki disease. It is characterized by systemic necrotizing vasculitis, primarily affecting small and medium arteries, especially the coronary, cranial, and cervical spinal meningeal arteries (Harcourt 1978; Burns *et al.* 1991; Felsburg *et al.* 1992; Snyder *et al.* 1995; Scott-Moncrieff *et al.* 1992). Although these non-murine models might in some cases provide advantages over mice, such as increased similarity to specific human vasculitides, most publications on these models are descriptive case reports, and there has been little use of such models to identify pathogenetic mechanisms or genetic susceptibility factors. This is probably because those conditions caused by viral infections have no known human counterpart, and those that do resemble a form of human vasculitis are so uncommon that it would be extremely difficult to identify a useful number of subjects.

Induced models of vasculitis

Serum sickness and the Arthus reaction

A wide variety of agents, including chemicals, infectious organisms or viruses, bacteria and yeast cell wall components, autoreactive antibodies and T cells, as well as many other immune or inflammatory stimuli, have been used to promote the development of vasculitis in experimental animals. The serum sickness model of immune complex-mediated vascular damage is one of the earliest reported models of experimentally induced vasculitis (Dixon *et al.* 1958). Many different variations of this model exist, but most involve injection of heterologous serum albumin into species such as rabbits or rats, which then leads to an antibody response to the foreign protein, circulating immune complex formation, deposition in vessel walls, complement activation, neutrophil adhesion and activation, and development of a necrotizing leukocytoclastic vasculitis. The Arthus and the reverse passive Arthus models are also commonly used models for immune-complex mediated vasculitis (Cochrane 1967). In the Arthus reaction model, immune complexes are formed at the vessel walls, which results in complement activation and a rapid neutrophil-mediated hemorrhagic vasculitis (Cochrane 1967). Rodents or rabbits are first immunized with a foreign antigen such as serum albumin to elicit antibody formation, followed later by direct injection of the antigen subcutaneously. In the reverse passive Arthus model, antibodies reactive against a foreign protein are injected into the skin, followed immediately by intravenous injection of the protein (Berden *et al.* 1983). These models have been used as tools to study mechanisms leading to vasculitic lesion formation in disease such as PAN, cutaneous leukocytoclastic angiitis, and SLE.

ANCA-associated vasculitides

Wegener's granulomatosis (WG), Churg–Strauss syndrome, and microscopic polyangiitis (MPA) are often referred to as

ANCA-associated vasculitic disorders. To date, many different studies have investigated the roles of ANCA (and AECA) in promoting development of vasculitis in rodents. Many different experimental protocols have been used, including immunization with MPO, apoptotic neutrophils, or human ANCA IgG from WG patients, and injection of ANCA- or AECA-positive IgG fractions from WG patients (Xiao *et al.* 2002; Little *et al.* 2005; Brouwer *et al.* 1993; Heeringa *et al.* 1997; Foucher *et al.* 1999; Rauova *et al.* 2002; Blank *et al.* 1995; Tomer *et al.* 1995; Damianovich *et al.* 1996; Weidebach *et al.* 2002). In most of these studies, the manipulations used either did not induce vasculitis consistently, or resulted primarily in perivascular accumulations of leukocytes with minimal evidence of endothelial or vessel wall damage. However, some reports describe development of vasculitis in lungs and kidneys, as well as alveolar hemorrhage and pulmonary granuloma formation, in rats subjected to various MPO immunization protocols (Brouwer *et al.* 1993; Foucher *et al.* 1999; Heeringa *et al.* 1997; Little *et al.* 2005; Xiao *et al.* 2002). The reason or reasons for the inconsistent induction of vasculitis in these studies is unknown, but it would appear that these models require further refinement, or that other models for ANCA-related vasculitides are needed.

Mercuric chloride-induced vasculitis

Treatment of Brown Norway (BN) rats with mercuric chloride (HgCl$_2$) results in the development of a Th2-associated autoimmune syndrome characterized by high IgE concentrations, antibodies to MPO, and inflammatory lesions in multiple organs (White *et al.* 2000). Vasculitis in this model was first reported by Mathieson *et al.* (Mathieson *et al.* 1992) who reported severe necrotizing vasculitis of submucosal vessels in the cecum appearing between 10 and 16 days in all HgCl$_2$-treated rats. Minimal or no vasculitis was evident in other organs. Interestingly, pretreatment of BN rats with broad spectrum antimicrobial agents inhibited development of vasculitis following HgCl$_2$ administration, suggesting that certain bacteria or other organisms are required for induction of vasculitis (Mathieson *et al.* 1992). Work on this model has largely come from Oliveira and colleagues, who have published several papers describing studies of the roles of various leukocyte populations and other inflammatory mediators in mediating vasculitis in the gut. Further studies showed that cecal vasculitis can occur as early as 24 hours following HgCl$_2$ administration (Qasim *et al.* 1995). Unlike vasculitis at later timepoints, acute vessel damage in this early form of the disease is not dependent on T cells and neutrophils but may primarily be mediated by mast cells (Vinen *et al.* 2004a). Finally, nitric oxide has been shown to partially contribute to vasculitis development in this model, while the complement system does not appear to play a major role (Woolfson *et al.* 1995; Mathieson *et al.* 1994). It has been suggested that this may serve as a model for Churg–Strauss syndrome and other ANCA-associated vasculitides (Vinen *et al.* 2004b).

Lactobacillus casei and *Candida albicans* cell wall-induced coronary arteritis

Lehman *et al.* (Lehman *et al.* 1985) described induction of coronary arteritis in mice by intraperitoneal injection of cell wall extracts of *Lactobacillus casei*. Lesions included extensive, asymmetric to circumferential, accumulation of mixed inflammatory cells in the adventitia, media, and intima, with various degrees of destruction of the media and intima, adventitial fibrosis, and intimal proliferation. Coronary arteritis was inducible in mice of A/J (C5 deficient), BALB/c, C57BL/6, and C3Heb/FeJ strains and in nude athymic mice of A/J and C57BL/6 strains, but not in C3H/HeJ mice, whose macrophages are Toll-like receptor 4 (TLR-4) deficient. The authors noted the similarity of the lesions to those of Kawasaki disease (KD) and suggested that *L. casei* cell wall-induced coronary arteritis could serve as a model for coronary arteritis in KD. The mechanisms of vasculitis in this model remain unclear, but recent reports present evidence that vasculitis induced by *L. casei* cell wall extracts is mediated by superantigen-induced responses (Duong *et al.* 2003) and is dependent on Toll-like receptor 2 (TLR-2) signaling (Rosenkranz *et al.* 2005). Similar lesions are induced in mice by injection of *Candida albicans* extracts (Takahashi *et al.* 2004). Susceptibility differs among strains, which has been used to identify susceptibility loci, including genes for cytokine receptors (Oharaseki *et al.* 2005). The etiology of KD has not been established, but many investigators now believe that infections, particularly with organisms expressing superantigens, could be causal or contributory factors in genetically susceptible patients (Wang *et al.* 2005). If that were the case, these models could provide valuable tools to help identify susceptibility loci as well as to study pathogenesis and potential treatments.

Adoptive transfer of lymphocytes cocultured with smooth muscle cells

Hart *et al.* (Hart *et al.* 1985) reported an interesting mouse model of vasculitis induced by transfer of splenic lymphocytes that had been cocultured with brain microvasculature smooth muscle cells. In this initial study, approximately 30% of the recipient mice developed vasculitis starting around 2–3 days post-transfer. The lesions were characterized primarily by mononuclear cell adhesion and infiltration into the media and adventitia of arterioles and venules. Treatment of donor and recipient mice with cyclophosphamide before coculture and lymphocyte transfer significantly increased the incidence to over 70%. Affected mice had vasculitis most frequently in the lungs and liver and occasionally in other organs. Some affected mice also had granulomatous vasculitis of the pulmonary arterioles. Further studies on this model showed that recipient mice develop autoantibodies reactive to smooth muscle antigens following lymphocyte transfer (Baiu *et al.* 2005). Passive transfer of serum from mice with active vasculitis to normal controls resulted in a high incidence of vasculitis a week after transfer. These investigations suggest that one of the mechanisms by which vasculitis may develop involves autoimmune responses to self-antigens in the vessel wall, including those expressed by smooth muscle cells. Further work on this model will be useful for studies of the roles of T and B cell autoimmune processes in vasculitis.

Cryoglobulin-mediated vasculitis

Serum cryoglobulins have been associated with a number of different diseases, including disorders that present with vasculitis as a primary or secondary manifestation, such as essential mixed cryoglobulinemia (MC), SLE, and rheumatoid arthritis (RA) (Ferri *et al.* 2002; Ferri and Mascia 2006). A murine model of cryoglobulin-induced vasculitis in mice has been used to study the role of cryoglobulins in initiating vasculitis (for review see Pastore *et al.* 2001). Gyotoku *et al.* (1987) developed a panel of IgG3 anti-IgG2a rheumatoid factor (RF) monoclonal antibodies having cryoglobulin activity from non-immunized MRL/MpJ-*Fas^lpr* mice. Several lines of hybridoma cells induced vasculitis and glomerulonephritis when injected into BALB/c mice. Further studies characterized the vasculitis as leukocytoclastic, with extensive neutrophil infiltration and extravasation of erythrocytes (Reininger *et al.* 1990). Other investigations using this model have shown an important role for neutrophils in the induction of skin vasculitis (Izui *et al.* 1998). Treatment of hybridoma-injected mice with anti-ICAM-1 or LFA-1 monoclonal antibodies significantly reduced neutrophil infiltration and development of skin lesions (Izui *et al.* 1998).

Summary

Studies using animal models, notably experimentally induced immune-complex disease and mice with SLE-like diseases, have led to identification of key mediators of vascular inflammation and have provided tools to evaluate potential treatments. Even so, animal models are sometimes criticized as not mimicking a particular form of human vasculitis closely enough. In our view, it is somewhat unrealistic to expect that inflammatory responses, even if closely similar in etiology and pathogenesis, be expressed identically in all species, especially species as phylogenetically distant as humans and mice. Furthermore, it must be considered that a particular clinicopathologic pattern of vasculitis, in either humans or animals, that is of unknown or unclear etiology and pathogenesis may be heterogeneous; that is, due to more than one combination of etiologic and genetic susceptibility factors. Pathogenetic pathways may differ in detail between humans and animals, but general mechanisms tend to be well conserved. Therefore, the power of animal model studies is less due to the ability to mimic specific human vasculitides than to its utility in identifying and analyzing pathogenetic pathways and their underlying genetic basis. The expanding knowledge of the mouse and human genomes, the ability to manipulate the mouse genome to create ever more sophisticated models, and the availability of a vast array of techniques and reagents with which to dissect murine immune and inflammatory responses in great detail assures that genetically engineered mouse models will be at the forefront of vasculitis research.

This is not to say that other animal models are not potentially useful. In our view, however, some of them have significant disadvantages, such as low incidence of vasculitis; the need for large sample sizes to achieve adequate statistical power; inconsistent expression of vasculitis among animals from different laboratories; technical complexity; occurrence only in an inbred strain unavailable to most investigators; and incomplete characterization of the incidence, type, distribution, and progression of vasculitis. Characterization of some models is complicated by lack of standardization of nomenclature for vasculitis among different authors, and in a few cases by apparent lack of knowledge of anatomic pathology, such as misinterpreting tangential sections through arterial branch points as aneurysms and classifying perivascular inflammatory cell accumulation without evidence of vessel wall injury as vasculitis.

The challenge is to identify, refine, or develop animal models of human vasculitides that probably have complex, multifactorial etiology and pathogenesis and for which there is poor understanding of the immune, inflammatory, genetic, and environmental factors leading to vasculitis. Use of tools such as array analysis to dissect inflammatory mechanisms in human vasculitides coupled with improvements in methods of genetic analysis may be expected to lead to new information about such factors that will lead in turn to generation of appropriate new animal models.

References

Alexander, E. L., Moyer, C., Travlos, G. S., Roths, J. B. and Murphy, E. D. (1985). Two histopathologic types of inflammatory vascular disease in MRL/Mp autoimmune mice. Model for human vasculitis in connective tissue disease. *Arthritis and Rheumatism*, **28**, 1146–55.

Arend, W. P., Malyak, M., Guthridge, C. J. and Gabay, C. (1998). Interleukin-1 receptor antagonist: role in biology. *Annual Review of Immunology*, **16**, 27–55.

Baiu, D. C., Barger, B., Sandor, M., Fabry, Z. and Hart, M. N. (2005). Autoantibodies to vascular smooth muscle are pathogenic for vasculitis. *American Journal of Pathology*, **166**, 1851–60.

Berden, J. H., Hang, L., McConahey, P. J. and Dixon, F. J. (1983). Analysis of vascular lesions in murine SLE. I. Association with serologic abnormalities. *Journal of Immunology*, **130**, 1699–705.

Bishop, S. P. (1989). Animal models of vasculitis. *Toxicologic Pathology*, **17**, 109–17.

Blank, M., Tomer, Y., Stein, M., *et al.* (1995). Immunization with anti-neutrophil cytoplasmic antibody (ANCA) induces the production of mouse ANCA and perivascular lymphocyte infiltration. *Clinical and Experimental Immunology*, **102**, 120–30.

Brouwer, E., Huitema, M. G., Klok, P. A., *et al.* (1993). Antimyeloperoxidase-associated proliferative glomerulonephritis: an animal model. *Journal of Experimental Medicine*, **177**, 905–14.

Burnet, F. M. and Holmes, M. C. (1965). The natural history of the NZB/NZW F1 hybrid mouse: a laboratory model of systemic lupus erythematosus. *Australasian Annals of Medicine*, **14**, 185–91.

Burns, J. C., Felsburg, P. J., Wilson, H., Rosen, F. S. and Glickman, L. T. (1991). Canine pain syndrome is a model for the study of Kawasaki disease. *Perspectives in Biology and Medicine*, **35**, 68–73.

Cochrane, C. G. (1967). The Arthus phenomenon–a mechanism of tissue damage. *Arthritis and Rheumatism*, **10**, 392–6.

Damianovich, M., Gilburd, B., George, J., *et al.* (1996). Pathogenic role of anti-endothelial cell antibodies in vasculitis. An idiotypic experimental model. *Journal of Immunology*, **156**, 4946–51.

Dimitriu-Bona, A., Matic, M., Ding, W., Yang, C. P. and Fillit, H. (1995). Cytotoxicity to endothelial cells by sera from aged MRL/lpr/lpr mice is associated with autoimmunity to cell surface heparan sulfate. *Clinical Immunology and Immunopathology*, **76**, 234–40.

Dixon, F. J., Andrews, B. S., Eisenberg, R. A., McConahey, P. J., Theofilopoulos, A. N. and Wilson, C. B. (1978). Etiology and pathogenesis of a spontaneous lupus-like syndrome in mice. *Arthritis and Rheumatism*, **21**, S64–7.

Dixon, F. J., Vazquez, J. J., Weigle, W. O. and Cochrane, C. G. (1958). Pathogenesis of serum sickness. *A. M. A. Archives of Pathology*, **65**, 18–28.

Duong, T. T., Silverman, E. D., Bissessar, M. V. and Yeung, R. S. (2003). Superantigenic activity is responsible for induction of coronary arteritis in mice: an animal model of Kawasaki disease. *International Immunology*, **15**, 79–89.

Felsburg, P. J., HogenEsch, H., Somberg, R. L., Snyder, P. W. and Glickman, L. T. (1992). Immunologic abnormalities in canine juvenile polyarteritis syndrome: a naturally occurring animal model of Kawasaki disease. *Clinical Immunology and Immunopathology*, **65**, 110–8.

Ferri, C. and Mascia, M. T. (2006). Cryoglobulinemic vasculitis. *Current Opinion in Rheumatology*, **18**, 54–63.

Ferri, C., Zignego, A. L. and Pileri, S. A. (2002). Cryoglobulins. *Journal of Clinical Pathology*, **55**, 4–13.

Foucher, P., Heeringa, P., Petersen, A. H., *et al.* (1999). Antimyeloperoxidase-associated lung disease. An experimental model. *American Journal of Respiratory and Critical Care Medicine*, **160**, 987–94.

Gyotoku, Y., Abdelmoula, M., Spertini, F., Izui, S. and Lambert, P. H. (1987). Cryoglobulinemia induced by monoclonal immunoglobulin G rheumatoid factors derived from autoimmune MRL/MpJ-lpr/lpr mice. *Journal of Immunology*, **138**, 3785–92.

Hamano, Y., Tsukamoto, K., Abe, M., *et al.* (2006). Genetic dissection of vasculitis, myeloperoxidase-specific antineutrophil cytoplasmic autoantibody production, and related traits in spontaneous crescentic glomerulonephritis-forming/Kinjoh mice. *Journal of Immunology*, **176**, 3662–73.

Harcourt, R. A. (1978). Polyarteritis in a colony of beagles. *Veterinary Record*, **102**, 519–22.

Harper, J. M., Thiru, S., Lockwood, C. M. and Cooke, A. (1998). Myeloperoxidase autoantibodies distinguish vasculitis mediated by anti-neutrophil cytoplasm antibodies from immune complex disease in MRL/Mp-lpr/lpr mice: a spontaneous model for human microscopic angiitis. *European Journal of Immunology*, **28**, 2217–26.

Hart, M. N., Tassell, S. K., Sadewasser, K. L., Schelper, R. L. and Moore, S. A. (1985). Autoimmune vasculitis resulting from in vitro immunization of lymphocytes to smooth muscle. The *American Journal of Pathology*, **119**, 448–55.

Heeringa, P., Foucher, P., Klok, P. A., *et al.* (1997). Systemic injection of products of activated neutrophils and H2O2 in myeloperoxidase-immunized rats leads to necrotizing vasculitis in the lungs and gut. *American Journal of Pathology*, **151**, 131–40.

Hewicker, M. and Trautwein, G. (1987). Sequential study of vasculitis in MRL mice. *Laboratory Animals*, **21**, 335–41.

Hicks, J. D. (1966). Vascular changes in the kidneys of NZB mice and F1 NZBxNZW hybrids. *Journal of Pathology and Bacteriology*, **91**, 479–86.

Horai, R., Saijo, S., Tanioka, H., *et al.* (2000). Development of chronic inflammatory arthropathy resembling rheumatoid arthritis in interleukin 1 receptor antagonist-deficient mice. *Journal of Experimental Medicine*, **191**, 313–20.

Ishida-Okawara, A., Ito-Ihara, T., Muso, E., *et al.* (2004). Neutrophil contribution to the crescentic glomerulonephritis in SCG/Kj mice. *Nephrology, Dialysis, Transplantation*, **19**, 1708–15.

Izui, S., Fulpius, T., Reininger, L., Pastore, Y. and Kobayakawa, T. (1998). Role of neutrophils in murine cryoglobulinemia. *Inflammation Research*, **47** (Suppl. 3), S145–50.

Kinjoh, K., Kyogoku, M. and Good, R. A. (1993). Genetic selection for crescent formation yields mouse strain with rapidly progressive glomerulonephritis and small vessel vasculitis. *Proceedings of the National Academy of Sciences of the United States of America*, **90**, 3413–7.

Kono, D. H., Park, M. S. and Theofilopoulos, A. N. (2003). Genetic complementation in female (BXSB x NZW)F2 mice. *Journal of Immunology*, **171**, 6442–7.

Lehman, T. J., Walker, S. M., Mahnovski, V. and McCurdy, D. (1985). Coronary arteritis in mice following the systemic injection of group B Lactobacillus casei cell walls in aqueous suspension. *Arthritis and Rheumatism*, **28**, 652–9.

Little, M. A., Smyth, C. L., Yadav, R., *et al.* (2005). Antineutrophil cytoplasm antibodies directed against myeloperoxidase augment leukocyte-microvascular interactions in vivo. *Blood*, **106**, 2050–8.

Luzina, I. G., Knitzer, R. H., Atamas, S. P., *et al.* (1999). Vasculitis in the Palmerston North mouse model of lupus: phenotype and cytokine production profile of infiltrating cells. *Arthritis and Rheumatism*, **42**, 561–8.

Mathieson, P. W., Qasim, F. J., Esnault, V. L. and Oliveira, D. B. (1993). Animal models of systemic vasculitis. *Journal of Autoimmunity*, **6**, 251–64.

Mathieson, P. W., Qasim, F. J., Thiru, S., Oldroyd, R. G. and Oliveira, D. B. (1994). Effects of decomplementation with cobra venom factor on experimental vasculitis. *Clinical and Experimental Immunology*, **97**, 474–7.

Mathieson, P. W., Thiru, S. and Oliveira, D. B. (1992). Mercuric chloride-treated brown Norway rats develop widespread tissue injury including necrotizing vasculitis. *Laboratory Investigation*, **67**, 121–9.

Matsuki, T., Isoda, K., Horai, R., *et al.* (2005). Involvement of tumor necrosis factor-alpha in the development of T cell-dependent aortitis in interleukin-1 receptor antagonist-deficient mice. *Circulation*, **112**, 1323–31.

McHale, J. F., Harari, O. A., Marshall, D. and Haskard, D. O. (1999). TNF-α and IL-1 sequentially induce endothelial ICAM-1 and VCAM-1 expression in MRL/*lpr* lupus-prone mice. *Journal of Immunology*, **163**, 3993–4000.

Mizutani, H., Engelman, R. W., Kinjoh, K. and Good, R. A. (1995). Gastrointestinal vasculitis in autoimmune-prone (NZW X BXSB)F1 mice: association with anticardiolipin autoantibodies. *Proceedings of the Society for Experimental Biology and Medicine*, **209**, 279–85.

Moyer, C. F. and Reinisch, C. L. (1984). The role of vascular smooth muscle cells in experimental autoimmune vasculitis. I. The initiation of delayed type hypersensitivity angiitis. *American Journal of Pathology*, **117**, 380–90.

Moyer, C. F., Strandberg, J. D. and Reinisch, C. L. (1987). Systemic mononuclear-cell vasculitis in MRL/Mp-lpr/lpr mice. A histologic and immunocytochemical analysis. *American Journal of Pathology*, **127**, 229–42.

Neumann, I., Birck, R., Newman, M., *et al.* (2003). SCG/Kinjoh mice: a model of ANCA-associated crescentic glomerulonephritis with immune deposits. *Kidney International*, **64**, 140–8.

Nicklin, M. J., Hughes, D. E., Barton, J. L., Ure, J. M. and Duff, G. W. (2000). Arterial inflammation in mice lacking the interleukin 1 receptor antagonist gene. *Journal of Experimental Medicine*, **191**, 303–12.

Nose, M., Terada, M., Nishihara, M., *et al.* (1998). Vasculitis-susceptible genes in mice with a deficit in Fas-mediated apoptosis. *International Journal of Cardiology*, **66** (Suppl. 1), S37–41.

Nose, M., Terada, M., Nishihara, M., *et al.* (2000). Genome analysis of collagen disease in MRL/lpr mice: polygenic inheritance resulting in the complex pathological manifestations. *International Journal of Cardiology*, **75** (Suppl. 1), S53–61.

Oharaseki, T., Kameoka, Y., Kura, F., Persad, A. S., Suzuki, K. and Naoe, S. (2005). Susceptibility loci to coronary arteritis in animal model of Kawasaki disease induced with Candida albicans -derived substances. *Microbiology and Immunology*, **49**, 181–9.

Pastore, Y., Lajaunias, F., Kuroki, A., Moll, T., Kikuchi, S. and Izui, S. (2001). An experimental model of cryoglobulin-associated vasculitis in mice. *Springer Seminars in Immunopathology*, **23**, 315–29.

Qasim, F. J., Thiru, S., Mathieson, P. W. and Oliveira, D. B. (1995). The time course and characterization of mercuric chloride-induced immunopathology in the brown Norway rat. *Journal of Autoimmunity*, **8**, 193–208.

Qu, W. M., Miyazaki, T., Terada, M., *et al.* (2000). Genetic dissection of vasculitis in MRL/lpr lupus mice: a novel susceptibility locus involving the CD72c allele. *European Journal of Immunology*, **30**, 2027–37.

Rauova, L., Gilburd, B., Zurgil, N., *et al.* (2002). Induction of biologically active antineutrophil cytoplasmic antibodies by immunization with human apoptotic polymorphonuclear leukocytes. *Clinical Immunology*, **103**, 69–78.

Reininger, L., Berney, T., Shibata T, Spertini F, Merino R and Izui S (1990). Cryoglobulinemia induced by a murine IgG3 rheumatoid factor: skin vasculitis and glomerulonephritis arise from distinct pathogenic mechanisms. *Proceedings of the National Academy of Sciences of the United States of America*, **87**, 10038–42.

Rosenkranz, M. E., Schulte, D. J., Agle, L. M., *et al.* (2005). TLR2 and MyD88 contribute to Lactobacillus casei extract-induced focal coronary arteritis in a mouse model of Kawasaki disease. *Circulation*, **112**, 2966–73.

Rossow, K. D., Collins, J. E., Goyal, S. M., Nelson, E. A., Christopher-Hennings, J. and Benfield, D. A. (1995). Pathogenesis of porcine reproductive and respiratory syndrome virus infection in gnotobiotic pigs. *Veterinary Pathology*, **32**, 361–73.

Scott-Moncrieff, J. C., Snyder, P. W., Glickman, L. T., Davis, E. L. and Felsburg, P. J. (1992). Systemic necrotizing vasculitis in nine young beagles. *Journal of the American Veterinary Medical Association*, **201**, 1553–8.

Shepherd, J., Little, M. C. and Nicklin, M. J. (2004). Psoriasis-like cutaneous inflammation in mice lacking interleukin-1 receptor antagonist. *Journal of Investigative Dermatology*, **122**, 665–9.

Shepherd, J. and Nicklin, M. J. (2005). Elastic-vessel arteritis in interleukin-1 receptor antagonist-deficient mice involves effector Th1 cells and requires interleukin-1 receptor. *Circulation*, **111**, 3135–40.

Snyder, P. W., Kazacos, E. A., Scott-Moncrieff, J. C., *et al.* (1995). Pathologic features of naturally occurring juvenile polyarteritis in beagle dogs. *Veterinary Pathology*, **32**, 337–45.

Staszak, C. and Harbeck, R. J. (1985). Mononuclear-cell pulmonary vasculitis in NZB/W mice. I. Histopathologic evaluation of spontaneously occurring pulmonary infiltrates. *American Journal of Pathology*, **120**, 99–105.

Takahashi, K., Oharaseki, T., Wakayama, M., Yokouchi, Y., Naoe, S. and Murata, H. (2004). Histopathological features of murine systemic vasculitis caused by Candida albicans extract–an animal model of Kawasaki disease. *Inflammation Research*, **53**, 72–7.

Theofilopoulos, A. N. and Dixon, F. J. (1985). Murine models of systemic lupus erythematosus. *Advances in Immunology*, **37**, 269–391.

Thibault, S., Drolet, R., Germain, M. C., D'Allaire, S., Larochelle, R. and Magar, R. (1998). Cutaneous and systemic necrotizing vasculitis in swine. *Veterinary Pathology*, **35**, 108–16.

Tomer, Y., Gilburd, B., Blank, M., *et al.* (1995). Characterization of biologically active antineutrophil cytoplasmic antibodies induced in mice. Pathogenetic role in experimental vasculitis. *Arthritis and Rheumatism*, **38**, 1375–81.

Vinen, C. S., Turner, D. R. and Oliveira, D. B. (2004a). A central role for the mast cell in early phase vasculitis in the Brown Norway rat model of vasculitis: a histological study. *International Journal of Experimental Pathology*, **85**, 165–74.

Vinen, C. S., Turner, D. R. and Oliveira, D. B. (2004b). Resistance to re-challenge in the Brown Norway rat model of vasculitis is not always complete and may reveal separate effector and regulatory populations. *Immunology*, **113**, 269–76.

Walker, S. E., Gray, R. H., Fulton, M., Wigley, R. D. and Schnitzer, B. (1978). Palmerston North mice, a new animal model of systemic lupus erythematosus. *Journal of Laboratory and Clinical Medicine*, **92**, 932–45.

Wang, C. L., Wu, Y. T., Liu, C. A., Kuo, H. C. and Yang, K. D. (2005). Kawasaki disease: infection, immunity and genetics. *Pediatric Infectious Disease Journal*, **24**, 998–1004.

Wang, Y., Nose, M., Kamoto, T., Nishimura, M. and Hiai, H. (1997). Host modifier genes affect mouse autoimmunity induced by the lpr gene. *American Journal of Pathology*, **151**, 1791–8.

Weidebach, W., Viana, V. S., Leon, E. P., *et al.* (2002). C-ANCA-positive IgG fraction from patients with Wegener's granulomatosis induces lung vasculitis in rats. *Clinical and Experimental Immunology*, **129**, 54–60.

White, K. L., David, D. W., Butterworth, L. F. and Klykken, P. C. (2000). Assessment of autoimmunity-inducing potential using the brown Norway rat challenge model. *Toxicology Letters*, **112–113**, 443–51.

Wigley, R. D. (1970). The aetiology of Polyareritis nodosa: A review. *New Zealand Medical Journal*, **71**, 151–8.

Wigley, R. D. and Couchman, K. G. (1966). Polyarteritis nodosa-like disease in outbred mice. *Nature*, **211**, 319–20.

Wigley, R. D., Couchman, K. G. and Maule, R. (1970). Polyarteritis nodosa: the natural history of a spontaneously occurring model in outbred mice. *Australasian Annals of Medicine*, **19**, 319–27.

Wigley, R. D., Craig, A. S., Williamson, K. I. and Couchman, K. G. (1975). Spontaneous arteritis and glomerulitis in mice. A comparison of light and electron microscopic renal changes in PN/n, NZB/BL, 101/MAC, and CBA/MAC mice. *Laboratory Investigation*, **33**, 8–15.

Woolfson, R. G., Qasim, F. J., Thiru, S., Oliveira, D. B., Neild, G. H. and Mathieson, P. W. (1995). Nitric oxide contributes to tissue injury in mercuric chloride-induced autoimmunity. *Biochemical and Biophysical Research Communications*, **217**, 515–21.

Xiao, H., Heeringa, P., Hu, P., *et al.* (2002). Antineutrophil cytoplasmic autoantibodies specific for myeloperoxidase cause glomerulonephritis and vasculitis in mice. *Journal of Clinical Investigation*, **110**, 955–63.

Yamada, A., Miyazaki, T., Lu, L. M., *et al.* (2003). Genetic basis of tissue specificity of vasculitis in MRL/lpr mice. *Arthritis and Rheumatism*, **48**, 1445–51.

Zhang, M. C., Misu, N., Furukawa, H., *et al.* (2006). An epistatic effect of the female specific loci on the development of autoimmune vasculitis and antinuclear autoantibody in murine lupus. *Annals of the Rheumatic Diseases*, **65**, 495–500.

CHAPTER 9

Pathologic features of vasculitis

Andrew Churg

Introduction and classification

This chapter presents a brief overview and illustrations of the pathologic features of vasculitis. Pathologic examination remains the gold standard for the diagnosis of vasculitis, but arriving at a definitive diagnosis on the basis of a biopsy (or autopsy) specimen alone is not always straightforward. For one thing, only a limited number of reaction patterns are seen in the vessels, but these identical reaction patterns can be found in a wide variety of conditions, some of which require vastly different treatment and have considerably different prognoses (Jennette and Falk 1997). Interpretation of biopsies for a diagnosis of vasculitis thus requires careful correlation with clinical information and a variety of laboratory data, such as ANCA status, to arrive at a precise diagnosis.

An additional problem is the wide range of pathologic findings that can be seen in some forms of vasculitis, some of which do not look vasculitic at all. Indeed, for purposes of pathologic diagnosis, it is crucial to recognize a broad spectrum of morphologic changes; insisting on a very narrow set of pathologic findings (particularly insisting on seeing "classic" lesions) before making a diagnosis of vasculitis leads to missed cases.

Sampling, both geographic and temporal, presents another problem. In some forms of vasculitis, such as giant cell arteritis (GCA), lesions are typically focal. They may be missed completely because of bad luck in the area biopsied, and may also be missed if the specimen is not sectioned completely. Similarly, the pathologist must be aware that vascular lesions change their appearance over time: necrotizing arteritis with fibrinoid necrosis is readily diagnosed, but it is easy to mistake old sclerosed arteritic lesions for non-specific thrombosis.

Lastly, as is true of many areas of pathology, understanding and diagnosing vasculitis is greatly facilitated by reference to a defined classification scheme. A variety of classification schemes have been proposed, some of them are contradictory, and application of different schemes place given patients into different diagnostic categories, including categories that may require different treatment. The discussion in this chapter follows the general scheme elucidated by the Chapel Hill Consensus conference (Jennette *et al.* 1994) (see Table 26.2 in Chapter 26) with subsequent modifications as noted (Jennette and Falk 2000a, 2000b), and as discussed in Chapter 1. This scheme classifies vasculitis primarily by the size of vessel involved.

Large-vessel vasculitis

The large-vessel vasculitides are defined as those that primarily involve the aorta and its major branches, particularly the branches to the head and neck and to the upper and lower limbs (Jennette *et al.* 1994; Jennette and Falk 1997, 2000b; Lie 1989), but also the coronary and pulmonary arteries. The primary entities included in this category are Takayasu's arteritis (TA) and GCA, both of which typically show a giant cell or granulomatous appearance. Both entities are relatively indolent processes that often have a long time course and often progress to vascular fibrosis or fibrotic obliteration, manifested clinically as reduced pulses (TA is frequently referred to as "pulseless disease"), bruits, and claudication. It should be noted that other types of vasculitis can involve the aorta and large vessels and have a granulomatous appearance (see below), and that a granulomatous reaction may be seen in forms of vasculitis that involve medium or small vessels (Table 9.1). Thus, the presence of giant cells by themselves is not diagnostic of giant cell or TA.

Table 9.1 Diseases that can show a giant cell or granulomatous pattern of vasculitis

In large vessels
Takayasu's arteritis
Giant cell (temporal) arteritis
Vasculitis associated with rheumatoid arthritis (uncommon)
Vasculitis associated with lupus (uncommon)

In medium and small vessels
Polyarteritis nodosa (PAN) (uncommon)
Kawasaki's disease (uncommon)
Vasculitis associated with rheumatoid arthritis (uncommon)
Vasculitis associated with tuberculous and fungal infections (common)
Sarcoidosis (common)
Buerger's disease (common)
Idiopathic granulomatous vasculitis (by definition)
Granulomatous vasculitis of the CNS (by definition)

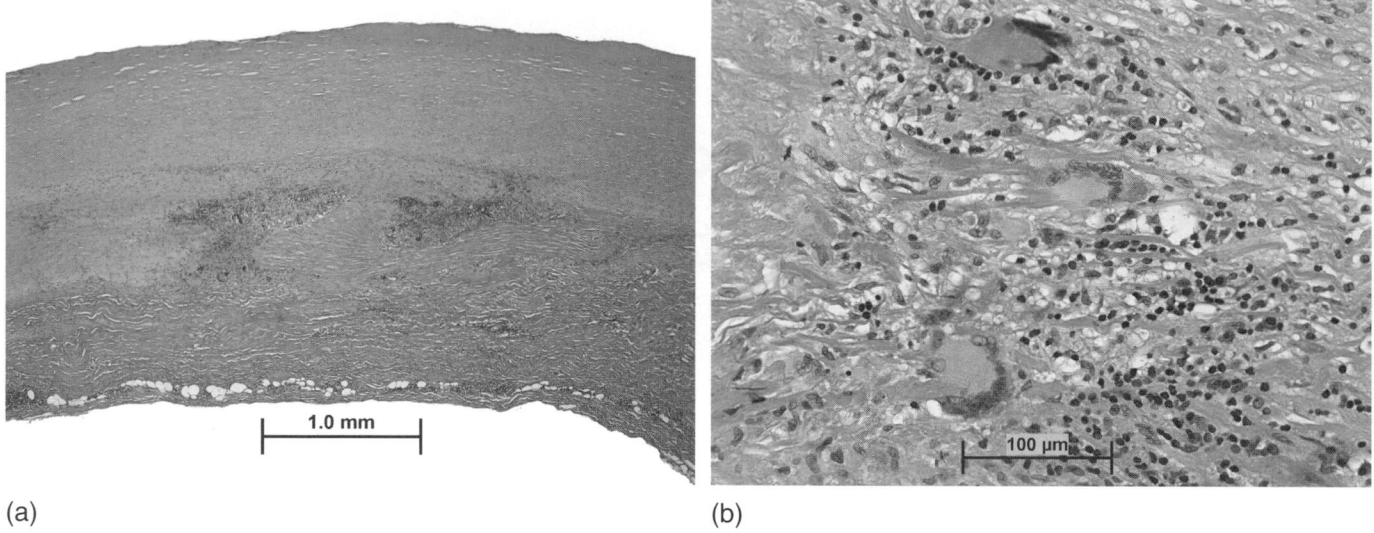

(a)   (b)

Figure 9.1 Takayasu's arteritis. Low power (A) and higher power (B) micrographs of the aorta showing a somewhat thickened wall and collections of inflammatory cells and characteristic giant cells. Courtesy of William D. Edwards, MD, Mayo Clinic, Rochester, Minnesota. (See Color Plate 5.)

The clinical features of GCA and TA are discussed in detail in Chapters 24 and 25. Because the morphology is essentially identical, separation is somewhat arbitrarily based on age (greater than 50 years of age for GCA, less than 50 years of age for TA); sex (predominantly female in TA); the frequent association of polymyalgia rheumatica with GCA; and to some extent the sites of involvement. TA tends to involve the extremities and abdominal aorta, while GCA commonly involves the temporal artery and other extracranial branches of the carotid, with only about 10 to 15% of cases having clinically overt disease outside this region (Lie 1991a).

In the acute phase, TA appears as a patchy inflammatory infiltrate that is predominantly lymphocytes and plasma cells, sometimes with an admixture of eosinophils and histiocytes (Figure 9.1). The number of giant cells is variable; in some cases they occur singly, and in others form poorly defined granulomas in the vessel wall (Lie 1991a). It has been claimed that the giant cells only occur in vessels that are calcified and are a form of foreign body reaction to

the calcium (Petursdottir *et al.* 1996). Infarct-like necrosis has been reported (Heggtveit *et al.* 1963). The inflammatory process occasionally extends into surrounding tissue such as retroperitoneal fat, mediastinal fat, and the vena cava (Kinare 1975).

The inflammatory reaction slowly destroys the elastic laminae of the vessel wall, and replaces the elastic tissue with fibrous tissue. The inflammatory infiltrate may largely or totally disappear, although if the disease recurs, both chronic inflammatory cells and giant cells reappear. The vessel wall in the chronic phase is typically thickened (Figures 9.2 and 9.3) and the lumen, particularly in limb vessels, coronary arteries, and pulmonary arteries, may be severely compromised (Figure 9.2). The severity of wall thickening appears to be proportional to the duration of disease (Lie 1991a). Thromboses may further occlude the lumen. Large-vessel ectasias/aneurysms

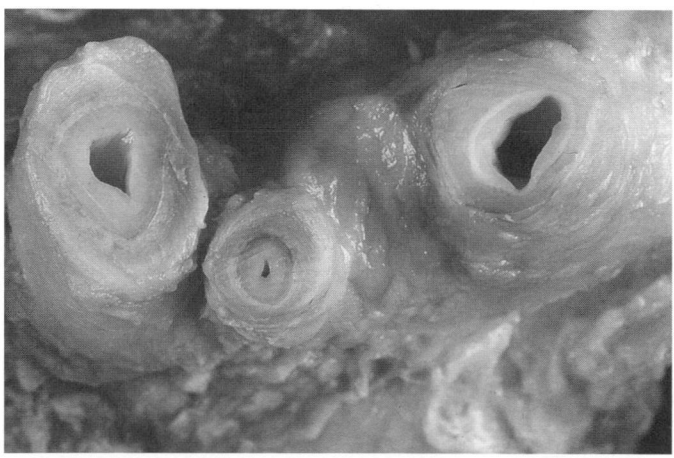

Figure 9.2 Takayasu's arteritis. Gross photograph of aortic arch branches showing marked lumenal narrowing and thickening of the arterial wall. Courtesy of William D. Edwards, MD, Mayo Clinic, Rochester, Minnesota. (See Color Plate 6.)

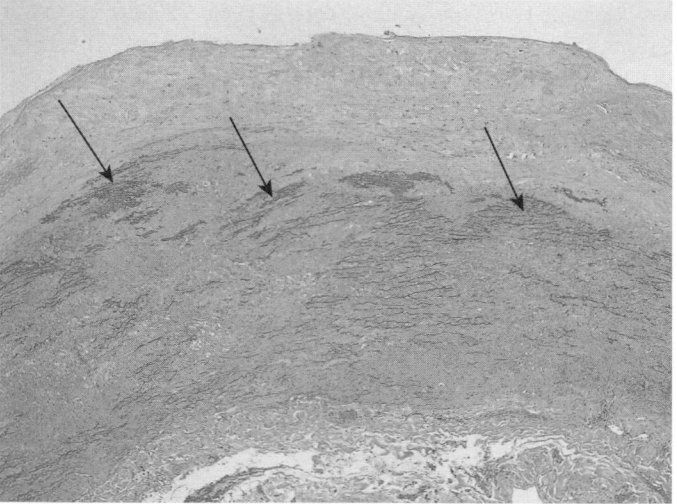

Figure 9.3 Takayasu's arteritis. In this example of long standing burnt out disease in the aorta, most of the elastica has disappeared and been replaced by fibrous tissue. (See Color Plate 7.)

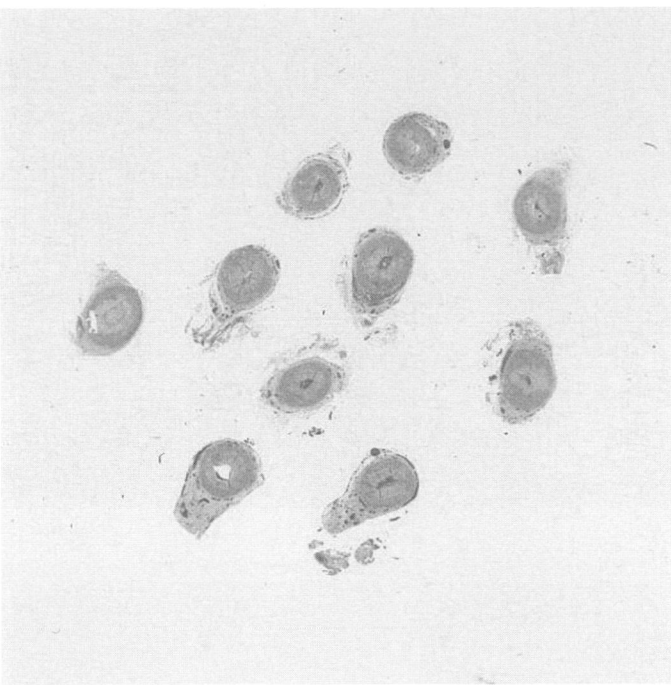

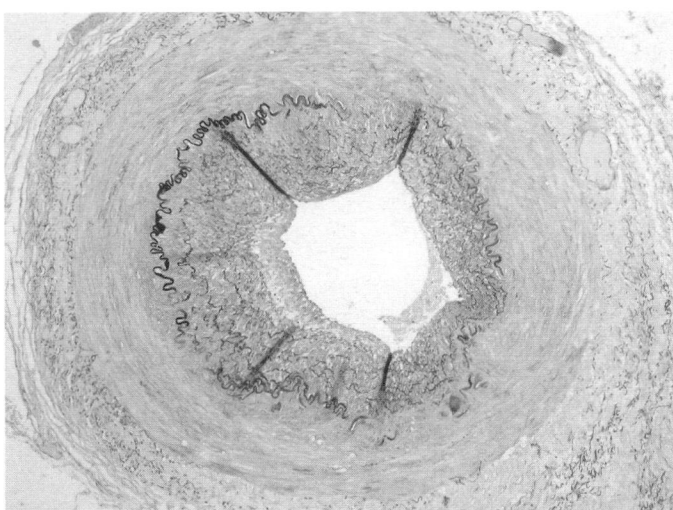

Figure 9.6 Giant cell arteritis. Elastic stain of one of the vessel segments illustrated in Figure 9.4. Note loss of elastic over most of the circumference of the vessel, a characteristic finding in many forms of vasculitis.

Figure 9.4 Giant cell arteritis. This figure shows the proper way to process temporal artery specimens for histology: the arterial segment is cut into numerous short pieces and all are embedded in one or more tissue blocks and then sectioned at multiple levels. (See Color Plate 8.)

and dissections also occur. Hypertensive and ischemic changes are typically seen in the kidney secondary to renal artery occlusion.

GCA, frequently called temporal arteritis (see Chapter 24), is morphologically similar to TA (Figures 9.4, 9.5, 9.6, and 9.7), but most cases involve the extracranial branches of the carotid artery, with the temporal, vertebral, ophthalmic, and posterior ciliary involved alone or in some combination in about 75% of cases (Wilkinson and Russell 1972). Clinically evident involvement of the aorta and large branches (Figure 9.7) is less common, although

clinically inapparent disease in these vessels can be demonstrated on angiography in some patients with otherwise typical temporal arteritis. Conversely, about 25% of patients with disease clinically located outside the head have radiographic evidence of temporal arteritis (Lie 1995b).

Arteritis of the temporal arteries has been studied in great detail and there are numerous morphologic variations. Giant cells are not always present, or may only be seen in small side branches, and occasionally only the temporal vein and not the artery is involved (Lie 1996a). Fibrinoid necrosis of the outer zone of the intima adjacent to the internal elastica has been reported by Lie (1996a) in 25% of a very large series of cases; however, its presence should raise the issue of whether the lesion is question is really GCA or another form of systemic vasculitis, as other systemic vasculitides can involve the temporal artery (Lie 1996a; Walz *et al.* 1994).

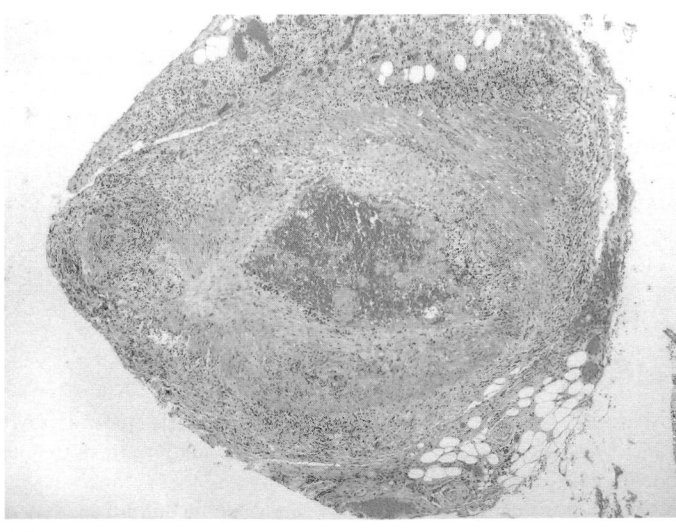

(a)

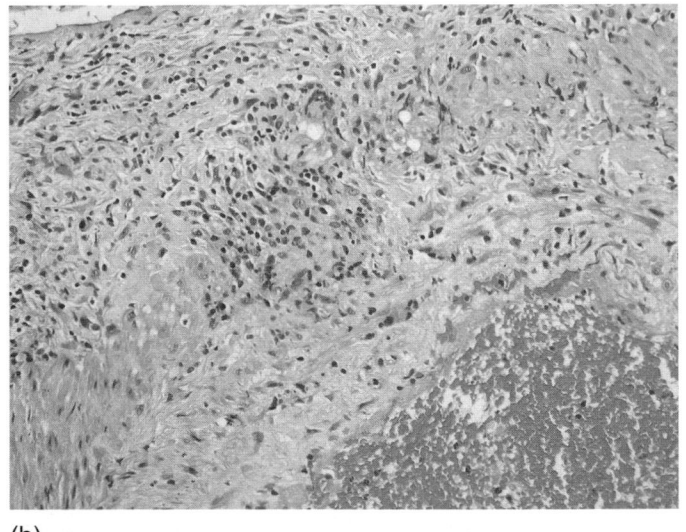

(b)

Figure 9.5 Giant cell arteritis. Low (a) and higher power (b) views of a temporal artery showing extensive inflammation involving largely the outer portion of the vessel wall; in (b) giant cells and inflammatory cells are seen to disrupt the muscularis. (See Color Plate 9.)

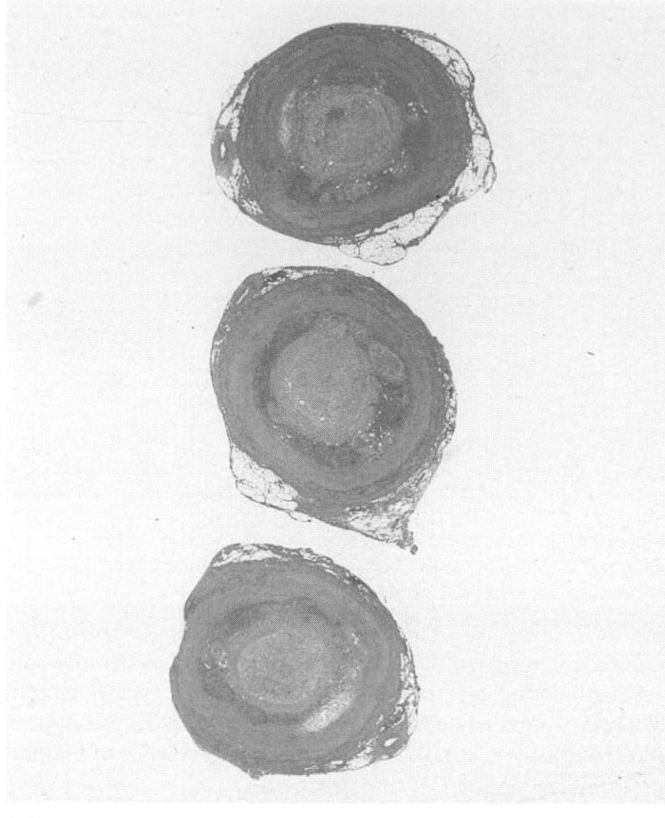

(a)

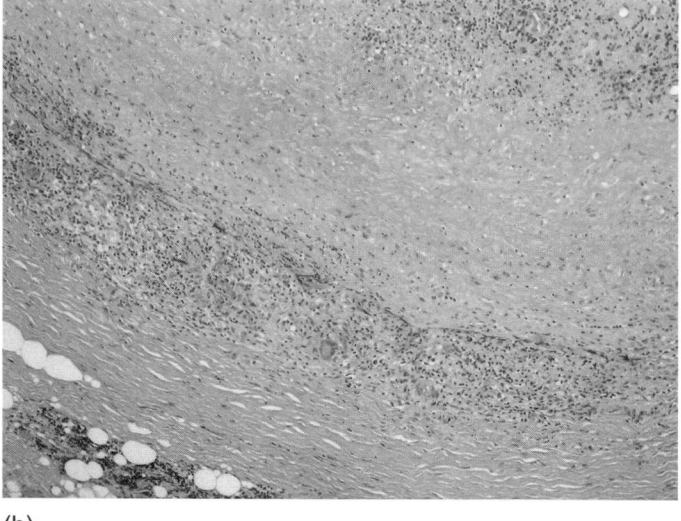

(b)

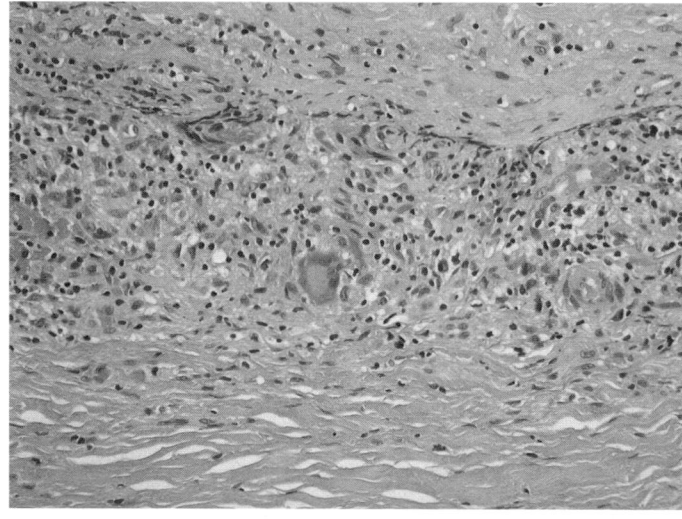

(c)

Figure 9.7 Giant cell arteritis involving a brachial artery. (a) This very low power view of a resected segment trisected shows complete luminal occlusion. Medium (b) and high power (c) views show inflammatory involvement of the arterial wall with giant cells, and fibrous obliteration (old thrombosis) of the lumen. (See Color Plate 10.)

In some instances the question arises of whether a fibrotic, pauci-inflammatory lesion is old (healed) GCA, or merely arteriosclerosis. Both can largely or completely obstruct the lumen. A useful rule of thumb is that arteriosclerosis produces minor loss or reduplication of elastica; however, if there is disorganization and loss of long elastic segments (Figure 9.6), this is more likely the residue of GCA (Ashton-Key and Gallagher 1991; Lie 1996a).

Because the temporal artery is amenable to biopsy, many pathologic specimens derive from this site. The reported sensitivity of temporal artery biopsy in the literature varies from 65 to 97% (Jacobs and Allen 1991) and bilateral biopsy is reported in some studies to considerably increase the yield (Ponge *et al.* 1988). Since the lesions are segmental, with skip areas, temporal artery and other putative GCA specimens need to be cut into short (1 to 2 mm) lengths, embedded completely, and then sectioned at multiple levels to ensure that a diagnostic area is not missed (Nordborg and Nordborg 1995; Lie 1996a) (Figure 9.4). It is not uncommon to receive biopsies after glucocorticoid therapy has been started, but Achkar *et al.* (1994) showed that even 14 days of steroid treatment does not affect the positive diagnosis rate in temporal artery specimens, although the morphologic appearances may be altered.

Vasculitis involving the aorta and its branches with a pathologic pattern of GCA has been reported to occur occasionally in patients with rheumatoid arthritis (RA) and systemic lupus erythematosus (SLE) (Lie 1989; Bahlas *et al.* 1998; Hall *et al.* 1983). Other types of vasculitic and primarily non-vasculitic disease can show a granulomatous vasculitic pattern in medium and small vessels, as listed in Table 9.1.

Medium-vessel vasculitis

Medium-vessel vasculitides, such as polyarteritis nodosa (PAN) and Kawasaki's disease (KD) (mucocutaneous lymph node syndrome), involve the main visceral arteries and their branches. They may involve smaller arteries as well; however, by definition, they do not involve arterioles, capillaries, or venules (Jennette and Falk 1997; Jennette and Falk 2000b). Medium-vessel vasculitides typically start with a necrotizing phase which often affects the vessel in an asymmetric fashion (Figure 9.8). In many instances the destructive process is manifest as so-called fibrinoid necrosis of the vessel wall, that is replacement of the wall by granular pink material that resembles fibrin on hematoxylin and eosin stain (Figure 9.8c), usually accompanied by an infiltrate of polymorphonuclear leukocytes. However, fibrinoid necrosis is not always present and the inflammatory infiltrate can be predominantly chronic inflammatory cells. The vasculitic process is segmental and may be focal. In fact it is characteristic to see acute lesions, healed or healing lesions, and totally uninvolved vessels in the same section (Figure 9.8a). This is the classic microscopic picture of vasculitis but its lack of diagnostic specificity for medium-vessel vasculitis must be stressed, since an identical picture can be seen in many forms of small-vessel vasculitis.

Inflammatory destruction of the wall can result in arterial rupture, thrombosis, and aneurysm formation. With time the inflammatory infiltrate becomes composed entirely of chronic inflammatory cells and then disappears, and the wall progressively scars, in some instances leading to fibrotic obliteration of the lumen (Figure 9.8d). At this stage there can be significant morphologic overlap with the changes seen in large-vessel vasculitis, and sometimes also difficulty in determining whether a vessel is merely thrombosed or the previous site of vasculitis. Elastic stains are very useful: loss of large portions of elastic laminae favor a diagnosis of vasculitis (Figure 9.8d), since ordinary bland thrombi do not destroy the elastica. Both PAN and KD can occasionally show a granulomatous arteritis (Lie 1989; Landing and Larson 1987).

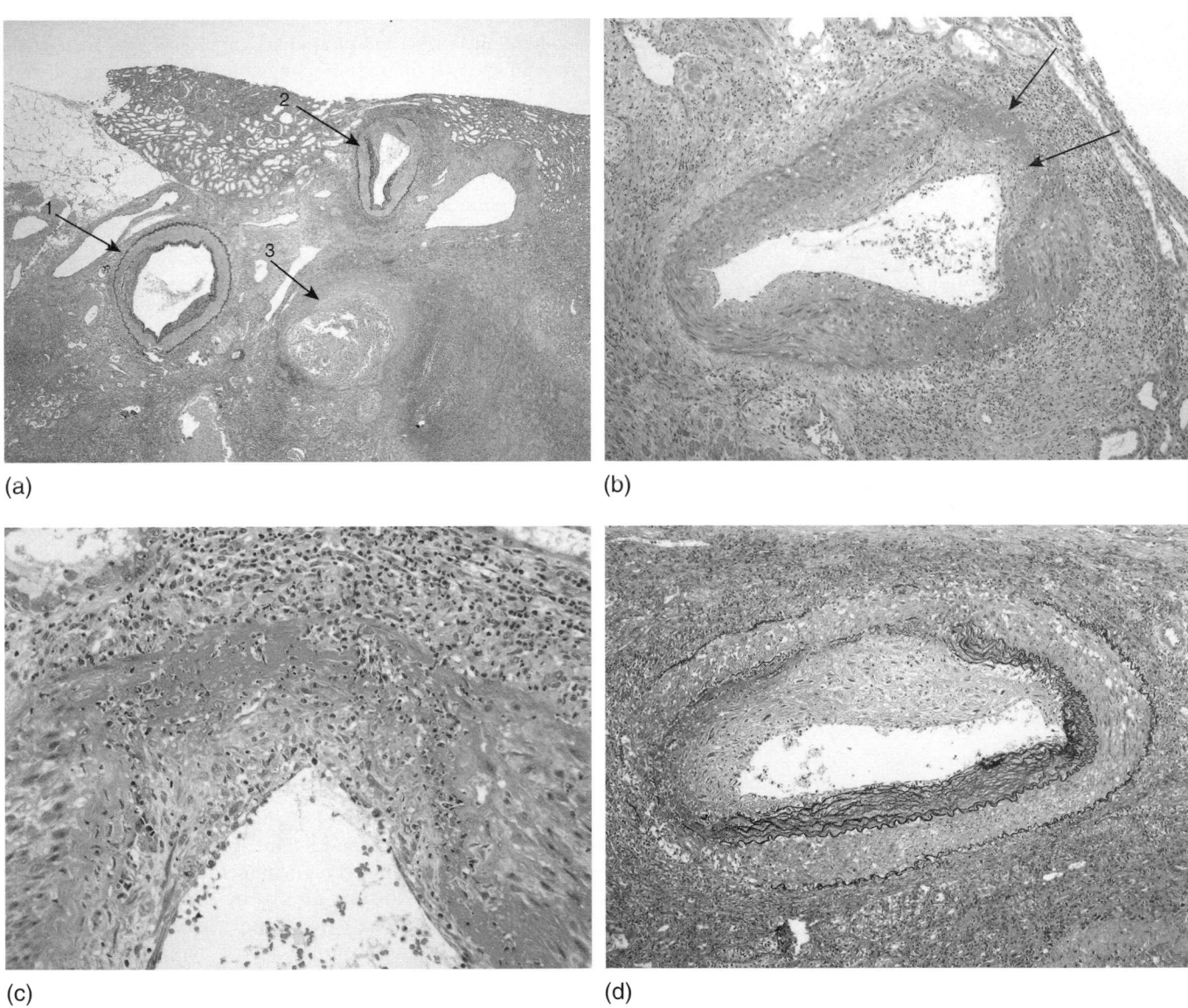

(a)

(b)

(c)

(d)

Figure 9.8 Polyarteritis nodosa involving relatively large intrarenal arteries. (a) Note the marked variation in degree of involvement in nearby vessels (probably all branches of the same artery). The branch on the left shows minimal damage, while the smaller branch on the right demonstrates loss of elastic over half of the perimeter. The lower shows nearly complete destruction of the wall. Elastic stain. Medium (b) and higher power (c) views of the vessel in (a). Note the characteristic focal necrosis which in (c) has the appearance of so-called fibrinoid. (d) Old healed lesion showing marked lumenal narrowing and loss of elastica in the same kidney. Loss of elastica indicates that this lesion did not result from bland thrombosis. Elastin stain. (See Color Plate 12.)

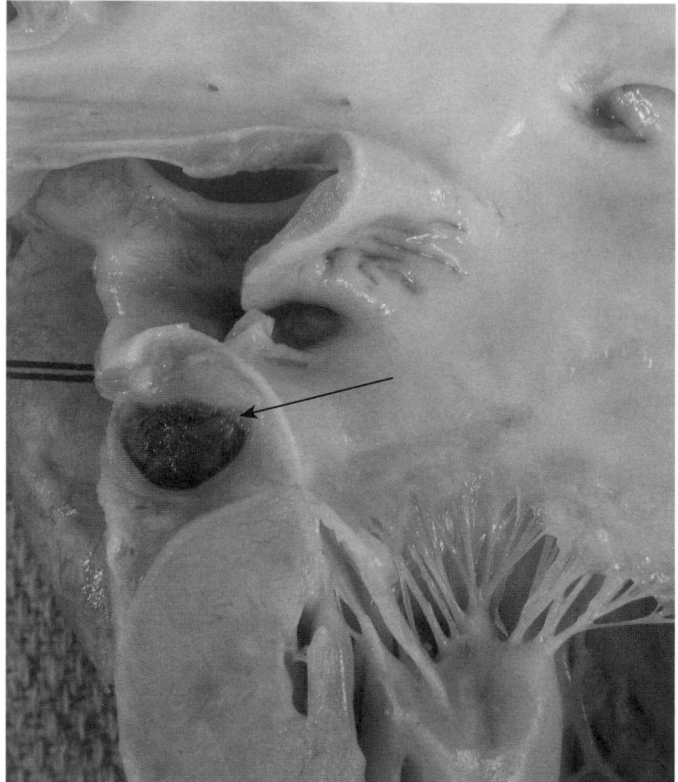

(a)

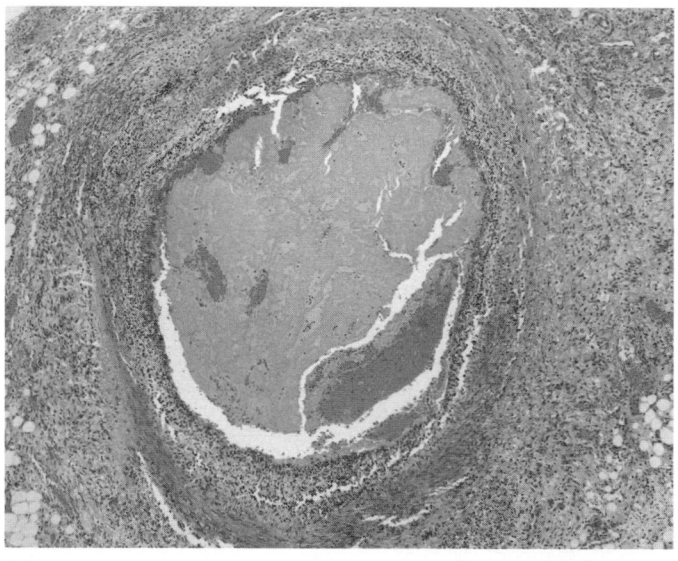

(b)

Figure 9.9 Kawasaki disease. (a) Gross photograph of heart of a child at autopsy showing aneurysmally dilated coronary artery with intralumenal thrombus. (b) Necrotizing arteritis involving a coronary artery. Courtesy of Glenn P. Taylor, MD, Division of Pathology, Hospital for Sick Children, Toronto, Ontario. (See Color Plate 11.)

The older literature is confusing because of the failure to separate PAN and MPA, and it is easy to find statements that polyarteritis causes a necrotizing glomerulonephritis. By current definitions such cases are labeled MPA, a form of small-vessel vasculitis.

Polyarteritis causes renal disease by occlusion of large vessels (Figure 9.8), leading to ischemia or infarction.

Although KD is morphologically similar to PAN (Figure 9.9), the clinical setting is quite different, since it affects largely children under 5, and starts as an acute febrile illness associated with mucosal changes, desquamation in the extremities, and enlarged lymph nodes (see Chapter 29). Small aneurysms are characteristic of both PAN and KD, but in the latter they commonly affect the coronary arteries (Figure 9.9), although other sites are involved as well (Landing and Larson 1987; Naoe *et al.* 1991). Veins appear to be involved fairly frequently in KD, and much less commonly in PAN.

Small-vessel vasculitides

Small-vessel vasculitides by definition involve arterioles, capillaries, and venules. Cutaneous leukocytoclastic vasculitis, various forms of glomerulonephritis, and pulmonary capillaritis with hemorrhage are characteristic findings in many different forms of small-vessel vasculitis, and they are not seen in medium and large-vessel vasculitides. These findings often go together to produce the dermal–renal syndrome (leukocytoclastic vasculitis and glomerulonephritis), typical of cryoglobulinemia and Henoch–Schönlein purpura (HSP), or the pulmonary–renal syndrome (glomerulonephritis with pulmonary hemorrhage) most commonly seen in Wegener's granulomatosis (WG), MPA, SLE, and occasionally in Churg–Strauss syndrome (CSS). In the past, the term hypersensitivity vasculitis, originally coined by Zeek *et al.* (1948), has been used for some forms of small-vessel vasculitis, but this term is not recommended because of its lack of specificity.

Most forms of small-vessel vasculitis can also involve medium or small arteries and produce necrotizing lesions (Figure 9.10) identical to those seen in PAN, so that biopsies showing only this pattern are difficult to classify without further information. By the definition given above, the vasculitides associated with collagen vascular diseases, notably SLE and RA, are designated as forms of small-vessel vasculitis, but they can involve much larger vessels, including the aorta (see below). This is true also of Behçet's syndrome (BS), where in fact large-vessel vasculitis is common (see below). Aneurysms have been viewed as pathognomonic of PAN, and are also common in KD (see above); however, aneurysms can be seen in small-vessel vasculitides (Jennette and Falk 2000b; Jennette *et al.* 2001; Lie 1989) and do not allow separation of medium and small-vessel diseases.

Information on ANCA status and the presence of immune complexes or circulating antibodies is extremely helpful in subclassifying small-vessel vasculitis (see Chapter 6). WG, CSS, and MPA are typically ANCA-positive and do not show deposition of immune complexes, whereas HSP, cryoglobulinemia, and vasculitis associated with collagen vascular disease are ANCA-negative (at least negative for myeloperoxidase and antiproteinase 3 ANCA) and are associated with immune complex deposition. Drugs can produce a picture of small-vessel vasculitis, most commonly cutaneous leukocytoclastic vasculitis, and may be associated with ANCA or immune complex formation or both (see below).

Cutaneous leukocytoclastic vasculitis involves primarily post-capillary venules in the upper dermis. The venules show endothelial swelling and, occasionally, actual fibrinoid necrosis (Figure 9.11). Most show an infiltrate of polymorphonuclear leukocytes, occasionally accompanied by eosinophils, and the neutrophils

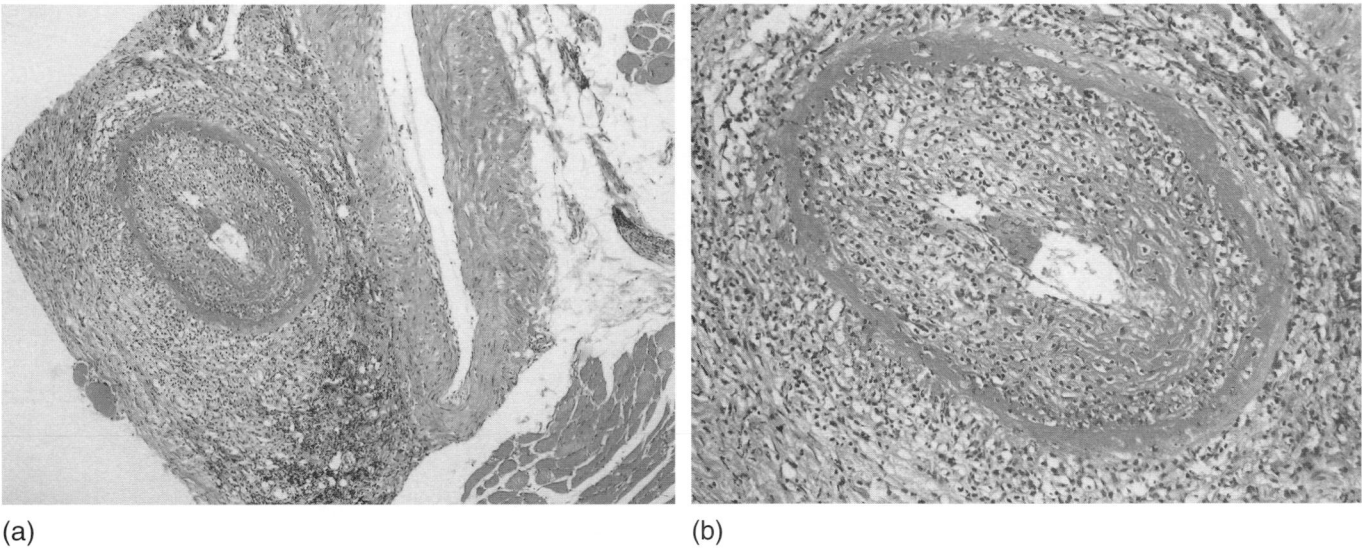

(a)

(b)

Figure 9.10 Microscopic polyangiitis. Low (a) and high (b) power views of necrotizing vasculitis involving a small artery in a muscle biopsy. The arterial wall is completely replaced by fibrinoid necrosis and an acute inflammatory infiltrate is present. This appearance can be seen in any form of small-vessel vasculitis and also in medium-vessel vasculitis (polyarteritis nodosa, Kawasaki disease) when it involves small arteries. (See Color Plate 13.)

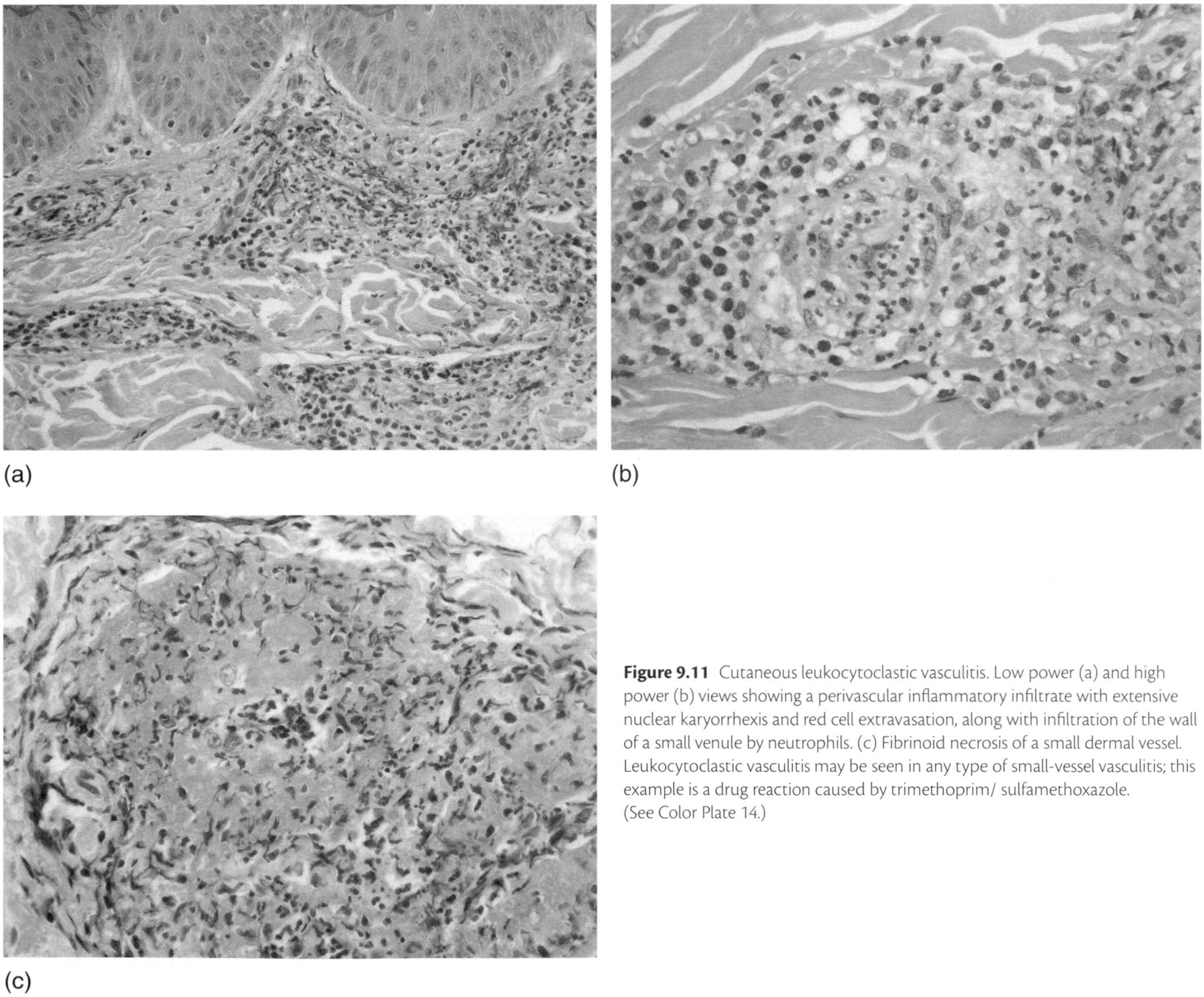

(a)

(b)

(c)

Figure 9.11 Cutaneous leukocytoclastic vasculitis. Low power (a) and high power (b) views showing a perivascular inflammatory infiltrate with extensive nuclear karyorrhexis and red cell extravasation, along with infiltration of the wall of a small venule by neutrophils. (c) Fibrinoid necrosis of a small dermal vessel. Leukocytoclastic vasculitis may be seen in any type of small-vessel vasculitis; this example is a drug reaction caused by trimethoprim/ sulfamethoxazole. (See Color Plate 14.)

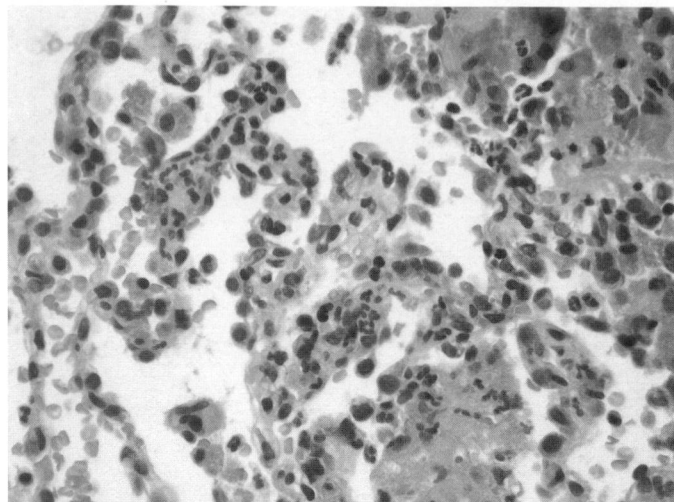

Figure 9.12 Pulmonary capillaritis. Characteristic pattern of neutrophils in alveolar walls and evidence of acute and chronic hemorrhage (hemosiderin-laden macrophages) in airspaces. This example is from a patient with rheumatoid arthritis and hemoptysis. (See Color Plate 15.)

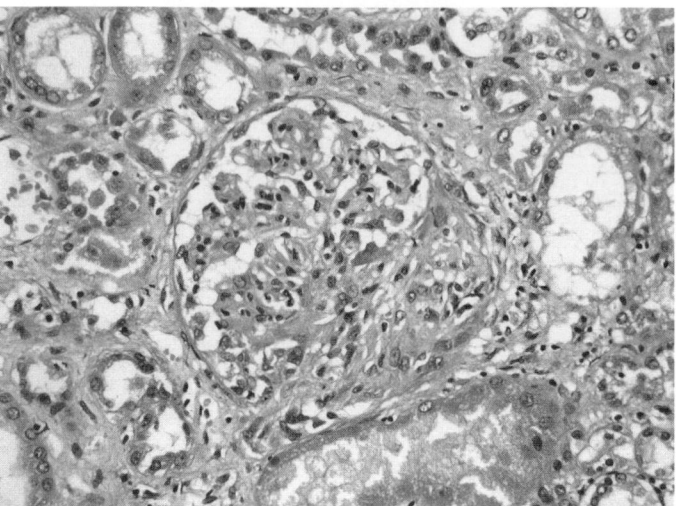

Figure 9.13 Crescentic glomerulonephritis from a case of microscopic polyangiitis. (See Color Plate 16.)

typically undergo karyorrhexis, so that nuclear fragments and extravasated red cells are found in the dermis around the affected vessels. In CSS, the infiltrate can be mostly or entirely composed of eosinophils. In some instances the infiltrate is composed of lymphocytes and plasma cells and there is minimal or no karyorrhexis. It is unclear whether this appearance represents a late or healing stage of the form with neutrophils, or has a different pathogenesis (Swerlick and Lawley 1991).

Pulmonary capillaritis consists of an infiltrate of neutrophils that remains largely confined to the interstitium of the alveolar walls (Figure 9.12), although there may be spillover into the alveoli. Capillaritis is usually accompanied by recent and old hemorrhage, the latter manifest as hemosiderin-laden macrophages in the air spaces (Figure 9.12). Although the process is referred to as capillaritis, involvement of small arterioles and venules is frequently seen (Myers and Katzenstein 1986). Foci of granulation tissue (bronchiolitis obliterans organizing pneumonia [BOOP]) are sometimes present and represent a response to hemorrhage.

Capillaritis can be very subtle, but one useful aid in histologic diagnosis is the presence of fibrin tufts attached to alveolar walls; careful examination, perhaps aided by elastic stains or stains for basement membrane, will reveal that the underlying alveolar wall is disrupted or actually necrotic. Many cases of pulmonary capillaritis are manifest clinically by massive hemoptysis. The presence of capillaritis in patients with hemoptysis is associated with a high mortality of up to 50% in patients with SLE (Zamora *et al.* 1997) and 31% in patients with MPA (Lauque *et al.* 2000). For this reason, such cases need to be reported by the pathologist in an emergent fashion and treated immediately. Necrotizing and crescentic (Figure 9.13) glomerulonephritis is characteristic of WG, MPASS, and, occasionally, CSS (Falk *et al.* 2000).

Specific forms of small-vessel vasculitis

Specific forms of small-vessel vasculitis are discussed below; Table 9.2 provides a scheme for separating the small-vessel vasculitides by morphology and laboratory findings.

ANCA-positive vasculitis
Wegener's granulomatosis

The classic formulation of WG involved a triad of upper airway lesions, necrotizing granulomatous vasculitis in the lung, and necrotizing glomerulonephritis (Godman and Churg 1954). Carrington and Liebow (1966) subsequently described what they labeled "limited Wegener's granulomatosis," in which other organs, particularly the skin, were involved. It is now recognized that WG can present in virtually any organ, and that the pattern of organ involvement frequently changes over time. It is in fact relatively uncommon to see the classic triad of involvement at the time of initial presentation. Thus a broader and more encompassing view of organ involvement by WG must be kept in mind. Active Wegener's granulomatosis is almost always cANCA (proteinase 3) positive.

The vascular lesions in WG are variable. In the lung the classic finding is basophilic necrosis with a surrounding palisade of

Table 9.2 Diagnostic separation scheme for small-vessel vasculitides

Pauci-immune (generally ANCA positive)	Immune complex positive
Wegener's granulomatosis granulomatous vasculitis with neutrophils	Collagen-vascular diseases immune complexes visible by light or electron microscopy
Churg–Strauss syndrome asthma, eosinophilia, eosinophilic vasculitis sometimes granulomas with eosinophilic necrosis	Henoch–Schönlein purpura complexes contain IgA
Microscopic polyangiitis no granulomas, no asthma or eosinophils	Cryoglobulinemic vasculitis circulating cryoglobulins
Some drug-induced vasculitis usually myeloperoxidase ANCA or atypical pANCA (other antigens)	Some drug-induced vasculitis

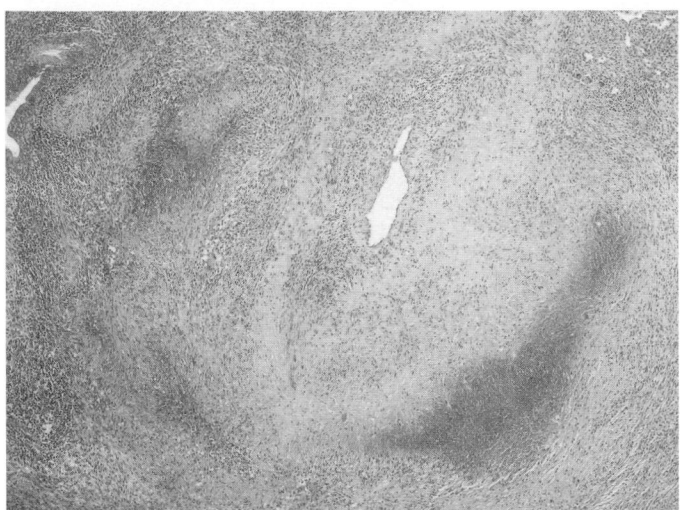

Figure 9.14 Wegener's granulomatosis. Characteristic pattern of 'geographic necrosis' (irregular necrosis); the surrounding palisade of epithelioid histiocytes, that is the 'granulomatosis', cannot be seen at this low power. (See Color Plate 17.)

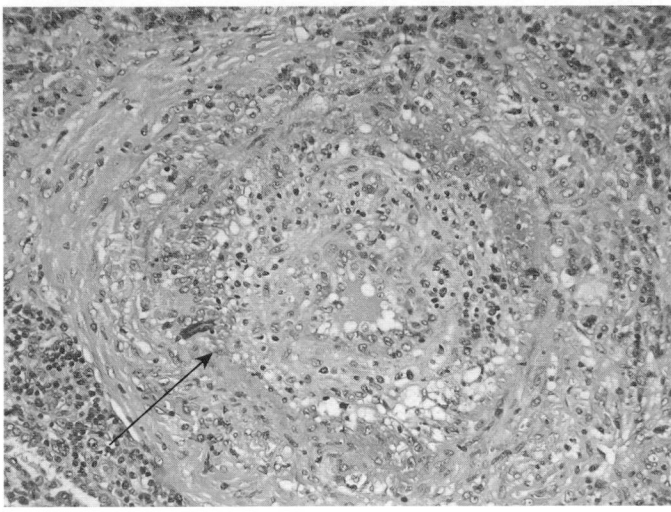

Figure 9.15 Wegener's granulomatosis. Small artery in lung showing necrotizing vasculitis. (See Color Plate 18.)

epithelioid histiocytes, that is granulomatosis, producing so-called geographic necrosis (Figure 9.14). This process may involve vessels or the parenchyma itself; however, the vasculitis in the lung may simply have giant cells with no necrosis, or fibrinoid necrosis (Figure 9.15), or sometimes just an infiltrate of chronic inflammatory cells. The vasculitis and necrosis are superimposed on a parenchymal background of individual giant cells and chronic inflammatory cells (Figure 9.16); however, sarcoid-type hard granulomas are not a feature of WG and their presence indicates an alternate diagnosis. Vasculitis is not always obvious, particularly in lung biopsies, but this does not change the diagnosis. Capillaritis with hemorrhage is common (Figure 9.17) and may be the sole manifestation of WG in the lung (Travis *et al.* 1987).

Early lesions of WG in the lung often show no vasculitis at all; rather there is necrosis of collagen with small neutrophilic abscesses

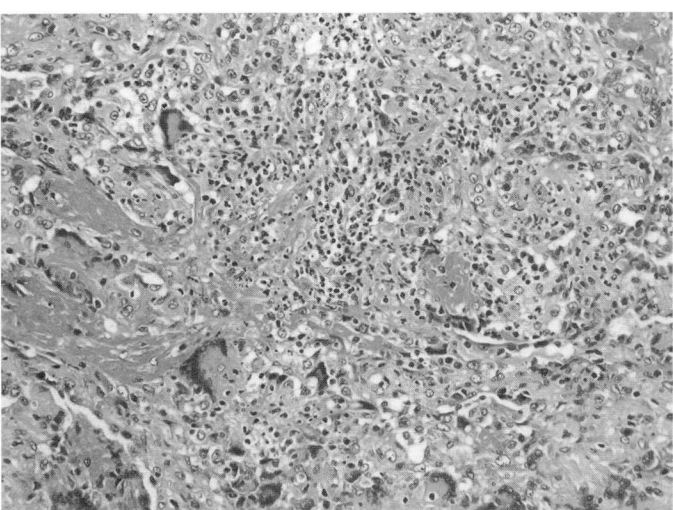

Figure 9.16 Wegener's granulomatosis. Typical inflammatory background seen in the lung, and composed of acute and chronic inflammatory cells and individual giant cells, but not hard granulomas. (See Color Plate 19.)

(Figure 9.18). Over time these become necrotic and develop the characteristic granulomatous response. This pattern is also seen in some examples of WG involving the orbit. Outside lung the granulomatous response is also much less frequent and the typical vasculitis shows neutrophils and fibrinoid necrosis (Figure 9.19), although, again, a wide range of patterns is seen. Infarcts are common when fairly large vessels are involved. In the upper respiratory tract, vasculitis is relatively uncommon, or at least hard to demonstrate on biopsy (Devaney *et al.* 1990), and most lesions appear as non-specific ulcers, sometimes containing giant cells (Figure 9.20). A positive proteinase 3 or myeloperoxidase ANCA is extremely helpful in making a diagnosis in this setting.

Churg–Strauss syndrome

Patients with CSS have asthma or allergic rhinitis and, usually, blood eosinophila. The original Churg-Strauss cases (Churg and Strauss 1951) all had a combination of eosinophilic tissue infiltration, necrotizing vasculitis, and granulomas with eosinophilic material in the centers. In practice this definition has proven to be much too restrictive, and few cases, at least on biopsy, show all three features (Lanham *et al.* 1984; Churg 2001).

A more realistic view, similar to that for WG, is that CSS is a vasculitis with variable manifestations. In practice, CSS can be divided into early or prevasculitic cases, cases with overt vasculitis, and cases with healed vasculitis (Churg 2001). These distinctions are of prognostic and treatment value, since early-phase disease responds well to glucocorticoids, but vasculitic-phase disease often requires addition of a cytotoxic agent and has associated mortality. CSS is typically pANCA (myeloperoxidase) positive.

In early-phase disease, vasculitis cannot be demonstrated clinically or on biopsy. Biopsy specimens typically show only an eosinophilic tissue infiltrate. In the lung this is identical to chronic eosinophilic pneumonia (Figure 9.21), but may also manifest as eosinophilic gastroenteritis or eosinophilic lymphadenitis.

In the vasculitic phase, the most characteristic lesion is a necrotizing vasculitis with fibrinoid necrosis that by itself cannot be distinguished from other small- and medium-sized vasculitides

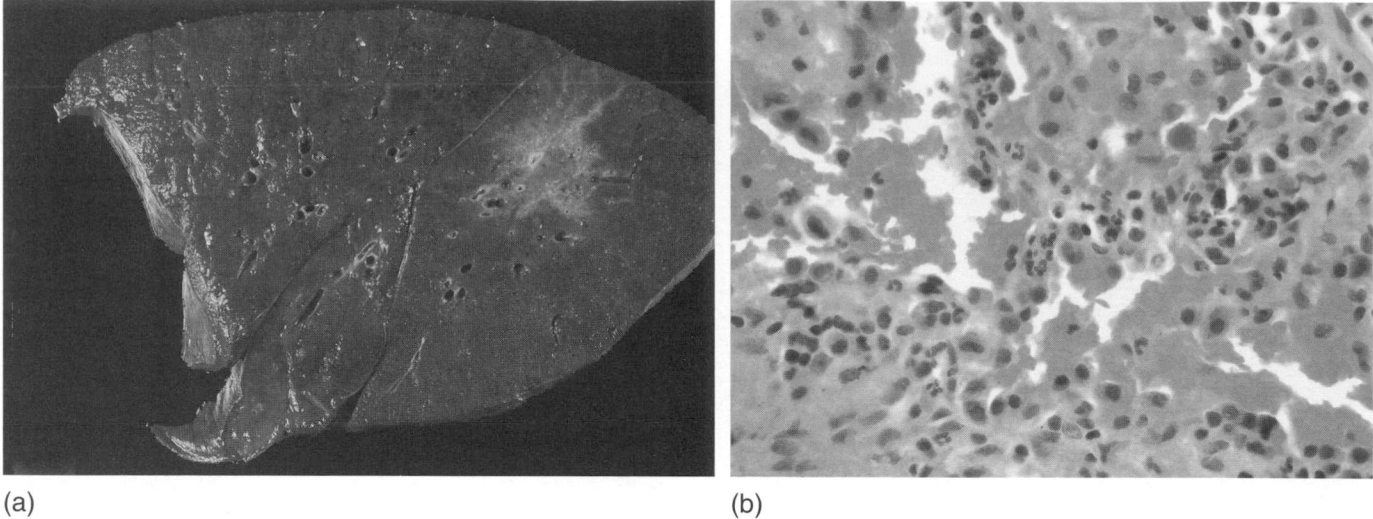

(a)

(b)

Figure 9.17 Wegener's granulomatosis. (a) Gross photograph showing extensive hemorrhage and an irregular upper lobe necrotizing mass lesion. (b) Microscopic pattern of capillaritis with hemorrhage, a frequent finding in the lung in Wegener's granulomatosis. (See Color Plate 20.)

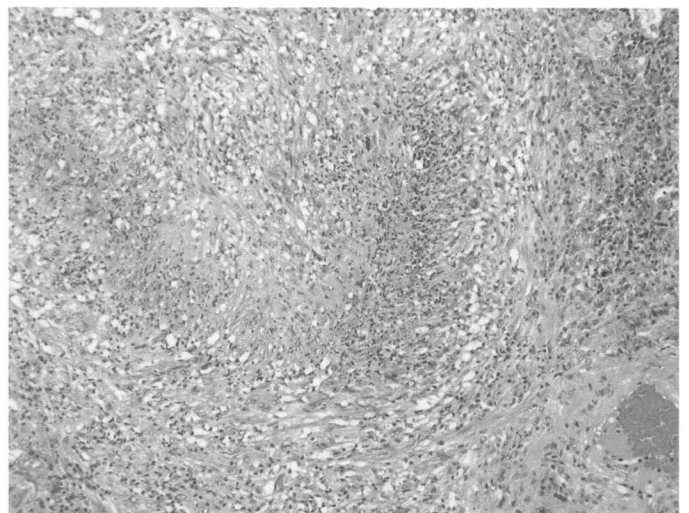

Figure 9.18 Wegener's granulomatosis. Early lesion consisting of a small neutrophilic abscess. In this example a palisade of epithelioid histiocytes is beginning to form; eventually such lesions end up as large or small areas of geographic necrosis. (See Color Plate 21.)

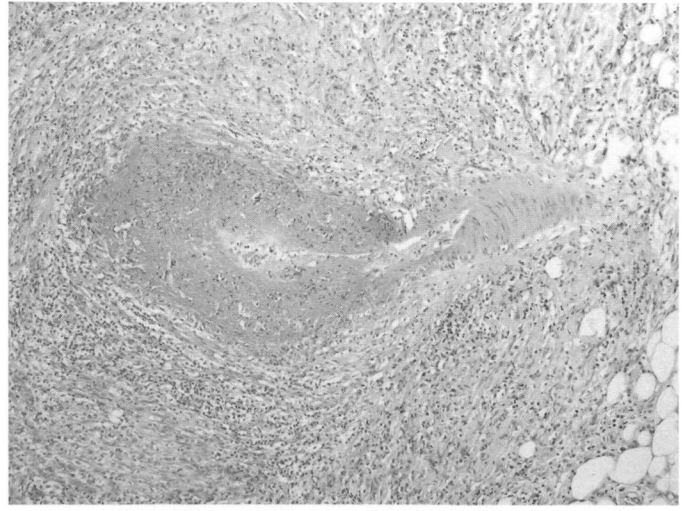

Figure 9.19 Wegener's granulomatosis. Necrotizing vasculitis with fibrinoid necrosis involving a mesenteric artery. (See Color Plate 22.)

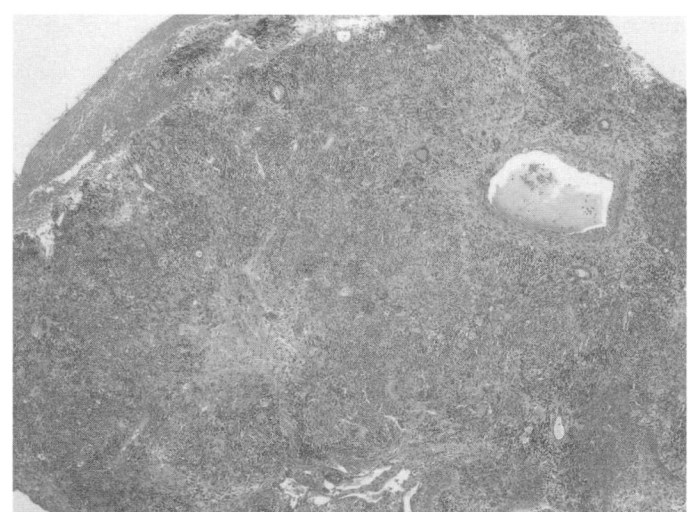

(a)

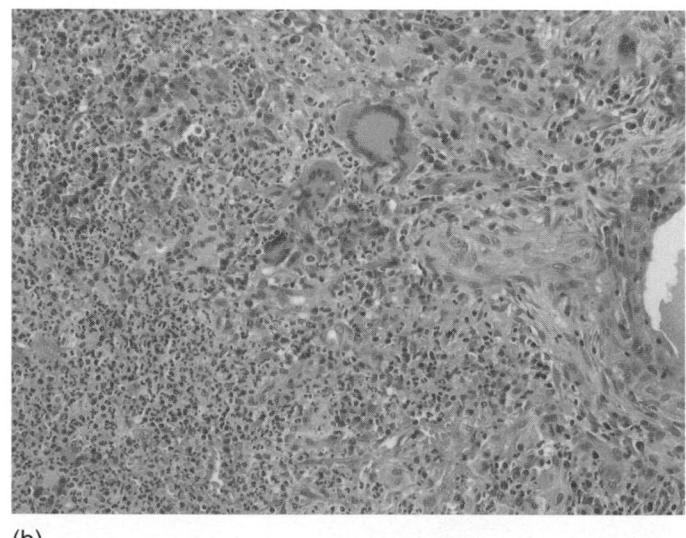

(b)

Figure 9.20 Wegener's granulomatosis. Biopsy of a nasal ulcer. (a) Most of the lesion is non-specific inflammation; a few giant cells are seen in the high power view (b). This appearance by itself is not diagnostic; however, if there is a positive cANCA, then these findings support a diagnosis of Wegener's granulomatosis. (See Color Plate 23.)

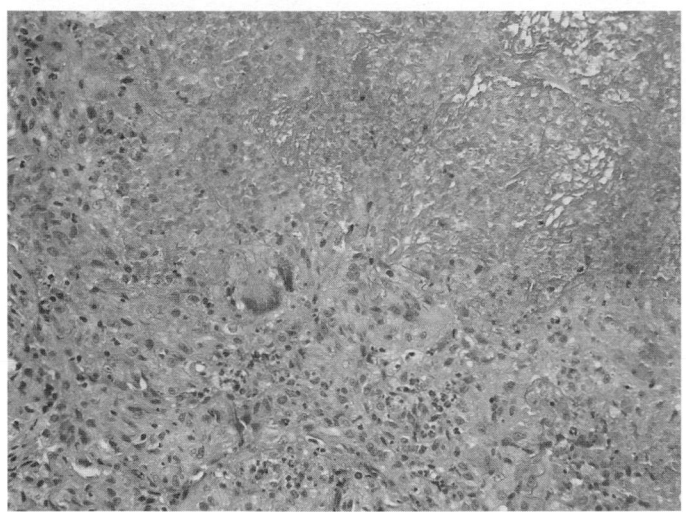

Figure 9.21 Churg–Strauss syndrome. Eosinophilic pneumonia-like area without vasculitis from a case of early phase (prevasculitic phase) disease. In this example there is eosinophilic necrosis, but this is a common finding in eosinophilic pneumonia of any cause and is not diagnostic of Churg–Strauss syndrome. (See Color Plate 24.)

except for the background eosinophil infiltrate in the surrounding tissue (Figure 9.22). The vasculitis need not be necrotizing; sometimes it simply consists of eosinophilic infiltration of vessels without necrosis (Figure 9.23), and it may also be granulomatous (Figure 9.24). Eosinophilic capillaritis can be seen in the lung (Figure 9.25) but it is relatively uncommon (about 3% of cases in the series of Guillevin *et al.* (1999a), and eosinophilic leukocytoclastic vasculitis in the skin (Figure 9.26). Eosinophilic infiltration of parenchymal tissues without vasculitis: for example, eosinophilic myocarditis, is common (Figure 9.27). Some cases show granulomas, typically formed on vessels, and containing eosinophilic necrotic centers (Figure 9.28), but the proportion of cases with granulomas in modern material is relatively small. In the postvasculitic phase the microscopic appearance is that of a burnt out vasculitis, typically with vascular occlusion and loss of elastica.

Microscopic polyangiitis

MPA is, by definition, an exclusionary diagnosis for a patient with a positive ANCA (either antiproteinase 3 or antimyeloperoxidase) and small-vessel vasculitis with no history of asthma/allergic rhinitis, no eosinophilia, and no granulomatous disease on biopsy. MPA again shows, in its most characteristic form, disseminated

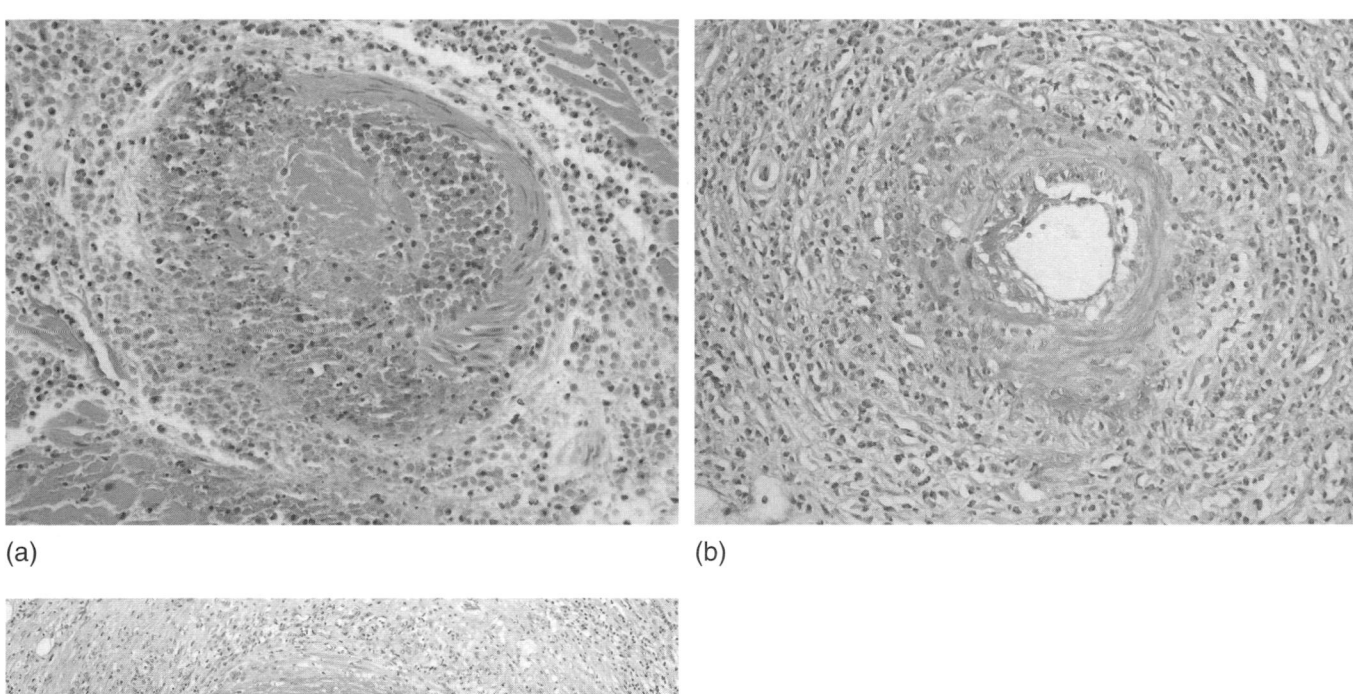

(a)

(b)

(c)

Figure 9.22 Churg–Strauss syndrome. Various appearances of necrotizing vasculitis in heart (a), nerve (b), and mesentery (c). Only the eosinophilic inflammatory infiltrate allows morphologic separation from other forms of small-vessel vasculitis. (See Color Plate 25.)

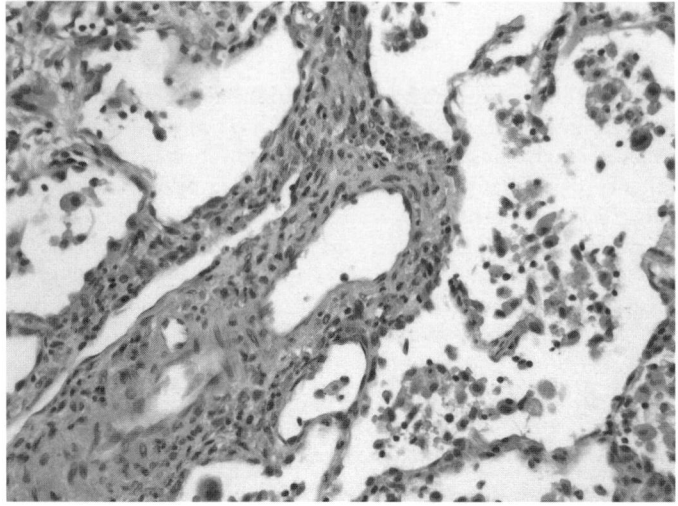

Figure 9.23 Churg–Strauss syndrome. Non-necrotizing eosinophilic vasculitis in the lung. (See Color Plate 26.)

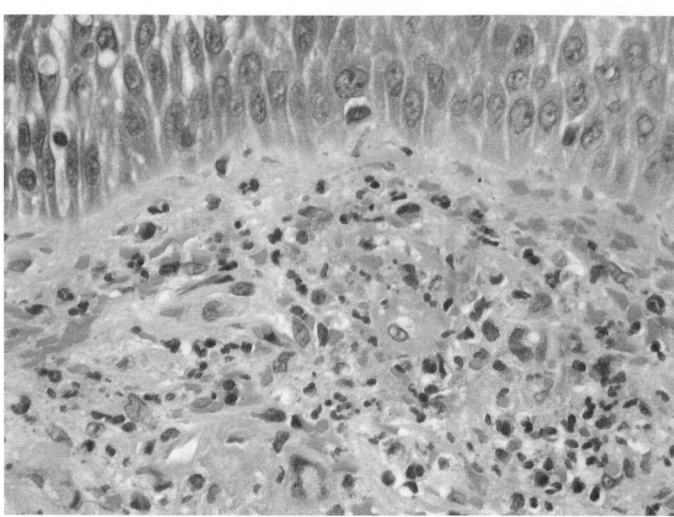

Figure 9.26 Churg–Strauss syndrome. Leukocytoclastic vasculitis in a patient with palpable purpura. Note the mixture of eosinophils and neutrophils, commonly seen in leukocytoclastic vasculitis in Churg–Strauss syndrome. (See Color Plate 29.)

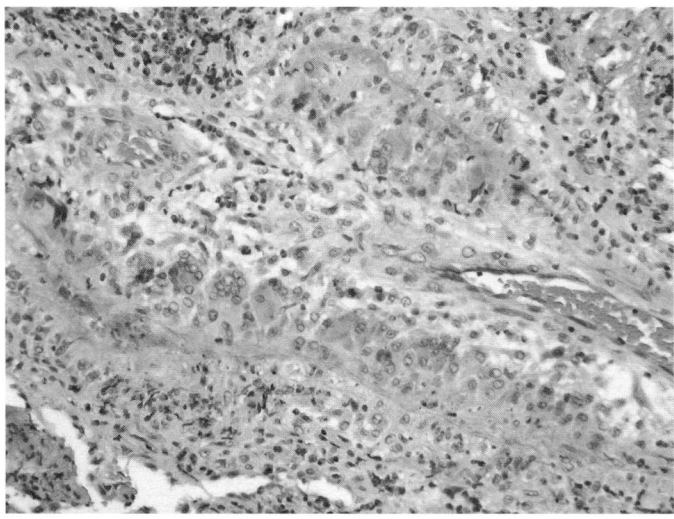

Figure 9.24 Churg–Strauss syndrome. Granulomatous eosinophilic vasculitis. (See Color Plate 27.)

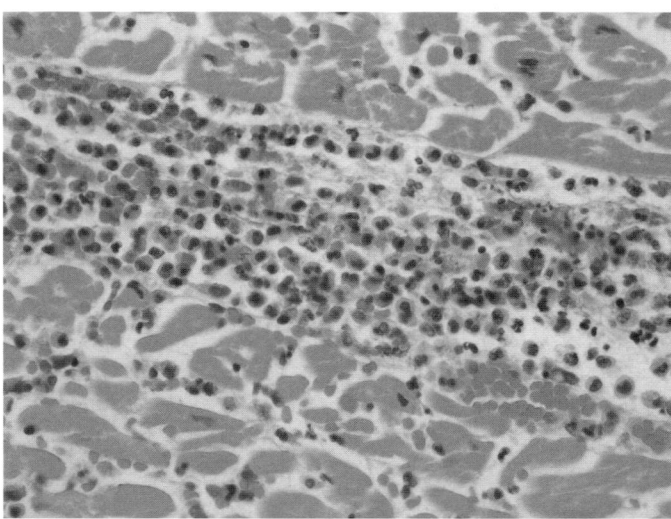

Figure 9.27 Churg–Strauss syndrome. Eosinophilic myocarditis. (See Color Plate 30.)

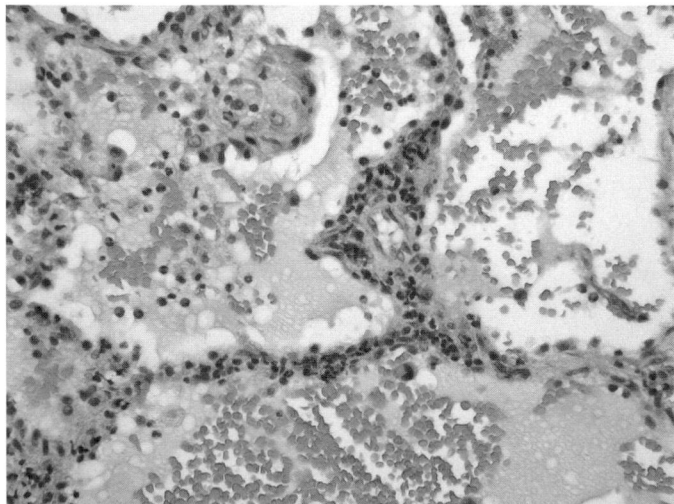

Figure 9.25 Churg–Strauss syndrome. Eosinophilic capillaritis in the lung. In Churg–Strauss syndrome the infiltrates in capillaritis may be only eosinophils or a mixture of eosinophils and neutrophils. (See Color Plate 28.)

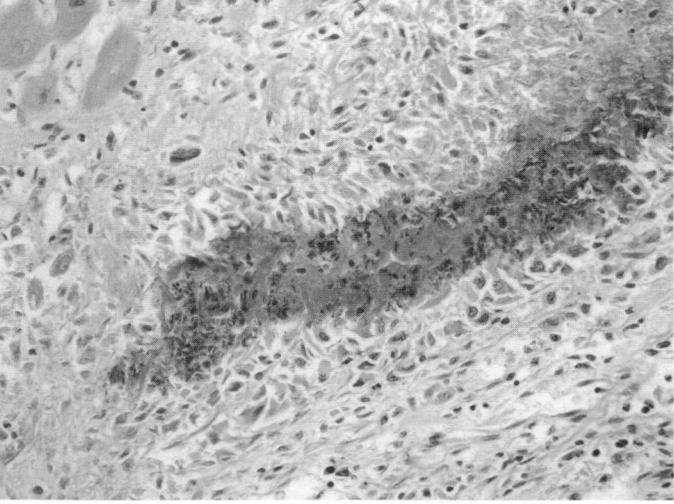

Figure 9.28 Churg–Strauss syndrome. Necrotizing granuloma with an eosinophilic center (so-called Churg–Strauss granuloma). Such lesions are relatively uncommon in modern pathologic specimens. (See Color Plate 31.)

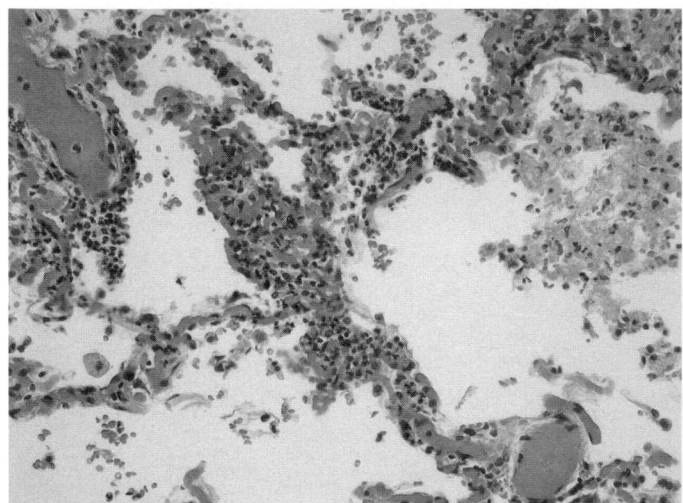

Figure 9.29 Microscopic polyangiitis. Capillaritis in lung. This is the most common pattern of lung involvement in microscopic polyangiitis. (See Color Plate 32.)

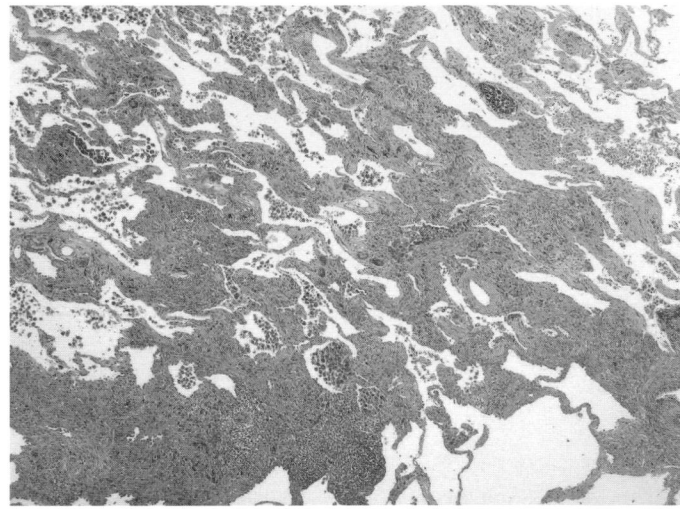

(a)

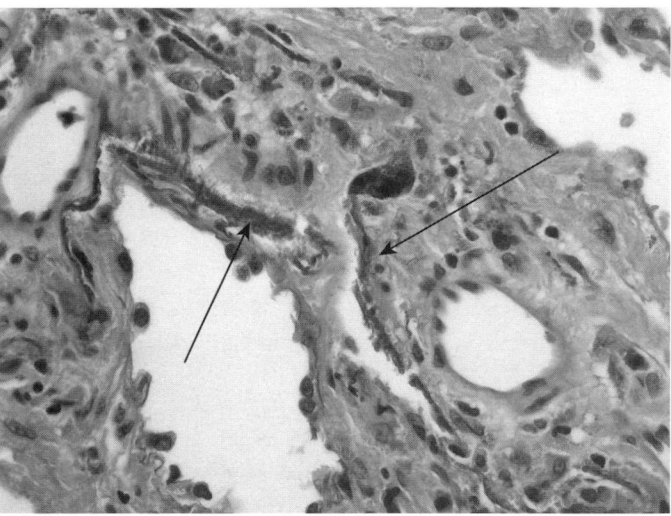

(b)

Figure 9.30 Microscopic polyangiitis. Interstitial fibrosis secondary to chronic pulmonary hemorrhage in a patient with microscopic polyangiitis. (a) Low power view showing diffuse interstitial fibrosis and masses of hemosiderin-laden macrophages in the airspaces. (b) High power view showing hemosiderin, indicative of old hemorrhage, in the interstitium, and encrustation of the vessel elastica by iron/calcium salts, a common finding in chronic hemorrhage. (See Color Plate 33.)

necrotizing vasculitis with fibrinoid necrosis (Figure 9.10), but may also be manifest as necrotizing and crescentic glomerulonephritis (seen in 90% or more of cases) (Jennette *et al.* 2001) (Figure 9.13), leukocytoclastic vasculitis in the skin, and capillaritis in the lung (Figure 9.29). MPA is the most common cause of the pulmonary–renal syndrome (Jennette *et al.* 2001).

Although most cases of MPA appear as relatively acute disease, in some instances the course is much more indolent (Guillevin *et al.* 1999b) and patients may report months to years of arthalgias or episodes of minor hemoptysis (Savage *et al.* 1985). Such patients sometimes develop interstitial pulmonary fibrosis secondary to chronic hemorrhage (Eschun *et al.* 2003; Nada *et al.* 1990; Burns 1998; Gaudin *et al.* 1995; Homma *et al.* 2004) (Figure 9.30).

Vasculitis associated with immune complex deposition
Vasculitis in collagen vascular disease
Vasculitis is reported to occur in 5 to 15% of all patients with RA (Danning *et al.* 1998) and is typically seen in patients with long-standing, severe disease and high titers of rheumatoid factor. Cutaneous leukocytoclastic vasculitis is common, but necrotizing vasculitis of larger vessels (Figure 9.31), including coronary or mesenteric arteries, and a form of GCA involving the aorta have all been reported (Bahlas *et al.* 1998; Hall *et al.* 1983), but some cases may represent the coexistence of GCA in a patient with RA (Hall *et al.* 1983; Bahlas *et al.* 1998). The medium and small-vessel vasculitis in RA is occasionally granulomatous (Lie 1989). Capillaritis may be seen in the lung (Figure 9.12), although it is relatively rare.

Vasculitis is reported in about one-third of patients with SLE (Drenkard *et al.* 1997). Cutaneous leukocytoclastic vasculitis is by far the most common presentation. Involvement of larger vessels in patterns similar to those in RA occurs but is much less frequent. More often SLE is associated with deposition of fibrinoid-like material, that is immune complexes, in vessels, but without an inflammatory response (Grishman and Spiera 1991). Pulmonary capillaritis with hemorrhage (Figure 9.32), as noted above, carries a high mortality. Deposition of immune complexes in the lung can be shown by immunofluoresence or electron microscopy.

Vasculitis in various sizes of vessels may also be seen in Sjögren's syndrome, systemic sclerosis, and relapsing polychondritis (see Chapter 34). Because the morphology is relatively non-specific, serologic testing is crucial to arriving at the correct diagnosis. It should be noted that patients with autoimmune disease may have a positive fluorescent ANCA, but by ELISA the ANCA are atypical; that is directed against an antigen other than myeloperoxidase or proteinase 3. Atypical ANCA against lactoferrin are probably the most common (see Chapter 6).

Henoch–Schonlein purpura
HSP is a small-vessel vasculitis characterized by deposition of IgA. The vasculitis is typically a combination of glomerulonephritis, which may take the form of mesangial proliferation or crescentic

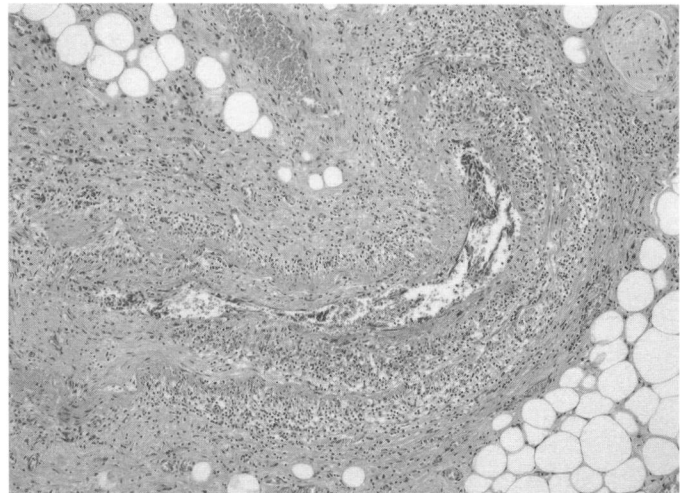

Figure 9.31 Rheumatoid vasculitis. Necrotizing vasculitis involving an artery in the peripancreatic fat. By itself this morphology could be seen in any form of small-vessel or medium-vessel vasculitis and further clinical/laboratory information is required for diagnosis. (See Color Plate 34.)

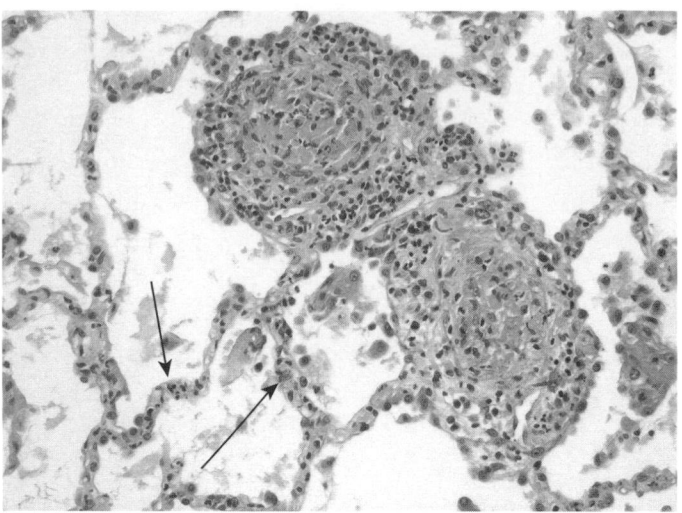

Figure 9.33 Cryoglobulinemia. Largely non-destructive vasculitis involving two small vessels in the lung; there is capillaritis as well. This combination of sizes of vessels involved is sometimes seen in small-vessel vasculitis. (See Color Plate 36.)

disease, and cutaneous leukocytoclastic vasculitis (White 1991). IgA can be demonstrated by immunofluorescence examination. Larger-vessel necrotizing arteritis also occurs but is less common and the same is true of pulmonary capillaritis (1.6% of patients in the large series of cases reported by Nadrous *et al.* 2004).

Cryoglobulinemia

Cryoglobulinemia is most often seen in patients with hepatitis C virus infection, and is characterized by the presence of circulating cryoglobulins that deposit in tissues. Cryoglobulinemic vasculitis typically involves the kidney and skin (as leukocytoclastic vasculitis) but may involve many other organs including the peripheral nervous system and the lung (Figure 9.33). Eosinophilic deposits of

cryoglobulins can be seen in vessel walls and appear to evoke a neutrophil response; the deposits are most often IgM. In the kidney the typical lesion is glomerulonephritis with mesangial proliferation and cryoglobulin deposition. Larger vessels are occasionally involved (Cacoub *et al.* 2002).

Drug-induced vasculitis

Drugs are a very common cause of small-vessel vasculitis, and the typical morphologic appearance is that of cutaneous leukocytoclastic vasculitis (Figure 9.11). Indeed it has been suggested that more than 95% of vasculitic skin lesions are drug-induced (Jennette and Falk 1997). Nevertheless, a wide variety of other organs as well as larger vessels may be involved (ten Holder *et al.* 2002). There is no morphologic specificity to drug-induced vasculitis, thus a history/timing of drug use is crucial to the diagnosis.

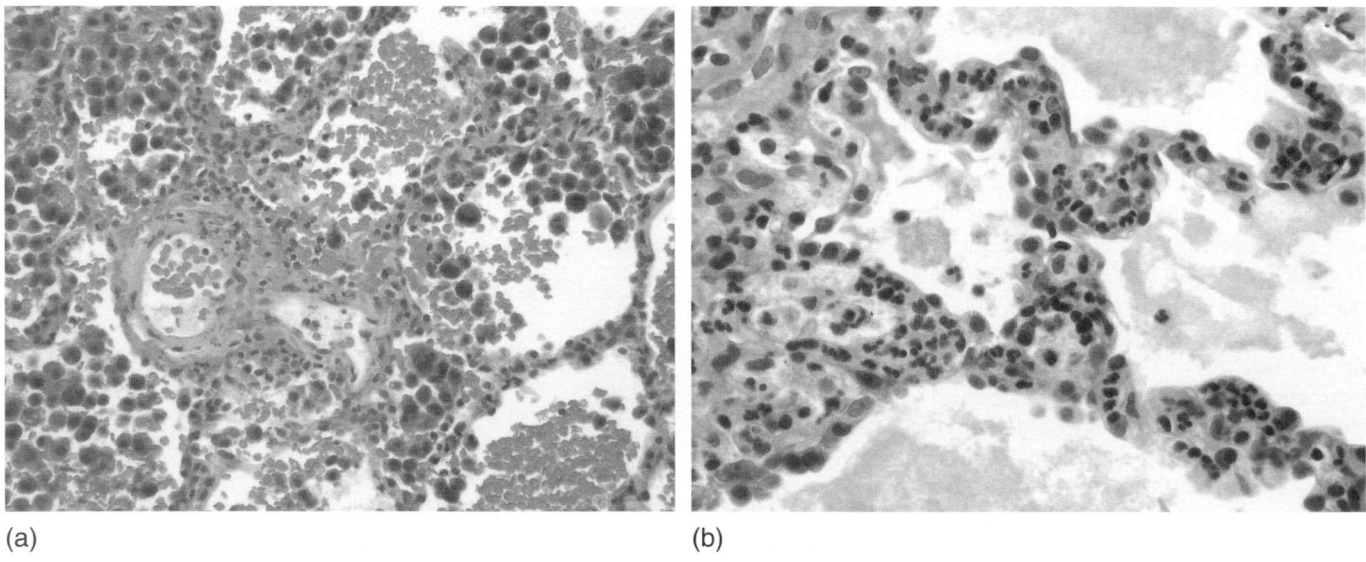

(a)   (b)

Figure 9.32 Pulmonary capillaritis with hemorrhage in lupus. (a) Medium power view showing acute hemorrhage (red blood cells) and hemosiderin laden macrophages; the latter are a useful finding that indicate the presence of real (as opposed to surgical) hemorrhage. (b) High power view of another area showing typical capillaritis. This biopsy also demonstrated immune complex deposits by immunofluorescence and electron microscopy. (See Color Plate 35.)

Drug-induced vasculitis may be associated with lupus-like serology (ANA, anti-dsDNA antibody), positive ANCA, or both (Choi *et al*. 2000). Of interest, the titer of myeloperoxidase ANCA is often extremely high in drug-associated vasculitis, much higher than in typical ANCA-positive vasculitides, and ANCA with unusual specificities including elastase and lactoferrin may also be found (Choi *et al*. 2000). Detailed listings of drugs known to induce vasculitis have recently been published (Doyle and Cuellar 2003; ten Holder *et al*. 2002).

Behçet's syndrome

BS was initially defined by the presence of oral and genital ulcers and uveitis. In fact, BS is a systemic disease associated with a variety of skin lesions; arthritis; gastrointestinal abnormalities including changes that can resemble those of chronic inflammatory bowel disease; CNS involvement; and pulmonary and cardiac disease. Vascular abnormalities typically appear late in the course, frequently 5 to 10 years after initial diagnosis (see Chapter 35).

BS is included among small-vessel vasculitides because it can involve arterioles and venules and produce leukocytoclastic vasculitis; however, there is a remarkably wide spectrum of vascular disease in BS (Koc *et al*. 1992). Both large arteries and veins are frequently involved, and venous thrombosis is, overall, the most common vascular abnormality. In the large series reported by Koc *et al*. (1992), significant venous thromboses were seen in 22% of cases and arterial disease in 12%. Some patients have antiphospholipid antibodies, although there is dispute about whether such antibodies are the cause of the thromboses (Fessler 1997).

BS may be associated with aortitis or inflammation of the pulmonary arteries, and with necrotizing medium-sized vessel disease (Lie 1988b; Lie 1989; Lakhanpal *et al*. 1985). Aneurysms are frequent sequelae in the aorta, and pulmonary artery aneurysms with thromboses or rupture are the most common form of pulmonary disease (Uzun 2005) (Figure 9.34). Microscopically there is an inflammatory infiltrate, most often of chronic inflammatory cells, with destruction of the elastica. The pulmonary changes are identical to those found in Hughes–Stovin syndrome (pulmonary artery

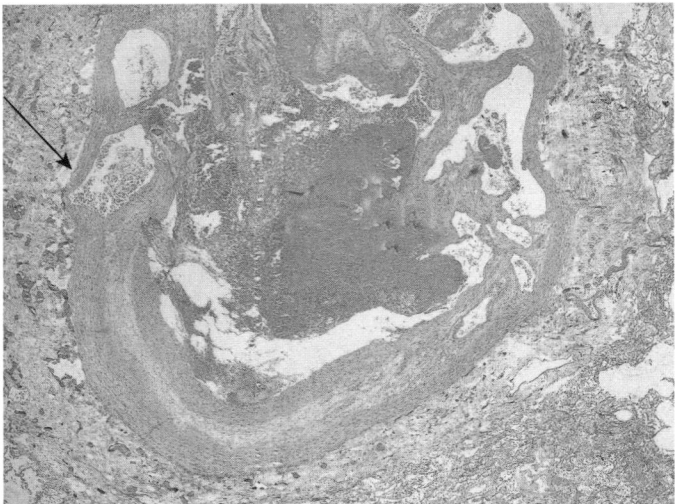

Figure 9.34 Behçet's syndrome. Low power view of an aneurysmally dilated and thrombosed pulmonary artery branch. Note the extreme thinning of the wall in some areas; such vessels are prone to rupture. (See Color Plate 37.)

aneurysms and systemic thromboses), and some authors believe that the latter is in fact a form of BS (Erkan *et al*. 2004; Slavin and DeGroot 1981; Durieux *et al*. 1981).

Other forms of vasculitis

Thromboangiitis obliterans (Buerger's disease)

Thromboangiitis obliterans (TAO) is a form of non-necrotizing vasculitis that affects primarily the upper and lower extremities (see Chapter 38). The disease is seen in cigarette smokers, predominantly young male smokers, and is characterized clinically by intermittent claudication of the arms and legs, migratory thrombophlebitis, and, often, Raynaud's phenomenon. In severe cases, Buerger's disease leads to ulcers and gangrene requiring amputation of digits, hands, feet, or distal extremities.

Pathologically, Buerger's disease affects medium and small-sized arteries and veins in the extremities (characteristically the posterior and anterior tibial, radial, ulnar, plantar, palmar, and digital vessels), and, rarely, visceral or cerebral sites (Lie 1988a, 1989, 1998). The lesions start as acute inflammatory infiltrates in the vessel walls and this process rapidly leads to the formation of morphologically unusual thrombi that are very cellular and may contain small collections of neutrophils resembling microabscesses (Figure 9.35). Over time the neutrophils are replaced, in both the vessel wall and the thrombi, by chronic inflammatory cells, and sometimes individual giant cells or granulomas are found in the thrombi (Figure 9.35). The process is focal and segmental, and is different from most forms of vasculitis in that there is no necrosis of the vessel walls, so that the underlying structure remains intact (Figure 9.35). The thrombi eventually undergo recanalization, and specific recognition of very old lesions as Buerger's disease versus thrombosis on some other basis is problematic; however, purely arteriosclerosic vessels usually do not become thrombosed (Lie 1988a).

Infectious vasculitis

Many types of infection can be associated with vasculitis (reviewed in Lie 1991b, 1996b; Oyoo and Espinoza 2005). Morphologically a variety of processes are seen, including direct or hematogenous spread of the organism into the vessel wall, leading in some instances to inflammatory destruction, often accompanied by: dilatation and spread into surrounding tissue (so-called mycotic aneurysm); overrunning of vessels by an infection-evoked inflammatory response; and granulomatous reactions, typical of mycobacterial and fungal diseases. In these settings the diagnosis is usually obvious from the accompanying pathologic processes. In some instances, indirect effects produce the morphologic picture of true fibrinoid necrosis or leukocytoclastic vasculitis, for example in hepatitis B infections where the immune response to the virus leads to immune complex formation and in hepatitis C infection resulting in cryoglobulinemia.

Apparently isolated vasculitis

Vasculitis is occasionally seen in small arteries, arterioles, and venules in pathologic specimens removed for some other reason. The most common sites are the appendix, gallbladder, female genital tract, breast, testis, and bladder. The process usually appears as a necrotizing lesion with fibrinoid necrosis (Figure 9.36), but occasionally is granulomatous. How often these findings represent a

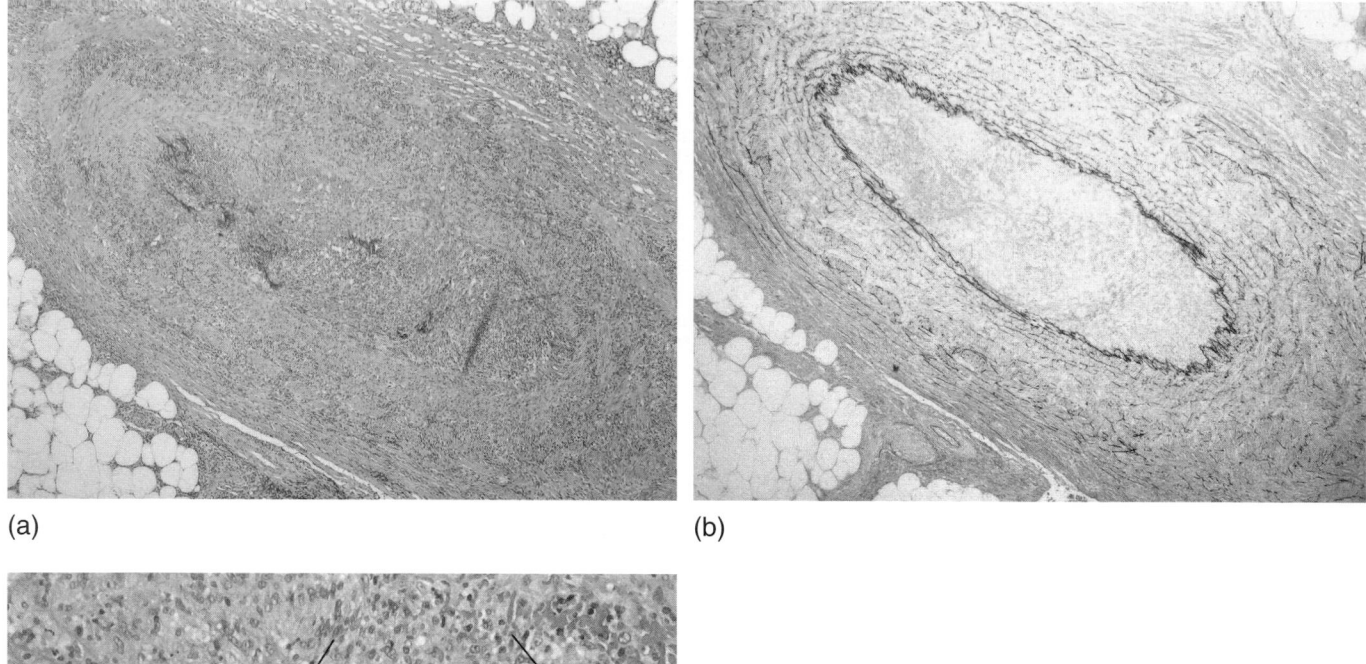

(a)

(b)

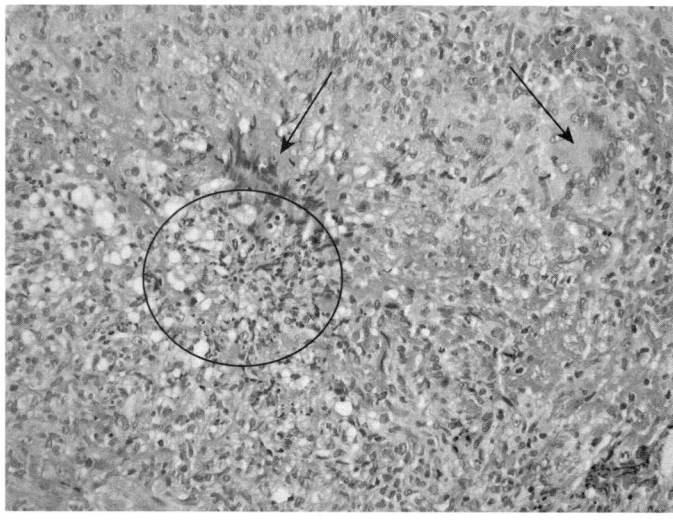

(c)

Figure 9.35 Thromboangiitis obliterans (Buerger's disease). Vasculitis involving a branch of the tibial artery. (a) Low power view showing a cellular thrombus and inflammatory cells in the vessel wall. (b) Elastic stain shows that, as opposed to most forms of vasculitis, the vessel wall is not destroyed in Buerger's disease. (c) High power view of the center of the thrombus shown in (a). Note the marked cellularity, presence of giant cells (upper right), and collections of neutrophils. These morphologic features are typical of Buerger's disease and are not seen in ordinary thrombi. (See Color Plate 38.)

true systemic vasculitis as opposed to a localized inflammatory process of no significance is disputed. Lie (1989) reviewed the literature and concluded that about one-third of cases were actually part of systemic disease; however, Ganesan *et al.* (2000) found evidence of systemic vasculitis in only four of 46 patients with isolated vasculitis in the female genital tract. In this situation, it is probably best to be very cautious about the significance of isolated vasculitis, and to suggest workup for systemic disease if clinically suspicious, rather than to make an outright pathologic diagnosis of vasculitis.

Selection of sites for biopsy

Selection of the proper site to biopsy greatly improves the diagnostic yield in vasculitis. The older notion that blind biopsies should be performed from muscle or nerve, regardless of symptoms, has clearly proven to be wrong (see Chapter 14). Lie (1989) cites overall true positive rates of 35% and false negative rates of 65% in cases of PAN for such biopsies. A general rule of thumb is to biopsy clinically affected sites such as kidney, skin, lung, and areas of muscle tenderness, or to biopsy electrophysiologically affected muscle

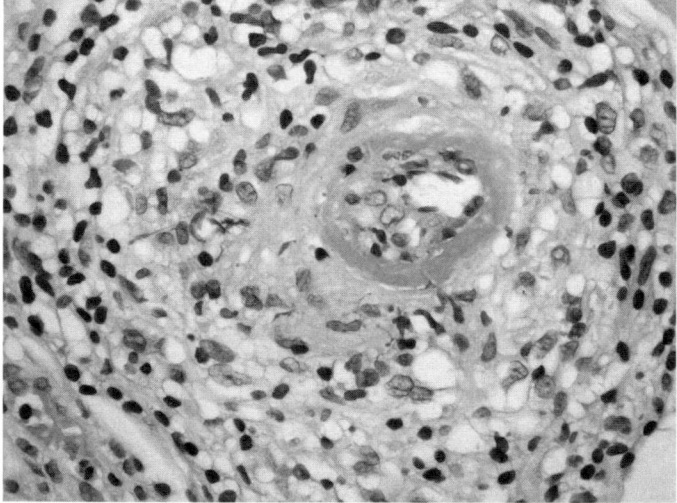

Figure 9.36 Isolated vasculitis. Necrotizing vasculitis in a small periappendiceal vessel in a case of acute appendicitis. In the majority of cases, this type of isolated vasculitis associated with inflammatory reactions is not indicative of systemic vasculitis. (See Color Plate 39.)

or nerve. The problems of sampling and focal lesions have been discussed above for temporal artery biopsies, and the same considerations hold true for other types of vasculitis: the specimen should be submitted for processing so as to maximize the amount of tissue examined and multiple levels obtained. Note that in the lung, however, large sections appear, empirically, much more useful for detecting capillaritis than are small sections.

Mimics of vasculitis

A number of other pathologic processes can mimic vasculitis microscopically (see Chapter 45). Most notably these include: pulmonary hypertension and malignant systemic hypertension, both of which can produce fibrinoid necrosis in small arteries; any type of inflammatory reaction which may overrun vessels; and some forms of lymphoma, particularly peripheral T-cell lymphomas and lymphomatoid granulomatosis, where the malignant cells infiltrate vascular walls. The antiphospholipid antibody syndrome is commonly associated with thromboses but sometimes also associated with a morphologic picture of vasculitis such as pulmonary capillaritis (Espinoza *et al.* 2002).

References

Achkar, A. A., Lie, J. T., Hunder, G. G., O'Fallon, W. M. and Gabriel, S. E. (1994). How does previous corticosteroid treatment affect the biopsy findings in giant cell (temporal) arteritis? *Annals of Internal Medicine*, **120**, 987–92.

Ashton-Key, M. and Gallagher, P. J. (1991). Surgical pathology of cranial arteritis and polymyalgia rheumatica. *Baillieres Clinical Rheumatology*, **5**, 387–404.

Bahlas, S., Ramos-Remus, C. and Davis, P. (1998). Clinical outcome of 149 patients with polymyalgia rheumatica and giant cell arteritis. *Journal of Rheumatology*, **25**, 99–104.

Burns, A. (1998). Pulmonary vasculitis. *Thorax*, **53**, 220–7.

Cacoub, P., Costedoat-Chalumeau, N., Lidove, O. and Alric, L. (2002). Cryoglobulinemia vasculitis. *Current Opinion in Rheumatology*, **14**, 29–35.

Carrington, C. B. and Liebow, A. (1966). Limited forms of angiitis and granulomatosis of Wegener's type. *American Journal of Medicine*, **41**, 497–527.

Choi, H. K., Merkel, P. A., Walker, A. M. and Niles, J. L. (2000). Drug-associated antineutrophil cytoplasmic antibody-positive vasculitis: prevalence among patients with high titers of antimyeloperoxidase antibodies. *Arthritis and Rheumatism*, **43**, 405–13.

Churg, J. and Churg, A. (1989). Primary and secondary vasculitis. *Modern Pathology*, **2**, 144–60.

Churg, A. (2001). Recent advances in the diagnosis of Churg-Strauss syndrome. *Modern Pathology*, **14**, 1284–93.

Churg, J. and Strauss, L. (1951). Allergic granulomatosis, allergic angiitis, and periarteritis nodosa. *American Journal of Pathology*, **27**, 277–301.

Danning, C. L., Illei, G. G. and Boumpas, D. T. (1998). Vasculitis associated with primary rheumatologic diseases. *Current Opinion in Rheumatology*, **10**, 58–65.

Devaney, K. O., Travis, W. D., Hoffman, G., Leavitt, R., Lebovics, R. and Fauci, A. S. (1990). Interpretation of head and neck biopsies in Wegener's granulomatosis. *American Journal of Surgical Pathology*, **14**, 555–64.

Doyle, M. K. and Cuellar, M. L. (2003). Drug-induced vasculitis. *Expert Opinion in Drug Safety*, **2**, 401–9.

Drenkard, C., Villa, A. R., Reyes, E., Abello, M. and Alarcon-Segovia, D. (1997). Vasculitis in systemic lupus erythematosus. *Lupus*, **6**, 235–42.

Durieux, P., Bletry, O., Huchon, G., Wechsler, B., Chretien, J. and Godeau, P. (1981). Multiple pulmonary arterial aneurysms in Behçet's disease and Hughes-Stovin syndrome. *American Journal of Medicine*, **71**, 736–41.

Erkan, D., Yazici, Y., Sanders, A., Trost, D. and Yazici, H. (2004). Is Hughes-Stovin syndrome Behçet's disease? *Clinical and Experimental Rheumatology*, **22** (Suppl. 34), S64–8.

Eschun, G. M., Mink, S. N. and Sharma, S. (2003). Pulmonary interstitial fibrosis as a presenting manifestation in perinuclear antineutrophilic cytoplasmic antibody microscopic polyangiitis. *Chest*, **123**, 297–301.

Espinosa, G., Cervera, R., Font, J. and Asherson, R. A. (2002). The lung in the antiphospholipid syndrome. *Annals of the Rheumatic Diseases*, **61**, 195–8.

Falk, R. J., Nachman, P. H., Hogan, S. L. and Jennette, J. C. (2000). ANCA glomerulonephritis and vasculitis: a Chapel Hill perspective. *Seminars in Nephrology*, **20**, 233–23.

Fessler, B. J. (1997). Thrombotic syndromes and autoimmune diseases. *Rheumatic Disease Clinics of North America*, **23**, 461–79.

Ganesan, R., Ferryman, S. R., Meier, L. and Rollason, T. P. (2000). Vasculitis of the female genital tract with clinicopathologic correlation: a study of 46 cases with follow-up. *International Journal of Gynecological Pathology*, **19**, 258–65.

Gaudin, P. B., Askin, F. B., Falk, R. J. and Jennette, J. C. (1995). The pathologic spectrum of pulmonary lesions in patients with anti-neutrophil cytoplasmic autoantibodies specific for anti-proteinase 3 and anti-myeloperoxidase. *American Journal of Clinical Pathology*, **104**, 7–16.

Grishman, E. and Spiera, A. (1991). Vasculitis in connective tissue diseases, including hypocomplementemic vasculitis. In *Systemic Vasculitides* (eds Churg, A. and Churg, J.), pp. 273–92. Igaku-Shoin Medical Publishers, New York.

Guillevin, L., Cohen, P., Gayraud, M., Lhote, F., Jarrousse, B. and Casassus, P. (1999a). Churg-Strauss syndrome. Clinical study and long-term follow-up of 96 patients. *Medicine* (Baltimore), **78**, 26–37.

Guillevin, L., Durand-Gasselin, B., Cevallos, R., Gayraud, M., Lhote, F., Callard, P., Amouroux, J., Casassus, P. and Jarrousse, B. (1999b). Microscopic polyangiitis: clinical and laboratory findings in eighty-five patients. *Arthritis and Rheumatism*, **42**, 421–30.

Godman, G. C. and Churg, J. (1954). Wegener's granulomatosis: pathology and review of the literature. *Archives of Pathology*, **58**, 533–53.

Hall, S., Ginsburg, W. W., Vollertsen, R. S. and Hunder, G. G. (1983). The coexistence of rheumatoid arthritis and giant cell arteritis. *Journal of Rheumatology*, **10**, 995–7.

Heggtveit, H. A., Hennigar, G. R. and Morrione, T. G. (1963). Panaortitis. *American Journal of Pathology*, **42**, 151–72.

Homma, S., Matsushita, H. and Nakata, K. (2004). Pulmonary fibrosis in myeloperoxidase antineutrophil cytoplasmic antibody-associated vasculitides. *Respirology*, **9**, 190–6.

Jacobs, M. R. and Allen, N. B. (1991). Giant cell arteritis. In *Systemic Vasculitides* (eds Churg, A. and Churg, J.), pp. 143–55. Igaku-Shoin Medical Publishers, New York.

Jennette, J. C., Falk, R. J., Andrassy, K., Bacon, P. A., Churg, J., Gross, W. L., et al. (1994). Nomenclature of systemic vasculitides. Proposal of an international consensus conference. *Arthritis and Rheumatism*, **37**, 187–92.

Jennette, J. C. and Falk, R. J. (1997). Small-vessel vasculitis. *New England Journal of Medicine*, **337**, 1512–23.

Jennette, J. C. and Falk, R. J. (2000a). Do vasculitis categorization systems really matter? *Current Rheumatology Reports*, **2**, 430–8.

Jennette, J. C. and Falk, R. J. (2000b). Overview of the nomenclature and diagnostic categorization of vasculitis. *Wien Klin Wochenschr*, **112**, 650–5.

Jennette, J. C., Thomas, D. B. and Falk, R. J. (2001). Microscopic polyangiitis (microscopic polyarteritis). *Seminars in Diagnostic Pathology*, **18**, 3–13.

Kinare, S. G. (1975). Nonspecific aortitis (Takayasu's disease). Autopsy study of 35 cases. *Pathologia et Microbiologia* (Basel), **43**, 134–9.

Koc, Y., Gullu, I., Akpek, G., Akpolat, T., Kansu, E., Kiraz, S., Batman, F., Kansu, T., Balkanci, F. and Akkaya, S. (1992). Vascular involvement in Behçet's disease. *Journal of Rheumatology*, **19**, 402–10.

Lakhanpal, S., Tani, K., Lie, J. T., Katoh, K., Ishigatsubo, Y. and Ohokubo, T. (1985). Pathologic features of Behçet's syndrome: a review of Japanese autopsy registry data. *Human Pathology*, **16**, 790–5.

Lauque, D., Cadranel, J., Lazor, R., Pourrat, J., Ronco, P., Guillevin, L. and Cordier, J. F. (2000). Microscopic polyangiitis with alveolar hemorrhage. A study of 29 cases and review of the literature. *Medicine* (Baltimore), **79**, 222–33.

Landing, B. H. and Larson, E. J. (1987). Pathological features of Kawasaki disease (mucocutaneous lymph node syndrome). *American Journal of Cardiovascular Pathology*, **1**, 218–29.

Lanham, J. G., Elkon, K. B., Pusey, C. D. and Hughes, G. R. (1984). Systemic vasculitis with asthma and eosinophilia: a clinical approach to the Churg-Strauss syndrome. *Medicine* (Baltimore), **63**, 65–81.

Lie, J.T. (1988a). Thromboangiitis obliterans (Buerger's disease) revisited. *Pathology Annual*, **23** (Pt 2), 257–91.

Lie, J. T. (1988b). Cardiac and pulmonary manifestations of Behcet syndrome. *Pathology, Research and Practice*, **183**, 347–55.

Lie, J. T. (1989). Systemic and isolated vasculitis. A rational approach to classification and pathologic diagnosis. *Pathology Annual*, 1989, **24**, 25–114.

Lie, J. T. (1991a). Takayasu's arteritis. In *Systemic Vasculitides* (eds Churg, A. and Churg, J.), pp. 159–80. Igaku-Shoin Medical Publishers, New York.

Lie, J. T. (1991b). Infection-related vasculitis. In *Systemic Vasculitides* (eds Churg, A. and Churg, J.), pp. 243–56. Igaku-Shoin Medical Publishers, New York.

Lie, J. T. (1995b). Aortic and extracranial large vessel giant cell arteritis: a review of 72 cases with histopathologic documentation. *Seminars in Arthritis and Rheumatism*, **24**, 422–31.

Lie, J. T. (1996a). Temporal artery biopsy diagnosis of giant cell arteritis: lessons from 1109 biopsies. *Anatomic Pathology* (Chicago, Ill. annual), **1**, 69–97.

Lie, J. T. (1996b). Vasculitis associated with infectious agents. *Current Opinion in Rheumatology*, **8**, 26–9.

Lie, J. T. (1998). Visceral intestinal Buerger's disease. *International Journal of Cardiology*, 66 (Suppl. 1), S249–56.

Myers, J. and Katzenstein, A. L.A. (1986). Microangiitis in lupus-induced pulmonary hemorrhage. *American Journal of Clinical Pathology*, **85**, 552–6.

Nada, A. K., Torres, V. E., Ryu, J. H., Lie, J. T. and Holley, K. E. (1990). Pulmonary fibrosis as an unusual clinical manifestation of a pulmonary-renal vasculitis in elderly patients. *Mayo Clinic Proceedings*, **65**, 847–56.

Nadrous, H. F., Yu, A. C., Specks, U. and Ryu, J. H. (2004). Pulmonary involvement in Henoch-Schonlein purpura. *Mayo Clinic Proceedings*, **79**, 1151–7.

Naoe, S., Takahashi, K., Masuda, H. and Tanaka, N. (1991). Kawasaki disease. With particular emphasis on arterial lesions. *Acta Pathologica Japonica*, **41**, 785–97.

Nordborg, E. and Nordborg, C. (1995). The influence of sectional interval on the reliability of temporal arterial biopsies in polymyalgia rheumatica. *Clinical Rheumatology*, **14**, 330–4.

Oyoo, O. and Espinoza, L. R. (2005). Infection-related Vasculitis. *Current Rheumatology Reports*, **7**, 281–7.

Petursdottir, V., Nordborg, E. and Nordborg, C. (1996). Atrophy of the aortic media in giant cell arteritis. *APMIS*, **104**, 191–8.

Ponge, T., Barrier, J. H., Grolleau, J. Y., Ponge, A., Vlasak, A. M. and Cottin, S. (1988). The efficacy of selective unilateral temporal artery biopsy versus bilateral biopsies for diagnosis of giant cell arteritis. *Journal of Rheumatology*, **15**, 997–1000.

Savage, C. O., Winearls, C. G., Evans, D. J., Rees, A. J. and Lockwood, C. M. (1985). Microscopic polyarteritis: presentation, pathology and prognosis. *Quarterly Journal of Medicine*, **56**, 467–83.

Slavin, R. E. and de Groot, W. J. (1981). Pathology of the lung in Behçet's disease. Case report and review of the literature. *American Journal of Surgical Pathology*, **5**, 779–88.

Swerlick, R. A. and Lawley, T. J. (1991). Small-vessel vasculitis and cutaneous vasculitis. In *Systemic Vasculitides* (eds Churg, A. and Churg, J.), pp. 193–201. Igaku-Shoin Medical Publishers, New York.

ten Holder, S. M., Joy, M. S. and Falk, R. J. (2002). Cutaneous and systemic manifestations of drug-induced vasculitis. *Annals of Pharmacotherapeutics*, **36**, 130–47.

Travis, W. D., Carpenter, H. A. and Lie, J. T. (1987). Diffuse pulmonary hemorrhage. An uncommon manifestation of Wegener's granulomatosis. *American Journal of Surgical Pathology*, **11**, 702–8.

Uzun, O., Akpolat, T. and Erkan, L. (2005). Pulmonary vasculitis in Behçet's disease: a cumulative analysis. *Chest*, **127**, 2243–53.

Walz LeBlanc, B. A., Keystone, E. C., Feltis, J. T., Geddie, W. R. and Lie, J. T. (1994). Polyarteritis nodosa clinically masquerading as temporal arteritis with lymphadenopathy. *Journal of Rheumatology*, **21**, 949–52.

White, R. H. R. (1991). Henoch-Schonlein purpura. In *Systemic Vasculitides* (eds Churg, A. and Churg, J.), pp. 203–18. Igaku-Shoin Medical (Chicago, Ill. annual) Publishers, New York.

Wilkinson, I. M. and Russell, R. W. (1972). Arteries of the head and neck in giant cell arteritis. A pathological study to show the pattern of arterial involvement. *Archives of Neurology*, **27**, 378–91.

Zamora, M. R., Warner, M. L., Tuder, R. and Schwarz, M. I. (1997). Diffuse alveolar hemorrhage and systemic lupus erythematosus. Clinical presentation, histology, survival, and outcome. *Medicine* (Baltimore), **76**, 192–202.

Zeek, P. M., Smith, C. C. and Weeter, J. C. (1948). Studies on periarteritis noduosa: the differentiation between the vascular lesions of periarteritis nodosa and of hypersensitivity. *American Journal of Pathology*, **24**, 889–917.

PART 3

Clinical manifestations common to vasculitis

CHAPTER 10

Cutaneous manifestations

Amy E. DeVore and Joseph L. Jorizzo

Introduction

Many of the systemic vasculitides have a cutaneous component. Patients with small, medium, or large-vessel disease may initially present to a dermatologist for diagnosis and management. Although the classic palpable purpura in dependent areas is more indicative of smaller vessel involvement, and necrotizing livedo reticularis and peripheral gangrene suggest larger vessel involvement, patients often present with multiple cutaneous manifestations requiring histopathologic correlation and systemic evaluation to determine the extent of disease. The various morphologies of vasculitic lesions in the skin will therefore be discussed prior to considering each of the specific disease entities.

General morphology

The multiple cutaneous morphologic forms include: palpable purpura; macular purpura; papules; nodules; plaques; pustules; necrotic lesions; ulcers; urticarial papules; and retiform (lace-like) lesions.

Palpable purpura is the most common form. Individual lesions are initially intensely erythematous to violaceous and gradually fade over days as the extravasated erythrocytes are degraded and resorbed. Purpuric lesions, by definition, are less than 10 mm in diameter. These do not blanch with firm pressure from an examiners palpating finger or microscope slide (diascopy), thus differentiating from simple inflammation or vasodilation in the skin. Pressure forces blood from dilated blood vessels leading to blanching, but no effect is seen on purpura since extravasated erythrocytes remain in the interstitium.

Papules are raised lesions measuring less than 10 mm in diameter. They are purpuric in patients with vasculitis. Nodules are also raised lesions but measure greater than 10 mm. They usually occur when the vasculitis has a deep component affecting the fat septae. Plaques occur when groups of papules enlarge and coalesce to form an elevated plateau-like skin lesion. The differential diagnosis of erythematous papules, nodules, and plaques is broad, but if vasculitis is suspected, biopsy should be performed to confirm their identity.

Pustules are palpable lesions due to intense neutrophil infiltration. Vasculitic pustules typically arise on a hemorrhagic base, and are not follicular, which can differentiate them from inflammatory pustules of other etiologies. Pustular lesions are classically seen in patients with Behçet's syndrome. Necrosis occurs when vascular damage is sufficient to cause hypoperfusion of tissue. A violaceous to dusky discoloration of the skin overlying the damaged vessel may herald ulceration or eschar formation. Ulceration in the absence of palpable purpura or other typical cutaneous vasculitic morphologies complicates a clinical picture, given the broad differential diagnosis of skin ulcers.

Urticarial lesions are a *sine qua non* of urticarial vasculitis. The lesions are erythematous papules or plaques similar to allergic urticaria, but when circled with ink can be shown to last longer than 24 hours. In contrast, lesions of urticaria, by definition, last less than 24 hours.

Retiform purpura, a lace-like violaceous, macular pattern in the skin with coexistent purpura, can be non-inflammatory or inflammatory. The majority of non-inflammatory causes include vascular occlusion states which are beyond the scope of this chapter; however, Wegener's granulomatosis (WG) and microscopic polyangiitis (MPA) are two vasculitic diseases which need to be considered in patients with this presentation. Erythema preceding the development of retiform lesions suggests inflammatory retiform purpura, whose causes include: polyarteritis nodosa (PAN); mixed cryoglobulinemia; vasculitides associated with connective tissue diseases; Churg–Strauss syndrome (CSS); WG; MPA; and livedoid vasculopathy (Piette 2003).

All of the specific types of vasculitis with cutaneous manifestations mentioned below are discussed in further detail in subsequent chapters within this text. We would refer the reader to those chapters for more in-depth discussions.

Cutaneous small-vessel vasculitis

In the past referred to as hypersensitivity vasculitis or preferably cutaneous leukocytoclastic vasculitis, cutaneous small-vessel vasculitis (CSVV) is the most common type of vasculitis. It is seen in both children and adults, and women more often than men, with ratios ranging from 2:1 to 3:1. In the majority of patients, the pathogenesis relates to circulating immune complexes (Dixon and Cochrane 1970) and the clinical manifestations reflect inflammation of postcapillary venules within the superficial dermis. A history of drug exposure or recent infection is often obtained.

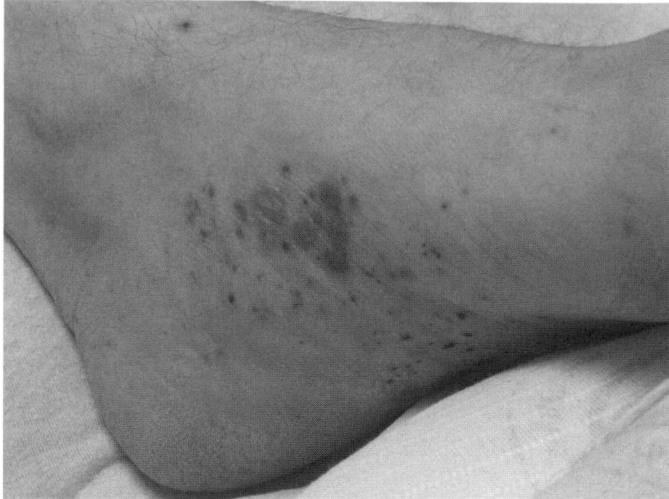

Figure 10.1 Palpable purpura concentrated around the ankle in a patient with CSVV. (See Color Plate 40.)

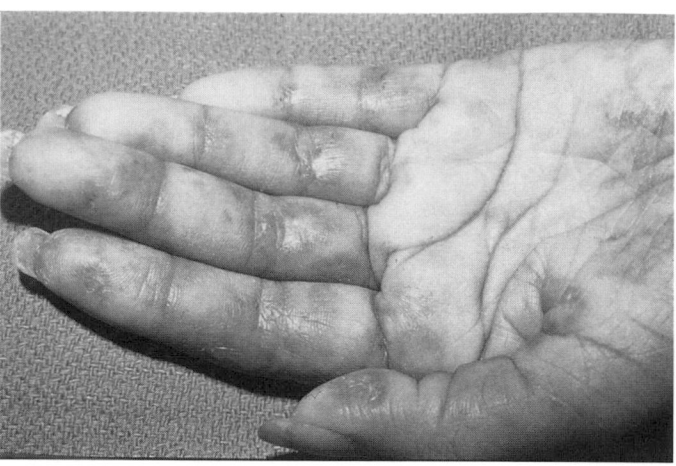

Figure 10.3 Systemic lupus erythematosus. Vasculitis in these patients may present as punctate lesions on the palms and fingers. Pain and disability is usually severe. Lesions heal with a white scar. (From Sams and Sams, Cutaneous manifestations. In: *Vasculitis* (G. V. Ball and S. L. Bridges, Jr, eds), 1st edn. Oxford University Press, 2002.) (See Color Plate 42.)

The typical presentation is palpable purpura in dependent areas prone to stasis (Figure 10.1) (Blanco *et al.* 1998; Dixon and Cochrane 1970; Martinez-Taboada *et al.* 1997; Sais *et al.* 1998). Lesions can begin as macules prior to becoming papules, nodules, vesicles, pustules, plaques, or bullae. Secondary changes might include ulceration, necrosis, edema, urticaria, and livedo reticularis. Lesions tend to occur as a single crop (Figure 10.2) and then resolve after weeks to months. Local symptoms include pruritus, pain or burning, and there may be systemic symptoms such as fever, arthralgias, and myalgias, but patients are often asymptomatic. In 90% of patients, CSVV is an isolated episode, but 10% of patients will have recurrent disease at intervals of up to several years (Fiorentino 2003).

A complete history and physical examination is mandatory for the correct diagnosis of CSVV. Screening for underlying malignancy, infection, connective tissue disease, and medication usage is also mandatory. Precipitating agents are reviewed in Chapter 39. CSVV may be a manifestation of a systemic small-vessel vasculitis syndrome. Patients with larger-vessel disease as in WG, PAN, or the vasculitis of rheumatoid arthritis, juvenile dermatomyositis, Sjögren's syndrome (SS), and systemic lupus erythematosus (SLE), may have classic clinicopathologic CSVV as well as larger-vessel lesions (Figure 10.3).

As isolated CSVV is usually self limited, treatment is optional. Measures to reduce stasis, such as compression hose and elevation, and use of non-steroidal anti-inflammatory drugs (NSAIDs) and antihistamines can reduce symptoms (Blanco *et al.* 1998; Lotti *et al.* 1998). Oral glucocorticoids in a tapering dose beginning with 60–80 mg prednisone and tapering over 2–3 weeks are often prescribed; however, no randomized, controlled trials have been performed to determine efficacy. Colchicine and dapsone have appeared to be effective in both open-label studies and small case series (Callen 1985; Fredenberg and Malkinson 1987; Hazen and Michel 1979; Plotnick *et al.* 1989). In refractory disease, immunosuppressive drugs may be considered (Callen *et al.* 1991; Heurkens *et al.* 1991; Jorizzo *et al.* 1991; Vena and Cassano 1999).

Henoch–Schönlein purpura

Henoch–Schönlein purpura (HSP), also termed anaphylactoid purpura or IgA immune complex vasculitis, is a subset of CSVV (see Chapter 40). Originally described as a tetrad of palpable purpura, gastrointestinal manifestations, arthritis, and glomerular involvement (Henoch 1874), HSP is defined as a small-vessel vasculitis due to deposition of IgA immune complexes in the skin, gastrointestinal system, and glomeruli, with or without joint involvement (Jennette *et al.* 1994). Seventy-five percent of cases occur in children under the age of 10 (Blanco *et al.* 1998). The disease usually follows an upper respiratory infection by 1 to 2 weeks. No single pathogenic agent, including group A beta-hemolytic streptococcus, has proven to be the major inciting factor (Saulsbury 1999).

Its most frequent initial symptoms are purpura, colicky abdominal pain, and arthralgias. Symmetric macular erythema or urticaria

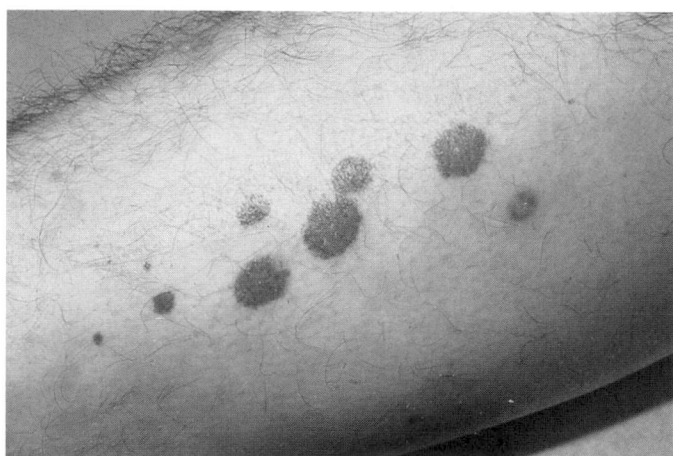

Figure 10.2 Cutaneous small-vessel (leukocytoclastic) vasculitis. Sharply demarcated palpable purpuric lesions. Note that the earliest visible lesion is a millimeter or two in diameter and that this individual lesion enlarges up to 10 mm in diameter. This is a lesion typical of cutaneous small-vessel (leukocytoclastic) vasculitis with inflammation in the postcapillary venules high in the dermis. (From Sams and Sams, Cutaneous manifestations. In: *Vasculitis* (G. V. Ball and S. L. Bridges, Jr, eds), 1st edn. Oxford University Press, 2002.) (See Color Plate 41.)

on the buttocks and extensor extremities may precede purpuric papules or plaques (Fiorentino 2003). Crops of lesions lasting 5–7 days can develop over a time period of 6–16 weeks prior to subsiding completely, although in 5–10% of patients the disease becomes chronic. Glomerulonephritis, usually mild, is found in 30–90% of patients, less than 5% of whom progress on to end-stage renal disease. Gastrointestinal bleeding (50–75% of patients) and arthritis of the knees and ankles (75%) are also typically present during the symptomatic time period.

HSP is a clinical diagnosis that can be supported by detecting IgA deposits on direct immunofluorescence in association with classic leukocytoclastic vasculitis on routine histopathology. Classification confusion exists because many published series label all childhood CSVV as HSP. Childhood CSVV occurs from other causes, that is, streptococcal infection or juvenile dermatomyositis, and adults may have HSP.

Treatment is largely supportive given the usual self-limiting nature of HSP (see Chapter 40). Oral glucocorticoids are given to decrease pain, arthritis, or renal involvement; however, no randomized controlled trials have validated this. Dapsone may shorten the duration of disease (Saulsbury 1999). High-dose glucocorticoids alone or with cyclophosphamide and dipyridamole may be beneficial for those with progressive renal involvement (Flynn *et al.* 2001; Iijima *et al.* 1998; Niaudet and Habib 1998; Saulsbury 1999). Intravenous immunoglobulin has been reported to lessen gastrointestinal, renal, and cutaneous disease (Lamireau *et al.* 2001; Rostoker *et al.* 1994; Saulsbury 1999).

Erythema elevatum diutinum

Erythema elevatum diutinum (EED) is a rare chronic disorder (see Chapter 42). This subset of cutaneous small-vessel vasculitis is seen predominantly in adults. The etiology is unknown but is thought by some clinicians to be secondary to immune complex deposition. EED has been described in association with the following: human immunodeficiency virus (HIV); IgA monoclonal gammopathy;

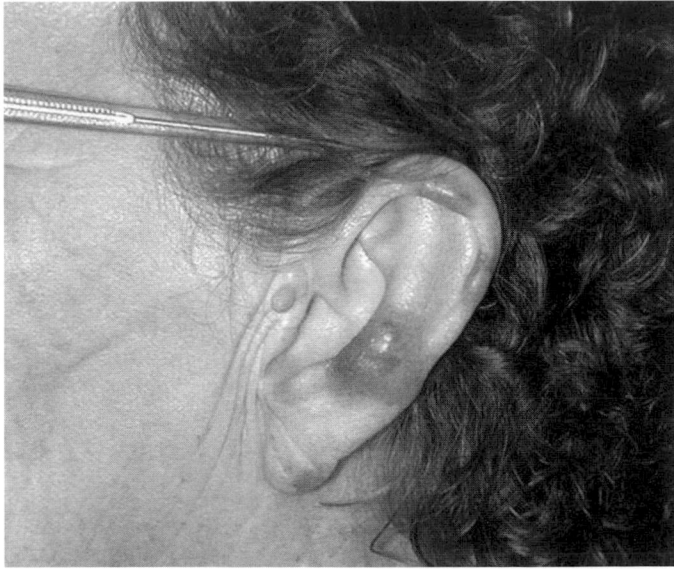

Figure 10.4 Violaceous nodules on the ear in a patient with erythema elevatum diutinum. (See Color Plate 43.)

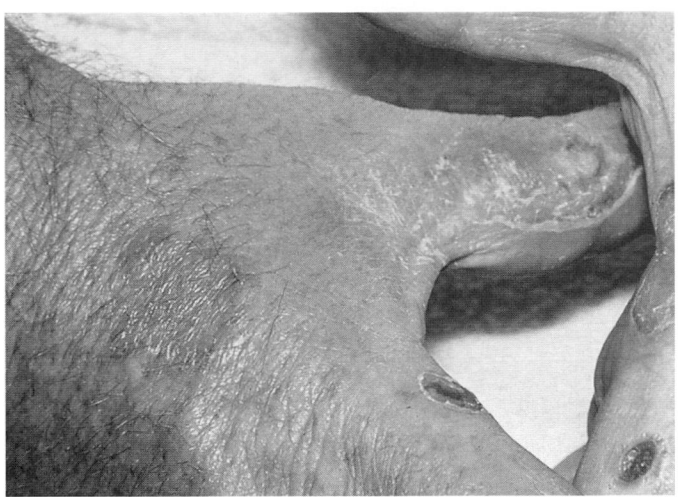

Figure 10.5 Erythema elevatum diutinum. Typical annular plaques on the thenar eminence, over the thumb and index finger. These lesions, in contrast to other forms of vasculitis, are strikingly static. (From Sams and Sams, Cutaneous manifestations. In: *Vasculitis* (G. V. Ball and S. L. Bridges, Jr, eds), 1st edn. Oxford University Press, 2002.) (See Color Plate 44.)

hypergammaglobulinemia; myelodysplasia; multiple myeloma; rheumatoid arthritis; relapsing polychondritis; celiac disease; inflammatory bowel disease; pyoderma gangrenosum; Hashimoto's thyroiditis; streptococcal infections; hepatitis; and syphilis (Chen *et al.* 2002; Cherif *et al.* 2005; Chowdhury *et al.* 2002; Delgado *et al.* 2001; Inoue *et al.* 1987; Martin *et al.* 2001; Morand *et al.* 2001; Planaguma *et al.* 1992; Tasanen *et al.* 1997; Walker and Badame 1990; Yamamoto *et al.* 2005; Yiannias *et al.* 1992).

Cutaneous lesions most commonly appear in a symmetric fashion on the dorsa of hands, knees, buttocks, and heels, and less often, face and ears (Figures 10.4 and 10.5). They are violaceous to red-brown papules, nodules, or plaques which may be painful or asymptomatic. The lesions typically become fibrotic and heal with atrophic scars. The course of disease ranges from 5–35 years with recurrent crops of new lesions developing over that time period. Histopathologic specimens reveal leukocytoclastic vasculitis and a mixed inflammatory infiltrate composed predominantly of neutrophils and eosinophils throughout the upper and mid dermis (Sangueza *et al.* 1997). Treatment has been successful with dapsone and niacinamide (Katz *et al.* 1977; Kohler and Lorincz 1980). High potency topical or intralesional corticosteroids may be beneficial in those with limited disease. For more refractory cases, other treatments as listed for CSVV may be considered.

Urticarial vasculitis

Urticarial vasculitis (UV) is a chronic disease, also considered to be a subset of cutaneous small-vessel vasculitis (see Chapter 42). A continuum of involvement exists, with hypocomplementemic UV and normocomplementemic UV being polar extremes. Hypocomplementemic UV is defined by the presence of anti-C1q precipitins with or without decreased C1 levels (Wisnieski *et al.* 1995; Wisnieski 2000). Patients at this end of the spectrum often have systemic involvement such as arthritis (50%), obstructive airway disease (20%), and gastrointestinal symptoms (20%) (Black 1999) and may meet criteria for SLE. UV can therefore be considered as a

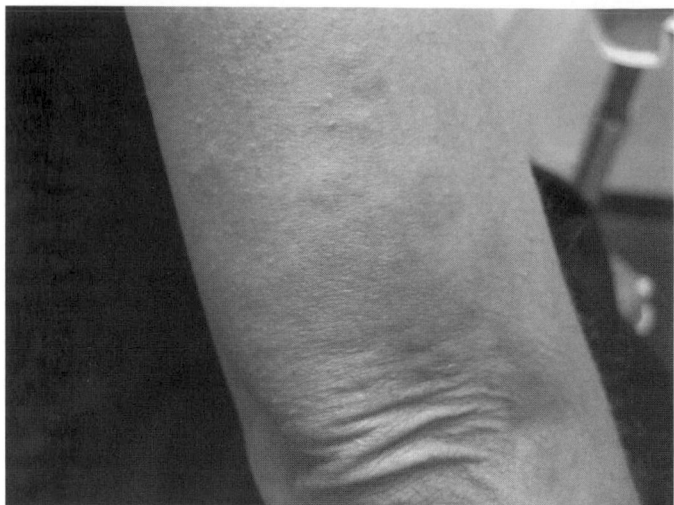

Figure 10.6 Urticarial vasculitis. Erythematous and violaceous papules and nodules on an upper extremity. (See Color Plate 45.)

continuum ranging from patients with cutaneous lesions alone, to cutaneous lesions with hypocomplementemia, and finally to patients who meet criteria for SLE (Barham *et al.* 2004).

Approximately 5–10% of patients with urticarial lesions will have UV (Black 1999). Skin lesions of UV consist of erythematous indurated wheals, angioedema, or macular erythema persisting longer than 24 hours, distinguishing these from allergic urticaria (Figures 10.6 and 10.7). Lesions tend to be more painful than pruritic and resolve with postinflammatory hyperpigmentation.

The etiology is often unknown; however, UV may accompany connective tissue disease, infections such as hepatitis B or C, gammopathies, drug ingestion, or malignancy (Black 1999). UV is thought to be an immune-complex-mediated disease, with circulating complexes demonstrable in up to 75% of patients

(Berg *et al.* 1988). Histopathologic examination confirms leukocytoclastic vasculitis.

There have been no controlled trials dedicated to treatment of UV. Oral glucocorticoids, hydroxychloroquine, colchicine, dapsone, NSAIDs, pentoxifylline, and mycophenolate mofetil may improve the disease (Fortson *et al.* 1986; Friedman *et al.* 2002; Lopez *et al.* 1984; Nurnberg *et al.* 1995; Saigal *et al.* 2003; Wiles *et al.* 1985; Worm *et al.* 2000). In addition, some patients require oral antihistamines to control the angioedema and urticaria-like lesions.

Acute hemorrhagic edema of childhood (Finkelstein's disease)

Acute hemorrhagic edema of childhood (AHEC) was first described in 1913. It is a rare disorder most commonly occurring in children under 2 years of age. A history of a preceding upper respiratory infection can often be elicited. AHEC has been described as a variant of CSVV (Cunningham *et al.* 1996; Legrain *et al.* 1991). Its initial sign may be facial edema followed by the abrupt onset of edematous petechiae and ecchymoses (Figure 10.8). Target-like, coin-shaped or annular purpuric lesions may be seen, sometimes progressing to bullae or necrosis. The edema may be asymptomatic and asymmetric, but the lesions themselves are often painful. Face, ears, and extremities are its most common locations. There is usually no extracutaneous involvement, but there may be rare associations with renal, gastrointestinal, or joint disease. The child may be febrile but does not appear to be toxic. The disease classically resolves in 1–3 weeks without sequelae. Important diagnoses to exclude are meningococcemia, Kawasaki disease, HSP, and erythema multiforme. The classic lesion is leukocytoclastic vasculitis. No treatment other than local wound care is indicated.

Essential mixed cryoglobulinemia

Cryoglobulins are circulating immunoglobulins that complex with proteins or other immunoglobulins and precipitate upon cold

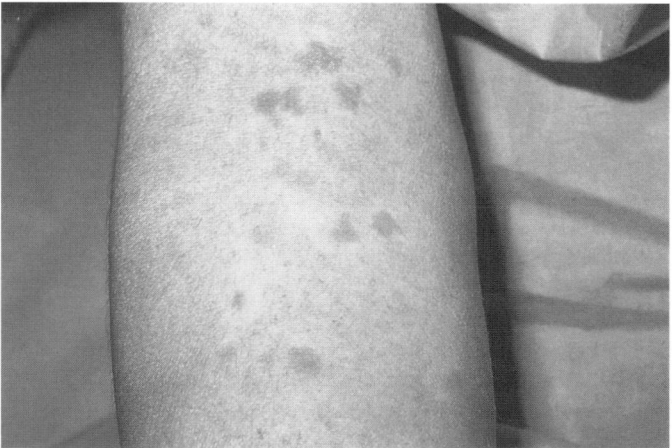

Figure 10.7 Urticarial lesions. Note that they are bright red and are surrounded by a pale halo. Light pressure with the palpating finger will cause blanching and diascopy with a clear microscope slide will often demonstrate tiny petechiae within the lesion. (From Sams and Sams, Cutaneous manifestations. In: *Vasculitis* (G. V. Ball and S. L. Bridges, Jr, eds), 1st edn. Oxford University Press, 2002.) (See Color Plate 46.)

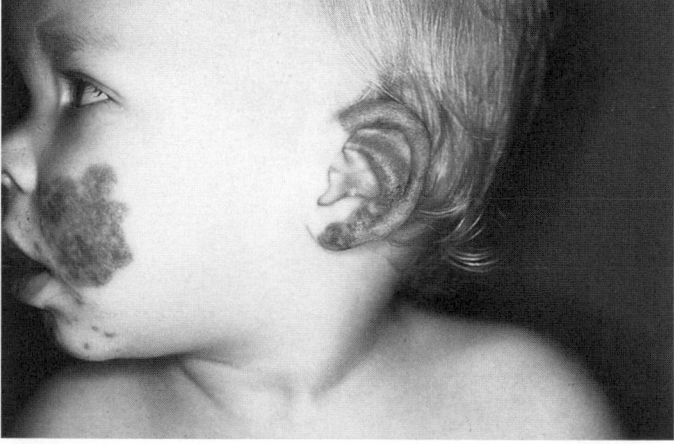

Figure 10.8 Acute hemorrhagic edema (Finkelstein's disease). This condition is characterized by the rapid onset of deep red to purple purpuric plaques on the cheeks, shoulders, and ears. In spite of the dramatic clinical appearance, lesions resolve spontaneously without sequelae. (From Sams and Sams, Cutaneous manifestations. In: *Vasculitis* (G. V. Ball and S. L. Bridges, Jr, eds), 1st edn. Oxford University Press, 2002.) (See Color Plate 47.)

exposure (see Chapter 41). Three types of cryoglobulins are described: type I is monoclonal IgM; type II is monoclonal IgM RF/IgG; and type III is polyclonal IgM RF/IgG (Brouet *et al.* 1974). Types II and III are referred to as mixed cryoglobulinemias because of the presence of both IgG and IgM. Type I cryoglobulinemia is associated with malignant hematologic disorders and its cutaneous manifestations are due to vascular obstruction rather than vasculitis. Types II and III are classified by some as a subtype of CSVV. Immune complexes deposit within vessel walls inciting complement activation and mediators of inflammation (Agnello *et al.* 1992).

Patients with mixed cryoglobulinemia often are infected with the hepatitis C virus (73–92%). Rather than being a distinct syndrome, this represents CSVV secondary to hepatitis C. Other associations include autoimmune diseases such as SS, SLE, PAN, systemic sclerosis, and antiphospholipid antibody syndrome (Ferri *et al.* 2004; Trejo *et al.* 2001).

The most common presenting sign in mixed cryoglobulinemia is palpable purpura, most often occurring on the extremities (Figures 10.9 and 10.10). Crops of lesions can appear after cold exposure, or prolonged sitting or standing, and typically last 3–10 days. Livedo reticularis, urticaria, urticarial vasculitis, digital ulceration, or gangrene also occur. Biopsy specimens show leukocytoclastic vasculitis (see Figure 9.11).

Systemic manifestations can be prominent with renal, hepatic, and neurologic disease causing morbidity or mortality. Fifteen per cent of patients will also develop malignancies such as B-cell lymphomas and less commonly hepatocellular carcinoma or thyroid cancer (Ferri *et al.* 2004). One study revealed an overall risk for development of non-Hodgkin lymphoma 35 times greater than the normal population (Monti *et al.* 2005).

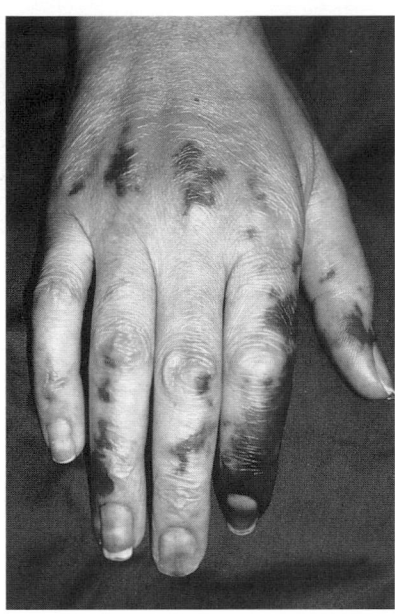

Figure 10.10 Cryoglobulinemia. Stellate shaped areas of purpura on the dorsum of the hand in a cool acral area. In this patient there is, in addition to occlusion of the vessels in the deep dermal plexus, occlusion of the digital arteries of the index finger. (From Sams and Sams, Cutaneous manifestations. In: *Vasculitis* (G. V. Ball and S. L. Bridges, Jr, eds), 1st edn. Oxford University Press, 2002.) (See Color Plate 49.)

In patients with underlying malignancy, autoimmune disease, or infection, treatment of the vasculitis is directed at the underlying disorder (see Chapter 41). Interferon-alpha with or without ribavirin has been successful in inducing partial or complete remission of cryoglobulinemia in those with underlying hepatitis C (Cresta *et al.* 1999; Donada *et al.* 1998; Rossi *et al.* 2003). Patients with severe mixed cryoglobulinemia not associated with hepatitis C may be candidates for therapy for CSVV.

Polyarteritis nodosa

PAN is a multisystem vasculitis affecting medium-sized vessels (see Chapter 26). Cutaneous manifestations are seen in 25–60% of patients with systemic PAN (Guillevin *et al.* 1997). Its pathogenesis has been linked to multiple infections and inflammatory conditions including streptococcal infection, hepatitis B and hepatitis C, SLE, inflammatory bowel disease and malignancy (Andreu *et al.* 2003; Garcia de La Pena Lefebvre *et al.* 2001; Lhote *et al.* 1998; Matsumara *et al.* 2000).

The distribution and appearance of vasculitic lesions in PAN is variable. Most commonly they present as a subcutaneous nodule or group of nodules coursing along a blood vessel on a lower extremity (Figure 10.11). The nodules may be painful, pulsatile, or secondarily ulcerated. Other findings include necrotizing livedo reticularis (Figure 10.12), with or without ulceration, and digital gangrene. Systemic symptoms are common and include fever, arthralgia, weight loss, and malaise.

Biopsy specimens reveal an inflammatory, necrotizing, and obliterative arteritis of small and medium-sized arteries. Aneurysms can form as blood vessels become weak and even necrotic due to focal vasculitis. The diagnosis of PAN is made by biopsy of muscle or sural nerve biopsy (Albert *et al.* 1988; Lightfoot *et al.* 1990) and

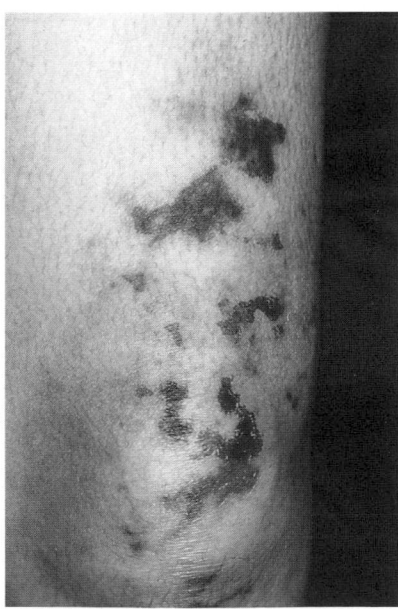

Figure 10.9 Typical lesions of cryoglobulinemia on the knee. Note the purpura and particularly the angulated lesions with sharp points indicative of occlusion in the deep dermal plexus prior to arborization. (From Sams and Sams, Cutaneous manifestations. In: *Vasculitis* (G. V. Ball and S. L. Bridges, Jr, eds), 1st edn. Oxford University Press, 2002.) (See Color Plate 48.)

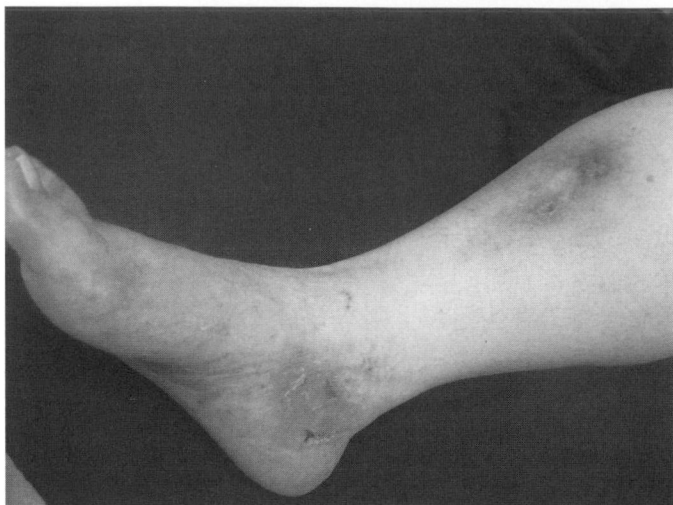

Figure 10.11 This patient with cutaneous PAN presented with ulcerated violaceous nodules coursing along a lower extremity vessel. (See Color Plate 50.)

visceral angiography or aortography demonstrating microaneurysms is also strongly suggestive of PAN.

Systemic PAN is life threatening but the advent of oral glucocorticoids has improved disease control. Patients with visceral involvement require months of oral glucocorticoid therapy at doses of 1–2 mg/kg/day of prednisone and slowly tapering thereafter. Adding cyclophosphamide may improve survival in those with severe systemic disease (Gayraud *et al.* 2001). In mild skin-limited disease, high-potency topical or intralesional glucocorticoids can be tried; however, for more severe or refractory localized disease oral glucocorticoids or low-dose weekly methotrexate may lead to improvement (Gayraud *et al.* 2001; Jorizzo *et al.* 1991).

Cutaneous polyarteritis nodosa (CPAN) (see Chapter 28) differs from systemic polyarteritis in its usual confinement to deep dermal small or medium-size arteries, most often sparing visceral organs. The lesions of CPAN are typically painful nodules on the lower

extremities, which may ulcerate. A distinctive feature is its chronic and relapsing nature. Some patients have been observed for more than 20 years without evidence of systemic disease.

Microscopic polyangiitis

MPA is a systemic necrotizing vasculitis involving vessels ranging in size from capillaries to arterioles (see Chapter 27). Its pathogenesis is poorly understood, and it is known as pauci-immune vasculitis because of the relative lack of immune deposits in vessel walls. Hepatitis B and C viral infections have been associated (Harper and Savage 2000).

Cutaneous lesions are seen in approximately 40% of patients with MPA. Palpable purpura is most common, but tender erythematous nodules, cutaneous ulcers, or necrotizing livedo reticularis can also be seen. The histopathology is similar to PAN, but confined to smaller vessels (Jennette *et al.* 2001), and biopsy specimens of palpable purpura will typically show leukocytoclastic vasculitis. Sixty per cent of patients with MPA have antibodies to myeloperoxidase (MPO) of pANCA (Guillevin *et al.* 1997; Jennette *et al.* 2001). See Chapter 27 for the treatment of MPA.

Wegener's granulomatosis

WG is classically described as a triad of systemic vasculitis, glomerulonephritis, and necrotizing granulomatous inflammation of the upper and lower respiratory tract (see Chapters 30, 31, and 32). WG only rarely initially presents with skin lesions (13%) or oral ulcers (6%) (Hoffman *et al.* 1992), but they appear eventually in 40% of patients. The most common lesion is palpable purpura, and others include tender subcutaneous nodules, papules, vesicles, petechiae, and pyoderma gangrenosum-like lesions. Patients may develop papulonecrotic lesions on the limbs (Figures 10.13 and 10.14), face, or scalp that may be mistaken for rheumatoid nodules. In contrast to rheumatoid nodules, these lesions ulcerate and are mobile in the dermis (Finan 1990). Oral ulcers are the second most common mucocutaneous sign, and gingival hyperplasia in the proper context is highly suggestive of WG (Knight *et al.* 2000).

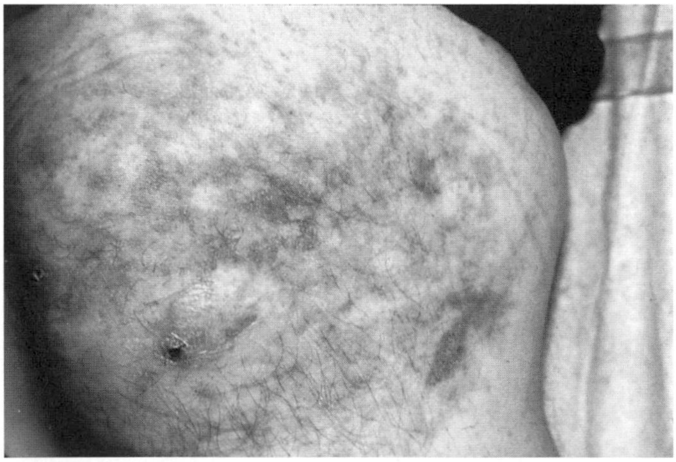

Figure 10.12 Polyarteritis nodosa. Reticulate purple discoloration about the knee. Many of these lesions will partially blanch indicating that at least some of the color is from vascular stasis rather than hemorrhage. (From Sams and Sams, Cutaneous manifestations. In: *Vasculitis* (G. V. Ball and S. L. Bridges, Jr, eds), 1st edn. Oxford University Press, 2002.) (See Color Plate 51.)

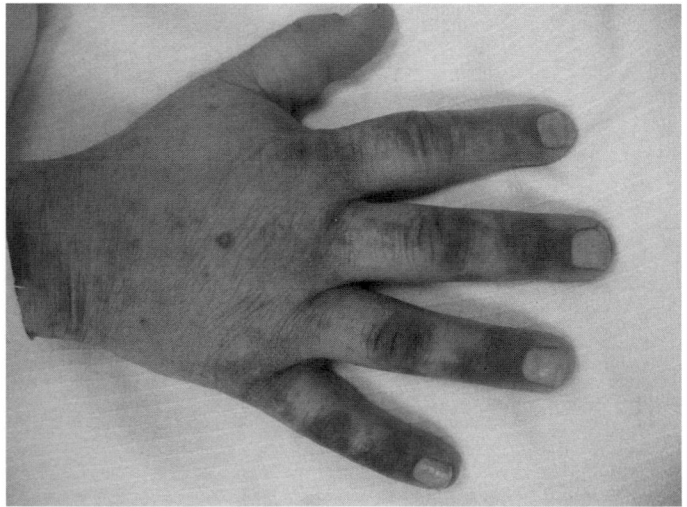

Figure 10.13 Distal extremity with necrotic papules and plaques in a patient with Wegener's granulomatosis. (See Color Plate 52.)

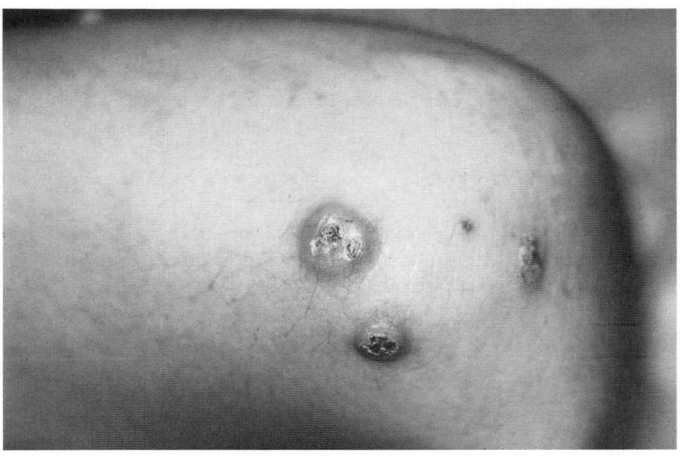

Figure 10.14 Wegener's granulomatosis. No cutaneous lesions are specific for this disease, as a wide range of presentations is possible. This patient had nodulopapules with necrotic centers. (From Sams and Sams, Cutaneous manifestations. In: *Vasculitis* (G. V. Ball and S. L. Bridges, Jr, eds), 1st edn. Oxford University Press, 2002.) (See Color Plate 53.)

Biopsy specimens from skin predominantly show non-specific histopathologic changes, including perivascular lymphocytic infiltrates, which may not be behind the pathophysiology of disease (Lie 1997). Fewer than 50% of skin biopsies will reveal leukocytoclastic vasculitis or granulomatous inflammation. See Chapter 32 for the treatment of WG.

Churg–Strauss syndrome

CSS is a systemic vasculitis characterized by a necrotizing vasculitis with extravascular granulomas, asthma, and eosinophilia (Chapter 33). Its etiology is unknown, although vaccination, desensitization, and rapid discontinuance of glucocorticoids in the treatment of asthma have been implicated (Guillevin *et al.* 1999).

Forty to 50% of patients have cutaneous manifestations (Davis *et al.* 1997; Guillevin *et al.* 1999), and up to 5% may present with

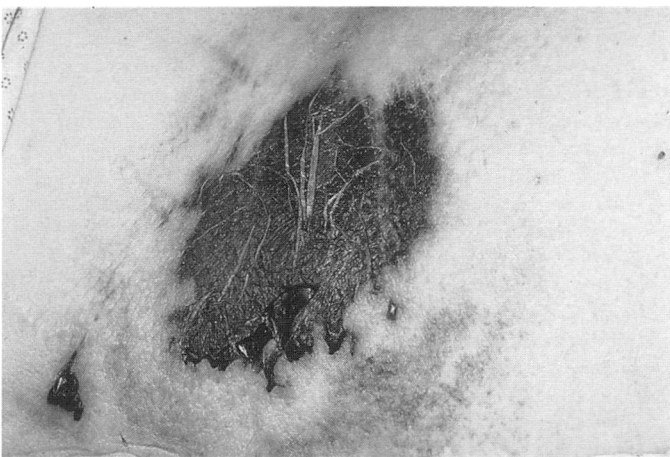

Figure 10.15 Churg-Strauss syndrome. A large purpuric plaque with stellate-shaped borders. Necrosis and ulcer formation occurred. (From Sams and Sams, Cutaneous manifestations. In: *Vasculitis* (G. V. Ball and S. L. Bridges, Jr, eds), 1st edn. Oxford University Press, 2002.) (See Color Plate 54.)

cutaneous vasculitis (Davis *et al.* 1997). The two most common skin manifestations are palpable purpura (Figure 10.15) and infiltrated nodules, typically on the scalp or limbs (Lhote *et al.* 1998). Livedo reticularis, migratory erythema, new-onset Raynaud's phenomenon with digital ischemia, aseptic pustules or vesicles, and infiltrated papules may also be seen.

Histopathologic specimens from skin lesions may reveal three key features: eosinophilic infiltration of tissue, formation of extravascular granulomas, and necrotizing vasculitis involving arteries and veins. Any or all of these features may be present in cutaneous specimens (Davis *et al.* 1997). See Chapter 33 for the treatment of CSS.

Giant cell arteritis

Giant cell arteritis (GCA) or temporal arteritis, is a granulomatous pan-arteritis that affects medium or large-sized arteries in patients over 50 years of age (see Chapter 24). The exact etiology of disease is unclear, but disease is three to four times more common in females and incidence is higher in those of northern European descent (Nordborg *et al.* 2000).

Cutaneous involvement is uncommon in GCA. Its most common skin manifestation is painful nodules over involved superficial arteries. Scalp ulcers occur rarely. The classic sign is a tender, swollen, nodular, pulseless temporal artery. Patients sometimes have tongue atrophy, edema, tenderness, and a cool sensation. Tongue necrosis and sloughing is rarely seen. Less specific findings are urticaria and panniculitis. Temporal artery biopsy is the gold standard for diagnosis of GCA. ESR is elevated greater than 40 mm/hour in 90–100% of patients. See Chapter 24 for the treatment of GCA.

Takayasu's arteritis

Takayasu's arteritis (TA) is a rare, chronic, recurrent vasculitis involving the aorta and great vessels. Etiology is unknown, but autoimmune disease and infections have been implicated. Disease is most common in young to middle-age women. TA progresses through two phases: an early, prepulseless systemic phase, and a late, pulseless disease phase. Cutaneous manifestations are seen in 15–20% of patients. Specific findings include erythema nodosum-like nodules or erythema induratum in the early phase, and pyoderma gangrenosum-like lesions or palpable purpura or granulomatous vasculitis in the late phase (Pascual-Lopez *et al.* 2004; Perniciaro *et al.* 1987). Urticarial lesions and livedo reticularis have also been described (Frances *et al.* 1990). Systemic manifestations are protean, and patients may present with hypertension, transient ischemic attacks, seizures, headaches, angina, congestive heart failure, pulmonary hypertension, and respiratory symptoms (Rizzi *et al.* 1999).

Imaging studies are the basis for diagnosis and for determining the extent of systemic involvement. Biopsy of an erythema nodosum-like lesion reveals leukocytoclastic vasculitis, granulomatous vasculitis, eosinophils, giant cells, and fibrinoid necrosis with or without lobular or septal panniculitis (Perniciaro *et al.* 1987). See Chapter 25 for the treatment of TA.

References

Agnello, V., Chung, R. T., and Kaplan, L. M. (1992). A role for hepatitis C virus infection in type II cryoglobulinemia. *New England Journal of Medicine*, **327**, 1490–5.

Albert, D. A., Rimon, D., and Silverstein, M. D. (1988). The diagnosis of polyarteritis nodosa. I. A literature-based decision analysis approach. *Arthritis and Rheumatism*, **31**, 1117–27.

Andreu, M., Gordien, E., Lhote, F., Andre, M. H., Deny, P., and Guillevin, L. (2003). [Simultaneous hepatitis B virus infection and polyarteritis nodosa. Three cases]. *Annales de Medecine Interne* (Paris), **154**, 205–8.

Barham, K. L, Jorizzo, J. L., Grattan B., and Cox, N. H. (2004). Vasculitis and neutrophilic vascular reactions. In *Rook's Textbook of Dermatology*, 7th edn (eds Burns, T. *et al.*), pp. 49.1–49.46. Blackwell Publishing, Oxford.

Berg, R. E., Kantor, G. R. and Bergfeld, W. F. (1988). Urticarial vasculitis. *International Journal of Dermatology*, **27**, 468–72.

Black, A. K. (1999). Urticarial vasculitis. *Clinical Dermatology*, **17**, 565–9.

Blanco, R., Martinez-Taboada, V. M., Rodriguez-Valverde, V., and Garcia-Fuentes, M. (1998). Cutaneous vasculitis in children and adults. Associated diseases and etiologic factors in 303 patients. *Medicine* (Baltimore), **77**, 403–18.

Brouet, J. C., Clauvel, J. P., Danon, F., Klein, M., and Seligmann, M. (1974). Biologic and clinical significance of cryoglobulins. A report of 86 cases. *American Journal of Medicine*, **57**, 775–88.

Callen, J. P. (1985). Colchicine is effective in controlling chronic cutaneous leukocytoclastic vasculitis. *Journal of the American Academy of Dermatology*, **13**, 193–200.

Callen, J. P., Spencer, L. V., Burruss, J. B., and Holtman, J. (1991). Azathioprine. An effective, corticosteroid-sparing therapy for patients with recalcitrant cutaneous lupus erythematosus or with recalcitrant cutaneous leukocytoclastic vasculitis. *Archives of Dermatology*, **127**, 515–22.

Chen, K. R., Toyohara, A., Suzuki, A., and Miyakawa, S. (2002). Clinical and histopathological spectrum of cutaneous vasculitis in rheumatoid arthritis. *British Journal of Dermatology*, **147**, 905–13.

Cherif, F., Abdelmoula, F. F., Smiri, W., Haouet, S., Azaiez, M. I., and Osman, A. D. (2005). [Erythema elevatum diutinum. A clinicopathologic study of 5 cases]. *Tunisie Médicale*, **83**, 123–6.

Chowdhury, M. M., Inaloz, H. S., Motley, R. J., and Knight, A. G. (2002). Erythema elevatum diutinum and IgA paraproteinaemia: 'a preclinical iceberg'. *International Journal of Dermatology*, **41**, 368–70.

Cresta, P., Musset, L., Cacoub, P., Frangeul, L., Vitour, D., Poynard, T., Opolon, P., Nguyen, D. T., Golliot, F., Piette, J. C., Huraux, J. M., and Lunel, F. (1999). Response to interferon alpha treatment and disappearance of cryoglobulinaemia in patients infected by hepatitis C virus. *Gut*, **45**, 122–8.

Cunningham, B. B., Caro, W. A., and Eramo, L. R. (1996). Neonatal acute hemorrhagic edema of childhood: case report and review of the English-language literature. *Pediatric Dermatology*, **13**, 39–44.

Dasgupta, B., Dolan, A. L., Panayi, G. S., and Fernandes, L. (1998). An initially double-blind controlled 96 week trial of depot methylprednisolone against oral prednisolone in the treatment of polymyalgia rheumatica. *British Journal of Rheumatology*, **37**, 189–95.

Davis, M. D., Daoud, M. S., McEvoy, M. T., and Su, W. P. (1997). Cutaneous manifestations of Churg-Strauss syndrome: a clinicopathologic correlation. *Journal of the American Academy of Dermatology*, **37**, 199–203.

Delgado, J., Gomez-Cerezo, J., Siguenza, M., Barbado, F. J., Dupond, J. L., and Vazquez, J. J. (2001). Relapsing polychondritis and erythema elevatum diutinum: an unusual association refractory to dapsone. *Journal of Rheumatology*, **28**, 634–5.

Della, R. A., Tavoni, A., Merlini, G., Baldini, C., Sebastiani, M., Lombardi, M., Neglia, D., and Bombardieri, S. (2005). Two Takayasu arteritis patients successfully treated with infliximab: a potential disease-modifying agent?. *Rheumatology* (Oxford), **44**, 1074–5.

Dixon, F. J. and Cochrane, C. G. (1970). The pathogenicity of antigen-antibody complexes. *Pathology Annual*, **5**, 355–79.

Donada, C., Crucitti, A., Donadon, V., Chemello, L., and Alberti, A. (1998). Interferon and ribavirin combination therapy in patients with chronic hepatitis C and mixed cryoglobulinemia. *Blood*, **92**, 2983–4.

Ferri, C., Sebastiani, M., Giuggioli, D., Cazzato, M., Longombardo, G., Antonelli, A., Puccini, R., Michelassi, C., and Zignego, A. L. (2004). Mixed cryoglobulinemia: demographic, clinical, and serologic features and survival in 231 patients. *Seminars in Arthritis and Rheumatism*, **33**, 355–74.

Finan, M. C. (1990). Rheumatoid papule, cutaneous extravascular necrotizing granuloma, and Churg-Strauss granuloma: are they the same entity? *Journal of the American Academy of Dermatology*, **22**, 142–3.

Fiorentino, D. F. (2003). Cutaneous vasculitis. *Journal of the American Academy of Dermatology*, **48**, 311–40.

Flynn, J. T., Smoyer, W. E., Bunchman, T. E., Kershaw, D. B., and Sedman, A. B. (2001). Treatment of Henoch-Schonlein purpura glomerulonephritis in children with high-dose corticosteroids plus oral cyclophosphamide. *American Journal of Nephrology*, **21**, 128–33.

Fortson, J. S., Zone, J. J., Hammond, M. E., and Groggel, G. C. (1986). Hypocomplementemic urticarial vasculitis syndrome responsive to dapsone. *Journal of the American Academy of Dermatology*, **15**, 1137–42.

Frances, C., Boisnic, S., Bletry, O., Dallot, A., Thomas, D., Kieffer, E., and Godeau, P. (1990). Cutaneous manifestations of Takayasu arteritis. A retrospective study of 80 cases. *Dermatologica*, **181**, 266–72.

Fredenberg, M. F. and Malkinson, F. D. (1987). Sulfone therapy in the treatment of leukocytoclastic vasculitis. Report of three cases. *Journal of the American Academy of Dermatology*, **16**, 772–8.

Friedman, E. S., LaNatra, N., and Stiller, M. J. (2002). NSAIDs in dermatologic therapy: review and preview. *Journal of Cutaneous Medicine and Surgery*, **6**, 449–59.

Garcia de La Pena Lefebvre, Mouthon, L., Cohen, P., Lhote, F., and Guillevin, L. (2001). Polyarteritis nodosa and mixed cryoglobulinaemia related to hepatitis B and C virus coinfection. *Annals of the Rheumatic Diseases*, **60**, 1068–9.

Gayraud, M., Guillevin, L., Le, T. P., Cohen, P., Lhote, F., Casassus, P., and Jarrousse, B. (2001). Long-term followup of polyarteritis nodosa, microscopic polyangiitis, and Churg-Strauss syndrome: analysis of four prospective trials including 278 patients. *Arthritis and Rheumatism*, **44**, 666–75.

Guillevin, L., Cohen, P., Gayraud, M., Lhote, F., Jarrousse, B., and Casassus, P. (1999). Churg-Strauss syndrome. Clinical study and long-term follow-up of 96 patients. *Medicine* (Baltimore), **78**, 26–37.

Guillevin, L., Lhote, F., and Gherardi, R. (1997). Polyarteritis nodosa, microscopic polyangiitis, and Churg-Strauss syndrome: clinical aspects, neurologic manifestations, and treatment. *Neurologic Clinics*, **15**, 865–86.

Harper, L. and Savage, C. O. (2000). Pathogenesis of ANCA-associated systemic vasculitis. *Journal of Pathology*, **190**, 349–59.

Hazen, P. G. and Michel, B. (1979). Management of necrotizing vasculitis with colchicine. Improvement in patients with cutaneous lesions and Behcet's syndrome. *Archives of Dermatology*, **115**, 1303–6.

Henoch, E. (1874). Uber ein eigentumliche Form von Purpura. *Berliner Klinische Wochenshrift*, **11**, 641–3.

Heurkens, A. H., Westedt, M. L., and Breedveld, F. C. (1991). Prednisone plus azathioprine treatment in patients with rheumatoid arthritis complicated by vasculitis. *Archives of Internal Medicine*, **151**, 2249–54.

Hoffman, G. S., Kerr, G. S., Leavitt, R. Y., Hallahan, C. W., Lebovics, R. S., Travis, W. D., Rottem, M., and Fauci, A. S. (1992). Wegener granulomatosis: an analysis of 158 patients. *Annals of Internal Medicine*, **116**, 488–98.

Iijima, K., Ito-Kariya, S., Nakamura, H., and Yoshikawa, N. (1998). Multiple combined therapy for severe Henoch-Schonlein nephritis in children. *Pediatric Nephrology*, **12**, 244–8.

Inoue, N., Ohtsuki, T., Mori, H., Sugihara, T., Yawata, Y., Takemoto, Y., Mannoji, M., and Togawa, A. (1987). [A case of multiple myeloma with erythema elevatum diutinum]. *Nippon Naika Gakkai Zasshi*, **76**, 588–9.

Jennette, J. C. and Falk, R. J. (1997). Small-vessel vasculitis. *New England Journal of Medicine*, **337**, 1512–23.

Jennette, J. C., Falk, R. J., Andrassy, K., Bacon, P. A., Churg, J., Gross, W. L., Hagen, E. C., Hoffman, G. S., Hunder, G. G., Kallenberg, C. G., and. (1994). Nomenclature of systemic vasculitides. Proposal of an international consensus conference. *Arthritis and Rheumatism*, **37**, 187–92.

Jennette, J. C., Thomas, D. B., and Falk, R. J. (2001). Microscopic polyangiitis (microscopic polyarteritis). *Seminars in Diagnostic Pathology*, **18**, 3–13.

Jorizzo, J. L., White, W. L., Wise, C. M., Zanolli, M. D., and Sherertz, E. F. (1991). Low-dose weekly methotrexate for unusual neutrophilic vascular reactions: cutaneous polyarteritis nodosa and Behcet's disease. *Journal of the American Academy of Dermatology*, **24**, 973–8.

Jover, J. A., Hernandez-Garcia, C., Morado, I. C., Vargas, E., Banares, A., and Fernandez-Gutierrez, B. (2001). Combined treatment of giant-cell arteritis with methotrexate and prednisone. a randomized, double-blind, placebo-controlled trial. *Annals of Internal Medicine*, **134**, 106–14.

Katz, S. I., Gallin, J. I., Hertz, K. C., Fauci, A. S., and Lawley, T. J. (1977). Erythema elevatum diutinum: skin and systemic manifestations, immunologic studies, and successful treatment with dapsone. *Medicine* (Baltimore), **56**, 443–55.

Knight, J. M., Hayduk, M. J., Summerlin, D. J., and Mirowski, G. W. (2000). Strawberry gingival hyperplasia: a pathognomonic mucocutaneous finding in Wegener granulomatosis. *Archives of Dermatology*, **136**, 171–3.

Kohler, I. K. and Lorincz, A. L. (1980). Erythema elevatum diutinum treated with niacinamide and tetracycline. *Archives of Dermatology*, **116**, 693–5.

Lamireau, T., Rebouissoux, L., and Hehunstre, J. P. (2001). Intravenous immunoglobulin therapy for severe digestive manifestations of Henoch-Schonlein purpura. *Acta Paediatrica*, **90**, 1081–2.

Lamprecht, P. (2005). TNF-alpha inhibitors in systemic vasculitides and connective tissue diseases. *Autoimmunity Reviews*, **4**, 28–34.

Legrain, V., Lejean, S., Taieb, A., Guillard, J. M., Battin, J., and Maleville, J. (1991). Infantile acute hemorrhagic edema of the skin: study of ten cases. *Journal of the American Academy of Dermatology*, **24**, 17–22.

Lhote, F., Cohen, P., and Guillevin, L. (1998). Polyarteritis nodosa, microscopic polyangiitis and Churg-Strauss syndrome. *Lupus*, **7**, 238–58.

Lie, J. T. (1997). Wegener's granulomatosis: histological documentation of common and uncommon manifestations in 216 patients. *Vasa*, **26**, 261–70.

Lightfoot, R. W., Jr., Michel, B. A., Bloch, D. A., Hunder, G. G., Zvaifler, N. J., McShane, D. J., Arend, W. P., Calabrese, L. H., Leavitt, R. Y., Lie, J. T., and. (1990). The American College of Rheumatology (1990 criteria for the classification of polyarteritis nodosa. *Arthritis and Rheumatism*, **33**, 1088–93.

Lopez, L. R., Davis, K. C., Kohler, P. F., and Schocket, A. L. (1984). The hypocomplementemic urticarial-vasculitis syndrome: therapeutic response to hydroxychloroquine. *Journal of Allergy and Clinical Immunology*, **73**, 600–3.

Lotti, T., Ghersetich, I., Comacchi, C., and Jorizzo, J. L. (1998). Cutaneous small-vessel vasculitis. *Journal of the American Academy of Dermatology*, **39**, 667–87.

Martin, J. I., Dronda, F., and Chaves, F. (2001). Erythema elevatum diutinum, a clinical entity to be considered in patients infected with HIV-1. *Clinical and Experimental Dermatology*, **26**, 725–6.

Martinez-Taboada, V. M., Blanco, R., Garcia-Fuentes, M., and Rodriguez-Valverde, V. (1997). Clinical features and outcome of 95 patients with hypersensitivity vasculitis. *American Journal of Medicine*, **102**, 186–91.

Matsumara, Y., Mizuno, K., Okamoto, H., and Imamura, S. (2000). A case of cutaneous polyarteritis nodosa associated with ulcerative colitis. *British Journal of Dermatology*, **142**, 561–2.

Monti, G., Pioltelli, P., Saccardo, F., Campanini, M., Candela, M., Cavallero, G., De, V. S., Ferri, C., Mazzaro, C., Migliaresi, S., Ossi, E., Pietrogrande, M., Gabrielli, A., Galli, M., and Invernizzi, F. (2005). Incidence and characteristics of non-Hodgkin lymphomas in a multicenter case file of patients with hepatitis C virus-related symptomatic mixed cryoglobulinemias. *Archives of Internal Medicine*, **165**, 101–5.

Morand, J. J., Lightburn, E., Richard, M. A., Hesse-Bonerandi, S., Carsuzaa, F., and Grob, J. J. (2001). [Skin manifestations associated with myelodysplastic syndromes]. *Revue de Medecine Interne*, **22**, 845–53.

Niaudet, P. and Habib, R. (1998). Methylprednisolone pulse therapy in the treatment of severe forms of Schonlein-Henoch purpura nephritis. *Pediatric Nephrology*, **12**, 238–43.

Nordborg, C., Nordborg, E., and Petursdottir, V. (2000). Giant cell arteritis. Epidemiology, etiology and pathogenesis. *APMIS*, **108**, 713–24.

Nordborg, E. and Nordborg, C. (2004). Giant cell arteritis: strategies in diagnosis and treatment. *Current Opinion in Rheumatology*, **16**, 25–30.

Nurnberg, W., Grabbe, J., and Czarnetzki, B. M. (1995). Urticarial vasculitis syndrome effectively treated with dapsone and pentoxifylline. *Acta Dermato-venereologica*, **75**, 54–6.

Pascual-Lopez, M., Hernandez-Nunez, A., ragues-Montanes, M., Dauden, E., Fraga, J., and Garcia-Diez, A. (2004). Takayasu's disease with cutaneous involvement. *Dermatology*, **208**, 10–5.

Perniciaro, C. V., Winkelmann, R. K., and Hunder, G. G. (1987). Cutaneous manifestations of Takayasu's arteritis. A clinicopathologic correlation. *Journal of the American Academy of Dermatology*, **17**, 998–1005.

Piette, W. (2003). Cutaneous manifestations of microvascular occlusion syndromes. *Dermatology*, **1**, 365–379.

Planaguma, M., Puig, L., Alomar, A., Matias-Guiu, X., and de Moragas, J. M. (1992). Pyoderma gangrenosum in association with erythema elevatum diutinum: report of two cases. *Cutis*, **49**, 201–6.

Plotnick, S., Huppert, A. S., and Kantor, G. (1989). Colchicine and leukocytoclastic vasculitis. *Arthritis and Rheumatism*, **32**, 1489–90.

Rizzi, R., Bruno, S., Stellacci, C., and Dammacco, R. (1999). Takayasu's arteritis: a cell-mediated large-vessel vasculitis. *International Journal of Clinical and Laboratory Research*, **29**, 8–13.

Rossi, P., Bertani, T., Baio, P., Caldara, R., Luliri, P., Tengattini, F., Bellavita, P., Mazzucco, G., and Misiani, R. (2003). Hepatitis C virus-related cryoglobulinemic glomerulonephritis: long-term remission after antiviral therapy. *Kidney International*, **63**, 2236–41.

Rostoker, G., svaux-Belghiti, D., Pilatte, Y., Petit-Phar, M., Philippon, C., Deforges, L., Terzidis, H., Intrator, L., Andre, C., Adnot, S., Bonin, P., Bierling, P., Remy, P., Lagrue, G., Lang, P., and Weil, B. (1994). High-dose immunoglobulin therapy for severe IgA nephropathy and Henoch-Schonlein purpura. *Annals of Internal Medicine*, **120**, 476–84.

Saigal, K., Valencia, I. C., Cohen, J., and Kerdel, F. A. (2003). Hypocomplementemic urticarial vasculitis with angioedema, a rare presentation of systemic lupus erythematosus: rapid response to rituximab. *Journal of the American Academy of Dermatology*, **49**, (Suppl.), S283–5.

Sais, G., Vidaller, A., Jucgla, A., Servitje, O., Condom, E., and Peyri, J. (1998). Prognostic factors in leukocytoclastic vasculitis: a clinicopathologic study of 160 patients. *Archives of Dermatology*, **134**, 309–15.

Sangueza, O. P., Pilcher, B., and Martin, S. J. (1997). Erythema elevatum diutinum: a clinicopathological study of eight cases. *American Journal of Dermatopathology*, **19**, 214–22.

Saulsbury, F. T. (1999). Henoch-Schonlein purpura in children. Report of 100 patients and review of the literature. *Medicine* (Baltimore), **78**, 395–409.

Shelhamer, J. H., Volkman, D. J., Parrillo, J. E., Lawley, T. J., Johnston, M. R., and Fauci, A. S. (1985). Takayasu's arteritis and its therapy. *Annals of Internal Medicine*, **103**, 121–6.

Stegeman, C. A. and Kallenberg, C. G. (2001). Clinical aspects of primary vasculitis. Springer *Seminars in Immunopathology*, **23**, 231–51.

Tasanen, K., Raudasoja, R., Kallioinen, M., and Ranki, A. (1997). Erythema elevatum diutinum in association with coeliac disease. *British Journal of Dermatology*, **136**, 624–7.

Tato, F., Rieger, J., and Hoffmann, U. (2005). Refractory Takayasu's arteritis successfully treated with the human, monoclonal anti-tumor necrosis factor antibody adalimumab. *International Angiology*, **24**, 304–7.

Trejo, O., Ramos-Casals, M., Garcia-Carrasco, M., Yague, J., Jimenez, S., de la, R. G., Cervera, R., Font, J., and Ingelmo, M. (2001). Cryoglobulinemia: study of etiologic factors and clinical and immunologic features in 443 patients from a single center. *Medicine* (Baltimore), **80**, 252–62.

Vena, G. A. and Cassano, N. (1999). Immunosuppressive therapy in cutaneous vasculitis. *Clinical Dermatology*, **17**, 633–40.

Walker, K. D. and Badame, A. J. (1990). Erythema elevatum diutinum in a patient with Crohn's disease. *Journal of the American Academy of Dermatology*, **22**, 948–52.

Wiles, J. C., Hansen, R. C., and Lynch, P. J. (1985). Urticarial vasculitis treated with colchicine. *Archives of Dermatology*, **121**, 802–5.

Wisnieski, J. J. (2000). Urticarial vasculitis. *Current Opinion in Rheumatology*, **12**, 24–31.

Wisnieski, J. J., Baer, A. N., Christensen, J., Cupps, T. R., Flagg, D. N., Jones, J. V., Katzenstein, P. L., McFadden, E. R., McMillen, J. J., and Pick, M. A. (1995). Hypocomplementemic urticarial vasculitis syndrome. Clinical and serologic findings in 18 patients. *Medicine* (Baltimore), **74**, 24–41.

Worm, M., Sterry, W., and Kolde, G. (2000). Mycophenolate mofetil is effective for maintenance therapy of hypocomplementaemic urticarial vasculitis. *British Journal of Dermatology*, **143**, 1324.

Yamamoto, T., Nakamura, S., and Nishioka, K. (2005). Erythema elevatum diutinum associated with Hashimoto's thyroiditis and antiphospholipid antibodies. *Journal of the American Academy of Dermatology*, **52**, 165–6.

Yi, E. S. and Colby, T. V. (2001). Wegener's granulomatosis. *Seminars in Diagnostic Pathology*, **18**, 34–46.

Yiannias, J. A., el-Azhary, R. A., and Gibson, L. E. (1992). Erythema elevatum diutinum: a clinical and histopathologic study of 13 patients. *Journal of the American Academy of Dermatology*, **26**, 38–44.

CHAPTER 11

Oral ulcers

Nadarajah Vigneswaran and Brad K. Rodu

Introduction

Oral ulcers are manifestations of diseases ranging from the mundane to the exotic. A discussion of oral ulcers is included in this text because of their prominence in the symptom complex of Behçet's syndrome (BS) and to a lesser degree in other forms of systemic vasculitis. The vast majority of ulcer patients have recurrent aphthous stomatitis (RAS), commonly known as canker sores, with single or multiple, recurrent, painful ulcers affecting the cheeks, lips, tongue, and soft palate. The term "aphthai," meaning a disorder affecting the mouth, was first introduced by Hippocrates between 460 BC and 370 BC (Sircus et al. 1957). Von Mikulicz and Kummel reported, in German, the first clinical description of RAS in 1888 in their textbook titled *Die Krankheiten des Mundes* (Mikulicz and Kummel 1898). The first English description of aphthous ulcers was published by Sibley in 1899 (Sibley 1899).

Worldwide RAS prevalence is generally around 15% but can reach 40–60% in selected groups (Jurge et al. 2006). About 1% of children in developed countries suffer from RAS, which begins around age 5 and peaks in the teenage years (Kleinman et al. 1994; Jurge et al. 2006). In children, the prevalence of RAS is higher in females (Field et al. 1992), and higher in groups with high socioeconomic status (Ship 1966; Crivelli et al. 1988). Most cases of RAS are self-limiting, with fewer and less severe outbreaks with increasing age.

Classification, diagnostic criteria, and natural history of RAS

Based on size, site, duration, and the tendency to heal with scarring (Cooke 1969; Jurge et al. 2006), RAS can be classified into three forms: minor (MiAU), major (MjAU), and herpetiform (HeAU). The term "herpetiform" is well established but unfortunate and misleading, since these ulcers are not associated with herpes viruses (Table 11.1).

MiAU, which are the most common form (80%), present as one to three small (<1.0 cm) discrete, shallow, oval to round ulcers (Bagan et al. 1991; Field and Allan 2003; Jurge et al. 2006). These painful ulcers consist of a yellow to tan, fibrinopurulent membrane with a slightly raised peripheral zone of erythema. MiAU occur most often in the anterior part of the mouth (Field and Allan 2003) and usually heal within 7–10 days without scarring. Recurrences are random, with ulcer-free intervals ranging from weeks to months (Figure 11.1a).

MjAU, first described by Sutton in 1911 as periadenitis mucosa necrotica recurrens, afflicts 10–15% of RAS patients (Figure 11.1b) (Sutton 1911; Bagan et al. 1991; Field and Allan 2003; Jurge et al. 2006). MjAU tend to occur throughout the mouth and oropharynx (Field and Allan 2003). These ulcers are larger (>1.0 cm), deeper, and heal more slowly (15–30 days), often with scarring.

HeAU, the third and least common variant (5%), presents as multiple clusters of small ulcers (1–2 mm) characteristically involving the lateral surfaces of the tongue and floor of the mouth (Figure 11.1c) (Field and Allan 2003). In later stages, these ulcers may fuse together forming large irregular lesions, which may heal with scarring.

RAS versus other ulcerative disorders

The differential diagnosis of RAS versus other ulcers is based on three criteria that are evaluated at patient presentation. The most important is whether the patient presents with a single ulcer, or whether there are multiple ulcers present. The second important distinguishing feature is whether the patient is experiencing a first ulcer episode or one of many recurrences. Finally, it is helpful to determine the duration of ulceration. In general, ulcers that have been present less than 3 weeks are considered acute, while those lasting over 3 weeks are considered chronic. Tables 11.2, 11.3,

Table 11.1 Clinical forms of recurrent aphthous stomatitis

	Minor aphthous ulcers (MiAU)	Major aphthous ulcers (MjAU)	Herpetiform aphthous ulcers (HeAU)
Size	<1.0 cm	>1.0 cm	0.1–0.2 cm
Number	1–3	1–10	10–100
Healing duration	7–10 days	15–30 days	10–30 days
Scarring	No	Yes	No/Yes
Percentage of RAS patients	80%	15%	5%

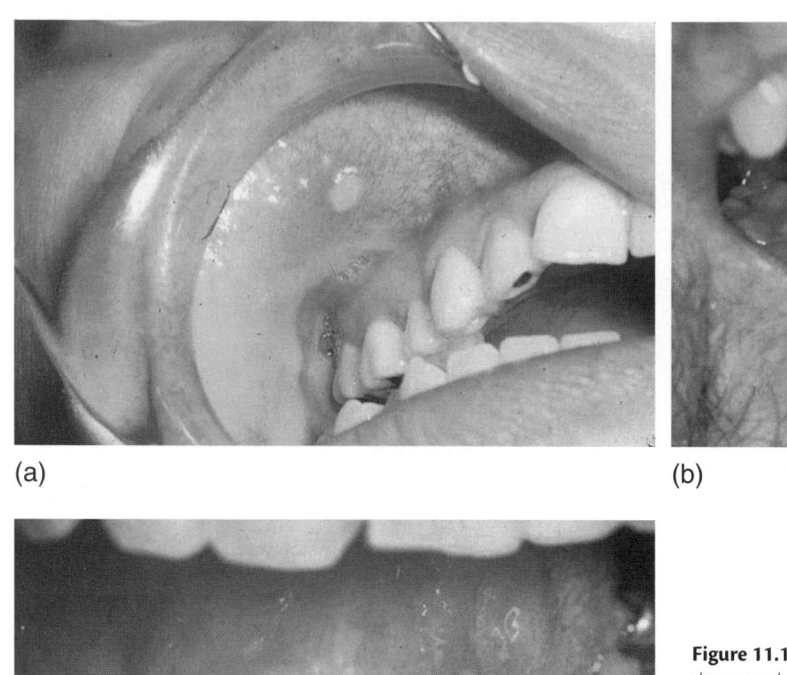

(a)

(b)

(c)

Figure 11.1 Clinical forms of RAS. (a) Minor aphthous ulcer (MiAU) of the upper labial mucosa presenting as a superficial, small (<1.0 cm) discrete, round to oval, shallow ulceration. The ulcer is covered by a yellow-tan fibrinopurulent membrane and is surrounded by an erythematous halo. (b) Major aphthous ulcer (MjAU) involving the ventral surface of the tongue as an irregular, large (>1.0 cm) deep ulceration. (c) Numerous herpetiform ulcers on the ventral surface of the tongue (Courtesy of Dr Craig B. Fowler). (See Color Plate 55.)

and 11.4 provide the array of potential diagnoses for oral ulcers, including vasculitis and other immune-mediated, inflammatory diseases, based on these diagnostic criteria.

Solitary ulcers appearing in a first episode

Acute ulcers

Traumatic ulcers and chemical/thermal burns

Traumatic ulcers and chemical/thermal wounds typically have an obvious history and are usually less painful than aphthous ulcers. Traumatic ulcers contain a yellow ulcer base surrounded concentrically by erythema and hyperkeratosis on the periphery. Thorough questioning of the patient often identifies the cause of these ulcers such as accidental biting or a poorly fitting denture. These ulcers frequently involve the lateral surface of the tongue, buccal mucosa, mucobuccal fold and lip – sites that are prone to accidental biting and denture irritation. Injury due to chemical, thermal, and electric burns commonly presents as a solitary necrotic ulcer or as a diffuse area of white necrotic epithelium. Most of these ulcers will heal within 3 weeks of removing the apparent cause.

Chronic ulcers

Traumatic ulcerative granuloma

On occasion, a traumatic ulcer of the tongue may not heal and persists to become a traumatic ulcerative granuloma with stromal eosinophilia. These ulcers are deeply cratered with raised indurated borders that are easily mistaken for a malignancy. Histologically, they demonstrate significant muscle degeneration and stromal eosinophilia. Most do not heal spontaneously and may require excision with adjacent intact mucosa. Incomplete excision of these ulcers may lead to recurrence.

Table 11.2 Differential diagnosis of solitary ulcers appearing in a first episode

	Local factors	Infectious	Immune mediated
Acute	Traumatic ulcer	None	None
	Chemical burn		
	Thermal burn		
Chronic	Squamous cell carcinoma	Tuberculosis ulcer	Chronic ulcerative stomatitis
	Traumatic ulcerative granuloma	Primary syphilis: Chancre	Wegener's granulomatosis
	Necrotizing sialometaplasia	Deep fungal infection (i.e. Histoplasmosis)	
	Ulcerated bony sequestrum	Cytomegalovirus infection	

Table 11.3 Differential diagnosis of multiple ulcers appearing in a first episode

	Local factors	Infectious	Immune mediated
Acute	None	Primary herpetic gingivostomatitis	Erythema multiforme
		Hand-foot-mouth disease	Reiter syndrome
		Herpangina	Sweet's syndrome
		Acute necrotizing ulcerative gingivitis	
Chronic	None	None	Contact mucositis

Table 11.4 Differential diagnosis of multiple ulcers appearing in recurrent episodes

	Local factors	Infectious	Immune mediated
Acute	None	Recurrent herpetic infection	Minor/Major aphthous ulcers
			Behçet's syndrome
			MAGIC syndrome
			PFAPA
			TRAPS
			Celiac disease
			Crohn's disease
			Cyclic neutropenia
			Erythema multiforme
Chronic	None	HSV infection in immunocompromised patients	Lichen planus
			Mucous membrane pemphigoid
			Pemphigus vulgaris

MAGIC: mouth and genital ulcers with inflamed cartilage.

PFAPA: periodic fever, aphthous stomatitis, pharyngitis, and cervical adenitis.

TRAPS: tumor necrosis factor receptor associated periodic syndrome.

Necrotizing sialometaplasia

Necrotizing sialometaplasia, a vascular disorder causing local ischemia and infarction of minor salivary glands, presents as a solitary, irregular, cratered ulcer that is not particularly painful. These ulcers heal on their own within 5 to 6 weeks.

Ulcerated bony sequestrum

These ulcers are frequently the result of traumatic injury to the tightly-bound mucoperiosteum leading to mucosal ulceration and bone sequestration overlying the mylohyoid ridge of the mandible, a torus, or an exostosis (Farah and Savage 2003). These ulcers are erythematous and edematous, with exposed yellowish-white, non-vital bone at their base. They are painful and may take many weeks or months to heal.

Malignant oral ulcers

Squamous cell carcinoma represents the most common malignant oral ulcer (>90%). This presents as a solitary, chronic, and indurated ulcer with raised margins and a red granular base. Salivary gland tumors involving the palate can also present as non-healing, chronic ulcers.

Infectious oral ulcers

Other less common causes of chronic oral ulcers include deep fungal (histoplasmosis, mucormycosis), bacterial (tuberculosis, primary syphilis), and viral infections (cytomegalovirus [CMV]). These ulcers are more frequently seen in HIV-infected and other immunosuppressed patients. More than 25% of persistent oral ulcers in AIDS patients are co-infected with CMV or HSV (Flaitz et al. 1996). Oral ulcers such as a chancre or deep fungal infection are likely to be indurated and deeply cratered, and they are often surprisingly painless. A biopsy is warranted for definitive diagnosis.

Chronic ulcerative stomatitis

Chronic ulcerative stomatitis (CUS) is a rare disorder that primarily involves the oral mucosa and, less frequently, the skin. The tongue is most commonly involved, followed by the buccal mucosa and gingiva (Solomon et al. 2003). CUS presents as non-healing, oral ulcers and erosions in middle-aged or elderly women (average age at diagnosis, 58.9 years). In fact, age at onset distinguishes CUS from RAS. CUS is also distinguished by a direct immunofluorescence pattern that is pathognomic (Lewis, Beutner et al. 1996). Importantly, CUS does not respond to topical or systemic glucocorticoids. Instead, hydroxychloroquine (200–400 mg/day) alone, or combined with low-dose glucocorticoids, is recommended to induce complete or long-lasting remission (Worle et al. 1997; Solomon et al. 2003).

Wegener's granulomatosis

Non-healing, progressively destructive oral ulcers on the palate may be a manifestation of Wegener's granulomatosis (WG) (Allen et al. 1991), a multisystem autoimmune disease characterized by necrotizing granulomatous vasculitis. Oral ulcers are seen in approximately 20% of patients who exhibit lesions primarily of the skin and mucosa, commonly known as superficial WG (Frances et al. 1994). In these patients, oral lesions can be the initial manifestation. The most specific oral manifestation of WG is the so-called "strawberry" gingivitis, characterized by localized or generalized hemorrhagic, friable, and hyperplastic gingiva showing a granular surface (Eufinger et al. 1992).

Multiple ulcers appearing in a first episode

Acute

Infectious oral ulcers

Patients with oral ulcers associated with primary herpetic gingivostomatitis, herpangina, and hand-foot-and-mouth disease have other constitutional symptoms of acute viral infection such as fever, malaise, headache, and sore throat. In addition, the diffuse nature of these lesions and the lack of previous episodes of similar lesions distinguish them from aphthous ulcers.

Acute necrotizing ulcerative gingivitis is a specific type of bacterial infection caused by *Borrelia vincentii* and *Fusobacterium fusiformis* that presents as "punched out", crater-like, necrotic ulcers exclusively on the marginal and interdental gingiva (Johnson and Engel 1986).

Erythema multiforme (EM)

Erythema multiforme (EM) is a self-limiting, mucocutaneous disorder of acute onset. EM presents orally as diffuse stomatitis, often extending onto the hard palate and the vermilion border of the lips. The large, irregular oral ulcers are often hemorrhagic. These ulcers are typically found on the non-keratinized mucosa, predominantly in the anterior parts of the mouth (Farthing *et al.* 2005).

Sweet's syndrome and Reiter's syndrome

Sweet's syndrome is characterized by an acute febrile neutrophilic dermatosis, presenting with fever, tender erythematous papules, and nodules on the skin, and aphthous-like oral ulcers (Notani, Kobayashi *et al.* 2000). Sweet's syndrome can be idiopathic, drug-induced, or associated with respiratory or gastrointestinal tract infections, inflammatory bowel disease, or internal malignancy (Cohen 2004). Juvenile Reiter's syndrome is a reactive process to gastrointestinal infection in children and exhibits a clinical triad of arthritis, conjunctivitis, and urethritis (Cuttica *et al.* 1992). Oral manifestations of Reiter's syndrome include aphthous-like oral ulcers (Liao *et al.* 2004).

Multiple ulcers appearing in recurrent episodes

Acute

Most of these ulcers represent either RAS or recurrent HSV ulcerations. Ulcers indistinguishable from RAS occur occasionally as a hypersensitivity reaction to certain drugs or as a manifestation of a systemic illness such as AIDS, BS, celiac disease, inflammatory bowel disease (Crohn's disease and ulcerative colitis), and PFAPA syndrome (periodic fever, aphthous ulcers, pharyngitis, adenitis). To complicate matters, several immunologic and allergic diseases result in oral ulcers that are frequently confused with RAS. Fortunately, it is usually easy to distinguish RAS from these diseases by careful history and clinical evaluation.

Recurrent HSV infection

These HSV ulcers are frequently confused with aphthous ulcers because of their recurrences and superficial similarities in clinical appearance (Weathers and Griffin 1970; Rodu and Mattingly 1992). In contrast to aphthous ulcers, recurrent herpetic ulcers are always preceded by vesicles and occur exclusively on keratinized mucosal surfaces such as gingiva and hard palate.

Drug-induced aphthous-like ulcers

Drug-induced aphthous-like oral ulcers are a recognized but under-diagnosed form of adverse drug reaction (McLeod 2000). Most involve older patients without a history of RAS after initiation of a new systemic or topical medication. These ulcers tend to heal spontaneously and recur with varying intervals, similar to RAS (McLeod 2000); however, these ulcers will undergo complete remission when the drug is withdrawn (McLeod 2000; Boulinguez *et al.* 2003).

Nicorandil, a potassium channel activator, is the drug most frequently cited as causing aphthous-like ulcerations (Agbo-Godeau *et al.* 1998; Cribier *et al.* 1998; Shotts *et al.* 1999). Non-steroidal anti-inflammatory drugs such as diclofenac and flurbiprofen have been reported to cause oral and genital ulcers (Healy and Thornhill 1995). The angiotensin-converting enzyme (ACE) inhibitor captopril and the ACE II antagonist losartan can also occasionally cause oral ulcers (Seedat 1979; Goffin *et al.* 1998). Frequent outbreaks of aphthous-like ulcers were noted after topical application of imiquimod to actinic cheilitis (Chakrabarty *et al.* 2005). Imiquimod stimulates a Th1-mediated proinflammatory immune response in these lesions, which may play a role in the pathogenesis of RAS, as discussed below.

AIDS

Oral ulcers with the appearance of MjAU and HeAU often appear in patients with later symptomatic stages of AIDS, with CD4 counts less than $100/mm^3$ (Margiotta *et al.* 1999; Kerr and Ship 2003). HIV-positive patients may also present with MjAU-like ulcers in the esophagus (known as idiopathic esophageal ulcers) and genital areas (Kerr and Ship 2003). Almost half of patients with ulcers have absolute $CD4^+$ T cell counts of less than $50/mm^3$ (MacPhail and Greenspan 1997). Outbreaks of RAS are significantly reduced with improvement in $CD4^+$ T cell counts following highly active antiretroviral therapy (HAART) (Kerr and Ship 2003). An association between immunosuppression and RAS further supports the notion that initiation and propagation of aphthous ulcers is caused by a deregulated proinflammatory cytokine response.

Behçet's syndrome

BS, a chronic multisystem disease in which oral ulcers are a prominent feature, is discussed comprehensively in Chapter 35. For a photograph of a BS-associated oral ulcer, see Figure 35.2. MAGIC (mouth and genital ulcers with inflamed cartilage) syndrome is a variant of BS, presenting with major aphthous ulcers, relapsing polychondritis, and in rare cases with multifocal neurologic abnormalities (Gertner 2004).

PFAPA syndrome

PFAPA is an acronym for the chief manifestations of this syndrome, namely: periodic fever (PF), aphthous stomatitis (A), pharyngitis (P), and cervical adenitis (A) (Marshall *et al.* 1989; Padeh *et al.* 1999; Thomas and Edwards 1999). PFAPA syndrome is a disorder seen exclusively in children younger than 5 years old. Typically, each episode lasts 5 to 7 days and recurs every 4 weeks. The children are otherwise healthy and exhibit no immune deficits. The only laboratory findings, mild leukocytosis and an increased erythrocyte sedimentation rate, are non-specific. PFAPA syndrome is a self-limiting disorder that usually resolves spontaneously by 10–15 years of age. A genetic basis for PFAPA has been suggested, but a mutation in the *MEFV* gene, which is responsible for familial Mediterranean fever, has been excluded as a possible cause (Cazeneuve *et al.* 2003). Most patients will respond to systemic glucocorticoids during acute episodes (Berlucchi *et al.* 2003). Regular intake of cimetidine has been shown to prevent recurrences in some children (Berlucchi *et al.* 2003). Elective tonsillectomy is also an effective therapeutic option (Berlucchi *et al.* 2003).

Aphthous ulcers can be a manifestation of another periodic fever syndrome known as TRAPS (tumor necrosis factor receptor associated periodic syndrome) (Saulsbury and Wispelwey 2005). TRAPS is caused by mutations in the gene encoding TNF-α receptor, and it presents with clinical findings similar to PFAPA (Saulsbury and Wispelwey 2005).

Gastrointestinal diseases

An association between gastrointestinal diseases and aphthous-type ulcers has been recognized for many years. In fact, the word sprue (celiac sprue, gluten-sensitive enteropathy, GSE) is derived from the Dutch word "spruw", meaning aphthous ulcer (Rogers 1997). The prevalence of ulcers associated with GSE varies from 4% to 17%, depending on geographic region (Ferguson *et al.* 1980; Wray 1981; Merchant *et al.* 1986). A recent case–control study documented that the prevalence of RAS in patients with celiac sprue did not differ significantly from matched controls (Sedghizadeh *et al.* 2002).

Aphthous-type ulcers may be a manifestation of Crohn's disease (CD) and, less frequently, ulcerative colitis (UC) (Furniss 1992; Rehberger *et al.* 1998; Sanchez *et al.* 2005). Oral ulcers were reported in 29% of patients with CD in one study (Plauth *et al.* 1991), but another study found ulcers in only 5.2% of CD patients and 5.8% of UC patients, which was similar to matched controls (Lisciandrano *et al.* 1996).

The association between gastrointestinal diseases and RAS, while not well characterized, may reflect associated vitamin and mineral deficiencies. Therefore, GSE, CD, and UC should be considered as risk indicators, but not necessarily as traditional risk factors, for RAS.

Cyclic neutropenia

Patients with cyclic neutropenia may experience recurrent aphthous-like ulcers approximately every 3 weeks (Field and Allan 2003; Jurge *et al.* 2006), often associated with other constitutional symptoms such as fever, malaise, and infections of the upper respiratory and gastrointestinal tracts. Although these ulcers occur mostly on the non-keratinized mucosa, they tend to be less painful and cause minimal discomfort to patients. Other functional neutropenic disorders, that is chronic granulomatous disease and benign familial neutropenia, also exhibit increased susceptibility to this type of oral ulceration (Field and Allan 2003).

Recurrent erythema multiforme (EM)

Intraoral EM may occasionally present as recurring acute ulcers, most often triggered by Herpes simplex virus (HSV) infection and therefore designated as Herpes-associated erythema multiforme or HAEM (Farthing *et al.* 1995; Farthing *et al.* 2005). These ulcers are frequently confused with MjAU because of their clinical resemblance and recurrent history. Patients typically have a history of HSV infections 1–2 weeks prior to the EM outbreak. Antiviral therapy prevents these EM recurrences in most cases.

Chronic

Mucocutaneous vesiculo-erosive diseases

The natural history and clinical appearance of mucocutaneous vesiculo-erosive disorders are often sufficient to differentiate them from RAS. Vesiculo-erosive diseases such as cicatricial pemphigoid and pemphigus vulgaris arise in older patients as blisters or bullae; these lesions subsequently break down into irregular erosions and ulcers. Vesiculo-erosive diseases do not spare the gingiva and hard palate. In these disorders, mucosal tissue becomes blistered following blunt trauma (Nikolsky sign). These ulcers are usually not confused with RAS because they are more diffuse and do not heal spontaneously. An exception is pemphigus, which in rare cases manifests MjAU- like oral ulcers that heal spontaneously and recur (Good and DiNubile 1993; Femiano *et al.* 2005). In the absence of cutaneous involvement, these ulcers can be misdiagnosed as RAS, leading to a delay in treatment for this potentially life-threatening disease. More than 60% of patients with pemphigus vulgaris have oral lesions, and in most of these cases they are the earliest manifestations.

The pathogenesis of RAS

Substantial evidence suggests that RAS arises in genetically susceptible individuals exposed to viral, bacterial, or environmental antigens, resulting in an autoimmune-like reaction or bystander effect associated with active chronic inflammation. In a normal, healthy individual, the oral mucosa is exposed to numerous antigens or insults, which can initiate an inflammatory cascade; however, a complex interaction between cytokines released from the cellular constituents of oral mucosa initiates immediate healing and return to normal function. Conversely, in RAS, a triggering agent or mild local trauma leads to mucosal damage and surface ulceration due to a deregulated immune response (Field and Allan 2003; Jurge *et al.* 2006). Furthermore, aphthous ulcers are more painful and heal more slowly than other mouth ulcers.

Abnormalities in the production of regulatory cytokines and antigen-induced signal transduction at the T-cell level play a role in the development and progression of aphthous ulcers (Field and Allan 2003; Jurge *et al.* 2006). The pattern of cytokine production in peripheral blood mononuclear cells, as well as the expression of epithelial and endothelial adhesion molecules and cytokines within the lesions, has been the focus of recent work.

Peripheral blood

RAS patients frequently show high serum IgM, IgA, IgD, and IgG levels compared with controls (Jurge *et al.* 2006). RAS patients also have lower serum levels of IgG_2 than controls, which are more pronounced during disease-free periods than in active stages (Vicente *et al.* 1996). Serum levels of acute phase C-reactive protein and β_2-microglobulin also increase during the preulcerative and ulcerative stages of RAS (Jurge *et al.* 2006).

Antiendothelial cell autoantibodies (AECA) are found in higher levels in RAS patients during the active ulcerative stage and between outbreaks (Healy and Thornhill 1999). AECA have been shown to play a significant role in antibody-mediated cellular cytotoxicity as well as up-regulation of the expression of leukocyte adhesion molecules (VCAM-1, ICAM-1, and E-selectin) in endothelial cells (Carvalho *et al.* 1996).

The major immunopathological differences that distinguish BS from RAS are the presence of circulating immune complexes and enhanced neutrophil migration (Ghate and Jorizzo 1999). Classic vasculitis is uncommon in RAS, whereas vasculitis mediated by these circulating immune complexes is present in BS (Frost *et al.* 1978; Reimer *et al.* 1983; Jorizzo *et al.* 1985; Rizzi *et al.* 1997).

The peripheral blood of RAS patients has decreased levels of CD4 and CD45R-positive naive Th cells (Bachtiar *et al.* 1998; Jurge *et al.* 2006). Furthermore, an increased number of activated CD4 and CDw29+ memory T-cells are noted in the peripheral blood of RAS patients during the early period of ulceration (Landesberg *et al.* 1990). Increased fractions of $\gamma\delta$ T cells (Pedersen and Ryder 1994) and natural killer (NK) cells (Pedersen *et al.* 1991) are noted in patients during the active stage of RAS compared with controls and patients in remission. During the exacerbation of aphthous ulcers, NK cell activity is substantially increased compared with the remission stage in the same patients (Sun *et al.* 1991).

A polarized proinflammatory Th1 immune response has been implicated in the pathophysiology of RAS and BS (Taylor *et al.* 1992; Lewkowicz *et al.* 2005). RAS as a Th1-dominant disease was further confirmed by a report that mitogen-activated peripheral blood mononuclear cells (PBMC) of RAS patients secrete three to five times higher levels of Th1-specfic proinflammatory cytokines, namely IFN-γ, TNF-α, IL-2, IL-5, and IL-6, compared to normal controls (Lewkowicz *et al.* 2005). Peripheral blood CD4+/CD25+ T-regulatory cells play an important role in maintaining the Th1/Th2 balance in the peripheral blood (Jonuleit 2001). These T-regulatory cells are markedly reduced in RAS patients, leading to a Th1-polarized immune response in these patients (Lewkowicz *et al.*, 2005).

Lesional tissue

A schematic model for the pathogenesis of aphthous ulcers is shown in Figure 11.2. The premonitory stage of RAS is characterized by infiltration of large granular lymphocytes (NK cells) (Mills *et al.* 1980) and CD4+ T cells into the lamina propria (Schroeder *et al.* 1983; Hayrinen-Immonen *et al.* 1991; Pedersen *et al.* 1992; Jurge *et al.* 2006). The number of CD4+ T cells continues to increase during the preulcerative stage. During the subsequent ulcerative stage CD8+ T cells appear within the epithelium and lamina propria,

and then disappear during the healing stage when the infiltrate consists of mostly CD4+ T cells (Savage *et al.* 1985). Neutrophils and mast cells are also recruited during the preulcerative and ulcerative stage (Dolby and Allison 1969; Schroeder *et al.* 1983, 1984). Mast cells frequently show membrane-to-membrane contact with substance P-containing nerve endings responsible for pain (Konttinen *et al.* 1994; Natah *et al.* 1998). Thus, accumulation and degranulation of mast cells in RAS is likely to be responsible for the pain associated with the lesions.

The recruitment of lymphocytes, neutrophils, and mast cells appears to be mediated by increased expression of cell-adhesion molecules in vascular endothelium and epithelial keratinocytes.

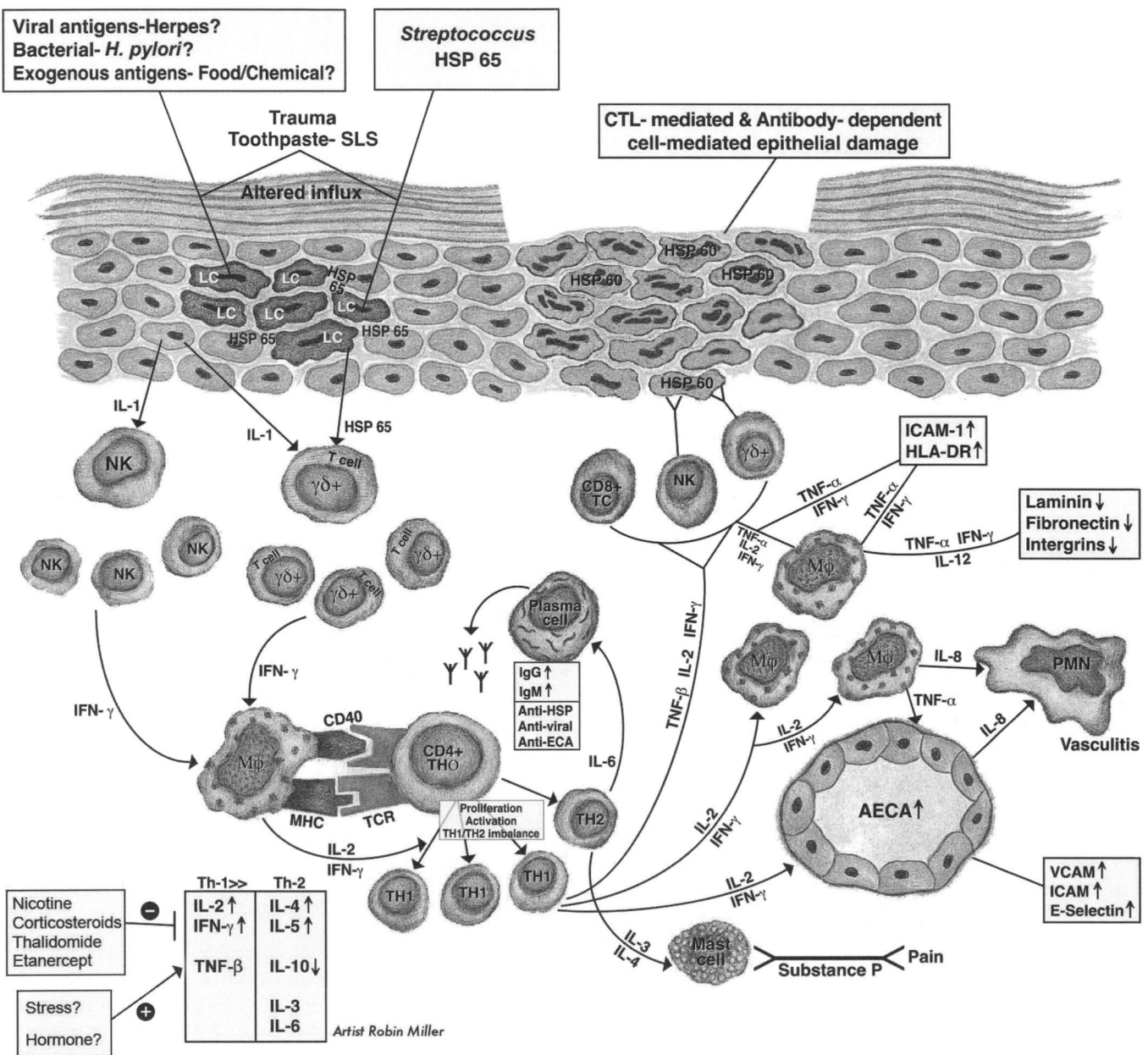

Figure 11.2 Schematic model for the pathogenesis of aphthous ulcers. Abbreviations: SLS, sodium lauryl sulfate; AECA, antiendothelial cell antibodies; VCAM, vascular cell adhesion molecule; ICAM, intercellular adhesion molecule; HSP, heat shock protein; MHC, major histocompatibility complex; TCR, T cell receptor; CTL, cytotoxic T lymphocyte; NK, natural killer cell; MΦ, macrophage; PMN, polymorphonuclear leukocyte (neutrophil).

Vascular endothelial cells in the lamina propria of aphthous ulcers show high expression of E-selectin, vascular cell adhesion molecule-1 (VCAM-1), and intracellular adhesion molecule (ICAM-1) (Healy and Thornhill 1999). Basal keratinocytes at the ulcer edge also demonstrate strong membrane expression of ICAM-1 (Healy and Thornhill 1999). Locally produced IL-I and TNF-α induce the expression of adhesion molecules in both vascular endothelium and keratinocytes (Li *et al.* 1996a, 1996b).

Elevated mRNA levels of proinflammatory cytokines IL-2, IL-4, IL-5, IFN-g, and TNF-a have been noted in RAS lesions (Buno *et al.* 1998). RAS lesions show lower levels of IL-10 than ulcers in non-RAS control patients (Buno *et al.* 1998). Recent microarray experiments comparing the gene expression profiles of RAS lesions and matched normal oral mucosa confirmed the up-regulation of Th1-specific genes and reduced expression of Th2-specific genes in aphthous ulcers (Borra *et al.* 2004). Increased levels of IL-2, IFN-γ and TNF-α, combined with low levels of IL-10 in aphthous ulcers indicate that Th1-polarized proinflammatory cytokines contribute to the pathogenesis of RAS (Buno *et al.* 1998; Borra *et al.* 2004).

Delayed healing response in aphthous ulcers

Re-epithelialization of aphthous ulcers is far slower than is seen in traumatic oral ulcers. This delay is attributed to the deficiency in expression of laminin, fibronectin- and epithelium-associated integrins at the healing front of these ulcers (Richards *et al.* 1996). Increased expression of proinflammatory cytokines in these ulcers may down-regulate the expression of keratinocyte integrins and their extracellular matrix receptors involved in re-epithelization.

Salivary epidermal growth factor (EGF) plays a crucial role in wound healing and re-epithelization of oral and gastrointestinal mucosa (Wright *et al.* 1990; Calabro *et al.* 1995). Prostaglandin E_2 (PGE_2), which has a cytoprotective effect on oral mucosa, is also found in high levels in normal saliva (Rigas and Levine 1983). Interestingly, salivary levels of EGF and PGE_2 are reduced to 25% and 50% of the normal range, respectively, in patients with active aphthous ulcers (Wu-Wang *et al.* 1995). Topical application of PGE_2 has been shown to reduce the recurrence of aphthous ulcers in susceptible patients (Taylor *et al.* 1993). It is possible that low salivary levels of EGF and PGE_2 contribute to the delayed healing of MjAU and HeAU. It should be noted that dry mouth (xerostomia) exacerbates RAS outbreaks.

Predisposing factors

Genetic basis

About 40% of patients who suffer from RAS have a positive family history (Sircus *et al.* 1957). These individuals usually develop oral ulcers at an earlier age and have a higher frequency of recurrence than RAS patients without a family history (Ship 1972).

RAS is highly correlated in monozygotic, but not dizygotic twins (Miller *et al.* 1977; Jurge *et al.* 2006). The genetic basis for RAS is further supported by its linkage with certain HLA subtypes which differ among different ethnic groups (Jurge *et al.* 2006). There were no specific IL-10, IL-12, and TNF-α gene polymorphisms that predicted an increased risk for RAS (Bazrafshani *et al.* 2000b, 2003). On the other hand, RAS showed a strong association with IL-1β and IL-6 gene polymorphisms (Bazrafshani *et al.* 2002a). These findings suggest that the dysregulated cytokine response in RAS may be genetically determined. Anxiety-related serotonin transporter gene

polymorphism (5-HTTLPR) also showed strong association with RAS (Victoria *et al.* 2005).

Potential role of microbial agents as cofactors in pathogenesis

Herpesviruses and bacterial organisms such as Streptococcus species and *Helicobacter pylori* have been implicated in the etiology and pathogenesis of RAS. Support for this finding is the detection of viral or bacterial genomic DNA in lesional tissue or peripheral blood mononuclear cells and the demonstration of an IgG or IgM antibody response to specific organisms.

Herpesviruses

The episodic and self-limited nature of RAS, the precipitation of ulcers by mechanical trauma, and anecdotal reports of RAS responding to acyclovir have prompted numerous attempts to associate herpesviruses with aphthous ulcers (Hooks 1978; Pedersen 1991, 1992; Pedersen *et al.* 1993). One difficulty in trying to associate RAS with viruses is that the prevalence of serum antibody positivity against different herpesviruses is very high (70–95%) among the adult population, indicating that most of the general population has been exposed to these viruses.

We believe it is highly unlikely that herpesviruses play a direct role in RAS for several reasons. First, no investigators have isolated or cultured any of the herpesviruses in aphthous ulcers. Positive serology and identification of viral DNA in RAS lesions could be a manifestation of coinfection or superinfection by viruses found in saliva. Secondly, aphthous ulcers do not spread by direct patient-to-patient contact. Finally, RAS lesions respond favorably to immuno-suppressive agents such as glucocorticoids and generally do not respond to antiviral medications. Thus, current data do not support a viral etiology of RAS (Jurge *et al.* 2006).

Helicobacter pylori (HP)

Following the discovery of its role in chronic gastritis and duodenal ulcers, several studies explored the potential role of *Helicobacter pylori* (*H. pylori*) in RAS (Leimola-Virtanen *et al.* 1995; Birek *et al.* 1999). *H. pylori* eradication in a group of *H. pylori*-antibody positive RAS patients in Greece significantly reduced the recurrence and symptoms of ulcers in these patients (Albanidou-Farmaki *et al.* 2005). On the other hand, no significant difference in the frequency of serum IgG response against *H. pylori* has been noted in RAS patients compared with patients who have other oral mucosal conditions and with healthy controls (Porter *et al.* 1997; Jurge *et al.* 2006). The prevalence of *H. pylori* infection in the oral cavity did not differ significantly between RAS and control patients (Fritscher *et al.* 2004). A study which attempted to isolate and culture *H. pylori* from aphthous ulcers was not successful (Chapman *et al.* 1998). In summary, there is no definitive evidence to support an etiologic role for *H. pylori* in RAS (Jurge *et al.* 2006).

Streptococcus sanguis

Numerous studies have investigated the relationship between the oral bacterium *Streptococcus sanguis* and RAS and BS (Kaneko *et al.* 1985, 1997). A search for this association was initiated primarily by observations showing a high incidence of tonsillitis and dental caries caused by *S. sanguis* in patients with BS (Kaneko *et al.* 1997). Moreover, various streptococcal antigens trigger a cutaneous hypersensitivity reaction and increased PBMC production of proinflammatory cytokines in BS (Kaneko *et al.* 1997). It has been postulated that 60–65 kD heat-shock proteins (Hsp) are common cross-reactive antigens between *S. sanguis* and oral epithelial cells (Lehner *et al.* 1991). Patients with RAS and BS have serum antibodies to mycobacterial Hsp65 and increases in Hsp65-reactive and T-cells (Hasan *et al.* 1995). Antibodies against mycobacterial Hsp65 have been shown to cross-react with *S. sanguis* Hsp, suggesting that they share a common antigenic determinant (Lehner *et al.* 1991). Thus, it has been hypothesized that microbial Hsp65 stimulates mucosal Langerhans cells, which in turn generate an autoreactive T-cell population primed against mitochondrial Hsp60 in oral epithelial cells(Hasan *et al.* 1995, 1996). The molecular mimicry between microbial 65 kD Hsp and the homologous human 60 kD Hsp peptide in the pathogenesis of RAS was substantiated further by defining their shared T-cell epitope (Hasan, Shinnick *et al.* 2002). This critical T-cell epitope stimulated the proliferation of a MHC class II-restricted subset of CD4+ T cells from RAS patients (Hasan *et al.* 2002).

In conclusion, there is no convincing data to support a bacterial or viral infectious etiology for RAS. But current evidence suggests that a molecular mimicry between bacterial Hsp and human mitochondrial Hsp may play a role in RAS pathogenesis.

Food hypersensitivity

Certain food products, as well as flavoring/ coloring agents and preservatives, have been implicated as precipitators of RAS (Table 11.5) (Hay and Reade 1984; Nolan *et al.* 1991). With the exception of GSE, a cause-and-effect relationship between a specific food substance and RAS has not been definitively proven (Jurge *et al.* 2006). Individuals with GSE manifest aphthous ulcers on introduction of gluten in their diet (Jurge *et al.* 2006). Elimination of these agents from the diet has, in some cases, been shown to cause remission of RAS (Jurge *et al.* 2006).

Effect of toothpaste detergents

Most toothpastes contain the anionic detergent sodium lauryl sulfate (SLS) at 1–3% of the total composition. The denaturing effect

Table 11.5 Food and chemical substances implicated as precipitating agents for RAS

Food items	
	Cereal, e.g. gluten
	Chocolate
	Dairy products, e.g. cheese
	Coffee
	Fruits, e.g. citrus, strawberry, tomato, pineapple, apple
	Nuts, e.g. walnuts
Chemical substances	
	Benzoate
	Cinnamaldehyde
	Nickel
	Paraben
	Dichromate
	Methyl methacrylate (from dentures)
	Sorbic acid

of SLS eliminates the protective mucosal layer, which leads to desquamation of the superficial epithelial cells and increased permeability to both water-soluble and fat-soluble molecules (Herlofson and Barkvoll 1996a). Thus, use of toothpastes containing SLS may facilitate the influx of exogenous ulcer-triggering antigens. RAS patients who use SLS-containing toothpaste experience more frequent ulcer outbreaks than those who use an SLS-free dentifrice (Herlofson and Barkvoll 1994, 1996b; Chahine *et al.* 1997).

Local trauma

Incidental local trauma resulting from: tooth brushing; flossing; chewing gum, nuts, candy, or other foods that have sharp surfaces; ill-fitting dental prostheses; local anesthetic injection; and dental treatments can precipitate aphthous ulcers (Field and Allan 2003). In normal patients, oral mucosal injury secondary to incidental trauma rapidly heals via a series of homeostatic repair mechanisms involving both mucosal and local immune responses. Conversely, incidental traumatic injury in RAS patients is complicated by immune-mediated tissue damage leading to ulceration (Buno *et al.* 1998). This phenomenon has been demonstrated experimentally using suture-induced mucosal trauma, which induces ulcers in RAS patients within 24 hours, compared with control subjects who suffer only a minimal inflammatory response (Buno *et al.* 1998).

Smoking cessation

Several studies have found that the prevalence of aphthous ulcers in cigarette smokers is significantly lower than in non-smokers (Chellemi *et al.* 1970; Shapiro *et al.* 1970; Axell and Henricsson 1985; Baron 1996). In fact, ex-smokers experience increased frequency and severity of aphthous ulcers (Baron 1996). Some reports have postulated that smoking induces increased epithelial keratinization, which protects against ulceration (Sallay and Banoczy 1968; Axell and Henricsson 1985). Other studies, however, have shown that smokeless tobacco use and nicotine replacement therapy have a similar effect on aphthous ulcers, suggesting that nicotine plays a key role (Sallay and Banoczy 1968; Axell and Henricsson 1985; Bittoun 1991; Grady *et al.* 1992). Nicotine inhibits the production of IL-2 and TNF-α by peripheral blood mononuclar cells (Madretsma *et al.* 1996; van Dijk *et al.* 1998), so it might lower the frequency of aphthous ulcers by modulating cytokine production.

Vitamin and mineral deficiency

Deficiencies in vitamins B_1, B_2, B_6, B_{12}, folic acid, and iron have been found in 3 to 18% of RAS patients (Jurge *et al.* 2006). In addition, a single case of RAS was attributed to zinc deficiency, as the patient subsequently responded to supplements of this mineral (Endre 1991). The association of RAS and nutrient deficiency may be sensitive to geographic or ethnic factors. Most studies showing an association originated in Europe or the Middle East, while a study from the US was entirely negative (Olson *et al.* 1982). It is possible that the reported deficiencies are secondary to inadequate nutritional intake in patients with large and painful oral ulcers and a pre-existing marginal diet.

Treatment

Although there is no cure for RAS, several treatment options afford periods of remission. Treatment is generally based on the severity of disease, the impact on the patient's quality of life and accompanying systemic medical conditions. Therapy should be tailored for the individual patient and follow a rational, stepwise progression, with an ultimate aim of achieving a most favorable risk: benefit ratio (Letsinger 2005). Categories of aphthous ulcer medications include: over-the-counter topical pain preparations, antimicrobial agents, topical and systemic anti-inflammatory drugs, and systemic immunomodulatory drugs. In addition, physical manipulation by surgery and cauterizing agents has been tried.

In evaluating efficacy of treatment, it is important to realize that MiAU heal spontaneously and that the frequency of recurrence, lesion duration, and degree of pain perception vary among patients. This makes it difficult to critically evaluate treatment regimens that claim a reduction in frequency of recurrence, pain, or time to healing. Furthermore, many treatment reports are little more than case studies without adequate controls, and thus are of questionable validity.

Over-the-counter medications

Patients with infrequent recurrences of small, mildly painful MiAU may not need any treatment or may be managed with over-the-counter products. Several available products act as surface-covering agents to reduce pain until the epithelium can regenerate (Rodu and Russell 1988; Rodu *et al.* 1988; Mahdi *et al.* 1996). These products may also contain the local anesthetic benzocaine to provide additional pain relief. Zilactin-B (Zila Pharmaceuticals) is a product that forms an adherent film that is impervious to irritants, thereby reducing pain and allowing patients to eat and drink (Rodu *et al.* 1988).

Regular use of a mouthwash containing chlorhexidine gluconate 0.12% (Peridex, Periogard) has been shown to reduce the frequency of recurrence, number of ulcers, and healing time, although some patients may experience more pain when using this medication due to its alcohol content (Hunter and Addy 1987). Regular use of chlorhexidine also leads to discoloration of teeth. Tetracycline mouth rinse has also reported to be beneficial in reducing the pain and accelerating the healing of aphthous ulcers (Graykowski and Kingman 1978).

Anti-inflammatory drugs

Amlexanox is an antiallergic and anti-inflammatory drug, which has been used in the treatment of bronchial asthma, allergic rhinitis, and conjunctivitis (Khandwala *et al.* 1997a, 1997b). A number of well-controlled clinical studies in the US have shown that topical application of 5% amlexanox (Aphthasol) reduces pain and accelerates ulcer healing (Jurge *et al.* 2006). This topical drug is well suited for patients who develop MiAU infrequently but have a low tolerance to pain.

In North America, topical glucocorticoids are the most commonly prescribed therapy for ulcers. Effective drug delivery by topical application to oral mucosa is limited by the continual movement of oral tissues and salivary flow. This problem may be partially overcome by the use of superpotent fluorinated glucocorticoid preparations such as fluocinonide (Lidex, Syntex) and clobetasol (Temovate, Glaxo) (Lo Muzio *et al.* 2001). We have found that application of these products to ulcers five times per day is very effective and minimizes systemic absorption and adverse effects. Topical glucocorticoids may be mixed with a cellulose compound such as Orabase (Colgate) or covered immediately by Zilactin-B.

Large MjAU on the soft palate, oropharyngeal region, and posterior ventral tongue can cause severe pain and interfere with food and fluid intake. These patients may benefit substantially from intralesional injection of triamcinolone acetonide (Kenalog-10, Bristol-Myers Squibb), which induces rapid healing and pain relief within 2 days. For patients with MjAU, we routinely prescribe systemic glucocorticoids. In our experience, RAS responds differently to various glucocorticoid preparations; triamcinolone and prednisone are not as effective as oral elixirs of betamethasone (0.6 mg/5 ml) (Celestone, Schering) and dexamethasone (0.5 mg/5 ml) (Decadron, Merck). For active lesions, we routinely prescribe a 10-day course of either medication, one teaspoon (5 ml) of which is to be rinsed throughout the mouth for 1 min, three times per day, and swallowed. This will induce remission in almost all patients, but those with a history of severe, debilitating RAS will invariably regress within 2 to 3 weeks. To avoid irregular and uncontrolled glucocorticoid use, we have employed a long-term tapering regimen of these agents. The initial 10-day period is followed by two teaspoons per day for 30 days, with further tapering as tolerated by the patient. The ultimate goal is the maintenance of a disease-free remission at the lowest possible glucocorticoid dose.

Immunomodulatory drugs

Due to the multiple side-effects of glucocorticoids, recent studies have focused on the use of immunomodulatory drugs.

Anti-TNF drugs

Since TNF-α plays an important role in the pathogenesis of RAS, use of anti-TNF agents can be effective for severe, recalcitrant RAS (Jurge *et al.* 2006). Drugs with anti-TNF properties include thalidomide, pentoxifylline and the biologic agents etanercept, infliximab, and adalimumab.

A multicenter, double-blind, randomized trial of oral and esophageal aphthous ulcers in AIDS patients found that oral ulcers healed within 4 weeks in 55% (16/29) of thalidomide-treated patients compared with 7% (2/28) in the placebo-treated group (Jacobson *et al.* 1997, 1999). When complete and partial responders were combined, almost 90% (26/29) of thalidomide-treated patients showed benefit compared with 25% (7/28) of controls. Thalidomide is also effective for RAS in immunocompetent patients (Bonnetblanc *et al.* 1996; Letsinger *et al.* 2005).

Because of the risk of birth defects, thalidomide use in either men or women of childbearing potential should be restricted to patients with severe RAS in whom continuous use of systemic glucocorticoids is either ineffective or contraindicated. Thalidomide should never be prescribed for women of childbearing age unless they use reliable contraception. Other potential side-effects of thalidomide are sedation, peripheral neuropathy, neutropenia, and skin rash (Tseng *et al.* 1996). Peripheral neuropathy may occur, but does not appear to be related to either cumulative dose or duration of therapy (Harland *et al.* 1995).

Pentoxifylline has been used to treat patients with chronic leukocytoclastic vasculitis and BS. A 1-month course of this drug (400 mg three times daily) resulted in either complete remission or less frequent episodes of RAS for as long as 9 months after therapy (Wahba-Yahav 1995; Letsinger *et al.* 2005; Jurge *et al.* 2006). With its minimal side-effects, pentoxifylline appears to have a promising therapeutic value in RAS (Chandrasekhar *et al.* 1999), but additional double-blind, randomized, placebo-controlled studies will be needed to confirm its efficacy. Etanercept is a recombinant fusion protein of the Fc portion of IgG and the TNFR2; it inhibits TNF-mediated cellular responses. Etanercept has been used successfully to treat severe RAS with minimal side-effects (Robinson and Guitart 2003).

Other immunomodulatory drugs

Other immunomodulatory drugs that have been reported to have therapeutic effect in RAS include azathioprine, levamisole, colchicine, and cyclosporin. However, most of these reports are either individual case studies or open trials involving only a few patients (Field and Allan 2003; Jurge *et al.* 2006). Thus, more extensive, controlled clinical trials are needed before any definitive judgment can be made about the effectiveness of these drugs for the treatment of RAS.

Surgery/cauterization

Surgical intervention is known to accelerate the healing of aphthous ulcers. Conversion of an aphthous ulcer to a wound may initiate a more regulated inflammatory response, which in turn increases the rate of healing. Low-power laser ablation and silver nitrate treatment of aphthous ulcers are two commonly used methods to convert them into wounds and accelerate healing (Colvard and Kuo 1991; Neiburger 1995). The cost: benefit ratio of laser ablation treatment for aphthous ulcers is, however, debatable. Silver nitrate is a dangerous cauterizing agent that may lead to a more extensive chemical burn if not carefully administered (Frost *et al.* 1978). We do not recommend its routine use by either health professionals or patients.

In summary, treatment of RAS patients is dictated by the severity of the disease. Most patients with moderate to severe RAS who seek medical attention can be treated with topical and/or systemic glucocorticoids. More aggressive treatment such as thalidomide should be restricted to patients who are unresponsive to glucocorticoid therapy or with adverse effects from glucocorticoids.

References

Agbo-Godeau, S., Joly, P., *et al.* (1998). Association of major aphthous ulcers and nicorandil. *Lancet*, **352**, 1598–9.

Albanidou-Farmaki, E., Giannoulis, L., *et al.* (2005). Outcome following treatment for Helicobacter pylori in patients with recurrent aphthous stomatitis. *Oral Diseases*, **11**, 22–6.

Allen, C. M., Camisa, C., *et al.* (1991). Wegener's granulomatosis: report of three cases with oral lesions. *Journal of Oral and Maxillofacial Surgery*, **49**, 294–8.

Axell, T. and Henricsson, V. (1985). Association between recurrent aphthous ulcers and tobacco habits. *Scandinavian Journal of Dental Research*, **93**, 239–42.

Bachtiar, E. W., Cornain, S., *et al.* (1998). Decreased CD4+/CD8+ ratio in major type of recurrent aphthous ulcers: comparing major to minor types of ulcers. *Asian Pacific Journal of Allergy and Immunology*, **16**, 75–9.

Bagan, J. V., Sanchis, J. M., *et al.* (1991). Recurrent aphthous stomatitis. A study of the clinical characteristics of lesions in 93 cases. *Journal of Oral Pathology and Medicine*, **20**, 395–7.

Baron, J. A. (1996). Beneficial effects of nicotine and cigarette smoking: the real, the possible and the spurious. *British Medical Bulletin*, **52**, 58–73.

Bazrafshani, M. R., Hajeer, A. H., *et al.* (2002a). IL-1B and IL-6 gene polymorphisms encode significant risk for the development of recurrent aphthous stomatitis (RAS). *Genes and Immunity*, **3**, 302–5.

Bazrafshani, M. R., Hajeer, A. H., *et al.* (2002b). Recurrent aphthous stomatitis and gene polymorphisms for the inflammatory markers TNF-alpha, TNF-beta and the vitamin D receptor: no association detected. *Oral Diseases*, **8**, 303–7.

Bazrafshani, M. R., Hajeer, A. H., *et al.* (2003). Polymorphisms in the IL-10 and IL-12 gene cluster and risk of developing recurrent aphthous stomatitis. *Oral Diseases*, **9**, 287–91.

Berlucchi, M., Meini, A., *et al.* (2003). Update on treatment of Marshall's syndrome (PFAPA syndrome, report of five cases with review of the literature. *Annals of Otology Rhinology and Laryngology*, **112**, 365–9.

Birek, C., Grandhi, R., *et al.* (1999). Detection of Helicobacter pylori in oral aphthous ulcers. *Journal of Oral Pathology and Medicine*, **28**, 197–203.

Bittoun, R. (1991). Recurrent aphthous ulcers and nicotine. *Medical Journal of Australia*, **154**, 471–2.

Bonnetblanc, J. M., Royer, C., *et al.* (1996). Thalidomide and recurrent aphthous stomatitis: a follow-up study. *Dermatology*, **193**, 321–3.

Borra, R. C., Andrade, P. M., *et al.* (2004). The Th1 /Th2 immune-type response of the recurrent aphthous ulceration analyzed by cDNA microarray. *Journal of Oral Pathology and Medicine*, **33**, 140–6.

Boulinguez, S., Sommet, A., *et al.* (2003). Oral nicorandil-induced lesions are not aphthous ulcers. *Journal of Oral Pathology and Medicine*, **32**, 482–5.

Buno, I. J., Huff, J. C., *et al.* (1998). Elevated levels of interferon gamma, tumor necrosis factor alpha, interleukins 2, 4, and 5, but not interleukin 10, are present in recurrent aphthous stomatitis. *Archives of Dermatology*, **134**, 827–31.

Calabro, A., Milani, S., *et al.* (1995). Role of epidermal growth factor in peptic ulcer healing. *Digestive Diseases and Sciences*, **40**, 2497–504.

Carvalho, D., Savage, C. O., *et al.* (1996). IgG antiendothelial cell autoantibodies from scleroderma patients induce leukocyte adhesion to human vascular endothelial cells in vitro. Induction of adhesion molecule expression and involvement of endothelium-derived cytokines. *Journal of Clinical Investigation*, **97**, 111–9.

Cazeneuve, C., Genevieve, D., *et al.* (2003). MEFV gene analysis in PFAPA. *Journal of Pediatrics*, **143**, 140–1.

Chahine, L., Sempson, N., *et al.* (1997). The effect of sodium lauryl sulfate on recurrent aphthous ulcers: a clinical study. *Compendium of Continuing Education in Dentistry (Jamesburg, NJ)*, **18**, 1238–40.

Chakrabarty, A. K., Mraz, S., *et al.* (2005). Aphthous ulcers associated with imiquimod and the treatment of actinic cheilitis. *Journal of the American Academy of Dermatology*, **52** (Suppl. 1), 35–7.

Chandrasekhar, J., Liem, A. A., *et al.* (1999). Oxypentifylline in the management of recurrent aphthous oral ulcers: an open clinical trial. *Oral Surgery, Oral Medicine, Oral Pathology, Oral Radiology, and Endodontics*, **87**, 564–7.

Chellemi, S. J., Olson, D. L., *et al.* (1970). The association between smoking and aphthous ulcers. A preliminary report. *Oral Surgery, Oral Medicine, Oral Pathology*, **29**, 832–6.

Cohen, P. R. (2004). Sweet's syndrome and relapsing polychondritis: is their appearance in the same patient a coincidental occurrence or a bona fide association of these conditions? *International Journal of Dermatology*, **43**, 772–7.

Colvard, M. and Kuo, P. (1991). Managing aphthous ulcers: laser treatment applied. *Journal of the American Dental Association*, **122**, 51–3.

Cooke, B. E. (1969). Recurrent oral ulceration. *British Journal of Dermatology*, **81**, 159–61.

Cribier, B., Marquart-Elbaz, C., *et al.* (1998). Chronic buccal ulceration induced by nicorandil. *British Journal of Dermatology*, **138**, 372–3.

Crivelli, M. R., Aguas, S., *et al.* (1988). Influence of socioeconomic status on oral mucosa lesion prevalence in schoolchildren. *Community Dentistry and Oral Epidemiology*, **16**, 58–60.

Cuttica, R. J., Scheines, E. J., *et al.* (1992). Juvenile onset Reiter's syndrome. A retrospective study of 26 patients. *Clinical and Experimental Rheumatology*, **10**, 285–8.

Dolby, A. E. and Allison, R. T. (1969). Quantitative changes in the mast cell population in Mikulicz's recurrent oral aphthae. *Journal of Dental Research*, **48**, 901–3.

Endre, L. (1991). Recurrent aphthous ulceration with zinc deficiency and cellular immune deficiency. *Oral Surgery, Oral Medicine, Oral Pathology*, **72**, 559–61.

Eufinger, H., Machtens, E., *et al.* (1992). Oral manifestations of Wegener's granulomatosis. Review of the literature and report of a case. *International Journal of Oral and Maxillofacial Surgery*, **21**, 50–3.

Farah, C. S. and Savage, N. W. (2003). Oral ulceration with bone sequestration. *Australian Dental Journal*, **48**, 61–4.

Farthing, P., Bagan, J. V., *et al.* (2005). Mucosal disease series. Number IV. Erythema multiforme. *Oral Diseases*, **11**, 261–7.

Farthing, P. M., Maragou, P., *et al.* (1995). Characteristics of the oral lesions in patients with cutaneous recurrent erythema multiforme. *Journal of Oral Pathology and Medicine*, **24**, 9–13.

Femiano, F., Gombos, F., *et al.* (2005). Pemphigus mimicking aphthous stomatitis. *Journal of Oral Pathology and Medicine*, **34**, 508–10.

Ferguson, M. M., Wray, D., *et al.* (1980). Coeliac disease associated with recurrent aphthae. *Gut*, **21**, 223–6.

Field, E. A. and Allan, R. B. (2003). Review article: oral ulceration–aetiopathogenesis, clinical diagnosis and management in the gastrointestinal clinic. *Alimentary Pharmacology and Therapeutics*, **18**, 949–62.

Field, E. A., Brookes, V., *et al.* (1992). Recurrent aphthous ulceration in children – a review. *International Journal of Paediatric Dentistry*, **2**, 1–10.

Flaitz, C. M., Nichols, C. M., *et al.* (1996). Herpesviridae-associated persistent mucocutaneous ulcers in acquired immunodeficiency syndrome. A clinicopathologic study. *Oral Surgery, Oral Medicine, Oral Pathology, Oral Radiology, and Endodontics*, **81**, 433–41.

Frances, C., Du, L. T., *et al.* (1994). Wegener's granulomatosis. Dermatological manifestations in 75 cases with clinicopathologic correlation. *Archives of Dermatology*, **130**, 861–7.

Fritscher, A. M., Cherubini, K., *et al.* (2004). Association between Helicobacter pylori and recurrent aphthous stomatitis in children and adolescents. *Journal of Oral Pathology and Medicine*, **33**, 129–32.

Frost, D. E., Barkmeier, W. W., *et al.* (1978). Aphthous ulcer–a treatment complication. Report of a case. *Oral Surgery, Oral Medicine, Oral Pathology*, **45**, 863–9.

Furniss, K. K. (1992). Aphthous ulcers seen with Crohn's disease [letter; comment]. *Nurse Practitioner*, **17**, 22.

Gertner, E. (2004). Severe recurrent neurological disease in the MAGIC syndrome. *Journal of Rheumatology*, **31**, 1018–9.

Ghate, J. V. and Jorizzo, J. L. (1999). Behçet's disease and complex aphthosis. *Journal of the American Academy of Dermatology*, **40**, 1–18; quiz 19–20.

Goffin, E., Pochet, J. M., *et al.* (1998). Aphtous ulcers of the mouth associated with losartan [letter]. *Clinical Nephrology*, **50**, 197.

Good, G. R. and DiNubile, M. J. (1993). Pemphigus presenting as oral ulcers refractory to acyclovir therapy. *New Jersey Medicine*, **90**, 667–70.

Grady, D., Ernster, V. L., *et al.* (1992). Smokeless tobacco use prevents aphthous stomatitis. *Oral Surgery, Oral Medicine, Oral Pathology*, **74**, 463–5.

Graykowski, E. A. and Kingman, A. (1978). Double-blind trial of tetracycline in recurrent aphthous ulceration. *Journal of Oral Pathology*, **7**, 376–82.

Harland, C. C., Steventon, G. B., *et al.* (1995). Thalidomide-induced neuropathy and genetic differences in drug metabolism. *European Journal of Clinical Pharmacology*, **49**, 1–6.

Hasan, A., Childerstone, A., *et al.* (1995). Recognition of a unique peptide epitope of the mycobacterial and human heat shock protein 65-60 antigen by T cells of patients with recurrent oral ulcers. *Clinical and Experimental Immunology*, **99**, 392–7.

Hasan, A., Fortune, F., *et al.* (1996). Role of gamma delta T cells in pathogenesis and diagnosis of Behcet's disease. *Lancet*, **347**, 789–94.

Hasan, A., Shinnick, T., *et al.* (2002). Defining a T-cell epitope within HSP 65 in recurrent aphthous stomatitis. *Clinical and Experimental Immunology*, **128**, 318–25.

Hay, K. D. and Reade, P. C. (1984). The use of an elimination diet in the treatment of recurrent aphthous ulceration of the oral cavity. *Oral Surgery, Oral Medicine, Oral Pathology*, **57**, 504–7.

Hayrinen-Immonen, R., Nordstrom, D., *et al.* (1991). Immune-inflammatory cells in recurrent oral ulcers (ROU). *Scandinavian Journal of Dental Research*, **99**, 510–8.

Healy, C. M. and Thornhill, M. H. (1995). An association between recurrent oro-genital ulceration and non-steroidal anti-inflammatory drugs. *Journal of Oral Pathology and Medicine*, **24**, 46–8.

Healy, C. M. and Thornhill, M. H. (1999). Induction of adhesion molecule expression on blood vessels and keratinocytes in recurrent oral ulceration. *Journal of Oral Pathology and Medicine*, **28**, 5–11.

Herlofson, B. B. and Barkvoll, P. (1994a). Sodium lauryl sulfate and recurrent aphthous ulcers. A preliminary study. *Acta Odontologica Scandinavica*, **52**, 257–9.

Herlofson, B. B. and Barkvoll, P. (1996a). The effect of two toothpaste detergents on the frequency of recurrent aphthous ulcers. *Acta Odontologica Scandinavica*, **54**, 150–3.

Herlofson, B. B. and Barkvoll, P. (1996b). Oral mucosal desquamation caused by two toothpaste detergents in an experimental model. *European Journal of Oral Sciences*, **104**, 21–6.

Hooks, J. J. (1978). Possibility of a viral etiology in recurrent aphthous ulcers and Behçet's syndrome. *Journal of Oral Pathology*, **7**, 353–64.

Jacobson, J. M., Greenspan, J. S., *et al.* (1997). Thalidomide for the treatment of oral aphthous ulcers in patients with human immunodeficiency virus infection. National Institute of Allergy and Infectious Diseases AIDS Clinical Trials Group. *New England Journal of Medicine*, **336**, 1487–93.

Jacobson, J. M., Spritzler, J., *et al.* (1999). Thalidomide for the treatment of esophageal aphthous ulcers in patients with human immunodeficiency virus infection. National Institute of Allergy and Infectious Disease AIDS Clinical Trials Group. *Journal of Infectious Diseases*, **180**, 61–7.

Johnson, B. D. and Engel, D. (1986). Acute necrotizing ulcerative gingivitis. A review of diagnosis, etiology and treatment. *Journal of Periodontology*, **57**, 141–50.

Jonuleit, H., Schmitt, E., Stassen, M., *et al.* (2001). Identification and functional characterization of human CD4(+)CD25(+) T cells with regulatory properties isolated from peripheral blood. *Journal of Experimental Medicine*, **193**, 1285–94.

Jorizzo, J. L., Taylor, R. S., *et al.* (1985). Complex aphthosis: a forme fruste of Behcet's syndrome? *Journal of the American Academy of Dermatology*, **13**, 80–4.

Jurge, S., Kuffer, R., *et al.* (2006). Number VI Recurrent aphthous stomatitis. *Oral Diseases*, **12**, 1–21.

Kaneko, F., Oyama, N., *et al.* (1997). Streptococcal infection in the pathogenesis of Behcet's disease and clinical effects of minocycline on the disease symptoms. *Yonsei Medical Journal*, **38**, 444–54.

Kaneko, F., Takahashi, Y., *et al.* (1985). Immunological studies on aphthous ulcer and erythema nodosum-like eruptions in Behcet's disease. *British Journal of Dermatology*, **113**, 303–12.

Kerr, A. R. and Ship, J. A. (2003). Management strategies for HIV-associated aphthous stomatitis. *American Journal of Clinical Dermatology*, **4**, 669–80.

Khandwala, A., Van Inwegen, R. G., *et al.* (1997a). 5% amlexanox oral paste, a new treatment for recurrent minor aphthous ulcers: I. Clinical demonstration of acceleration of healing and resolution of pain. *Oral Surgery, Oral Medicine, Oral Pathology, Oral Radiology, and Endodontics*, **83**, 222–30.

Khandwala, A., Van Inwegen, R. G., *et al.* (1997b). 5% amlexanox oral paste, a new treatment for recurrent minor aphthous ulcers: II. Pharmacokinetics and demonstration of clinical safety. *Oral Surgery, Oral Medicine, Oral Pathology, Oral Radiology, and Endodontics*, **83**, 231–8.

Kleinman, D. V., Swango, P. A., *et al.* (1994). Epidemiology of oral mucosal lesions in United States schoolchildren: 1986–87. *Community Dentistry and Oral Epidemiology*, **22**, 243–53.

Konttinen, Y. T., Hayrinen-Immonen, R. H., *et al.* (1994). Innervation of recurrent aphthous ulcers. *Oral Microbiology and Immunology*, **9**, 60–4.

Landesberg, R., Fallon, M., *et al.* (1990). Alterations of T helper/inducer and T suppressor/inducer cells in patients with recurrent aphthous ulcers. *Oral Surgery, Oral Medicine, Oral Pathology*, **69**, 205–8.

Lehner, T., Lavery, E., *et al.* (1991). Association between the 65-kilodalton heat shock protein, Streptococcus sanguis, and the corresponding antibodies in Behcet's syndrome. *Infection and Immunity*, **59**, 1434–41.

Leimola-Virtanen, R., Happonen, R. P., *et al.* (1995). Cytomegalovirus (CMV) and Helicobacter pylori (HP) found in oral mucosal ulcers. *Journal of Oral Pathology and Medicine*, **24**, 14–7.

Letsinger, J. A., McCarty, M. A., *et al.* (2005). Complex aphthosis: a large case series with evaluation algorithm and therapeutic ladder from topicals to thalidomide. *Journal of the American Academy of Dermatology*, **52**, 500–8.

Lewis, J. E., Beutner, E. H., *et al.* (1996). Chronic ulcerative stomatitis with stratified epithelium-specific antinuclear antibodies. *International Journal of Dermatology*, **35**, 272–5.

Lewkowicz, N., Lewkowicz, P., *et al.* (2005). Predominance of Type 1 cytokines and decreased number of CD4(+)CD25(+high) T regulatory cells in peripheral blood of patients with recurrent aphthous ulcerations. *Immunology Letters*, **99**, 57–62.

Li, J., Farthing, P. M., *et al.* (1996a). IL-1 alpha and IL-6 production by oral and skin keratinocytes: similarities and differences in response to cytokine treatment in vitro. *Journal of Oral Pathology and Medicine*, **25**, 157–62.

Li, J., Mahiouz, D. L., *et al.* (1996b). Heterogeneity of ICAM-1 expression, and cytokine regulation of ICAM-1 expression, in skin and oral keratinocytes. *Journal of Oral Pathology and Medicine*, **25**, 112–8.

Liao, C. H., Huang, J. L., *et al.* (2004). Juvenile Reiter's syndrome: a case report. *J Microbiol Immunol Infect*, **37**, 379–81.

Lisciandrano, D., Ranzi, T., *et al.* (1996). Prevalence of oral lesions in inflammatory bowel disease. *American Journal of Gastroenterology*, **91**, 7–10.

Lo Muzio, L., della Valle, A., *et al.* (2001). The treatment of oral aphthous ulceration or erosive lichen planus with topical clobetasol propionate in three preparations: a clinical and pilot study on 54 patients. *Journal of Oral Pathology and Medicine*, **30**, 611–7.

MacPhail, L. A. and Greenspan, J. S. (1997). Oral ulceration in HIV infection: investigation and pathogenesis. *Oral Diseases*, **3** (Suppl.1), S190–3.

Madretsma, G. S., Donze, G. J., *et al.* (1996). Nicotine inhibits the in vitro production of interleukin 2 and tumour necrosis factor-alpha by human mononuclear cells. *Immunopharmacology*, **35**, 47–51.

Mahdi, A. B., Coulter, W. A., *et al.* (1996). Efficacy of bioadhesive patches in the treatment of recurrent aphthous stomatitis. *Journal of Oral Pathology and Medicine*, **25**, 416–9.

Margiotta, V., Campisi, G., *et al.* (1999). HIV infection: oral lesions, CD4+ cell count and viral load in an Italian study population. *Journal of Oral Pathology and Medicine*, **28**, 173–7.

Marshall, G. S., Edwards, K. M., *et al.* (1989). PFAPA syndrome [letter; comment]. *Pediatric Infectious Disease Journal*, **8**, 658–9.

McLeod, R. I. (2000). Drug-induced aphthous ulcers. *British Journal of Dermatology*, **143**, 1137–9.

Merchant, N. E., Ferguson, M. M., *et al.* (1986). The detection of IgA-reticulin antibodies and their incidence in patients with recurrent aphthae. *Journal of Oral Medicine*, **41**, 31–4.

Mikulicz, J. v. and Kummel, W. (1898). *Die Krankheiten des Mundes*. Jena.

Miller, M. F., Garfunkel, A. A., *et al.* (1977). Inheritance patterns in recurrent aphthous ulcers: twin and pedigree data. *Oral Surgery, Oral Medicine, Oral Pathology*, **43**, 886–91.

Mills, M. P., Mackler, B. F., *et al.* (1980). Quantitative distribution of inflammatory cells in recurrent aphthous stomatitis. *Journal of Dental Research*, **59**, 562–6.

Natah, S. S., Hayrinen-Immonen, R., *et al.* (1998). Quantitative assessment of mast cells in recurrent aphthous ulcers (RAU). *Journal of Oral Pathology and Medicine*, **27**, 124–9.

Neiburger, E. J. (1995). The effect of low-power lasers on intraoral wound healing. *New York State Dental Journal*, **61**, 40–3.

Nolan, A., Lamey, P. J., *et al.* (1991). Recurrent aphthous ulceration and food sensitivity. *Journal of Oral Pathology and Medicine*, **20**, 473–5.

Notani, K., Kobayashi, S., *et al.* (2000). A case of Sweet's syndrome (acute febrile neutrophilic dermatosis) with palatal ulceration. *Oral Surgery, Oral Medicine, Oral Pathology, Oral Radiology, and Endodontics*, **89**, 477–9.

Olson, J. A., Feinberg, I., *et al.* (1982). Serum vitamin B12, folate, and iron levels in recurrent aphthous ulceration. *Oral Surgery, Oral Medicine, Oral Pathology*, **54**, 517–20.

Padeh, S., Brezniak, N., *et al.* (1999). Periodic fever, aphthous stomatitis, pharyngitis, and adenopathy syndrome: clinical characteristics and outcome. *Journal of Pediatrics*, **135**, 98–101.

Pedersen, A. (1991). Are recurrent oral aphthous ulcers of viral etiology? *Medical Hypotheses*, **36**, 206–10.

Pedersen, A. (1992). Acyclovir in the prevention of severe aphthous ulcers [letter]. *Archives of Dermatology*, **128**, 119–20.

Pedersen, A., Hougen, H. P., *et al.* (1992). T-lymphocyte subsets in oral mucosa of patients with recurrent aphthous ulceration. *Journal of Oral Pathology and Medicine*, **21**, 176–80.

Pedersen, A., Klausen, B., *et al.* (1991). Peripheral lymphocyte subpopulations in recurrent aphthous ulceration. *Acta Odontologica Scandinavica*, **49**, 203–6.

Pedersen, A., Madsen, H. O., *et al.* (1993). Varicella-zoster virus DNA in recurrent aphthous ulcers. *Scandinavian Journal of Dental Research*, **101**, 311–3.

Pedersen, A. and Ryder, L. P. (1994). Gamma delta T-cell fraction of peripheral blood is increased in recurrent aphthous ulceration. *Clinical Immunology and Immunopathology*, **72**, 98–104.

Plauth, M., Jenss, H., *et al.* (1991). Oral manifestations of Crohn's disease. An analysis of 79 cases. *Journal of Clinical Gastroenterology*, **13**, 29–37.

Porter, S. R., Barker, G. R., *et al.* (1997). Serum IgG antibodies to Helicobacter pylori in patients with recurrent aphthous stomatitis and other oral disorders. *Oral Surgery, Oral Medicine, Oral Pathology, Oral Radiology, and Endodontics*, **83**, 325–8.

Rehberger, A., Puspok, A., *et al.* (1998). Crohn's disease masquerading as aphthous ulcers. *European Journal of Dermatology*, **8**, 274–6.

Reimer, G., Luckner, L., *et al.* (1983). Direct immunofluorescence in recurrent aphthous ulcers and Behcet's disease. *Dermatologica*, **167**, 293–8.

Richards, D. W., MacPhail, L. A., *et al.* (1996). Expression of laminin 5, fibronectin, and epithelium-associated integrins in recurrent aphthous ulcers. *Journal of Dental Research*, **75**, 1512–7.

Rigas, B. and Levine, L. (1983). Concentrations of arachidonic-acid metabolites in human mixed saliva are independent of flow rate. *Archives of Oral Biology*, **28**, 1135–7.

Rizzi, R., Bruno, S., *et al.* (1997). Behcet's disease: an immune-mediated vasculitis involving vessels of all sizes. *International Journal of Clinical and Laboratory Research*, **27**, 225–32.

Robinson, N. D. and Guitart, J. (2003). Recalcitrant, recurrent aphthous stomatitis treated with etanercept. *Archives of Dermatology*, **139**, 1259–62.

Rodu, B. and Mattingly, G. (1992). Oral mucosal ulcers: diagnosis and management. *Journal of the American Dental Association*, **123**, 83–6.

Rodu, B. and Russell, C. M. (1988). Performance of a hydroxypropyl cellulose film former in normal and ulcerated oral mucosa. *Oral Surgery, Oral Medicine, Oral Pathology*, **65**, 699–703.

Rodu, B., Russell, C. M., *et al.* (1988). Clinical and chemical properties of a novel mucosal bioadhesive agent. *Journal of Oral Pathology*, **17**, 564–7.

Rogers, R. S., 3rd (1997). Recurrent aphthous stomatitis: clinical characteristics and associated systemic disorders. *Seminars in Cutaneous Medicine and Surgery*, **16**, 278–83.

Sallay, K. and Banoczy, J. (1968). Remarks on the possibilities of the simultaneous occurrence of hyperkeratosis of the mucous membrane and recurrent aphthae. *Oral Surgery, Oral Medicine, and Oral Pathology*, **25**, 171–175.

Sanchez, A. R., Rogers, 3rd, R. S., *et al.* (2005). Oral ulcerations are associated with the loss of response to infliximab in Crohn's disease. *Journal of Oral Pathology and Medicine*, **34**, 53–5.

Saulsbury, F. T. and Wispelwey, B. (2005). Tumor necrosis factor receptor-associated periodic syndrome in a young adult who had features of periodic fever, aphthous stomatitis, pharyngitis, and adenitis as a child. *Journal of Pediatrics*, **146**, 283–5.

Savage, N. W., Seymour, G. J., *et al.* (1985). T-lymphocyte subset changes in recurrent aphthous stomatitis. *Oral Surgery, Oral Medicine, Oral Pathology*, **60**, 175–81.

Schroeder, H. E., Muller-Glauser, W., *et al.* (1983). Stereologic analysis of leukocyte infiltration in oral ulcers of developing Mikulicz aphthae. *Oral Surgery, Oral Medicine, Oral Pathology*, **56**, 629–40.

Schroeder, H. E., Muller-Glauser, W., *et al.* (1984). Pathomorphologic features of the ulcerative stage of oral aphthous ulcerations. *Oral Surgery, Oral Medicine, Oral Pathology*, **58**, 293–305.

Sedghizadeh, P. P., Shuler, C. F., *et al.* (2002). Celiac disease and recurrent aphthous stomatitis: a report and review of the literature. *Oral Surgery, Oral Medicine, Oral Pathology, Oral Radiology, and Endodontics*, **94**, 474–8.

Seedat, Y. K. (1979). Aphthous ulcers of mouth from captopril [letter]. *Lancet*, **2**, 1297–8.

Shapiro, S., Olson, D. L., *et al.* (1970). The association between smoking and aphthous ulcers. *Oral Surgery, Oral Medicine, Oral Pathology*, **30**, 624–30.

Ship, II (1966). Socioeconomic status and recurrent aphthous ulcers. *Journal of the American Dental Association*, **73**, 120–3.

Ship, II (1972). Epidemiologic aspects of recurrent aphthous ulcerations. *Oral Surgery, Oral Medicine, Oral Pathology*, **33**, 400–6.

Shotts, R. H., Scully, C., *et al.* (1999). Nicorandil-induced severe oral ulceration: a newly recognized drug reaction. *Oral Surgery, Oral Medicine, Oral Pathology, Oral Radiology, and Endodontics*, **87**, 706–7.

Sibley, W. K. (1899). Ulcus neuroticum mucosae oris. *British Medical Journal*, **1**, 900.

Sircus, W., Church, R., *et al.* (1957). Recurrent aphthous ulcerations of the mouth. *Quarterly Journal of Medicine*, **26**, 235–249.

Solomon, L. W., Aguirre, A., *et al.* (2003). Chronic ulcerative stomatitis: clinical, histopathologic, and immunopathologic findings. *Oral Surgery, Oral Medicine, Oral Pathology, Oral Radiology, and Endodontics*, **96**, 718–26.

Sun, A., Chu, C. T., *et al.* (1991). Mechanisms of depressed natural killer cell activity in recurrent aphthous ulcers. *Clinical Immunology and Immunopathology*, **60**, 83–92.

Sutton, J. L. (1911). Periadenitis mucosa necrotica recurrens. *Journal of Cutaneous Disease*, **29**, 65–71.

Taylor, L. J., Bagg, J., *et al.* (1992). Increased production of tumour necrosis factor by peripheral blood leukocytes in patients with recurrent oral aphthous ulceration. *Journal of Oral Pathology and Medicine*, **21**, 21–5.

Taylor, L. J., Walker, D. M., *et al.* (1993). A clinical trial of prostaglandin E2 in recurrent aphthous ulceration. *British Dental Journal*, **175**, 125–9.

Thomas, K. T. and Edwards, K. M. (1999). Periodic fever syndrome. *Pediatric Infectious Disease Journal*, **18**, 68–9.

Tseng, S., Pak, G., *et al.* (1996). Rediscovering thalidomide: a review of its mechanism of action, side effects, and potential uses. *Journal of the American Academy of Dermatology*, **35**, 969–79.

van Dijk, A. P., Meijssen, M. A., *et al.* (1998). Transdermal nicotine inhibits interleukin 2 synthesis by mononuclear cells derived from healthy volunteers. *European Journal of Clinical Investigation*, **28**, 664–71.

Vicente, M., Soria, A., *et al.* (1996). Immunoglobulin G subclass measurements in recurrent aphthous stomatitis. *Journal of Oral Pathology and Medicine*, **25**, 538–40.

Victoria, J. M., Correia-Silva Jde, F., *et al.* (2005). Serotonin transporter gene polymorphism (5-HTTLPR) in patients with recurrent aphthous stomatitis. *Journal of Oral Pathology and Medicine*, **34**, 494–7.

Wahba-Yahav, A. V. (1995). Pentoxifylline in intractable recurrent aphthous stomatitis: an open trial. *Journal of the American Academy of Dermatology*, **33**, 680–2.

Weathers, D. R. and Griffin, J. W. (1970). Intraoral ulcerations of recurrent herpes simplex and recurrent aphthae: two distinct clinical entities. *Journal of the American Dental Association*, **81**, 81–7.

Worle, B., Wollenberg, A., *et al.* (1997). Chronic ulcerative stomatitis. *British Journal of Dermatology*, **137**, 262–5.

Wray, D. (1981). Gluten-sensitive recurrent aphthous stomatitis. *Digestive Diseases and Sciences*, **26**, 737–40.

Wright, N. A., Pike, C., *et al.* (1990). Induction of a novel epidermal growth factor-secreting cell lineage by mucosal ulceration in human gastrointestinal stem cells. *Nature*, **343**, 82–5.

Wu-Wang, C. Y., Patel, M., *et al.* (1995). Decreased levels of salivary prostaglandin E2 and epidermal growth factor in recurrent aphthous stomatitis. *Archives of Oral Biology*, **40**, 1093–8.

CHAPTER 12

Ocular manifestations of systemic vasculitis

Sumru Onal and C. Stephen Foster

Blood vessel inflammation and necrosis are the main pathological features associated with vasculitis. The vasculitides include a wide range of heterogeneous disorders in which specific vessels in the body are the target of an abnormal immune response causing pathological changes. The term vasculitis is used to describe inflammation and resultant damage of the vascular endothelium with consequent necrosis of the blood vessel wall. This may lead to vessel destruction or occlusion and local ischemia to the affected organs. For this reason, the clinical features of the vasculitides vary immensely and are dependent on the site, type, size, and distribution of the vessels involved by the inflammatory process.

Vasculitides also affect the vessels of the eye, sometimes as the initial presentation. The ocular manifestations of the disease may be the feature that leads the patient to seek medical care, and the eye may be one of the most exquisitely sensitive indications for ominous, otherwise silent, subclinical disease activity. Ocular signs of systemic vasculitides present in many forms, including proptosis; orbititis; conjunctivitis; episcleritis; scleritis; peripheral ulcerative keratitis; retinal vasculitis; uveitis; and neuro-ophthalmologic disease. Prompt recognition and association of ocular symptoms with a diagnosis of systemic vasculitis can be life-saving. Diagnosis and institution of appropriate therapy will help to control the ocular disease and, more importantly, the systemic disease.

Ophthalmic examination can be vital in the diagnosis and treatment of systemic vasculitis. The ophthalmologist will be involved in the evaluation of patients with vasculitis who present for the first time with ocular symptoms or who are referred with a known diagnosis of vasculitis for an ophthalmic examination and determination of disease activity and extension. In patients presenting for the first time with only ocular symptoms, the role of the ophthalmologist is crucial in making a diagnosis or providing the internist with the information necessary to create a focused differential diagnosis and treatment plan. The ophthalmic evaluation of patients with a known vasculitis is of value in their management.

A complete ophthalmic evaluation should include a detailed medical history, with history of present illness, past medical history, and a thorough review of systems, in addition to the ocular history. The patient's previous history of infection, neoplasm, drug-sensitivity, and rheumatological disease must be especially carefully elicited in an effort to distinguish between primary and secondary vasculitis. The ophthalmic examination must be complemented with the examination of the skin, joints, extremities, nasal and oral mucosa, and neurologic system to determine the systemic extension of the disease.

Classification

The Chapel Hill Conference in 1992 revised criteria and created uniform terminology to name, define, classify, and diagnose the systemic vasculitides, including immunodiagnostic markers and histological characteristics specific for some of the diseases (Jennette *et al.* 1994) (see Table 26.2 in Chapter 26). Classification of vasculitis syndromes is discussed in Chapter 1. The anatomic classification of the vessels is as follows. Large vessel refers to the aorta and the largest branches directed towards major body regions namely the extremities and the head and neck. Medium-sized vessel refers to the main visceral arteries such as the renal, hepatic, coronary, and mesenteric arteries. Finally, small vessel refers to venules, capillaries, arterioles, and the intraparenchymal distal arterial radicals that connect the arterioles. Some small and large vessel vasculitides may involve medium-sized arteries, but large- and medium-sized vessel vasculitides do not involve vessels smaller than arteries.

There is a group of secondary vasculitides that are caused by exogenous factors that have the capacity to trigger a vasculitic process. These secondary vasculitides include those due to infections or neoplasm, and drug-induced vasculitis. Secondary vasculitis also occurs in certain autoimmune disorders, such as systemic lupus erythematosus, Behçet's disease, and sarcoidosis.

Systemic lupus erythematosus is an autoimmune disorder characterized by the production of numerous autoantibodies. Systemic clinical manifestations are diverse and include cutaneous disease, arthritis, renal involvement, cardiac involvement, neuropsychiatric manifestations, and hematologic abnormalities. Ocular manifestations of the disease include eyelid lesions of discoid lupus erythematosus; episcleritis; scleritis; keratoconjunctivitis sicca; keratopathy; uveitis; retinal and choroidal microangiopathy; retinal vasculitis; papillitis; and neuro-ophthalmic disease (Uy and Chan 2002; Poole and Graham 1999).

Behçet's syndrome (BS) is an inflammatory disorder of unknown cause characterized by oral and genital ulceration associated with uveitis, skin lesions, neurologic complications, and arthritis (Chapter 35). The underlying pathology in BS is an obliterative and necrotizing vasculitis that affects both the arteries and the veins in all organ systems (Mochizuki *et al.* 1996). The frequency of ocular involvement in patients with BS is around 70% (Mochizuki *et al.* 1996). The typical form of ocular involvement is a relapsing remitting uveitis of explosive nature. Less commonly it may present in the form of conjunctivitis; conjunctival ulcers; keratitis; episcleritis; scleritis; and extraocular muscle paralysis from neurologic involvement of Behçet's syndrome (Matsuo *et al.* 2002; Colvard *et al.* 1977; Zamir *et al.* 2003). Uveitis may involve the anterior or posterior segment or more commonly both. The mean age at onset of uveitis is around 30 years. Males are more frequently involved with an earlier disease onset and more severe ocular disease. The most frequent type of ocular involvement is panuveitis with retinal vasculitis and vitritis. Other manifestations are retinitis, hypopyon uveitis, and papillitis (Tugal-Tutkun *et al.* 2004). Retinal vascular occlusions are particularly associated with Behçet's syndrome. Branch retinal vein occlusions or even central retinal vein occlusions are more common in Behçet's syndrome than in any other retinal vasculitis (Chee 1998).

Sarcoidosis is a multisystem systemic disease characterized by non-caseating granulomatous infiltration of affected tissues and occasionally vasculitis (see Chapter 42). The frequency of ocular involvement in sarcoidosis ranges from 26% to 50%. Anterior segment pathology is the most common ocular manifestation and can be seen in 85% of patients with ocular sarcoidosis. Anterior segment findings are granulomas and cicatrizing conjunctivitis; anterior uveitis, usually granulomatous and chronic; iris nodules; band keratopathy; and scleritis. The posterior segment may be involved in 25% of patients with ocular sarcoidosis and include vitritis, intermediate uveitis, posterior uveitis, and panuveitis. Periphlebitis is a hallmark, although not pathognomonic, of sarcoidosis and may be associated with yellow perivenous exudates. Other manifestations include choroidal nodules and exudative retinal detachment, which may result in ocular phthisis (loss of function and shrinkage in size of the eye) (Stavrou and Foster 2002; Poole and Graham 1999).

Ocular manifestations of the primary systemic vasculitides

Small-vessel vasculitis

Wegener's granulomatosis (WG)

Clinical manifestations

Wegener's granulomatosis is an autoimmune vasculitis that affects small arteries and veins (see Chapters 30, 31, and 32). Sites including the eye and orbit may be affected by vasculitis, producing clinically obvious inflammation. Ocular involvement does not differ in frequency or severity between classic and limited WG (Stavrou *et al.* 1993).

Ocular manifestations

The incidence of ocular involvement in WG ranges between 29% and 58%, and it has been shown to be the presenting feature in 15% of patients (Bullen *et al.* 1983; Fauci *et al.* 1983). WG can affect any ocular or periocular tissue. The eye may be secondarily involved due to contiguous granulomatous paranasal sinus disease, which can cause orbital inflammation; obstruction of the nasolacrimal duct; ocular muscle involvement; and optic neuropathy. In addition, WG may present as dacryoadenitis, dacryocystitis, and eyelid

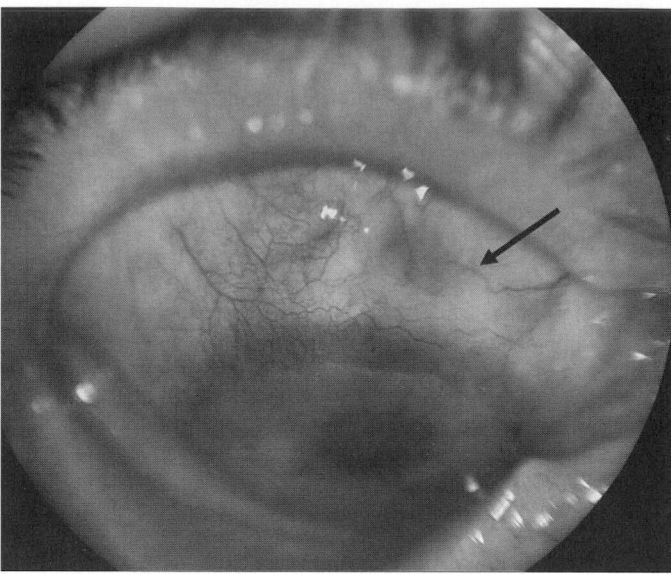

Figure 12.1 Peripheral ulcerative keratitis involving the superior peripheral cornea, arrow showing an area of sclera and peripheral cornea with ischemia and non-perfusion. (See Color Plate 56.)

granulomas (Bullen *et al.* 1983; Holds *et al.* 1989; Kopstein *et al.* 1999). Patients may develop peripheral ulcerative keratitis; corneal granuloma; episcleritis; necrotizing scleritis; or uveitis (Perez *et al.* 2004). Retinitis, occlusive retinal vasculitis, choroiditis, posterior scleritis, and ischemic optic neuritis have also been reported. Horner's syndrome, cranial nerve palsy, and cavernous sinus thrombosis are the neuro-ophthalmologic presentations of WG (Perez *et al.* 2004); however, the optic nerve, retina, and the uveal tract may be less frequently involved (Jampol *et al.* 1978; Bullen *et al.* 1983; Jaben and Norton 1982).

Peripheral ulcerative keratitis (Figure 12.1) and necrotizing scleritis (Figure 12.2), often bilateral, are common lesions and peripheral

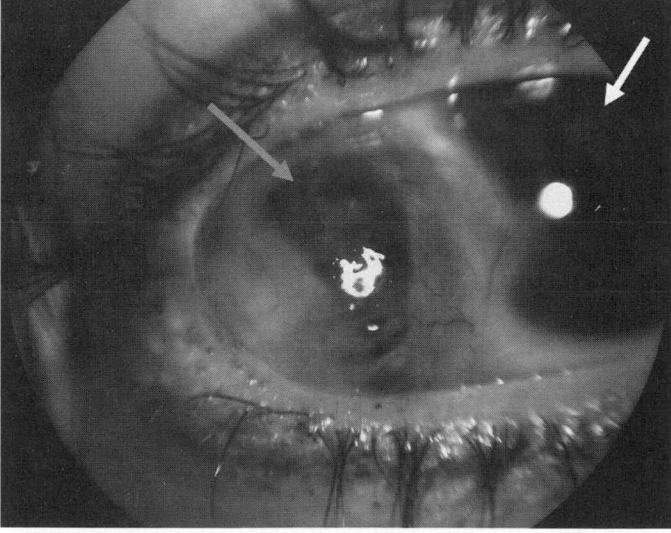

Figure 12.2 Sequelae of necrotizing scleritis in a patient with Wegener's granulomatosis. Red arrow shows a large area of scleral loss with uveal show that is covered only with a thin layer of overlying epithelium. White arrow points to the cornea and the anterior chamber. (See Color Plate 57.)

ulcerative keratitis, necrotizing scleritis, or both are reported with increasing frequency as the initial clinical sign of WG (Foster 2004). Focal ocular involvement of the peripheral cornea and sclera, in contrast to contiguous involvement, is caused by a small-vessel vasculitis of the intrascleral portions of the anterior cilliary arteries or perilimbal arteries or both (Austin *et al.* 1978; Cogan 1955; Frayer 1960). The peripheral ulcerative keratitis is frequently preceded by localized conjunctivitis or episcleritis, followed by the onset of true scleritis and paralimbal infiltrates which lead to epithelial and stromal necrosis with subsequent furrow-like ulceration. The crescentic peripheral corneal ulcer may extend concentrically to form a ring ulcer or may progress centrally. Scleral inflammation is invariably present, ranging from redness to localized necrotizing scleritis. The biomicroscopic appearance of the ulcer may be quite similar to that of Mooren's ulcer, except that the sclera is never involved in the latter.

Most patients with WG are cANCA positive. A specificity of approximately 90% has been claimed for cANCA in biopsy-proven WG (van der Woude *et al.* 1985). The sensitivity of the cANCA is close to 100% for patients with active generalized disease (Nölle *et al.* 1989). In the limited form of the disease pANCA may be prominent (Soukiasian *et al.* 1992). In general, ANCA titers have imperfect correlation with the disease activity. Power and associates have demonstrated that a relapse of scleritis is not preceded by a significant rise in ANCA titer. Following treatment, a failure of ANCA titers to return to normal levels may be associated with relapse in patients with limited ophthalmic WG (Power *et al.* 1995).

The corneal and scleral destruction progresses, often slowly but relentlessly, in spite of medical and surgical ocular treatment: topical and systemic glucocorticoids are notably ineffective. WG-associated peripheral ulcerative keratitis and necrotizing scleritis resolve only after institution of systemic immunosuppressive therapy (Foster 2004).

Churg–Strauss syndrome (CSS)
Clinical manifestations
CSS, initially described as allergic granulomatosis and angiitis, is a systemic "allergic" disease characterized by eosinophil-rich granulomatous inflammation involving the respiratory tract, and necrotizing vasculitis affecting small- to medium-sized vessels (Jennette *et al.* 1994) (see Chapter 33). ANCA (usually pANCA) are detected in approximately 50% of patients with CSS (Seo and Stone 2004). The presence of ANCA was shown to more closely correlate with ischemic vasculitic type of ocular involvement, which includes amaurosis fugax, ischemic optic neuropathy, central retinal artery occlusion, and branch retinal vein occlusion, than with manifestations of orbital inflammation. A positive ANCA may also be a risk factor for sudden visual loss even in patients with no established ocular involvement (Takanashi *et al.* 2001).

Ocular manifestations
CSS can present with various ocular manifestations, but this is rare. Multiple ocular lesions have been reported: orbital inflammatory pseudotumor; conjunctival granuloma; episcleritis; peripheral ulcerative keratitis; uveitis; uveoscleritis; amaurosis fugax; retinal artery occlusion; ischemic optic neuropathy; and multifocal choroidal ischemia (Takanashi *et al.* 2001). Patients with CSS may also have cranial nerve neuropathies, especially oculomotor nerve palsy and superior oblique palsy (Weinstein *et al.* 1983).

Microscopic polyangiitis (MPA)
Clinical manifestations
MPA is characterized by a systemic necrotizing vasculitis affecting small vessels (see Chapter 27).

Ocular manifestations
Although MPA can affect all ocular and orbital tissues, the most common ocular finding of the disease is peripheral ulcerative keratitis. A peripheral ulcerative keratitis morphologically similar to Mooren's ulcer has been observed as the presenting manifestation. Involvement of the adjacent sclera clearly distinguishes peripheral ulcerative keratitis in WG, polyarteritis nodosa, microscopic polyangiitis, or CSS syndrome from Mooren's ulcer. Although ocular and systemic signs and symptoms usually coincide, ocular findings can precede the onset of systemic disease. Hence ocular inflammation may be the presenting clinical manifestation of MPA, leading the patient to seek medical attention initially from an ophthalmologist (Foster 1980; Lhote *et al.* 1996; Wise 1951). Darlington and associates described a healthy 16-year-old girl who presented with unilateral peripheral ulcerative keratitis and 5 months later experienced renal failure. Renal biopsy and serologic tests confirmed the diagnosis of MPA (Darlington *et al.* 2001). Milhara and associates reported two patients with MPA and different presentations: one of the patients with hypopyon uveitis and cotton wool spots in one eye, and the other with bilateral scleritis associated with peripheral ulcerative keratitis (Milhara *et al.* 2004). MPA with eyelid and conjunctival involvement has also been reported (Caster *et al.* 1996). Biopsy of the conjunctival nodule was consistent with non-granulomatous small-vessel vasculitis. Patients with retinal vasculitis due to MPA have also been described (Akova *et al.* 1993; Gallagher *et al.* 2004).

Henoch–Schönlein purpura (HSP)
Clinical manifestations
Henoch–Schönlein purpura (HSP), also known as anaphylactoid purpura, is an acute vasculitis that most commonly affects children (Saulsbury 1999) (see Chapter 40).

Ocular manifestations
Involvement of the eye is a rare complication of HSP (Saulsbury 2001). Recurrent episcleritis was the first ocular manifestation to be described. This correlated in one patient with her skin and joint symptoms, all of which responded simultaneously to systemic treatment with prednisone. The other two reported ocular manifestations of HSP are anterior uveitis and keratitis (Yamabe 1988).

Cryoglobulinemic vasculitis
Clinical manifestations
Cryoglobulinemia has been defined most succinctly as the presence of circulating immunoglobulins that precipitate at temperatures below 37°C and redissolve on rewarming (Meltzer *et al.* 1966; Brouet *et al.* 1974; Gorevic *et al.* 1980; Gorevic and Frangione 1991; Ferri *et al.* 1991) (see Chapter 41).

Ocular manifestations
Corneal deposits of immunoglobulins have been observed in essential mixed cryoglobulinemia. When vision is disturbed, superficial keratectomy and excimer laser phototherapeutic keratectomy have been reported to be successful in its management (Kremer and Blumenthal 1997; Kremer *et al.* 1989). Posterior segment involvement has also been described in essential mixed

cryoglobulinemia: Purtscher-like retinopathy, retinal vasculitis, and serous retinal and retinal pigment epithelium detachment (Cohen *et al.* 1996; Myers *et al.* 2001; Treister and Machemer 1977).

Cutaneous small-vessel vasculitis (CSVV)
Clinical manifestations
Cutaneous small-vessel vasculitis, also known as cutaneous leukocytoclastic vasculitis, hypersensitivity vasculitis, allergic vasculitis, and necrotizing vasculitis, is an immune complex-mediated, neutrophil-induced, small-vessel vasculitis (Jennette *et al.* 1994) (see Chapter 39).

Ocular manifestations
Eye lesions in patients with CSVV occur rarely. One report identified a patient with biopsy-proven CSVV limited to the skin, with bilateral anterior uveitis and "mutton-fat" keratitic precipitates (Corwin and Baum 1982). The uveitis occurred after the onset of the skin manifestations and it responded to topical and systemic glucocorticoids. Tsai and associates described a patient with CSVV and limited skin involvement who presented with panuveitis and active multifocal retinitis and vasculitis (Tsai *et al.* 1993). Fluorescein angiography was characteristic of vasculitis, and an extensive workup ruled out a systemic condition. Treatment with systemic glucocorticoids was sufficient to control skin and ocular symptoms.

Ocular involvement has been reported in a few patients with erythema elevatum diutinum (see Chapter 42). Casanova and associates described a 64-year-old man with an unusual granulomatous pattern of erythema elevatum diutinum associated with autoimmune keratolysis (Casanova *et al.* 2001). The patient presented with bilateral superior corneal melting with perforation in the left eye. Histopathologic examination of the conjunctiva was consistent with granulomatous vasculitis with neutrophilic infiltrates, giant cells, and fibroblastic proliferation. Shimazaki and associates reported a 27-year-old woman with Terrien marginal degeneration and erythema elevatum diutinum (Shimazaki *et al.* 1998). Takiwaki and associates noted peripheral ulcerative keratitis and erythema elevatum diutinum in three patients. All three had high titers of rheumatoid factor. Both peripheral ulcerative keratitis and the skin disease were successfully controlled with dapsone (Takiwaki *et al.* 1998). Similarly, Aldave and associates described erythema elevatum diutinum associated with peripheral keratitis that responded well to dapsone (Aldave *et al.* 2003). Mitamura and associates (Mitamura *et al.* 2004) reported a 22-year-old woman with nodular scleritis and panuvetis and erythema elevatum diutinum in whom skin and ocular disease were treated with systemic diaminodiphenyl sulfone and glucocorticoids.

Medium-sized vessel vasculitis

Polyarteritis nodosa (PAN)
Clinical manifestations
PAN is a rare, subacute or chronic disorder characterized by focal and episodic necrotizing inflammation of the wall of medium-sized muscular arteries (see Chapter 26).

Ocular manifestations
Ocular involvement is present in 10–20% of patients with PAN and it can be the first manifestation (Perez *et al.* 2004). Anterior segment signs of PAN include: conjunctival infarction; keratoconjunctivitis sicca; episcleritis; scleritis; and sclerokeratitis. Necrotizing scleritis, often associated with peripheral ulcerative keratitis, is the

most frequent type of scleritis in patients with PAN. The scleritis is extremely painful and destructive unless the correct diagnosis is made and control of the underlying disease has been achieved. The peripheral ulcerative keratitis is progressive, both circumferentially and centrally, with undermining of the central edge of the ulcer that results in an overhanging lip of the cornea; however, scleral involvement helps to distinguish Mooren's ulcer from the sclerokeratitis associated with systemic vasculitides (Messmer and Foster 1999; Soheilian 2002). Cogan's syndrome has also been described in association with PAN (Gilbert and Talbot 1969).

Involvement of the iris vasculature may produce acute, nongranulomatous iritis as well as vitritis. Diffuse bilateral nongranulomatous panuveitis associated with retinal vasculitis has also been described in PAN. The most common ocular findings in polyarteritis nodosa are choroidal and retinal vasculitis (Figure 12.3). Choroidal vasculitis is the most common histologic abnormality; the presence of yellow subretinal patches is less often appreciated clinically (Perez *et al.* 2004; Soheilian 2002; Morgan *et al.* 1986). Choroidal infarcts and exudative retinal detachments occur secondary to involvement of posterior ciliary arteries and choroidal vessels (Cynthia *et al.* 2001; Perez *et al.* 2004); choroidal vascular insufficiency can also produce transient ischemic attacks. Elschnig spots scattered throughout the posterior pole result from choroidal ischemia secondary to poor perfusion of the affected areas of the choroid. The presence of Elschnig spots is not specific for PAN; they can occur in a variety of systemic vasculitic syndromes, but their presence is an ominous prognostic sign (Klien 1968). Subhyaloid hemorrhage; retinal hemorrhages; edema; lipid exudates; cotton-wool spots; marked irregularity of the caliper of retinal vessels, and exudative retinal detachment have all been described as has vascular occlusion (particularly central retinal artery occlusion) (Soheilian 2002; Cynthia *et al.* 2001).

Orbital involvement may produce exophthalmos or pseudotumor as a result of inflammation of the orbital vessels (Soheilian 2002). Optic nerve involvement takes several different forms, such as papilledema or papillitis due to optic nerve vasculitis. In one study, papilledema was present in 10% of patients (Ford and Siekert 1965; Soheilian 2002). Arteritis of the posterior ciliary vessels with intermittent choroidal vascular insufficiency may be responsible for recurrent episodes of monocular constrictions of the visual field with sparing of central vision. Other neuro-ophthalmologic

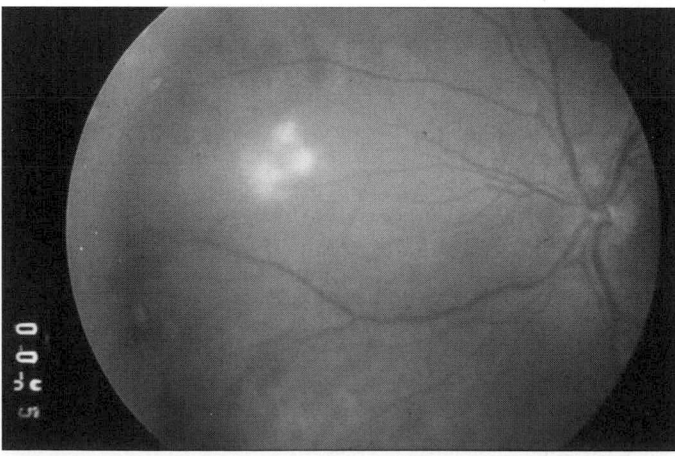

Figure 12.3 Perivascular exudation indicating retinal vasculitis in a patient with polyarteritis nodosa. (See Color Plate 58.)

findings of the disease may evolve secondary to vasculitic involvement of the central or peripheral nervous system manifesting as third, fifth, sixth, and seventh nerve palsies; hemianopia; nystagmus; amaurosis fugax; diplopia; and Horner syndrome (Ford and Siekert 1965; Soheilian 2002).

Kawasaki's disease (KD)
Clinical manifestations
KD, also known as acute infantile febrile mucocutaneous lymph node syndrome, affects infants and young children (see Chapter 29).

Ocular manifestations
Self-limited conjunctivitis is the most frequent, if not constant, feature of KD. In addition, bilateral iridocyclitis; superficial punctate keratitis; vitreous opacity; papilledema; orbital myositis; and extraocular muscle palsy have been described (Bligard 1987; Lin et al. 1999; Sheard et al. 2000; Ohno et al. 1982; Jacob et al. 1982). Dacryocystitis has been reported as late sequelae of KD (Mauriello et al. 1986). In a post-mortem study, inner retinal ischemia has been documented (Font et al. 1983).

Large-vessel vasculitis

Giant cell arteritis (GCA)
Clinical manifestations
GCA is a systemic necrotizing vasculitis with a predilection for large- and medium-sized vessels, most commonly of the head and neck (Barchuk et al.1997; Poole and Graham 1999; Zaman et al. 1997; Bhatti and Tabandeh 2001) (see Chapter 24). GCA is usually, but not always, preceded by systemic symptoms. Hayreh et al. noted that about 50% of patients had both ocular and extraocular symptoms, whereas 21.2% presented with ocular involvement only (occult giant cell arteritis) (Hayreh et al. 1998b).

Ocular manifestations
GCA is an ophthalmic emergency, since it can rapidly progress to unilateral or bilateral, profound and permanent vision loss (Tovilla-Canales 1998). In a series of 170 patients with biopsy-proven GCA, 50% presented with ocular involvement (Hayreh et al. 1998a). Ocular symptoms were visual loss of varying severity in 83 (97.7%), amaurosis fugax in 26 (30.6%), diplopia in five (5.9%), and eye pain in seven (8.2%). Ocular ischemic lesions consisted of arteritic anterior ischemic optic neuropathy in 69 (81.2%); central retinal artery occlusion in 12 (14.1%); cilioretinal artery occlusion in 12 (of 55 patients with satisfactory fluorescein angiography [21.8%]); posterior ischemic optic neuropathy in six (7.1%); and ocular ischemia in one (1.2%) (Hayreh et al. 1998a). Permanent visual loss often was preceded for several days or weeks by systemic or transient visual symptoms (Hayreh et al. 1998a; Font et al. 1997). If untreated, unilateral visual loss may progress to bilateral involvement within days to weeks. Bilateral loss of vision occurs in approximately one-third of patients with GCA (Hayreh et al. 1998a). Permanent visual loss is more frequent in patients with transient visual loss, transient diplopia, and jaw claudication (Cid et al. 1998; Gonzalez-Gay et al. 1998, 2000). Transient visual loss may be the harbinger of permanent visual loss in as many as 50% of patients (Gonzalez-Gay et al. 2000). Cerebrovascular accidents caused by GCA are more frequently associated with permanent visual loss or jaw claudication (Gonzalez-Gay et al. 1998, 2000). The risk of ischemic complications appears to be higher in the absence of constitutional symptoms and blunted inflammatory response as evidenced by lower ESR, suggesting that patients with a paucity of systemic signs and symptoms (occult GCA) are at a higher risk for ocular involvement and visual loss (Cid et al. 1998).

In most patients the cause of visual loss is anterior ischemic optic neuropathy. Pallid or chalky white swelling of the optic nerve head is highly suggestive of GCA, representing infarction of the optic nerve head caused by severe vasculitis (Hayreh et al. 1998a). Arteritic anterior ischemic optic neuropathy occurs in 81–94% of GCA patients. Other causes of visual loss include posterior ischemic optic neuropathy; central retinal artery occlusion; choroidal ischemia; and posterior visual pathway infarctions. Ocular motility disturbances reflect ischemia of extraocular muscles, ocular motor nerves, or the brainstem (Ghanchi and Dutton 1997).

Takayasu's arteritis (TA)
Clinical manifestations
Takayasu's arteritis was first described by Takayasu in 1908 (see Chapter 25).

Ocular manifestations
Ophthalmic manifestations of TA include visual disturbance (35%) and transient blindness (8%) (Kerr et al. 1994). Amaurosis fugax may be related to transient retinal, choroidal, or optic nerve ischemia of an embolic nature, or more likely of hemodynamic origin due to obliteration of the carotid arteries. In mild ocular ischemia, retinal vessels develop generalized vasodilation with capillary microaneurysms. As the disease advances, arteriovenous anastomosis, capillary dropout, and eventually complications such as cataract, neovascular glaucoma, vitreous hemorrhages, retinal detachment, and optic atrophy can develop. Fluorescein angiograpy may show acute retinal and choroidal hypoperfusion, in particular, the arm-to-retina circulation time can be prolonged. Delayed arteriovenous filling time on the fluorescein angiogram is mainly an indicator of chronic, moderate to severe retinal ischemia. Disease of the descending aorta may lead to hypertension of the upper extremities, and eventually hypertensive retinopathy. In a series of 78 patients with Takayasu arteritis, hypertensive retinopathy was found in approximately 30% (Chun et al. 2001). Patients with Takayasu arteritis can also present with retinal vasculitis or anterior ischemic optic neuropathy. The latter is associated with a worse prognosis (Karam et al. 1999; Kiyosawa and Baba 1998).

Diagnostic approach to vasculitis in patients with inflammatory ocular disease

A comprehensive ocular and systemic history with extensive review of medical system is essential in the evaluation of all patients with ocular inflammatory disease as well as in patients with systemic vasculitides. A multidisciplinary approach is generally needed in the evaluation of a patient with vasculitis and should include specialists on internal medicine, dermatology, neurology, ophthalmology, radiology, otorhinolaryngology, and possibly other specialties.

Ophthalmoscopic evaluation of retinal vessels and fluorescein angiography can be extremely valuable in demonstrating the presence of retinal vasculitis. Three recent studies have addressed the issue of performing unilateral or bilateral temporal artery biopsies in patients with suspected GCA (Boyev et al. 1999; Danesh-Meyer et al. 2000; Pless et al. 2000). The probability of obtaining a positive result in the setting of a contralateral negative biopsy was determined to be 1 to 5%. Despite the relatively low added yield of performing bilateral biopsies, the argument has been made that because the risk of surgery is relatively small and the added diagnostic benefits profound, the technique should be considered in all patients strongly suspected to have giant cell arteritis (Miller 2000; Savino 2000). However, the final decision to perform bilateral biopsies should be made on a case-by-case basis (Lessell 2000).

In patients with ocular involvement, the ophthalmologist can provide useful and important specimens for analysis. Ocular tissues affected by vasculitis accessible for biopsy include the conjunctiva, sclera, and orbital tissue. Retina and choroid, which usually become available after enucleation or post-mortem, may also be available for histopathologic evaluation. In patients with necrotizing scleritis, the finding of necrotizing granuloma with or without inflammatory microangiopathy is very suggestive of WG even if classic necrotizing granulomatous vasculitis is not seen.

The diagnostic evaluation of patients with vasculitis should not be limited to searching only for systemic primary vasculitides. Secondary etiologies must be considered, specifically other autoimmune disorders and infectious diseases (see Chapters 24 and 42). One must remember that patients with vasculitis are at a high risk of rapidly developing life-threatening complications of systemic involvement; prompt diagnosis affords the initiation of appropriate systemic, life-saving treatment.

Treatment

See the chapters on individual diseases for detailed discussions of therapeutic approaches. The treatment of systemic vasculitis can be life-saving, but the medications employed for this purpose all have potential side-effects, some of which can be life-threatening. Consequently, the prescribing and monitoring of such medications must be performed by an individual who is, by virtue of training and experience, truly expert in such matters. Ophthalmologists lacking special training in this area must refer patients with systemic vasculitis to specialists familiar with use of chemotherapeutic immunosuppressive agents and monitoring for efficacy, toxicity, and complications. Conversely, the active participation of the ophthalmologist in monitoring the ocular manifestations of systemic vasculitis is essential to the care of the patient. Only the ophthalmologist can assess the degree of active inflammation, information critical in managing immunosuppressive therapy by a rheumatologist.

References

Akova, Y. A., Jabbur, N. S. and Foster, C. S. (1993). Ocular presentation of polyarteritis nodosa. Clinical course and management with steroid and cytotoxic therapy. *Ophthalmology*, **100**, 1775–81.

Aldave, A. J., Shih, J. L., Jovkar, S. and McLeod, S. D. (2003). Peripheral keratitis associated with erythema elevatum diutinum. *American Journal of Ophthalmology*, **135**, 389–90.

Austin, P., Green, W. R., Sallyer, D. C., Walsh, F. B. and Kleinfelter, H. T. (1978). Peripheral corneal degeneration and occlusive vasculitis in Wegener's granulomatosis. *American Journal of Ophthalmology*, **85**, 311–17.

Barchuk, W. T., Centeno, L.,. Frohman, L. and Bielory, L. (1997). Immunology and ocular manifestations of giant cell arteritis. *Ocular Immunology and Inflammation*, **5**, 141–6.

Bhatti, M. T. and Tabandeh, H. (2001). Giant cell arteritis: diagnosis and management. *Current Opinion in Ophthalmology*, **12**, 393–9.

Bligard, C. A. (1987). Kawasaki disease and its diagnosis. *Pediatric Dermatology*, **4**, 75–84.

Boyev, L. R., Miller, N. R. and Green, W. R. (1999). Efficacy of unilateral versus bilateral temporal artery biopsies for the diagnosis of giant cell arteritis. *American Journal of Ophthalmology*, **128**, 211–5.

Brouet, J. C., Clouvel, J. P., Danon, F., Klein, M. and Seligman, M. (1974). Biologic and clinical significance of cryoglobulins. *American Journal of Medicine*, **57**, 775–88.

Bullen, C. L., Liesegang, T. J., McDonald, T. J. and DeRemee, R. A. (1983). Ocular complications of Wegener's granulomatosis. *Ophthalmology*, **90**, 279–90.

Casanova, F. H.C., Meirelles, R. L., Tojar, M., Martins, N. C., Rigueiro, M. P. and de Freitas, D. (2001). Autoimmune keratolysis in a patient with leukocytoclastic vasculitis. *Cornea*, **20**, 329–32.

Caster, J. C., Shetlar, D. J., Pappolla, M. A. and Yee, R. W. (1996). Microscopic polyangiitis with ocular involvement. *Archives of Ophthalmology*, **114**, 346–8.

Chee, S. P. (1998). Retinal vasculitis associated with systemic disease. *Ophthalmology Clinics of North America*, **11**, 655.

Chun, Y. S., Park, S. J., Park, I. K., Chung, H. and Lee, J. (2001). The clinical and ocular manifestations of Takayasu arteritis. *Retina*, **21**, 132–40.

Cid, M. C., Font, C., Oristrell, J., *et al.*(1998). Association between strong inflammatory response and low risk of developing visual loss and other cranial ischemic complications in giant cell (temporal) arteritis. *Arthritis and Rheumatism*, **41**, 26–32.

Cogan, D. G. (1955). Corneoscleral lesions in periarteritis nodosa and Wegener's granulomatosis. *Transaction of the American Ophthalmological Society*, **53**, 321–44.

Cohen, S. M., Kokame, G. T. and Gass, J. D. (1996). Paraproteinemias associated with serous detachments of the retinal pigment epithelium and neurosensory retina. *Retina*, **16**, 467–73.

Colvard, D. M., Robertson, D. M. and O'Duffy, J. D. (1977). The ocular manifestations of Behçet's disease. *Archives of Ophthalmology*, **95**, 1813–7.

Corwin, J. M. and Baum, J. (1982). Iridocyclitis in two patients with hypocomplementemic cutaneous vasculitis. *American Journal of Ophthalmology*, **94**, 111–3.

Cynthia, T. H., Kerrison, J. B., Miller, N. R. and Goldberg, M. F. (2001). Choroidal infarction, anterior ischemic neuropathy, and central retinal artery occlusion from polyarteritis nodosa. *Retina*, **21**, 348–51.

Danesh-Meyer, H. V., Savino, P. J., Eagle, R. C. Jr, Kubis, K. C. and Sergott, R. C. (2000). Low diagnostic yield with second biopsies in suspected giant cell arteritis. *Journal of Neuroophthalmology*, **20**, 213–5.

Darlington, J. K., Mannis, M. J., Sefal, W. A., Feiz, V. and Klug, D. E. (2001). Peripheral nonulcerative keratitis as a presenting sign of microscopic polyangiitis. *Cornea*, **20**, 522.

Ewert, B. H., Jennette, J. C. and Falk, R. J. (1992). Anti-myeloperoxidase antibodies stimulate neutrophils to damage human endothelial cells. *Kidney International*, **41**, 373–83.

Fauci, A. S., Haynes, B. F., Katz, P. and Wolff, S. M. (1983). Wegener's granulomatosis: prospective clinical and therapeutic experience with 85 patients for 21 years. *Annals of Internal Medicine*, **98**, 76–85.

Ferri, C., Greco, F., Longombardo, G., *et al.* (1991). Antibodies to hepatitis C virus in patients with mixed cryoglobulinemia. *Arthritis and Rheumatism*, **34**, 1606–10.

Font, C., Cid, M. C., Coll-Vinent, B., *et al.* (1997). Clinical features in patients with permanent visual loss due to biopsy- proven giant cell arteritis. *British Journal of Rheumatology*, **36**, 251–4.

Font, R. L., Mehta, R. S., Streusand, S. B., *et al.* (1983). Bilateral retinal ischemia in Kawasaki disease. Postmortem findings and electron microscopic observations. *Ophthalmology*, **90**, 569–77.

Ford, R. G. and Siekert, R. G. (1965). Central nervous system manifestations of periarteritis nodosa. *Neurology*, **15**, 114.

Foster, C. S. (2004). Connective tissue/collagen vascular diseases. In *The Cornea* (eds Foster, C. S., Azar, D. T., and Dohlman, C. H.), pp. 515–50. Lippincott Williams and Wilkins.

Foster, C. S. (1980). Immunosuppressive therapy for external ocular inflammatory disease. *Ophthalmology*, **87**, 140–50.

Frayer, W. C. (1960). The histopathology of perilimbal ulceration in Wegener's granulomatosis. *Archives of Ophthalmology*, **64**, 58–64.

Frohnert, P. P. and Sheps, S. G. (1967). Long-term follow-up study of periarteritis nodosa. *American Journal of Medicine*, **43**, 8–14.

Gallagher, M. H., Ooi, K. G.J. and Thomas, M., *et al.* (2004). ANCA associated pauci-immune retinal vasculitis. *British Journal of Ophthalmology*, **89**, 608.

Ghanchi, F. D. and Dutton, G. N. (1997). Current concepts in giant cell (temporal) arteritis. *Survey of Ophthalmology*, **42**, 99–123.

Gilbert, W. S. and Talbot, F. J. (1969). Cogan's syndrome. Signs of polyarteritis nodosa and cerebral venous sinus thrombosis. *Archives of Ophthalmology*, **82**, 633.

Gonzalez-Gay, M. A., Blanco, R., Rodriguez-Valverde, V., *et al.* (1998). Permanent visual loss and cerebrovascular accidents in giant cell arteritis: predictors and response to treatment. *Arthritis and Rheumatism*, **41**, 1497–504.

Gonzalez-Gay, M. A., Garcia-Porrua, C., Llorca, J., *et al.* (2000). Visual manifestations of giant cell arteritis: trends and clinical spectrum in 161 patients. *Medicine* (Baltimore), **79**, 283–92.

Gorevic, P. D. and Frangione, B. (1991). Mixed cryoglobulinemia cross-reactive idiotypes: implication for relationship of MC to rheumatic and lymphoproliferative diseases. *Seminars on Hematology*, **28**, 79–94.

Gorevic, P. D., Kassab, H. J., Levo, Y., *et al.* (1980). Mixed cryoglobulinemia: clinical aspects and long-term follow-up of 40 patients. *American Journal of Medicine*, **69**, 287–308.

Hayreh, S. S., Podhajsky, P. A. and Zimmerman, B. (1998a). Ocular manifestations of giant cell arteritis. *American Journal of Ophthalmololgy*, **125**, 509–20.

Hayreh, S. S., Podhajsky, P. A. and Zimmerman, B. (1998b). Occult giant cell arteritis: ocular manifestations. *American Journal of Ophthalmology*, **125**, 521–6.

Holds, J. B., Anderson, R. L. and Wolin, M. J. (1989). Dacryocystectomy for the treatment of dacryocystitis patients with Wegener's granulomatosis. *Ophthalmic Surgery*, **20**, 443–4.

Jaben, S. L. and Norton, E. W. D. (1982). Exudative retinal detachment in Wegener's granulomatosis. *Annals of Ophthalmology*, **14**, 717.

Jacob, J. L., Polomeno, R. C., Chad, Z. and Lapointe, N. (1982). Ocular manifestations of Kawasaki disease (mucocutaneous lymph node syndrome). *Canadian Journal of Ophthalmology*, **17**, 199–202.

Jampol, L. M., West, C. and Goldberg, M. F. (1978). Therapy of scleritis with cytotoxic agents. *American Journal of Ophthalmology*, **86**, 266.

Jennette, J. C., Falk, R. J., Andrassy, K., *et al.* (1994). Nomenclature of systemic vasculitides. Proposal of an international consensus conference. *Arthritis and Rheumatism*, **37**, 187–92.

Karam, E. Z., Muci-Mendoza, R. and Hedges, T. R. (1999). Retinal findings in Takayasu's arteritis. *Acta Ophthalmologica Scandinavica*, **77**, 209–13.

Kerr, G. S., Hallahan, C. W., Giordano, J., *et al.* (1994). Takayasu arteritis. *Annals of Internal Medicine*, **120**, 919–29.

Kiyosawa, M. and Baba, T. (1998). Ophthalmological findings in patients with Takayasu disease. *International Journal of Cardiology*, **66** (Suppl.), S141–7.

Klien, B. A. (1968). Ischemic infarcts of the choroid (Elschinig spots). A cause of retinal separation in hypertensive disease with renal insufficiency. A clinical and histopathologic study. *American Journal of Ophthalmology*, **66**, 1069–74.

Kopstein, A. B., Kristopaitis, T., Gujrati, T. M., *et al.* (1999). Orbital Wegener granulomatosis without systemic findings. *Ophthalmic Plastic Reconstructive Surgery*, **15**, 467–9.

Kremer, I. and Blumenthal, M. (1997). Excimer phototherapeutic keratectomy for corneal subepithelial cryoglobulin deposits. *Journal of Cataract and Refractive Surgery*, **23**, 1119–21.

Kremer, I., Wright, P., Merin, S., *et al.* (1989). Corneal subepithelial monoclonal kappa IgG deposits in essential cryoglobulinaemia. *British Journal of Ophthalmology*, **73**, 669–73.

Lessell, S. (2000). Bilateral temporal artery biopsies in giant cell arteritis. *Journal of Neuroophthalmology*, **20**, 220–1.

Lhote, F., Cohen, P., Généreau, T., *et al.* (1996). Microscopic polyangiitis: clinical aspects and treatment. *Annales de Medicine Interne* (Paris), **147**, 165–77.

Lin, H., Burton, E. M. and Felz, M. W. (1999). Orbital myositis due to Kawasaki's disease. *Pediatric Radiology*, **29**, 634–6.

Matsuo, T., Itami, M. and Nakagawa, H. (2002). The incidence and pathology of conjunctival ulceration in Behçet's syndrome. *British Journal of Ophthalmology*, **86**, 140–3.

Mauriello, J. A., Stabile, C. and Wagner, R. S. (1986). Dacryocystitis following Kawasaki's disease. *Ophthalmic Plastic and Reconstructive Surgery*, **2**, 209–11.

Meltzer, M., Franklin, E. C., Elias, K., *et al.* (1966). Cryoglobulinemia: a clinical and laboratory study. II: Cryoglobulins with rheumatoid factor activity. *American Journal of Medicine*, **40**, 837–56.

Messmer, E. M. and Foster, C. S. (1999). Vasculitic peripheral ulcerative keratitis. *Survey of Ophthalmology*, **43**, 379–96.

Milhara, M., Hasayaka, S., Watanabe, K. *et al.* (2004). Ocular manifestations in patients with microscopic polyangiitis. *European Journal of Ophthalmology*, **15**, 138.

Miller, N. R. (2000). Giant cell arteritis. *Journal of Neuroophthalmology*, **20**, 219–220.

Mitamura, Y., Fujiwara, O., Miyanishi, K., Sato, H., Saga, K. and Ohtsuka, K. (2004). Nodular scleritis with erythema elevatum diutinum. *American Journal of Ophthalmology*, **137**, 368–70.

Mochizuki, M., Akduman, L. and Nussenblatt, R. B. (1996). Behçet's disease. In *Ocular Infection and Immunity* (Pepose, J. S., Holland, G. N., and Wilhelmus, K. R., eds), pp. 663–75. Mosby, St Louis.

Morgan, C. M., Foster, C. S., D'Amico, J. D., *et al.* (1986). Retinal vasculitis in polyarteritis nodosa. *Retina*, **6**, 205–9.

Myers, J. P., Di Bisceglie, A. M. and Mann, E. S. (2001). Cryoglobulinemia associated with Purtscher-like retinopathy. *American Journal of Ophthalmology*, **131**, 802–4.

Nölle, B., Specks, U., Lüdemann, J., *et al.* (1989). Anticytoplasmic autoantibodies: their immunodiagnostic value in Wegener's granulomatosis. *Annals of Internal Medicine*, **64**, 28–36.

Ohno, S., Miyajima, T., Higuchi, M., *et al.* (1982). Ocular manifestations of Kawasaki's disease (mucocutaneous lymph node syndrome). *American Journal of Ophthalmology*, **93**, 713–7.

Perez, V. L., Chavala, S. H., Ahmed, M. *et al.* (2004). Ocular manifestations and concepts of systemic vasculitides. *Survey of Ophthalmology*, **49**, 399–418.

Pless, M., Rizzo, J. F. III, Lamkin, J. C., *et al.*(2000) Concordance of bilateral temporal artery biopsy in giant cell arteritis. *Journal of Neuroophthalmology*, **20**, 216–8.

Poole, T. R. and Graham, E. M. (1999). Ocular manifestations of rheumatologic disorders. *Current Opinion in Ophthalmology*, **10**, 458–63.

Power, W. J., Rodriguez, A., Neves, R. A., *et al.* (1995). Disease relapse in patients with ocular manifestations of Wegener granulomatosis. *Ophthalmology*, **102**, 154–60.

Saulsbury, F. T. (2001). Henoch-Schönlein purpura. *Current Opinion in Rheumatology*, **13**, 35–40.

Saulsbury, F. T. (1999). Henoch-Schönlein purpura in children. Report of 100 patients and review of the literature. *Medicine* (Baltimore), **78**, 395–409.

Savino, P. J. (2000). Giant cell arteritis. *Journal of Neuroophthalmology*, **20**, 221.

Seo, P. and Stone, J. H. (2004). The antineutrophil cytoplasmic antibody-associated vasculitides. *American Journal of Medicine*, **117**, 39–50.

Sheard, R. M., Pandey, K. R., Barnes, N. D. and Vivian, A. J. (2000). Kawasaki disease presenting as orbital cellulitis. *Journal of Pediatric Ophthalmology and Strabismus*, **37**, 123–5.

Shimazaki, J., Yang, H. Y., Shimmura, S., *et al.* (1998). Terrien's marginal degeneration associated with erythema elevatum diutinum. *Cornea*, **17**, 342–4.

Soheilian, M. (2002). Polyarteritis nodosa. In *Diagnosis and Treatment of Uveitis* (Foster, C. S. and Vitale, A. T. eds), pp. 653–60. W. B. Saunders Company, Philadelphia.

Stavrou, P., Deutsch, J., Rene, C. *et al.* (1993). Ocular manifestations of classical and limited Wegener's granulomatosis. *Quarterly Journal of Medicine*, **86**, 719–25.

Stavrou, P. and Foster, C. S. (2002). Sarcoidosis. In *Diagnosis and Treatment of Uveitis* (Foster, C. S. and Vitale, A. T. eds), pp.710–25. W. B. Saunders Company, Philadelphia.

Soukiasian, S. H., Foster, C. S., Niles, J. L. and Raizman, M. B. (1992). Diagnostic value of antineutrophil cytoplasmic antibodies in scleritis associated with Wegener's granulomatosis. *Ophthalmology*, **99**, 125–32.

Takanashi, T., Uchida, S., Arita, M., Okada, M. and Kashii, S. (2001). Orbital inflammatory pseudotumor and ischemic vasculitis in Churg-Strauss syndrome. Report of two cases and review of the literature. *Ophthalmology*, **108**, 1129–33.

Takiwaki, H., Kubo, Y., Tsuda, H., *et al.* (1998). Peripheral ulcerative keratitis associated with erythema elevatum diutinum and a positive rheumatoid factor: a report of three cases. *British Journal of Dermatology*, **138**, 893–7.

Tervaert, J. W., Goldschmeding, R., Elema, H. D., *et al.* (1990). Association of autoantibodies to myeloperoxidase with different forms of vasculitis. *Arthritis and Rheumatism*, **33**, 1264–72.

Tovilla-Canales, J. L. (1998). Ocular manifestations of giant cell arteritis. *Current Opinion in Ophthalmology*, **9**, 73–9.

Treister, G. and Machemer, R. (1977). Results of vitrectomy for rare proliferative and hemorrhagic diseases. *American Journal of Ophthalmology*, **84**, 394–412.

Tsai, J. C., Forster, D. J., Ober, R. R. and Rao, N. A. (1993). Panuveitis and multifocal retinitis in a patient with leucocytoclastic vasculitis. *British Journal of Ophthalmology*, **77**, 318–20.

Tugal-Tutkun, I., Onal, S., Altan-Yaycioglu, R., Altunbas, H. H. and Urgancioglu, M. (2004). Uveitis in Behçet's disease: an analysis of 880 cases. *American Journal of Ophthalmology*, **138**, 373–80.

Uy, H. S. and Chan, P. S. (2002). Systemic lupus erythematosus. In *Diagnosis and Treatment of Uveitis* (Foster, C. S. and Vitale, A. T. eds), pp.601–9. W. B. Saunders Company, Philadelphia.

van der Woude, F. J., Rasmussen, N., Lobatto, S., *et al.* (1985). Autoantibodies against neutrophils and monocytes: tools for diagnosis and marker of disease activity in Wegener's granulomatosis. *Lancet*, **1**, 425–9.

Weinstein, J. M., Chui, H., Lane, S., *et al.* (1983). Churg-Strauss syndrome (allergic granulomatous angiitis). Neuro-ophthalmologic manifestations. *Archives of Ophthalmology*, **101**, 1217–20.

Wise, G. N. (1951). Ocular periarteritis nodosa. Report of two cases. *Archives of Ophthalmology*, **45**, 1–11.

Yamabe, H., Ozawa, K., Fukushi, K., *et al.* (1988). IgA nephropathy and Henoch-Schönlein purpura nephritis with anterior uveitis. *Nephron*, **50**, 368–70.

Zaman, F., Granville, L. and Trocme, S. D. (1997). Ocular manifestations of immunologic and rheumatologic inflammatory disorders. *Current Opinion in Ophthalmology*, **8**, 81–4.

Zamir, E., Bodaghi, B., Tugal-Tutkun, I., *et al.*(2003). Conjunctival ulcers in Behçet's disease. *Ophthalmology*, **110**, 1137–41.

CHAPTER 13

Cardiopulmonary manifestations of vasculitis

Stephen K. Frankel and Marvin I. Schwarz

Introduction

Cardiopulmonary disease in vasculitis is frequent and contributes significantly to both morbidity and mortality. Cardiopulmonary manifestations in vasculitis are quite diverse (Table 13.1), ranging from an asymptomatic patient with an abnormal chest radiograph to a catastrophic event such as diffuse alveolar hemorrhage (DAH) or sudden death. Since patients can first present with isolated (or seemingly isolated) pulmonary or cardiac events, there is often confusion with more common entities such as malignancy, infection, connective tissue disease, drug toxicity, and embolic phenomena. Alternatively, a patient with known disease can develop cardiopulmonary disease following diagnosis, or there can be a simultaneous onset of cardiopulmonary manifestations with other systemic manifestations of disease.

The scope of cardiopulmonary complications

Upper respiratory tract disease

Chronic rhinitis and sinusitis are common problems and are usually due to allergic, infectious, or anatomic causes. Nevertheless, in patients with refractory, ulcerative or destructive disease, or in whom other more common causes have been excluded, the possibility of vasculitis, and in particular, ANCA-associated vasculitis, should be considered.

Most patients (>90%) with Wegener's granulomatosis (WG) will develop upper respiratory tract disease and present with rhinorrhea, epistaxis, septal perforation, nasal pain, congestion, otitis, ear pain, hearing loss, mastoiditis, sinusitis, or ulcerations, bony destruction, and deformities involving the nose, ears, or sinuses (Reinhold-Keller 2000; Specks 2003; Anderson 1992) (see Chapter 31). Sinus imaging will reveal abnormalities in 85% of patients (Fauci 1983; Hoffman et al.1992; Lynch et al. 2004). Furthermore, upper and lower respiratory tract disease are independent risk factors for disease relapse after remission (Hogan et al. 2005). Upper respiratory tract disease is also characteristic of Churg–Strauss syndrome (CSS), seen in approximately 70% of patients, presenting as allergic or eosinophilic rhinitis or sinusitis (Guillevin 1988, 1999a; Lanham et al. 1984). Upper respiratory tract involvement is less common in microscopic polyangiitis (MPA), occurring in 0–15% of patients.

Asthma and airways disease

Asthma occurs in all patients with CSS. While the duration and severity of the asthma is variable, it generally precedes the onset of the systemic vasculitis by several years. Asthma that precedes CSS is typically difficult to treat, often requiring courses of oral glucocorticoids to maintain disease control and is indistinguishable from other cases of chronic asthma. Status asthmaticus results in increased morbidity and mortality in patients with CSS.

In WG, involvement of the trachea and bronchi occurs in approximately 60% of patients. This includes granulomatous airway lesions, subglottic, tracheal or bronchial stenosis, tracheo- or bronchomalacia, ulcerations, hemorrhage, pseudotumor, or segmental or lobar collapse from airway narrowing or occlusion (Daum et al. 1995). Patients report shortness of breath, wheezing, exercise intolerance, voice change, hoarseness, difficulty speaking or swallowing, hemoptysis, and chest discomfort. Subglottic or tracheal stenosis may present as a threatened airway and can be fatal (Figure 13.1). Pulmonary function testing may be helpful in establishing large airway involvement. Truncation of the inspiratory, expiratory, or both portions of the flow volume loop may represent variable extrathoracic, variable intrathoracic, or fixed obstruction respectively; however, diagnostic sensitivity of the flow volume loop is limited. Flexible fiberoptic bronchoscopy with direct visualization is the single most useful test for evaluation of the airway. Depending upon the location and severity of the airway complication, a combination of immunosuppressive therapy, interventional pulmonary techniques such as laser ablation, dilatation, local glucocorticoid injection and airway stenting, and surgery may be considered (Utzig et al. 2002; Hoffman et al. 2003).

Parenchymal lung disease

Pulmonary infiltrates in vasculitis may represent primary vasculitic inflammation and necrosis, such as the granulomatous inflammation and necrotizing vasculitis of WG or the eosinophilic pneumonia and necrotizing vasculitis of CSS. Infection, DAH, heart failure/pulmonary edema, and drug-induced lung disease may also occur. While the specific radiographic pattern may suggest one of the above (diffuse alveolar filling would be more suggestive of DAH while focal reticulonodular infiltrates would suggest infection or primary vasculitic involvement), all possibilities should be considered.

Table 13.1 Cardiopulmonary manifestations of selected vasculitides

	WG	MPA	CSS	KD	PAN	TA	BS
Upper airway disease	+++	++	+++	–	–	–	–
Asthma and airways disease	+++	–	+++	–	–	–	–
Infiltrates	+++	++	+++	–	+	+	+
Nodules and cavities	+++	+	++	–	–	–	+
Alveolar hemorrhage	++	++	+	–	–	–	+
Pulmonary artery abnormalities	–	+	–	–	–	+++	++
Pleural disease	++	++	++	–	+	+	+
Thromboembolic disease	++	–	–	–	–	+	++
Arrhythmias and conduction delays	++	+	++	++	+	+	+
Cardiomyopathy, myocarditis, and heart failure	++	++	++	++	++	++	+
Coronary arteritis	++	++	++	++	++	++	+
Pericardial disease	++	++	++	++	+	+	+
Infection	++	++	++	++	++	++	++
Drug toxicity	++	++	++	++	++	++	++

WG, Wegener's granulomatosis; MPA, microscopic polyangiitis; CSS, Churg–Strauss syndrome; KD, Kawasaki's disease; PAN, polyarteritis nodosa; TA, Takayasu's arteritis; BS, Behçet's syndrome.

– Not reported or data unavailable; + rare, but reported; ++ well characterized and accepted disease manifestation; +++ characteristic and frequent disease manifestation.

Lung disease is common in WG (80%), and the chest radiograph may reveal diffuse infiltrates, focal consolidation, nodules, cavities, or atelectasis from bronchial involvement. It is most often bilateral, and the infiltrates change and evolve over time. Computed tomography (CT) gives a more detailed and comprehensive characterization of the infiltrates and may show a variety of changes including focal consolidation, ground glass attenuation, cavitary disease, nodular or micronodular disease, septal thickening, bronchovascular cuffing, pleural disease, and tracheobronchial complications (Reuter *et al.* 1998; Aberle *et al.* 1990; Maskell *et al.* 1993; Sheehan

et al. 2003; Papiris *et al.* 1992; Weir *et al.* 1992). Similarly, 40–75% of patients with CSS have infiltrates on chest radiographs and up to 90% have abnormal CT imaging (Chumbley *et al.* 1977; Buschman *et al.* 1990; Choi *et al.* 2000; Worthy *et al.* 1998; Guillevin *et al.* 1999a; Abu-Shakra *et al.* 1994; Lanham *et al.* 1984). The most common presentation on chest imaging is bilateral, heterogenous, patchy disease with ground glass attenuation with or without areas of focal consolidation and pleural effusion. MPA may also present with diffuse pulmonary infiltrates representative of DAH in up to 30% of patients. Likewise, other vasculitides, including giant cell

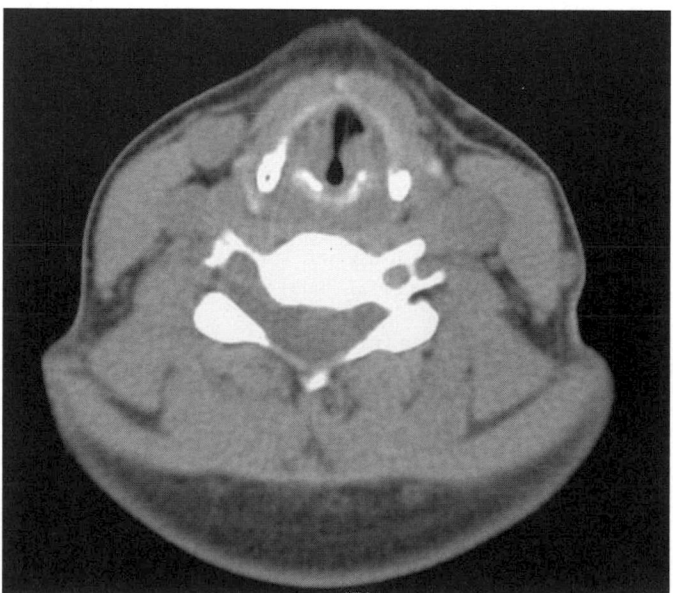

Figure 13.1 CT image of tracheal stenosis in a patient with Wegener's granulomatosis.

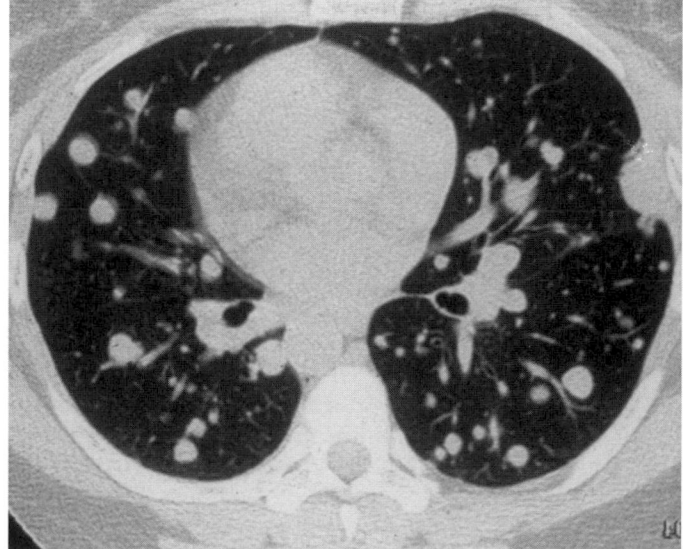

Figure 13.2 CT image of multiple, bilateral nodules in a patient with Wegener's granulomatosis.

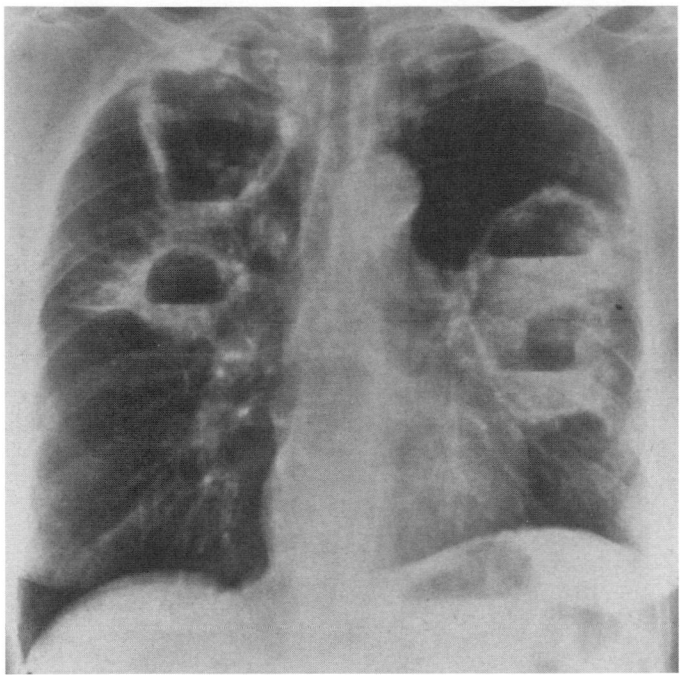

(a)

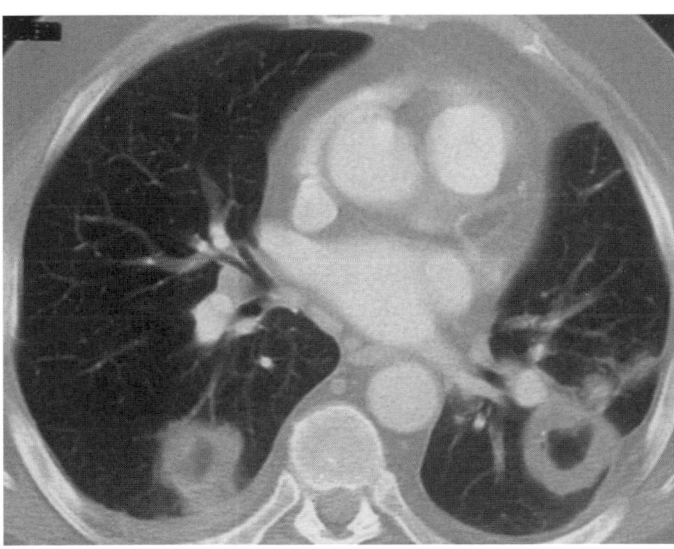

(b)

Figure 13.3 (a) Chest radiograph and (b) CT image of cavitary lesions in a patient with Wegener's granulomatosis.

arteritis, Takayasu's arteritis, Henoch–Schönlein purpura, cryoglobulinemia, and Behçet's syndrome may cause pulmonary infiltrates (see below).

Nodules and cavities

The appearance of lung nodules and cavitary disease evokes a differential diagnosis that includes malignancy, infection (in particular atypical infections), septic emboli, sarcoidosis, connective tissue disease (the necrobiotic nodules of rheumatoid arthritis), and ANCA-associated vasculitis (Figures 13.2 and 13.3). A study by Cordier *et al.* of 77 patients with WG found nodular disease in 69% of patients, and in 43% cavities were detected (Cordier *et al.* 1990).

Another CT study of patients with WG found nodular disease in 90%, with cavitation in 48% (Lee *et al.* 2003). The nodules vary in size (0.3–10 cm), can be limited in number or multiple and bilateral (Cordier *et al.* 1990).

Diffuse alveolar hemorrhage (DAH)

DAH is a serious complication of vasculitis and an independent risk factor for poor outcome (Hogan 1996). Classically, patients with DAH present with hemoptysis, radiographic alveolar infiltrates, and anemia (Figure 13.4). Patients report shortness of breath and hemptysis (although up to one-third of patients will not complain of hemoptysis at the time of presentation). Other symptoms include chest discomfort, cough, fatigue, malaise, and fever. The chest radiograph demonstrates patchy, bilateral, alveolar infiltrates producing ground glass attenuation, and sometimes alveolar consolidation, on CT imaging. The infiltrates are usually diffuse, but may have a lower lobe predilection. Unilateral or focal infiltrates may be seen initially, but ultimately evolve into the diffuse pattern. With recurrent DAH, fibrosis may produce reticular infiltrates and septal line thickening. An elevated diffusing capacity of carbon monoxide (DL_{CO}) >30% above normal predicted values also suggests the diagnosis of DAH. The differential diagnosis includes pneumonia, drug reaction, pulmonary edema, acute pneumonitis, and acute respiratory distress syndrome.

The diagnosis of DAH is made at bronchoscopy when serial aliquots of lavage fluid demonstrate a persistently bloody return on aspiration (Figure 13.5). Pathologically, DAH may represent pulmonary capillaritis (a small vessel vasculitis of the lung), bland hemorrhage, or diffuse alveolar damage with hemorrhage, but distinguishing among these requires surgical lung biopsy.

The differential diagnosis for DAH is extensive but focuses upon vasculitis (Table 13.2). Pulmonary–renal syndrome refers to those patients with both DAH and glomerulonephritis, and 80% of these patients will ultimately be diagnosed with an ANCA-associated vasculitis or antiglomerular basement membrane disease (Goodpasture's syndrome). The remaining patients have connective tissue diseases, cryoglobulinemia, Henoch–Schönlein purpura, and infection or postinfectious complications (Jayne 1998; Niles 1996). Goodpasture's syndrome mimics the ANCA-associated vasculitides limited to the lungs and kidneys, as it is characterized by DAH and crescentic glomerulonephritis, and in 10–20% of cases is pANCA positive (Rodriguez *et al.* 2002).

Treatment of DAH secondary to vasculitis includes supportive care (including mechanical ventilation if necessary), correction of coagulation abnormalities, and treatment of the underlying vasculitis. Intravenous, high-dose glucocorticoids are recommended, as is early introduction of plasmapheresis for severe or refractory disease (Nachman 1996; Klemmer *et al.* 2003; Gaskin and Pusey 2001). Cyclophosphamide (or if contraindicated, azathioprine) may also be initiated; however, given the slow onset of action of cyclophosphamide and the potential for serious complications (bone marrow toxicity, infection), some experts defer the initiation of cyclophosphamide in critically-ill patients (Lee and Specks 2004). Respiratory failure and the need for mechanical ventilation is a poor prognostic factor (Guillevin *et al.* 1999a; Lauque *et al.* 2000). The literature reports several cases in which recombinant factor VII was used successfully for hemostasis in patients with severe, uncontrolled alveolar hemorrhage (Betensley and Yankaskas 2002; Henke *et al.* 2004).

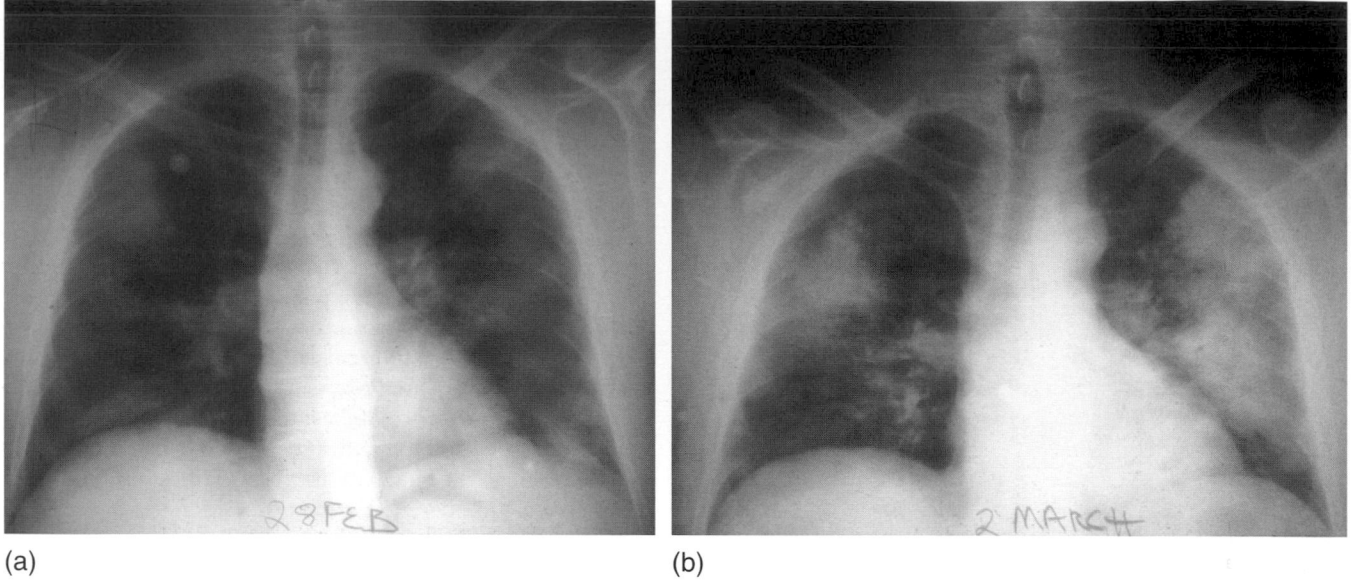

(a)   (b)

Figure 13.4 Chest radiographs of a patient with diffuse alveolar hemorrhage. (a) On admission with hemoptysis and (b) 3 days later with fulminant disease and respiratory distress.

Pulmonary artery aneurysms, pseudoaneurysms, stenoses, and occlusions

Medium and large-vessel vasculitis can affect the vessels of the heart and lungs, as well as the aorta and its branches, often with catastrophic results. Pulmonary artery aneurysms are unusual. When these occur and are not the result of trauma or a complication of right heart catheterization, then Behçet's syndrome, Hughes–Stovin syndrome, and, to a lesser extent, Takayasu's arteritis should be considered. Stenoses and occlusions of the pulmonary arteries are more commonly seen with Takayasu's arteritis. The most common early symptom of pulmonary artery aneurysm is hemoptysis, but patients may present with an abnormal radiograph, signs and symptoms of a mass effect of the aneurysm, or a

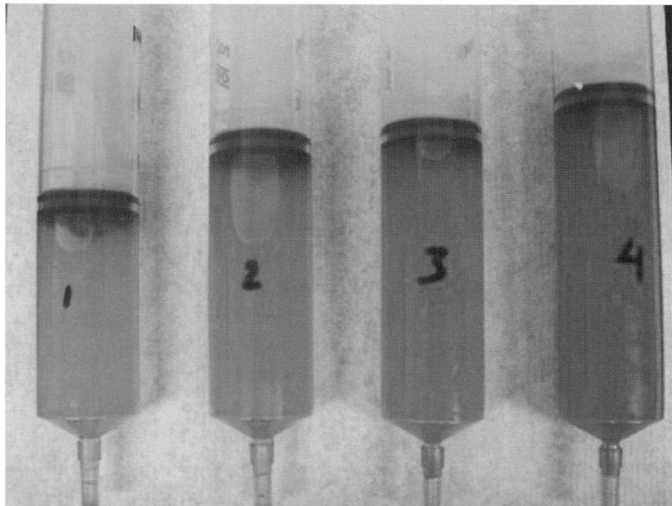

Figure 13.5 Diffuse alveolar hemorrhage is diagnosed during bronchoscopy when serial aliquots of lavagate demonstrate a persistently bloody return. Photograph courtesy of Gregory P. Cosgrove, MD. (See Color Plate 59).

more fulminant bleeding complication. Pulmonary artery aneurysms range in size from 1–10 cm and can be single or multiple. Angiography is effective for the imaging of pulmonary artery aneurysms, but it carries some risk. Thus, CT angiography and MRI have largely replaced direct angiography (Berkmen 1998).

There are no randomized, controlled trials which evaluate medical treatment of pulmonary artery aneurysms secondary to vasculitis, but immunosuppression (glucocorticoids and cytotoxic agents), embolization, surgery, anticoagulation, and antiplatelet therapies have all been tried (Uzun *et al.* 2005). Of these, immunosuppression seems to confer the greatest benefit, and, in the setting of massive hemoptysis, embolization of the feeding vessel is indicated. While thrombus formation may be common within pulmonary artery aneurysms, anticoagulation carries considerable risk, and inasmuch as the thrombi are often adherent and organized, it is often reasonable to avoid the use of anticoagulants (Uzun *et al.* 2005).

Pulmonary hypertension

Primary pulmonary arterial hypertension is a rare complication of vasculitis but there are case reports (Lie 1996; Roncoroni *et al.* 1992). Primary plexogenic arteriopathy, thromboembolic disease, pulmonary hypertension secondary to parenchymal lung disease, constrictive pericarditis, tamponade, restrictive cardiomyopathy and heart failure should all be considered as potential causes of pulmonary hypertension in the patient with vasculitis.

Venous thromboembolic disease

Venous thromboembolic disease (VTE) is well-described in antiphospholipid syndrome and the primary connective tissue diseases, most often in systemic lupus erythematosus (SLE). Similarly, excess cases of VTE occur in WG as reported by the WeCLOT investigators in conjunction with the WGET trial; 29 cases of VTE were found among 180 patients with WG. This is an incidence of 7.0 per 100 person-years which is comparable to patients with a known history of prior VTE and more than 20 times that of the general

Table 13.2 Differential diagnosis of diffuse alveolar hemorrhage

Capillaritis
Pauci-immune disease/ ANCA-associated vasculitides
Wegener's granulomatosis
Microscopic polyangiitis
Churg–Strauss syndrome
Idiopathic pauci-immune pulmonary capillaritis
Immune complex-mediated disease
Goodpasture's syndrome
Essential cryoglobulinemia
Henoch–Schönlein pupura
Behçet's syndrome
Primary connective tissue diseases
Systemic lupus erythematosus
Rheumatoid arthritis
Scleroderma
Polymyositis/ dermatomyositis
Antiphospholipid syndrome
Mixed connective tissue disease
Drug-induced lung injury
Penicillamine
Chemotherapeutic agents
Propylthiouracil
Bland hemorrhage
Idiopathic pulmonary hemosiderosis
Sleep apnea (severe)
Coagulopathies
Cardiac disease
Mitral stenosis
Heart failure
Drug and inhalation-induced lung injury
Chemotherapeutic agents
Trimellitic anhydride
Amiodarone
Nitrofurantoin
Pulmonary veno-occlusive disease
Diffuse alveolar damage

population (Merkel *et al.* 2005; WGET Investigators 2005). Venous and arterial thromboembolic disease is also common in Behçet's syndrome. The Italian Behçet's syndrome cohort found deep venous thrombosis in 21% of patients and superficial thrombophlebitis in 10.9% (Pipitone *et al.* 2004). Intracardiac (right-sided) thrombus is an uncommon but reported complication of Behçet's syndrome (Mogulkoc *et al.* 2000).

Pleural disease

Pleural effusions have been reported in the ANCA-associated vasculitides, polyarteritis nodosa (PAN), Behçet's syndrome, and giant cell arteritis. If present, they are of small volume (Cordier *et al.* 1990; James 1988). If a pleural effusion is identified in a patient with vasculitis,

other considerations for its origin include infection (i.e. a parapneumonic effusion or empyema), heart failure, or thromboembolic disease.

Infection

Infection, particularly pneumonia and sepsis, are important causes of morbidity and mortality in patients with vasculitis. The diagnosis is frequently delayed or missed because of overlap between the signs and symptoms of infection, disease activity, and drug toxicity. This is most likely in patients receiving immunosuppressive therapy in whom severe disease, atypical organisms, and atypical presentations can be expected. Glucocorticoids have been shown to independently increase the risk of infectious complications (Stuck 1989). A retrospective analysis of 595 vasculitis patients found that 26% of deaths were caused by infection and that this was second only to complications of the vasculitic syndrome (58%) (Bourgarit *et al.* 2005). A smaller study reported that 12.9% of deaths in treated vasculitis patients were due to infection (Gayraud 2001).

Drug toxicity

As with infection, drug toxicity can often be mistaken for vasculitic disease activity. Methotrexate is associated with a drug-induced pneumonitis in 2–10% of patients, but pulmonary complications have also been reported with other immunosuppressive agents (Frankel 2003).

Conduction abnormalities, arrhythmia, and sudden death

Conduction delay, bundle branch block, sinus node dysfunction, and heart block are complications of vasculitis and are presumed due to endomyocardial or coronary vasculitis (Wilcke *et al.* 2003; Handa *et al.* 1997; Yokoi *et al.* 1992). Moreover arrhythmias may occur, most frequently sinus tachycardia and supraventricular tachycardia (Mirone *et al.* 1997; Schiavone *et al.* 1985). More serious arrhythmias such as ventricular tachycardia and sudden death have been reported occasionally (Nakada 1996; Haney *et al.* 1995; Siburian *et al.* 1993; Fong *et al.* 1992; Hosenpud *et al.* 1986). Treatment requires therapy directed at the vasculitis as well as the conduction disorder or arrhythmia itself.

Systolic and diastolic dysfunction, cardiomyopathy, and heart failure

Primary vasculitic involvement of the myocardial arterioles and venules may accompany inflammation and granuloma formation within the heart muscle resulting in (endo)myocarditis (Pagnoux and Guillevin 2005). While it may be asymptomatic, it can lead to systolic or diastolic dysfunction, cardiomyopathy, and heart failure. Ischemic cardiomyopathy and heart failure may also occur as a result of vasculitis-associated coronary artery disease (see below). Other causes of heart failure in vasculitis include valvular heart disease, aortic arch disease, or long-standing vasculitis-induced hypertension. Cardiomyopathy has been shown to correlate with poor outcomes (Guillevin 1996). Given the high morbidity and mortality associated with cardiac vasculitis, a more intensive immunosuppressive regimen such as cyclophosphamide plus glucocorticoids is recommended.

Valvular heart disease

While unusual in small vessel vasculitis, cases of valvular heart disease have been described but are more common with large vessel disease, particularly Takayasu's arteritis. In Takayasu's arteritis, 17–55% of patients will develop aortic insufficiency (Maksimowicz-McKinnon and Hoffman 2004; Numano and Kobayashi 1999).

Coronary artery disease

Coronary arteritis (primary vasculitic involvement of the coronary arteries) is most often seen in vasculitis that affects the medium sized vessels. Coronary artery aneurysms or ectasia have been found in 15–25% of untreated children with Kawasaki's disease (Newburger *et al*. 2004). Approximately 10% of patients with PAN will develop clinically-significant coronary arteritis, although autopsy studies reveal a 50–62% incidence of coronary artery involvement (Schrader *et al*. 1985; Holsinger *et al*. 1962). Similarly, 5–25% of patients with Takayasu's arteritis develop coronary arteritis (Lie 1998). Coronary arteritis involves the epicardial portion of the vessel or the smaller myocardial intramural portion of the vessel and may produce myocardial infarction, ischemic cardiomyopathy, and heart failure (Pagnoux and Guillevin 2005). It should also be noted that glucocorticoids may accelerate underlying atherosclerosis. Therefore, atherosclerotic heart disease must also be considered in the differential diagnosis of patients with vasculitis and coronary artery disease.

Pericardial disease

Pericarditis may occur with any form of vasculitis, and is one of the more common cardiac manifestations of the ANCA-associated vasculitic syndromes. It is more common in the primary connective tissue diseases, especially SLE. While pericarditis is often an incidental finding, clinically-significant pericarditis and pericardial effusions, and less commonly, constrictive pericarditis, hemorrhagic pericarditis, and cardiac tamponade have all been described (Grant *et al*. 1994).

The great vessels

The large vessel vasculitides and Behçet's syndrome affect the great vessels of the chest leading to aneurysm formation, dissection, thrombosis, stenosis, rupture, or occlusion with systemic emboli from *in situ* thrombi. Stenotic lesions of the aorta or its main branches are common in Takayasu's arteritis, at times with incidental limb claudication, syncope or near-syncope, visual disturbances, hypertension, bruits, or diminished or absent pulses (Mwipatayi *et al*. 2005; Kerr *et al*. 1994; Hall *et al*.1985; Lupi-Herrera *et al*. 1977; Nakao *et al*. 1967; Sharma *et al*. 1996). CT and MRI are the imaging modalities of choice to identify and characterize great and large vessel vasculitides (Choe and Lee 1998). Positron emission tomography (PET) is still at an investigational stage, but appears to provide considerable information regarding inflammation and disease activity in the vessel wall (Kissin and Merkel 2004) (see Chapter 20).

Hypertension

Hypertension results from lesions such as renal artery stenosis and glomerulonephritis. It is common in PAN and Takayasu's arteritis.

Clinical evaluation

History and physical

The cardiopulmonary manifestations of vasculitis will often be evinced as general chest symptoms such as shortness of breath, cough, hemoptysis, chest pain or discomfort, wheezing or asthma, tachypnea, increased work of breathing, or reduced exercise tolerance. Alternatively, there can be general cardiovascular symptoms: lightheadedness, syncope, hypertension, tachycardia, or, in catastrophic cases, heart failure or sudden death. A detailed and thorough history and physical examination is central to the cardiopulmonary evaluation. Careful attention to seemingly unrelated complaints, a review of systems, and the physical examination may reveal evidence of extrathoracic disease that suggests that the presenting cardiopulmonary complaint is caused by an underlying vasculitis, primary connective tissue disease, or other systemic autoimmune disease.

Laboratory testing

Laboratory testing is useful for diagnostic purposes and for characterizing the extent and severity of a known case of vasculitis. Recommended studies often include routine screening laboratories such as a complete blood count (CBC); metabolic panel; blood urea nitrogen; serum creatinine; urinalysis with microscopic sediment examination; liver function tests; erythrocyte sedimentation rate; and C-reactive protein. Determination of ANCA status, including anti-PR3 and anti-MPO ELISA testing is often indicated (see Chapters 6 and 21). If the differential diagnosis includes one of the primary connective tissue diseases, antiphospholipid syndrome or cryoglobulinemia, appropriate tests are ordered (see Chapters 34, 44, and 41). If Goodpasture's syndrome is a consideration, serum should be tested for the presence of antiglomerular basement membrane antibodies and renal biopsy considered urgently. Patients with confirmed vasculitis should also have a baseline electrocardiogram as part of their diagnostic evaluation.

Pulmonary function testing and arterial blood gas analysis

Measurement of lung function by physiologic testing and gas exchange are necessary to assess the integrity of the respiratory system and characterize and quantify impairment, both initially and longitudinally. Lung volumes, spirometry, bronchodilator response, DL_{CO}, and blood gas analysis on room air form the core physiologic assessment. Given the wide array of potential pulmonary manifestations of vasculitis, obstructive, restrictive, or mixed patterns of ventilatory impairment with an increased, decreased, or normal DL_{CO} are all potentially consistent with an underlying vasculitis. The tests, however, cannot mandate a diagnosis of vasculitis, nor do they permit a specific pulmonary manifestation to be attributed to vasculitis.

Imaging studies

Imaging studies are a key component of the initial cardiopulmonary evaluation and longitudinal monitoring of the disease. Chest radiographs, and particularly CT scanning of the chest, may identify clinically silent pulmonary disease and reveal its extent. CT of the sinuses is helpful in characterizing upper respiratory tract involvement. While MRI is not useful for lung imaging, it is ideal for imaging of the pulmonary arteries and great vessels of the chest (Chapter 19). CT angiography is an alternative means for examining the pulmonary arteries. Direct catheter-guided pulmonary angiography is performed on occasion, but carries risks.

With regard to cardiac imaging, echocardiography is useful for suspected cardiac involvement and may detect systolic or diastolic dysfunction, prior myocardial infarction, cardiomyopathy, valvular heart disease, coronary artery aneurysms, or pericardial disease, but, its sensitivity is limited. While cardiac MRI to look for cardiac vasculitis is promising, its role remains unclear (Manning *et al.* 2002). Coronary angiography will accurately assess the coronary vessels, but is invasive and does not reliably detect disease in smaller branches.

Invasive studies and biopsy

Although the diagnosis of vasculitis may be established on clinical grounds supported by characteristic radiographic or serologic testing, tissue acquisition is frequently necessary for definitive diagnosis. In patients with skin or upper airway involvement, easy access and low morbidity make these a reasonable choice for initial biopsy in spite of limited diagnostic yields. Biopsy of involved upper airways is diagnostic in 21–70% of patients; sinus tissue is more likely to be diagnostic than nasal tissue (Devaney *et al.* 1990; Colby *et al.* 1991; Del Buono and Flint 1991).

Bronchoscopy is the procedure of choice for the evaluation and diagnosis of DAH and it may also be useful to exclude infection and focal airway lesions. Airway lesions are relatively common in WG but are rarely seen in other vasculitic disorders. Biopsy of visualized endobronchial lesions yields diagnostic tissue in only 18% of patients (Daum *et al.* 1995). Transbronchial biopsies are rarely useful in pulmonary vasculitis (Schnabel *et al.* 1997).

Percutaneous renal biopsy establishes the existence of rapidly progressive glomerulonephritis (Chapter 16). A histopathologic diagnosis of pauci-immune necrotizing glomerulonephritis reflects an ANCA-positive vasculitis in the majority of cases (Hauer *et al.* 2002; Weiss and Crissman 1985). Surgical open lung biopsy, if necessary, usually establishes a definitive diagnosis in the patient suspected of having vasculitis (Travis *et al.* 1991; Specks 2003; Frankel *et al.* 2005). Tissue should be formalin-fixed for hematoxylin and eosin staining and special stains, frozen for immunofluorescence studies, and cultured for microbial agents. Endomyocardial biopsies are occasionally done, but given the potential risks and low diagnostic yield, it is used sparingly.

Specific vasculitides

Wegener's granulomatosis (Chapters 30, 31, and 32)

WG involves the upper airways, tracheobronchial tree, pleural space, pulmonary vasculature, and pulmonary parenchyma. Approximately 10% of patients with WG will have disease limited to the lung at the time of presentation. Cardiac complications, while uncommon, occur in 5–15% of patients, and include coronary arteritis, (endo-)myocarditis, cardiomyopathy, valvular heart disease, conduction abnormalities, arrhythmia, and pericardial disease (Korantzopoulos *et al.* 2004; Goodfield *et al.* 1995; Lynch *et al.* 2004; Grant *et al.* 1994). A literature review by Forstot *et al.* (1980) found that the most common manifestations of cardiac disease in WG are pericarditis (50%), coronary arteritis (50%), myocarditis (25%), valvulitis or endocarditis (21%), conduction system granulomas (17%), AV node arteritis (13%), sinus node arteritis (13%), and myocardial infarction (11%).

Microscopic polyangiitis (MPA) (Chapter 27)

Pulmonary disease occurs in 20–30% of patients with DAH being the most common manifestation (Lane *et al.* 2005; Collins and Quismorio 2005; Lauque *et al.* 2000). Other rare lung complications include isolated radiographic infiltrates, pulmonary arterial aneurysms, pulmonary fibrosis, and bronchiolitis, though it is likely that at least some of these are the result of recurrent and chronic alveolar hemorrhage (Collins and Quismorio 2005; Brugiere *et al.* 1997; Homma *et al.* 2004). Although cardiac involvement is considered uncommon in MPA, a study of 85 patients with MPA revealed heart failure in 17.6% and pericarditis in 10% (Guillevin *et al.* 1999b).

Churg–Strauss syndrome (Chapter 33)

CSS must be differentiated from other eosinophilic lung diseases associated with asthma such as chronic eosinophilic pneumonia, allergic bronchopulmonary mycosis, drug reactions, hypereosinophilic syndrome, parasitic infection, and simple asthma/atopic disease. Moreover, CSS may present as atopy with gastrointestinal (perforation, ischemia, bleeding) or cardiac disease (cardiomyopathy, conduction abnormalities).

Recently, a number of case series and individual reports suggested a possible relationship between the use of leukotriene inhibitors for therapy of asthma and the development of CSS (Weschler 1998; Weschler 2000). The question remains as to whether leukotriene inhibitors could promote the biologic conversion of a subset of severe asthma patients to CSS (Weller 2001). To date, it has been difficult to demonstrate a causal link, and it is more likely that the introduction of leukotriene inhibitors permits dose reductions in oral glucocorticoids in severe asthma patients, and that this in turn unmasks previously treated but unrecognized CSS (Jamaleddine *et al.* 2002).

Cardiac disease accounts for 33–83% of deaths due to CSS (Chumbley *et al.* 1977; Lanham *et al.* 1984; Bourgarit *et al.* 2005). Cardiac involvement in CSS is often expressed as a cardiomyopathy as a result of either endomyocarditis with myocardial eosinophilic infiltrates or coronary arteritis with ischemic injury to the myocardium. Myocardial fibrosis, congestive heart failure, valvular heart disease, myocardial infarction, conduction delays, arrhythmias, pericardial disease, and sudden death have all been described (Kozak *et al.* 1995). Interestingly, a recent study by Fourtassou and colleagues found that patients with cardiac involvement in CSS were more likely to be ANCA-negative than those without cardiac complications (Sable-Fourtassou *et al.* 2005).

Polyarteritis nodosa (Chapter 26)

As noted above, coronary arteritis is common in PAN and can result in myocardial infarction, ischemic cardiomyopathy, or death. Pulmonary involvement with classic PAN is rare but DAH, radiographic infiltrates and pleural effusion have been seen.

Kawasaki's disease (Chapter 29)

Among children with Kawasaki's disease, 15–25% will develop coronary artery aneurysms if diagnosis and treatment are delayed (Newburger *et al.* 2004). A significant percentage of patients with cardiac involvement will subsequently develop myocarditis, conduction delays, arrhythmia or pericarditis. Mitral regurgitation and aortic regurgitation also occur. While in general the prognosis for Kawasaki's disease is excellent, myocardial infarction, heart failure, and sudden death represent catastrophic complications, and the majority of deaths are due to coronary complications (Kato *et al.* 1986).

Takayasu's arteritis (Chapter 25)

Takayasu's arteritis affects the pulmonary arteries in approximately 50% of patients (Vanoli *et al.* 1999; Yamada *et al.* 2000), potentially causing pulmonary artery stenosis, occlusion, aneurysm with rupture, or pulmonary hypertension. Takayasu's arteritis affects the coronary arteries in 5–25% of patients, most commonly at the level of the coronary ostitia where they arise from the aorta; such involvement may lead to myocardial infarction or sudden death (Lie 1987, 1998). Dilatation of the aortic root and aortic insufficiency are relatively common. An echocardiographic study of 78 patients with Takayasu's arteritis and giant cell arteritis identified left ventricular systolic dysfunction in 18% of patients (Pfizenmaier *et al.* 2004). It is of interest that left ventricular dysfunction did not correlate with hemodynamic variables, aortic regurgitation, or systemic hypertension, suggesting that primary cardiac inflammation was responsible for a significant proportion of the cases. Finally, thoracic and abdominal aortic aneurysm, stenosis, dissection, rupture, coarctation, and occlusion are hallmarks of Takayasu's arteritis.

Giant cell arteritis (Chapter 24)

GCA involves the thoracic aorta in 8–10% of patients and can cause serious or fatal complications (Evans *et al.* 1994). Aortitis with aortic aneurysm formation, ectasia, rupture, and dissection occur, and aneurysmal dilatation of the aortic root may lead to aortic regurgitation and congestive heart failure (Gelsomino *et al.* 2005; Nesi *et al.* 2002; Evans *et al.* 1994, 1995; Klein *et al.* 1975). Lung involvement is unusual, but there are reports of cough; hoarseness; sore throat; radiographic infiltrates (including one instance of with multiple pulmonary nodules); pleural effusions; granulomatous lung disease; pulmonary artery stenosis; obstruction and thrombosis; DAH; and multiple pulmonary infarctions (Olopade *et al.* 1997; Karam and Fulmer 1982; Ladanyi and Fraser 1987; Bradley *et al.* 1984; Huong Dle *et al.* 2003; Radhamanohar 1991). Coronary arteritis secondary to GCA has also been reported (Kumar *et al.* 2002).

Behçet's syndrome (Chapter 35)

Pulmonary artery aneurysms are the most common lung complication of Behçet's syndrome, occurring in 1–8% of patients (Erkan *et al.* 2001) (Figure 13.6). Pulmonary artery aneurysms affect predominantly young men and convey a 50% mortality rate (Hamuryudan *et al.* 1994). Other pulmonary signs of Behçet's syndrome include atelectasis; organizing pneumonia; thromboembolic disease; DAH due to capillaritis; pleural effusions; abnormal pulmonary function tests; and pneumonia (Uzun *et al.* 2005).

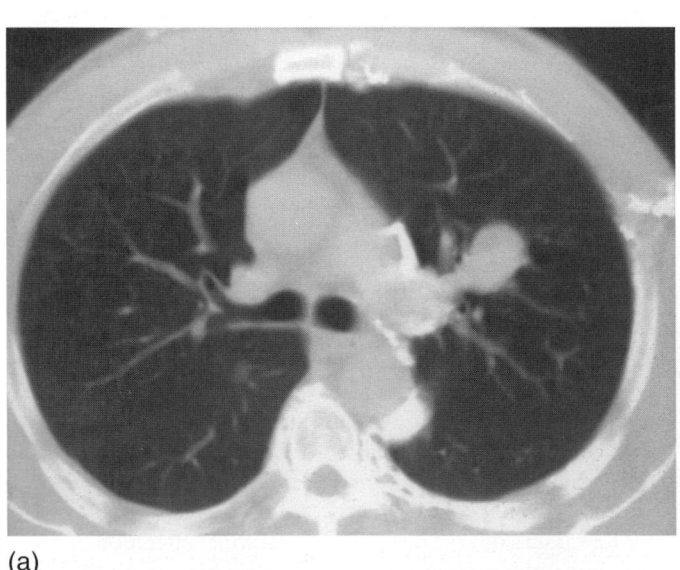

(a)

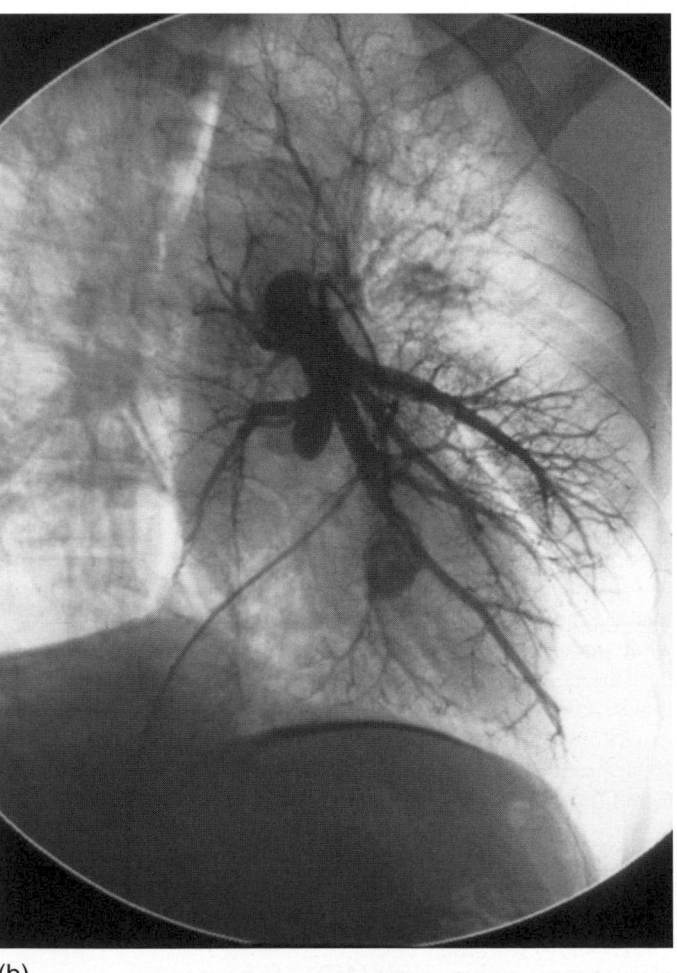

(b)

Figure 13.6 (a) CT image and (b) angiography of pulmonary artery aneurysms in a patient with Behçet's syndrome.

There is a long list of possible cardiovascular complications: great or large vessel aneurysms with rupture, thrombosis, and dilatation; coronary artery disease; myocardial infarction; endocarditis; myocarditis; cardiomyopathy; heart failure; pericardial disease; repolarization abnormalities; arrhythmias; mitral valve prolapse; aortic valve prolapse; mitral regurgitation; aneurysms of the sinus of Valsalva; interatrial septal aneurysms; and endomyocardial fibrosis (Atzeni *et al.* 2005; Gurgun *et al.* 2002; Mirone *et al.* 1997).

Henoch–Schönlein purpura (Chapter 40)

A retrospective study of HSP found that 2.4% of patients, all adults, had pulmonary disease (Nadrous *et al.* 2004). Based upon this and previously reported cases, DAH appears to be the most pulmonary common manifestation of HSP, although in one case pulmonary fibrosis was identified (Nadrous *et al.* 2004; Vats *et al.* 1999; Olson *et al.* 1992).

Mixed cryoglobulinemia (Chapter 41)

Pulmonary involvement is rare with cryoglobulinemic vasculitis, although case reports of DAH and acute lung injury are recorded (Suzuki *et al.* 2003; Gomez-Tello *et al.* 1999). Infiltrates and mild lung function abnormalities have been recognized as well (Viegi *et al.* 1989; Ferri *et al.* 1998). Congestive heart failure, myocardial infarction, pericardial disease and valvular heart disease have been reported with cryoglobulinemia.

Secondary vasculitis in primary connective tissue diseases (Chapter 34)

Connective tissue diseases cause a variety of cardiopulmonary disorders and are present in approximately 20% of patients with a primary CTD. These include interstitial lung disease; pulmonary hypertension; pleural disease; airways disease; thromboembolic disease; diaphragmatic and respiratory muscle weakness; diffuse alveolar hemorrhage; pericardial disease; myocarditis; valvular heart disease; cardiomyopathy; coronary arteritis; conduction delays; and arrhythmias.

References

Aberle, D. R., Gamsu, G. and Lynch, D. (1990). Thoracic manifestations of Wegener granulomatosis: diagnosis and course. *Radiology*, **174**, 703–9.

Abu-Shakra, M., Smythe, H., Lewtas, J., Badley, E., Weber, D. and Keystone, E. (1994). Outcome of polyarteritis nodosa and Churg-Strauss syndrome. An analysis of twenty-five patients. *Arthritis and Rheumatism*, **37**, 1798–803.

Anderson, G., Coles, E. T., Crane, M., Douglas, A. C., Gibbs, A. R., Geddes, D. M., *et al.* (1992). Wegener's granulomatosis: a series of 265 British cases seen between 1975 and 1985. A report by a sub-committee of the British Thoracic Society Research Committee. *Quarterly Journal of Medicine*, **83**, 427–38.

Atzeni, F., Sarzi-Puttini, P., Doria, A., Boiardi, L., Pipitone, N. and Salvarani, C. (2005). Behçet's disease and cardiovascular involvement. *Lupus*, **14**, 723–6.

Berkmen, T. (1998). MR angiography of aneurysms in Behçet disease: a report of four cases. *Journal of Computer Assisted Tomography*, **22**, 202–6.

Betensley, A. D. and Yankaskas, J. R. (2002). Factor viia for alveolar hemorrhage in microscopic polyangiitis. *American Journal of Respiratory and Critical Care Medicine*, **166**, 1291–2.

Bourgarit, A., Le Toumelin, P., Pagnoux, C., Cohen, P., Mahr, A., Le Guern, V., *et al.* (2005). Deaths occurring during the first year after treatment onset for polyarteritis nodosa, microscopic polyangiitis, and Churg-Strauss syndrome: a retrospective analysis of causes and factors predictive of mortality based on 595 patients *Medicine (Baltimore)*, **84**, 323–30.

Bradley, J. D., Pinals, R. S., Blumenfeld, H. B. and Poston, W. M. (1984). Giant cell arteritis with pulmonary nodules. *American Journal of Medicine*, **77**, 135–40.

Brugiere, O., Raffy, O., Sleiman, C., Groussard, O., Rothchild, E., Mellot, F., *et al.* (1997). Progressive obstructive lung disease associated with microscopic polyangiitis. *American Journal of Respiratory and Critical Care Medicine*, **155**, 739–42.

Buschman, D. L., Waldron, J. A. and King, T. E. (1990). Churg Strauss pulmonary vasculitis: high resolution computed tomography scanning and pathologic findings. *American Review of Respiratory Disease*, **142**, 458–461.

Choe, Y. H. and Lee, W. R. (1998). Magnetic resonance imaging diagnosis of Takayasu arteritis. *International Journal of Cardiology*, **66**, S175–9.

Choi, Y. H., Im, J.-G., Han, B. K., Kim, J.-H., Lee, K. Y. and Myong, N. H. (2000). Thoracic manifestations of churg-strauss syndrome. *Chest*, **117**, 117–24.

Chumbley, L. C., Harrison, E. G., Jr. and DeRemee, R. A. (1977). Allergic granulomatosis and angiitis (Churg-Strauss syndrome). Report and analysis of 30 cases. *Mayo Clinic Proceedings*, **52**, 477–84.

Colby, T. V., Tazelaar, H. D., Specks, U. and DeRemee, R. A. (1991). Nasal biopsy in Wegener's granulomatosis *Human Pathology*, **22**, 101–4.

Collins, C. E. and Quismorio, F. P., Jr. (2005). Pulmonary involvement in microscopic polyangiitis *Current Opinion in Pulmonary Medicine*, **11**, 447–51.

Cordier, J.-F., Valeyre, D., Guillevin, L., Loire, R. and Crechot, J.-M. (1990). Pulmonary wegener's granulomatosis. A clinical and imaging study of 77 cases. *Chest*, **97**, 906–12.

Daum, T. E., Specks, U., Colby, T. V., Edell, E. S., Brutinel, M. W., Prakash, U. B., *et al.* (1995). Tracheobronchial involvement in Wegener's granulomatosis. *American Journal of Respiratory and Critical Care Medicine*, **151**, 522–6.

Del Buono, E. A. and Flint, A. (1991). Diagnostic usefulness of nasal biopsy in Wegener's granulomatosis. *Human Pathology*, **22**, 107–10.

Devaney, K. O., Travis, W. D., Hoffman, G., Leavitt, R., Lebovics, R. and Fauci, A. S. (1990). Interpretation of head and neck biopsies in Wegener's granulomatosis. A pathologic study of 126 biopsies in 70 patients. *American Journal of Surgical Pathology*, **14**, 555–64.

Erkan, F., Gul, A. and Tasali, E. (2001). Pulmonary manifestations of Behçet's disease. *Thorax*, **56**, 572–8.

Evans, J. M., Bowles, C. A., Bjornsson, J., Mullany, C. J. and Hunder, G. G. (1994). Thoracic aortic aneurysm and rupture in giant cell arteritis. A descriptive study of 41 cases. *Arthritis and Rheumatism*, **37**, 1539–47.

Evans, J. M., O'Fallon, W. M. and Hunder, G. G. (1995). Increased incidence of aortic aneurysm and dissection in giant cell (temporal) arteritis. A population-based study. *Annals of Internal Medicine*, **122**, 502–7.

Fauci, A. S., Haynes, B. F., Katz, P., and Wolff, S. M. (1983). Wegener's granulomatosis: propsective clinical and therapeutic expeience with 85 patients for 21 years. *Annals of Internal Medicine*, **98**, 76–85.

Ferri, C., La Civita, L., Longombardo, G., Zignego, A. L. and Pasero, G. (1998). Mixed cryoglobulinaemia: a cross-road between autoimmune and lymphoproliferative disorders. *Lupus*, **7**, 275–9.

Fong, C., Schmidt, G., Cain, N., Cranswick, P. and Tonkin, A. M. (1992). Churg-Strauss syndrome, cardiac involvement and life threatening ventricular arrhythmias. *Australian and New Zealand Journal of Medicine*, **22**, 167–8.

Forstot, J. Z., Overlie, P. A., Neufeld, G. K., Harmon, C. E. and Forstot, S. L. (1980). Cardiac complications of Wegener granulomatosis: a case report of complete heart block and review of the literature. *Seminars in Arthritis and Rheumatism*, **10**, 148–54.

Frankel, S. K. (2003). Drug-induced lung disease. In *Current Diagnosis and Treatment in Pulmonary Medicine* (eds, Hanley, M. E. and Welsh, C. H.), pp. 337–47. Lange Medical Books/McGraw-Hill, New York.

Frankel, S. K., Cosgrove, G. P. and Brown, K. K. (2005). Small vessel vasculitis of the lung. *Chronic Respiratory Disease*, **2**, 75–84.

Gaskin, G. and Pusey, C. (2001). Plasmapheresis in antineutrophil cytoplasmic antibody-associated systemic vasculitis. *Therapeutic Apheresis*, **5**, 176–81.

Gayraud, M., Guillevin, L., le Toumelin, P., Cohen, P., Lhote, F., Casassus, P. and Jarrousse, B. (2001). Long-term followup of polyarteritis nodosa, microscopic polyangiitis, and Churg-Strauss syndrome: analysis of four prospective trials including 278 patients. *Arthritis and Rheumatism*, **44**, 666–75.

Gelsomino, S., Romagnoli, S., Gori, F., Nesi, G., Anichini, C., Sorbara, C., *et al.* (2005). Annuloaortic ectasia and giant cell arteritis. *Annals of Thoracic Surgery*, **80**, 101–5.

Gomez-Tello, V., Onoro-Canaveral, J. J., de la Casa Monje, R. M., Gomez-Casero, R. B., Moreno Hurtrez, J. L., Garcia-Montes, M., *et al.* (1999). Diffuse recidivant alveolar hemorrhage in a patient with hepatitis C virus-related mixed cryoglobulinemia. *Intensive Care Medicine*, **25**, 319–22.

Goodfield, N. E., Bhandari, S., Plant, W. D., Morley-Davies, A. and Sutherland, G. R. (1995). Cardiac involvement in Wegener's granulomatosis. *British Heart Journal*, **73**, 110–5.

Grant, S. C., Levy, R. D., Venning, M. C., Ward, C. and Brooks, N. H. (1994). Wegener's granulomatosis and the heart. *British Heart Journal*, **71**, 82–86.

Guillevin, L., Cohen, P., Gayraud, M., Lhote, F., Jarrousse, B., and Casassus, P. (1999a). Churg-Strauss syndrome. Clinical study and long-term follow-up of 96 patients. *Medicine*, **78**, 26–37.

Guillevin, L., Durand-Gasselin, B., Cevallos, R., Gayraud, M., Lhote, F., Callard, P., *et al.* (1999b). Microscopic polyangiitis: clinical and laboratory findings in eighty-five patients. *Arthritis and Rheumatism*, **42**, 421–30.

Guillevin, L., Houng Du, L. T., Godeau, P., Jais, P., and Wechsler, B. (1988). Clinical findings and prognosis of polyarteritis nodosa and Churg-Strauss angiitis: A study in 165 patients. *British Journal of Rheumatology*, **27**, 258–64.

Guillevin, L., Lhote, F., Gayraud, M., Cohen, P., Jarrousse, B., Lortholary, O., Thibult, N., and Casassus, P. (1996). Prognostic factors in polyarteritis nodosa and churg-strauss syndrome. A prospective study in 342 patients. *Medicine*, **75**, 17–28.

Gurgun, C., Ercan, E., Ceyhan, C., Yavuzgil, O., Zoghi, M., Aksu, K., *et al.* (2002). Cardiovascular involvement in Behçet's disease. *Japanese Heart Journal*, **43**, 389–98.

Hall, S., Barr, W., Lie, J. T., Stanson, A. W., Kazmier, F. J., and Hunder, G. G. (1985). Takayasu's arteritis: a study of 32 North American patients. *Medicine*, **64**, 89–99.

Hamuryudan, V., Yurdakul, S., Moral, F., Numan, F., Tuzun, H., Tuzuner, N., *et al.* (1994). Pulmonary arterial aneurysms in Behçet's syndrome: a report of 24 cases. *British Journal of Rheumatology*, **33**, 48–51.

Handa, R., Wali, J. P., Aggarwal, P., Wig, N., Biswas, A. and Kumar, A. K. (1997). Wegener's granulomatosis with complete heart block. *Clinical and Experimental Rheumatology*, **15**, 97–9.

Haney, I., Beghetti, M., McCrindle, B. W. and Gow, R. M. (1995). Ventricular arrhythmia complicating Kawasaki disease *Canadian Journal of Cardiology*, **11**, 931–3.

Hauer, H. A., Bajema, I. M., van Houwelingen, H. C., Ferrario, F., Noel, L. H., Waldherr, R., *et al.* (2002). Renal histology in ANCA-associated vasculitis: differences between diagnostic and serologic subgroups. *Kidney International*, **61**, 80–9.

Henke, D. C., Falk, R. J. and Gabriel, D. A. (2004). Successful treatment of diffuse alveolar hemorrhage with activated factor VII. *Annals of Internal Medicine*, **140**, 493–4.

Hoffman, G. S., Kerr, G. S., Leavitt, R. Y., Hallahan, C. W., Lebovics, R. S., Travis, W. D., Rottem, M., and Fauci, A. S. (1992). Wegener's granulomatosis: An analysis of 158 patients. *Annals of Internal Medicine*, **116**, 488–98.

Hoffman, G. S., Thomas-Golbanov, C. K., Chan, J., Akst, L. M. and Eliachar, I. (2003). Treatment of subglottic stenosis, due to Wegener's granulomatosis, with intralesional corticosteroids and dilation. *Journal of Rheumatology*, **30**, 1017–21.

Hogan, S. L., Falk, R. J., Chin, H., Cai, J., Jennette, C. E., Jennette, J. C., *et al.* (2005). Predictors of relapse and treatment resistance in antineutrophil cytoplasmic antibody-associated small-vessel vasculitis. *Annals of Internal Medicine*, **143**, 621–31.

Hogan, S. L., Nachman, P. H., Wilkman, A. S., Jennette, J. C., and Falk, R. J. (1996). Prognostic markers in patients with antineutrophil cytoplasmic autoantibody-associated microscopic polyangiitis and glomerulonephritis. *Journal of the American Society for Nephrology*, **7**, 23–32.

Holsinger, D. R., Osmundson, P. J. and Edwards, J. E. (1962). The heart in periarteritis nodosa. *Circulation*, **25**, 610–8.

Homma, S., Matsushita, H. and Nakata, K. (2004). Pulmonary fibrosis in myeloperoxidase antineutrophil cytoplasmic antibody-associated vasculitides. *Respirology*, **9**, 190–6.

Hosenpud, J. D., McAnulty, J. H. and Niles, N. R. (1986). Unexpected myocardial disease in patients with life threatening arrhythmias. *British Heart Journal*, **56**, 55–61.

Huong Dle, T., Andreu, M. R., Duhaut, P., Godeau, P. and Piette, J. C. (2003). Intra-alveolar haemorrhage in temporal arteritis. *Annals of the Rheumatic Diseases*, **62**, 189–90.

Jamaleddine, G., Diab, K., Tabbarah, Z., Tawil, A. and Arayssi, T. (2002). Leukotriene antagonists and the Churg-Strauss syndrome. *Seminars in Arthritis and Rheumatism*, **31**, 218–27.

James, D. G. (1988). 'Silk route disease' (Behçet's disease). *Western Journal of Medicine*, **148**, 433–7.

Jayne, D. R. (1998). Pulmonary-renal syndrome. *Seminars in Respiratory and Critical Care Medicine*, **19**, 69–77.

Karam, G. H. and Fulmer, J. D. (1982). Giant cell arteritis presenting as interstitial lung disease. *Chest*, **82**, 781–4.

Kato, H., Ichinose, E. and Kawasaki, T. (1986). Myocardial infarction in Kawasaki disease: clinical analyses in 195 cases. *Journal of Pediatrics*, **108**, 923–7.

Kerr, G. S., Hallahan, C. W., Giordano, J., Leavitt, R. Y., Fauci, A. S., Rottem, M., and Hoffman, G. S. (1994). Takayasu's arteritis. *Annals of Internal Medicine*, **120**, 919–29.

Kissin, E. Y. and Merkel, P. A. (2004). Diagnostic imaging in Takayasu arteritis. *Current Opinion in Rheumatology*, **16**, 31–7.

Klein, R. G., Hunder, G. G., Stanson, A. W. and Sheps, S. G. (1975). Large artery involvement in giant cell (temporal) arteritis. *Annals of Internal Medicine*, **83**, 806–12.

Klemmer, P. J., Chalermskulrat, W., Reif, M. S., Hogan, S. L., Henke, D. C. and Falk, R. J. (2003). Plasmapheresis therapy for diffuse alveolar hemorrhage in patients with small vessel vasculitis. *American Journal of Kidney Diseases*, **42**, 1149–53.

Korantzopoulos, P., Papaioannides, D. and Siogas, K. (2004). The heart in Wegener's granulomatosis. *Cardiology*, **102**, 7–10.

Kozak, M., Gill, E. A. and Green, L. S. (1995). The Churg-Strauss syndrome. A case report with angiographically documented coronary involvement and a review of the literature. *Chest*, **107**, 578–80.

Kumar, P., Velissaris, T., Sheppard, M. N. and Pepper, J. R. (2002). Giant cell arteritis confined to intramural cornary arteries. Unforseen hazards myocardial protection. *Journal of Cardiovascular Surgery (Torino)*, **43**, 647–9.

Ladanyi, M. and Fraser, R. S. (1987). Pulmonary involvement in giant cell arteritis. *Archives of Pathology and Laboratory Medicine*, **111**, 1178–80.

Lane, S. E., Watts, R. A., Shepstone, L. and Scott, D. G. (2005). Primary systemic vasculitis: clinical features and mortality. *Quarterly Journal of Medicine*, **98**, 97–111.

Lanham, J., Elkon, K., Pusey, C. and Hughes, G. (1984). Systemic vasculitis with asthma and eosinophilia: a clinical approach to the Churg-Strauss syndrome. *Medicine*, **63**, 65–81.

Lauque, D., Cadranel, J., Lazor, R., Pourrat, J., Ronco, P., Guillevin, L., *et al.* (2000). Microscopic polyangiitis with alveolar hemorrhage. A study of 29 cases and review of the literature. Groupe d'Etudes et de Recherche sur les Maladies "Orphelines" Pulmonaires (GERM"O"P). *Medicine* (Baltimore), **79**, 222–33.

Lee, A. S. and Specks, U. (2004). Pulmonary capillaritis. *Seminars in Respiratory and Critical Care Medicine*, **25**, 547–55.

Lee, K. S., Kim, T. S., Fujimoto, K., Moriya, H., Watanabe, H., Tateishi, U., *et al.* (2003). Thoracic manifestation of Wegener's granulomatosis: CT findings in 30 patients. *European Radiology*, **13**, 43–51.

Lie, J. T. (1987). Coronary vasculitis. *Archives of Pathology and Laboratory Medicine*, **111**, 224–233.

Lie, J. T. (1996). Isolated pulmonary Takayasu arteritis: clinicopathologic characteristics. *Modern Pathology*, **9**, 469–74.

Lie, J. T. (1998). Pathology of isolated nonclassical and catastrophic manifestations of Takayasu arteritis. *International Journal of Cardiology*, **66**, S11–S21.

Lupi-Herrera, E., Sanchez-Torres, G., Marchushamer, J., Mispireta, J., Horwitz, S., and Vela, J. E. (1977). Takayasu's arteritis. Clinical study of 107 cases. *American Heart Journal*, **93**, 94–103.

Lynch, J. P., 3rd, White, E., Tazelaar, H. and Langford, C. A. (2004). Wegener's granulomatosis: evolving concepts in treatment. *Seminars in Respiratory and Critical Care Medicine*, **25**, 491–521.

Maksimowicz-McKinnon, K. and Hoffman, G. S. (2004). Large-vessel vasculitis. *Seminars in Respiratory and Critical Care Medicine*, **25**, 569–79.

Manning, W. J., Stuber, M., Danias, P. G., Botnar, R. M., Yeon, S. B. and Aepfelbacher, F. C. (2002). Coronary magnetic resonance imaging: current status. *Current Problems in Cardiology*, **27**, 275–333.

Maskell, G. F., Lockwood, C. M. and Flower, C. D. (1993). Computed tomography of the lung in Wegener's granulomatosis. *Clinical Radiology*, **48**, 377–80.

Merkel, P. A., Lo, G. H., Holbrook, J. T., Tibbs, A. K., Allen, N. B., Davis, J. C., Jr., *et al.* (2005). Brief communication: high incidence of venous thrombotic events among patients with Wegener granulomatosis: the Wegener's Clinical Occurrence of Thrombosis (WeCLOT) Study. *Annals of Internal Medicine*, **142**, 620–6.

Mirone, L., Altomonte, L., Ferlisi, E. M., Zoli, A. and Magaro, M. (1997). Behçet's disease and cardiac arrhythmia. *Clinical Rheumatology*, **16**, 99–100.

Mogulkoc, N., Burgess, M. I. and Bishop, P. W. (2000). Intracardiac thrombus in Behçet's disease: a systematic review. *Chest*, **118**, 479–87.

Mwipatayi, B. P., Jeffery, P. C., Beningfield, S. J., Matley, P. J., Naidoo, N. G., Kalla, A. A., *et al.* (2005). Takayasu arteritis: clinical features and management: report of 272 cases. *Australian and New Zealand Journal of Surgery*, **75**, 110–7.

Nachman, P. H., Hogan, S. L., Jennette, J. C., and Falk, R. J. (1996). Treatment response and relapse in antineutrophil cyctoplasmic autoantibody-associated microscopic polyangiitis and glomerulonephritis. *Journal of the American Society for Nephrology*, **7**, 33–39.

Nadrous, H. F., Yu, A. C., Specks, U. and Ryu, J. H. (2004). Pulmonary involvement in Henoch-Schonlein purpura. *Mayo Clinic Proceedings*, **79**, 1151–7.

Nakada, T. (1996). Ventricular arrhythmia and possible myocardial ischemia in late stage Kawasaki disease: patient with a normal coronary arteriogram. *Acta Paediatrica Japonica*, **38**, 365–9.

Nakao, K., Ikeda, M., Kimata, S-I., Niitani, H., Miyahara, M., Ishimi, Z-I., Hashiba, K., Takeda, Y., Ozawa, T., Matsushita, S., and Kuramochi, M. (1967). Takayasu's arteritis: clinical report of eight-four cases and immunological studies of seven cases. *Circulation*, **35**, 1141–1155.

Nesi, G., Anichini, C., Pedemonte, E., Tozzini, S., Calamai, G., Montesi, G. F., *et al.* (2002). Giant cell arteritis presenting with annuloaortic ectasia. *Chest*, **121**, 1365–7.

Newburger, J. W., Takahashi, M., Gerber, M. A., Gewitz, M. H., Tani, L. Y., Burns, J. C., *et al.* (2004). Diagnosis, treatment, and long-term management of Kawasaki disease: a statement for health professionals from the Committee on Rheumatic Fever, Endocarditis, and Kawasaki Disease, Council on Cardiovascular Disease in the Young, American Heart Association. *Pediatrics*, **114**, 1708–33.

Niles, J. L., Bottinger, E. P., Saurina, G. R., Kelly, K. J., Pan, G., Collins, A. B. and McCluskey, R. T. (1996). The syndrome of lung hemorrhage and nephritis is usually an ANCA-associated condition. *Archives of Internal Medicine*, **156**, 440–5.

Numano, F. and Kobayashi, Y. (1999). Takayasu arteritis–beyond pulselessness. *Internal Medicine*, **38**, 226–32.

Olopade, C. O., Sekosan, M. and Schraufnagel, D. E. (1997). Giant cell arteritis manifesting as chronic cough and fever of unknown origin. *Mayo Clinic Proceedings*, **72**, 1048–50.

Olson, J. C., Kelly, K. J., Pan, C. G. and Wortmann, D. W. (1992). Pulmonary disease with hemorrhage in Henoch-Schoenlein purpura. *Pediatrics*, **89**, 1177–81.

Pagnoux, C. and Guillevin, L. (2005). Cardiac involvement in small and medium-sized vessel vasculitides. *Lupus*, **14**, 718–22.

Papiris, S. A., Manoussakis, M. N., Drosos, A. A., Kontogiannis, D., Constantopoulos, S. H. and Moutsopoulos, H. M. (1992). Imaging of thoracic Wegener's granulomatosis: the computed tomographic appearance. *American Journal of Medicine*, **93**, 529–36.

Pfizenmaier, D. H., Al Atawi, F. O., Castillo, Y., Chandrasekaran, K. and Cooper, L. T. (2004). Predictors of left ventricular dysfunction in patients with Takayasu's or giant cell aortitis. *Clinical and Experimental Rheumatology*, **22**, S41–5.

Pipitone, N., Boiardi, L., Olivieri, I., Cantini, F., Salvi, F., Malatesta, R., *et al.* (2004). Clinical manifestations of Behçet's disease in 137 Italian patients: results of a multicenter study. *Clinical and Experimental Rheumatology*, **22**, S46–51.

Radhamanohar, M. (1991). Multiple pulmonary infarctions caused by giant cell arteritis. *Postgraduate Medical Journal*, **67**, 491.

Reinhold-Keller, E., Beuge, N., Latza, U., DeGroot, K., Rudert, H., Nolle, B., Heller, M., and Gross, W. (2000). An interdisciplinary approach to the care of patients with wegener's granulomatosis. *Arthritis and Rheumatism*, **43**, 1021–32.

Reuter, M., Schnabel, A., Wesner, F., Tetzlaff, K., Risheng, Y., Gross, W. L., and Heller, M. (1998). Pulmonary Wegener's granulomatosis: correlation between high-resolution CT findings and clinical scoring of disease activity. *Chest*, **114**, 500–6.

Rodriguez, W., Hanania, N., Guy, E. and Guntupalli, J. (2002). Pulmonary-renal syndromes in the intensive care unit. *Critical Care Clinics*, **18**, 881–95, x.

Roncoroni, A. J., Alvarez, C. and Molinas, F. (1992). Plexogenic arteriopathy associated with pulmonary vasculitis in systemic lupus erythematosus. *Respiration*, **59**, 52–6.

Sable-Fourtassou, R., Cohen, P., Mahr, A., Pagnoux, C., Mouthon, L., Jayne, D., *et al.* (2005). Antineutrophil cytoplasmic antibodies and the Churg-Strauss syndrome. *Annals of Internal Medicine*, **143**, 632–8.

Schiavone, W. A., Ahmad, M. and Ockner, S. A. (1985). Unusual cardiac complications of Wegener's granulomatosis. *Chest*, **88**, 745–8.

Schnabel, A., Holl-Ulrich, K., Dalhoff, K., Reuter, M. and Gross, W. L. (1997). Efficacy of transbronchial biopsy in pulmonary vaculitides. *European Respiratory Journal*, **10**, 2738–43.

Schrader, M. L., Hochman, J. S. and Bulkley, B. H. (1985). The heart in polyarteritis nodosa: a clinicopathologic study. *American Heart Journal*, **109**, 1353–9.

Sharma, B. K., Jain, S., and Sagar, S. (1996). Systemic manifestations of Takayasu arteritis: the expanding spectrum. *International Journal of Cardiology*, **54**, S149–54.

Sheehan, R. E., Flint, J. D. and Muller, N. L. (2003). Computed tomography features of the thoracic manifestations of Wegener granulomatosis. *Journal of Thoracic Imaging*, **18**, 34–41.

Siburian, G., Hashimoto, Y. and Numano, F. (1993). Ventricular arrhythmias in Takayasu arteritis. *International Journal of Cardiology*, **40**, 243–9.

Specks, U. (2003). Pulmonary vasculitis. *Interstitial Lung Disease* (eds, Schwarz, M. I. and King, T. E.), pp. 599–631. B. C. Decker, Hamilton.

Stuck, A. E., Minder, C. E., and Frey, F. J. (1989). Risk of infectious complications in patients taking glucocorticoids. *Review of Infectious Diseases*, **11**, 954–963.

Suzuki, R., Morita, H., Komukai, D., Hasegawa, T., Nakao, N., Ideura, T., *et al.* (2003). Mixed cryoglobulinemia due to chronic hepatitis C with severe pulmonary involvement. *Internal Medicine*, **42**, 1210–4.

Travis, W. D., Hoffman, G. S., Leavitt, R. Y., Pass, H. I. and Fauci, A. S. (1991). Surgical pathology of the lung in Wegener's granulomatosis. *American Journal of Surgical Pathology*, **15**, 315–33.

Utzig, M. J., Warzelhan, J., Wertzel, H., Berwanger, I. and Hasse, J. (2002). Role of thoracic surgery and interventional bronchoscopy in Wegener's granulomatosis. *Annals of Thoracic Surgery*, **74**, 1948–52.

Uzun, O., Akpolat, T. and Erkan, L. (2005). Pulmonary vasculitis in Behçet's disease: A cumulative analysis. *Chest*, **127**, 2243–53.

Vanoli, M., Castellani, M., Bacchiani, G., Cali, G., Mietner, B., Origgi, L., *et al.* (1999). Non-invasive assessment of pulmonary artery involvement in Takayasu's arteritis. *Clinical and Experimental Rheumatology*, **17**, 215–8.

Vats, K. R., Vats, A., Kim, Y., Dassenko, D. and Sinaiko, A. R. (1999). Henoch-Schonlein purpura and pulmonary hemorrhage: a report and literature review. *Pediatric Nephrology*, **13**, 530–4.

Viegi, G., Fornai, E., Ferri, C., Di Munno, O., Begliomini, E., Vitali, C., *et al.* (1989). Lung function in essential mixed cryoglobulinemia: a short-term follow-up. *Clinical Rheumatology*, **8**, 331–8.

Weir, I. H., Muller, N. L., Chiles, C., Godwin, J. D., Lee, S. H. and Kullnig, P. (1992). Wegener's granulomatosis: findings from computed tomography of the chest in 10 patients. *Canadian Association of Radiologists Journal*, **43**, 31–4.

Weiss, M. A. and Crissman, J. D. (1985). Segmental necrotizing glomerulonephritis: diagnostic, prognostic, and therapeutic significance. *American Journal of Kidney Diseases*, **6**, 199–211.

Weller, P. F., Plaut, M., Taggart, V. and Trontell, A. (2001). The relationship of asthma therapy and Churg-Strauss syndrome: NIH workshop summary report. *Journal of Allergy and Clinical Immunology*, **108**, 175–83.

Weschler, M. E., Finn, D., Gunawardena, D., Westlake, R., Barker, A., Haranath, S. P., Pauwels, R. A., Kips, J. C. and Drazen, J. M. (2000). Churg-Strauss syndrome in patients receiving montelukast as treatment for asthma. *Chest*, **117**, 708–13.

Weschler, M. E., Garpestad, E., Flier, S. R., Kocher, O., Weiland, D. A., Polito, A. J., Klinek, M. M., Bigby, T. D., Wong, G. A., Helmers, R. A., and Drazen, J. M. (1998). Pulmonary infiltrates, eosinophilia, and cardiomyopathy following corticosteroid withdrawal in patients with asthma receiving zafirlukast. *JAMA*, **279**, 455–7.

WGET Investigators (2005). Etanercept plus standard therapy for Wegener's granulomatosis. *New England Journal of Medicine*, **352**, 351– 61.

Wilcke, J. T., Nielsen, P. K. and Jacobsen, T. N. (2003). Reversible complete heart block due to Wegener's granulomatosis. *International Journal of Cardiology*, **89**, 297–8.

Worthy, S. A., Muller, N. L., Hansell, D. M. and Flower, C. D. (1998). Churg-Strauss syndrome: the spectrum of pulmonary CT findings in 17 patients. *AJR American Journal of Roentgenology*, **170**, 297–300.

Yamada, I., Nakagawa, T., Himeno, Y., Kobayashi, Y., Numano, F. and Shibuya, H. (2000). Takayasu arteritis: diagnosis with breath-hold contrast-enhanced three-dimensional MR angiography. *Journal of Magnetic Resonance Imaging*, **11**, 481–7.

Yokoi, K., Akaike, M., Nishiuchi, T., Kawai, H. and Saito, S. (1992). Scar formation in the cardiac conduction system of a patient with Takayasu's arteritis. *Cardiology*, **81**, 378–83.

CHAPTER 14

Vasculitic neuropathy

Shin J. Oh

Introduction

Peripheral neuropathy is a common and important clinical manifestation of systemic necrotizing vasculitis (SNV). Peripheral neuropathy due to necrotizing vasculitis is called vasculitic neuropathy and is the result of ischemic damage due to occlusion of blood vessels associated with an inflammatory process in the vessel walls of the vasa nervorum. Vasculitic neuropathy can occur either as a manifestation of multisystem involvement or as an independent disease process, such as non-systemic vasculitic neuropathy. Though vasculitic neuropathy is relatively rare, its recognition is important because it is potentially treatable. In the past few decades, remarkable progress has been made in various aspects of vasculitic neuropathy. This chapter presents an overview of the classical concepts.

Vulnerability of peripheral nerves to vasculitic neuropathy

The hallmark of all SNV is inflammation and necrosis of the blood vessels, typically involving medium- and small-sized arteries. Since the vasa nervorum in the peripheral nerves fall into the spectrum of small-sized arteries and arterioles, it is not surprising that peripheral neuropathy is a common manifestation of SNV. The vessels responsible for vasculitic neuropathy are predominantly the arterioles of the epineurium, which typically have a diameter ranging from 30 to 300 micrometers (μm) (Conn and Dyck 1984; Dyck et al. 1972). Typical lumina measure 10–25 μm for transperineurial arterioles and 10–20 μm for epineurial capillaries (Beggs et al. 1991; Dyck et al. 1985; Giannini and Dyck 1993).

The microvasculature of peripheral nerves has several unique features (McManis et al. 1993). There is a rich anastomotic blood supply through two functionally distinct vascular systems: the extrinsic system composed of the epineurial vessels and regional arteries, arterioles, and venules, and the intrinsic system of the longitudinal microvessels within the fascicles themselves. These two systems are linked by a complex system of interconnecting vessels that provide high blood flow in the baseline state (McManis et al. 1993; Slady et al. 1985). This rich blood supply, along with the capacity of nerves to function relatively well with anaerobic metabolism, makes peripheral nerves relatively resistant to ischemia. Only with intensive involvement of the vasa nervorum does ischemic damage occur.

On the other hand, some characteristics of the endoneurial vessels actually render nerves susceptible to ischemia. The endoneurial capillaries are larger and more widely spaced, particularly in the central fascicular regions, than in other tissues (Bell and Weddell 1984a, 1984b). In addition, there is a poorly developed smooth muscle layer (McManis et al. 1993), so peripheral nerve tissue is virtually incapable of autoregulating blood flow and is susceptible to the small changes in perfusion pressure that may occur with a vasculitic process. Because of this vulnerability, a central fascicular fiber loss does occur in vasculitic neuropathy and is regarded as a typical pathological feature of ischemic neuropathy (Dyck et al. 1972).

Dyck et al. (1972) found that, in patients with vasculitic neuropathy associated with rheumatoid arthritis (RA), the most vulnerable area of the major nerves is in the mid-upper arm and mid-thigh levels, presumably because they are in a watershed zone of poor perfusion. At these levels, they found focal areas of nerve fiber degeneration largely in the centers of fascicles (central fascicular degeneration). Distal to these levels, central fascicular degeneration became more pronounced, with more fascicles becoming affected and broadening of the lesions in the fascicles already damaged. In view of the striking similarity between central fascicular degeneration in vasculitic neuropathy and that seen in diabetic ophthalmoplegia, in which ischemia is also implicated, this pattern of fiber degeneration may be typical of ischemic lesions in the nerve.

Pathology of vasculitic neuropathy

To render a definite diagnosis of vasculitic neuropathy, the unmistakable histological features of vasculitis must be present: active, inactive, or healed necrotizing changes and infiltration of inflammatory cells within the vessel wall. Several histological types of arterial changes are described in vasculitic neuropathy, including Type I (active vasculitis), Type II (inactive [or healed] vasculitis), and Type III (probable vasculitis) (Table 14.1). These are described below.

Perivascular infiltration of inflammatory mononuclear cells

This process is an early and mild arterial insult according to Dyck et al. (1972) and occurs without any intramural necrosis or cellular infiltration (Figure 14.1a). This alone is not enough to be diagnostic of vasculitis because a similar finding is observed in inflammatory neuropathies, especially in acute forms. However, there are some histological features that are helpful in differentiating these

Table 14.1 Pathological criteria of definite and probable vasculitis

	Definite	Probable
Wees *et al.* (1981)	Type I: active vasculitis – definite fibrinoid necrosis with infiltration of inflammatory cells within the vessel wall, or Type II: inactive (or healed) vasculitis – concentric fibrous scarring and intramural thickening of the vessel walls, and minimal intramural and perivascular infiltration of inflammatory cells.	Type III: the presence of perivascular infiltration of inflammatory cells and active axonal degeneration without any definite intramural infiltration of inflammatory cells.
Dyck *et al.* (1987)	1. Inflammation of the vessel wall and 2. Necrosis of the wall	1. Mural or perivascular inflammation without tissue necrosis, with or without intimal proliferation, or 2. Evidence of necrosis or previous necrosis of the arterioles wall without inflammation, with or without intimal pr oliferation and with or without focal or multifocal fiber degeneration.
Hawke *et al.* (1991)	1. Vessel wall necrosis and an inflammatory cell reaction	An inflammatory reaction in or around a vessel with a diameter greater than 30 μm.
Davies *et al.* (1996)	1. Vessel wall necrosis with perivascular or transmural infiltration of inflammatory cells, or 2. Perivascular inflammatory infiltrates with evidence of previous vessel wall necrosis (fibrous obliteration with or without recanalization, disruption of the internal elastic lamina or hemosiderin within the vessel wall).	1. Perivascular inflammatory cell in the medium sized (>120 μm) vessels with prominent acute axonal degeneration or focal nerve damage with aberrant regenerating nerve cell clusters, or 2. Small-vessel cuffing with segmental fiber degeneration or acute axonal degeneration in 40% of fibers in the teased nerve.
Collins *et al.* (2000)	1. Transmural inflammatory cell infiltration in at least one blood vessels combined with signs of vascular injury such as fibrinoid necrosis, endothelial disruption, fragmentation of the internal elastic lamina, lumen, or hemorrhage into the vessel wall.	1. Perivascular inflammatory cells and at least one other supportive pathological features: vascular thickening and sclerosis, narrowing or obliteration of the lumen, thrombosis with or without recanalization, epineurial capillary proliferation, periadventitial hemosiderin, asymmetric nerve fiber loss, or Wallerian-like degeneration.

Criteria of Said (1988b) include: transmural infiltration of small epineurial; perineurial arteries with inflammatory cells; leukocytoclasia; fibrinoid necrosis; destruction of the internal elastic lamina; occlusion of the lumen; and the usual sparing of adjacent venules.

Criteria of Kissel *et al.* (1985) include: segmental wall necrosis and transmural inflammatory cell infiltration in at least one epineurial blood vessel (perivascular inflammation, central fiber atrophy or selective fascicular atrophy are excluded).

disorders. In vasculitic neuropathies, axonal degeneration is the predominant finding, whereas in inflammatory neuropathies, segmental demyelination and endoneurial inflammatory cells are typical findings. An exception has been found in vasculitic neuropathy associated with HIV, in which inflammatory cells are often present in the endoneurial space and small endoneurial blood vessels are affected (Said 1995). Thus, we make a diagnosis of probable vasculitis when perivascular infiltrates of inflammatory cells are present together with axonal degeneration and there is a decreased population of myelinated fibers with clinical findings compatible with vasculitis (Wees *et al.* 1981). This is a Type III lesion according to our classification (Wees *et al.* 1981) (Table 14.1).

Active vasculitis

This is represented by acute changes including fibrinoid necrosis of the media with intramural and perivascular infiltrates of inflammatory cells, polymorphonuclear leukocytes, lymphocytes, and eosinophils (Figures 14.1b and 14.1c). Polymorphonuclear leukocytes may be prominent, but usually lymphocytes predominate in the vessel wall and perivascular area. Eosinophils are present in vasculitis of various etiologies but marked eosinophilic infiltration suggests Churg–Strauss syndrome (Midroni and Bilbao 1995; Oh *et al.* 1986). Together with these cardinal findings, dissolution of the internal elastic membrane and edema or thickening of the adventitia are typically noted. Active vasculitis represents a Type I lesion in our classification (Wees *et al.* 1981). With active vasculitis, hemorrhage into surrounding tissue may occur, sometimes in a perineurial or subperineurial crescentic pattern.

Inactive vasculitis

This is manifested by chronic changes including concentric fibrous scarring and thickening of the intima and media with minimal intramural and perivascular infiltrates of inflammatory cells, lymphocytes, and plasma cells (Figure 14.1d). Splitting and actual overgrowth of the internal elastic membrane usually accompany this lesion, which is Type II in our classification (Wees *et al.* 1981).

Healed vasculitic lesions

These are indicative of previous severe injury to the arterial wall. They are characterized by perivascular and intramural fibrosis with

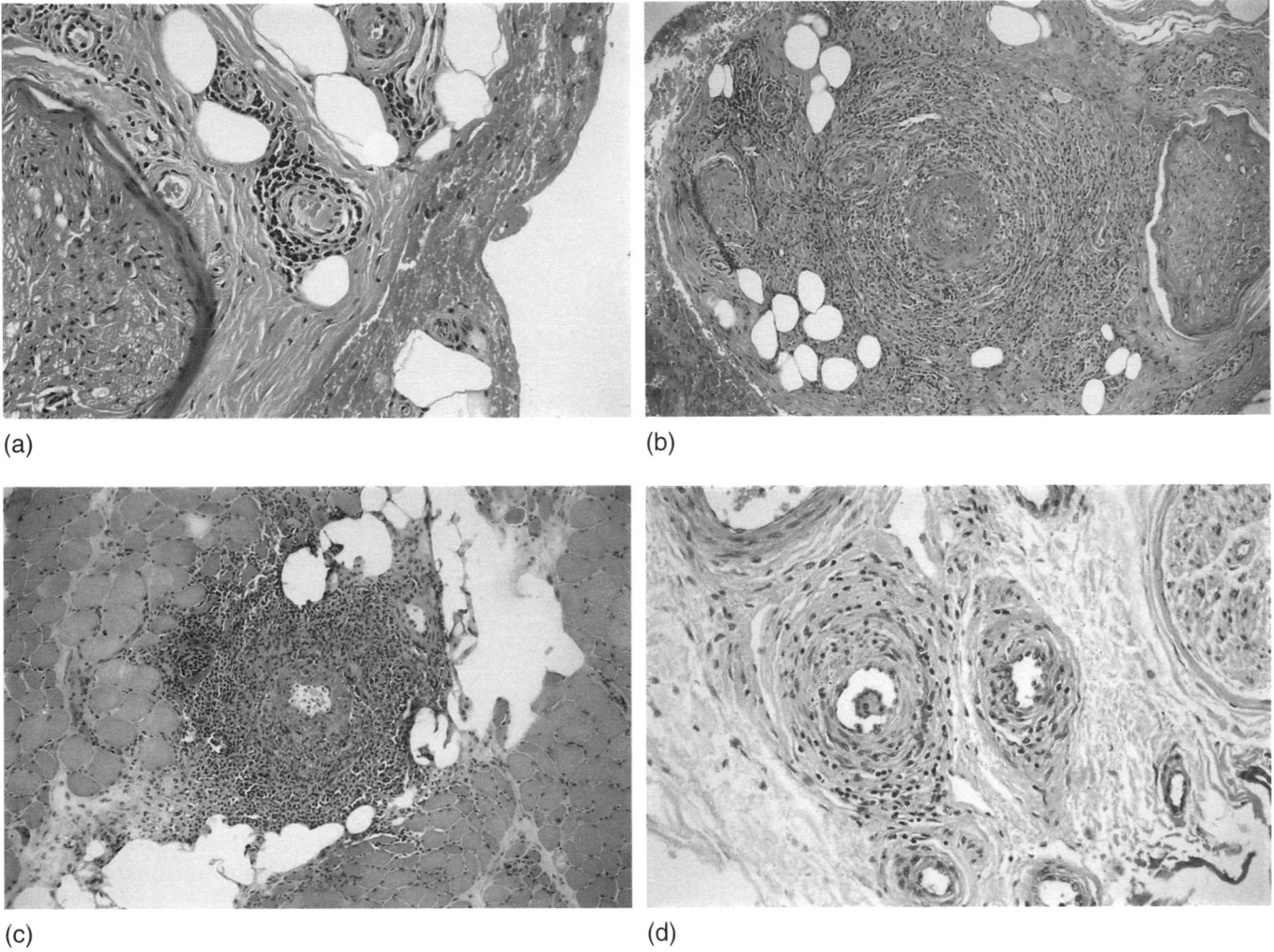

(a)

(b)

(c)

(d)

Figure 14.1 (a) Perivascular collection of mononuclear inflammatory cells (Type III) in the small arteriole in the epineurial space. There is no intramural infiltration of inflammatory cells or fibrinoid necrosis. Paraffin section H & E, magnification 250 ×. (b) Active vasculitis (Type I) in the larger arteriole in the epineurial space. There is intramural infiltration of mononuclear cells and fibrinoid necrosis of muscular and adventitial layers and near occlusion due to intimal thickening. The arteriole is enlarged due to active vasculitic process. Paraffin section. H & E, magnification 100 ×. (c) Active vasculitis (Type I) in the arteriole in the perimysial space in muscle. Intimal thickening, intramural infiltrations of mononuclear inflammatory cells, and fibrinoid necrosis of muscular and adventitial layers of arteriole are seen. The arteriole is enlarged due to active vasculitic process. Frozen section. H & E, magnification 100 ×. (d) Inactive vasculitis (Type II). Thick intimal layer and scattered intramural inflammatory cells in the muscular and adventitial layers of small arteriole in the epineurial space are present. Paraffin section H & E, magnification 100 ×. (See Color Plate 60.)

fragmentation of the internal elastic membrane and narrowing, occlusion, and calcification of the lumen or recanalization of the previously occluded lumen. Hemosiderin-laden macrophages, indicative of old hemorrhage, may cluster in a periadvential location. There are no perivascular or intramural inflammatory cells. This lesion may mimic atherosclerotic changes; however, careful study of the vessels with connective tissue and elastin stains helps differentiate these two different processes. Fragmentation of the internal elastic membrane is suggestive of healed vasculitis. Midroni and Bilbao (1995) occasionally observed miniature bundles of aberrant regenerating axons, reminiscent of a traumatic neuroma. Schroder (1986) has drawn attention to the reactive proliferation of capillaries that can occur in the epineurium after a vascular insult, although this observation is not specific to vasculitis. Thus, these findings

should be regarded as clues suggestive of the presence of remote vasculitis, but not indicative or diagnostic of vasculitis.

Axonal degeneration

Axonal degeneration is the predominant pattern and is due to the ischemic damage of the nerve (Figure 14.1e) (Hawke *et al.* 1991; Loveshin and Kernohan 1948; Wees *et al.* 1981). Said *et al.* (1988b) observed axonal degeneration in an average of 65% of nerve fibers. The degree of axonal degeneration depends on the activity of the vasculitic process. Prominent axonal degeneration is invariably seen with active vasculitic lesions and is best observed in the longitudinal cuts on frozen sections. Late in the disease, the process of axonal degeneration is more complete and few, if any, fibers remain.

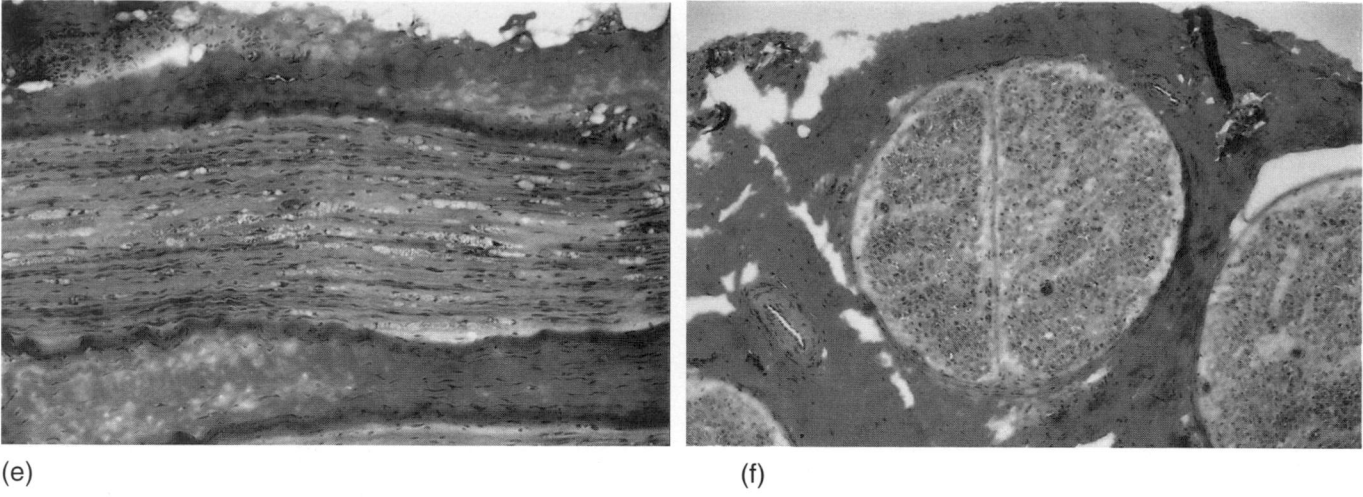

(e)   (f)

Figure 14.1 (e) Prominent myelin-digestion chambers (vacuoles) such as these are indicative of axonal degeneration in one nerve fascicle. Myelin remnants (ovoids) are stained as red. Frozen section. Modified trichrome, magnification 100 ×.
(f) Selective fascicular atrophy indicative of ischemic neuropathy. Loss of myelinated fibers in the right half of fascicle is due to occlusion of vasa nervorum supplying blood to this section of fascicle. Myelinated fibers are stained as "red", magnification 100 ×. (See Color Plate 60).

Patterns of degeneration

Various patterns of degeneration of fibers are noted, ranging from central fascicular degeneration to total fascicular atrophy, depending on the severity of neuropathy (Figure 14.1f). Although central fascicular degeneration is typical of ischemic neuropathy, total fascicular atrophy is also typical as a result of the total occlusion of arterioles that supply blood to the involved fascicle.

It should be emphasized that any combination of these changes may be found in a single sural nerve biopsy, indicating an ongoing process (Hawke *et al.* 1991). In most cases, the nerve lesions appear to result from the summation of vascular lesions of different ages (Fujimura *et al.* 1991). In autopsy series (Dyck *et al.* 1982; Loveshin and Kernohan 1948), all these changes could be seen along the course of an involved peripheral nerve. Dyck *et al.* (1972) stated that chronic changes are usually seen in nerves of patients with long-standing, non-progressive neuropathy, and acute lesions in patients with clinically acute neuropathy.

It is not possible to diagnose specific vasculitic syndromes from nerve biopsy specimens. In general, the caliber of involved vessels may allow one to assign a given biopsy to one of two broad groups (Chalk *et al.* 1993a). Vasculitic involvement of larger (100–250 μm) epineurial arterioles is a typical feature of Churg–Strauss syndrome (CSS), Wegener's granulomatosis (WG), rheumatoid vasculitis, and microscopic polyangiitis (MPA). Predominant involvement of smaller (<100 μm) epineurial arterioles is more suggestive of Sjögren's syndrome, systemic lupus erythematosus (SLE), and non-systemic vasculitis of nerves (Chalk *et al.* 1993a). Involvement of epineurial veins occurs more commonly in WG and CSS than in PAN (Lie 1990). Vasculitis of endoneurial vessels is uncommon and would theoretically be classified with leukocytoclastic (hypersensitivity) vasculitis according to Midroni and Bilbao (1995). In HIV-induced vasculitic neuropathy, mononuclear cells are often present in the endoneurial space and vasculitic change is seen more often in endoneurial vessels (Calabrese *et al.* 1989; Said *et al.* 1987).

Although a definite histological diagnosis of vasculitis in the nerve should be based on the demonstration of active or inactive vasculitis (Type I and II lesions, respectively), the concept of probable vasculitis in the nerve is introduced because the definite criteria of vasculitis are too stringent to be clinically useful in vasculitic neuropathy (Table 14.1). In about one-quarter of patients with vasculitic neuropathy, the criteria for definite vasculitic neuropathy are lacking (Table 14.2). This is most likely due to the absence of medium- and small-sized arteries in the nerve, which are often involved in SNV. Although the criteria for probable vasculitis differ from author to author, perivascular infiltration (cuffing) of inflammatory cells must be present. This finding alone is not sufficient for the diagnosis of vasculitis because it is a non-specific finding

Table 14.2 Distribution of definite and probable vasculitis

	Type of vasculitis	No. of cases	Definite	Probable
Wees *et al.* (1981)	Systemic	17	15[1]	1
Dyck *et al.* (1987)	Systemic	45	26	13[2]
	Non-systemic	20	5	15
Hawke *et al.* (1991)	Systemic	34	30	3[3]
Davies *et al.* (1996)	Systemic	76	57	19
	Non-systemic	25	19	6
Claussen *et al.* (2000)	Systemic	45	33[4]	12
Collins *et al.* (2000)	Systemic	25	15	10
	Non-systemic	11	7	4

[1] Type I in 14 cases and Type II in 1 case. In 1 case, vasculitis in muscle biopsy.

[2] In 6, nerve biopsy is non-diagnostic. Definite vasculitis in other tissues.

[3] In 1 case, nerve biopsy is non-diagnostic. However, autopsy showed definite vasculitis in other tissues.

[4] Type I, in 27 cases and Type II in 6 cases.

in nerve pathology. This is especially true in the context of chronic inflammatory demyelinating polyneuropathy (CIDP). Predominant axonal degeneration favors vasculitis, whereas segmental demyelination and endoneurial inflammatory cells favor CIDP. Because of this, we recommend that perivascular infiltration of inflammatory cells and axonal degeneration be considered as the minimal diagnostic criteria for probable vasculitis.

The criteria for probable vasculitic neuropathy are appropriate to use in the clinical diagnosis of patients with suspected vasculitic neuropathy. Three studies showed that all patients with probable vasculitis on nerve biopsy were proven to have systemic vasculitis by other means. In the Wees *et al.* report (1981) of one patient with Type III nerve biopsy, angiography of the celiac axis showed typical microaneurysms of PAN. In Dyck's 13 cases of probable vasculitic neuropathy, vasculitis was confirmed by liver and kidney biopsies and post-mortem findings (Dyck *et al.* 1987). In Hawke's series, vasculitis was confirmed in each case by muscle biopsy, kidney biopsy, or autopsy (Hawke *et al.* 1991).

Pathogenesis of vasculitic neuropathy

It is generally accepted that the nerve fiber degeneration in this disorder is ischemic secondary to vasculitis in the vasa nervorum (Asbury and Johnson 1978; Dyck *et al.* 1972); however, there are different opinions with regard to the appearance of the consequent nerve alteration following ischemia. Dyck *et al.* (1972) did not believe that infarction occurs in nerve. Their view was based on a detailed study of the involved nerves in rheumatoid vasculitic neuropathy, which did not reveal any evidence of infarction (defined as a circumscribed area of necrosis of all cellular elements leading to liquefaction with a border of macrophages, such as occurs in the brain). They maintained that the infarcts of nerves described by Kernohan and Woltman (1938) were not infarcts, but probably Renault's corpuscles. On the other hand, Asbury and Johnson (1978) believe that frank infarct necrosis of the nerve does occur in vasculitic, amyloid, and diabetic neuropathies.

The pattern of neuropathic involvement in vasculitic neuropathy depends on the extent and temporal progression of the ischemic changes (Fathers and Fuller 1996). Mononeuropathy multiplex, the classical pattern of neuropathy in vasculitic neuropathy, is due to lesions in larger vessels, leading to whole nerve trunk infarction in nerves scattered throughout the body (Figure 14.2). On the other hand, asymmetrical polyneuropathy (overlapping mononeuropathy multiplex) results from a confluence of patchy discrete infarction of smaller vessels in many individual peripheral nerves, together with superimposed mononeuropathy from damage of whole nerve trunks. Symmetrical polyneuropathy is a consequence of a more diffuse peripheral nerve ischemia due to multiple small lesions, which are more likely to affect longer nerves.

The classical theory of the pathogenesis of immune-mediated vasculitis is that immune complex deposition in blood vessel walls leads to inflammation and infiltration of polymorphonuclear leukocytes with subsequent tissue necrosis producing the pathological picture of leukocytoclasis (Fauci *et al.* 1978). Recent studies confirmed that this mechanism is also operative in vasculitic neuropathy. Kissel *et al.* (1989) found immunofluorescent evidence for immune complex involvement in 85% of biopsies in their series, and only in those vessels that also had intense cellular infiltrates. In Hawke's series (1991), immunofluorescent staining was positive

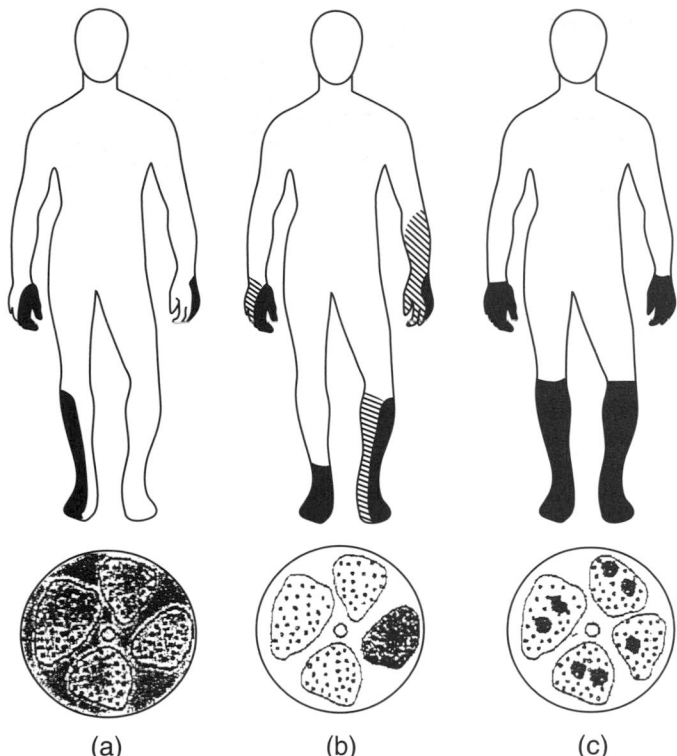

Figure 14.2 (a) Mononeuropathy multiplex: right peroneal, left ulnar, and right superficial radial sensory radial neuropathy, occurring due to ischemic degeneration of whole nerve of these individual nerves. Shaded area of the nerve represents the ischemic degeneration. (b) Asymmetrical polyneuropathy due to more patch damage in the scattered many nerves, but not corresponding to the named nerves. Lined areas represent milder degree of involvement. (c) Symmetrical polyneuropathy due to multiple small lesions in the nerve fascicles, which are more likely to affect longer nerves.

on nerves in 100% of 20 patients. In 16 cases, immunoglobulin, complement C3, and fibrinogen were present in endoneurial or perineurial blood vessels. In four cases, only C3 and fibrinogen were found. In control nerves, occasional faint fluorescence was detected with C3 on endoneurial capillaries, but there was no fluorescent staining of larger epineurial or perineurial vessels. There were four cases without cellular invasion of the sural nerve in which there was immunofluorescent evidence of immune complex deposition. Panegyres *et al.* (1990) also observed immune complex deposits in 13 (72%) of 18 cases.

Kissel *et al.* (1989) have questioned the role of immune complexes, as they found that cellular infiltrates in vascular lesions were composed predominantly of T cells (71 %) and macrophages (27%). Two-thirds of the T cells were of the CD8[+] subset. In contrast, B cells and polymorphonuclear leukocytes were extremely rare, and a leukocytoclastic reaction was never observed. In contrast, Panegyres *et al.* (1990) found the ratio of lymphocytes to macrophages to vary from 3:1 to 1:23, with substantial numbers of B lymphocytes in the three nerves in which lymphocyte subtyping was performed. Neither group found any correlation between the types of inflammatory cells and the presence or type of associated systemic disease. On the basis of these findings, Kissel *et al.* (1989) suggested a cytotoxic T cell-mediated process as a primary mechanism of vascular damage in peripheral nerve vasculitis.

Biopsy diagnosis of vasculitic neuropathy

Nerve biopsy in diagnosis of vasculitic neuropathy

Nerve biopsy is often indicated in vasculitis and vasculitic neuropathy for three reasons (Oh 1990). First, peripheral nerves, including the sural nerve, are commonly involved in vasculitic neuropathy (Wees *et al.* 1981). Second, the diagnostic yield is high when the sural nerve conduction is abnormal (Claussen *et al.* 2000; Wees *et al.* 1981). Finally, vasculitis and vasculitic neuropathy are treatable. In Oh's series of 385 nerve biopsies over a 16-year period, vasculitic neuropathy was the most commonly diagnosed specific form of neuropathy, accounting for 12% (Oh 1990). When clinical features suggest the possibility of systemic vasculitis, detailed neurological and electrophysiological tests are mandatory. Asymptomatic peripheral neuropathy was detected by the nerve conduction study (NCS) in an average of 10% of patients with vasculitic neuropathy (see below) (Claussen *et al.* 2000). When the patient has vasculitic neuropathy by neurological and electrophysiological tests, nerve biopsy is definitely indicated if obtaining other tissues for diagnosis is not feasible or warranted. Three nerves are most suitable for biopsy: the sural, superficial peroneal, and superficial radial nerves. The sural nerve is most commonly biopsied because it is easily identifiable, is commonly involved in vasculitic neuropathy, and can reliably be tested electrophysiologically. On the other hand, Said and Kissel recommend superficial peroneal nerve biopsy because it allows simultaneous muscle biopsy from the adjacent peroneus brevis muscle through a single incision on the lateral aspect of the leg (Kissel and Mendell 1992; Said *et al.* 1988b). Oh and colleagues prefer sural nerve biopsy because they have found the superficial peroneal nerve to be less reliable in nerve conduction testing and much harder to locate anatomically than the sural nerve.

To increase the diagnostic yield in vasculitic neuropathy, the following guidelines and precautions are recommended.

First, the sural nerve should be tested electrophysiologically and the more impaired sural nerve biopsied. In one report, vasculitic neuropathy was diagnosed by sural nerve biopsy in 100% of 15 patients with sural nerve conduction abnormalities. Of these, 14 had vasculitis and one had probable vasculitis (Wees *et al.* 1981). Based on this finding, Wees *et al.* (1981) stated that abnormality in the sural nerve conduction was prerequisite to the demonstration of vasculitis on biopsy, but this concept has been challenged: seven cases of sural nerve biopsy-proven vasculitis with normal sensory nerve conduction have been reported (Davidson and Sundstrom 1988; Hawke *et al.* 1991; Midroni and Bilbao 1995). In a recent series of 44 confirmed cases of vasculitis, NCS on the biopsied sural nerve were abnormal in 38 of 39 patients tested. One patient with vasculitis had nerve conduction velocities (NCV) within the normal range (± 2 standard deviations from the mean), but a relatively decreased amplitude in sensory compound nerve action potential (CNAP) when compared with the same nerve on the other side. Among the three other cases with normal NCS of the sural nerve that was biopsied, there was no evidence of vasculitis (Claussen *et al.* 2000). Thus, abnormal sural nerve conduction strongly correlates with the finding of vasculitis, suggesting that this test can be used to estimate the likelihood of a positive nerve biopsy.

Normal sural nerve conduction does not preclude the diagnosis of vasculitis on the sural nerve biopsy, but does decrease the likelihood of a positive biopsy. Thus, when the sural nerve conduction is normal, we recommend electrophysiological testing on the superficial peroneal and superficial radial sensory nerves, as these alternative nerves may be biopsied. We have successfully used this approach to confirm vasculitis in two patients. Kissel and Mendell (1992) had to perform only two superficial radial nerve biopsies over a 15-year period, both of which proved sufficient for diagnosis. In regard to the superficial peroneal nerve, there are no published data that correlate the nerve conduction data and nerve biopsy findings.

The second recommendation is that a biopsy specimen of the entire cross-section of the nerve should be obtained. There is no role for fascicular nerve biopsy in suspected vasculitic neuropathy because the vasa nervorum are located in the epineurial and perineurial space, which may not be obtained by fascicular biopsy. This was unquestionably documented in the study by Dyck *et al.* (1972); all eight whole nerve biopsies demonstrated vasculitic neuropathy while three of six fascicular biopsies failed to show vasculitic change.

Third, although this is not well-documented, it seems prudent to perform the sural nerve biopsy early because glucocorticoid treatment may alter the histological features of vasculitis.

Fourth, it is necessary to cut multiple sections from different levels of the specimen since vasculitis is multifocal and segmental. It has been our repeated experience that only a few sections of the biopsied nerve show the diagnostic change. According to Said (1995), characteristic lesions may be present on segments of the arteries as short as to 50 mm. Thus, in cases of suspected vasculitic neuropathy, one should cut and stain as many sections of the biopsied nerve as possible.

Muscle biopsy in diagnosis of vasculitic neuropathy

Muscle was the first tissue chosen for diagnosis of vasculitis and was the favored diagnostic biopsy site until nerve biopsy was introduced in 1968 (Dyck and Lofren 1968). In 1952, Maxeiner *et al.* reported a diagnostic sensitivity for vasculitis of 13% in 136 muscles biopsies among 106 cases suspected of PAN and a diagnostic sensitivity of 35% in 26 cases of documented PAN. They also stated that the likelihood of positive biopsy was higher when a local lesion (nodule or tenderness) was present, compared with random sampling (30% versus 8%, respectively). In 1955, Garcia *et al.* (1955) reported seven cases of polyarteritis diagnosed by calf muscle biopsy, all of which were later confirmed at autopsy. In the 1960s, Bleehen and Lovelace *et al.* described the technique of superficial peroneal sensory nerve and peroneus brevis muscle biopsy in polyarteritis (Bleehan *et al.* 1963; Lovelace 1964). Despite the general availability of nerve biopsy, muscle biopsy remained the main diagnostic procedure for vasculitis at some medical centers until the 1980s.

Dhalberge *et al.* (1989) compared various diagnostic tests in 40 cases of suspected SNV and reported a diagnostic sensitivity of 19% among 26 muscle biopsies. Among 10 patients with proven SNV, they found 50% sensitivity and concluded that the muscle biopsy was the most valuable of the relatively safe procedures. They did not utilize nerve biopsy in any of their cases. Dyck *et al.* (1987) reported a diagnostic sensitivity of 25% in muscle biopsy of 12 cases of proven vasculitis neuropathy. Said *et al.* (1988b) reported that peroneus brevis muscle biopsy had a diagnostic sensitivity of 75% among 83 proven cases of vasculitic neuropathy. This figure was exceptionally high and defied explanation. It is worth noting, however, that the same authors recently reported that muscle biopsy had a diagnostic sensitivity of 54%, a figure more in agreement with the consensus of other reports. At the University of Alabama at Birmingham, a 17% diagnostic sensitivity of muscle biopsy was found among 115 cases of suspected SNV and 42% sensitivity among 45 cases of proven vasculitic neuropathy (Claussen *et al.* 2000). Among six studies, five (all except Said *et al.* 1988b) have shown that nerve biopsy has a higher diagnostic sensitivity than does muscle biopsy.

Thus, in general, the diagnostic value of muscle biopsy in patients with suspected SNV is disappointingly low, indicating that this should not be the first choice of biopsy. If clinical findings and electrophysiological studies on the sural, superficial peroneal, and superficial radial nerves are normal and an affected nerve is not accessible for biopsy, then muscle biopsy may be the only choice for tissue diagnosis.

In selecting a muscle for biopsy, clinical and needle electromyography (EMG) data are useful. In one series, abnormal needle EMG findings in the biopsied muscle did not discriminate between positive and negative biopsies, but a trend was noted between the presence of fibrillation and positive sharp waves and vasculitis on the muscle biopsy (Claussen *et al.* 2000). On this basis, it is preferable to biopsy a muscle that shows fibrillation and positive sharp waves on the needle EMG study.

Diagnostic sensitivity of simultaneous nerve and muscle biopsy

The diagnostic sensitivity of simultaneously obtained nerve and muscle biopsy depends solely on the criteria used for patient selection. Among those with suspected SNV or vasculitic neuropathy, the diagnostic sensitivity averages 30% for the nerve biopsy in contrast to 16% for the muscle biopsy (Table 14.3). Among patients with confirmed vasculitic neuropathy, the diagnostic sensitivity averages 71% for the nerve biopsy and 45% for the muscle biopsy. These findings indicate the superiority of nerve biopsy over muscle biopsy. Our data strongly support the higher sensitivity of nerve biopsy (39% of all cases) compared with muscle biopsy (17% of all cases) for patients with suspected and definite vasculitis. In none of our cases was the muscle biopsy positive for vasculitis when the nerve biopsy was negative, but in three cases the muscle biopsy was more specific and resulted in a definite diagnosis, increasing the diagnostic yield from 29% to 31%. Thus our results support the notion that muscle biopsy is complementary to nerve biopsy in the detection of vasculitis. Previous studies also found that adding muscle biopsy to the nerve biopsy increased the positive diagnostic yield by 6 to 25% (Hawke *et al.* 1991; Said *et al.* 1988b). On the basis of these findings, the combined biopsy of nerve and muscle is widely advocated when considering vasculitis in the differential diagnosis. We usually do the sural nerve biopsy together with biopsy of the anterior tibialis or gastrocnemius muscle. Another method is to perform the nerve biopsy first and,

Table 14.3 Diagnostic sensitivity of nerve and muscle biopsies in vasculitic neuropathy

Authors	Patients	No. cases	Nerve biopsy	Muscle biopsy	Comments
Dyck *et al.* (1987)	SNV, biopsy-proven VN	45	58% (26/45)	25% (3/12)	Sural/gastrocnemius
Said *et al.* (1988b)	SNV, biopsy-proven VN	83	51%	75%	Superficial peroneal/peroneus brevis
Said (1995)	SNV, biopsy-proven VN	?	62%	54%	Same as above?
Claussen *et al.* (2000)	SNV, suspected[3]	115	39%	17%	Sural in all /anterior tibialis in 2/3 of cases
	SNV, biopsy-proven VN	45	100%	42%	
Collins *et al.* (2000)	SNV,[4] suspected	70	27%	16%	Superficial peroneal/peroneus brevis
	SNV, biopsy-proven VN	22	90%	50%	
Said (1995)	SNV, biopsy-proven VN	425	76.5%	59.5%	Superficial peroneal/peroneus brevis
Maxeiner *et al.* (1952)	SNV, suspected	136[1]		13%	
	SNV, biopsy-proven	26	35%		
Dahlberg *et al.* (1989)	SNV, suspected	26[2]	1	9%	
Cruz Martinez *et al.* (1988)	SNV, biopsy-proven VN	14	86%	79%	
Dyck *et al.* (1987)	NSV, biopsy-proven VN	20	100%		All by sural nerve biopsy
Davies *et al.* (1996)	NSV; biopsy-proven VN	25	100%		All by sural nerve biopsy
Collins *et al.* (2003)	NSV, biopsy-proven VN	48	100%		Sural in 30; SP/PB in 19; Sup radial in 2
Kararizou (2005)	NSV, biopsy-proven VN	22	100%		All by sural nerve biopsy

[1] 136 muscle biopsies from 106 cases suspected of polyarteritis nodosa.

[2] 26 muscle biopsies.

[3] Neuropathy/myopathy in 66 and no neuromuscular syndromes in 15.

Others: no clinical information.

[4] Including 7 cases of NSV.

Abbreviations: SNV, systemic necrotizing vasculitis; NSV, non-systemic vasculitis; VN, vasculitic neuropathy.

depending on the findings in the nerve, consider performing muscle biopsy later.

Vasculitic neuropathy in systemic necrotizing vasculitis

Incidence and risk factors

The exact incidence and prevalence of vasculitic neuropathy are unknown. An approximation of the frequency of vasculitic neuropathy can be ascertained from a report of the American College of Rheumatology subcommittee on classification of vasculitis (Bloch *et al.* 1990; Hunder *et al.* 1990). In this study, 1000 new cases of vasculitis were detected at 48 medical centers over a 5.5-year period. Since peripheral neuropathy occurs in up to 70% of patients with primary vasculitic syndromes, approximately 700 new cases of vasculitis neuropathy were estimated at 48 medical centers over the study period, or three cases per year per center. This figure closely approximates that of several published series (Table 14.4).

Vasculitic neuropathy is rare compared with other types of peripheral neuropathy. The most common cause for neuropathy in the US is diabetes mellitus. One study showed that 35% of 100 elderly (over 65 years of age) patients with disabling neuropathy had one form or another of vasculitic neuropathy proved by nerve biopsy (Chia *et al.* 1996).

The frequency of peripheral neuropathy in SNV syndromes ranges from 25% in CSS to 70% in PAN (Table 14.5). Peripheral neuropathy can be the initial manifestation of PAN. The frequency of peripheral neuropathy in the primary rheumatic diseases ranged from 1.5% in scleroderma to 18% in SLE. Most, though not all, cases of peripheral neuropathy in primary rheumatic diseases are due to vasculitic neuropathy.

Clinical manifestations

Clinical clues and laboratory features suggesting vasculitis in adults are discussed in Chapter 21. Vasculitic neuropathy affects males

Table 14.4 Frequency of cases with vasculitic neuropathy

Authors	Sources	No of cases	Years[1]	Cases/ year
Wees *et al.* (1981)	Nerve/muscle biopsy	17	5	3.4
Dyck *et al.* (1987)	Medical record/nerve biopsy	65[2]	22	2.9
Said *et al.* (1988b)	Nerve/muscle biopsy	100	15	6.6
Oh (1990)	385 nerve/muscle biopsy	46	16	2.9
Hawke *et al.* (1991)	1024 nerve biopsy	34	12	2.8
Kissel (1994)	350 nerve biopsy	16	10	1.6
Davies *et al.* (1996)	1559 nerve biopsy	25[3]	9	2.7
Collins *et al.* (2000)	SPN/PBM biopsy[4]	22	10	2.2
Collins *et al.* (2003)	Nerve/muscle biopsy	48[3]	20	2.4
Kararizou *et al.* (2005)	Nerve biopsy	22[3]	20	1.1
Said (1995)	Nerve biopsy	425	34	12.5

[1] Duration of years these cases were collected.

[2] 45 systemic necrotizing vasculitic neuropathy and 20 non-systemic necrotizing vasculitic neuropathy.

[3] Non-systemic vasculitic neuropathy.

[4] SPN/PBM, superficial peroneal nerve/peroneal brevis muscle biopsy.

Table 14.5 Systemic diseases associated with vasculitic neuropathy

	Prevalence of disease	Frequency of vasculitic neuropathy (%)
Primary vasculitic diseases		
Polyarteritis nodosa	Rare	50–70
Churg–Strauss syndrome	Rare	64
Wegener's granulomatosis	Rare	25
Giant cell arteritis	Common in elderly	5–14
Microscopic polyangiitis	Rare	Uncertain
Rheumatoid diseases		
Rheumatoid arthritis	Common	10
Systemic lupus erythematosus	Common	2–18
Sjögren's syndrome	Common	9
Progressive systemic sclerosis	Uncommon	1.5
Behçet's syndrome	Rare	5
Hypereosinophilic syndrome	Rare	14
Hypersensitivity vasculitis	Common	10
Other conditions with vasculitis		
Cryoglobulinemia	Rare	50
Malignancy	Common	Rare
HIV infection	Variable	2
Lyme disease	Variable	<1

and females equally and is most common in older individuals. The time course of disease varies from a rapid onset over days to weeks (25% develop in less than 4 weeks) to a more gradual evolution over many months (50% more than 2 months) (Hawke *et al.* 1991). When onset of disease is acute, it may mimic Guillian–Barré syndrome (GBS) (Suggs *et al.* 1992). In vasculitic neuropathy due to SNV, it is rare to have a disease course longer than 1 year (Hawke *et al.* 1991; Kissel *et al.* 1985; Wees *et al.* 1981) but in non-systemic vasculitic neuropathy, a period of more than 12 months before diagnosis is not uncommon (Davies *et al.* 1996). In general, patients with mononeuropathy multiplex have symptoms for a shorter period (mean 9.2 weeks) than patients with either an asymmetrical neuropathy (mean 32 weeks) or a symmetrical neuropathy (mean 20 weeks) (Hawke *et al.* 1991). This is likely due to clinicians' higher index of suspicion of vasculitic neuropathy in a setting of rapidly evolving mononeuropathy multiplex than in one of slowly progressing asymmetrical or symmetrical polyneuropathy.

Vasculitis-induced ischemic changes in the nerve are not a selective process, and so both sensory and motor fibers are usually affected. All patients in Hawke's series (1991) had a sensorimotor peripheral neuropathy; however, pure sensory neuropathy has also been reported (see below), so sensory neuropathy alone does not rule out vasculitic neuropathy. Nerves in the legs are affected more often than nerves in the arms. Pain and dysesthesia are present in 53–70% of patients with vasculitic neuropathy (Hawke *et al.* 1991; Kissel *et al.* 1985). A typical clinical picture is deep aching pain in the affected limb with subsequent development of unpleasant paresthesia in the cutaneous distribution of the affected nerve. In vasculitic neuropathy due to SNV, common systemic symptoms are fever, anorexia, weight loss, and fatigue (Kissel *et al.* 1985; Wees *et al.* 1981). Systemic symptoms usually develop at the same time as vasculitic neuropathy but may precede it by more than 6 months (Hawke *et al.* 1991). In non-vasculitic neuropathy, systemic features are absent (Davies *et al.* 1996; Dyck *et al.* 1987; Kissel *et al.* 1985).

In 1981, Wees *et al.* published the first paper reporting asymmetrical and symmetrical polyneuropathy as manifestations of vasculitic neuropathy, and polyneuropathy as the most common form of vasculitic neuropathy. Since then it has been well accepted that there are three main patterns of neuropathy though the relative frequency varies from study to study (Table 14.6). A review of the literature confirms the finding that polyneuropathy (asymmetrical or symmetrical) is common, being observed in 55% of cases. The classical pattern of mononeuropathy multiplex was seen only in one-third of patients. Recognition of this concept is important; one should not exclude the possibility of vasculitic neuropathy because of the absence of mononeuropathy multiplex.

Mononeuropathy multiplex

Mononeuropathy multiplex has been touted as a classic manifestation of vasculitic neuropathy and the most common neurologic manifestation in PAN. Mononeuropathy multiplex is defined as the involvement of two or more individual nerves in more than one extremity, for example the ulnar nerve in one arm and the peroneal nerve in a leg. In vasculitic neuropathy, this is due to lesions in larger arterioles or small arteries, leading to whole-nerve trunk infarction. True mononeuropathy multiplex is thought to be the most distinctive pattern in vasculitic neuropathy (Kissel and Mendell 1992). Chalk *et al.* (1993) wrote the following: "Usually, vasculitic neuropathy presents as the syndrome of multiple mononeuropathies, in which single peripheral nerves or cranial nerves are affected in succession. Abrupt onset of weakness, prickling paresthesia, or sensory loss, often associated with local pain, is characteristic. Occasional patients develop a flurry of neuropathic deficits in several limbs during a single day."

In Ford and Siekert's series (1965), 54% of patients had mononeuropathy multiplex. In Guillevin's series (Guillevin *et al.* 1992), mononeuropathy multiplex was reported in 70% of 182 cases of PAN. Cohen *et al.* (1980) used mononeuropathy multiplex as a criterion for the diagnosis of PAN. Since mononeuropathy multiplex can be due to multiple causes, including multifocal motor and motor-sensory demyelinating neuropathies, this is no longer justifiable (Table 14.7). Of note, multifocal demyelinating neuropathy is more common than vasculitic mononeuropathy multiplex in our clinic.

Mononeuropathy

Mononeuropathy multiplex, by definition, requires the involvement of at least two nerves. There have been several reports of mononeuropathy as a manifestation of vasculitic neuropathy (Bouche *et al.* 1986; Said *et al.* 1988b; Wees *et al.* 1981). Two cases of mononeuropathy were found among 17 patients with systemic vasculitic neuropathy: peroneal neuropathy in a patient with RA, and anterior interosseous neuropathy in a patient with PAN (Wees *et al.* 1981). In both cases, NCS showed diffuse neuropathy and abnormal sural nerve conduction. One group found five (11%) cases of mononeuropathy among 44 cases of vasculitic neuropathy (Claussen *et al.* 2000). Said *et al.* (1988b) reported 13 cases of mononeuropathy among 100 cases of vasculitic neuropathy: peroneal neuropathy in 11, femoral neuropathy in one, and ulnar neuropathy in one. Bouche *et al.* (1986) also reported three cases of mononeuropathy: one sciatic neuropathy, one peroneal nerve palsy, and one ulnar neuropathy. This indicates that mononeuropathy is a manifestation of vasculitic neuropathy in about 10% of patients with systemic necrotizing vasculitis.

Asymmetrical polyneuropathy

Asymmetrical polyneuropathy is characterized by an asymmetrical distribution of motor and sensory deficits between two limbs, for example symmetrical sensory polyneuropathy with left peroneal neuropathy. Kissel and Mendell (1992) termed such a pattern overlapping mononeuropathy multiplex. In their series, this was the most common clinical presentation in vasculitic neuropathy, but in a compiled series it was seen in 23% of cases (Table 14.6). Many clinicians, usually non-neurologists, have labeled this pattern mononeuropathy multiplex, using this term loosely. Thus, confusion has resulted as to the frequency of mononeuropathy multiplex in vasculitic neuropathy. Asymmetric polyneuropathy should not be confused with true mononeuropathy multiplex, which has a distinct list of differential diagnoses (Table 14.7). Asymmetrical polyneuropathy results from simultaneous, patchy, discrete infarctions of smaller vessels in many individual peripheral nerves, together with superimposed mononeuropathies due to damage of whole nerve trunks.

Symmetrical polyneuropathy

Symmetrical polyneuropathy is characterized by an ascending and distal, symmetrical, stocking–glove type sensory loss with flaccid distal weakness. The classical examples of symmetrical polyneuropathy are metabolic and alcoholic neuropathies. Thus, vasculitic neuropathy has not usually been considered in the differential diagnosis of this clinical finding. Since the 1980s, however, several studies have shown that vasculitis can cause symmetrical polyneuropathy (Table 14.6). In fact, a symmetrical polyneuropathy pattern is seen in one-third of patients with vasculitic neuropathy. Because most of such patients do not have a history of extensive mononeuropathy multiplex, symmetrical polyneuropathy is likely a consequence of more diffuse peripheral nerve ischemia due to multiple small lesions affecting longer nerves. Presentation of vasculitis neuropathy as a symmetrical polyneuropathy represents the most difficult diagnostic challenge for clinicians because of a low index of suspicion. In Hawke's series (1991), patients with mononeuropathy multiplex had a shorter period (mean 9.2 weeks) before diagnosis than did patients with symmetrical polyneuropathy (mean 20.4 weeks), or asymmetrical polyneuropathy (31.6 weeks). Most patients with vasculitic symmetrical polyneuropathy have mixed sensorimotor findings. However, pure sensory symmetrical polyneuropathy has been reported in a few cases (see below). A pure motor symmetrical polyneuropathy, classically seen in acute or chronic inflammatory demyelinating polyneuropathy, has not been reported in vasculitic neuropathy.

Sensory neuropathy

It has been claimed that in RA, sensory polyneuropathy is not due to vasculitis (Conn and Dyck 1984); however, Wees *et al.* (1981) described one RA patient with symmetrical sensory polyneuropathy who had a definite vasculitis on sural nerve biopsy. Moore and Fauci (1981) reported one patient with sensory polyneuropathy and two patients with cutaneous sensory neuropathy. Subsequently, Dyck *et al.* (1987) described one case of sensory neuropathy with non-systemic vasculitis neuropathy (NSVN) and Lacomis *et al.* (1997) reported one case of sensory neuropathy and vasculitis. In a recent analysis of a series of SNV, there were 10 (23%) examples of sensory polyneuropathy among 44 vasculitic neuropathy cases. Puechal *et al.* (1995) reported 15 patients with sensory neuropathy among 32 with vasculitic neuropathy and RA. These findings indicate that sensory polyneuropathy may be

Table 14.6 Distribution of neuropathy patterns in the vasculitic neuropathy[1]

	1981 Wees et al. SNV	1985 Kissel et al. SNV	1991 Hawke et al. SNV	1986 Bouche et al. SNV	1995 Midroni and Bilbao SNV	2000 Claussen et al. SNV	2000 Collins et al. S/NSNV[3]	1987 Dyck et al. NSVN	1996 Davies et al. NSVN	2003 Collins et al. NSDN	2005 Kararizou et al. NSVN	Total SNV	Total NSVN	Total
Mononeuropathy multiplex	3	2	16	9	12	10	3[4]	12	10	6	9	55 (29%)	37 (32%)	92 (30%)
Mononeuropathy	(2)[2]					(5)						(7)	(7)	(14)
Asymmetrical polyneuropathy	4	8	10	7	5	4	18[4]	4	7	37	4	56 (30%)	52 (45%)	108 (36%)
Symmetrical polyneuropathy	3	6	8	3	14	21	1	4	8	5	8	56 (30%)	25 (22%)	81 (27%)
Sensory	(1)					(8)	(2)	(1)				(11)	(1)	(13)
Asymptomatic neuropathy	7	0	3	1	9							20 (12%)	0	20 (7%)
Myopathy	(2)					(3)						(5)	0	(5)
Total cases	17	16	34	22	32	44	22	20	25	48	22	187	115	302

Abbreviations: SNV, systemic necrotizing vasculitic neuropathy; NSNV, non-systemic necrotizing vasculitic neuropathy.

[1] These are compiled from the reports which classified the neuropathy patterns into three categories: mononeuropathy multiplex, asymmetrical polyneuropathy, and symmetrical polyneuropathies. Said et al. (1988b) and Cruz Martinez et al. (1988) series are excluded.

Said: 13 mononeuropathy, 62 mononeuropathy multiplex, 19 symmetrical neuropathy, and 6 no neuropathy.

Cruz Martinez: 5 mononeuropathy multiplex, 7 symmetrical polyneuropathy, 3, asymptomatic.

[2] 2 cases are included in 3 cases of mononeuropathy multiplex.

[3] 7 cases had NSVN.

[4] This includes asymmetrical lumbar plexopathy.

Table 14.7 Various diseases with mononeuropathy multiplex

Category	Diseases
Ischemic	Vasculitic neuropathy
	Diabetic neuropathy
	Amyloid neuropathy
Inflammatory	Multifocal motor sensory demyelinating neuropathy
	Multifocal motor neuropathy
	Sarcoidosis
	Brachial plexus neuropathy
	Lumbosacral plexus neuropathy
	Lymphomatoid granulomatosis
Infectious	Leprosy
	Lyme disease
	HIV
Hereditary	Hereditary liability to pressure palsy
Malignant disease	Lymphomatous neuropathy

present as a manifestation of vasculitic neuropathy, contrary to previous claims.

Collins *et al.* (2000) reported pure or predominant sensory neuropathy in 10% of 36 cases with histologically proven vasculitis by the superficial peroneal nerve and peroneal brevis muscle biopsy. Collins *et al.* (2003) also reported predominantly sensory findings in 13% of 48 patients with NSVN. We reported 17 (16%) cases of sensory vasculitic neuropathy among 106 cases with histologically proven vasculitic neuropathy. In 65% of cases, sensory vasculitic neuropathy was associated with systemic vasculitis. The most common clinical presentation was symmetrical polyneuropathy, in 53% of cases. The most common nerve conduction pattern was diffuse neuropathy of axonal degeneration. Sural nerve biopsy was diagnostic in 88% of cases. In two cases, muscle biopsy was necessary for the definite diagnosis of vasculitis. Non-systemic sensory vasculitic neuropathy is usually benign. Of 11 patients followed for longer than 2 years, none developed motor weakness due to neuropathy. Kararizou *et al.* (2005) reported eight cases of sensory neuropathy among 22 patients with NSVN. These studies indicate that sensory vasculitic neuropathy does exist and can be due to vasculitic neuropathy.

Asymptomatic vasculitic neuropathy

Subclinical involvement detected only by nerve conduction studies, called asymptomatic vasculitic neuropathy, was described in 1981 (Wees *et al.* 1981). Among 17 patients with SNV, there were seven (41%) who did not show any clinical signs of peripheral neuropathy: two had myopathy, three had generalized weakness, and two had complaints of weakness. Systemic symptoms and laboratory findings were suggestive of PAN, which led to NCS. In all these patients, a diffuse neuropathy was detected by the NCS and vasculitis was confirmed by the sural nerve biopsy. Subsequent studies confirmed the existence of asymptomatic vasculitic neuropathy. Among 22 patients with vasculitic neuropathy, Bouche *et al.* (1986) found three (14%) with myalgia, but no definite clinical sign of peripheral nerve involvement, who had a neuropathic pattern on the electrophysiological study. Cruz Martinez *et al.* (1988) reported

similar findings in their series of 15 patients with biopsy-proven vasculitis: two patients had electrophysiological but not clinical evidence of neuropathy. Said *et al.* (1988b) reported six patients with no clinical neuropathy but with spontaneous pain in muscles, among 100 biopsy-proven cases of vasculitic neuropathy. Among 81 suspected cases of SNV, Claussen *et al.* 2000 found seven (9%) who had systemic features without neuropathy; in all five patients who underwent NCS there was evidence of neuropathy. Four (57%) of these seven patients were found to have vasculitis on nerve biopsy. These studies suggest that it is useful to evaluate patients suspected of SNV by an electrophysiological study, even if there is no clinical evidence of neuropathy. The electrophysiological tests should include NCS in the lower extremities, since these tests are extremely sensitive. If neuropathy is found, then biopsy of the involved nerve can follow immediately and frozen sections can confirm the diagnosis of vasculitic neuropathy.

Electrophysiological findings

NCS play three important roles in the diagnosis of peripheral nerve vasculitis. The first is to detect peripheral neuropathy among patients suspected of SNV but who do not have neurologic symptoms. Adequate NCS were able to detect asymptomatic peripheral neuropathy among such patients in 6–41% of cases, as discussed above. The second important role relates to the selection of a nerve for biopsy. When sural nerve conduction is normal, electrophysiological testing of the superficial peroneal and superficial radial sensory nerves is recommended. If the testing is abnormal, these nerves may be biopsied. Studies comparing the nerve conduction abnormalities and the diagnostic yield of superficial peroneal nerve and superficial radial nerve are not available at this time. The third important role is detection of asymptomatic nerve involvement not obvious by the clinical evaluation among individuals with neurologic or muscular disease. Wees *et al.* (1981) identified diffuse neuropathy by NCS in two patients with mononeuropathy, in one patient with mononeuropathy multiplex, and in two cases of myopathy. In four of five patients with mononeuropathy multiplex, Cruz Martinez *et al.* (1988) found more diffuse signs of neuropathy than suggested by clinical findings. Bouche *et al.* (1986) reported a similar observation in patients with mononeuropathy multiplex. In our experience, the most common nerve conduction abnormality in patients with vasculitic neuropathy is diffuse neuropathy, rather than mononeuropathy multiplex. For this reason, the lack of clear-cut mononeuropathy multiplex on nerve conduction studies cannot be used to exclude a vasculitic neuropathy.

Nerve conduction abnormalities in vasculitic neuropathies are typical of axonal degeneration (Bouche *et al.* 1986; Cruz Martinez *et al.* 1988; Dyck *et al.* 1987; Hawke *et al.* 1991; Kissel *et al.*; Wees *et al.* 1981). NCS were found to be abnormal in all patients with evidence of vasculitic neuropathy on physical examination. The most common nerve conduction abnormality was abnormal sensory nerve conduction (79–100% of patients), with absent compound muscle action potential (CMAP) being most frequently observed. Sural nerve conduction abnormality was common, seen in 80–100% of cases. Sensory nerve conduction in median and ulnar nerves was abnormal in 70% of cases. Mixed nerve conduction was abnormal in the median nerves in 30% and in the ulnar nerves in 40% of the cases. Motor nerve conduction was less affected than sensory nerve conduction. NCV was slow in median and ulnar nerves in 8%, in peroneal nerves in 83%, and in posterior tibial nerves in 53% of cases. Motor NCV was either normal or minimally slow, suggesting axonal neuropathy. As expected with axonal degeneration, the CMAP amplitude was typically reduced. Bouche *et al.* (1986) found reduced CMAP amplitude in all of his reported cases. Compared with the upper extremities, the lower extremities were more often involved, with the most commonly affected nerves being the peroneal and sural. In the upper extremities, the ulnar nerves were much more commonly involved than the median nerves. This suggests that the distribution of nerve infarction in mononeuropathy multiplex is not random.

The needle EMG classically shows a denervation process in the distal muscles in diffuse neuropathy. In cases of mononeuropathy or mononeuropathy multiplex, this was confined to the involved muscles. Fibrillations and positive sharp waves (PSW) were most commonly observed, as expected in axonal degeneration. Motor unit potentials (MUP) were relatively normal with little evidence of the high-amplitude long duration MUPs that characterize reinnervation. Most patients had a strikingly reduced motor unit recruitment pattern in clinically affected muscles, with sparse numbers of MUPs firing in isolation at a rapid rate on maximum effort. Conduction block, an electrophysiological hallmark of segmental demyelination, has rarely been reported in vasculitic neuropathy. Among 65 cases, Dyck *et al.* (1987) reported mild focal conduction block in two. We found conduction block in one nerve in nine of 47 cases. In none of these cases was a multifocal conduction block observed, nor was any other electrophysiological manifestation of demyelination found. Hawke *et al.* observed conduction block in three patients, two of whom had mononeuropathy multiplex. Ropert and Metral (1990) reported five cases of conduction block in necrotizing vasculitis; however, their data were not conclusive in view of the extremely low distal CMAP in four cases. Jamieson *et al.* (1991) reported a patient with necrotizing vasculitis who showed a multifocal conduction block in the first study but classic axonal neuropathy in a later study. These findings suggest that conduction block may be present in a few nerves transiently during the acute denervating stage of vasculitic neuropathy. Widespread asymmetrical conduction block in the presence of relatively well-preserved distal CMAP is strongly suggestive of an inflammatory demyelinating neuropathy.

The needle EMG can also detect myopathy, either symptomatic or asymptomatic, in some patients with vasculitic neuropathy. This is because myositis or myopathy is not uncommon in many rheumatic diseases. Wees *et al.* (1981) found a myopathic pattern (many small-amplitude and short-duration MUPs with early recruitment) in two patients with clinical evidence of myopathy, in two patients with generalized weakness, and in one patient with mononeuropathy. Bouche *et al.* (1986) found a myopathic pattern in one case of mononeuropathy multiplex, in six cases of diffuse neuropathy, and in one patient without clinical signs of neuropathy. Needle EMG findings may be helpful in selecting the specific muscle for biopsy. In the article by Claussen *et al.* (2000), abnormal needle EMG findings in biopsied muscle did not allow discrimination between biopsy-positive and biopsy-negative vasculitis cases. There was, however, a trend toward correlation between the presence of fibrillation and positive sharp waves and vasculitis in the muscle biopsy, suggesting that selection of a muscle on this basis may result in a higher diagnostic yield of vasculitis.

Laboratory findings

There is no specific laboratory marker for vasculitic neuropathy (Table 14.8). Thus, the laboratory evaluation is directed toward identifying the underlying causes of vasculitis or a serologic abnormality that may point toward a specific vasculitic syndrome. The most important laboratory test in SNV is the erythrocyte sedimentation rate (ESR), because an elevated ESR is its most consistent and common abnormality. It is almost invariably elevated in PAN, WG, and giant cell arteritis and therefore is useful diagnostically in these disorders (Haynes *et al.* 1986). Cryoglobulin assays may be useful, as vasculitic neuropathy is common in all forms of cryoglobulinemia (Garcia *et al.* 1988; Nemni *et al.* 1988). This is especially true in patients with hepatitis C virus-associated cryoglobulinemia (Khella *et al.* 1995). In HIV patients, vasculitic neuropathy is rare, usually occurring before the development of AIDS (Calabrese *et al.* 1989; Fuller *et al.* 1993). A few patients with Lyme disease have also been reported to have mononeuropathy multiplex with a vasculitis demonstrated pathologically (Meier *et al.* 1989). Thus, if clinical findings are compatible, HIV or Lyme titers should be ordered.

CSF is usually normal in vasculitic neuropathy except for mild elevation of protein in one-third of patients. On the other hand, abundant cells and high protein are the classical CSF pattern in HIV vasculitic neuropathy (Said 1995).

Sakai *et al.* (2005) reported that the mean plasma VEGF level in five patients with vasculitic neuropathy (one patient with NSVN) was significantly higher than in healthy controls, or in patients with GBS, CIDP, or amyotrophic lateral sclerosis. In view of small numbers, further studies with a larger study population are necessary.

Sanada *et al.* (2003) suggested MRA of the lower limb as a potential tool for the follow-up evaluation of vasculitic neuropathy. MR angiography of the lower limb in one case of NSVN showed arterial occlusion at the distal level of both tibial and peroneal arteries, which were nutrient arteries of the sural nerve. After 6 weeks of glucocorticoid therapy, MRA of the lower limbs showed marked improvement of arterial occlusion. This coincided with neurologic and electrophysiologic improvement.

Diagnosis

In NSVN, a definite diagnosis of vasculitic neuropathy is based on the nerve biopsy (Table 14.9) because, by definition, no other organ is involved. There is, however, a huge difference between two series with regard to the ratio of definite vasculitis to probable vasculitis in the nerve biopsy. In the series of Dyck *et al.* (1987), definite vasculitis was found in only 25% of cases, whereas in Davies's series (Davies *et al.* 1996), it was identified in 76% of cases. This difference between the two figures is not easily explained. The histological diagnosis of vasculitic neuropathy was confirmed by nerve biopsy in 82–100% of patients with systemic necrotizing neuropathy. The next most productive tissue was muscle biopsy. In rare cases, the tissue diagnosis was made by the liver or kidney biopsy or at autopsy. In a few cases, celiac angiography was used to diagnose vasculitic neuropathy (Table 14.9). Though Said (1995) stated that the tissue diagnosis of vasculitis was easily made by specific skin biopsy, the consensus is that this is less diagnostic and not necessarily indicative of systemic involvement (Lie 1990).

Table 14.8 Laboratory findings in vasculitic neuropathy

Laboratory test	Systemic necrotizing vasculitis			Non-systemic necrotizing vasculitis				
	1981 Wees et al. (n=17)	1985 Kissel et al. (n=16)	1991 Hawke et al. (n=14)	1986 Bouche et al. (n=22)	2000 Collins et al. (n=25)	1987 Dyck et al. (n=20)	1996 Davies et al. (n=25)	2003 Collins et al. (n=48)
High sedementation rate	14 (82%)	14 (87%)	6 (43%)	19 (86%)	17/22 (77%)	8 (40%)	10 (40%)	22 (25%)
Leukocytosis	6			14	14/23 (61%)	0		11 (23%)
Leukopenia	3							
Anemia	9				14/22 (64%)			15 (31%)
Rheumatiod factor (+)	9	4	7	2/11[1]	10/18 (55%)	1/6	2/18	10 (20%)
Low complement	5/10				4/19 (21%)			5 (11%)
Eosinophilia	3			8				
Hypergammaglobulinemia	3	4/13		13/18				
High creatine kinase	3							
Hepatitis B antigen	1/5		3/9	6/18				
Antinuclear antibody titer (+)	4	3	8		7/20 (35%)	3/11	4/20	19 (39%)
High serum creatinine	1	3						
Proteinuria	2							
Cryoglobulin	1					0/7		
Cerebrospinal fluid								
high protein			1/7 (14%)	4/9 (44%)		8/17 (47%)		5/19 (26%)
elevated cell count			0			0		1/19
oligoclonal band			1	1				

[1] 2/11, positive in 2 cases out of 11 tested cases.

Treatment

There have been no prospective, randomized controlled trials of therapy in vasculitic neuropathy, and present therapies are based therefore on collective experience in vasculitis in general. In SNV, the treatment of choice has been combined cyclophosphamide and glucocorticoids. In patients with neurologic involvement of vasculitis (10 CNS and 15 peripheral neuropathy), Moore and Fauci (1981) reported that virtually no extension or progression of disease activity was seen in any patient receiving an adequate course of cyclophosphamide for a reasonable duration of time. In systemic rheumatoid vasculitis, Scott and Bacon (1984) reported more frequent healing of vasculitic lesions including leg ulcers and neuropathy, a lower incidence of relapse, fewer serious complications, and a lower mortality rate with intermittent cyclophosphamide plus methylprednisolone than with other treatments.

The precise regimen for an individual patient depends on the extent, severity, and tempo of the vasculitic neuropathy and other organ involvement. Usually, a combination of prednisone 60 mg a day and oral cyclophosphamide 150 mg a day is recommended as the initial regimen. The combined therapy is continued until significant improvement occurs and the clinical condition stabilizes. This may take 6 to 12 months. At this point, prednisone is slowly tapered and a switch from cyclophosphamide to azathioprine

2 mg/kg per day is recommended, following the current practice in ANCA-associated vasculitis (Jayne et al. 2003). Azathioprine is then slowly tapered. Following treatment with cyclophosphamide (Langford and Sneller 1997; Rasmussen et al. 1996), it is reasonable to continue azathioprine treatment up to 1 year after all signs of the disease have subsided. This optimistic goal may not easily be achievable in vasculitic neuropathy, in which many symptoms and signs may persist. Thus, the recommendation is to continue the maintenance dose of azathioprine for 1 year after vasculitic neuropathy becomes inactive or maximum improvement has been achieved. If relapse occurs, either during tapering or maintenance of prednisone or azathioprine, the drugs must be increased to the previous dose. According to Hawke (1991), vasculitic neuropathy is generally treated for more than 2 years.

The recovery of function in vasculitic neuropathy is slow and lags considerably behind control of the vasculitis because axonal regeneration must occur. In some patients with systemic vasculitides, serum markers such as the ESR, complement levels, or ANCA titers can be followed. These markers are useful for therapeutic control of vasculitis, but are not necessarily beneficial as a diagnostic index for vasculitic neuropathy. The role of NCS in this regard has not been assessed. Therefore, a careful neurological evaluation is the best measure available for the determination of disease status

Table 14.9 Diagnostic methods for vasculitic neuropathy

Authors	Total cases	Nerve biopsy[1]	Muscle biopsy	Other
Wees et al. 1981	17	15 (82%)	3	1 celiac angiography[2]
Kissel et al. 1985	16	16	0	
Dyck et al. 1985	45	39 (87%)	3 (7%)	16: liver, kidney, post-mortem
				13 had probable vasculitis
Said et al. 1988b	95	42 (44%)	53[3]	0
Hawke et al. 1991				
	34	33 (97%)	2 (6%)	3 based on probable vasculitis[4]
				One renal biopsy; one autopsy
Claussen et al. 2000	45	45 (100%)	3 (7%)	9 based on Type III
Collins et al. 2000	22[5]	19 (86%)	4(18%)	

[1] This includes the definite and probable vasculitis by the pathology criteria except Kissel and Said series in which the definite vasculitis criteria was only used.

[2] Type III.

[3] In 16, muscle was the only tissue biopsied.

[4] Probable vasculitic neuropathy in 3. Diagnosis is confirmed by muscle biopsy in 2 and renal biopsy in 1.

[5] 7 cases with NSVN were included. In 3 cases with SVN, diagnosis is confirmed by muscle biopsy: nerve biopsy was negative in 2 and nerve was not found in 1. One additional case with NSVN had definite vasculitis in muscle.

in vasculitic neuropathy. In addition to immunosuppressive treatment, aggressive physical and occupational therapy is usually indicated during the recovery stage of the disease, to improve the patient's range of motion of joints, optimize functional status, and maintain strength. To manage neuropathic pain, the use of gabapentin, clonazepam, carbamazepine, or amitriptyline may be required.

There is no convincing evidence that plasma exchange benefits patients with vasculitis or vasculitic neuropathy (Guillevin et al. 1988; Winkelstein et al. 1984). In an open trial of eight patients with rheumatoid vasculitis, a course of plasma exchange given with conventional immunosuppressive agents resulted in more rapid healing of skin lesions than in patients treated with immunosuppressive agents alone (Winkelstein et al. 1984). The peripheral neuropathy in these patients, however, did not improve. In 165 patients with either PAN or CSS (67% of whom had peripheral neuropathy), the effect of plasma exchange on patients given prednisone alone or a combination of prednisone and cyclophosphamide was examined. The survival curves were not significantly influenced by plasma exchange (Guillevin et al. 1988).

The role of intravenous immunoglobulin (IVIg) in the treatment of vasculitis is still controversial. Though several uncontrolled investigations have demonstrated the efficacy of high-dose IVIg (0.4 gm/kg per d for 5 days) in the treatment of ANCA-associated vasculitis (Klassen et al. 1996; Levy et al. 1999; Lockwood 1996), another study failed to demonstrate its benefit (Richter et al. 1994). There has been only one report of a favorable outcome with IVIg in vasculitic neuropathy (Schifitto et al. 1997). In a patient with HIV-related vasculitic mononeuropathy multiplex, clinical improvement was achieved and maintained for 19 months with combined treatment with high-dose glucocorticoids and monthly IVIg for 4 months.

Prognosis

Studies of the prognosis in vasculitic neuropathy are limited. Several studies of PAN did not find that peripheral neuropathy was associated with a poorer outcome (Cohen et al. 1980; Fronert and Sheps 1967; Sack et al. 1975). Among the various factors analyzed, the only significant prognostic factor identified in vasculitic neuropathy was age: older age predicts a worse outcome (Hawke 1991). Chang et al. (1984) found that patients with no recurrence of systemic vasculitis within 18 months of initial appearance of mononeuropathy multiplex have a good prognosis. Puechal et al. (1995) showed that vasculitic neuropathy in RA is an indicator of poor prognosis: the overall survival rate at 5 years was 57%. They also found that cutaneous vasculitis, extensive mononeuropathy multiplex (more than three limbs involved), and depressed C4 level are indicators of a poor prognosis.

Three studies have addressed the issue of long-term survival in vasculitic neuropathy. The survival rate was found to be 37% (Hawke 1991), 57% (Puechal et al. 1995), and 60% at 5 years (Chang et al. 1984), and 71% at 6 years (Dyck et al. 1987). Death was usually attributed to vasculitis (Dyck et al. 1987) and usually occurred within 6 months after onset of illness (Hawke 1991). There is no good explanation for the markedly different survival rates between Hawke's series and Dyck's series, except that in the former most deaths were due to non-vasculitic causes, and in Dyck's series most were due to vasculitis. With treatment, vasculitic neuropathy has been found to have a good prognosis in terms of functional recovery. Moore and Fauci (1981) reported that even those patients with severe peripheral neuropathies improved greatly over time with treatment of the underlying diseases, physical therapy, and rehabilitation. Dyck et al. (1987) reported that two-thirds of living patients were better than at their first evaluation. Complete recovery was reported in 11% (Hawke 1991) to 21% (Chang et al. 1984) over a 3- to 5-year follow-up period. On recovery, patients were able to ambulate without assistance in 58% (Chang et al. 1984) to 84% of cases (Hawke). Relapse was reported in 25% of cases in Chang's series and in 0% in Hawke's series. Relapse was most likely due to premature cessation of prednisone or cytotoxic medications or treatment with suboptimal doses of these drugs. Despite reasonable functional recovery, many patients had persistent sensory symptoms, especially in the lower limbs (Davies 1994).

Non-systemic vasculitic neuropathy

Vasculitis confined to peripheral nerves is termed non-systemic vasculitic neuropathy (NSVN) (Dyck et al. 1987). Though this entity was described first in 1938 by Keroohan and Woltman in a 48-year-old man with necrotizing vasculitis restricted to the peripheral nervous system at autopsy, the concept of localized peripheral nerve system vasculitis was reintroduced in 1985 when Kissel et al. reported seven cases of NSVN among 16 cases of biopsy-proven vasculitic neuropathy. None of their cases had any other organ involvement or abnormal serological tests. Dyck et al. (1987) reported 20 patients with NSVN among 65 cases of necrotizing vasculitis. Davies et al. (1996) reported their experience with 25 patients with NSVN. Said et al. (1988b) reported 32 cases of peripheral neuropathy alone among 100 patients with necrotizing vasculitis. Collins et al. (2003) described 48 patients with NSVN at presentation. Unlike other groups, this group includes patients with constitutional symptoms such as weight loss and unexplained fever. Weight loss was observed in 35% of cases and unexplained fever in 15%. This raises a question whether all of Collins' cases represent pure NSVN. Kararizou *et al.* (2005) reported 22 cases of NSVN. It is worth noting that patients with NSNV, because of the absence of systemic symptoms or other organ involvement, are likely to see a neurologist. This is in contrast to SVN patients who are likely to be seen by a primary care physician or rheumatologist.

NSVN represents about 25% of cases of vasculitic neuropathy (Davies *et al.* 1996; Dyck *et al.* 1987; Said *et al.* 1988b). In NSVN, there are no signs of systemic or organ involvement, such as weight loss, fever, anorexia, or kidney failure (Table 14.10). There is no difference in the types of neuropathy, but Dyck *et al.* (1987) observed that there are some differences between NSVN and SVN at the microscopic level. In NSVN, smaller perineurial arterioles were more often involved, the severity of pathology was less, and probable vasculitis (perivascular infiltration of cells without intramural infiltration of cells or fibrinoid necrosis) was more common in NSVN.

Dyck *et al.* (1987) believed that an underlying indolent necrotizing vasculitis of the small epineurial arterioles was responsible; Davies *et al.* (1996) observed the vasculitic features predominantly in the epineurial arterioles, not very different from SVN. Both showed axonal degeneration as the predominant pathological finding and selective fascicular atrophy or central atrophy as ischemic changes. Immune complexes in the vessel walls were observed as commonly in NSVN as in SVN (Davies *et al.* 1996). High ESR

Table 14.10 Pathological, clinical, and laboratory differences between systemic necrotizing (SNV) and non-systemic necrotizing (NSNV) vasculitic neuropathies

	SNV	NSNV
Pathological features		
Commonly involved	Epineurial arteriole	Perineurial smaller arteriole
Types of vasculitis	More often definite	More common "probable"
Severity	More severe	Less severe
Axonal degeneration	No difference	No difference
Ischemic change	No difference	No difference
Clinical features	Essentially the same	Essentially the same
Laboratory features		
Elevated ESR	Common	Rare
Positive ANA	Common	Extremely rare
Positive RF	Common	Extremely rare
Hepatitis B surface antigen	20%	None
Diagnosis	Can be diagnosed from other tissue	Nerve biopsy is sine qua non
Duration of disease	Weeks to months	Months to years
Treatment	Cyclophosphamide	Glucocorticoids alone?
Prognosis	Serious	Benign

(>40 mm/h) was noted in 25–50% of cases (Collins *et al.* 2003; Kissel *et al.* 1985). Hepatitis B antigen, monoclonal gammopathy and cryoglobulin were absent in NSVN (Dyck *et al.* 1987). Collins *et al.* (2003) reported monoclonal gammopathy in three (8%; 3/37 cases) patients older than 50 years. Nerve biopsy is necessary for diagnosis of NSVN; without it, vasculitis cannot be reliably differentiated from other rapidly progressive neuropathies because many cases of NSVN appear symmetrical and serological markers are usually absent.

In contrast to SNV, NSVN is relatively benign: the disease is indolent and protracted over years and appears not to be life-threatening (Dyck *et al.* 1987). Davies *et al.* (1996) observed that only one of their 25 patients died during the 3-year follow-up period. The majority had a monophasic course, but 32% had at least one relapse during the follow-up period. Said (1995) followed 29 patients over an average of 6 years; 37% of these developed systemic manifestations, 37% died an average of 3.3 years after the onset of neuropathy (eight from systemic manifestations and three from infection) and 24% had one or more relapses of neuropathy. Among 48 cases of NSVN cases with longer than 6 months follow-up period, Collins *et al.* (2003) noted relapse of neuropathy in 38% of cases, spread of vasculitis to skin in 6%, and death in 21%. Only half of the deaths were due to vasculitis. Five-year survival rate was 85–87% in Said's and Collins' series. Patients in these two series had a worse prognosis than did those in Dyck's series, perhaps due to inclusion of some cases of SVN.

With glucocorticoid treatment in all cases and additional immunosuppressive medications in half the cases, there was significant improvement in the disability scale in the report by Davie *et al.* (1996). In several of the case reported by Dyck *et al.* (1987), prednisone appeared to halt progression of the disease. On this basis, Chalk *et al.* (1993) stated that, in a substantial number of patients with NSVN, the relatively favorable outlook might make the risks of immunosuppressive therapy difficult to justify. Kissel and Mendell (1992) also stated that treatment with glucocorticoids alone may be appropriate. On the other hand, Collins *et al.* compared the outcomes between 28 patients treated with glucocorticoids alone and 20 with combination therapy (glucocorticoids and cyclophosphamide). They found the combination therapy was more effective than glucocorticoid monotherapy in inducing remission (95% versus 61%) and improving disability (85% versus 57%), with trends towards reduced relapse rate (29% versus 59%), chronic pain (44% versus 71%), and 5-year mortality. Based on this one study, it seems prudent to treat NSVN with glucocorticoids first and add cyclophosphamide if the patient does not respond well.

There is controversy as to the nature of NSVN: an organ-specific vasculitis (Davies *et al.* 1996; Dyck 1987) versus a mild form of systemic vasculitis (Kissel *et al.* 1989; Said *et al.* 1988b). Said (1988b) and Collins *et al.* (2003) argued against an organ-specific vasculitis because of the demonstration of necrotizing arteritis in muscle specimens of 81% of his patients with peripheral neuropathy alone and the development of systemic manifestations in 37% during the follow-up period. His argument may be tainted by the fact that not all his patients had NSVN, as discussed above. Davies *et al.* (1996) supported an organ-specific vasculitis theory. Many of their NSVN patients had a very severe neuropathy, whereas many patients with severe SNV had a relatively mild neuropathy or none at all.

Paraneoplastic vasculitic neuropathy

Paraneoplastic vasculitis (PV) is rare and usually presents as cutaneous leukocytoclastic vasculitis in association with leukemia and lymphomas (Sanche-Guerrero *et al.* 1990) (see Chapter 42). Paraneoplastic vasculitic neuropathy (PVN) is even less common. Fifteen patients with PVN have been reported in the literature thus far (Oh 1997; Turner *et al.* 2003; Ansari *et al.* 2004). At UAB, only two (1.3%) among 151 patients with biopsy-proven vasculitic neuropathy over the past 25 years had PVN. Diverse cancers have been reported in association with PV, the most common being small cell lung cancer (SCLC) and lymphoma, which accounted for 54% of cases (Table 14.11). Malignancy was found 1–18 months before neuropathy in 42% of cases and 2–29 months after the diagnosis of neuropathy in another 42% of cases. PV is generally a disease of the older population. The neuropathy is usually subacute and progressive, ranging from a few days to 8 months. Symmetrical polyneuropathy is the most common pattern; asymmetrical polyneuropathy and mononeuropathy multiplex are less common. PV is invariably characterized by mixed motor and sensory neuropathy. Systemic symptoms are lacking. The most prominent abnormal laboratory findings were high ESR (80% of cases) and high cerebrospinal fluid protein content (91%). Anti-Hu antibodies were noted in three patients, prompting a search for occult SCLC in both, which was found in one. NCS were typical of axonal

Table 14.11 Differential diagnosis between paraneoplastic and systemic vasculitic neuropathy

	Paraneoplastic	Systemic[1]
Sex	Male predominance	Equal
Age	51–78 years (mean 58)	19–84 years (mean 62)
Associated disease	SCLC and lymphoma 50%	Rheumatological disease 35%
Onset	Subacute	Subacute
Clinical features	Mixed neuropathy; varied; symmetrical po lyneuropathy to mononeuropathy	Mostly mixed; varied; symmetrical polyneuropathy to mononeuropathy multiplex
Systemic symptoms and signs	Rare	Common
CNS symptoms and signs	Rare	Rare
Laboratory	High ESR	High ESR
Anti-Hu antibody	Rare	None
CSF findings	High protein with normal cells	Usually normal
EMG/NCV	Axonal neuropathy	Axonal neuropathy
Biopsy	Microvasculitis Nerve: muscle (70%)[2]	Necrotizing vasculitis Nerve: muscle (42%)[1]
Immunotherapy	Moderately effective	Moderately effective
Tumor therapy	Some benefit	N.A.

[1] From Claussen *et al.* (2000).

[2] 70% of muscle biopsies showed vasculitis.

degeneration. The diagnosis of vasculitis was made in all cases by inspection of a peripheral nerve biopsy that showed microvasculitis (nine cases), or necrotizing vasculitis (four cases). Vasculitis was also common (70%) on muscle biopsy. Chemotherapy and cyclophosphamide with or without glucocorticoids alone were associated with improvement in two-third of patients.

Vasculitic neuropathy in HIV

Vasculitic neuropathy is rare in HIV, occurring in 0.1–3% of patients with AIDS-related complex or AIDS (see Chapter 42). Prior to 1997, 27 cases were reported (Brannagan 1997). It was at times the first manifestation of HIV (Lange 1988). The predominant manifestation of HIV vasculitic neuropathy was distal and symmetric polyneuropathy (eight of 18 cases) and asymmetrical polyneuropathy (six cases) with weight loss, myalgia, weakness, and leg tenderness (Gehardi 1993; Said *et al.* 1988); mononeuritis multiplex was least common. In most patients, vasculitic neuropathy was not associated with other organ involvement and was usually monophasic without relapse or remission. Histopathological studies showed inflammation and fibrinoid necrosis of arteries smaller than those typically affected in SNV. Endoneurial inflammatory cells were prominent. Active necrotizing lesions on biopsy did not coexist with healed lesions. Necrotizing vasculitis may occur with CD4[+] T cell counts ranging from 14 to 540. The ESR is usually elevated and CSF is usually characterized by increased protein content and pleocytosis. Cryoglobulinemia has also been described in several patients with HIV infection and mononeuropathy multiplex. Clinical improvement followed glucocorticoid therapy in nine of 11 cases (Gisselbrecht *et al.* 1997). Plasmapheresis followed by zidovudine (AZT) was effective in three patients (Bradley *et al.* 1984). There are also some data to suggest that AZT may be prophylactic for HIV vasculitic neuropathy.

Vasculitic neuropathy with diabetes mellitus

In recent years, there has been a flurry of reports of inflammatory vasculopathy in diabetes mellitus. In 1984, Bradley *et al.* reported six patients (three of whom were diabetic) with painful lumbosacral plexopathy, elevation of ESR, and epineurial lymphocyte infiltration. Prednisone, alone or in conjunction with cyclophosphamide, led to eventual improvement in these patients. None had systemic vasculitis or cancer. Younger *et al.* (1986) found microvasculitis (inflammatory infiltration of the walls of blood vessels measuring 70 μm or less) with scattered cells in the endoneurium in the sural nerve biopsy in 12 (60%) of 20 patients (four with distal peripheral neuropathy, six with proximal diabetic neuropathy, and two with mononeuropathy multiplex). Perivascular lymphocytic infiltration alone was seen in eight (40%) patients (two with distal and six with proximal diabetic neuropathy). In addition, three patients had focal ischemia. Axonal degeneration was seen in 10 tested nerves. In eight patients (seven with microvasculitis and one with severe perivasculitis), clinical improvement was obtained with IVIg. Said *et al.* (1994) reported endoneurial inflammatory cells in four patients and vasculitis in the epi- or perineurial vessels and ischemic changes in two of 10 patients with painful diabetic proximal neuropathy who had biopsy of the intermediate femoral cutaneous nerve. The two patients with vasculitis improved with prednisone therapy. In 10 patients with proximal diabetic neuropathy, Krendal *et al.* (1995) reported perivascular lymphocytic infiltrates in the epineurial small vessels, in either the femoral cutaneous nerve (two patients) or the sural nerve (three patients). Neurological improvement with immunosuppressive therapy (often including IVIg) was noted.

Llewelyn *et al.* (1998) asserted that, in 15 cases of diabetic amyotrophy, biopsy of the intermediate cutaneous nerve of the thigh (a sensory branch of the femoral nerve) showed epineurial microvasculitis in three cases and nonvasculitic epineurial inflammatory infiltrate in another case. In one other patient, microvasculitis was found in both the sural nerve and a quadriceps muscle biopsy specimen. Dyck *et al.* (1999) found the following in distal nerve biopsy of 33 patients with diabetic lumbosacral radiculo-plexopathy (diabetic amyotrophy): epineurial perivascular inflammation in all; microvasculitis (transmural infiltration of inflammatory cells without fibrinoid necrosis) in 13; necrotizing vasculitis in two; and evidence of previous bleeding in 19 (58%). They concluded that the primary event in diabetic amyotrophy is a microscopic vasculitis, and weight loss may be a constitutional symptom of necrotizing vasculitis. In 15 patients with diabetic amyotrophy undergoing nerve biopsy (13 intermediate femoral cutaneous nerve and two sural nerve), Kelker *et al.* (2000) found healed vasculitis in one, microvasculitis in the epineurial space in four, and perivascular inflammatory cells in six. In 15 muscle biopsies (14 rectus femoris and one gastrocnemius muscle), neurogenic atrophy was observed in all cases and inflammatory myopathy in one case.

These studies showed that inflammatory vasculopathy is observed in 20–100% of nerve biopsies in diabetic neuropathy, especially in patients with proximal diabetic neuropathy (diabetic amyotrophy), and that microvasculitis seems to be a common feature. These studies also suggested that prednisone or IVIg is effective therapy in these patients. The consensus opinion is that inflammatory vasculopathy, possibly immune mediated, plays an important role in the pathogenesis of diabetic amyotrophy.

Vasculitic neuropathy with hepatitis C virus infection

Hepatitis C virus (HCV) infection is associated with cryoglobulinemia and associated vasculitis (see Chapter 41). Recently, Apartis *et al.* (1996) studied 15 patients with mixed cryoglobulinemia and peripheral neuropathy, 10 of whom had distal symmetric polyneuropathy and five of whom had mononeuropathy multiplex. Of these, seven with distal symmetric polyneuropathy and three with mononeuropathy multiplex had positive HCV serology. Necrotizing vasculitis was found in two of nine nerve biopsies from the HCV-positive patients, and interferon-α apparently improved peripheral neuropathy in two. Khella *et al.* (1995) described a patient with mononeuropathy multiplex, HCV virus infection, and mixed cryoglobulinemia who had axonal degeneration by EMG and vasculitis of the epineurial vessels on sural nerve biopsy. High-dose prednisone and one course of plasmapheresis were tried with minimal symptomatic improvement. Interferon-α was started at a dose of 3 million units three times per week. Nine months later, the patient was free from neuropathy. David *et al.* (1996) described a person with non-systemic vasculitic mononeuropathy multiplex, cryoglobulinemia, and HCV infection which was stabilized with prednisone, cyclophosphamide, and interferon-α treatment. Initially, immunosuppressive therapy was selected over interferon-α alone; this drug was added 2–3 months later, in part as an adjunct therapy for neuropathy. It was during these few months that the patient's condition stabilized and subsequently improved. It seems that interferon-α is the treatment of choice for vasculitic neuropathy associated with HCV infection.

Vasculitic neuropathy associated with other diseases (see Chapter 42)

Malignant atrophic papulosis (Kohlmcicr–Dcgos arteritis, Degos' disease) is a rare, often fatal, systemic vasculitis, primarily involving the skin, gastrointestinal tract, and brain. Ahbury and Johnson (1978) reported a case in which skin, brain, and peripheral nerves were the primary targets, and sural nerve biopsy showed perineurial small arteries with subintimal proliferation, vessel wall thickening, luminal narrowing, and minimal perivascular inflammation.

Schoene *et al.* (1981) reported a patient with Creutzfeldt–Jakob disease and typical spongioform encephalopathy, but with unusual clinical manifestations including a purpuric, non-pruritic papular rash, and polyneuropathy; sural nerve biopsy showed subacute vasculitis.

Oh reported sarcoid polyneuropathy showing granulomatous vasculitis in epineurial small arteries, which produced almost complete occlusion of the lumen. Perivascular infiltrate of lymphocytes and perineurial granulomata were also found (Oh 1979). Granulomatous vasculitis in sarcoid neuropathy was reported in three additional cases (Vital *et al.* 1982; Gelassi *et al.* 1984; Iwada *et al.* 1993). Said *et al.* (2002) observed necrotizing vasculitis in the nerve biopsy in seven of 11 cases of sarcoid neuropathy and suggested the possibility of ischemic nerve lesions as its cause.

Human T-lymphotrophic virus I (HTLV-I) can cause T cell leukemia, myelopathy, and polymyositis. The pathology of HTLV-I myclopathy is charactcrizcd by pcrivascular inflammation, but vasculitis is not seen. Similar perivascular inflammation is seen in some patients with peripheral neuropathy (Said *et al.* 1988a). A single paper described three patients with HTLV-I and biopsies showing necrotizing vasculitis (Vernat *et al.* 1990). Neuropathy occurs in 36–40% of patients with symptomatic late Lyme disease. Sural nerve biopsy in this disorder is characterized by perivascular collections of inflammatory cells and axonal degeneration in a majority of cases (Halpern *et al.* 1987; Vallat *et al.* 1987). A few patients with Lyme disease had mononeuropathy multiplex with vasculitis demonstrated pathologically (Camponovo and Meier 1986; Meier *et al.* 1989). Characteristic nerve biopsy findings include perivascular infiltration of inflammatory cells in the epineurial arterioles and veins and axonal degeneration without necrotizing lesions of the vessel walls (Meier *et al.* 1989). Active leprous neuropathy, once the most common cause of neuropathy in the world, is invariably associated with non-necrotizing lymphocytic vasculitis (Said 1994). In patients with multibacillary leprosy, vasculitis is associated with infection of the endothelial cells by *Mycobacterium leprae*.

References

Ansari, J., Nagabhushan, N., Syed, R., Bomanji, J., Bacon, C. M. and Lee, S. M. (2004). Small cell lung cancer associated with anti-Hu paranoeplastic sensory neuropathy and peripehral nerve microvasculitis: case report and literature review. *Clinical Oncology*, **16**, 71–6.

Apartis, E., Leger, J. M., Musset, L., *et al.* (1996). Peripheral neuropathy associated with essential mixed cryoglobulinaemia: a role for hepatitis C virus infection? *Journal of Neurology, Neurosurgery and Psychiatry,* **60,** 661–6.

Asbury, A. K. and Johnson, P. C. (1978). *Pathology of peripheral nerve.* W. B. Saunders, Philadelphia.

Beggs, J., Johnson, P. C., Olafsen, A., *et al.* (1991). Transperineurial arterioles in human sural nerve. *Journal of Neuropathology and Experimental Neurology,* **50,** 704–18.

Bell, M. A. and Weddell, A. G.M. (1984a). A descriptive study of the blood vessels of the sciatic nerve in the rat, man and other mammals. *Brain,* **107,** 871–98.

Bell, M. A. and Weddell, A. G.M. (1984b). A morphometric study of intrafascular vessels of mammalian sciatic nerve. *Muscle Nerve,* **7,** 524–34.

Bleechen, S. S., Lovelace, R. E. and Cotton, R. E. (1963). Mononeuritis multiplex in polyarteritis nodosa. *Quarterly Journal of Medicine,* **32,** 193–209.

Bloch, D. A., Michael, B. A., Hunder, G. G., *et al.* (1990). The American College of Rheumatology 1990 criteria for the classification of vasculitis. Patients and methods. *Arthritis and Rheumatism,* **33,** 1068–73.

Bouche, P., Leger, J. M., Travers, M. A., Cathala, H. P. and Castaigne, P. (1986). Peripheral neuropathy in systemic vasculitis: clinical and electrophysiologic study of 22 cases. *Neurology,* **36,** 1598–602.

Bradley, W. G., Chad, D., Verghese, J. P., *et al.* (1984). Painful lumbosacral plexopathy with elevated erythrocyte sedimentation ratre: A treatable inflammatory syndrome. *Annals of Neurology,* **15,** 457–64.

Brannagan, T. H. (1997). Retroviral-associated vasculitis of the nervous system. *Neurologic Clinics,* **15,** 927–44.

Calabrese, L. H., Estes, M., Yen-Lieberman, B., *et al.* (1989). Systemic vasculitis in association with human immunodeficiency virus infection. *Arthritis and Rheumatism,* **32,** 569–76.

Camponovo, F. and Meier, C. (1986). Neuropathy of vasculitic origin in a case of Garin-Boujadour-Bannwarth syndrome with positive borrelia antibody response. *Journal of Neurology,* **233,** 69–72.

Chalk, C. H., Dyck, P. J. and Conn, D. L. Dyck P. J. and Thomas P. K. (eds.) (1993a). Vasculitic neuropathy. In *Diseases of peripheral nervous system,* pp. 1424–36. W. B. Saunders, Philadelphia.

Chalk, C. H., Hamburger, H. A. and Dyck, P. J. (1993b). Antineutrophil cytoplasmic antibodies in vasculitis peripheral neuropathy. *Neurology,* **43,** 1826–7.

Chang, R. W., Bell, C. L. and Hallett, M. (1984). Clinical characteristics and prognosis of vasculitic mononeurpathy multiplex. *Archives in Neurology,* **41,** 618–21.

Chia, L. A. F., Lacroix, C., Adams, D., Plante, V. and Said, G. (1996). Contribution of nerve biopsy findings to the diagnosis of disabling neuropathy in the elderly. A retrospective review of 100 consecutive patients. *Brain,* **119,** 1091–8.

Claussen, G. C., Thomas, T. D., Goyne, C., Vazquez, L. G., and Oh, S. J. (2000). Diagnostic value of nerve and muscle biopsy in suspected vasculitis cases. *Journal of Clinical Neuromuscular Disease,* **1,** 117–23.

Cohen, R. D., Conn, D. L. and Ilstrup, D. M. (1980). Clinical features, prognosis, and response to treatment in polyarteritis. *Mayo Clinic Proceedings,* **55,** 146–55.

Collins, M. P., Mendell, J. R., Periquet, M. I., *et al.* (2000). Superficial peroneal nerve/poeroneus brevis muscle biopsy in vasculitic neuropathy. *Neurology,* **55,** 636–43.

Collins, M. P., Periquet, M. I., Mendell, J. R., Sahenk, Z., Nagaraja, H. N. and Kissel, J. T. (2003). Nonsystemic vasculitic neuropathy: insights from a clinical cohort. *Neurology,* **61,** 623–30.

Conn, D. L. and Dyck, P. J. (1984). Angiopathic neuropathy in connective tissue disease. In *Peripheral neuropathy* (eds, Dyck, P. J., Thomas, P. K., Lambert, E. H. and Bunge, R.), pp. 2027–43. W. B. Saunders, Philadelphia.

Cruz Martinez, A., Barbado, F. J., Ferrer, M. T., *et al.* (1988). Electrophysiological study in systemic necrotizing vasculitis of the polyarteritis nod as a group. *Electromyography and Clinical Neurophysiology,* **28,** 167–73.

Dahlberg, P., Lockhart, J. and Overholt, E. (1989). Diagnostic studies for systemic necrotizing vasculitis: sensitivity, specificity, and predictive value in patients with multisystem disease. *Archives of Internal Medicine,* **149,** 161–5.

David, W. S., Peine, C., Schlesinger, P. and Smith, S. A. (1996). Nonsystemic vasculitic mononeuropathy multiplex, cryoglobulinemia, and hepatitis C. *Muscle and Nerve,* **19,** 1596–602.

Davidson, J. R. and Sundstrom, W. R. (1988). Sural nerve biopsy in systemic necrotizing vasculitis. *Arthritis and Rheumatism,* **31,** 149–50.

Davies, L. (1994). Vasculitic neuropathy. *Baillière's Clinical Neurology* 3:193–210.

Davies, L., Spies, J., Pollard, J. and McLeod, J. (1996). Vasculitis confined to peripheral nerves. *Brain,* **119,** 1441–8.

Dyck, P. J. and Lofgren, E. P. (1968). Nerve biopsy. Choice of nerve, method, symptoms and usefulness. *Medical Clinics of North America,* **52,** 885–93.

Dyck, P. J., Benstead, T. J., Conn, D. L., Stevens, J. C. and Windebank, A. J. (1987). Non-systemic vasculitic neuropathy. *Brain,* **110,** 843–54.

Dyck, P. J., Conn, D. L. and Okazaki, H. (1972). Necrotizing angiopathic neuropathy: three dimensional morphology of fiber degeneration related to sites of occluded vessels. *Mayo Clinics Proceedings,* **47,** 461–75.

Dyck, P. J., Hansen, S., Karnes, J., *et al.* (1985). Capillary number and percentage closed in human diabetic sural nerve. *Proceedings of the National Academy of Science USA,* **82,** 2513–17.

Dyck, P. J., Norell, J. E. and Dyck, P. J. (1999). Microvasculitis and ischemia in diabetic lumbosacral radiculoplexus neuropathy. *Neurology,* **53,** 2113–21.

Fathers, E. and Fuller, G. N. (1996). Vasculitic neuropathy. *British Journal of Hospital Medicine,* **55,** 643–7.

Fauci, A. S., Haynes, B. F. and Katz, P. (1978). The spectrum of vasculitis: clinical, pathologic, immunologic and therapeutic considerations. *Annals of Internal Medicine,* **89,** 660–76.

Ford, R. and Sickert, R. (1965). Central nervous system manifestations of periarteritis nodosa. *Neurology,* **15,** 114–22.

Fronert, P. P. and Sheps, S. G. (1967). Long-term follow-up study of periarteritis nodosa. *American Journal of Medicine,* **43,** 8–14.

Fujimura, H., Lacroix, C. and Said, G. (1991). Vulnerability of nerve fibers to ischemia. A quantitative light and electron microscope study. *Brain,* **114,** 731–3.

Fuller, G. N., Jacobs, J. M. and Guiloff, R. J. (1993). Nature and incidence of peripheral nerve syndromes in HIV infection. *Journal of Neurology, Neurosurgery and Psychiatry,* **56,** 372–81.

Garcia, R., Godlewski, W., Gruner, J., *et al.* (1955). Sur les formes multinevritiques *et* polynevritiques de la perarterite noueuse; Etude de 7 observations inedites. *Annals of Medicine,* **56,** 113–47.

Gelassi, G., Gibertoni, M., Mancini, A., *et al.* (1984). Sarcoidosis of the peripheral nerve: Clinical, electrophysiological and histological study of two cases. *European Neurology,* **23,** 459–65.

Giannini, C. and Dyck, P. J. (1993). Ultrastructural morphometric features of human sural nerve endoneurial microvessels. *Journal of Neuropathology and Experimental Neurology,* **52,** 361–9.

Gisselbrecht, M., Cohen, O., Lortholary, O., *et al.* (1997). HIV -related vasculitis: Clinical presentation and therapeutic approach on six patients (letter). *AIDS,* **11,** 121–3.

Guillevin, L., Du, L. T.H., Godeau, P., *et al.* (1988). Clinical findings and prognosis of polyarteritis nodosa and ChurgStrauss angiitis. A study of 165 patients. *British Journal of Rheumatology,* **27,** 258–64.

Guillevin, L., Lhote, F., Jarrousse, B., *et al.* (1992). Treatment of polyarteritis nodosa and Churg-Strauss syndrome. A meta-analysis of 3 prospective controlled trials including 182 patients over 12 years. *Annales de Medecine Interne* (Paris), **143,** 405–16.

Halpern, J. J., Little, B. W., Coyle, P. K. and Dattwyler, R. J. (1987). Lyme disease: cause of treatable peripheral neuropathy. *Neurology*, **37**, 1700–6.

Hawke, S. H.B., Davies, L., Pamphlett, R., Guo, Y. P., Pollard, J. D. and McLeod, J. G. (1991). Vasculitic neuropathy. A clinical and pathological study. *Brain*, **114**, 2175–90.

Haynes, B. F., Allen, N. B. and Fauci, A. S. (1986). Diagnostic and therapeutic approach to the patient with vasculitis. *Medical Clinics of North America*, **70**, 355–68.

Hunder, G. G., Arend, W. P., Bloch, D. A., *et al.* (1990). The American College of Rheumatology 1990 criteria for the classification of vasculitis. *Arthritis and Rheumatism*, **33**, 1065–7.

Iwata, M., Kondo, M., Ando, M., *et al.* (1993). [Peripheral polyneuropathy due to sarcoidosis in a patient with intrathoracic, ocular and skin lesions]. [Japanese]. Nihon Kyobu Shikkan Gakkai Zasshi. *Japanese Journal of Thoracic Diseases*, **31**, 1050–5.

Jamieson, P., Giuliani, M. and Martinez, J. (1991). Necrotizing angiopathy presenting with multifocal conduction blocks. *Neurology*, **41**, 442–4.

Jayne, D. J., Rasmussen, N., Andrassy, K., Bacon, P., *et al.* (2003). A randomized trial of maintenance therapy for vasculitis associated with antineutrophil cytoplasmic autoantiobides. *New England Journal of Medicine*, **349**, 36–44.

Kararizou, E., Davaki, P., Karandreas, N., Davou, R. and Vassilopoulos, D. (2005). Nonsystemic vasculitic neuropathy: a clinicopathological study of 22 cases. *Journal of Rheumatology*, **32**, 853–8.

Kelkar, P., Masood, M. and Parry, G. J. (2000). Distinctive pathologic findings in proximal diabetic neuropathy (diabetic amyotrophy). *Neurology*, **55**, 83–8.

Kernahan, J. W. and Woltman, H. W. (1938). Periarteritis nodosa: a clinicopathologic study with special reference to nervous system. *Archives of Neurological Psychiatry*, **39**, 655–86.

Khella, S. L., Frost, S., Hermann, G. A., *et al.* (1995). Hepatitis C infection, cryoglobulinemia, and vasculitic neuropathy. Treatment with interferon alpha: case report and literature review. *Neurology*, **45**, 407–11.

Kissel, J. T. and Mendell, J. R. (1992). Vasculitic neuropathy. *Neurology Clinics*, **10**, 761–81.

Kissel, J. T. (1994). Vasculitis of the peripheral nervous system. *Seminars in Neurology*, **14**, 361–9.

Kissel, J. T., Eiethman, J. L., Omerza, J., Rammohan, K. W. and Mendell, J. R. (1989). Peripheral nerve vasculitis: immune characterization of the vascular lesions. *Annals of Neurology*, **25**, 291–7.

Kissel, J. T., Slivka, A. P., Warmolts, J. R. and Mendell, J. R. (1985). The clinical spectrum of necrotizing angiopathy of the peripheral nervous system. *Annals of Neurology*, **18**, 251–7.

Klassen, L. W., Calabrese, L. H. and Laxer, R. M. (1996). Intravenous immunglobulin in rheumatic disease. *Rheumatic Disease Clinics of North America*, **22**, 155–73.

Krendal, D. A., Costigan, D. A. and Hopkins, L. C. (1995). Successful treatment of neuropathy in patients with diabetes mellitus. *Archives of Neurology*, **52**, 1053–61.

Krendal, D. A., Zacharias, A. and Younger, D. S. (1997). Autoimmune diabetic neuropathy. *Neurologic Clinics*, **15**, 959–71.

Lacomis, D., Giuliani, M. J., Steen, V. and Powell, H. C. (1997). Small fiber neuropathy and vasculitis. *Arthritis and Rheumatism*, **40**, 1173–7.

Langford, C. and Sneller, M. C. (1997). New developments in the treatment of Wegener's granulomatosis, polyarteritis nodosa, microscopy polyarteritis and Churg-Strauss. *Current Opinion in Rheumatology*, **7**, 26–30.

Levy, Y., George, J., Fabbrizzi, F., Rotman, P., Paz, Y. and Shoenfeld, Y. (1999). Marked improvement of ChurgStrauss vasculitis with intravenous gammaglobulins. *Southern Medical Journal*, **92**, 412–14.

Lie, J. (1990). Illustrated histopathologic classification criteria for selected vasculitis syndromes. *Arthritis and Rheumatism*, **33**, 1074–87.

Llewelyn, J. G., Thomas, P. K. and King, R. H. (1998). Epineurial microvasculitis in proximal diabetic neuropathy. *Journal of Neurology*, **245**, 159–65.

Lockwood, C. M. (1996). New treatment strategies for systemic vasculitis: the role of intravenous immune globulin therapy. *Clinical and Experimental Immunology*, **1**, 77–82.

Lovelace, R. E. (1964). Mononeuritis multiplex in polyarteritis nodosa. *Neurology*, **14**, 434–42.

Loveshin, L. L. and Kernahan, J. W. (1948). Peripheral neuritis in periarteritis nodosa: a clinocopathological study. *Archives of Internal Medicine*, **82**, 321–38.

Maxeiner, S., McDonald, J. and Kirklin, J. (1952). Muscle biopsy in the diagnosis of periarteritis nodosa: an evaluation. *Surgical Clinics of North America*, **32**, 1223–35.

McManis, P. G., Low, P. A. and Lagerlund, T. D. (1993). Microenvironment of nerve: blood flow and ischemia. In *Peripheral neuropathy* (eds Dyck, P. J. and Thoma, P. R.), pp. 453–75, 3rd edn. W. B. Saunders, Philadelphia.

Meier, C., Grahmann, F., Engelhat, A. and Dumas, M. (1989). Peripheral nerve disorders in lyme borreliosis: nerve biopsy studies in eight cases. *Acta Neuropathologica* (Berlin), **79**, 271–8.

Midroni, G. and Bilbao, J. M. (1995). *Biopsy diagnosis of peripheral neuropathy.* Butterworth-Heinemann, Boston.

Moore, P. M. and Fauci, A. S. (1981). Neurologic manifestations of systemic vasculitis. *American Journal of Medicine*, **71**, 517–24.

Nemni, R., Corbo, M., Fazio, R., Quattrini, A., Comi, G. and Canal, N. (1988). Cryoglobulinaemic neuropathy: a clinical, morphological and immunocytochemical study of eight cases. *Brain*, **111**, 541–52.

Oh, S. J. (1990). Diagnostic usefulness and limitations of the sural nerve biopsy. *Yonsei Medical Journal*, **31**, 1–26.

Oh, S. J. (1997). Paraneoplastic vasculitis of the peripheral nervous system. *Neurologic Clinics*, **15**, 849–63.

Oh, S. J., Herrara, G. and Spalding, D. M. (1986). Eosinophilic vasculitic neuropathy in the Churg-Strauss syndrome. *Arthritis and Rheumatism*, **29**, 1173–5.

Panegyres, P. K., Iumbergs, P. E., Leong, A. S.Y. and Bourne, A. J. (1990). Vasculitis of peripheral nerve and skeletal muscle: clinopathological correlation and immunopathic mechanisms. *Journal of Neurological Science*, **100**, 193–202.

Puechal, X., Said, G., Hilliquin, P., *et al.* (1995). Peripheral neuropathy with necrotizing vasculitis in rheumatoid arthritis. A clinicopathologic and prognosis study of thirty-two patients. *Arthritis and Rheumatism*, **38**, 1618–29.

Rasmussen, N., Jayne, D. R.W., Abramowicz, D., *et al.* (1996). European therapeutic trials in ANCA associated systemic vasculitis: Disease scoring, consensus regimens and proposed clinical trials. *Sarcoidosis*, **13**, 29–34.

Richter, E., Schanbel, E., Csernok, E., *et al.* (1994). Treatment of ANCA-associated systemic vasculitis with high-dose intravenous immunoglobulin. *Arthritis and Rheumatism*, **37**, S3S3.

Ropert A. and Metral S. (1990). Conduction block in neuropathies with necrotizing vasculitis. *Muscle and Nerve*, **13**, 102–105.

Sack, M., Cassidy, J. T. and Bole, G. G. (1975). Prognostic factors in polyarteritis. *Journal of Rheumatology*, **2**, 411–20.

Said, G. (1994). Inflammatory neuropathies associated with known infections (HIV, leprosy, Chagas's disease, Lyme disease). *Bailieres Clinical Neurology*, **3**, 149–71.

Said, G. (1995). Vasculitic neuropathy. *Bailieres Clinical Neurology*, **4**, 489–503.

Said, G., Goulon-Goeau, E., Lacroix, E., *et al.* (1988a). Inflammatory lesions of peripheral nerve in a patient with human T-lymphotrophic virus type I-associated myelopathy. *Annals of Neurology*, **24**, 275–7.

Said, G., Goulon-Goeau, E., Lacroix, E. and Moulonguer, A. (1994). Nerve biopsy findings in different patterns of proximal diagetic neuropathy. *Annals of Neurology*, **35**, 559–69.

Said, G., Lacroix, E., Andrieu, J. M., *et al.* (1987). Necrotizing arteritis in patients with inflammatory neuropathy and immunodeficiency virus infection. *Neurology*, **37** (Suppl.), 176 (abstract).

Said, G., Lacroix-Ciaudo, E., Fujimura, H., Bias, E. and Faux, N. (1988b). The peripheral neuropathy of necrotizing arteritis: a clinicopathological study. *Annals of Neurology*, **23**, 461–5.

Said, G., Lacroix, C., Plante-Bordeneuve, V., *et al.* (2002). Nerve granulomas and vasculitis in sarcoid peripheral neuropathy: a clinicopathological study of 11 patients. *Brain*, **125**, 264–75.

Sakai, K., Komai, K., Yanase, D. and Yamada, M. (2005). Plasma VEGF as a marker for the diagnosis and treatment of vasculitic neuropathy. *Journal of Neurology, Neurosurgery and Psychiatry*, **76**, 296.

Sanada, M., Terada, M., Suzuki, E., Kashiwagi, A. and Yasuda, H. (2003). MR angiography for the evaluation of non-systemic vasculitic neuropathy. *Acta Radiologica*, **44**, 316–8.

Sanche-Guerrero, J., Gutrre-Urena, S., Vidaller, A., *et al.* (1990). Vasculitis as a paraneoplastic syndrome. Report of 11 cases and review of the literature. *Journal of Rheumatology*, **17**, 1458–62.

Schifitto, G., Barbano, R. L., Kieburtz, K. D., Cohn, S. E. and Zwillich, S. H. (1997). HIV related vasculitic mononeuropathy multiplex: a role for IVIG? (letter). *Journal of Neurology, Neurosurgery and Psychiatry*, **63**, 255–6.

Schoene, W. E., Masters, E. L., Gibbs, E., Gajdusek, D. E., Tyler, H. R., Moore, F. D. and Dammin, G. (1981). Transmissible spongiform encephalopathy (CreutzfeldJakob disease). Atypical clinical and pathological findings. *Archives in Neurology*, **38**, 473–7.

Schroder, J. M. (1986). Proliferation of epineural capillaries and smooth muscle cells in angiopathic peripheral neuropathy. *Acta Neuropathology*, **72**, 29–37.

Scott, D. G.I. and Bacon, P. A. (1984). Intravenous cyclophosphamide and methylprednisolone in treatment of systemic rheumatoid vasculitis. *American Journal of Medicine*, **76**, 377–84.

Seo, J. H., Ryan, H. F., Claussen, G. C., Thomas, T. D. and Oh, S. J. (2004). Sensory neuropathy in vasculitis. A clinical, pathlogic, and electrophysiologic study. *Neurology*, **63**, 874–8.

Slady, T., Greenberg, H. and Brown, M. (1985). Regional perfusion in normal and ischemic rat sciatic nerves. *Annals of Neurology*, **17**, 191–5.

Suggs, S. J. Thomas, I. N. Joy, S. J. Lopez-Mendez, A. and Oh, S. J. (1992). Vasculitic neuropathy mimicking Guillain-Barre syndrome. *Arthritis and Rheumatism*, **35**, 975–8.

Turner, M. R., Warren, J. D., Jacobs, J. M., *et al.* (2003). Microvasculitic paraproteinemic polyneuropathy and B-cell lymphoma. *J Peripher Nerve Syst*, **8**, 100–7.

Vallat, J. M., Hugon, P., Lubveau, M., Lebourtet, M. P., Dumas, M. and Desproges-Gottgeron, R. (1987). Tickbite meningoradiculoneuritis: clinical, electrophysiolgic, and histologic findings in 10 cases. *Neurology*, **37**, 749–53.

Vital, C., Aubertin, J., Ragnault, M., Amigues, H., Mouton, L. and Bellance, R. (1982). Sarcoidosis of the peripheral nerve: a histological and ultastructural study of two cases. *Acta Neuropathologica*, **58**, 111–4.

Wees, S. J., Sunwoo, I. N. and Oh, S. J. (1981). Sural nerve biopsy in systemic necrotizing vasculitis. *American Journal of Medicine*, **71**, 525–32.

Winkelstein, A., Starz, T. W. and Agarwal, A. (1984). Efficacy of combined therapy with plasmapheresis and immunosuppressants in rheumatoid vasculitis. *Journal of Rheumatology*, **11**, 162–6.

Younger, D. S., Rosoklija, G., Hays, A. P., Trojaborg, W. and Latov, N. (1986). Diabetic peripheral neuropathy: a clinicopathologic and immunohistochemical analysis of sural nerve biopsies. *Muscle and Nerve*, **19**, 722–7.

CHAPTER 15

Vasculitic manifestations in the gastrointestinal tract

Gaafar Ragab

In order to better understand the manifestations and consequences of vasculitic lesions in the gastrointestinal (GI) tract, and the different approaches to diagnosis, it is necessary to briefly review the anatomy and physiology of the GI tract. It is also important to understand the various pathogenetic mechanisms causing bowel ischemia, and the wide range of differential diagnoses.

Anatomic considerations

The blood supply of the GI system has intramural and extramural components. The intramural vascular distribution is generally well-developed with plexuses in the different layers of the bowel wall, and with distinctive features in the liver, small intestine, and gastroesophageal junction which are adapted to their function (Geboes et al. 2001). The extramural arterial supply for the esophagus is derived from the thoracic aorta or its major branches. Blood supply to the abdominal organs is provided by three major, unpaired vessels arising from the abdominal aorta, namely the celiac trunk and the superior and inferior mesenteric arteries. There is individual variability in the anatomy of the gastrointestinal vasculature (Geboes et al. 2001).

The celiac trunk provides the blood supply from the distal esophagus to the descending duodenum (Geboes et al. 2001). The stomach is vascularized by four well-anastomosed main arteries: the right and left gastric arteries and the right and left gastroepiploic arteries. Other important vessels include the gastroduodenal arteries, the short gastric arteries, a posterior gastric artery, an accessory left gastric artery, and supraduodenal arteries. The main vessels give rise to some specific collaterals, for example the omental arteries that may form an omental arcade as well as other branches (Vandamme and Bonte 1988). The blood supply to the cardia, fundus, and body of the stomach is excellent, due to anastomotic connections, but it is not as good at the antral curvatures, and is poor at the anterior and posterior walls of this area due to poor anastomosis (Liebermann-Meffert et al. 1984). The gastroduodenal artery provides an important connection between the celiac trunk and the superior mesenteric artery (SMA) (Geboes et al. 2001).

The SMA supplies the transverse and ascending duodenum, the jejunum and ileum, and the large bowel to the splenic flexure. With variations in the branching pattern, it gives off the inferior pancreaticoduodenal, the middle colic, the right colic, the ileocoecal, and

intestinal branches. The ileum and jejunum are supplied by the SMA and its intestinal branches. The middle, right, and ileocoecal branches of the SMA anastomose with each other to form the marginal artery of Drummond, along the inner border of the colon. This artery is completed by branches of the left colic which arises from the inferior mesenteric artery (IMA). This provides an important anastomosis between the superior and inferior mesenteric arteries (Geboes et al. 2001; Fisher and Fry 1987). The IMA supplies the colon from the splenic flexure to the rectum. It forms several anastomotic connections to the lumbar branches of the abdominal aorta, the sacral artery, and the internal iliac arteries (Geboes et al. 2001; Fisher and Fry 1987).

The liver has a double blood supply. The portal vein brings venous blood from the intestine and spleen, and the hepatic artery coming from the celiac axis supplies the liver with arterial blood. The venous drainage from the liver is into the right and left hepatic veins, which enter the inferior vena cava (Sherlock and Dooley 2002). The superior and inferior mesenteric veins parallel their arteries and drain the respective territories of the GI tract. The inferior mesenteric vein drains into the splenic, which joins the superior mesenteric vein to form the portal vein. The mesenteric veins are connected by collateral vessels and they anastomose with the caval venous system through the esophageal plexus, the rectal plexus, and the paraumbilical veins (Geboes et al. 2001).

The bowel vasculature should be viewed as a single functional unit. Whether ischemia develops depends mainly on the amount of blood that flows into a diseased artery from other arteries (Cognet et al. 2002). Multiple visceral arterial lesions may be found in patients without symptoms, while others with a single lesion have pain (Roobottom and Dubbins 1993). The occurrence of painful ischemia will depend upon the site of the lesion, for example whether it is down stream from an anastomosis or not. The ability of the patient to develop collaterals may be compromised in patients with other vascular abnormalities. The tempo of progression of the lesion will also play a role. For example in Takayasu's arteritis, severe occlusion may occur before there is a chance for anastomotic collaterals to develop (Cognet et al. 2002). Thanks to lavish collateral connections, proximal mesenteric venous occlusion does not usually result in severe bowel ischemia, unlike occlusion of distal mesenteric veins, which causes infarction of the bowel wall with serious consequences (Rademaker 1998).

Pathophysiology of GI tract circulation

The GI tract receives around one-fifth of resting cardiac output, most of which supplies the intestinal mucosa (Gallavan *et al.* 1989; Quamar and Read 1985). Autoregulatory mechanisms can significantly increase this figure postprandially (Gallavan *et al.* 1989; Reilly and Bulkley 1993). When systemic blood pressure is below 40 mmHg, local autoregulation is overruled by systemic autoregulation, and local protective mechanisms fail (Mathews and Parks 1976a, 1976b). Non-occlusive mesenteric ischemia can thus occur with patent mesenteric arteries, accounting for 20–30% of all cases of acute mesenteric ischemia (with a mortality rate in the order of 50%). Mesenteric vasospasm persists even after correction of the precipitating event (Trompeter *et al.* 2002).

Whether ischemia is precipitated by underperfusion or occlusion, the initial lesions are followed by an inflammatory response due to the release of mediators such as platelet-activating factor and cytokines, including tumor necrosis factor (TNF)-α (Bradbury *et al.* 1993; Kuroda *et al.* 1994), from activated neutrophils, macrophages, platelets, mast cells, and endothelium. They result in further damage to the bowel wall.

Acute bowel ischemia passes through three stages. The first stage, referred to as reversible ischemic enteritis or colitis, is characterized by mucosal necrosis, erosions, ulcerations, and sometimes hemorrhage (Haglund and Bergqvist 1999). The second stage shows deeper damage with necrosis reaching the deep submucosa. Stricture formation may ensue from healing by fibrosis (Whitehead 1976). The third stage is transmural bowel wall necrosis or infarction and is associated with a high mortality rate. Superinfection after the breakdown of the mucosal barrier will further contribute to the process of wall necrosis (Musemeche *et al.* 1986; Quellet *et al.* 1988).

Toxic proteases, bacteria and their toxins, as well as free radicals produced in the reperfusion phase will contribute to severe intestinal necrosis. Serious systemic effects may result, including hepatic and renal dysfunction; myocardmial and circulatory changes; bone marrow failure; and increased risk of sepsis; disseminated intravascular coagulation; and multiple organ failure (Harward *et al.* 1993; Jamieson *et al.* 1993; Fontes *et al.* 1994; Landow and Anderson 1994; Smith *et al.* 1994).

Manifestations of GI tract vasculitis

Few of the classification criteria and diagnostic guidelines of nine identified vasculitic syndromes refer to a part of the GI tract other than the oral cavity. In Henoch–Schönlein purpura (HSP), there is bowel angina (one of four criteria); in polyarteritis nodosa (PAN), arteriographic abnormalities of the visceral arteries (one of 10 criteria); but there are no GI criteria in Takayasu's arteritis, giant cell arteritis, Kawasaki's disease, Wegener's granulomatosis, Churg–Strauss syndrome, leukocytoclastic (hypersensitivity) vasculitis, or Behçet's syndrome (Mills *et al.* 1990; Lightfoot *et al.* 1990; Arend *et al.* 1990; Hunder *et al.* 1990; Kawasaki 1974; Leavitt *et al* 1990; Masi *et al.* 1990; Calabrese *et al.* 1990; International Study Group for Behçet's Disease 1990). It is understood that the classification criteria are not meant for diagnosis of these diseases, rather for classification when the vasculitic entity has been established, yet this absence signifies the limited repertoire of clinical symptoms and signs of GI tract vasculitis and the non-specificity of diagnostic findings.

The extent and clinical course of disease depend on the size and location of the affected vessel and the histological characteristics of the lesion. Radiological findings in various types of vasculitis often overlap considerably and therefore have limited value in making a specific diagnosis. Nevertheless, the possibility of vasculitis should be considered whenever mesenteric ischemic changes occur in young patients; are noted at unusual sites such as stomach, duodenum, or rectum; concomitantly involve the small and large intestine; or are associated with genitourinary involvement. Knowledge of systemic clinical manifestations in affected patients may suggest a specific diagnosis (Ha *et al.* 2000).

Acute bowel ischemia with transmural infarction causes local complications such as bleeding, perforation, abscess formation, and peritonitis. It is clear that partial mural bowel ischemia may also result in similar consequences upon disruption of the mucosal barrier. Whether arterial or venous, other causes of mesenteric ischemia must be kept in mind (Tables 15.1 and 15.2). Causes of non-occlusive reduction of mesenteric blood supply must be appreciated as well (Table 15.3).

Table 15.1 Causes of acute occlusion of the superior mesenteric artery

Thromboembolism: of left atrial origin
Atherosclerosis
Thromboembolism: of aortic origin
Mesenteric arterial thrombosis
Aortic or mesenteric dissection
Cholesterol embolization (spontaneous or postoperative)
Aortic surgery
Stent placement
Therapeutic embolization to treat hemorrhage
Antiphospholipid antibody syndrome
Systemic vasculitis
Takayasu arteritis
Giant cell arteritis
Polyarteritis nodosa
Systemic lupus erythematosus
Henoch Schönlein purpura
Wegener's granulomatosis
Churg–Strauss syndrome
Thromboangiitis obliterans
Rheumatoid vasculitis
Behçet's syndrome
Thrombotic thrombocytopenic purpura
Hemolytic-uremic syndrome
Fibromuscular dysplasia
Miscellaneous
Diabetes mellitus
Amyloidosis
Oxalosis

Table 15.2 Causes of occlusion of mesenteric veins

Venous thrombosis due to
Infiltrative conditions
Neoplastic conditions
Inflammatory conditions
Abdominal infectious conditions
Hypercoagulable conditions
Polycythemia vera
Sickle cell disease
Thrombocytosis
Antithrombin III, protein C and protein S deficiency
Carcinoma
Pregnancy
Drugs
Systemic vasculitis
Wegener's granulomatosis
Systemic lupus erythematosus
Behçet's syndrome
Enterocolic lymphocytic phlebitis
Complicated bowel obstruction
Strangulated hernia
Strangulated closed loop obstruction
Volvulus
Intussusception
Intestinal overdistention

Table 15.3 Causes of non-occlusive reduction of mesenteric blood supply

Shock bowel
Familial dysautonomia
Pheochromocytoma
High-endurance athletes
Chronic renal failure
Trauma
Radiation
Corrosive injury
Iatrogenic
Immunotherapy
Chemotherapy
Vasoconstriction
Digitalis
Ergotamine
Vasopressin
Epinephrine
Hypotension
Antihypertensive drugs
Diuretics
Antidepressants
Prostaglandin antagonists
Narcotics
Cocaine
Heroin

Symptoms of GI tract vasculitis include: abdominal angina, defined as postprandial abdominal pain with weight loss and anorexia; changes in bowel habits and vomiting are less common. In the stomach, vasculitis may present as incapacitating gastroparesis with vomiting, postprandial heaviness, and delayed gastric emptying. Casey *et al.* (1993) advised investigating the visceral arteries, at least with Doppler ultrasound, in patients with chronic gastric symptoms unresponsive to pharmacotherapy. Cachexia suggesting a malignancy can occur with severe malabsorption or if the patient eats less to avoid triggering the pain. As these symptoms are not uncommon, and tend to develop insidiously, the diagnosis may be delayed.

Pagnoux *et al.* (2005) reviewed the medical records of 62 patients with systemic small and medium-sized vessel vasculitides and GI tract involvement followed between 1981 and 2002. Vasculitides were distributed as follows: 38 PAN (21 related to hepatitis B virus); 11 Churg–Strauss syndrome; six Wegener's granulomatosis; four microscopic polyangitis; and three rheumatoid arthritis associated vasculitis. GI tract manifestations were present at, or occurred within 3 months of, diagnosis in 50 (81%) patients. Symptoms were abdominal pain in 61 (97%); nausea or vomiting in 21 (34%); diarrhea in 17 (27%); hematochezia or melena in 10 (16%); and hematemesis in four (6%). Endoscopic detection of gastroduodenal ulcerations was noted in 17 (27%) patients, esophageal ulcerations in seven (11%) patients, and colorectal ulcerations in six (10%) patients, but histologic signs of vasculitis were found in

only three colon biopsies. Twenty-one (34%) patients had a surgical abdomen; 11 (18%) developed peritonitis; nine (15%) had bowel perforations; 10 (16%) bowel ischemia/infarction; four (6%) intestinal occlusion; six (10%) acute appendicitis; five (8%) cholecystitis; and three (5%) acute pancreatitis. Some patients had more than one condition, and 16 (26%) patients died. The respective 10-month and 5-year survival rates were 71% and 56% for the 21 surgical patients, whereas they rose to 94% and 82% for the 41 patients without surgical abdomen. Peritonitis, perforations, ischemia or infarctions, and intestinal occlusion were the only GI tract manifestations significantly associated with increased mortality in multivariate analysis. For the 15 patients with these conditions, 6-month and 5-year survival rates were 60% and 46%, respectively. None of the other GI tract or extraintestinal vasculitis-related symptoms or angiographic abnormalities was predictive of surgical complications or poor outcome. They noted, however, that prognosis has dramatically improved over the 30-year period represented by this study, and attributed this to better management with prompt surgical intervention when indicated, and the combined use of glucocorticoids and immunosuppressive drugs.

Imaging

Despite the technical developments of non-invasive imaging modalities such as CT, MRI, and ultrasound (see Chapter 19), selective angiography of mesenteric arteries is still the gold standard in diagnosing peripheral splanchnic vessel disease (Trompeter *et al.* 2002). It is believed that arterial occlusions caused by non-atheromatous lesions, including vasculitis, is more prevalent in the visceral arteries than at other sites (Cognet *et al.* 2002). The diagnosis of chronic mesenteric ischemia requires confident elimination of other conditions because this condition often does not manifest as one or more arterial stenoses on vascular imaging. Barium enema may show thumbprinting due to submucosal edema or hemorrhage. This sign is fairly specific for ischemic bowel (Sultan *et al.* 1999). Contrast-enhanced CT of the entire abdominal cavity may provide useful information on inflammatory, neoplastic, and vascular diseases of the abdomen. If pain is alleviated by meals, endoscopy is in order to look for an ulcer of the stomach or duodenum. If liver function tests show abnormalities (cholestasis in particular), ultrasound or MR cholangiography should be considered to look for biliary obstruction. When the main non-vascular causes of abdominal pain have been ruled out, the bowel vasculature should be studied (Cognet *et al.* 2002).

Duplex ultrasound is an accurate screening test for proximal arterial stenosis or occlusion. A peak systolic velocity greater than 275 cm/sec seems to be highly specific for significant SMA stenosis (Moneta *et al.* 1993) and an end-diastolic velocity greater than 45 cm/sec may be even more accurate (Perko 2001). Blunting of fasting and postprandial differences in peak systolic velocity in the SMA (as assessed by ultrasound duplex scanning) was reported in patients with high-grade stenosis (Gentile *et al.* 1995) suggesting failure of the mesenteric blood flow to adapt to meal-related circulatory needs.

Siğirci *et al.* (2003) examined mesenteric artery flow using Doppler sonography in patients with Behçet's syndrome. They found that symptomatic patients with Behçet's syndrome involving the GI tract had a significantly increased flow in both the superior and inferior mesenteric arteries, whereas Behçet's syndrome patients without GI tract involvement did not differ from controls. Ripollés *et al.* (2005) studied sonographic findings in 58 patients with proven ischemic colitis, and reported a prospective sensitivity of sonography for the characterization of colonic abnormalities of 93.5% (58/62 patients). Segmental involvement was observed in 28%. Altered pericolic fat was the only sonographic variable significantly associated with the presence of transmural necrosis. Contrast-enhanced MR angiography has been useful for detection of significant arterial stenosis (Meaney *et al.* 1997). An important advantage, compared to CT angiography, is that it is entirely safe even when there is severe renal disease.

Assessment of emergent abdominal vascular conditions is possible today with the use of multidetector row CT angiography. The techniques of three-dimensional image reconstruction (shaded surface display, maximum intensity projection, and volume rendering) may permit their use as the initial or only imaging methods for surgical planning in emergent vascular conditions (Frauenfelder *et al.* 2004) and for planning of angiographic interventional treatments.

Arterial-phase CT scans and CT angiograms are of great value in the assessment of mesenteric arteries. They are helpful in identifying the site, level, and cause of bowel ischemia. Portal venous scans have additional advantages of depicting mesenteric veins, allowing better assessment of the bowel wall itself, and providing greater accuracy in the detection of perforation, abscess formation, and

peritonitis (Wiesner *et al.* 2003). Acute bowel ischemia may cause various morphological changes, including: homogenous or heterogenous hypo- or hyperattenuating wall thickening; dilatation; abnormal or absent wall enhancement; mesenteric stranding; vascular engorgement; ascites; pneumatosis; and portal venous gas (Bartnicke and Balfe 1994; Ha *et al.* 2000). Acute bowel ischemia may affect the small or large bowel and may be diffuse or localized, segmental or focal, and superficial or transmural; therefore it can mimic various diseases (Horton *et al.* 1999, 2000).

Byun *et al.* (1999) accepted the presence of at least three of the following signs on abdominal CT as diagnostic of ischemic bowel disease: bowel wall thickening; a target sign; dilation of intestinal segments; engorgement of vessels; and increased attenuation of mesenteric fat. There are three major pitfalls by which CT detection of bowel ischemia may be missed. First, a colonic segment with superficial mucosal ischemia may react with spasticity, which may be misinterpreted as simple contraction. Second, bowel wall thickness is different in a widely distended ischemic colonic segment than it is in a less distended, normal colonic segment. Thus, a bowel wall thickness of 3–5 mm in a distended colonic segment, which would be normal for a non-distended segment, should be interpreted as thickened. Third, there is a tendency to misinterpret bowel wall dilatation and air–fluid levels as ileus or pseudo-obstruction (Wiesner *et al.* 2003). In spite of these pitfalls, the sensitivity of CT for the diagnosis of acute bowel ischemia (82%) was comparable to that of angiography (87.5%) when the two modalities were compared directly (Klein *et al.* 1995).

Although non-invasive diagnostic investigations are very helpful, and increasingly promising, they may better be used as screening tests for avoiding unnecessary angiograms. The diagnosis of ischemia continues to rest on a careful medical history. Prompt surgical or interventional decisions should not be delayed.

Takayasu's arteritis

In Takayasu's arteritis (TA), non-specific gastrointestinal symptoms, such as anorexia, nausea, vomiting, and loss of weight, may take place during the prepulseless phase. True gastrointestinal morbidity resulting from arterial stenosis (Hall *et al.* 1985) and organ ischemia is rare. Acute abdominal signs as the first manifestation, although unusual, have been reported (Hands and Murie 1991; Cornejo *et al.* 2002). Chronic mesenteric ischemia presenting with weight loss and postprandial pain has also been reported (Bongard *et al.* 1992; Vega Saenz *et al.* 1995; Tyagi *et al.* 1997; Rajiv *et al.* 2004; Desai *et al.* 2004). The pain is typically postprandial, gradually increasing in severity, and then slowly resolving, and may be relieved by vomiting. There is sometimes significant weight loss, and the patient may develop a fear of eating (Rajiv *et al.* 2004). Angeli *et al.* (2001) reviewed the literature for the prevalence of main aortic branch involvement (stenosis or occlusion) at angiography and cited the following in descending order: superior mesenteric (17–29%), inferior mesenteric (4–27%), and celiac (9–18%) (see Figure 15.1). Koyama and his team (1995) reported a case of proper hepatic artery aneurysm. Sonographic exploration of the aorta and its major branches may have limitations. Even with the Doppler technique, minor stenotic changes and subtle mural irregularities can be missed. Nevertheless, it is considered an excellent screening modality for primary diagnosis (see Figure 15.2), and,

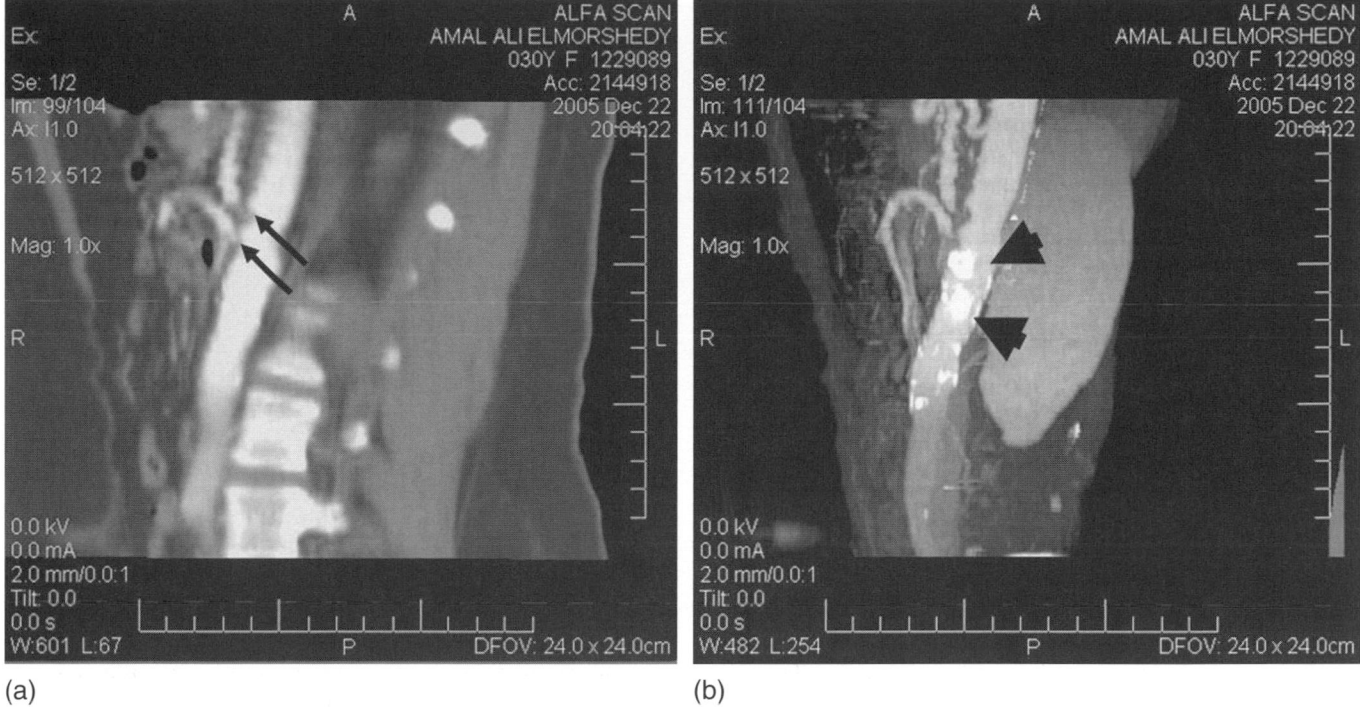

(a)   (b)

Figure 15.1 CT scan of the aorta, celiac artery, and superior mesenteric arteries in a case of TA. (a) Oblique parasagittal reformatted image using maximum intensity projection technique for the abdominal aorta showing significant narrowing at the origin of the celiac axis and superior mesenteric arteries (black arrows). (b) CT angiogram using volume-rendering technique for the abdominal aorta showing medial patchy calcifications (arrowheads).

thanks to its low invasiveness and cost, can be used for long-term follow-up of patients (Angeli *et al.* 1999).

Intervention in cases with significant vessel involvement is usually multidisciplinary. Several approaches include surgery (Esato *et al.* 1982; Koyama *et al.* 1995; Desai *et al.* 2004) and radiological intervention (Bongard *et al.* 1992; Tyagi *et al.* 1997; Rajiv *et al.* 2004). Glucocorticoids should be used judiciously in the perioperative or peri-interventional period (Vega Sanez *et al.* 1995; Rajiv *et al.* 2004).

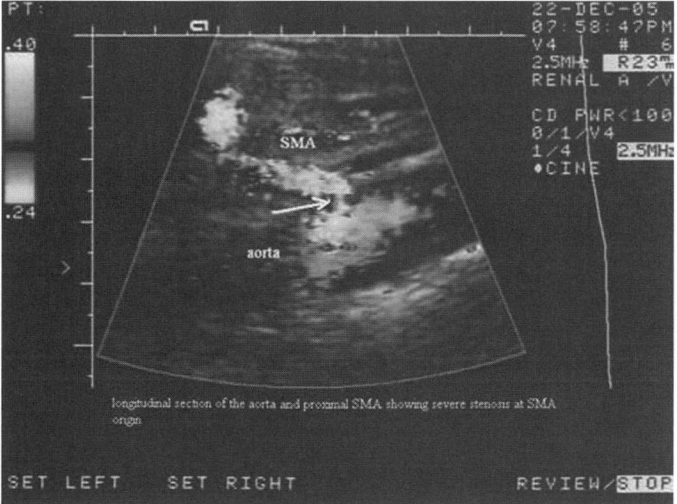

Figure 15.2 Arterial duplex examination of the aorta, celiac artery, and superior mesenteric arteries in a case of TA showing narrowing of SMA (arrow). (See Color Plate 61).

Giant cell arteritis

Extracranial vessel involvement is not an uncommon finding in patients with giant cell arteritis (GCA) at autopsy. Clinical manifestations due to such involvement are rare (Phelan *et al.* 1993) and it appears that GI vasculitis is less common in GCA than in other vasculitides (Strigley and Gardiner 1980). Most reports of GCA involving the GI tract are of small intestinal disease, in the form of infarction or perforation (Strigley and Gardiner 1980; Krant and Ross 1992; Smith *et al.* 1988). Lockhart and Robbin (2003) described a case of abdominal angina with diarrhea and weight loss of 4 months duration. The pain was initially episodic and diffuse, with subsequent development of postprandial cramps that were relieved after a bowel movement. The patient had an antecedent history of vasculitis suggestive of GCA. Her physical examination was unremarkable, without abdominal tenderness, peritoneal sounds, or bowel sounds. Angiogram suggested diffuse arterial abnormalities including those in the SMA. An intraoperative ultrasonography (US) image of the SMA demonstrated marked narrowing with near occlusion as it divided into its branches, and a thick hypoechoic wall, referred to as a halo, where thickening was diffuse and symmetric. This halo is similar to that described by Schmidt (2000) and Schmidt *et al.* (1999). Trimble and Weisz (2002) reported an 87-year-old male with infarction of the sigmoid colon secondary to GCA. The patient had an acute surgical abdomen and at surgery the colon was markedly distended, and an ischemic segment of the sigmoid colon was resected. Microscopic examination showed early infarction and GCA was noted throughout the sections of the associated mesocolon. De Winter and his coworkers (2000) reported a 63-year-old man with pyrexia of unknown origin who had increased ^{18}F-fluorodeoxyglucose uptake on positron emission tomography (PET) scan in the major thoracic vessels and abnormal splenic accumulation. Eventually, temporal artery biopsy confirmed the diagnosis of GCA. A follow-up PET scan after 6 weeks of glucocorticoid treatment showed a marked reduction of the vascularity and splenic uptake, prompting the authors to conclude that GCA can involve the spleen.

Polyarteritis nodosa

GI tract involvement has been reported in polyarteritis nodosa (PAN) by many investigators, with percentages ranging from 14 to 53% (Frohnert and Sheps 1967; Fortin *et al.* 1992; Guillevin *et al.* 1995). Most older series have included patients with MPA and CSS as well as those with PAN. GI tract manifestations are among the most serious expressions of PAN. Guillevin *et al.* 1995 studied the nature and incidence of GI manifestations in 53 patients with PAN and CSS. Eighteen of the 53 cases (34%) had GI tract manifestations; these were considered among the symptoms revealing PAN in seven (13.2%) of the 53 cases. Six of the 18 patients with GI tract manifestations had definite organ involvement related to vasculitis. Abdominal pain without characteristic organ involvement or surgical abdomen was present in 12 of 18 patients. Furthermore, among the subgroup of patients with GI hemorrhage, perforation, digestive tract surgery due to PAN, intractable abdominal pain, and weight loss greater than 20% of normal weight attributable to GI tract ischemia, there was a significantly lower 10-year survival rate compared to patients without GI tract manifestations (Guillevin *et al.* 1995).

Guillevin and his group included GI involvement among the items constituting the five-factor score, which can predict the 5-year survival rate of patients with PAN. Stanson and his coworkers (2001) reviewed the positive angiographic findings in 56 consecutive patients with PAN. They reported the following arterial bed distribution: gastric 33%, gastroduodenal 8%, hepatic 89%, SMA 97%, and inferior mesenteric artery (IMA) 100%. Angiographic findings included aneurysms, ectasia, or occlusive disease. The true frequency is difficult to determine because of the non-specificity of findings and small sampling size. Jee *et al.* (2000) described multiple aneurysms at the jejunal, ileal, right colic and mid colic branches of the SMA, IMA, hepatic, and left gastric arteries. Mesenteric infarction, perforation or aneurysmal rupture in PAN is disastrous, and relapses after treatment can take place (Guillevin *et al.* 1995; Levine *et al.* 2002; Travers *et al.* 1979; Fauci 1978). Gastric and esophageal perforations are rare (Gourgoutis *et al.* 1971). Histologic changes in the affected arteries in PAN may include aneurysms with hyalinosis, focal neovascularization, infiltration of mononuclear cells and neutrophils, and focal capillaritis (Figure 15.3) (see Chapter 9).

Involvement of the gallbladder (Blidi *et al.* 1996; Gorgun *et al.* 2002; Anon 1938; Parangi *et al.* 1991; Ito *et al.* 1991), the pancreas (Griffith and Vural 1951; Ito *et al.* 1991), and the appendix (Moyana 1988; Ozcay *et al.* 2003) have all been reported. PAN may be detected at cholecystectomy or appendectomy in the absence of other disease manifestations (Blidi *et al.* 1996). This apparently isolated vasculitis usually appears as a necrotizing lesion with fibrinoid necrosis but occasionally is granulomatous (see Chapter 9). How often these findings represent a true systemic vasculitis as opposed to a localized inflammatory process of no significance is disputed (see Chapter 9). Vasculitis in an organ removed for reasons other

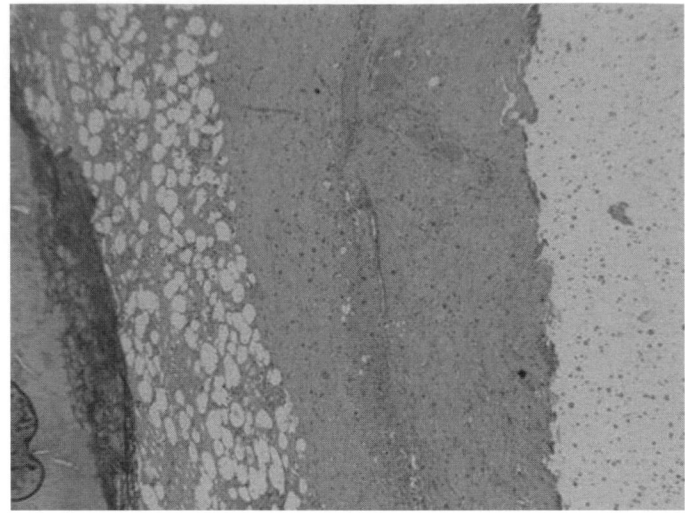

Figure 15.3 Polyarteritis nodosa. Microscopic examination (H and E staining) of celiac artery aneurysm, surgically removed from a patient with polyarteritis nodosa. (See Color Plate 62).

than systemic vasculitis should be interpreted cautiously and should prompt further history and workup for systemic disease if clinically suspicious.

The liver is a common site of involvement in PAN. The vascular changes result in aneurysm formation, or rupture, infarction, or interstitial hepatitis. Hekali *et al.* (1991) compared the angiographically observed visceral aneurysms in 71 PAN patients to those of other diseases with similar findings (seven from severe arterial hypertension and three from rheumatoid arthritis). The mean number of hepatic aneurysms was higher in PAN patients, and five of 17 PAN patients had numerous and large aneurysms. In spite of its common involvement, hepatic disease may remain undetected (Morway 1954). A constellation of presentations betraying hepatic disease was, nonetheless, cited: hematoma (Fitchett and Oakley 1975; Ayers and Fitchett 1992); intrahepatic bleeding and hemobilia (Yazici *et al.* 1997); and hemorrhage (Brandstetter *et al.* 1995; Ozcay *et al.* 2003). These may be further complicated by peritonitis or intestinal hemorrhage. Hepatic sequelae of HBV infection are well appreciated. The incidence of HBV infection is decreasing and this is reflected in its diminishing role as a causative agent in PAN.

Endoscopy may detect ischemic areas and ulcers. Total abdominal angiography leads to a more accurate appraisal of organ involvement (Ewald 1987), especially of occult aneurysms. This intervention should be considered in anticipation of the risk of rupture of large aneurysms (Stanson *et al.* 2001). CT and MR imaging may show bowel wall thickening with the so-called target sign, mesenteric vessel engorgement and haziness, ascites, or small-bowel obstruction, which may give a beak-like luminal narrowing (Jee *et al.* 2000).

Surgery is obligatory in cases of perforation, hemorrhage, infarction, pancreatitis, appendicitis, or cholecystitis. Not infrequently, multiple perforations are found. Relapses are frequent, and immunosuppressive therapy may increase the likelihood of infections and delayed healing. Intensive medical management is necessary. Glucocorticoid doses should not be lowered, nor should cyclophosphamide administration be postponed in the perioperative period.

Intravenous pulse cyclophosphamide is preferable to oral treatment because of its more rapid onset of action, and its reliable delivery to the blood. Its administration is recommended intraoperatively or immediately postoperatively to control the disease at the time of surgery (Guillevin 1999).

Kawasaki's disease

The GI manifestations of Kawasaki's disease (KD) have been described as early or late (Zulian et al. 2003). Diagnosis may be challenging in patients with atypical or incomplete KD (Zulian et al. 2003). GI tract involvement may include small bowel obstruction (Murphy et al. 1987; Mele and Evans 1996), focal colitis (Chung et al. 1996), bowel infarction (Mercer and Carpenter 1981), intestinal pseudo-obstruction (Akikusa et al. 2004), and hepatobiliary disease (Cody et al. 1996). Zulian and his group (2003) described 10 children (4.6%) among a cohort of 219 KD patients who had severe abdominal complaints coincident with their disease onset. The most common symptoms at onset were acute abdominal pain and distension, vomiting, hepatomegaly, and jaundice. Hematemesis was present in one; toxic shock syndrome requiring intensive care admission occurred in four. Five patients had laparotomy, three had percutaneous transhepatic biliary drainage, and one needed GI endoscopy. Postoperative diagnosis was gallbladder hydrops with cholestasis in five, paralytic ileus in three, appendicular vasculitis in one, and hemorrhagic duodenitis in one. All patients completely recovered, but 50% developed coronary aneurysm despite early intravenous gammaglobulin (IVIg) treatment.

Intestinal pseudo-obstruction has been reported to occur in 2–3% of children with KD (Miyake et al. 1987; Wheeler et al. 1990). Persistent vomiting, which is uncommon in KD, may be a clue to diagnosis (Akikusa et al. 2004). It tends to be seen early in pseudo-obstruction (Miyake et al. 1987), in contrast to mechanical bowel obstruction due to strictures, where vomiting generally appears 2–4 weeks after the acute illness (Murphy et al. 1987; Mele and Evans 1996). The pathogenesis of this entity is felt to relate to mesenteric vasculitis with ischemia and associated dysfunction of the myenteric plexus. The absence of mesenteric vessel abnormalities upon imaging suggests small vessel disease (Miyake et al. 1987; Franken et al. 1979). The treatment varies from simple bowel rest (Wheeler et al. 1990) to intravenous glucocorticoids (Miyake et al. 1987). In three cases, IVIg was given for pseudo-obstruction. In two cases, it was administered concomitant with bowel symptoms, and in both there seems to have been a subsequent rapid resolution of symptoms (Zulian et al. 2003; Fang et al. 2001). In the third case, the intestinal symptoms had resolved with conservative management by the time the child was recognized as having KD and given IVIg (Akikusa 2004). Pseudo-obstruction raises concern for coronary artery disease, since in the study of Miyake et al. (1987), five of the seven cases who developed this were found to have coronary artery disease. Similarly, Zulian and his group (2003) detected coronary artery aneurysm in one-half of their 10 cases presenting with a surgical abdomen, of whom three were felt to have pseudo-obstruction. The two groups suggested pseudo-obstruction as a marker of significant vasculitis. Abnormal liver function tests seem to be a common theme among studies examining potential predictors of IVIg failure (Fukunishi et al. 2000; Han et al. 2000; Durongpisitkul et al. 2003).

Wegener's granulomatosis

The frequency of GI involvement in Wegener's granulomatosis (WG) is uncertain as the few well-documented cases are selectively biased towards more aggressive cases (Haworth and Pusey 1984; Storesund et al. 1998). In the early autopsy study conducted by Walton (1958), necrotizing intestinal arteriolitis was found in 24% of 56 cases. Hoffman et al. (1992) analyzed 158 patients and reported no intestinal manifestations. Haworth and Pusey (1984) found abdominal symptoms in four of 45 patients in their records. Storesund et al. (1998) discussed the clinical and pathological presentations of severe intestinal involvement in WG. They found two females and four males, one of whom developed two episodes of bowel manifestations necessitating immediate surgical interventions. The average age at onset of intestinal symptoms was 43.3 years (26–55 years) and the first signs of their manifestations developed within the first 2 year of illness. Acute pain, peritonitis, or distention was the main clinical picture in six of the seven events, whereas the seventh presented with profuse diarrhea with blood and mucus. The small bowel was involved in two, the large intestine in three, and both in two of the seven episodes.

Histologically, vasculitis, ischemia, inflammation, and ulceration predominated, while granulomas were rarely identified. Surgery was performed in six episodes, and perforation was seen four times. The authors believed that the manifestations were associated with the disease process rather than related to the preceding treatment with immunosuppressive drugs. Pickhardt and Curran (2001) described a case of fulminant enterocolitis initially suspected to represent *Clostridium difficile* colitis that proved to be due to WG. Their patient was also exceptional in having severe GI disease without concomitant renal involvement. Steele and his coworkers (2001) described a young woman who presented initially to hospital with GI symptoms and then developed severe colitis and hemorrhage prior to the occurrence of respiratory tract symptoms, rapidly progressive renal failure, and nasal septal perforation. Sokol et al. (1984) noted an unusual presentation of WG disease in a 16-year-old black woman with diarrhea, fever, weight loss, abdominal pain, arthralgias, and mouth ulcers, suggesting the diagnosis of inflammatory bowel disease. Biopsy specimens of rectal mucosa, oro-and nasopharynx, and skin conclusively established the diagnosis of WG. The authors emphasized the value of taking biopsy specimens of oral lesions.

The CT findings of WG of the bowel are not unique to the disease. They share features with other small-vessel vasculitides, such as multifocal or diffuse bowel wall thickening, abnormal wall enhancement, mesenteric vascular engorgement, and ascites (Figure 15.4). Nonetheless, establishing the diagnosis of progressive vasculitis through CT is useful in directing therapy (Pickhard and Curran 2001).

Churg–Strauss syndrome

The GI tract is the third most common site of involvement in Churg–Strauss syndrome (CSS) (~50% of patients), after lung and skin (Kurita et al. 1994). Pathologic findings include multiple intestinal ulcerations with or without perforation, ischemic change, intestinal obstruction, and ileus (Kurita et al. 1994; Sharma et al. 1996). Intestinal perforation has been reported as a rare complication of CSS (Sharma et al. 1996). In Japan, however, intestinal perforation is frequently reported, with the small intestine being

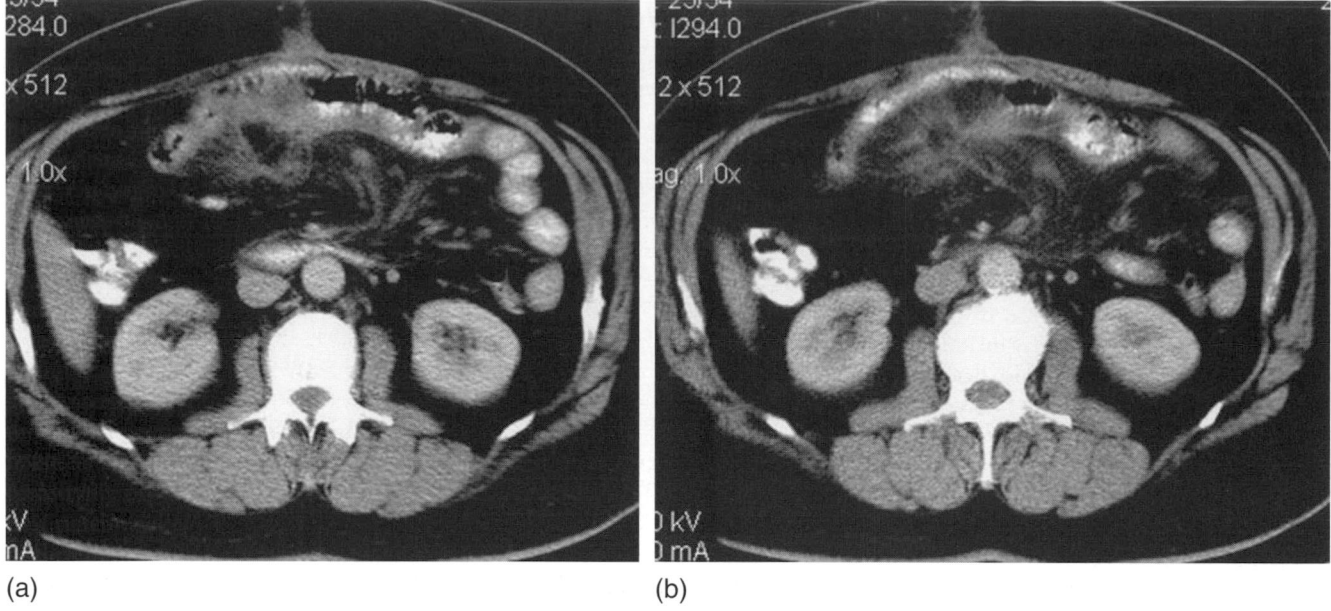

(a)   (b)

Figure 15.4 CT scan of abdomen in a case of acute mesenteric ischemia in a case of Wegener's granulomatosis. (a and b) Two contiguous axial CT sections through the umblical region demonstrating irregular mural thickening of one of the small intestinal loops with multiple air fluid levels. It is seen adherent to the anterior abdominal wall.

the most common site (Shimamoto *et al.* 1990). Histologically, CSS can be differentiated from PAN by the presence of extravascular granulomas and heavy eosinophilic infiltration in the small and medium-sized arteries and veins, whereas eosinophilic gastroenteritis is distinguished from CSS by the lack of vasculitis.

The clinical picture consists of pain, ileus, ischemic bowel disease, bleeding ulcers, and bloody diarrhea. It may be so severe as to cause acute abdomen necessitating surgical interference (Kurita *et al.* 1994; Sharma *et al.* 1996; Kaneki *et al.* 1998). The small intestine is the most common site of involvement (Sharma *et al.* 1996; Nakamura *et al.* 2002). Involvement of the colon has also been reported (Ohwada *et al.* 1997; Kim *et al.* 2000; Suzuki *et al.* 2005), and the duodenum can be the site of inflammation detected by upper endoscopy (Nishie *et al.* 2003). Suzuki and his group (2005) reported a case of colon erosion, acalculous cholecystitis, and liver abscesses that responded to antibiotic therapy. In the review of literature in this report, only six cases of cholecystitis, and one of liver abscesses were cited. Nakamura *et al.* (1991) reported melena caused by ruptured hepatic aneurysm into the intrahepatic bile ducts. The occurrence of pancreatitis, hemorrhage, or perforation is predictive of a poor outlook (Guillevin *et al.* 1999). Although abdominal complaints rarely appear as initial symptoms, this entity should be considered when the patient with abdominal pain presents with eosinophilia, asthma, or allergic rhinitis (Nisihe *et al.* 2003), or during glucocorticoid withdrawal in asthmatic patients when the so-called "forme frustes" CSS may be encountered (Churg 2001). Intensive perioperative management is essential to ensure a favorable clinical outcome.

Microscopic polyangiitis

GI symptoms of microscopic polyangiitis (MPA) were identified when this entity was recognized as distinct from PAN. Lhote *et al.* (1996) reported abdominal pain in 32–58% and digestive tract

bleeding in 29% of cases. In 1999, Guillevin *et al.* retrospectively analyzed 85 MPA patients and reported GI involvement in 30.6%. They believed that MPA is often a generalized disease characterized by multivisceral involvement. In their study, GI tract involvement was as frequent as in patients with PAN and CSS. It may be severe, and in two patients was responsible for death. Guillevin and his coworkers reported abdominal pain in 23 patients, melena in four, hematemesis in three, bowel perforation in one, cholecystitis in two, appendicitis in one, and pancreatitis in one, and death occurred in two patients. When HBV or HCV infection was present, there was no clinical evidence that the viral infection was responsible for the vasculitis. Patients with elevated transaminase levels had no detectable viral antigens, antibodies to virus, or molecular biologic evidence of virus replication. MPA has been cited as a cause of oral lesions (Shiboski *et al.* 2002), massive intestinal bleeding (Ueda *et al.* 2001), extended colonic ulcerations and hemorrhage, with crypt abscess formation (Tsai *et al.* 2004), as well as focal rectal capillaritis manifesting as painless rectal bleeding (Komanduri *et al.* 2002).

Henoch–Schönlein purpura

GI involvement occurs in approximately two-thirds of children with Henoch–Schönlein purpura (HSP) (Katz *et al.* 1991; Ajitha 2001; Tizard 1979). It usually is evident as abdominal pain. Abdominal symptoms precede the typical rash in ~36% of cases (Lanzkowsky 1992; Choong and Beasley 1998). Other presenting symptoms include nausea, vomiting, and diarrhea, which may be accompanied by melena that is believed to be associated with increased risk of renal disease (Tizard 1999). The importance of GI manifestations led to the inclusion of bowel angina among the American College of Rheumatology 1990 criteria for the classification of HSP (Mills *et al.* 1990). HSP is believed to be triggered by a respiratory tract infection; however, there are reports that incriminate GI tract pathogens in that role. The list includes Shigella (Roza et al. 1983), Yersinia (Rasmussen 1982), Campylobacter (Lind et al. 1994) and Clostridium difficile enteritis (Boey et al. 1997). Chen et al. (2005) described characteristic endoscopic findings in a patient with HSP. These included discrete coin-like petechiae, hemorrhagic erosions, and skip hyperemic and ecchymotic lesions, seen in the gastric antrum, cecum, ileocecal valve, and sigmoid colon.

In their review of intra-abdominal manifestations of HSP, Choong and Beasley (1998) found that major complications of abdominal involvement develop in 4.6% (range 1.3–13.6%), citing intussusception as by far the most common complication. It is confined to the small bowel in 58% of cases. Bowel ischemia and infarction; intestinal perforation; fistula formation; late ileal stricture; acute appendicitis; massive upper GI bleeding; pancreatitis; hydrops of the gallbladder; and pseudomembranous colitis are infrequent. Involvement of the ileum or ascending colon can mimic acute appendicitis and leads to unnecessary appendectomy (Katz et al. 1991). Kim et al. (2005) reviewed three cases of appendicitis and reported a fourth case, where fibrinoid necrosis and neutrophilic infiltrations could be demonstrated in the small vessels of the appendix.

Factor XIII activity has been reported to be low in HSP, especially with severe GI disease (De Mattia et al. 1995). Ultrasound may reveal generalized thickening of intestinal wall, ascites, intussusception (Chen et al. 2005), distended appendix surrounded by hyperechoic inflamed fat (Kim 2004), or features consistent with acalculous cholecystitis (Hoffman et al. 2004). Ultrasonography complements serial clinical assessment, clarifies the nature of involvement, and reduces the risk of unnecessary surgery (Choong and Beasley 1998). The hallmarks of HSP on CT are multiple focal areas of bowel thickening, mesenteric edema, vascular engorgement, and non-specific lymphadenopathy (Jeong et al. 1997).

In the study of Ajitha and his group (2001), four of their seven patients on glucocorticoids had no recurrence, and in two the GI symptoms were milder. Parenteral glucocorticoids have been advocated for severe abdominal pain, but they should be used with caution if there is active GI bleeding (Chen et al. 2005).

Behçet's syndrome

The frequency of GI tract involvement in Behçet's syndrome (BS) varies in different countries: Turkey 2.8–5%, Israeli Arabs 0%, Egypt 20%, Kuwait 21%, Scotland 50%, and Japan 50–60% (Yazici et al. 1980; Jankowski et al. 1992; Abdel-Monem 2004; Jaber et al. 2002; Mousa et al. 1986; Shimizu et al. 1979; Oshima et al. 1963).

Symptoms of GI involvement of BS are mainly dysphagia, abdominal pain, nausea, vomiting, flatulence, and diarrhea, sometimes with blood (see Chapter 35). Esophageal involvement is reported to range from 2–11% of cases, although this may be an underestimate (Bayraktar et al. 2000). Esophageal lesions include ulcers (linear, oval, or round), usually in the middle third of the esophagus (Ozenc et al. 1990; Yashiro et al. 1986), fistulae (Asaoka et al. 1990); pseudomembranous esophagitis (Bottomley et al. 1992); or varices related to portosystemic anastomoses (Bayraktar 1995). The gastric mucosa appears to be the least affected part of the GI tract; the most frequent gastric lesions are aphthous ulcers (Kasahara et al. 1981; Lakhanpal et al. 1985). In the duodenum, aphthous ulcers have been described both clinically

(Ozenc et al. 1990) and in post-mortem studies (Kasahara et al. 1981). Resistance to medical treatment is remarkable, and perforation may complicate these ulcers (Testini et al. 1996). Although gastric outlet obstruction can occur, there is not usually a deformity of the duodenum (Ozenc et al. 1990). Kandilci et al. (1992) described four cases of endoscopic bulbitis with microthrombi of mucosal vessels detected microscopically. Intestinal BS occurs in two forms: mucosal inflammation and ischemia. Small-vessel disease underlies ulceration, whereas large-vessel involvement of a mesenteric artery or its major branches leads to ischemia and infarction (Bayraktar et al. 2000). The small intestine is the most frequently involved extraoral part of the GI tract in BS (Kasahara et al. 1981). The lesions are most commonly found in the terminal ileum and the cecum, and less frequently in the colon. The lesions are commonly aphthous ulcers, or they may be deep round or oval ulcers with a punched-out appearance, whereas longitudinal ulcers are rare. Lee et al. (1997) reported 37 persons with intestinal BS, of whom 26 were surgically managed. A solitary ulcer was observed in 22 cases (60%) while multiple ulcers were present in 15 cases. Chang et al. (2000) described a case of ileocecal ulcer and cecocecal fistula. Bowel perforation is unusual but serious (Kaklamani et al. 1998; Ghate and Jorizzo 1999).

Rectal and anal involvement are quite rare, and may share features with ulcerative colitis, both clinically and histopathologically (Hamza 1993) (Figure 15.5). Vasculitis of small veins and venules is common, characterized by lymphocytic infiltration. Focal rectal colitis characterized by the presence of crypt abscesses, submucosal fibrosis, and an inflammatory reaction with an intact mucosa was described, despite an intact mucosa (Sayek et al. 1991).

The differential diagnosis of intestinal BS includes Crohn's disease, ulcerative colitis, cecal tuberculosis, cecal amebiasis, benign tumors, and drug-induced damage. It is often difficult to distinguish between BS and inflammatory bowel disease, as they share common extraintestinal features: oral ulcers, uveitis, erythema nodosum, and arthritis (Sakane 1999). BS can be distinguished from Crohn's disease by having ulcers that, characteristically, do not show a granuloma. Ulcers in BS are deep and associated with a vasculitis that is usually a venulitis. Fistula formation and perforation tend to occur early in the course of BS. The colonic ulcers of BS are deeper than those of ulcerative colitis.

The ileocecal region is the most frequently involved location; while in ulcerative colitis the disease usually starts at the rectum and moves proximally (Bayraktar et al. 2000). Acute pancreatitis was reported by Houng (1992), and Lakhanpal et al. (1985) described pathologic features of pancreatitis in five cases of a large Japanese autopsy registry (170 cases). Biochemical evidence of pancreatitis is a relatively common finding in BS, even in the absence of other diagnostic clues (Bayraktar et al. 2000).

The most common hepatic complication of BS is Budd–Chiari syndrome (BCS) (Bayraktar et al. 1993; Bizmuth et al. 1990). BS accounts for 42.4% of the cases of BCS with recognizable underlying disease in Turkey (Bayraktar et al. 1993). Goubran et al. (1999) reported 30 cases of BCS; in 25 an etiologic factor could be identified. Four patients (16%) had BS (one with a concomitant protein C deficiency). BCS presents with hepatomegaly, leg edema, ascites, and venous dilatation over the trunk. With thrombosis involving a long segment of inferior vena cava (IVC), the outcome is much worse than when it involves the hepatic portion of IVC. Other hepatobiliary conditions reported in BS include: hepatomegaly due to

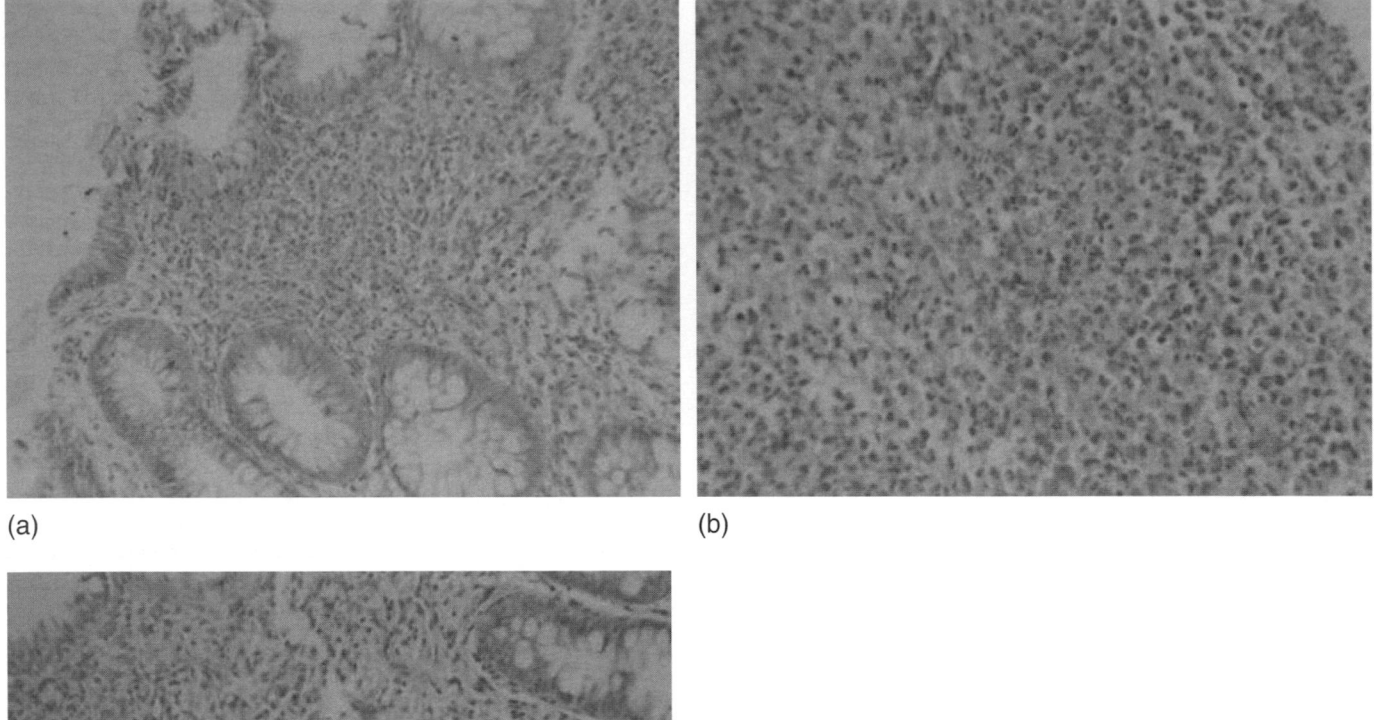

(a)

(b)

(c)

Figure 15.5 Behçet's syndrome. Portions of colonic mucosa showing focal crypt distortion, surface mucosal erosions (a), and necrotic debris heavily infiltrated by neutrophils (b). The mucosal tissue shows focal crypt distortion and moderate infiltration of the lamina propria by neutrophils and mononuclear cells (c). (See Color Plate 63).

steatosis or congestion; cirrhosis; acute and chronic hepatitis; cholelisthiasis; acute cholecystitis; toxic hepatitis; hepatic abscess (Lakhanpal 1985; Manna *et al.* 1985); and primary biliary cirrhosis (Jankowski *et al.* 1992). Aphthous lesions on the hepatic capsule (Barrier 1982) and a case with resemblance to small duct primary sclerosing cholangitis (Hisaoka 1994) were reported. Splenomegaly is noted in 20% of patients even in the absence of portal hypertension (Soysal *et al.* 1990). Lakhanpal *et al.* (1985) discovered 37 cases of splenic involvement in a total of 170 studied at autopsy. They reported splenitis, congestion, splenomegaly, hemosiderosis, infarction, and autosplenectomy in order of descending frequency. Peritonitis may be encountered in BS. Saccular and fusiform arterial aneurysms of medium-sized arteries as well as arterial occlusions, stenosis, and arteriovenous fistula have been described (Bayraktar *et al.* 1993). Intestinal amyloidosis may be responsible for diarrhea and malabsorption. The amyloid present is type AA. It tends to occur about a decade after the disease onset (Melikoglu *et al.* 2001).

Upper GI tract radiological examination is helpful in showing deep ulcers, intestinal stenoses, or fistulas (Asaoka *et al.* 1990).

Pyloric stenosis in the absence of duodenal deformity is characteristic. The colonic lesions of BS can be seen using double contrast barium studies. Colonic haustrations are well preserved in BS and ulcers can be detected (Bayraktar *et al.* 2000). Intestinal BS is treated with sulfasalazine, systemic or local glucocorticoids, and thalidomide. Cyclosporin has proven to be ineffective (Kaklamani *et al.* 1998; Bayraktar *et al.* 2000). There is a report of successful use of the anti-TNF-α antibody infliximab) to treat ileocolitis of BS (Kram *et al.* 2003).

Surgery is considered for perforation and persistent bleeding. Invasive surgical procedures often result in excessive inflammatory cell infiltration into the treated tissues, with subsequent anastomotic leakage. Intermediate doses of glucocorticoids are given to the patients for several days postoperatively (Sakane *et al.* 1999). The creation of a stoma is preferred over primary anastomosis because of the high rate of intestinal leak, perforation, and fistulation at anastomotic sites (Bayraktar *et al.* 2000). Lee *et al.* (1997), commenting on the high recurrence rate (46.1%), strongly recommended periodic follow-up with radiography and endoscopy. They advised examination of the entire bowel at the time of operation, and that bowel resection should include a generous normal margin.

Thromboangiitis obliterans (Buerger's disease)

Although some authors claim that GI manifestations in thromboangiitis obliterans (TAO), especially early in the disease, are misdiagnosed (Adam *et al.* 2002), there is some controversy about whether TAO causes GI problems (Hassoun *et al.* 2001). Intestinal TAO occurs mostly in men, but there are reports of it affecting women (Raat *et al.* 1993; Lie 1998). Visceral involvement may appear simultaneously with limb ischemia (Cho *et al.* 2005) or may precede it (Broide *et al.* 1993; Adam *et al.* 2002), which suggests that TAO should be considered in young male smokers with unexplained abdominal pain. Multiple sites are often involved, and there is a tendency to recur (Pfitzmann *et al.* 2002; Siddiqui *et al.* 2001), or have occlusion of vascular grafts (Schellong *et al.* 1994). The SMA, followed by the celiac trunk, is the artery most frequently involved (Ito *et al.* 1993; Pfitzmann *et al.* 2002; Raat *et al.* 1993; Schellong *et al.* 1994; Hassoun *et al.* 2001), although the IMA (Garcia *et al.* 1998) and hepatic artery (Adam *et al.* 2002) can also be affected. Attention to the possibility and prompt intervention is required to avoid this potentially life-threatening complication of visceral TAO (Deitch *et al.* 1981; Siddiqui *et al.* 2001).

Vasculitis of rheumatoid arthritis

Rheumatoid vasculitis is a relatively uncommon complication of rheumatoid arthritis (RA). Pagnoux *et al.* (2005) reported three RA-associated vasculitis patients among their series of 62 patients (5%). Rheumatoid vasculitis has been reported to cause: multiple, small bowel ulcerations (Takeuchi and Kuroda 2000); pancolitis and discrete colonic ulcerations following glucocorticoid treatment (Burt *et al.* 1983); appendicitis (Van Laar *et al.* 1998); and widespread microaneurysms of celiac and extra-intestinal small and medium-sized vessels (Hitter *et al.* 1988). Achkar *et al.* (1995) described a patient with serious intra-abdominal hemorrhage from a ruptured aneurysm of the inferior pancreaticoduodenal artery in the setting of rheumatoid vasculitis. Jacobsen *et al.* (1985) reported a case of mesenteric arteritis complicated by perforation of the ileum with generalized peritonitis. Perforation due to intestinal infarction was also reported in the small intestine (Tsai 1980), and in a combined ileal and sigmoid infarction (Babian *et al.* 1998). Another complication of rheumatoid vasculitis is stricture formation in the small bowel (Kuehne *et al.* 1992), or the colon (Keating 1998). Marcolongo *et al.* (1979) studied gastric, colonic, and rectal biopsies obtained from patients with RA. Histologic changes were characterized by partial or complete loss of superficial epithelium, inflammatory cellular infiltrate, and the presence of vasculitic lesions. McCurley and Collins (1984) described three patients with complicated RA and bowel infarction in which the distal mesenteric vessels were occluded by endarteritis characterized by intimal proliferation without vessel wall necrosis or inflammation. These vascular lesions were progressive and rendered the patients vulnerable to infarction during periods of decreased cardiac output. Okuda *et al.* (1990) reported two patients with RA complicated by severe attacks of enterocolitis, presumably due to mesenteric vasculitis.

Systemic lupus erythematosus

Lupus enteritis is a serious presentation of systemic lupus erythematosus (SLE), with a prevalence rate ranging between 0.2 and 5.3% (Medina *et al.* 1997; Drenkard *et al.* 1997). Lee *et al.* (2002) retrospectively studied 175 SLE patients, 38 (22%) of whom had at least one episode of acute abdominal pain. Lupus enteritis, based on CT findings, was found in 17 patients, comprising 45% of those presenting with acute abdominal pain. Histologic findings may include inflammatory infiltrates or hyalinization of capillary walls with a wire-loop appearance reminiscent of lupus nephritis (Figure 15.6). The spectrum of lupus enteritis included pain and hemorrhage with gastritis, diarrhea, hemorrhage, perforation,

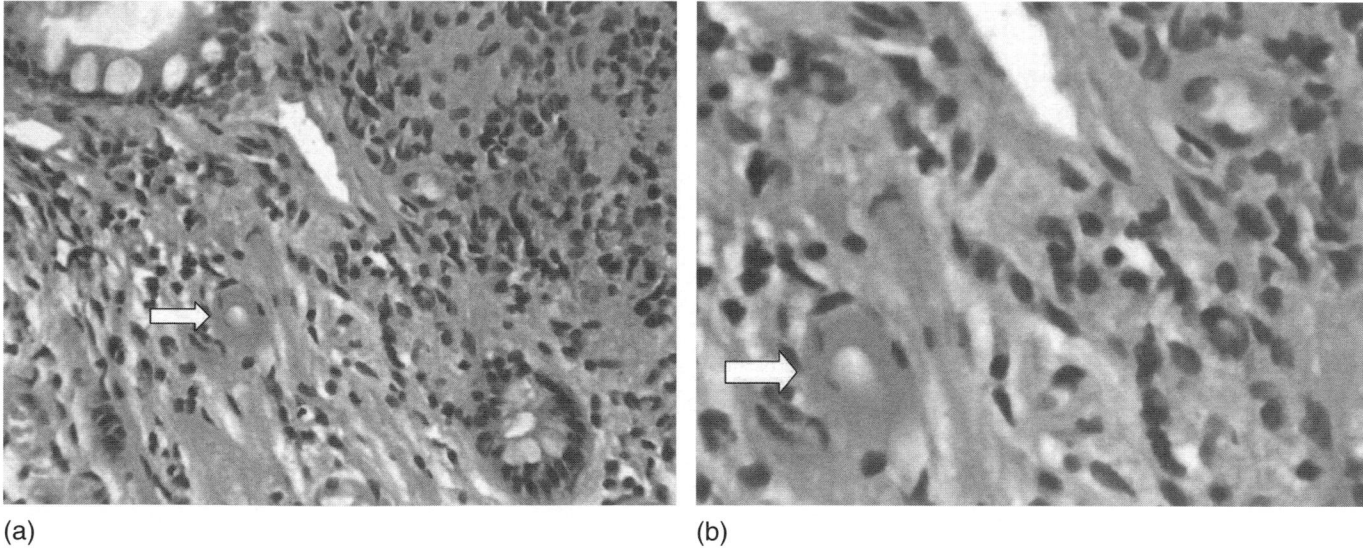

(a)   (b)

Figure 15.6 Endoscopically obtained section of ileum in a case of systemic lupus erythematosus (H and E staining), showing infiltration by inflammatory cells. Note hyalinization of the capillary wall with an appearance reminiscent of the "wire-loop" in lupus nephritis (white arrow). The patient was diagnosed with lupus enteritis. (a) × 400; (b) × 800. (See Color Plate 64).

infarction, and ileus with ileitis. Colitis presents with similar changes, as well as intussusception leading to pain and obstruction (Hoffman and Katz 1980). Other less frequent manifestations include: esophageal dysmotility and arteritis (Gastrucci *et al.* 1990; Harvey *et al.* 1954); protein-losing enteropathy (Pelletier *et al.* 1992); massive ischemic colitis (Kistin *et al.* 1978); and perforated colonic diverticulae (Zizic *et al.* 1997). The rectum can be involved in: gangrenous ischemic colitis (Reissman *et al.* 1994); stenosis (Palvio and Christensen 1987); ulceration (Amit *et al.* 1999); and perforation with necrosis of the rectosigmoid (Lazaris *et al.* 2003), although rectal involvement is rare (14% of cases) owing to its rich blood supply (Lee *et al.* 2002). Lee and his group (2002) found lupus enteritis to be the most common cause of acute abdominal pain. It was the initial manifestation of SLE in six of 17 cases (35.3%). The jejunum and the ileum were the sites most commonly affected, being involved in 80% and 85% of cases, respectively; 90% of cases had involvement in multiple vascular territories, and four cases relapsed.

There is disagreement in the literature regarding the association between intestinal infarction and presence of antiphospholipid antibodies (Medina *et al.* 1997; Sanchez-Guerrero *et al.* 1992; Lee *et al.* 2002) and its relationship to lupus activity (Medina *et al.* 1997; Lee *et al.* 2002). Leukopenia is frequently reported to correlate with the occurrence of lupus enteritis (Lee *et al.* 2002; Sultan *et al.* 1999). Macroscopically, there are no pathognomonic findings suggestive of SLE; the appearance varies from segmental edema to discrete ulceration, gangrene and perforation (Sasamura *et al.* 1991; Grimbacher *et al.* 1998). Histologically, both small-vessel arteritis and venulitis have been described. Associated findings include atrophy and degeneration of the media of small arteries, fibrinoid necrosis of vessel walls, old thrombosis, phlebitis, and monocyte infiltrate in the lamina propria. Acute and chronic inflammatory infiltrate and punched out ulcers with edematous mucosa can be detected on colonoscopy (Grimbacher *et al.* 1998). Pneumatosis cystoides intestinalis may also occur (Cabrera *et al.* 1994) although it is a non-specific finding. Plain radiography may show intraperitoneal free air, pneumatosis cystoide intestinalis, ileus, or a pseudo-obstruction pattern. Barium enema may show thumbprinting due to submucosal edema or hemorrhage, which is fairly specific for ischemic bowel (Sultan *et al.* 1999). With insidious onset of symptoms, evaluation should incorporate ultrasound and abdominal CT. Abdominal ultrasound may show bowel wall thickening (Shiohira 1993). Abdominal CT may show changes diagnostic of ischemic bowel disease as noted above, including bowel wall thickening, target sign, dilation of intestinal segments, engorgement of vessels, and increased attenuation of mesenteric fat. Angiography is not useful as the disease affects the small vessels. Endoscopy may be helpful and radioisotopic scanning using gallium and indium[111] white cell scanning has been used to highlight areas of inflammation and sepsis (Sultan *et al.* 1999). Laparoscopy or laparotomy may be considered (Al-Hakeem 1998).

Medical treatment was successfully reported in intestinal vasculitis with high-dose prednisolone (Medina *et al.* 1997; Cabrera *et al.* 1994; Turner *et al.* 1996) and intravenous cyclophosphamide (Grimbacher *et al.* 1998; Turner *et al.* 1996). Small intestinal ischemia, infarction, and perforation of any segment require emergency surgery. Large bowel ischemia may be treated conservatively, and laparoscopy may be considered, as it is less invasive, and less consequential when compared to open surgery (Medina *et al.* 1997).

Miscellaneous forms of vasculitis

Lopez *et al.* (1980) studied leukocytoclastic (hypersensitivity) vasculitis (LCV) on skin biopsy in 18 patients with who were younger than 16 years of age and 75 older patients with LCV. Significant GI manifestations at presentation or exacerbation of vasculitis were more frequent in the younger age group (66%), compared to the older ones (26%). No consistent radiologic findings were noted. Duodenal and peritoneal biopsies suggested vasculitis in six patients. Four patients needed exploratory laparotomy. Only one patient had intestinal infarction, and two patients with acute abdomen responded promptly to intravenous glucocorticoids. They suggested that early recognition and treatment with glucocorticoids could avoid surgery. Vlahos *et al.* (2005) presented a case of localized LCV of the left colon with megacolon. Diffuse mucosal thickening of the antrum, duodenum and jejunum were reported in a person with LCV (Nagarajan *et al.* 2005). Histopathologic examination of tissue from patients with LCV and GI involvement may reveal non-specific findings of vasculitis (Figure 15.7).

Gaburri *et al.* (2004) reported finding colonic ulcers in a 48-year old woman treated with propylthiouracil. She had ANCA-positive vasculitis with a perinuclear pattern with secondary antiphospholipid syndrome. Cogan syndrome was reported to present with refractory aortitis and mesenteric vasculitis (Andrey *et al.* 1995). Endoscopy was normal and the diagnosis was confirmed by angiography. Immunosuppressive agents were unsuccessful. Dermatomyositis was reported to cause vasculitis involving small arteries and capillaries, resulting in ischemia and necrosis in any part of the GI tract with serious consequences (Eshraghi *et al.* 1998). Cytomegalovirus (CMV) vasculitis in the intestine of a patient with acquired immune deficiency syndrome (AIDS) (Shintaku *et al.* 1991); CMV vasculitis causing middle and left colic vein thrombosis and ischemic colitis in a renal transplant patient (Muldoon *et al.* 1996); and *Rickettsia* (now *Orientia) tsutsugamushi*-induced vasculitic lesions (scrub typhus) detected by upper GI endoscopy (Kim *et al.* 2000) have all been described.

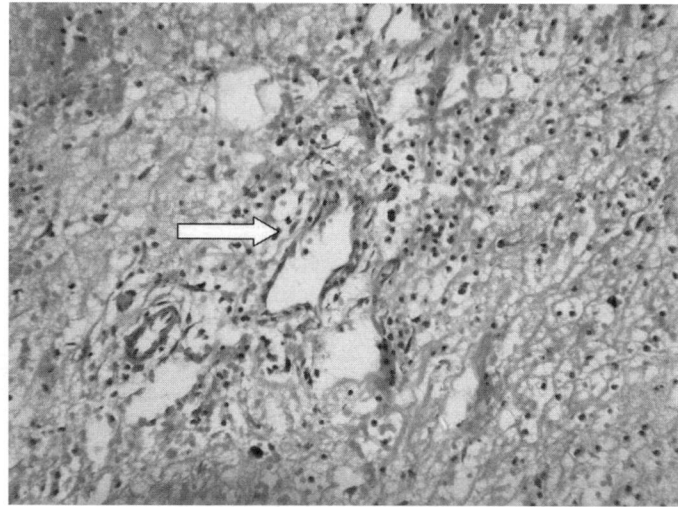

Figure 15.7 Findings of non-specific vasculitis. Surgically obtained section of ileum in a case of leucocytoclastic vasculitis (H and E staining). Small vessels show wall infiltration with mononuclear cells and neutrophils (white arrow). × 200. (See Color Plate 65).

As an example of vasculitis associated with lymphoproliferative disease, Laberge and Kerlan (2002) reported a case of lymphocytic lymphoma presenting with vasculitis. Their patient died of diffuse bowel ischemia several days after laparotomy. Enterocolic lymphocytic phlebitis (ELP) is a rare cause of GI tract ischemia, involving only the mural and mesenteric veins, which are surrounded by a lymphocytic and sometimes granulomatous infiltrate. The mesenteric arterial system and the systemic vasculature are characteristically spared (Abraham *et al.* 2004). Regional vasculitis describes an entity of isolated lesion, where no underlying connective tissue disease can be found. This entity has an excellent prognosis when compared to systemic variants after treatment with glucocorticoids and selective surgery, and attention to the possibility saves the patient the risk of unnecessary cytotoxic therapy.

References

Abdel-Monem, M. (2001). *Behçet's disease in Egypt*. The National Congress on Rheumatic Disease, Allied Conditions-Rehabilitation.

Abraham, S. C., Solem, C. A., Hauser, S. C., *et al.* (2004). Chronic antral ulcer associated with gastroduodenal lymphocytic phlebitis. *American Journal of Surgical Pathology*, **28**, 1695–63.

Achkar, A. A., Stanson, A. W., Johnson, C. M., *et al.* (1995). Rheumatoid vasculitis manifesting as intraabdominal hemorrhage. *Mayo Clinic Proceedings*, **70**, 565–9.

Adam, C., Benamouzig, R., Royer, I., *et al.* (2002). Buerger's disease or thromboangiitis obliterans revealed by an enteric ischemia. Case report and literature review. *Gastroenterologie Clinique et Biologique*, **26**, 409–11.

Ajitha, B., Sandra, A., Shuthakirthi, D. S., *et al.* (2001). Evaluation and therapeutic outcome of palpable purpura. *Indian J Derm. Venereol Leprol*, **67**, 320–3

Akikusa, J. D., Laxer, R. M. and Friedman, J. N. (2004). Intestinal pseudoobstruction in Kawasaki disease. *Pediatrics*, **113**, e504–6.

Al-Hakeem, M. S. and McMillen, M. A. (1998). Evaluation of abdominal pain in systemic lupus erythematosus. *American Journal of Surgery*, **176**, 291–4.

Amit, G., Stalnikowicz, R., Ostrovsky, Y., *et al.* (1999). Rectal ulcer: a rare Gastrointestinal Manifestation of systemic lupus erythematosus. *Journal of Clinical Gastroenterology*, **29**, 200–2.

Angeli, E., Salvioni, M. and Venturini, M. (1999). Diagnosis of takayasu's arteritis with color Doppler sonography comparison with angiographic findings. In *11th European Congress of Radiology*. Vienna.

Angeli, E., Vanzulli, A., Venturini, M., *et al.* (2001). The role of radiology in the diagnosis and management of Takayasu arteritis. *Journal of Nephrology*, **14**, 514–4.

Arend, W. P., Michel, B. A., Bloch, D. A., *et al.* (1990). The American College of Rheumatology 1990. Criteria for the classification of Takayasu arteritis. *Arthritis and Rheumatism*, **33**, 1129–32.

Asaoka, M., Sakai, Y., Kimura, J., *et al.* (1990). A case of tracheaesophageal fistula in Behçet's disease repaired with pericardial patch and gastric roll (Japanese). *J Jpn Assoc Thoracic Surg*, **38**, 1549–53.

Audrey, C. H.O., Melvin, I., Roat, A. V., *et al.* (1999). Cogan's syndrome with refractory abdominal aortitis and mesenteric vasculitis. *Journal of Rheumatology*, **26**, 1404–7.

Ayers, A. B. and Fitchett, D. H. (1992). Hepatic hematoma in polyarteritis nodosa. *British Journal of Radiology*, **49**, 184–5.

Babian, M., Nasef, S. and Soloway, G. (1998). Gastrointestinal infarction as a manifestation of rheumatoid vasculitis. *American Journal of Gastroenterology*, **93**, 119–20.

Barrier, J., Cerbeland, P., Raffi, F., *et al.* (1982). Aphthous hepatic lesions and Behçet's syndrome. *La semaine des hôpitaux: organe fondé par l'Association d'enseignement médical des hôpitaux de Paris*, **58**, 2395–6.

Bartnicke, B. J. and Balfe, D. M. (1994). CT appearance of intestinal ischaemia and intramural haemorrhage. *Radiology Clinics of North America*, **32**, 845–60.

Bayraktar, Y., Balkanei, F., Kansu, F., *et al.* (1993). Budd-Chiari syndrome: analysis of 30 cases. *Angiology*, **44**, 541–51.

Bayraktar, Y., Balkani, F., Kansu, E., *et al.* (1995). Cavernous transformation of the portal vein: a common manifestation of Behçet's disease. *American Journal of Gastroenterology*, **90**, 1476–9.

Bayraktar, Y., Ozaslan, E. and Van Threl, D. H. (2000). Gastrintestinal manifestations of Behçet's disease. *Journal of Clinical Gastroenterology*, **3**, 144–54.

Bizmuth, E., Hadenque, A., Hammel, P., *et al.* (1990). Hepatic vein thrombosis in Behçet's disease. *Hepatology*, **11**, 968.

Blidi, M., Quang, T., Cassan, P., *et al.* (1996). Cholecystite aigues de la periarterite noueuse: huit observations. *Annales Medecine Interne* (Paris), **147**, 304.

Boey, C. C., Ramanujam, T. M. and Looi, L. M. (1997). Clostridium difficile-related necrotizing pseudomembranous enteritis in association with Henoch-Schonlein purpura. *Journal of Pediatric Gastroenterology and Nutrition*, **24**, 426–9.

Bongard, O., Schneider, P. A., Krahenbuhl, B. and Bounameaux, H. (1992). Transluminal angioplasty of the aorta, renal and mesenteric arteries in Takayasu arteritis: report of two cases. *European Journal of Vascular Surgery*, **6**, 567–71.

Bottomley, W. W., Dakkak, M., Walton, S., *et al.* (1992). Esophageal involvement in Behçet's disease. Is endoscopy necessary? *Digestive Diseases and Sciences*, **37**, 594–7.

Bradbury, A. W., Murie, J. A. and Ruckley, C. V. (1993). Role of the leucocyte in the pathogenesis of vascular disease. *British Journal of Surgery*, **80**, 1503–12.

Brandstetter, K., Shroeder, W. and Bautz, W. (1995). Massive intrahepatic hemorrhage as the initial manifestation of panarteritis nodosa. *Roentgenpraxis*, **48**, 209–11.

Broide, E., Scapa, E., Peer, A., *et al.* (1993). Buerger's disease presenting as acute small bowel ischemia. *Gastroenterology*, **104**, 1192–5.

Burt, R. W., Berenson, M. M., Samuelson, C. O., *et al.* (1983). Rheumatoid vasculitis of the colon presenting as pancolitis. *Digestive Diseases and Sciences*, **28**, 183–8.

Byun, J. Y., Ha, H. K., Yu, S. Y., *et al.* (1999). CT Features of systemic lupus erythematosus in patients with acute abdominal pain: Emphasis on ischemic bowel disease. *Radiology*, **211**, 203–9.

Cabrera, G. E., Scopelitis, E., Cuellar, M. L., *et al.* (1994). Pneumatosis cystoides intestinalis in systemic lupus erythematosus with intestinal vasculitis: treatment with high dose prednisone. *Clinical Rheumatology*, **13**, 312–6.

Calabrese, L. H., Michel, B. A., Bloch, D. A., *et al.* (1990). The American College of Rheumatology 1990. Criteria for the classification of Hypersensitivity vasculitis. *Arthritis and Rheumatism*, **33**, 1108–13.

Case Records of the Massachussetts General Hospital (1938). Case 242–01. *New England Journal of Medicine*, **218**, 838–43.

Casey, K. M., Quigley, T. M., Kozarek, R. A. and Racker, E. J. (1993). Lethal nature of ischemic gastropathy. *American Journal of Surgery*, **165**, 646–9.

Chan, J. C., Li, P. K., Lai, F. M., *et al.* (1992). Fatal adult Henoch-Schonlein purpura due to small intestinal infarction. *Journal of Internal Medicine*, **232**, 181–4.

Chang, H., Kim, J. and Chung, H. (2000). Ileo-cecal ulcer with a cecocecal fistula in Behçet's disease. *Korean Journal of Internal Medicine*, **15**, 99–101.

Chen, M.-J., Wang, T.-E., Chang, W.-H., *et al.* (2005). Endoscopic findings in a patient with Henoch-Schonlein purpura. *World Journal of Gastroenterology*, **11**, 2354–6.

Cho, Y. P., Kang, G. H., Han, M. S., *et al.* (2005). Mesenteric involvement of acute stage Buerger's disease as the initial clinical manifestation: report of a case. *Surgery Today*, **35**, 499–501.

Choong, C. K. and Beasley, S. W. (1998). Intra-abdominal manifestations of Henoch-Schonlein purpura. *Journal of Pediatrics and Child Health*, **34**, 405–9.

Chung, C. J., Rayder, S., Meyers, W., *et al.* (1996). Kawasaki disease presenting as focal colitis. *Pediatric Radiology*, **26**, 455–7.

Churg, A. (2001). Recent advances in the diagnosis of Churg-Strauss Syndrome. *Modern Pathology*, **14**, 1284–93.

Cognet, F., Ben Salem, D., Dranssart, M., *et al.* (2002). Chronic mesenteric ischemia: imaging and percutaneous treatment. *Radiographics*, **22**, 863–79.

Conron, M. and Beynon, H. L.C. (2000). Rare diseases. 11 Churg Strauss syndrome. *Thorax*, **55**, 870–7.

Cornejo, R., Gatica, H., Segovia, E., *et al.* (2002). Intestinal necrosis as clinical presentation of Takayasu arteritis. *Revista Medica de Chile*, **130**, 1159–64.

De Mattia, D., Penza, R., Giordano, P., *et al.* (1995). Von Willebrand factor and factor XIII in children with Henoch-Schonlein purpura. *Pediatric Nephrology*, **9**, 603–5.

De Winter, F., Petrovic, M., Van de Wiele, C., Vogelaers, D., Afschrift, M., Dierckx, R. A. (2000). Imaging of giant cell arteritis: Evidence of splenic involvement using FDG positron emission tomography. *Clinical Nuclear Medicine*, **25**, 633–4.

Deitch, E. A. and Sikkema, W. W. (1981). Intestinal manifestation of Buerger's disease: case report and literature review, **47**, 326–8.

Desai, K. A., Cotter, M. M., Doucet, L., *et al.* (2004). Pathology case of the month. 39-year-old woman with abdominal pain and weight loss. Takayasu arteritis (TA). *Journal of the Louisiana State Medical Society*, **156**, 230–4.

Drenkard, C., Villa, A. R., Reyes, E., *et al.* (1997). Vasculitis in systemic lupus erythematosus. *Lupus*, **6**, 235–42.

Durongpisitkul, K., Soongswang, J., Laohaprasitiporn, D., *et al.* (2003). Immunoglobulin failure and Retreatment in Kawasaki Disease. *Pediatric Cardiology*, **89**, 916–22.

Eshraghi, N., Farahmand, M., Maerz, L. L., *et al.* (1998). Adult-onset dermatomyositis with severe gastrointestinal manifestations: case report and review of the literature. *Surgery*, **123**, 356–8.

Esato, K., Norma, F. and Kurata, S. (1982). Mesenteric infarction in takayasu's arteritis treated by thromboendarterectomy and intestinal resection. *Japanese Journal of Surgery*, **12**, 130–4.

Evans, D. J., Wilkins, M. J., Wazir, J. F. and Rosin, D. (1998). Extracranial giant cell arteritis. *Journal of the Royal College of Surgeons Edinburgh*, **43**, 207–8.

Ewald, E. A., Griffin, D. and Mccuue, W. J. (1987). Correlation of angiographic abnormalities with disease manifestations and disease severity in polyarteritis nodosa. *Journal of Rheumatology*, **14**, 952–6.

Fang, S. B., Lee, H. C., Huang, F. Y., *et al.* (2001). Intestinal pseudoobstruction followed by major clinical features of Kawasaki disease: report of one case. *Acta Paediatrica Taiwanica*, **42**, 111–4.

Fauci, A. S., Haynes, B. F. and Katz, P. (1978). The spectrum of vasculitis: clinical, pathologic, immunologic and therapeutic considerations. *Annals of Internal Medicine*, **89**, 660–77.

Fisher, D. F. and Fry, W. J. (1987). Collateral mesenteric circulation. *Surgery Gynecology and Obstetrics*, **164**, 487–92.

Fitchett, D. H. and Oakley, C. M. (1975). Perihepatic hematoma in polyarteritis nodosa. *Proceedings of the Royal Society of Medicine*, **68**, 805–6.

Fontes, B., Moore, F. A., Moore, E. E., *et al.* (1994) Gut ischemia induces bone marrow failure and increases risk of infection. *Journal of Surgical Research*, **57**, 505–9.

Fortin, P. R., Larson, M. G., Watters, A. K., *et al.* (1995). Prognostic factors in systemic necrotizing vasculitis of the polyarteritis nodosa group-a review of 45 cases. *Journal of Rheumatology*, **22**, 78–84.

Franken, E. A. Jr, Kleiman, M. B., Norins, A. L., *et al.* (1979). Intestinal pseudoobstruction in mucocutaneous lymph-node syndrome. *Radiology*, **130**, 649–51.

Frauenfelder, T., Wildermuth, S., Marincek, B. and Boehm, T. (2004). Non-traumatic emergent abdominal vascular conditions: advantages of multi-detector row CT and three-dimensional imaging. *RadioGraphics*, **24**, 481–96.

Frohnert, P. and Sheps, S. (1967). Long-term follow-up study of polyarteritis nodosa. *American Journal of Medicine*, **48**, 8–14.

Fukunishi, M., Kikkawa, M., Hamana, K., *et al.* (2000). Prediction of non-responsiveness to intravenous high-dose gammaglobulin therapy in patients with Kawasaki disease at onset. *Journal of Pediatrics*, **137**, 172–6.

Gaburri, P. D., Chebli, J. M.F., Attalla, A., *et al.* (2005). Colonic ulcers in propylthiouracil induced vasculitis with secondary antiphospholipid syndrome. *Postgraduate Medical Journal*, **81**, 338–40.

Gallavan, R. H., Jr, Parks, D. A. and Jacobson, E. D. (1989). The gastrointestinal system: pathophysiology of the gastrointestinal circulation. In *Handbook of physiology* (eds Schulz, S. and Woods, J.), pp. 1713–32. American Physiological Society, Bethesda.

Garcia, A. N., Cubero, L. L., Zolba, L. R., *et al.* (1998). Thromboangiitis obliterans (Buerger's disease) with intestinal involvement. A case report. *Angiology*, **49**, 489–92.

Gastrucci, G., Alimandi, L., Fichera, A., *et al.* (1990). Changes in esophageal motility in patients with systemic lupus erythematosus: an esophago-manometric study. *Minerva Diet Gastro*, **36**, 3–7.

Geboes, K., Geboes, K. P. and Maleux, G. (2001). Vascular anatomy of the gastrointestinal tract. *Baillieres Best Practice and Research in Clinical Gastroenterology*, **1**, 1–14.

Gentile, A. T., Moneta, G. L., Lee, R. W., Masser, P. A., Taylor, L. M. and Porter, J. M. (1995). Usefulness of fasting and postprandial duplex ultrasound examination for predicting high-grade superior mesenteric artery stenosis. *American Journal of Surgery*, **169**, 476–9.

Ghate, J. and Jorizzo, J. (1999). Behçet's disease and complex aphthosis. *Journal of the American Academy of Dermatology*, **40**, 1–18.

Gorgun, E. and Ozmen, V. (2002). Acalculous gangrenous cholecystitis in a young adult: a gastrointestinal manifestation of polyarteritis nodosa. *Surgical Laparoscopy, Endoscopy and Percutaneous Techniques*, **12**, 359–61.

Goubran, H. A., Omar, A. A., El-Maghallawy, A. A., *et al.* (1999). A look into the etiology of 30 adults with Budd-Chiari syndrome. *Hepatology*, **30**, 573A.

Gourgoutis, G., Paguirigan, A. and Berzins, T. (1971). Gastric perforation in polyarteritis nodosa. *American Journal of Digestive Diseases*, **16**, 171–7.

Griffith, G. C. and Vural, I. L. (1951). Polyarteritis nodosa: a correlation of clinical and postmortem findings in seventeen cases. *Circulation*, **3**, 481–94.

Grimbacher, B., Huber, M., Kempis, J., *et al.* (1998). Successful treatment of gastrointestinal vasculitis due to systemic lupus erythematosus with intravenous pulse cyclophosphamide: a clinical case report and review of the literature. *British Journal of Rheumatology*, **37**, 1023–8.

Guillevin, L. (1999). Treatment of classic polyarteritis nodosa in 1999. (Editorial comments) *Nephrology Dialysis Transplantation*, **14**, 2077–9.

Guillevin, L., Cohen, P., Gayraud, M., *et al.* (1999). Churg-Strauss syndrome clinical study and long term follow up of 96 patients. *Medicine* (Baltimore) **78**, 26–37.

Guillevin, L., Durand-Gasselin, B., Cevallos, R., *et al.* (1999). Microscopic polyangiitis: clinical and laboratory findings in eighty-five patients. *Arthritis and Rheumatism*, **42**, 421–30.

Guillevin, L., Lhote, F., Gallais, V., *et al.* (1995). Gastrointestinal tract involvement in polyarteritis nodosa and Churg-Strauss syndrome. *Annales de Medecine Interne*, (Paris), **146**, 206–7.

Ha, H. K., Lee, S. H., Rha, S. E., *et al.* (2000). Radiologic features of vasculitis involving the gastrointestinal tract. *Radiographics*, **20**, 779–94.

Ha, H. K., Rha, S. E., Kim, A. Y., Auh, Y. H. (2000). CT and MR diagnosis of intestinal ischaemia. *Seminars in Ultrasound CT and MR*, **21**, 40–55.

Hagland, U. and Bergqvist, D. (1999). Intestinal ischemia: the basics. *Langenbecks Archives of Surgery*, **384**, 233–8.

Hall, S., Barr, W. and Lie, J. T. (1985). Takayasu arteritis. A study of 32 North American patients. *Medicine*, **64**, 89.

Hamza, M. (1993). Proctitis in Behçet's disease: study of 6 cases. *Revue du Rhumatisme*, **60**, 925–7.

Han, R. K., Silverman, E. D., Newman, A., *et al.* (2000). Management and outcome of persistent or recurrent fever after initial intravenous Gammagloublin therapy in acute Kawasaki disease. *Archives of Pediatric and Adolescent Medicine*, **154**, 694–9.

Hands, L. and Murie, J. A. (1991). Takayasu arteritis: a rare cause of acute abdomen in a Caucasian male. *European Journal of Vascular Surgery*, **5**, 217–9.

Harvey, A., Shulman, L., Tumulty, P., *et al.* (1954). Systemic lupus erythematosus: review of the literature and clinical analysis of 138 cases. *Medicine*, **33**, 291–437.

Harward, T. R., Brooks, D. L., Flynn, T. C. and Seeger, J. M. (1993). Mutliple organ dysfunction after mesenteric artery revascularization. *Journal of Vascular Surgery*, **18**, 459–67, discussion 467–9.

Hassan, W. U. and Daymond, T. J. (1993). Small bowel infarction in association with giant cell arteritis. *British Journal of Rheumatology*, **32**, 942.

Hassoun, Z., Lacross, M. and De Ronde, T. (2001). Intestinal involvement in Buerger's disease. *Journal of Clinical Gastroenterology*, **32**, 85–9.

Haworth, S. J. and Pusey, C. D. (1984). Severe intestinal involvement in Wegener's granulomatosis. *Gut*, **25**, 1296.

Hekali, P., Kajander, H., Pajarti, R., *et al.* (1991). Diagnostic significance of angiographically observed visceral aneurysms with regard to polyarteritis nodosa. *Acta Radiology*, **32**, 143–8.

Hisaoka, M., Haratake, J. and Nakamura, T. (1994). Small bile duct abnormalities and chronic intrahepatic cholestasis in Behçet's syndrome. *Hepatol-Gastroenterol*, **41**, 267–70.

Hitter, E., William, L., Chappel, R., *et al.* (1988). Abdominal microaneurysms in rheumatoid arthritis. *British Journal of Rheumatology*, **27**, 239–40.

Hoffman, B. I. and Katz, W. A. (1980). The gastrointestinal manifestations of systemic lupus erythematosus: a review of the literature. *Seminars in Arthritis and Rheumatism*, **9**, 237–47.

Hoffman, G. S., Kerr, G. S., Leavitt, R. Y., *et al.* (1992). Wegener granulomatosis: an analysis of 158 patients. *Annals of Internal Medicine*, **116**, 488–98.

Hoffmann, J. C., Cremer, P., Preiss, J. C., *et al.* (2004). Gallbladder involvement of Henoch-Schonlein purpura mimicking acute acalculous cholecystitis. *Digestion*, **70**, 45–8.

Horton, K. M., Corl, F. M. and Fishman, E. K. (1999). CT of nonneoplastic diseases of the small bowel: spectrum of disease. *Journal of Computer Assisted Tomography*, **23**, 417–28.

Horton, K. M., Corl, F. M. and Fishman, E. K. (2000). CT evaluation of the colon: inflammatory disease. *RadioGraphics*, **20**, 399–418.

Houng, D. L.T., Wechsler, B., Bruno, D. I., *et al.* (1992). Acute pancreatitis in Behçet's disease. *Digestive Diseases and Sciences*, **37**, 1452–3.

Hunder, G. G., Bloch, D. A., Michel, B. A., *et al.* (1990). The American College of Rheumatology. Criteria for the classification of Giant Cell arteritis. *Arthritis and Rheumatism*, **33**, 1122–8.

International Study Group for Behçet's Disease (1990). Criteria for diagnosis of Behçet's disease. *Lancet*, **335**, 1078–80.

Ito, M., Nihei, Z., Ichikawa, W., *et al.* (1993). Intestinal ischemia resulting from Buerger's disease: report of a case. *Surgery Today,* **23**, 988–92.

Ito, M., Sano, K., Inaba, H., *et al.* (1991). Localized necrotizing arteritis. A report of two cases involving the gallbladder and pancreas. *Archives of Pathology and Laboratory Medicine*, **115**, 780–3.

Jaber, J., Milo, G., Halpera, G. J., *et al.* (2002). Prevalence of Behçet's disease in an Arab community disease in Israel. *Annals of the Rheumatic Diseases*, **16**, 365–6.

Jacobsen, S. E., Petersen, P. and Jensen, P. (1985). Acute abdomen in rheumatoid arthritis due to mesenteric arteritis. A case report and review. *Dan Med Bull*, **32**, 191–3.

Jamieson, W. G., De Rose, G., Harris, K. A., Pliagus, G. and Stafford, L. (1993). Myocardial and circulatory performance during the ischemic phase of superior mesenteric artery occlusion. *Canadian Journal of Surgery*, **36**, 435–9.

Jankowski, J., Crombie, I. and Jankowski, R. (1992). Behçet's disease in Scotland. *Postgraduate Medical Journal*, **68**, 566–70.

Jee, K. N., Ha, H. K., Lee, I. J., *et al.* (2000). Radiologic findings of abdominal polyarteritis Nodosa. *American Journal of Roentgenology*, **174**, 1675–9.

Jeong, Y. K., Ha, H. K., Yoon, C. H., *et al.* (1997). Gastrointestinal involvement in Henoch-Schonlein syndrome: CT findings AJR. *American Journal of Roentgenology*, **168**, 965–8.

Kaklamani, V., Vaiopoulos, G. and Kaklamani, P. (1998). Behçet's disease. *Seminars in Arthritis and Rheumatism*, **27**, 197–217.

Kandilci, U., Gurer, M. A., Turner, C., *et al.* (1992). Gastrointestinal manifestations in Behçet's disease. *Turkish Journal of Gastroenterology*, **3**, 238–43.

Kaneki, T., Kawashima, A., Hayano, T., *et al.* (1998). Churg-Strauss syndrome (allergic granulomatous angiitis presenting with ileus caused by ischemic ileal ulcer). *Journal of Gastroenterology,* **33**, 112–6.

Kasahara, Y., Tanaka, S., Nishimo, M., *et al.* (1981). Intestinal involvement in Behçet's disease: review of 136 surgical cases in the Japanese literature. *Diseases of the Colon and Rectum*, **24**, 103–6.

Kawasaki, T., Kosaki, T., Okawa, S., *et al.* (1974). A new infantile acute febrile mucocutaneous lymph node syndrome (MLNS) prevailing in Japan. *Pediatrics*, **54**, 271–6.

Keating, J. P., King, B. R., Kenwright, D. N., *et al.* (1998). Vasculitis-induced colonic strictures: report of two cases. *Diseases of the Colon and Rectum*, **41**, 1316–21.

Kim, C. J., Chung, H. Y., Kim, S. Y., *et al.* (2005). Acute appendicitis in Henoch-Schonlein purpura: a case report. *Journal of Korean Medical Science*, **20**, 899–900.

Kim, S., Chung, I., Chung, I. K., *et al.* (2000). The clinical significance of upper gastrointestinal endoscopy in gastrointestinal vasculitis related to Scrub Typhus. *Endoscopy*, **32**, 950–5.

Kim, Y. B., Choi, S. W., Park, I. S., *et al.* (2000). Churg-Strauss syndrome with perforating ulcers of the colon. *Journal of Korean Medical Science*, **15**, 580–8.

Kistin, M. G. Kaplan, M. M. and Harrington, J. T. (1978). Diffuse ischemic colitis associated with systemic lupus erythematosus—response to subtotal colectomy. *Gastroenterology*, **75**, 1147–51.

Klein, H. M., Lensing, R., Klosterhalfen, C. T. and Gunther, R. W. (1995). Diagnostic imaging of mesenteric infacrction. *Radiology*, **197**, 79–82.

Komanduri, S., Shriram, J. and Keshavarzian, A. (2002). Focal Rectal Capillaritis: Microscopic Polyangiitis Presenting as Painless Rectal Bleeding. *Journal of Clinical Gastroenterology*, **35**, 157–9.

Koyama, M., Tanaka, M., Shimizu, M., *et al.* (1995). Surgical treatment of mesenteric infarction, thoracoabdominal aortic aneurysm, and proper hepatic aneurysm in a middle-aged woman with Takayasu's arteritis. *Journal of Cardiovascular Surgery* (Torimo), **36**, 337–41.

Kram, M. T., May, L. D., Goodman, S., *et al.* (2003). Behçet's ileocolitis: successful treatment with tumor necrosis factor-alpha antibody (Infliximab) therapy report of a case. *Diseases of the Colon and Rectum*, **46**, 118–21.

Krant, J. D. and Ross, J. M. (1992). Extracranial giant cell arteritis restricted to the small bowel. *Arthritis and Rheumatism*, **35**, 603–4.

Kuehne, S. E., Gauvin, G. P. and Shortsleeve, M. J. (1992). Small bowel stricture caused by rheumatoid vasculitis. *Radiology*, **184**, 215–6.

Kurita, M., Niwa, Y., Hamada, E., *et al.* (1994). Churg-Strauss syndrome (allergic granulomatous angiitis) with multiple perforating ulcers of the small intestine, multiple ulcers of the colon and mononeuritis multiplex. *Gastroenterology*, **29**, 208–13.

Kuroda, T., Shiohara, E., Homma, T., Furukawa, Y. and Chiba, S. (1994). Effects of leucocyte and platelet depletion on ischemia-reperfusion injury to the dog pancreas. *Gastroenterology*, **107**, 1125–34.

LaBerge, J. M. and Kerlau, R. K. (2002). Vasculitis associated with lymphoproliferative disease (case 1). *The Society of Cardiovascular Interventional Radiology Annual Meeting.*

Lakhanpal, S., Tani, K., Lie, J. T., *et al.* (1985). Pathologic features of Behçet's syndrome: a review of Japanese autopsy registry data. *Human Pathology*, **16**, 790–5.

Landow, L. and Andersen, L. W. (1994). Splanchnic ischemia and its role in multiple organ failure. *Acta Anaesthesiologica Scandinavica*, **38**, 626–39.

Lanzkowsky, S., Lanzkowsky, L. and Lanzkowsky, P. (1992). Henoch-Schonlein purpura. *Pediatric Review*, **13**, 130–7.

Lazaris, A. Ch., Papanikolaou, I. S., Theodoropoulos, G. E., *et al.* (2003). Ischaemic necrosis of the rectum and sigmoid colon complicating systemic lupus erythematosus. *Acta Gastro-Enterologica Belgica*, **66**, 191–4.

Leavitt, R. Y., Fauci, A. S., Bloch, D. A., *et al.* (1990). The American College of Rheumatology 1990. Criteria for the classification of Wegener's granulomatosis. *Arthritis and Rheumatism*, **33**, 1101–7.

Lee, C.-K., Ahn, M. S., Lee, E. Y., *et al.* (2002). Acute abdominal pain in systemic lupus erythematosus: focus on lupus enteritis (gastrointestinal vasculitis). *Annals of the Rheumatic Diseases*, **61**, 547–50.

Lee, K. S., Kim, S. J., Lee, B. C., *et al.* (1997). Surgical treatment of intestinal Behcet's disease. *Yonsei Medical Journal*, **38**, 455–60.

Levrine, S. M., Hellmann, D. B. and Stone, J. H. (2002). Gastrointestinal involvement in polyarteritis nodosa (1986–2000): presentation and outcome in 24 patients. *American Journal of Medicine*, **112**, 386–91.

Lhote, F., Cohen, P., Genereau, T., *et al.* (1996). Microscopic polyangiitis: clinical aspects and treatment. *Annales de Medecine Interne* (Paris), **147**, 165–77.

Lie, J. T. (1998). Visceral intestinal Buerger's disease. *International Journal of Cardiology*, **66** (Suppl. 1), S 249–56.

Liebermann-Meffert, D., Neff, U., Marti, W., Vosmeer, S. and Allgower, M. (1984). The muscles and blood supply of the stomach. *Schweizerische Medizinische Wochenschrift*, **114**, 711–3.

Lightfoot, R. W. Jr, Michel, B. A., Bloch, D. A., *et al* (1990). The American College of Rheumatology. Criteria for the classification of polyarteritis nodosa. *Arthritis and Rheumatism*, **33**, 1088–93.

Lind, K. M., Gaub, J. and Pedersen, R. S. (1994). Henoch Schonlein purpura associated with Campylobacter jejuni enteritis. *Scandinavian Journal of Urology and Nephrology*, **28**, 179–81.

Ljungstrom, K. G., Strandberg, O. and Sandstedt, B. (1989). Infarction of the small bowel caused by giant cell arteritis: case report. *Acta Chirurgica Scandinavica*, **155**, 361–3.

Lockhart, M. E. and Robbin, M. L. (2003). Case 58: Giant cell arteritis. *Radiology*, **227**, 512–5.

Lopez, L. R., Schocket, A. L., Stanford, R. E., *et al.* (1980). Gastrointestinal involvement in leukocytoclastic vasculitis and polyarteritis nodosa. *Journal of Rheumatology*, **7**, 677–84.

Manna, R., Ghirlanda, G., Bochicchio, G. B., *et al.* (1985). Chronic active hepatitis and Behcet's syndrome. *Clinical Rheumatology*, **4**, 93–6.

Marcolongo, R., Boyeli, P. F. and Montagnani, M. (1979). Gastrointestinal involvement in rheumatoid arthritis: a boipsy study. *Journal of Rheumatology*, **6**, 163–73.

Masi, A. T., Hunder, G. G., Lie, J. T., *et al.* (1990). The American College of Rheumatology 1990. Criteria for the classification of Churg-Strauss syndrome (allergic granulomatosis and angitis). *Arthritis and Rheumatism*, **33**, 1094–100.

Mathews, J. G. and Parks, T. G. (1976a). Ischemic colitis in the experimental animal I. Comparison of the effects of acute and subacute vascular occlusion. *Gut*, **17**, 671–6.

Mathews, J. G. and Parks, T. G. (1976b). Ischemic colitis in the experimental animal II. Role of hypovolemia in the production of the disease. *Gut*, **17**, 677–84.

McCurley, T. L. and Collins, R. D. (1984). Intestinal infarction in rheumatoid arthritis. Three cases due to unusual obliterative vascular lesions. *Archives of Pathology and Laboratory Medicine*, **108**, 125–8.

Meaney, J. F., Prince, M. R., Nostrant, T. T. and Stanley, J. C. (1997). Gadolinium-enhanced MR angiography of visceral arteries in patients with superior chronic mesenteric ishaemia. *Journal of Magnetic Resonance Imaging*, **7**, 171–6.

Medina, F., Ayala, A., Jara, L. J., *et al.* (1997). Acute abdomen in systemic lupus erythematosus: the importance of early laparotomy. *American Journal of Medicine*, **103**, 1000–5.

Mele, T. and Evans, M. (1996). Intestinal obstruction as a complication of Kawasaki disease. *Journal of Pediatric Surgery*, **31**, 985–6.

Melikoglu, M., Altiparmak, M., Fresko, I., *et al.* (2001). A reappraisal of amyloidosis in Behcet's syndrome. *Rheumatology (Oxford)*, **40**, 212–5.

Mercer, S. and Carpenter, B. (1981). Surgical complications of Kawasaki disease. *Journal of Pediatric Surgery*, **16**, 444–8.

Mills, J. A., Michel, B. A., Bloch, D. A., *et al.* (1990). The American college of rheumatology criteria for the classification of Henoch-Schonlein purpura. *Arthritis and Rheumatism*, **33**, 1114–21.

Mills, J. A., Michel, B. A., Bloch, D. A., *et al.* (1990). The American College of Rheumatology 1990. Criteria for the classification of Henoch-Schonlein purpura. *Arthritis and Rheumatism*, **33**, 1114–21.

Miyake, T., Kawamori, J., Yoshida, T., *et al.* (1987). Small bowel pseudoobstruction in kawasaki disease. *Pediatric Radiology*, **17**, 383–6.

Mohan, N., Gomes, M. N. and Cupps, T. R. (2002). Isolated superior mesenteric artery vasculitis with response to glucocorticoids. *Journal of Clinical Rheumatology*, **8**, 94–8.

Moneta, G. L., Lee, R. W., Yeager, R. A., Taylor, L. M. and Porter, J. M. (1993). Mesenteric duplex scanning: a blinded prospective study. *Journal of Vascular Surgery*, **17**, 79–84.

Morway, F. H. and Lundberg, E. A. (1954). The clinical manifestations of essential polyarteritis nodosa (periarteritis nodosa) with emphasis on the hepatic manifestations. *Annals of Internal Medicine*, **40**, 1145–64.

Mousa, A. R., Marafy, A. A., Rifai, K. M., *et al.* (1986). Behcet's disease in Kuwait: a report of 29 cases and a review. *Scandinavian Journal of Rheumatology*, **15**, 310–2.

Moyona, T. N. (1988). Necrotizing arteritis of vermiform appendix: a clinicopathologic study of 12 cases. *Archives of Pathology and Laboratory Medicine*, **112**, 738–41.

Muldoon, J., O'Riordan, K., Rao, S., *et al.* (1996). Ischemic colitis secondary to venous thrombosis: a rare presentation of cytomegalovirus vasculitis following renal transplantation. *Transplantation*, **61**, 11.

Murphy, D. J. Jr, Morrow, W. R., Harberg, F. J., *et al.* (1987). *Clinical Pediatrics*, **26**, 193–6.

Musemeche, C. A., Kosloske, A. M., Borlow, S. A. and Umland, E. T. (1986). Comparative effects of ischemia, bacteria and substrate on the pathogenesis of intestinal necrosis. *Journal of Pediatric Surgery*, **21**, 536–8.

Nagarajan, S., Friedrich, T., Garcia, M., *et al.* (2005). Gastrointestinal leukocytoclastic vasculitis: an adverse effect of sirolimus. *Pediatric Transplantation*, **9**, 97.

Nakamura, S., Yokoi, Y., Suzuki, S., *et al.* (1991). A case of melena caused by hepatic aneurysm ruptured into the intrahepatic bile duct in a patient with Allergic Granulomatous Angiitis. *Journal of Surgery*, **21**, 471–5.

Nakamura, Y., Sakurai, Y., Matsubara, T., *et al.* (2002). Multiple perforated ulcers of the small intestine associated with allergic granulomatous angiitis: report of a case. *Surgery Today*, **32**, 541–6.

Nakazawa, K., Itah, N. and Duan, H. S. (1992). Polyarteritis nodosa with artrophy of the left hepatic lobe. *Acta Pathologica Japonica* **42**, 662–6.

Nathan, K., Gunasekaran, T. S. and Berman, J. H. (1999). Recurrent gastrointestinal Henoch-Schonlein purpura. *Journal of Clinical Gastroenterology*, **29**, 86–9.

Nishie, M., Tomiyama, M., Kamijo, M., *et al.* (2003). Acute cholecystitis and duodenitis associated with Churg-Strauss syndrome. *Hepatogastroenterology*, **50**, 998–1002.

Ohwada, S., Yanagisawa, A., Joshita, T., *et al.* (1997). Necrotizing granulomatous vasculitis of transverse colon and gall bladder. *Hepatogastroenterology*, **44**, 1090–4.

Okuda, Y., Takasugi, K. and Imai, A. (1990). Two cases of rheumatoid arthritis complicated with vasculitis–induced ischemic enterocolitis [Japanese]. *Ryumachi*, **30**, 403–8.

Oshima, Y., Shimizu, T., Yokohari, R., *et al.* (1963). Clinical studies on Behcet's syndrome. *Annals of the Rheumatic Diseases*, **22**, 36–45.

Ozcay, N., Arda, K., Sugunes, T., *et al.* (2003). Polyarteritis nodosa presenting with necrotizing appendicitis and hepatic aneurysm rupture. *Turkish Journal of Gastroenterology*, **14**, 68–70.

Ozenc, A., Bayraktar, Y. and Baykal, A. (1990). Pyloric stenosis with esophageal lesions in intestinal Behçet's syndrome. *American Journal of Gastroenterology*, **85**, 727–8.

Pagnoux, C., Mahr, A., Cohen, P., Guillevin, L., *et al*. (2005). Presentation and outcome of gastrointestinal involvement in systemic necrotizing vasculitides: Analysis of 62 patients with polyarteritis nodosa, microscopic polyangiitis, Wegener granulomatosis, Churg-Strauss syndrome, or rheumatoid arthritis-associated vasculitis. *Medicine*, **84**, 115–28.

Palvio, D. H. and Christensen, K. S. (1987). Systemic lupus erythematosus with rectal stenosis simulating tumour or diverticlosis. Case report. *Acta Chirurgica Scandinavica*, **153**, 63–5.

Parangi, S., Oz, M. C., Blume, R. S., *et al*. (1991). Hepatobiliary complications of polyarteritis nodosa. *Archives of Surgery*, **126**, 909–12.

Patterson, A., Scully, C., Barnard, N., *et al*. (1992). Necrosis of the tongue in a patient with intestinal infarction. *Oral Surgery, Oral Medicine, Oral Pathology*, **74**, 582–6.

Pelletier, S., Ekert, P., Landi, B., *et al*. (1992). Exudative enteropathy in disseminated lupus erythematosus. *Am Gastroenterol Hepatol*, **28**, 259–62.

Perko, M. J. Duplex ultrasound for assessment of superior mesenteric artery blood flow. (2001). *European Journal of Vascular and Endovascular Surgery*, **21**, 106.

Pfitzmann, R., Nussler, N. C., Heise, M., *et al*. (2002). Mesenteric artery occlusion as a rare complication of thromboangiitis obliterans. *Chirurg*, **73**, 742.

Phelan, M. J., Kok, K., Burrow, C., *et al*. (1993). Small bowel infarction in association with giant cell arteritis. *British Journal of Rheumatology*, **32**, 63–5.

Pickhardt, P. J. and Curran, V. W. (2001). Case report: Fulminant enterocolitis in Wegener's granulomatosis, CT findings with pathologic correlation. *American Journal of Roentgenology*, **177**, 1335–7.

Quamar, M. I. and Read, A. E. (1985). Intestinal blood flow. *Quarterly Journal of Medicine*, **56**, 417–9.

Quellet, J. Y., Duprat, G. Jr, Lapuriere, J., Gregoire, A. and Fontaine, A. (1988). Pyocolon: an unusual manifestation of colon ischemia. *Canadian Association of Radiologists Journal*, **39**, 235–7.

Raat, H., Stock, L., Broeckaert, L., *et al*. (1993). Mesenteric involvement of thromboangiitis obliterans (Buerger's disease) in a woman. *J Belge Radiol*, **76**, 245–6.

Rademaker, J. (1998). Veno-occlusive disease of the colon: CT findings. *European Radiology*, **8**, 1420–1.

Rajive, M., Deepak, S. and Anil, J. (2004). Takayasu arteritis presenting as chronic mesenteric ischemia. *Indian Journal of Gastrenterology*, **23**, 73–4.

Rasmussen, N. H. (1982). Henoch-Schonlein purpura after Yersiniosis. *Archives of Disease in Childhood*, **57**, 322–3.

Reilly, P. M. and Bulkley, G. B. (1993). Vasoactive mediators and splanchnic perfusion. *Critical Care Medicine*, **21**, 55–68.

Reissman, P., Weiss, E. G., Teo, T. A., *et al*. (1994). Gangrenous ischemic colitis of the rectum a rare complication of systemic lupus erythematosus. *American Journal of Gastroenterology*, **89**, 2234–6.

Ripollés, T., Suno, L., Martinez-Pérez, M., Pastor, M. R., Igual, A. and López, A. (2005). Sonographic findings in ischaemic colitis in 58 patients. *American Journal of Roentgenology*, **184**, 777–185.

Roobottom, C. A. and Dubbins, P. A. (1993). Significant disease of the celiac and superior mesenteric arteries in asymptomatic patients: predictive value of Doppler sonography. *American Journal of Roentgenology*, **161**, 985–8.

Roza, M., Galbe, M., Gonzalez Baschwirtz, C., *et al*. (1983). Henoch Schonlein purpura after shigellosis. *Clinical Nephrology*, **20**, 269.

Sakane, T., Takeno, M., Suzuki, N., *et al*. (1999). Behçet's disease. *New England Journal of Medicine*, **341**, 1284–91.

Sanchez-Guerrero, J., Reyes, E. and Alarcon-Segovia, D. (1992). Primary anti-phospholipid syndrome as a cause of intestinal infarction. *Journal of Rheumatology*, **19**, 623–5.

Sasamura, H., Nakamoto, H., Ryuzaki, M. T., *et al*. (1991). Repeated intestinal ulcerations in a patient with systemic lupus erythematosus and high serum antiphosphipid antibody levels. *Southern Medical Journal*, **84**, 515–7.

Sayek, I., Aran, O., Uzunalimoglu, B., *et al*. (1991). Intestinal Behçet's disease: surgical experience in seven cases. *Hepatogastroenterol*, **38**, 81–3.

Schellong, S. M., Bernhards, J., Ensslen, F., *et al*. (1994). Intestinal type of thromboangiitis obliterans (Buerger's disease). *Journal of Internal Medicine*, **235**, 69–73.

Schmidt, W. A. (2000). Doppler ultrasound in the diagnosis of giant cell arteritis. *Clinical and Experimental Rheumatology*, **18**, s40–2.

Schmidt, W. A., Kraft, H. E., Brokowski, A., *et al*. (1999). Color duplex ultrasonography in large vessel giant cell arteritis. *Scandinavian Journal of Rheumatology*, **9, 28**, 374–6.

Sharma, M. C., Safaya, R. and Sidhu, B. S. (1996). Perforation of the small intestine caused by Churg Strauss syndrome. *Journal of Clinical Gastroenterology*, **23**, 232–5.

Sherlock, S. and Dooley, J. (2002). Chapter 1. Anatomy and function. In: *Diseases of the liver and biliary system*, 11th Edition. pp. 1–18. Blackwell Publishing Company, Oxford, UK.

Shiboski, C. H., Regezy, J. A., Sanchez, H. C., *et al*. (2002). Oral lesions as the first clinical sign of microscopic polyangiitis: a case report. *Oral Surgery, Oral Medicine, Oral Pathology, Oral Radiology, and Endodontics*, **94**, 707–11.

Shimamoto, C., Hirata, I., Ohshiba, S., *et al*. (1990). Syndrome (allergic granulomatous angiitis) with peculiar multiple colonic ulcers. *American Journal of Gastroenterology*, **85**, 316–9.

Shimizu, T., Ehrlich, G. E., Inaba, G., *et al*. (1979). Behçet's disease (Behçet's syndrome). *Seminars in Arthritis and Rheumatism*, **8**, 223–60.

Shintaku, M., Inoue, N., Sasaki, M., *et al*. (1991). Cytomegalo virus vasculitis accompanied by an exuberant fibroblastic reaction in the intestine of an AIDS patient. *Acta Pathologica Japonica*, **41**, 900–4.

Shiohira, Y., Uehara, H., Miyazato, F., *et al*. (1993). Vasculitis-related acute abdomen in systemic lupus erythematosus–ultrasound appearances in lupus patients with intraabdominal vasculitis. *Rheumatology*, **33**, 235–41.

Siddiqui, M. Z., Reis, E. D., Soundararajan, K., *et al*. (2001). MD. Buerger's disease affecting mesenteric arteries: a rare cause of intestinal ischemia-a case report. *Vascular Surgery*, **35**, 235–8.

Siğirci, A., Senol, M., Aydin, E., Kultur, R., Alkan, A., Altinok, M. T., *et al*. (2003). doppler waveforms and blood flow parameters of the superior and inferior mesenteric arteries in patients having Behçet's disease with and without gastrointestinal symptoms. *Journal of Ultrasound in Medicine*, **22**, 449–57.

Smith, F. C., Gosling, P., Sanghera, K., Green, M. A., Patersen, I. S. and Shearman, C. P. (1994). Microproteinuria predicts the severity of systemic effects of reperfusion injury following infra renal aortic aneurysm repair. *Annals of Vascular Surgery*, **8**, 1–5.

Smith, J. A.E., O'sullivan, M., Gough, J., *et al*. (1988). Small-intestinal perforation secondary to localized giant cell arteritis of the mesenteric vessels. *British Journal of Rheumatology*, **27**, 236–8.

Sokol, R. J., Farrell, M. K. and McAdams, A. J. (1984). An unusual presentation of Wegener's granulomatosis mimicking inflammatory bowel disease. **87**, 246–32.

Soysal, M., Denizci, U., Alhan, S., *et al*. (1990). Splenic size in Behçet's syndrome. *British Journal of Rheumatology*, **29**, 497–8.

Srigley, J. R. and Gardiner, G. W. (1980). Giant cell arteritis with small bowel infarction. *American Journal of Gastroenterology*, **73**, 157–61.

Stanson, A. W., Friese, J. L., Johnson, C. M., *et al*. (2001). Polyarteritis nodosa: spectrum of angiographic findings. *Radiographics*, **21**, 151–9.

Steele, C., Bohra, S., Broe, P., *et al*. (2001). FE. Acute upper gastrointestinal haemorrhage and colitis: an unusual presentation of Wegener's granulomatosis. *European Journal of Gastroenterology and Hepatology*, **13**, 993–9.

Stenwig, J. T. (1976). Intestinal gangrene due to giant cell arteritis: report of a case. *Journal of the Oslo City Hospitals*, **26**, 49–55.

Storesund, B., Gran, J. T. and Koldingsnes, W. (1998). Severe intestinal involvement in Wegener's granulomatosis: report of two cases and review of the literature. *British Journal of Rheumatology*, **37**, 387–90.

Sultan, S. M., Ioannou, Y. and Isenberg, D. A. (1999). A review of gastrointestinal manifestations of systemic lupus erythematosus (Review). *Rheumatology*, **38**, 917–32.

Suzuki, M., Nabeshima, K., Miyazaki, M., *et al.* (2005). Churg-Strauss syndrome complicated by colon erosion, acalculous cholecystitis and liver abscess. *World Journal of Gastroenterology*, **11**, 5248–50.

Takeuchi, K. and Kuroda, Y. (2000). Rheumatoid vasculitis with multiple intestinal ulcerations: report of a case (Japanese). *Ryumachi*, **40**, 639–43.

Testini, M., Verzillo, F., Paradiso, V., *et al.* (1996). The surgical treatment of vascular and gastrointestinal implications in Behçet's disease. Report of four cases. *Panminerva Medica*, **38**, 185–9.

Tizard, E. J. (1999). Henoch-Schonlein purpura. *Archives of Disease in Childhood*, **80**, 380–3.

Trimble, M. A. and Weisz, M. A. (2002). Letters to the editor: Infarction of the sigmoid colon secondary to giant cell arteritis. *Rheumatology*, **41**, 108–10.

Trompeter, M., Brazda, T., Remy, C. T., Vestring, T. and Reimer, P. (2002). Non-occlusive mesenteric ischemia: etiology, diagnosis, and interventional therapy. *European Radiology*, **12**, 1179–87.

Tsai, C. N., Chang, C. M., Chuang, C. H., *et al.* (2004). Extended colonic ulcerations in a patient with microscopic polyangiitis. *Annals of the Rheumatic Disease*, **63**, 1521–2.

Tsai, J. T. (1980). Perforation of the small bowel with rheumatoid arthritis. *Southern Medical Journal*, **73**, 939–40.

Turner, H. E., Myszor, M. F., Bradlow, A., *et al.* (1996). Lupus or lupoid hepatitis with mesenteric vasculitis (clinical conference). *British Journal of Rheumatology*, **35**, 1309–11.

Tyagi, S., Verma, P. K., Kumar, N., *et al.* (1997). Stent angioplasty for relief of chronic ischemia in Takayasu arteritis. *Indian Heart Journal*, **49**, 315–8.

Ueda, S., Matsumoto, M., Ahm, T., *et al.* (2001). Microscopic polyangiitis complicated with massive intestinal bleeding. *Journal of Gastroenterology*, **36**, 264–70.

Van Laar, J. M., Smit, V. T., de Beus, W. M., *et al.* (1998). Rheumatoid vasculitis presenting as appendicitis. *Clinical and Experimental Rheumatology*, **16**, 736–6.

Vandamme, J. P. and Bonte, J. (1988). The blood supply of the stomach. *Acta Anatomica* (Basel), **131**, 89–96.

Vega Saenz, J. L., Barajas Martinez, J. M. and Torres Almendros, M. (1995). Ischemic colitis as manifestation of Takayasu arteritis. *Gastroenterologia hepatalogia*, **18**, 326–9.

Vlahos, K., Theodoropoulos, G. E., Lazaris, A. Ch., *et al.* (2005). Isolated colonic leukocytoclastic vasculitis causing segmental megacolon: report of a rare case. *Disease of the Colon and Rectum*, **48**, 167–71.

Wheeler, R. A., Najmaldin, A. S., Soubra, M., *et al.* (1990). Surgical presentation of Kawasaki disease (mucocutaneous lymph node syndrome). *British Journal of Surgery*, **77**, 1273–4.

Whitehead, R. (1976). The pathology of ischemia of the intestines. *Pathology Annual*, **11**, 1–52.

Wiesner, W., Khurana, B., Ji, H. and Ros, P. R. (2003). CT of acute bowel ischaemia. *Radiology*, **226**, 635–50.

Winter, H. S. (1987). Steroid effects on the course of abdominal pain in children with Henoch-Schonlein purpura. *Pediatrics*, **79**, 1018–21.

Yazici, H., Tuzun, Y., Pazarh, *et al.* (1980). Behçet's disease as seen in Turkey. *Haematologica*, **65**, 381–3.

Yazici, Z., Savci, G., Parlak, M., *et al.* (1997). Polyarteritis nodosa presenting with hemobilia and intestinal hemorrhage. *European Radiology*, **7**, 1059–61.

Yashiro, K., Nagasako, K., Hasegawak, *et al.* (1986). Esophageal lesions in intestinal Behçet's disease. *Endoscopy*, **18**, 57–60.

Zizic, T. M., Shulman, L. E. and Stevens, M. B. (1997). Colonic perforations in systemic lupus erythematosus. *Lupus*, **6**, 235–42.

Zulian, F., Falcini, F., Zancan, L., *et al.* (2003). Acute surgical abdomen as presenting manifestation of Kawasaki disease. *Journal of Pediatrics*, **142**, 731–5.

CHAPTER 16

Renal manifestations

Cees G. M. Kallenberg and Jan W. Cohen Tervaert

Renal involvement is common in both secondary and primary vasculitides, particularly the antineutrophil cytoplasmic antibody (ANCA)-associated primary vasculitides, in which it is one of the major manifestations and has a great impact on prognosis. Vasculitis may even be restricted to the kidneys as in idiopathic ANCA-associated necrotizing crescentic glomerulonephritis. In this chapter, the renal manifestations of the primary vasculitides are discussed. In addition, the clinical course, histopathologic findings, and pathogenesis, as well as prognosis and treatment of renal involvement are described.

Renal involvement in large-vessel vasculitides

Giant cell arteritis

Giant cell arteritis (GCA) is defined, according to the Chapel Hill Consensus Conference (Jennette et al. 1994), as a granulomatous arteritis of the aorta and its major branches, with a predilection for the extracranial branches of the carotid arteries (see Chapter 24). It often involves the temporal artery, occurs in patients generally older than 40 years, and is frequently associated with polymyalgia rheumatica. Mild proteinuria and microscopic hematuria (sometimes with red cell casts) have been described in less than 10% of patients (Klein et al. 1975); renal insufficiency is rare in GCA. Secondary renal amyloidosis has been described in a few cases of GCA and should be suspected in persons with a long history of GCA who develop proteinuria and renal failure (Escriba et al. 2000).

Overlapping syndromes of GCA with other forms of systemic vasculitis do occur. Cases of GCA in conjunction with ANCA-positive crescentic glomerulonephritis have been described (Logar et al. 1994; Muller et al. 2004). Classical polyarteritis nodosa (PAN) affecting the kidney has also been documented together with GCA (O'Neill et al. 1976). It is not clear at present whether the occurrence of other forms of vasculitis in patients with GCA is based on a pathophysiologically relevant association. The distinction made between the different forms of vasculitis is somewhat arbitrary and overlapping forms do frequently occur.

What conclusion can be drawn? Renal involvement is not a characteristic finding of GCA. When signs of renal involvement, such as proteinuria, hematuria, or renal insufficiency, are present or develop in patients with GCA, other conditions should be suspected.

Diagnostic work-up, including ANCA testing and a renal biopsy, if indicated, should be performed in order to reveal the underlying cause of the observed renal abnormalities. Treatment should be directed at the underlying cause or condition.

Takayasu's arteritis

Takayasu's arteritis (TA) has been defined as a granulomatous inflammation of the aorta and its major branches (see Chapter 25). In contrast to GCA, patients are generally younger than 40 years and female (Jennette et al. 1994). The arteritis in its acute stage is characterized by infiltration of the vessel wall with mononuclear cells, granulocytes, and, sometimes, giant cells. The inflammatory process leads to obstructive changes due to intimal proliferation and medial fibrosis. Although the vessels in the upper part of the body are affected more frequently, extension of the disease process to the abdominal vessels occurs. Extension to the level of the renal arteries may result in renovascular hypertension and renal insufficiency, generally mild, due to obstruction of the ostia of the renal arteries or involvement of the renal arteries themselves (Lagneau and Michel 1985). Hypertension, although difficult to detect in cases of pulseless disease, and renal insufficiency, should raise suspicion of involvement of the renal arteries.

Mild proteinuria and hematuria may occur, but overt glomerular or interstitial disease is uncommon. Secondary AA amyloidosis has been described in a few cases (Wada et al. 1999). In addition, a few cases of concomitant IgA nephropathy have been described but this may be only coincidental (Cavatorta et al. 1995). Signs of glomerular or interstitial disease suggest the coexistence of another condition necessitating diagnostic work-up.

The active stage of Takayasu's arteritis, in which CRP levels are generally elevated, is treated with glucocorticoids, sometimes in combination with immunosuppressive drugs. Renal artery stenosis can be treated by interventional radiology techniques, such as percutaneous transluminal renal angioplasty with or without stent placement (Lovaria et al. 1999), or by reconstructive surgery. Results of surgery are usually satisfactory, although complex and repeat revascularization procedures are often needed. One series reported cure of hypertension in 12 of 19 patients (63%), improvement in six (31%), and no change in one patient (6%); one of these 19 patients died due to a complication of the procedure (Kieffer et al. 1990). A recent study on 27 patients with TA-induced renal artery stenosis demonstrated patency of the grafts in 90% of patients after 5 years, making renal revascularization the treatment of choice in this condition (Weaver *et al.* 2004).

Renal involvement in medium-vessel vasculitides

Kawasaki's disease

Kawasaki's disease (KD) is a form of arteritis involving large, medium-sized, and small arteries (see Chapter 29). Primary renal involvement is rare, but there may be acute renal failure, either due to fluid exudation from the intravascular to the extravascular space (prerenal insufficiency) or nephritis, which has not been well defined (Senzaki *et al.* 1994). Ultrasonography showed enlarged kidneys with increased cortical echogenicity in a few cases (Nardi *et al.* 1985). Histological findings in three cases suggested immune complex disease (Salcedo *et al.* 1988), interstitial nephritis (Veiga *et al.* 1992), and mesangial sclerosis (Joh *et al.* 1997), respectively. Post-mortem studies on 18 patients who died of acute KD showed infiltration of IgA plasma cells in different organs, including the kidney, suggesting a triggering agent from the respiratory tract inducing a systemic IgA response (Rowley *et al.* 2000). Taken together, renal pathology in KD has not been well defined.

Classic polyarteritis nodosa

Classic polyarteritis nodosa (PAN) is characterized by necrotizing inflammation of medium-size or small arteries; glomerulonephritis or vasculitis in arterioles, capillaries, or venules is absent (see Chapter 26). Tests for antineutrophil cytoplasmic antibodies (ANCA) are generally negative. Classic PAN affects muscular arteries, frequently at bifurcations and in a segmental distribution. Necrotizing arteritis occurs in the acute stage with infiltration of the vessel wall with neutrophils, monocytes, and lymphocytes, and sometimes eosinophils. The lesions differ in age, varying from fibrinoid necrosis, which is frequent in the acute stage, to obliterative changes due to intimal and medial proliferation in the healing stages. Cortical infarcts result from ischemia due to acute or chronic obliteration. In necrotic areas, aneurysms may occur and rupture, resulting in renal, perirenal, and retroperitoneal hemorrhage (Chandrakantan and Kaufman 1999).

Hypertension, of renovascular origin, is present in at least 50% of patients (Cohen *et al.* 1980). Furthermore, there may be symptoms, such as flank pain and hematuria, related to hemorrhage from ruptured microaneurysms. Hematuria is present in most of the cases and some degree of proteinuria (mostly mild) and renal insufficiency is frequent. A renal biopsy may show characteristic findings in intrarenal arteries. Due to the risk of hemorrhage from rupturing aneurysms, a renal biopsy is not advocated as a first choice for diagnosis. Renal angiography can detect aneurysms as well as non-aneurysmal lesions such as perfusion defects, collateral arteries, and delayed emptying of small renal arteries. The sensitivity and specificity of renal aneurysms for a diagnosis of PAN were 43% and 69%, respectively, as shown in a study of 25 children with PAN (Brogan *et al.* 2002). When non-aneurysmal lesions were included in the analysis sensitivity rose to 80% but specificity fell to 50%.

Treatment of classic PAN with major organ involvement, such as the kidneys, consists of glucocorticoids (prednisone, 1 mg/kg/d) accompanied by cyclophosphamide (2–3 mg/kg/d) (see Chapter 26).

Milder cases, with musculoskeletal involvement only, can be treated with oral glucocorticoids, such as prednisone, alone. Hypertension must be treated, but one should be watchful for the development of acute renal failure induced by ACE-inhibitors (Wang *et al.* 1996). Major hemorrhages can be treated by interventional radiology techniques such as embolization (Schouffoer *et al.* 1998).

ANCA-associated small-vessel vasculitides

Antineutrophil cytoplasmic antibodies were first described as sensitive and specific markers for active Wegener's granulomatosis (WG) by van der Woude *et al.* (1985). The autoantibodies in WG produce a characteristic cytoplasmic staining pattern (cANCA) by indirect immunofluorescence (IIF) on ethanol-fixed neutrophils (see Chapter 6). The target antigen of cANCA is proteinase 3, a third serine protease (in addition to elastase and cathepsin G) from azurophilic granules (Goldschmeding *et al.* 1989). Shortly after the detection of cANCA in WG, it was found that many patients with related conditions, such as microscopic polyangiitis (MPA), Churg–Strauss syndrome (CSS), and idiopathic necrotizing crescentic glomerulonephritis (NCGN), had autoantibodies that produced a perinuclear staining pattern (pANCA) on ethanol-fixed neutrophils. The target antigen of pANCA in those conditions is myeloperoxidase (MPO) (Kallenberg *et al.* 1994). The specificity of autoantibodies to either proteinase 3 (PR3) or MPO in the aforementioned conditions, as well as the similarity of their renal histopathological findings (see below), justify their classification as ANCA-associated vasculitides (Kallenberg *et al.* 1994).

We discuss the renal manifestations of this group of disorders, then deal with their pathophysiology, especially the role of ANCA, and finally review treatment of their renal manifestations.

Wegener's granulomatosis

Wegener's granulomatosis (WG) is defined by the Chapel Hill Consensus Conference as a granulomatous inflammation involving the respiratory tract and necrotizing vasculitis affecting small to medium-sized vessels (see Chapters 30, 31, and 32). Renal involvement occurs frequently in WG and necrotizing glomerulonephritis is common (Jennette *et al.* 1994). At first presentation, approximately 50% of patients show clinical signs of renal involvement such as proteinuria, urinary sediment abnormalities, and diminished renal function. The remaining patients present with extrarenal granulomatous inflammation, with more or less overt vasculitis, particularly in the upper airways. More than 50% of the patients who present without renal manifestations develop clinical evidence of renal involvement during the course of their disease (Hoffman *et al.* 1992; Reinhold-Keller *et al.* 2000). Although the clinical course of renal involvement in WG is highly variable, the typical presentation of a patient with WG consists of a period of insidious onset with upper airway symptoms, general malaise, myalgias, and arthralgias. This stage may last for months to years, after which a more acute phase may occur with systemic vasculitis particularly manifested in the kidneys. Clinically, this course is described as rapidly progressive glomerulonephritis (RPGN). RPGN is characterized by a rapid decline in renal function together with signs of glomerulonephritis (proteinuria that generally does not progress to nephrotic syndrome), and microscopic hematuria with cellular casts (Fauci *et al.* 1983; Hoffman *et al.* 1992).

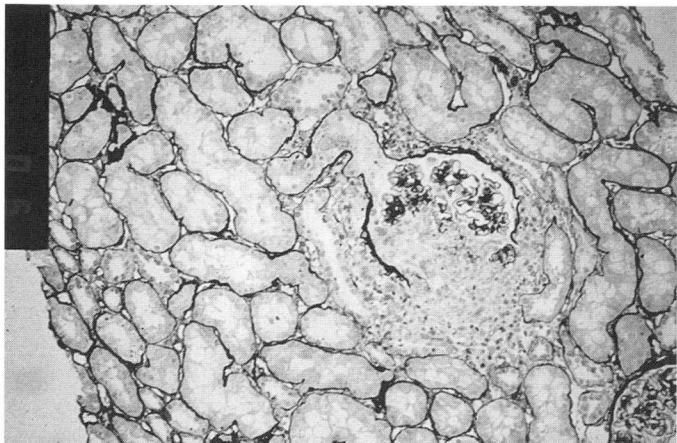

Figure 16.1 Wegener's granulomatosis in a 72-year-old male, admitted with fever, multiple pulmonary nodules on chest radiograph, microscopic hematuria, mild proteinuria, and a serum creatinine concentration of 135 µmol/l. Renal biopsy shows a periglomerular round cell infiltration, destruction of Bowman's capsule, and an extracapillary crescent. Silvermethenamine, HE, × 50. (See Color Plate 66).

Histopathologically, the initial phase is characterized by endothelial swelling with infiltration of polymorphonuclear granulocytes followed by fibrinoid necrosis of the capillary wall and intracapillary thrombosis. Next, cellular crescents develop along with extension of the vasculitic process. Crescents mature and lead to destruction of Bowman's capsule (Figure 16.1). Periglomerular inflammation follows, not infrequently accompanied by pseudo-granuloma formation. The interstitium is also involved in most cases, with infiltration of lymphocytes, monocytes, plasma cells and polymorphonuclear leukocytes. Granuloma formation occurs, particularly in the interstitium, in about 10% of the cases. Necrotizing vasculitis is seen at times in the interstitial small arteries and in more advanced stages, sclerosis. Crescents become fibrous and global, or diffuse glomerulosclerosis develops. Most importantly, direct immunofluorescence studies do not clearly demonstrate immune deposits along the glomerular capillary wall. Some IgM and C3 deposits can be seen, particularly in Bowman's space, but a typical granular or linear staining pattern of the glomerular capillary wall is lacking. Based on these findings, the renal histology has been described as pauci-immune glomerulonephritis. By electron microscopy, however, (Haas and Eustace 2004) immune complex deposits are found in over half of renal biopsies suggesting that immune complexes may play a role in initiation of the disease process (Brons *et al.* 2001).

This immunofluorescence pattern contrasts with the linear staining seen in patients with RPGN as part of antiglomerular basement membrane (anti-GBM) disease, and with the granular staining seen in RPGN as part of immune-complex-mediated glomerulonephritis seen in systemic autoimmune diseases and infection-related conditions (Jennette and Falk 1994; Jennette *et al.* 1989; Ronco *et al.* 1983). In some cases, IgA nephropathy appears late in the course of the disease (Andrassy *et al.* 1992).

Microscopic polyangiitis

Microscopic polyangiitis (MPA) has been defined as necrotizing vasculitis with few or no immune deposits affecting small vessels of all types (see Chapter 27). Necrotizing glomerulonephritis is common, as is pulmonary capillaritis. MPA is distinguished from classic PAN. In MPA, the major sites of the vasculitic process are arterioles, capillaries, and venules. ANCA are present in most instances and are directed to MPO in about 70% of the cases, while only 20% of cases have antibodies to PR3, and around 10% are ANCA-negative (Kallenberg *et al.* 1994). MPA frequently presents as a renal–pulmonary syndrome in which rapidly progressive glomerulonephritis occurs together with lung hemorrhage that may lead to pulmonary insufficiency (Jennette 1991). Other organ systems may be involved as well, particularly the skin, evident as palpable purpura. Mononeuropathy multiplex may also occur. Renal lesions cause proteinuria, which is generally mild; hematuria with red cell casts; and varying degrees of renal insufficiency. Renal insufficiency may appear rapidly, particularly in cases with a renal-pulmonary syndrome, but in many cases there is an insidious onset of renal insufficiency, especially in anti-MPO associated disease (Franssen *et al.* 1995). Differences in the clinical course between patients with anti-PR3 associated disease versus those with anti-MPO-associated NCGN are discussed below.

In patients with MPA, histopathological renal lesions resemble those in patients with WG. Granuloma formation is, however, unusual in renal biopsies from patients with MPA. In addition, the more insidious clinical course of renal lesions in patients with MPA versus those with WG is reflected in a larger number of chronic lesions, such as glomerulosclerosis and interstitial fibrosis, at presentation (Franssen *et al.* 1995). As in NCGN that is part of WG, immune deposits are scarce in renal biopsies from patients with MPA. As such, the condition is designated as pauci-immune NCGN (Stilmant *et al.* 1979).

Churg–Strauss syndrome

Churg–Strauss syndrome (CSS) has been defined by the Chapel Hill Group as an eosinophil-rich inflammation with granulomatous inflammation involving the respiratory tract and necrotizing vasculitis affecting small to medium-sized vessels, in association with asthma and blood eosinophilia (Jennette *et al.* 1994) (see Chapter 33). Renal involvement occurs in about 50% of CSS patients. The clinical presentation of renal disease is not different from that in MPA and WG: microscopic hematuria with cellular casts, proteinuria, and varying degrees of renal insufficiency (Eustace *et al.* 1999; Lanham *et al.* 1984). The most striking histologic finding is the widespread infiltration of activated eosinophils, particularly in the interstitium, accompanied by granuloma formation. In the majority of cases, glomeruli show focal or diffuse necrotizing and crescentic glomerulonephritis. By direct immunofluorescence, immune deposits are generally absent, which classifies glomerulonephritis in CSS as pauci-immune (Clutterbuck *et al.* 1990; Gaskin *et al.* 1991). In some cases, however, there are findings more consistent with classical PAN, such as necrotizing arteritis of medium-sized arteries and aneurysm formation.

There is no consensus on the role of ANCA in CSS. In general, about 50–60% of patients are ANCA-positive. Of those positive for ANCA, most have autoantibodies to MPO (Cohen *et al.* 1995; Cohen Tervaert *et al.* 1991a; Eustace *et al.* 1999). ANCA-negative CSS patients tend to present with limited disease, whereas CSS patients positive for ANCA usually present with major organ involvement, frequently including the kidneys (Cohen Tervaert *et al.*

1991a, 1991b). The dichotomy of CSS as an ANCA-negative disease connected with the hypereosinophilic syndrome, and an ANCA-positive disease with small-vessel vasculitis including the kidneys has recently been highlighted (Sinico *et al.* 2005; Kallenberg 2005).

Idiopathic necrotizing and crescentic glomerulonephritis (NCGN)

As already discussed, NCGN is the characteristic renal histopathological manifestation in ANCA-associated small vessel vasculitides. A number of patients present with pauci-immune NCGN without extrarenal manifestations of systemic vasculitis. In most of these, ANCA are positive and directed against MPO. This condition, therefore, can be considered as a form of MPA limited to the kidney. Patients present with the characteristic findings of NCGN: rapidly progressive glomerulonephritis with hematuria and cellular casts, mild proteinuria and renal insufficiency. In addition, arthralgia, myalgia and general malaise are common. Signs of systemic vasculitis may develop later on, but the majority of patients with NCGN do not develop systemic vasculitis. The histopathological findings in the kidneys are indistinguishable from those observed in patients with MPA. This fact also underscores that idiopathic NCGN can be considered as a renal limited form of MPA (Jennette 1998; Jennette *et al.* 1989; Stilmant *et al.* 1979).

Anti-PR3 versus anti-MPO associated glomerulonephritis

Are there clinically relevant differences between anti-PR3 and anti-MPO associated glomerulonephritis? Franssen *et al.* (1995) retrospectively analyzed clinical features, pattern of pretreatment renal function loss, renal morphology and outcome in a series of 46 patients with anti-PR3 associated disease and 46 patients with anti-MPO associated disease. The mean number of affected organs in the anti-PR3 group exceeded that of the anti-MPO group (3.9 versus 1.4). Granuloma formation occurred more frequently in anti-PR3 patients (Franssen *et al.* 1998). More relapses are seen in anti-PR3 patients compared to anti-MPO patients (Franssen *et al.* 1995, 1998; Booth *et al.* 2003). Although the prevalence of renal disease did not differ between both groups, pretreatment renal function deteriorated significantly faster in anti-PR3 patients than in anti-MPO patients. Also, the activity index of the renal biopsies was higher in the anti-PR3 patients, whereas the chronicity index was lower. Kidney survival was not different between the groups. Slot *et al.* (2003) observed differences during follow-up: in anti-PR3 patients, long-term renal survival is determined by the occurrence of renal relapses, whereas in anti-MPO patients long-term renal survival is determined by slow progressive renal failure related to persistent proteinuria (Franssen *et al.* 1998). In order to find an explanation for these differences, these investigators studied the neutrophil activating potential of IgG fractions from their anti-PR3 and anti-MPO patients (see below) (Franssen *et al.* 1999). They found that the anti-PR3 containing fractions had a significantly higher potential to induce neutrophil activation than the anti-MPO fractions. These data suggest that the presence of anti-PR3 induces a more acute inflammatory response compared with anti-MPO. Their data (reviewed in Franssen *et al.* 2000) argue for a distinction between anti-PR3-associated vasculitis and anti-MPO-associated vasculitis.

Pathophysiology of the ANCA-associated glomerulonephritides

Data supporting a pathophysiological role for ANCA are discussed extensively in Chapter 7. As discussed above, ANCA directed to either MPO or PR3 are closely associated with pauci-immune necrotizing crescentic glomerulonephritis, either idiopathic or as part of WG, MPA, and CSS (Kallenberg *et al.* 1994). Longitudinal observations point to a relationship between changes in level of the autoantibodies and changes in disease activity of the associated disorders, as rises in titers of ANCA appear to precede clinical disease activity (Cohen Tervaert *et al.* 1989; Egner and Chapel 1990; Jayne *et al.* 1995). Treatment based on changes in ANCA titers resulted in the prevention of disease relapses (Cohen Tervaert *et al.* 1990). These studies, generally based on small series of patients, used ANCA titration in the indirect immunofluorescence test for quantifications, which is not the most accurate way of quantifying levels of autoantibodies. Indeed, other authors could not confirm a strong correlation between rising titers and ensuing relapses (Kerr *et al.* 1993). Boomsma *et al.*, in a 2-year prospective study, have analyzed this relationship in 85 patients with anti-PR3-associated glomerulonephritis/vasculitis, using ELISA for quantification of the autoantibodies. They found that 27 out of the 33 relapses that occurred during the study period were preceded by a significant rise in PR3-ANCA levels, whereas 11 rises in PR3-ANCA were not followed by a relapse (Boomsma *et al.* 2000). It has also been shown that patients with anti-PR3-associated disease have an eight-fold increased risk for relapse once ANCA is persistently or intermittently positive after induction of remission (Stegeman *et al.* 1994). These data suggest that ANCA are involved in the pathophysiology of PR3-ANCA/ MPO-ANCA-associated pauci-immune glomerulonephritis.

What other data support a pathophysiological role for ANCA? ANCA are able to activate neutrophils *in vitro* to produce reactive oxygen species and to release lytic enzymes such as elastase and PR3 (Falk *et al.* 1990). Neutrophils must be in a state of preactivation (primed) to be activated by ANCA. Priming occurs in the presence of low amounts of proinflammatory cytokines such as tumor necrosis factor-α (TNFα) or interleukin-1 (IL-1). During priming, the target antigens of ANCA, that is PR3 and MPO, are expressed at the cell surface and are therefore accessible for interaction with ANCA. Interestingly, neutrophils, *ex vivo*, can also express PR3 on their surface, but not MPO, in a resting state without priming (mPR3). Percentages of mPR3-expressing neutrophils differ between individuals and seem genetically determined (Schreiber *et al.* 2003). High levels of mPR3-expressing neutrophils are found in patients with WG and are associated with relapsing disease (Rarok *et al.* 2002). *In vitro*, mPR3-expressing neutrophils can be stimulated by anti-PR3 antibodies without priming (van Rossum 2004). The interaction between neutrophils and ANCA occurs only when neutrophils are adherent to a surface, a process in which β_2-integrins are involved (Reumaux *et al.* 1995). This process is assumed to occur *in vivo* at the endothelial surface. Indeed, activated neutrophils adherent to the endothelium are observed in renal biopsies from patients with ANCA-associated NCGN (Brouwer *et al.* 1994). ANCA-induced neutrophil activation involves not only binding of the antibodies via their F(ab)$_2$-fragments to surface expressed PR3 or MPO, but also interaction of their Fc regions with Fc receptors on neutrophils, particularly with the FcgRIIa (Porges *et al.* 1994).

FcgRIIa is the only Fc receptor that interacts with IgG_2, but it also has a particular affinity for the IgG_3-subclass. Interestingly, the increase in neutrophil activating capacity of serum IgG fractions from remission to relapse in patients with PR3-ANCA-positive WG correlates with increases of the IgG_3 subclass of ANCA in those fractions, and not with that of the other subclasses (Mulder *et al.* 1995). In addition, renal relapses of WG are particularly associated with increases of the IgG_3 subclass of ANCA, although IgG_1 and IgG_4-subclasses of ANCA are present as well (Brouwer *et al.* 1991). These data suggest that the IgG_3 subclass of ANCA plays an important role in neutrophil activation via Fcg receptor interactions.

In vitro studies using endothelial monolayers have also shown that neutrophils, in the presence of ANCA, are able to adhere to and lyse endothelial cells (Ewert *et al.* 1992; Savage *et al.* 1992). Elegant studies by Savage and colleagues demonstrated that ANCA are able to induce stable adherence of rolling neutrophils to layers expressing adhesion molecules (Radford *et al.* 2000). Whether endothelial cells themselves express ANCA antigens, such as PR3, has been a subject of controversy. Data from Mayet *et al.* (1993, 1996) suggest that endothelial cells express PR3, particularly when activated, and that ANCA can bind to surface PR3 resulting in up-regulation of adhesion molecules and further cellular activation. Others, however, have not been able to confirm PR3 expression by endothelial cells (King *et al.* 1995), but have demonstrated that PR3 binds to endothelial cells via a specific receptor (Taekema-Roelvink *et al.* 2000).

More definite evidence for a pathophysiological role of ANCA may come from animal models. Passive transfer of ANCA in primates or the induction of an autoimmune response to MPO in rats does not result in renal lesions (Brouwer *et al.* 1993). When, however, the products of activated neutrophils (lytic enzymes, MPO, and its substrate H_2O_2) are perfused into the renal artery in rats immunized with MPO, severe pauci-immune NCGN develops (Brouwer *et al.* 1993). These studies suggest that, initially, cationic proteins such as MPO and PR3 from activated neutrophils adhere to the glomerular capillary wall and are bound by their cognate antibodies. The immune complexes activate the complement system resulting in attraction of neutrophils. Those neutrophils are subsequently activated by ANCA and degrade the immune complexes that were initially present.

The potential of ANCA to augment an inflammatory *in vivo* reaction has been demonstrated by Heeringa *et al.* (1996) in an animal model of antiglomerular basement membrane (anti-GBM) disease. They injected a subclinical dose of heterologous anti-GBM antibodies in rats, which resulted in deposition of immunoglobulins along the GBM without severe glomerulonephritis. In rats immunized with human MPO, which develop anti-MPO antibodies cross-reactive to their own MPO, severe necrotizing and crescentic glomerulonephritis developed after injection of a subclinical dose of anti-GBM antibody. These experiments show the phlogistic potential of ANCA. The most convincing model for the pathogenicity of ANCA comes from studies in MPO-deficient mice. These mice were immunized with mouse MPO and their splenocytes were transferred to immunodeficient mice, which develop severe necrotizing and crescentic glomerulonephritis, granulomatous inflammation, and systemic necrotizing vasculitis (Xiao *et al.* 2002). Passive transfer of anti-MPO IgG alone also resulted in focal NCGN with a paucity of Ig deposition. Lesions in the latter model could be aggravated by injection of lipopolysaccharide (Huugen *et al.* 2005). These data demonstrate the pathogenic potential of MPO-ANCA.

A comparable approach using PR3-deficient mice did not result in necrotizing systemic vasculitis (Pfister *et al.* 2004). Thus, a satisfactory model for PR3-ANCA-associated vasculitis is still lacking.

Renal biopsy in ANCA-associated (renal) vasculitides

Before renal biopsy is considered, the involvement of the kidneys and the degree of disease activity should be assessed. Tests necessary to assess renal involvement include serum creatinine and creatinine clearance, urinalysis to determine if proteinuria is present, and examination of urinary sediment to look for cellular casts. A renal biopsy should be strongly considered in cases in which a specific diagnosis has not yet been made and renal involvement is evident. Even if a diagnosis of WG has been made, a renal biopsy is strongly advocated if the laboratory abnormalities mentioned above are present, in order to look for evidence of vasculitis, to assess activity and damage due to scarring.

Outcome of ANCA-associated renal vasculitis is variable. In a series of 246 new patients with this condition, 28% reached end-stage renal failure, of whom 47% died. Cumulative patient survival in this cohort of 246 patients was 82% at 1 year and 76% at 5 years. Mortality was associated with older age, initial creatinine level greater than 200 mmol/l, and sepsis (Booth *et al.* 2003). Renal outcome is related to initial creatinine level and to the presence or absence of tubular atrophy, normal glomeruli, fibrinoid necrosis, extracapillary proliferation, and age (Vergunst *et al.* 2003). For treatment recommendations, see chapters dealing with the specific diseases.

Other forms of small vessel vasculitis with renal involvement

Henoch–Schönlein purpura (HSP) was defined by the Chapel Hill Consensus Conference (Jennette *et al.* 1994) as vasculitis with IgA-dominant immune deposits affecting small vessels (capillaries, venules, or arterioles). Renal involvement has been reported in 33% of children with HSP and in 63% of adults (Rieu and Noel 1999). The disease is usually self-limiting and without serious sequelae, but in a minority of patients, particularly adults, renal lesions may progress to end-stage renal disease (Fogazzi *et al.* 1989). The diagnosis of HSP is made on clinical grounds together with characteristic small vessel vasculitis with IgA-dominant immune deposits. The classification criteria of the American College of Rheumatology, to be applied for the classification of patients with already-proven vasculitis, include palpable purpura, an age of less than 20 years at onset, bowel angina, and wall granulocytes on biopsy (Mills *et al.* 1990), but, remarkably, do not include IgA deposits.

Renal involvement is characterized by granular mesangial IgA deposits, frequently in combination with complement C3 and fibrinogen. IgA deposits are predominantly of the IgA_1 subclass, the IgA is polymeric, and both light chains are present. In view of the relation between upper respiratory tract infections and relapses of HSP, it has been suggested that dysregulation in IgA-class immune responsiveness is basic to the pathogenesis of HSP. The pathogenesis of HSP has not yet been fully elucidated (Feehally and Allen 1999). Varying degrees of glomerular injury are present: in some cases, there are only minimal abnormalities at light microscopy in the presence of typical immunofluorescence findings (Heaton *et al.*

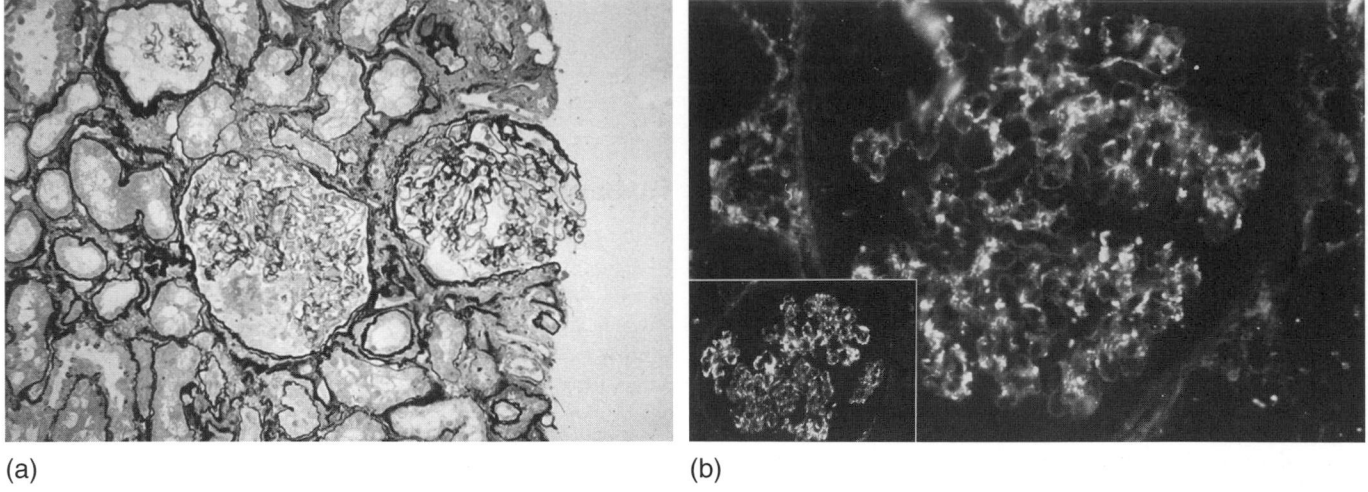

(a) (b)

Figure 16.2 Henoch–Schönlein nephritis. (a) Renal biopsy of a 45-year-old female with recurrent cutaneous vasculitis and episodes of gastrointestinal vasculitis of 2 years' duration, which was taken because of recent onset hematuria and severe proteinuria. Renal biopsy shows a focal and segmental extracapillary crescentic glomerulonephritis of recent origin. Silvermethenamine, HE, × 50. (b) Staining with monoclonal anti-IgA1 antibodies shows diffuse glomerular, granular, deposits in the mesangia and locally in the capillary wall. Insert: staining for C3 shows a similar pattern. Immunofluorescence, anti-IgA, × 125.

1977; Meadow *et al.* 1972). Mesangial proliferation without endocapillary proliferation and crescent formation is present in 25% of biopsies. The remaining ~75% show more extensive mesangial proliferation with focal to diffuse endocapillary proliferation accompanied by crescents and membranoproliferative glomerulonephritis (Figure 16.2). Results of histopathologic examination of renal lesions in HSP are important because the severity of the lesions is a major prognostic determinant. Large proportions of glomeruli with crescents correlates with increased risk for developing end-stage renal disease (Yoshikawa *et al.* 1981).

Permanent renal impairment does not develop if urinalysis is normal during the first 6 months after presentation, as deduced from a systemic review covering 12 studies of 1133 children. Renal impairment, however, occurred in 1.6% of patients with isolated urinary abnormalities during this period, and in 19.5% of patients who developed a nephritic or nephrotic syndrome (Narchi 2005).

Cryoglobulinemic renal vasculitis

In the Chapel Hill Consensus Conference, cryoglobulinemic vasculitis was classified as one of the primary vasculitides (Jennette *et al.* 1994). Many cases of Type II and III cryoglobulinemic vasculitis are related to infection with hepatitis C virus (HCV) (Johnson *et al.* 1994;

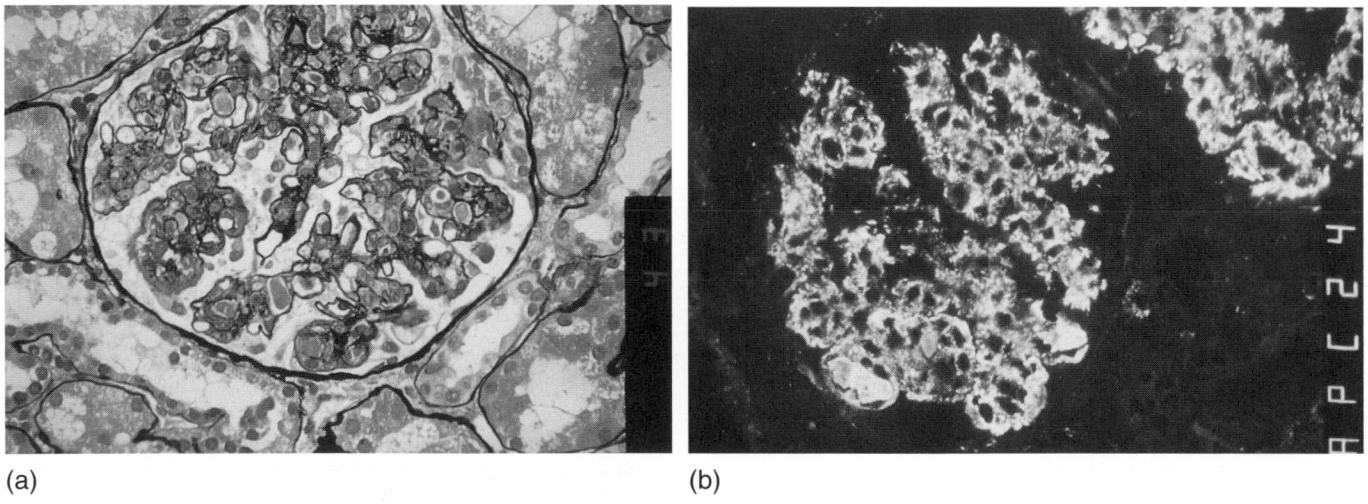

(a) (b)

Figure 16.3 Essential Type II cryoglobulinemia. (a) Diffuse proliferation of mesangial cells and subendothelial deposition of eosinophilic material with or without mesangial (matrix) interposition is shown. Silvermethenamine, HE, × 125. (b) Anti-C3 polyclonal antibodies. Diffuse glomerular granular deposition of immune complexes consisting of IgG, IgM, and Clq (not shown) and C3 in the mesangial area is seen as well as subendothelial deposition and occasionally intracapillary aggregates. Immunofluorescence × 125.

Misiani *et al.* 1992) and HCV-related proteins or RNA are present not only in the cryoglobulins but also in the vessel wall (Dammacco and Sansonno 1997). Thus, in most cases, cryoglobulinemic vasculitis is a secondary vasculitis.

Cryoglobulinemic vasculitis is a prototype of an immune-complex-mediated vasculitis, in which circulating cryoglobulins are demonstrable in serum, complement C3, and, particularly, C4 are decreased in serum, and immune deposits are present in the vessel walls (Gorevic *et al.* 1980) (see Figure 16.3). The kidneys are involved in 25–50% of patients with this disorder. Cryoglobulinemic membranoproliferative glomerulonephritis is particularly prevalent in patients with Type II mixed cryoglobulins (D'Amico *et al.* 1989). By light microscopy, eosinophilic deposits are visible within the glomerular capillaries, together with massive infiltration of monocytes and polymorphonuclear leukocytes. Extracapillary proliferation may occur. Direct immunofluorescence reveals deposits of IgM, IgG, C1q, and C3 (D'Amico *et al.* 1989); vasculitis of the small and medium-sized renal arteries may be present.

Conclusion

In the large vessel vasculitides, renal involvement is relatively rare. Vasculitis of medium-sized arteries may affect the kidneys at the level of the renal artery and its bifurcations. When the glomerular capillaries are involved, vasculitis is classified as small-vessel vasculitis. Small-vessel ANCA-associated diseases frequently show renal involvement, which is a major factor in outcome. Kidney disease is also frequent in Henoch–Schönlein purpura and cryoglobulinemic vasculitis. Classification of the renal vasculitis is important for prognosis and treatment. Treatment is based on glucocorticoids with or without immunosuppressive drugs, but new, hopefully less toxic, treatment modalities are being explored.

Acknowledgements

The authors acknowledge Professor van Breda Vriesman, and Henk van Rie (both of the Department of Clinical Immunology, University Hospital Maastricht, Maastricht, The Netherlands) for providing the figures of renal biopsies.

References

Andrassy, K., Waldherr, R., Erb, A. and Ritz, E. (1992). De novo glomerulonephritis in patients during remission from Wegener's granulomatosis. *Clinical Nephrology*, **38**, 295–8.

Boomsma, M. M., Stegeman, C. A., van der Leij, M. J., Oost, W., Herman, S. J., Kallenberg, C. G.M., Limburg, P. C. and Cohen Tervaert, J. W. (2000). Prediction of relapses in Wegener's granulomatosis by measurement of anti neutrophil cytoplasmic antibody levels; a prospective study. *Arthritis and Rheumatism*, **43**, 2025–33.

Booth, A. D., Almond, M. K., Burns, A., Ellis, P., Gaskin, G., Neild, G. H., Plaisance, M., Pusey, C. D. and Jayne, D. R. (2003). Outcome of ANCA-associated renal vasculitis: a 5-year retrospective study. *American Journal of Kidney Diseases*, **41**, 776–84.

Brogan, P. A., Davies, R., Gordon, I. and Dillon, M. J. (2002). Renal angiography in children with polyarteritis nodosa. *Pediatric Nephrology*, **17**, 277–83.

Brons, R. H., Kallenberg, C. G. and Tervaert, J. W. (2001). Are antineutrophil cytoplasmic antibody-associated vasculitides pauci-immune? *Rheumatic Disease Clinics of North America*, **27**, 833–48.

Brouwer, E., Cohen Tervaert, J. W., Horst, G., Huitema, M. C., Giessen, M. van der, Limburg, P. C. and Kallenberg, C. G. M. (1991). Predominance of IgG4 subclass of anti-neutrophil cytoplasmic autoantibodies in patients with Wegener's Granulomatosis and clinically related disorders. *Clinical and Experimental Immunology*, **83**, 379–86.

Brouwer, E., Huitema, M. G., Klok, P. A., Cohen Tervaert, J. W., Weening, J. J. and Kallenberg, C. G.M. (1993). Anti-myeloperoxidase associated proliferative glomerulonephritis: an animal model. *Journal of Experimental Medicine*, **177**, 905–14.

Brouwer, E., Huitema, M. G., Mulder, A. H.L., Heeringa, P., van Goor, H., Cohen Tervaert, J. W., Weening, J. J. and Kallenberg, C. G. M. (1994). Neutrophil activation in vitro and in vivo in Wegener's granulomatosis. *Kidney International*, **45**, 1120–31.

Cavatorta, F., Campisi, S., Trabassi, E., Zollo, A. and Salvidio, G. (1995). IgA nephropathy associated with Takayasu's arteritis: report of a case and review of the literature. *American Journal of Nephrology*, **15**, 165–7.

Chandrakantan, A. and Kaufman, J. (1999). Renal hemorrhage in polyarteritis nodosa: diagnosis and management. *American Journal of Kidney Disease*, **33**, e8.

Clutterbuck, E. J., Evans, D. J. and Pusey, C. D. (1990). Renal involvement in Churg-Strauss syndrome. *Nephrology, Dialysis, Transplantation*, **5**, 161–7.

Cohen Tervaert, J. W., Woude, F. J. van der, Fauci, A. S., Ambrus, J. L., Velosa, J., Keane, W. F., Meijer, S., Giessen, M. van der, The, T. H., Hem, G. K. van der and Kallenberg, C. G. M. (1989). Association between active Wegener's granulomatosis and anticytoplasmic antibodies. *Archives of Internal Medicine*, **149**, 2461–5.

Cohen Tervaert, J. W., Huitema, M. G., Hené, R. J., Sluiter, W. J., The, T. H., van der Hem, G. K. and Kallenberg, C. G. M. (1990). Prevention of relapses in Wegener's granulomatosis by treatment based on antineutrophil cytoplasmic antibody titre. *Lancet*, **336**, 709–11.

Cohen Tervaert, J. W., Goldschemeding, R., Borne, A. E.G.Kr von dem and Kallenberg, C. G. M. (1991a). Anti-myeloperoxidase antibodies in the Churg Strauss syndrome. *Thorax*, **46**, 70–1.

Cohen Tervaert, J. W., Limburg, P. C., Elema, J. D., Huitema, M. G., Horst, G., The, T. H. and Kallenberg, C. G. M. (1991b). Detection of autoantibodies against myeloid lysosomal enzymes: a useful adjunct to classification of patients with biopsy-proven necrotizing arteritis. *American Journal of Medicine*, **91**, 59–66.

Cohen, P., Guillevin, L., Baril, L., Lhote, F., Noel, L. H. and Lesavre, P. (1995). Persistence of antineutrophil cytoplasmic antibodies (ANCA) in asymptomatic patients with systemic polyarteritis nodosa or Churg-Strauss syndrome: follow up of 53 patients. *Clinical and Experimental Rheumatology*, **13**, 193–8.

Cohen, R. D., Conn, D. L. and Ilstrup, D. M. (1980). Clinical features, prognosis and response to treatment in polyarteritis. *Mayo Clinic Proceedings*, **55**, 146–55.

D'Amico, G., Colasanti, G., Ferrario, F. and Sinico, R. A. (1989). Renal involvement in essential mixed cryoglobulinemia. *Kidney International*, **35**, 1004.

Dammacco, F. and Sansonno, D. (1997). Mixed cryoglobulinemia as a model of systemic vasculitis. *Clinical Reviews in Allergy and Immunology*, **15**, 97–119.

Egner, W. and Chapel, H. M. (1990). Titration of antibodies against neutrophil cytoplasmic antigens is useful in monitoring disease activity in systemic vasculitides. *Clinical and Experimental Immunology*, **82**, 244–9.

Escriba, A., Morales, E., Albizua, E., Herrero, J. C., Ortuno, T., Carreno, A., Dominguez-Gil, B. and Praga, M. (2000). Secondary (AA-type) amyloidosis in patients with polymyalgia rheumatica. *American Journal of Kidney Disease*, **35**, 137–40.

Eustace, J. A., Nadasdy, T. and Choi, M. (1999). The Churg Strauss syndrome. *Journal of the American Society of Nephrology*, **10**, 2048–55.

Ewert, B. H., Jennette, J. C. and Falk, R. J. (1992). Anti-myeloperoxidase antibodies stimulate neutrophils to damage human endothelial cells. *Kidney International*, **41**, 375–83.

Falk, R. J., Terrell, R. S., Charles, L. A., Jennette, J. C. (1990). Anti-neutrophil cytoplasmic autoantibodies induce neutrophils to degranulate and produce oxygen radicals in vitro. *Proceedings of the National Academy of Sciences of the United States of America*, **87**, 4115–9.

Fauci, A., Haynes, B. F., Katz, P. and Wolff, S. (1983). Wegener's granulomatosis: prospective clinical and therapeutic experience with 85 patients for 21 years. *Annals of Internal Medicine*, **98**, 76–85.

Feehally, J. and Allen, A. C. (1999). Pathogenesis of IgA nephropathy. *Annals Medicine Interne* (Paris), **150**, 91–8.

Fogazzi, G. B., Pasquali, S., Moriggi, M., Casanova, S., Damilano, I., Mihatsch, M. J., Zuccheli, P. and Ponticelli, C. (1989). Long-term outcome of Schönlein-Henoch nephritis in the adult. *Clinical Nephrology*, **31**, 60–6.

Franssen, C. F. M., Gans, R. O. B., Arends, B., Hageluken, C., Wee, P. M. ter, Gerlag, P. G. G. and Hoorntje, S. J. (1995). Differences between anti-myeloperoxidase and anti-proteinase 3 associated renal disease. *Kidney International*, **47**, 193–9.

Franssen, C. F. M., Gans, R., Kallenberg, C. G. M., Hageluken, C. and Hoorntje, S. J. (1998). Disease spectrum of patients with antineutrophil cytoplasmic autoantibodies of defined specificities: distinct differences between patients with anti-proteinase 3 and anti-myeloperoxidase autoantibodies. *Journal of Internal Medicine*, **244**, 209–16.

Franssen, C. F., Stegeman, C. A., Oost-Kort, W. W., Kallenberg, C. G., Limburg, P. C., Tiebosch, A., De Jong, P. E. and Tervaert, J. W. (1998). Determinants of renal outcome in anti-myeloperoxidase-associated necrotizing crescentic glomerulonephritis. *Journal of the American Society of Nephrology*, **9**, 1915–23.

Franssen, C. F. M., Huitema, M. G., Muller Kobold, A. C., Oost-Kort, W., Limburg, P. C., Tiebosch, A., *et al.* (1999). In vitro neutrophil activation by antibodies to proteinase 3 and myeloperoxidase from patients with crescentic glomerulonephritis. *Journal of the American Society of Nephrology*, **10**, 1506–15.

Franssen, C. F. M., Stegeman, C. A., Kallenberg, C. G. M., Gans, R. O.B., de Jong, P. E., Hoorntje, S. J. and Cohen Tervaert, J. W. (2000). Antiproteinase 3-and anti-myeloperonidase-associated vasculitis. *Kidney International*, **57**, 2195–206.

Gaskin, G., Clutterbuck, E. J. and Pusey, C. D. (1991). Renal disease in the Churg-Strauss syndrome. *Contributions to Nephrology*, **94**, 58–65.

Goldschmeding, R., van der Schoot, C. E., ten Bokkel Huinink, D., Hack, C. E., van den Ende, M. E., Kallenberg, C. G. M. and von dem Borne, A. E. G. Kr. (1989). Wegener's Granulomatosis autoantibodies identify a novel diisopropylfluorophosphate-binding protein in the lysosomes of normal human neutrophils. *Journal of Clinical Investigation*, **84**, 1577–87.

Gorevic, P. D., Kassab, H. J., Levo, Y., *et al.* (1980). Mixed cryoglobulinemia: clinical aspects and long-term follow-up of 40 patients. *American Journal of Medicine*, **69**, 287.

Haas, M. and Eustace, J.A., (2004). Immune complex deposits in ANCA-associated crescentic glomerulonephritis: A study of 126 cases. *Kidney International*, **65**, 2145–52.

Heaton, J. M., Turner, D. R. and Cameron, J. S. (1977). Localization of glomerular 'deposits' in Henoch-Schönlein nephritis. *Histopathology*, **1**, 93–104.

Heeringa, P., Brouwer, E., Klok, P. A., Huitema, M. G., Born, J. van den, Weening, J. J. and Kallenberg, C. G. M. (1996). Autoantibodies to myeloperoxidase aggravate mild anti-glomerular-basement-membrane-mediated glomerular injury in the rat. *American Journal of Pathology*, **149**, 1695–706.

Hoffman, G. S., Kerr, G. S., Leavitt, R. Y., *et al.* (1992). Wegener's granulomatosis: an analysis of 158 patients. *Annals of Internal Medicine*, **116**, 488–98.

Huugen, D., Xiao, H, van Esch, A., Falk, R. J., Peutz-Kootstra, C. J., Buurman, W. A., Tervaert, J. W., Jennette, J. C. and Heeringa, P. (2005). Aggravation of anti-myeloperoxidase antibody-induced glomerulonephritis by bacterial lipopolysaccharide: role of tumor necrosis factor-alpha. *American Journal of Pathology*, **167**, 47–58.

Jayne, D. R.W., Gaskin, G., Pusey, C. D. and Lockwood, C. M. (1995). ANCA and predicting relapse in systemic vasculitis. *Quarterly Journal of Medicine*, **88**, 127–33.

Jennette, J. C. (1991). Antineutrophil cytoplasmic autoanti-body-associated disease: a pathologist's perspective: *American Journal of Kidney Disease*, **18**, 164–70.

Jennette, J. C. (1998). Crescentic glomerulonephritis. In *Heptinstall's pathology of the kidney* (eds J. C. Jennette, J. L. Olson, M. M., Schwartz and F. G. Silva), pp. 625–56. Lippincott-Raven, Philadelphia.

Jennette, J. C. and Falk, R. J. (1994).. The pathology of vasculitis involving the kidney. *American Journal of Kidney Disease*, **24**, 130.

Jennette, J. C., Falk, R. J., Andrassy, K., Bacon, B. A., Churg, J., Gross, W. L., Hagen, E. C., Hoffmann, G. S., Hunder, G. G., Kallenberg, C. G. M., McCluskey, R. T., Sinico, R. A., Rees, A. J., van Es, L. A., Waldherr, R. and Wiik, A. (1994). Nomenclature of systemic vasculitides: the proposal of an international consensus conference. *Arthritis and Rheumatism*, **37**, 187–92.

Jennette, J. C., Wilkman, A. S. and Falk, R. J. (1989). Anti-neutrophil cytoplasmic autoantibody-associated glomerulonephritis and vasculitis. *American Journal of Pathology*, **135**, 921–30.

Joh, K., Kanetsuna, Y., Ishikawa, Y., Aizawa, S., Naito, L. and Sado, Y. (1997). Diffuse mesangial sclerosis associated with Kawasaki disease: analysis of alpha chains (alpha 1-alpha 6) of human type 1 in the renal basement membrane. *Virchows Archiv*, **430**, 489–94.

Johnson, R. J., Willson, R., Yamabe, K., *et al.* (1994). Renal manifestations of hepatitis C virus infection. *Kidney International*, **46**, 1255.

Kallenberg, C. G. M., Brouwer, E., Weening, J. J. and Cohen Tervaert, J. W. (1994). Anti-neutrophil cytoplasmic antibodies: current diagnostic and pathophysiological potential. *Kidney International*, **46**, 1–15.

Kallenberg, C. G. M. (2005). Churg Strauss syndrome: just one disease entity? *Arthritis and Rheumatism*, **52**, 2589–93.

Kerr, G. R., Fleischer, T. H. A., Hallahan, C. D., *et al.* (1993). Limited prognostic value of changes in antineutrophil cytoplasmic antibody titer in patients with Wegener's granulomatosis. *Arthritis and Rheumatism*, **36**, 365–71.

Kieffer, E., Piquois, A., Bertal, A., Bletry, O. and Godeau, P. (1990). Reconstructive surgery of the renal arteries in Takayasu's disease. *Annals of Vascular Surgery*, **4**, 156–65.

King, W. J., Adu, D., Daha, M. R., *et al.* (1995). Endothelial cells and renal epithelial cells do not express the Wegener's autoantigen, proteinase 3. *Clinical and Experimental Immunology*, **102**, 98–105.

Klein, R. G., Hunder, G. G., Stanson, A. W. and Sheps, S. C. (1975). Large artery involvement in giant cell (temporal) arteritis. *Annals of Internal Medicine*, **83**, 806.

Lagneau, P. and Michel, J. B. (1985). Renovascular hypertension and Takayasu's disease. *Journal of Urology*, **134**, 876.

Lanham, J. G., Elkon, K. B., Pusey, C. D. and Hughes, G. R. (1984). Systemic vasculitis with asthma and eosinophilia: a clinical approach to the Churg-Strauss syndrome. *Medicine*, **63**, 65.

Logar, D., Rozman, B., Vizjak, A., Ferluga, D., Mulder, A. H. L. and Kallenberg, C. G. M. (1994). Arteritis of both internal carotid arteries in a patient with focal crescentic glomerulonephritis and antineutrophil cytoplasmic antibodies (c-ANCA). *British Journal of Rheumatology*, **33**, 167–9.

Lovaria, A., Nicolini, A., Meregaglia, D., Saccheri, S., Rivolta, R., Montanari, E., Morganti, A. and Rossi, P. (1999). Interventional radiology in the treatment of renal artery stenosis. *Annals of Urology*, **33**, 146–55.

Mayet, W. J., Csernok, E., Szymkowiak, C., Gross, W. L. and Meyer zum Büschenfelde, K. H. (1993). Human endothelial cells express proteinase 3, the target antigen of anti-cytoplasmic antibodies in Wegener's granulomatosis. *Blood*, **82**, 1221–9.

Mayet, W. J., Schwarting, A., Orth, T., Duchmann, R. and Meyer zum Büschenfelde, K. H. (1996). Antibodies to proteinase 3 mediate expression of vascular cell adhesion molecule-1 (VCAM-1). *Clinical and Experimental Immunology*, **103**, 259–67.

Meadow, S. R., Glasgow, E. F., White, R. H., Moncrieff, M. W., Cameron, J. S. and Ogg, C. S. (1972). Schönlein-Henoch nephritis. *Quarterly Journal of Medicine*, **41**, 241–58.

Mills, J. A., Michel, B. A., Bloch, D. A., *et al.* (1990). The American College of Rheumatology 1990 criteria for the classification of Henoch-Schonlein purpura. *Arthritis and Rheumatism*, **33**, 1114–21.

Misiani, R., Bellavita, P., Fenili, D., *et al.* (1992). Hepatitis C virus infection in patients with essential mixed cryoglobulinemia. *Annals of Internal Medicine*, **117**, 573.

Mulder, A. H., Stegeman, C. A. and Kallenberg, C. G. M. (1995). Activation of granulocytes by anti-neutrophil cytoplasmic antibodies (ANCA) in Wegener's granulomatosis: a predominant role for the IgG3 subclass of ANCA. *Clinical and Experimental Immunology*, **101**, 227–32.

Muller, E., Schneider, W., Kettritz, U., Schmidt, W. A., Luft, F. C. and Gobel, U. (2004). Temporal arteritis with pauci-immune glomerulonephritis: a systemic disease. *Clinical Nephrology*, **62**, 384–6.

Narchi, H. (2005). Risk of long term renal impairment and duration of follow-up recommended for Henoch-Schönlein purpura with normal or minimal urinary findings: a systematic review. *Archives of Diseases in Children*, **90**, 916–20.

Nardi, P. M., Haller, J. O., Friedman, A. P., Slovis, T. L. and Schaffer, R. M. (1985). Renal manifestations of Kawasaki's disease. *Pediatric Radiology*, **15**, 116–18.

O'Neill, Jr. W. M., Hammar, S. A. and Bloomer, H. A. (1976). Giant-cell arteritis with visceral angiitis. *Archives of Internal Medicine*, **136**, 1157.

Pfister, H., Ollert, M., Frohlich, L. F., Quintanilla-Martinez, L., Colby, T. V., Specks, U. and Jenne, D. E. (2004). Antineutrophil cytoplasmic autoantibodies against the murine homolog of proteinase 3 (Wegener autoantigen) are pathogenic in vivo. *Blood*, **104**, 1411–18.

Porges, A. J., Redecha, P. B., Kimberly, W. T., Csernok, E., Gross, W. L. and Kimberly, R. P. (1994). Anti-neutrophil cytoplasmic antibodies engage and activate human neutrophils via Fc gamma RIIa. *Journal of Immunology*, **153**, 1271–80.

Radford, D. J., Savage, C. O. S. and Nash, G. B. (2000). Treatment of rolling neutrophils with antineutrophil cytoplasmic antibodies causes conversion to firm integrin-mediated adhesion. *Arthritis and Rheumatism*, **43**, 1337–45.

Rarok, A. A., Stegeman, C. A., Limburg, P. C. and Kallenberg, C. G. M. (2002). Neutrophil membrane expression of proteinase 3 is related to relapse in PR3-ANCA-associated vasculitis. *Journal of the American Society of Nephrology*, **13**, 2232–8.

Reinhold-Keller, E., Beuge, N., Latza, U., de Groot, K., Rudert, H., Nolle, B., Heller, M. and Gross, W. L. (2000). An interdisciplinary approach to the care of patients with Wegener's granulomatosis: long-term outcome in 155 patients. *Arthritis and Rheumatism*, **43**, 1021–32.

Reumaux, D., Vossebeld, P. J., Roos, D. and Verhoeven, A. J. (1995). Effect of tumor necrosis factor-induced integrin activation on Fc gamma receptor II-mediated signal transduction: relevance for activation of neutrophils by anti-proteinase 3 or anti-myeloperoxidase antibodies. *Blood*, **86**, 3189–95.

Rieu, P. and Noel, L. H. (1999). Henoch/Schönlein nephritis in children and adults: morphological features and clinico-pathological correlations. *Annals Medicine Interne (Paris)*, **150**, 151–9.

Ronco, P., Verroust, P., Mignon, F., *et al.* (1983). Immunopathologic studies of polyarteritis nodosa and Wegener's granulomatosis: A report of 43 patients with 51 renal biopsies. *Quarterly Journal of Medicine*, **52**, 212–23.

Rossum, A. P. van, Rarok, A. A., Huitema, M. G., Fassina, G., Limburg, P. C. and Kallenberg, C. G. M. (2004). Constitutive membrane expression of proteinase 3 and neutrophil activation by anti-PR3 antibodies. *Journal of Leukocyte Biology*, **76**, 1162–70.

Rowley, A. H., Shulman, S. T., Mask, C. A., Finn, L. S., Terai, M., Baker, S. C., Galliani, C. A., Takahashi, Naoe, S., Kalelkar, M. B. and Crawford, S. E. (2000). IgA plasma cell infiltration of proximal respiratory tract, pancreas, kidney, and coronary artery in acute kawasaki disease. *Journal of Infectious Diseases*, **182**, 1183–91.

Salcedo, J. R., Greenberg, L. and Kapur, S. (1988). Renal histology of mucocutaneous lymph node syndrome (Kawasaki disease). *Clinical Nephrology*, **29**, 47–51.

Savage, C. O., Pottinger, B. E., Gaskin, G., Pusey, C. D. and Pearson, J. D. (1992). Autoantibodies developing to myeloperoxidase and proteinase 3 in systemic vasculitis stimulate neutrophil cytotoxicity toward cultured endothelial cells. *American Journal of Pathology*, **141**, 335–42.

Schouffoer, A. A., Siegert, C. E., Arend, S. M., Thompson, J. and van Oostaijen, J. A. (1998). Embolization of a ruptured aneurysm in classic polyarteritis presenting as perirenal hematoma. *Archives of Internal Medicine*, **158**, 1466–8.

Schreiber, A., Busjahn, A., Luft, F. C. and Kettritz, R. (2003). Membrane expression of proteinase 3 is genetically determined. *Journal of the American Society of Nephrology*, **14**, 68–75.

Senzaki, H., Suda, M., Noma, S., Kawaguchi, H., Sakakihara, Y. and Hishi, T. (1994). Acute heart failure and acute renal failure in Kawasaki disease. *Acta Paediatrica Japonica*, **36**, 443–7.

Sinico, R. A., DiToma, L., Maggiore, U., Bottera, P., Radice, A., Tosoni, C., Grasselli, C., Pavone, L., Gregorini, G., Monti, S., Frassi, M., Vecchio, F., Corace, C., Venegoni, E. and Buzio, C. (2005). Prevalence and clinical significance of antineutrophil cytoplasmic antibodies in Churg-Strauss syndrome. *Arthritis and Rheumatism*, **52**, 2926–35.

Slot, M., Cohen Tervaert, J. W., Franssen, C. and Stegeman, C. (2003). Renal survival and prognostic factors in patients with PR3-ANCA associated vasculitis with renal involvement. *Kidney International*, **63**, 670–7.

Stegeman, C. A., Cohen Tervaert, J. W., Sluiter, W. J., Manson, W. L., de Jong, P. E. and Kallenberg, C. G. M. (1994). Association of nasal carriage of *Staphylococcus aureus* and higher relapse rate in Wegener's granulomatosis. *Annals of Internal Medicine*, **120**, 12–17.

Stilmant, M. M., Bolton, W. K., Sturgill, B. C., *et al.* (1979). Crescentic glomerulonephritis without immune deposits: clinicopathologic features. *Kidney International*, **15**, 184–95.

Taekema-Roelvink, M. E., Van Kooten, C., Heemskerk, E., Schroeijers, W. and Daha, M. R. (2000). Proteinase 3 interacts with a 111-KD membrane molecule of human umbilical vein endothelial cells. *Journal of the American Society of Nephrology*, **11**, 640–8.

van der Woude, F. J., Rasmussen, N., Lobatto, S., Wiik, A., Permin, H., Es, L. A. van, Giessen, M. van der, Hem, G. K. van der and The, T. H. (1985). Autoantibodies to neutrophils and monocytes: tool for diagnosis and marker of disease activity in Wegener's granulomatosis. *Lancet*, **ii**, 425–9.

Veiga, P. A., Pieroni, D., Baier, W. and Feld, L. G. (1992). Association of Kawasaki disease and interstitial nephritis. *Pediatric Nephrology*, **6**, 421–3.

Vergunst, C. E., van Gurp, E., Hagen, E. C., van Houwelingen HC, Hauer HA, Noel LH, *et al.* (2003). An index for renal outcome in ANCA-associated glomerulonephritis. *American Journal of Kidney Diseases*, **41**, 532–8.

Wada, Y., Nishida, H., Kohno, K., Tamai, O., Fujisawa, M., Katoh, S., Morimatsu, M. and Okuda, S. (1999). AA amyloidosis in Takayasu's arteritis-long-term survival on maintenance haemodialysis. *Nephrology, Dialysis, Transplantation*, **14**, 2478–81.

Wang, A. Y., Lai, K. N., Li, P. K., Leung, C. B. and Lui, S. F. (1996). Acute renal failure induced by angiotensin converting enzyme inhibitor in a patient with polyarteritis nodosa. *Renal Failure*, **18**, 293–8.

Weaver, F. A., Kumar, S. R., Yellin, A. E., Anderson, S., Hood, D. B., Rowe, V. L., Kitridou, R. C., Kohl, R. D. and Alexancer, J. (2004). Renal revascularization in Takayasu arteritis-induced renal artery stenosis. *Journal of Vascular Surgery*, **3**, 749–57.

Xiao, H., Heeringa, P., Hu, P., Liu, Z., Zhao, M., Aratani, Y., Maeda, N., Falk, R. J. and Jennette, J. C. (2002). Antineutrophil cytoplasmic autoantibodies specific for myeloperoxidase cause glomerulonephritis and vasculitis in mice. *Journal of Clinical Investigation*, **110**, 955–63.

Yoshikawa, N., White, R. H. and Cameron, J. S. (1981). Prognostic significance of the glomerular changes in Henoch Schönlein nephritis. *Clinical Nephrology*, **16**, 223–9.

CHAPTER 17

Digital ischemia and Raynaud's phenomenon

K. Kwasind Huston, John H. Stone, and Fredrick M. Wigley

Introduction

Insufficient blood flow to the distal extremities often constitutes a patient's first clear indication of an underlying illness. The severity of this process can range from a mild nuisance to critical ischemia and tissue destruction. For patients, even mild symptoms can cause great emotional distress, especially in the setting of diagnostic uncertainty. For physicians, digital ischemia poses a diagnostic challenge with high stakes. Failure to diagnose the cause promptly and institute effective therapy prolongs the patient's discomfort and leads to the loss of tissue viability. Few clinical events are more painful to observe than the slow death of a digit or limb stricken with insufficient blood flow, awaiting either autoamputation or surgical removal. The urgency of digital ischemia often dictates that treatment based on the proper interpretation of clinical clues must begin before the definitive diagnosis is secure. Accurate knowledge of disease mechanisms allows rational treatment decisions even when diagnostic information is incomplete.

For general practitioners, few clinical findings are more strongly associated with rheumatic disease than digital ischemia and Raynaud's phenomenon. At the same time, few syndromes are the source of greater confusion regarding terminology, etiology, and management. More than 130 years after Maurice Raynaud first described "l'asphyxie locale et de la gangréne symétrique des extrémités" (local asphyxia and symmetrical gangrene of the digits) (Raynaud 1862), there remains a tendency to lump many forms of digital ischemia under the rubric of Raynaud's disease. Because all etiologies of digital ischemia are not alike, and because therapeutic approaches to this problem vary according to the precise cause, an essential step in patient management is distinguishing between vasculitic, vasospastic, thrombotic, and other causes of digital ischemia.

In this chapter, the focus is on digital ischemia and Raynaud's phenomenon related to systemic rheumatic conditions, particularly vasculitis and the connective tissue diseases (scleroderma, systemic lupus erythematous [SLE], and related conditions). There has been dramatic progress in defining the pathophysiologic events leading to vasospasm and vasculopathy over the last several years. This knowledge has led to many exciting and new treatment modalities for Raynaud's phenomenon and digital ischemia.

Definitions

Historical perspective

In 1862, Raynaud described a condition "which in the ordinary language is designated under the name of *dead finger*". He described 31 patients who suffered from varying combinations and degrees of digital pallor, cyanosis, and symmetrical gangrene, all of which he attributed to prolonged vasospasm. To Raynaud, the symmetry of the process that he observed strongly implicated hyperactivity of the sympathetic nervous system as its cause. On inspection of the cases, it is clear that substantial heterogeneity existed within this group of patients. Whereas some suffered extensive gangrene, others experienced only a "slight inconvenience ... which often passes unperceived so that it does not require any treatment" (Raynaud 1862).

The malady first described by Raynaud became known as Raynaud's disease. This unfortunate label persists today in medical jargon, albeit with a variety of usages. In the late 1800s, Hutchinson noted that there were several distinct causes of symmetrical gangrene, including heart failure and senile atherosclerosis (Hutchinson 1901). He was the first to note the development of scleroderma several years after the onset of Raynaud's disease (Hutchinson 1896). In view of the varied causes of Raynaud's disease, Hutchinson suggested Raynaud's phenomenon as an alternative term. He wrote: "All who have studied in any detail the cases which have been grouped together under the name of Raynaud's malady will admit that the time has arrived when they ought to be classified. They are not all alike, nor do they tend to the same results" (Hutchinson 1901).

Over the ensuing decades, other influential medical thinkers addressed the issue initially framed by Raynaud. Allen and Brown (1932a) noted that Raynaud had recanted the strong association between "local asphyxia" of the digits and symmetrical gangrene in his later writings. Specifically, Raynaud had characterized asphyxia and gangrene as two degrees of the same malady, with gangrene often absent. In 1932, they defined Raynaud's disease by the following criteria: (1) intermittent attacks of color changes in the acral regions; (2) symmetrical or bilateral involvement; (3) absence of clinical evidence of occlusive lesions in the peripheral arteries; (4) minimal trophic changes or gangrene; (5) presence of the disorder for at least 2 years; and (6) no evidence of a secondary cause.

In a description of 265 patients diagnosed with Raynaud's disease at the Mayo Clinic, Allen and Brown concluded that only 147 met their criteria for this diagnosis. In addition to the relative lack of gangrene in the disorder they called Raynaud's disease, they also commented on a characteristic absence of pain "ordinary of no significance" (Allen and Brown 1932b). Raynaud's disease as delineated by Allen and Brown corresponds to primary Raynaud's phenomenon in today's nomenclature (see below).

Lewis and Pickering, contemporaries of Allen and Brown, believed that consensus on a definition for Raynaud's disease could never be achieved and proposed that the term be discarded (Lewis and Pickering 1933). In its place, they proposed the consideration of two major categories of digital ischemia: (1) Raynaud's phenomenon (corresponding to Allen and Brown's criteria for Raynaud's disease); and (2) gangrene/necrosis, an entirely separate (but non-uniform) entity. To Lewis and Pickering, Raynaud's phenomenon signified "active and intermittent closure of small arteries of the order of those supplying the digits, a closure manifesting itself clinically in a pallid or fully cyanotic state of the affected skin" (Lewis and Pickering 1933). The authors emphasized that this phenomenon (illustrated in Figure 17.1) should not be regarded as the result of only one set of circumstances.

In contrast, with regard to the second major category, digital gangrene/necrosis, Lewis and Pickering stated that digital artery vasospasm was "not an essential or even a usual precursor of" that condition (Lewis and Pickering 1933). Rather, they asserted, digital gangrene/necrosis stemmed from a permanent structural change, resulting in "plugging" of the culprit arteries. Though lacking proof, Lewis and Pickering (1933) hypothesized that "intimal changes, including thrombosis, are usually or always responsible for the obliteration of small arteries leading to necrosis".

Under the heading of conditions associated with gangrene, Lewis and Pickering included not only disorders leading to major digital infarction (Figure 17.2a and 17.2b), but also the minute necrotic foci that we now term digital pitting (Figure 17.3). In making these distinctions, they anticipated the modern definitions of primary and secondary Raynaud's phenomenon.

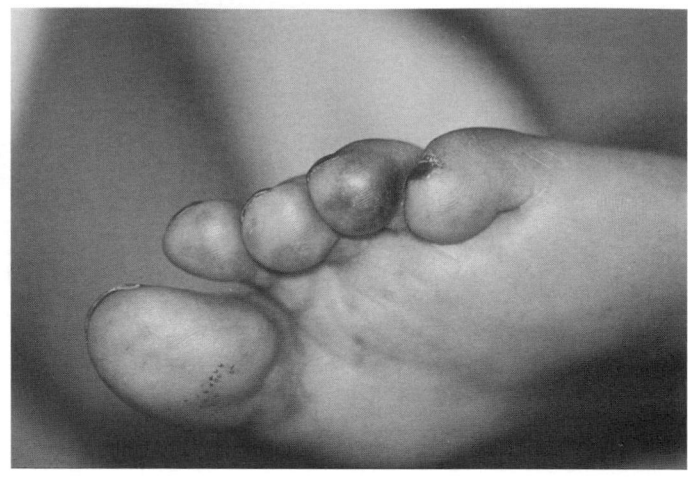

(a)

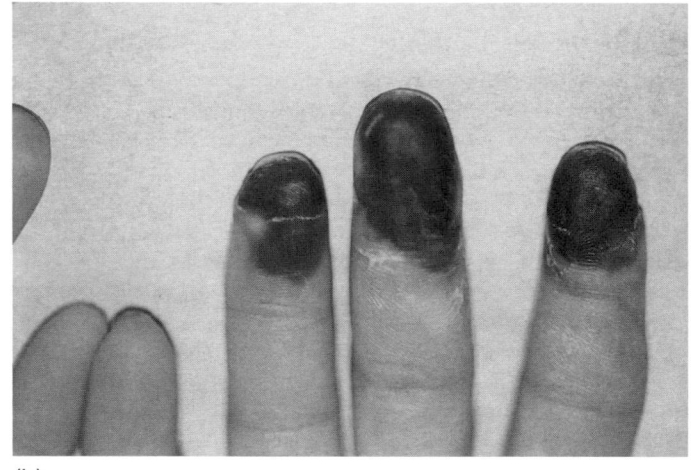

(b)

Figure 17.2 Digital infarctions occurring in Wegener's granulomatosis and Buerger's disease. (a) Wegener's granulomatosis. (b) Thromboangiitis obliterans (Buerger's disease). (See Color Plate 68).

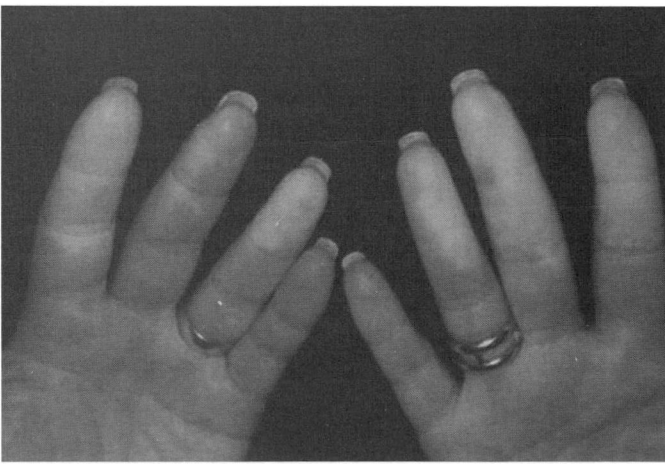

Figure 17.1 Raynaud's phenomenon, representing digital artery vasospasm leading to pallor. In prolonged vasospasm, pallor gives way to cyanosis, followed by rubor as circulation is restored. (See Color Plate 67).

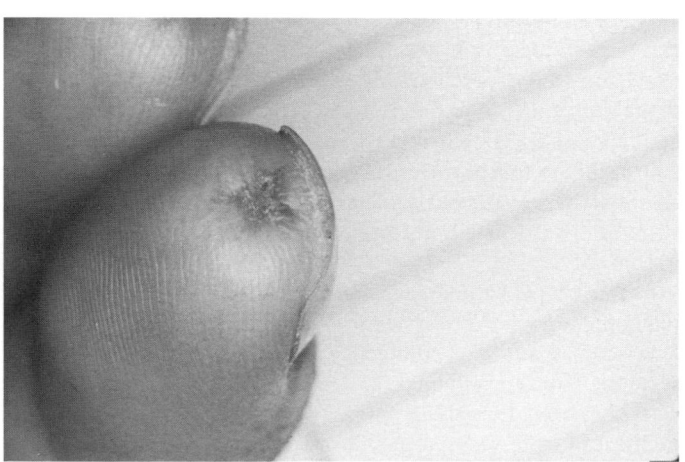

Figure 17.3 Digital pitting in a patient with diffuse systemic sclerosis. (See Color Plate 69).

Table 17.1 Nomenclature schemes for Raynaud's phenomenon

Underlying disorder	United States	Europe
No	Primary Raynaud's phenomenon	Primary Raynaud's disease
Yes	Secondary Raynaud's phenomenon	Raynaud's syndrome

Current nomenclature

At least two parallel systems of nomenclature exist in the classification of Raynaud's phenomenon (Table 17.1). In the United States, objection has existed to use of the stigma "Raynaud's *disease*" for patients in whom vasospasm is the principal pathophysiologic mechanism. Thus, primary Raynaud's *phenomenon* is the preferred designation for the occurrence of cold-induced vasospasm that is not associated with a disease or known cause (LeRoy and Medsger 1992). Secondary Raynaud's phenomenon is the term of vasospasm induced by cold in the setting of an underlying disorder. In Europe, Raynaud's phenomenon is the blanket term for any type of cold-induced digital vasospasm (Belch 1990), and the concept of Raynaud's phenomenon is divided into Raynaud's syndrome (associated with an underlying condition) and primary Raynaud's disease (where no underlying condition is present).

Lack of consensus regarding these issues will probably persist until the precise causes of cold-induced vasospasm (likely multifactorial) are defined more clearly. Another source of confusion results from the imprecise application of the moniker Raynaud's (whether disease, syndrome, or phenomenon) to conditions in which vasospasm is not the principal event – or perhaps not even a minor one. Most forms of vasculitis fall under this category. Although some degree of vasospasm may be present in the vasculitic disorders, the principal event is narrowing of the blood vessel lumen by necrotizing inflammation, frequently complicated by the occurrence of thrombi in the microvasculature. The importance of this distinction is not semantic: digital ischemia resulting from vasculitic inflammation requires drastically different therapy than does vasospasm due to primary or secondary Raynaud's phenomenon.

Epidemiology

Most studies of Raynaud's phenomenon have been conducted at academic medical centers, and thus the prevalence data are biased toward patients with more severe illnesses. Only recently have population-based surveys estimated the prevalence of Raynaud's phenomenon in the general population. The data vary depending on the diagnostic criteria, the survey technique, and the particular characteristics of the population surveyed.

Population-based surveys estimate the prevalence of Raynaud's phenomenon to be between 4.9% and 20.1% in women, and between 3.8% and 13.5% in men (Maricq *et al.* 1993). Surveys across different ethnic groups consistently report figures in the range of 3–5%: from Spain, 3.2–4.7% (Riera *et al.* 1993); from the Netherlands, 2.9% (Bartelink *et al.* 1992); from Japan, 3.0–3.4% (Inaba *et al.* 1993); from Turkey, 5.9% (Onbasi *et al.* 2005); from the United States, 4.3–5.7% (Maricq *et al.* 1989); and among urban-dwelling African-Americans, 4.0% (Gelber *et al.* 1999). Outlying estimates include those from France, 13.5–20.1% (Marciq *et al.* 1993); Sweden, 15.9% (Leppert *et al.* 1987); and Estonia, 7.9–8.3% (Valter and Maricq 1997). The prevalence of Raynaud's phenomenon is higher among young women, among family members of people with Raynaud's phenomenon, and in geographic areas with cold temperatures.

A recent study focused on the incidence and natural history of Raynaud's phenomenon in a community based population derived from the Framingham Offspring Study Cohort (Suter *et al.* 2005). In that report of 717 women and 641 men, the incidence, over a period of 7 years, was 2.2% in women and 1.5% in men. Interestingly, the symptoms of Raynaud's rarely interfered with daily activities and remitted in 64% of affected patients.

Many case reports document that Raynaud's phenomenon can be associated with vasculitis or be a presenting sign of a disease process with vasculitis (Andreu-Sanchez *et al.* 1991). Furthermore, most review articles list vasculitis as a cause of Raynaud's phenomenon; however, few surveys have measured the true frequency of vasculitis as the cause of Raynaud's phenomenon in patients presenting with that complaint. Most reports of associations between vasculitis and Raynaud's phenomenon must be regarded with caution because of the failure to obtain definitive diagnoses of vasculitis; loose usage of the term vasculitis (in particular, a tendency for certain connective tissue disorders, for example scleroderma and SLE, to be labeled as such); confusion resulting from alterations in vasculitis classification schemes (Jennette *et al.* 1994; Lie 1994); and imprecise definitions of what is meant by Raynaud's phenomenon.

Primary Raynaud's phenomenon is the most common diagnosis in most surveys. Raynaud's phenomenon associated with a connective tissue disease (scleroderma, SLE, inflammatory myopathies) is the second most common category reported. Among 100 patients presenting to an academic center with Raynaud's phenomenon, Porter *et al.* reported vasculitis principally in conjunction with connective tissue diseases (Porter *et al.* 1976). A tabulation of 631 cases seen at the same institution found that 37.4% had primary Raynaud's phenomenon, 37.2% had a connective tissue disease, 3.5% had hypersensitivity angiitis, 1.9% had Buerger's disease, and 20% had other disorders not associated with vasculitis (Friedman *et al.* 1988). Thus, in that study, Raynaud's phenomenon was attributed to vasculitis in fewer than 5% of the patients.

Similarly, another survey from 50 Italian medical centers found that among 761 patients with Raynaud's phenomenon, scleroderma was the most common cause (28.4%). Vasculitis, in contrast, was reported in less than 5% of cases (Grassi *et al.* 1998). A population-based survey in South Carolina found that 32% of patients had primary Raynaud's phenomenon, 60% had Raynaud's phenomenon and other health problems, and 8% had evidence of a connective tissue disease (Maricq *et al.* 1990). Vasculitis was not reported in any of the patients who described symptoms compatible with Raynaud's phenomenon in that study. Finally, a study of 118 patients assessed the prevalence of secondary disorders in patients with Raynaud's phenomenon that were referred to a rheumatology center in Italy (De Angelis *et al.* 2003). Of the 118 patients, 52% had a secondary disorder (47% with scleroderma) but none had vasculitis.

In summary, the existing studies of Raynaud's phenomenon document a moderately high prevalence of this condition. Estimates of the prevalence of Raynaud's phenomenon are stable across many populations. The true prevalence of vasculitis among patients with symptoms of Raynaud's, although not well known, is probably less than 5%. As discussed below, many characteristics of vasculitis-associated digital ischemia differ from those of vasospasm-induced Raynaud's phenomenon.

Pathogenesis

This section focuses on the pathogenesis of primary and secondary Raynaud's phenomenon. Specific information about vascular dysfunction in the vasculitides is found elsewhere in this text.

Physiologic control of blood vessel caliber

Maintenance of core body temperature is achieved partly by alteration of blood flow to the skin surface through a dense array of arterio-venous (AV) shunts. During local or whole body cooling, blood flow to the skin is reduced via vasoconstriction of these shunts. In contrast, warm temperatures cause vasodilatation, thereby fostering heat exchange. The thermoregulatory vessels, which also provide nutritional support to the digits, are influenced not only by changes in temperature, but also by emotional stress and a variety of other environmental factors.

These changes in blood flow are mediated primarily by reflex increases in sympathetic tone. Regulation of regional blood flow is complex, altered not only by neural signals, but also by hormonal influences and mediators released by both the endothelium and circulating cells. Certain autonomic nerve endings release a group of neurotransmitters that mediate vasodilation. These include nitric oxide, vasoactive intestinal peptide, and acetylcholine. Cutaneous vasculature is also sensitive to mediators released from sensory fibers, including calcitonin gene related peptide (CGRP), substance P, neurokinin A, and neuropeptide Y (Generini *et al.* 2005).

Cutaneous blood vessels are richly innervated by a variety of neuron subtypes. The most potent influences on the digital circulation are the α_2-adrenergic receptors, with vasoconstriction of small arteries under α_2-adrenergic tone. The expression of α_2-adrenergic receptors is influenced by temperature. At cold temperatures, *in vitro* studies demonstrate up-regulation of α_2-adrenergic receptors, as well as an increased affinity of α-adrenoceptors for norepinephrine, the major sympathetic neurotransmitter (Flavahan *et al.* 1985). Studies in human volunteers have confirmed the role of α_2-adrenoceptors in mediating cold-induced vasoconstriction (Coffman and Cohen 1988; Ekenvall *et al.* 1988). There are now at least three known α_2-adrenergic receptor subtypes, α_{2A}, α_{2B}, and α_{2C} (Philipp *et al.* 2002). Interestingly, the α_{2C} adrenergic receptor remains localized to intracellular compartments under normal conditions where it is unavailable for binding to its ligand; however, upon exposure to cold, the α_{2C} receptor translocates from the Golgi network to the cell surface where it is available for agonist-induced activation (Jeyaraj *et al.* 2001). Receptor translocation is mediated by the Rho/Rho kinase signaling pathway, possibly in response to stimulation by reactive oxygen species generated by smooth muscle cell mitochondria (Bailey *et al.* 2004, 2005). Furthermore, inhibition of the α_{2C} receptor has been shown to prevent cold-induced vasoconstriction, highlighting the importance of specific receptor subtypes in normal physiologic mechanisms of thermoregulation (Chotani *et al.* 2000). These mechanistic insights may have direct implications for treatment of Raynaud's phenomenon.

The endothelium of cutaneous blood vessels also influences local blood flow in response to a variety of stimuli. The endothelium of the vessel can be activated by a number of mechanisms, including: changes in the physical environment of the cell, such as shear stress altered by local blood flow; alterations in the biochemical milieu, such as regional hypoxia; circulating hormones; neurotransmitters released by autonomic or sensory nerves; autocoids from the vessels themselves, such as bradykinin; mediators released from circulating cells, such as platelet-derived serotonin and thromboxane A; and endothelial released factors such as prostacyclin or endothelin.

Primary Raynaud's phenomenon

The pathophysiology of Raynaud's phenomenon remains incompletely understood. The factors contributing to this condition are complex, and are probably different for the primary and secondary forms of Raynaud's phenomenon. As suggested by Lewis and Pickering (1933), most of the current evidence implicates a local vascular defect rather than a central nervous system abnormality as the principal problem, with a resulting unfavorable balance between vasodilatory and vasoconstrictive stimuli.

Familial aggregation occurs in primary Raynaud's phenomenon (Freedman *et al.* 1999); approximately 30% of patients with primary Raynaud's phenomenon have first-degree family members with the condition. This finding suggests the possibility of a specific gene defect(s) among patients with primary Raynaud's phenomenon. Indeed, it has been suggested that primary Raynaud's phenomenon is a trait rather than a disorder (Hadler 1998).

In primary Raynaud's phenomenon, exaggerated cold sensitivity of the α_2-adrenoceptors is thought to be a major factor in patients' symptoms, possibly via cold-induced translocation of the α_{2C} adrenergic receptor to the plasma membrane of regulatory cells. This hypothesis is supported by the inhibition of vasospastic attacks by selective α_2-adrenoceptor antagonists and increased sensitivity to agonists in patients with primary Raynaud's phenomenon (Freedman *et al.* 1993, 1995). Additional studies with more specific agonists and antagonists of α_2-adrenoceptors may elucidate the defect(s) present in primary Raynaud's phenomenon.

Non-adrenergic defects in control of regional blood flow may also contribute to primary Raynaud's phenomenon. Non-adrenergic mechanisms may modulate the α_2-adrenergic response by increasing the number of receptors, or they may alter the activity of receptors by changes in the intercellular signal-transduction pathway. Increased production of endothelin-1 (Zamora *et al.* 1990), decreased production of CGRP (perhaps secondary to loss of cutaneous innervation) (Bunker *et al.* 1990), and impaired endothelial function (Bedarida *et al.* 1993) have all been reported in primary Raynaud's phenomenon.

Recent attention has focused on the protein tyrosine kinase signal transduction pathway. Blood vessels taken from patients with primary Raynaud's phenomenon showed increased tyrosine phosphorylation in response to cold-induced contraction compared to control blood vessels (Furspan *et al.* 2004). Both vessel contraction and tyrosine phosphorylation could be inhibited by a protein tyrosine kinase inhibitor leading to the conclusion that tyrosine phosphorylation mediates blood vessel reactivity in Raynaud's patients.

An epidemiological survey reports that women using unopposed estrogen are more likely to have Raynaud's phenomenon, suggesting a negative influence of estrogen on digital vessels (Fraenkel *et al.* 1998);

however, others have demonstrated that the acute infusion of estrogen improves cutaneous blood flow in Raynaud's phenomenon (Lekakis *et al.* 1998). There is increasing *in vitro* and *in vivo* evidence to support the vasodilatory properties of estrogen via the nitric oxide pathway (Generini *et al.* 2005). At this point, the interaction between estrogen and Raynaud's remains unclear.

Secondary Raynaud's phenomenon

Endothelial dysfunction and smooth muscle defects have also been implicated in secondary Raynaud's phenomenon. Depending on the specific disease or type of vascular injury, there may be several reasons for disruption of normal vascular tone. A disease process leading to injury of the endothelium potentially diminishes production of vasodilators such as nitric oxide. Dysfunctional endothelial cells also promote intravascular thrombosis; enhance the release of mediators that activate vascular smooth muscle cells; and promote inflammatory responses by increased expression of adhesion molecules.

Most of the studies investigating the role of the endothelium in secondary Raynaud's phenomenon have been performed in scleroderma, a disease associated with a profound vasculopathy and repeated digital ischemic events that often lead to digital ulcers and amputation. In the digital arteries of scleroderma patients, there is luminal narrowing of more than 75% caused by intimal fibrosis and occlusion of the lumen by thrombi. Evidence of endothelial cell activation is reported in cutaneous vessels (Freemont *et al.* 1992; Prescott *et al.* 1992). These findings suggest the presence of endothelial dysfunction (Pearson 1991).

Platelet activation is also evident in scleroderma, with increased systemic release of thomboxane, a potent vasoconstricting prostaglandin (Reilley *et al.* 1986). Increased platelet adhesion, decreased storage of von Willebrand factor, and decreased adenosine uptake are all manifestations of endothelial damage in scleroderma (Herrick *et al.* 1996). Infusion of L-arginine, the substrate for nitric oxide production, can reverse the vasospasm in the hands of scleroderma patients (Freedman *et al.* 1999), suggesting that defects in nitric oxide production may also exist in scleroderma, but work by Flavahan reports normal endothelial function of scleroderma blood vessels using cutaneous arteries isolated from biopsies of clinically uninvolved skin (Flavahan *et al.* 2000). These *in vitro* studies of scleroderma vessels demonstrate a profound increase in sensitivity (up to 300-fold) to α_2-adrenoceptor-mediator vasoconstriction of smooth muscle, independent of endothelial mechanisms. This study suggests that an early defect in scleroderma may exist in the vascular smooth muscle response, while later the endothelial cell damage occurs, causing a vasculopathy with progressive ischemia that results from an imbalance between vessel loss and angiogenesis.

The vasculopathy in scleroderma is characterized by intimal proliferation thought to be associated with vascular smooth muscle cells having a synthetic or "dedifferentiated" phenotype. It is hypothesized that these cells differ from the normal "differentiated" vascular smooth muscle cell responsible for vascular tone in that they produce extracellular matrix proteins and are involved in vessel remodeling (Flavahan *et al.* 2003). It is also possible that circulating stem cells enter the vessel and differentiate into myofibroblasts with synthetic capacity. The mechanisms involved in vessel remodeling are incompletely understood but likely involve an interplay between extracellular matrix proteins such as elastin and fibrillin-1, various cytokines including transforming growth factor-β, members of the matrix metalloproteinase family of proteases, and reactive oxygen species (Flavahan *et al.* 2003; Bou-Gharios *et al.* 2004; Filippov *et al.* 2005; Su *et al.* 2001). There is phenotypic alteration of the vascular smooth muscle cells with migration to the vascular intima, proliferation, and enhanced extracellular matrix protein secretion with subsequent vessel dysfunction resulting in ischemic damage to underperfused tissue.

These blood vessel lesions occur in the setting of inadequate new blood vessel formation despite elevated circulating levels of vascular endothelial growth factor (Flavahan *et al.* 2003). This suggests additional defects in downstream regulation of angiogenesis but whether this is due to defects in the endothelial cell response to angiogenic stimuli or the presence of inhibitors of angiogenesis is currently not known. Increased levels of the angiogenesis inhibitors endostatin and thrombospondin-1 have been reported in scleroderma (Hebbar *et al.* 2000; Macko *et al.* 2002). In addition, recent studies suggest that there are inadequate numbers of circulating bone marrow-derived endothelial precursors in scleroderma. These cells are normally capable of repairing or remodeling damaged vessels and loss of this function could cause a defect in vasculogenesis (Kuwana *et al.* 2004).

While few studies have investigated directly the mediators of digital ischemia and vasospasm in vasculitis, it is likely that a complex series of events occurs after direct injury to the endothelium, with profound disturbances in normal regulatory mechanisms. Vascular occlusion and damage reduce tissue perfusion, creating ischemia. While ischemia releases potent vasodilators, damaged vessels are unlikely to have normal responses. Thus, it is not surprising to see secondary vasospasm and Raynaud's phenomenon in vasculitic diseases.

Clinical evaluation

Differential diagnosis

Primary Raynaud's is typically elicited by patient history but on occasion the stress associated with a medical visit or entrance into a cold examination room will precipitate an attack. This is especially true for those patients who are more prone to frequent vasospasm. The physician often has the luxury of time when considering potential diagnostic and treatment modalities in these patients. In contrast, the occurrence of critical digit ischemia is a medical emergency. This condition requires a swift diagnostic evaluation and the prompt institution of treatment, usually before the work-up is complete. Before narrowing the focus to the rheumatic conditions, a wide array of diagnostic categories must be excluded (Table 17.2).

An exhaustive description of the clinical evaluation for all causes of digital ischemia is beyond the scope of this chapter, but the following points are pertinent. First, the clinical evaluation begins with a careful history. Following completion of the history, the possibility of an underlying systemic inflammatory condition should be apparent to the examiner. During the physical examination, particular attention may then be directed toward narrowing the differential diagnosis and determining the severity of the disorder. A history of cigarette smoking, particularly when heavy, is relevant to not only to atherosclerosis, but also to Buerger's disease (thromboangiitis obliterans). Obstetrical histories of second

Table 17.2 Differential diagnosis of digital ischemia

Primary Raynaud's phenomenon	Antiphospholipid syndrome
Secondary Raynaud's phenomenon	Blood dyscrasias
Systemic sclerosis	Cryoglobulinemia
Systemic lupus erythematosus	Paraproteinemias
Inflammatory myopathy	Cold agglutinins
Rheumatoid arthritis	Polycythemia vera
Sjögren's syndrome	
Mixed connective tissue disease	
Undifferentiated connective tissue disease	
Vasculitides	Drugs and toxins
Buerger's disease	Ergotamines
Wegener's granulomatosis	Vinblastine
Polyarteritis nodosa	Bleomycin
Microscopic polyangiitis	Amphetamines
Churg–Strauss syndrome	Vinyl chloride exposure
Cryoglobulinemic vasculitis	Clonidine
Takayasu's arteritis	Carboplatin
Giant cell arteritis	Gemcitabine
Structural arterial disease	Occupational
	Hand–arm vibration syndrome
	Hypothenar hammer syndrome
	Other
	Atherosclerosis
	Thoracic outlet syndrome
	Reflex sympathetic dystrophy
	Hypothyroidism
	Cold injury (frostbite)
	Paraneoplastic

or third trimester miscarriages may indicate the antiphospholipid antibody (aPL) syndrome. Occupational histories may reveal risk factors for mechanically-induced digital ischemia, such as the hypothenar hammer syndrome (Pineda *et al.* 1985). Other forms of trauma, such as extreme cold exposure, also constitute information that must be elicited in the patient's history. A history of weight loss or cachexia may provide a clue to an unrecognized malignancy.

Among systemic inflammatory illnesses leading to vessel occlusion, four major disease processes (often not mutually exclusive) pertain. These are: (1) necrotizing inflammation; (2) vasospasm; (3) non-inflammatory vasculopathy; and (4) thrombus formation. In approaching the patient, these four processes may be viewed broadly as corresponding to vasculitic diseases, primary Raynaud's phenomenon, connective tissue diseases, and clotting diatheses (particularly aPL-associated disorders), respectively. This construct is useful, because recognition of the underlying mechanism will allow a logical approach to diagnosis and treatment decisions. Because issues related to thrombosis are covered elsewhere in this text, the following sections focus on the clinical evaluation of patients with digital ischemia caused by the primary mechanisms of vasculitis, vasospasm, and vasculopathy.

Interpreting the color changes

Primary Raynaud's phenomenon is generally mild in nature. Exposure to cold triggers pallor that extends from the digital tip to its middle or base. Sharp color demarcation indicates virtually complete closure of the digital artery and cutaneous arterioles. The pallor remains for a short period of time before cyanosis (a blue/gray or even blackish discoloration) appears, caused by the pooling of slow-flowing, deoxygenated blood. The digital skin and other areas exposed to cold (hands, arms, face, nose, ears, knees, feet) may appear mottled, and remain cyanotic for approximately 15–20 minutes after rewarming. Following reversal of the vasoconstriction, an erythematous blush occurs, caused by hyperemic reperfusion of the digit.

Many patients recall the cyanotic phase of Raynaud's phenomenon vividly but overlook the other phases, particularly the pallor phase. Throughout the attack, patients feel symptoms of numbness, "pins and needles", and discomfort, sometimes accompanied by a sense of limb clumsiness. As noted by Allen and Brown, pain is uncommon in primary Raynaud's phenomenon (Allen and Brown 1932a).

Not every patient reports the classic triphasic color changes (white, blue, and red). Thus, a history of unusual sensitivity to cold and episodic white and blue discoloration of the digital skin in response to cold is sufficient for a diagnosis of Raynaud's phenomenon. A typical attack begins asymmetrically, in one or two fingers. On continued exposure to cold, patients with primary Raynaud's phenomenon may develop pallor of all of the fingers of both hands.

The criteria for diagnosis of primary Raynaud's include symmetric vasospastic attacks precipitated by cold or emotional stress in the absence of tissue necrosis. Patients with this disorder should have no evidence of an underlying secondary cause for Raynaud's and normal laboratory testing including autoantibodies and erythrocyte sedimentation rate. In addition, these patients should have normal nailfold capillaries. Cutaneous capillaries can be examined by placing a drop of immersion oil at the base of the patient's fingernail and viewing the nailfold with an ophthalmoscope set to 10 to 40 diopters or with a stereoscopic microscope. Abnormal capillaries with vessel dilatation or loss of capillary loops suggest a secondary cause of Raynaud's such as scleroderma, dermatomyositis, or systemic lupus erythematosus (Wigley 2002).

Persistent asymmetric attacks, particularly if associated with pain, prolonged ischemia, or tissue ulceration, also suggest secondary Raynaud's phenomenon. These findings are suggestive of a more dramatic disease process affecting blood vessels. In contrast to the findings in primary Raynaud's phenomenon, vessels in patients with secondary causes such as scleroderma are chronically ill with multiple abnormalities (see Pathogenesis section) even in the absence of acute vasospasm. Spasm of these narrowed, fibrotic vessels leads to more startling perfusion deficits in these patients. The index and middle fingers are usually more sensitive to attacks than the other fingers. The thumb is the least sensitive digit. Toes as well as fingers may be affected, but finger involvement is usually more intense. Rarely, a patient with secondary Raynaud's phenomenon has attacks only in the feet.

In vasculitis, the presentation of digital ischemia differs strikingly from primary Raynaud's phenomenon, but may be similar in appearance to secondary Raynaud's phenomenon. Vasculitis patients with digital ischemia present with acutely painful, swollen fingers, and signs of tissue ischemia. The process is usually symmetrical, but often there is a marked disparity between involvement of the upper and lower extremities. The digit is often reddened secondary to the dilatation of small blood vessels, an attempt to foster collateral flow. The fingertips or the sites of subsequent tissue infarction are initially pale, with rims of cyanosis mixed with erythema. The involved digits are exquisitely tender to touch. Pain often extends into the deep tissues of the fingers, hands, and, occasionally, the arms. The pain may be so intense that the patient is unable to sleep, pacing the floor or hanging the ischemic limb over the edge of the bed in an attempt to improve local blood flow. Although the ischemia may wax and wane, it persists without complete recovery, even with prolonged exposure to warmth. If digital ischemia is not reversed by prompt, effective treatment, tissue infarction and gangrene ensue.

Patients with vasculitis-associated digital ischemia seldom recall any pallor phase, noting instead the onset of pain followed by the rapid onset of cyanosis and progression to gangrene. In vasculitis, digital ulceration is a consequence of vascular occlusion, complicated by elements of vasoconstriction.

Physical examination clues

The presence of specific findings on physical examination often differentiate the four major pathophysiologic processes in digital ischemia (vasculitis, vasospasm, vasculopathy, and thrombosis) with a high degree of specificity. Although the entire patient must be considered and examined thoroughly, careful attention to the hands may be particularly instructive:

♦ Patients with primary Raynaud's typically have normal appearing digits in the absence of acute vasospasm.

♦ Connective tissue disorders associated with digital ischemia can result in marked cyanosis (Figure 17.4).

♦ Patients with scleroderma-spectrum illnesses may have sclerodactyly, telangiectasias, hypopigmentation (in dark-skinned individuals), or calcinosis cutis (Figure 17.5).

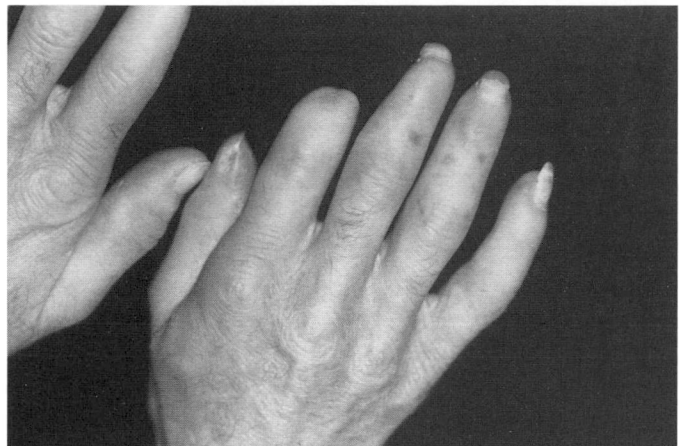

Figure 17.5 Patient with limited systemic sclerosis, sclerodactyly, and telangiectasias.

♦ Capillary loop dilatations, often visible to the naked eye (Figure 17.6), firmly place the underlying illness in the spectrum of connective tissue disease. Normal capillary architecture suggests primary Raynaud's phenomenon.

♦ The loss of digital pulp attests to previous digital infarctions (Figure 17.7), but this may occur in many connective tissue disorders as well as in the vasculitides. Thus, digital pulp atrophy does not distinguish ischemia due to vasculitis from that caused by connective tissue diseases.

♦ A positive Allen's test or the absence of pulses in the wrists or feet suggests the presence of a process involving medium-sized arteries.

♦ In contrast to the vasospasm associated with connective tissue diseases, necrotizing vasculitis commonly causes splinter hemorrhages (Figure 17.8).

Specific clinical testing

Several days elapse before results of most serologic analyses are available and so treatment must begin before the entire diagnostic

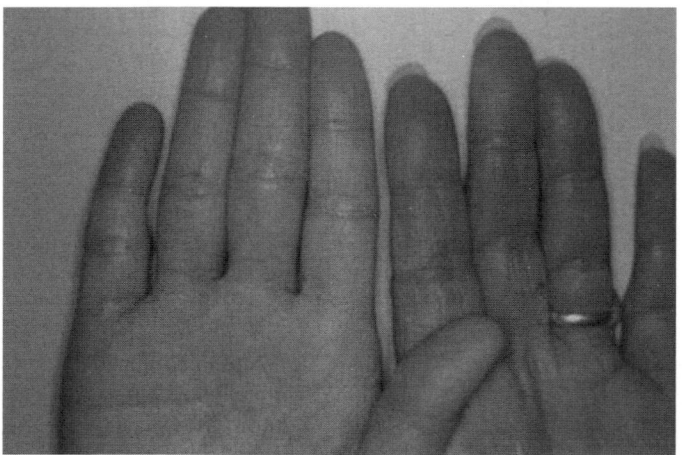

Figure 17.4 Cyanosis in a patient with systemic sclerosis. (See Color Plate 70).

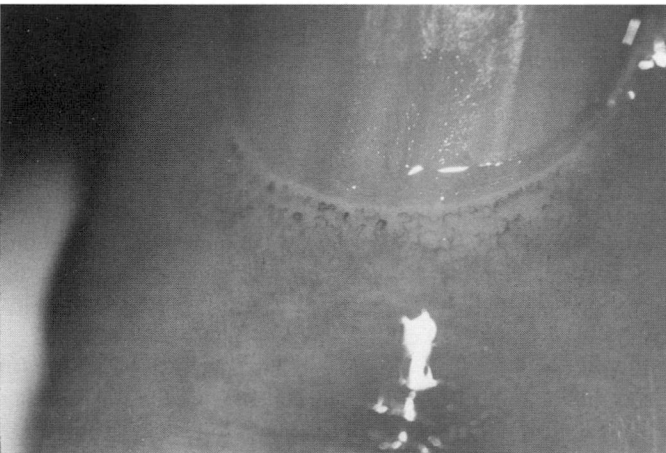

Figure 17.6 Capillary loop dilatation in a patient with systemic sclerosis. (See Color Plate 71).

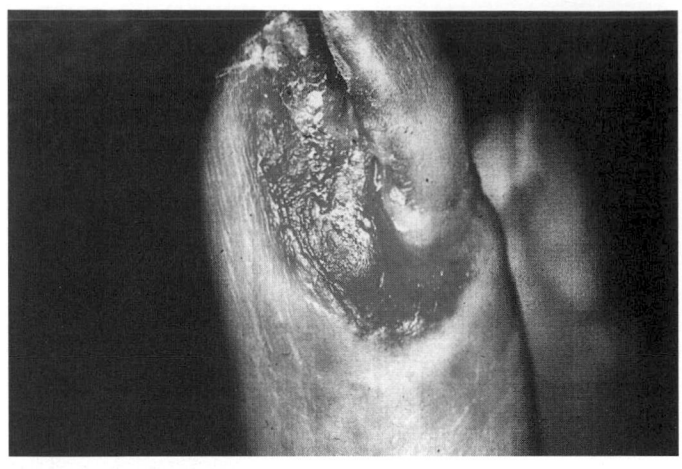

(a)

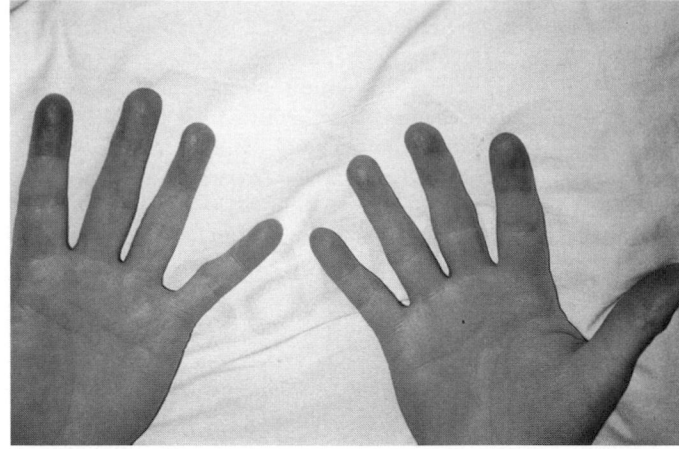

(a)

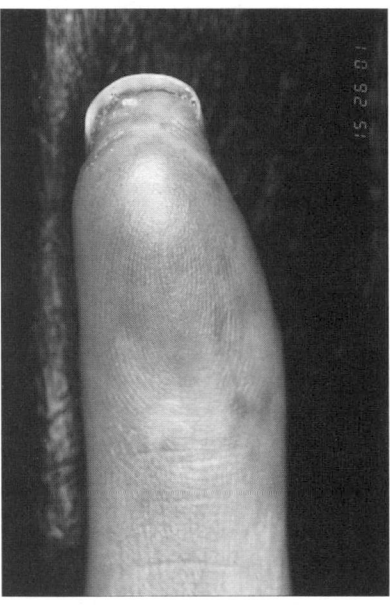

(b)

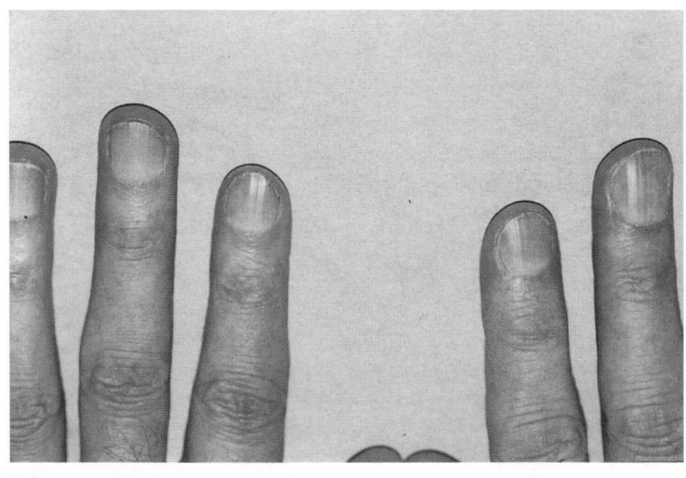

(b)

Figure 17.7 Digital infarction (a), with subsequent loss of digital pulp (b). (See Color Plate 72).

evaluation is complete, but a full work-up is essential to knowledgeable patient management beyond the first few days. The battery of blood and urine tests that is useful in the initial assessment of patients with digital ischemia is displayed in Table 17.3. Selected imaging studies (particularly chest radiography), directed by findings in the history, physical examination, and other evaluations, may also be instructive. Increased acute phase proteins, as indicated by an elevated erythrocyte sedimentation rate or C-reactive protein, are very helpful in distinguishing digital ischemia due to inflammatory causes, that is systemic necrotizing vasculitis or vasculitis associated with a connective tissue disease, from the vasculopathy characterized by intimal fibrosis and vasospasm associated with Raynaud's phenomenon in scleroderma. The presence of a secondary disorder will dictate further diagnostic evaluation.

(c)

Figure 17.8 Digital ischemia in a patient with vasculitis. (a) Purple, cyanotic discoloration on the palmar side. (b) Splinter hemorrhages. (c) Normal fingers again, several months after start of treatment. The splinter hemorrhages have nearly grown out. (See Color Plate 73).

Table 17.3 Useful blood and urine tests in the evaluation of digital ischemia

Blood	
	Complete blood count with differential
	Serum electrolytes and chemistries
	Thyroid-stimulating hormone
	Lipid profile
	Erythrocyte sedimentation rate (or C-reactive protein)
	Antinuclear antibody screen
	Assays for precipitins: anti-Ro, -La, -Sm, -RNP
	C3 and C4 complement levels
	Topoisomerase III (Scl-70) antibodies
	Antineutrophil cytoplasmic antibody assays (positive immunofluorescence tests followed by ELISA for proteinase-3 and myeloperoxidase antibodies)
	Antiphospholipid antibody tests (anticardiolipin antibodies, anti- β_2-glycoprotein I antibodies, assays to detect lupus anticoagulants, rapid plasma reagin)[1]
	Cryoglobulins
	Serum protein electropheresis
Urine	
	Urinalysis with microscopy
	Urine protein electropheresis

[1] Additional investigations may be required if a primary thrombotic process is suspected.

Utility of angiography

The usefulness of angiogram was studied in a group of 103 patients who presented with bilateral Raynaud's phenomenon and had no obvious underlying disease process (Van Vugt *et al.* 2003). Angiography revealed vasospasm in 44 patients, peripheral embolism in eight patients, and vasculitis in six patients (three with Buerger's disease). Somewhat surprisingly, 44 patients had evidence of atherosclerotic disease despite a mean age of 46.7 years. Of these patients, 47% had laboratory evidence of dyslipidemia. These results suggest a high prevalence of atherosclerosis in patients with Raynaud's and this finding requires further investigation.

Angiography is not required for all patients with digital ischemia. In many cases, angiography only serves to confirm what both the patient and clinician already know (that the patient has insufficient blood flow to the extremities) but fails to clarify the cause (Figure 17.9). In general, the careful, astute performance of a history and physical examination, supplemented by selected diagnostic tests of the blood and urine, are more reliable than angiographic procedures in making these distinctions.

The presence of corkscrew-shaped collateral blood vessels at the levels of the wrists or ankles suggests Buerger's disease (thromboangiitis obliterans) (see Chapter 38) in a patient with a compatible history, but the specificity of this finding is imperfect. In the proper clinical setting, angiography of other vascular beds (mesenteric or renal blood vessels) may confirm the diagnosis of polyarteritis nodosa. Finally, angiography of the extremities sometimes provides

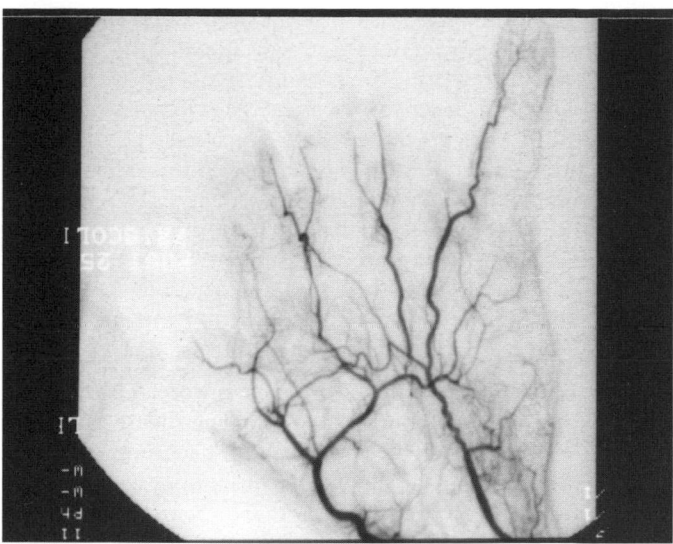

Figure 17.9 Angiogram of a 59-year-old man with severe digital ischemia caused by vasculitis. His digital ischemia resolved entirely with immunosuppression (cyclophosphamide and glucocorticoids). The sharp "cut-off" appearance to the blood vessels cannot be distinguished from thrombosis.

useful information by indicating the extent of disease: substantial territory at risk may support more aggressive treatment with immunosuppressive drugs. The extent of vessel involvement, however, correlates imperfectly with the likelihood of treatment response. In the setting of vasculitis, the decision to add a cytotoxic agent is probably founded more securely on evidence of disease in vital organs or an inadequate response of the digital ischemia to the initial use of glucocorticoids, rather than to the extent of vessel involvement.

Treatment

The principal mode of therapy in digital ischemia associated with rheumatic conditions is predicated on the perceived pathophysiology in each individual patient. Several guidelines are useful in designing the approach to treatment:

♦ For primary Raynaud's phenomenon or for Raynaud's phenomenon caused by a connective tissue disease, treatment should be directed toward reversing vasospasm. An algorithm for the treatment of vasospasm is described below.

♦ In some patients with connective tissue diseases (particularly SLE, dermatomyositis, mixed connective tissue disease, and undifferentiated connective tissue disease), necrotizing vasculitis may be superimposed on a predisposition to vasospasm. In SLE, for example, episodes of Raynaud's phenomenon are usually similar to those that occur in primary Raynaud's phenomenon: relatively painless, uncomplicated, and not associated with ischemia-induced tissue injury. When such a patient develops severe Raynaud's attacks with threatened digital infarction, one must consider the possibility of vasculitis (or thrombotic vascular occlusion secondary to the aPL syndrome). Glucocorticoids alone are usually sufficient to control vasculitis associated with a connective tissue disease.

◆ For patients with digital ischemia caused by a primary systemic necrotizing vasculitis (Wegener's granulomatosis, polyarteritis nodosa, the Churg–Strauss syndrome, or others), immunosuppression is the cornerstone of treatment. In addition to glucocorticoids, these patients often require a cytotoxic agent, usually cyclophosphamide. In such patients, trials of vasodilators may be attempted, but such modalities are unlikely to achieve the dramatic effect they sometimes have in disorders in which vasospasm is the principal mechanism. Furthermore, the use of vasodilators in vasculitis may lead to a steal phenomenon in which the healthy blood vessels dilate but inflamed vessels cannot, which exacerbates ischemia in inflamed tissues.

◆ In the acute setting, thrombosis of the microvasculature may complicate digital ischemia caused by either intense vasospasm or necrotizing vasculitis. Treatment with heparin in the acute phase (while waiting for vasodilators or immunosuppression to take effect) may be prudent, even though few studies provide unequivocal support for this practice. Obviously, anticoagulation should not be employed in patients with pulmonary capillaritis, mesenteric hemorrhage, bleeding into the central nervous system, or other such precarious clinical situations. Long-term anticoagulation with coumadin or low molecular-weight heparin is usually unnecessary.

◆ Finally, certain specific forms of vasculitis, such as Buerger's disease and cryoglobulinemia, may require additional treatment strategies (smoking cessation or antiviral therapy). Approaches to these individual types of vasculitis are discussed elsewhere in this textbook.

Below, we discuss separately the two major therapeutic approaches, vasodilation and immunosuppression.

Treatment of Raynaud's phenomenon

The treatment of Raynaud's phenomenon consists of both pharmacological and non-pharmacological therapies. Avoidance of the cold and other triggering factors are usually sufficient to ameliorate the problem in primary Raynaud's phenomenon. The maintenance of a warm core body temperature (in addition to warm extremities) is a critical element in the treatment of this condition.

Non-pharmacologic interventions are important in secondary Raynaud's phenomenon as well. Indeed, such strategies are the cornerstone of day-to-day management of this problem. Patients with severe Raynaud's phenomenon must reduce any undue demands on the peripheral circulation. Resting the involved limb, reducing repetitive motion or local trauma, and controlling environmental factors such as ambient temperature and emotional stress are essential supporting measures. Patients with severe Raynaud's phenomenon should also modify their work environments to avoid cold temperatures, undue stress, or repeated digital trauma. Although relaxation and behavior modification (cold avoidance and stress management), are important, these measures are unlikely to be curative in patients with secondary Raynaud's phenomenon. Biofeedback plays no important role in the treatment of severe Raynaud's phenomenon (Raynaud's Treatment Study Investigators 2000).

The importance of smoking cessation was addressed by a study of patients with Raynaud's secondary to occupational exposure to a vibratory stimulus (Cherniack *et al.* 2000). In a cross sectional examination of 601 current and former vibratory tool users, symptoms were found to be more severe in those who smoked compared to non-smokers. In a long-term follow-up study of 199 affected individuals who were all removed from the vibration exposure for 2 years, smokers were twice as likely as non-smokers to have continued, severe vasospasm. Thus, even after removal from the stimulus that caused Raynaud's, smokers experienced a delayed improvement in vasospasm compared with non-smokers. It is likely that smoking cessation is beneficial for patients with other forms of Raynaud's phenomenon as well.

Calcium-channel blockers constitute the first-line pharmacologic treatment for patients with Raynaud's phenomenon. A meta-analysis of 18 trials examining calcium channel blockers for primary Raynaud's was published in 2005 (Thompson and Pope 2005). The majority of trials used nifedipine compared with placebo and an overall reduction in both frequency and severity of symptoms was demonstrated. Although improvements were statistically significant, the clinical efficacy was felt to be relatively small. Another meta-analysis has been performed in patients with Raynaud's secondary to scleroderma (Thomopson *et al.* 2001). This study included six randomized, controlled trials of calcium channel blockers (mostly nifedipine) versus placebo. Similar to the analysis of primary Raynaud's patients, this study demonstrated a significant reduction in frequency and severity of symptoms which was determined to be of moderate clinical utility.

Although few studies have used the sustained release preparations of nifedipine, these agents or other newer dihydropyridine calcium channel blockers are the initial pharmacologic treatment of choice in practice, because of their greater ease of use (Sturgill and Seibold 1998). Long-acting dihydropyridine calcium-channel blockers, for example amlopidine, isradipine, and felodipine, have not been rigorously tested, but might be preferable to shorter-acting agents in scleroderma patients because they have less negative inotropic effects (La Civita *et al.* 1993).

If sustained-release calcium-channel blockers are ineffective, a reasonable second approach is to try intermittent dosing with shorter-acting preparations of the same agent, or to switch to a different calcium-channel blocker. The calcium-channel blocker dose must be maximized before an agent is declared a failure. Some clinicians recommend combining different calcium-channel blockers, in recognition of the fact that there are distinct categories of these agents (Spedding and Vanhoutte 1993), but this strategy has not been subjected to a therapeutic trial.

A host of other vasodilating drugs, including nitrates (topical and oral) and sympatholytic agents (reserpine, guanethidine, methyldopa, prazosin, phenoxybenzamine, phentolamine, and others) have been employed in Raynaud's phenomenon (Coffman and Cohen 1987; McFayden *et al.* 1973; Russell and Lessard 1985; Varadi and Lawrence 1969). Although many of these agents have not been studied thoroughly, in general they are less useful than calcium-channel blockers and often have substantial side-effects. Nevertheless, in critical situations, we sometimes combine one of these agents, for example prazosin, with a calcium-channel blocker. A systematic review examining the efficacy of prazosin over placebo reported a modest treatment effect with this drug (Pope *et al.* 1998).

For patients with Raynaud's phenomenon that is refractory to non-pharmacologic measures and to calcium-channel blockers there are now several options including prostaglandins, phosphodiesterase inhibitors, selective serotonin reuptake inhibitors, angiotensin II receptor inhibitors, and angiotensin-converting enzyme inhibitors.

Results with an intravenous prostacyclin analogue (iloprost) have been encouraging. A double-blind, placebo-controlled study of 131 scleroderma patients found that the weekly attack rate decreased by 39% in iloprost-treated patients, compared with a 22% decrease in the placebo group (P = 0.005) (Wigley et al. 1994). A Raynaud's phenomenon severity score decreased by 35% in the iloprost group, compared with 20% in the placebo group (P = 0.011). The results of a 12-month randomized trial comparing cyclic intravenous iloprost with nifedipine were reported in 2001 (Scorza et al. 2001). Iloprost was given as an 8-hour infusion daily for 5 days and subsequently as an 8-hour infusion every 6 weeks. The authors reported significant improvements in skin score and Raynaud's severity in the iloprost group versus the nifedipine group. Intravenous iloprost is currently unavailable in the United States, and two placebo-controlled trials of oral iloprost in scleroderma patients did not reveal statistically significant differences between the treatment and placebo groups (Belch et al. 1995; Wigley et al. 1998a).

Sildenafil is a type 5 phosphodiesterase inhibitor that promotes smooth muscle cell relaxation and vasodilatation. It has recently been shown to be efficacious in a randomized placebo controlled trial of pulmonary hypertension which included scleroderma patients (Galie et al. 2005). There are also now two small studies reporting the efficacy of this agent in treating patients with Raynaud's phenomenon (Fries et al. 2005; Gore and Silver 2005).

Serotonin is released by activated platelets as well as nerve endings and is a potent vasoconstrictor. There have been several case reports of serotonin reuptake inhibitors in the treatment of Raynaud's as well as a recent randomized trial of fluoxetine compared with nifedipine (Rey et al. 2003; Garcia-Porrua et al. 2004; Coleiro et al. 2001). Fluoxetine resulted in significantly improved frequency and severity of Raynaud's symptoms but nifedipine showed only a trend towards improvement. Follow up studies are clearly indicated for these agents.

Angiotensin converting enzyme inhibitors have demonstrated mixed results in several studies of these agents (Hummers and Wigley 2003). Only one of two placebo controlled trials reported benefit. The angiotensin II receptor blocker losartan has shown efficacy in primary Raynaud's but less so in scleroderma patients. These agents have been used at our institution with mixed results.

Endothelin is a small peptide produced by endothelial cells which has potent vasoconstrictive properties. The endothelin receptors can be found on various cell types including endothelial cells, smooth muscle cells, and fibroblasts, and this peptide may play a role in vascular remodeling and disease pathogenesis. Bosentan, an endothelin receptor antagonist, is effective in treating pulmonary hypertension associated with scleroderma (Rubin et al. 2002). In addition, this drug is effective in preventing new digital ulcers and improving hand function in scleroderma patients (Korn et al. 2004). Despite this finding, Bosentan did not improve symptoms of Raynaud's phenomenon.

In addition to drug therapy for Raynaud's phenomenon, there has been increased interest in low-level laser therapy as a non-pharmacologic modality for primary and secondary Raynaud's. Two short-term, randomized, placebo controlled trials of low-level laser therapy applied to the hands of patients reported improvements in both frequency and severity of Raynaud's (Al-Awami et al. 2004; Hirschl et al. 2004). Longer-term trials are needed to confirm the benefit of laser treatment but the results to date are intriguing. The biological mechanism of laser therapy is currently unclear but may deserve more attention.

In severe cases of Raynaud's phenomenon that are refractory to oral agents, the use of intravenous prostacyclin (PGI$_2$, Flolan), approved for use in primary pulmonary hypertension, may be considered (Wigley et al. 1998b). This agent was beneficial for scleroderma-associated pulmonary hypertension in a randomized controlled trial that also showed trends towards improved Raynaud's severity in these patients (Badesch et al. 2000).

Some cases of Raynaud's phenomenon are complicated by digital ulcerations, with critical ischemia and demarcation of the involved digit(s). These patients may require hospitalization. Attempts to maximize blood flow to the involved extremity should include all of the modalities described for the treatment of Raynaud's phenomenon. Maintenance of rest in a warm environment is essential. In addition to calcium-channel blockers, we treat patients who have ischemic digital ulcers with aspirin, 325 mg/day. Surgical interventions may include temporary lumbar, cervical, or digital sympathetic blocks, to determine the potential of sympathectomy for reversing acute vasospasm (Flatt 1983). We often employ repeated digital nerve blocks in the acute setting, using bupivicaine every 12 hours. Permanent sympathectomies may be attempted if the temporary blocks are successful. Digital sympathectomies are safer and may be more useful than more proximal procedures (Zachary et al. 1997). Finally, even if the condition progresses to digital gangrene, surgical amputation of digits should be avoided acutely, and autoamputation should be allowed to occur.

Future therapies will likely be directed against more selected targets. A recent, small study of an investigational agent has focused treatment on advances in the pathophysiology of cold-induced vasospasm (Wise et al. 2004). This study examined the time to recovery of skin temperature after a cold challenge in scleroderma patients given a selective inhibitor of the α_{2C} receptor. As discussed in the Pathogenesis section of this chapter, the α_{2C} adrenergic receptor is thought to mediate vasoconstriction in response to cold. Patients given the study drug had shorter temperature recovery times compared to patients given placebo. Larger studies are needed to define the role of this agent in Raynaud's phenomenon, but this represents a potential advance in selective targeting of drugs to the relevant disease causing mechanism. Inhibitors of the Rho/Rho kinase system that allows translocation of the α_{2C} receptor to the cell surface are currently under investigation. Lastly, antioxidants may be helpful in that oxidative stress stimulates Rho/Rho kinase signaling and mobilization of α_{2C} to the cell surface (Bailey et. al. 2005). Preliminary studies with probucol (Denton et al. 1999) and N-acetylcysteine (Sambo et al. 2001) suggest benefit of antioxidant therapy.

Treatment of digital ischemia caused by systemic necrotizing vasculitis

Patients presenting with digital ischemia of a suspected inflammatory cause should be hospitalized. Analogous to the treatment of myocardial infarction, the first 24 hours after presentation to a physician may be critical in determining outcome. In addition to the attention that must be directed to treatment of the digital ischemia and to pain control, patients must be carefully assessed for the extent and severity of disease in other organs. Patients presenting with digital ischemia often have rapidly progressive disease of the kidneys, lungs, nerves, and gastrointestinal tract.

The non-pharmacological treatments discussed with regard to the treatment of secondary Raynaud's phenomenon are directly applicable to the management of digital ischemia in vasculitis as well. A warm environment is essential, and substantial narcotic analgesia may be required for some weeks. The first line of treatment for digital ischemia associated with systemic necrotizing vasculitis is high-dose glucocorticoid therapy. In practice, we employ 3-day intravenous pulses of methylprednisolone in patients with severe, digit- or limb-threatening ischemia. In patients with less severe ischemia and no evidence of other critical organ involvement, we sometimes give lower glucocorticoid doses, such as methylprednisolone, 1 mg/kg/day, or oral daily prednisone. As a rule, in the absence of significant contraindications to high doses of glucocorticoids, it is proper to err on the side of administering too much glucocorticoid treatment in the first few days, because the side-effects of such therapy are usually well-tolerated (or manageable) in the short-term and are unlikely to be lasting. However, careful attention must be paid to the management of potential side-effects of longer-term glucocorticoid treatment such as osteoporosis prevention, careful glucose and blood pressure monitoring, and prompt treatment of infections.

Some patients with necrotizing vasculitis, particularly those whose disease involvement is limited to the extremities, respond well to glucocorticoids alone. These patients typically have dramatic responses within 24 hours of glucocorticoid administration. Others, however, manifest only moderate responses to glucocorticoids and, at the completion of a 3-day methylprednisolone pulse, fail to demonstrate sustained improvement. These patients, as well as those with evidence of organ- or life-threatening disease in other systems, should be treated with cyclophosphamide, in addition to glucocorticoids. For vasculitis patients receiving the combination of glucocorticoids and cyclophosphamide, we routinely administer trimethoprim-sulfamethoxazole (TMP/SMZ) (one double-strength tablet by mouth each day) as prophylaxis against *Pneumocystis carinii* pneumonia. Patients who are allergic to TMP/SMZ may receive instead dapsone 100 mg daily.

Regardless of their initial response to glucocorticoids, all patients with digital ischemia must be followed carefully until their disease is under good control. Digital ischemia may herald organ-threatening vasculitis in other systems that require cyclophosphamide, and such organ involvement may not be evident at presentation. Consequently, we re-evaluate patients not longer than 1 week following discharge from the hospital. The duration of immunosuppressive therapy for each patient must be individualized, but may be predicted in large measure from the precise type of underlying vasculitis. Whereas the ANCA-associated vasculitides generally require concomitant glucocorticoids and cyclophosphamide therapy, other forms of vasculitis may respond adequately to prednisone alone. These issues are discussed in other chapters of this book.

In the weeks after the initiation of treatment, assessment of disease activity in patients with digital vasculitis presents a challenging task. Blood vessels damaged by the acute vasculitic injury may never return to their premorbid condition. Fingers involved by the inflammation become cyanotic when exposed to cold for months afterward, and even in normal temperatures may remain cool to touch for years, without advancement of the ischemic process or further threats to tissue viability. In such cases, a stable pattern of digital coolness, that is involvement of the same fingers or toes from one visit to the next, rather than spread of involvement to previously uninvolved digits, is reassuring.

Necrotic fingertips and toes may require many months for the painful process of auto-amputation to occur. Months after the inflammatory process has been arrested, selected patients with digital necrosis secondary to vasculitis may be candidates for surgical removal of necrotic tissue. This procedure provides substantial pain relief and causes little loss of viable tissue, provided that the process of autoamputation has advanced sufficiently.

References

Al-Awami, M., Schillinger, M., Maca, T., Polanz, S. and Minar, E. (2004). Low level laser therapy for treatment of primary and secondary Raynaud's phenomenon. *VASA. Zeitschrift Für Uefäskrankheiten. Journal for Vascular Diseases*, **33**, 25–9.

Aldoori, M., Bruce, W. and Dieppe, P. (1986). Nifedipine in the treatment of Raynaud's syndrome. *Cardiovascular Research*, **20**, 466–9.

Allen, E. and Brown, G. (1932a). Raynaud's disease: a critical review of minor requisites for diagnosis. *American Journal of the Medical Sciences*, **183**, 187–200.

Allen, E and Brown, G. (1932b). Raynaud's disease: A clinical study of one hundred and forty-seven cases. *Journal of the American Medical Association*, **99**, 1472–8.

Andreu-Sanchez, J., Martin-Santos, J., Isasi-Zaragoza, C., Trujillo-Castellanos, A., Cuende-Quintana, E. and Mulero, J. (1991). Raynaud's phenomenon as initial manifestation of cutaneous polyarteritis nodosa. *Annals of the Rheumatic Diseases*, **50**, 48–50.

Badesch, D. B., Tapson, V. F., McGoon, M. D., *et al.* (2000). Continuous intravenous epoprostenol for pulmonary hypertension due to the scleroderma spectrum of disease. *Annals of Internal Medicine*, **132**, 425–34.

Bailey S. R., Eid, A. H., Mitra, S., Flavahan, S. and Flavahan, N. A. (2004). Rho kinase mediates cold-induced constriction of cutaneous arteries. *Circulation Research*, **94**, 1367–74.

Bailey S. R., Mitra, S., Flavahan, S. and Flavahan, N. A. (2005). Reactive oxygen species from smooth muscle mitochondria initiate cold-induced constriction of cutaneous arteries. *American Journal of Physiology – Heart and Circulatory Physiology*, **289**, 243–50.

Bartelink, M., Wollersheim, H., van de Lisdonk, E. *et al.* (1992). Prevalence of Raynaud's phenomenon. *Netherlands Journal of Medicine*, **41**, 149–52.

Bedarida, G., Kim, D., Blaschke, T. *et al.* (1993). Venodilation in Raynaud's disease. *Lancet*, **342**, 1451–4.

Belch, J. (1990). The phenomenon, syndrome and disease of Maurice Raynaud. *British Journal of Rheumatology*, **29**, 162–5.

Belch, J., Capell, H., Cooke, E. *et al.* (1995). Oral iloprost as a treatment for Raynaud's syndrome: A double-blind multicentre placebo-controlled study. *Annals of the Rheumatic Diseases*, **54**, 197–200.

Bombardier, C., Gladman, D., Urowitz, M., Caron, D., Chang, C. *et al.* (1989). Derivation of the SLEDAI: A disease activity index for lupus patients. *Arthritis and Rheumatism*, **35**, 630–40.

Bou-Gharios, G., Ponticos M., Rajkumar, V. and Abranham, D. (2004). Extra-cellular matrix in vascular networks. *Cell Proliferation*, **37**, 207–20.

Bunker, C., Terenghi, G., Springall, D. *et al.* (1990). Deficiency of calcitonin gene-related peptide in Raynaud's phenomenon. *Lancet*, **336**, 1530–3.

Cherniack, M., Clive, J., and Seidner, A. (2000). Vibration exposure, smoking, and vascular dysfunction. *Occupational and Environmental Medicine*, **57**, 341–47.

Chotani, M., Flavahan, S., Mitra, S., *et al.* (2000). Silent alpha(2C)-adrenergic receptors enable cold-induced vasoconstriction in cutaneous arteries. *American Journal of Physiology – Heart and Circulatory Physiology*, **278**, H1075–83.

Coffman, J. and Cohen, R. (1987). Intra-arterial vasodilator agents to reverse finger vasoconstriction. *Clinical Pharmacological Therapy*, **41**, 574–88.

Coffman, J. and Cohen, R. (1988). Role of alpha-adrenoceptor subtypes mediating sympathetic vasoconstriction in human digits. *European Journal of Clinical Investigation*, **18**, 309–13.

Coleiro, B., Marshall, S. E., Denton, C. P., *et al.* (2001). Treatment of Raynaud's phenomenon with the selective serotonin reuptake inhibitor fluoxetine. *Rheumatology*, **40**, 1038–43.

De Angelis, R., Del Medico, P., Blasetti, P. and Cervini, C. (2003). Raynaud's phenomenon: clinical spectrum of 118 patients. *Clinical Rheumatology*, **22**, 279–84.

Denton C. P., Bunce T. D., Darado M. B., *et al.* (1999). Probucol improves symptoms and reduces lipoprotein oxidation susceptibility in patients with Raynaud's phenomenon. *Rheumatology*, **38**, 309–15.

Ekenvall, L., Lindblad, L., Norbreck, O. *et al.* (1988). α-Adrenoceptors and cold-induced vasoconstriction in human finger skin. *American Journal of Physiology*, **255**, H1000–3.

Filippov, S., Koenig, G. C., Chun, T., *et al.* (2005). MT1-matrix metalloproteinase directs arterial wall invasion and neointima formation by vascular smooth muscle cells. *Journal of Experimental Medicine*, **202**, 663–71.

Finch, M., Dawson, J., Johnston, G. *et al.* (1986). The peripheral vascular effects of nifedipine in Raynaud's syndrome associated with scleroderms: A double-blind crossover study. *Clinical Rheumatology*, **5**, 493.

Flatt, A. (1983). Digital arterial sympathectomy. *Journal of Hand Surgery* [American], **8**, 283–8.

Flavahan, N. A., Lindblad, L. E., Verbeuren, T. J. *et al.* (1985). Cooling and α_1- and α_2-adrenergic responses in cutaneous veins: Role of receptor-reserve. *American Journal of Physiology*, **249**, H950–5.

Flavahan, N. A., Flavahan, S., Liu, Q., Wu, S., Tidmore, W., Wiener, C. M., Spence, R. J., and Wigley, F. M. (2000). Increased α_2-adrenergic constriction of isolated arterioles in diffuse scleroderma. *Arthritis and Rheumatism*, **43**, 1886–90.

Flavahan, N. A., Flavahan, S., Mitra, S., and Chotani, M. (2003). The vasculopathy of Raynaud's phenomenon and scleroderma. *Rheumatic Disease Clinics of North America*, **29**, 275–91.

Fraenkel, L. Zhang, Y., Chaisson, C. E., *et al.* (1998). The association of estrogen replacement therapy and the Raynaud's phenomenon in postmenopausal women. *Annals of Internal Medicine*, **129**, 208–11.

Freedman, R., Moten, M., Migaly, P. *et al.* (1993). Cold-induced potentiation of α_2-adrenergic vasoconstriction in primary Raynaud's disease. *Arthritis and Rheumatism*, **36**, 685–90.

Freedman, R., Baer, R. and Mayes, M. (1995). Blockade of vasospastic attacks by a$_2$-adrenergic but not a$_1$-adrenergic antagonists in idiopathic Raynaud's disease. *Circulation*, **92**, 1448–51.

Freedman, R., Girgis, R. and Mayes, M. (1999). Acute effect of nitric oxide on Raynaud's phenomenon in scleroderma. *Lancet*, **354**, 739.

Freemont, A., Hoyland, J., Fielding, P. *et al.* (1992). Studies of microvascular endothelium in uninvolved skin of patients with systemic sclerosis: Direct evidence for a generalized microangiopathy. *British Journal of Dermatology*, **126**, 561–8.

Friedman, E. I., Taylor, L. M. Jr, and Porter, J. M. (1988). Late-onset Raynaud's syndrome: Diagnostic and therapeutic considerations. *Geriatrics*, **43**, 59–70.

Fries, R., Shariat, K., von Wilmowsky, H. and Bohm, M. (2005). Sildenafil in the treatment of Raynaud's phenomenon resistant to vasodilatory therapy. *Circulation*, **112**, 2980–5.

Furspan, P. B., Chatterjee, S. and Freedman, R. R. (2004). Increased tyrosine phosphorylation mediates the cooling-induced contraction and increased vascular reactivity of Raynaud's disease. *Arthritis and Rheumatism*, **50**, 1578–85.

Galie, N., Ghofrani, H. A., Torbicki, A., *et al.* (2005). Sildenafil citrate therapy for pulmonary arterial hypertension. *New England Journal of Medicine*, **353**, 2148–57.

Garcia-Porrua, C., Margarinos, C. C. and Gonzalez-Gay, M. A. (2004). Raynaud's phenomenon and serotonin reuptake inhibitors. *Journal of Rheumatology*, **31**, 2090–1.

Gelber, A., Wigley, F., Stallings, R., Bone, L., Barker, A., Baylor, I. *et al.* (1999). Raynaud's phenomenon in an inner-city African American community: Prevalence of symptoms, health status, and co-morbid cardiovascular disease. *Journal of Clinical Epidemiology*, **52**, 441–6.

Generini, S., Seibold, J. and Matucci-Cerinic, M. (2005). Estrogens and neuropeptides in Raynaud's phenomenon. *Rheumatic Disease Clinics of North America*, **31**, 177–86.

Gore, J. and Silver, R. (2005). Oral sildenafil for the treatment of Raynaud's phenomenon and digital ulcers secondary to systemic sclerosis. *Annals of Rheumatic Disease*, **64**, 1387.

Grassi, W., De Angelis, R., Lapadula, G., Leardini, G. and Scarpa, R. (1998). Clinical diagnosis found in patients with Raynaud's phenomenon: a multicenter study. *Rheumatology International*, **18**, 17–20.

Hadler, N. (1998). 'Primary Raynaud's' is not a disease or even a disorder; It's a trait. *Journal of Rheumatology*, **25**, 2291–4.

Hebbar, M., Peyrat, J. P., Hornez, L., *et al.* (2000). Increased concentrations of the circulating angiogenesis inhibitor endostatin in patients with systemic sclerosis. *Arthritis and Rheumatism*, **43**, 889–93.

Herrick, A., Illingworth, K., Blann, A. *et al.* (1996). Von Willebrand factor, thrombomodulin thromboxane, B-thromboglobulin, and markers of fibrinolysis in primary Raynaud's phenomenon and systemic sclerosis. *Annals of the Rheumatic Diseases*, **55**, 122–7.

Hirschl, M., Katzenschlager, R., Francesconi, C. and Kundi, M. (2004). Low level laser therapy in primary Raynaud's phenomenon – results of a placebo controlled double blind intervention study. *Journal of Rheumatology*, **31**, 2408–12.

Hummers, L. K. and Wigley, F. M. (2003). Management of Raynaud's phenomenon and digital ischemic lesions in scleroderma. *Rheumatic Disease Clinics of North America*, **29**, 293–313.

Hutchinson, J. (1896). Acro-scleroderma following Raynaud's phenomenon. *Clinical Journal*, **7**, 240.

Hutchinson, J. (1901). Raynaud's phenomenon. *Medical Press*, **123**, 403–5.

Inaba, R., Maeda, M., Fujita, S., Kashiki, N., Komura, Y., Nagata, C. *et al.* (1993). Prevalence of Raynaud's phenomenon and specific clinical signs related to progressive systemic sclerosis in the general population of Japan. *International Journal of Dermatology*, **32**, 652–5.

Jennette, J., Falk, R., Andrassy, K. *et al.* (1994). Nomenclature of systemic vasculitides. Proposal of an international consensus conference. *Arthritis and Rheumatism*, **37**, 187–92.

Jeyaraj, S. C., Chotani, M. A., Mitra, S., Gregg, H. E., Flavahan, N. A. and Morrison, K. J. (2001). Cooling evokes redistribution of α_{2C}-adrenoceptors from golgi to plasma membrane in transfected human embryonic kidney 293 cells. *Molecular Pharmacology*, **60**, 1195–200.

Korn, J. H., Mayes, M., Cerinic, M. M., *et al.* (2004). Digital ulcers in systemic sclerosis. *Arthritis and Rheumatism*, **50**, 3985–93.

Kuwana, M., Okazaki, Y., Yasuoka, H., Kawakami, Y. and Ikeda, Y. (2004). Defective vasculogenesis in systemic sclerosis. *Lancet*, **364**, 603–10.

La Civita, L., Pitaro, N., Rossi, M. *et al.* (1993). Amlodipine in the treatment of Raynaud's phenomenon. *British Journal of Rheumatology*, **32**, 524–5.

Lekakis, J. Mavrikakis, M., Papamichael, C. *et al.* (1998). Short-term estrogen administration improves abnormal endothelial function in women with systemic sclerosis and Raynaud's phenomenon. *American Heart Journal*, **136**, 905–12.

Leppert, J., Aberg, H., Ringqvist, I. and Sorensson, S. (1987). Raynaud's phenomenon in a female population: Prevalence and association with other conditions. *Angiology*, **38**, 871–7.

LeRoy, E. and Medsger, T. (1992). Raynaud's phenomenon: A proposal for classification. *Clinical and Experimental Rheumatology*, **10**, 485–8.

Lewis, T. and Pickering, G. (1933). Observations upon maladies in which the blood supply to digits ceases intermittently or permanently, and upon bilateral gangrene of digits; observations to so called 'Raynaud's disease'. *Clinical Science*, **1**, 327–66.

Lie, J. (1994). Nomenclature and classification of vasculitis: Plus ca change, plus c'est la meme chose. *Arthritis and Rheumatism*, **37**, 181–6.

Macko, R. F., Gelber, A. C., Young, B. A., et al. (2002). Increased circulating concentrations of the counteradhesive proteins sparc and thrombospondin-1 in systemic sclerosis (scleroderma). Relationship to platelet and endothelial cell activation. *Journal of Rheumatology*, **29**, 2565–70.

Maricq, H., Weinrich, M., Keil, J. et al. (1989). Prevalence of scleroderma spectrum disorders in the general population of South Carolina. *Arthritis and Rheumatism*, **32**, 998–1006.

Maricq, H., McGregor, A., Diat, F., Smith, E., Maxwell, D., LeRoy, C. et al. (1990). Major clinical diagnoses found among patients with Raynaud's phenomenon from the general population. *Journal of Rheumatology*, **17**, 1171–6.

Maricq, H., Carpentier, P., Weinrich, M. et al. (1993). Geographic variation in the prevalence if Raynaud's phenomenon: Charleston, SC, USA, versus Tarentaise, Savoie, France. *Journal of Rheumatology*, **20**, 70–6.

McFayden, I., Housley, E. and Macherson, A. (1973). Intra-arterial reserpine administration on Raynaud's syndrome. *Archives of Internal Medicine*, **132**, 256–60.

Mohrland, J., Porter, J., Smith, E. et al. (1985). A multiclinic, placebo-controlled, double-blind study of prostaglandin E_1 in RP. *Annals of the Rheumatic Diseases,*, **44**, 754–60.

Onbasi, K., Sahin, I., Onbasi, O., Ustun, Y. and Koca, D. (2005). Raynaud's phenomenon in a healthy Turkish population. *Clinical Rheumatology*, **24**, 365–9.

Pearson, J. (1991). The endothelium: Its role in scleroderma. *Annals of the Rheumatic Diseases*, **50**, 866–71.

Philipp, M., Brede, M. and Hein, L. (2002). Physiological significance of α_2-adrenergic receptor subtype diversity: one receptor is not enough. *American Journal of Physiology – Regulatory, Integrative, and Comparative Physiology*, **283**, R287–95.

Pineda, C., Weisman, M., Bookstein, J. and Saltzstein, S. (1985). Hypothenar hammer syndrome. Form of reversible Raynaud's phenomenon. *American Journal of Medicine*, **79**, 561–70.

Pope, J., Fenlon, D., Thompson, A., et al. (1998). Prazosin for Raynaud's phenomenon in progressive systemic sclerosis. *Cochrane Database of Systematic Reviews*, **2**, CD000956.

Porter, J., Bardana, E., Baur, G. et al. (1976). The clinical significance of Raynaud's syndrome. *Surgery*, **80**, 756–64.

Prescott, R., Freemont, A., Jones, C. et al. (1992). Sequential dermal microvascular and perivascular changes in the development of scleroderma. *Journal of Pathology*, **166**, 255–63.

Rademaker, M., Cooke, E., Almond, N. et al. (1989). Comparison of intravenous infusions of iloprost and oral nifedipine in the treatment of RP in patients with systemic sclerosis. *British Medical Journal*, **298**, 561–3.

Raynaud, M. (1862). *De l'asphyxie locale et de la gangréne symétrique des extrémités*. Rignoux, Paris. [Raynaud's Treatment Study Investigators (2000). Comparison of sustained-released nifedipine and temperature biofeedback for treatment of primary Raynaud phenomenon: Results from a randomized clinical trial with 1-year follow-up. *Archives of Internal Medicine*. **160**, 1101–8.]

Reilly, I., Roy, L. and Fitzgerald, G. (1986). Biosynthesis of thromboxane in patients with systemic sclerosis and Raynaud's phenomenon. *British Medical Journal*, **292**, 1037–9.

Rey, J., Cretel, E., Jean, R., Pastor, M. J. and Durand, J. M. (2003). Serotonin reuptake inhibitors, Raynaud's phenomenon and erythromelalgia. *Rheumatology*, **42**, 601–2

Riera, D., Vilardell, M., Vaque, J. et al. (1993). Prevalence of Raynaud's phenomenon in a healthy Spanish population. *Journal of Rheumatology*, **20**, 66–9.

Rodeheffer, R., Rommer, J., Wigley, F. et al. (1983). Controlled double-blind trial of nifedipine in the treatment of Raynaud's phenomenon. *New England Journal of Medicine*, **308**, 880–5.

Rubin, L. J., Badesch, D. B., Barst, R. J., et al. (2002). Bosentan therapy for pulmonary arterial hypertension. *New England Journal of Medicine*, **346**, 896–903.

Russell, L. and Lessard, J. (1985). Prazosin treatment of Raynaud's phenomenon: A double-blind single crossover study. *Journal of Rheumatology*, **12**, 94–102.

Sambo P., Amico D., Giacomelli R., et al. (2001). Intravenous N-acetylcysteine for treatment of Raynaud's phenomenon secondary to systemic sclerosis: a pilot study. *Journal of Rheumatology*, **28**, 2257–62.

Sauza, J., Kraus, A., Gonzales-Amaro, R. et al. (1984). Effect if the calcium channel blocker nifedipine in Raynaud's phenomenon: A double-blind trial. *Journal Rheumatology*, **11**, 362–8.

Scorza, R., Caronni, M., Mascagni, B., et al. (2001). Effects of long-term cyclic iloprost therapy in systemic sclerosis with Raynaud's phenomenon. A randomized, controlled study. *Clinical and Experimental Rheumatology*, **19**, 503–8.

Smith, D. and McKendry, R. (1982). Controlled trial of nifedipine in the treatment of Raynaud's phenomenon. *Lancet*, **2**, 1299.

Spedding, M. and Vanhoutte, P. (1993). Nomenclature of calcium channel and channel modulators. *Journal of Cardiovascular Pharmacology*, **22**, 906–8.

Sturgill, M. and Seibold, J. (1998). Rational use of calcium-channel antagonists in Raynaud's phenomenon. *Current Opinion in Rheumatology*, **10**, 584–8.

Su, B., Mitra, S., Gregg, H., et al. (2001). Redox regulation of vascular smooth muscle cell differentiation. *Circulation Research*, **89**, 39–46.

Suter, L. G., Murabito, J. M., Felson, D. T., Fraenkel, L. (2005). The incidence and natural history of Raynaud's phenomenon in the community. *Arthritis and Rheumatism*, **52**, 1259–63.

Thompson, A. E., Shea, B., Welch, V., Fenlon, D. and Pope, J. E. (2001). Calcium-channel blockers for Raynaud's phenomenon in systemic sclerosis. *Arthritis and Rheumatism*, **44**, 1841–7.

Thompson, A. E. and Pope, J. E. (2005). Calcium-channel blockers for Primary Raynaud's phenomenon: a meta-analysis. *Rheumatology*, **44**, 145–50.

Valter, I, and Maricq, H. (1997). Prevalence of Raynaud phenomenon in Tartu and Tartumaa, southern Estonia. *Scandinavian Journal of Rheumatology*, **26**, 117–24.

Van Vugt, R. M., Kater, L., Dijkstra, P. F., Schardijn, G. H.C., Kastelein, J. J.P. and Bijlsma, J. W.J. (2003). The outcome of angiography in patients with Rayndaud's phenomenon: An unexpected role for atherosclerosis and hypercholesterolemia. *Clinical and Experimental Rheumatology*, **21**, 445–50.

Varadi, D. and Lawrence, A. (1969). Suppression of Raynaud's phenomenon by methyldopa. *Archives of Internal Medicine*, **124**, 13.

Wigley, F., Wise, R., Seibold, J. et al. (1994). Intravenous iloprost onfusion in patients with RP secondary to systemic sclerosis. *Annals of Internal Medicine*, **120**, 199–206.

Wigley, F., Badesch, D., Rubin, L. et al. (1998a). The effect of epoprostenol (E) on Raynaud's phenomenon (RP) in patients with scleroderma spectrum of disease (SSD) and pulmonary hypertension (PH). *Arthritis and Rheumatism*, **41**, S1243.

Wigley, F., Korn, J., Csuka, M., Medsger, T., Rothfield, N., Ellman, M. et al. (1998b). Oral iloprost in patients with Raynaud phenomenon secondary to systemic sclerosis: A multicenter, placebo-controlled, double-blind study. *Arthritis and Rheumatism*, **41**, 670–7.

Wigley, F. (2002). Raynaud's phenomenon. *New England Journal of Medicine*, **347,** 1001–8.

Wise, R. A., Wigley, F. M., White, B., *et al.* (2004). Efficacy and tolerability of a selective α_{2C}-adrenergic receptor blocker in recovery from cold-induced vasospasm in scleroderma patients. *Arthritis and Rheumatism*, **50,** 3994–4001.

Zachary, L., Rice-Puoci, F. and Ellman, M. (1997). Digital sympathectomy for fingertip ulcerations/infarctions in scleroderma patients. *Arthritis and Rheumatism*, **40,** S1339.

Zamora, M., O'Brien, R., Rutherford, R. *et al.* (1990). Serum endothelin-1 concentrations and cold provocation in primary Raynaud's phenomenon. *Lancet*, **336,** 1144–7.

PART 4

Imaging and percutaneous interventions

Angiography has long been established as the imaging modality allowing high resolution detail of the lumen of vessels; however, it is increasingly replaced by non-invasive cross-sectional imaging studies in the evaluation of vasculitis. These newer techniques are less invasive than conventional angiography, and can portray the lumen and changes occurring within the vessel wall, often at an early stage of disease when medical intervention is most effective. Unlike conventional angiography, cross-sectional imaging can also disclose changes in affected organs.

Choosing between invasive and non-invasive imaging studies may be influenced by availability of equipment and radiologists skilled in the performance and interpretation of the procedures. Other factors which may dictate choice of procedures include concern for exposure to ionizing radiation, particularly in childhood, and the desirability of follow-up imaging to determine the course of disease and its treatment. In the last few years, cross-sectional imaging procedures have evolved more than angiography, which nevertheless still provides superior resolution of small and peripheral vessels. The more static nature of angiographic techniques compared to cross-sectional imaging is evident in a comparison between the relevant chapters in the first edition of this text, and their present form, which shows only slight changes in the chapter on conventional angiography (Chapter 18), and impressive advances in the chapter on cross-sectional imaging (Chapter 19) as well as a new chapter on positron emission tomography (Chapter 20).

CHAPTER 18

Angiography and percutaneous interventions

Souheil Saddekni, Larry Horesh, Robert Leonardo, and Saravanan Kasthuri

Introduction

The end result of the inflammatory process in vasculitis is a broad range of vascular changes including stenoses, occlusions, aneurysms, and pseudoaneurysms. The arterial vasculitides are classified based on their etiology or their anatomical vessel involvement (see Chapter 1). The anatomic classification adopted for angiographic purposes divides vasculitis into three categories: (1) large vessels, (2) small and medium vessels, and (3) vessels of all sizes. Most vasculitis involving predominantly large vessels are one of two types: Takayasu's arteritis and giant cell arteritis. Vasculitis of medium and small vessels include polyarteritis nodosa/ microscopic angiitis and Buerger's disease (thromboangiitis obliterans). Many vasculitides involve vessels of all sizes, including connective tissue diseases, substance abuse vasculitis, Behçet's syndrome, and infection-related arteritis.

Diagnosis of these vascular inflammatory disorders is sometimes difficult. The clinical features are variable and are often the result of an occlusive process and abnormal blood flow through the affected vessels, which may cause organ ischemia, organ damage and, less frequently, vessel rupture. The occlusive process is not unique to these disorders; in fact, it is more commonly encountered in atherosclerosis. Therefore, the clinical presentation, laboratory results, type and pattern of vascular involvement, and angiographic features are all important for definitive diagnosis and treatment.

Certain characteristic patterns are highly specific and nearly diagnostic. For example, when stenoses or occlusions of the aortic arch or arch vessels are encountered, the only major diagnostic considerations are atherosclerotic disease (see Chapter 45), giant cell arteritis (GCA) (see Chapter 24), and in younger individuals, Takayasu's arteritis (TA) (see Chapter 25). Other characteristic findings are multiple pulmonary aneurysms with large vein thrombosis in Behçet's syndrome (BS) (see Figure 18.11). A relatively young male smoker with lower extremity ischemia, and certain arteriographic changes, is most likely to have thromboangiitis obliterans (TAO). Multiple small aneurysms in the renal or mesenteric circulation are most commonly associated with polyarteritis nodosa (PAN). Large vessel saccular aneurysms, especially with surrounding fluid, are characteristic of mycotic aneurysms. Linear dystrophic (tree-bark) calcifications in the ascending aorta characterize syphilitic aneurysms, and may be found in patients with negative syphilis serology.

Interventional radiology techniques

Over the past two decades, the advent and refinement of interventional radiology has made an impact on treatment, as well as diagnosis, of particular complications of vasculitides. Chronic occlusive lesions are now sometimes treated with percutaneous balloon angioplasty (PTA) and stenting. This treatment offers an attractive non-surgical alternative for dilating certain lesions in TA for relief of cerebral, upper extremity, or renal ischemia. Newer stent grafts are being placed with increasing safety and anatomic reconstructive options. These will undoubtedly have a great impact on large vessel (aortic, subclavian, iliac, and femoral artery) reconstruction and revascularization, whereas finer instruments and techniques such as those used in the coronary circulation will allow safer and more widespread use of these modalities in smaller and more peripheral vessels.

When acute arterial occlusions are encountered, thrombolytic therapy may reveal a focal underlying stenosis amenable to angioplasty in a medium-size vessel occlusion; thrombolysis may offer the only therapeutic option available for small-vessel thrombotic occlusions. Embolization techniques have been used to occlude BS-associated pulmonary aneurysms not responsive to immunosuppression. Traditional surgical intervention for thoracic and abdominal aneurysms in BS is associated with high morbidity since many patients are on active drug therapy. Suture line pseudoaneurysm formation and thrombosis are frequent. In regards to PAN, microcatheters and microcoils have been used for selective embolization in what might have been catastrophic renal or gastrointestinal microaneurysmal rupture.

As the role of interventional radiology in the management of local complications of systemic vasculitides becomes more established, future interventions will hopefully complement and benefit from immunologic and cellular advances in treating this set of disorders. Immunosuppressive drugs or monoclonal antibodies can perhaps be delivered locally (for example, loaded on a balloon catheter) to certain lesions to suppress hyperplasia and reduce the likelihood of recurrent stenosis. Alternatively, these agents may be injected in a concentrated form through microcatheters into a limited arterial bed for regional treatment. These technical feats are, however, yet to prove their clinical usefulness.

For the purpose of this chapter, we focus on current angiography and intervention in vasculitis syndromes encountered in a vascular and interventional radiology practice. Patients undergo angiography either to establish a diagnosis, to document the extent of involvement, or perhaps to treat the disease. These are more applicable to large and medium vessel diseases than to the small vessel varieties such as Wegener's granulomatosis (WG), Churg–Strauss syndrome (CSS), microscopic polyangiitis (MPA), Henoch-Schönlein purpura (HSP), cryoglobulinemic vasculitis and cutaneous small-vessel (leukocytoclastic) vasculitis. The diagnosis and treatment in these small-vessel diseases is usually established on clinical, laboratory, and pathologic grounds rather than by angiography, and they are not discussed in this chapter.

Some non-inflammatory syndromes present with a clinical picture similar to vasculitis, such as acute ischemic symptoms in the upper extremities. For example, patients with a clinical history of Raynaud's phenomenon and no evidence of systemic disease can have peripheral small-vessel occlusions angiographically indistinguishable from those of TAO or connective tissue disease (see Figure 18.21). Treatment in these patients is directed towards relief of acute ischemia (anticoagulation, thrombolysis, PTA, or surgical intervention) (see Figure 18.21). At times, it is quite difficult to establish a final diagnosis.

Takayasu's arteritis

Takayasu's arteritis (TA) is a non-specific inflammation of unknown etiology affecting the aorta, its branches, and occasionally the pulmonary arteries (see Chapter 25). The end result is marked fibrosis and thickening of the arterial wall, which most often results in stenosis or occlusion and occasionally aneurysm formation (Lupi-Herrera et al. 1977; Strachnan 1964).

Patients with TA have a diverse course. Some patients already have advanced arterial obstruction and collateral circulation when they first develop constitutional symptoms. At times, the presentation is during a "burned-out" phase with stenoses and occlusions but without evidence of active inflammation (Hall et al. 1985). In late stages, inflammatory aortic lesions resemble the more common atherosclerotic disease, which often gets superimposed and obscures the original inflammatory lesions. The diagnosis can be confirmed with arterial biopsy, but biopsy is positive in only 35% of cases.

Angiographic evaluation of Takayasu's arteritis

Angiographic abnormalities appear to follow certain patterns of involvement. TA has been classified by Lupi-Herrera et al. (1975) into four categories, based on anatomic distribution of the disease. Type I involves the aortic arch and its branches and Type II the descending thoracic and abdominal aorta without the arch. Types III and IV are combinations of Types I and II either without or with pulmonary arterial involvement, respectively.

Inflammation is most prominent in the outer media and adventitia (Nasu 1976), with progressive fibrosis and thickening occurring in these layers. Aneurysms form when disruption of the vessel wall is extensive and the adventitia is weakened (Figure 18.1).

The most common angiographic abnormalities of the aorta and its branches are stenoses (Nasu 1976) (Figure 18.2). Skip lesions occur often and the transition from normal vessel to diseased is often abrupt. The contour of the stenoses is smooth in two-thirds of the cases. In the active phase, however, inhomogenous thickening and contour irregularities occur because the degree of destruction of the arterial wall is not uniform (Lande and Berkman 1986).

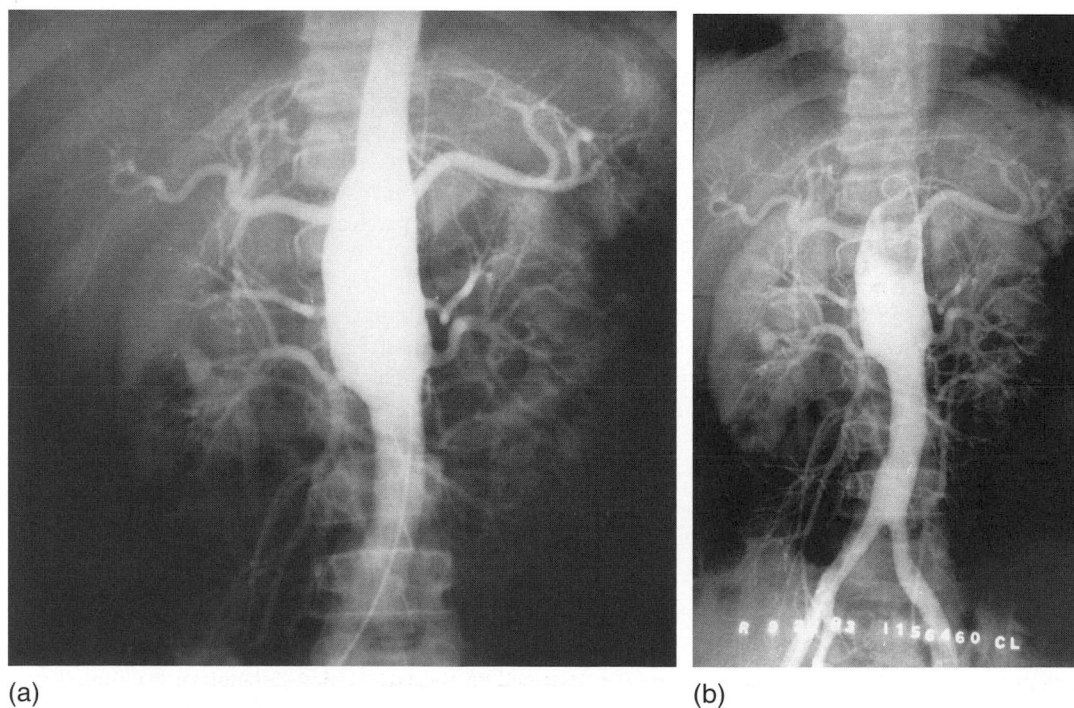

(a)   (b)

Figure 18.1 Takayasu's arteritis – aneurysmal form. A 12-year-old child presented with abdominal pain and was found to have an elevated ESR. Anteroposterior projections of the upper (a) and lower (b) abdominal aorta show a fusiform aneurysm of the upper abdominal aorta involving the origin of the celiac, superior mesenteric, and renal arteries. (c) Lateral view.

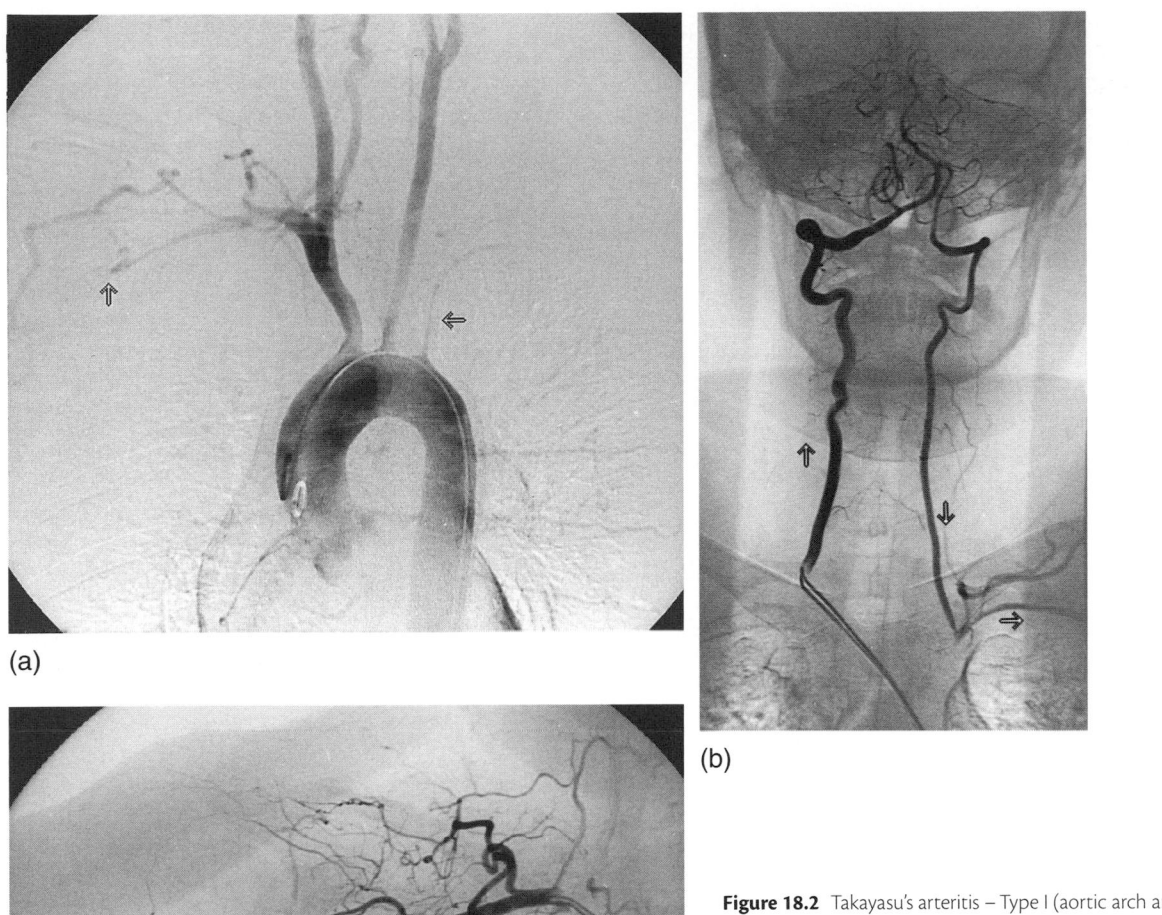

(a)

(b)

(c)

Figure 18.2 Takayasu's arteritis – Type I (aortic arch and its branches). A 35-year-old female presented with claudication in both upper extremities. Physical examination revealed weak pulses in both upper extremities and carotid bruits. (a) Arch aortogram shows almost complete occlusion of the proximal left subclavian artery (horizontal arrow) and complete occlusion of the right subclavian artery (vertical arrow). (b) Antegrade filling of the right vertebral and the posterior circulation. There is reversed flow in the left vertebral artery, which fills the left subclavian artery (subclavian steal syndrome). White arrows denote the direction of blood flow. (c) Diffuse narrowing of right subclavian artery and complete occlusion of the right axillary artery (vertical arrow). The right brachial artery is reconstituted (horizontal arrow).

Long-segment stenoses (more than 5 cm) are more common than short ones (Yamato *et al.* 1986). Within the thorax, the left subclavian artery is most often involved. The carotid arteries are the next most commonly involved (Figure 18.3). Coronary artery involvement is seen in approximately 10% of cases. Dilation of the ascending aorta can lead to aortic insufficiency. Serpiginous, fine vessels are seen in the wall of the aortic arch and the descending aorta, which represent enlarged vaso vasorum providing collateral blood flow. Within the abdomen, stenoses occur most often in the abdominal aorta and next most often in the renal arteries. The superior mesenteric artery is the most frequently involved visceral artery (Park *et al.* 1989). Stenoses in mesenteric vessels lead to abdominal pain, hypertension, or visceral organ ischemia, which may require

intervention. In the pulmonary arteries, stenoses and occlusions are seen in any of the branch vessels, but most often in the upper lobes. Systemic collaterals provide flow to the lungs at times and dilation of the pulmonary arteries is rare. Pulmonary involvement is asymptomatic in many patients, although some demonstrate right heart strain (Lupi-Herrera *et al.* 1977). There is no correlation between the extent of the pulmonary arterial lesions and the extent of systemic arteritis.

Interventional radiographic treatment in TA

Operative intervention in TA has been employed mainly to relieve brain ischemia due to aortic arch syndrome and to relieve renovascular hypertension caused by stenosis of the aorta or renal arteries

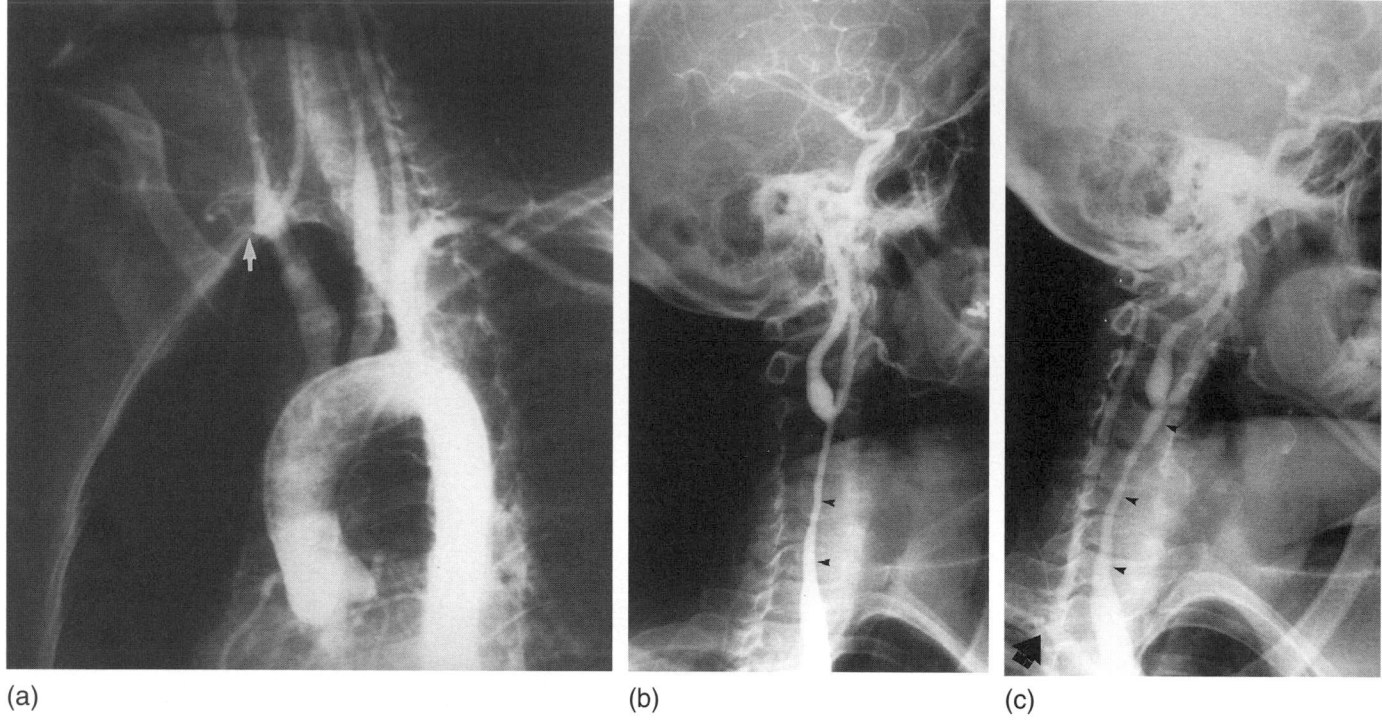

(a) (b) (c)

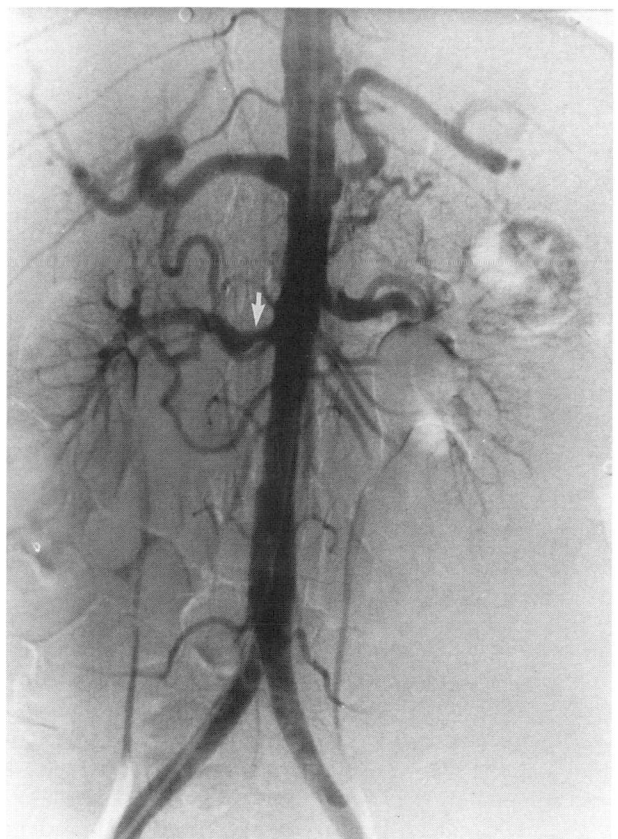

(c)

Figure 18.3 Takayasu's arteritis – Type III. A 31-year-old female with pulse discrepancy, bilateral carotid bruits, and elevated ESR. (a) Aortic arch study demonstrates bilateral diffuse disease in the great vessels. There is complete occlusion of the right subclavian artery (white arrow). Selective left carotid (b) and innominate artery (c) injections illustrate diffuse, severe, long segment stenosis (black arrowheads) of the common carotid arteries. The black arrow in (c) points to occluded right subclavian artery distal to the origin of the vertebral artery. (d) Manual subtraction abdominal aortogram shows stenosis of the proximal right renal artery (vertical white arrow) and narrowing of the infra-renal aorta.

(Inada *et al.* 1970; Kimoto 1979; Kusaba *et al.* 1973). Arterial aneurysms or aortic regurgitation may require surgical intervention. Bypass grafts usually yield better outcome than endarterectomy procedures (Pajari *et al.* 1986). The most important determinant of 5-year patency of a graft is whether it was placed during active inflammation; treatment with warfarin or platelet inhibitors plays a minor role in outcome (Pajari *et al.* 1986). The 5-year patency rate was 50% when grafts were placed during active inflammation and 88% when placed during quiescent intervals. Angioplasty can supplant surgery as the primary treatment of stenotic occlusive disease. Serial arteriography is often used to evaluate disease progression; once stenoses develop they do not resolve and they most often worsen.

The first PTA in TA was reported in 1980 by Saddekni *et al.* in a patient with renovascular hypertension. Despite resistance to balloon inflation of the affected renal artery, the final result of this PTA was successful. This initial experience has been extended in India, where TA is more prevalent. Sharma and colleagues have explored some of the technical features involved in PTA of TA (Sharma *et al.* 1990). They found that the stenoses in TA were non-compliant and resistant. The patients frequently complained of extreme pain with dilation. The minimal involvement of the intima makes the passage of a guide wire feasible, but the fibrotic element of the lesions creates significant resistance to balloon dilation (Castaneda-Zuniga *et al.* 1981; Rao *et al.* 1993; Srur *et al.* 1985). Prolonged dilation is often required for TA. Immediate results of PTA of fibroplastic lesions may not appear satisfactory; however, delayed response and improvement due to remodeling has been noted (Park *et al.* 1989; Srur *et al.* 1985) (Figure 18.4). Since the lesions in TA are often progressive, repeated percutaneous treatment for stenotic disease is preferred over surgery. Neither angioplasty nor operative intervention is recommended when there is evidence of active inflammation. Some studies show that PTA is successful in 90% of TA cases (Tyagi *et al.* 1993), with long-term primary patency rates in excess of 60% (Rao *et al.* 1993). Recurrent lesions can often be treated easily with repeat angioplasty, with markedly prolonged secondary patency rates. Occluded segments often contain thrombus within the arterial lumen, and thrombolysis may reveal underlying stenosis amenable to angioplasty (Rao *et al.* 1993).

Angioplasty/stenting can play a complementary role to surgery in some cases (Figure 18.5). While aortobifemoral bypass can be performed in cases where percutaneous treatment is not feasible, focal lesions involving the renal or visceral arteries can be treated through interventional radiology (Rozenblit and Saddekni 1999). This can be done prior to surgery in an attempt to decrease the morbidity of surgery or after bypass to treat newly developed focal lesions or recurrences.

Giant cell arteritis

Giant cell arteritis (GCA) and TA both affect large vessels (see Chapter 24). GCA frequently, but not universally, affects the temporal arteries (Jennette *et al.* 1994). Temporal artery involvement can also be seen in PAN and WG (Jennette *et al.* 1994). The defining feature of GCA is the initial active inflammatory process, which involves the inner media and inner elastic lamina (Jennette *et al.* 1994). Age at onset is useful in differentiating between TA and GCA; GCA is a much more common disease than TA in persons beyond 50 years of age. Angiography in GCA is performed with special attention to the large arteries known to be favored sites of involvement. This disease has a predilection for the aorta and its major branches, along with the extracranial branches of the carotid artery (Klein *et al.* 1975) (Figure 18.6). Approximately 14% of patients with GCA demonstrate large artery involvement (Hamrin 1972; Klein *et al.* 1975). When there is involvement of only large vessels, it is difficult to differentiate between GCA and TA based on angiographic features; it is practically impossible if the aorta and large vessels are both involved.

Polyarteritis nodosa

Polyarteritis nodosa (PAN) is a systemic, necrotizing, predominantly medium-sized vessel vasculitis that classically involves the renal and visceral arteries (Bron *et al.* 1995) (see Chapter 26). Coronary arteries are the next most commonly involved vessels; microscopic arteries are not involved. Since no diagnostic serological test exists, angiography can have an important role in the diagnosis of PAN. Organs involved with PAN may be inaccessible for biopsy and the biopsy of uninvolved sites has a poor yield (Provenzale and Allen 1996). The angiographic diagnosis of PAN has a sensitivity and specificity of approximately 90%, a positive predictive value (PPV) of 55%, and a negative predictive value (NPV) of 98% (Hekali *et al.* 1991). The "gold standard" for the diagnosis of PAN is demonstration of necrotizing inflammation of medium-sized arteries (Easterbrook 1980).

Renal artery involvement (Figure 18.7), seen in 70% of patients, often causes hypertension and hematuria. Gastrointestinal manifestations include abdominal pain, GI bleeding, and bowel infarction. In PAN, the elastic lamina is destroyed and the media undergoes fibrinoid necrosis. Microaneuryms (1–5 mm) arise from weakened, necrotic portions of the arterial wall. Aneurysms are not pathognomonic of PAN and not all PAN patients have microaneurysms. Small vessels tend to thrombose and can be seen as occlusions in arteriography. Focal lesions tend to occur at vessel bifurcations. PAN is the most common cause of microaneurysms. Aneurysms of visceral arteries have been demonstrated in 60–90% of PAN patients (Figure 18.8), but some patients with visceral aneurysms have diagnoses other than PAN (Bron *et al.* 1995; Fleming and Stern 1965). The mean number of visceral aneurysms in PAN is higher than in other disorders. Glucocorticoid treatment can result in resolution of aneurysms. In PAN, healing lesions, chronic stenoses, and acute aneurysm formation can all coexist (Hekali *et al.* 1991).

Spontaneous hemorrhage from a ruptured aneurysm in PAN is seen most often in young men with a history of hypertension who develop sudden, severe flank or abdominal pain (Capps and Klein 1970; Chandrakantan and Kaufman 1999). Transcatheter selective embolization can be life saving and preserve renal function at the same time. Angiographic embolization of hemorrhage in the gastrointestinal tract has also been performed and can avert catastrophe (Herskowitz *et al.* 1993). At times, the culprit vessel resulting in hemorrhage is not found, and more non-selective embolization based on CT scan findings is indicated (Chandrakantan and Kaufman 1999; Smith and Wernick 1989). Coronary arterial involvement includes thrombosis, aneurysms, and irregularity. Approximately 60% of patients with clinical cardiac symptoms had large vessel coronary involvement and 40% had small vessel involvement at autopsy (Przybojewski 1981). Patients with PAN have a short duration of preinfarct angina, suggesting rapid progression of the lesion.

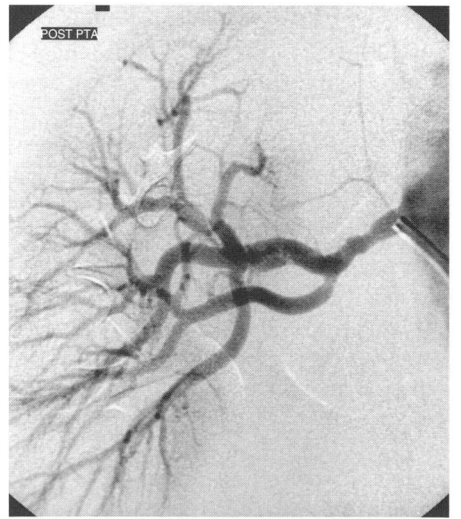

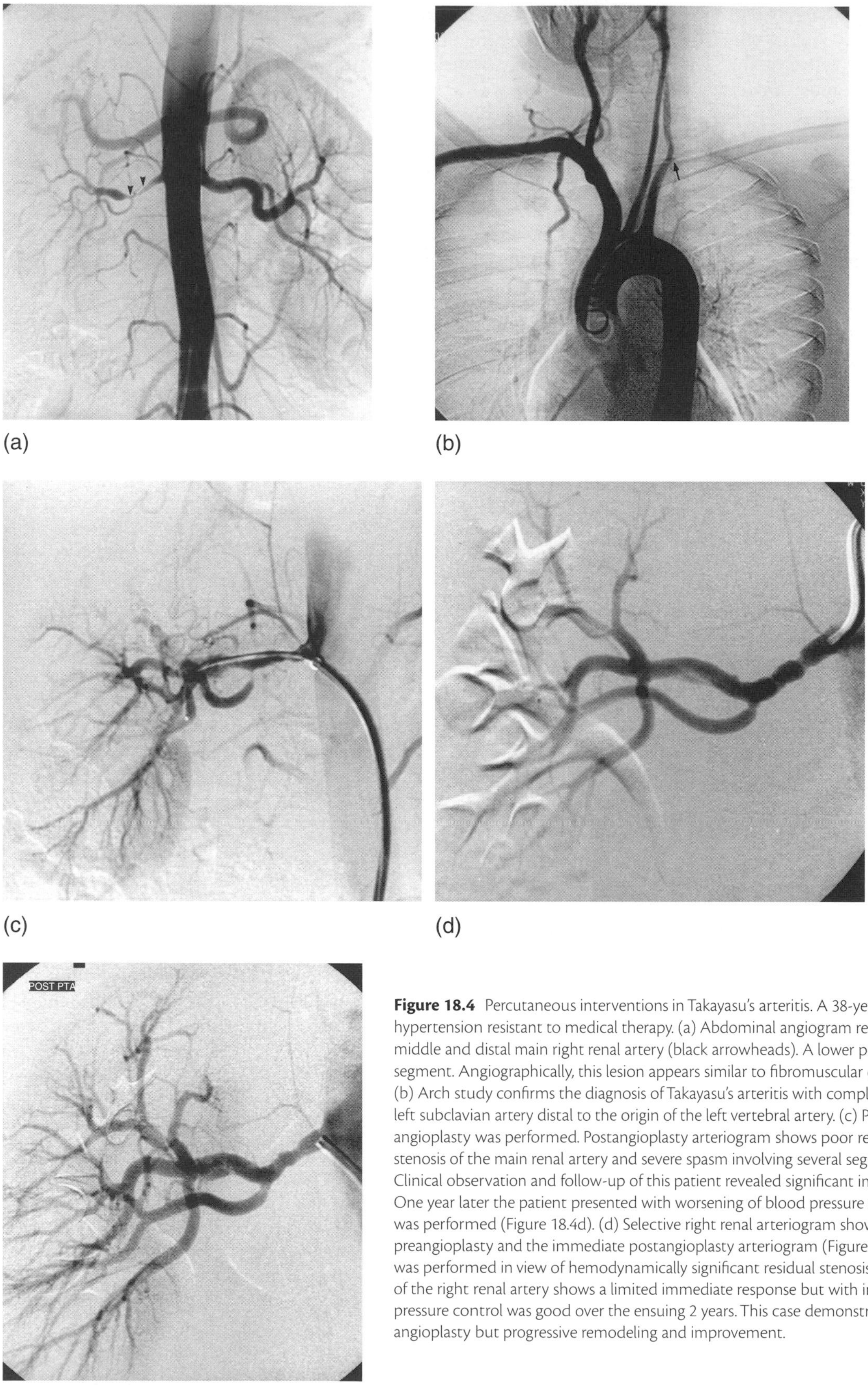

Figure 18.4 Percutaneous interventions in Takayasu's arteritis. A 38-year-old female who has severe hypertension resistant to medical therapy. (a) Abdominal angiogram reveals a long tubular stenosis in the middle and distal main right renal artery (black arrowheads). A lower pole branch arises from the stenotic segment. Angiographically, this lesion appears similar to fibromuscular dysplasia (see Figure 18.18). (b) Arch study confirms the diagnosis of Takayasu's arteritis with complete occlusion (black arrow) of the left subclavian artery distal to the origin of the left vertebral artery. (c) Percutaneous transluminal renal angioplasty was performed. Postangioplasty arteriogram shows poor results with persistent, significant stenosis of the main renal artery and severe spasm involving several segmental branches of the renal artery. Clinical observation and follow-up of this patient revealed significant improvement in her hypertension. One year later the patient presented with worsening of blood pressure control. Repeat angiography was performed (Figure 18.4d). (d) Selective right renal arteriogram shows improvement over the initial preangioplasty and the immediate postangioplasty arteriogram (Figures 18.4a and 18.4c). Repeat angioplasty was performed in view of hemodynamically significant residual stenosis (Figure 18.4e). (e) Repeat angioplasty of the right renal artery shows a limited immediate response but with improvement of the stenosis. Blood pressure control was good over the ensuing 2 years. This case demonstrates limited immediate response to angioplasty but progressive remodeling and improvement.

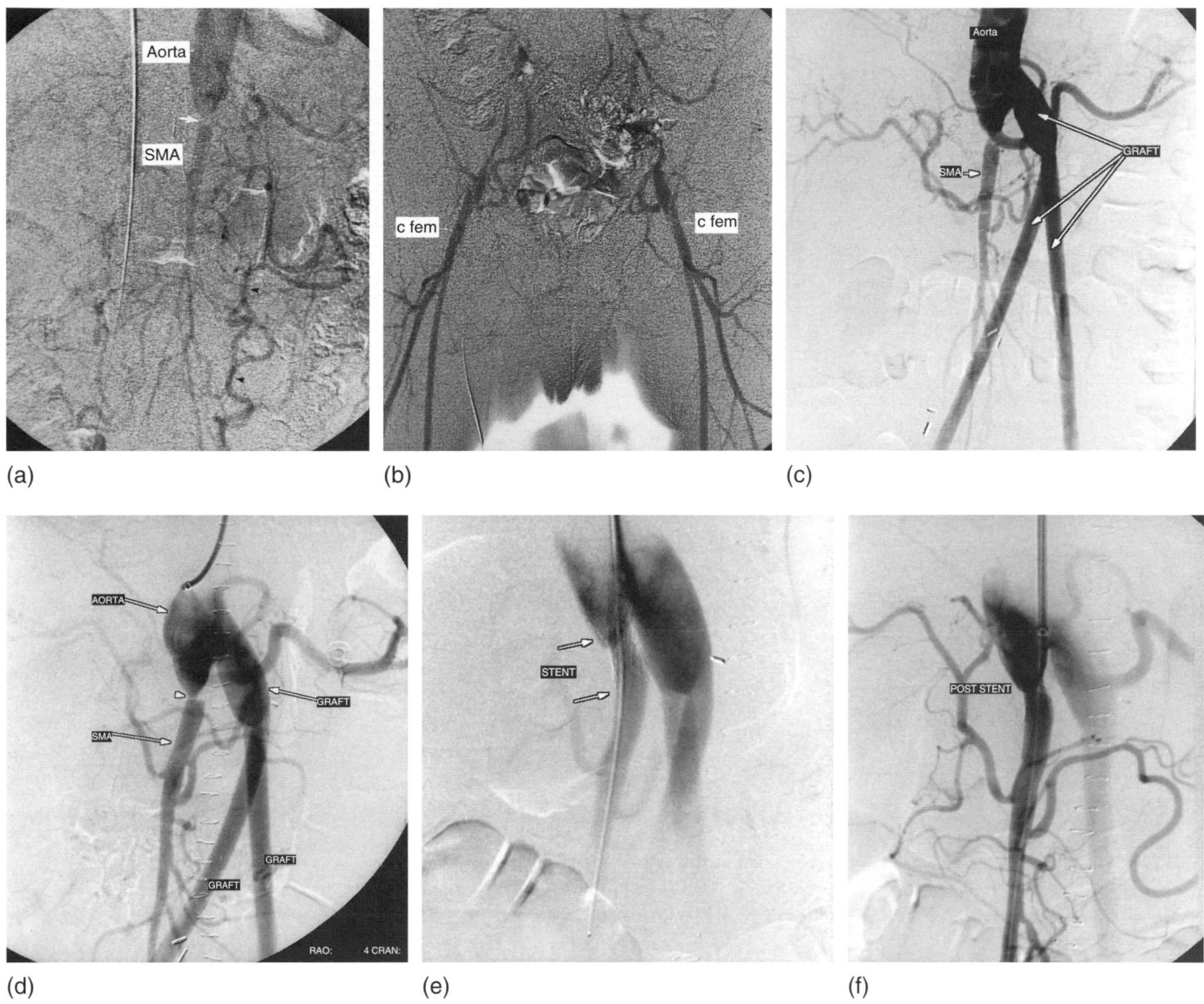

Figure 18.5 Surgical and percutaneous interventions in Takayasu's arteritis – Type II. A 40-year-old male presented with renal failure and bilateral lower extremity claudication. (a) IVDSA (intravenous digital subtraction angiography) shows that the abdominal aorta is patent to the level of the origin of the superior mesenteric artery (SMA), but is totally occluded distally. There is probably proximal stenosis in the SMA (white arrow). Note the prominent retroperitoneal collaterals (black arrowheads) and occluded renal arteries. (b) Reconstitution of normal appearing common femoral arteries (c fem). A supra-celiac aorto-bifemoral graft was performed with satisfactory flow in the celiac and SMA. Intraoperative examination of the abdominal aorta, adjacent lymph nodes, and soft tissues was consistent with aortitis. (c) Abdominal aortogram showing proximal anatomosis of the aorto-bifemoral graft to the supra-celiac aorta. The proximal splenic artery overlaps to obscure the stenosis at the origin of the SMA. The replaced right hepatic artery arising from the SMA, a normal anatomical variant. (d) Oblique projection of the abdominal aorta shows severe stenosis at the origin of the SMA (arrow head). (e) Angioplasty followed by stenting of the SMA ostial stenosis was performed. Arrows indicate stent. (f) After stenting, there is excellent flow through the SMA and replaced right hepatic artery.

Many of the myocardial infarctions in PAN patients are large but silent. In several cases, the infarction occurred shortly after glucocorticoids were started. It has been suggested that the reparative process led to fibrosis occluding the culprit vessels.

Kawasaki's disease

Kawasaki's disease (KD) is an acute inflammatory disease causing systemic vasculitis, which primarily affects infants and young children.

The diagnosis is established on clinical grounds and, importantly, angiography and echocardiography. Cardiovascular involvement is frequent, with coronary artery aneurysms the most predominant vascular abnormality, occurring in 15–20% of cases. Aneurysms may also involve other medium-sized vessels such as the axillary, iliac or renal arteries. For more details, see Chapter 29. Cross-sectional imaging studies can be used advantageously for diagnosis and follow-up of these patients, obviating the need for invasive angiography.

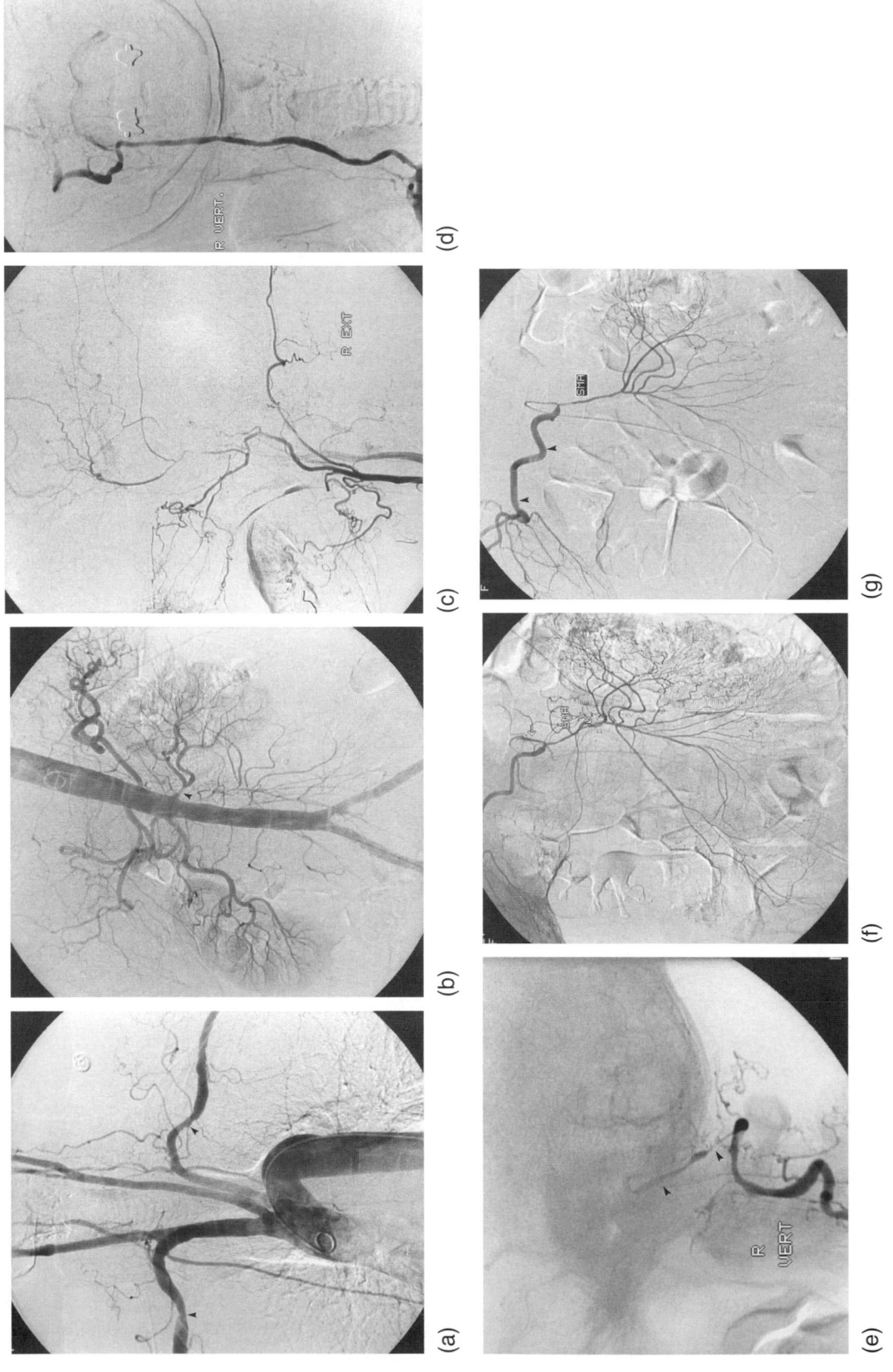

Figure 18.6 *Giant cell arteritis (GCA). (a) Arch aortogram illustrates irregularities involving both subclavian arteries (black arrowheads). (b) Abdominal aortogram shows proximal left renal artery stenosis (black arrowhead). (c) Diffuse disease in branches of the external carotid artery. (d) Diffuse irregular narrowing of the vertebral artery. (e) Diffuse, severe stenosis of the intracranial segment of the right vertebral artery (arrowheads). (f) Diffuse, severe, tubular stenosis of the proximal half of the SMA (white arrows). (g) The replaced right hepatic artery (black arrowheads) is a normal variation arising from the proximal SMA and is free of disease.*

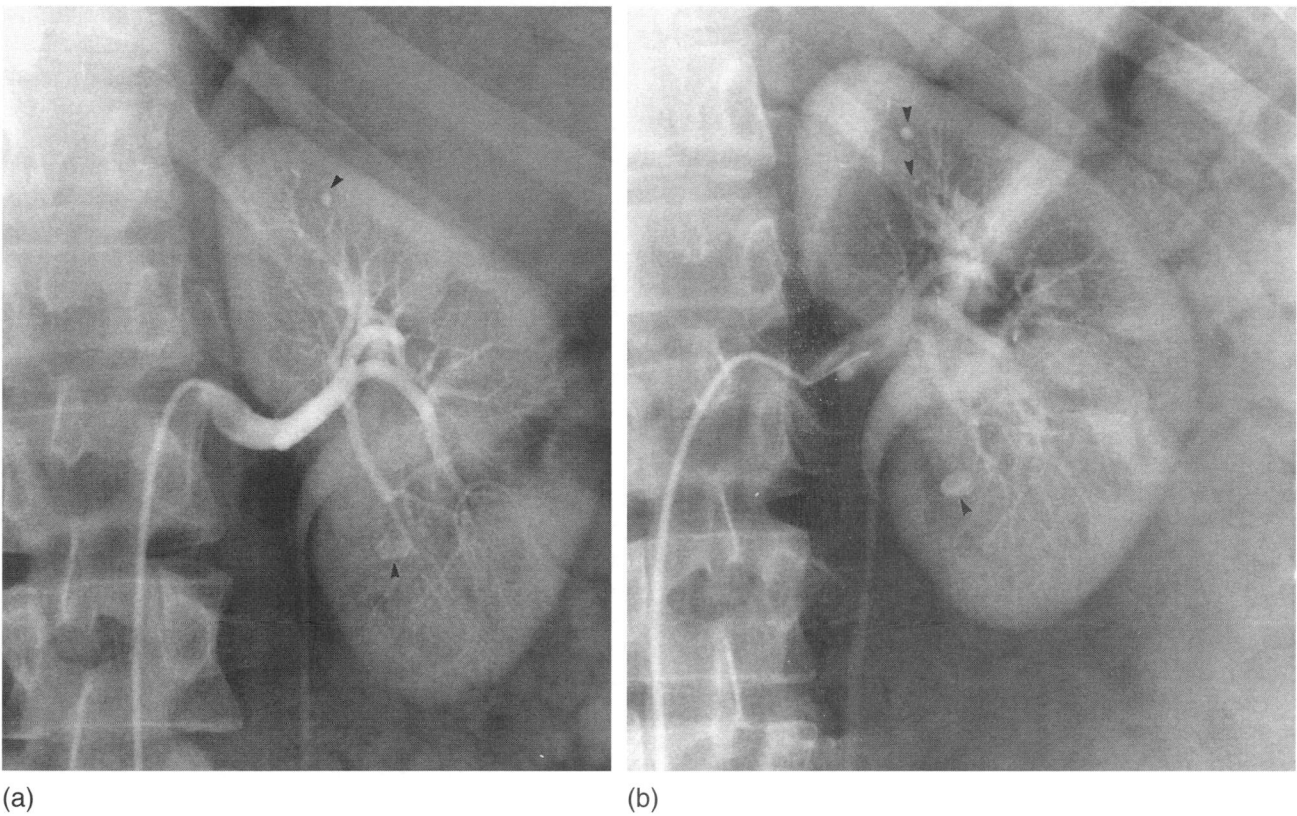

(a)   (b)

Figure 18.7 Polyarteritis nodosa (PAN) in the kidney. An 18-year-old female presents with cutaneous and nasal mucosal lesions suspicious for systemic vasculitis. Early (a) and late (b) arterial phase of selective left renal arteriogram. Note the multiple, small, round aneurysms (arrows) characteristic of PAN.

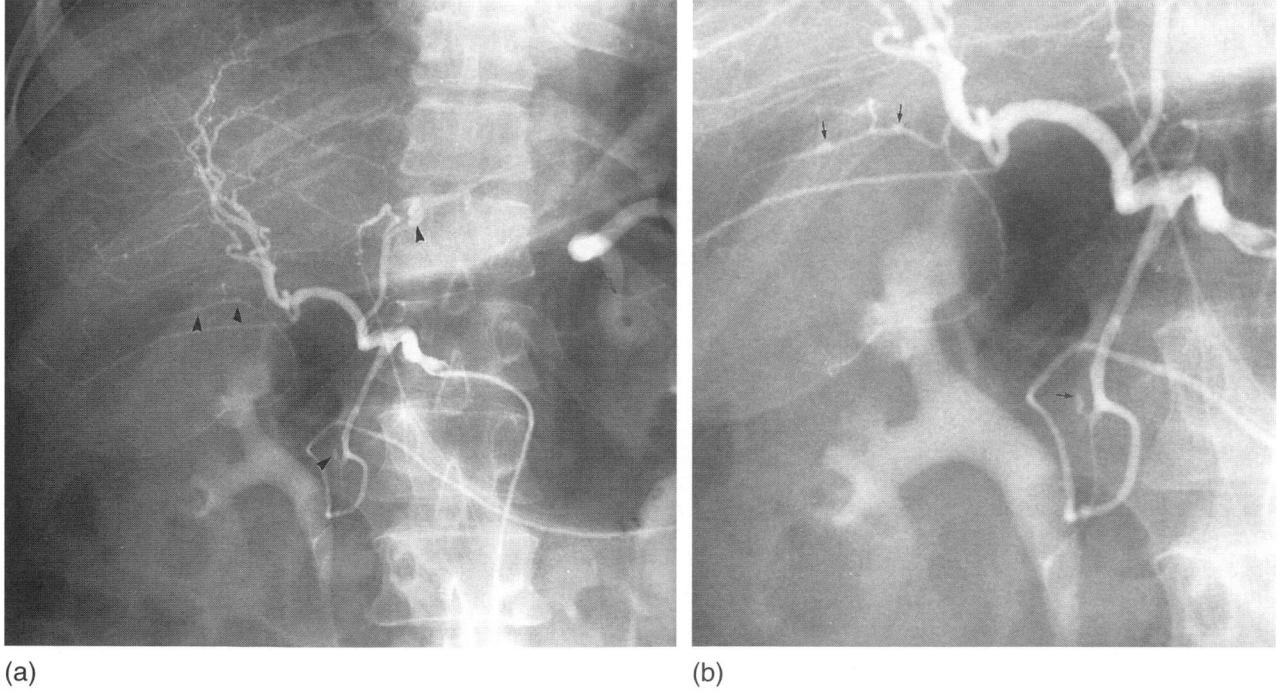

(a)   (b)

Figure 18.8 Visceral PAN. A 50-year-old male with abdominal pain suspected to have vasculitis. (a) Multiple small aneurysms are seen in the cystic artery branch arising from the right hepatic artery, pancreaticoduodenal branches of the gastroduodenal artery, and the left hepatic artery (black arrowheads). (b) Magnified view of the cystic artery aneurysms.

Thromboangiitis obliterans

Thromboangiitis obliterans, also referred to as Buerger's disease, is a distinct vasculitis of medium and small-sized arteries and veins, which initially involves the distal vessels of the legs and arms and progresses proximally, either in a contiguous or skip-zone fashion. The first case was described in 1879 by Feliz von Winiwarter, an Austrian surgeon. Leo Buerger published his first group of patients, which served as the cornerstone for subsequent study, in 1908.

The prevalence of TAO has decreased since its first description, but has remained fairly constant over the past few decades. This may represent a refinement in diagnosis rather than a true decrease in prevalence. There is greater incidence of the disease in eastern Europe, Asia, and the Middle East. Some series have estimated its prevalence among women as high as 20% (Olin *et al.* 1990; Yorukoglu *et al.* 1993), most likely reflective of the increased prevalence of smoking among women. When present, the severity of the disease is equal in both sexes (Lie 1987). For more details, see Chapter 38.

Histologically, vessels affected by Buerger's disease vary according to the chronologic age of the lesion. Acutely, vessels show severe inflammation involving all three layers of the vessel wall. In the subacute phase, there is progressive organization of an occlusive thrombus; in the chronic phase, there is complete organization of an occlusive thrombus with extensive recanalization, and adventitial and perivascular fibrosis. These chronic occlusions are almost always accompanied by extensive collateral circulation, which accounts for some of the characteristic angiographic findings of the disease (Tanaka 1998).

Although there is no single angiographic feature specific for TAO, a typical constellation of radiologic findings, in the proper clinical setting, is diagnostic (Hagen and Lohse 1984; Rivera 1973; Suzuki *et al.* 1996). The main angiographic findings are multiple, bilateral focal areas of stenosis or occlusion, with normal proximal and intervening vessels. The patient is normally free of atherosclerotic changes and uninvolved vessels demonstrate smooth lamina. The occlusions are usually of the cut-off variety. Corkscrew collaterals often develop in TAO, but are not specific, as they are also often seen in atherosclerotic disease. However, direct collaterals, which arise either from adjacent uninvolved vessels, or from the proximal segment of an occluded vessel, are thought to be fairly characteristic of TAO. These collaterals can be seen to run directly along a thrombosed segment of artery in a direct network of collaterals. This unusual pattern of collateral vessels has been hypothesized to represent dilated vasa vasorum (Figures 18.9 and 18.10). A second pattern of collateral vessels was described to resemble a "tree root" or "spider's leg". These collateral vessels originate from distally occluded vessels and can either re-open as direct collaterals distally, or terminate within the soft tissues. In the early stages of TAO, a "corrugated" pattern is noted, which involves a short segment of a peripheral vessel. This is felt to either represent alterations in a vessel prior to thrombotic occlusion, or a recanalized vessel.

The standing-wave pattern has a reported prevalence up to 75% in TAO (Hagen and Lohse 1984). This is characterized by a "goose-trachea" change in the outline of a larger arterial trunk, most notably in the femoralpopliteal segment, and was originally postulated to represent a preobstruction lesion with intimal hyperplasia that was specific for TAO (Shionoya *et al.* 1978). However, it has also been shown that standing waves can be seen with any distal obstruction, and represent flow phenomena relating to inflow obstruction and the creation of backflow waves (Lehrer 1967). Thus while this may be a helpful sign in diagnosing TAO, it is not specific.

Behçet's syndrome

Behçet's syndrome (BS) is a multisystemic disorder affecting young adults mostly from the Middle East and Far East (see Chapter 35). Any large or small artery, vein, or organ may be involved in an unpredictable combination (Chajek and Fainaur 1975). Venous lesions are more common than large artery involvement, causing thrombosis of veins such as the superior vena cava or inferior vena cava. Arterial manifestations are rare, occurring in approximately 2.5% of patients with longstanding disease. Arterial involvement can be divided into three groups: the first group involves arterial occlusions, the second group arterial aneurysms, and the third group pulmonary artery aneurysms (Park *et al.* 1984). BS is virtually the only vasculitis leading to pulmonary arterial aneurysms (Lacombe *et al.* 1985), which are usually multiple (Figure 18.11). In general, invasive angiography should be avoided in BS, since vessel (artery and vein) punctures can lead to thrombosis (Tunaci *et al.* 1995) or aneurysms.

Pulmonary artery aneurysms in BS may rupture, with significant morbidity; they may be treated successfully with medications. Transcatheter embolization has been performed for patients with symptomatic aneurysms that do not regress with glucocorticoid treatment. Surgical bypass is complicated at times by aneurysm formation at the anastomosis (Hamza 1987). Thus, as noted above, angiography should generally be avoided in BS. Caval thrombosis is also frequent and may preclude transcatheter pulmonary arterial intervention (Tunaci *et al.* 1995).

Infection-related vasculitis

Inflammation of the arterial wall due to infection leads to various manifestations, which depend largely on the size of the affected vessel. Virtually all infectious organisms have been implicated in this form of vasculitis (see Chapters 42 and 45). Aneurysms or pseudoaneurysms, typically called mycotic aneurysms, can be seen in infection of vessels of all sizes.

There are several routes of infection of the vessel wall: (1) direct extension from an intravascular source (endocarditis); (2) hematogenous seeding to diseased intima or vaso vasorum (bacteremia from any source); (3) direct extension from an extravascular source (abscess, osteomyelitis); (4) lymphangitic spread; and (5) direct contamination from trauma, intravenous drug abuse, and instrumentation.

Infectious aortitis

Some infectious agents preferentially involve large vessels such as the aorta and pulmonary arteries. *Salmonella* can cause infectious aortitis, but staphylococcal and streptococcal aortitis (Bronze *et al.* 1999) are more common. Treponemes and mycobacteria also have a predilection for the aorta (see Chapter 42).

Salmonella aortitis

Salmonella aortitis is typically seen in elderly patients with pre-existing atherosclerosis, aortic aneurysm, or a vascular graft. It typically causes aneurysms of the thoracic (20%) or abdominal

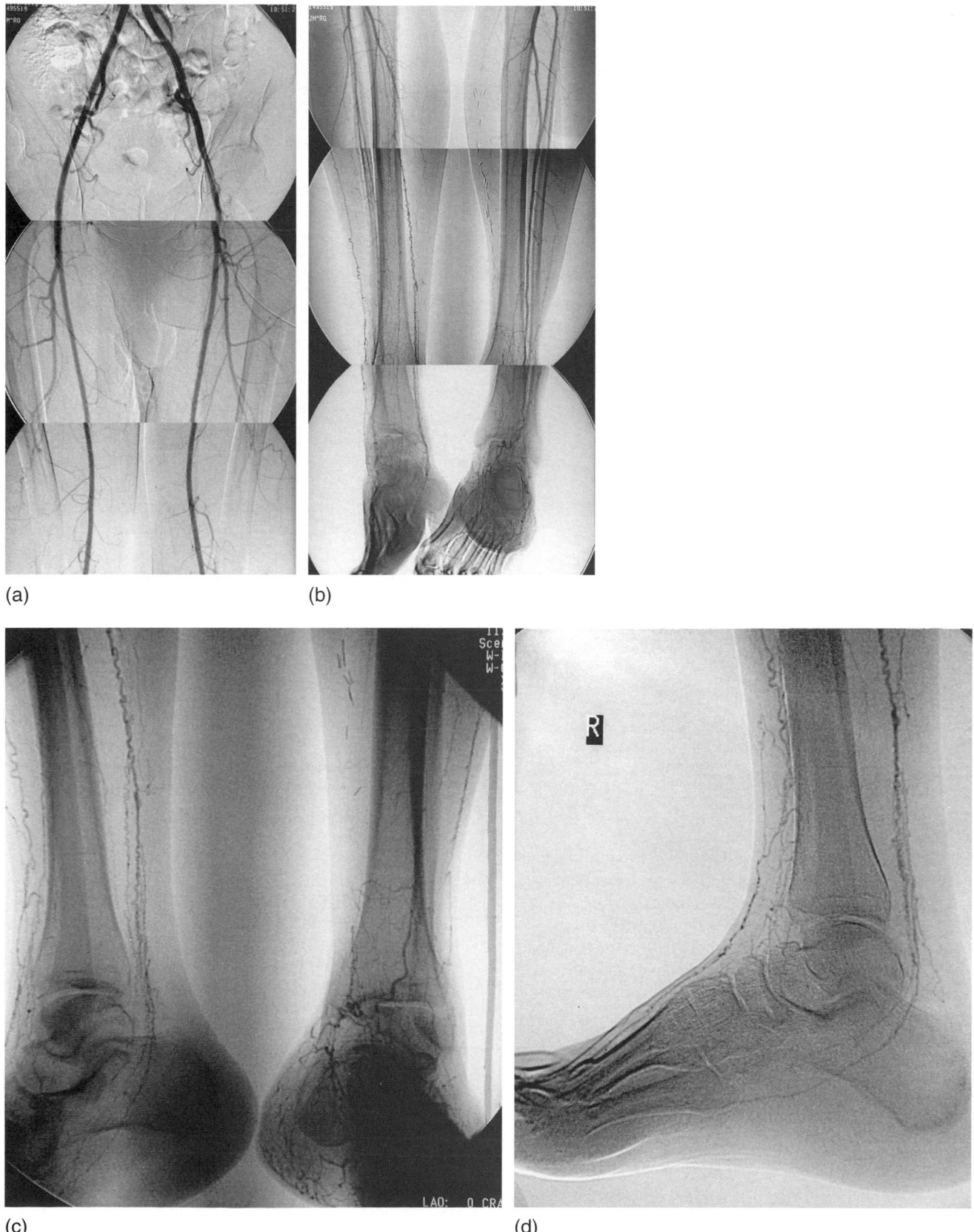

Figure 18.9 Thromboangiitis obliterans (TAO). A 42-year-old male smoker with a long history of bilateral calf claudication, presents with new onset, right foot rest pain. Pathologic examination of an amputated toe was consistent with TAO. (a) Normal-appearing vessels are seen above the knee. (b) Below the knee, there is severe occlusive disease of all tibio-peroneal vessels. Only the left peroneal artery is patent. (c) Classic corkscrew collaterals. (d) Magnified view of the corkscrew collaterals.

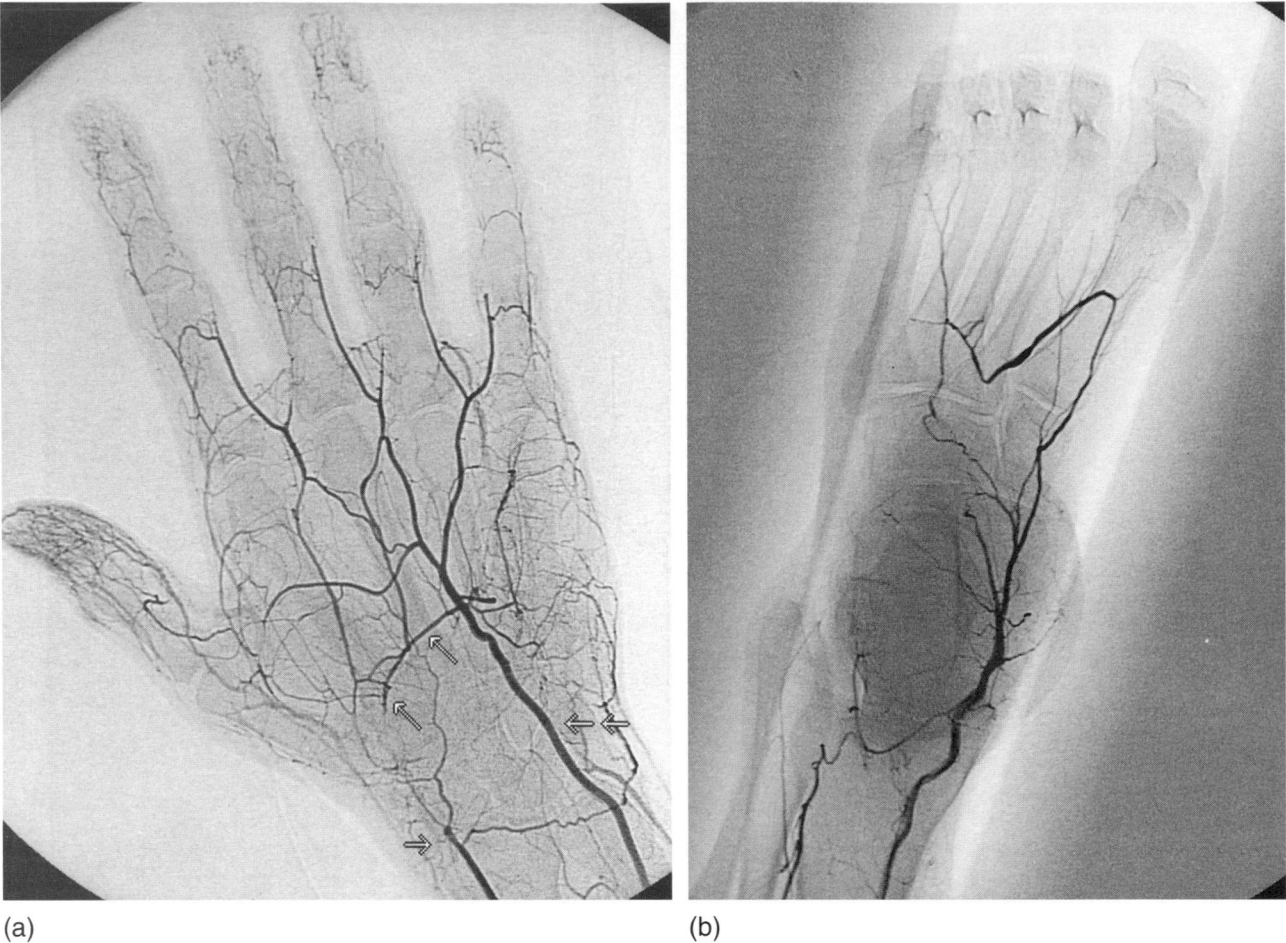

(a)   (b)

Figure 18.10 Raynaud's phenomenon in thromboangiitis obliterans. A 29-year-old female, heavy smoker with history of recurrent Raynaud's phenomenon presents with coldness and numbness in the extremities. Clinical evaluation revealed no evidence of systemic vasculitis. (a) Right hand arteriogram demonstrates occlusion of the distal radial artery and all distal proper digital arteries. Similar findings were seen in the left hand. (b) Left foot arteriogram (anteroposterior projection) demonstrates occlusion of the anterior tibial, dorsalis pedis, and multiple digital arteries.

aorta (80%) (Oskoui *et al.* 1993) (Figure 18.12). The clinical presentation is often misleading and rupture is a frequent complication (Flamand *et al.* 1992; Katz *et al.* 1992). The clinical diagnosis of an infectious aneurysm is difficult unless it is very large or develops a complication such as rupture. More than 90% of patients present with fever and non-specific back and abdominal pain (Flamand *et al.* 1992). These patients need to be identified as early as possible to avoid complications. Treatment includes long-term antibiotics and surgical resection of the aneurysm and extra-anatomic bypass (Katz *et al.* 1992). Surgical procedures may be difficult and only 50% of patients survive the perioperative period.

Syphilitic aortitis

Syphilitic aortitis is initiated by hematogenous spread of treponemes and is a manifestation of tertiary syphilis. The ascending aorta and the aortic arch are typically involved. The vaso vasorum is destroyed by perivascular inflammation, which ultimately leads to fibrosis of the aortic media. Syphilitic aortitis causes aortic aneurysms with or without valvular incompetence and coronary ostial stenosis. Linear calcification is present in 70% of patients. Diagnosis can be difficult as there may be no reliable history of syphilis and serologic studies may be negative.

Drug abuse

Intravenous drug abuse may lead to vascular complications related to local injury or infections from unclean needles. Pseudoaneurysms or arteriovenous fistulae may form. Accidental injection of hypertonic solution containing powder, or other foreign substances, into the arterial system can result in multiple occlusions of digital arteries (Figure 18.13). Raynaud's phenomenon may follow this form of injury (Yao *et al.* 1972). Long-term ingestion of certain compounds, most notably ergotamine, causes diffuse arterial spasm reminiscent of vasculitis.

Vasculitis secondary to connective tissue diseases

Inflammatory vascular disease can occur with systemic lupus erythematosus, rheumatoid arthritis, and scleroderma (see Chapter 34). Angiographic appearances of these entities overlap and definite diagnosis cannot be made on the basis of angiographic features alone, though it provides corroborative information.

Systemic lupus erythematosus

Raynaud's phenomenon is present in up to 30% of patients with systemic lupus erythematosus (SLE). Vasculitis in patients with

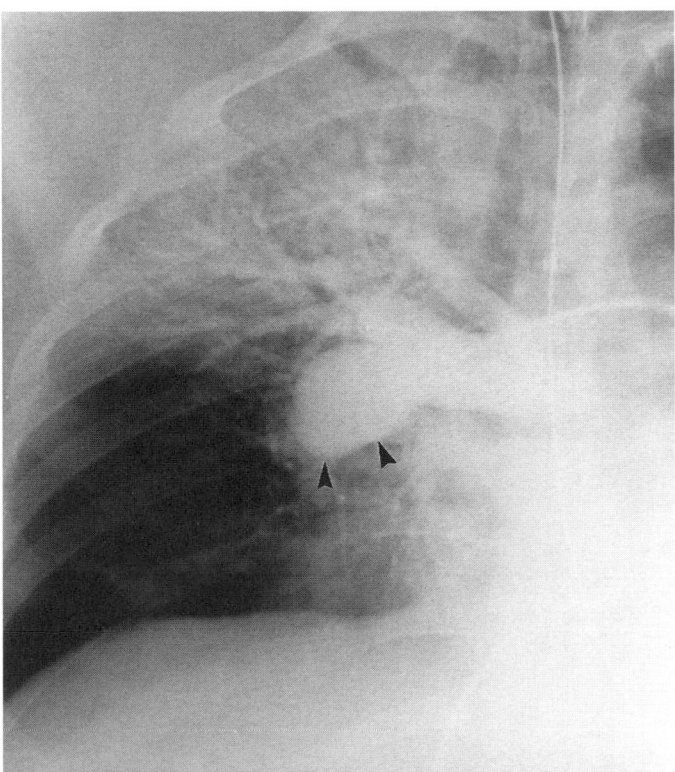

Figure 18.11 Behçet's syndrome. A large aneurysm (black arrowheads) is seen in the right lower pulmonary artery, with occlusion of its segmental branches consistent with thrombosis.

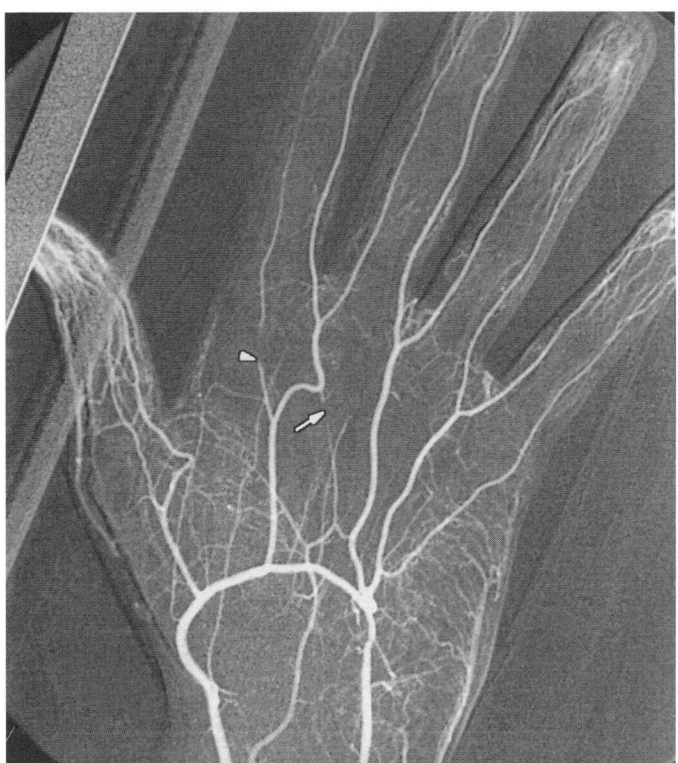

Figure 18.13 Drug abuse vasculitis. An 18-year-old male with history of IV drug abuse presents with severe pain in the fingertips immediately after attempted intravenous injection of a street drug. An arteriogram of the left hand shows focal embolic occlusion in the proper digital (arrowhead) and common digital arteries (arrow).

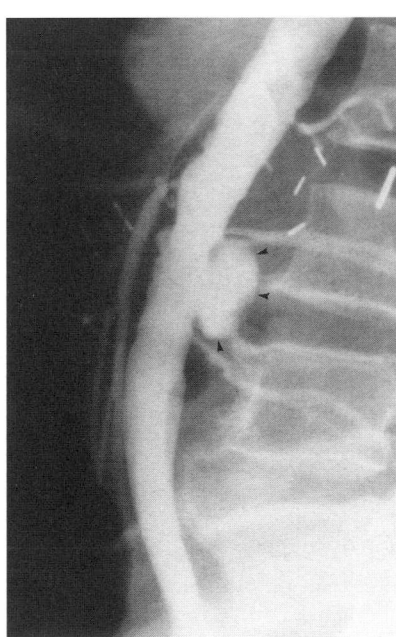

Figure 18.12 Salmonella aortitis. A 62-year-old male with fever and *Salmonella* osteomyelitis of the right ilium, presents with lower abdominal pain. Findings on abdominal CT scan prompted aortogram. Abdominal aortogram (lateral projection) shows a saccular aneurysm from the posterior wall of the infrarenal aorta (black arrowheads). The patient was treated with resection of the aneurysm and left axillary artery to bifemoral bypass graft.

SLE typically involves medium- and small-sized vessels, although large vessels can also be involved. Angiographically, small and medium-sized vessels show tapered or abrupt occlusions with sparse formation of collateral vessels (Figure 18.14). Since hypercoagulability is common in SLE due to the presence of antiphospholipid antibodies and other factors, arterial occlusions may be due to thrombosis or to vasculitis. The two etiologies may be indistinguishable in a given patient (Figure 18.15). Renal artery thrombosis or stenosis can occur in primary or secondary antiphospholipid syndrome.

Rheumatoid arthritis

Vasculitis is seen in small number of patients with long-standing, severe rheumatoid arthritis (RA). Angiographic examinations show either occlusive or hyperemic arterial abnormalities (Laws *et al.* 1963). Most of the occlusive lesions occur at the level of the digital arteries, although medium-sized vessels are also involved (Figure 18.16). Hyperemic changes tend to occur around regions of synovial proliferation.

Scleroderma

In scleroderma, small vessels of the digits, kidneys, and heart show intimal thickening with fibrous deposition and occlusion. Over 80% of patients have a history of Raynaud's phenomenon. Angiography demonstrates multiple focal stenoses and occlusion, especially in small vessels. Arteriography of the hand shows severe

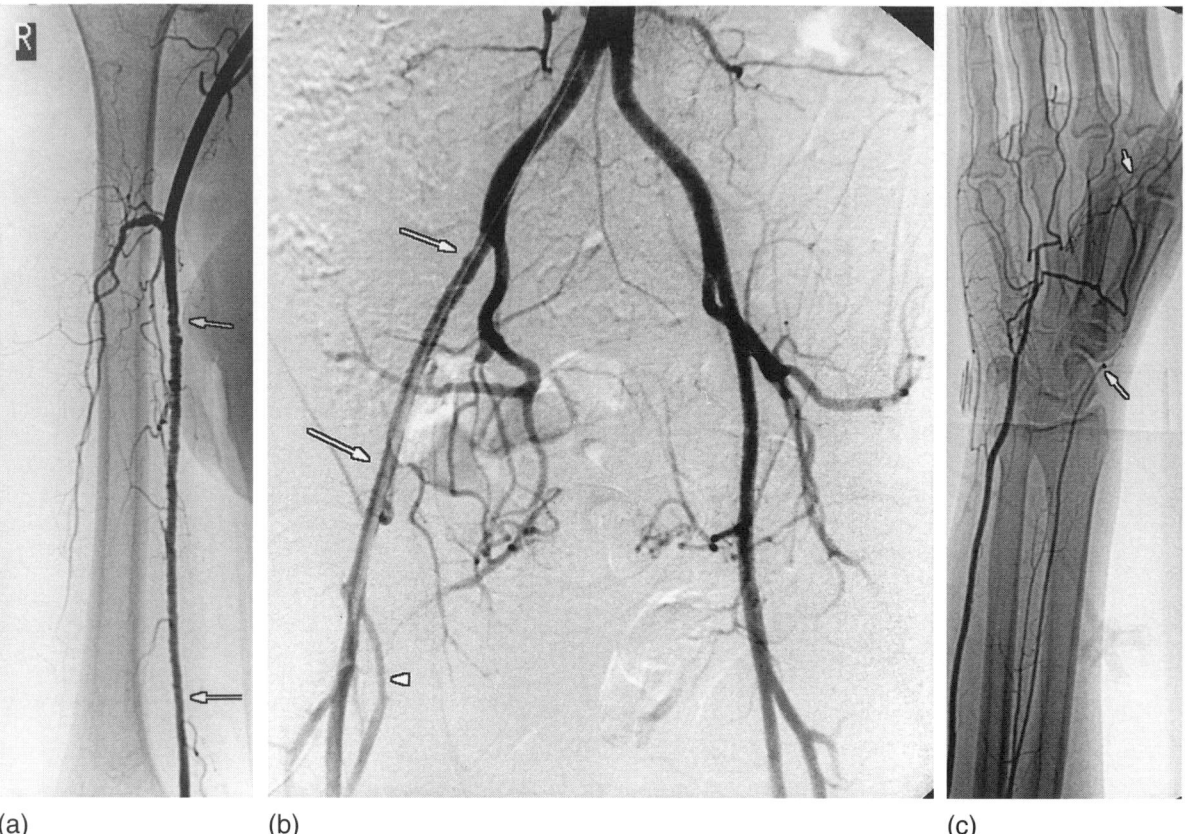

(a)   (b)   (c)

Figure 18.14 Systemic lupus erythematosus (SLE). A 30-year-old white female with SLE presents with numb, cold hands and feet. (a) Luminal irregularity of the entire brachial artery (white arrows). (b) Pelvic arteriogram shows luminal irregularity involving right external iliac artery (white arrows). (c) Occluded radial artery at the wrist (large white arrow).

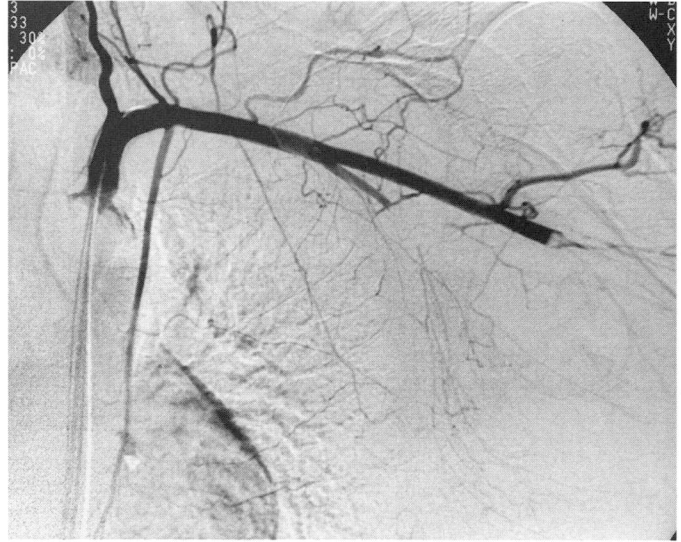

Figure 18.15 Systemic lupus erythematosus. A 39-year-old female with a history of lupus vasculitis presented with left upper extremity ischemic symptoms. Selective left subclavian arteriogram shows abrupt cut-off in upper brachial artery with poor collateral flow consistent with acute thrombosis. She underwent thrombolysis with tissue plasminogen activator infusion with complete resolution of symptoms.

involvement of proper digital arteries, generally in the mid- or distal portion of the vessel (Dabich *et al.* 1972).

Mimickers of vasculitis

A multitude of conditions may imitate vasculitis (see Chapter 45). Hypothenar hammer syndrome (Figure 18.17) and other occupational injuries, neurofibromatosis (Figure 18.18), thoracic outlet syndrome, radiation injury, frostbite, and drug abuse can produce vascular changes mimicking vasculitis. Three disorders are commonly seen and merit brief discussion.

Fibromuscular dysplasia

Arterial fibrous lesions are often detected during angiography of practically all branches of the aorta, particularly the renal and carotid arteries. The etiology is fibromuscular dysplasia is unknown. It is usually associated with renovascular hypertension and predominantly occurs in young Caucasian women. Harrison and McCormack (1971) developed a pathologic classification based on the arterial layer involved. The most common type is known as "medial fibroplasia with mural aneurysm" and has the classic "string of beads" appearance (Figure 18.19). This appearance is

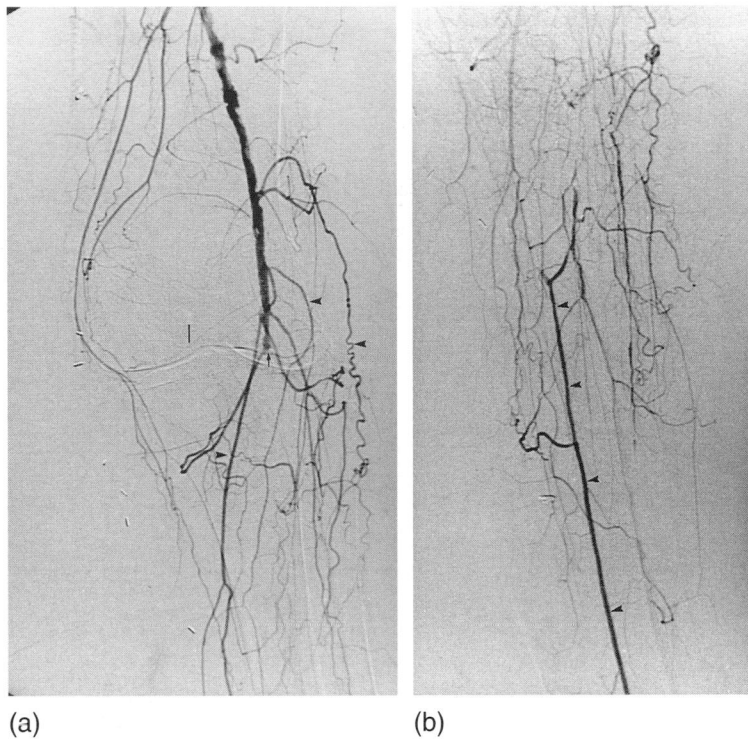

(a)   (b)

Figure 18.16 Rheumatoid arthritis. A 49-year-old female with rheumatoid arthritis presents with symptoms of ischemia in the lower extremities. (a) Complete occlusion of the popliteal artery at the level of joint line (black arrow) with collaterals (black arrowheads). (b) Reconstitution of the posterial tibial artery (black arrowheads), which is the only run-off vessel to the foot.

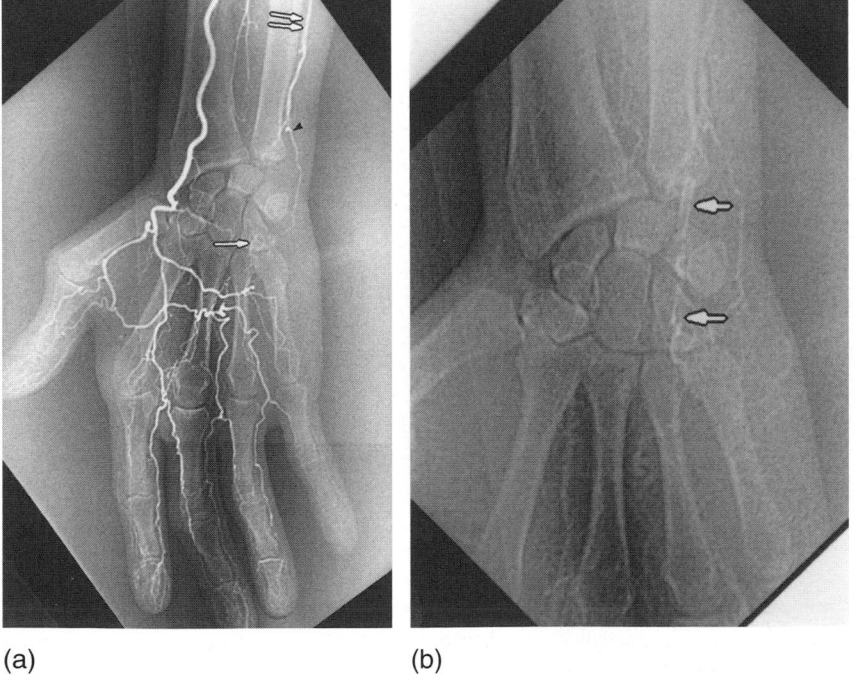

(a)   (b)

Figure 18.17 Trauma: hypothenar hammer syndrome. A construction worker presented with numbness of the right ring and little fingers. He had classic history of repetitive trauma to the right hypothenar eminence. (a) Right hand arteriogram shows occlusion of the distal ulnar artery (double arrows). The single arrow points to the hook of the hamate bone where occlusion of the ulnar artery begins. Retrograde thrombosis has occurred to the first significant collateral vessel (black arrowhead). The radial artery fills the deep and superficial palmar arches and digital arteries. (b) Magnified view of the late arterial phase shows the shadow of the distal ulnar artery filled with thrombus (arrows).

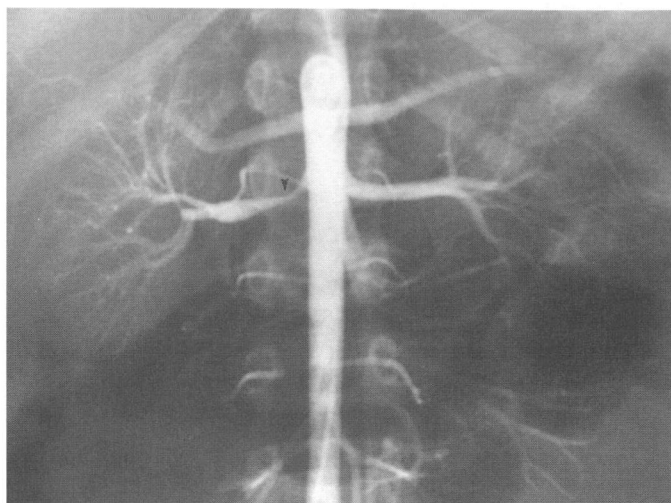

Figure 18.18 Neurofibromatosis, Type I: tubular stenoses. A 3-year-old male child presented with hypertension underwent abdominal aortogram. The patient had *café au lait* spots consistent with Type I neurofibromatosis. Abdominal aortogram shows severe tubular stenosis of the right main renal artery (black arrowhead). A similar appearance can be seen in intimal fibroplasia and large vessel vasculitides.

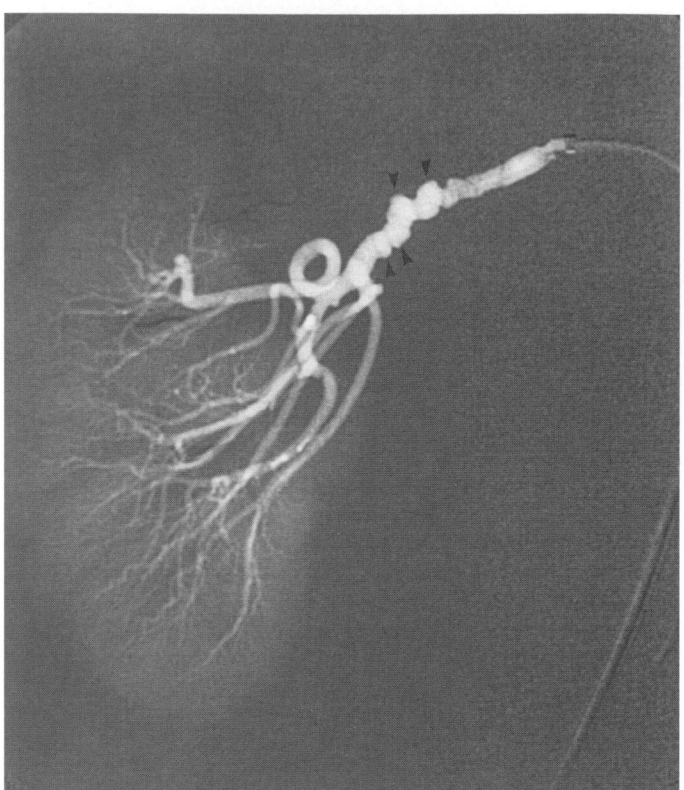

Figure 18.19 Fibromuscular dysplasia: medial fibroplasia with mural aneurysm. A 55-year-old white female with long history of poorly controlled hypertension underwent angiography to rule out renal artery stenosis. Selective right lower renal artery injection demonstrates the characteristic corrugated or "string of beads" appearance (black arrowheads) involving the distal portion of the main renal artery prior to branching. Upper renal artery injection revealed similar pathology (not shown). Angioplasty of both renal arteries was performed and the patient remained normotensive.

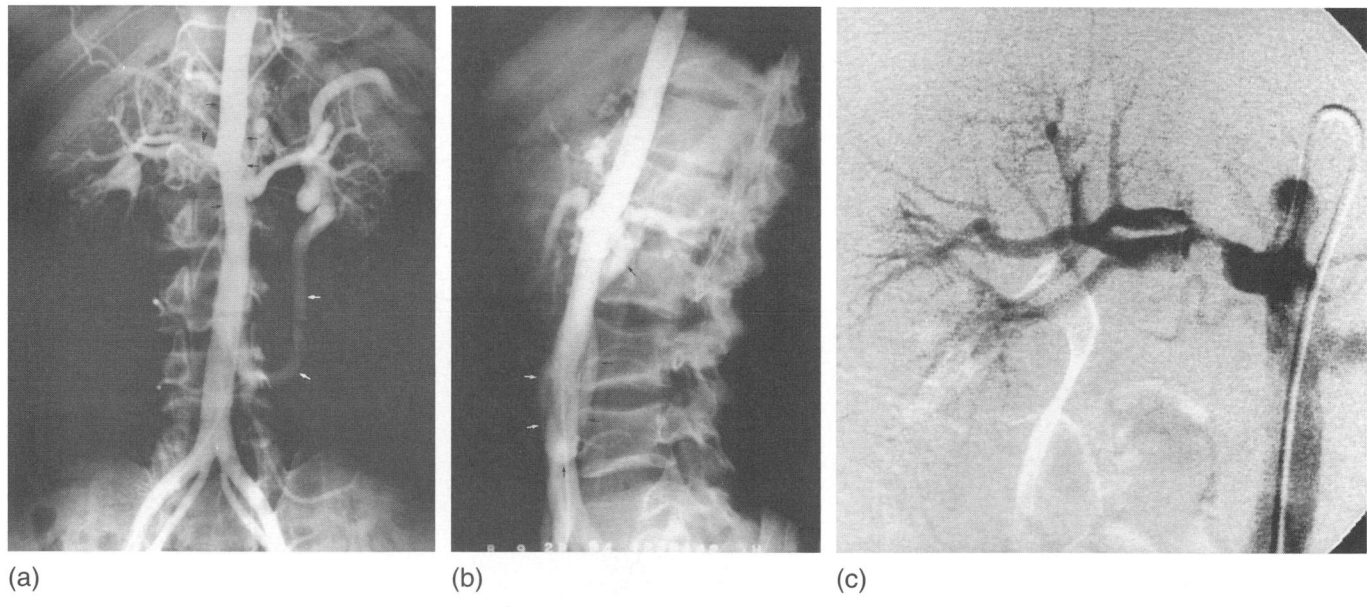

(a)   (b)   (c)

Figure 18.20 Midaortic syndrome. A 19-year-old male with hypertension. Evaluation for systemic vasculitis was negative. Findings in this syndrome are similar to Takayasu's arteritis, but are seen only in the mid-abdominal aorta. (a and b) Anteroposterior and lateral views of the abdominal aortogram show nearly complete occlusion of the celiac and superior mesenteric arteries with stenotic suprarenal and renal segments of the abdominal aorta (black arrows). Note the huge inferior mesenteric artery (black and white arrows) providing collateral supply to branches of the superior mesenteric artery and stenosis in the right main renal artery (black arrowhead). (c) Selective right renal arteriogram shows severe stenosis of the right main renal artery with extension to the ostia of the anterior and posterior divisions.

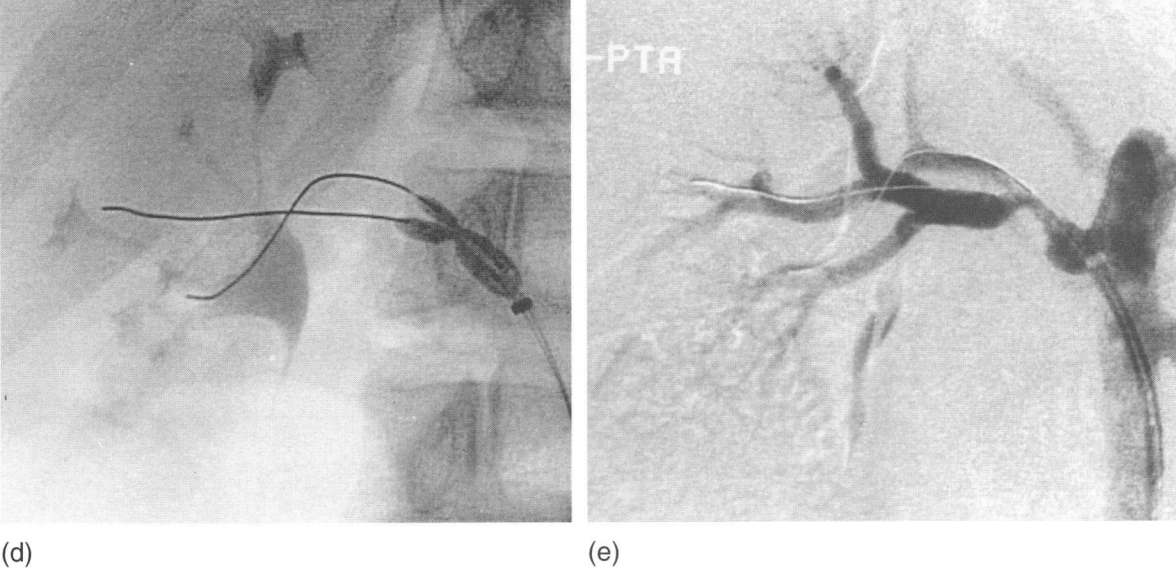

(d)   (e)

Figure 18.20 (cont.) (d) Right renal artery angioplasty. Note the simultaneous angioplasty, after placing a balloon catheter in each division of the right main renal artery (the so-called "kissing balloon technique"). (e) After angioplasty, the right renal arteriogram shows limited immediate success, as is common in Takayasu's arteritis.

diagnostic and requires no further investigation. The other types, typically lumped under the term "intimal", (Figure 18.4a) may have short or long tubular stenoses that are impossible to differentiate angiographically from vasculitic lesions. Fibromuscular dysplasia is not a systemic disease.

Midaortic syndrome

Developmental narrowing of the abdominal aorta, also known as abdominal coarctation, with ostial stenoses of the renal and or visceral arteries, is occasionally seen during evaluation of renovascular hypertension (Figure 18.20). The appearance is similar to the

abdominal form of Takayasu's arteritis (Lewis *et al.* 1988). This problem is usually discovered in childhood or adolescence (Stanley *et al.* 1981). Major vascular reconstruction is often required.

Raynaud's phenomenon

Raynaud's phenomenon (Raynaud 1862) is episodic spasm of small vessels of upper extremity precipitated by cold temperatures. Its classic clinical features are blanching of the hand leading to bluish discoloration, followed by pink coloration with symptoms of numbness, tingling, and pain on recovery (Klippel 1991). Angiographically, this is characterized by multiple areas of segmental but reversible

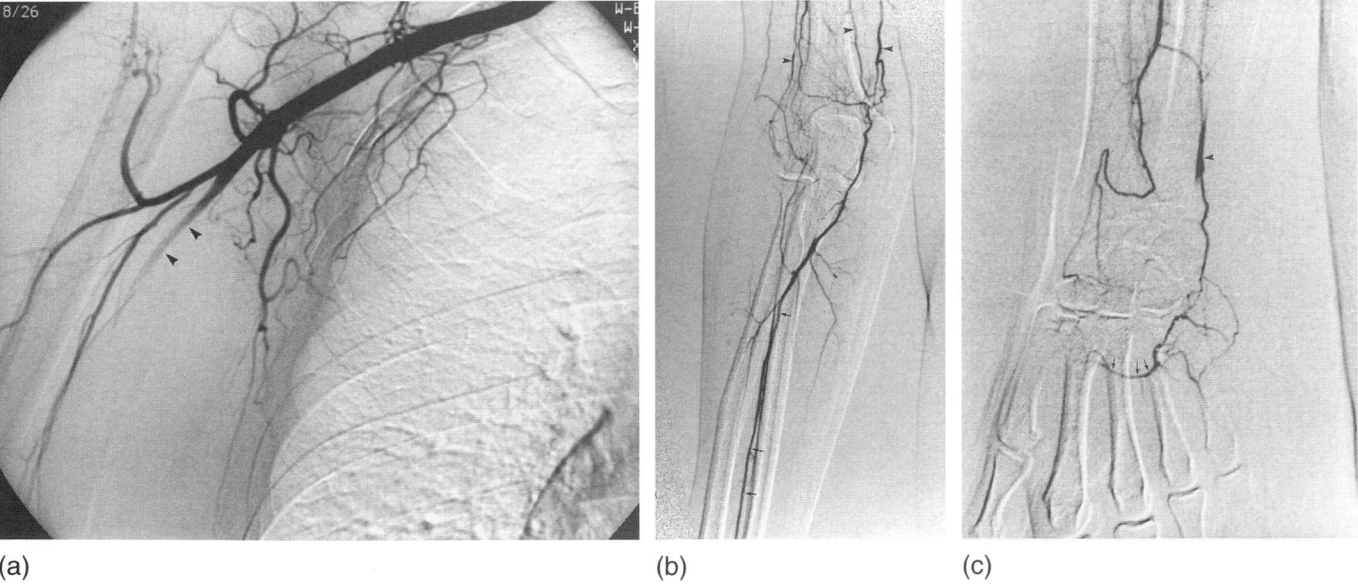

(a)   (b)   (c)

Figure 18.21 Raynaud's phenomenon. A 49-year-old female patient with a history of recurrent Raynaud's phenomenon presented with acute ischemia of the right upper extremity. (a) Selective right subclavian artery injection shows complete occlusion of the upper right brachial artery (black arrowheads). (b) Occlusion of the brachial, radial, and ulnar arteries. Small collaterals (black arrowheads) reconstitute the interosseous artery (black arrows). (c) Arteriogram showing circulation to the distal right forearm and wrist demonstrates an occluded ulnar artery and partial reconstitution of the radial artery (black arrowhead). Collaterals reconstitute part of the deep palmar arch (black arrows). The patient underwent thrombolysis with intra-arterial urokinase infusion overnight. The patient improved clinically, with no signs of residual ischemia.

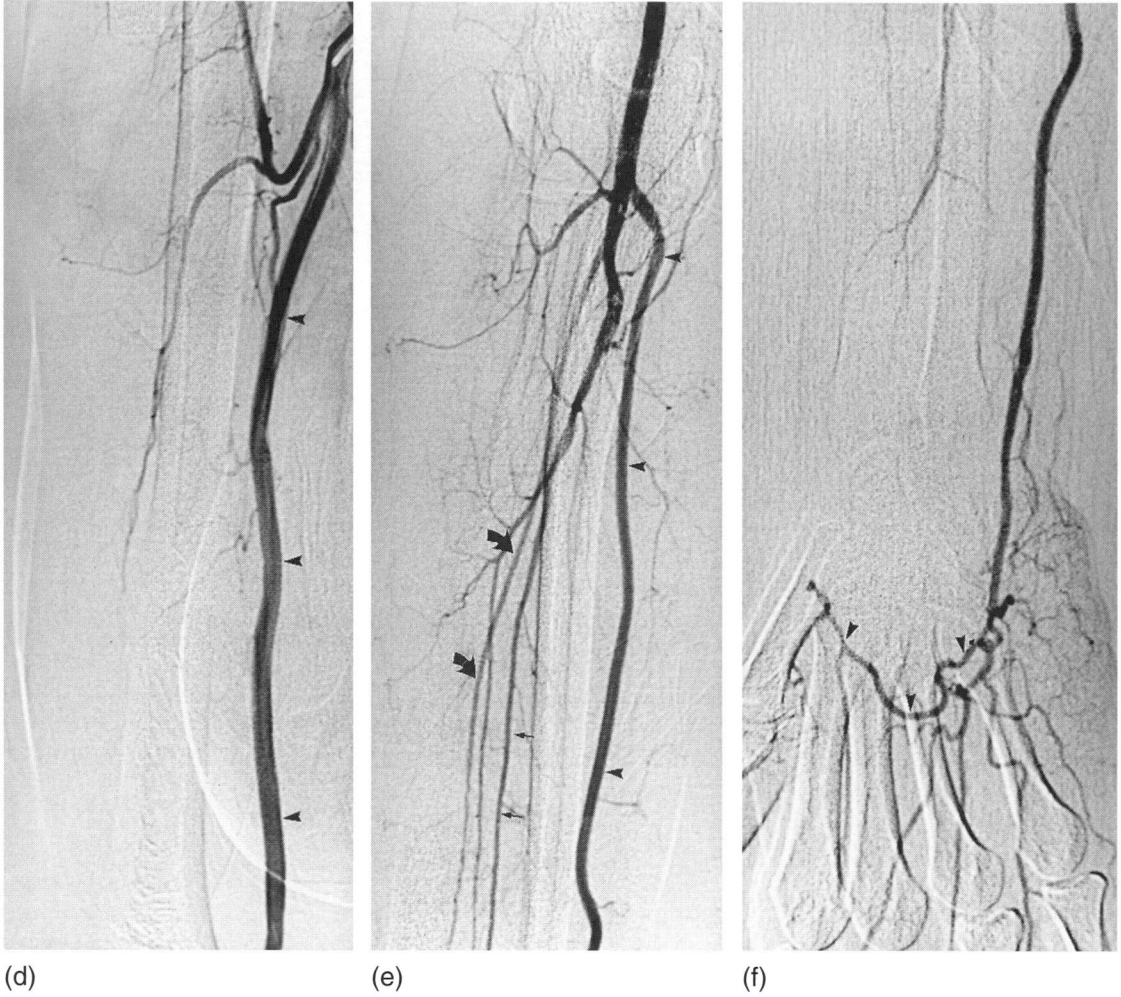

(d)   (e)   (f)

Figure 18.21 (*cont*) (d, e, f) Post-thrombolysis arteriogram demonstrated complete resolution of the thrombosis within the right brachial artery (black arrowheads in d). Other widely patent vessels (e) include the radial (black arrowheads), ulnar (curved arrows), and interrosseous arteries (black arrows). The deep palmar arch (black arrowheads) and its branches are well visualized (f). There is no significant underlying arterial disease. Evaluation of this patient over a period of several years consistently failed to reveal an etiology for recurrent Raynaud's phenomenon and arterial thrombosis.

spasm that improves with vasodilators or poststress maneuver. Patients with Raynaud's phenomenon may have severe ischemia and arterial thrombosis, but it is debatable whether this represents a separate, but related, problem (see Figure 18.21 and Chapter 17).

References

Bron, K. M., Strott, C. A. and Shapiro, A. P. (1995). The diagnostic value of angiographic observations in polyaarteritis nodosa. A case of multiple aneurysms in the visceral organs. *Archives of Internal Medicine*, **116**, 450.

Bronze, M. S., Shirwany, A., Corbett, C. and Schaberg, D. R. (1999). Infectious aortitis: an uncommon manifestation of infection with *Streptococcus pneumoniae*. *American Journal of Medicine*, **107**, 627–30.

Buerger, L. (1908). Thrombo-angiitis obliterans: A study of the vascular lesion leading to pre-senile spontaneous gangrene. *American Journal of the Medical Sciences*, **136**, 567–80.

Capps, J. H. and Klein, R. M. (1970). Polyarteritis nodosa as a cause of perirenal and retroperitoneal hemorrhage. *Radiology*, **94**, 143.

Castaneda-Zuniga, W. R., Formanek, A., Lillehei, R. C., Tadavarthy, M. and Amplatz, K. (1981). Non-surgical treatment of Takayasu's disease. *Cardiovascular and Interventional Radiology*, **4**, 245–8.

Chajek, T. and Fainaur, M. (1975). Behçet's disease. Report of 41 cases and review of the literature. *Medicine*, **S4**, 179–96.

Chandrakantan, A. and Kaufman, J. (1999). Clinical nephrology teaching case-renal hemorrhage in polyarteritis nodosa: Diagnosis and management. *American Journal of Kidney Diseases*, **33**, 1–3.

Dabich, L., Bookstein, J. J., Zweifler, A. and Zarafonetis, C. J.D. (1972). Digital arteries in patients with scleroderma. *Archives of Internal Medicine*, **130**, 708.

Easterbrook, J. S. (1980). Renal and hepatic microaneurysms: Report of a new entity simulating polyarteritis nodosa. *Radiology*, **137**, 629.

Flamand, F., Harris, K. A., DeRose, G., Karam, B. and Jamieson, W. G. (1992). Arteritis due to Salmonella with aneurysm formation: two cases. *Canadian Journal of Surgery*, **35**, 248–52.

Fleming, R. J. and Stern, L. Z. (1965). Multiple intraparenchymal renal aneurysms in polyarteritis nodosa. *Radiology*, **84**, 100.

Hagen, B. and Lohse, S. (1984). Clinical and radiologic aspects of Buerger's disease. *Cardiovascular and Interventional Radiology*, **7**, 283–93.

Hall, S., Barr, W., Lie, J. T., Stanson, A. W., Kazmier, F. J. and Hunder, G. G. (1985). Takayasu artertis. A study of 32 North American patients. *Medicine*, **64**, 89–99.

Hamrin, B. (1972). Polymyalgia arteritica. *Acta Medica Scandinavica*, **533** (Suppl.), 1–131.

Hamza, M. (1987). Large artery involvement in Behçet's disease. *Journal of Rheumatology*, **14**, 554–9.

Harrison, E. G., Jr and McCormack, L. J. (1971). Pathologic classifications of renal arterial disease in renovascular hypertension. *Mayo Clinic Proceedings*, **46**, 161–7.

Hekali, P., Kajander, H., Pajari, R., Stenman, S. and Somer, T. (1991). Diagnostic significance of angiographically observed visceral aneurysms with regard to polyarteritis nodosa. *Acta Radiologica*, **32**, 143–8.

Herskowitz, M. M., Flyer, M. A. and Sclafani, S. J.A. (1993). Percutaneous transhepatic coil embolization of a ruptured intrahepatic aneurysm in polyarteritis nodosa. *Cardiovascular and Interventional Radiology*, **16**, 254–6.

Inada, K., Katsummura, T., Hirai, J. and Sunada, T. (1970). Surgical treatment in the aortitis syndrome. *Archives of Surgery*, **100**, 220–4.

Iwia, T. (1998). Buerger's disease with intestinal involvement. *Internal Journal of Cardiology*, **66** (Suppl. 1), S257–63.

Jennette, J. C., Falk, R. J., Andrassy, K., Bacon, P. A., Churg, J., Gross, W. L., Hagen, E. C., Hoffman, G. S., Hunder, G. G., Kallenberg, C. G.M., McCluskey, R. T., Sinico, R. A., Rees, J., van Es, L. A., Waldherr, R. and Wiik, A. (1994). Nomenclature of systemic vasculitides, proposal of an international consensus conference. *Arthritis and Rheumatism*, **37**, 187–92.

Katz, S. G., Andros, G. and Kohl, R. D. (1992). Salmonella infection of the abdominal aorta. *Surgery Gynaecology and Obstetrics*, **175**, 102–6.

Kimoto, S. (1979). The history and present status of aortic surgery in Japan particularly for aortitis syndrome. *Journal of Cardiovascular Surgery*, **20**, 107–28.

Klein, R. G., Hunder, G. G., Stanson, A. W. and Sheps, S. G. (1975). Large artery involvement in giant cell (temporal) arteritis. *Annals of Internal Medicine*, **83**, 806–12.

Klippel, J. H. (1991). Raymond's phenomenon: the French tri-color. *Archives of Internal Medicine*, **151**, 2389–93.

Kusaba, A., Inokuchi, K., Kiyose, T. and Oka, N. (1973). Carotid reconstruction for Takayasu's (pulseless) disease using open thromboendarterectomy at aortocarotid Junction. *Japanese Journal of Surgery*, **3**, 91–7.

Lacombe, P., Frija, G., Parlier, H., Lang, F., Hamza, R. and Bismuth, V. (1985). Transcatheter embolization of multiple pulmonary artery aneurysms in Behçet's syndrome. *Acta Radiologica Diagnosis*, **26**, 251–3.

Lande, A. and Berkman, Y. M. (1986). Radiologic aspects of aortitis. In *Aortitis: clinical, pathologic, and radiographic aspects*, (eds Lande, A., Berkman, Y. M. and McAllister, H. A. Jr.), pp. 81–143. Raven Press, New York.

Laws, J. W., Lillie, J. G. and Scott, J. T. (1963). Arteriographic appearances in rheumatoid arthritis and other disorders. *British Journal of Radiology*, **36**, 477.

Lehrer, H. (1967). The physiology of angiographic arterial waves. *Radiology*, **89**, 11.

Lewis, III, V. D., Meranze, S. G., McLean, G. K., O'Neill, Jr., J. A., Berkowitz, Henry D. and Burke, D. R. (1988). The midaortic syndrome: Diagnosis and treatment. *Cardiovascular Radiology*, **167**, 111–13.

Lie, J. T. (1987). Thromboangiitis obliterans (Buerger's disease) in women. *Medicine*, **66**, 65–72.

Lupi-Herrera E., Sanchez-Torres, G., Marcushamer, J., Mispireta, J., Horwitz, S. and Vela, J. E. (1977). Takayasu's arteritis. Clinical study of 107 cases. *American Heart Journal*, **93**, 94–103.

Lupi-Herrera E., Sanchez-Torres, G., Horwitz, S. and Gutierrez, F. E. (1975). Pulmonary artery involvement in Takayasu's arteritis. *Chest*, **67**, 69.

Nasu, T. (1976). Aortitis syndrome: pathologic aspect. *Gendai Iryo*, **8**, 1143–50.

Olin, J., Young, J., Graor, R., Ruschhaupt, W. and Bartholomew, J. (1990). The changing clinical spectrum of thromboangiitis obliterans (Buerger's disease). *Circulation*, **82** (Suppl. IV), 3–8.

Oskoui R., Davis W. A. and Gomes M. N. (1993). Salmonella aortitis: a report of a successfully treated case with a comprehensive review of the literature. *Archives of Internal Medicine*, **153**, 517–25.

Pajari, R., Hekali, P. and Harjola, P. T. (1986). Treatment of Takayasu's arteritis: An analysis of 29 operated patients. *Thoracic and Cardiovascular Surgeon*, **34**, 176–81.

Park, J. H., Han, M. C., Kim, S. H., Oh, B. H., Park, Y. B. and Seo, J. D. (1989). Takayasu arteritis: Angiographic findings and results of angioplasty. *American Journal of Roentgenology*, **153**, 1069–74.

Park, J. H., Han, M. C. and Bettmann, M. A. (1984). Arterial manifestations of Behçet disease. *American Journal of Radiology*, **143**, 821–5.

Przybojewski, J. Z. (1981). Polyarteritis nodosa in the adult- report of a case with repeated myocardial infarction and a review of cardiac involvement. *South African Medical Journal*, **26**, 512–18.

Provenzale, J. M. and Allen, N. B. (1996). Neuroradiologic findings in polyarteritis nodosa. *American Journal of Neuroradiology*, **17**, 1119–26.

Rao, S. A., Mandalam, K. R., Rao, V. R., Gupta, A. K., Joseph, S., Unni, M. N., Subramanyan, R. and Neelakandhan, K. S. (1993). Takayasu Arteritis: Initial and long-term follow-up in 16 patients after percutaneous transluminal angioplasty of the descending thoracic and abdominal aorta. *Radiology*, **189**, 173–9.

Raynaud, A. G.M. (1862). De l'asphyxie locale et de la gangrene symetrique des extremities. (Translated by T. Barlow, New Sydenham Society, London, 1888). In *Textbook of angiography of vascular disease* (eds Neiman, H. L. and Yao, J. S.T.), p. 365. Churchill Livingstone, New York.

Rivera, R. (1973). Roentgenographic diagnosis of Buerger's disease. *Journal of Cardiovascular Surgery*, **14**, 40–6.

Rozenblit, G. N. and Saddekni, S. (1999). Percutaneous renal revascularization in children and adolescents with reno- vascular hypertension. *Techniques in Vascular and Interventional Radiology*, **2**, 84–90.

Saddekni, S., Sniderman, K. W., Hilton, S. and Sos, T. A. (1980). Percutaneous transluminal angioplasty in non-atherosclerotic lesions. *American Journal of Roentgenology*, **135**, 975–82.

Sharma, S., Rajani, M., Kaul, U., Talwar, K. K., Dev, V. and Shrivastava, S. (1990). Initial experience with percutaneous transluminal angioplasty in the management of Takayasu's arteritis. *British Journal of Radiology*, **63**, 517–22.

Shionoya, S., Ban, J., Nakata, G., Matsubara, J., Hirai, M. and Kawai, S. (1978). Involvement of the iliac artery in Buerger's disease. *Journal of Cardiovascular Surgery*, **19**, 69–76.

Smith, D. and Wernick, R. (1989). Spontaneous rupture of a renal artery aneurysm in polyarteritis nodosa: Critical review of the literature and report of a case. *American Journal of Medicine*, **87**, 464–7.

Stanley, J. C., Graham, L. M., Whitehouse, W. M., Jr., Zelenock, G. B., Erlandson, E. E., Cronenwett, J. L. and Lindenauer, S. M. (1981). Developmental occlusive disease of the abdominal aorta and the splanchnic and renal arteries. *American Journal of Surgery*, **142**, 190–6.

Strachnan, R. W. (1964). The natural history of Takayasu's arteriopathy. *Quarterly Journal of Medicine*, **33**, 57.

Srur, M. F., Sos, T. A., Saddekni, S., Cohn, D. J., Rozenblit, G. and Wetter, E. B. (1985). Intimal fibromuscular dysplasia and Takayasu's arteritis: delayed response to percutaneous transluminal renal angioplasty. *Radiology*, **157**, 657–60.

Suzuki, S., Yamada, I. and Himeno, Y. (1996). Angiographic findings in Buerger Disease. *Internal Journal of Cardiology*, **54** (Suppl.), S189–95.

Tanaka, K. (1998). Pathology and pathogenesis of Buerger's disease. *Internal Journal of Cardiology*, **66** (Suppl. 1), S237–42.

Tunaci, A., Berkmen, Y. M. and Gokmen, E. (1995). *American Journal of Roentgenology*, **164**, 51–6.

Tyagi, S., Singh, B., Kaul, U. A., Sethi, K. K., Arora, R. and Khalilullah, M. (1993). Balloon angioplasty for renovascular hypertension in Takayasu's arteritis. *American Heart Journal*, **125**, 1386–93.

von Winiwarter, F. (1879). Ueber eine eigenthumliche Form von Endarteritis und Endophlebitis mit Gangren des Fusses. *Archiv für Klinische Chirurgie*, **23**, 202–26.

Yamato, M., Lecky, J. W., Hiramatsu, K. and Kohda, E. (1986). Takayasu arteritis: Radiographic and angiographic findings in 59 patients. *Radiology*, **161**, 329–34.

Yao, J. S.T., Goodwin, D. P., and Kenyon, J. R. (1970). Case of ergot poisoning. *British Medical Journal*, **3**, 86.

Yorukoglu, Y., Ilgit, E., Zengin, M., Nazleil, K., Salman, E. and Yucel, E. (1993). Thromboangiitis obliterans (Buerger's disease in women – a reevaluation). *Angiology*, **44**, 527–32.

CHAPTER 19

Cross-sectional imaging in vasculitis

Enrique A. Sabater and Anthony W. Stanson

Introduction

The established gold-standard imaging test for the diagnosis of vasculitis is angiography, and angiographic findings are included in the diagnostic criteria of multiple vasculitides. While angiography allows high-resolution detail of changes affecting the lumen of vessels, one of its main limitations is the inability to visualize the actual changes occurring in the walls of blood vessels where the pathologic changes affecting the lumen of the vessel are occurring. More importantly, mural changes may precede luminal changes, making angiography abnormal only at later stages of disease. For these reasons, the non-invasive cross sectional imaging modalities of ultrasonography (US), computed tomography (CT), and magnetic resonance imaging (MRI) are assuming a more important role in the diagnosis and follow-up of vasculitis, sometimes suggesting the diagnosis at earlier stages of disease when early treatment may have greater impact on disease progression.

All three of these modalities, and in particular CT and MRI, have seen recent advances, now allowing faster and higher-resolution scanning. With these improvements, CT and MRI can be used to obtain high-quality angiographic images with minimally invasive techniques. CT angiography can now match the angiographic images obtained for evaluation of large and medium-size vessel vasculitis with the new multidetector scanners that allow reformatting images in any plane and three-dimensional (3D) reconstructions. Conventional angiography, however, provides better resolution than CT and MRI for imaging of peripheral vessels. Ultrasound provides excellent vessel detail to assess luminal and mural changes in peripheral and superficial vessels.

The cross sectional imaging modalities are also useful for demonstrating the end-organ effects and complications of the vasculitic process. Depending on the specific vasculitis, abnormalities can be demonstrated in any organ, most commonly in the lungs, heart, liver, kidneys, bowel, and brain.

The non-specific clinical features of many vasculitides often lead to differential diagnoses that include infectious or malignant processes. Cross-sectional imaging is frequently initially performed with these diagnoses in mind. It is important to be cognizant of the potential findings in vasculitis in order to recognize them and facilitate early treatment of the disease.

Ultrasonography

Ultrasonography (US) uses high frequency sound waves transmitted through the patient's tissues and generates an image from the echoes reflected by the tissues and their interfaces. Gray scale or B-mode images provide anatomical detail and characterization of the tissues. Beyond anatomical imaging, Doppler ultrasonography uses the Doppler principle to analyze the ultrasound waves reflected by moving blood, and generate blood velocity waveforms. This can be used to assess vascular hemodynamics, allowing quantitative assessment of flow direction and velocity, and qualitative assessment of flow waveforms for indirect evidence of proximal or distal disease.

Advantages of US include its widespread availability, low-cost, exam speed, and absence of contraindications. US avoids the need for ionizing radiation or IV contrast injection. It allows multiplanar real-time imaging and, for superficial vessels, excellent detail of the vessel walls with better resolution than CT or MRI. Disadvantages of ultrasound for vascular imaging are due mostly to the difficulty in visualizing certain vessels adequately, either because of body habitus, depth of the vessel, or intervening anatomical structures blocking the vessel from an appropriate imaging window. In addition, the quality of the examination and demonstration of findings is heavily dependent on the skill and diligence of the sonographer, compared to the more reproducible and relatively operator-independent images obtained by CT or MRI.

Computed tomography

Computed tomography (CT) generates a cross sectional image of the body from a computer reconstruction of measurements of X-ray transmission through a thin slice of tissue. CT has continued to evolve from conventional scanners, to faster helical scanners and the new generation of multidetector scanners, which allow even faster imaging with greater scan coverage. With the latest generation of multidetector scanners, an isovolumetric piece of the anatomy is imaged at the highest resolution of the scanner (0.6 mm for a 64 slice scanner), allowing reconstruction of the images in any imaging plane while preserving the same spatial resolution (Figure 19.1). This advancement has led to the virtual replacement of the majority of diagnostic angiography with CT angiography (CTA). For CTA, scanning is performed in the transverse (axial) plane after a bolus infusion of contrast, and three-dimensional

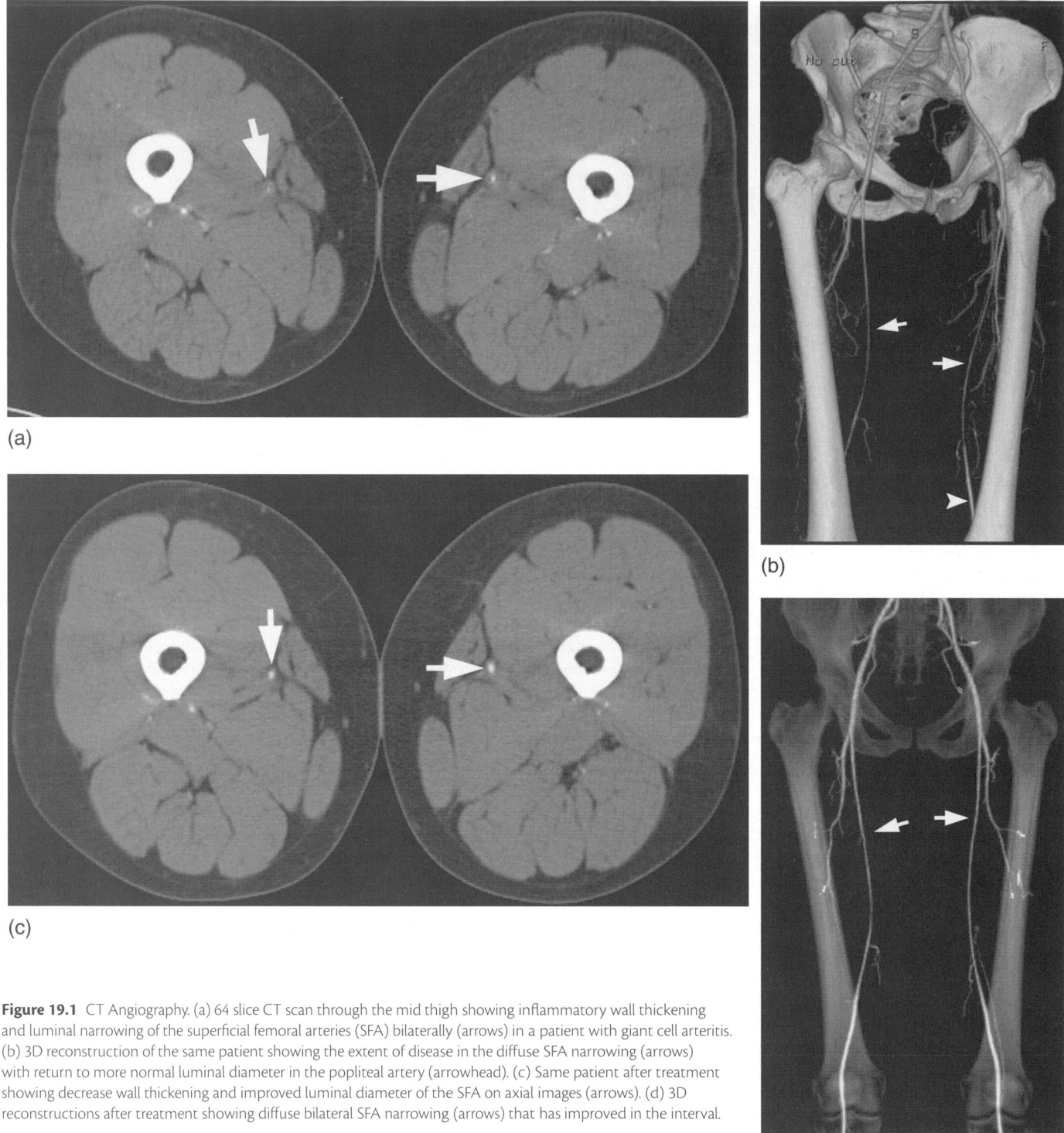

Figure 19.1 CT Angiography. (a) 64 slice CT scan through the mid thigh showing inflammatory wall thickening and luminal narrowing of the superficial femoral arteries (SFA) bilaterally (arrows) in a patient with giant cell arteritis. (b) 3D reconstruction of the same patient showing the extent of disease in the diffuse SFA narrowing (arrows) with return to more normal luminal diameter in the popliteal artery (arrowhead). (c) Same patient after treatment showing decrease wall thickening and improved luminal diameter of the SFA on axial images (arrows). (d) 3D reconstructions after treatment showing diffuse bilateral SFA narrowing (arrows) that has improved in the interval.

images are generated from software reconstructions of the axial scans. Conventional catheter angiography is mostly performed for resolving questionable findings on CTA, imaging small vessel disease, obtaining physiologic data such as pressure measurements to determine severity of disease, and for treatment of disease.

Advantages of CT include its widespread availability, rapid scan acquisition, good spatial resolution, excellent demonstration of calcifications and bone detail, excellent imaging of parenchymal changes and complications of vasculitis, and reproducible results. The examination is well tolerated by most patients. CTA only needs a peripheral IV for the contrast bolus administration, which is a great advantage over catheter-based conventional angiography by avoiding the risk of complications at the arterial puncture site and at the arteries traversed with the catheters and wires. Disadvantages of CT in comparison with MRI and US include the use of ionizing radiation, which is less than the radiation dose from angiography, and the need to use iodinated contrast for CTA for adequate tissue contrast. Iodinated contrast has potential detrimental effect on renal function and the potential for allergic reactions. CT is limited to acquiring images in the axial orientation while MRI has unlimited scan orientation possibilities; however, the new generation of multidetector scanners allows reconstruction of the axially obtained data in any plane without loss of resolution. Software improvements allow the reconstructions to be done quickly to aid in the detection of disease.

Ideally, CT scanning in vasculitis should be performed first without contrast, to improve detection of calcium and of increased attenuation, as is seen in hemorrhage or hematoma. Contrast enhanced images should then be obtained in the arterial phase, to allow CTA reconstructions during peak vessel enhancement. A third acquisition should be obtained after a time delay from the contrast injection to demonstrate the enhancement of organ parenchyma and arterial walls. Despite performing these three acquisitions, exam times are considerably faster than with MRI. The disadvantage of this approach is the amount of radiation given to the patient, which can have long-term effects, especially in younger patients.

Magnetic resonance imaging

MRI uses the magnetic properties of hydrogen atoms in body tissues to generate an image. In general, MRI has limited spatial resolution when compared to CT but superior contrast resolution. That is, imaging sequences can be obtained to bring out the difference between normal and diseased tissue and between tissues of different composition. MRI also has the advantage of allowing imaging in any plane, as mentioned above. Subtle changes in some arteries, particularly mural changes, are best demonstrated by imaging perpendicular to the long axis of the arterial wall, which can be done with MRI. This advantage of MRI can now be matched by CTA using the newer multidetector scanners.

Standard imaging sequences for MRI include the conventional T1 weighted spin echo sequence, which is well suited for evaluating anatomy because of its better spatial resolution, and T2 weighted spin echo sequence, which is more time-consuming but provides excellent tissue contrast without intravenous contrast. Intravenous contrast is occasionally used with T1 weighted sequences to demonstrate abnormal vascularity in soft tissues or organs, including arterial walls. This requires low doses of gadolinium and, usually, a delay before the start of imaging. Cardiac gating is used with spin echo techniques to eliminate artifacts from cardiac motion and best depict anatomic abnormalities in the thoracic aortic region and arch branches. Fast spin echo techniques are available to obtain T2-like information with faster scan times, but these techniques often have reduced spatial resolution and the quality is unpredictable.

MRI has continued to evolve with the development of faster equipment and imaging sequences, which have allowed quicker examinations, improved spatial resolution, and the development of contrast-enhanced magnetic resonance angiography (MRA) using an intravenous bolus of gadolinium. Vascular imaging is often possible with non-invasive MRA time-of-flight or phase-contrast techniques. In many centers, contrast MRA, although invasive, has replaced non-contrast MRA, since it provides the best arterial detail without the artifacts of non-contrast techniques, thus facilitating faster and more accurate exams. Contrast MRA images are obtained with precise timing after a fast bolus of larger amounts of gadolinium, which is different from the contrast enhanced MRI approach for organ parenchyma enhancement described above. Images are obtained in a three-dimensional acquisition which allows viewing of the data in any desired plane, optimizing detection of abnormalities and depiction of anatomy (Hartnell 1999). Functional information, as in cardiac function and valve function, can be demonstrated with gradient echo cine techniques.

Advantages of MRI include its versatile orientation of the imaging plane, use of non-ionizing radiation, lack of significant nephrotoxicity of gadolinium, and excellent tissue contrast. Disadvantages include the length of time of the exam, its poor imaging of calcium/ calcifications, reduced spatial resolution, expense, more limited availability, potential for claustrophobia limiting the tolerability of the exam, and contraindication of the exam in patients with pacemakers and other implantable devices.

Role of cross-sectional imaging in vasculitis

Vascular changes

Cross sectional imaging can be used to image the arterial and venous changes of vasculitis, by demonstrating the lumen of the vessel and mural changes. Vessel luminal changes can be demonstrated with angiographic techniques and include irregularity, stenosis, occlusion, ectasia, aneurysm, and dissection. Mural changes can also be demonstrated, including wall thickening, calcifications, hematomas, and mural thrombus. The ability to image the vessel wall and to provide non- or minimally-invasive angiographic images are the key advantages of cross-sectional imaging. Luminal and mural changes can also be characterized as to distribution, location, and morphology, which may provide clues for suggesting the differential diagnosis of the disease process. Mural changes can also be followed on repeat studies to assess response to treatment or progression of disease (Figure 19.2).

Some vasculitides have a significant component of venous involvement. Ultrasonography is well established as the imaging method of choice for extremity deep venous thrombosis, with magnetic resonance venography (MRV) and CT venography also being used at some centers. Conventional venography is rarely used today, such as when the calf veins cannot be adequately seen by other methods and suspicion is high for thrombosis. MRI best demonstrates occlusion of the venous drainage of the brain. Evaluation of intestinal or solid organ venous drainage and superior vena cava (SVC) or inferior vena cava (IVC) is best demonstrated by cross sectional techniques of CT or MRI.

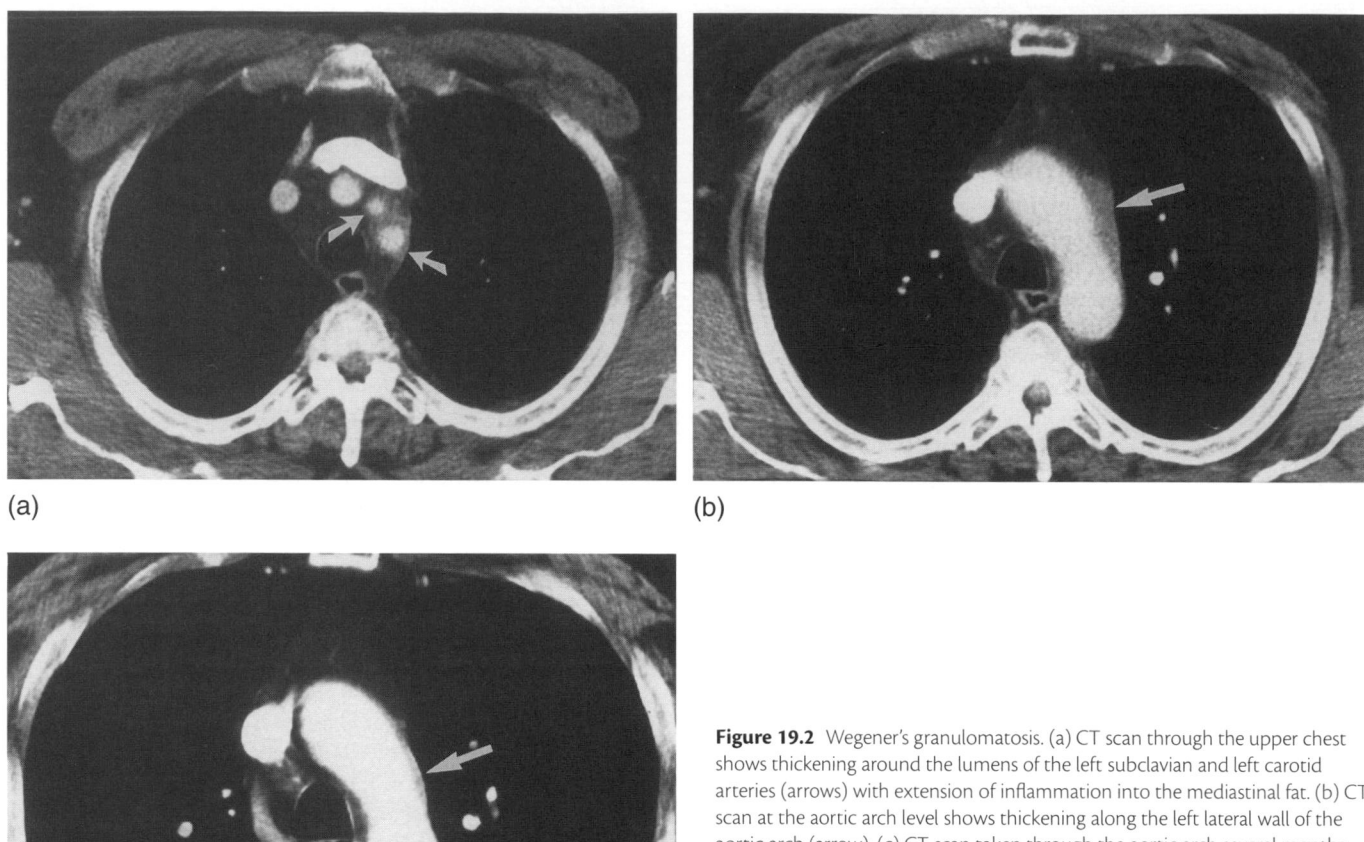

Figure 19.2 Wegener's granulomatosis. (a) CT scan through the upper chest shows thickening around the lumens of the left subclavian and left carotid arteries (arrows) with extension of inflammation into the mediastinal fat. (b) CT scan at the aortic arch level shows thickening along the left lateral wall of the aortic arch (arrow). (c) CT scan taken through the aortic arch several months after therapy shows reduction in the degree of thickening of the left wall of the aortic arch (arrow).

Organ changes and complications

Cross sectional imaging can provide additional insight into the diagnosis of vasculitis by demonstrating characteristic changes and distribution of involvement of organs affected. In smaller-vessel vasculitides where vessel changes are not detectable, the parenchymal effects of the vasculitis are most often the only findings on cross-sectional imaging. Compromise of arterial flow may be evident as ischemic changes or infarcts in the affected organs. Venous outflow compromise will also result in ischemic changes and congestion. Arterial aneurysms may rupture, appearing as intraparenchymal or subcapsular hemorrhage. The perivascular inflammatory process may also extend to the organ parenchyma and become prominent as areas of abnormal CT attenuation or MRI signal. Nodules and masses may be seen in vasculitides associated with granuloma formation. CT and MRI may detect perivascular inflammation as infiltrative changes in the fat surrounding vessels, most commonly seen in the mediastinum, retroperitoneum, and mesentery. Rupture

of aneurysms and bleeds from infarcted organs may present as free hemorrhage or focal hematomas anywhere in the body.

The optimal cross-sectional imaging modality for a particular patient depends on the body part to be imaged and the advantages of each modality. Certain modalities are well established as providing the best information for a specific body part. For example, MRI is the modality of choice for imaging the brain and central nervous system for changes of vasculitis. CT, including regular thickness scanning and high-resolution thin section scans, is the established best modality for studying lung disease. In most cases, neither of these examples requires contrast administration. Other areas can be imaged with either modality, depending on the situation. For example, the abdomen is frequently screened with ultrasound, which can be definitive for some organ lesions, but often additional information is needed from CT or MRI. CT is excellent for abdominal disease and is often also used for screening, but lesions can be missed without intravenous contrast administration. MRI can then be used to demonstrate abdominal disease in patients with renal insufficiency or severe iodinated contrast allergy. In the orbit, CT best demonstrates bone changes, such as the destructive lesions found in Wegener's granulomatosis. On the other hand, MRI best demonstrates the soft tissue extension of disease and best characterizes the abnormalities by its signal characteristics. Radiologists are trained in how to choose the best imaging modality for the clinical situation and indication and can help other physicians in obtaining a thorough, efficient, and safe imaging evaluation.

Imaging of specific types of vasculitis

Takayasu's arteritis

Takayasu's arteritis (Chapter 25) is the ideal vasculitis for MRI and CT imaging with cross-sectional images and angiographic techniques. Since large elastic arteries, including the aorta, its major branches, and the pulmonary arteries are affected, mural changes are well within the spatial resolution of CT and MRI, which gives these imaging modalities an important role in early diagnosis. The large caliber of the thoracic aorta and its orientation perpendicular to the axial scanning plane make this artery ideally suited for CT evaluation (Chung et al. 1996). In the affected population, which is generally young, atherosclerotic changes in the vessel wall are usually not present to confuse the diagnosis. The main advantage of cross-sectional imaging over conventional angiography is the demonstration of mural changes, which have been noted to be more frequent than luminal changes and would be usually missed by conventional angiography (Yamada et al. 1998). In addition, the potential complications of conventional angiography are avoided with cross-sectional imaging.

The significant feature of early disease is thickening of the aortic or great vessel wall. At this stage of the disease, conventional angiography relies on detecting descending aortic wall thickening as a subtle increase in the distance between the intraluminal contrast and the air in the lung. Since the luminal diameter is not affected, angiography can easily miss the subtle mural changes of early disease. The aorta and innominate artery are the most common sites for mural changes in the presence of a normal appearing angiogram (Park et al. 1997). Normally, the aortic wall is less than 1 mm in thickness and the outer edge of the aorta is sharply defined. In patients with Takayasu's arteritis, this sharp vessel definition is lost. CT without contrast may demonstrate higher attenuation thickened arterial walls (Park 1996). This high attenuation may be due to proliferation of fibrous and connective tissue and increased calcium content in the media and adventitia (Sharma et al. 1996). A "double ring" pattern of aortic wall thickening has been described in CT with intravenous contrast (Figure 19.3) (Park 1996; Hayashi et al. 1991). An inner, poorly-enhancing ring is thought to represent mucoid or gelatinous swelling of the intima (Hayashi et al. 1991) or the low attenuation intima trapped between the increased attenuation of the lumen and the media/adventitia (Sharma et al. 1996). The outer and thicker, well-enhanced ring is thought to represent active medial and adventitial inflammation probably with enlarged vasa vasorum. Enhancement may occur in the early arterial phase or may be delayed (Park et al. 1997). With proper timing of the scanning during the contrast bolus in the arterial phase, subtle thickening can be detected with high sensitivity by CT (Matsunaga et al. 1997). Timing is important since non-contrast or delayed images after contrast cannot reliably identify the aortic wall separate from the lumen. MRI can also detect wall thickening with the advantage that no contrast is needed to distinguish between the wall and the lumen of the artery (Figures 19.4 and 19.5) (Matsunaga et al. 1998). For evaluating the aortic arch and pulmonary arteries, MRI allows imaging in the best plane to see the wall changes, which can now also be achieved with reformatted images from multidetector CTA. Wall enhancement has been demonstrated with gadolinium. Infiltration of the adjacent mediastinal fat can sometimes be observed with CT and MRI, corresponding to the perivascular infiltration by various cells occasionally seen around the vasa vasorum.

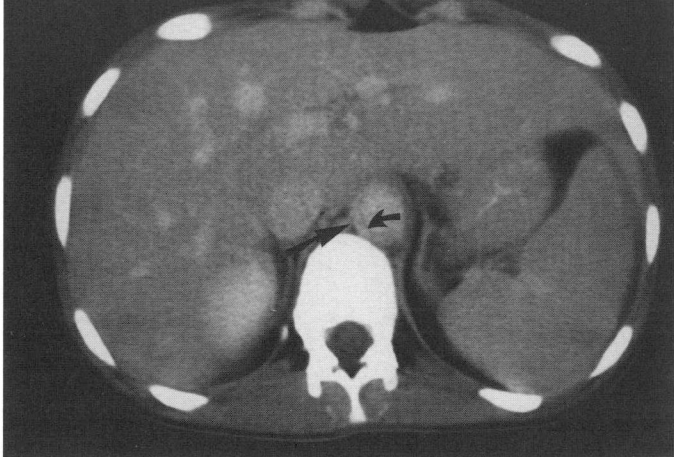

Figure 19.3 Takayasu's arteritis. CT scan through the upper abdomen shows thick, contrast enhancing wall of the aorta (arrow) and an inner ring of low density (curved arrow) indicating the inner wall.

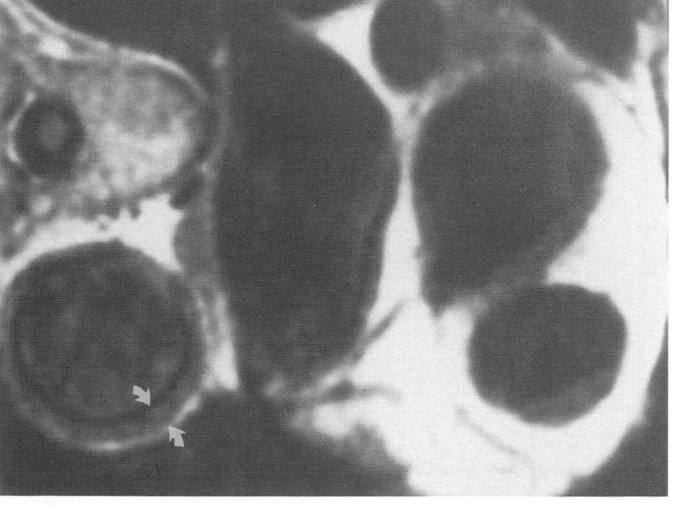

Figure 19.4 Takayasu's arteritis. MRI cross section through the mid chest shows wall thickening (between the arrows) of the descending thoracic aorta.

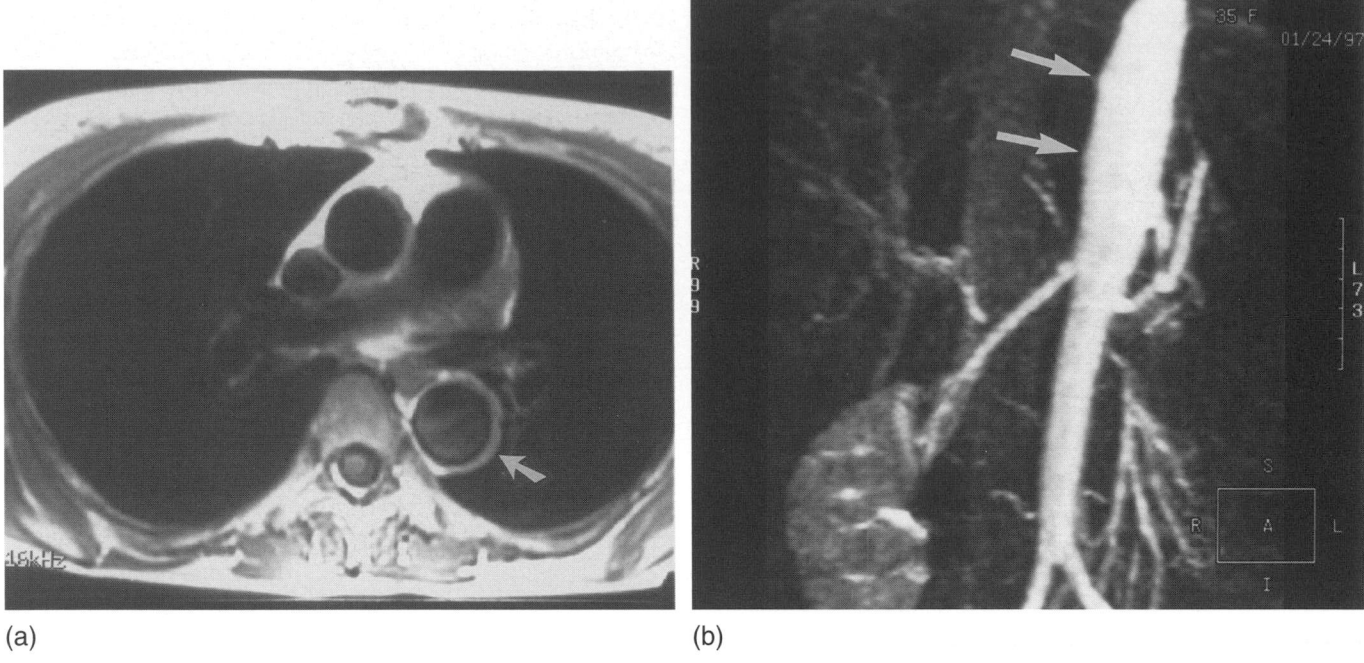

Figure 19.5 Takayasu's arteritis. (a) Transverse MRI through the mid-chest shows thickening of the wall of the descending thoracic aorta (arrow) with high signal intensity. (b) MRA coronal view of the abdominal aorta with gadolinium enhancement shows subtle irregularity of the suprarenal aortic lumen (arrows) in addition to slight expansion of the diameter.

CT and MRI findings have been used to document response to treatment and therefore to predict which early lesions may progress to stenosis. Based on a small number of patients, MRI studies have shown resolution of arterial wall contrast enhancement, edema, and thickening after treatment, which may correlate with prevention of stenotic lesions (Aluquin *et al.* 2002; Andrews *et al.* 2004). The largest series following CT findings before and after treatment showed that

about half the patients had absence of arterial wall enhancement and decrease in amount of wall thickening after treatment. In this study, thickening progressed in 25% of patients (Paul *et al.* 2001).

Ultrasound can also demonstrate the mural and luminal changes of Takayasu's arteritis. In a study evaluating the brachiocephalic vessels, all patients had subclavian artery involvement (one-third of them bilaterally), and the majority (69%) had common carotid artery involvement, which was always bilateral. The mural thickening

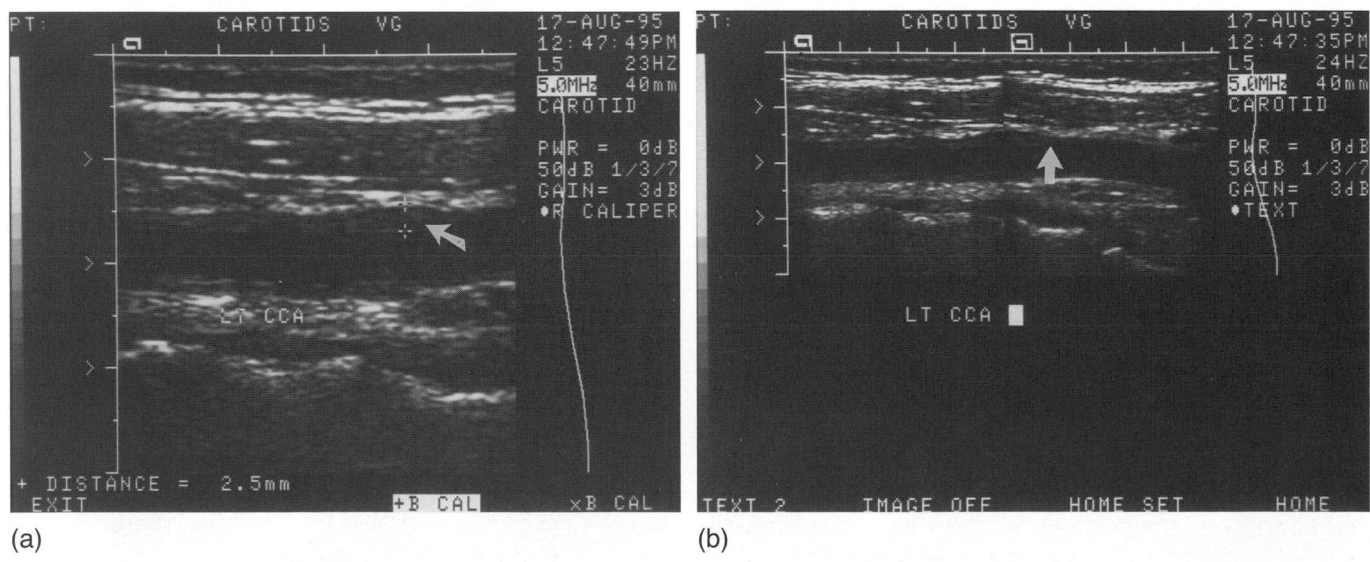

Figure 19.6 Takayasu's arteritis. (a) Ultrasound examination in longitudinal view of the common carotid artery shows circumferential, hypoechoic wall thickening measured at 2.5 mm (arrow). Normal thickness is less than 0.8 mm. (b) This larger field of view shows the segmental distribution of disease. There is sharp cut-off of the wall thickening involving the left half of the image (arrow) while there is no evidence of wall thickening to the right of the arrow.

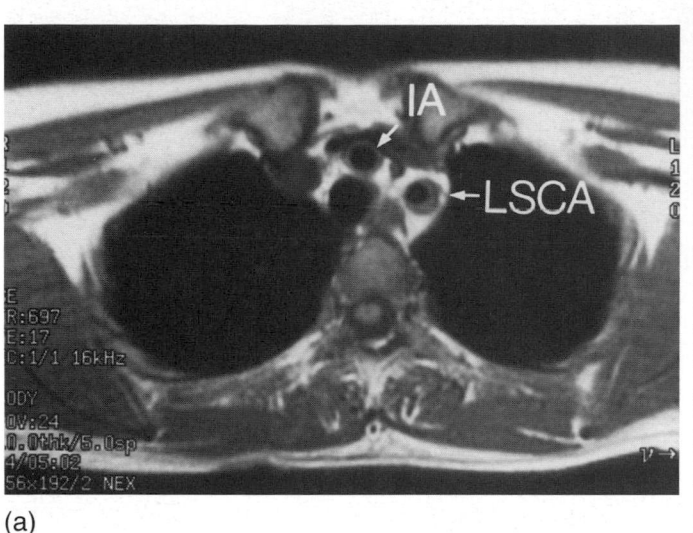

(a)

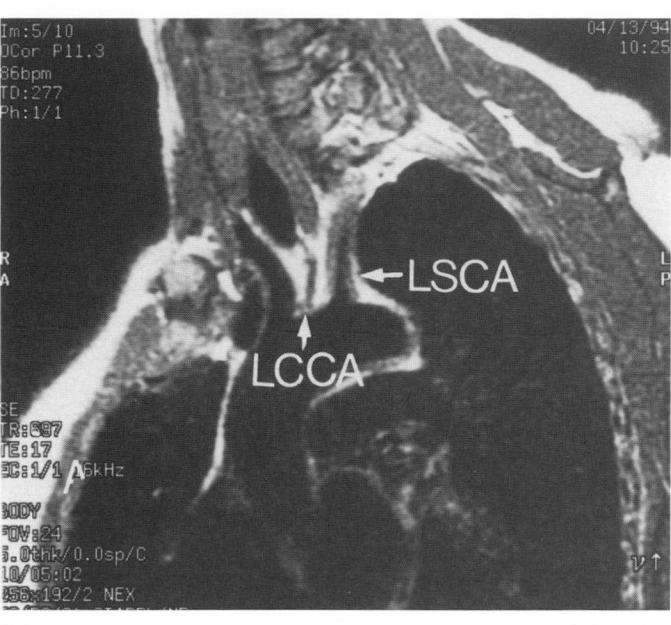

(b)

Figure 19.7 Takayasu's arteritis. (a) MRI through the upper chest shows wall thickening of the innominate artery (arrow IA) and of the left subclavian artery (arrow LSCA). Between these two is a stenotic remnant of the left common carotid artery. (b) MRI with oblique sagittal view shows stenosis of the left subclavian artery (arrow LSCA) with circumferential wall thickening and severe stenosis of the left common carotid artery (arrow LCCA) from its origin.

tends to be homogeneous, circumferential, iso- or hyperechoic, and typically involves the proximal half to two-thirds of the common carotid arteries. When affected, there is a sharp distal cut-off for the wall changes (Figure 19.6). Rarely, patients may have internal carotid artery involvement. Doppler evaluation is useful to demonstrate the hemodynamic effects of the stenotic disease. Disadvantages of US include underestimation of subclavian artery disease and difficulty imaging the proximal subclavian artery, which may result in a false-negative exam (Sun *et al.* 1996).

During the late phase, or pulseless stage, of the disease, occlusive arterial changes predominate as a result of pronounced fibrotic thickening of the adventitia and intima. The diagnosis of Takayasu's arteritis is most often made during this stage of the disease, and is frequently confirmed by angiography. CTA and MRA provide excellent angiographic images of the aorta and major branches to make the diagnosis non- or minimally-invasively (Figure 19.7). Sensitivity and specificity for luminal changes in the thoracic aorta and major branches has been shown to be 93% or greater by CT when compared to angiography (Yamada *et al.* 1998). Takayasu's arteritis is the only aortitis resulting in stenosis or occlusion of the aorta (Figure 19.8). As in conventional angiography, findings include long and diffuse, or short and segmental, irregular stenosis or occlusions of major branches of the aorta near their origins. Skip areas of involvement are common when imaging lumen irregularity or stenosis, but more diffuse mural involvement has been demonstrated in the angiographically normal areas (Sharma *et al.* 1996). Commonly involved are the left subclavian artery, left common carotid artery (CCA), innominate artery, renal artery, celiac artery, superior mesenteric artery, and the pulmonary artery (Figure 19.9). Stenotic lesions are more common in the thoracic aorta than in the abdominal aorta. Skip areas of involvement and abundant collateralization are frequently seen. Fusiform or sacular

true aneurysms, ectasia, and post-stenotic aneurysms can be seen, most commonly in the aorta and its branches (Figures 19.10 and 19.11). Ruptures have also been reported (Regina *et al.* 1998). Cine MRI can accurately depict the aortic regurgitation that often accompanies dilatation of the ascending aorta (Matsunaga *et al.* 1998). Dissections have been reported in the descending thoracic

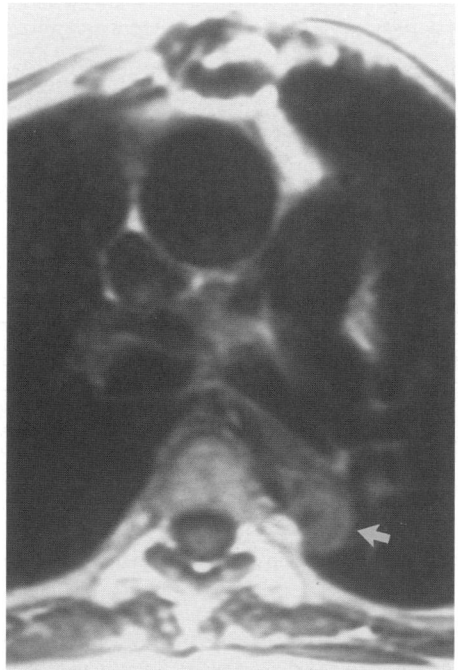

Figure 19.8 Takayasu's arteritis. MRI through the mid-chest shows the descending thoracic aorta (arrow) to have a small caliber and to be occluded.

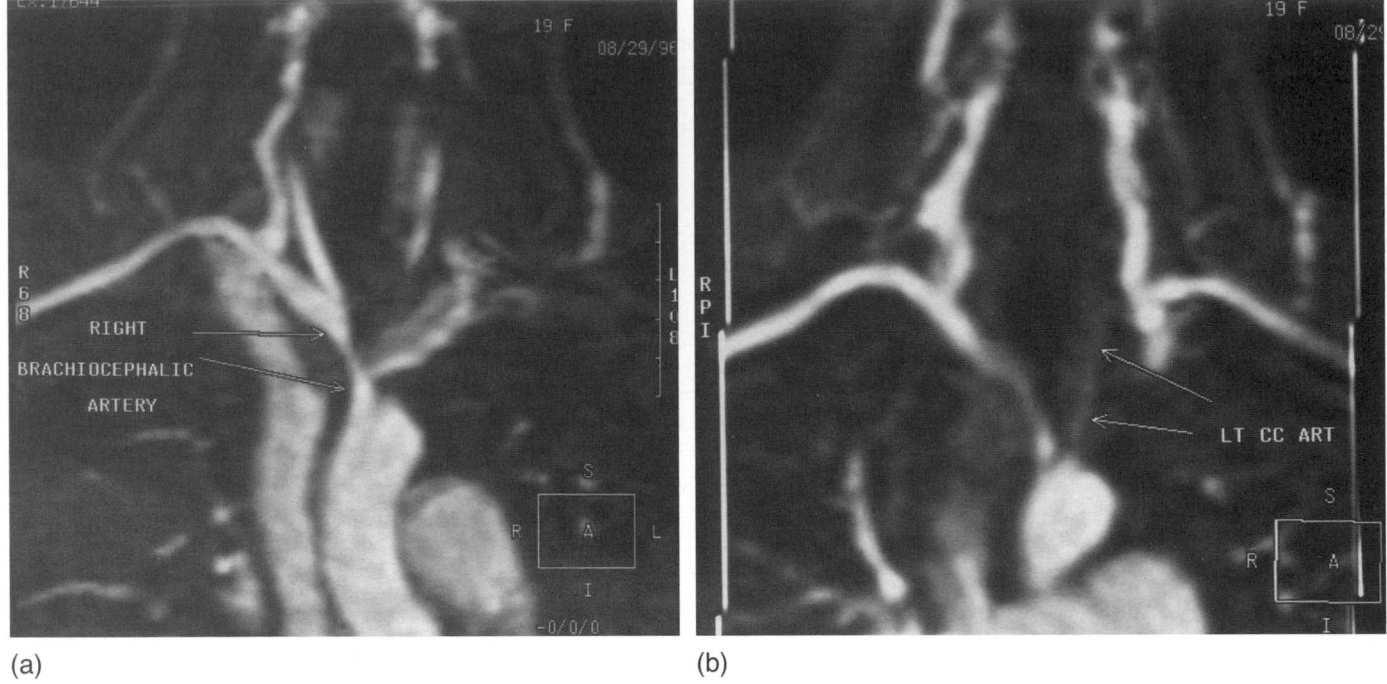

Figure 19.9 Takayasu's arteritis. Coronal view of MRA with gadolinium injection shows: (a) segmental stenosis of the innominate (brachiocephalic) artery (arrows); (b) the left common carotid artery (arrows LT CC ART) has marked narrowing of its lumen, as seen in a different projection.

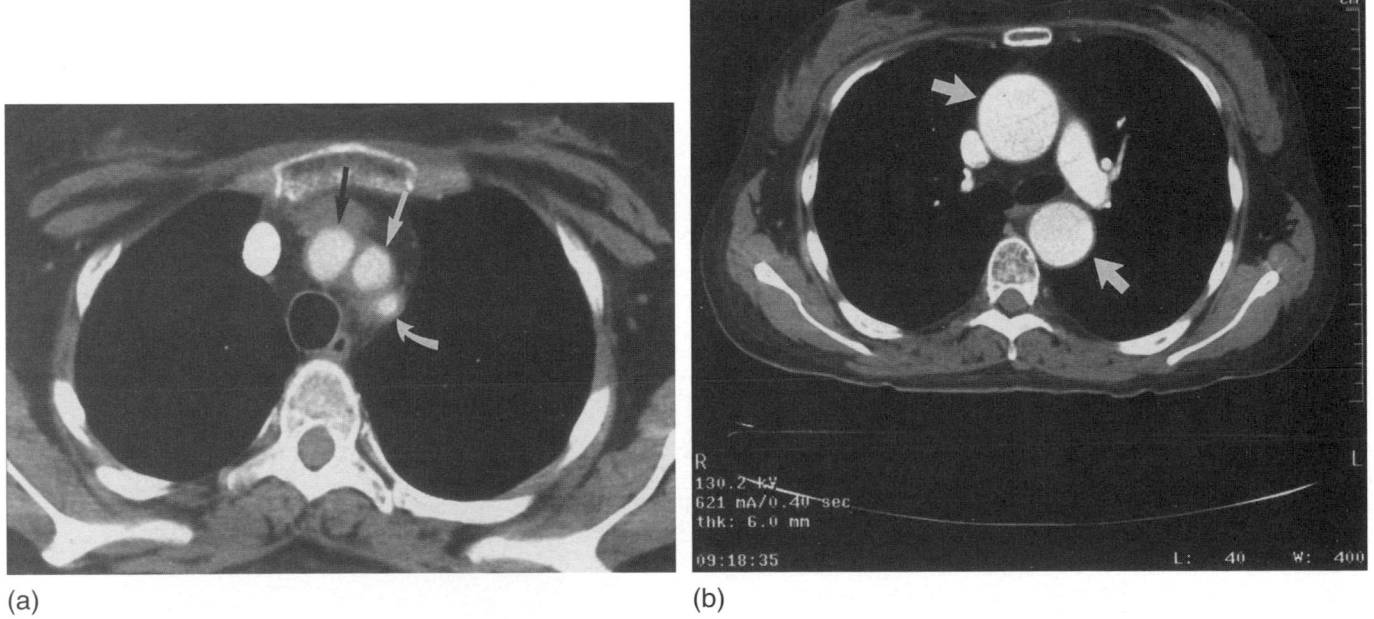

Figure 19.10 Takayasu's arteritis. (a) CT scan through the upper chest shows expansion of the innominate artery (black arrow) and left common carotid artery (white arrow) with surrounding thickening of the arterial walls. The left subclavian artery has a much smaller caliber (curved arrow) and its wall is also thickened. (b) CT scan through the chest taken at the level below the aortic arch shows ectasia of the ascending and descending segments of the thoracic aorta (arrows). There is slight wall thickening in the descending segment.

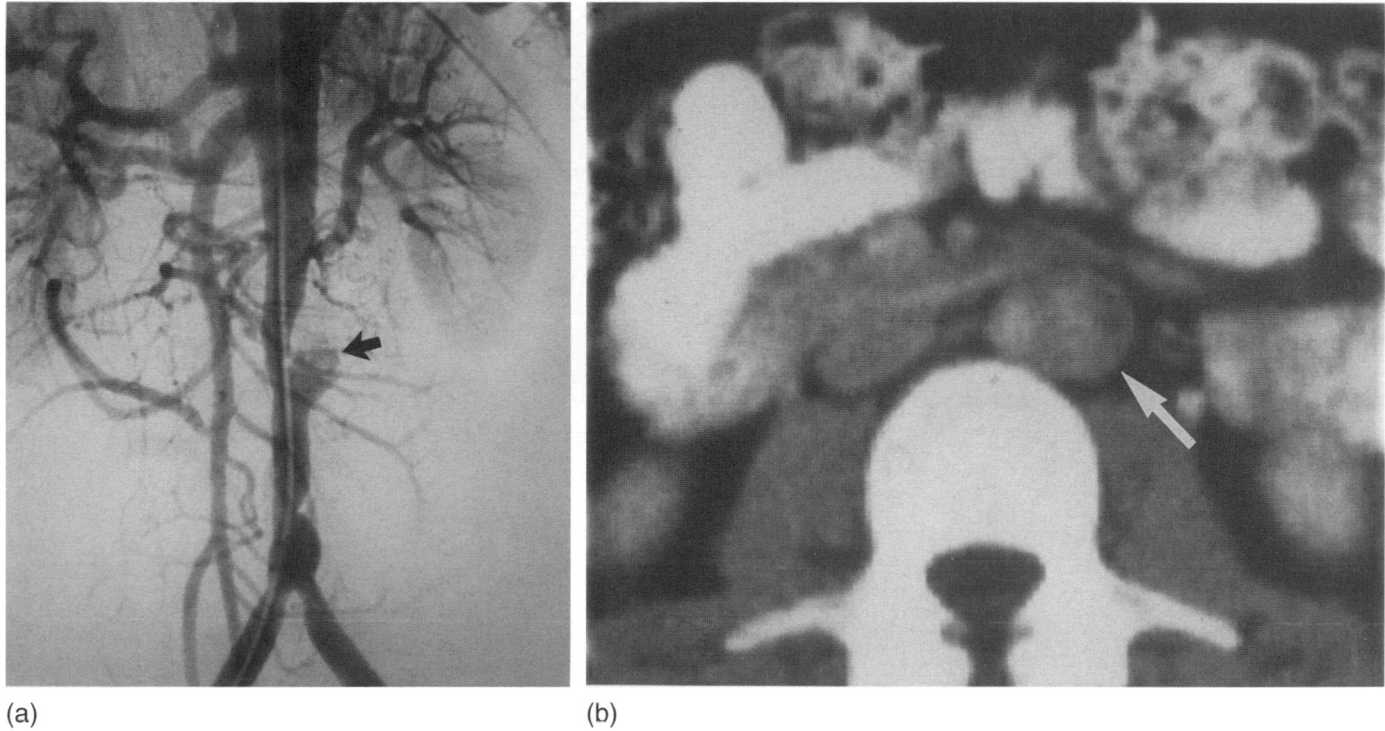

Figure 19.11 Takayasu's arteritis. (a) Abdominal aortogram shows marked irregularity of the infrarenal aorta and a small saccular aneurysm on the left side (arrow). (b) CT scan through the infrarenal aorta at the level of the eccentric saccular aneurysm (arrow).

aorta but are rare, and all reported cases had associated hypertension in addition to the media degeneration of the disease (Matsunaga *et al.* 1997). US can show diffuse homogeneous circumferential thickening of the vessel wall in the proximal CCA, with Doppler findings of increased flow velocity and turbulence through the involved segments if they are stenotic. The distal common, internal and external carotid arteries are spared and demonstrate dampened waveforms.

Another finding during the late stage of the disease is aortic wall calcification, which occurs after 5 years of disease (Figure 19.12).

CT best demonstrates this, since MRI misses subtle calcifications due to the lack of signal. Calcification is usually fine, sharp, and pencil-like and involves the arch and descending thoracic aorta. This is consistent with the dystrophic type of calcifications seen from deposits of calcium in scarred media and intima. Takayasu's arteritis should be strongly suspected when a relatively young female patient is found to have this type of arterial calcifications. "Degenerative" calcifications may also be seen when secondary atherosclerosis develops, and is demonstrated by rough, irregular, and heavy deposits in the damaged intima (Matsunaga *et al.* 1997).

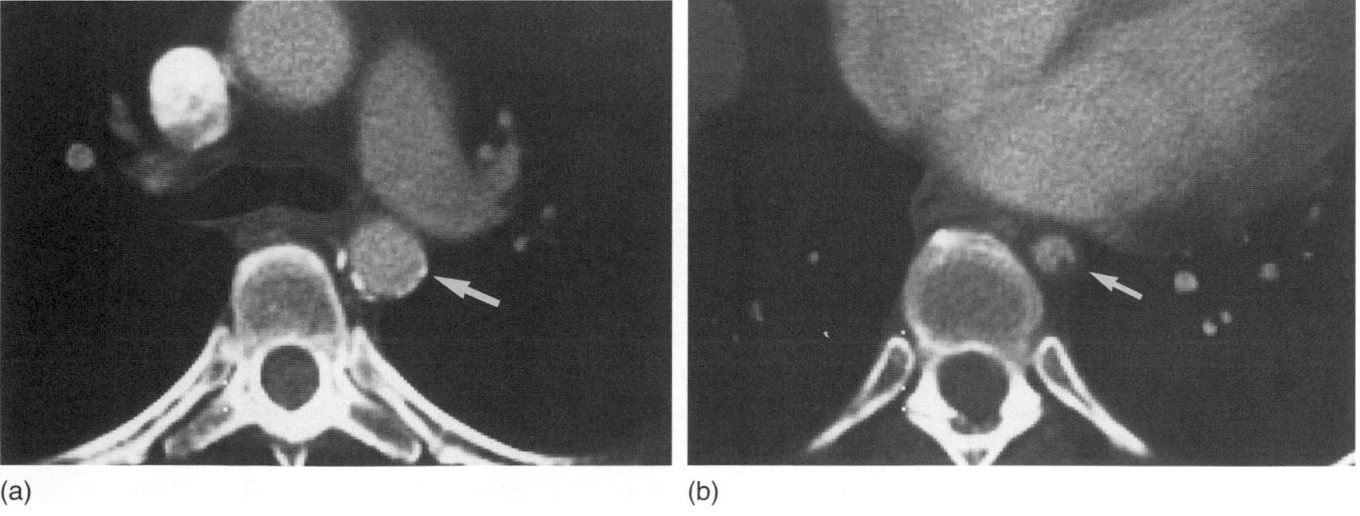

Figure 19.12 Takayasu's arteritis. (a) CT scan through the upper chest shows scattered calcification in the wall of the descending thoracic aorta (arrow) indicating endstage Takayasu's arteritis. (b) CT scan through the lower chest shows high-grade stenosis of the aorta (arrow).

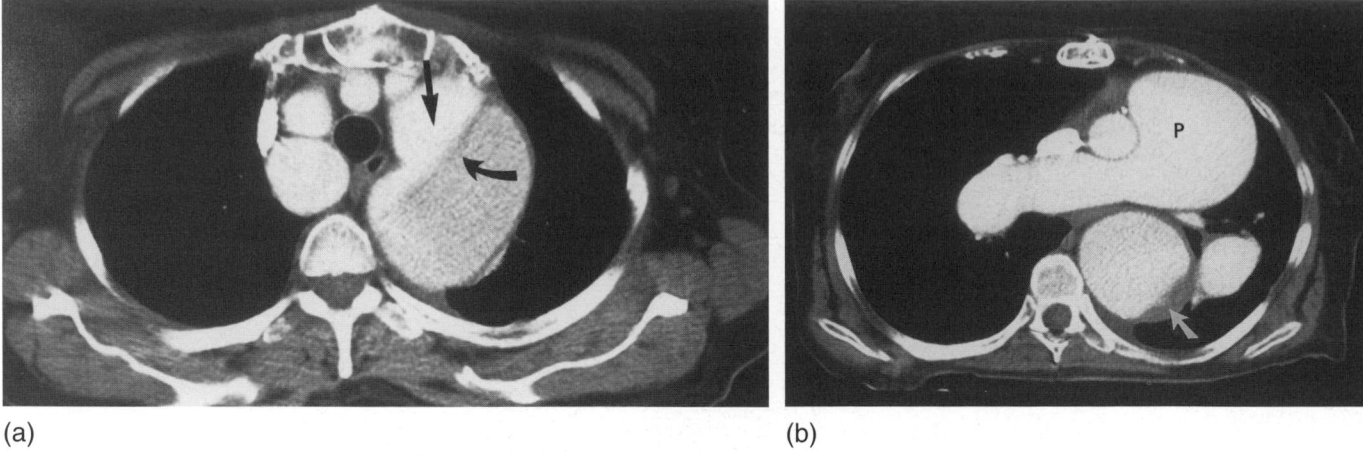

(a)   (b)

Figure 19.13 Giant cell arteritis with late development of aneurysm and dissection. (a) CT scan through the aortic arch shows a dissecting aneurysm with the true lumen anterior (arrow) and false lumen posterior (curved arrow). (b) CT scan through the mid-chest level shows an aneurysm of the descending aortic segment at the caudal end of the dissection (arrow). The pulmonary artery (P) is also aneurysmal.

It has been suggested that early and delayed mural enhancement on CT represents active disease, while lack of mural enhancement, high precontrast attenuation, and wall calcifications are more common in inactive disease (Antoniou *et al.* 1998).

Pulmonary arterial stenoses are specific for Takayasu's arteritis versus other forms of arteritis and can be demonstrated by CT or MRI. In the early phase of the disease, wall thickening has been detected in cases where conventional angiography demonstrates a normal lumen. Involvement is more frequent in upper lobe pulmonary arteries and in segmental branches, but can be seen in subsegmental branches (Park *et al.* 1995). The main differential diagnosis for these findings is chronic thromboembolic disease and, therefore, abnormal findings in systemic arteries should be sought to differentiate TA from this condition. Late findings in Takayasu's arteritis include dilatation of the central pulmonary arteries and a "pruned tree" appearance of peripheral pulmonary arteries. CT may show a flame-shaped termination of the pulmonary artery (Matsunaga *et al.* 1997), which is also seen in aortic branches. Enlarged collateral communication between the systemic and pulmonary arterial circulation should be sought as indirect evidence of hemodynamically significant involvement of the pulmonary artery. Chest CT, particularly high resolution CT, may demonstrate mosaic attenuation of the pulmonary parenchyma, which is seen as patchy areas of low attenuation thought to represent regional hypoperfusion. Pulmonary vessels within these areas of low attenuation may show reduced caliber and number compared to the surrounding lung. These parenchymal findings correlate with the presence of pulmonary arteritis on angiography. Subpleural reticulolinear changes and pleural thickening may be seen, but these findings do not correlate with the presence of angiographic findings of arteritis (Takahashi *et al.* 1996). Also reported are bilateral, small, poorly marginated centrilobular nodules, and branching linear opacities that resolve with treatment and recur with recurrence of symptoms. These may represent distended pulmonary arteries receiving high-pressure systemic flow from bronchial artery collaterals (Hara *et al.* 1998).

Giant cell arteritis

Giant cell arteritis (GCA) (Chapter 24), as is the case with Takayasu's arteritis, produces changes in the arterial wall and lumen that may be demonstrated by CT, MRI, and US. The arterial segments involved are more distal in GCA than in Takayasu's arteritis, which requires higher resolution scanning for their detection. For evaluation of luminal arterial changes in the thorax and upper extremities, high-resolution multidetector CTA with 3D reconstructions and 3D MRA are suitable, rather than conventional angiography. Typical findings are the same as in conventional angiography with stenosis, occlusions, and skip lesions. The typical long, smooth stenosis of the distal subclavian and axillary arteries seen with this vasculitis can be clearly demonstrated with CTA and MRA. CT and MRI are the best modalities for demonstrating aortic involvement in GCA, both for the initial diagnosis and to follow patients for complications such as aneurysms and dissections (Figure 19.13). A population-based cohort study demonstrated marked increased risk of aortic aneurysm in GCA patients compared to matched controls (Evans *et al.* 1995). Aneurysms were more commonly late sequelae of the disease. Thoracic aortic aneurysms developed at a median of 5.8 years after the initial diagnosis, while abdominal aortic aneurysms were noted at a median of

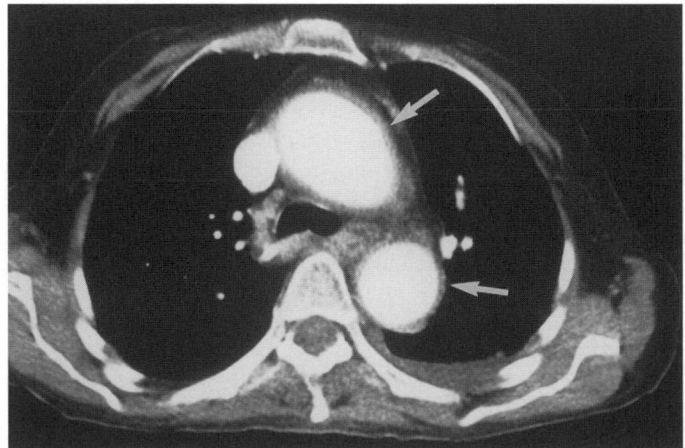

Figure 19.14 Giant cell arteritis. CT scan through the upper chest below the level of the aortic arch shows ectasia of the ascending and descending segments and thickening of the wall of the aorta (arrows).

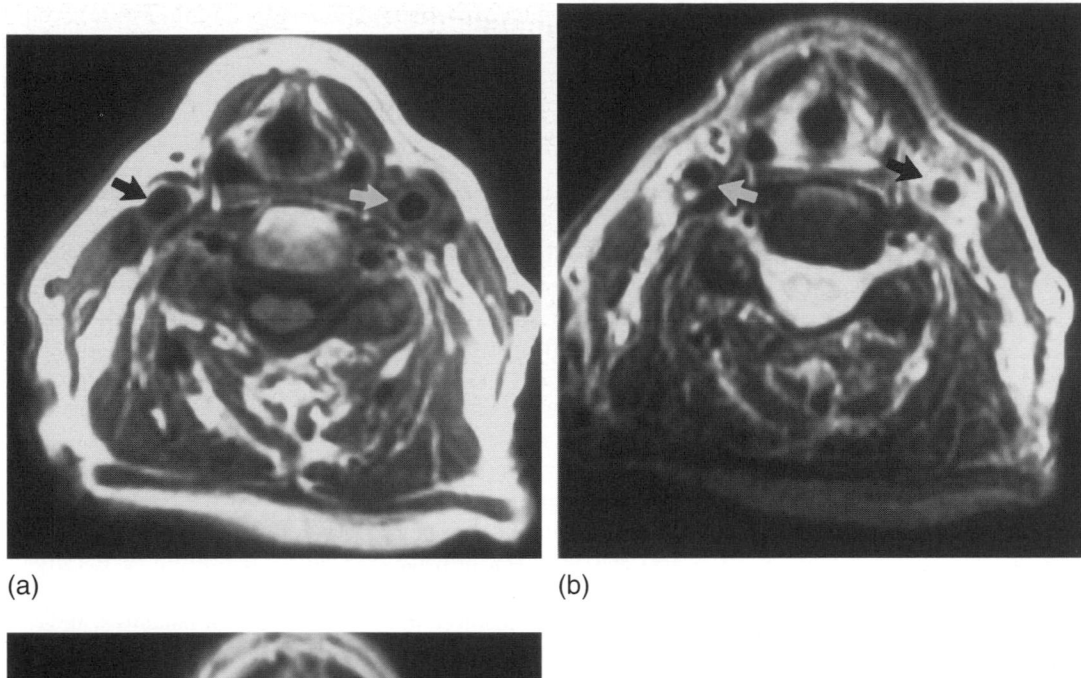

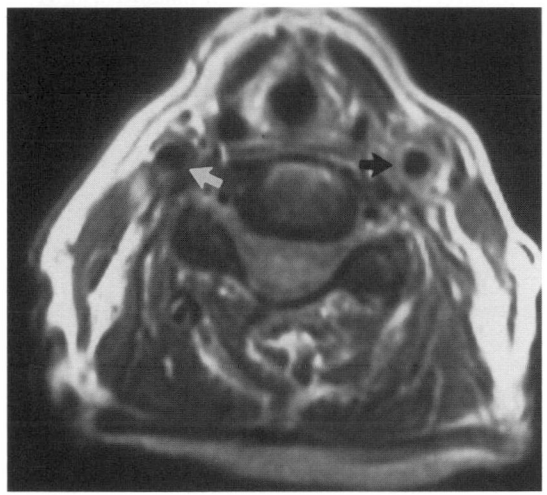

Figure 19.15 Giant cell arteritis. MR scans through the neck with three different sequences. (a) T1 sequence shows circumferential thickening of the left common carotid artery (LCCA) wall (white arrow) compared to the normal imperceptible wall of the right common carotid artery (RCCA, black arrow). Low signal around the LCCA represents inflammation extending into the perivascular fat. Normal, high T1 signal fat is seen around the RCCA. (b) T2 sequence shows markedly increased signal intensity of the LCCA wall (black arrow) from inflammation compared to the normal RCCA (white arrow). (c) Gadolinium enhancement of the LCCA wall (black arrow) is best appreciated by comparing with the precontrast image (a). Notice no significant enhancement of the normal RCCA (white arrow).

2.5 years after diagnosis. When aortic root dilatation is present, cine MRI techniques may demonstrate the commonly associated aortic valve insufficiency.

Thickening of the wall of the aorta or proximal arch vessels in GCA is well demonstrated by CT or MRI (Figures 19.14 and 19.15). The more typical involvement of medium-sized arteries can be diagnosed with the higher resolution CT and MR scanners, but smaller arteries may not be imaged with enough resolution to exclude the diagnosis reliably. The main differential diagnosis for mural changes in these vessels in the older patient population typically affected by GCA is atherosclerosis. Differentiation of atherosclerosis from GCA remains a challenge in the early stages of the disease. Features that suggest GCA include circumferential wall thickening, the distribution of the vessels affected, and inflammatory changes in the surrounding fat. CT has an advantage over MRI in the detection of wall calcifications seen as part of atherosclerosis.

The superficial temporal artery is commonly involved with GCA and represents an opportunity to make the diagnosis. Although this artery can be easily biopsied for diagnosis, the biopsy requires a long segment of artery, potential bilateral biopsies, and proper timing relative to the course of the disease (Hunder and Weyand 1997). Investigators have used high-frequency US examination of this artery to make the diagnosis or to improve the utility of the biopsy by identifying a shorter, ultrasonographically abnormal arterial segment. Studies have looked at wall thickening (Figure 19.16), luminal irregularity, stenosis or occlusions, and changes in blood flow velocity, with conflicting results. The main challenge remains in distinguishing vasculitis from atherosclerosis. One study reported the presence of a hypoechoic halo around the lumen of the temporal artery as a characteristic finding in temporal arteritis not seen with atherosclerosis (Figure 19.17) (Schmidt *et al.* 1997). The halo disappeared after a mean of 16 days of treatment with glucocorticoids and was thought to represent wall edema, rather than cellular

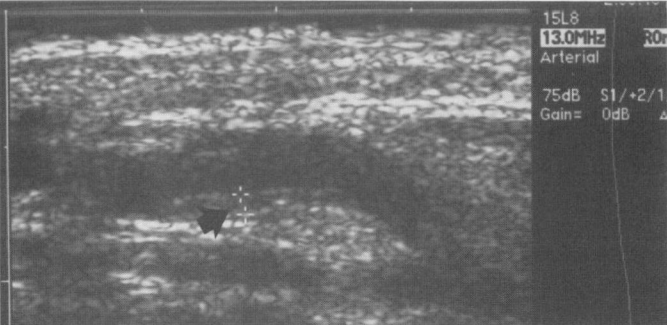

Figure 19.16 Giant cell arteritis. Longitudinal ultrasound view of the superficial temporal artery shows marked wall thickening (arrow).

infiltrate. In this study, 12 of 16 biopsies that included the arterial segment with a halo were positive (Schmidt *et al.* 1997). In another study, all of the six positive biopsies had halos while two patients with halos had negative biopsies (Venz *et al.* 1998). A more recent study of 32 patients with suspected GCA showed that absence of the halo sign or inflammatory stenosis predicted with certainty a negative biopsy, which could reduce the high percent of negative biopsies being performed (LeSar *et al.* 2002). Similar halos have also been reported in arteries in the upper extremity and neck of patients with GCA (Schmidt *et al.* 1999; Skopinski *et al.* 1999). Other studies have found wall thickening or presence of a halo to be uncommon and have focused on evaluation of blood flow velocity by Doppler examination (Lauwerys *et al.* 1997; Barrier *et al.* 1982; Puechal *et al.* 1995). One such study demonstrated that a low distal temporal artery velocity best distinguishes between GCA and polymyalgia rheumatica or normal controls (Lauwerys *et al.* 1997). Conflicting results have been reported on the positive or negative predictive value of Doppler studies. To improve sensitivity and specificity, some investigators have included examination of multiple arteries (temporal, facial, and ophthalmic) to obtain a combined score (Puechal *et al.* 1995). Additional studies with larger numbers of

patients and different conditions are needed. In the future, a combination of anatomical and Doppler ultrasound findings of multiple extracranial arteries may prove more reliable for determining the absence or presence of disease and aid in the decision whether of not to perform a biopsy.

Polyarteritis nodosa and microscopic polyangiitis

Vascular changes in polyarteritis nodosa (PAN) (Chapter 26) involve mostly medium-sized arteries, while microscopic polyangiitis (MPA) (Chapter 27) involves small arteries, venules and capillaries. Considerable overlap in imaging findings is seen with other necrotizing vasculitis such as Wegener's granulomatosis (Figure 19.2) (see Chapter 31) and systemic lupus erythematosus (Chapter 34). Spatial resolution limits the capacity of cross sectional imaging to detect subtle arterial changes of stenosis, occlusions, and dilatations often seen by conventional angiography in these smaller arteries. With more advanced disease, CTA and MRA can frequently detect arterial abnormalities (Figures 19.18a, c, d, and f). CT mainly, but also MRI and US, provide excellent visualization of the organ changes and complications accompanying PAN or MPA.

The kidney is involved in more than 85% of patients with PAN and MPA, and multiple findings have been described. CTA and MRA fail to demonstrate the typical intrarenal microaneurysms but may demonstrate larger intra and extrarenal aneurysms as well as stenosis and occlusion of the renal artery and its branches. CT or MRI can demonstrate multiple peripheral, wedge-shaped areas of cortical ischemia or infarction (Figures 19.18b, 19.18e, and 19.19) (Moss and Bush 1992). An uncommon presentation of PAN is a perinephric subcapsular hemorrhage or a retroperitoneal hemorrhage from rupture of a renal artery aneurysm. US virtually always detects a perirenal abnormality but often cannot distinguish hemorrhage from tumor or abscess. CT and MRI are helpful in detecting the abnormality and excluding common potential causes, including tumors and polycystic kidney disease. If no underlying disease is identified, angiography should be the next step to exclude vasculitis. If CT or MRI identifies multiple aneurysms and cortical infarcts, a necrotizing vasculitis should be highly suspected, PAN being the most common (Brkovic *et al.* 1996).

The chest is the next most common area involved in MPA. Possible findings include wedge-shaped or round, peripheral pulmonary infiltrates of non-segmental distribution simulating thromboembolic disease with infarction. Cavitation may be seen with these infiltrates. Massive pulmonary edema may be the result of congestive heart failure from cardiac involvement in PAN. These pulmonary changes are best demonstrated by CT. Cardiac involvement may present with cardiac enlargement and pericardial thickening or effusion, suggesting pericarditis (Gunal *et al.* 1997). Cardiac involvement can be assessed by echocardiography, MRI, or CT.

The liver and mesenteric arteries are commonly involved with PAN and are a major cause of morbidity and mortality. Aneurysms in the liver can be detected by cross-sectional imaging, and are most often seen at arterial branching points (Figure 19.20). As in the kidneys, peripheral areas of infarction may be seen. Spontaneous rupture of aneurysms may occur, resulting in contained intraparenchymal or subcapsular hematomas, or free intraperitoneal hemorrhage. Cross-sectional imaging is again helpful to exclude malignancy, adenoma, or trauma as the cause of hemorrhage (Holzknecht *et al.* 1997). The jejunum is the segment of bowel most commonly involved and CT may demonstrate bowel wall thickening and

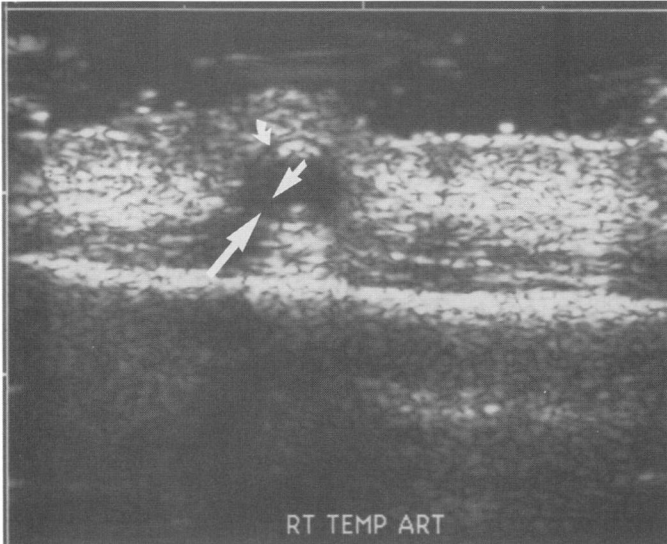

Figure 19.17 Giant cell arteritis. Transverse ultrasound examination of the superficial temporal artery shows circumferential wall thickening (between the arrows) and an hypoechoic halo (curved arrow).

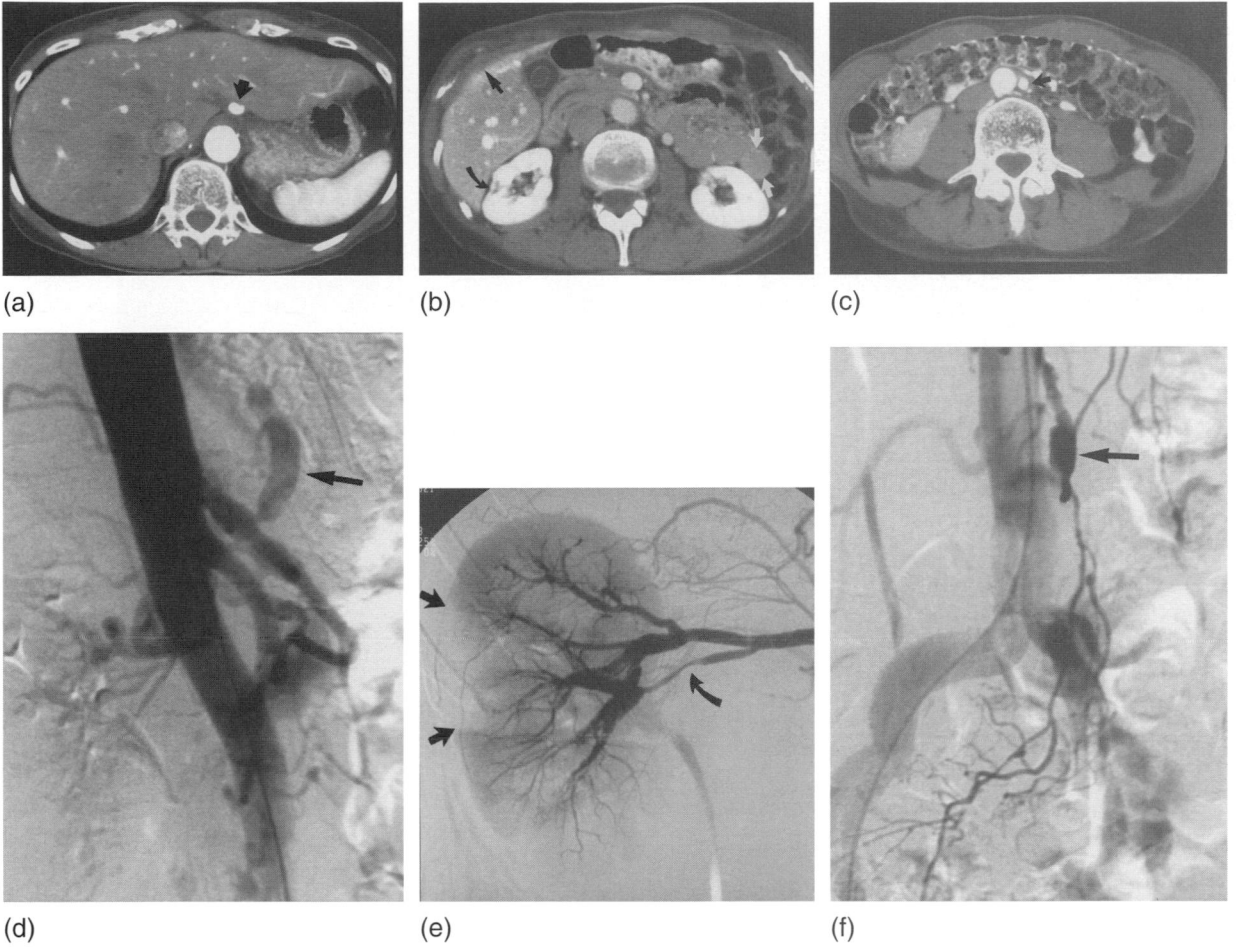

Figure 19.18 Polyarteritis nodosa with multiorgan involvement. CT scans through the upper and mid abdomen shows: (a) aneurysm of left gastric artery (arrow); (b) small cortical infarction of the right kidney (curved arrow), small subcapsular hepatic hematoma (arrow), and small bowel wall thickening from ischemia (between white arrows); (c) aneurysm of the inferior mesenteric artery with perivascular inflammatory changes (arrow). Abdominal angiograms show: (d) Lateral aortogram shows a fusiform aneurysm of the left gastric artery (arrow); (e) Renal arteriogram shows zone of infarction in the mid-right kidney (between the arrows) and diffuse narrowing of a primary branch of the right renal artery (curved arrow), additional irregularities of the renal artery are also noted; (f) Fusiform aneurysm of the inferior mesenteric artery (arrow), multiple smaller aneurysms and luminal irregularities are present in the distribution of the IMA.

edema from ischemia/infarction (Figure 19.18b). CT is also the best imaging modality to detect pneumoperitoneum, which can be seen when infarction results in bowel perforation.

Kawasaki's disease

Kawasaki's disease (KD) has a definite predilection for the coronary arteries (Chapter 29). Coronary angiography has been the gold standard for diagnosis of coronary disease and echocardiography is the most used non-invasive imaging modality for diagnosis and follow-up. Cardiac-gated MRI and multidetector coronary CTA are capable of evaluating coronary pathology and cardiac function abnormalities, and can be used to replace coronary angiography for the diagnosis and late evaluation of this disease. Ideally, non-invasive imaging can replace higher risk invasive procedures in this young population.

Echocardiography can help establish the diagnosis of KD by detecting coronary artery dilatation or aneurysms. It has also been used to follow regression of the disease after treatment has been initiated. Ischemic changes can also be indirectly assessed by evaluation of regional wall motion (Takahashi 1997). Echocardiography has limitations in detecting distal aneurysms, detecting stenosis, or thrombosis. It is also more difficult to consistently perform in older children (Duerinckx *et al.* 1997). Transesophageal echocardiography has been used for the diagnosis and follow-up of adult KD when transthoracic echocardiography is unable to detect the aneurysms (Habon *et al.* 1998).

MRI has many advantages for cardiac imaging. It can visualize the arterial lumen, the presence of intimal proliferation or thrombus, and detect flow. It also offers better visualization of distal aneurysms than echocardiography and better measurement of total length of long aneurysms, thereby stratifying patients with regard to treatment regimens and follow-up schedules (Duerinckx *et al.* 1997). Advances in MRI technology, such as faster speeds of image acquisition, have led to increasing use of MRI for diagnosis and

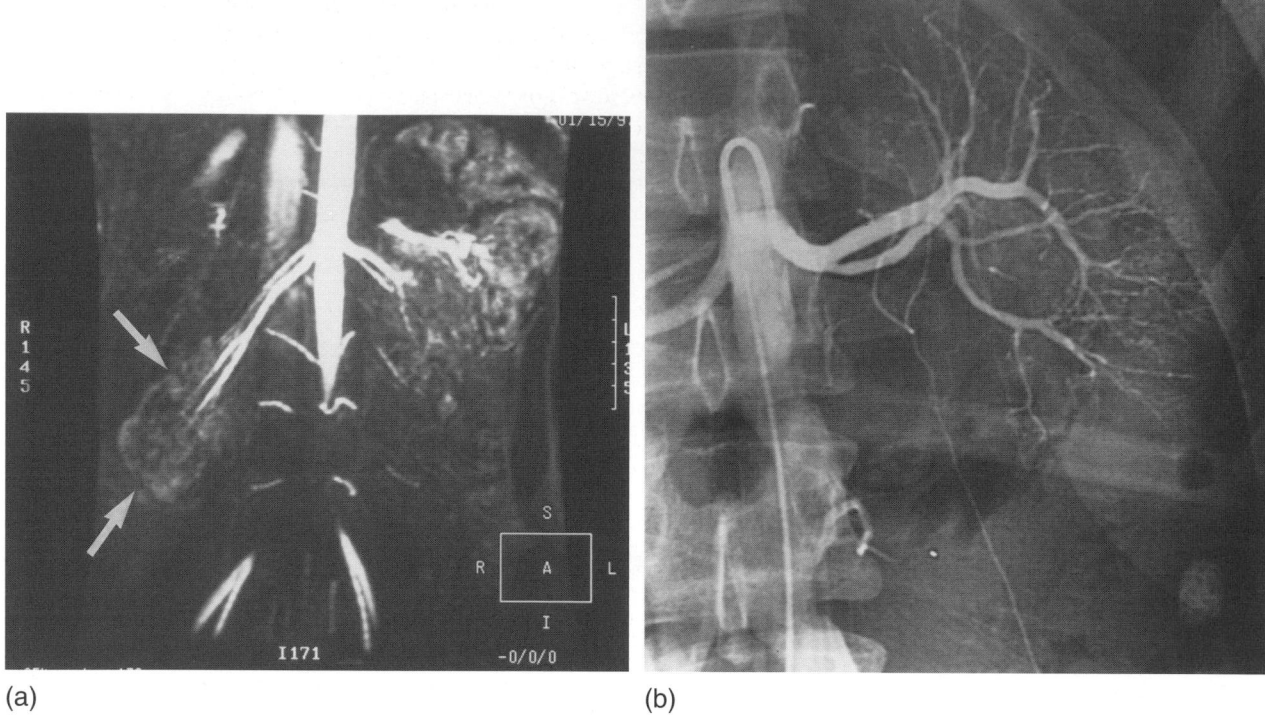

Figure 19.19 Polyarteritis nodosa. (a) MRA with gadolinium coronal view shows irregularity of the renal parenchyma on the right (arrows). The left kidney has similar disease but is not well identified because it is only partially included in the section. (b) Left renal arteriogram shows diffuse irregularity and stenosis of the renal artery branches.

evaluation of KD of the coronary arteries. The largest series comparing MRI to conventional angiography showed complete agreement of findings between the two modalities in 13 pediatric patients, ages 3 to 8 years (Mavrogeni *et al.* 2004). Although multidetector CTA can be used to evaluate the coronary arteries in early disease, MRI has the significant advantage of avoiding ionizing radiation exposure in this young patient population. MRI can also demonstrate active inflammation and edema in the walls of the vessels (McMahon *et al.* 2005). For diagnosis of early disease, coronary

angiography can be supplanted by the combination of echocardiography and MRI.

Multidetector CTA has been used in the evaluation of late findings of coronary KD in adolescents and young adults and has been shown to have excellent correlation with findings on coronary angiography (Kanamaru *et al.* 2005). CT is the best imaging modality for determining aneurysm size and for follow-up of thrombus formation and calcifications associated with these aneurysms (Fuyama *et al.* 1996). CTA has better resolution than MRI for detecting changes in peripheral arteries in the later stages of the disease. Kawasaki disease can also result in aneurysms in the aorta and other major arteries, including iliac, axillary, and renal arteries. Pericarditis can also occur with this disease. All cross sectional imaging modalities may detect these changes. For diagnosis of late KD changes, the cross sectional imaging modalities, particularly CTA, can replace coronary angiography and therefore avoid the risks of an invasive procedure in these young patients.

Rheumatoid arthritis

Rheumatoid arthritis (RA) may be complicated by vasculitis that can resemble the changes described above for PAN (Chapter 34). CT can detect visceral arterial involvement with aneurysms, stenosis, and occlusions, and the complications of infarctions, hemorrhage, and bowel perforations. Aortitis can also be seen with CT or MRI, with predilection for the ascending aorta and development of aortic valve insufficiency. Changes of pericarditis with pericardial thickening and effusions may be demonstrated with CT, MRI, or US.

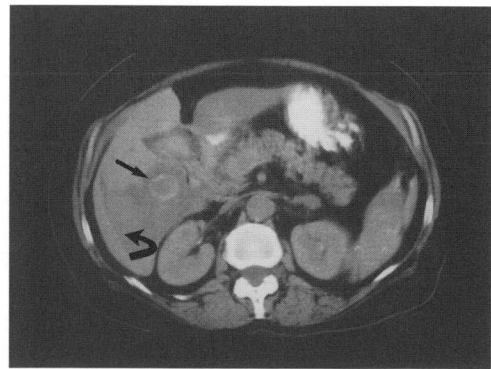

Figure 19.20 Polyarteritis nodosa with ruptured aneurysm in the liver. CT scan through the upper abdomen without contrast enhancement shows a large aneurysm of a hepatic artery branch (arrow) with surrounding hematoma (curved arrow) in the posterior aspect of the right lobe of the liver.

Systemic lupus erythematosus and antiphospholipid syndrome

Systemic lupus erythematosus (SLE) causes arterial or venous thrombotic changes in a significant number of patients (Chapter 34). Venous thrombosis is most common in the deep venous system of the extremities, where vascular ultrasound plays a primary role for detection. Venous thrombosis can also occur more centrally, characteristically involving the renal veins, and has also been reported in the vena cava, mesenteric vein, superior sagittal sinus, and other sites (Si-Hoe et al. 1997; Flusser et al. 1996). CT and MRI are well-suited for detection of renal vein or vena cava thrombosis. CT findings of renal vein thrombosis include: a dilated renal vein containing thrombus; IVC thrombus in 40 to 50% of patients; presence of pericapsular venous collaterals (when changes are chronic); and renal enlargement and abnormal parenchymal enhancement pattern (Si-Hoe et al. 1997). MRI can also demonstrate these findings, and is particularly useful when iodinated contrast cannot be used due to renal failure. Central venous thrombosis in the thorax from SLE or antiphospholipid syndrome (APS) (Chapter 44) can be detected by CT or MRI (Alcazar-Ramirez et al. 1997). MRI has the advantage of detecting abnormalities without contrast by using gradient echo sequences. Color Doppler ultrasound is not useful for detecting SVC thrombosis and may be misleading when evaluating the subclavian and brachiocephalic veins because they cannot be compressed.

Aortitis has been reported in cases of APS (Seror et al. 1998). These cases involved the infrarenal abdominal aorta and showed segmental, circumferential aortic wall thickening with high attenuation on CT and also with infiltration of the para-aortic fat. In one case, MRI showed aortic wall thickening with enhancement after gadolinium, while conventional angiography and ultrasound were negative. The usefulness of cross sectional imaging for treatment follow-up was shown when CT demonstrated resolution of changes after 6 to 8 weeks of glucocorticoid therapy. Two cases of aortic thrombosis, one infrarenal and one supraceliac, have been reported. Renal artery thrombosis or stenosis can occur in primary or secondary APS.

SLE commonly affects the kidneys. CT detects severe disease by demonstrating diffuse enlargement or diminution in renal size. CT may also demonstrate renal vein thrombosis and other potentially treatable causes of renal failure, including ureteral obstruction and abscesses. Spontaneous subcapsular renal hematomas secondary to vasculitis have also been reported.

In SLE patients presenting with abdominal pain, CT plays a key role in excluding a surgical abdomen and preventing unnecessary exploratory laparotomy when the symptoms are due to mesenteric vasculitis and serositis. Lupus mesenteric vasculitis may mimic other more common lesions, and often presents with severe, disabling abdominal pain. Delayed recognition is potentially fatal if it leads to infarction and perforation. If instituted early, glucocorticoid treatment may stop progression. Abdominal radiographs are not helpful and barium studies are non-specific. The key CT finding for this diagnosis is a palisade-like prominence of the mesenteric vessels leading to the involved bowel loop. Mesenteric vessels are seen as thickened, non-tapering vessels which appear increased in number because of their increased prominence (the comb sign) (Ko et al. 1997; Si-Hoe et al. 1997). These findings may correlate with inflammatory cell infiltration in the wall of vessels and perivascular edema resulting in vessel engorgement. The involved bowel loop is usually in the superior mesenteric artery distribution and most often demonstrates symmetrical and circumferential bowel wall thickening (between 3 and 10 mm), with a low attenuation middle layer between higher attenuation inner and outer layers (double halo or target sign). Specific CT findings for bowel infarction should be sought to avoid delay of surgical treatment. These findings include pneumatosis intestinalis and air in the mesenteric veins or portal veins. Infarction may progress to perforation, which can be seen by CT as free fluid or abscess formation with or without pneumoperitoneum.

Behçet's syndrome

Behçet's syndrome (BS) lends itself to diagnostic imaging with CT, MRI, and US due to its involvement of large veins and arteries (Chapter 35). This is a disease where conventional angiography should be avoided if possible due to the higher risk of aneurysm formation at arterial puncture sites. Venous punctures also carry the risk of initiating venous thrombosis. Both US and non-contrast MRA techniques can be performed without puncture of the vascular system.

Veins are involved more frequently than arteries in BS (25%). Findings include a wide range of lesions, from subcutaneous thrombophlebitis, to DVT, to large vein occlusion. Among large veins, the IVC is most frequently involved followed by the SVC, common iliac veins, and hepatic veins (Terzioglu et al. 1998). Dural sinus thrombosis may occur. Venous occlusion may be accompanied by varix formation. The most common lesion is superficial thrombophlebitis of the lower extremity. Extremity DVT is best evaluated by ultrasound, including compression images. If US is indeterminate due to poor visualization of extremity veins, MR venography techniques can be performed without the need for contrast. CT venography techniques can also be performed but require intravenous injection of iodinated contrast. CT or MR produces the best images of larger thoracic, abdominal, and pelvic veins. One limitation of MR venographic techniques is difficulty distinguishing between absence of flow due to occlusion and very slow flow due to severe stenosis. Other MR sequences may be employed to determine if the vein lumen is filled with thrombus.

Arterial involvement in BS includes arterial occlusions and aneurysm formation. Aneurysms occur more frequently than occlusions and carry a poor prognosis. They are often multiple and may show rapid progression leading to pseudoaneurysm formation and rupture, which is the leading cause of death in BS. Aneurysms are difficult to treat since they tend to recur after surgical repair at the anastomotic sites (Akiyama et al. 1998; Berkmen 1998). With MRI, T1 spin echo sequences are used to show the anatomy, locate the aneurysm; and evaluate the surrounding area for lesions. Non-contrast MRA techniques may then be performed, including time-of-flight and gradient echo sequences. The time-of-flight technique may underestimate the size of the aneurysm due to artifact produced by saturation of flow in areas of high turbulence, but this is overcome by the information from the T1 spin-echo images (Berkmen 1998). If findings are not clear, gadolinium MRA or CTA may be used for improved visualization of luminal abnormalities.

Arterial lesions occur most frequently in the aorta, followed in frequency by the pulmonary, femoral, popliteal, subclavian, and carotid arteries, with occasional coronary artery involvement

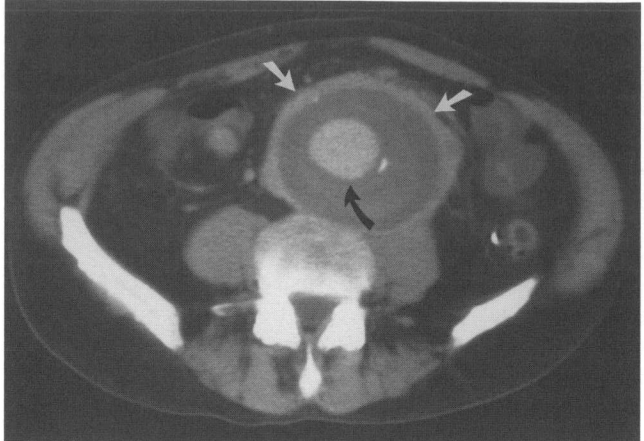

Figure 19.21 Inflammatory aneurysm of the abdominal aorta. There is considerable thickening of the wall (arrows) of the infrarenal aortic aneurysm. Note there is relative sparing of the posterior wall. There is also considerable thrombus between the opacified lumen (curved arrow) and the thickened inflamed wall.

(Berkmen 1998; Park *et al.* 1984). BS is the only known acquired disorder that causes pulmonary artery aneurysms, which are best demonstrated by pulmonary CTA or MRA (Greene *et al.* 1998). CT has the advantage of also demonstrating associated lung parenchymal abnormalities, including regional differences in perfusion, air space nodules, and pleural-based, wedge-shaped masses that may result from pulmonary infarction. The lobar arteries are involved half the time, and the main pulmonary arteries and segmental branches are each involved approximately 25% of the time (Tunaci *et al.* 1999). Aneurysms tend to disappear or at least regress after several months to years. Visceral artery involvement is rare but has been reported, including a renal artery aneurysm rupture identified by CT (Sueyoshi *et al.* 1996). Mesenteric vascular engorgement, similar to SLE changes described above, has also been seen (Ha *et al.* 1998).

A case of internal carotid artery dissection imaged by color-flow Doppler US has been reported (Pannone *et al.* 1998). The authors postulate that arterial dissections in BS may be due to the same vasa vasorum vasculitis suspected as the basis of aneurysm formation.

Thromboangiitis obliterans

Thromboangiitis obliterans (TAO) or Buerger's disease affects small- and medium-sized arteries and veins, primarily in the extremities (Chapter 38). Conventional angiography is frequently used to confirm the diagnosis and establish the extent of the disease, however, few reports discuss cross sectional imaging of TAO. Multidetector CTA can demonstrate the occlusive pattern suggestive of TAO in the extremity arterial supply with better resolution than previous CT scanners or MRA. MRA techniques with time-resolved contrast enhancement have improved visualization of arteries supplying blood to the feet and hands and are capable of suggesting the diagnosis from the disease pattern. Conventional angiography is still used when evaluating for possible distal target vessels for revascularization. US can be used in the diagnosis of extremity venous thrombosis and Doppler ultrasonography can demonstrate tapered narrowing and occlusions of extremity arteries. Findings are often bilateral and one of the key observations is the absence of atheromatous plaque at or proximal to the sites of occlusion (Fiessinger 1997). Other sites of arterial involvement besides the extremities have been reported, including mesenteric and renal arteries (Iwai 1998; Gomi *et al.* 1978); these would be amenable to diagnosis with MRA and CTA.

Chronic periaortitis

Chronic periaortitis is caused by lymphocytic inflammation of the adventitia of the aorta and occurs most frequently in the infrarenal abdominal aorta. Patients present with pain (which may mimic a rupturing aneurysm), generalized malaise, and elevated erythrocyte sedimentation rate. Different disorders have been reported which involve the same inflammatory process but with varying degrees of inflammation and fibrosis, frequencies of aneurysms, and involvement of adjacent organs. These disorders are idiopathic retroperitoneal fibrosis, or mediastinal fibrosis, and inflammatory aneurysm. CT is well-established as the preferred modality for making the diagnosis, since US may miss the findings. CT shows a thick, enhancing rind of soft tissue around the aorta (Figures 19.21 and 22).

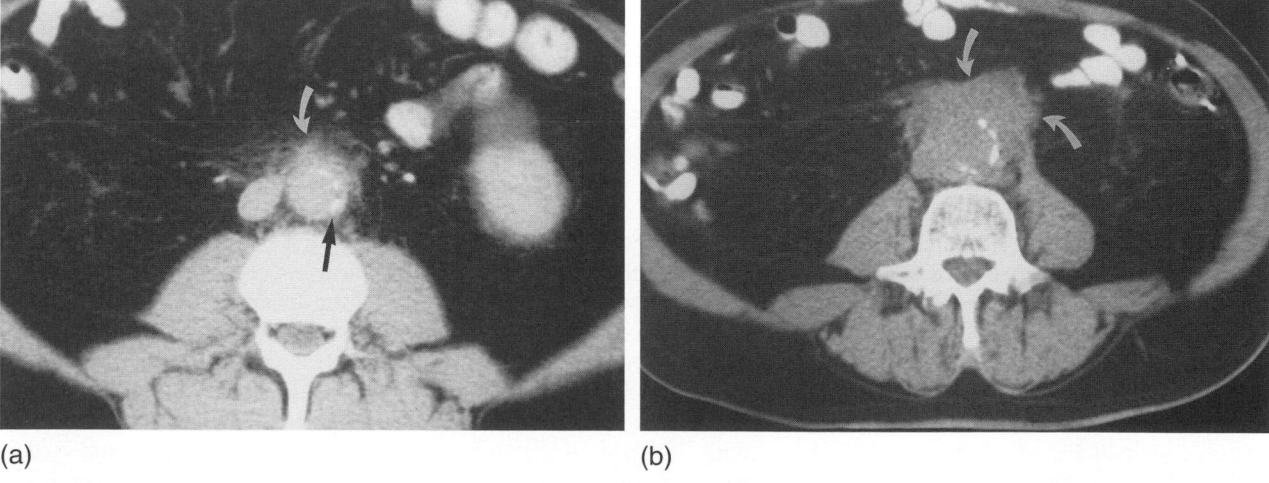

(a)   (b)

Figure 19.22 Periaortitis with progression. (a) The aortic lumen is demarcated by calcification (arrow). The irregular thick wall beyond this is inflammation (curved arrow). (b) Three months later there is marked increase in the degree of wall thickening (curved arrows).

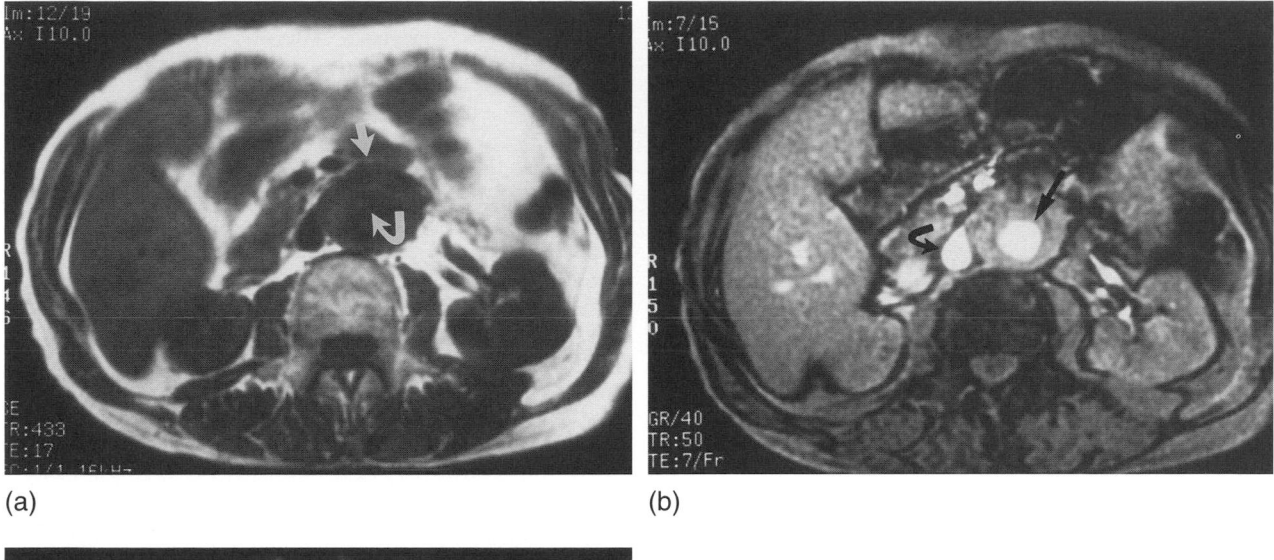

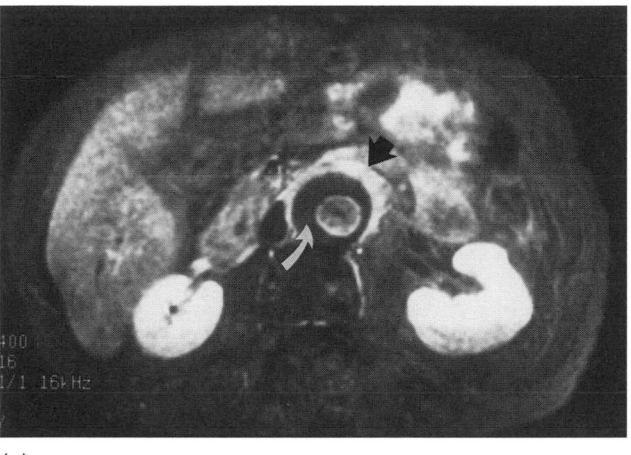

Figure 19.23 Inflammatory aneurysm. (a) MRI T1 shows aneurysm of the infrarenal aorta. The thick rind (arrow) is difficult to distinguish from the lumen (curved arrow). (b) MRI through the same level but with a sequence of gradient recalled echo shows high signal intensity of the lumens of the aorta (arrow) and IVC (curved arrow). There is not clear distinction of the thick wall of the aorta from thrombus in the aneurysm. (c) MRA with gadolinium enhancement in the late phase shows high signal intensity of the wall thickening (arrow). The lumen of the aorta, in the center of the aneurysm, is partially enhanced and can be distinguished from the low signal intensity mural thrombus (curved arrow).

In inflammatory aneurysms, this confluent soft tissue thickening is located primarily anterolateral with posterior sparing. Other types of retroperitoneal fibrosis tend to produce more circumferential involvement around the aorta and more irregular periaortic extension of the process. Chronic periaortitis is almost always associated with calcified atheromatous changes of the infrarenal abdominal aorta. Assessment of aneurysmal dilatation requires measuring the luminal diameter (inside the intima) of the aorta rather than the outer diameter of the lesion, since the outer diameter includes inflammatory thickening that does not correlate with the risk of aortic rupture. Periaortitis may not be associated with aneurysmal dilatation of the lumen, defined as one and one-half times the normal diameter of the aorta, but usually presents with luminal ectasia. MRI has also been used to image periaortitis and different sequences are needed to delineate the lumen, arterial wall and periaortic soft tissue rind (Figure 19.23). In inflammatory aneurysms, T2 weighted images may demonstrate a multilayered, or "onion skin", appearance with variable signal intensities for the aneurysm and the adjacent inflammation. CT and MRI can also delineate adjacent organ involvement, in particular vena cava stenosis or occlusion and ureteral obstruction with hydronephrosis (Tennant *et al.* 1993; Arrive *et al.* 1995).

References

Akiyama, K., Hirota, J., Ohkado, A. and Shiina, Y. (1998). Multivarious clinical manifestations of multiple pseudoaneurysms in Behçet's disease. *Journal of Cardiovascular Surgery*, **39,** 175–8.

Alcazar-Ramirez, J. D., Fernandez-Nebro, A., Abarca, M., Salgado, F., De Haro-Liger, M., Rodriguez-Andreu, J., *et al.* (1997). Central vein thrombosis in the antiphospholipid syndrome. *Lupus*, **6,** 549–51.

Aluquin, V. P. R., Albano, S. A., Chan, F., Sandborg, C., Pitlick, P. T. (2002). Magnetic resonance imaging in the diagnosis and follow up of Takayasu's arteritis in children. *Annals of the Rheumatic Diseases*, **61,** 526–9.

Andrews, J., Al-Nahhas, A., Pennell, D. J., Hossain, M. S., Davies, K. A., Haskard, D. O. and Mason, J. C. (2004). Non-invasive imaging in the diagnosis and management of Takayasu's arteritis. *Annals of the Rheumatic Diseases*, **63,** 995–1000.

Antoniou, A., Vlahos, L. and Mourikis, D. (1998). Abdominal Takayasu's arteritis: imaging with color duplex sonography. *European Radiology*, **8,** 547–9.

Arrive, L., Correas, J. M., Leseche, G. and Ghebontni, L. (1995). Inflammatory aneurysms of the abdominal aorta: CT findings. *American Journal of Roentgenology*, **165,** 1481–4.

Barrier, J., Potel, G., Renaut-Hovasse, H., Hanh, T. H., Peltier, P., Chamary, V., *et al.* (1982). The use of Doppler flow studies in the diagnosis of giant cell arteritis. Selection of temporal artery biopsy site is facilitated. *Journal of the American Medical Association*, **248,** 2158–9.

Berkmen, T. (1998). MR angiography of aneurysms in Behçet's disease: a report of four cases. *Journal of Computer Assisted Tomography*, **22**, 202–6.

Brkovic, D., Moehring, K., Doersam, J., Pomer, S., Kaelble, T. and Riedasch, G. (1996). Aetiology, diagnosis and management of spontaneous perirenal haematomas. *European Urology*, **29**, 302–7.

Chung, J. W., Park, J. H., Im, J. G., Chung, M. J., Han, M. C. and Ahn, H. (1996). Spiral CT angiography of the thoracic aorta. *Radiographics*, **16**, 811–24.

Duerinckx, A. J., Troutman, B., Allada, V. and Kim, D. (1997). Coronary MR angiography in Kawasaki disease. *American Journal of Roentgenology*, **168**, 114–6.

Evans, J. M., O'Fallon, W. M. and Hunder, G. G. (1995). Increased incidence of aortic aneurysm and dissection in giant cell (temporal) arteritis. *Annals of Internal Medicine*, **122**, 502–7.

Fiessinger, J. N. (1997). Thromboangiitis obliterans (Buerger's disease). *Revue du Rhumatisme, English Edition*, **64**, 281–2.

Flusser, D., Abu-Shakra, M., Baumgarten-Kleiner, A., Flusser, G. and Sukenik, S. (1996). Superior sagittal sinus thrombosis in a patient with systemic lupus erythematosus. *Lupus*, **5**, 334–6.

Fuyama, Y., Hamada, R., Uehara, R., Yano, I., Fujiwara, M., Matoba, M., *et al.* (1996). Long-term follow up of abdominal aortic aneurysm complicating Kawasaki disease: comparison of the effectiveness of different imaging methods. *Acta Paediatrica Japonica*, **38**, 252–5.

Gomi, T., Ikeda, T. and Yuhara, M. (1978). Renovascular hypertension due to Buerger's disease. *Japanese Heart Journal*, **19**, 308–14.

Greene, R. M. E., Saleh, A., Taylor, A. K. M., Callaghan, M., Addis, B. J., Nzewi, O. C., *et al.* (1998). Non-invasive assessment of bleeding pulmonary artery aneurysms due to Behçet's disease. *European Radiology*, **8**, 359–63.

Gunal, N., Kara, N., Cakar, N., Kocak, H., Kahramanyol, O. and Cetinkaya, E. (1997). Cardiac involvement in childhood polyarteritis nodosa. *International Journal of Cardiology*, **60**, 257–62.

Ha, H. K., Lee, H. J., Yang, S. K., Ki, W. W., Yoon, K. H., Shin, Y. M., *et al.* (1998). Intestinal Behcet syndrome: CT features of patients with and patients without complications. *Radiology*, **209**, 449–54.

Habon, T., Toth, K., Keltai, M., Lengyel, M. and Palik, I. (1998). An adult case of Kawasaki disease with multiplex coronary aneurysms and myocardial infarction: the role of transesophageal echocardiography. *Clinical Cardiology*, **21**, 529–32.

Hara, M., Sobue, R., Ohba, S., Kitase, M., Sasaki, S., Ogino, H., *et al.* (1998). Diffuse pulmonary lesions in early phase Takayasu arteritis predominantly involving pulmonary artery. *Journal of Computer Assisted Tomography*, **22**, 801–3.

Hartnell, G. G. (1999). Great vessels of the chest. In *Magnetic resonance of the heart and great vessels: clinical applications*, (eds Bogaert, J., Duerinckx, A. J. and Rademakers, F. E.), pp. 246–8. Springer-Verlag.

Hayashi, H., Katayama, N., Takagi, R., Matsuoka, Y. and Matsunaga, N. (1991). CT analysis of vascular wall during the active phase of Takayasu's aortitis (abstr.) *European Radiology*, **1** (Suppl.), S239.

Holzknecht, N., Gauger, J., Helmberger, T., Stabler, A. and Reiser, M. (1997). Cross-sectional imaging findings in a case of polyarteritis nodosa with ruptured hepatic artery aneurysm. *American Journal of Roentgenology*, **169**, 1317–9.

Hunder, G. G. and Weyand, C. M. (1997). Sonography in giant-cell arteritis. *New England Journal of Medicine*, **337**, 1385–6.

Iwai, T. (1998). Buerger's disease with intestinal involvement. *International Journal of Cardiology*, **66**, S257–63.

Kanamaru, H., Sato, Y., Takayama, T., Ayusawa, M., Karasawa, K., Sumitomo, N. and Harada, K. (2005). Assessment of coronary artery abnormalities by multislice spiral computed tomography in adolescents and young adults with Kawasaki disease. *American Journal of Cardiology*, **95**, 522–5.

Ko, S. F., Lee, T. Y., Cheng, T. T., Ng, S. H., Lai, H. M., Cheng, Y. F., *et al.* (1997). CT findings at lupus mesenteric vasculitis. *Acta Radiologica*, **38**, 115–20.

Lauwerys, B. R., Puttemans, T., Houssiau, F. A. and Devogelaer, J. P. (1997). Color Doppler sonography of the temporal arteries in giant cell arteritis and polymyalgia rheumatica. *Journal of Rheumatology*, **24**, 1570–4.

LeSar, C.J., Meir, G.H., DeMasi, R.J., Sood, J., Nelms, C.R., Carter, K.A., *et al.* (2002) The utility of color duplex ultrasonography in the diagnosis of temporal arteritis. *Journal of Vascular Surgery*, **36**, 1154–60.

Matsunaga, N., Hayashi, K., Sakamoto, I., Matsuoka, Y., Ogawa, Y., Honjo, K., *et al.* (1998). Takayasu arteritis: MR manifestations and diagnosis of acute and chronic phase. *Journal of Magnetic Resonance Imaging*, **8**, 406–14.

Matsunaga, N., Hayashi, K., Sakamoto, I., Ogawa, Y. and Matsumoto, T. (1997). Takayasu arteritis: protean radiologic manifestations and diagnosis. *Radiographics*, **17**, 579–94.

Mavrogeni, S., Papadopoulos, G., Douskou, M., Kaklis, S., Seimenis, I., Baras, P., *et al.* (2004). Magnetic resonance angiography is equivalent to x-ray coronary angiography for the evaluation of coronary arteries in Kawasaki disease. *Journal of the American College of Cardiology*, **43**, 649–52.

McMahon, C. J., Su, J. T., Taylor, M. D., Krishnamurthy, R., Muthupillai, R., Kovalchin, J. P., *et al.* (2005). Detection of active coronary arterial vasculitis using magnetic resonance imaging in Kawasaki disease. *Circulation*, **112**, e315–6.

Moss, A. A. and Bush, W. H. (1992). The kidneys. In *Computed tomography of the body with magnetic resonance imaging*, (eds Moss, A. A., Gamsu, G. and Genant, H. K.), pp.1003–5. W. B. Saunders Company.

Pannone, A., Lucchetti, G., Stazi, G., Corvi, F., Ferguson, T. L., Massucci, M., *et al.* (1998). Internal carotid artery dissection in a patient with Behçet's syndrome. *Annals of Vascular Surgery*, **12**, 463–7.

Park, J. H. (1996). Conventional and CT angiographic diagnosis of Takayasu arteritis. *International Journal of Cardiology*, **54**, S165–71.

Park, J. H., Chung, J. W., Im, J. G., Kim, S. K., Park, Y. B. and Han, M. C. (1995). Takayasu arteritis: evaluation of mural changes in the aorta and pulmonary artery with CT angiography. *Radiology*, **196**, 89–93.

Park, J. H., Chung, J. W., Lee, K. W., Park, Y. B. and Han, M. C. (1997). CT angiography of Takayasu arteritis: comparison with conventional angiography. *Journal of Vascular and Interventional Radiology*, **8**, 393–400.

Park, J. H., Han, M. C. and Bettmann, M. A. (1984). Arterial manifestations of Behçet's disease. *American Journal of Roentgenology*, **143**, 821–5.

Paul, J. F., Fiessinger, J. N., Sapoval, M., Hernigou, A., Mousseaux, E., Emmerich, J. and Piette, J. C. (2001). Follow-up electron beam CT for the management of early phase Takayasu arteritis. *Journal of Computed Assisted Tomography*, **25**, 924–31.

Puechal, X., Chauveau, M. and Menkes, C. J. (1995). Temporal Doppler-flow studies for suspected giant-cell arteritis. *Lancet*, **345**, 1437–8.

Regina, G., Fullone, M., Testini, M., Todisco, C., Greco, L., Rizzi, R., *et al.* (1998). Aneurysms of the supra-aortic trunks in Takayasu's disease. Report of two cases. *Journal of Cardiovascular Surgery*, **39**, 757–60.

Schmidt, W. A., Kraft, H. E., Borkowski, A. and Gromnica-Ihle, E. J. (1999). Color duplex ultrasonography in large-vessel giant cell arteritis. *Scandinavian Journal of Rheumatology*, **28**, 374–6.

Schmidt, W. A., Kraft, H. E., Vorpahl, K., Volker, L. and Gromnica-Ihle, E. J. (1997). Color duplex ultrasonography in the diagnosis of temporal arteritis. *New England Journal of Medicine*, **337**, 1336–42.

Seror, O., Fain, O., Dordea, M., Ghenassia, C., Coderc, E. and Sellier, N. (1998). Aortitis with antiphospholipid antibodies: CT and MR findings. *European Radiology*, **8**, 1373–5.

Sharma, S., Sharma, S., Taneja, K., Gupta, A. K. and Rajani, M. (1996). Morphologic mural changes in the aorta revealed by CT in patients with nonspecific aortoarteritis (Takayasu's arteritis). *American Journal of Roentenology*, **167**, 1321–5.

Si-Hoe, C. K., Thng, C. H., Chee, S. G., Teo, E. K. and Chng, H. H. (1997). Abdominal computed tomography in systemic lupus erythematosus. *Clinical Radiology*, **52**, 284–9.

Skopinski, S., Constans, J., Cherifi, H., Midy, D., Jarnier, P., Le Metayer, P., et al. (1999). Inflammatory arteriopathy of the arms in the course of Horton disease. Report of six cases. *Journal des Maladies Vasculaires*, **24**, 45–8.

Sueyoshi, E., Sakamoto, I., Hayashi, N., Fukuda, T., Matsunaga, N., Hayashi, K., et al. (1996). Ruptured renal artery aneurysm due to Behçet's disease. *Abdominal Imaging*, **21**, 166–7.

Sun, Y., Yip, P. K., Jeng, J. S., Hwang, B. S. and Lin, W. H. (1996). Ultrasonographic study and long-term follow-up of Takayasu's arteritis. *Stroke*, **27**, 2178–82.

Takahashi, K., Honda, M., Furuse, M., Yanagisawa, M. and Saitoh, K. (1996). CT findings of pulmonary parenchyma in Takayasu arteritis. *Journal of Computer Assisted Tomography*, **20**, 742–8.

Takahashi, M. (1997). Kawasaki disease. *Current Opinion in Pediatrics*, **9**, 523–9.

Tennant, W. G., Hartnell, G. G., Baird, R. N. and Horrocks, M. (1993). Radiologic investigation of abdominal aortic aneurysm disease: comparison of three modalities in staging and the detection of inflammatory change. *Journal of Vascular Surgery*, **17**, 703–9.

Terzioglu, E., Kirmaz, C., Uslu, R., Sin, A., Kokuludag, A., Sagduyu, A., et al. (1998). Superior vena cava syndrome together with multiple venous thrombosis in Behçet's disease. *Clinical Rheumatology*, **17**, 176–7.

Tunaci, M., Ozkorkmaz, B., Tunaci, A., Gul, A., Engin, G. and Acunas, B. (1999). CT findings of pulmonary artery aneurysms during treatment for Behcet's disease. *American Journal of Roentgenology*, **172**, 729–33.

Venz, S., Hosten, N., Nordwald, K., Lemke, A. J., Schroder, R., Bock, J. C., et al. (1998). Use of high resolution color Doppler sonography in diagnosis of temporal arteritis. *Rofo. Fortschritte auf dem Gebiete der Rontgenstrahlen und der Neuen Bildgebenden Verfahren*, **169**, 605–8.

Yamada, I., Nakagawa, T., Himeno, Y., Numano, F. and Shibuya, H. (1998). Takayasu arteritis: evaluation of the thoracic aorta with CT. *Radiology*, **209**, 103–9.

CHAPTER 20

PET imaging in vasculitis

Adil Al-Nahhas and Myles Webb

Positron emission tomography (PET) is now firmly established as an important imaging modality in the management and follow-up of patients with a variety of ailments. Although PET has been used as a research tool for over 25 years, it has only recently been introduced into clinical practice where its role is evolving with impressive speed.

Basic principles of PET imaging

PET involves the use of short-lived radionuclides that are positron-emitters, commonly produced in a cyclotron, with half-lives (time for the radionuclide to decay to half its activity) ranging from a few minutes to 2 hours. They are in a constant state of radioactive decay, resulting in the emission of positively charged particles (positrons). Following its emission, the positron can travel for only a short distance of few millimeters in tissues, before interacting violently with an electron (a negatively charged particle), in what is termed an annihilation reaction. This results in disappearance of both particles and their replacement by two gamma rays traveling at 180° to each other and coincident in time. The detection and registration of these pairs of gamma rays is done by a PET scanner, commonly comprised of a full ring of detectors that surround the patient, with associated photomultipliers and electronic circuitry that help to identify and augment the signals. The arrival of the two gamma rays at the detectors within a fraction of microseconds allows the software to recognize them as arising from the same interaction, and locates the site of that interaction to somewhere along the line joining them. After millions of such coordinates have been drawn, mapping of the distribution of the radionuclide in the body becomes possible.

This coincidence detection ability is unique to PET, resulting in significant improvement in spatial resolution (the power to discriminate between two objects) over standard nuclear medicine imaging. The currently available scanners have a favorable spatial resolution of 5 mm.

Radionuclides used in PET imaging

Fluorine-18 (^{18}F) is the most commonly used positron-emitting radionuclide and has a half-life of 110 minutes. Others include nitrogen-13 (^{13}N), carbon-11 (^{11}C) and oxygen-15 (^{15}O) (Table 20.1). These radionuclides are attached to biochemical compounds or ligands that facilitate their transport to areas of the human body to which the ligands bind to or associate with. An example is the combination of ^{18}F with a sugar to make ^{18}F-fluorodeoxyglucose (^{18}F-FDG) which is taken up by tissues using glucose as their metabolic substrate. FDG is phosphorylated via hexokinase to FDG-6-phosphate, which cannot be metabolized further and is trapped inside cells. Metabolically active cells, such as cancer cells, thus trap large amounts of ^{18}F, which enables them to be imaged and identified.

In the human body, ^{18}F-FDG is preferentially distributed to metabolically active tissues (brain and myocardium) with less uptake in the liver and spleen (Figure 20.1). It is excreted through the urinary tract and therefore the kidneys and bladder also demonstrate high uptake of ^{18}F-FDG. Doses of radionuclides given for PET scanning are expressed in million disintegrations (or million coincidences) per second, defined as million Becquerel (MBq). The average effective radiation dose in Sievert (Sv) units to the patient from a dose of 200 MBq ^{18}F-fluordeoxyglucose (FDG) is 5 mSv (the comparable dose from a standard chest CT scan is 8 mSv).

The early observation that tumors utilize more glucose than normal tissue helped to establish the role of ^{18}F-FDG PET in the evaluation of malignancies (Warburg 1956). Highly metabolic tumors show intense ^{18}F-FDG uptake (Figure 20.2). The fact that most available positron-emitters are isotopes of the basic components of our internal biological milieu such as oxygen, carbon, and nitrogen allows imaging of the inner environment of the human body (Table 20.1). Unfortunately, these positron-emitters have very short half-lives that restrict their use to research performed in centers

Table 20.1 Common positron-emitters with corresponding half-lives and methods of production

Isotope	Half-life (minutes)	Production method
Carbon-11	20.5	Cyclotron
Nitrogen-13	10.0	Cyclotron
Oxygen-15	2.1	Cyclotron
Fluorine-18	110	Cyclotron
Gallium-68	68	In-house generator
Rubidium-82	1.3	In-house generator

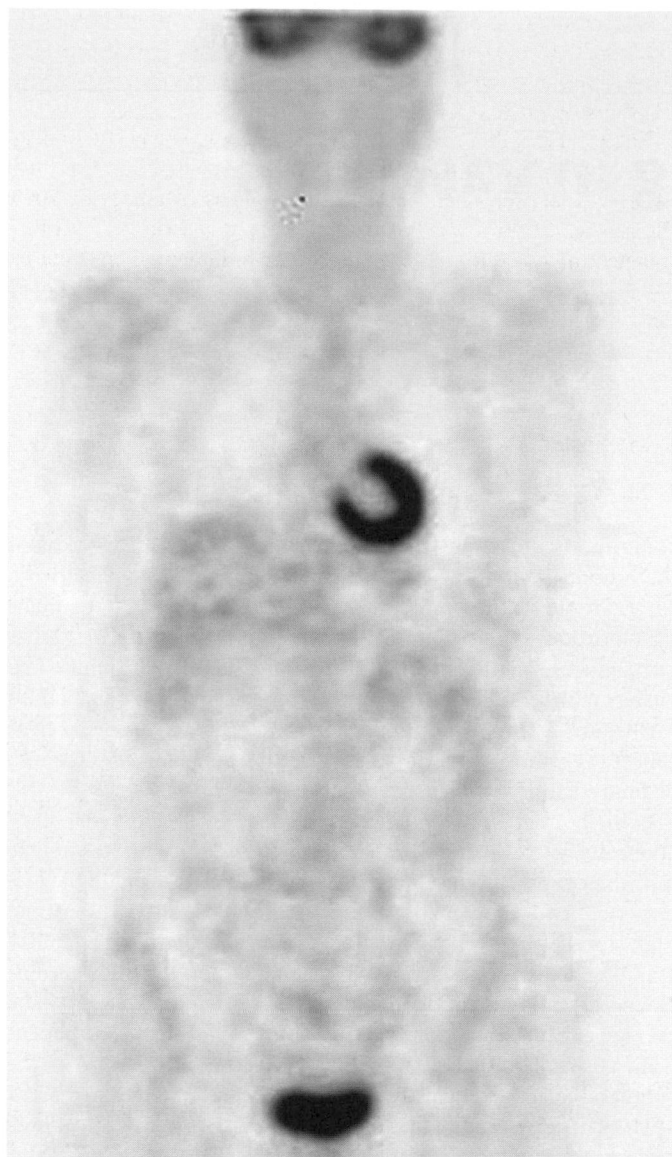

Figure. 20.1 Normal distribution of ¹⁸F–FDG. Note uptake in the metabolically active cerebral cortex and myocardium. The tracer is excreted through the renal pathway and some activity is usually seen in the kidneys or bladder.

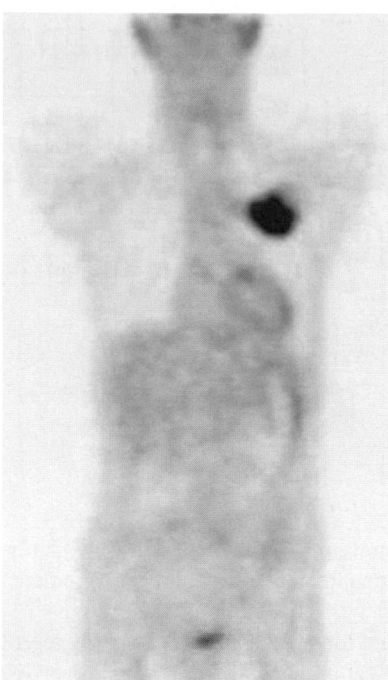

Figure. 20.2 Intense ¹⁸F–FDG uptake in non-small cell lung carcinoma in the left upper lobe. The excellent resolution is demonstrated by the difference of uptake in the tumor compared to adjacent normal lung tissue.

that are very close to a cyclotron. Our discussion in this chapter will therefore be limited to the use of ¹⁸F-FDG.

Clinical application of PET

The major clinical applications of PET are in oncology (85–90% of PET imaging), cardiology, and neuropsychiatry. ¹⁸F-FDG is predominantly used, as it has very high sensitivity in the detection of a large variety of cancers when compared to other PET radiopharmaceuticals (Hustinx *et al.* 2002). In particular, it is a good marker of proliferative potential and aggressiveness in lung cancer (Higashi *et al.* 2003), lymphoma (Spaepen *et al.* 2002), brain (Benard *et al.* 2003), and soft tissue tumors (Ioannidis and Lau 2003).

The metabolic activity of tumors fluctuates throughout the course of the disease, being modulated by the immune system responses as well as the effect of chemoradiotherapy. Such responses

may escape detection by CT or MRI due to absence of structural changes in the early stages. The detection by ¹⁸F-FDG PET of early response to therapy plays a significant role in the management of cancer and has been termed functional imaging, as compared to anatomical imaging with CT and MRI. Functional imaging is now considered vital in the assessment of disease response to therapy in many tumors, particularly in lymphoma.

Infectious and inflammatory lesions also demonstrate high uptake of ¹⁸F-FDG (due to highly metabolically active cells), which lowers the specificity of PET scanning for cancer. Microautoradiography has shown high levels of accumulation of ¹⁸F-FDG within macrophages, activated lymphocytes, and granulation tissue (Kubota *et al.* 1992; Ishimori *et al.* 2002) and this may relate to increased oxidative metabolism in these cells (Rudd *et al.* 2002). A good clinical example of the sensitivity of ¹⁸F-FDG PET in the detection of inflammation/infection is in colitis. In a small series of patients with colitis, Kresnik and coworkers showed that ¹⁸F-FDG PET was able to detect the disease in an early clinical stage, when morphological imaging methods and colonoscopy were non-diagnostic (Kresnik *et al.* 2002).

Other infectious/inflammatory conditions associated with increased ¹⁸F-FDG uptake include abscesses (Tahara *et al.* 1989), herpetic encephalitis (Meyer *et al.* 1994), human immunodeficiency virus (HIV) disease (O'Doherty *et al.* 1997), sarcoidosis (Brudin *et al.* 1994), granulomas (Naumann *et al.* 2002), musculoskeletal infection (Guhlmann *et al.* 1998; Kalicke *et al.* 2000; Stumpe *et al.* 2000; Cook and Fogelman 2001) and others. In fact, the ability of ¹⁸F-FDG to detect both malignant and infectious/inflammatory lesions has been used favorably in the management of patients with fever of unknown origin (FUO) (O'Dohorty *et al.* 1997; Meller *et al.* 2000; Blockmans *et al.* 2001). The use of ¹⁸F-FDG PET to detect and characterize infection and inflammation continues to expand, as its unique abilities become better known (Zhuang *et al.* 2005).

Use of ¹⁸F-FDG PET in vasculitis

In routine ¹⁸F-FDG PET scans, the aorta and its immediate branches usually demonstrate only background uptake of activity (Figure 20.1). This is due to the low numbers of metabolically active cells, specifically fibroblasts and smooth muscle cells, dispersed between the many elastic layers of the arterial wall. The muscular arteries of the abdomen and lower limbs can demonstrate mildly increased uptake of activity in a linear and continuous distribution due to the dynamic activity of large numbers of smooth muscle cells utilizing glucose (Yun *et al.* 2001).

Abnormal uptake of ¹⁸F-FDG may also occur within arterial walls affected by atherosclerosis and aging, due to increased numbers of smooth muscle and inflammatory cells within vessel walls. As a result, the ¹⁸F-FDG PET scan will demonstrate increased vascular wall uptake that is especially noticeable in patients over 60 years of age, where the pattern of activity is focal and non-linear (Yun *et al.* 2001).

The pattern of uptake of ¹⁸F-FDG PET in vascular walls becomes distinctly abnormal in large-vessel vasculitis. Published case reports have demonstrated the value of ¹⁸F-FDG PET scan in diagnosing vasculitis associated with systemic lupus erythematosus (SLE) (Hiraiwa *et al.* 1983), neuro-Behçet's syndrome (Wildhagen *et al.* 1989), Takayasu's arteritis (TA) (Hara *et al.* 1999), giant cell arteritis (GCA) (Turlakow *et al.* 2001), and idiopathic periaortitis (Brodmann *et al.* 2003). These studies describe abnormal, increased uptake of ¹⁸F-FDG, extending in a linear pattern, along the walls of the involved vessels. Subsequent, larger studies have confirmed that this is the typical distribution of ¹⁸F-FDG in large-vessel arteritis.

Of particular note is a study by Blockmans and colleagues who compared the findings of ¹⁸F-FDG PET in 25 subjects with GCA or polymyalgia rheumatica (PMR) with those of 44 age-matched control subjects. They detected vascular uptake in the vessels of the thorax and legs in 76% of the affected group compared to 23% of normal controls (p <0.0001). They concluded that ¹⁸F-FDG PET had a sensitivity of 56%, specificity of 98%, positive predictive value of 93% and a negative predictive value of 80% in the diagnosis of vasculitis associated with GCA (Blockmans *et al.* 2000). This study also demonstrated that the ¹⁸F-FDG PET scan was a valuable, non-invasive modality for early diagnosis and was capable of determining the extent of disease and response to therapy.

Additional studies have compared the ¹⁸F-FDG PET scan with other diagnostic modalities in vasculitis. Meller *et al.* compared ¹⁸F-FDG PET and MRI in 15 patients presenting with FUO or elevated ESR/CRP and a diagnosis of vasculitis (Meller *et al.* 2003b). Of the 15 patients, 14 had GCA and one had TA. The study demonstrated that the ¹⁸F-FDG PET scan better identified the extent of the vasculitis and was more sensitive in monitoring disease activity and the response to immunosuppressive therapy than MRI, and correlated well with clinical and laboratory findings in all patients. An interesting outcome of this study was the demonstration of a higher frequency of aortic involvement in GCA compared to the published reports of 3–15%, which required a different approach to treatment to prevent life-threatening complications. The authors concluded that a traditional angiographic approach to diagnosing vasculitis in this setting would have missed the diagnosis in all cases, the reason being that ¹⁸F-FDG PET scan can diagnose early

disease in the absence of late complications such as stenosis, aneurysmal dilatation, or occlusive disease. Similar conclusions were drawn by our group in a study of six newly diagnosed TA patients (Andrews *et al.* 2004).

The ¹⁸F-FDG PET scan has also been shown to be useful in diagnosing vasculitis in the setting of non-specific symptoms such as fever, malaise, weight loss, and arthralgias (Malik *et al.* 2003; Fletcher and Espinola 2004). The high sensitivity of ¹⁸F-FDG PET in detecting vasculitis has been used as an argument to characterize PMR as a form of vasculitis (Blockmans *et al.* 1999; Moosig *et al.* 2004).

Takayasu's arteritis has been the subject of more studies with ¹⁸F-FDG PET than other large vessel diseases and some detailed discussion may serve as an example of the utility of PET in this category of vasculitis.

¹⁸F-FDG PET in Takayasu's arteritis

Takayasu's arteritis (TA) is a rare, chronic inflammatory arteritis affecting large vessels, predominantly the aorta and its main branches (see Chapter 25). The condition was named for Professor Mikito Takayasu who, in the early nineteenth century, presented the case of a 21-year-old woman with characteristic fundal arteriovenous anastomoses (Numano 2002). TA typically affects young women and may present early with vague constitutional symptoms including anemia, arthralgia, fever, and weight loss, and elevated acute phase reactants. Unfortunately, TA often presents late in the course of the disease with symptoms of end organ ischemia. This is related to occlusive vasculopathy secondary to vessel wall thickening, fibrosis, stenoses, thromboses, or aneurysm formation. (Kerr 1995).

TA typically affects the aortic arch and descending aorta, subclavian, and pulmonary arteries. The American College of Rheumatology has developed criteria for the classification of TA (see Chapter 25). Diagnosis is based on three out of six of these features being present, which yields a sensitivity of 90.5% and a specificity of 97.8% among patients with systemic vasculitis (Arend *et al.* 1990). As can be seen from these criteria, clinical assessment plays a large role in the diagnosis and management of TA; however, clinical assessment alone may underestimate disease activity (Arend *et al.* 1990; Johnston *et al.* 2002; Kerr 1995). In approximately 50% of patients, serological acute phase reactants do not correlate with clinical features or the degree of clinical activity (Kerr *et al.* 1994). Further, at the time of surgical bypass for patients with critical stenoses, 40% of patients in clinical remission have histological evidence of active disease (Lagneau *et al.* 1987).

Angiography is regarded as the gold standard technique for investigating TA and plays a prominent role in the diagnostic algorithm (see Chapter 18). Nevertheless, it is known to have low sensitivity in detecting early arterial wall changes, which characterize the early phase of TA. It has therefore been suggested that non-invasive imaging such as MRI and MR angiography (MRA) (see Chapter 19), and ¹⁸F-FDG PET, may be more reliable than conventional angiography in the investigation of TA (Choe *et al.* 1999; Matsunaga *et al.* 1998; Derdelinckx *et al.* 2000; Andrews *et al.* 2004).

The use of ¹⁸F- FDG PET in TA is based on its ability to detect active glucose turnover within inflamed vascular walls. In the acute phase of TA, the media is infiltrated by lymphocytes and occasional giant cells with neovascularization. Mucopolysaccharides, smooth muscle cells, and fibroblasts induce thickening of the intima. In addition, T cells and dendritic cells, along with few B cells, granulocytes, and macrophages surround the neovascularization of the deep intima (Johnston *et al.* 2002). It is currently believed that the large number of inflammatory cells utilizing glucose is the major factor accounting for the ^{18}F–FDG PET scan findings in TA (Yun *et al.* 2001). In particular, glucose utilization is increased via cellular glucose transporters, especially GLUT-1, which is over-expressed in inflammatory cells due to both cytokine stimulation and a gene-dependent mechanism that is up-regulated in chronic inflammation (Meller *et al.* 2003a).

The first indication of the value of ^{18}F-FDG in TA was the report of a 20-year-old female presenting with fatigue, weight loss, night sweats, and diminished left radial pulse. The scan showed intense and abnormal ^{18}F-FDG uptake in the aorta, brachiocephalic, common carotid and proximal subclavian arteries. This report suggested the use of ^{18}F-FDG in the prestenotic phase of the disease to allow for treatment that may prevent progression (Hara *et al.* 1999).

This and other studies established the pattern of [18]F -FDG PET uptake in active TA, showing mild to severely increased accumulation of tracer in larger arterial walls in a continuous linear distribution that may outline the artery as a tubular structure (Figure 20.3). The activity may also be patchy but always conforms to known arterial territories. Smaller arterial branches may not be visualized due to the resolution limits of ^{18}F-FDG PET scan. The degree of activity can be numerically measured with the standardized uptake value (SUV). This is an index of tracer uptake and is dependant on the dose injected, its timing, and the patient's body mass. The upper range of normal SUV in the assessment of tumors is around 2.5; however, in TA, this value does not necessarily reflect disease severity. Even in highly active disease, the SUV may be low (Kobayashi *et al.* 2005; Webb *et al.* 2004). It is more useful to note a relative increase in activity when compared to background in an arterial territory than rely solely on the SUV as an indicator of disease severity or alternatively to adopt a grading system of vessel wall uptake (Walter *et al.* 2005). SUV is more useful in the follow-up of the same patient.

The above criteria were used in our study of 18 patients with known TA, in which ^{18}F-FDG PET results were compared with angiography and clinical scoring. We documented a sensitivity of 92% and specificity of 100% for ^{18}F-FDG PET in identifying disease activity (Figure 20.4), with negative and positive predictive values of 85% and 100% respectively. We found that performing the ^{18}F-FDG PET scans helped in the management of TA and assessing response to therapy (Figure 20.5), in particular by reducing the need to perform arterial biopsies or repeat angiography (Webb *et al.* 2004).

There is limited experience of the utility of ^{18}F-FDG in detecting brain involvement in TA. Most studies are performed as whole-body scans with exclusion of the head from the field of view due to the high metabolic rate in the brain causing intense ^{18}F-FDG uptake. However, a recent study has clearly demonstrated the value of ^{18}F-FDG in detecting brain abnormalities in four out of five patients with TA (Weiner *et al.* 2004).

When comparing ^{18}F-FDG PET with MRA, MRI, and conventional angiography, it has been demonstrated that the ^{18}F-FDG PET scan detects more lesions and is the best modality to detect early-stage disease (Andrews *et al.* 2004; Webb *et al.* 2004; Meller *et al.* 2003b). This is extremely important as the earlier the diagnosis, the better the outcome. Additionally, the ^{18}F-FDG PET scan can assess the whole body and is non-invasive, unlike conventional angiography, which carries a significant risk of morbidity and mortality (Meller *et al.* 2003a). ^{18}F-FDG PET is also more sensitive than MRI in detecting resolution of the inflammation during immunosuppressive therapy (Meller *et al.* 2003b).

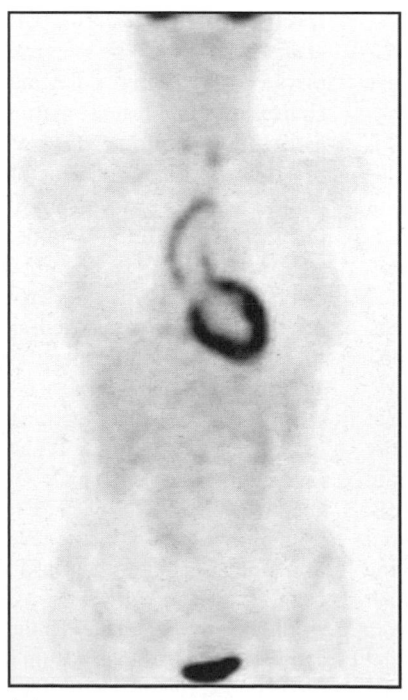 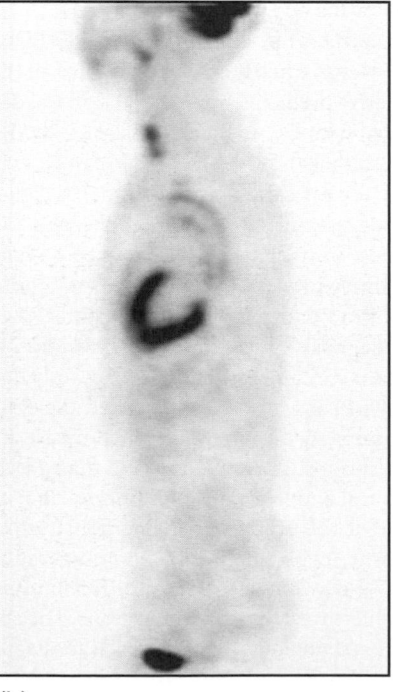

Figure 20.3 Coronal (a) and saggital (b) sections of ^{18}F-FDG PET scan showing tubular uptake in active Takayasu's arteritis involving entire aorta and proximal common carotid arteries. This appearance has become the classic hallmark of large-vessel arteritis.

(a)   (b)

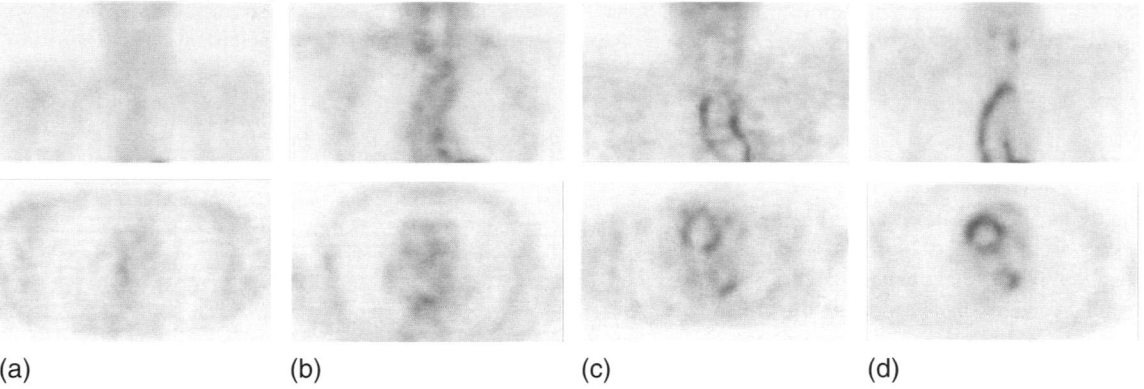

Figure 20.4 Different grades of ¹⁸F-FDG uptake, reflecting levels of disease activity, demonstrated in coronal (top) and transverse (bottom) sections in the same patients. (a) Normal uptake with SUV of 1.5. (b) Minimally increased uptake with SUV of 2.3. (c) Moderately increased uptake with SUV of 3.1. (d) Severely increased uptake with SUV of 4.5.

Although highly sensitive and specific, the ¹⁸F-FDG PET scan may be falsely positive in the presence of atherosclerosis. This is due to the large number of fibroblasts and smooth muscle cells in atherosclerotic lesions. Differentiating the two conditions is easy in young patients, newly diagnosed with TA, who are not prone to extensive atherosclerotic lesions. Even in older patients in whom atherosclerotic lesions are more common, the differentiation between the two conditions is facilitated by the pattern of activity; atherosclerotic lesions tend to be more focal and non-linear. Correlation with other imaging such as CT or performing PET/CT can provide supportive information (Kobayashi *et al.* 2005).

Limitations

The diagnostic utility of ¹⁸F -FDG PET in vasculitis is not without limitations, of which the most vital is the unavailability of PET scanners throughout the world. Hopefully, the increasing awareness of the important role of this imaging modality will cause health care providers to reverse this situation in the near future.

False-negative results

Small-vessel vasculitis is difficult to detect due to limited spatial resolution. This fact, coupled with the intense signal of ¹⁸F-FDG from normal brain tissue, makes the detection of giant cell arteritis (GCA) rather difficult, forcing reliance on the presence of associated large-vessel involvement. Likewise, the detection of coronary vasculitis is impeded by intense myocardial uptake and constant motion.

Uptake of ¹⁸F-FDG can vary according to blood glucose levels, posing a particular problem in diabetic patients, and treatment with glucocorticoids may cause false-negative results (Dunphy *et al.* 2005). In false-negative cases, identification can be enhanced by delaying imaging to more than the standard 1 hour postinjection to improve the target-to-background ratio. This is supported by *in vitro* studies showing persistent accumulation of FDG by macrophages over 3 hours (Deichen *et al.* 2003). Another approach to reduce false-negative results was suggested by Walter and colleagues in a study of 26 patients with GCA and TA and age-matched controls. Correlating their visual grading of vessel wall uptake with CRP and ESR, they found reduced diagnostic sensitivity (<50%) in patients with CRP <12 mg/l or an ESR <12 mm/h. They suggested limiting ¹⁸F-FDG scans to patients with active inflammation and, if possible, after withdrawal of glucocorticoid treatment (Walter *et al.* 2005). However, inflammatory markers may prove unreliable (Webb *et al.* 2004) while stopping glucocorticoids in a critically ill patient is viewed as a suboptimal approach by both doctors and patients.

In difficult cases, various quantification methods, including the calculation of SUV and measurement of target/non-target ratio may reduce subjective bias.

False-positive results

As discussed above, confusion may arise with extensive atherosclerosis and, undoubtedly, with small mediastinal tumors, and lymph nodes. The size and location of these abnormalities and the pattern of uptake (tubular vs. focal) can help in the differentiation of these conditions. The increasing use of hybrid PET/CT scanners, capable

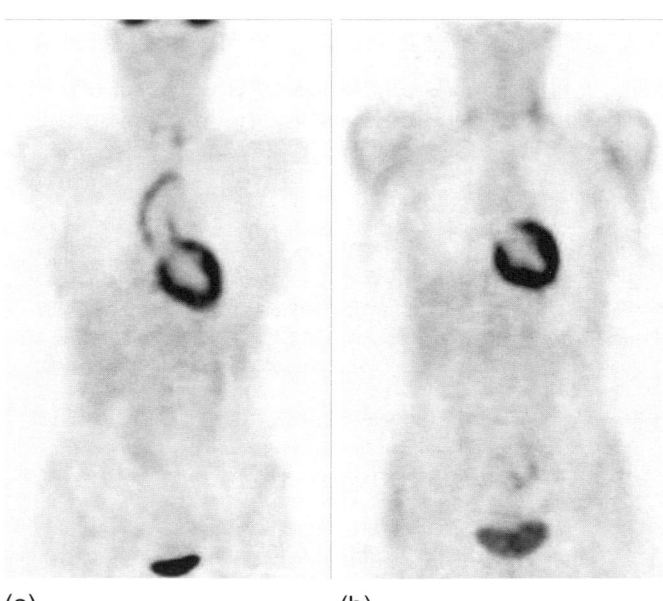

Figure 20.5 Coronal sections of pretherapy (a) and post-therapy (b) ¹⁸F-FDG PET scan of same TA patient as in Figure 20.3. There is clear reduction uptake coinciding with clinical remission and reduction in acute phase response.

of superimposing areas of ^{18}F-FDG uptake on corresponding CT maps, will significantly improve the overall diagnostic power. This has been confirmed in a group of 16 patients with TA (Kobayashi *et al.* 2005).

Summary

^{18}F-FDG PET scan is a highly sensitive, specific, and non-invasive diagnostic tool in large vessel vasculitis, particularly in TA but also in GCA. It is more sensitive than other diagnostic modalities and clinical assessment, and can be used in all stages of the disease, to accurately assess disease activity and monitor the effectiveness of treatment. The facility of whole-body imaging makes it easy to detect unsuspected vascular involvement. Its value is limited in coronary vasculitis, temporal arteritis, and small vessel disease and in the presence of widespread atherosclerotic disease. However, the frequency of false-negative or false-positive results can be minimized with appropriate measures.

References

Andrews, J., Al-Nahhas, A., Pennell, D. J., *et al.* (2004). Non-invasive imaging in the diagnosis and management of Takayasu's arteritis. *Annals of the Rheumatic Diseases*, **63**, 995–1000.

Arend, W., Michel, B., Bloch, D., *et al.* (1990). The American College of Rheumatology 1990 criteria for the classification of Takayasu arteritis. *Arthritis and Rheumatism*, **33**, 1129–34.

Benard, F., Romsa, J. and Hustinx, R. (2003). Imaging gliomas with positron emission tomography and single-photon emission computed tomography. *Seminars in Nuclear Medicine*, **33**, 148–62.

Blockmans, D., Maes, A., Stroobants, S., *et al.* (1999). New arguments for a vasculitic nature of polymyalgia rheumatica using positron emission tomography. *Rheumatology* (Oxford), **38**, 444–7.

Blockmans, D., Stroobants, S., Maes, A., Mortelmans, L. (2000). Positron emission tomography in giant cell arteritis and polymyalgia rheumatica: evidence for inflammation of the aortic arch. *American Journal of Medicine*, **108**, 246–9.

Blockmans, D., Knockaert, D., Maes, A., *et al.* (2001). Clinical value of [(18)F]fluoro-deoxyglucose positron emission tomography for patients with fever of unknown origin. *Clinical Infectious Diseases*, **32**, 191–6.

Brodmann, M., Lipp, R. W., Aigner, R., *et al.* (2003). Positron emission tomography reveals extended thoracic and abdominal peri-aortitis. *Vascular Medicine*, **8**, 127–8.

Brudin, L. H., Valind, S. O., Rhodes, C. G., *et al.* (1994). Fluorine-18 deoxyglucose uptake in sarcoidosis measured with positron emission tomography. *European Journal of Nuclear Medicine*, **21**, 297–305.

Choe, Y. H., Kim, D. K., Koh, E. M., Do, Y. S. and Lee, W. R. (1999). Takayasu arteritis: diagnosis with MR imaging and MR angiography in acute and chronic active stages. *Journal of Magnetic Resonance Imaging*, **10**, 751–7.

Cook, G. J. and Fogelman, I. (2001). The role of positron emission tomography in skeletal disease. *Seminars in Nuclear Medicine*, **31**, 50–61.

Deichen, J. T., Prante, O., Gack, M., Schmiedehausen, K. and Kuwert, T. (2003). Uptake of [18F]fluorodeoxyglucose in human monocyte-macrophages in vitro. *European Journal of Nuclear Medicine*, **30**, 267–73.

Derdelinckx, I., Maes, A., Bogaert, J., Mortelmans, L., Blockmans, D. (2000). Positron emission tomography scan in the diagnosis and follow up of aortitis of the thoracic aorta. *Acta Cardiologica*, **55**, 193–5.

Dunphy, M. P., Freiman, A., Larson, S. M. and Strauss, H. W. (2005). Association of Vascular 18F-FDG Uptake with Vascular Calcification. *Journal of Nuclear Medicine*, **46**, 1278–84.

Fletcher, T. M. and Espinola, D. (2004). Positron emission tomography in the diagnosis of giant cell arteritis. *Clinical Nuclear Medicine*, **29**, 617–9.

Guhlmann, A., Brecht-Krauss, D., Suger, G., *et al.* (1998). Chronic osteomyelitis: detection with FDG PET and correlation with histopathologic findings. *Radiology*, **206**, 749–54.

Hara, M., Goodman, P. C., Leder, R. A. (1999). FDG-PET finding in early-phase Takayasu arteritis. *Journal of Computer Assisted Tomography*, **23**, 16–18.

Higashi, K., Matsunari, I., Ueda, Y., *et al.* (2003). Value of whole-body FDG PET in management of lung cancer. *Annals of Nuclear Medicine*, **17**, 1–14.

Hiraiwa, M., Nonaka, C., Abe, T. and Iio, M. (1983). Positron emission tomography in systemic lupus erythematosus: relation of cerebral vasculitis to PET findings. *American Journal of Neuroradiology*, **4**, 541–3.

Hustinx, R., Benard, F. and Alavi, A. (2002). Whole-body FDG-PET in the management of patients with cancer. *Seminars in Nuclear Medicine*, **32**, 35–46.

Ioannidis, J. P. and Lau, J. (2003). 18F-FDG PET for the diagnosis and grading of soft-tissue sarcoma: a meta-analysis. *Journal of Nuclear Medicine*, **44**, 717–24.

Ishimori, T., Saga, T., Mamede, M., *et al.* (2002). Increased (18)F-FDG uptake in a model of inflammation: concanavalin A-mediated lymphocyte activation. *Journal of Nuclear Medicine*, **43**, 658–63.

Johnston, S., Lock, R. and Gompels, M. (2002). Takayasu arteritis: a review. *Journal of Clinical Pathology*, **55**, 481–6.

Kalicke, T., Schmitz, A., Risse, J. H., *et al.* (2000). Fluorine-18 fluorodeoxyglucose PET in infectious bone diseases: results of histologically confirmed cases. *European Journal of Nuclear Medicine*, **27**, 524–8.

Kerr, G., Hallahan, C., Giordano, J., *et al.* (1994). Takayasu arteritis. *Annals of Internal Medicine*, **120**, 919–29.

Kerr, G. S. (1995). Takayasu's arteritis. *Rheumatic Disease Clinics of North America*, **21**, 1041–58.

Kobayashi, Y., Ishii, K., Oda, K., *et al.* (2005). Aortic wall inflammation due to Takayasu arteritis imaged with 18F-FDG PET co registered with enhanced CT. *Journal of Nuclear Medicine*, **46**, 917–22.

Kresnik, E., Gallowitsch, H. J., Mikosch, P., *et al.* (2002). (18)F-FDG positron emission tomography in the early diagnosis of enterocolitis: preliminary results. *European Journal of Nuclear Medicine Molecular Imaging*, **29**, 1389–92.

Kubota, R., Yamada, S., Kubota, K., Ishiwata, K., Tamahashi, N. and Ido, T. (1992). Intratumoral distribution of fluorine-18-fluorodeoxyglucose in vivo: high accumulation in macrophages and granulation tissues studied by microautoradiography. *Journal of Nuclear Medicine*, **33**, 1972–80.

Lagneau, P., Michel, J. and Vuong, P. (1987). Surgical treatment of Takayasu's disease. *Annals of Surgery*, **205**, 157–66.

Malik, I. S., Harare, O., Al-Nahhas, A., Beatt, K. and Mason, J. (2003). Takayasu's arteritis: management of left main stem stenosis. *Heart*, **89**, e9.

Matsunaga, N., Hayashi, K., Sakamoto, *et al.* (1998). Takayasu arteritis: MR manifestations and diagnosis of acute and chronic phase. *Magnetic Resonance Imaging*, **8**, 406–14.

Meller, I., Altenvoerde, G., Munzel, U., Jauho, A., Behe, M., Gratz, S., *et al.* (2000). Fever of unknown origin: prospective comparison of [18F] FDG imaging with a double-head coincidence camera and gallium-67 citrate SPET. *European Journal of Nuclear Medicine*, **27**, 1617–25.

Meller, J., Grabbe, E., Becker, W. and Vosshenrich, R. (2003a). Value of F-18 FDG hybrid camera PET and MRI in early takayasu aortitis. *European Radiology*, **13**, 400–5.

Meller, J., Strutz, F., Siefker, U., Scheel, A., Sahlmann, C. O., Lehmann, K., *et al.* (2003b). Early diagnosis and follow-up of aortitis with [18F]FDG PET and MRI. *European Journal of Nuclear Medicine Molecular Imaging*, **30**, 730–6.

Meyer, M. A., Hubner, K. F., Raja, S., Hunter, K. and Paulsen, W. A. (1994). Sequential positron emission tomographic evaluations of brain metabolism in acute herpes encephalitis. *Journal of Neuroimaging*, **4**, 104–5.

Moosig, F., Czech, N., Mehl, C., *et al.* (2004). Correlation between 18-fluorodeoxyglucose accumulation in large vessels and serological markers of inflammation in polymyalgia rheumatica: a quantitative PET study. *Annals of the Rheumatic Diseases*, **63**, 870–3.

Naumann, R., Beuthien-Baumann, B., Fischer, R., *et al.* (2002). Simultaneous occurrence of Hodgkin's lymphoma and eosinophilic granuloma: a potential pitfall in positron emission tomography imaging. *Clinical Lymphoma*, **3**, 121–4.

Numano, F. (2002). The story of Takayasu arteritis. *Rheumatology*, **41**, 103–6.

O'Doherty, M. J., Barrington, S. F., Campbell, M., Lowe, J. and Bradbeer, C. S. (1997). PET scanning and the human immunodeficiency virus-positive patient. *Journal of Nuclear Medicine*, **38**, 1575–83.

Rudd, J. H.F., Warburton, E. A., Fryer, T. D., *et al.* (2002). Imaging atherosclerotic plaque inflammation with 18F-fluorodeoxyglucose positron emission tomography. *Circulation*, **105**, 2708–11.

Spaepen, K., Stroobants, S., Dupont, P., *et al.* (2002). Early restaging positron emission tomography with (18)F-fluorodeoxyglucose predicts outcome in patients with aggressive non-Hodgkin's lymphoma. *Annals of Oncology*, **13**, 1356–3.

Stumpe, K. D., Dazzi, H., Schaffner, A. and von Schulthess, G. K. (2000). Infection imaging using whole-body FDG-PET. *European Journal of Nuclear Medicine*, **27**, 822–32.

Tahara, T., Ichiya, Y., Kuwabara, Y., *et al.* (1989). High [18F]-fluorodeoxyglucose uptake in abdominal abscesses: a PET study. *Journal of Computer Assisted Tomography*, **13**, 829–31.

Turlakow, A., Yeung, H. W., Pui, J., *et al.* (2001). Flurodeoxyglucose positron emission tomography in the diagnosis of giant cell arteritis. *Archives of Internal Medicine*, **161**, 1003–7.

Walter, M. A., Melzer, R. A., Schindler, C., Muller-Brand, J., Tyndall, A. and Nitzsche, E. U. (2005). The value of [18F]FDG-PET in the diagnosis of large-vessel vasculitis and the assessment of activity and extent of disease. *European Journal of Nuclear Medicine Molecular Imaging*, **32**, 674–81.

Warburg, O. (1956). On the origin of cancer cells. *Science*, **123**, 309–14.

Webb, M., Chambers, A., Al-Nahhas, A., Mason, J. C., Maudlin, L., Rahman, L. and Frank, J. (2004). The role of 18F-FDG PET in characterising disease activity in Takayasu arteritis. *European Journal of Nuclear Medicine Molecular Imaging*, **31**, 627–34.

Weiner, S. M., Vaith, P., Walker, U. A. and Brink, I. (2004). Detection of alterations in brain glucose metabolism by positron emission tomography in Takayasu's arteritis. *European Journal of Nuclear Medicine Molecular Imaging*, **31**, 300–2.

Wildhagen, K., Meyer, G. J., Stoppe, G., Heintz, P., Deicher, H. and Hundeshagen, H. (1989). PET and MR imaging in a neuro-Behcet syndrome. *European Journal of Nuclear Medicine*, **15**, 764–6.

Yun, M., Yeh, D., Araujo, L., Jang, S., Newberg, A. and Alavi, A. (2001). F-18 FDG uptake in the large arteries. A new observation. *Clinical Nuclear Medicine*, **26**, 314–9.

Zhuang, H., Yu, J. Q. and Alavi, A. (2005). Applications of fluorodeoxyglucose-PET imaging in the detection of infection and inflammation and other benign disorders. *Radiologic Clinics of North America*, **43**, 121–34.

PART 5

Vasculitic diseases and syndromes and related disorders

CHAPTER 21

Approach to the diagnosis of vasculitis in adult patients

Barri J. Fessler

Introduction

The diagnosis of vasculitis is one of the most challenging tasks in the practice of medicine. Non-specific symptoms, overlapping syndromes, lack of highly sensitive or specific diagnostic tests, and the absence of generally accepted diagnostic criteria are issues that plague even the most experienced clinicians. While classification criteria for the different vasculitic syndromes have been proposed for research purposes (Arend *et al.* 1990; Bloch *et al.* 1990; Calabrese *et al.* 1990; Hunder *et al.* 1990; Jennette *et al.* 1994; Leavitt *et al.* 1990; Lightfoot, Jr *et al.* 1990; Masi *et al.* 1990; Mills *et al.* 1990), the application of these criteria for diagnosis is not useful in the clinical setting (Rao *et al.* 1998; Sorensen 2000) (see Chapter 1). Unfortunately, at this time there is no evidence-based algorithm for the diagnosis of vasculitis. To complicate matters further, there are numerous conditions which can mimic primary vasculitic syndromes (Table 21.1; discussed further in Chapter 45). The diagnosis of a specific form of vasculitis ultimately depends on the identification of particular patterns of clinical, radiographic, laboratory, and histopathologic features.

The evaluation of a patient with symptoms suggestive of a vasculitic syndrome must be individually tailored, based on the extent of organ involvement and tempo of the disease manifestations. Early in the disease course, a vasculitic syndrome may present with vague constitutional symptoms or involve one organ system, making the timely diagnosis especially challenging. As other disease manifestations evolve over time, morbidity and mortality associated with the syndrome increase; therefore, aggressive evaluation and prompt treatment is critically important in improving outcomes. The demonstration of vasculitis on tissue biopsy remains the gold standard for diagnosis. However, in situations where the pretest probability of a vasculitic syndrome is high and biopsies cannot be obtained or are negative, either due to sampling error or prior treatment, surrogate markers of vasculitis along with serology and imaging can support a diagnosis. Understanding the usefulness and limitations of serologies, imaging studies, and biopsies is important in establishing a correct diagnosis. This chapter will focus on the approach to the diagnosis of vasculitis in adults and will discuss emerging technologies that can be helpful in supporting the diagnosis.

Initial approach to the diagnosis

The recognition that certain signs and symptoms may be due to an underlying inflammatory vascular process is the first step in establishing a diagnosis of vasculitis. Clinical manifestations, including rapidly progressive multisystem inflammatory disease, constitutional symptoms, chronic fevers, symptoms of tissue ischemia (especially in unusual patient populations such as in a young woman), neuropathy, or suspicious skin lesions such as palpable purpura, should heighten suspicion for vasculitis. The patient's history and physical examination remain the most powerful diagnostic tools available to the clinician. There is no single typical presentation for vasculitis; therefore recognition of patterns or clusters of signs and symptoms is critically important. Complaints of headaches, scalp tenderness, jaw claudication, vision loss, and muscle pain/stiffness raise the possibility of giant cell arteritis (Weyand and Goronzy 2003). New-onset cough with hemoptysis and hematuria suggests the development of a pulmonary–renal syndrome (Gallagher *et al.* 2002). Coupled with the presence of chronic sinus involvement or asthma and eosinophilia, diagnoses such as Wegener's granulomatosis and Churg–Strauss syndrome, respectively, emerge as possibilities (Lane *et al.* 2005). The absence of a pulse or blood pressure in an arm suggests an occlusive vascular process such as Takayasu's arteritis (Park *et al.* 2005). The presence of Raynaud's phenomenon and palpable purpura in a patient with hepatitis C virus (HCV) infection raises the possibility of cryoglobulinemic vasculitis (Schott *et al.* 2001). Age of syndrome onset can also be informative. Giant cell arteritis generally develops in patients over 50 years of age (Machado *et al.* 1988) whereas Kawasaki's disease occurs almost exclusively in children (Lane *et al.* 2005).

A thorough history can help identify risk factors associated with the development of certain vasculitides, such as smoking or exposure to second-hand smoke and Buerger's disease, blood transfusions and HCV-associated cryoglobulinemia, or underlying diseases which can mimic vasculitis such as atherosclerosis or malignancy. Information that should be specifically sought includes: illicit drug use; high risk sexual behavior; prior thromboses; miscarriages; travel history; prior malignancies; operations; invasive procedures; dental work; medications; over the counter supplements or herbal

Table 21.1 Primary and secondary vasculitides

Primary	Secondary and mimics
Large vessel involvement	**Infections**
Giant cell arteritis	Subacute bacterial endocarditis
Takayasu's arteritis	Syphilis
Behçet's syndrome	Hepatitis B
Medium and small vessel involvement	Hepatitis C
Polyarteritis nodosa	CMV
Cutaneous polyarteritis	EBV
Wegener's granulomatosis	HIV
Churg–Strauss syndrome	Meningococcemia
Microscopic polyangiitis	Tuberculosis
Buerger's disease	Brucella
Cryoglobulinemia	Salmonella
Kawasaki disease	Rocky Mountain spotted fever
Behçet's syndrome	**Medications**
Primary angiitis of the CNS	β-lactams
Cogan's syndrome	Sulfonamides
Predominately small vessel involvement	Quinolones
Cutaneous leukocytoclastic vasculitis	Macrolides
Urticarial vasculitis	Thiazides
Behçet's syndrome	Loop diuretics
Henoch–Schönlein purpura	Beta blockers
	Phenytoin
	Propylthiouracil
	Selective serotonin reuptake inhibitors
	NSAIDs
	Anti-tumor necrosis factor antibodies
	Colony stimulating factors (GM-CSF, G-GSF)
	Drugs
	Cocaine
	Amphetamines
	Heroin
	Connective tissue diseases
	Rheumatoid arthritis
	Systemic lupus erythematosus
	Sjögren's syndrome
	Polymyositis
	Dermatomyositis
	Other
	Malignancy
	Thrombotic thrombocytopenic purpura
	Cardiac myxoma
	Cholesterol emboli syndrome
	Atherosclerosis
	Calciphylaxis
	Amyloidosis
	Moyamoya disease
	Ehlers–Danlos syndrome
	Fibromuscular dysplasia
	Antiphospholipid antibody syndrome

preparations; occupation; hobbies, and medication and chemical exposures.

Physical examination may provide clues to the presence of vasculitis or one of its mimics. It can also help to delineate the extent of clinical organ involvement and provide a framework for further diagnostic testing. A thorough vascular exam including palpation of arterial pulses, auscultation for bruits, and blood pressure measurements in all four extremities should be performed in all patients suspected of vasculitis. There are four forms of vasculitis that cause bruits: Takayasu's arteritis, giant cell arteritis, Behçet's syndrome, and Cogan's syndrome. Three forms of vasculitis lead to loss of a pulse: Takayasu's arteritis, giant cell arteritis, and Buerger's disease (Stone *et al.* 2001). Even in a patient who presents with "only a rash," all systems must be examined to look for early or occult involvement. As outlined in Table 21.2, any organ system can be involved and the clinical expression of vasculitis is diverse. Many of these findings, when viewed in isolation, are non-specific but, when interpreted in the context of the history and laboratory findings, can help to establish a diagnosis. For example, the finding of new-onset hypertension is a frequent finding in the general population, but when coupled with abdominal pain and

Table 21.2 Physical examination findings that may suggest an underlying vasculitis

Vital signs:	New onset hypertension, lack of a pulse or blood pressure in an extremity, fever, unintentional weight loss
Head:	Scalp tenderness, swollen nodular and tender temporal artery, scalp necrosis
Eyes:	Retinal vasculitis, embolic phenomenon, episcleritis, scleritis, dacrocystitis, visual field deficits, vision loss
Ears:	Chondritis, otitis media, hearing loss
Nose:	Friable mucosa, ulcerations, septal perforation, cobblestone changes, swelling or collapse of the nasal bridge (saddle nose deformity)
Oropharynx:	Mucosal ulcerations, hoarseness, stridor
Pulmonary:	Wheezing, crackles, dullness to percussion, pleural rub
Cardiac:	New or worsening heart murmur, decreased intensity of heart sounds, pericardial rub, irregular rhythm
Abdomen:	Tenderness, decreased bowel sounds, bruits, stool hemoccult positivity
Genital:	Testicular tenderness, ulcerations on penis/scrotum or vulva/vagina
Vascular:	Bruits in the subclavian, carotid, axillary, brachial, abdominal, femoral and/or popliteal arteries; absence of pulses in arms or legs
Skeletal:	Joint pain and/or synovitis
Neurologic:	Muscle pain or weakness, single or multiple mononeuropathy, polyneuropathy, mononeuritis multiplex, headaches, change in mental status, seizures, cranial neuropathy
Skin:	Petechial or purpuric rashes, cutaneous ulcerations, nodules, digital infarcts, periungual erythema or infarcts, splinter hemorrhages under fingernails, gangrene, erythema nodosa, pseudofolliculitis, livedo reticularis, Raynaud's phenomenon, urticaria (especially if it lasts >24 hours)

mononeuropathy multiplex, it suggests the possibility of polyarteritis nodosa. Therefore, familiarity with the patterns of symptomatology in vasculitic syndromes is essential.

Laboratory testing

Initially, basic laboratory tests consisting of a complete blood count, serum creatinine, transaminases (ALT, AST), urinalysis, and erythrocyte sedimentation rate (ESR) should be obtained. Normochromic, normocytic anemia is common in vasculitic syndromes. In addition, thrombocytosis is frequently seen and is reflective of the acute phase response. In contrast, thrombocytopenia and leukopenia are not expected in primary vasculitic syndromes and would suggest an alternate diagnosis. Eosinophilia may be observed in several of the vasculitic syndromes as well as vasculitis mimics. The presence of hematuria (with dysmorphic red blood cells on microscopic examination) or proteinuria can indicate glomerular involvement prior to a rise in serum creatinine. Microscopic examination of the urine should be performed on a fresh urine specimen to increase the potential to observe cellular casts which degrade over time. Elevated transaminases may indicate liver involvement and would lead to supplemental testing for hepatitis B virus and HCV infection, both of which can be associated with polyarteritis nodosa or cryoglobulinemia. Hepatitis B surface antigen can be seen in up to 10% of patients with polyarteritis nodosa; however, elevated transaminases are not specific to liver involvement and can also be seen in muscle inflammation or infarction and hemolysis. Creatine kinase and aldolase should be checked if muscle involvement is suspected or if elevated transaminases are not felt to be related to liver inflammation. An elevated ESR is frequently observed in vasculitis, but a normal or low ESR does not rule out a diagnosis of vasculitis. An elevated ESR is non-specific, also being observed in malignancies and infections. Up to 24% of patients with giant cell arteritis have a normal ESR (Salvarani and Hunder 2001; Weyand et al. 2000; Zweegman et al. 1993).

There are no specific laboratory tests to diagnose vasculitis. Neither antineutrophil cytoplasmic antibodies (ANCA) nor complement levels should be used as screening tests. Proposed indications for ANCA testing by indirect immunofluorescence include the presence of glomerulonephritis (especially if rapidly progressive); pulmonary hemorrhage; cutaneous vasculitis with systemic features; multiple lung nodules; chronic destructive disease of the upper airways; long-standing sinusitis or otitis; subglottic or tracheal stenosis; peripheral neuropathy; and retro-orbital mass (Hagen et al. 1998; Mandl et al. 2002). A cytoplasmic staining pattern (cANCA) is seen most commonly in generalized Wegener's granulomatosis (WG) and the perinuclear staining (pANCA) is seen most commonly in microscopic polyangiitis (MPA).

Taken in isolation, a positive ANCA test does not establish a diagnosis of vasculitis; ANCAs can be seen in a diverse spectrum of conditions including inflammatory bowel disease, infections, and systemic lupus erythematosus (Radice and Sinico 2005). If the ANCA immunofluorescence test is positive, then enzyme-linked immunosorbent assays (ELISA) testing for antibodies to serine proteinase 3 (PR3) and myeloperoxidase (MPO) are necessary. These assays have a significantly higher positive predictive value than the immunofluorescence ANCA test (83% versus 45%). The results of the ANCA test and anti-PR3/MPO antibodies should be interpreted together to increase their usefulness. If both sets of tests (cANCA and anti-PR3 antibodies; and pANCA and anti-MPO antibodies) are positive, this is highly suggestive of WG and MPA, respectively (Stone et al. 2000). However, between 10–20% of patients with classical WG will have pANCA and anti-MPO antibodies and some patients with MPA or Churg–Strauss syndrome have cANCA positivity. To further complicate the usefulness of the test, 10–50% of patients with biopsy-proven vasculitis will not have any positive serologies (Radice and Sinico 2005).

ANCA testing should not take the place of tissue confirmation of a diagnosis of WG or MPA unless the clinical findings are overwhelmingly classical and infection has been thoroughly excluded. Complement levels are useful in the differential diagnosis of glomerulonephritis; C3 and C4 levels are usually decreased in lupus nephritis, cryoglobulinemia, or endocarditis but are typically normal in many vasculitic syndromes such as WG or MPA (Hebert et al. 1991). Antiglomerular basement membrane (GBM) antibodies should be obtained in the evaluation of alveolar hemorrhage, normocomplementemic glomerulonephritis, or a pulmonary–renal syndrome (Herody et al. 1993).

Antinuclear antibodies (ANA) and rheumatoid factor (RF) are also not useful screening tests for vasculitis because they can be observed in any of the vasculitic syndromes and many of its mimics. The ANA should only be ordered if the diagnosis of systemic lupus erythematosus is being entertained based on history and physical examination findings. Similarly, the RF should only be obtained if an underlying diagnosis of rheumatoid arthritis is suspected based on physical examination. The RF can be significantly elevated in patients with cryoglobulinemia, Sjögren's syndrome, and subacute bacterial endocarditis (Dorner et al. 2004).

Laboratory tests are useful in excluding some of the secondary causes of vasculitis or its mimics. At least three sets of blood cultures should be obtained in any febrile patient with multiorgan system involvement to evaluate for endocarditis. If the clinical suspicion for endocarditis is high, then echocardiography should also be performed, despite negative blood cultures. In the appropriate clinical setting, specific serologic tests for organisms can be helpful, such as tests for syphilis in the evaluation of aortitis.

Diagnostic tests to confirm suspicions of vasculitis

After initial evaluation by history, physical examination, and basic laboratory testing, the distribution of organ involvement should suggest a differential diagnosis. However, this process is not static; new clinical manifestations can develop at any time and may change the diagnostic pathway. Secondary testing (Table 21.3) should focus on providing supportive evidence for a vasculitic process and excluding mimics. For example, in a patient presenting with prominent symptoms of peripheral neuropathy or myopathy, electrodiagnostic tests (electromyography and nerve conduction tests) should be obtained. If a neuropathy is documented, the distinctions among infection, toxin, malignancy, metabolic, and inflammatory etiologies need to be considered. If vasculitis remains in the differential, then a nerve/muscle biopsy would be considered if an accessible nerve is affected (see Chapter 14). As noted above, demonstration of vasculitis on tissue biopsy is preferred to establish the diagnosis. However, if tissue cannot be obtained (or is unrevealing) then directed imaging is indicated.

Table 21.3 Diagnostic tests used in evaluation of suspected vasculitis

Chest radiograph and high-resolution CT scan
Sinus radiograph and CT scan
Orbital CT scan or MRI
Electromyography and nerve conduction tests
Echocardiography
Ultrasound of temporal arteries
Brain MRI with angiogram
Angiography
MRI angiogram of aorta and branches
CT Angiography
PET scan
Tissue biopsy: skin, nerve, muscle, lung, kidney, temporal artery

To delineate areas of suspected organ involvement, imaging studies such as CT or MRI are frequently obtained (see Chapter 19). In addition, they can be used to direct the site of tissue biopsy for focal lesions. MRI or CT are used for evaluation of ears, eyes, nose, and throat involvement in a suspected vasculitic syndrome. MRI can delineate mucosal inflammation, air–fluid levels, cavitary lesions, and retro-orbital inflammatory or fibrotic masses. CT scans can demonstrate mucosal thickening, air–fluid levels, sclerosing osteitis, bone thickening, and bone destruction (Lohrmann et al. 2006). In a patient with central nervous system involvement, MRI of the brain with gadolinium can demonstrate areas of ischemia, infarcts, mass lesions, and meningeal enhancement. MR imaging of the brain is abnormal in >90% of patients with histologically proven angiitis of the central nervous system (Calabrese et al. 1997), but a normal MRI does not rule out central nervous system vasculitis. Further evaluation of the central nervous system includes a lumbar puncture, cerebral angiogram, and brain biopsy. In the setting of a normal MRI and normal cerebrospinal fluid, central nervous system vasculitis is rare (Calabrese et al. 1997).

In a patient with suspected pulmonary involvement, a radiograph of the chest can be informative if it demonstrates nodules, opacities, or infiltrates; however, if it is normal, it does not exclude a pulmonary process. High-resolution CT (HRCT) scanning of the chest is much more sensitive, unmasking pulmonary abnormalities in patients with WG whose chest radiographs are normal (Reuter et al. 1998) (Chapters 13 and 31). HRCT can help to make the distinction between active inflammation ("ground glass changes") and fibrosis. However, it cannot accurately make the distinction between infiltrates due to alveolar bleeding from vasculitis, infection, or medication toxicity. Biopsy of focal lesions in the lung should be pursued.

Tissue biopsy

Ideally, tissue biopsy should be performed prior to treatment initiation; however, if there is critical organ involvement, treatment should never be delayed for diagnostic purposes. The location of a biopsy is determined by suspicion for clinical involvement and accessibility of tissue, for example biopsy of one of the aortic branches would not be feasible; therefore, an imaging study would be utilized in place of biopsy. If several organ systems are involved, choice of biopsy site is determined by the morbidity of the procedure and the likelihood of obtaining disease-specific information. Whereas a skin biopsy demonstrating leukocytoclastic vasculitis confirms the presence of vasculitis, it does not narrow the differential diagnosis with respect to the specific type of vasculitis present, such as polyarteritis nodosa, WG, etc. In contrast, a lung biopsy showing vasculitis, geographic necrosis, and palisading granulomas would suggest WG (Travis et al. 1991). When biopsies reveal classic vasculitic changes, they are very informative; however, a normal biopsy does not exclude a diagnosis of vasculitis. Factors that can influence biopsy positivity include inadequate tissue sample and prior immunosuppressive treatment. Certain vasculitides, such as giant cell arteritis, are characterized by patchy vascular inflammation which results in normal areas of vessel wall scattered between areas of vasculitis (skip lesions); if insufficient tissue is obtained, the vasculitis can be missed (Albert et al. 1976). Blind tissue biopsies, that is sampling of tissue which is not clinically involved, have a low diagnostic yield for vasculitis (19% for nerve and 29% for muscle) (Albert et al. 1988). The demonstration of vasculitis in a tissue specimen is not a final diagnosis. It should be viewed as a sign of an underlying process which must be interpreted in the context of the clinical, serologic, and imaging studies to establish a final diagnosis.

Temporal artery biopsy

In a patient presenting with symptoms suggestive of giant cell arteritis, the diagnostic procedure of choice is the temporal artery biopsy. However, giant cell arteritis can sometimes present with vague signs and symptoms such as fevers, myalgias, and anemia in the absence of headaches, jaw claudication, etc. (Calamia and Hunder 1981; Gonzalez-Gay et al. 2005). In patients over the age of 65 years, giant cell arteritis is the etiology for 16% of fevers of unknown origin (FUO) (Esposito and Gleckman 1978). Therefore, a temporal artery biopsy may also be considered in the evaluation of FUOs in this older population (after malignancy and infections have been excluded).

The decision regarding whether to perform unilateral or bilateral temporal artery biopsy is controversial. Some advocate unilateral biopsy with a contralateral biopsy if the initial biopsy is negative. A large section of artery (~3–4 cm) needs to be removed to increase the diagnostic yield. Others perform routine bilateral biopsies in all patients. Clinical findings that predict a high probability of a positive temporal artery biopsy include jaw claudication, new headaches, eye symptoms, and tender temporal artery (Smetana and Shmerling 2002). Nevertheless, approximately 10% of patients with the clinical diagnosis of giant cell arteritis have normal biopsies (Hall et al. 1983).

Skin biopsy

In patients with cutaneous involvement, a skin biopsy is easy to obtain and has low morbidity. A skin biopsy can easily demonstrate vasculitis. Direct immunofluorescence of skin can reveal IgA deposits in patients with Henoch–Schönlein purpura (Van Hale et al. 1986) or prominent IgG deposition around blood vessels and the basement membrane zone in hypocomplementemic urticarial vasculitis (Mehregan *et al.* 1992). Still, skin biopsies typically provide a general diagnosis of inflammatory vascular disease rather than a precise disease entity.

Lung biopsy

When lower respiratory tract abnormalities are present, obtaining lung tissue is often essential. Transbronchial biopsy has a low diagnostic yield for demonstrating vasculitis (Schnabel *et al.* 1997) but is useful in confirming the presence of pulmonary hemorrhage and evaluating for infectious or malignant etiologies. Open lung biopsy is highly sensitive and specific for confirming a diagnosis of WG (Hoffman *et al.* 1992; Mark *et al.* 1988), but there is substantial morbidity and mortality associated with the procedure. Video-assisted thoracic surgery (VATS) for obtaining lung tissue may provide an excellent alternative to open lung biopsy due to its low morbidity and mortality (Ooi *et al.* 2005).

Nerve and muscle biopsy

In patients suspected of having nerve involvement, a nerve biopsy should be considered (see Chapter 14). The yield of a nerve biopsy is higher with site selection guided by clinical and electrodiagnostic findings. The diagnostic yield from a nerve and muscle biopsy that is not clinically involved is only 19% and 29% respectively (Albert *et al.* 1988). However, despite having abnormal electrodiagnostic findings, up to 45% of nerve biopsies can reveal no diagnostic pathology (Pioro and Calabrese 1995; Rappaport *et al.* 1993). Biopsy of skeletal muscle along with nerve biopsy can increase the diagnostic yield for vasculitis (Collins *et al.* 2000; Stone *et al.* 2001). The sural and superficial peroneal nerves are the most commonly biopsied nerves, but the radial sensory nerve is also amenable to biopsy. The morbidity associated with nerve biopsy is not trivial; infection, non-healing ulcers, and chronic pain at the incision site have been observed (Gabriel *et al.* 2000; Rappaport *et al.* 1993).

Nasal or sinus biopsy

In patients with symptoms suggestive of WG or Churg–Strauss syndrome, a sample of nasal or sinus tissue can be examined although the diagnostic yield is very low. Acute and chronic inflammation is frequently observed and is completely non-diagnostic. Vasculitis and granulomas are very rarely demonstrated; therefore, it is of limited diagnostic value for vasculitis.

Renal biopsy

In patients with multisystem disease and a rising creatinine or in the setting of proteinuria of unexplained etiology or cellular casts, a renal biopsy should be considered for diagnostic and prognostic purposes (see Chapter 16). Standard stains (hematoxylin and eosin, silver, trichrome), immunofluorescence, and electron microscopy should be performed on all specimens. Most commonly, the renal biopsy reveals glomerular disease, for example focal segmental necrotizing glomerulonephritis or crescentic glomerulonephritis. True necrotizing arteritis or granulomas are rarely seen on renal biopsy. In a patient with symptoms suggestive of generalized WG, the biopsy site of choice would be lung rather than kidney because there is a higher likelihood of finding vasculitis and granulomas in the lung.

Vascular imaging studies

Angiography

Traditionally, angiography has been the diagnostic procedure of choice for detecting arterial stenoses, occlusions, and aneurysms in large and medium-sized vessels within the central nervous system, chest, and abdomen (see Chapter 18). In addition, angiography may be used when biopsies are not feasible or are unrevealing. The presence of multiple saccular aneurysms in more than one organ is highly suggestive of vasculitis. However, a multitude of other conditions can mimic angiographic vasculitic changes including: atherosclerosis; amyloidosis; vasospasm; infection; fibromuscular dysplasia; Ehlers–Danlos syndrome; atrial myxoma; pheochromocytoma; use of sympathomimetic drugs; and malignancy (see Chapter 45). Therefore, the results of the imaging study must be interpreted in the context of the clinical setting. The specificity of brain angiography in differentiating vasculitis mimics from histologically defined angiitis of the central nervous system is less than 30% (Duna and Calabrese 1995). Several other caveats exist when interpreting angiographic results. Angiography does not have adequate resolution for small vessels; therefore, conditions characterized predominantly by small-vessel inflammation, such as Henoch–Schönlein purpura, may be overlooked. In addition, aneurysms take time to develop and consequently they may not be demonstrated when the angiogram is performed early in the disease course. Similarly, traditional angiography only visualizes the lumen of the vessel; thickening of the vessel wall which may occur prior to the development of stenoses or aneurysms would not be demonstrated on routine angiography. Limiting factors for performing angiography include the presence of compromised renal function which could be worsened following infusion of contrast dye, as well as risk for ischemic complications. In patients with Behçet's syndrome, angiography is not recommended due to increased risk for aneurysm formation at arterial puncture sites (Kingston *et al.* 1979).

Magnetic resonance imaging

For the evaluation of the aorta and its primary branches, magnetic resonance imaging (MRI) is being performed more commonly now in place of traditional angiography (see Chapter 19). There is no risk for ionizing radiation or iodinated contrast material; therefore, it can be used for serial imaging. It provides visualization of the vessel lumen and also demonstrates vessel wall edema and thickness (Flamm *et al.* 1998). Although MRI is felt to have excellent sensitivity and specificity for large-vessel vasculitis (Yamada *et al.* 2000) it is not without limitations. It may overestimate vascular occlusions, it does not image small branch vessels and vascular calcifications are poorly visualized (Yamada *et al.* 2000). In addition, disease activity as measured by vessel wall edema on MRI does not consistently correlate with symptoms, acute phase reactants, or occurrence of new anatomic changes on subsequent exams (Tso *et al.* 2002). The incorporation of angiography into MR imaging allows for more detailed vascular characterization (Narvaez *et al.* 2005).

Computed tomography

Computed tomography (CT) scanning can provide details regarding the degree and nature of vessel wall thickening, for example calcification and extent of disease (see Chapter 19). The addition of three-dimensional reconstruction techniques contributes angiogram-like images, highlighting areas of stenosis, occlusion, and aneurysmal dilation.

Ultrasound

Color duplex ultrasonography provides better resolution than MRI or CT scan for medium sized peripheral arteries such as temporal, carotid, axillary, and femoral arteries (see Chapter 19). Blood flow, wall thickening, and plaques can be visualized. Findings suggestive of vasculitis include hypoechoic dark wall swelling (halo sign), increased flow velocity due to stenosis, and acute occlusion (Schmidt et al. 1997; Schmidt et al. 2003; Nesher et al. 2002). These findings reflect inflamed arterial walls and are not specific for giant cell arteritis. In a meta-analysis of studies using ultrasonography for giant cell arteritis, the sensitivity of the halo sign was 69% and specificity was 82% compared with temporal artery biopsy (Karassa et al. 2005). Rarely, other entities such as polyarteritis nodosa, Churg–Strauss syndrome, WG, or amyloidosis can cause temporal artery inflammation. Ultrasound is most effective in diagnosing new cases of giant cell arteritis; it is much less effective in detecting cases of recurrent disease.

PET scanning

Positron emission tomography (PET) is a non-invasive, metabolic imaging modality based on the regional distribution of ^{18}F-fluorodeoxyglucose, which has been used extensively in the management of oncology patients. It is now emerging as a promising tool in the diagnosis of large-vessel vasculitis (Blockmans et al. 2000; Walter et al. 2005) (see Chapter 20). It visualizes the entire body in a single image and can demonstrate the distribution of vascular involvement. The PET signal is weak for small arteries such as temporal arteries but strong for branches extending from the aorta. The main application of the PET scan will likely be in the evaluation of atypical presentations of vasculitis and monitoring response to therapy. Additional studies are needed to evaluate the sensitivity and specificity of PET scanning in large-vessel vasculitis (Belhocine et al. 2003).

Conclusions

Diagnosis of vasculitis is challenging. It first requires familiarity with the clinical features of the different syndromes and narrowing down the differential diagnosis based on the patient's history and physical examination. The next requirement is selection of appropriate tests to delineate areas of disease involvement with focus on demonstrating vasculitis, either through tissue biopsy or imaging studies. Choice of biopsy site is determined by the morbidity of the procedure and the likelihood of obtaining disease-specific information. The type of imaging study is chosen based on size and location of vessels involved. At the same time, secondary causes of vasculitis and mimics of vasculitis must be excluded. Because systemic vasculitis can be life threatening if untreated, a clinician oftentimes must institute several treatments concurrently, directed towards the suspected vasculitis as well as its mimics, while the investigation is in progress. If the clinical presentation is atypical, and tissue biopsy or imaging is not obtained early in the disease course, a definitive diagnosis may never be established, leading to confusion about long-term treatment and prognosis.

Editors' note

A study of ^{18}F-fluorodeoxyglucose positron tomography (PET) in 35 patients with GCA was done between May 2000 and July 2003 by Blockmans and colleagues (Blockmans et al. (2006) Arthritis and Rheumatism (Arthritis Care and Research), 55, 131–7). They found FDG uptake in 29 patients at the time of diagnosis. Vascular uptake at diagnosis was not related to the presence or absence of clinical or laboratory findings except for jaw claudication, which resulted in a lower incidence of uptake. The uptake was almost always bilateral, was greatest in the subclavian arteries, and the abdominal and thoracic aorta were visualized in about one-half of patients. Increased FDG uptake in the shoulders correlated well with symptoms of polymyalgia rheumatica. Repeat scans were done 3 and 6 months after beginning treatment with prednisolone, and although the total vascular score fell significantly after 3 months of treatment, from 3 to 6 months there was no further decrease in uptake. The primary objective of the study was to determine whether repeated FDG PET scans would differentiate patients who were prone to relapse and those who were not. The results did not allow this differentiation. The authors concluded that the use of FDG-PET scintigraphy in GCA lay in the diagnostic investigation of its atypical presentations.

References

Albert, D. A., Rimon, D., and Silverstein, M. D. (1988). The diagnosis of polyarteritis nodosa. I. A literature-based decision analysis approach. Arthritis and Rheumatism, 31, 1117–27.

Albert, D. M., Ruchman, M. C., and Keltner, J. L. (1976). Skip areas in temporal arteritis. Archives of Ophthalmology, 94, 2072–7.

Arend, W. P., Michel, B. A., Bloch, D. A., Hunder, G. G., Calabrese, L. H., Edworthy, S. M., Fauci, A. S., Leavitt, R. Y., Lie, J. T., Lightfoot, R. W., Jr., et al. (1990). The American College of Rheumatology 1990 criteria for the classification of Takayasu arteritis. Arthritis and Rheumatism, 33, 1129–34.

Belhocine, T., Blockmans, D., Hustinx, R., Vandevivere, J., and Mortelmans, L. (2003). Imaging of large vessel vasculitis with (18).FDG PET: illusion or reality? A critical review of the literature data. European Journal of Nuclear Medicine and Molecular Imaging, 30, 1305–13.

Bloch, D. A., Michel, B. A., Hunder, G. G., McShane, D. J., Arend, W. P., Calabrese, L. H., Edworthy, S. M., Fauci, A. S., Fries, J. F., and Leavitt, R. Y. (1990). The American College of Rheumatology 1990 criteria for the classification of vasculitis. Patients and methods. Arthritis and Rheumatism, 33, 1068–73.

Blockmans, D., Stroobants, S., Maes, A., and Mortelmans, L. (2000). Positron emission tomography in giant cell arteritis and polymyalgia rheumatica: evidence for inflammation of the aortic arch. American Journal of Medicine, 108, 246–9.

Calabrese, L. H., Duna, G. F., and Lie, J. T. (1997). Vasculitis in the central nervous system. Arthritis and Rheumatism, 40, 1189–201.

Calabrese, L. H., Michel, B. A., Bloch, D. A., Arend, W. P., Edworthy, S. M., Fauci, A. S., Fries, J. F., Hunder, G. G., Leavitt, R. Y., Lie, J. T., et al. (1990). The American College of Rheumatology 1990 criteria for the classification of hypersensitivity vasculitis. Arthritis and Rheumatism, 33, 1108–13.

Calamia, K. T. and Hunder, G. G. (1981). Giant cell arteritis (temporal arteritis) presenting as fever of undetermined origin. Arthritis and Rheumatism, 24, 1414–18.

Collins, M. P., Mendell, J. R., Periquet, M. I., Sahenk, Z., Amato, A. A., Gronseth, G. S., Barohn, R. J., Jackson, C. E., and Kissel, J. T. (2000). Superficial peroneal nerve/peroneus brevis muscle biopsy in vasculitic neuropathy. Neurology, 55, 636–43.

Dorner, T., Egerer, K., Feist, E., and Burmester, G. R. (2004). Rheumatoid factor revisited. *Current Opinion in Rheumatology*, **16**, 246–53.

Duna, G. F. and Calabrese, L. H. (1995). Limitations of invasive modalities in the diagnosis of primary angiitis of the central nervous system. *Journal of Rheumatology*, **22**, 662–7.

Esposito, A. L. and Gleckman, R. A. (1978). Fever of unknown origin in the elderly. *Journal of the American Geriatrics Society*, **26**, 498–505.

Flamm, S. D., White, R. D., and Hoffman, G. S. (1998). The clinical application of 'edema-weighted' magnetic resonance imaging in the assessment of Takayasu's arteritis. *International Journal of Cardiology*, **66** (Suppl. 1), S151–9.

Gabriel, C. M., Howard, R., Kinsella, N., Lucas, S., McColl, I., Saldanha, G., Hall, S. M., and Hughes, R. A. (2000). Prospective study of the usefulness of sural nerve biopsy. *Journal of Neurology Neurosurgery and Psychiatry*, **69**, 442–6.

Gallagher, H., Kwan, J. T., and Jayne, D. R. (2002). Pulmonary renal syndrome: a 4-year, single-center experience. *American Journal of Kidney Diseases*, **39**, 42–7.

Gonzalez-Gay, M. A., Lopez-Diaz, M. J., Barros, S., Garcia-Porrua, C., Sanchez-Andrade, A., Paz-Carreira, J., Martin, J., and Llorca, J. (2005). Giant cell arteritis: laboratory tests at the time of diagnosis in a series of 240 patients. *Medicine* (Baltimore), **84**, 277–90.

Hagen, E. C., Daha, M. R., Hermans, J., Andrassy, K., Csernok, E., Gaskin, G., Lesavre, P., Ludemann, J., Rasmussen, N., Sinico, R. A., Wiik, A., and van der Woude, F. J. (1998). Diagnostic value of standardized assays for anti-neutrophil cytoplasmic antibodies in idiopathic systemic vasculitis. EC/BCR Project for ANCA Assay Standardization. *Kidney International*, **53**, 743–53.

Hall, S., Persellin, S., Lie, J. T., O'Brien, P. C., Kurland, L. T., and Hunder, G. G. (1983). The therapeutic impact of temporal artery biopsy. *Lancet*, **2**, 1217–20.

Hebert, L. A., Cosio, F. G., and Neff, J. C. (1991). Diagnostic significance of hypocomplementemia. *Kidney International*, **39**, 811–21.

Herody, M., Bobrie, G., Gouarin, C., Grunfeld, J. P., and Noel, L. H. (1993). Anti-GBM disease: predictive value of clinical, histological and serological data. *Clinical Nephrology*, **40**, 249–55.

Hoffman, G. S., Kerr, G. S., Leavitt, R. Y., Hallahan, C. W., Lebovics, R. S., Travis, W. D., Rottem, M., and Fauci, A. S. (1992). Wegener granulomatosis: an analysis of 158 patients. *Annals of Internal Medicine*, **116**, 488–98.

Hunder, G. G., Bloch, D. A., Michel, B. A., Stevens, M. B., Arend, W. P., Calabrese, L. H., Edworthy, S. M., Fauci, A. S., Leavitt, R. Y., Lie, J. T., *et al.* (1990). The American College of Rheumatology 1990 criteria for the classification of giant cell arteritis. *Arthritis and Rheumatism*, **33**, 1122–8.

Jennette, J. C., Falk, R. J., Andrassy, K., Bacon, P. A., Churg, J., Gross, W. L., Hagen, E. C., Hoffman, G. S., Hunder, G. G., Kallenberg, C. G., *et al.* (1994). Nomenclature of systemic vasculitides. Proposal of an international consensus conference. *Arthritis and Rheumatism*, **37**, 187–92.

Karassa, F. B., Matsagas, M. I., Schmidt, W. A., and Ioannidis, J. P. (2005). Meta-analysis: test performance of ultrasonography for giant-cell arteritis. *Annals of Internal Medicine*, **142**, 359–69.

Kingston, M., Ratcliffe, J. R., Alltree, M., and Merendino, K. A. (1979). Aneurysm after arterial puncture in Behçet's disease. *British Medical Journal*, **1**, 1766–7.

Lane, S. E., Watts, R., and Scott, D. G. (2005). Epidemiology of systemic vasculitis. *Curr. Rheumatol Rep.*, **7**, 270–5.

Lane, S. E., Watts, R. A., Shepstone, L., and Scott, D. G. (2005). Primary systemic vasculitis: clinical features and mortality. *Quarterly Journal of Medicine*, **98**, 97–111.

Leavitt, R. Y., Fauci, A. S., Bloch, D. A., Michel, B. A., Hunder, G. G., Arend, W. P., Calabrese, L. H., Fries, J. F., Lie, J. T., Lightfoot, R. W., Jr., *et al.* (1990). The American College of Rheumatology 1990 criteria for the classification of Wegener's granulomatosis. *Arthritis and Rheumatism*, **33**, 1101–7.

Lightfoot, R. W., Jr., Michel, B. A., Bloch, D. A., Hunder, G. G., Zvaifler, N. J., McShane, D. J., Arend, W. P., Calabrese, L. H., Leavitt, R. Y., Lie, J. T., *et al.* (1990). The American College of Rheumatology 1990 criteria for the classification of polyarteritis nodosa. *Arthritis and Rheumatism*, **33**, 1088–93.

Lohrmann, C., Uhl, M., Warnatz, K., Kotter, E., Ghanem, N., and Langer, M. (2006). Sinonasal computed tomography in patients with Wegener's granulomatosis. *Journal of Computer Assisted Tomography*, **30**, 122–5.

Machado, E. B., Michet, C. J., Ballard, D. J., Hunder, G. G., Beard, C. M., Chu, C. P., and O'Fallon, W. M. (1988). Trends in incidence and clinical presentation of temporal arteritis in Olmsted County, Minnesota, 1950–1985. *Arthritis and Rheumatism*, **31**, 745–9.

Mandl, L. A., Solomon, D. H., Smith, E. L., Lew, R. A., Katz, J. N., and Shmerling, R. H. (2002). Using antineutrophil cytoplasmic antibody testing to diagnose vasculitis: can test-ordering guidelines improve diagnostic accuracy? *Archives of Internal Medicine*, **162**, 1509–14.

Mark, E. J., Matsubara, O., Tan-Liu, N. S., and Fienberg, R. (1988). The pulmonary biopsy in the early diagnosis of Wegener's (pathergic) granulomatosis: a study based on 35 open lung biopsies. *Human Pathology*, **19**, 1065–71.

Masi, A. T., Hunder, G. G., Lie, J. T., Michel, B. A., Bloch, D. A., Arend, W. P., Calabrese, L. H., Edworthy, S. M., Fauci, A. S., Leavitt, R. Y., *et al.* (1990). The American College of Rheumatology 1990 criteria for the classification of Churg-Strauss syndrome (allergic granulomatosis and angiitis). *Arthritis and Rheumatism*, **33**, 1094–100.

Mehregan, D. R., Hall, M. J., and Gibson, L. E. (1992). Urticarial vasculitis: a histopathologic and clinical review of 72 cases. *Journal of the American Academy of Dermatology*, **26**, 441–8.

Mills, J. A., Michel, B. A., Bloch, D. A., Calabrese, L. H., Hunder, G. G., Arend, W. P., Edworthy, S. M., Fauci, A. S., Leavitt, R. Y., Lie, J. T., *et al.* (1990). The American College of Rheumatology 1990 criteria for the classification of Henoch-Schönlein purpura. *Arthritis and Rheumatism*, **33**, 1114–21.

Narvaez, J., Narvaez, J. A., Nolla, J. M., Sirvent, E., Reina, D., and Valverde, J. (2005). Giant cell arteritis and polymyalgia rheumatica: usefulness of vascular magnetic resonance imaging studies in the diagnosis of aortitis. *Rheumatology* (Oxford), **44**, 479–83.

Nesher, G., Shemesh, D., Mates, M., Sonnenblick, M., and Abramowitz, H. B. (2002). The predictive value of the halo sign in color Doppler ultrasonography of the temporal arteries for diagnosing giant cell arteritis. *Journal of Rheumatology*, **29**, 1224–6.

Ooi, A., Iyenger, S., Ferguson, J., and Ritchie, A. J. (2005). VATS lung biopsy in suspected, diffuse interstitial lung disease provides diagnosis, and alters management strategies. *Heart Lung Circ.*, **14**, 90–2.

Park, M. C., Lee, S. W., Park, Y. B., Chung, N. S., and Lee, S. K. (2005). Clinical characteristics and outcomes of Takayasu's arteritis: analysis of 108 patients using standardized criteria for diagnosis, activity assessment, and angiographic classification. *Scandinavian Journal of Rheumatology*, **34**, 284–92.

Pioro, M. and Calabrese, L. H. (1995). How useful is sural nerve biopsy in the diagnosis of systemic vasculitis? *Arthritis and Rheumatism*, **38**, S339.

Radice, A. and Sinico, R. A. (2005). Antineutrophil cytoplasmic antibodies (ANCA). *Autoimmunity*, **38**, 93–103.

Rao, J. K., Allen, N. B., and Pincus, T. (1998). Limitations of the 1990 American College of Rheumatology classification criteria in the diagnosis of vasculitis. *Annals of Internal Medicine*, **129**, 345–52.

Rappaport, W. D., Valente, J., Hunter, G. C., Rance, N. E., Lick, S., Lewis, T., and Neal, D. (1993). Clinical utilization and complications of sural nerve biopsy. *American Journal of Surgery*, **166**, 252–6.

Reuter, M., Schnabel, A., Wesner, F., Tetzlaff, K., Risheng, Y., Gross, W. L., and Heller, M. (1998). Pulmonary Wegener's granulomatosis: correlation between high-resolution CT findings and clinical scoring of disease activity. *Chest*, **114**, 500–6.

Salvarani, C. and Hunder, G. G. (2001). Giant cell arteritis with low erythrocyte sedimentation rate: frequency of occurence in a population-based study. *Arthritis and Rheumatism*, **45**, 140–5.

Schmidt, D., Hetzel, A., Reinhard, M., and Auw-Haedrich, C. (2003). Comparison between color duplex ultrasonography and histology of the temporal artery in cranial arteritis (giant cell arteritis). *European Journal of Medicinal Research*, **8**, 1–7.

Schmidt, W. A., Kraft, H. E., Vorpahl, K., Volker, L., and Gromnica-Ihle, E. J. (1997). Color duplex ultrasonography in the diagnosis of temporal arteritis. *New England Journal of Medicine*, **337**, 1336–42.

Schnabel, A., Holl-Ulrich, K., Dalhoff, K., Reuter, M., and Gross, W. L. (1997). Efficacy of transbronchial biopsy in pulmonary vaculitides. *European Respiratory Journal*, **10**, 2738–43.

Schott, P., Hartmann, H., and Ramadori, G. (2001). Hepatitis C virus-associated mixed cryoglobulinemia. Clinical manifestations, histopathological changes, mechanisms of cryoprecipitation and options of treatment. *Histology and Histopathology*, **16**, 1275–85.

Smetana, G. W. and Shmerling, R. H. (2002). Does this patient have temporal arteritis? *Journal of the American Medical Association*, **287**, 92–101.

Sorensen, S. F., Slot, O., Tvede, N., and Petersen, J. (2000). A prospective study of vasculitis patients collected in a five year period: evaluation of the Chapel Hill nomenclature. *Annals of the Rheumatic Diseases*, **59**, 478–82.

Stone, J. H., Calabrese, L. H., Hoffman, G. S., Pusey, C. D., Hunder, G. G., and Hellmann, D. B. (2001). Vasculitis. A collection of pearls and myths. *Rheumatic Disease Clinics of North America*, **27**, 677–728.

Stone, J. H., Talor, M., Stebbing, J., Uhlfelder, M. L., Rose, N. R., Carson, K. A., Hellmann, D. B., and Burek, C. L. (2000). Test characteristics of immunofluorescence and ELISA tests in 856 consecutive patients with possible ANCA-associated conditions. *Arthritis Care Research*, **13**, 424–34.

Travis, W. D., Hoffman, G. S., Leavitt, R. Y., Pass, H. I., and Fauci, A. S. (1991). Surgical pathology of the lung in Wegener's granulomatosis. Review of 87 open lung biopsies from 67 patients. *American Journal of Surgical Pathology*, **15**, 315–33.

Tso, E., Flamm, S. D., White, R. D., Schvartzman, P. R., Mascha, E., and Hoffman, G. S. (2002). Takayasu arteritis: utility and limitations of magnetic resonance imaging in diagnosis and treatment. *Arthritis and Rheumatism*, **46**, 1634–42.

Van Hale, H. M., Gibson, L. E., and Schroeter, A. L. (1986). Henoch-Schönlein vasculitis: direct immunofluorescence study of uninvolved skin. *Journal of the American Academy of Dermatology*, **15**, 665–70.

Walter, M. A., Melzer, R. A., Schindler, C., Muller-Brand, J., Tyndall, A., and Nitzsche, E. U. (2005). The value of [18F]FDG-PET in the diagnosis of large-vessel vasculitis and the assessment of activity and extent of disease. *European Journal of Nuclear Medicine and Molecular Imaging*, **32**, 674–81.

Weyand, C. M., Fulbright, J. W., Hunder, G. G., Evans, J. M., and Goronzy, J. J. (2000). Treatment of giant cell arteritis: interleukin-6 as a biologic marker of disease activity. *Arthritis and Rheumatism*, **43**, 1041–8.

Weyand, C. M. and Goronzy, J. J. (2003). Giant-cell arteritis and polymyalgia rheumatica. *Annals of Internal Medicine*, **139**, 505–15.

Yamada, I., Nakagawa, T., Himeno, Y., Kobayashi, Y., Numano, F., and Shibuya, H. (2000). Takayasu arteritis: diagnosis with breath-hold contrast-enhanced three-dimensional MR angiography. *Journal of Magnetic Resonance Imaging*, **11**, 481–7.

Zweegman, S., Makkink, B., and Stehouwer, C. D. (1993). Giant-cell arteritis with normal erythrocyte sedimentation rate: case report and review of the literature. *Netherlands Journal of Medicine*, **42**, 128–31.

CHAPTER 22

Vasculitis in infancy, childhood, and adolescence

Ross E. Petty

The spectrum of vasculitis varies with age. The most common vasculitides of infancy and childhood are all but unknown in the adult population; those that are common in the aging population do not occur in young children. Most forms of vasculitis are uncommon or rare in childhood. The exceptions are Henoch–Schönlein purpura (HSP) and Kawasaki disease (KD), which are not only the most common vasculitides of childhood, but are probably the most common systemic vasculitides in any age group. This chapter will focus on vasculitides that occur predominantly in children, and on the features of childhood onset of vasculitis that also occur in the adult population.

Classification of vasculitis in childhood

Until recently, classifications of childhood vasculitis have been modifications of those used in adult populations (Jennette *et al.* 1994; Hunder *et al.* 1990). The Pediatric Rheumatology European Society (PRES) proposed a classification that was age-appropriate and arrived at by consensus of an international committee of pediatric rheumatologists and nephrologists (Table 22.1) (Ozen *et al.* 2006). Like others before it, this classification is based primarily on size of the affected vessels, but is adapted to fit current knowledge of vasculitides as they occur in childhood and adolescence.

Takayasu arteritis (TA) is the only vasculitis of childhood affecting large arteries. KD is the most common of the medium-sized vasculitides. The small-vessel vasculitides are classified as granulomatous or non-granulomatous. Wegener's granulomatosis (WG) is the only significant granulomatous, small-vessel vasculitis seen in childhood; HSP is the major non-granulomatous, small-vessel vasculitis. Other vasculitides occur in childhood, but they are extremely rare, and from our limited knowledge of their characteristics, appear to be similar to the disease in adults.

Common vasculitides of childhood

HSP and KD, two vasculitides that are predominantly diseases of childhood, account for more than 90 percent of all cases of vasculitis in this age group.

Henoch–Schönlein purpura

HSP is the most commonly reported vasculitis in children in Europe, North America, and India and is discussed extensively in Chapter 40. Data from other parts of the world are lacking, and in Japan, where Kawasaki disease (KD) is common, HSP may be the second most common vasculitis of childhood. J.L. Schönlein described the triad of arthritis, purpura, and abnormalities of the renal sediment in 1837 (Schönlein 1837). Henoch added the fourth important element, abdominal pain, in 1974 (Henoch 1974). Recently proposed classification criteria (Ozen *et al.* 2006) are shown in Table 22.2.

Epidemiology and genetics

HSP occurs most commonly between the ages of 5 and 7 years (Yang *et al.* 2005; Trapani *et al.* 2005), but may occur in infancy and adulthood. It is somewhat more common in boys than girls (1.2:1.0). Estimates of the annual incidence range from 2.5 to more than 20 per 100,000, with the highest incidence in the winter months.

Familial HSP is observed occasionally, although no consistent genetic marker has been identified. Motoyama and Iitaka (2005) recently reported eight of 428 families in which two members had HSP (seven sets of siblings and a mother–daughter pair). In three pairs, HSP occurred within 1 month of each other. Possible genetic associations include heterozygous deficiency of C2, and, in those with nephritis, increased frequency of HLA B35 and DRB1*01 (Amoli *et al.* 2002). An increased frequency of the C4B*Q0 null allele reported in Icelandic children with HSP suggests that inadequate functioning of the complement pathway in elimination of immune complexes may predispose to HSP (Steffanson *et al.* 2005).

Etiology and pathogenesis

The cause of HSP is unknown; however, clinical evidence of a preceding upper respiratory tract infection and occasional reports of associations with streptococci, mycoplasma, *Bartonella henselae*, and with a variety of viruses suggest an infectious etiology. The high levels of serum IgA (Trygstad *et al.* 1971; Saulsbury 1999) and the characteristic predominance of IgA in the vasculitic lesions (Baart de la Faille-Kuyper *et al.* 1973) also suggest the possibility of a transmucosal infectious etiology. However, no organism has been consistently linked to the occurrence of HSP, and the wide variety of bacterial and viral infections that have been reported suggest that the effect of infection in general, rather than a specific infection, may be of more pathogenic significance.

Table 22.1 Pediatric Rheumatology European Society (PRES) classification of childhood vasculitis (from Ozen *et al.* 2006)

1. Predominantly large-vessel vasculitis

    Takayasu's arteritis

2. Predominantly medium-sized vessel vasculitis

    Childhood polyarteritis nodosa

    Cutaneous polyarteritis nodosa

    Kawasaki disease

3. Predominantly small-sized vessel vasculitis

    Granulomatous

        Wegener's granulomatosis

        Churg–Strauss syndrome

    Non-granulomatous

        Microscopic polyangiitis

        Henoch–Schönlein purpura

        Isolated cutaneous leukocytoclastic vasculitis

        Hypocomplementemic urticarial vasculitis

4. Other Vasculitides

    Behçet's syndrome

    Vasculitis secondary to infection (including Hepatitis B-associated PAN), malignancies and drugs

    Vasculitis associated with connective tissue diseases

    Isolated vasculitis of the central nervous system

    Cogan's syndrome

    Unclassified

Diagnosis

According to the proposed diagnostic criteria shown in Table 22.2, the diagnosis can be made on the basis of the presence of palpable purpura, with one or more of the following criteria: arthralgia or arthritis; abdominal pain; and hematuria. Occasionally, however, biopsy of skin or kidney is necessary to confirm the diagnosis. The differential diagnosis includes microscopic polyangiitis (MPA) and polyarteritis nodosa (PAN).

Clinical manifestations

The signs and symptoms of HSP usually become evident over the course of a few days or a week. The child may be quite well, or have low-grade fever and malaise. The frequency of clinical characteristics is listed in Table 22.3. Palpable purpura predominates on the buttocks and lower extremities. Lesions range in size from petechiae to coalescent purpura several centimeters in diameter. Larger lesions may ulcerate. Edema may occur over the dorsum of the hands and feet and is a characteristic finding in the scalp, where it

Table 22.2 Classification criteria for Henoch–Schönlein purpura (from Ozen *et al.* 2006)

Palpable purpura in the presence of at least one of:
  diffuse abdominal pain
  any biopsy showing predominant IgA deposition
  arthralgia or arthritis
  any hematuria and/or proteinuria

Table 22.3 Common manifestations of Henoch–Schönlein purpura (from Saulsbury 1999)

Purpura	100%
Arthritis	82%
Abdominal pain	63%
Gastrointestinal bleeding	33%
Occult	23%
Gross	10%
Glomerulonephritis	40%
Hematuria	40%
Gross hematuria	7%
Proteinuria	25%
Nephrotic syndrome	3%
Other	
Orchitis	9%[1]
Seizures	2%
Duodenal obstruction	1%

[1] Percent of boys.

may be most evident on a dependent area of the head, particularly in very young children. Scrotal edema is a rare occurrence.

Arthralgias or arthritis occur in approximately 80% of patients. It is usually oligoarticular and affects predominantly large joints. In the series reported by Saulsbury (1999), the feet and ankles were affected in 72%, the knees in 50%, hands and wrists in 26%, and elbows in 10%. The swelling is characteristically periarticular, and the joint is painful on motion. The entire course of joint disease usually begins within a week of development of purpura, is usually limited to a few days to a week, and resolves completely.

Abdominal pain occurs in two-thirds of children. It usually occurs early in the disease course, and may be the initial manifestation, preceding other signs by days. Colicky abdominal pain may be severe and be accompanied by vomiting and occult or, less frequently, gross blood in the stools. Bowel obstruction, infarction, and perforation may ensue. The small bowel is most frequently affected by these complications. Intussusception is a rare (~1 in 250) but serious complication (Chang *et al.* 2004). It is reported to be ilioileal in more than two-thirds and ileocolic in the remainder (Chang *et al.* 2004; Szer 1996). Ulceration of the stomach or duodenum has been reported (Fu *et al.* 2005).

Renal disease manifested by hematuria and proteinuria occurs in 40–50% of patients, usually within the first month after onset of rash. In the large series reported by Chang *et al.* (2005), microscopic hematuria occurred in 14.2% and gross hematuria in 4.6%. Nephrotic syndrome occurred in less than 1%.

Pathology

The characteristic lesion is leukocytoclastic vasculitis of small capillaries and postcapillary venules in the skin, and focal or diffuse proliferative glomerulonephritis. Deposition of IgA in affected vessels is highly characteristic (Ferrario and Rastaldo 2005).

Laboratory investigations

Leukocytosis and thrombocytosis are present. Erythrocyte sedimentation rate (ESR) and C-reactive protein (CRP) are usually elevated, and serum IgA levels are elevated in half of patients. Components of the complement system are usually normal, although early in the disease course activation of the alternative complement pathway is common. In general there is no increased prevalence of autoantibodies, although IgA antibodies to endothelial surface antigens may be detected using human umbilical cord endothelial cells (Yang *et al.* 2002). It has been reported that antibodies to neutrophil cytoplasmic antigens (ANCA) of the IgA, but not IgG, isotype are associated with early HSP, but disappear in the convalescent stage of the disease (Ozaltin *et al.* 2004).

Treatment

In most patients, supportive treatment, including analgesia, is all that is required. Although glucocorticoids may rapidly reduce the severity of the joint and skin disease, they are seldom required for the management of these manifestations. There is no strong evidence to suggest that early treatment with glucocorticoids reduces the risk of renal or gastrointestinal disease. In a double-blind, placebo-controlled study, Huber *et al.* (2004) studied the effect of prednisone on development of renal and gastrointestinal disease at 1 year. The treatment group consisted of 20 children with HSP seen in the emergency room of a tertiary care pediatric hospital given oral prednisone (2 mg/kg/day for 1 week followed by a weaning dose for a second week), which was compared to a similar group of children who received supportive therapy only (nasogastric suction, parenteral nutrition). There was no significant difference in the rate of renal disease at 1 year, or in the rate of gastrointestinal complications, although two children in the placebo group had intussusceptions compared to none in the prednisone treated group.

In the face of established renal disease, the value of glucocorticoids is controversial. Renal disease is usually self-limited, but some evidence suggests that the early use of high-dose methylprednisolone may minimize the effects of renal disease (Niaudet and Habib 1998).

A number of case series document the effectiveness of cyclosporine in children with HSP complicated by nephritic syndrome (Shin *et al.* 2005a). In a small non-randomized study, azathioprine together with glucocorticoids was shown to improve renal outcome of children with HSP and nephritic syndrome compared to treatment with glucocorticoids alone (Shin *et al.* 2005b). Experience with other drugs including anticoagulants and intravenous immunoglobulin is very limited, but has not shown any dramatic effect. Renal transplantation has been required in a few patients with HSP, and the rate of recurrence in the transplanted kidney is approximately one in three (Meulders *et al.* 1994).

Outcome

The long-term prognosis is usually excellent, but HSP may have a monocyclic or polycyclic course, and recurrences (usually purpura and abdominal pain) occur in one-third to one-half of children. Hematuria and proteinuria may persist for well over a year in up to half of patients (Chang *et al.* 2005). The development of chronic renal failure in 5% may be predicted by the presence of hypertension and nephritic or nephrotic syndrome at onset. In such patients, progressive renal dysfunction may occur over a period of many years. In children with normal urinalysis and blood pressure at diagnosis, the risk of developing hypertension as a late sequela is low (Nussinovitch *et al.* 2005).

Kawasaki's disease

Kawasaki's disease (KD) is discussed extensively in Chapter 29. The description by Kawasaki (1967) of the febrile exanthematous illness which now bears his name, marked an important milestone,

Table 22.4 Proposed classification criteria for Kawasaki's disease (from Ozen *et al.* 2006)

Abnormality	Characteristics
Fever	High, spiking, poorly responsive to antipyretics
Rash	Polymorphous, not vesicular or crusting Desquamates in perineum (early) and palms and soles (later)
Extremity changes	Swelling of hands or feet often with purple discoloration of palms or soles
Adenitis	Cervical, usually unilateral, may appear to be a single node
Conjunctivitis	Bulbar, non-suppurative, bilateral
Mucosal changes	Red, swollen vertically cracked lips, erythema of oropharynx, "strawberry" tongue

Classification criteria are fulfilled in the presence of fever for at least 5 days plus four of the other criteria. In the presence of fever and coronary artery involvement (demonstrated by echocardiography), fewer than four of the remaining criteria are needed to fulfill the classification requirements.

although isolated examples of this disease had been previously recognized, often diagnosed as fatal infantile polyarteritis nodosa (Munro-Faure 1959). The epidemics of KD in Japan, and subsequently in other countries, have been of great interest, and this disease now constitutes one of the most important exanthematous illnesses of infancy and childhood, the second most common childhood vasculitis world-wide, and the most common cause of acquired heart disease in childhood in the industrialized world. Proposed classification criteria are shown in Table 22.4.

Epidemiology and genetics

KD is a disease of young children; the peak age at onset in North America is about 2 years of age, (Holman *et al.* 2003a) and more than 80% have onset under the age of 5 years. Occasionally older children and adolescents have KD. Boys are affected more commonly than girls (1.4:1.0). The incidence of KD varies widely throughout the world, being highest in Japan. Although it has been reported that the incidence in the United States is increasing (Chang 2002), re-evaluation of this study discounted this finding because the study did not use the recommended weighting technique to account for the differences in stratified sampling across different years (Chang 2003; Holman *et al.* 2003b). However, detailed epidemiologic studies in Japan demonstrated a steady increase in the incidence over the past 14 years to 140 per 100,000 children under age 5 and it has been suggested that at present rates, 1 in every 150 children in Japan will suffer from this disease (Burns *et al.* 2005a).

Japanese studies demonstrated that 1% of children with KD had affected siblings (Yanagawa *et al.* 1995). In twins, concordance was 14% (Harada *et al.* 1986) Interestingly, most affected twins developed the disease within 2 weeks of each other, suggesting an important role for an environmental agent. In North America, children of Japanese, Southeast Asian, and Chinese ancestry are particularly at risk to develop KD. African Americans may have a lower frequency of KD than Americans of Asian ancestry, but a higher frequency than is seen in American Caucasians (Davis *et al.* 1995). There is a suggestion that African Americans with KD have a lower incidence of coronary artery disease (Porcalla *et al.* 2005).

Distinct epidemics of KD were recorded in Japan in 1982 and 1986 (Yanagawa *et al.* 2001; Yanagawa *et al.* 1999). Although such striking epidemics have not been observed since, there is good evidence for a seasonal occurrence of the disease throughout Japan (Burns *et al.* 2005a). A less striking seasonality in occurrence has been observed in North America with more cases seen in the winter months (Bell *et al.* 1983).

Etiology and pathogenesis

The cause of KD is unknown, but its epidemiologic characteristics suggest that it represents a response to a communicable agent, involving a specific organism or a superantigen (Yeung 2005). Although many viruses and bacteria have been linked to KD, no consistent association has been demonstrated (Yeung 2004). It seems more likely that some property common to many viruses and bacteria, that is a superantigen, is the inciting agent, a finding supported by restricted T cell receptor variable region gene segment usage (Abe *et al.* 1992). This superantigen theory is also supported by evidence derived from a *Lactobacillus caseii*-induced murine model of KD (Duong *et al.* 2003).

Clinical manifestations

KD begins as a febrile illness. Its manifestations can be roughly divided into three phases, although there is great variability in the sequence of clinical findings (Table 22.4). The first phase is characterized by the abrupt onset of fever of 39–40°C, lasting for 10–14 days (untreated) and often preceded or accompanied by symptoms of an upper respiratory tract or gastrointestinal infection. The younger child is usually intensely irritable. During this time, conjunctivitis, rash, cervical adenitis, and arthritis may develop. A subacute phase lasts for 2–4 weeks if untreated, and is characterized by gradual normalization of fever, disappearance of the mucosal changes, conjunctivitis, adenitis and arthritis, and desquamation of the skin of the palms and soles. It is during the subacute phase that coronary artery aneurysms most often make their appearance. The third, convalescent phase may last months during which time the inflamed arteries heal, other manifestations of KD disappear, and there is normalization of the acute phase response.

Clinical evidence of cardiac disease is usually absent, although sinus tachycardia is present. In some children, congestive heart failure occurs early in the disease course as a result of myocarditis. Obstruction of aneurysms (especially those >8 mm in diameter) may result in myocardial infarction, arrhythmias, or sudden death.

In addition to the signs and symptoms encompassed in the classification criteria, children with KD frequently have: arthralgia or arthritis; coryza (usually in the early stages of the disease); anterior uveitis (associated with conjunctivitis) (Smith *et al.* 1989); mild diarrhea; and abdominal pain, sometimes with hydrops of the gallbladder (Suddleson *et al.* 1987). Typical KD is usually readily recognizable; incomplete KD presents a difficult diagnostic challenge. The characteristics of the classification criteria are discussed below.

- *Fever.* A persistent fever of 40°C or higher that is minimally responsive to antipyretics is present in all children with KD. It is usually accompanied, in young patients in particular, by marked irritability, and does not respond to antibiotic therapy.
- *Conjunctivitis.* Bilateral bulbar, non-suppurative conjunctivitis, sometimes with perilimbal sparing, is present in about 90%

of patients. It is often accompanied by anterior uveitis, demonstrable on slit-lamp, and in 10–20% of instances by keratitis, vitreous opacities, or papilledema (Kumagai *et al.* 1996).

- *Changes in lips and oral mucosa.* Red, swollen, vertically cracked lips, erythema of the oropharynx, or strawberry tongue occur in 85–90%. The throat may be sore, but an exudate is not present.
- *Rash.* The exanthem of KD is polymorphic, usually macular or maculopapular, but not vesicular or crusting. It may occur anywhere, and is often accentuated in the perineal area. Desquamation occurs earliest in the perineum (often within the first 7–10 days), but is usually most dramatic on the palms and soles where sheet-like desquamation begins at the tips of the digits and around the nails in the second to fourth weeks of illness.
- *Lymphadenopathy.* By history, transient unilateral cervical adenopathy is quite common, but it is often an early feature and disappears before the child is seen by a physician. Ultrasonography reveals the presence of two or more nodes in a single mass.
- *Extremity changes.* The palms and soles may be bright red, and the dorsum of the hands and feet are often edematous.

Other clinical abnormalities include arthritis, usually in the knees or ankles, most often occurring in the recovery phase of the disease. There are no sequelae. Transient sensorineural deafness has been reported (Knott *et al.* 2001).

Differential diagnosis

Classical KD is usually easily recognizable. However, in children in whom all classification criteria are not met (incomplete KD) or in whom there are unusual manifestations (atypical KD), a number of viral or bacterial illnesses may be considered, including adenovirus, parvovirus, herpesvirus, leptospirosis, streptococcal, and staphylococcal infections. Toxic shock syndrome is rarely a consideration. In the child with protracted disease, systemic juvenile idiopathic arthritis and PAN should be considered. Since many febrile children are treated with antibiotics, a drug reaction may be confused with incomplete KD.

Pathology

Medium-sized arteries, particularly (but not exclusively) the coronary arteries, are the site of inflammation characterized by fibrinoid necrosis (Fujiwara *et al.* 1978). IgA producing B lymphocytes and macrophages are the characteristic infiltrating cells (Rowley *et al.* 1997). Later, aneurysms, thrombosis, and stenosis develop. Inflammation of the myocardium, endocardium, and pericardium is common in the early stages of the disease; fibrosis occurs later.

Laboratory investigations

Marked elevation of the ESR and serum CRP, and elevation of the white blood cell count are characteristic in the acute phase of the disease. The platelet count is initially normal, or occasionally subnormal, but becomes markedly elevated in the subacute phase of the disease when counts exceeding one million are not unusual. Urinalysis may reveal sterile pyuria. Mild elevations of liver enzymes are common. The irritability and headache so frequently observed in children with KD is reflected by increased protein and cells and decreased glucose in the cerebrospinal fluid (Dengler *et al.* 1998). Autoantibodies including those to endothelial antigens and ANCAs are not characteristic of KD, at least early in the disease course (Guzman *et al.* 1994; Nash *et al.* 1995).

Echocardiography is most commonly used to evaluate the coronary arteries for the presence of abnormalities, which include increased vessel wall echogenicity, dilatation, aneurysms, thrombosis, and stenosis. Electrocardiography may demonstrate evidence of pericarditis, myocarditis, or myocardial ischemia. It is recommended (Dijani *et al.* 1994) that it be performed at the time of diagnosis and again 6 to 8 weeks later. In untreated patients, coronary artery aneurysms develop in 25%, almost always between the second and eighth weeks of disease, although they occasionally develop earlier.

Treatment

Treatment of KD is initiated in hospital with intravenous immunoglobulin (IVIg) and aspirin. Currently it is recommended that IVIg be given in a dose of 2 g/kg together with anti-inflammatory doses of aspirin (80–100 mg/kg/d) (American Academy of Pediatrics 2003). There is usually a prompt response to this treatment with immediate fall in fever, and improvement in sense of well-being, and disappearance of other signs over a few days. IVIg has also been shown to lower the incidence of coronary artery aneurysms (Newburger *et al.* 1986). High-dose aspirin therapy is continued until the platelet count begins to return to normal at which time the dose is reduced to 2–3 mg/kg/day until the platelet count normalizes. Ordinarily, a single dose of IVIg suffices. Occasionally, however, the initial IVIg infusion has no effect, or the fever or other signs of systemic inflammation return 24–36 hours later. In such instances, it is appropriate to retreat with the same dose of IVIg. Children who do not respond to a second dose of IVIg should be given intravenous methylprednisolone (30 mg/kg to a maximum of 1 g/day for 1–3 consecutive days). Failure to maintain a response to this regimen should prompt use of oral prednisone (2 mg/kg/day in divided doses) until evidence of inflammation has disappeared. Although early studies of the treatment of KD suggested that glucocorticoids were contraindicated, this is clearly not the case (Sundel *et al.* 2003; Lang *et al.* 2006).

The administration of the anti-TNF biologic infliximab to 17 children with KD with either persistent arthritis or persistent or recrudescent fever following two IVIg infusions, and in nine patients, IV methylprednisolone, resulted in rapid cessation of fever in 14 of 15 patients (Burns *et al.* 2005b). Full delineation of the role of infliximab will require prospective evaluation. Other approaches such as plasmapheresis and the use of cytotoxic agents have been little studied and their role is probably minimal.

Follow-up

Monitoring of children with KD is important in the acute and convalescent phases of the disease. In those with coronary artery abnormalities, much longer follow-up is needed. In the absence of coronary aneurysms, the child with KD can be considered to have recovered when clinical signs and symptoms have disappeared, and laboratory abnormalities, especially platelet count and ESR, have returned to normal. Until that time they should receive low-dose aspirin, and be evaluated every 2–4 weeks. The presence of coronary artery changes necessitates more intensive observation. Depending on the severity of the arterial lesion, patients may need restriction of physical activities, repeated echocardiography, or cardiac stress tests or coronary angiography (Newburger *et al.* 2004).

Outcome

With the exception of coronary artery disease, enduring complications of KD are rare. The outcome of KD has been dramatically improved by treatment with IVIg, aspirin, and, when necessary, glucocorticoids. Treatment with IVIg has reduced the incidence of coronary artery aneurysms to <5%. Most aneurysms eventually disappear, but it is likely that abnormalities of the endothelium persist, perhaps for decades. Aneurysms rarely rupture, but occlusion with thrombosis is an important sequel, especially in the child with giant aneurysms (>8 mm in diameter), and may result in myocardial infarction or sudden death, even years after the initial illness.

Long-term studies of mortality in patients who had KD are beginning to emerge. A Japanese study of more than 6000 individuals who had KD between 1982 and 1992 and who were followed until 2001, showed that although early death occurred in 29 patients during the acute phase, later deaths were not significantly increased (Nakamura *et al.* 2005).

Uncommon vasculitides of childhood

Primary vasculitis other than HSP and KD is rare in childhood, although somewhat more common in adolescence. The diseases discussed in this section usually present as a fever of unknown origin, failure to thrive, or with cutaneous, cardiovascular, central nervous system, or bronchopulmonary signs and symptoms. Because of their rarity, recognition of the diagnosis may be delayed, resulting in morbidity and increased mortality. In most ways, diseases such as TA, WG, PAN, and MPA closely resemble the same diseases in adults.

Takayasu's arteritis

Takayasu's arteritis (TA) is an uncommon inflammatory disease that affects the aorta and its major branches (see Chapter 25). It follows HSP and KD as the third most common vasculitis in childhood and adolescence world-wide. The proposed criteria for the diagnosis of TA in children and adolescents are shown in Table 22.5.

Epidemiology and genetics

TA is rare in infancy, and most common in adolescence. It occurs world-wide but is most commonly reported from Japan, Southeast Asia, and the Indian subcontinent although the incidence and prevalence are uncertain. It is the most common cause of renovascular hypertension in Asian children (Chugh *et al.* 1992). It is twice as common in girls as in boys in most series. Although TA has been reported in twins and other family members, it is seldom familial. HLA B-52 has been associated with TA in Japan, Korea, and India (Yajima *et al.* 1994).

Table 22.5 Criteria for diagnosis of Takayasu's arteritis in childhood (from Ozen *et al.* 2006)

Angiographic abnormalities of the aorta or its main branches demonstrated by conventional angiography, CT, or MRI, plus at least 1 of the following:
1. Decreased peripheral artery pulse(s) and/or claudication of extremity(ies)
2. Blood pressure difference of >10 mmHg
3. Bruits over aorta and/or its major branches
4. Hypertension (compared to age-matched normal values)

Etiology, pathogenesis, and pathology

The etiology is unknown but an immune pathogenesis is likely. In acute disease there is $\gamma\delta$ T cell, cytotoxic T cell and natural killer (NK) cell infiltration of the vasa vasorum and destruction of the media and adventia through release of perforin, with intimal hyperplasia resulting in stenosis (Seko 2000). With time the elastic fibers of the media are destroyed (leading to aneurysms) and fibrosis replaces the smooth muscle of the media (leading to stenosis). Granulomas with giant cells are present (Kothari 2002).

Clinical manifestations

Symptoms and signs of TA reflect the pattern of vessel involvement. Hypertension and its manifestations are the most common presenting features, occurring in 21 of 23 children in a recent series (Stanley et al. 2003). Fever, weight loss, anorexia, night sweats, headache, claudication, chest wall pain, and myalgias are common presenting features. A neurologic event such as a cerebrovascular accident may be the initial manifestation of the disease, and occurs at some time during the course of the disease in one-quarter to one-half of patients (Kothari 2002). On examination, hypertension, absence of one or more peripheral pulses, tenderness of major vessels, and the presence of bruits over the aorta or its main branches support the diagnosis. The characteristic wreath-like retinal vascular pattern originally described by Takayasu is rare, although other retinal changes, resulting from ischemia, are present in up to one-half of patients (Chun et al. 2001).

Laboratory investigations

The acute phase response is usually markedly abnormal. Antinuclear antibody, rheumatoid factor, and ANCA are negative, although antibodies to endothelial cell antigens and anticardiolipin antibodies may be present (Eichorn et al. 1996). It is a difficult challenge to determine the presence and degree of active inflammation in a child with TA. Aside from signs and symptoms, and abnormalities of acute phase reactants, which may not reliably reflect the extent of active disease, imaging studies are probably the best way to monitor disease activity by the demonstration of new lesions.

Imaging studies (arteriography or magnetic resonance imaging) provide the definitive diagnosis (Kothari 2002; Stanley et al. 2003). TA is classified according to the distribution of aneurysms and stenosis in vessels into: Type I (aortic arch and its branches, ~60%); Type II (thoracoabdominal aorta and its branches, ~40%); Type III (lesions of both aortic arch and thoracoabdominal aorta and its branches, <1%); and Type IV (with pulmonary vessel involvement, <1%). In most children, Types II and III distribution predominate. Renal artery stenosis is present in about three-quarters (Kothari 2002).

Treatment

Studies of the treatment of TA in adults have been the guide for management of the disease in children and adolescents. Treatment is initiated with prednisone in doses of 1–2 mg/kg/day, usually in divided doses. Cyclophosphamide is added at a dose of 2 mg/kg/day orally, or given monthly for 4–6 months in a dose of 0.5–1.0 g/m^2. The cyclophosphamide is then replaced by oral or subcutaneous methotrexate (0.35–0.65 mg/kg/week) (Shelhamer et al. 1985). There is evidence that methotrexate can be successfully used instead of cyclophosphamide in glucocorticoid-resistant patients (Hoffman et al. 1994). Preliminary studies of the use of anti-TNF agents in conjunction with glucocorticoids are encouraging (Hoffman et al. 2004).

Unfortunately, there are no prospective controlled trials comparing these regimens and the data in children are very limited. Aggressive management of hypertension is essential. Antiplatelet doses of aspirin may be useful in preventing intravascular clotting, particularly if anticardiolipin antibodies are present. Surgical stenting or bypassing of severely stenotic areas of artery may be required in the child with uncontrolled hypertension or vascular compromise of the central nervous system. The subject of treatment has been recently reviewed by Liang and Hoffman (2004).

Outcome

Hypertension, cerebrovascular accident, and renal failure are major long-term complications. In most children and adolescents, TA is a chronic or life-long illness, with periods of quiescence punctuated by signs or symptoms of vascular insufficiency, or laboratory evidence of active disease. Outcome is probably significantly improved in those who receive early treatment, before fibrosis has led to stenosis, which is not responsive to medical treatment. Long-term anti-inflammatory treatment is usually necessary. Mortality in reported studies ranges from 10% (Shrivastava 1995) to 31% (Dabague and Reyes 1996). Causes of death in adults with TA include cardiac failure, renal failure, ruptured aneurysms, and stroke. Studies of long-term survival of juvenile-onset TA have not been reported.

Wegener's granulomatosis

Wegener granulomatosis (WG) is a granulomatous vasculitis affecting vessels of the respiratory tract, kidneys, and occasionally other sites (see Chapters 30, 31, and 32). It is an important cause of pulmonary hemorrhage in children and adolescents. The proposed criteria for the diagnosis of WG in children and adolescents are shown in Table 22.6.

Epidemiology and genetics

WG is a rare disease, but there is evidence that it may be increasing in frequency (Watts et al. 2000; Koldingsnes et al. 2000). It appears to be more common in northern than southern Europe (Watts et al. 1997). There are no incidence and prevalence data for this disease in childhood and adolescence, and its greatest frequency is in late adulthood. In reported series, boys slightly outnumber girls. There are no genetic studies of childhood-onset WG.

Etiology, pathogenesis, and pathology

Although the cause of WG is unknown, increasing interest in a possible role of environmental factors is reflected in recent publications. The histological picture is that of a granulomatous vasculitis affecting small and medium-sized arteries, in the upper and lower airways, the kidneys, and occasionally other sites.

Table 22.6 Classification criteria for Wegener's granulomatosis in childhood (from Ozen et al. 2006)

Three of the following criteria should be present::
1. Abnormal urinalysis
2. Granulomatous inflammation on biopsy
3. Nasal and/or sinus inflammation
4. Subglottic, tracheal, or endobronchial stenosis
5. Characteristic abnormalities on chest radiography or CT
6. Presence of cANCA (anti-PR3)

Clinical manifestations

Constitutional symptoms such as fever and weight loss, coupled with evidence of sinopulmonary or renal disease, and laboratory evidence of inflammation should raise the question of a systemic vasculitis such as WG. Sinopulmonary disease and renal disease are characteristic of WG, but the clinical manifestations are varied (Rottem *et al.* 1993; Stegmayr *et al.* 2000; Belostotsky *et al.* 2002; Frosch *et al.* 2004) (Table 22.7). Signs and symptoms reflecting inflammation of the sinuses, nose, and ears are the most common presenting features. Subglottic stenosis is quite characteristic of childhood-onset WG, occurring in up to 50%, but is usually not manifested until later in the disease course. Pulmonary infiltrates, nodules, and hemoptysis are sometimes present at onset, but increase in frequency with duration of disease. Glomerulonephritis occurs in almost two-thirds. Cutaneous granulomas, often over the elbow or knee, may ulcerate. In some children, inflammation of the nose results in a saddle nose deformity and perforation of the nasal septum.

Laboratory investigations

Elevated ESR, platelet count, and white blood cell count are all non-specific but common findings in WG. Elevation of Factor VIII related antigen (von Willebrand Factor antigen) suggests the

presence of active inflammation of blood vessels. The presence of ANCA, chiefly cANCA directed at proteinase-3 (PR-3), is highly suggestive of the diagnosis. Other autoantibodies, including antinuclear antibodies, are usually not present.

Chest radiographs show a range of abnormalities, from pleural effusions, to infiltrates, nodules, and cavitating lesions, even in the absence of pulmonary symptoms or signs. Thin-section computed tomography more clearly delineates these lesions. Radiographs of the sinuses often reveal widespread inflammation.

Treatment

This is a life-threatening disease, and early therapy with cyclophosphamide (2 mg/kg/day orally or 0.75 g/m^2/month intravenously) and prednisone (1 mg/kg/day orally) is the initial treatment of choice. Glucocorticoids can be administered as intravenous methylprednisolone (30 mg/kg/day on 1–5 consecutive days), followed by oral prednisone in the very sick child.

Outcome

The outcome of patients with WG has dramatically improved since the institution of treatment with cyclophosphamide; however, long-term outcome studies in children are lacking. The major long-term morbidities of the disease include subglottic stenosis, nasal deformity, and renal insufficiency.

Polyarteritis nodosa

Polyarteritis (PAN) is a relapsing necrotizing vasculitis affecting small and medium-sized muscular arteries and resulting in formation of aneurysms. The proposed classification criteria are given in Table 22.8.

Epidemiology and genetics

This rare disease occurs world-wide, but is most commonly reported from Japan and Turkey (Ozen *et al.* 2004; Maeda *et al.* 1997). It affects males and females with equal frequency and, in childhood, appears to be most common in the late childhood, preteen years.

Etiology, pathogenesis, and pathology

The etiology of PAN is unknown. A limited form of the disease, cutaneous polyarteritis, is often associated with preceding infection with group A streptococci (Sheth *et al.* 1994). The associations of PAN with hepatitis B and C, reported in adults (Guillevin *et al.* 1995), do not appear to be a factor in childhood-onset disease. Familial occurrence is rare and no genetic markers have been identified.

Table 22.7 Manifestations of Wegener's granulomatosis in childhood (data from 23 patients reported by Rottem *et al.* 1993)

Manifestations	Percent of patients affected	
	At onset	Total
Ear, nose, throat	87	91
Sinusitis	61	83
Nasal disease	48	65
Otitis media	39	48
Subglottic stenosis	4	48
Ear pain	22	22
Oral and tongue lesions	4	9
Arthralgia/arthritis	30	78
Pulmonary disease	22	74
Infiltrates	9	61
Nodules	13	43
Hemoptysis	9	26
Pleuritis	9	13
Glomerulonephritis	9	61
Rash	9	52
Ocular disease	13	48
Dacryocystitis	4	26
Eye pain	4	17
Proptosis	0	17
Scleritis/episcleritis	4	13
Conjunctivitis	0	9
Visual loss	0	9
Corneal ulcers	0	4
Fever	22	43
Weight loss	13	26
CNS disease	4	17
Peripheral neuropathy	0	9
Pericarditis	9	9

Table 22.8 Classification criteria for childhood polyarteritis nodosa

Biopsy showing small and mid-sized artery necrotizing vasculitis OR angiographic abnormalities (aneurysms or occlusions)[1] plus at least 2 of the following criteria:
1. Skin involvement (livedo reticularis, subcutaneous nodules, other vasculitis lesions)
2. Muscle pain or tenderness
3. Systemic hypertension (relative to normal age matched values)
4. Mononeuropathy or polyneuropathy
5. Abnormal urinalysis and/or impaired renal function
6. Testicular pain or tenderness
7. Signs or symptoms suggesting vasculitis of any other major organ system (gastrointestinal, cardiac, pulmonary, or central nervous system)

[1] Should include conventional angiography if MRI is normal.

Table 22.9 Clinical abnormalities in 81 children with polyarteritis nodosa

Fever	84%
Arthritis/arthralgia	74%
Abdominal pain	68%
Myalgia	67%
Skin abnormalities	
Rash	69%
Edema	20%
Petechiae	17%
Mucous membrane abnormalities	9%
Nervous system abnormalities	
Seizures	16%
Other, e.g., peripheral neuropathy	10%
Cardiac disease	21%
Pulmonary disease	7%
Renal disease	25%

From Cassidy, J.T. and Petty, R.E. (2005). Polyarteritis and related vasculitides. In *Textbook of pediatric rheumatology*, (eds Cassidy, J.T., Petty, R.E., Laxer, R.M., and Lindsley, C.B.), 5th edn, pp. 512–20. Saunders/Elsevier, New York.

The histopathology is characterized by segmental necrotizing vasculitis of small and medium-sized arteries with fibrinoid necrosis. Destruction of the internal elastic lamina results in aneurysm formation which is most common in bifurcations in the mesenteric and renal vasculature.

Clinical manifestations

Fever, weight loss, abdominal pain (reflecting ischemia), muscle pain and tenderness, livedo reticularis, and painful subcutaneous nodules, typically in the calves or soles of the feet herald the onset of the disease (Cassidy *et al.* 2005) (Table 22.9). Arthritis occurs in up to two-thirds of patients. Peripheral neuropathy or central nervous system disorders occur in approximately two-thirds. Highly suggestive, but rare, manifestations include episcleritis, and scrotal pain secondary to vasculitis involving the testis.

Laboratory investigations

Markers of the acute phase response are abnormal. Autoantibodies are usually absent, although ANCA are occasionally present, usually reacting with myeloperoxidase (perinuclear immunofluorescence pattern, pANCA). Arteriography or magnetic resonance angiography confirm the presence of aneurysms involving the renal, celiac, or mesenteric arteries. Excisional biopsy of a subcutaneous nodule reveals the typical necrotizing fibrinoid necrosis of a small muscular artery.

Treatment and outcome

Prednisone (1–2 mg/kg/day) in split doses is usually sufficient to control this inflammatory vasculitis. Failure to respond within a few weeks should prompt the addition of azathioprine (2 mg/kg/day) or cyclophosphamide (2 mg/kg/day). Most disease is monophasic, and most children with PAN do well, although myocardial infarction, persistent peripheral neuropathy, renal failure, and hypertension may occur.

Cutaneous polyarteritis is limited to fever, skin, and joints. The cutaneous findings, including livedo and subcutaneous nodules may be striking, but the outcome after treatment with prednisone (0.5–1.0 mg/kg/day) is usually very favorable.

Microscopic polyangiitis

Microscopic polyangiitis (MPA) is a necrotizing vasculitis of small vessels (primarily in the kidney and lung) characterized by few or no immune deposits (pauci-immune), and by the presence of ANCA which react with myeloperoxidase (pANCA) (Savage *et al.* 1985; Peco-Antic *et al.* 2006; Hattori *et al.* 2001; Besbas *et al.* 2000).

Epidemiology and genetics

MPA is rare in childhood, and there are no valid incidence and prevalence data. It appears to be more common in girls and occurs predominantly in the second decade of life. It is reported worldwide, and the most recent large series have been reported from Serbia (Peco-Antic *et al.* 2006), Japan (Hattori *et al.* 2001), and Turkey (Besbas *et al.* 2000). No genetic markers have been identified.

Etiology, pathogenesis, and pathology

The etiology is unknown; some reports identify increased incidence in winter and early spring, suggesting a possible infectious cause (Hattori *et al.* 2001).

Clinical manifestations

Constitutional manifestations (fever, weight loss) may be present for months before renal or pulmonary disease becomes evident. Renal involvement at onset ranges from asymptomatic microscopic hematuria and proteinuria to glomerulonephritis, nephritic syndrome, and renal failure. Hypertension occurs in at least one-half of patients. Pulmonary disease presents as hemoptysis and chest radiographs show infiltrates. Rashes, including purpura, occur in almost all patients. Headache and seizures may occur, and may reflect cerebral vasculitis.

Laboratory investigations

Inflammatory indices are increased non-specifically. pANCA with specificity for myeloperoxidase is usually detected in significant titer. Renal histopathology shows focal segmental glomerular necrosis with fibrous and fibrocellular crescents (Peco-Antic *et al.* 2006). The lesions are pauci-immune; that is, immunofluorescence studies of immunoglobulin are negative.

Treatment and outcome

In addition to prednisone (IV methylprednisolone 30 mg/kg/day on 1–3 consecutive days) or oral prednisone (1–2 mg/kg/day), and cyclophosphamide (2 mg/kg/day), azathioprine, mycophenolate mofetil, and cyclosporine A have been occasionally used (Peco-Antic *et al.* 2006). The outcome is variable, with many patients requiring dialysis or renal transplantation.

Other rare vasculitides of childhood

There are isolated case reports of other vasculitides in childhood which resemble their counterparts in adult life. These include Churg–Strauss syndrome (CSS), of which there are 10 reported childhood or adolescent cases (Lindsley *et al.* 2005), a non-giant cell non-necrotizing vasculitis of the temporal artery, which has been reported in a few children (Lie 1995), and central nervous system vasculitis. The latter disorder has been thought to be very rare, but recent reports (Benseler *et al.* 2006) suggest that it may have been under-diagnosed. More detailed descriptions of these and other vasculitides are provided in the text edited by Cassidy *et al.* (Cassidy *et al.* 2005).

References

Abe, J., Kotzin, B. L., Jujo, K., Melish, M. E., Glode, M. P., Kohsaka, T. and Leung, D. Y. (1992). Selective expansion of T cells expressing T-cell receptor variable regions V beta 2 and V beta 8 in Kawasaki disease. *Proceedings of the National Academy of Sciences USA*, **89**, 4066–70.

American Academy of Pediatrics (2003). Kawasaki syndrome. In *Red Book: Report of the Committee on Infectious Diseases* (Pickering, L. K. ed.), pp. 392–5. American Academy of Pediatrics, Elk Grove Village, Il.

Amoli, M. M., Thomson, W., Hajeer, A. H., *et al.* (2001). HLA DRB1*01 association with Henoch Schonlein purpura in patients in northwest Spain. *Journal of Rheumatology*, **28**, 1266–70.

Amoli, M. M., Thomson, W., Hajeer, A. H., *et al.* (2002). HLA B35 association with nephritis in Henoch Shönlein purpura. *Journal of Rheumatology*, **29**, 948–9.

Baart de la Faille-Kuyper, E. H.Y., Kater, L., Kooiker, C. J. and Dorhout Mees, E. J. (1973). IgA deposits in cutaneous blood vessel walls and mesangium in Henoch-Schönlein syndrome. *Lancet*, 1, 892–3.

Bell, D. M., Morens, D. M., Holman, R. C., *et al.* (1983). Kawasaki syndrome in the United States 1976–1980. *American Journal of Diseases of Childhood*, **137**, 211–4.

Belostotsky, V. M., Shah, V. and Dillon, M. J. (2002). Clinical features in 17 paediatric patients with Wegener granulomatosis. *Pediatric Nephrology*, **17**, 754–61.

Benseler, S. M., Silverman, E., Aviv, R. I., *et al.* (2006). Primary central nervous system vasculitis in children. *Arthritis and Rheumatism*, **54**, 1291–7.

Besbas, N., Ozen, S., Saatchi, U., *et al.* (2000). Renal involvement in polyarteritis nodosa: evaluation of 26 Turkish children. *Pediatric Nephrology*, **14**, 325–7.

Burns, J. C., Cayan, D. R., Tong, G., *et al.* (2005a). Seasonality and temporal clustering of Kawasaki syndrome. *Epidemiology*, **16**, 220–5.

Burns, J. C., Mason, W. H., Hauger, S. B., *et al.* (2005b). Infliximab treatment for refractory Kawasaki syndrome. *Journal of Pediatrics*, **146**, 662–7.

Cassidy, J. T. and Petty, R. E. (2005). Polyarteritis nodosa and related vasculitides. In *Textbook of pediatric rheumatology* (Cassidy, J. T., Petty, R. E., Laxer, R. M., and Lindsley, C. B. eds.), 5th edn, pp. 512–20. Saunders/Elsevier, Philadelphia.

Cassidy, J. T., Petty, R. E., Laxer, R. M. and Lindsley, C. B. (2005). *Textbook of pediatric rheumatology*, 5th edn. Saunders/Elsevier, Philadelphia.

Chang, R.-K. R. (2002). Hospitalizations for Kawasaki disease among children in the United States, 1988–1997. *Pediatrics*, **109**, e87.

Chang, R. K. (2003). The incidence of Kawasaki disease in the United States did not increase between 1988 and 1997. *Pediatrics*, **111**, 1124–5.

Chang, W. L., Yang, Y. H., Lin, Y. T. and Chiang, B. L. (2004). Gastrointestinal manifestations in Henoch-Schönlein purpura: a review of 261 patients. *Acta Paediatrica*, **93**, 1427–31.

Chang, W.-L., Yang, Y.-S., Wang, L.-C., *et al.* (2005). Renal manifestations in Henoch-Schönlein purpura: a 10-year study. *Pediatric Nephrology*, **20**, 1269–72.

Chugh, K. S. and Sakhuja, V. (1992). Takayasu's arteritis as a cause of renovascular hypertension in Asian countries. *American Journal of Nephrology*, **306**, 464–5.

Chun, Y. S., Park, S.-J., Park, I. K., *et al.* (2001). The clinical and ocular manifestations of Takayasu arteritis. *Retina*, **21**, 132–40.

Dabague, J. and Reyes, P. A. (1996). Takayasu arteritis in Mexico. A 38-year clinical perspective through literature review. *International Journal of Cardiology* 54 (Suppl.), S103–9.

Davis, R. L., Waller, P. L., Mueller, B. A., *et al.* (1995). Kawasaki syndrome in Washington State. Race-specific incidence rates and residential proximity to water. *Archives of Pediatric and Adolescent Medicine*, **149**, 66–9.

Dengler, L. D., Capparelli, E. V., Bastian, J. F., *et al.* (1998). Cerebrospinal fluid profile in patients with acute Kawasaki Disease. *Pediatric Infectious Diseases Journal*, **17**, 478–81.

Dijani, A. S., Taubert, E. A., Takahashi, M., *et al.* (1994). Guidelines for long-term management of patients with Kawasaki disease. Report from the Committee on Rheumatic Fever, Endocarditis and Kawasaki Disease. Council on Cardiovascular Diseases in the Young. American Heart Association. *Circulation*, **89**, 916–22.

Duong, T. T., Silverman, E. D., Bissessar, M. V. and Yeung, R. S. (2003). Superantigenic activity is responsible for induction of coronary arteritis in mice: An animal model of Kawasaki disease. *International Immunology*, **15**, 79–89.

Eichorn, J., Sima, D., Thiel, B., *et al.* (1996). Anti-endothelial cell antibodies in Takayasu arteritis. *Circulation*, **94**, 2396–401.

Ferrario, F. and Rastaldo, M. P. (2005). Henoch-Schönlein nephritis. *Journal of Nephrology*, **18**, 637–41.

Frosch, M. and Foell, D. (2004). Wegener granulomatosis in childhood and adolescence. *European Journal of Pediatrics*, **163**, 425–34.

Fu, K. I., Yagi, S., Mashimo, Y., Sugitani, K., *et al.* (2005). Regression of Helicobacter pylori-negative duodenal ulcers complicated by Schönlein-Henoch purpura with H. pylori eradication therapy: the first report. *Digestive Diseases and Sciences*, **50**, 381–4.

Fujiwara, H. and Hamashima, Y. (1978). Pathology of the heart in Kawasaki disease. *Pediatrics*, **61**, 100–7.

Guillevin, L., Lhote, F., Cohen, P., *et al.* (1995).Polyarteritis nodosa related to hepatitis B virus. A prospective study with long-term observation of 41 patients. *Medicine* (Baltimore), **74**, 238–53.

Guzman, J., Fung, M. and Petty, R. E. (1994). Diagnostic value of anti-neutrophil and anti-endothelial cello antibodies in early Kawasaki Disease. *Journal of Pediatrics,* **124**, 917–20.

Harada, F., Sada, M., Kamiya, T., *et al.* (1986). Genetic analysis of Kawasaki syndrome. *American Journal of Human Genetics*, **39**, 537–9.

Hattori, M., Kurayama, H. and Koitabashi, Y. (2001). Antineutrophil cytoplasmic autoantibody-associated glomerulonephritis in children. *Journal of the American Society for Nephrology*, **12**, 1493–500.

Henoch, E. H. (1974). About a peculiar form of purpura. Berlin. [Reprinted in *American Journal of Diseases of Childhood*, **128**, 78–89.]

Hoffman, G. S., Leavitt, R. Y., Kerr, G. S., *et al.* (1994).Treatment of glucocorticoid-resistant or relapsing Takayasu arteritis with methotrexate. *Arthritis and Rheumatism*, **37**, 578–82.

Hoffman, G. S., Merkel, P. A., Brasington, R. D., *et al.* (2004). Anti-tumor necrosis factor therapy in patients with difficult to treat Takayasu arteritis. *Arthritis and Rheumatism*, **50**, 2296–304.

Holman, R. C., Curns, A. T., Belay, E. D., *et al.* (2003a). Kawasaki syndrome hospitalizations in the United States 1997 and 2000. *Pediatrics*, **112**, 495–501.

Holman, R. C., Belay, E. D., Curns, A. T., Schonberger, L. B., Steiner, C. and Chang, R.-K. R. (2003b). Kawasaki syndrome hospitalizations among children in the United States, 1988–1997 [letter]. *Pediatrics*, **111**, 448.

Huber, A. M., King, J., McLaine, P., *et al.* (2004).A randomized placebo-controlled trial of prednisone in early Henoch Schönlein purpura. *BMC Medicine*, **2**, 7–14.

Hunder, G. G., Arend, W. P., Bloch, D. A., *et al.* (1990). The American College of Rheumatology 1990 criteria for the classification of vasculitis. Introduction. *Arthritis and Rheumatism*, **33**, 1065–7.

Jennette, J. C., Falk, R. J., Andrassy, K., *et al.* (1994). Nomenclature of systemic vasculitides. Proposal of an international consensus conference. *Arthritis and Rheumatism*, **37**, 187–92.

Kawasaki, T. (1967). Acute febrile mucocutaneous syndrome with lymphoid involvement with specific desquamation of the fingers and toes in children. *Arerugi*, **16**, 178–222.

Knott, P. D., Orloff, L. A., Harris, J. P., *et al.* (2001). Sensorineural hearing loss and Kawasaki disease: a prospective study. *American Journal of Otolaryngology*, **22**, 343–8.

Koldingsnes, W. and Nossent, H. (2000). Epidemiology of Wegener's granulomatosis in northern Norway. *Arthritis and Rheumatism*, **43**, 2481–7.

Kothari, S. S. (2002). Takayasu's arteritis in children – a review. *Images Pediatric Cardiology*, **9**, 4–23.

Kumagai, N. and Ohno, S. (1996). Kawasaki disease. In *Ocular immunity and infection* (Pepose, J. S., Holland, G. M. and Wilhelmus, K. R., eds), pp. 391–6. Mosby, St. Louis.

Lang, B. A., Yeung, R. S., Oen, K. G., *et al.* (2006). Corticosteroid treatment of refractory Kawasaki disease. *Journal of Rheumatology*, **33**, 803–9.

Liang, P. and Hoffman, G. S. (2004). Advances in the medical and surgical treatment of Takayasu arteritis. *Current Opinion in Rheumatology*, **17**, 16–24.

Lie, J. T. (1995). Bilateral juvenile temporal arteritis. *Journal of Rheumatology*, **22**, 774–6.

Lindsley, C. B. and Laxer, R. M. (2005). Granulomatous vasculitis, giant cell arteritis, and sarcoidosis. In *Textbook of pediatric rheumatology* (Cassidy, J. T., Petty, R. E., Laxer, R. M. and Lindsley, C. B., eds), 5th edn, pp. 539–60. Saunders/Elsevier, Philadelphia.

Maeda, M., Kobayahi, M., Okamoto, S., *et al.* (1997). Clinical observation of 14 cases of childhood polyarteritis nodosa in Japan. *Acta Paediatrica Japonica*, **39**, 277–9.

Meulders, Q., Pirson, Y., Cosyns, J. P., *et al.* (1994). Course of Henoch-Schönlein nephritis after renal transplantation. Report of ten patients and review of the literature. *Transplantation*, **58**, 1179–86.

Motoyama, O. and Iitaka, K. (2005). Familial cases of Henoch-Schönlein purpura in eight families. *Pediatrics International*, **47**, 612–15.

Munro-Faure, H. (1959). Necrotizing arteritis of the coronary vessels in infancy. *Pediatrics*, **23**, 914–26.

Nakamura, Y., Aso, E., Yashiro, M., *et al.* (2005). Mortality among persons with a history of Kawasaki disease in Japan: can paediatricians safely discontinue follow-up of children with a history of the disease but without cardiac sequelae? *Acta Paediatrica*, **94**, 429–34.

Nash, M. C., Shah, V., Reader, J. A. and Dillon, M. J. (1995). Anti-neutrophil cytoplasmic antibodies and anti-endothelial cell antibodies are not increased in Kawasaki disease. *British Journal of Rheumatology*, **34**, 882–7.

Newburger, J. W., Takahashi, M., Burns, J. C., Beiser, A. S., Chung, K. J., Duffy, C. E., Glode, M. P., Mason, W. H., Reddy, V., Sanders, S. P., *et al.* (1986). The treatment of Kawasaki syndrome with intravenous gamma globulin. *New England Journal of Medicine*, **315**, 341–7.

Newburger, J. W., *et al.* (2004). Diagnosis, treatment and long-term management of Kawasaki disease: a statement for health professionals from the Committee on Rheumatic Fever, Endocarditis and Kawasaki Disease. Council on Cardiovascular Disease in the Young. American Heart Association. *Pediatrics*, **114**, 1708–33.

Niaudet, P. and Habib, R. (1998). Methylprednisolone pulse therapy in the treatment of severe forms of Schönlein-Henoch purpura nephritis. *Pediatric Nephrology*, **12**, 238–43.

Nussinovitch, N., Elishkevitz, K., Volovitz, B. and Nussinovitch, M. (2005). Hypertension as a late sequela of Henoch-Schönlein purpura. *Clinical Pediatrics* (Phila), **44**, 543–7.

Ozaltin, F., Bakkaloglu, A., Ozen, S., *et al.* (2004). The significance of IgA class of antineutrophil cytoplasmic antibodies (ANCA) in childhood Henoch-Schönlein purpura. *Clinical Rheumatology*, **23**, 426–9.

Ozen, S., Anton, J., Arisoy, N., *et al.* (2004). Juvenile polyarteritis: results of a multicenter survey of 110 children. *Journal of Pediatrics*, **145**, 517–22.

Ozen, S., Ruperto, N., Dillon, M. J., *et al.* (2006). EULAR/PReS endorsed consensus criteria for the classification of childhood vasculitides. *Annals of the Rheumatic Diseases*, **65**, 936–41.

Peco-Antic, A., Bonaci-Nikolic, B., Basta-Jovanovic, G., *et al.* (2006). Childhood microscopic polyangiitis associated with MPO-ANCA. *Pediatric Nephrology*, **21**, 46–53.

Porcalla, A. R., Sable, C. A., Patel, K. M. *et al.* (2005). The epidemiology of Kawasaki disease in an urban hospital: does African American race protect against coronary artery aneurysms? *Pediatric Cardiology*, **26**, 775–81.

Rottem, M., Fauci, A. S., Hallahan, C. W., *et al.* (1993). Wegener granulomatosis in children and adolescents: Clinical presentation and outcome. *Journal of Pediatrics*, **122**, 26–31.

Rowley, A. H., Eckerley, C. A., Jack, H. M. *et al.* (1997). IgA plasma cells in vascular tissue of patients with Kawasaki syndrome. *Journal of Immunology*, **159**, 5946–55.

Saulsbury, F. T. (1999). Henoch-Schonlein purpura in children: Report of 100 patients and review of the literature. *Medicine* (Baltimore), **78**, 395–409.

Savage, C. O., Winearls, C. G., Evans, D. J., *et al.* (1985). Microscopic polyarteritis: presentation, pathology and prognosis. *Quarterly Journal of Medicine*, **56**, 467–83.

Schönlein, J. L. (1837). *Allegemeine und Specielle Pathologie und Therapie*, 3rd edn. Literatur-Vomptoinr, Herisau, Germany.

Seko, Y. (2000). Takayasu arteritis. Insights into immunopathology. *Japanese Heart Journal*, **41**, 15–26.

Shelhamer, J. H., Volkman, D. J. and Parrillo, J. E. (1985). Takayasu's arteritis and its therapy. *Annals of Internal Medicine*, **103**, 121–6.

Sheth, A. P., Olson, J. C. and Esterly, N. B. (1994). Cutaneous polyarteritis nodosa of childhood. *Journal of the American Academy of Dermatology*, **31**, 561–6.

Shin, J. I., Park, J. M., Shin, Y. H., *et al.* (2005a). Cyclosporin A therapy for severe Henoch-Schönlein nephritis with nephrotic syndrome. *Pediatric Nephrology*, **20**, 1093–7.

Shin, J. I., Park, J. M., Kim, J. H., *et al.* (2005b). Can azathioprine and steroids alter the progression of severe Henoch-Schönlein nephritis in children? *Pediatric Nephrology*, **20**, 1087–92.

Shrivastava, S. (1995). Takayasu's arteritis. *American Heart Journal*, **129**, 1228–9.

Smith, L. B., Newburger, J. W. and Burns, J. C. (1989). Kawasaki syndrome and the eye. *Pediatric Infectious Diseases*, **8**, 116–8.

Stanley, P., Roebuck, D., Barboza, A., *et al.* (2003). Takayau's arteritis in children. *Techniques in Vascular and Interventional Radiology*, **6**, 158–68.

Steffanson, T. V., Kolka, R. S., Sigurdardottir, S. L., *et al.* (2005). Increased frequency of C4B*Q0 alleles in patients with Henoch-Schönlein purpura. *Scandinavian Journal of Immunology*, **61**, 274–8.

Stegmayr, B. G., Gothefors, L., Malmer, B., *et al.* (2000). Wegener granulomatosis in children and young adults. A case study of ten patients. *Pediatric Nephrology*, **14**, 208–13.

Suddleson, E. A., Reid, B., Woolley, M. M. and Takahashi, M. (1987). Hydrops of the gallbladder associated with Kawasaki syndrome. *Journal of Pediatric Surgery*, **22**, 956–9.

Sundel, R. P., Baker, A. L., Fulton, D. R. and Newburger, J. W. (2003). Corticosteroids in the initial treatment of Kawasaki disease: report of a randomized trial. *Journal of Pediatrics*, **142**, 611–16.

Szer, I. (1996). Henoch Schönlein purpura: When and how to treat. *Journal of Rheumatology*, **23**, 1661–5.

Trapani, S., Micheli, A., Grisolia, F., *et al.* (2005). Henoch Schonlein purpura in childhood: Epidemiological and clinical analysis of 150 cases over a 5-year period and review of literature. *Seminars in Arthritis and Rheumatism*, **35**, 143–53.

Trygstad, C. W. and Stiehm, E. R. (1971). Elevated IgA globulin in anaphylactoid purpura. *Pediatrics*, **47**, 1023–8.

Watts, R. A. and Scott, D. G. (1997). Classification and epidemiology of the vasculitides. *Baillieres Clinical Rheumatology*, **11**, 191–217.

Watts, R. A., Lane, S. E., Bentham, G. and Scott, D. G. I. (2000). Epidemiology of systemic vasculitis. *Arthritis and Rheumatism*, **43**, 414–19.

Yajima, M., Numsno, F., Park, Y. B. and Sagar, S. (1994). Comparative studies of patients with Takayasu arteritis in Japan, Korea and India. Comparison of clinical manifestations, angiography, and HLA-B antigen. *Japanese Circulation Journal*, **58**, 9–14.

Yanagawa, H., Yashiro, M., Nakamura, Y., *et al.* (1995). Nationwide surveillance of Kawasaki disease in Japan, 1984 to 1993. *Pediatric Infectious Diseases Journal*, **14,** 69–71.

Yanagawa, H., Nakamura, Y., Yashiro, M., *et al.* (2001). Incidence survey of Kawasaki disease in 1997 and 1998 in Japan. *Pediatrics*, **107**, E33.

Yanagawa, H., Nakamura, Y., Ojima, T., *et al.* (1999). Changes in epidemic patterns of Kawasaki disease in Japan. *Pediatric Infectious Diseases Journal*, **18,** 64–6.

Yang, Y. H., Hung, C. F., Hsu, C. R., *et al.* (2005). A nationwide survey on epidemiological characteristics of childhood Henoch-Schönlein purpura in Taiwan. *Rheumatology* (Oxford), **44,** 618–22.

Yang, Y.-H., Wang, S. J., Chuang, Y.-H., *et al.* (2002). The level of IgA antibodies to human umbilical vein endothelial cells can be enhanced by TNF-α treatment in children with Henoch-Schönlein purpura. *Clinical and Experimental Immunology*, **130**, 352–7.

Yeung, R. S. M. (2005). Pathogenesis and treatment of Kawasaki's disease. *Current Opinion in Rheumatology*, **17,** 617–23.

Yeung, R. S. M. (2004). The etiology of Kawasaki disease: a superantigen-mediated process. *Progress in Pediatric Cardiology*, **19,** 109–13.

CHAPTER 23

Assessment of disease activity and damage

Raashid A. Luqmani and Paul A. Bacon

Introduction

Purpose of assessment

In systemic vasculitis, assessment is important in order to define the severity of disease and to form a rational basis for a treatment strategy. The vasculitides represent a group of heterogeneous disorders with potential to present to a number of different specialists depending on the clinical manifestations. The manifestations change over time as the disease evolves and also change in response to therapy. The original descriptions of systemic vasculitis were of life-threatening, acute illnesses with little hope of improvement. However, the increasing use of immunosuppressive therapy, particularly cyclophosphamide, has converted this set of diseases into chronic relapsing disorders which require long-term care and follow-up (Hoffman *et al.* 1992; Gordon *et al.* 1993; Hogan *et al.* 2005; Booth *et al.* 2003). Our current therapeutic strategies can achieve short-term control of disease rather than curing it. The result is a dramatic improvement in mortality but a subsequent increase in disease burden through chronic, grumbling disease, a significant incidence of relapse, and accumulating drug toxicity. Disease assessment in this context provides the ability to clarify the status of individual patients using a standardized approach to define the amount of current disease activity as well as its extent in different organ systems. A vigilant, serial approach to documenting disease activity has provided a greater understanding of the patterns of disease and the nature of disease evolution in the context of systemic vasculitis. In turn, these observations have allowed improvements in the design of prospective studies of current and new therapeutic interventions in the management of vasculitis. A consequence of standardized assessment is the ease with which such trials can now be conducted across multiple centers by providing consensus definitions of disease status and response to therapy.

Concepts of assessment

Disease severity, especially in the case of chronic disease, represents a broad description of the disease and its effects on the individual. In acute presentations of vasculitis, disease activity is the main concern and dictates how treatment regimens should be applied. If patients survive the initial episode of disease activity, and this is increasingly the case, they are faced with the longer-term problems of the accumulation of disease activity, the development of scars representing disease damage, and the influence of drugs causing significant morbidity. The therapeutic plan for managing such different aspects of vasculitis needs to be more detailed and different from the initial disease control. Severity of disease is influenced not only by initial and subsequent disease activity but also the accumulating damage (Exley *et al.* 1997a; Exley 1998). Damage is therefore emerging as an important concept in chronic diseases such as vasculitis and must be differentiated from disease activity. Both activity and damage may contribute to prognosis (Luqmani 2004). The number of organ systems affected by the disease is a further important factor associated with an adverse long-term prognosis (Exley 1997b). An examination of the extent of disease involvement, both of activity and of damage, can give deeper insights into overall severity compared to a consideration of the degree of involvement of a single major organ such as the kidney. Finally, the impact on a patient's well-being is influenced by factors specific to the individual patient as well as to disease activity and damage. The patient's perception of their health is an important but somewhat overlooked aspect of the overall disease morbidity. It should be seen as an area for future development in clinical trials of vasculitis since it may provide an important insight into the patient's perspective on disease outcome in response to therapy. In a number of chronic diseases, the patient's perceptions are recorded as a measure of the effect or impact of a disease on his or her function and quality of life. All these concepts, namely the degree and extent of disease activity, disease damage, and quality of life, are important to provide an overall understanding of the patient's current clinical status. Each of these aspects of disease may contribute to overall prognosis.

Clinical assessments can be used to measure morbidity in vasculitis and provide an effective surrogate. A number of robust clinical instruments have been developed with the same rigor applied to the development of a laboratory assay. These clinical tools may be used as the basis of comparison when developing new laboratory assays or testing existing laboratory-based investigations aimed at providing further information about disease status in systemic vasculitis. The clinical status of a patient typically remains the gold standard for deciding on any therapeutic change and should remain at the forefront of disease assessment in systemic vasculitis. Serological tests can support the suspicion that a patient has changed their clinical state and may suggest that a change in therapy is needed, but assessment of the overall clinical situation is needed to ratify such a change.

Benefits of assessment

Patients with vasculitis have a complicated and potentially life-threatening set of problems. It is very important to undertake a detailed clinical assessment before commencing therapy, which can then be specifically tailored to the individual patient. While we still struggle to define precisely the specific type of vasculitis we are dealing with, the generic, detailed assessments of the patient's clinical status will yield essential information on how to manage that patient. There is considerable overlap between clinical assessment instruments for vasculitis and we favor the use of a generic instrument. Some disease activity assessments have been produced specifically for one particular disease, such as such as the Disease Extent Index (DEI) for Wegener's granulomatosis (WG) (De Groot *et al.* 2001; see Table 31.3 in Chapter 31) or the Birmingham Vasculitis Activity Score (BVAS) for WG (BVAS/WG) (Stone *et al.* 2001). These two disease-specific instruments were introduced for different reasons. The DEI was developed for long-term outcome studies to include the full extent of WG that, unlike other forms of ANCA-associated vasculitides, has important granulomatous manifestations in addition to vascular inflammation. The BVAS/WG was developed as a result of the need for a simplified instrument to use in shorter-term clinical trials. These instruments are of value for their specific purposes but within the wider context of patients with systemic vasculitis, the overlap of clinical features means that such focused instruments are of less value than the generic ones which provide the ability to study related diseases such as other ANCA-associated vasculitides. The generic instruments also allow description of patients where the precise subset of vasculitis remains uncertain. This is particularly important in patients presenting at an early stage, when assessment of severity and initiation of treatment is required before the characteristic severe features develop. Given that early diagnosis is increasingly going to be the case due to our greater understanding of vasculitis, generic instruments are likely to be more useful than disease-specific ones.

The criticism against the use of such generalized clinical assessments can be addressed by looking at the practical reality of assessing and managing vasculitis. In general, we would predict that the quantitative scores from activity indices will be greater in patients with a larger number of systems involved compared to those with more limited disease. For example, patients with giant cell arteritis would be unlikely to achieve very high scores on a disease activity index compared to patients with multiorgan involvement from WG. The Takayasu's form of aortoarteritis is another form of vasculitis where the distribution of involved vessels is so different from the small vessel vasculitides that the clinical expression of disease also varies markedly. A disease-specific index tailored to the specific features, using the same concept as the DEI, would aid understanding of Takayasu's arteritis and its epidemiology across different continents. The initial development of such an index has been reported by the Indian Rheumatology vasculitis study group and it is currently being validated (Sivakumar 2005). It is possible to combine a core generic instrument with a smaller module that includes specific items for individual diseases, and this topic is being actively discussed within the context of the OMERACT (Outcome Measures in Rheumatology) group (Merkel *et al.* 2005).

In designing therapeutic trials for systemic vasculitis it is a prerequisite to standardize assessment of disease prior to initiating the trial. In part this reflects the complexity of vasculitis but also the rarity of this disease, which imposes the need for clinical studies of vasculitis to be multicenter by their nature. Provision of a standardized assessment tool for vasculitis offers a training opportunity for physicians in different specialties who may see very little vasculitis, so that they can appreciate the diversity of the disease and achieve a greater understanding of strategies of management. We would strongly recommend that any clinicians contemplating a clinical trial of systemic vasculitis use one of the validated instruments. They should also ensure adequate training and quality control by members of their group to assure that the data being collected for the trial will avoid the problem of interobserver variability (Luqmani 2004).

Uses of disease activity indices

The primary use of a disease activity index has been to provide a detailed description of the state of activity of a patient with vasculitis according to the opinion of the clinician looking after that individual patient. It is clear, however, that such an index would have multiple functions beyond simply describing the state of the patient's disease. It is important to remember that the data from which a disease activity index derives depends entirely on the expert assessment of the patient by the clinician, and is supported by the clinician's experience in managing vasculitis. When an activity index is applied to patients it is important that the clinician using the instrument has some experience in managing vasculitis but also, and crucially, has been trained in the use of the instrument. The latter becomes even more important when we consider the potential role of such an index in clinical trials of systemic vasculitis involving multiple centers.

While it might initially seem that disease-specific measures would be preferable in clinical trials and for individual patients, the overlap in clinical features of different types of related small-vessel vasculitis means that a precise label of a specific type of vasculitis may not be possible for many patients. The sharing of clinical features would support the use of a generic instrument such as the Birmingham Vasculitis Activity Score (BVAS) (Luqmani *et al.* 1994) or its subsequent versions (Luqmani *et al.* 1997). The BVAS is a clinical index of disease activity based on symptoms and signs in nine categories: systemic signs; skin; mucous membranes and eyes; ear, nose, and throat (ENT); chest; heart, and vessels; GI tract; kidney; and nervous system. Maximum points are accorded to each category; the maximum score is 63. Disease features are scored only when they are attributable to active vasculitis. In addition to the (BVAS/WG) (Stone *et al.* 2001), the DEI is also specific for WG (see Table 31.3 in Chapter 31) and may prove a useful measure of prognosis (de Groot *et al.* 2001). For multicenter, randomized clinical trials of therapy, BVAS is the most widely adopted disease assessment tool, and the items in its current version are listed in Table 23.1.

Laboratory tests

There is no gold standard clinical or laboratory test for measuring disease status in systemic vasculitis. Serological tests can prove unreliable in evaluating patients with vasculitis. Serum C-reactive protein (CRP) is affected by disease activity but also by the presence of infection or other inflammatory causes (Luqmani *et al.* 1994).

Table 23.1 Criteria included in current version of the Birmingham Vasculitis Activity Score

1. General	Maximum scores
Myalgia	Pain in the muscles
Arthralgia or arthritis	Pain in the joints or joint inflammation
Fever ≥38.0°C	Documented oral/axillary temperature elevation. Rectal temps are 0.5°C higher
Weight Loss	At least 2 kg loss of body weight (not fluid) having occurred since last assessment or in 4 weeks not as a consequence of dieting
2. Cutaneous	**Maximum scores**
Infarct	Area of tissue necrosis or splinter hemorrhages
Purpura	Petechiae (small red spots), palpable purpura, or ecchymoses (large plaques) in skin or oozing (in the absence of trauma) in the mucous membranes
Ulcer	Open sore in a skin surface
Gangrene	Extensive tissue necrosis, e.g. digit
Other skin vasculitis	Livedo reticularis, subcutaneous nodules, erythema nodosum, etc.
3. Mucous membranes/eyes	**Maximum scores**
Mouth ulcers/ granulomata	Aphthous stomatitis, deep ulcers and/or "strawberry" gingival hyperplasia, excluding lupus erythematosus, and infection
Genital ulcers	Ulcers localized in the genitalia or perineum, excluding infections
Adnexal inflammation	Salivary (diffuse, tender swelling unrelated to meals) or lacrimal gland inflammation; exclude other causes (infection); specialist opinion preferable
Significant proptosis	Protrusion of the eyeball due to significant amounts of inflammation in the orbit; if unilateral, there should be a difference of 2 mm between one eye and the other; this may be associated with diplopia due to infiltration of extraocular muscles; developing myopia (measured on best visual acuity, see later) can also be a manifestation of proptosis
Red eye (epi)scleritis	Inflammation of the sclerae (specialist opinion usually required); can be heralded by photophobia
Red eye conjunctivitis	Inflammation of the conjunctivae (exclude infectious causes and excluding uveitis as cause of red eye, also exclude conjunctivitis sicca which should not be scored as this is not a feature of active vasculitis); specialist opinion not usually required
Blepharitis	Inflammation of eyelids; exclude other causes (trauma, infection); usually no specialist opinion is required
Keratitis	Inflammation of central or peripheral cornea as evaluated by specialist
Blurred vision	Altered measurement of best visual acuity from previous or baseline, requiring specialist opinion for further evaluation
Sudden visual loss	Sudden loss of vision requiring ophthalmological assessment
Uveitis	Inflammation of the uvea (iris, ciliary body, choroid) confirmed by ophthalmologist
Retinal vasculitis	Retinal vessel sheathing on examination by specialist or confirmed by retinal fluoroscein angiography
Retinal vessel thrombosis	Arterial or venous retinal blood vessel occlusion
Retinal exudates	Any area of soft retinal exudates (exclude hard exudates) seen on ophthalmoscopic examination
Retinal hemorrhages	Any area of retinal hemorrhage seen on ophthalmoscopic examination
4. ENT	**Maximum scores**
Bloody nasal discharge/nasal crusts/ulcers and/or granulomata	Bloody, mucopurulent, nasal secretion, light or dark brown crusts frequently obstructing the nose, nasal ulcers and/or granulomatous lesions observed by rhinoscopy
Paranasal sinus involvement	Tenderness or pain over paranasal sinuses usually with pathologic imaging (CT, MR, x-ray, ultrasound)
Subglottic stenosis	Stridor and hoarseness due to inflammation and narrowing of the subglottic area observed by laryngoscopy
Conductive hearing loss	Hearing loss due to middle ear involvement confirmed by otoscopy and/or tuning fork examination and/or audiometry
Sensorineural hearing loss	Hearing loss due to auditory nerve or cochlear damage confirmed by audiometry
5. Chest	**Maximum scores**
Wheeze	Wheeze on clinical examination
Nodules or cavities	New lesions, detected by chest radiography
Pleural effusion/pleurisy	Pleural pain and/or friction rub on clinical assessment or new onset of radiologically confirmed pleural effusion; other causes, e.g. infection, malignancy, should be excluded

Table 23.1 (*cont.*)

Infiltrate	Detected by chest radiography or CT scan; other causes (infection) should be excluded
Endobronchial involvement	Endobronchial pseudotumor or ulcerative lesions. Other causes such as infection or malignancy should be excluded. Note: Smooth stenotic lesions are to be included in VDI; subglottic lesions are to be recorded in the ENT section.
Massive hemoptysis/ alveolar hemorrhage	Major pulmonary bleeding, with shifting pulmonary infiltrates; other causes of bleeding should be excluded if possible
Respiratory failure	Dyspnea which is sufficiently severe as to require artificial ventilation
6. Cardiovascular	**Maximum scores**
Loss of pulses	Loss of pulses in any vessel detected clinically; this may include loss of pulses leading to threatened loss of limb
Valvular heart disease	Significant valve abnormalities in the aortic mitral or pulmonary valves detected clinically or echocardiographically
Pericarditis	Pericardial pain and/or friction rub on clinical assessment
Ischemic cardiac pain	Typical clinical history of cardiac pain leading to myocardial infarction or angina; consider the possibility of more common causes (e.g. atherosclerosis)
Cardiomyopathy Congestive cardiac failure	Significant impairment of cardiac function due to poor ventricular wall motion confirmed on echocardiography Heart failure by history or clinical examination
7. Abdominal	**Maximum scores**
Peritonism/peritonitis	Acute abdominal pain with peritonism/peritonitis due to perforation/ infarction of small bowel, appendix or gallbladder etc., or acute pancreatitis confirmed by radiology/surgery/elevated amylase
Bloody diarrhea	Of recent onset; inflammatory bowel disease and infectious causes excluded
Ischemic abdominal pain	Severe abdominal pain with typical features of ischemia confirmed by imaging or at surgery, with typical appearances of aneursyms or abnormal vasculature characteristic of vasculitis
8. Renal	**Maximum scores**
Hypertension	Diastolic BP >95 mm Hg, accelerated or not, with or without retinal changes
Proteinuria	>1+ on urinalysis; >0.2 g/24 hours; infection should be excluded
Hematuria	10 or more RBC per high power field, excluding urinary infection and urinary lithiasis (stone)
Creatinine 125–249	Serum creatinine values 125–249 μmol/l (1.41–2.81 mg/dl) at first assessment only
Creatinine 250–499	Serum creatinine values 250–499 μmol/l (2.82–5.64 mg/dl) at first assessment only
Creatinine ≥500	Serum creatinine values 500 μmol/l (5.65 mg/dl) or greater at first assessment only
Rise in creatinine >30% or creatinine clearance fall >25%	Significant deterioration in renal function attributable to active vasculitis
9. Nervous system	**Maximum scores**
Headache	New, unaccustomed and persistent headache
Meningitis	Severe headache with neck stiffness ascribed to inflammatory meningitis after excluding infection/bleeding
Organic confusion	Impaired orientation, memory or other intellectual function in the absence of metabolic, psychiatric, pharmacological, or toxic causes
Seizures (not hypertensive)	Paroxysmal electrical discharges in the brain and producing characteristic physical changes including tonic and clonic movements and certain behavioral changes
Stroke	Cerebrovascular accident resulting in focal neurological signs such as paresis, weakness, etc; a stroke due to other causes, e.g. atherosclerosis, should be considered and appropriate neurological advice is recommended
Cord lesion	Transverse myelitis with lower extremity weakness or sensory loss (usually with a detectable sensory level) with loss of sphincter control (rectal and urinary bladder)
Cranial nerve palsy	Facial nerve palsy, recurrent nerve palsy, oculomotor nerve palsy, etc. excluding sensorineural hearing loss and ophthalmic symptoms due to inflammation
Sensory peripheral neuropathy	Sensory neuropathy resulting in glove and/or stocking distribution of sensory loss. Other causes, e.g. idiopathic, metabolic, vitamin deficiencies, infectious, toxic, and hereditary, should be excluded
Motor mononeuritis/ multiplex	Simultaneous neuritis of single or many peripheral nerves, only scored if motor involvement; other causes, e.g. diabetes, sarcoidosis, carcinoma, and amyloidosis, should be excluded

If **all** the above abnormalities are due to low grade grumbling disease and not due to new/worse disease, then record as persistent disease. Otherwise, all items are scored as new/worse.

Thus, the CRP cannot be used to distinguish between these clinical problems. Unfortunately the coexistence of infection and active vasculitis is common, partly because infection is likely to trigger episodes of active vasculitis. The presence of high titers of circulating ANCA may support a diagnosis of active vasculitis but in patients with established ANCA-related disease, variation in ANCA titer occurs in the absence of clinical manifestations in 29 to 43% of cases (Boomsma *et al.* 2000). Some previous suggestions of more precise measurement of subtypes of ANCA as being helpful in measuring disease activity have not proven universally useful. We would advise against the suggestion that treatment should be based solely on a change in ANCA status, although such a change may increase clinical watchfulness. However, there is good evidence that the presence of persistently positive ANCA in a patient who is otherwise in clinical remission is associated with an increased incidence of clinical relapse and thus may be an indication to continue induction therapy rather than switch to maintenance therapy (Slot *et al.* 2004). A variety of other markers of endothelial damage, including endothelial microparticles or molecules released from endothelium, have been measured in patients with systemic vasculitis (Brogan and Dillon 2004). There is evidence that endothelial microparticle levels increase with disease activity in childhood vasculitis (Brogan *et al.* 2004). Some correlations exist between disease activity and elevations of von Willebrand factor or intracellular adhesion molecules but it would be difficult to conclude that any single marker or combination of markers currently offers a robust measure with which to guide treatment (Di Lorenzo *et al.* 2004; Janssen *et al.* 1994).

Disease damage: clinical assessment

Damage is defined as "the accumulation of irreversible scars which have arisen since the onset of a diagnosis of vasculitis" (Exley *et al.* 1997a). It is a measure of both the impact of the disease and its treatment on the patient's physiological status. Conceptually, a scar is a permanent change to the patient even if the resulting clinical problem appears to resolve or is compensated for. The current concept of damage is that it does represent an accumulation of morbidity suffered by the patient and should be regarded as a permanent change to their status. The Vasculitis Damage Index (VDI), the most widely used measure of disease damage in vasculitis, is a reflection of multiorgan multisystem scarring (see criteria in Table 23.2). The VDI (Exley *et al.* 1997a) is the only currently validated measure of permanent scarring in patients with vasculitis. It is based on multiorgan involvement and collects information on all potentially damage-related items, evaluated from the onset of the vasculitis. This includes the effects of disease and its treatment, as well as intercurrent (sometimes coincidental) events that may be unrelated to the vasculitis or its treatment. There is no attempt to attribute cause. This might initially seem unscientific but in practice it is often difficult or impossible to precisely attribute causation to events such as the development of pulmonary fibrosis. They may be due to either the vasculitis or its treatment or to intercurrent comorbidity which has worsened since vasculitis was diagnosed and its treatment was established. From the patient's perspective, all of these problems are part of the total disease burden and this is encapsulated by the VDI. The items included in the VDI were selected by consensus from physicians managing systemic vasculitis. The VDI has been validated and is an effective means of documenting disease morbidity in vasculitis; it also has prognostic value. It could serve as a surrogate outcome measure for clinical trials as well as an important factor for long-term outcome studies.

Uses of a damage index

Regular application of the VDI to vasculitis patients demonstrates that accumulation of damage often occurs early in the disease process and does have a significant impact on later mortality (Exley *et al.* 1997b). In a large study of WG patients, damage accumulated despite effective disease control in the vast majority of patients (Seo *et al.* 2005). Both of these studies support the concept that damage actually occurs early in the disease process, unlike the perception in many rheumatic diseases where damage tends to occur towards the end of the disease. In 120 patients studied from Birmingham, UK, one-third had already sustained damage before presenting to hospital and by 6 months of follow-up most patients already had between two and four items of damage; 95% of patients had at least one item of damage and some patients had several items of damage in multiple organs. In two-thirds of patients, two or more organ systems were involved (Exley *et al.* 1997b). The initial rate of damage accumulation is more rapid than during subsequent follow-up but further damage may accumulate following a relapse. Nevertheless, relapses are not associated with as much damage accumulation compared to initial presentation. The implications for therapy are clear. The initial phase of disease is often the worst; more effective disease control at the early stage may prevent accumulation of serious damage with irreversible effects.

Predicting prognosis and outcome

Providing a prognosis for patients with vasculitis is an important part of their management. In clinical trials it is very useful to know what the likely prognosis is for a particular disease so that the effects of therapy can be more accurately measured. In addition, trials can be designed with the knowledge that drugs and therapy should be aiming to improve on the existing likely prognosis. Prognosis should be examined not only from the point of view of mortality but also from good or poor outcome in terms of quality of life. This becomes a more challenging, but also potentially more useful, aspect of measuring disease status in vasculitis because survival rates are now very high and chronic morbidity and disease scarring are very common.

The Five Factor Score (Guillevin *et al.* 1988; Gayraud *et al.* 2001; Bourgarit *et al.* 2005) (see Table 23.3) is a simple prognostic tool which has been found to be effective for patients with polyarteritis nodosa (PAN) and Churg–Strauss Syndrome (CSS). It is based on the extent of serious organ involvement. This has allowed the development and testing of trial protocols dependent on disease severity and has resulted in some useful advances in managing vasculitis, but it is unfortunately limited to use in PAN and CSS. BVAS can also provide prognostic information at onset; this has been shown in two large studies of disease activity in cohorts of patients with vasculitis (Luqmani *et al.* 1994; Gayraud *et al.* 2001). A high BVAS at diagnosis is predictive of subsequent poor outcome. In one study however, there was no evidence of a prognostic value to BVAS (Koldingsnes and Nossent 2003).

Table 23.2 Criteria included in the Vasculitis Damage Index (VDI)

Musculoskeletal

a. *Significant muscle atrophy or weakness:* Demonstrated on clinical examination (not attributable to CVA)

b. *Deforming or erosive arthritis:* Deformities on clinical examination confirmed by radiographs (excluding avascular necrosis), on clinical examination and radiographs.

c. *Osteoporosis with fractures or vertebral collapse:* By history confirmed on X ray film (excluding avascular necrosis).

d. *Avascular necrosis:* Demonstrated by appropriate radiological techniques.

e. *Osteomyelitis:* Documented clinically, confirmed by X-ray and/or culture.

Skin/mucous membranes

a. *Alopecia:* Major (e.g. requiring wig) chronic hair loss with or without scars, documented clinically.

b. *Cutaneous ulcers:* Open sore on skin surface, excluding that caused by venous thrombosis.

c. *Mouth ulceration:* Recurrent crops or persistent mouth ulcers requiring therapy.

Ocular

a. *Cataract:* A lens opacity (cataract) in either eye documented by ophthalmoscopy.

b. *Retinal change:* Any significant change documented by ophthalmoscopic examination; may result in field defect, legal blindness.

c. *Optic atrophy:* Documented by ophthalmoscopic examination.

d. *Visual impairment/diplopia:* Restricted eye movements (not due to nerve palsies), reduced visual acuity, double vision or tunnel vision.

e. *Blindness:* Complete loss of vision in one or both eyes.

f. *Orbital wall destruction:* Significant bone destruction as documented on radiographs/CT/MRI.

ENT

a. *Hearing loss:* Any hearing loss due to middle ear involvement or to auditory nerve/cochlear damage, preferably confirmed by audiometry.

b. *Nasal blockage/chronic discharge/crusting:* Difficulties with breathing through the nose and/or with purulent discharge and/or with crust formation usually requiring nasal lavage.

c. *Nasal bridge collapse/septal perforation:* Saddle nose deformity and/or perforation of nasal septum.

d. *Chronic sinusitis/radiological damage:* Chronic purulent nasal discharge with sinus pain and/or radiological evidence of sinusitis with or without bone destruction.

e. *Subglottic stenosis with or without surgery:* Persistent hoarseness and/or stridor preferably confirmed by endoscopy and/or radiographs.

Pulmonary

a. *Pulmonary hypertension:* Right ventricular prominence or loud P2 (confirmed by cardiac investigation if appropriate).

b. *Pulmonary fibrosis:* According to physical signs and radiographs (confirmed by relevant tests if necessary); this may include patients who require pulmonary resection.

c. *Pulmonary infarction:* According to chest radiographs or ventilation/perfusion scan.

d. *Pleural fibrosis:* According to chest radiographs.

e. *Chronic asthma:* Significant reversible airways obstruction.

f. *Chronic breathlessness:* Significant symptomatic breathing difficulties and/or shortness of breath without hard signs on radiographs or pulmonary function tests.

g. *Impaired lung function:* Significant abnormality of pulmonary function.

Cardiovascular

a. *Angina/angioplasty/coronary artery bypass:* On history confirmed at least by ECG changes.

b. *Myocardial infarction:* On history confirmed at least by ECG changes or cardiac enzyme elevation.

c. *Cardiomyopathy:* Chronic ventricular dysfunction documented clinically or on appropriate investigation.

d. *Valvular disease:* Significant diastolic or systolic murmur confirmed by cardiac tests if appropriate.

e. *Pericarditis:* Symptomatic pericardial inflammation or constriction for at least 3 months or pericardiectomy.

f. *Hypertension:* Diastolic BP >95 or requiring antihypertensive drugs.

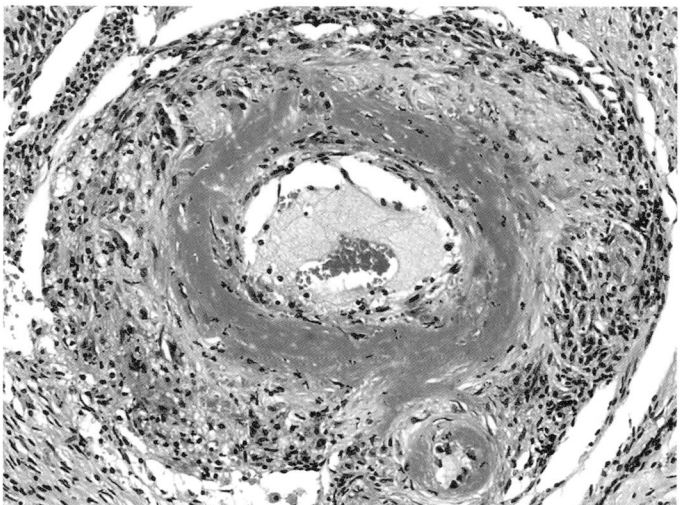

Plate 1 Severe necrotizing arteritis, muscular artery, uterus. HE. Original magnification 20×.

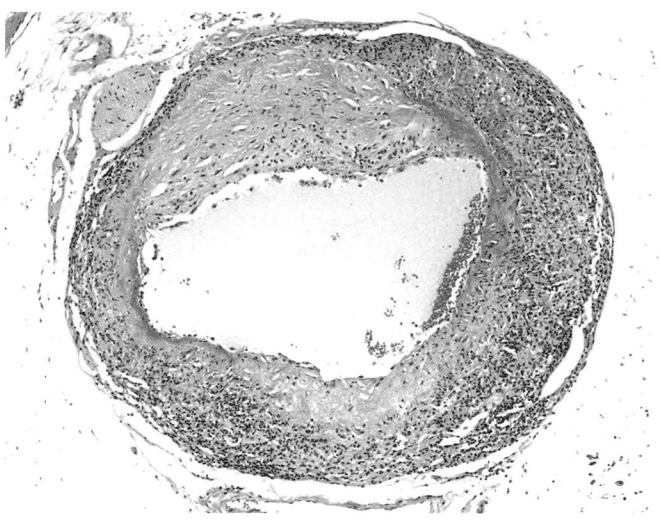

Plate 2 Severe chronic active arteritis, external carotid artery. HE. Original magnification 10×.

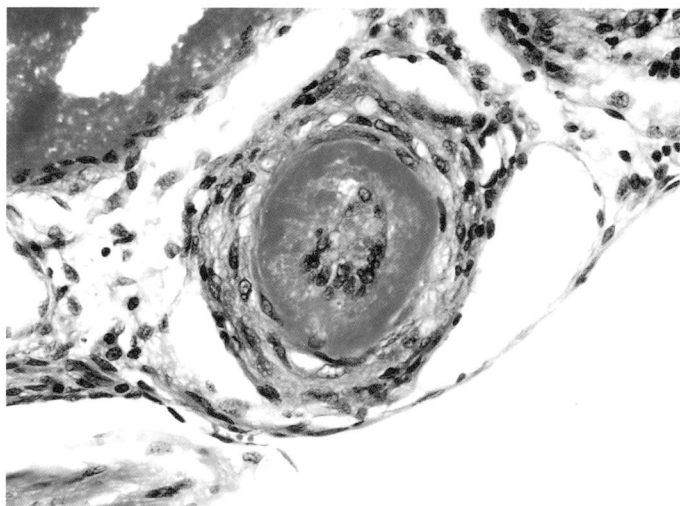

Plate 3 Medial necrosis, muscular artery, uterus. HE. Original magnification 40×.

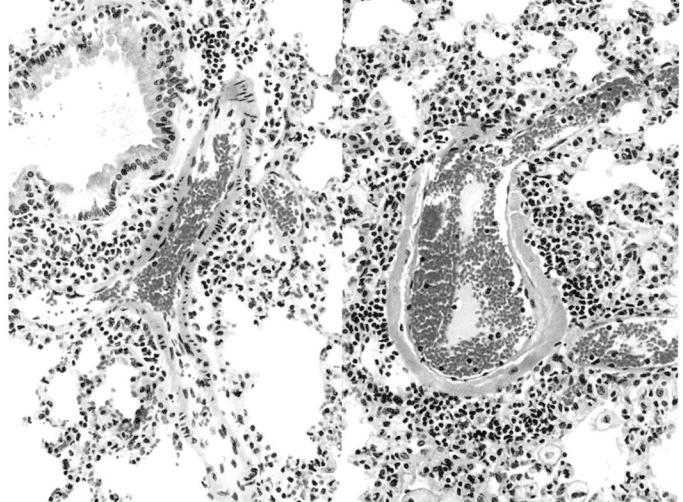

Plate 4 Perivascular lymphocyte accumulation without vasculitis; left, pulmonary artery; right, pulmonary vein. HE. Original magnification 20×.

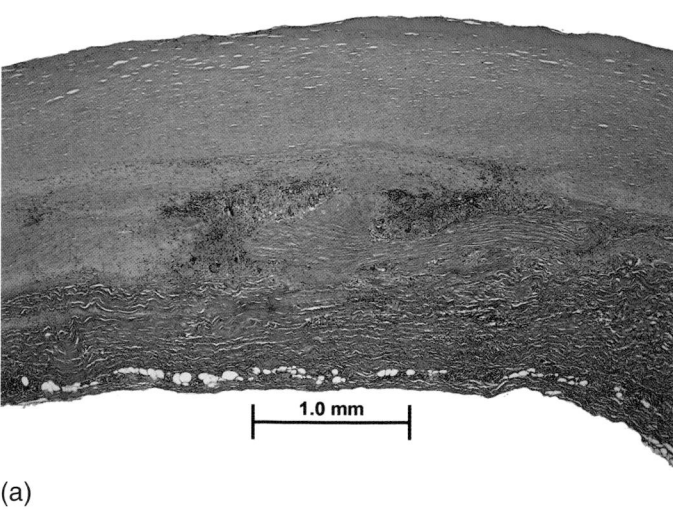

(a)

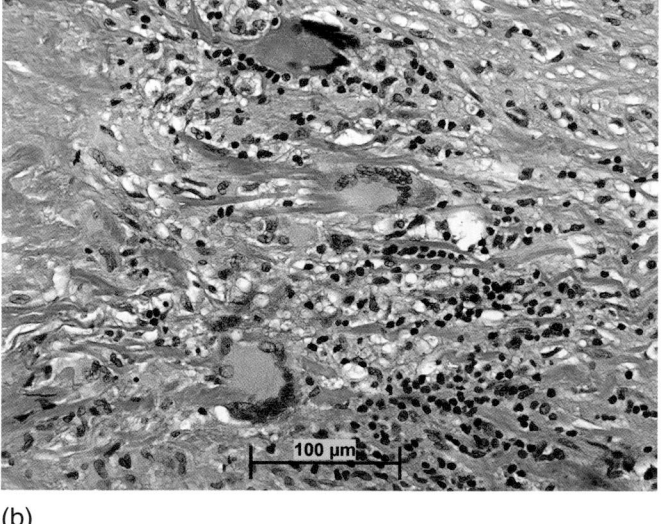

(b)

Plate 5 Takayasu's arteritis. Low power (a) and higher power (b) micrographs of the aorta showing a somewhat thickened wall and collections of inflammatory cells and characteristic giant cells. Courtesy of William D. Edwards, MD, Mayo Clinic, Rochester, Minnesota.

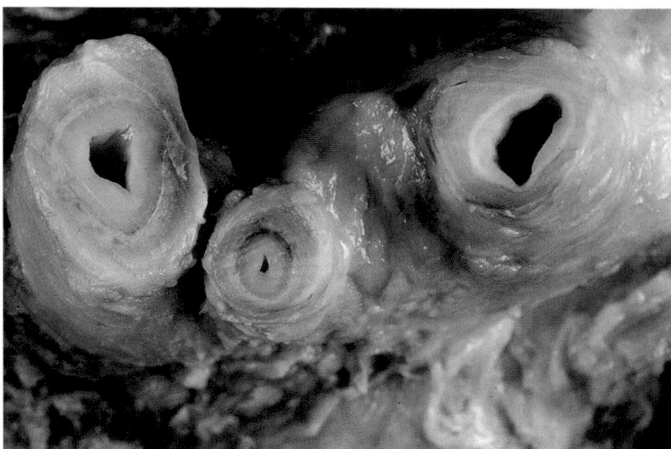

Plate 6 Takayasu's arteritis. Gross photograph of aortic arch branches showing marked lumenal narrowing and thickening of the arterial wall. Courtesy of William D. Edwards, MD, Mayo Clinic, Rochester, Minnesota.

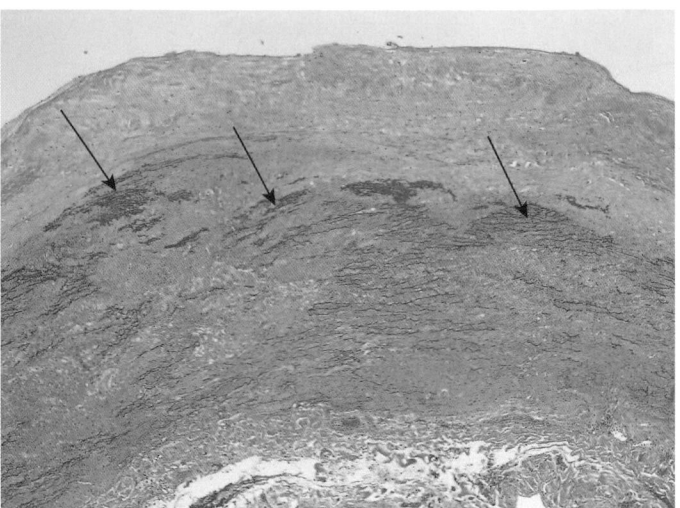

Plate 7 Takayasu's arteritis. In this example of long standing burnt out disease in the aorta, most of the elastica has disappeared and been replaced by fibrous tissue.

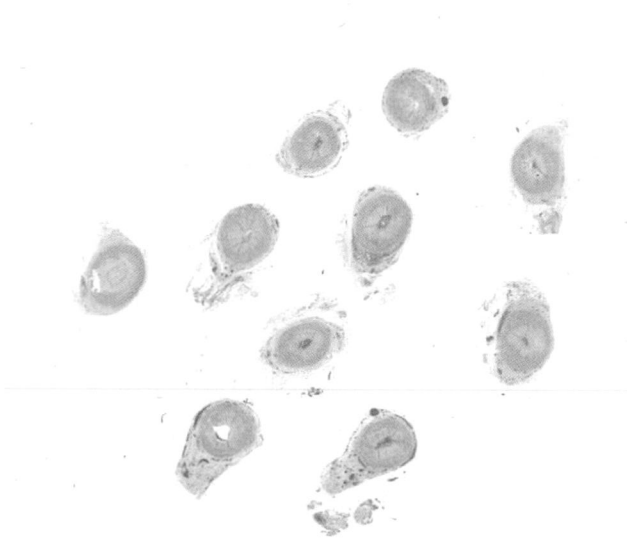

Plate 8 Giant cell arteritis. This figure shows the proper way to process temporal artery specimens for histology: the arterial segment is cut into numerous short pieces and all are embedded in one or more tissue blocks and then sectioned at multiple levels.

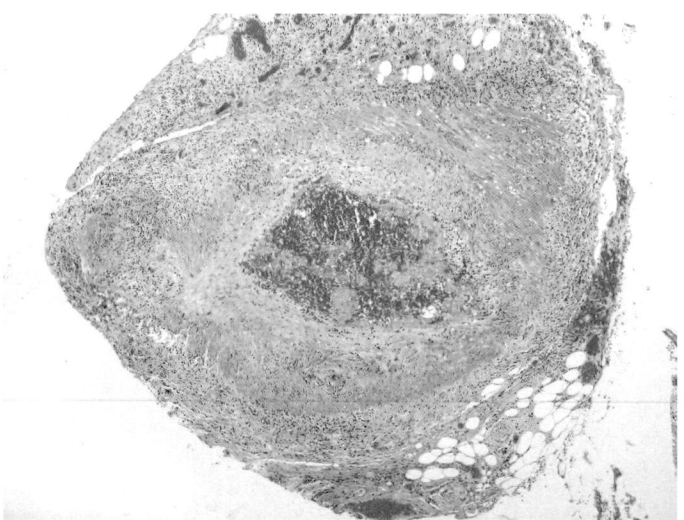

(a)

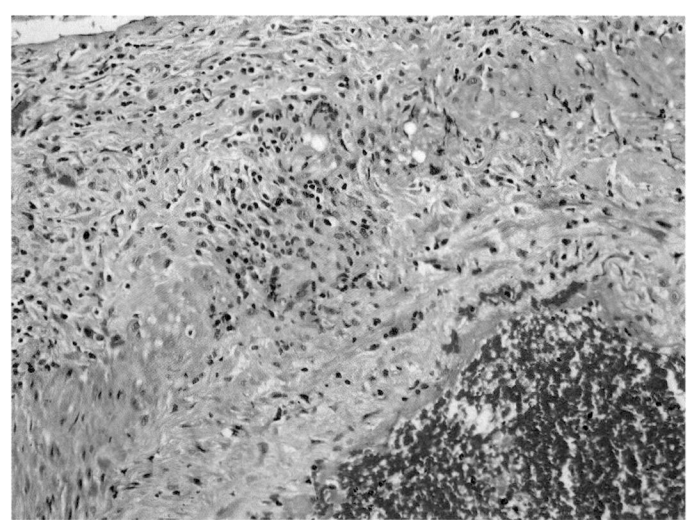

(b)

Plate 9 Giant cell arteritis. Low (a) and higher power (b) views of a temporal artery showing extensive inflammation involving largely the outer portion of the vessel wall; in B giant cells and inflammatory cells are seen to disrupt the muscularis.

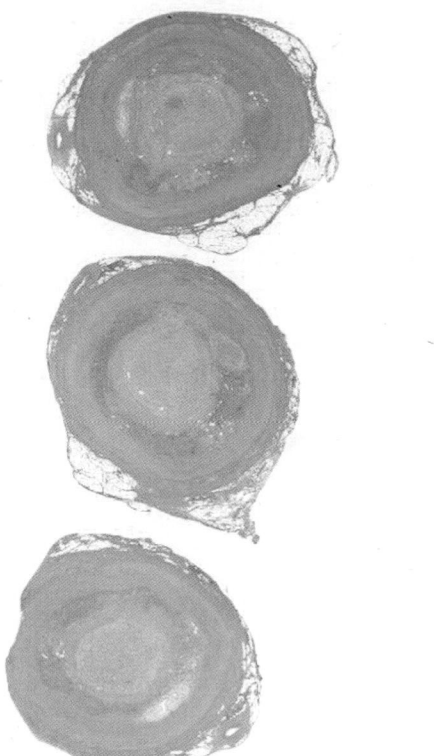

(a)

Plate 10 Giant cell arteritis involving a brachial artery. (a) This very low power view of a resected segment trisected shows complete luminal occlusion. Medium (b) and high power (c) views show inflammatory involvement of the arterial wall with giant cells, and fibrous obliteration (old thrombosis) of the lumen.

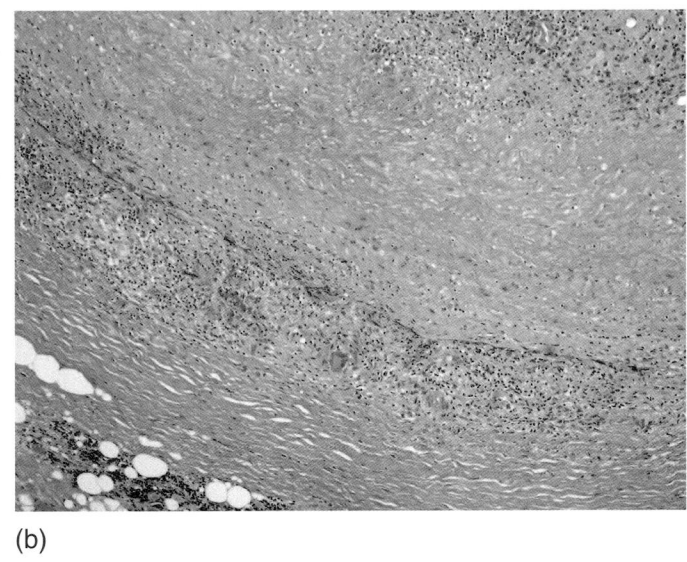

(b)

(c)

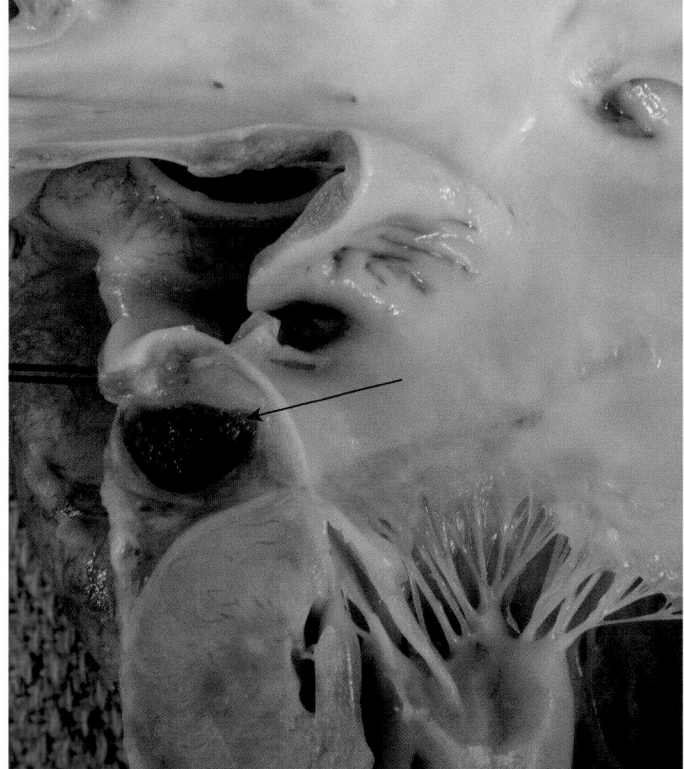

(a)

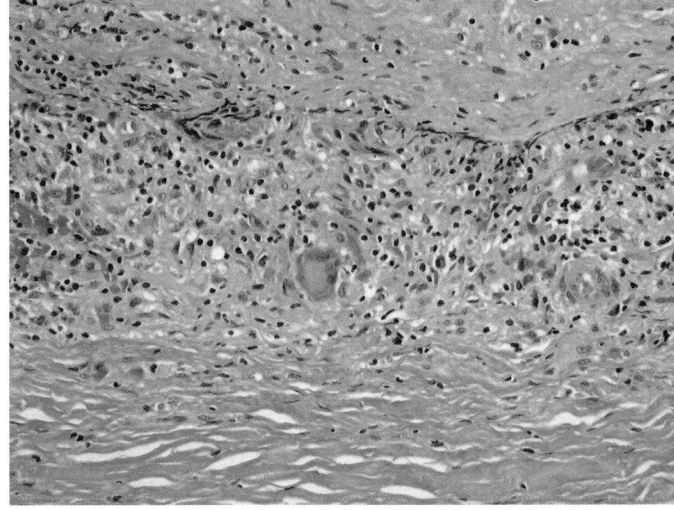

(b)

Plate 11 Kawasaki disease. (a) Gross photograph of heart of a child at autopsy showing aneurysmally dilated coronary artery with intralumenal thrombus. (b) Necrotizing arteritis involving a coronary artery. Courtesy of Glenn P. Taylor, MD, Division of Pathology, Hospital for Sick Children, Toronto, Ontario.

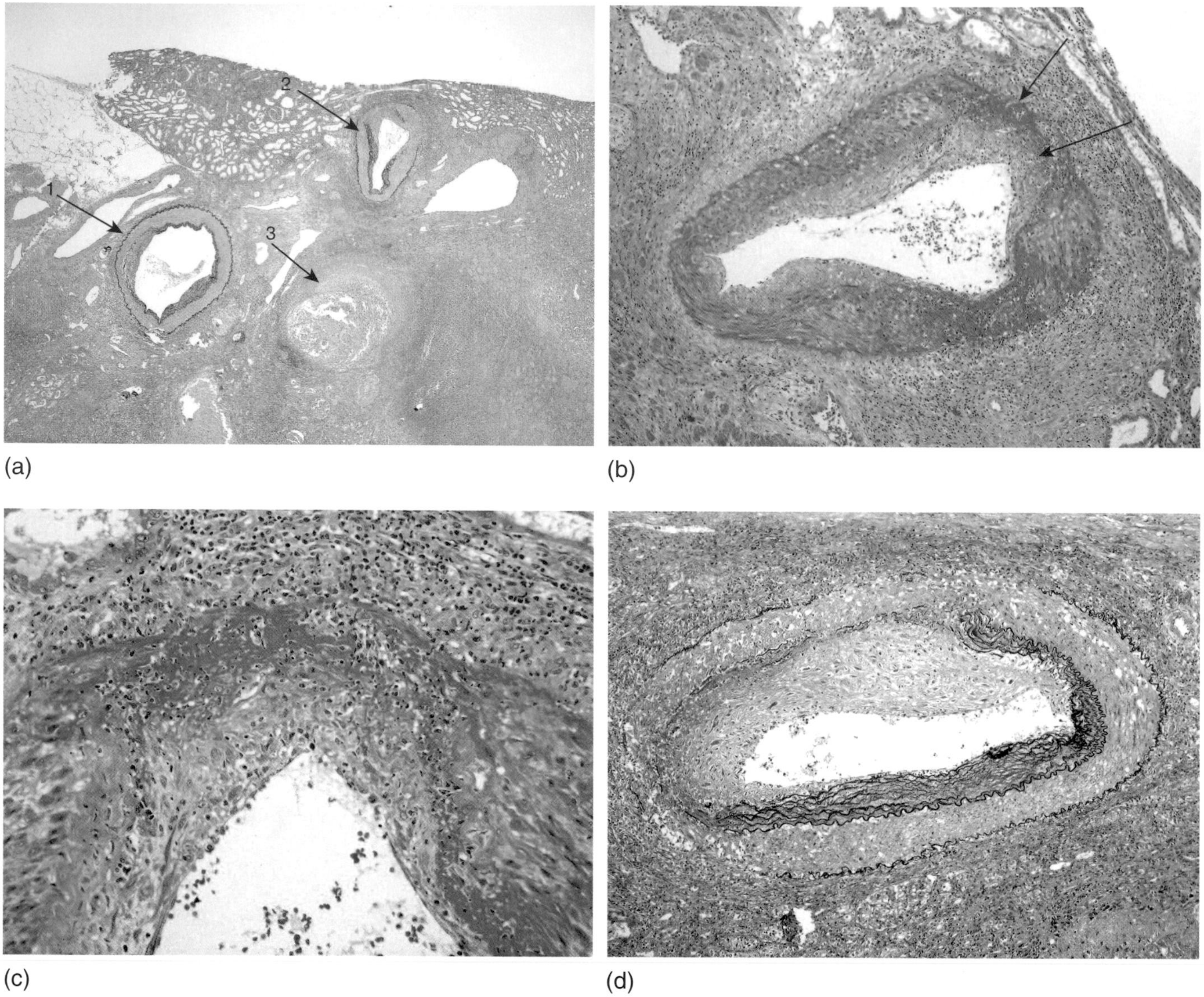

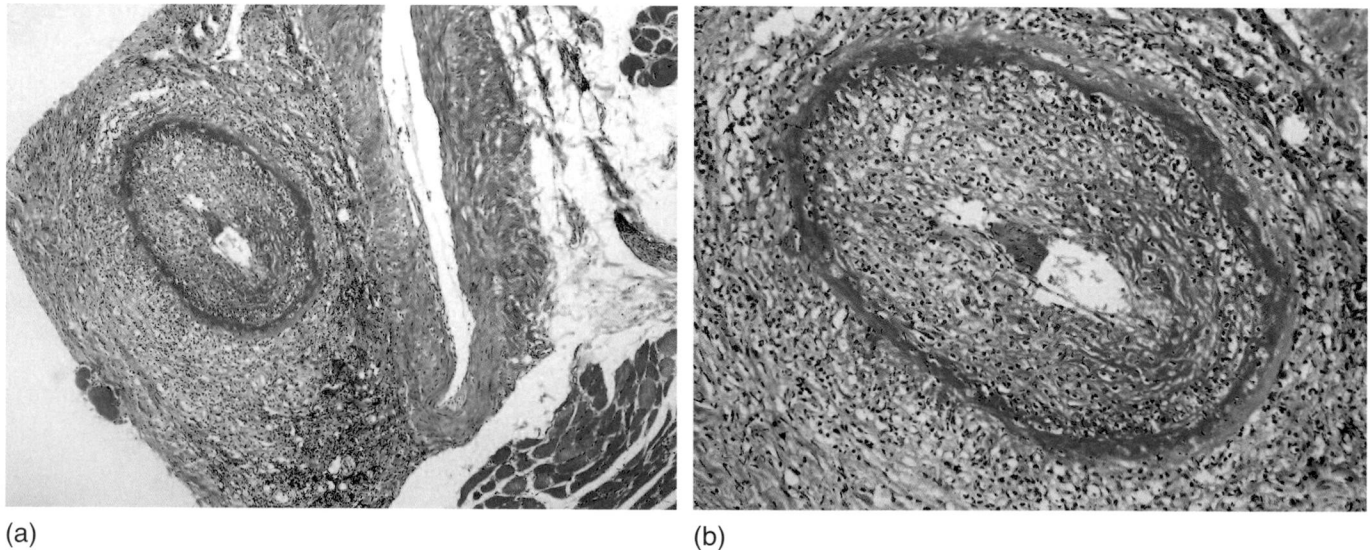

Plate 12 Polyarteritis nodosa involving relatively large intrarenal arteries. (a) Note the marked variation in degree of involvement in nearby vessels (probably all branches of the same artery). The branch on the left shows minimal damage, while the smaller branch on the right demonstrates loss of elastic over half of the perimeter. The lower shows nearly complete destruction of the wall. Elastic stain. Medium (b) and higher power (c) views of the vessel in (a). Note the characteristic focal necrosis which in (c) has the appearance of so-called fibrinoid. (d) Old healed lesion showing marked lumenal narrowing and loss of elastica in the same kidney. Loss of elastica indicates that this lesion did not result from bland thrombosis. Elastin stain.

Plate 13 Microscopic polyangiitis. Low (a) and high (b) power views of necrotizing vasculitis involving a small artery in a muscle biopsy. The arterial wall is completely replaced by fibrinoid necrosis and an acute inflammatory infiltrate is present. This appearance can be seen in any form of small-vessel vasculitis and also in medium-vessel vasculitis (polyarteritis nodosa, Kawasaki disease) when it involves small arteries.

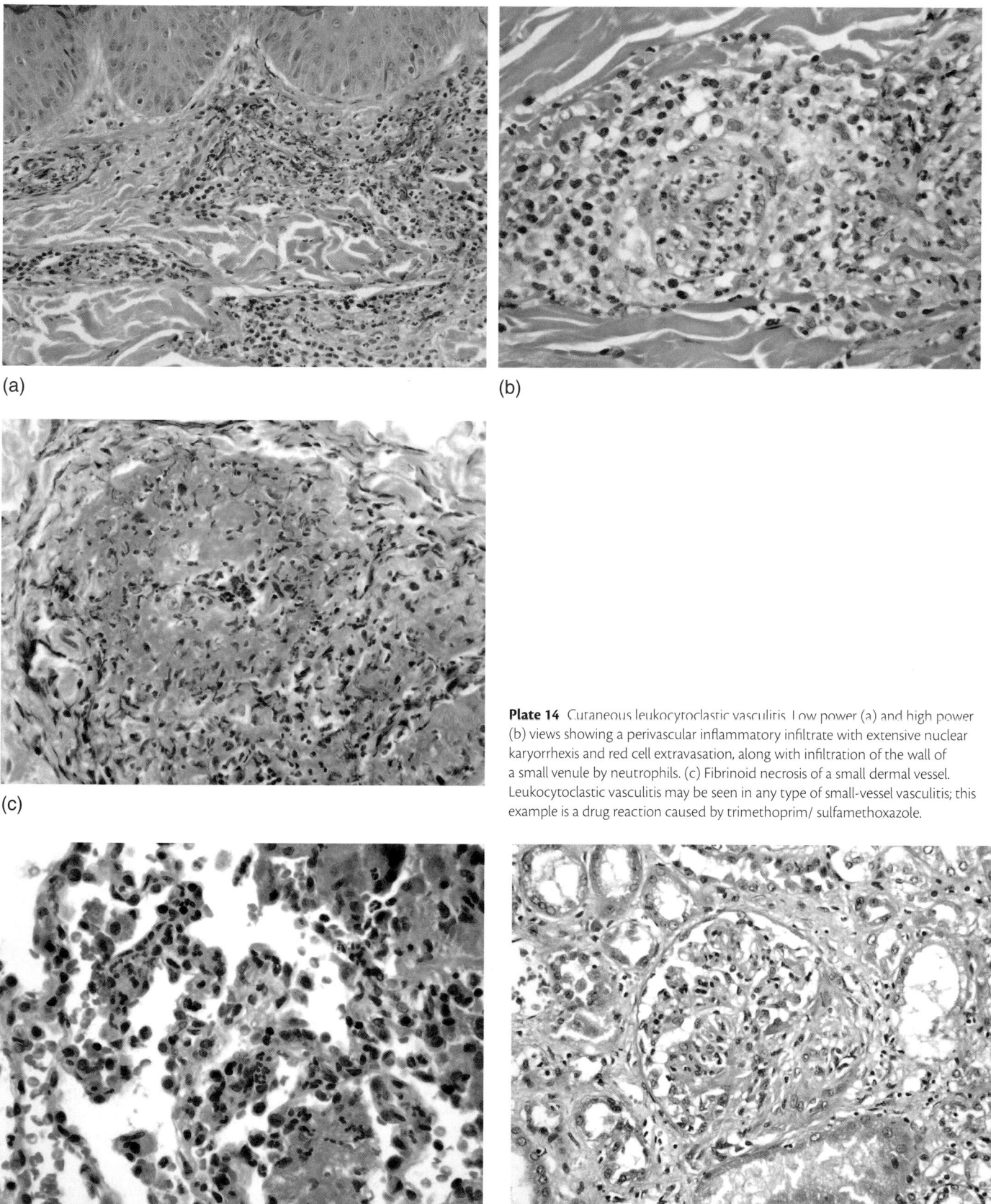

(a)

(b)

(c)

Plate 14 Cutaneous leukocytoclastic vasculitis. Low power (a) and high power (b) views showing a perivascular inflammatory infiltrate with extensive nuclear karyorrhexis and red cell extravasation, along with infiltration of the wall of a small venule by neutrophils. (c) Fibrinoid necrosis of a small dermal vessel. Leukocytoclastic vasculitis may be seen in any type of small-vessel vasculitis; this example is a drug reaction caused by trimethoprim/ sulfamethoxazole.

Plate 15 Pulmonary capillaritis. Characteristic pattern of neutrophils in alveolar walls and evidence of acute and chronic hemorrhage (hemosiderin-laden macrophages) in airspaces. This example is from a patient with rheumatoid arthritis and hemoptysis.

Plate 16 Crescentic glomerulonephritis from a case of microscopic polyangiitis.

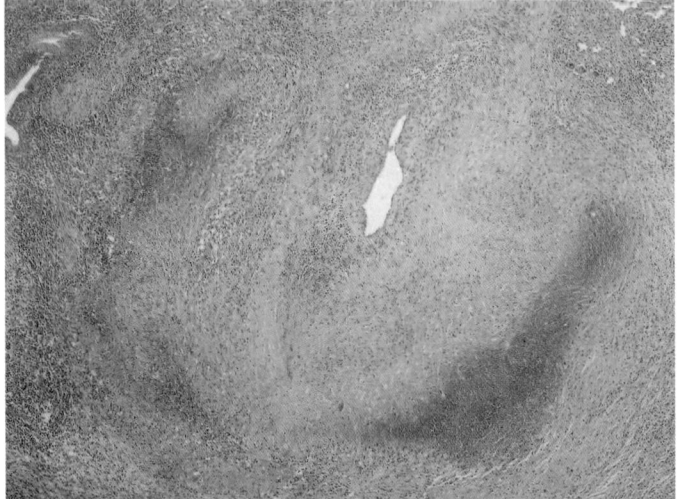

Plate 17 Wegener's granulomatosis. Characteristic pattern of 'geographic necrosis' (irregular necrosis); the surrounding palisade of epithelioid histiocytes, that is the 'granulomatosis', cannot be seen at this low power.

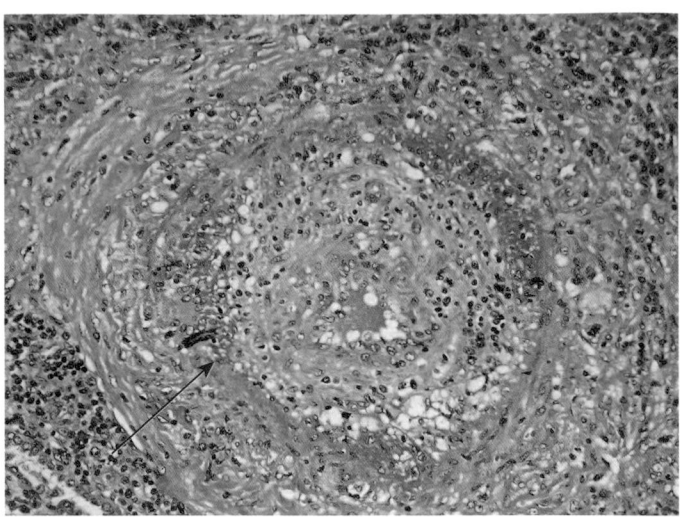

Plate 18 Wegener's granulomatosis. Small artery in lung showing necrotizing vasculitis.

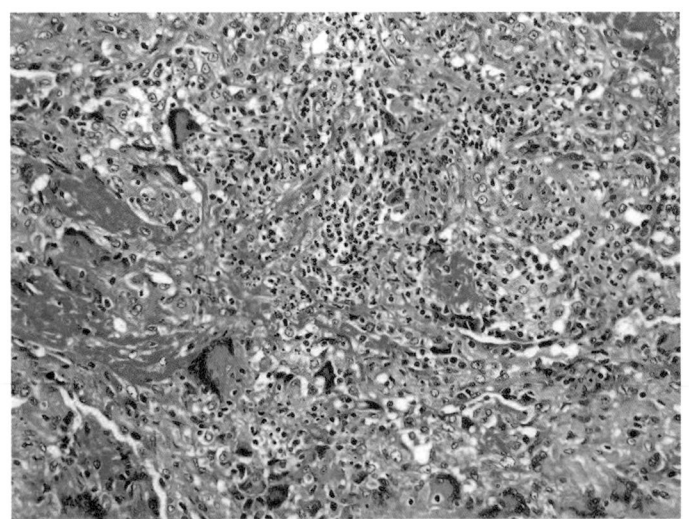

Plate 19 Wegener's granulomatosis. Typical inflammatory background seen in the lung, and composed of acute and chronic inflammatory cells and individual giant cells, but not hard granulomas.

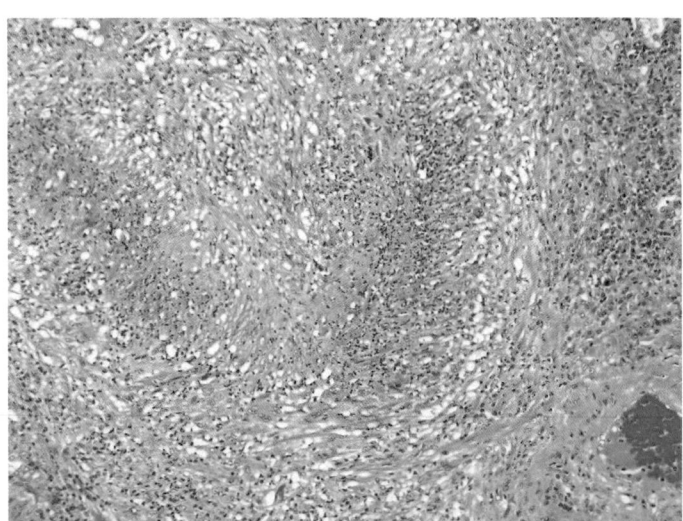

Plate 21 Wegener's granulomatosis. Early lesion consisting of a small neutrophilic abscess. In this example a palisade of epithelioid histiocytes is beginning to form; eventually such lesions end up as large or small areas of geographic necrosis.

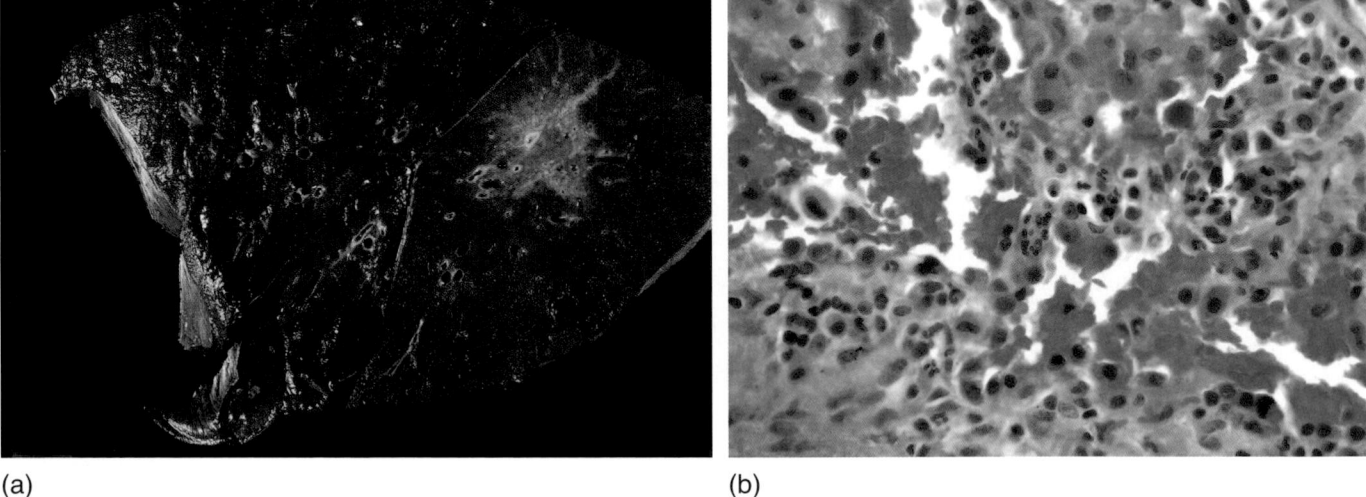

(a)   (b)

Plate 20 Wegener's granulomatosis. (a) Gross photograph showing extensive hemorrhage and an irregular upper lobe necrotizing mass lesion. (b) Microscopic pattern of capillaritis with hemorrhage, a frequent finding in the lung in Wegener's granulomatosis.

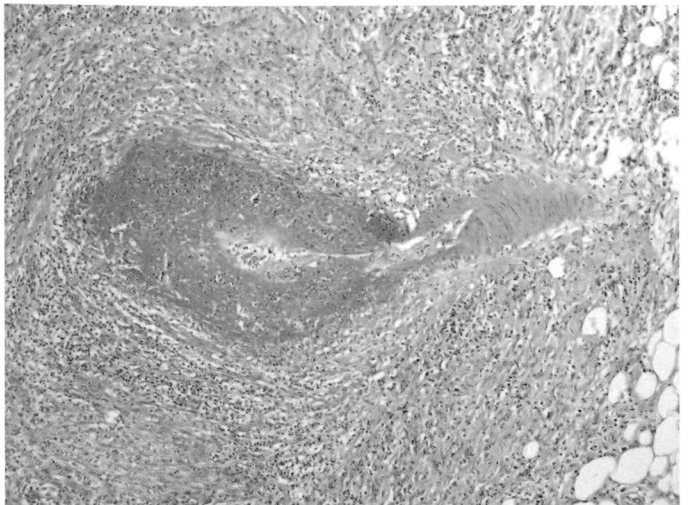

Plate 22 Wegener's granulomatosis. Necrotizing vasculitis with fibrinoid necrosis involving a mesenteric artery.

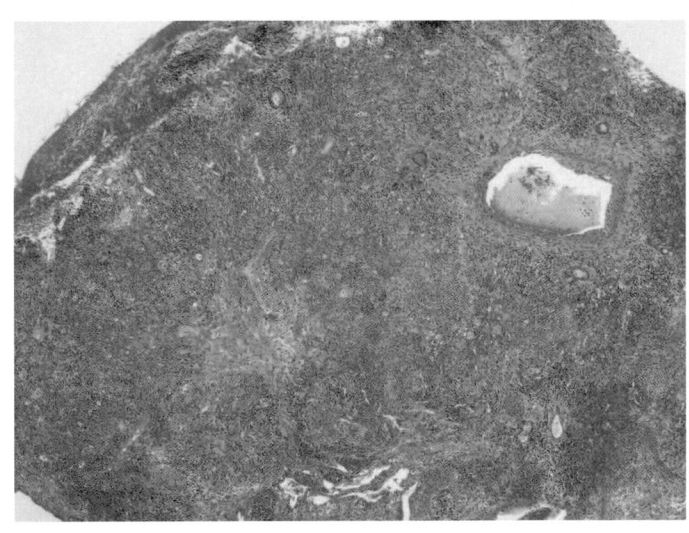

(a)

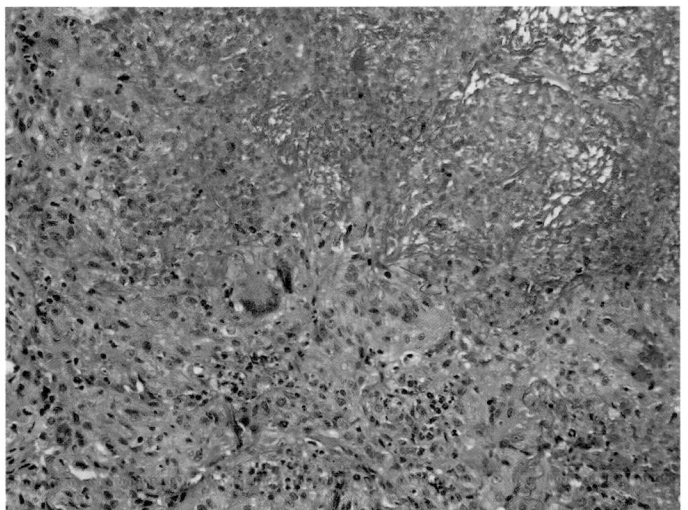

Plate 24 Churg–Strauss syndrome. Eosinophilic pneumonia-like area without vasculitis from a case of early phase (prevasculitic phase) disease. In this example there is eosinophilic necrosis, but this is a common finding in eosinophilic pneumonia of any cause and is not diagnostic of Churg–Strauss syndrome.)

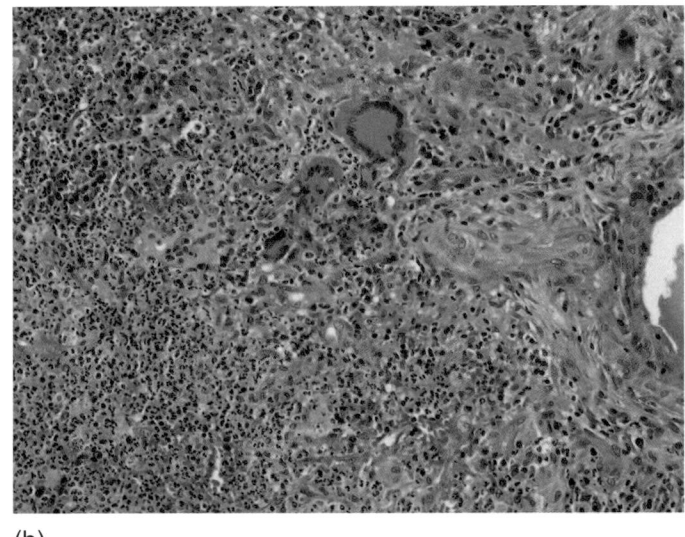

(b)

Plate 23 Wegener's granulomatosis. Biopsy of a nasal ulcer. (a) Most of the lesion is non-specific inflammation; a few giant cells are seen in the high power view (b). This appearance by itself is not diagnostic; however, if there is a positive cANCA, then these findings support a diagnosis of Wegener's granulomatosis.

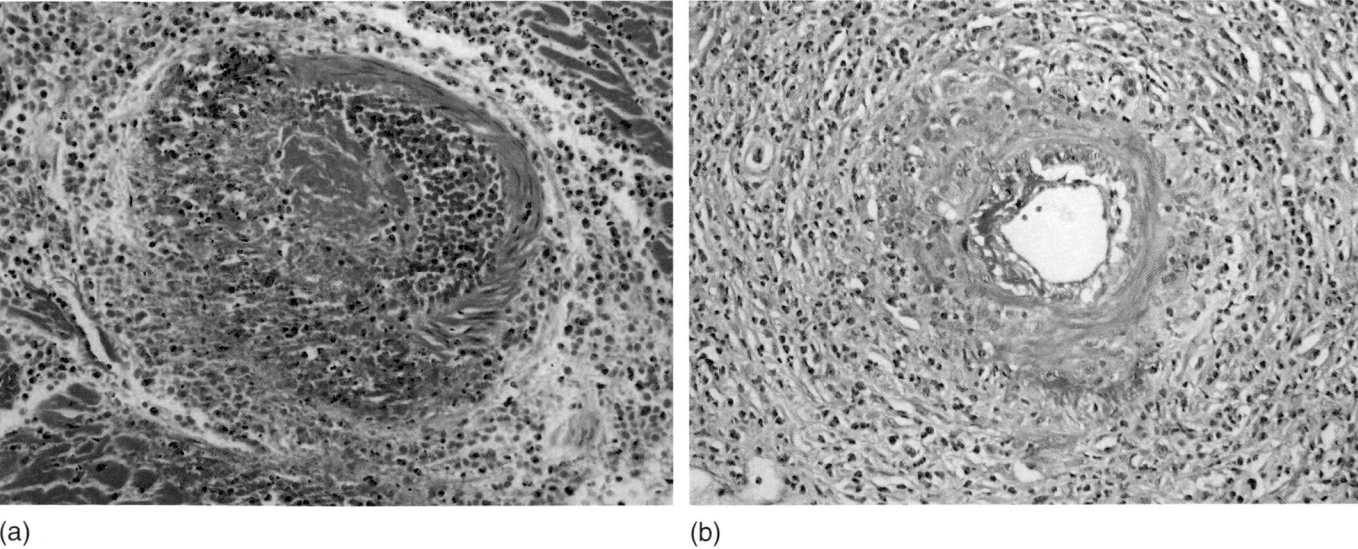

(a)

(b)

Plate 25 Churg–Strauss syndrome. Various appearances of necrotizing vasculitis in heart (a), nerve (b), and mesentery (c). Only the eosinophilic inflammatory infiltrate allows morphologic separation from other forms of small-vessel vasculitis.

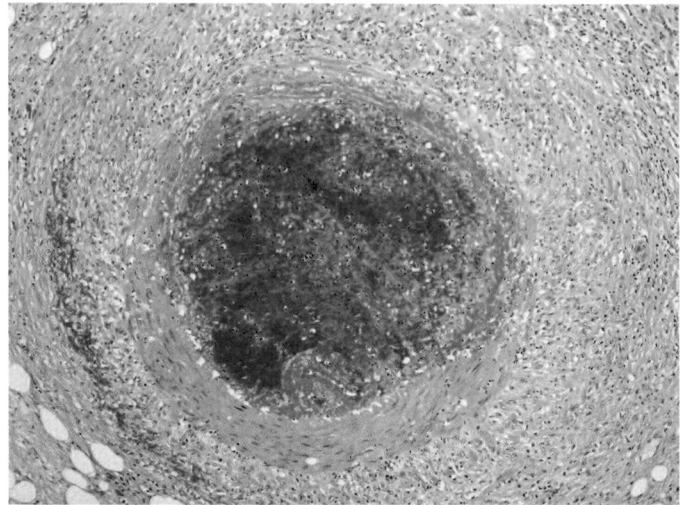

(c)

Plate 25 (*cont.*)

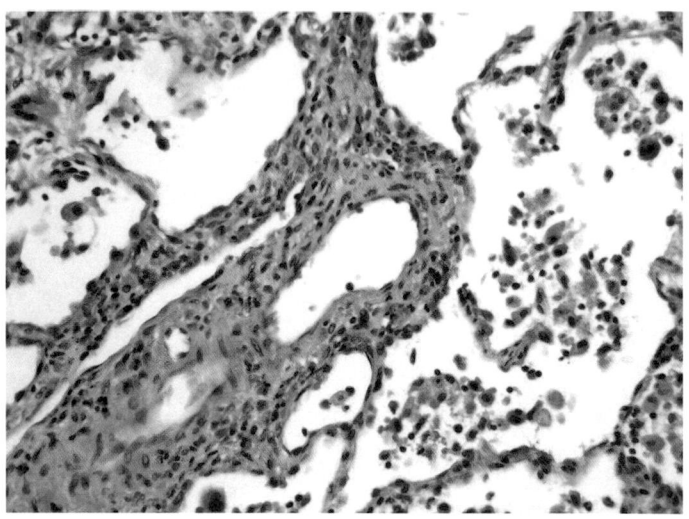

Plate 26 Churg–Strauss syndrome. Non-necrotizing eosinophilic vasculitis in the lung.

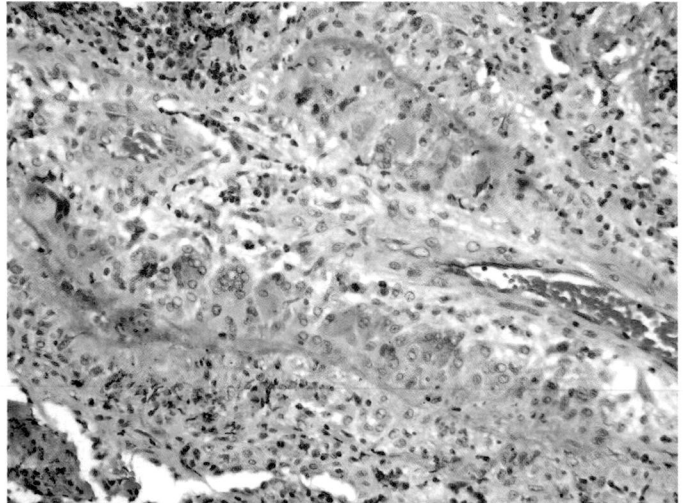

Plate 27 Churg–Strauss syndrome. Granulomatous eosinophilic vasculitis.

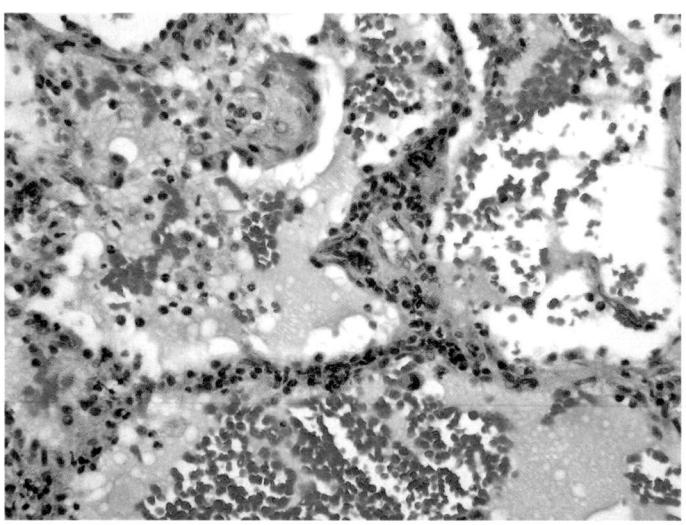

Plate 28 Churg–Strauss syndrome. Eosinophilic capillaritis in the lung. In Churg–Strauss syndrome the infiltrates in capillaritis may be only eosinophils or a mixture of eosinophils and neutrophils.

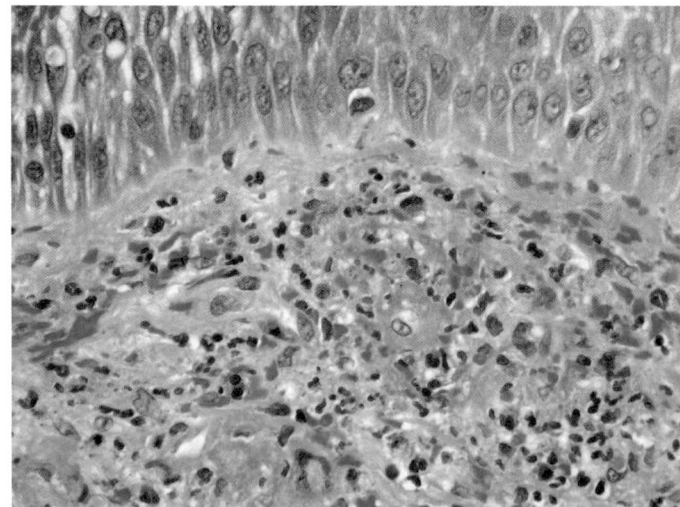

Plate 29 Churg–Strauss syndrome. Leukocytoclastic vasculitis in a patient with palpable purpura. Note the mixture of eosinophils and neutrophils, commonly seen in leukocytoclastic vasculitis in Churg–Strauss syndrome.

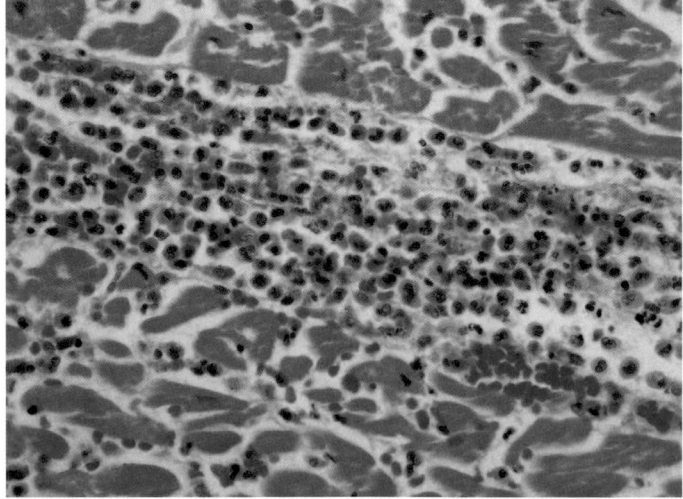

Plate 30 Churg–Strauss syndrome. Eosinophilic myocarditis.

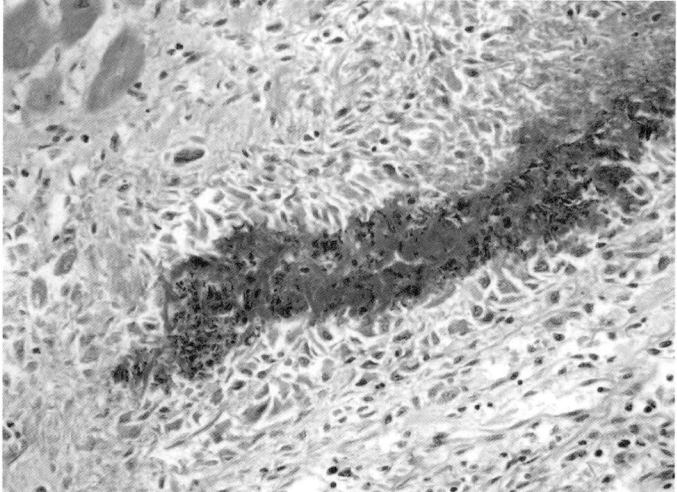

Plate 31 Churg–Strauss syndrome. Necrotizing granuloma with an eosinophilic center (so-called Churg–Strauss granuloma). Such lesions are relatively uncommon in modern pathologic specimens.

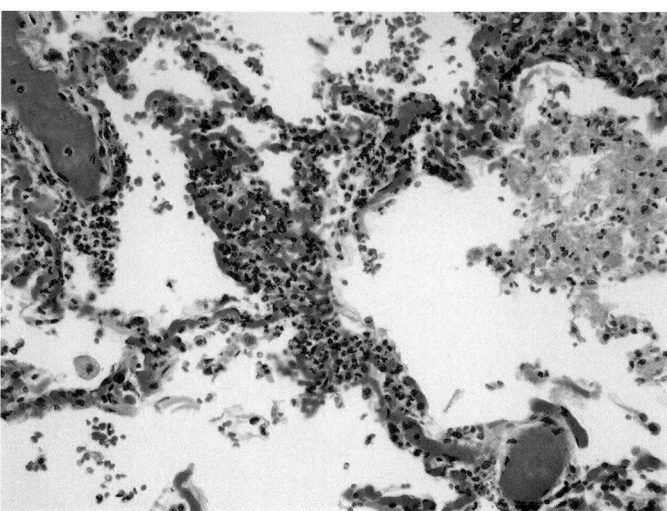

Plate 32 Microscopic polyangiitis. Capillaritis in lung. This is the most common pattern of lung involvement in microscopic polyangiitis.

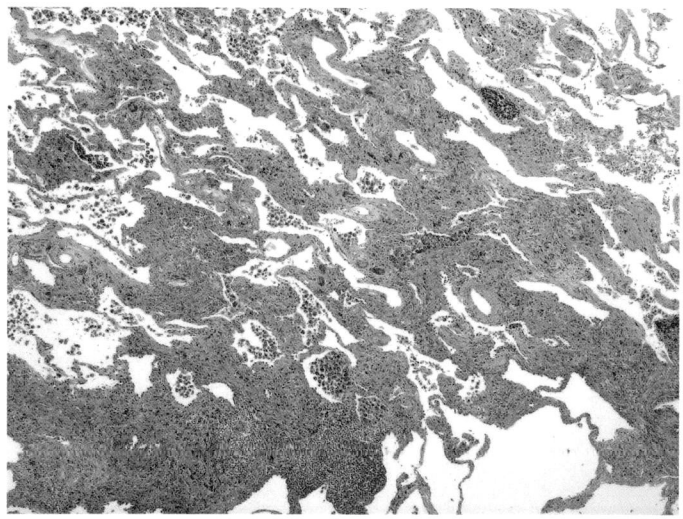

(a)

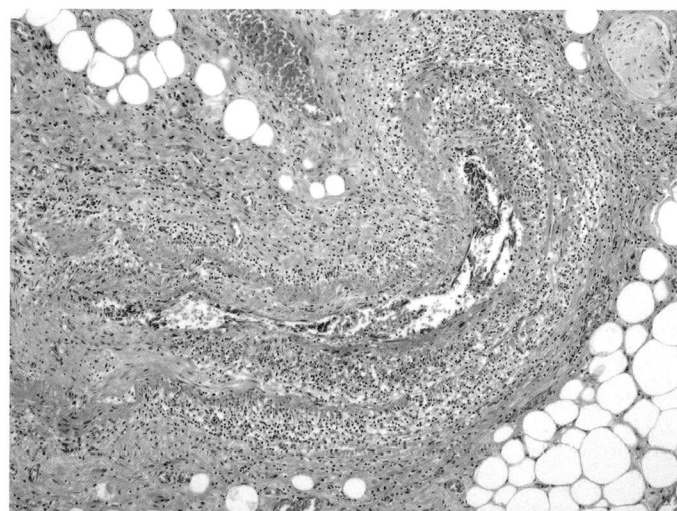

Plate 34 Rheumatoid vasculitis. Necrotizing vasculitis involving an artery in the peripancreatic fat. By itself this morphology could be seen in any form of small-vessel or medium-vessel vasculitis and further clinical/laboratory information is required for diagnosis.

(b)

Plate 33 Microscopic polyangiitis. Interstitial fibrosis secondary to chronic pulmonary hemorrhage in a patient with microscopic polyangiitis. (a) Low power view showing diffuse interstitial fibrosis and masses of hemosiderin-laden macrophages in the airspaces. (b) High power view showing hemosiderin, indicative of old hemorrhage, in the interstitium, and encrustation of the vessel elastica by iron/calcium salts, a common finding in chronic hemorrhage.

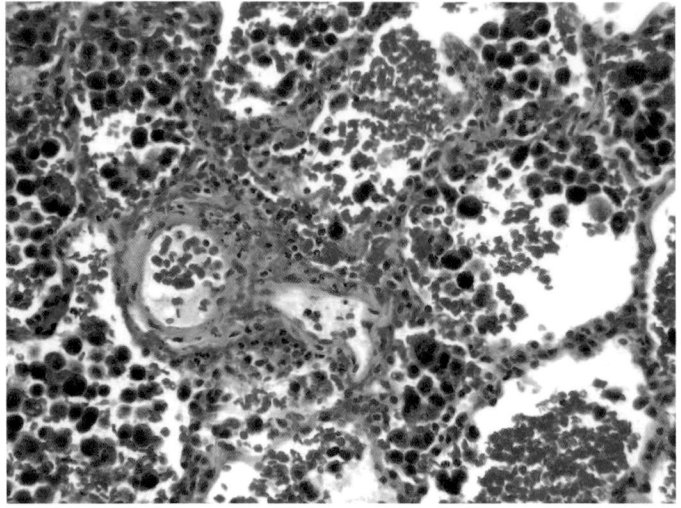

(a)

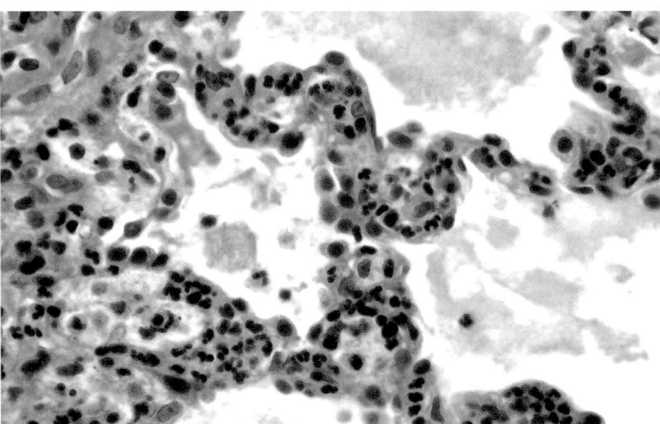

(b)

Plate 35 Pulmonary capillaritis with hemorrhage in lupus. (a) Medium power view showing acute hemorrhage (red blood cells) and hemosiderin laden macrophages; the latter are a useful finding that indicate the presence of real (as opposed to surgical) hemorrhage. (b) High power view of another area showing typical capillaritis. This biopsy also demonstrated immune complex deposits by immunofluorescence and electron microscopy.

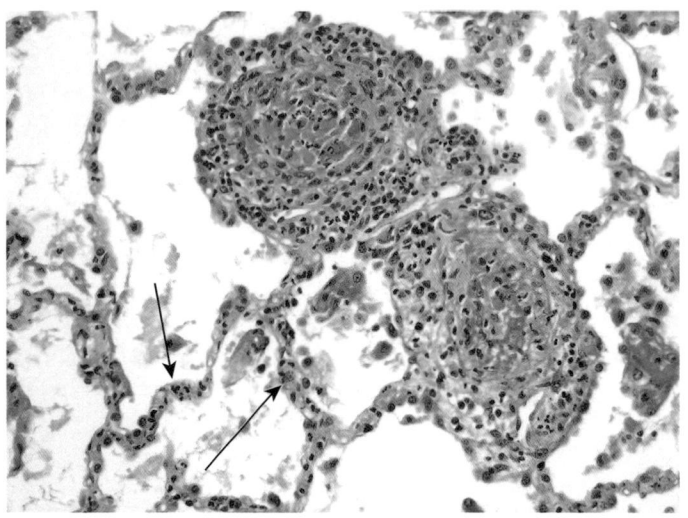

Plate 36 Cryoglobulinemia. Largely non-destructive vasculitis involving two small vessels in the lung; there is capillaritis as well. This combination of sizes of vessels involved is sometimes seen in small-vessel vasculitis.

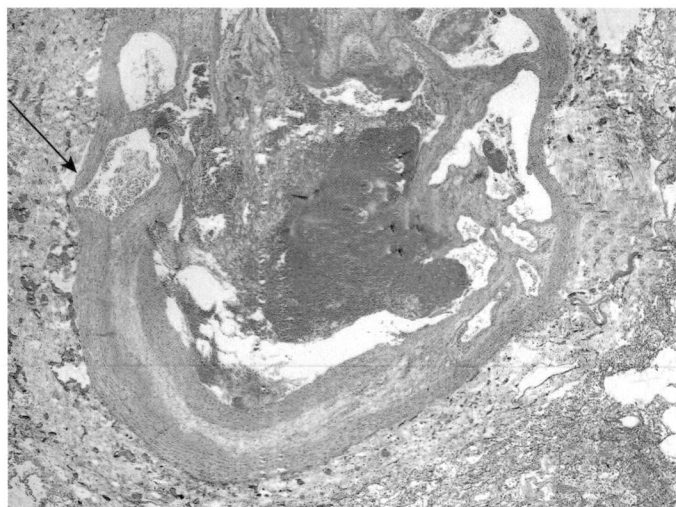

Plate 37 Behçet's syndrome. Low power view of an aneurysmally dilated and thrombosed pulmonary artery branch. Note the extreme thinning of the wall in some areas; such vessels are prone to rupture.

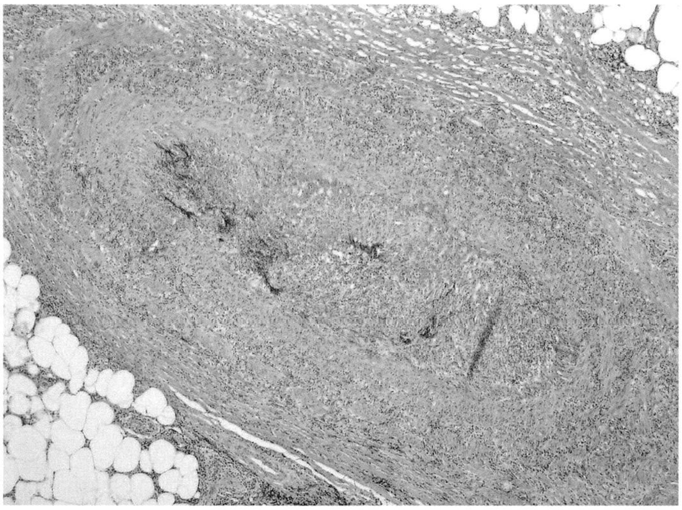

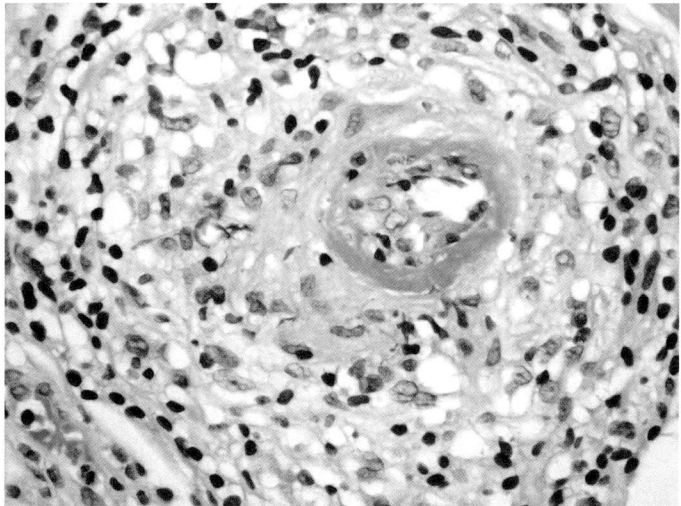

(a)

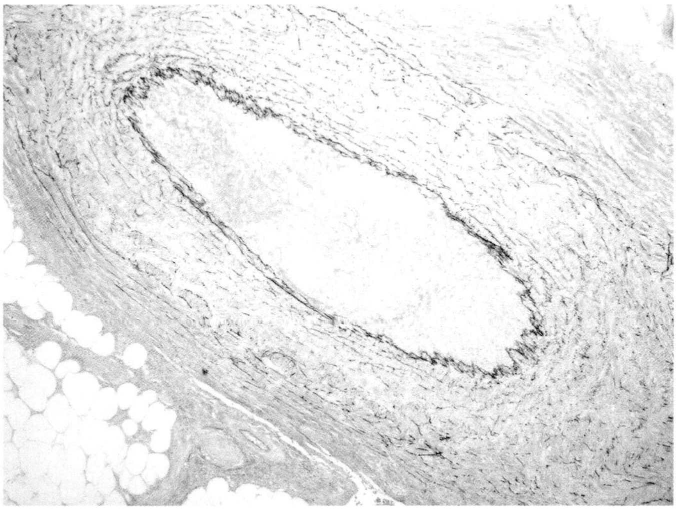

(b)

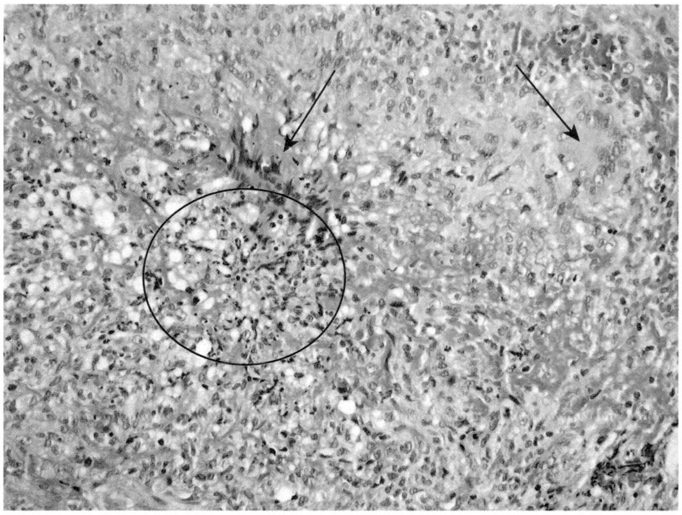

(c)

Plate 38 Thromboangiitis obliterans (Buerger's disease). Vasculitis involving a branch of the tibial artery. (a) Low power view showing a cellular thrombus and inflammatory cells in the vessel wall. (b) Elastic stain shows that, as opposed to most forms of vasculitis, the vessel wall is not destroyed in Buerger's disease. (c) High power view of the center of the thrombus shown in (a). Note the marked cellularity, presence of giant cells (upper right), and collections of neutrophils. These morphologic features are typical of Buerger's disease and are not seen in ordinary thrombi.

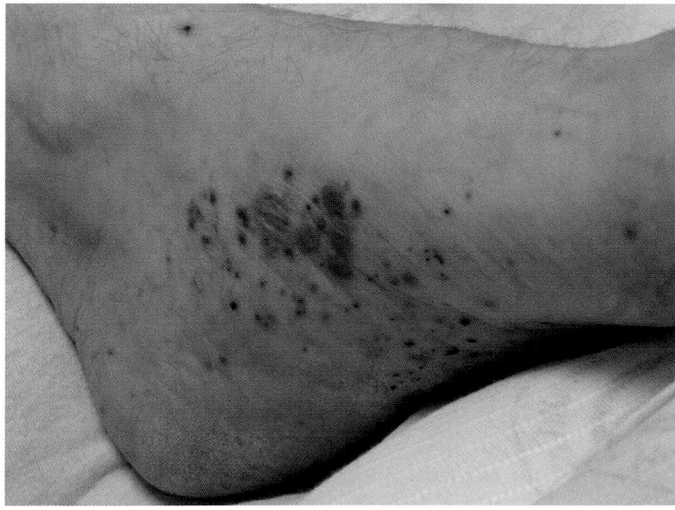

Plate 39 Isolated vasculitis. Necrotizing vasculitis in a small periappendiceal vessel in a case of acute appendicitis. In the majority of cases, this type of isolated vasculitis associated with inflammatory reactions is not indicative of systemic vasculitis.

Plate 40 Palpable purpura concentrated around the ankle in a patient with cutaneous small-vessel vasculitis.

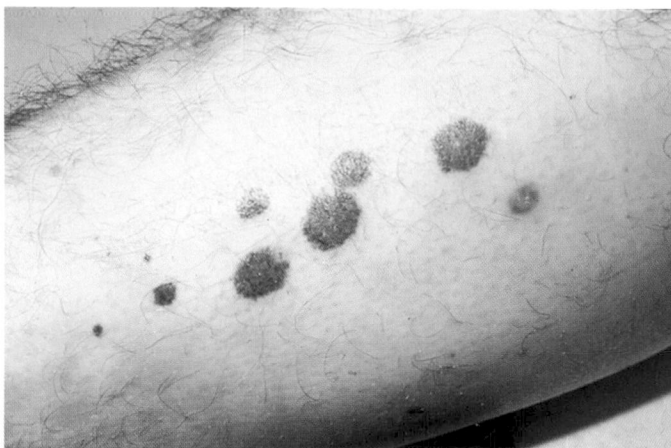

Plate 41 Cutaneous small-vessel (leukocytoclastic) vasculitis. Sharply demarcated palpable purpuric lesions. Note that the earliest visible lesion is a millimeter or two in diameter and that this individual lesion enlarges up to 10 mm in diameter. This is a lesion typical of cutaneous small-vessel (leukocytoclastic) vasculitis with inflammation in the postcapillary venules high in the dermis. (From Sams and Sams, Cutaneous Manifestations. In: *Vasculitis* (G. V. Ball and S. L. Bridges, Jr, eds), 1st edn. Oxford University Press, 2002.)

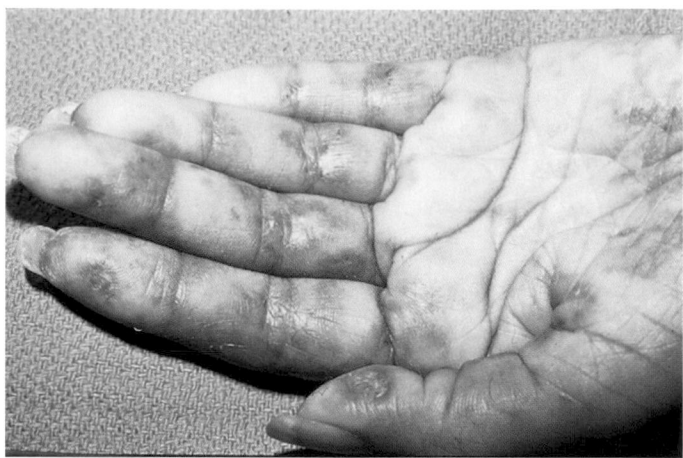

Plate 42 Systemic lupus erythematosus. Vasculitis in these patients may present as punctate lesions on the palms and fingers. Pain and disability is usually severe. Lesions heal with a white scar. (From Sams and Sams, Cutaneous Manifestations. In: *Vasculitis* (G. V. Ball and S. L. Bridges, Jr, eds), 1st edn. Oxford University Press, 2002.)

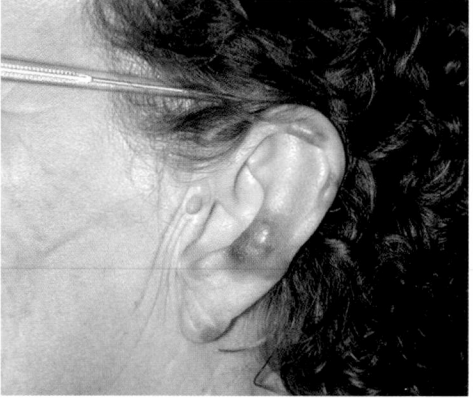

Plate 43 Violaceous nodules on the ear in a patient with erythema elevatum diutinum.

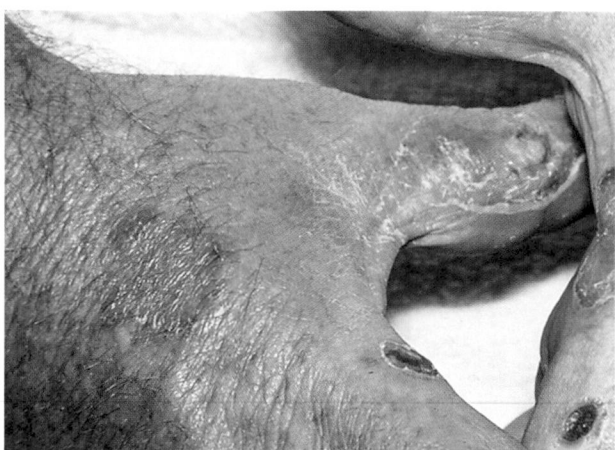

Plate 44 Erythema elevatum diutinum. Typical annular plaques on the thenar eminence, over the thumb and index finger. These lesions, in contrast to other forms of vasculitis, are strikingly static. (From Sams and Sams, Cutaneous Manifestations. In: *Vasculitis* (G. V. Ball and S. L. Bridges, Jr, eds), 1st edn. Oxford University Press, 2002.)

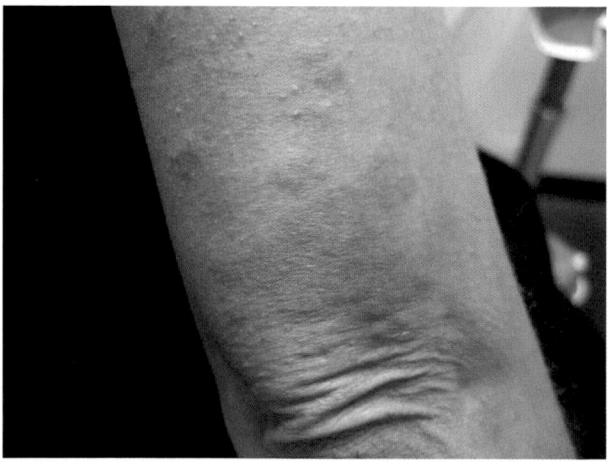

Plate 45 Urticarial vasculitis. Erythematous and violaceous papules and nodules on an upper extremity.

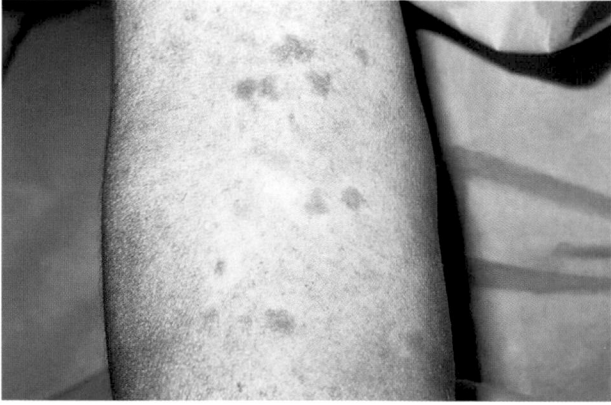

Plate 46 Urticarial lesions. Note that they are bright red and are surrounded by a pale halo. Light pressure with the palpating finger will cause blanching and diascopy with a clear microscope slide will often demonstrate tiny petechiae within the lesion. (From Sams and Sams, Cutaneous Manifestations. In: *Vasculitis* (G. V. Ball and S. L. Bridges, Jr, eds), 1st edn. Oxford University Press, 2002.)

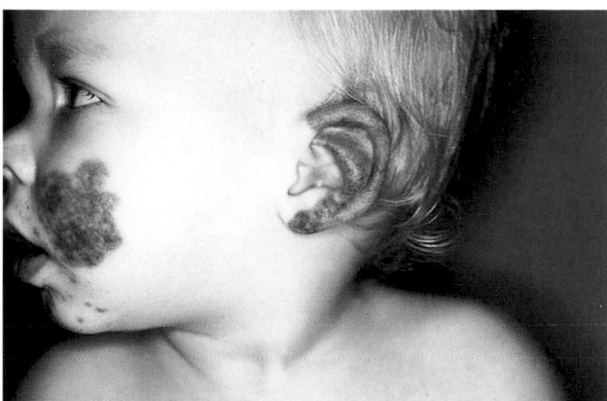

Plate 47 Acute hemorrhagic edema (Finkelstein's disease). This condition is characterized by the rapid onset of deep red to purple purpuric plaques on the cheeks, shoulders, and ears. In spite of the dramatic clinical appearance, lesions resolve spontaneously without sequelae. (From Sams and Sams, Cutaneous Manifestations. In: *Vasculitis* (G. V. Ball and S. L. Bridges, Jr, eds), 1st edn. Oxford University Press, 2002.)

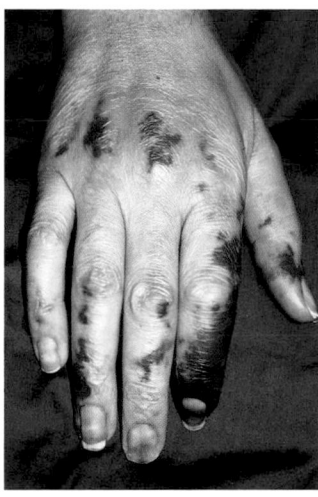

Plate 49 Cryoglobulinemia. Stellate shaped areas of purpura on the dorsum of the hand in a cool acral area. In this patient there is, in addition to occlusion of the vessels in the deep dermal plexus, occlusion of the digital arteries of the index finger. (From Sams and Sams, Cutaneous Manifestations. In: *Vasculitis* (G. V. Ball and S. L. Bridges, Jr, eds), 1st edn. Oxford University Press, 2002.)

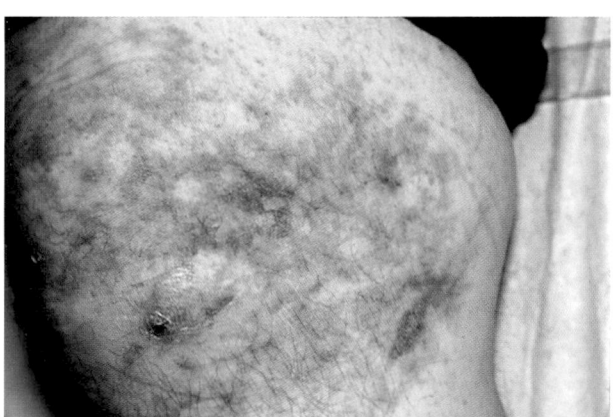

Plate 51 Polyarteritis nodosa. Reticulate purple discoloration about the knee. Many of these lesions will partially blanch indicating that at least some of the color is from vascular stasis rather than hemorrhage. (From Sams and Sams, Cutaneous Manifestations. In: *Vasculitis* (G. V. Ball and S. L. Bridges, Jr, eds), 1st edn. Oxford University Press, 2002.)

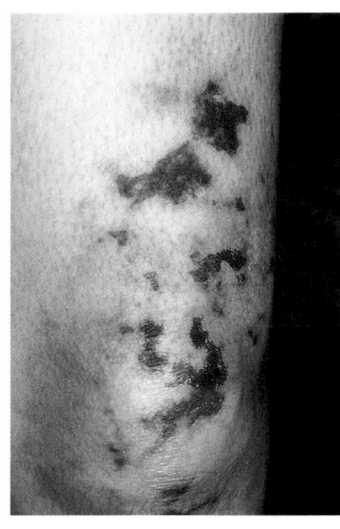

Plate 48 Typical lesions of cryoglobulinemia on the knee. Note the purpura and particularly the angulated lesions with sharp points indicative of occlusion in the deep dermal plexus prior to arborization. (From Sams and Sams, Cutaneous Manifestations. In: *Vasculitis* (G. V. Ball and S. L. Bridges, Jr, eds), 1st edn. Oxford University Press, 2002.)

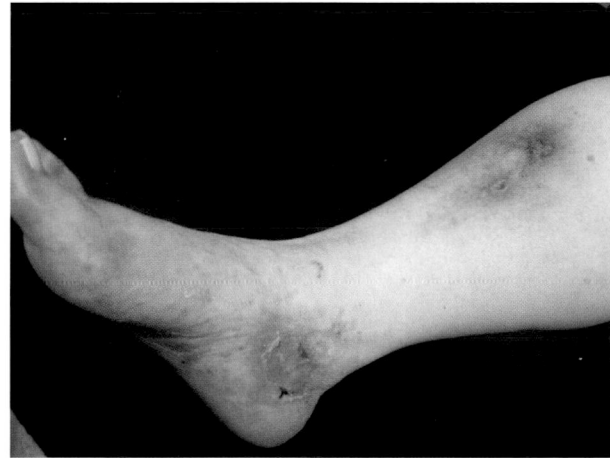

Plate 50 This patient with cutaneous polyarteritis nodosa presented with ulcerated violaceous nodules coursing along a lower extremity vessel.

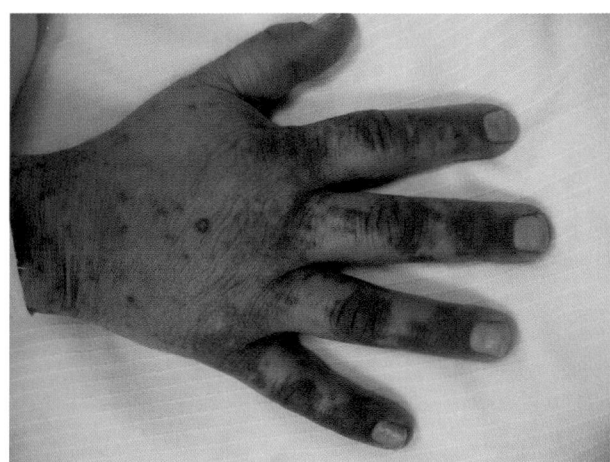

Plate 52 Distal extremity with necrotic papules and plaques in a patient with Wegener's granulomatosis.

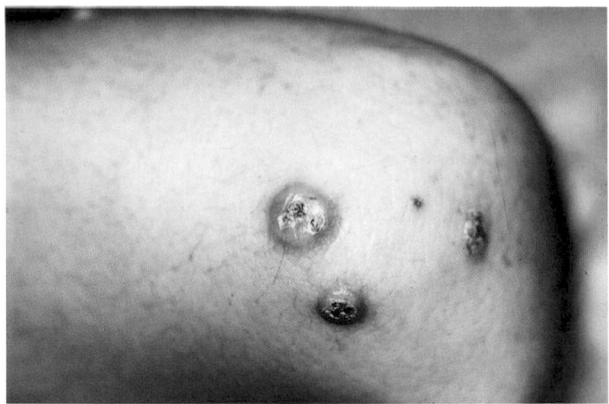

Plate 53 Wegener's granulomatosis. No cutaneous lesions are specific for this disease, as a wide range of presentations is possible. This patient had nodulopapules with necrotic centers. (From Sams and Sams, Cutaneous Manifestations. In: *Vasculitis* (G. V. Ball and S. L. Bridges, Jr, eds), 1st edn. Oxford University Press, 2002.)

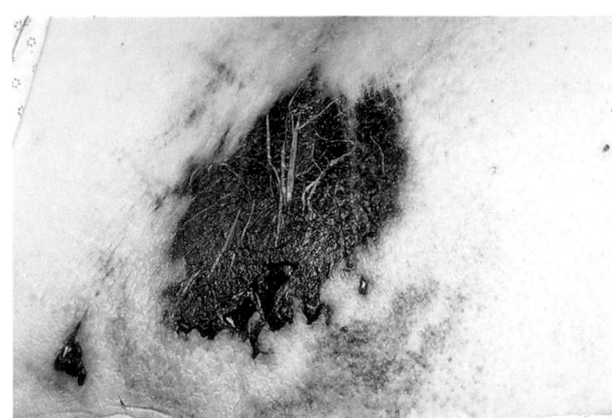

Plate 54 Churg–Strauss syndrome. A large purpuric plaque with stellate-shaped borders. Necrosis and ulcer formation occurred. (From Sams and Sams, Cutaneous Manifestations. In: *Vasculitis* (G. V. Ball and S. L. Bridges, Jr, eds), 1st edn. Oxford University Press, 2002.)

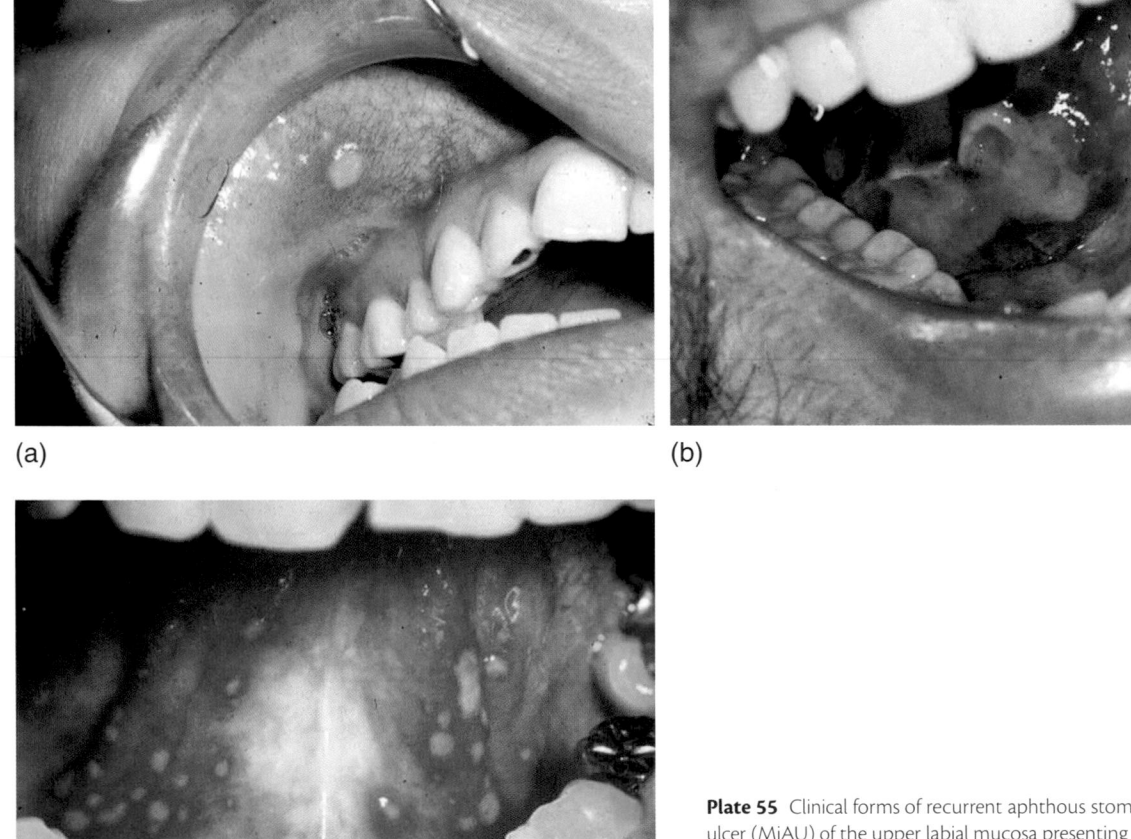

(a)

(b)

(c)

Plate 55 Clinical forms of recurrent aphthous stomatitis (RAS). (a) Minor aphthous ulcer (MiAU) of the upper labial mucosa presenting as a superficial, small (<1.0 cm) discrete, round to oval, shallow ulceration. The ulcer is covered by a yellow-tan fibrinopurulent membrane and is surrounded by an erythematous halo. (b) Major aphthous ulcer (MjAU) involving the ventral surface of the tongue as an irregular, large (>1.0 cm) deep ulceration. (c) Numerous herpetiform ulcers on the ventral surface of the tongue (Courtesy of Dr Craig B. Fowler).

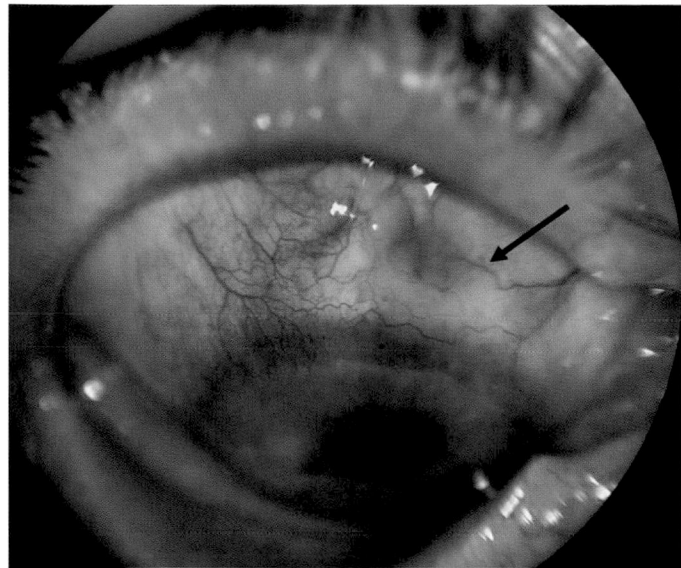

Plate 56 Peripheral ulcerative keratitis involving the superior peripheral cornea, arrow showing an area of sclera and peripheral cornea with ischemia and non-perfusion.

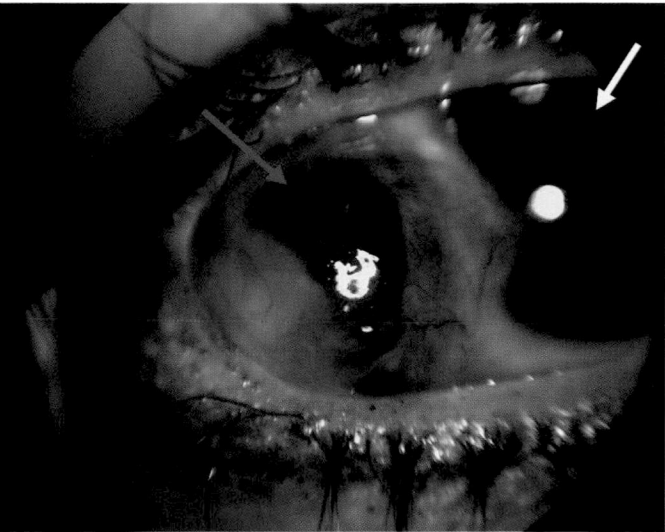

Plate 57 Sequelae of necrotizing scleritis in a patient with Wegener's granulomatosis. Red arrow shows a large area of scleral loss with uveal show that is covered only with a thin layer of overlying epithelium. White arrow points to the cornea and the anterior chamber.

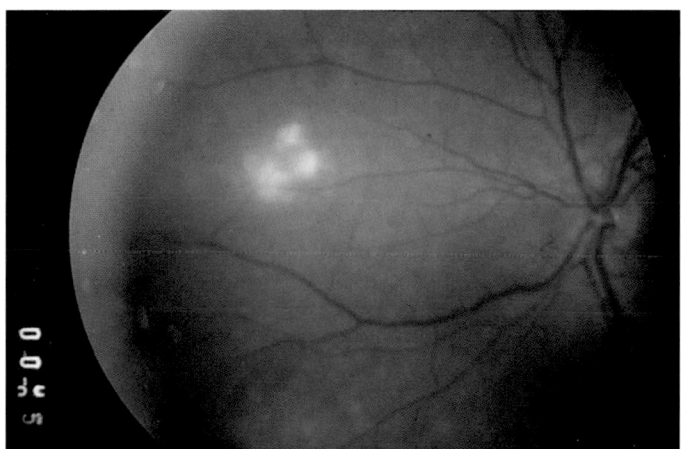

Plate 58 Perivascular exudation indicating retinal vasculitis in a patient with polyarteritis nodosa.

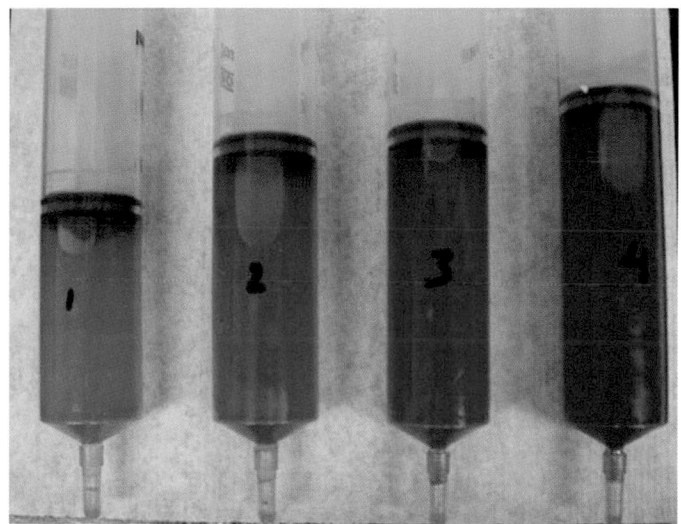

Plate 59 Diffuse alveolar hemorrhage is diagnosed during bronchoscopy when serial aliquots of lavagate demonstrate a persistently bloody return. Photograph courtesy of Gregory P. Cosgrove, MD.

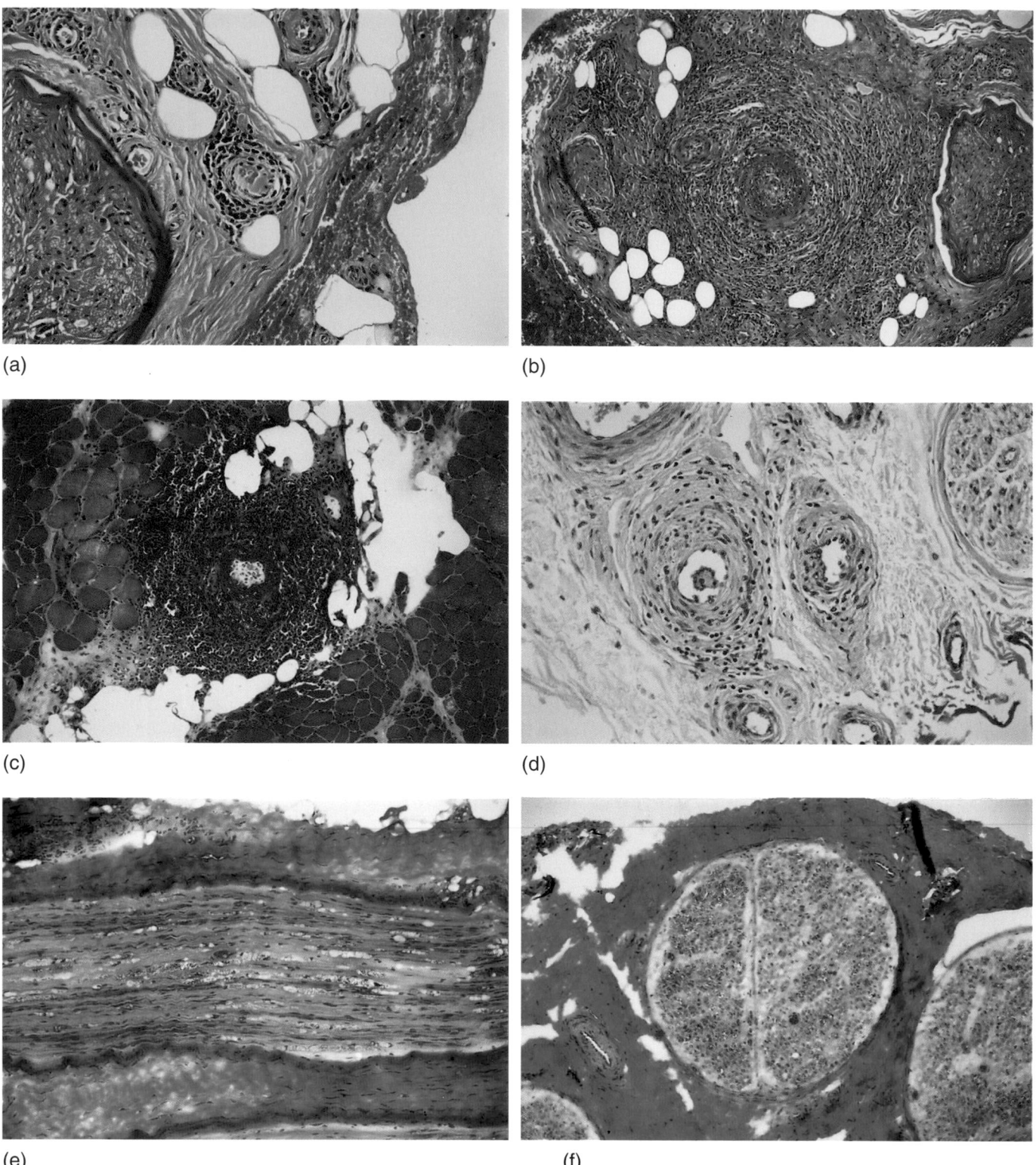

Plate 60 (a) Perivascular collection of mononuclear inflammatory cells (Type III) in the small arteriole in the epineurial space. There is no intramural infiltration of inflammatory cells or fibrinoid necrosis. Paraffin section H & E, magnification 250×. (b) Active vasculitis (Type I) in the larger arteriole in the epineurial space. There is intramural infiltration of mononuclear cells and fibrinoid necrosis of muscular and adventitial layers and near occlusion due to intimal thickening. The arteriole is enlarged due to active vasculitic process. Paraffin section. H & E, magnification 100×. (c) Active vasculitis (Type I) in the arteriole in the perimysial space in muscle. Intimal thickening, intramural infiltrations of mononuclear inflammatory cells, and fibrinoid necrosis of muscular and adventitial layers of arteriole are seen. The arteriole is enlarged due to active vasculitic process. Frozen section. H & E, magnification 100×. (d) Inactive vasculitis (Type II). Thick intimal layer and scattered intramural inflammatory cells in the muscular and adventitial layers of small arteriole in the epineurial space are present. Paraffin section H & E, magnification 100×. (e) Prominent myelin-digestion chambers (vacuoles) such as these are indicative of axonal degeneration in one nerve fascicle. Myelin remnants (ovoids) are stained as red. Frozen section. Modified trichrome, magnification 100×. (f) Selective fascicular atrophy indicative of ischemic neuropathy. Loss of myelinated fibers in the one half of fascicle (arrow) is due to occlusion of vasa nervorum supplying blood to this section of fascicle. Myelinated fibers are stained as 'red', magnification 100×.

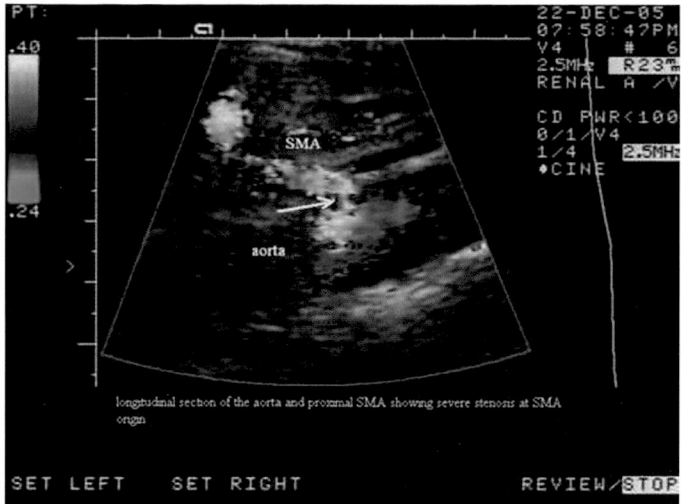

Plate 61 Arterial duplex examination of the aorta, celiac artery, and superior mesenteric arteries in a case of Takayasu's arteritis showing narrowing of superior mesenteric artery (arrow).

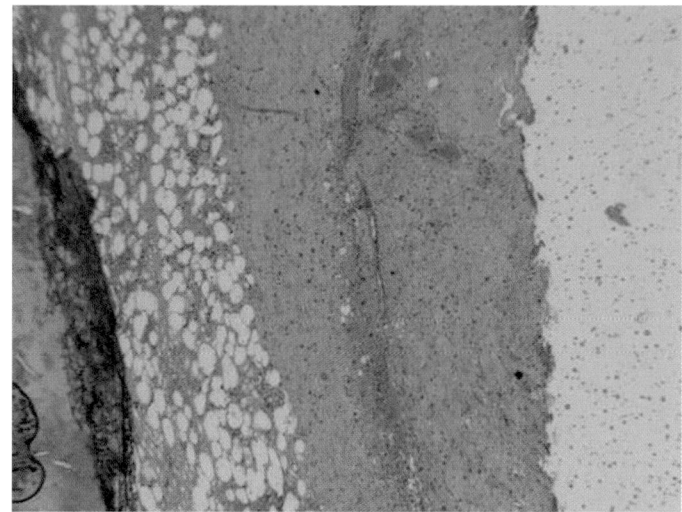

Plate 62 Polyarteritis nodosa. Microscopic examination (H and E staining) of celiac artery aneurysm, surgically removed from a patient with polyarteritis nodosa.

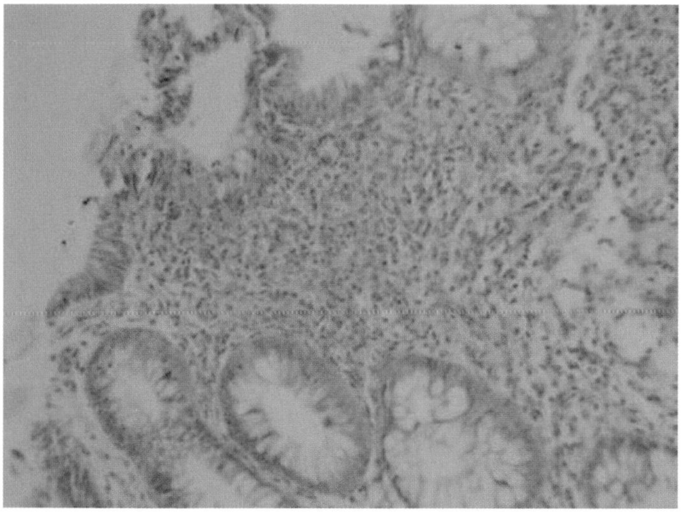

(a)

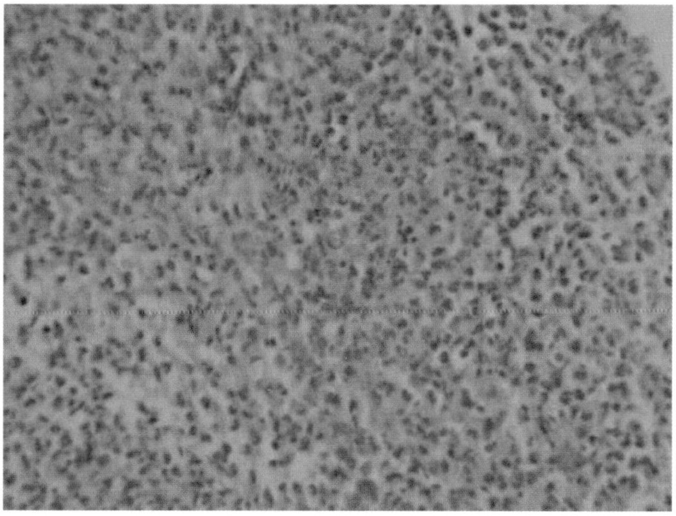

(b)

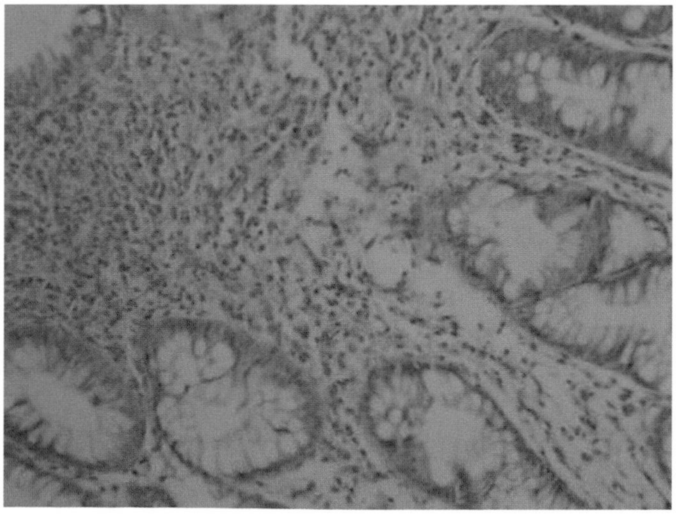

(c)

Plate 63 Behçet's syndrome. Portions of colonic mucosa showing focal crypt distortion, surface mucosal erosions (a), and necrotic debris heavily infiltrated by neutrophils (b). The mucosal tissue shows focal crypt distortion and moderate infiltration of the lamina propria by neutrophils and mononuclear cells (c).

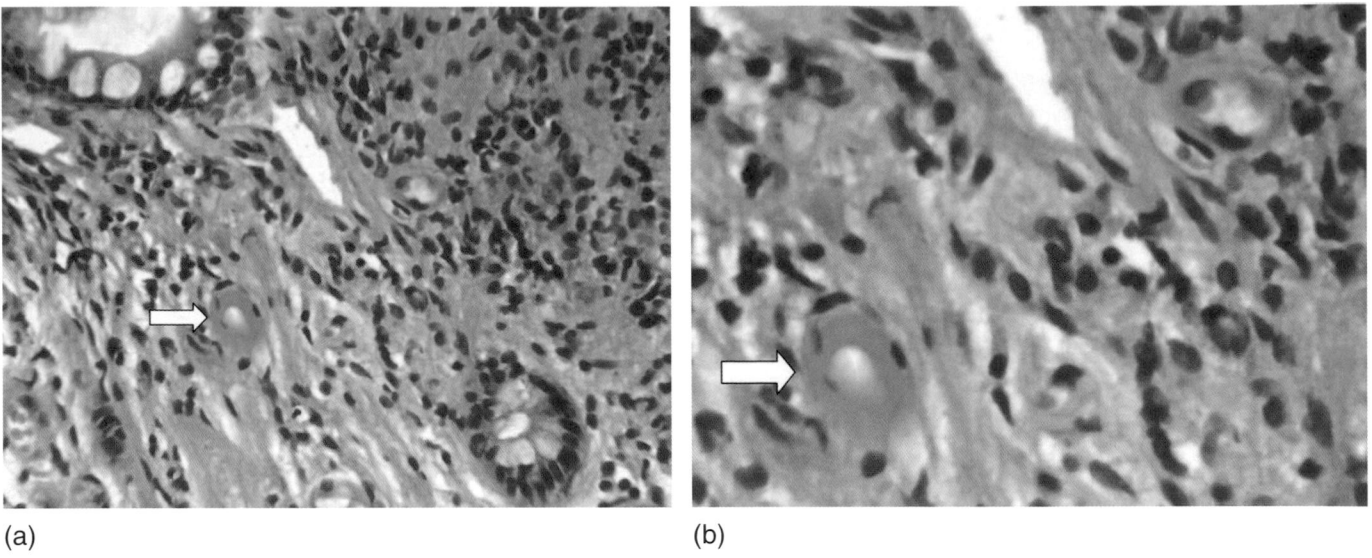

(a)　　　　　　　　　　　　　　　(b)

Plate 64 Findings of non-specific vasculitis. Surgically obtained section of ileum in a case of leucocytoclastic vasculitis (H and E staining). Small vessels show wall infiltration with mononuclear cells and neutrophils (white arrow). × 200.

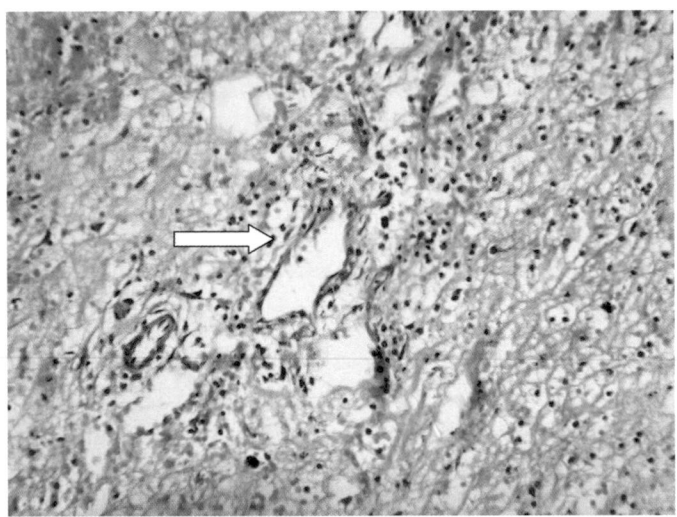

Plate 65 Endoscopically obtained section of ileum in a case of systemic lupus erythematosus (H and E staining), showing infiltration by inflammatory cells. Note hyalinization of the capillary wall with an appearance reminiscent of the 'wire-loop' in lupus nephritis (white arrow). The patient was diagnosed with lupus enteritis. (a) × 400; (b) × 800.

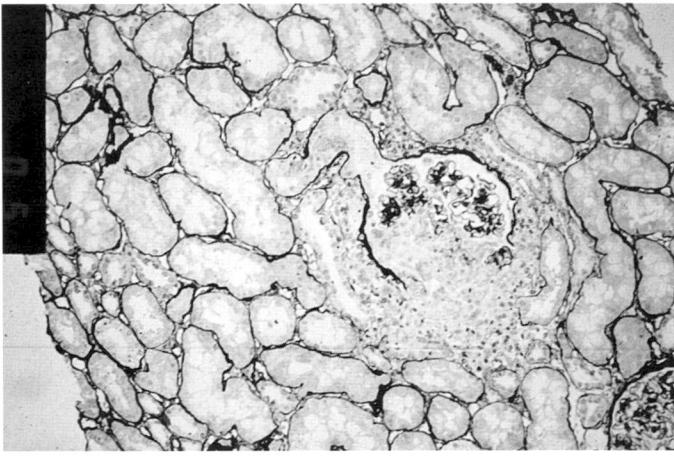

Plate 66 Wegener's granulomatosis in a 72-year-old male, admitted with fever, multiple pulmonary nodules on chest radiograph, microscopic hematuria, mild proteinuria, and a serum creatinine concentration of 135 μmol/L. Renal biopsy shows a periglomerular round cell infiltration, destruction of Bowman's capsule, and an extracapillary crescent. Silvermethenamine, HE, × 50.

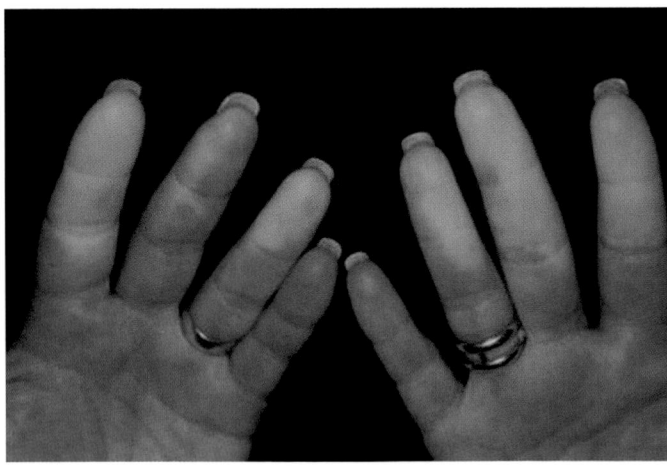

Plate 67 Raynaud's phenomenon, representing digital artery vasospasm leading to pallor. In prolonged vasospasm, pallor gives way to cyanosis, followed by rubor as circulation is restored.

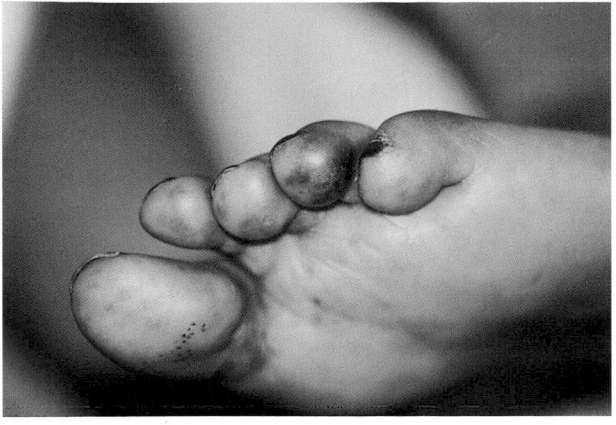

(a)

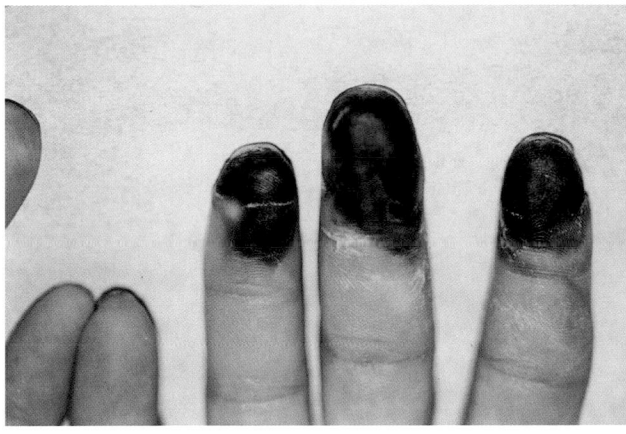

(b)

Plate 68 Digital infarctions occurring in Wegener's granulomatosis and Buerger's disease. (a) Wegener's granulomatosis. (b) Thromboangiitis obliterans (Buerger's disease).

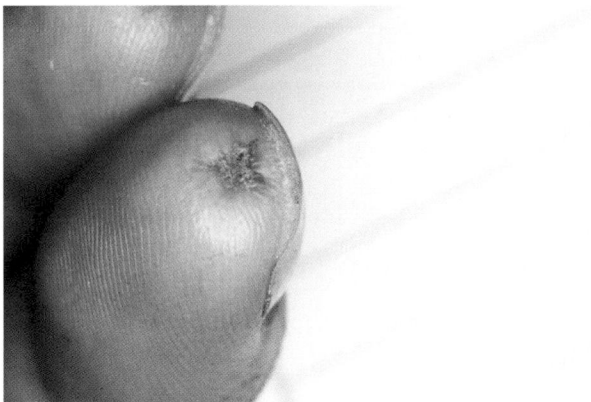

Plate 69 Digital pitting in a patient with diffuse systemic sclerosis.

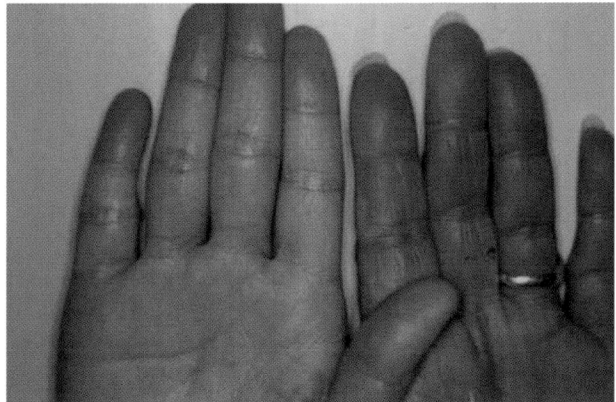

Plate 70 Cyanosis in a patient with systemic sclerosis.

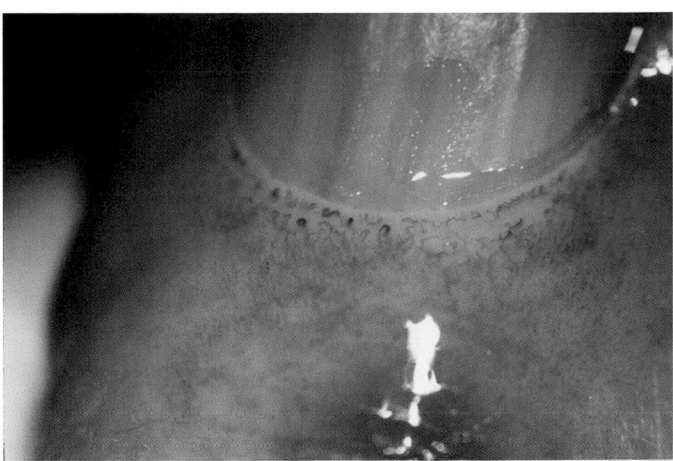

Plate 71 Capillary loop dilatation in a patient with systemic sclerosis.

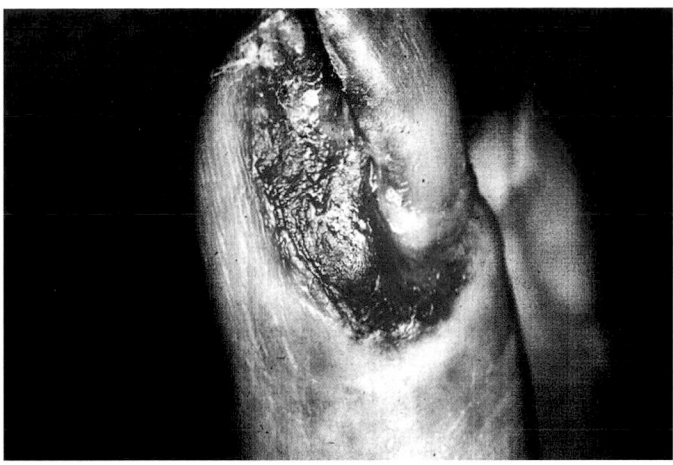

(a)

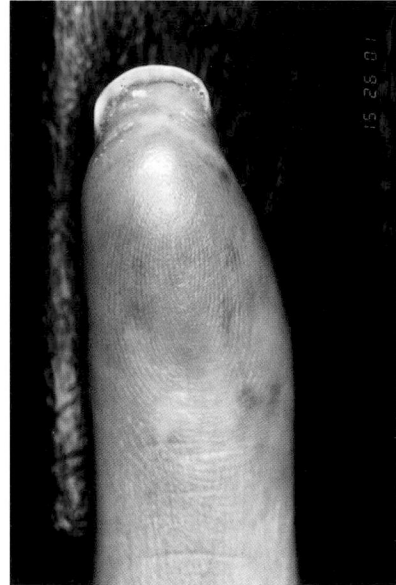

(b)

Plate 72 Digital infarction (a), with subsequent loss of digital pulp (b).

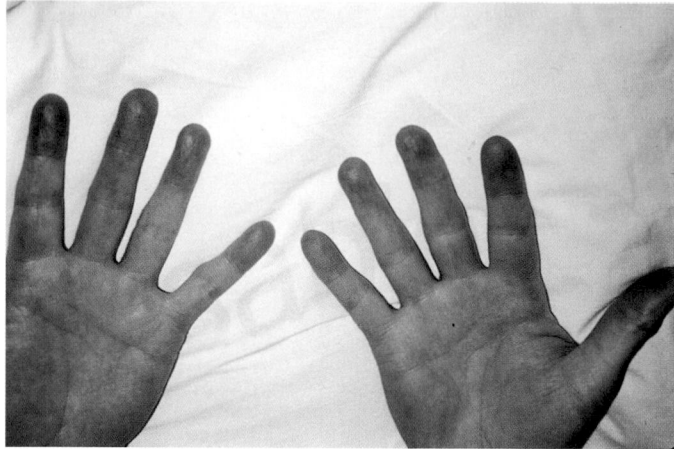

(a)

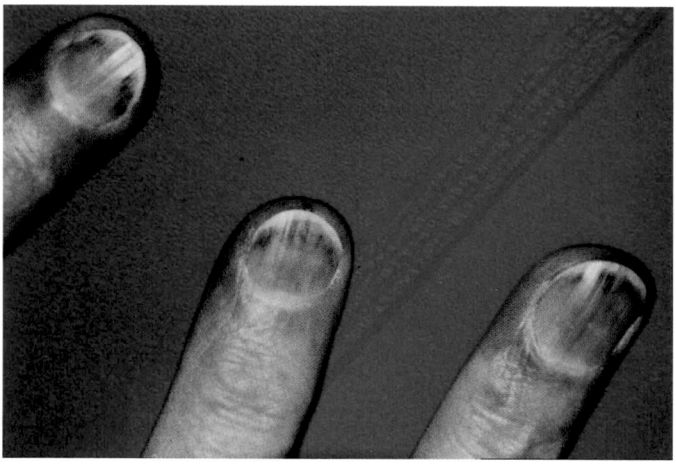

(b)

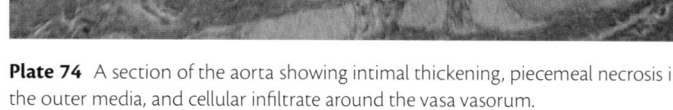

Plate 74 A section of the aorta showing intimal thickening, piecemeal necrosis in the outer media, and cellular infiltrate around the vasa vasorum.

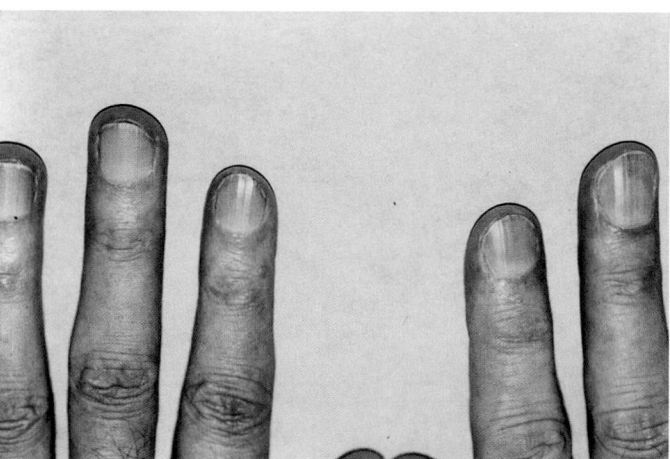

(c)

Plate 73 Digital ischemia in a patient with vasculitis. (a) Purple, cyanotic discoloration on the palmar side. (b) Splinter hemorrhages. (c) Normal fingers again, several months after start of treatment. The splinter hemorrhages have nearly grown out.

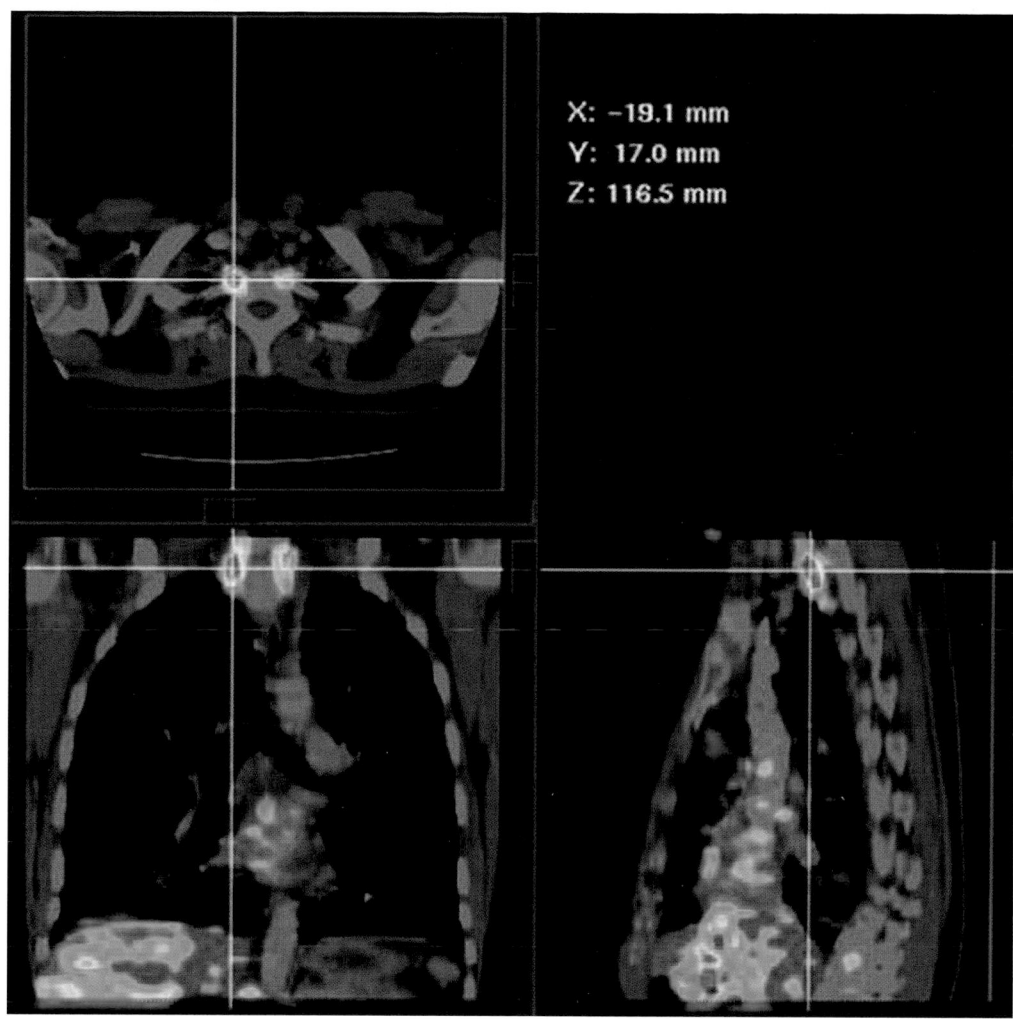

Plate 75 ¹⁸F-FDG PET image coimaged with enhanced CT showed active inflammation in both vertebral arteries.

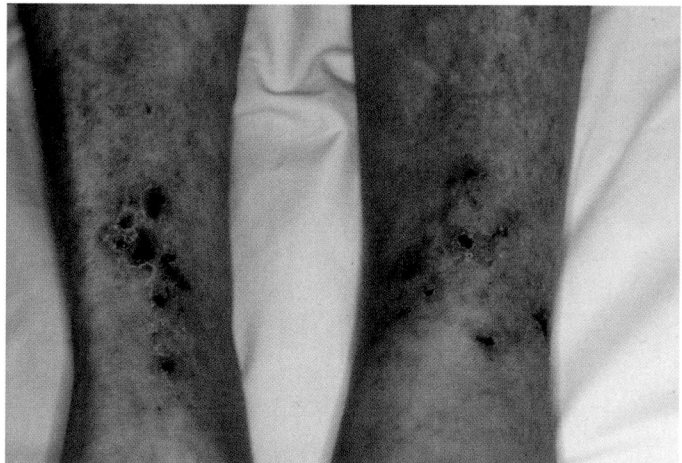

Plate 76 Necrotic purpura of the legs and ankles in a polyarteritis nodosa patient.

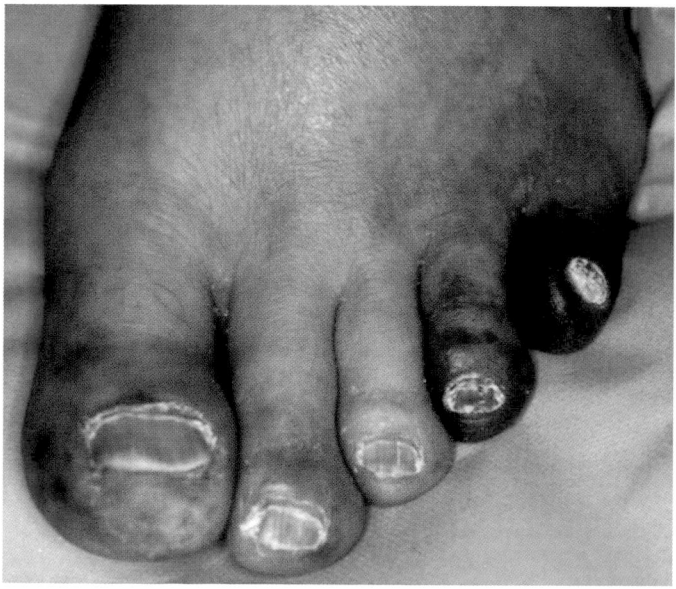

Plate 77 Toe ischemia in a polyarteritis nodosa patient.

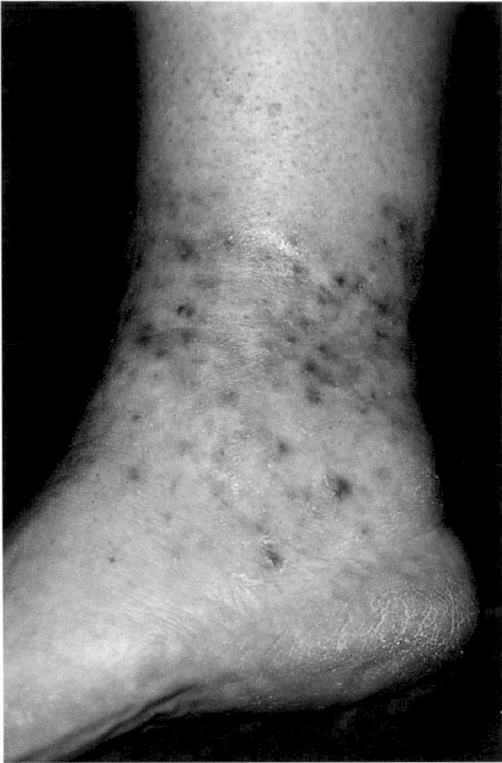

Plate 78 Tender nodules and livedo reticularis about the left ankle of a woman with cutaneous polyarteritis.

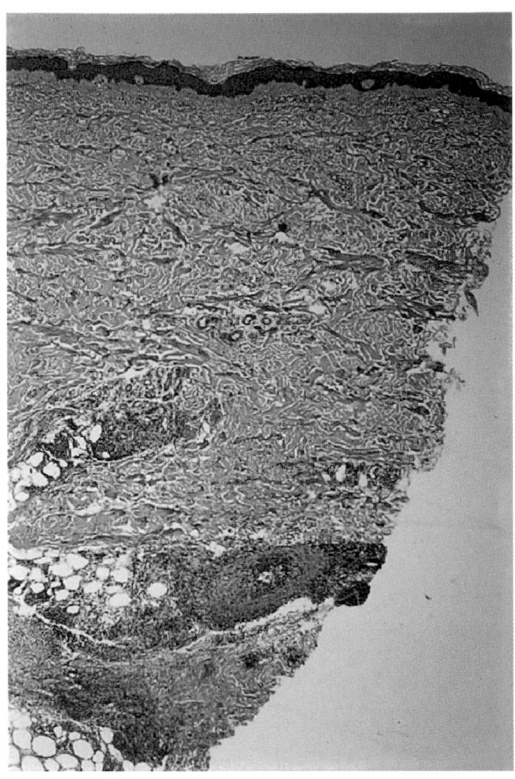

Plate 79 Cutaneous polyarteritis. Skin punch biopsy. Inflammatory cells infiltrating the medium sized arteries of the deep reticular dermis. (H & E stain.)

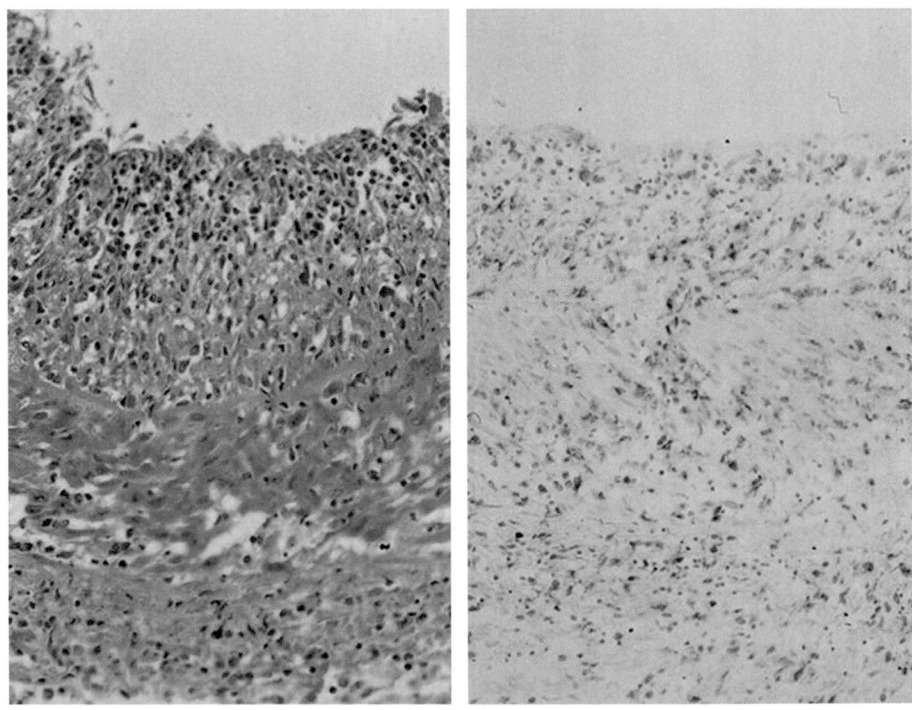

Plate 80 Panarteritis, inflammation of all layers of the artery, of a coronary artery in a patient who died 10 days after the onset of Kawasaki's disease. (a) Hematoxylin and eosin stain; (b) immunohistochemical study using anti-CD68 antibody.

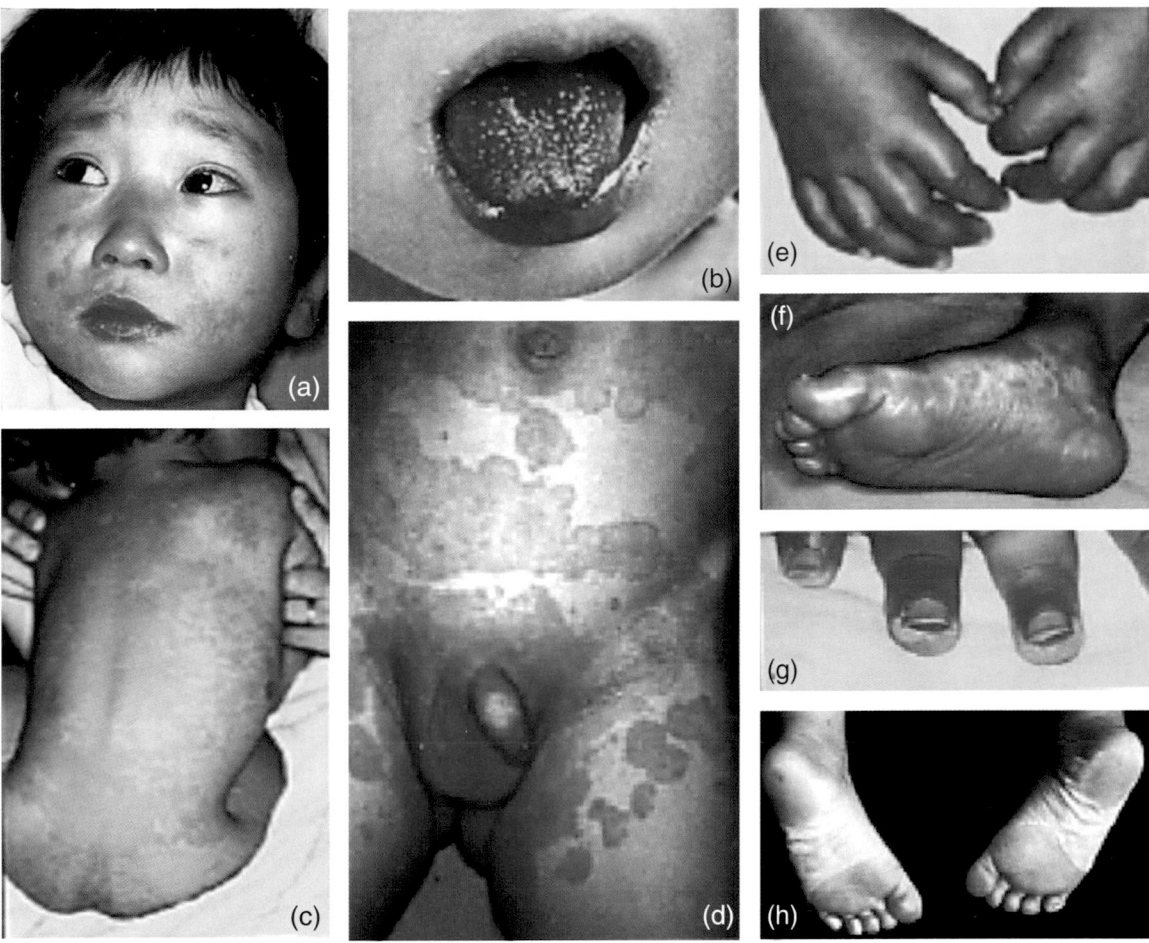

Plate 81 Clinical manifestations of Kawasaki's disease. (a) Typical appearance of Kawasaki face, bilateral conjunctival congestion, and reddening and fissuring of lips. (b) Strawberry tongue. (C and D) Polymorphous exanthema. (e) Indurative edema of the hands. (f) Redness and swelling of the sole. (G and H) Desquamation of fingers and foot.

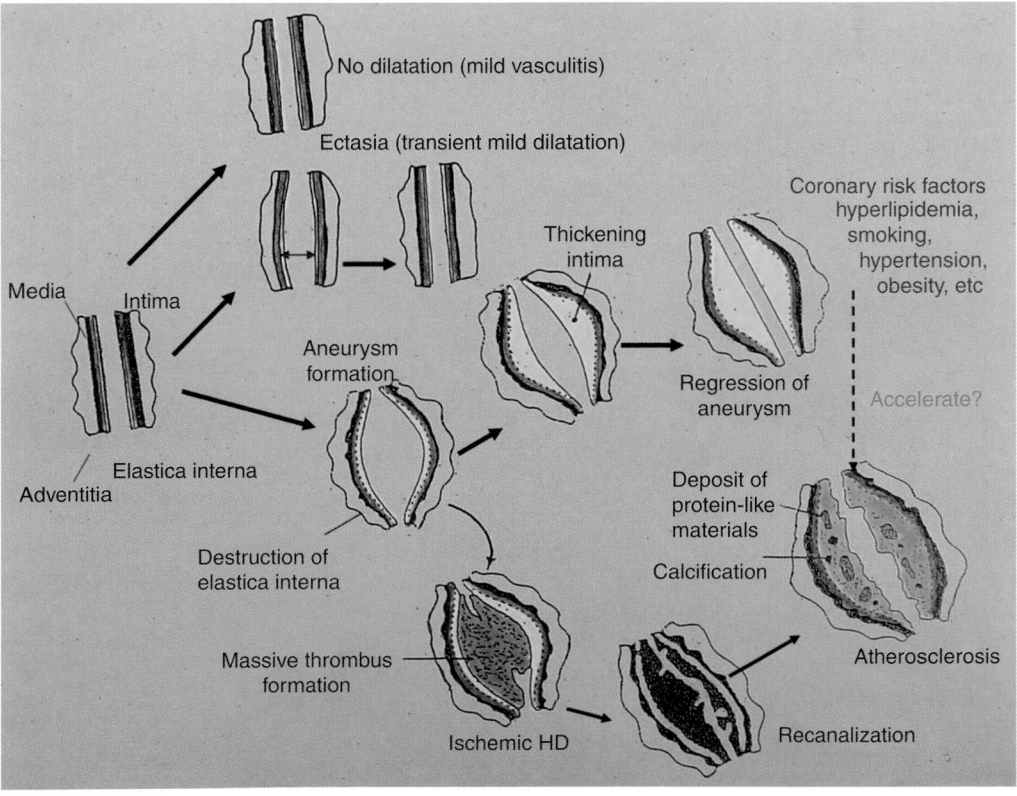

Plate 82 Pathological sequences of coronary aneurysms.

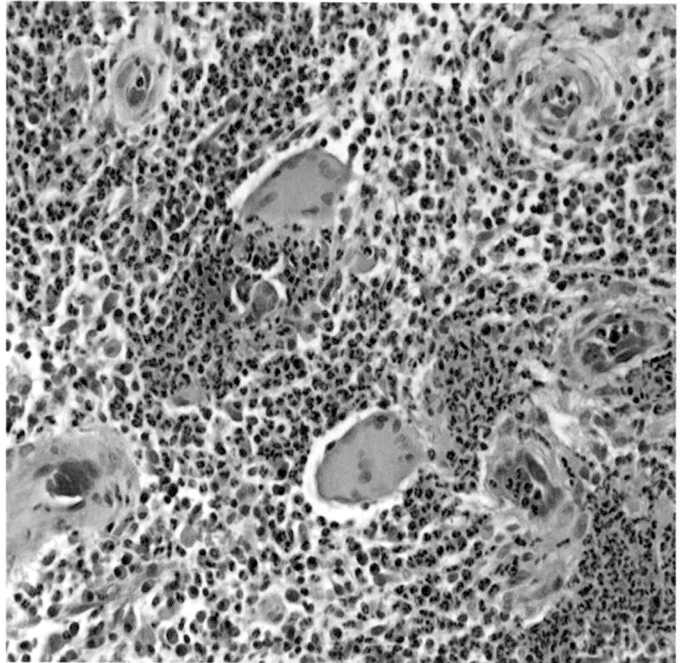

Plate 83 Wegener's granulomatosis—granulomatous lesions in nasal biopsy: typical ill-defined epitheloid cell granulomas with several multinucleated giant cells and neutrophilic microabscesses.

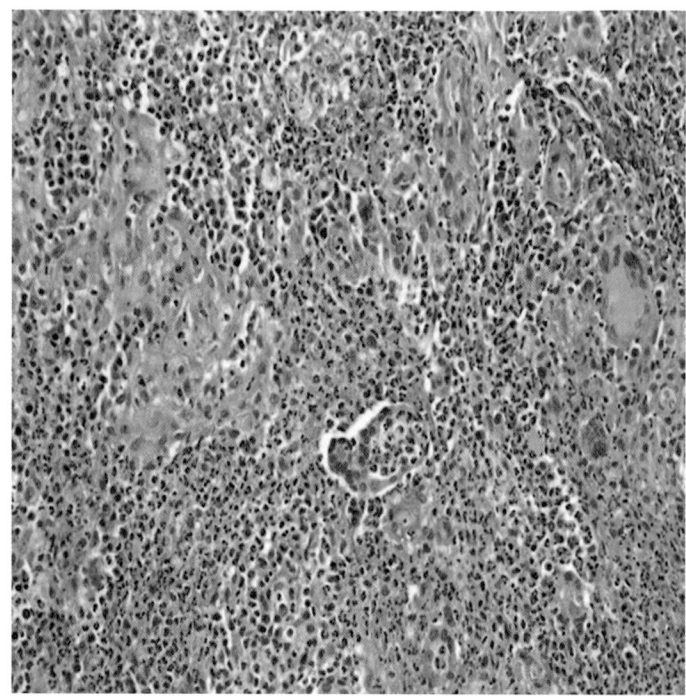

Plate 84 Wegener's granulomatosis—granulomatous and vasculitic lesions in nasal biopsy: diffuse granulomatous tissue, several dispersed multinucleated giant cells, and neutrophilic microabscesses. Vasculitis of small venule (upper right) with onion-skin appearance of vessel wall and intramural inflammatory infiltrates.

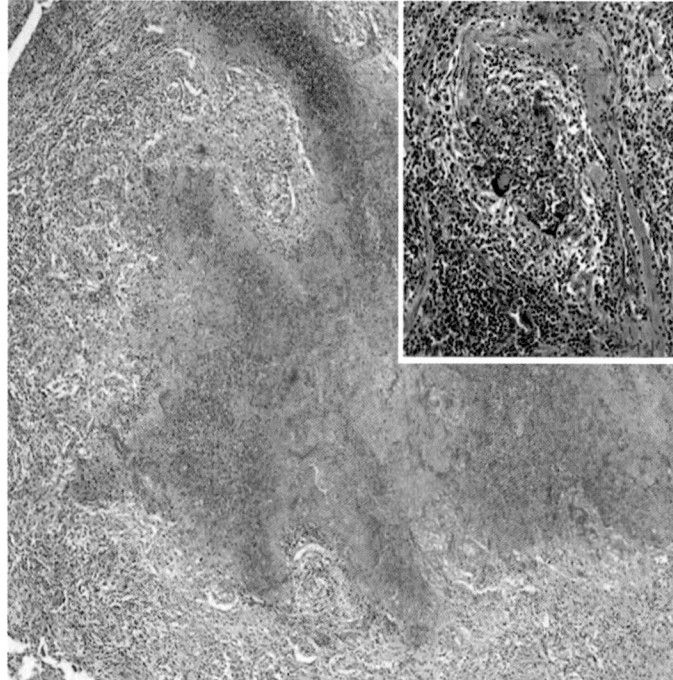

Plate 85 Wegener's granulomatosis—granulomatous lesions in nasal biopsy: Destruction of nasal cartilage (a) and bone (b) by inflammatory granulomatous tissue.

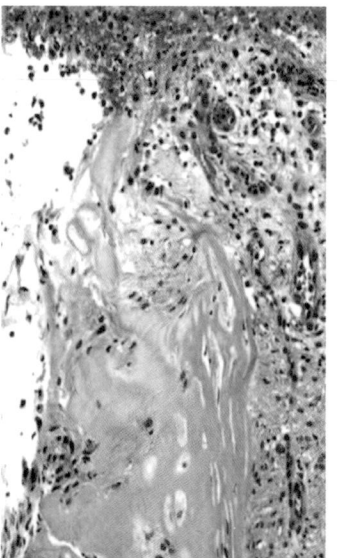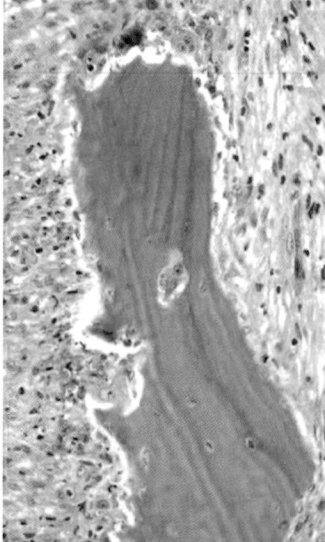

Plate 86 Wegener's granulomatosis—granulomatous lesions in lung biopsy: large necrotizing granuloma with palisading histiocytes and large central geographical necrosis. Inset: granulomatous vasculitis of lung (medium-sized vessel) with obliteration of vessel lumen and dense intramural inflammatory infiltrates, including numerous multinucleated giant cells.

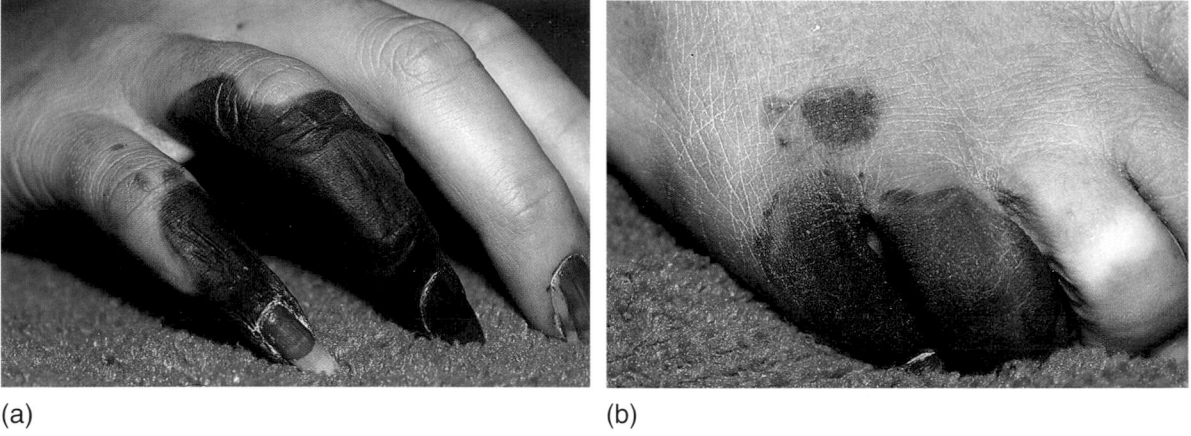

(a)   (b)

Plate 87 Hand (a) and foot (b) of an 18-year-old woman with digital necrosis due to Wegener's granulomatosis. (Courtesy of Dr Gene Ball.)

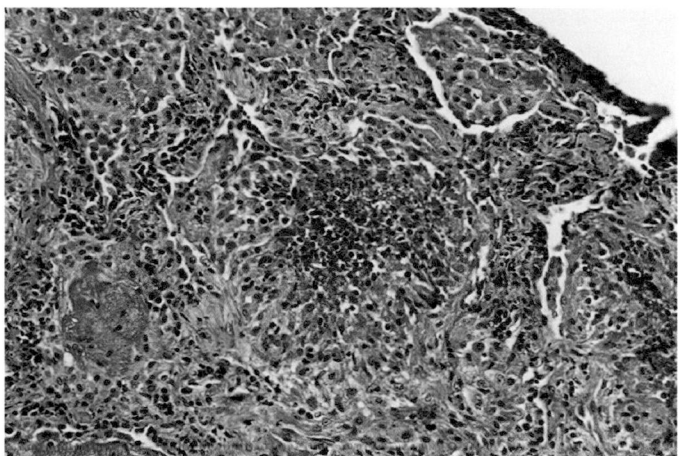

Plate 88 Extravascular granuloma in the lung, also referred to as the Churg–Strauss or allergic granuloma. (Courtesy of Dr Jeffrey L. Myers). From: R. A. DeRemee. Churg–Strauss Syndrome. In: *Vasculitis*, 1st edn, G. V. Ball and S. L. Bridges, Jr, eds. Oxford University Press, 2002.

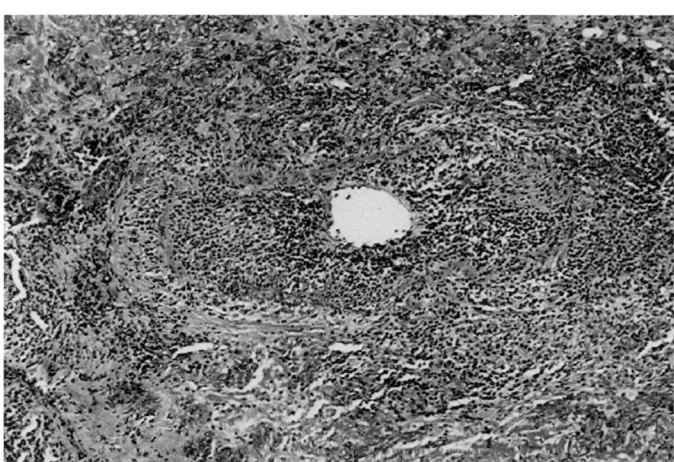

Plate 89 Churg–Strauss syndrome. Necrotizing vasculitis of a small pulmonary artery with prominent eosinophilic infiltration. (Courtesy of Dr Jeffrey L. Myers). From: R. A. DeRemee. Churg–Strauss Syndrome. In: *Vasculitis*, 1st edn, G. V. Ball and S. L. Bridges, Jr, eds. Oxford University Press, 2002.

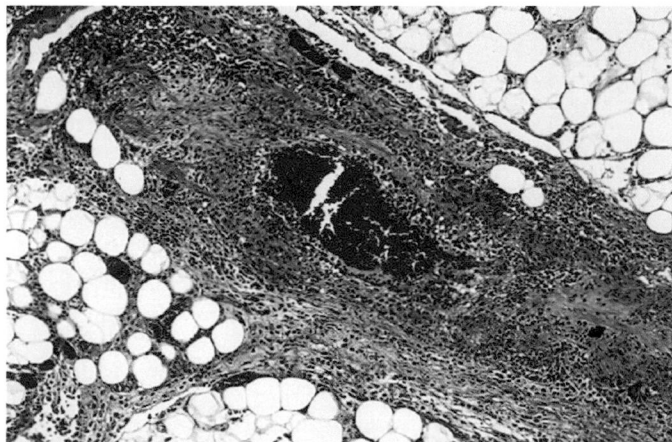

Plate 90 Churg–Strauss syndrome. Necrotizing vasculitis of a small extrapulmonary artery. (Courtesy of Dr Jeffrey L. Myers). From: R. A. DeRemee. Churg–Strauss Syndrome. In: *Vasculitis*, 1st edn, (G. V. Ball and S. L. Bridges, Jr, eds). Oxford University Press, 2002.

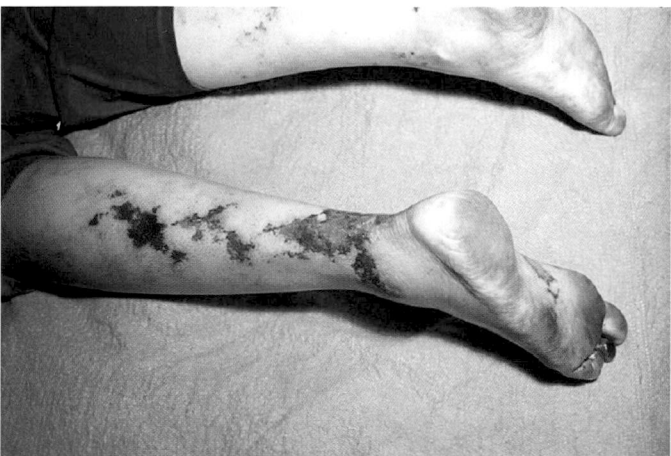

Plate 91 Extensive, rapidly developing, necrosis due to rheumatoid vasculitis in a 60-year-old woman, who subsequently died with inflammation in the coronary arteries as well. (Courtesy of Dr Gene Ball.) From: R. Jones and L. Moreland. Vasculitis in Primary Connective Tissue Diseases. In: *Vasculitis*, 1st edn. (G. V. Ball and S. L. Bridges, Jr., eds). Oxford University Press, 2002.

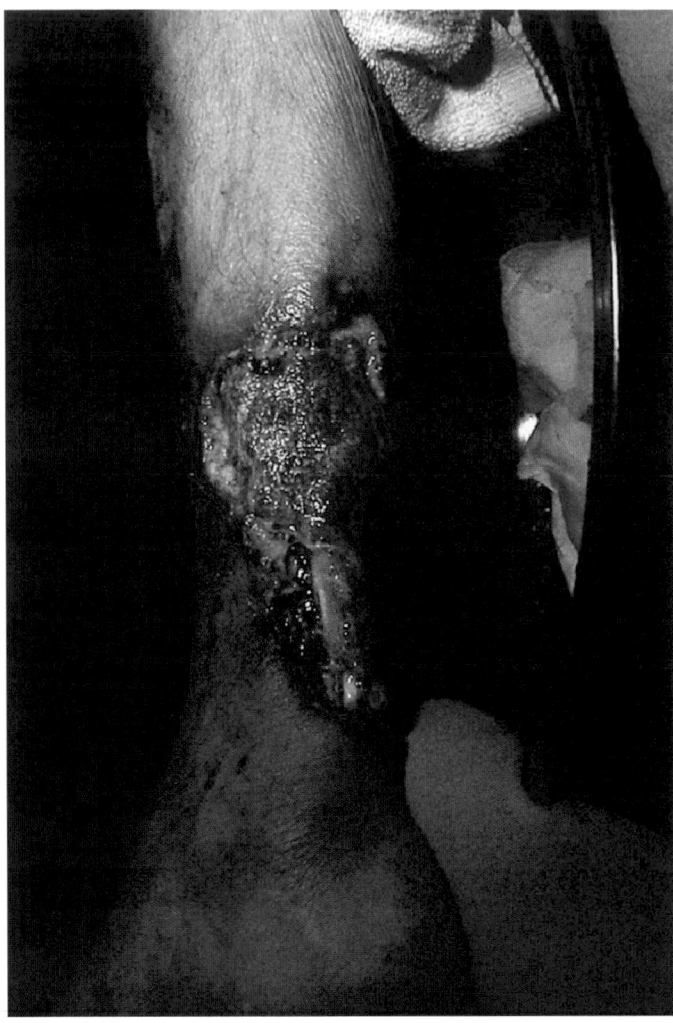

Plate 92 Vasculitis in a young woman with systemic lupus erythematosus. (Courtesy of Dr Gene Ball.) From: R. Jones and L. Moreland. Vasculitis in Primary Connective Tissue Diseases. In: *Vasculitis*, 1st edn. (G. V. Ball and S. L. Bridges, Jr., eds). Oxford University Press, 2002.

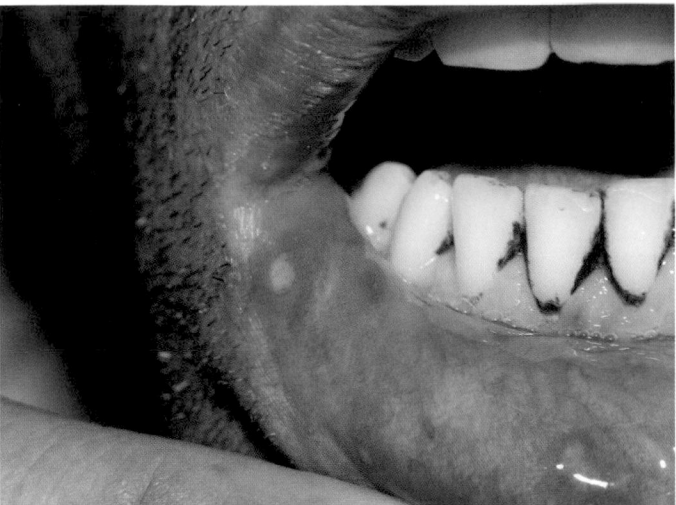

Plate 93 Behçet's syndrome. Oral ulcers.

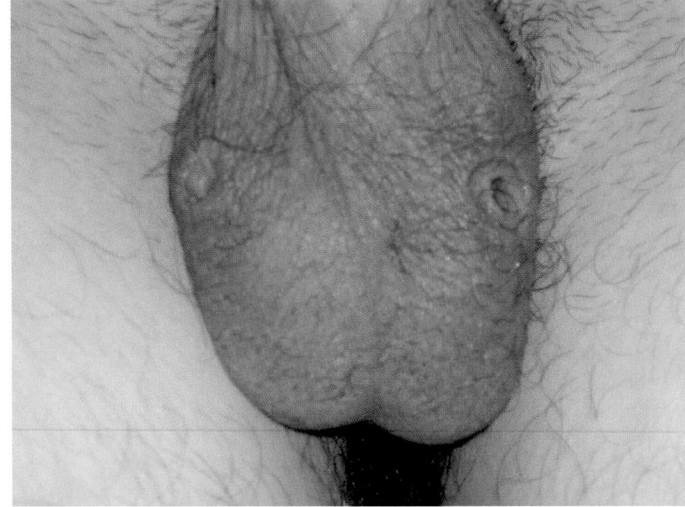

Plate 94 Behçet's syndrome. Genital ulcers.

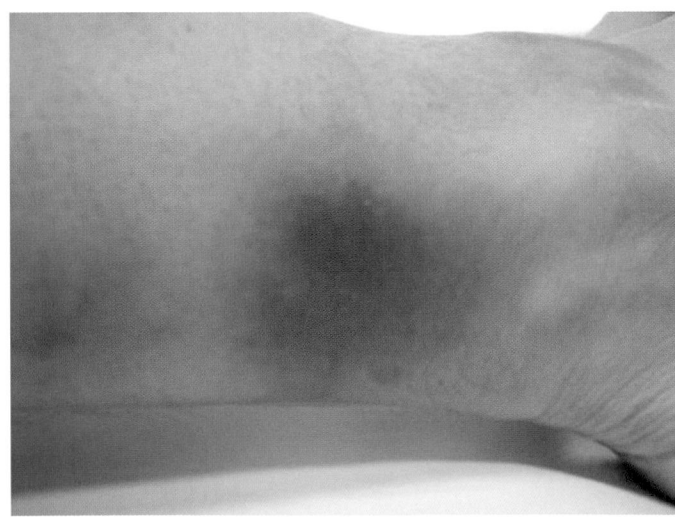

Plate 95 Behçet's syndrome. Erythema nodosum-like lesion.

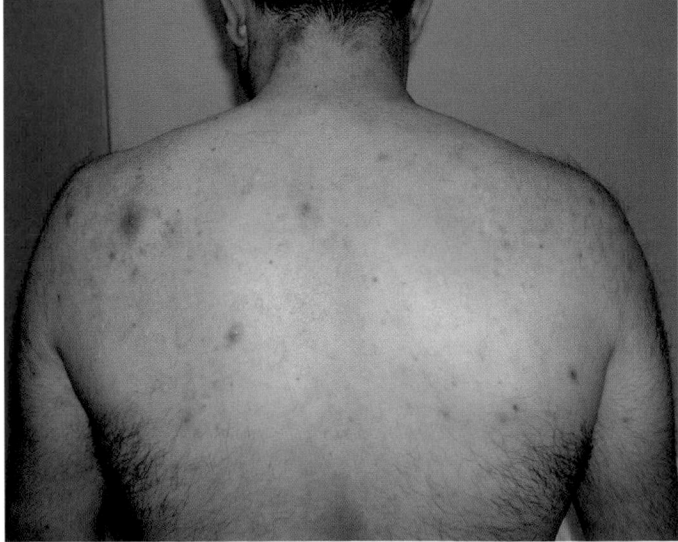

Plate 96 Behçet's syndrome. Osteofollicular (acne)-like lesions.

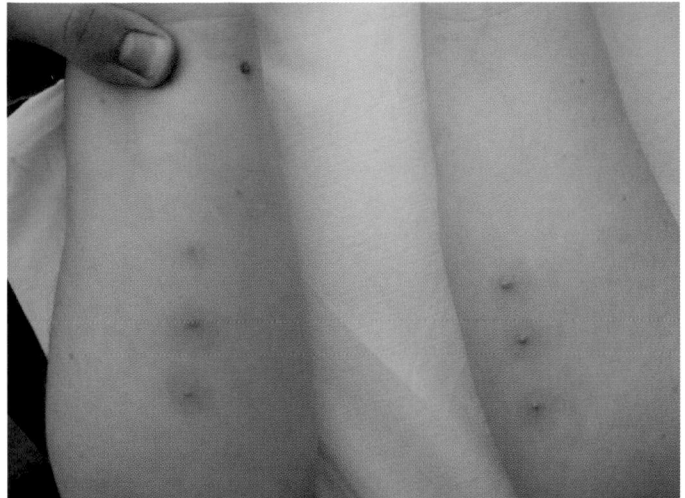

Plate 97 Behçet's syndrome. Positive pathergy reaction.

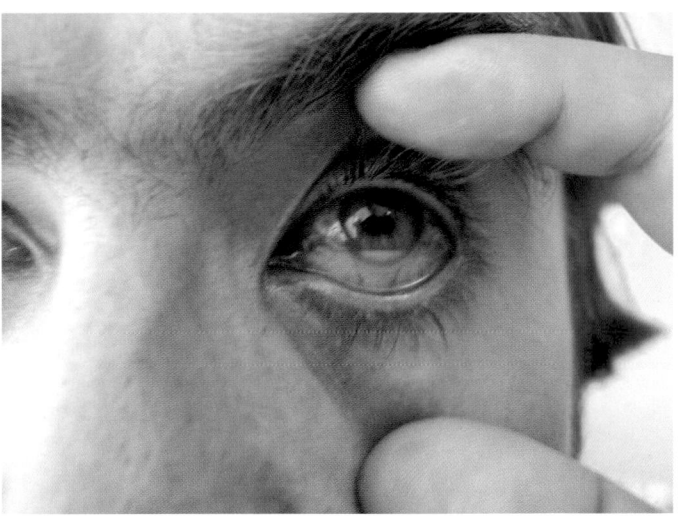

Plate 98 Behçet's syndrome. Hypopyon uveitis.

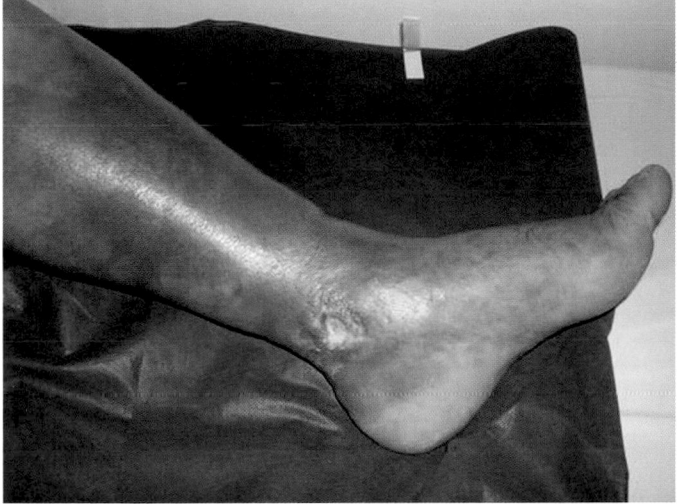

Plate 99 Behçet's syndrome. Chronic thrombosis of the leg veins with hyperpigmentation and a skin ulcer.

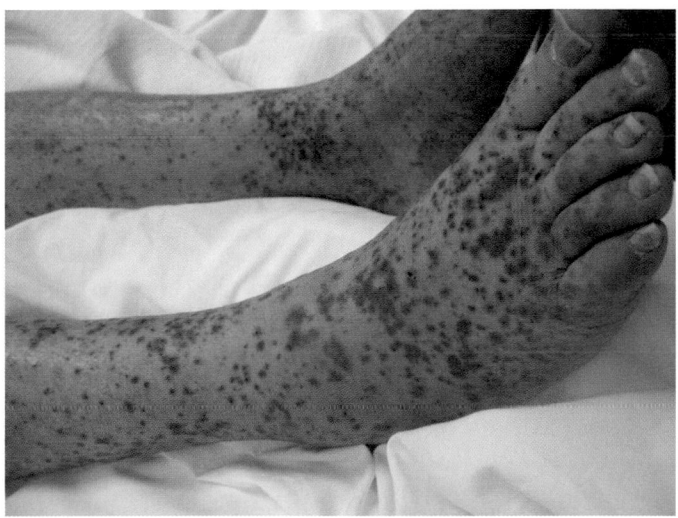

Plate 100 Diffuse palpable purpura on the bilateral lower extremities representing cutaneous small-vessel vasculitis.

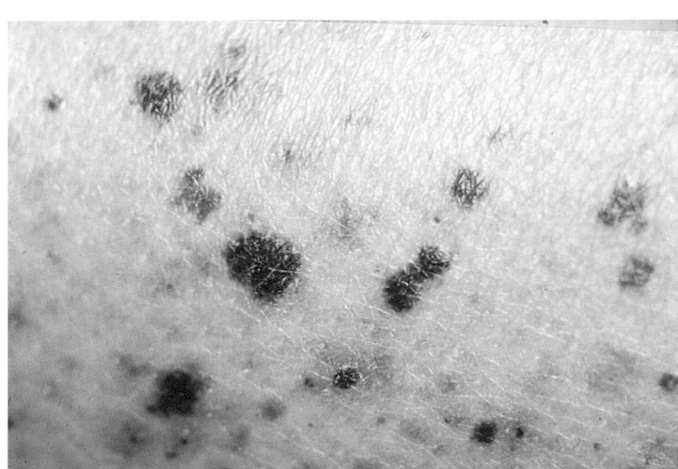

Plate 101 Cutaneous small-vessel vasculitis. Individual lesions are usually less than 1 cm diameter and demonstrate sharply demarcated margins. (From Sams, H. H. and Sams, W. M. Jr (2002). Cutaneous leukocytoplastic vasculitis. In *Vasculitis* (Ball, G. V. and Bridges, S. L. Jr, eds), 1st edn, pp. 467–75. Oxford University Press, New York.)

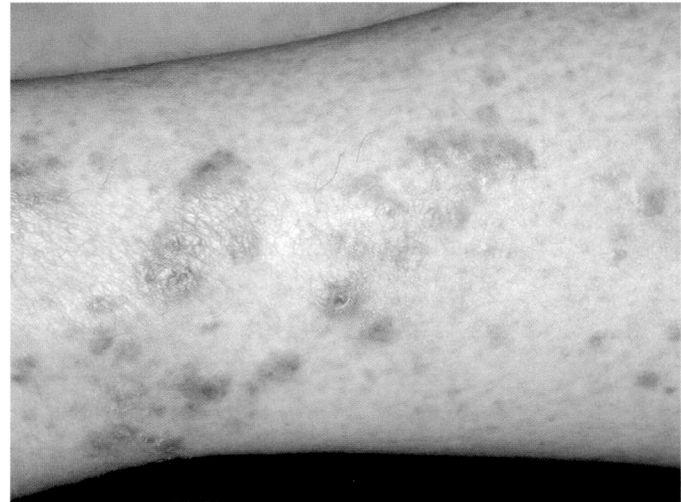

Plate 102 Cutaneous small-vessel vasculitis. Individual lesions may coalesce to larger plaques.

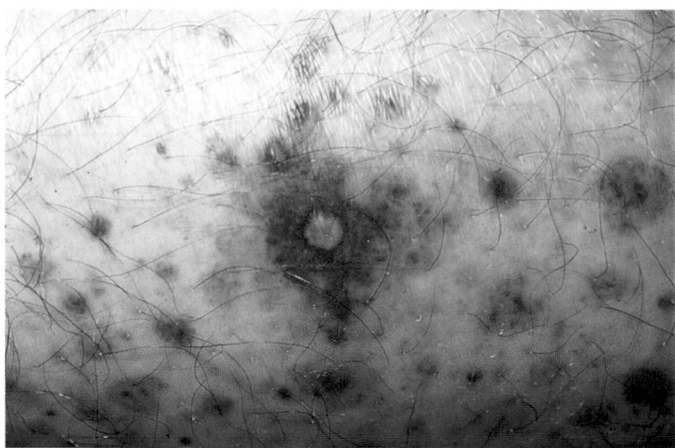

Plate 103 Cutaneous small-vessel vasculitis. Intense neutrophilic infiltrate may lead to pustule formation on a hemorrhagic base. (From Sams, H. H. and Sams, W. M. Jr (2002). Cutaneous leukocytoplastic vasculitis. In *Vasculitis* (Ball, G. V. and Bridges, S. L. Jr, eds), 1st edn, pp. 467–75. Oxford University Press, New York.)

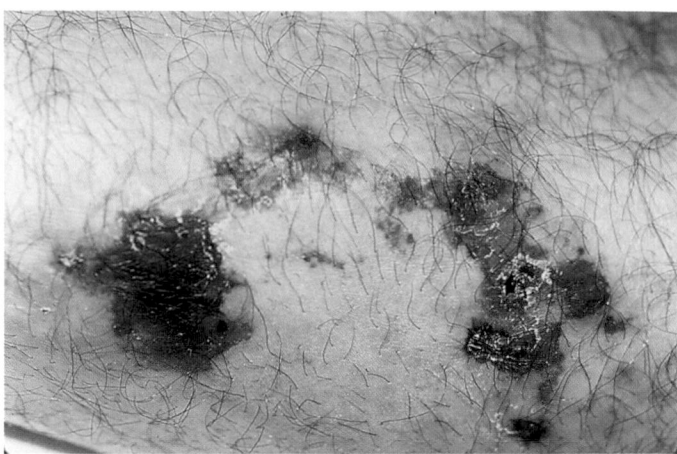

Plate 104 Cutaneous small-vessel vasculitis. With sufficient vascular destruction, necrosis ensues, often with irregular borders. (From Sams, H. H. and Sams, W. M. Jr (2002). Cutaneous leukocytoplastic vasculitis. In *Vasculitis* (Ball, G. V. and Bridges, S. L. Jr, eds), 1st edn, pp. 467–75. Oxford University Press, New York.)

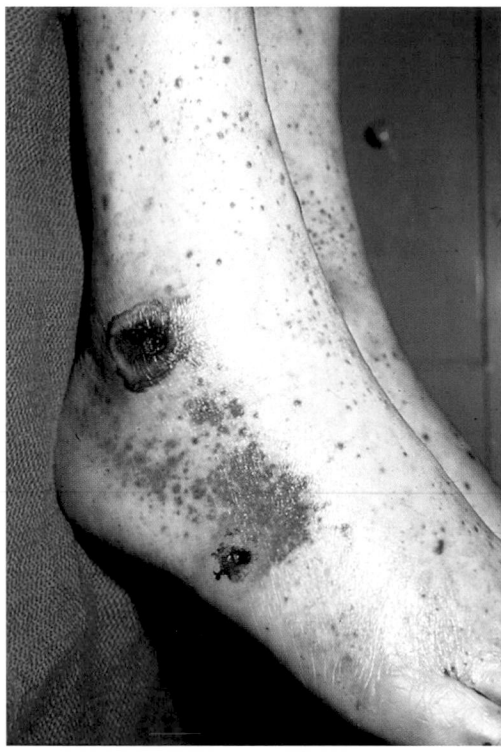

Plate 105 Cutaneous small-vessel vasculitis. Necrosis and blister formation may occur, as this example proximal to the lateral malleolus. (From Sams, H. H. and Sams, W. M. Jr (2002). Cutaneous leukocytoplastic vasculitis. In *Vasculitis* (Ball, G. V. and Bridges, S. L. Jr, eds), 1st edn, pp. 467–75. Oxford University Press, New York.)

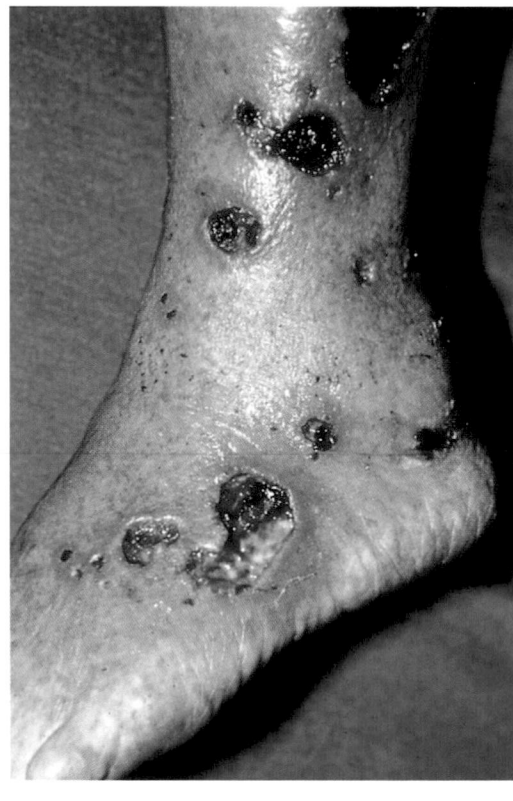

Plate 107 Severe ulcers may form in cutaneous small-vessel vasculitis. (From Sams, H. H. and Sams, W. M. Jr (2002). Cutaneous leukocytoplastic vasculitis. In *Vasculitis* (Ball, G. V. and Bridges, S. L. Jr, eds), 1st edn, pp. 467–75. Oxford University Press, New York.)

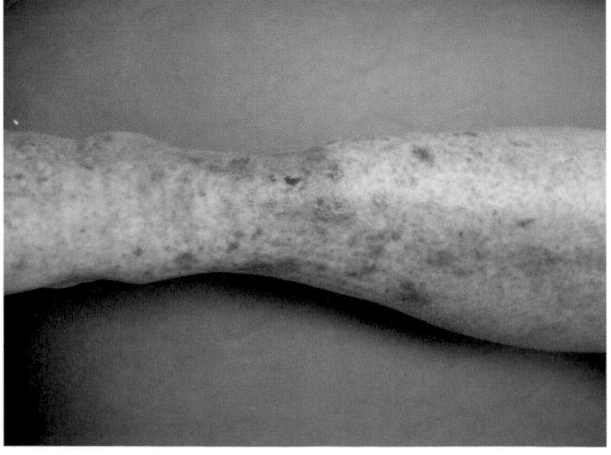

Plate 106 This patient with cutaneous small-vessel vasculitis had palpable purpura complicated by ulceration.

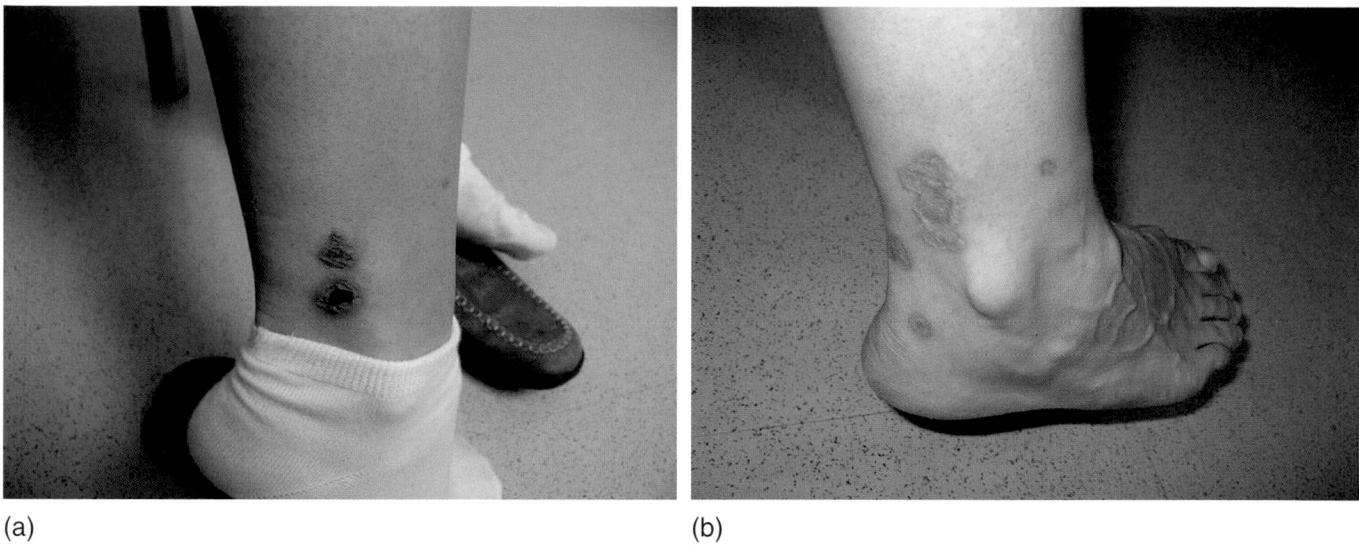

(a) (b)

Plate 108 Ulcerations (a) may heal with scar formation (b), as seen in this 40-year-old woman who had resolution of cutaneous small-vessel vasculitis. (Courtesy of Dr Lou Bridges.)

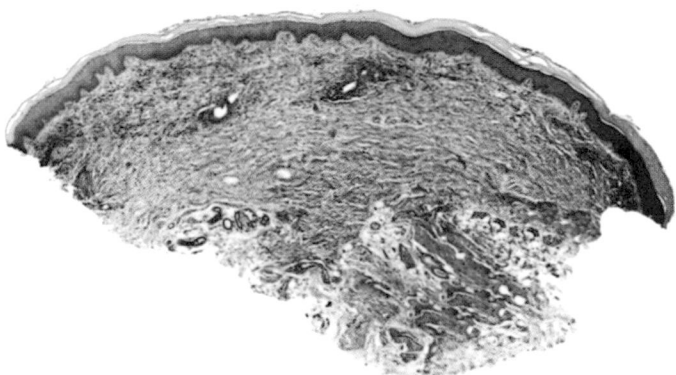

Plate 109 Cutaneous small-vessel vasculitis. Low power histopathologic skin specimen showing dense superficial perivascular inflammation. (Courtesy of Dr Omar Sangueza.)

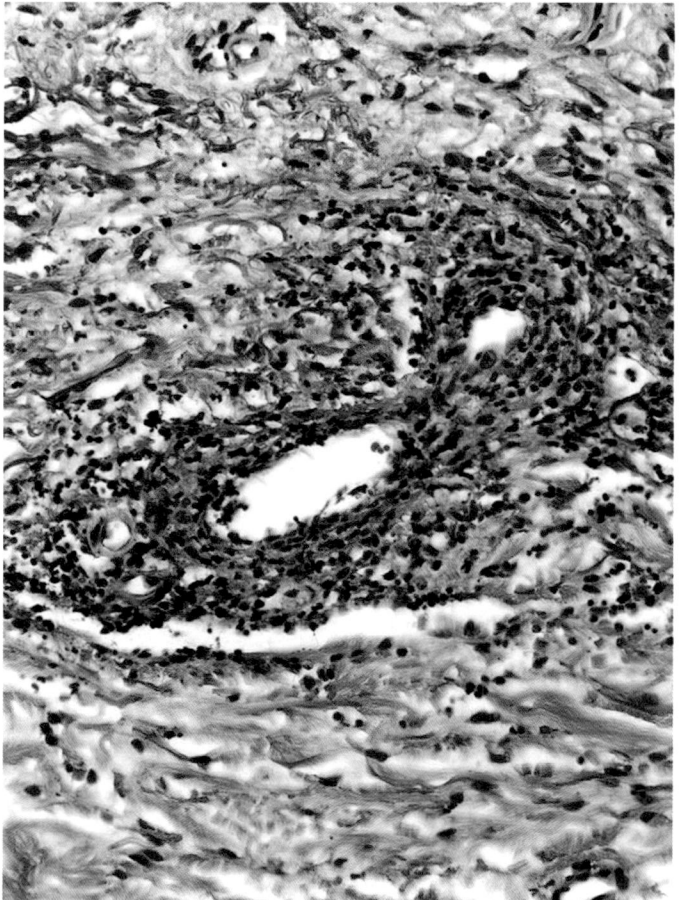

Plate 110 Cutaneous small-vessel vasculitis. The affected small vessel demonstrates fibrinoid necrosis of the wall, neutrophilic infiltration with nuclear dust, and extravasation of red blood cells. (Courtesy of Dr Omar Sangueza.)

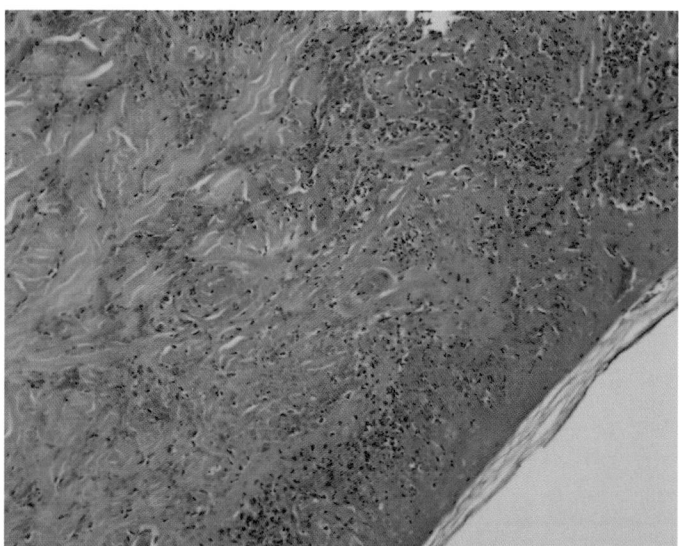

Plate 111 Skin biopsy of a patient with Henoch–Schönlein purpura showing dermal vascular neutrophilic inflammatory infiltration, leukocytoclasia, vessel wall fibrinoid necrosis, and hematic extravasation (Hematoxylin and eosin × 100.)

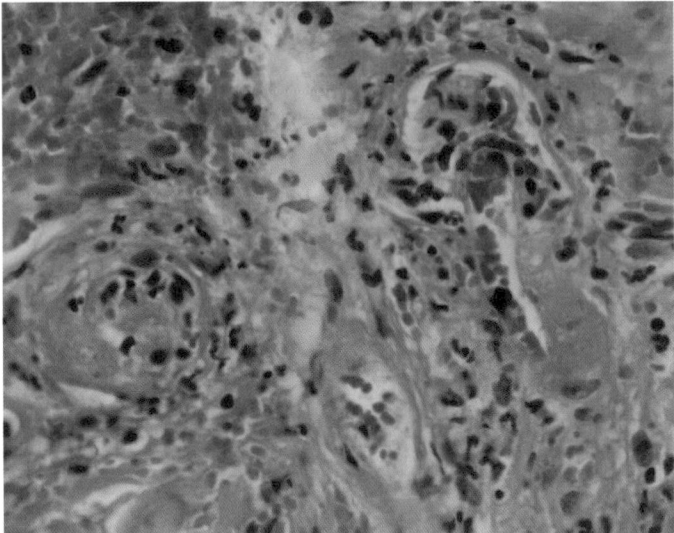

Plate 112 Henoch–Schönlein purpura. Skin biopsy disclosing small-sized blood vessel vasculitis with two vessels showing peripheral leukocytoclasia, fibrin thrombosis, fibrinoid necrosis, and red cell extravasation consistent with leukocytoclastic vasculitis. (Hematoxylin and eosin × 400.)

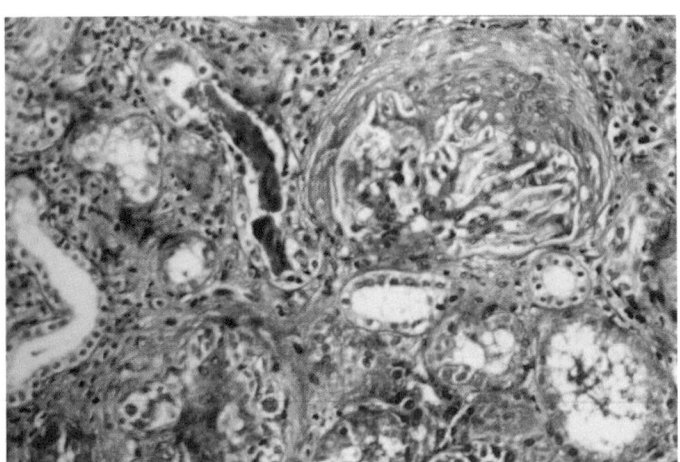

Plate 113 Henoch–Schönlein purpura. Kidney biopsy showing glomerular sclerosis and crescent formation. (Masson × 400.)

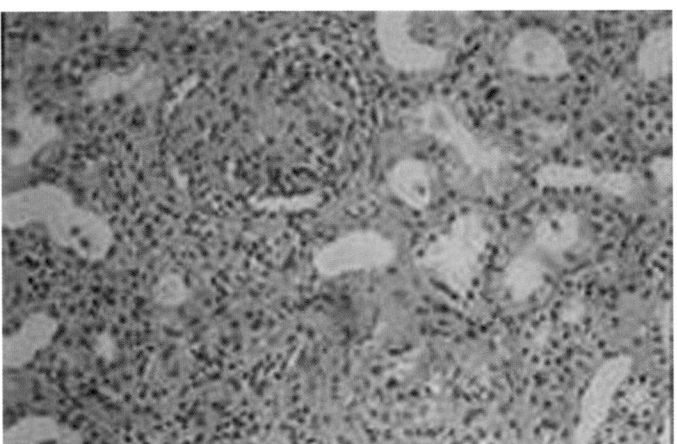

Plate 114 Henoch–Schönlein purpura. Renal biopsy showing two glomeruli. One of them has an extracapillary proliferative crescent that obliterates the glomerular tuft. The other glomerulus shows diffuse mesangial proliferative involvement. (Hematoxylin and eosin × 100.)

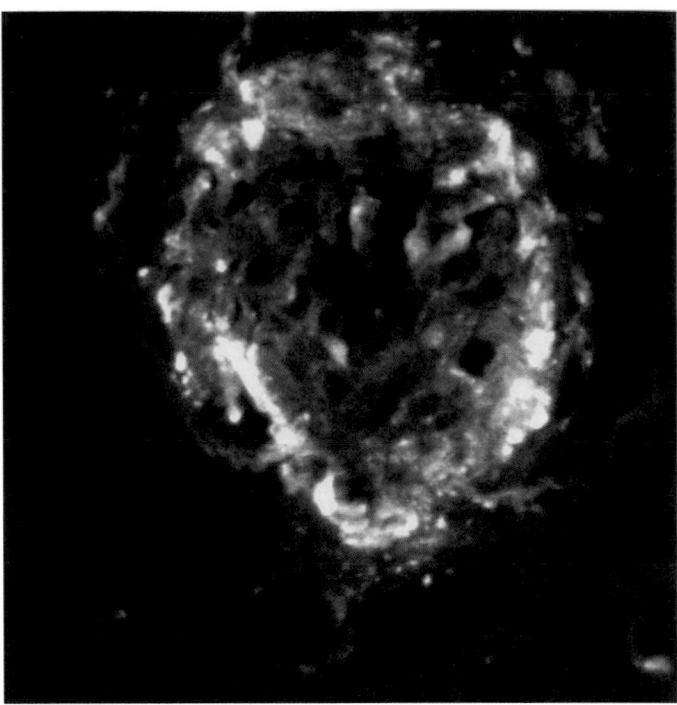

Plate 115 Glomerulus from a patient with Henoch–Schönlein purpura and proliferative mesangial glomerulonephritis with granular mesangial deposits of IgA. (IgA immunofluorescence × 400.)

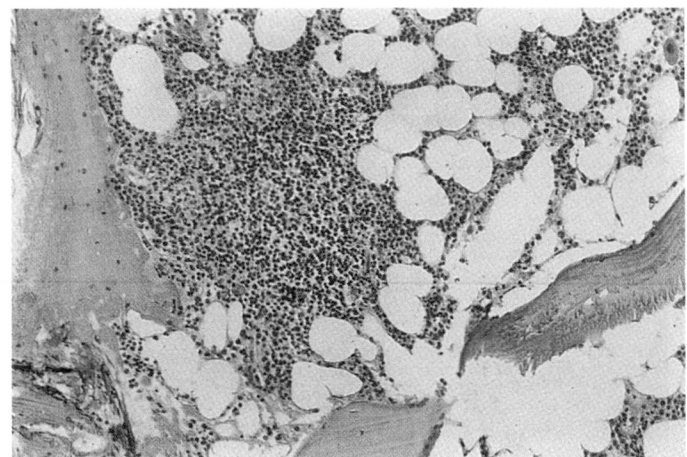

Plate 116 Bone marrow biopsy of a patient with type II HCV-related cryoglobulinemia showing a nodular infiltrate consisting of small lymphocytes, lymphoplasmacytoid elements, and plasma cells (Giemsa, 250 × magnification).

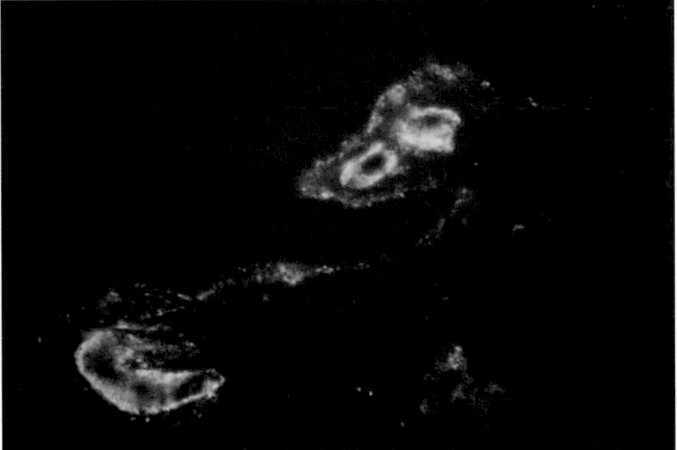

Plate 117 Cryoglobulinemic vasculitis. Immune complex deposits at the level of the basal membrane of dermal vessels. Immunofluorescence staining with anti-IgM antiserum of a cutaneous purpuric lesion (320 × magnification).

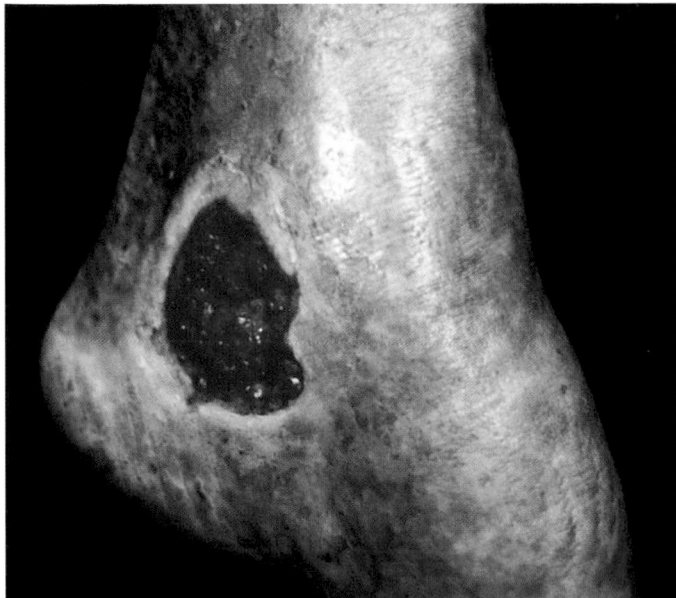

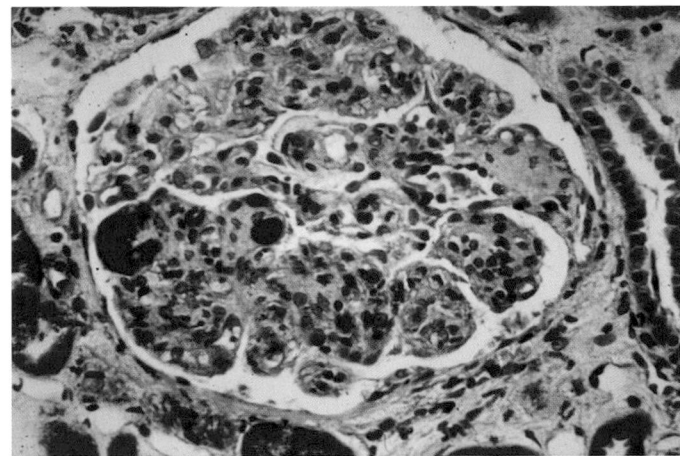

Plate 119 Kidney biopsy in a patient with type II HCV-related cryoglobulinemia showing membranoproliferative glomerulonephritis with mononuclear cell infiltration and intraluminal thrombi (PAS, 320 × magnification).

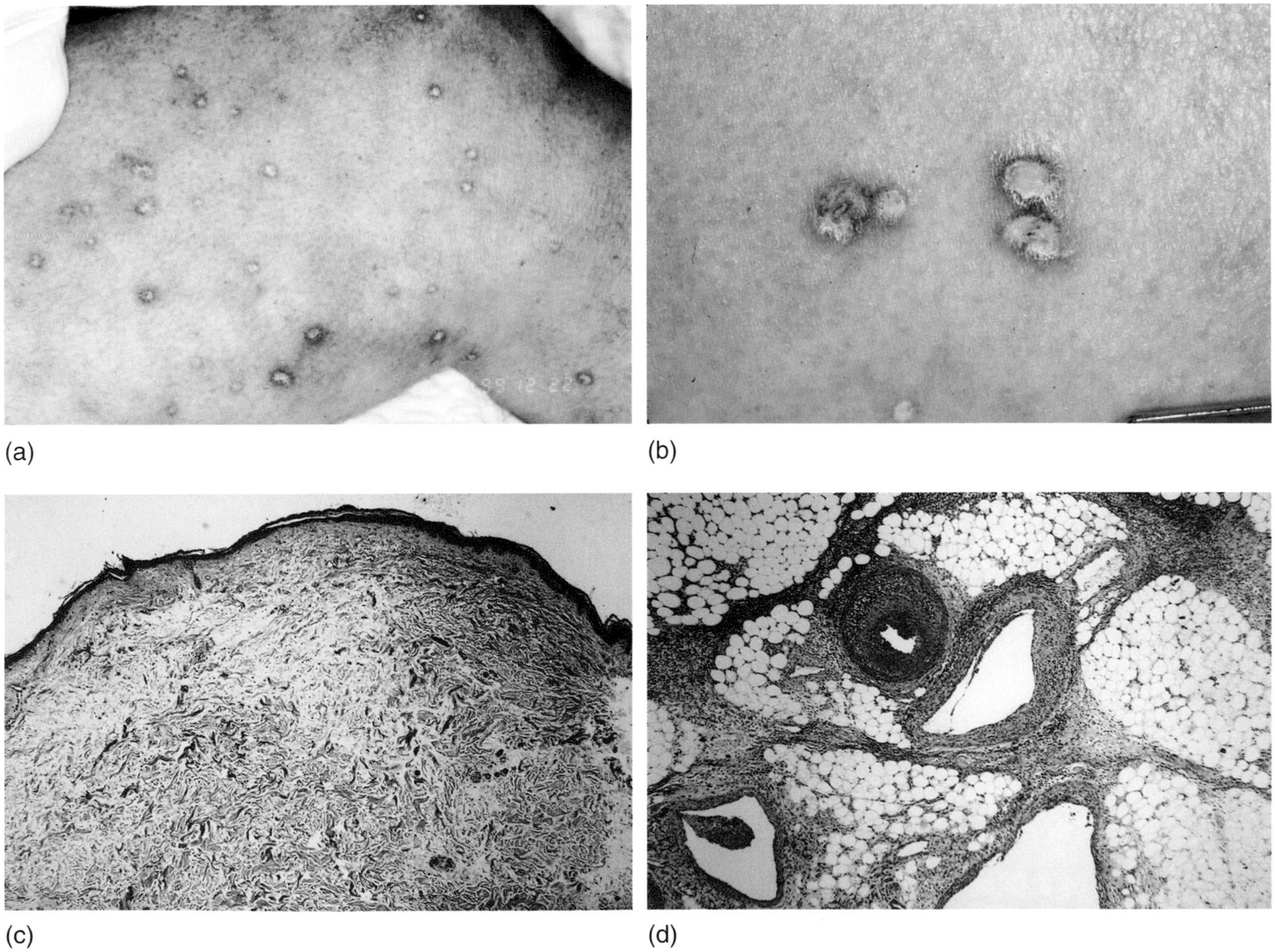

Plate 118 Malleolar ulcer in a patient with cutaneous type III HCV-related cryoglobulinemia. The surrounding skin shows aeas of ocherous pigmentation due to longstanding cryoglobulinemic purpura.

(a)

(b)

(c)

(d)

Plate 120 Cutaneous lesions of Degos' syndrome. (a) Skin lesions on the thigh of an affected individual. (b) Close-up view of lesions demonstrating pale yellow papules with violaceous margins; lesion on the left has overlying scale. (c) Photomicrograph of skin lesion demonstrating edematous, relatively acellular dermis. (d) Involved arteriole and vein in subjacent pannicular tissue demonstrating perivascular lymphoid infiltrates, proliferation of endothelium, and arteriolar thrombus. (Courtesy of Dr M. K. Abele.)

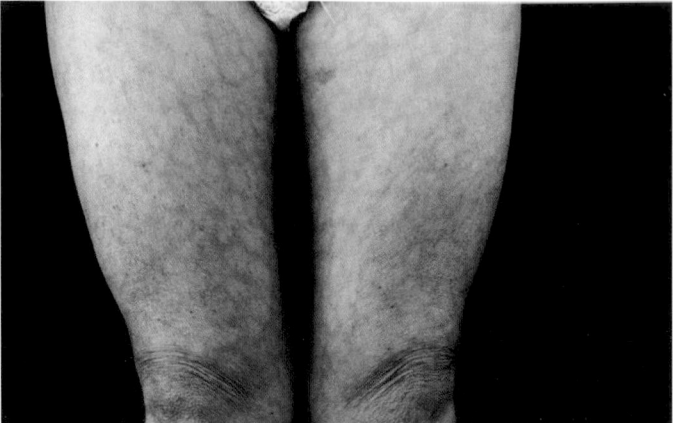

Plate 121 Livedo reticularis in a patient with systemic lupus erythematosus.

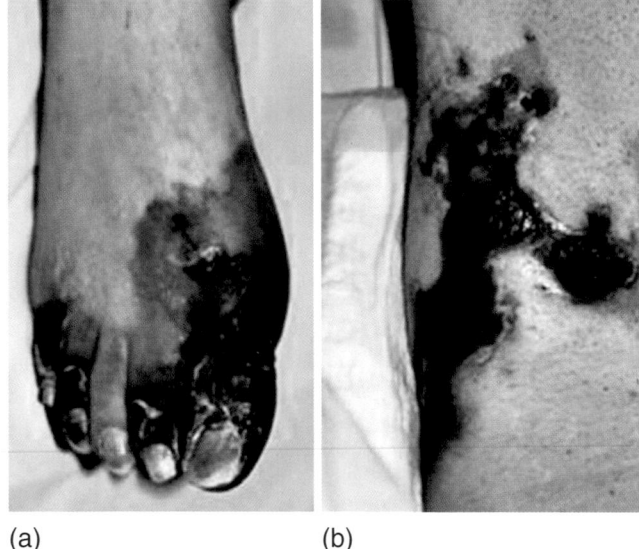

(a)   (b)

Plate 123 (A and B) Catastrophic antiphospholipid syndrome in a patient with severe skin necrosis and gangrene from widespread thrombosis.

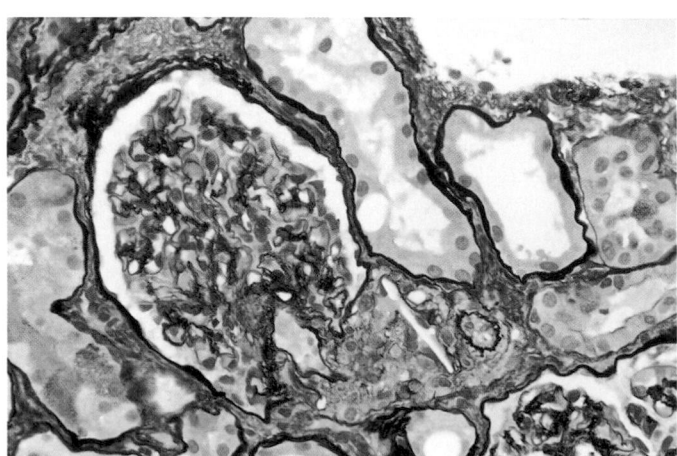

Plate 124 Atheromatous embolus lodged in an afferent renal arteriole.

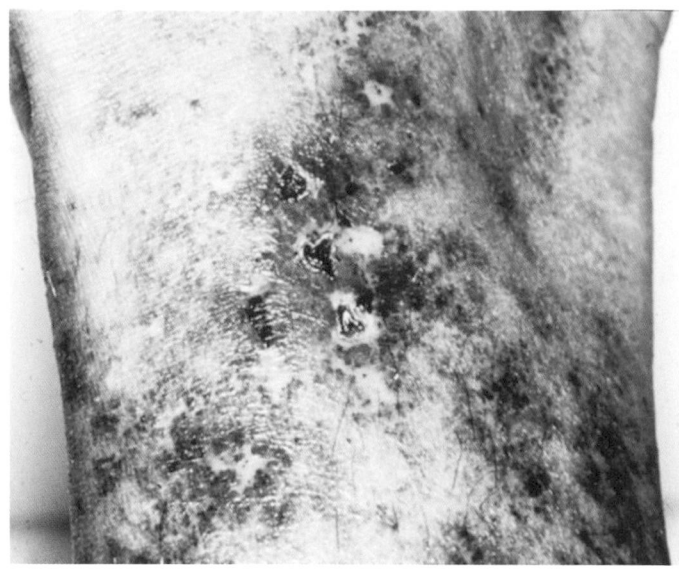

Plate 122 Livedo vasculitis. Characteristic lesions on the medial lower leg showing stellate shaped areas of necrosis and stellate white scars (atrophie blanche) surrounded by macular purpura and secondary hemosiderin pigmentation. (From Sams and Sams (2002) Cutaneous manifestations. In *Vasculitis*, (Ball, G. V. and Bridges, S. L. Jr, eds), 1st edn, Oxford University Press.)

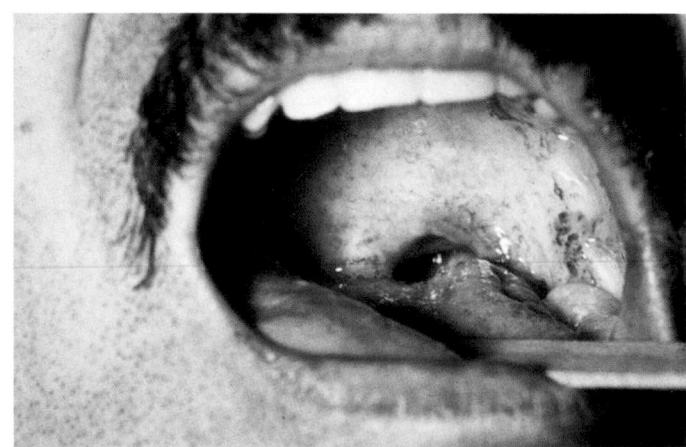

(a)

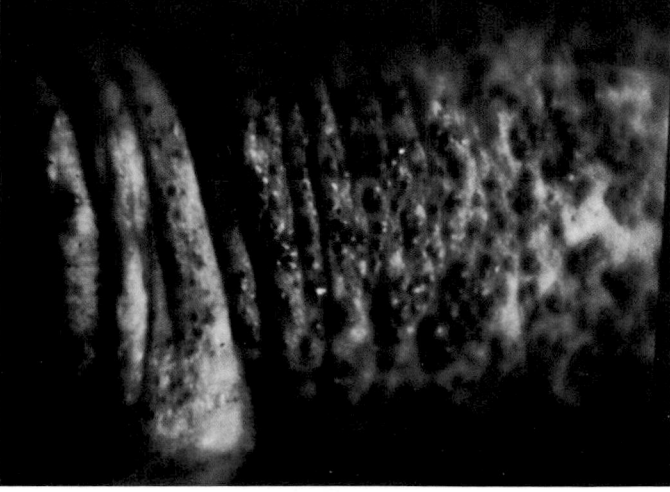

(b)

Plate 125 Angiokeratomas in the mouth (a) and on the penis (b) of a young man with Anderson–Fabry disease

Peripheral vascular disease

a. Absent pulses in one limb: Detected clinically.

b. Second episode of absent pulses in one limb: Detected clinically.

c. Major vessel stenosis: For example, carotid or renal stenosis, documented on Doppler or angiography.

d. Claudication: Exercise related ischemic pain in peripheral large vessel present for at least 3 months.

e. Minor tissue loss: For example, loss of finger tip pulp space.

f. Major tissue loss: For example, the loss of digit(s) or limb(s), including by surgical resection.

g. Complicated venous thrombosis: With persistent swelling, ulceration, or clinical evidence of venous stasis.

Gastrointestinal

a. Gut infarction/resection: Infarction or resection of bowel below duodenum; or of gallbladder, spleen, or liver.

b. Mesenteric insufficiency/pancreatitis: Typical abdominal pain confirmed on angiography or enzyme changes.

c. Chronic peritonitis: Typical abdominal pain and peritoneal irritation on clinical examination.

d. Esophageal stricture or surgery: On history or by further appropriate tests.

Renal

a. Estimated or measured GFR <50%: By any locally used method.

b. Proteinuria of >0.5 g/24 hours: By any locally used method.

c. End stage renal failure: Failure of native kidneys regardless of subsequent dialysis or transplantation.

Neuropsychiatric

a. Cognitive impairment: Memory deficit, difficulty with calculation, poor concentration, difficulty in spoken or written language, impaired performance level, documented on clinical examination (e.g. short mental test score) or by formal neurocognitive testing.

b. Major psychosis: Altered ability to function in normal activity due to psychiatric reasons. Severe disturbance of the perception of reality characterized by the following features: delusions, hallucinations (auditory, visual), incoherence, marked loose associations, impoverished thought content, marked illogical thinking, bizarre, disorganized, or catatonic behavior.

c. Seizures: Paroxysmal electrical discharge occurring in the brain and producing characteristic physical changes including tonic and clonic movements, and certain behavioral disorders. Only seizures requiring therapy for more than 3 months are counted as damage.

d. Cerebrovascular accident: CVA resulting in focal findings such as paresis, weakness, etc., OR surgical resection for causes other than malignancy.

e. Cranial nerve lesion: Cranial neuropathy, excluding optic nerve or sensorineural deafness.

f. Peripheral neuropathy: Peripheral neuropathy resulting in either motor or sensory dysfunction.

g. Transverse myelitis: Lower extremity weakness or sensory loss with loss of sphincter control (rectal and urinary bladder).

Other

a. Gonadal failure: Premature secondary amenorrhoea or azoospermia.

b. Bone marrow failure: Leukopenia (WBC <4000/mm^3), or thrombocytopenia (platelets <140,000) or anemia (hemoglobin <10 g/dL) preferably confirmed by bone marrow aspiration.

c. Diabetes mellitus: Requiring any type of therapy.

d. Chemical cystitis: Persistent hematuria or shrunken bladder. This does not include acute hemorrhagic cystitis which should be scored as an adverse drug reaction ADR.

e. Malignancy: Documented by pathology, excluding dysplasias.

f. Other: Any feature considered by patient or doctor to be an important scar or consequence which has arisen since onset of disease.

The VDI is a cumulative assessment of organ dysfunction, damage, or scarring; a score of damage rather than active vasculitis. Damage is defined as having ever been present for at least 3 months and occurring since the onset of vasculitis.

The VDI is probably the most effective predictor of poor outcome currently available. Multiorgan, multisystem involvement, as measured by the VDI, in patients within the first two years of disease is predictive of subsequent increased risk of death. This is particularly the case when critical systems are involved such as the cardiovascular system or the neurological system (Exley *et al.* 1998). This might suggest that there should be different weighting applied to different sections of the VDI just as applies currently to the BVAS, but the important factor again seems to be the extent of organ involvement. Comparing VDI scores in patients who subsequently died with those who subsequently survived at least 5 years, the former patients had higher numbers of VDI items and more organ systems involved by damage than the group who survived (Exley *et al.* 1997a). The rate of accumulation of new items was also

Table 23.3 The Five Factor Score

Criteria:

Renal insufficiency (serum creatinine ≥1.58 mg/dl (150 micromol/l))
Proteinuria (≥1 g/24 hours)
Central nervous system involvement
Cardiomyopathy
Severe gastrointestinal involvement (GI bleeding, infaction, or pancreatitis)

The FFS is based on the five clinical items above, with the presence of each given 1 point for a maximum score of 5.

more rapid in the patients who died compared to those who did not die (Exley *et al.*1997b). Risks for mortality can be predicted from the VDI at 2 years; clearly this is preliminary, but the findings are being re-evaluated in larger numbers of patients with vasculitis through the European Vasculitis Study Group. This should provide a more refined approach to outcome prediction in the future.

Disease states

Definitions of disease status are invaluable in clinical trial work: they allow patients to be more precisely described in categorical states of active disease, relapse, remission, or partial remission. Definitions of response to treatment may provide a further indication of success or failure of specific therapies. Such definitions have currently been used in different ways by different groups and there is an attempt to co-ordinate this through OMERACT (Merkel *et al.* 2005). Once agreed upon, these should provide the basis of further validation studies and subsequent use on a more practical level for clinical trials. It is likely that OMERACT definitions of disease states will be based largely on the clinical tools for assessment of vasculitis described in this chapter.

Further assessment of systemic vasculitis

Clinical assessment of vasculitis for disease activity and damage is primarily done by the physician evaluating the patient at one interaction; this assessment can be repeated as required. On occasions further investigations are required in order to make the diagnosis, examine the possibility that disease is active, or determine that a complication has arisen. This additional radiological, histological, or serological information complements the clinical information but does not replace the value of the clinical evaluation. The composite description of the patient's state, both from a clinical and a laboratory aspect, will allow us to learn more about the disease and the effectiveness of therapy. In this way we can follow the progress of individual patients and ensure that they are given appropriate therapy to limit disease activity and drug-related damage.

Long-term outcome of vasculitis

With the change in prognosis of systemic vasculitis we are now witnessing the evolution of the disease from a life-threatening, short-lived illness into one characterized by chronic morbidity and in some cases long-term mortality. In other inflammatory connective tissue diseases such as SLE, there is a known risk of endothelial dysfunction and damage associated with long-term disease and this clinically manifests as ischemic heart disease occurring at a premature age. Patients with vasculitis may be at premature risk of accelerated atheroma and there is considerable evidence that endothelial dysfunction is common among patients with active vasculitis to a degree that is similar to patients who have had ischemic cardiac events (Raza *et al.* 2000; Filer *et al.* 2003; Booth *et al.* 2004; Raza *et al.* 2005). There is some evidence that the likelihood of cardiovascular and cerebrovascular events is higher in patients with vasculitis than in their non-affected counterparts but the evidence is accumulating slowly. The use of chemotherapy drugs does cause long-term concern about the potential risk of developing cancer, particularly bladder carcinoma as a result of exposure to long-term cyclophosphamide. However, it is becoming clear that patients with vasculitis actually have an increased risk in cancer compared to non-vasculitic individuals and that this is not related to their drug therapy (Hellmich *et al.* 2004; Pankhurst *et al.* 2004). Only by undertaking large, long-term studies of patients with systemic vasculitis will we learn more about the link between vasculitis and its treatment and the subsequent development of some of these more common clinical problems. Although a number of patients with vasculitis are elderly and may be at high risk of developing cardiovascular disease and cancer, younger patients may be suffering premature events directly as a result of vasculitis. This issue needs to be further evaluated and is currently the subject of investigation by the European Vasculitis Study Group.

Function/patient perspective

The impact of a diagnosis of vasculitis and its treatment on individual patients is variable. The amount of distress and harm to the overall lifestyle of individuals can be huge. The importance of individual aspects of disease or their treatment on patients may be very different from the perspective of the clinician. Conventionally, disease status is measured in vasculitis by the clinician deciding on whether the patient is doing well or not well and providing accurate clinical tools to describe this in more detail. However, from the patient's perspective this approach may not be the most satisfactory way of describing the impact of disease. For example, some aspects of damage which clinicians may regard as relatively trivial, such as hair loss or development of hypertension requiring antihypertensive medication, may in fact have a disproportionately high impact on the patient's perception of how successful their treatment has been. The value of recording the patient's perceptions of their disease status is very high and has been developed successfully in many fields. Satisfactory assessment of patient-related quality of life assessment in vasculitis remains suboptimal. Measuring the impact, or burden, of disease in different disease entities may have some advantages; instruments such as the Short Form 36 provide a broad overview of the patient's functioning and well-being (Newall *et al.* 2005; Koutantji *et al.* 2003; Reinhold-Keller *et al.* 2002). There is a growing interest in developing disease-specific functional indices which would have advantages if they were applicable to different forms of vasculitis. However, a functional index for specific disease entities within vasculitis might suffer from too much variation when measuring general morbidity. Use of the Short Form 36 in these patients suggests that it may provide a different, patient-centered view of disease severity rather than a medical model of outcome. One survey of a large cohort of patients with vasculitis demonstrated that while the majority of patients had good control of the disease as measured by BVAS, the majority rated themselves as having very high disability (mainly physical), which did not correlate with disease activity (Raza *et al.* 1999). Short Form 36 values improve over time in these patients but the rate of improvement falls significantly behind the rate of clinician-measured improvement in disease state. These studies are based on limited numbers of patients and there is a plan to evaluate the Short Form 36 in a larger group of patients (using the European Vasculitis Study Group trial data).

New developments in disease assessment

Disease states

A refinement of the clinical status of patients with vasculitis requires a standardized agreement on what constitutes relapse, remission, and states in between these extremes. Definitions of partial improvement or partial deterioration may also need to be more carefully explored. These disease states are essential for clinical trial development but would also serve a function in clinical practice. This would give a context to measures of disease activity by providing the framework in which these tools can be applied. The OMERACT group is currently developing this area and this will need to be followed by clinical studies to ensure the robustness of these disease definitions (Merkel *et al.* 2005).

Quality control of indices to measure activity and damage in vasculitis

All clinical tools measuring disease activity are to some extent flawed; they cannot be gold standards and will always be imperfect. Each activity or damage tool must be viewed as the best compromise between current evidence and clinical practice. With usage each tool's flaws will become apparent, so these assessments should be regularly reviewed and revised. This process of audit applies to any assessment whether it is clinical or laboratory based, and should be regarded as part of the natural maintenance required to ensure that these tools serve their intended purpose. Maintenance implies that there may be a change in some aspects of the measurement tools to improve their robustness but this does not necessarily imply a change in the underlying principles. As part of this development we may expect new and improved versions of existing tools and possibly the development of related, perhaps more disease focused, assessments to be fully validated prior to application in practice or in clinical trials. We look forward to a collaborative approach with an internationally agreed set of standards useful in undertaking measurement of disease activity and damage both in practice and in clinical trials. For example, the European League against Rheumatism has recently prepared a set of recommendations for conducting clinical trials in ANCA-associated vasculitis (Hellmich *et al.* 2006). Many of the items discussed in this chapter are part of that document.

Standardization

Development of standardized training packages for disease activity and damage assessments must become routine to ensure a valid use, particularly in multicenter clinical trials in which clinicians do not have experience with these instruments. Training packages are expected to improve this situation and also provide an excellent opportunity for less experienced clinicians and trainees to learn more about vasculitis. These can be prepared as distance learning packages, based on paper cases carefully prepared from real life examples.

Summary

Assessment of the systemic vasculitides is an integral part of their management and is directly linked to treatment decisions. A structured approach to evaluation of patients has allowed us to describe in detail disease flares, chronic grumbling disease and chronic scars, and poor functioning. Detailed description of patient morbidity is a new aspect to management of vasculitis as a result of improved patient survival. The instruments described in this chapter provide a collective picture of disease burden, offering qualitative and quantitative information on disease status which can facilitate therapeutic decision making. Such instruments are recommended for use both in clinical practice and in clinical trials. These tools should form an integral part of any new clinical trial design in systemic vasculitis, as they represent the best available measure of disease morbidity in conjunction with basic laboratory markers for disease diagnosis. Design of studies which employ disease activity and damage markers should now be the norm.

Acknowledgements

Kathryn Cook for secretarial support.

References

Boomsma, M. M., Stegeman, C. A., van der Leij, M. J., *et al.* (2000). Prediction of relapses in Wegener's Granulomatosis by measurement of antineutrophil cytoplasmic antibody levels: a prospective study. *Arthritis and Rheumatism*, **43**, 2025–33.

Booth, A. D., Jayne, D. R., Kharbanda, R. K., McEniery, C. M., Mackenzie, I. S., Brown, J. and Wilkinson, I. B. (2004). Infliximab improves endothelial dysfunction in systemic vasculitis: a model of vascular inflammation. *Circulation*, **109**, 1718–23.

Booth, A. D., Almond, M. K., Burns, A., Ellis, P., Gaskin, G., Neild, G. H., Plaisance, M., Pusey, C. D., Jayne, D. R.; Pan-Thames Renal Research Group (2003). Outcome of ANCA-associated renal vasculitis: a 5-year retrospective study. *American Journal of Kidney Diseases*, **41**, 776–84.

Bourgarit, A., Le Toumelin, P., Pagnoux, C., *et al.* (2005). French Vasculitis Study Group. Deaths occurring during the first year after treatment onset for polyarteritis nodosa, microscopic polyangiitis, and Churg-Strauss syndrome: a retrospective analysis of causes and factors predictive of mortality based on 595 patients. *Medicine* (Baltimore), **84**, 323–30.

Brogan, P. A. and Dillon, M. J. (2004). Endothelial microparticles and the diagnosis of the vasculitides. *Internal Medicine*, **43**, 1115–9.

Brogan, P. A., Shah, V., Brachet, C., *et al.* (2004). Endothelial and platelet microparticles in vasculitis of the young. *Arthritis and Rheumatism*, **50**, 927–36.

De Groot, K., Gross, W. L., Herlyn, K. and Reinhold-Keller, E. (2001). Development and Validation of a Disease Extent Index for Wegener's Granulomatosis. *Clinical Nephrology*, **55**, 31–8.

Di Lorenzo, G., Pacor, M. L., Mansueto, P., *et al.* (2004). Circulating levels of soluble adhesion molecules in patients with ANCA-associated vasculitis. *Journal of Nephrology*, **17**, 800–7.

Exley, A. R., Bacon, P. A., Luqmani, R. A., *et al.* (1997a). Development and Initial Validation of the Vasculitis Damage Index (VDI) for the Standardised Clinical Assessment of Damage in the Systemic Vasculitides. *Arthritis and Rheumatism*, **40**, 371–80.

Exley, A. R., Bacon, P. A., Luqmani, R. A., Kitas, G. D., Carruthers, D. M. and Moots, R. (1998). Examination of disease severity in systemic vasculitis from the novel perspective of damage using the vasculitis damage index (VDI). *British Journal of Rheumatology*, **37**, 57–63.

Exley, A., Carruthers, D. M., Luqmani, R. A., *et al.* (1997b). Damage occurs early in systemic vasculitis and is an index of outcome. *Quarterly Journal of Medicine*, **90**, 391–9.

Filer, A. D., Gardner-Medwin, J. M., Thambyrajah, J., Raza, K., Carruthers, D. M., Stevens, R. J., Liu, L., Lowe, S. E., Townend, J. N. and Bacon, P. A. (2003). Diffuse endothelial dysfunction is common to ANCA associated systemic vasculitis and polyarteritis nodosa. *Annals of the Rheumatic Diseases*, **62**, 162–7.

Gayraud, M., Guillevin, L., le Toumelin, P., *et al.* (2001). French Vasculitis Study Group. Long-term followup of polyarteritis nodosa, microscopic polyangiitis, and Churg-Strauss syndrome: analysis of four prospective trials including 278 patients. *Arthritis and Rheumatism*, **44**, 666–75.

Gordon, M., Luqmani, R. A., Adu, D., *et al.* (1993). Relapses in patients with a systemic vasculitis. *Quarterly Journal of Medicine*, **86**, 779–89.

Guillevin, L., Le Thi Huong, D., Godeau, P., Jais, P. and Wechsler, B. (1988). Clinical findings and prognosis of polyarteritis nodosa and Churg-Strauss angiitis: a study in 165 patients. *British Journal of Rheumatology*, **27**, 258–64.

Hellmich, B., Kausch, I., Doehn, C., Jocham, D., Holl-Ulrich, K. and Gross, W. L. (2004). Urinary bladder cancer in Wegener's Granulomatosis: is it more than cyclophosphamide? *Annals of the Rheumatic Diseases*, **63**, 1183–5.

Hellmich, B., Flossmann, O., Gross, W. L., *et al.* (2006). EULAR recommendations for conducting clinical studies and/or clinical trials in systemic vasculitis: Focus on ANCA-associated vasculitis. *Annals of the Rheumatic Diseases*.

Hoffman, G. S., Kerr, G. S., Leavitt, R. Y., *et al.* (1992). Wegener's granulomatosis: an analysis of 158 patients. *Annals of Internal Medicine*, **116**, 488–98.

Hogan, S. L., Falke, R. J., Chin, H., *et al.* (2005). Predictors of relapse and treatment resistance in anti-neutrophil cytoplasmic antibody associated small vessel vasculitis. *Annals of Internal Medicine*, **143**, 621–31.

Janssen, B., Luqmani, R. A., Gordon, C., *et al.* (1994). Correlation of blood levels of soluble vascular cell adhesion molecule-1 with disease activity in systemic lupus erythematosus and vasculitis. *British Journal of Rheumatology*, **33**, 1112–6.

Koldingsnes, W. and Nossent, J. C. (2003). Baseline features and initial treatment as predictors of remission and relapse in Wegener's Granulomatosis. *Journal of Rheumatology*, **30**, 80–8.

Koutantji, M., Harrold, E., Lane, S. E., Pearce, S., Watts, R. A. and Scott, D.G. (2003). Investigation of quality of life, mood, pain, disability and disease status in primary systemic vasculitis. *Arthritis and Rheumatism*, **49**, 826–37.

Luqmani, R. (2004). Disease assessment in systemic vasculitis. *Journal of Rheumatology*, **7**, 172–9.

Luqmani, R. A., Bacon, P. A., Moots, R. J., *et al.* (1994). Birmingham vasculitis activity score (BVAS) in systemic necrotizing vasculitis. *Quarterly Journal of Medicine*, **87**, 671–8.

Luqmani, R. A., Exley, A. R., Kitas, G. D. and Bacon, P. A. (1997). Disease assessment and management of the vasculitides. *Baillieres Clinical Rheumatology*, **11**, 422–47.

Merkel, P., Seo, P., Aries, P., *et al.* for the Vasculitis Clinical Research Consortium (2005). Current status of outcome measures in vasculitis: focus on Wegener's granulomatosis and microscopic polyangiitis. Report from OMERACT 7. *Journal of Rheumatology*, **32**, 2488–95.

Newall, C., Schinke, S., Savage, C. O., Hill, S. and Harper, L. (2005). Impairment of lung function, health status and functional capacity in patients with ANCA-associated vasculitis. *Rheumatology* (Oxford), **44**, 623–8.

Pankhurst, T., Savage, C. O., Gordon, C. and Harper, L. (2004). Malignancy is increased in ANCA-associated vasculitis. *Rheumatology* (Oxford), **43**, 1532–5.

Raza, K., Wilson, A., Carruthers, D. M., *et al.* (1999). Impaired SF 36 in patients with primary systemic vasculitis: influence of factors besides disease activity and damage. *Arthritis and Rheumatism*, 42 (Suppl.), S315.

Raza, K., Thambyrajah, J., Townend, J. N., Exley, A. R., Hortas, C., Filer, A., Carruthers, D. M. and Bacon, P. A. (2000). Suppression of inflammation in primary systemic vasculitis restores vascular endothelial function: lessons for atherosclerotic disease? *Circulation*, **102**, 1470–2.

Raza, K., Carruthers, D. M., Stevens, R., Filer, A. D., Townend, J. N. and Bacon, P. A. (2005). Infliximab leads to a rapid but transient improvement in endothelial function in patients with primary systemic vasculitis. *Annals of the Rheumatic Diseases*.

Reinhold-Keller, E., Herlyn, K., Wagner-Bastmeyer, R., *et al.* (2002). Effect of Wegener's Granulomatosis on work disability, need for medical care, and quality of life in patients younger than 40 years at diagnosis. *Arthritis and Rheumatism*, **47**, 320–5.

Seo, P., Min, Y. I., Holbrook, J. T., *et al.* for the WGET Research Group. (2005). Damage caused by Wegener's granulomatosis and its treatment: prospective data from the Wegener's Granulomatosis Etanercept Trial (WGET). *Arthritis and Rheumatism*, **52**, 2168–78.

Sivakumar, M. R., Misra, R. N., Bacon, P. A., for the Indian Rheumatology Association Vasculitis Study Group. (2005). Development of a disease extent index to assess Takayasu arteritis. *Rheumatology*, **44**, (S3) 6–7.

Slot, M. C., Tervaert, J. W., Boomsma, M. M. and Stegeman, C. A. (2004). Positive classic antineutrophil cytoplasmic antibody (C-ANCA) titer at switch to azathioprine therapy associated with relapse in proteinase 3-related vasculitis. *Arthritis and Rheumatism*, **51**, 269–73.

Stone, J. H., Hoffman, G. S., Merkel, P. A. *et al.* (2001). A disease-specific activity index for Wegener's granulomatosis: modification of the Birmingham Vasculitis Activity Score. International Network for the Study of Systemic Vasculitides. *Arthritis and Rheumatism*, **44**, 912–20.

CHAPTER 24

Giant cell arteritis and polymyalgia rheumatica

Gideon Nesher and Ronit Nesher

Giant-cell arteritis (GCA) is an arteritis of the major branches of the aorta with a predilection for the extracranial branches of the carotid artery, and the aorta itself. It occurs in patients older than 50 years, and often involves the temporal arteries (Jennette *et al.* 1994). GCA is often associated with polymyalgia rheumatica (PMR), a clinical syndrome characterized by aching and morning stiffness in the shoulder or hip girdles. PMR may present without any clinical evidence of GCA.

Epidemiology

GCA and PMR are more common among people of North European descent than among Mediterranean people, and are rare among African Americans, native Americans, and Asians (Baldursson *et al.* 1994; Boesen and Sorensen 1987; Franzen *et al.* 1991; Gilbert *et al.* 1999; González-Gay *et al.* 2001a; Gran and Myklebust 1997; Haugberg *et al.* 2000; Kobayashi *et al.* 2003; Petursdottir *et al.* 1999; Salvarani *et al.* 1991, 2004; Smith *et al.* 1983; Sonnenblick *et al.* 1994). Table 24.1 shows the incidence rates in various parts of the world.

The incidence of GCA increases with age. The age-specific incidence rates per 100,000 population increase from 2 in the age group 50–59 years, to 52 in the age group 80 and older (Salvarani *et al.* 2004). GCA incidence is reported to be rising (González-Gay *et al.* 2001; Petursdottir *et al.* 1999). In a 50-year observation period in the population of Olmsted County, Minnesota, the incidence rate increased from the 1950s to the 1970s, but has been stable since then (Salvarani *et al.* 2004). Seasonal variations and a cyclic pattern of annual incidence rates were reported by several groups (Elling *et al.* 1996; Petursdottir *et al.* 1999; Salvarani *et al.* 2004; Sonnenblick *et al.* 1994), but such fluctuations were not observed by others.

The actual prevalence of GCA is unknown, but an estimate of its prevalence can be based on a large-scale post-mortem study in Sweden. It disclosed signs of active or healed GCA in 1.6% of 849 autopsies of individuals who were older than 50 years (Ostberg 1973). This is considerably higher than the estimated prevalence of 1:750 persons older than 50 years in Olmsted County, Minnesota, and Ribe County, Denmark (Huston *et al.* 1978; Boesen and Sorensen 1987).

PMR is more common than GCA (Table 24.1). Similar to GCA, the highest annual incidence rates were observed in northern Europe (Boesen and Sorensen 1987; Doran *et al.* 2002; Gran and Myklebust 1997; González-Gay *et al.* 1999; Salvarani *et al.* 1991). The estimated prevalence in Minnesota was 1 in 200 persons older than 50 years (Chuang *et al.* 1982). A population-based survey of individuals older than 65 years in Cambridge, UK, reported a higher prevalence of 1:30 (Kyle *et al.* 1985). In both PMR and GCA, women are more commonly affected than men.

Etiology

The high incidence rates of GCA and PMR in northern Europe and among people of north European descent suggests a genetic predisposition. Studies of HLA antigens in different populations showed that HLA-DR4 was over-represented (Combe *et al.* 1998; Dababneh *et al.* 1998; Weyand *et al.* 1992). It was found that 60% of GCA patients from Minnesota expressed the DRB*0401 or DRB*0404/8 alleles of the HLA-DR4 haplotype, and that the remaining HLA-DRB1*04-negative patients expressed one of the following alleles: DRB*03, DRB*08, DRB*13, or DRB*15/16 (Weyand *et al.* 1992). All of these GCA patients shared a sequence motif spanning the amino acid positions 28–31 of the HLA-DRB1 chain, which maps to the second hypervariable region located in the antigen binding site of the HLA-DR molecule.

Table 24.1 Annual incidence of GCA and PMR in various parts of the world; rates per 100,000 persons older than 50 years

	Giant cell arteritis	Polymyalgia rheumatica
Northern Europe and northern USA	32.8 (Norway)	112.6 (Norway)
	25.4 (Iceland)	68.3 (Denmark)
	23.3 (Denmark)	58.7 (Minnesota, USA)
	22.7 (Finland)	50.0 (Sweden)
	22.2 (Sweden)	
	18.8 (Minnesota, USA)	
Mediterranean countries	10.2 (Israel)	
	10.2 (Spain)	13.5 (Spain)
	6.9 (Italy)	12.7 (Italy)
Southern USA	1.6 (Tennessee, USA)	
Asia, Far East	1.5 (Japan)	

Such a genetic element predisposing to GCA might affect antigen presentation and recognition, which can be a critical event in the pathogenesis of GCA; however, it is not yet clear whether this genetic factor is relevant for all populations. Although European studies found over-representation of B1*0401 and B1*0404/8 in PMR and GCA, the frequency of the shared epitope in amino acid positions 28–31 was not increased when compared with controls (Combe *et al.* 1998; Dababneh *et al.* 1998; Martinez-Taboada *et al.* 2004).

Polymorphisms in several genes have been found to be associated with increased susceptibility or with disease severity. These include variations in the genes encoding intercellular adhesion molecule-1 (ICAM-1), interferon-gamma (IFN-γ), vascular endothelial growth factor (VEGF), and endothelial nitric oxide synthase, as well as in the interleukin (IL)-1 cluster and the IL-6 promoter (Amoli *et al.* 2003; Boiardi *et al.* 2003; González-Gay *et al.* 2003, 2004a; Salvarani *et al.* 2003). Therefore it is apparent that susceptibility to GCA and PMR is polygenic.

The link between aging and disease onset is a striking feature of both GCA and PMR. It seems likely that physiologic aging of the arterial walls causes degenerative changes in the elastic tissue (Lie *et al.* 1970). In susceptible individuals, this may result in autoimmune reaction to an altered antigen. Immunosenescence may also be an important factor in the preferential onset of GCA and PMR in old age. Possible mechanisms are breakdown in immune tolerance or increased susceptibility to infectious triggers.

Infectious agents have been suggested as causal factors. A prospective French study reported that PMR and GCA patients were two to three times more likely to have IgM antibodies against parainfluenza virus type 1 at the time of diagnosis, when compared with age-matched controls (Duhaut *et al.* 1999a). Since most elderly individuals are exposed to this virus earlier in life, this might suggest a reinfection. A study of 13 counties in Denmark documented annual variation of PMR and GCA incidence rates, clustering in five peaks over a period of 13 years (Elling *et al.* 1996). There was close association between these peaks and epidemics of *Mycoplasma pneumoniae*, *Chlamydia pneumoniae*, and parvovirus B19. However, a study from Sweden found no evidence for recent infection with *Chlamydia* (Uddhammar *et al.* 1997).

Attempts have been made to detect viral DNA in temporal artery biopsy specimens. In some studies parvovirus was more prevalent in GCA compared to controls (Gabriel *et al.* 1999; Alvarez-Lafuente *et al.* 2005); however, this was not corroborated by others (Rodriguez-Pla *et al.* 2004).

The significance of these observations is unclear, but it is possible that a variety of infectious agents-related antigens may trigger the development of PMR and GCA in genetically predisposed, elderly individuals.

Histopathology

Almost any artery can be affected in GCA (Ostberg 1972). In autopsy studies, the most commonly involved arteries in the head and neck were the temporal, vertebral, ophthalmic, and posterior ciliary (Wilkinson and Russell 1972). Other cranial, cervical, thoracic, abdominal, and peripheral arteries were involved less commonly (Lie 1995). The arteries were affected in a segmental fashion.

The histopathologic findings in GCA are shown in Figures 9.4–9.7 in Chapter 9. They typically consist of transmural lymphocyte and macrophage infiltrates, which may be confined to the region of the internal or external lamina or the adventitia (Ashton-Key and Gallagher 1991; Lie 1995). The internal elastic lamina is fragmented and surrounded by inflammatory cells. Foci of calcification may be present. There is patchy degeneration and dropout of smooth muscle cells in the media. Multinucleated giant cells are often present, mostly adjacent to the fragmented elastic lamina or degenerated smooth muscle cells. The presence of giant cells is not required for the diagnosis if other features are compatible. Granulomas and fibrinoid necrosis are rare, and their presence should alert the clinician to search for another type of vasculitis. Concentric intimal thickening, partly due to edema, may narrow or even completely occlude the vessel, and luminal thrombosis may occur.

It should be noted that there may be foci of fragmented and reduplicated internal elastic lamina in the temporal arteries in healthy elderly individuals (Lie *et al.* 1970). Patchy and mild thickening of the intima may be seen, but inflammatory infiltrates and giant cells are not present, and intimal thickening is often not concentric. In healed temporal arteritis, the characteristic feature is medial scarring, often with neovascularization. Mild inflammation may persist. The intima contains irregularly arranged fibrous tissue, and the elastic lamina remains fragmented for the most part.

Periarterial lymphocytic infiltration is noted occasionally in the absence of arteritis (Chakrabarty and Franks 2000; Corcoran *et al.* 2001). The significance of this lymphocytic infiltrate is uncertain. It is regarded by some as associated with aging, and not indicative of an inflammatory process. However, it may occur during the phase of healing following the start of glucocorticoid therapy, and it may be a marker of associated vasculitis by proximity to an active lesion. Indeed, in some cases of periarterial lymphocytic infiltration, further examination of the biopsy specimen at multiple levels disclosed arteritis (Chakrabarty and Franks 2000).

At times, small-vessel vasculitis surrounding a spared temporal artery is noted, and 19 such cases have been studied extensively. Twelve were eventually diagnosed as GCA, while three patients had evidence of systemic necrotizing vasculitis, and four had evidence of peripheral neuropathy (Esteban *et al.* 2001). Histologic features associated with GCA were: extension of the inflammatory infiltrate toward the adventitia of the temporal artery; involvement of its vasa vasorum; and the absence of fibrinoid necrosis in the small vessels.

Ultrastructural studies (Ashton-Key and Gallagher 1991) have not found evidence of phagocytosis of elastic tissue, but material resembling basement membrane was identified in vacuoles in the cytoplasm of macrophages. Immunohistochemical findings are conflicting, but immunoglobulin and complement deposits reported in some cases probably reflect non-specific diffusion through the damaged endothelium.

In PMR, histopathologic findings have little to contribute to diagnosis or understanding of symptoms. Muscle biopsy may show atrophy of muscle fibers, but no signs of myositis (Uddhammar *et al.* 1998a). Synovial biopsies of affected joints often show non-specific low-grade synovitis (Chou and Schumacher 1984).

Pathogenesis

Evidence suggests that cellular immunity plays the major role in the pathogenesis of GCA and PMR. In both conditions, the majority of circulating monocytes are activated, secreting IL-1 and IL-6 (Wagner *et al.* 1994). Serum IL-6 levels were increased and correlated with disease activity; in contrast, levels of tumor necrosis factor-α (TNF-α) were not increased (Roche *et al.* 1993; Uddhammar *et al.* 1998b). Some studies reported that the fraction of circulating CD8+ T-cells was reduced, but this was not corroborated by others (Macchioni *et al.* 1993; Martinez-Taboada *et al.* 2001).

The role of humoral immunity in GCA and PMR is less certain. Lymphocytes infiltrating the temporal artery wall do not include B cells or plasma cells; however, circulating immune complexes were detected in patients during periods of active disease (Smith *et al.* 1987). There have been reports on the occurrence of various auto-antibodies, especially antiphospholipid antibodies (Chakravarty *et al.* 1995; Duhaut *et al.* 1998; Espinoza *et al.* 1991), but their significance in regard to the pathogenesis of GCA is not clear.

In the arterial lesions of GCA, localization of the inflammatory cells and multinucleated giant cells around the fragmented internal elastic lamina at the intima–media junction is suggestive of an autoimmune reaction against elastin or adjacent macromolecules. In one study, a proliferative response of peripheral blood cells from patients with GCA mononuclear cells was observed following incubation with elastin peptides (Gillot *et al.* 1997).

The inflammatory reaction in the vessel wall consists mainly of CD4+ T lymphocytes and macrophages (Cid *et al.* 1989). In inflamed arteries, HLA-DR is most highly expressed in adventitial microvessels (vasa vasorum), suggesting that this is the site of entry of inflammatory cells into the arterial wall (Nordborg and Nordborg 1998). These microvessels produce a variety of adhesion molecules that regulate transport of inflammatory cells (Cid *et al.* 2000).

The CD4+ T lymphocytes are attracted by activated arterial wall dendritic cells. Immature dendritic cells are scattered throughout tissues and act as sentinels that sample the antigenic environment. Normal temporal arteries contain immature dendritic cells, located at the media–adventitia junction. These dendritic cells have a unique surface receptor profile, including a series of Toll-like receptors (TLR). Ligands of TLR4 are able to start maturation of these dendritic cells (Ma-Krupa 2005).

In GCA dendritic cells are activated, producing proinflammatory cytokines such as IL-6 and IL-18, and expressing CD-86, which is critical for interaction with T cells through binding to CD28 on T cell membranes. However, instead of migrating towards lymphoid organs as they do in most instances, dendritic cells in GCA are trapped in the vessel wall, attracting T lymphocytes and activating them (Ma-Krupa 2002; Weyand and Goronzy 2003).

The reason for entrapment of dendritic cells is probably related to the coproduction of both chemokines and their chemokine receptors by the same cells. The homing chemokines CCL18, CCL19, and CCL21 are produced by activated dendritic cells, but the chemokine receptor CCR7 that binds those chemokines is also produced. These chemokines are normally produced in lymphoid tissues, and they direct activated dendritic cells towards those tissues. The result of this abnormal signaling is trapping of dendritic cells in the arterial wall and attraction of T cells (Ma-Krupa 2002; Weyand and Goronzy 2003).

The infiltrating CD4+ T cells colocalize with dendritic cells in the vessel wall. Confocal microscopy study confirmed their cell–cell interaction (Wagner 2003). Inflammatory cells then migrate through the media. Macrophages infiltrating the arterial wall

exhibit topographical and functional diversity (Weyand *et al.* 1996). Cells producing transforming growth factor-beta (TGF-β), IL-1, and IL-6 preferentially localize in the adventitia. Another subgroup producing nitric oxide synthetase (NOS) is found in the intima. The intima–media junction is the preferred site for macrophages expressing matrix metalloproteinases (MMP) and platelet-derived growth factor (PDGF) (Kaiser *et al.* 1998; Weyand *et al.* 1996). MMP may facilitate movement of transformed smooth muscle cells to the subendothelial layer where they proliferate, causing intimal hyperplasia and narrowing of the lumen.

A small fraction of the tissue-infiltrating CD4+ T cells in GCA express IL-2 receptor, the hallmark of recent activation (Cid *et al.* 1989; Wagner *et al.* 1996). Most of these cells express mRNA specific for IL-2 and for IFN-γ, markers of the Th1 lymphocyte subset (Weyand *et al.* 1994a). Most of the IFN-γ producing T cells are aggregated in the adventitia (Wagner *et al.* 1996). High transcription of IFN-γ mRNA is associated with the formation of giant cells, and with evidence of cranial ischemic symptoms (Weyand *et al.* 1997). Ischemic complications also correlate with the degree of intimal hyperplasia and the accumulation of PDGF-producing macrophages at the media–intima junction (Kaiser *et al.* 1998).

Sequence analysis of the T cell receptor (TCR) V-beta elements demonstrated that several individual TCR specificities were present in multiple copies in artery specimens, indicating clonal expansion (Weyand *et al.* 1994b). Moreover, T cells with identical beta-chains were isolated from distinct inflammatory foci in the same arterial specimen, suggesting that these cells were disease-relevant. This is consistent with *in situ* T cell activation in response to contact with disease-specific antigens. One of these T-cell clonotypes was shown to proliferate in response to extracts from temporal arteries obtained from GCA and PMR patients (Martinez-Taboada *et al.* 1996).

A proposed hypothesis (Weyand and Goronzy 2003) suggests that initially arterial wall dendritic cells become activated by unknown stimulus, and recruit lymphocytes. A group of CD4+ T cells undergo *in situ* clonal expansion in response to those unknown antigens, producing IL-2 and IFN-γ. T cells and macrophages probably cross-stimulate each other to amplify the immune response. Monocyte-macrophages become multinucleated giant cells following exposure to IFN-γ. In addition to recruiting lymphocytes, the macrophages produce MMP, which facilitate the movement of inflammatory cells and transformed myocytes (myofibroblasts) through the vessel wall towards the intima. Macrophages also produce PDGF which stimulates intimal proliferation, and VEGF which stimulates neoangiogenesis in the media and in the thickened intima. The combination of destruction and repair mechanisms causes the typical histopathologic changes and may result in severe narrowing of the arterial lumen, which produces symptoms of ischemia.

PMR patients share many pathogenetic features with GCA (Ma-Krupa 2004; Weyand and Goronzy 2003). In both conditions, the majority of circulating monocytes are activated, and serum IL-6 concentration is elevated (Roche *et al.* 1993; Uddhammar *et al.* 1998b). Morphologic analysis of non-inflamed vascular segments revealed greater atrophy of the media smooth muscle and larger calcifications of the internal elastic lamina in both PMR and GCA compared with controls (Nordborg *et al.* 1991).

There is evidence for vascular inflammation in the temporal arteries of PMR patients, without histologic evidence of arteritis. Using fluorodeoxyglucose (FDG) positron emission tomography (PET) scanning, increased uptake was documented in thoracic and upper leg vessels in both GCA and PMR patients (see also Chapter 20). This is suggestive of inflammation in these vessels (Blockmans *et al.* 1999, 2000; Moosig *et al.* 2004). In addition, in temporal arteries from PMR patients the dendritic cells are activated, and there is local expression of IL-1, IL-2, and TGF-β (Weyand *et al.* 1994a; Weyand and Goronzy 2003). However, in contrast to GCA, T cells producing IFN-γ are not attracted to the vessel wall. This lack of IFN-γ expression in temporal arteries from PMR patients suggests that its production is crucial to the development of overt vasculitis and that a TH1 response may be suppressed in PMR, possibly by anti-inflammatory cytokines such as IL-10 (Straub *et al.* 1999), or by other mechanisms.

Clinical features

The signs and symptoms of GCA can be classified into four subsets (Table 24.2). Patients may develop any combination of these manifestations. The onset may be abrupt, but in most instances symptoms are insidious, and develop gradually over a period of several weeks.

Table 24.2 Classification of clinical features of giant cell arteritis

	Symptom	Frequency[1]
Cranial arteritis	Headache, scalp tenderness	Very common
	Prominent temporal arteries	Common
	Jaw claudication	Common
	Vision loss and other ophthalmic manifestations	Uncommon
	Cerebrovascular accidents/ transient ischemic attacks	Uncommon
	Vestibuloauditory manifestations	Uncommon
	Trismus, dysphagia	Uncommon
	Neuropsychiatric manifestations	Rare
	Scalp or tongue infarction	Rare
	Facial pain, carotidynia	Rare
Extracranial arteritis	Respiratory symptoms	Uncommon
	Peripheral neuropathies	Uncommon
	Aortic arch syndrome, aortic valve insufficiency, aortic aneurysm and dissection	Uncommon
	Angina pectoris, myocardial infarction	Rare
	Abdominal angina, bowel infarction	Rare
	Leg claudication, infarction	Rare
	Renal failure, nephrotic syndrome	Rare
Systemic symptoms	Fever	Common
	Malaise, fatigue, anorexia, weight loss	Common
Musculoskeletal symptoms	Polymyalgia rheumatica	Common
	Peripheral synovitis	Uncommon

[1] very common = more than 60% of the patients; common = 30–60% of the patients; uncommon = 5–29% of the patients; rare = less than 5% of the patients.

Craniofacial symptoms

Headache is a frequent presenting symptom and is typically felt over one or both temporal areas, although generalized or occipital headaches have been reported. Severity is variable, and the headache may be continuous or paroxysmal. Removal of the temporal artery may ameliorate the headaches in some cases. The origin of the pain is believed to be the inflamed arteries, which may be swollen and tender. The headache is probably mediated by nerve growth factor, which is increased in inflamed tissues and acts on nociceptor fibers to produce hyperalgesia (Saldanha *et al.* 1999).

Scalp tenderness is seen most often in patients with headaches. It also can be localized to the temporal or occipital areas, but may be diffuse. Wearing a hat or glasses, or combing the hair may be uncomfortable. In extreme cases, involvement of the scalp arteries may lead to segmental scalp necrosis (Dudenhoefer *et al.* 1998).

Pain in the tongue or jaw during mastication, which resolves with rest (jaw claudication), is common. One study reported reduction of jaw opening in 7% of GCA patients (Nir-Paz *et al.* 2002). Facial pain has also been reported. Rarely, ischemia may result in tongue infarction (Hellmann 2002). Some patients experience pain and tenderness over the carotid arteries (González-Gay and Garcia-Porrua 1998).

Neurologic manifestations

GCA patients may present with various neurologic manifestations (Caselli *et al.* 1988a). Cerebrovascular accidents (CVA) are uncommon, occurring in 3–7% of GCA patients (Caselli *et al.* 1988a; Nesher *et al.* 2004a). This may be an underestimate, since it is sometimes difficult to decide whether a CVA in an elderly patient is related to GCA or to atherosclerotic vascular disease although strokes in uncommon vascular distributions are among the leading causes of GCA-related morbidity and mortality (Graham *et al.* 1981; Save-Soderbergh *et al.* 1986).

Involvement of the vertebrobasilar system is relatively more common in GCA-related CVA than in atherosclerotic CVA (Nesher *et al.* 2004a; Ruegg *et al.* 2003). It is important to note that CVA may still develop after glucocorticoid therapy is begun, either within the first 2 weeks or while tapering the dose (González-Gay *et al.* 1998a; Nesher *et al.* 2004a; Staunton *et al.* 2000).

Rare neuropsychiatric manifestations include dementia, psychotic features, and depression (Caselli 1990; Johnson *et al.* 1997; Pascuzzi *et al.* 1989). These complications may be secondary to multiple brain infarcts (Ely 1998). Metabolic causes should always be considered in elderly GCA patients with confusion and deterioration of mental status. Several cases have been described with disorientation and weakness related to severe hyponatremia due to the syndrome of inappropriate secretion of antidiuretic hormone (SIADH). This probably reflects ischemia of the posterior pituitary gland. The symptoms and hyponatremia improved following glucocorticoid therapy (Gentric *et al.* 1988).

Visual hallucinations have also been reported, but these are not true psychiatric manifestations since they occur in individuals with intact cognition, and always in association with visual loss (Nesher *et al.* 2001). In such cases, even slight deterioration of visual acuity may result in decreasing stimuli to the visual cortex, leading to increased autonomous cortical activity manifesting as visual hallucinations. These visions are typically vivid and pleasant, and the patients are aware of their unreal nature. They resolve within a few weeks, probably reflecting cortical adaptation to the reduced visual acuity.

Peripheral neuropathies are uncommon (Caselli *et al.* 1988b). The pathogenesis of this type of neuropathy probably relates to inflammation of nutrient arteries, causing mononeuropathies or symmetric polyneuropathy. Other possible mechanisms of nerve injury include extension of the inflammatory process from adjacent arteries, such as in brachial plexopathy with its proximity to the subclavian artery (Nesher *et al.* 1987), and compression by adjacent synovitis causing carpal tunnel syndrome (Healey 1984). Symptoms improved with treatment in most patients.

Glucocorticoid treatment of GCA patients presenting with dementia or psychosis can improve or stabilize the symptoms (Johnson *et al.* 1997; Pascuzzi *et al.* 1989), but it may initially worsen the psychotic features. In such cases, glucocorticoid treatment should be combined with antipsychotic therapy.

Ophthalmic manifestations

Ophthalmic manifestations are common, and may cause blindness (Miller 2001). Arteritic anterior ischemic optic neuropathy (AION) is the leading cause of blindness in GCA (González-Gay *et al.* 2000a; Hayreh *et al.* 1998; Miller 2001). It may be the presenting manifestation of GCA. Arteritic AION results from vasculitis of the short posterior ciliary arteries, branches of the ophthalmic artery, which supply the optic nerve head and the choroid. Vasculitis in these arteries is apparently common, occurring in almost all autopsied GCA patients (Wilkinson and Russell 1972); however, it is clinically silent in most.

In the general population, AION occurs much more commonly as a result of atherosclerosis, embolic disease, or transient hypotension (defined as non-arteritic AION). In general, only about 5% of patients with AION have GCA (Miller 2001). Examination of the fundus at the time of the acute event may not distinguish between arteritic and non-arteritic AION. Other symptoms, signs, and laboratory parameters suggestive of inflammation may help distinguish between the two etiologies. In addition, there may be some clues in the ophthalmological work-up.

In many patients with GCA, fluorescein angiography of the fundus discloses occlusive disease of the short posterior ciliary arteries, seen as a delay of the filling of choroidal vessels around the optic disc (Hayreh *et al.* 1998; Siatkowski *et al.* 1993). This may serve to distinguish cases of arteritic AION from non-arteritic AION, since in the latter, choroidal non-perfusion is uncommon. Similar findings of involvement of ophthalmic vessels have been reported with color Doppler imaging of the eye and orbital arteries (Ghanchi *et al.* 1996). Choroidal ischemia itself may cause some blurry vision, which probably precedes arteritic AION and can be reversible with prompt therapy (Quillen *et al.* 1993; Siatkowski *et al.* 1993).

Arteritic AION may also be distinguished from non-arteritic AION after the acute phase. Using fundus photographs, it was found that the end-stage optic disc appearance in arteritic AION showed cupping (excavation) of the disc, present in 92% of the cases. In contrast, only 2% of cases with non-arteritic AION had cupping of the disc (Danesh-Meyer *et al.* 2001). This different outcome was corroborated using imaging of the optic disc with the Heidelberg Retinal Tomograph (Danesh-Meyer *et al.* 2005b).

Less common causes of visual loss are central retinal artery occlusion, posterior ischemic optic neuropathy, and cortical blindness. The frequency of acute visual loss in GCA fell dramatically following the introduction of glucocorticoid therapy for this disease. It has continued to decrease since the 1980s, probably due to increasing awareness of physicians and earlier diagnosis of GCA patients (Nesher *et al.* 1996). Nevertheless, it still occurs in as many as 20% of GCA patients (González-Gay *et al.* 2000a; Liu *et al.* 1994; Nesher *et al.* 2004a). AION is unilateral in most cases, and occurs most often prior to the commencement of glucocorticoid therapy. However, new or recurrent AION in the other eye may appear simultaneously, during the first few days of therapy, or while the dose is being tapered (Aiello *et al.* 1993; Chan *et al.* 2005; Cornblath and Eggenberger 1997; González-Gay *et al.* 1998a; Hayreh *et al.* 1998; Liu *et al.* 1994; Nesher *et al.* 2004a).

Vision loss in GCA is sudden. However, several studies reported that 50% or more of GCA patients with irreversible visual loss had premonitory visual symptoms, such as blurry vision, amaurosis fugax, visual hallucinations, or diplopia (Font *et al.* 1997; González-Gay *et al.* 2000a; Nesher *et al.* 2004a). Amaurosis fugax is probably the most ominous sign of impending visual loss. If left untreated, the likelihood of developing permanent loss of vision is about 50% (Hayreh *et al.* 1998; González-Gay *et al.* 2000a). These premonitory symptoms may precede vision loss by several days, and should be considered a medical emergency in GCA as prompt treatment may prevent the development of irreversible complications (González-Gay *et al.* 1998a; Hayreh *et al.* 1998).

Following vision loss, the visual outcome is poor, even in patients treated with high-doses of glucocorticoids following the acute event. Only 5% had some improvement of both visual acuity and central visual field (Danesh-Meyer *et al.* 2005a; Hayreh *et al.* 2002). Timing of treatment was important: there was a shorter interval between onset of visual loss and start of therapy in the few patients that improved. There is no valid evidence that intravenous mega-dose glucocorticoid therapy is more effective than oral therapy in improving vision or preventing visual deterioration (Hayreh and Zimmerman 2003). The main reason for immediate treatment with glucocorticoids following vision loss is to prevent further deterioration of vision, and blindness of the fellow eye (Hayreh 1991).

Other manifestations of ophthalmic involvement in GCA are rare, and include orbital pseudotumor (characterized by proptosis), ocular hypotony, and ptosis (Miller 2001). In some cases these may improve with glucocorticoid therapy.

Risk factors for cranial ischemic complications

Cranial ischemic complications, mainly stroke and vision loss, are the most dreaded manifestations of GCA. In recent years there have been attempts by several groups of researchers to evaluate individual risk factors for these complications (Cid *et al.* 1998; Duhaut *et al.* 1998; González-Gay *et al.* 1998a, 2000a, 2004b; Hayreh *et al.* 1998; Liozon *et al.* 2001; Nesher *et al.* 2004a; Salvarani *et al.* 2005a).

Although results of these studies were not unanimous, it appears that any sign or symptom of permanent or transient cranial ischemia is a risk factor for vision loss or CVA. In addition, the presence of traditional risk factors for atherosclerosis seemed to increase the risk of CVA and vision loss. The presence of thrombocytosis and antiphospholipid antibodies may also contribute to the increased risk. On the other hand, it has been suggested that GCA patients with strong systemic inflammatory responses, and those with PMR symptoms, have a low risk of developing cranial ischemic complications.

This paradoxical protective effect of the intense inflammatory syndrome is possibly related to the effect of a certain cytokine profile. There is a correlation between the intensity of the systemic inflammatory response and production of IL-1, TNF-α, and IL-6 in the temporal artery (Hernandez-Rodriguez *et al.* 2004). Specifically, increased production of IL-6 was associated with lower incidence of ischemic complications, possibly mediated by its ability to stimulate endothelial cell proliferation (Hernandez-Rodriguez *et al.* 2003).

Vestibuloauditory manifestations

Vestibuloauditory manifestations probably result from deprivation of blood supply to the terminal cochleovestibular vessels. These manifestations were uncommon in retrospective observations, but more common in prospective studies (Amor-Dorado *et al.* 2003; Caselli *et al.* 1988a). Symptoms are unilateral or bilateral hearing loss, vertigo, and tinnitus (Amor-Dorado *et al.* 2003; Hausch and Harrington 1998). Onset is usually insidious. In a prospective study, 89% of GCA patients had abnormal vestibular tests, 64% had subjective hearing impairment, 52% had vertigo, and 50% had tinnitus. These were reversible in most cases following steroid therapy. After 3 months of treatment only 30% remained with abnormal vestibular tests, 16% still had hearing impairment, 14% had tinnitus, and 2% had vertigo.

Involvement of thoracoabdominal and peripheral arteries

Signs of occlusive changes in large arteries of the chest and upper extremities are uncommon, but can be the earliest sign of the disease (Brack *et al.* 1999; Evans *et al.* 1994; Lie 1995). The clinical findings are those of the aortic arch syndrome, indistinguishable from those of Takayasu arteritis: intermittent arm claudication, Raynaud's phenomenon, absent or decreased pulses, and bruits over the involved arteries (subclavian, axillary, and brachial). Angiograms show smooth stenoses or obliteration of the involved vessels. Non-invasive imaging can also be used to document vasculitic involvement (Blockmans *et al.* 2000; Schmidt *et al.* 2002).

These manifestations may occur in any GCA patient as part of the disease. There is a subset of GCA patients characterized by those presenting features (Brack *et al.* 1999). These patients are relatively young (mean 66 years), cranial symptoms are less frequent, the ESR less elevated, and the rate of positive temporal artery biopsies tends to be lower. The response to therapy is favorable in most cases.

Clinical signs of aortitis are uncommon in GCA (Evans *et al.* 1995; González-Gay *et al.* 2004c; Lie 1995; Neunninghoff *et al.* 2003); however, this condition may be underdiagnosed, since symptoms are frequently mild and insidious. Involvement of the aorta is more common in the thoracic segment. Thoracic aortic aneurysm or dissection was reported in 10% of GCA patients (two cases per 100 person-years at risk) (González-Gay *et al.* 2004c; Neunninghoff *et al.* 2003). In most GCA patients with aortic abnormalities, symptoms occur late in the course of the disease, sometimes years after completion of the course of glucocorticoid treatment (Evans *et al.* 1994).

Aside from patients in whom the aortic abnormality was discovered on a routine chest radiograph, the most common initial symptom of aortic involvement was dyspnea on exertion due to incompetence of the aortic valve (Evans *et al.* 1994). Other presentations are chest pain and sudden death. Dissection of the thoracic aorta occurred in 50% of these patients and was fatal in half of them. Hyperlipidemia and hypertension were associated with aortic involvement (González-Gay *et al.* 2004c; Neunninghoff *et al.* 2003). The outcome of surgical procedures (aortic valve replacement and resection of thoracic aortic aneurysm) was often favorable.

Involvement of the coronary, mesenteric, and other visceral and peripheral arteries is supposedly rare (Lie 1995). It is difficult to determine clinically whether a coronary event is related to GCA or atherosclerosis (Nordborg and Bengtsson 1989). Coronary and mesenteric arteritis can be clinically silent, or present as angina pectoris and acute myocardial infarction, or as abdominal angina and bowel infarction, respectively (Srigley and Gardiner 1980). Lower limb arteritis is rare, but may result in severe ischemia (Le Hello *et al.* 2001; Lie 1995). In contrast to most other vasculitides, GCA infrequently affects the kidneys (Truong *et al.* 1985).

Respiratory manifestations

Respiratory manifestations are uncommon (Larson *et al.* 1984). Their cause is undetermined, but they are possibly associated with vasculitis involving the respiratory tract. Symptoms include nonproductive cough, sore throat, and hoarseness. Lung infiltrates, interstitial lung disease, nodules or pleural effusion have been seen on chest radiographs (Kramer *et al.* 1987).

Systemic manifestations

Systemic manifestations such as fever, malaise, fatigue, anorexia, and weight loss occur often in GCA patients. In some cases, these are the only symptoms of the disease (the occult presentation of GCA), and a high index of suspicion is needed to make the diagnosis. Fever is usually low-grade, but temperatures may exceed 39°C. The presence of intense systemic manifestations seems to be paradoxically protective against cranial ischemic complications (see above), but is also associated with more disease flares and a need for relatively higher glucocorticoid doses and prolonged duration of therapy (Hernandez-Rodriguez *et al.* 2002). The presence of intense systemic inflammatory manifestations has been associated with developing aortic aneurysm at a later stage (González-Gay *et al.* 2004c).

Polymyalgia rheumatica symptoms

The typical symptoms of PMR are aching and stiffness, which may develop abruptly or insidiously over several weeks (Salvarani *et al.* 1997a). Night pain is common. In the majority of patients, the shoulder girdle is the first to become involved. Involvement of the neck and the hip girdle may follow. Symptoms are symmetric, or become symmetric within a couple of weeks, and may extend to the proximal parts of the limbs. These symptoms are probably related to inflammation of the subacromial, subdeltoid, and trochanteric bursae, and the glenohumeral or hip joints (Salvarani *et al.* 1997b; Cantini *et al.* 2005).

Although muscle testing is difficult due to pain with movement, strength seems to be unimpaired; however, patients with long-standing, untreated disease may develop disuse muscle atrophy and frozen shoulders (adhesive capsulitis). One-third of PMR patients without evidence of GCA have systemic manifestations such as fever, malaise, and anorexia, but these are often milder than systemic symptoms in GCA patients (Salvarani et al. 1997a).

A subgroup of PMR patients has synovitis of peripheral joints (Gran and Mykelbust 2000; Healey 1984; Salvarani et al. 1998). The only finding might be arthralgia or slight puffiness (Salvarani et al. 1999) but some patients present with symmetric synovitis with pitting edema and some develop carpal tunnel syndrome (Navarez et al. 2001; Olivieri et al. 1997; Salvarani et al. 1996, 1998). The peripheral arthritis is non-erosive, predominantly affecting the knees, wrists, and metacarpophalangeal joints, and the synovial fluid is mildly inflammatory. PMR patients with peripheral arthritis have more severe disease, with more relapses and longer duration of treatment, but concurrence with GCA was less common. It is difficult at times to distinguish between these patients and patients with elderly-onset rheumatoid arthritis (RA) (Pease et al. 2005).

Laboratory investigations

Erythrocyte sedimentation rate (ESR) and C reactive protein (CRP) are elevated in almost all patients with PMR or GCA (Table 24.3). Levels of other acute phase reactants, such as fibrinogen and haptoglobin, are also elevated in the majority of patients. It is controversial whether initial levels of ESR and CRP predict the subsequent disease course (González-Gay et al. 1997b; Pountain and Hazleman 1997). Another matter of uncertainty is which of these two tests correlates better with disease activity at presentation or during relapses (Hayreh et al. 1997; Kyle et al. 1989; Mallya et al. 1985). CRP levels respond faster to changes in disease activity, but in most patients, both CRP and ESR decrease to normal levels after 4 weeks of treatment with glucocorticoids. Some patients may have persistently elevated levels of CRP, and in one study of PMR, this was associated with increased risk of relapse (Salvarani et al. 2005b). The reliability of ESR and CRP as indicators of relapse is not clear, since levels are often normal during relapses, or may be increased due to other causes (Kyle et al. 1989). It has been suggested that IL-6 may serve as a better marker of disease activity (Salvarani et al. 2005b; Uddhammar et al. 1998b; Weyand et al. 2000).

Table 24.3 Abnormalities in common laboratory tests in polymyalgia rheumatica and giant cell arteritis

Test		Frequency[1]
Acute phase reactants	Elevated ESR	Very common
	Elevated CRP	Very common
	Others (fibrinogen, etc.)	Very common
Blood count	Anemia	Very common
	Thrombocytosis	Common[2]
	Leukocytosis	Uncommon
Liver function tests	Elevated alkaline phosphatase	Common
	Elevated transaminases	Uncommon
	Low albumin	Uncommon
Urinalysis	Proteinuria, hematuria	Uncommon [2]

[1] very common = more than 60% of the patients, common = 30–60% of the patients, uncommon = 5–29% of the patients, rare = less than 5% of the patients.

[2] less frequent in polymyalgia rheumatica.

A small group of patients (about 5–10% with GCA and 5–20% with PMR) may present with typical features of the disease but without elevation of the ESR (Cantini et al. 2000; Martinez-Taboada et al. 2000; Proven et al. 1999; Salvarani and Hunder 2001). CRP levels were elevated in 80–90% of the patients who had normal ESR (Cantini et al. 2000; Salvarani et al. 2005b). In many patients with normal ESR at presentation, the levels decreased in response to glucocorticoid therapy. Systemic manifestations and anemia were less frequent compared with those of patients with elevated ESR, but other clinical features and the course of the disease were not significantly different in most of the reports.

Mild to moderate normochromic normocytic anemia is observed in 50–75% of patients with GCA and PMR. Thrombocytosis and leukocytosis are less common, occurring in 30–50% and 15–30% of patients, respectively. All improve following therapy and remission of the disease. Globulin levels may be elevated, especially the alpha-2 and gamma fractions.

Abnormalities in liver function tests occur frequently (Kyle 1991). Modest elevation of alkaline phosphatase is most common, followed by increased transaminases and low albumin levels. All return to normal following treatment. Liver scan may be normal, or show slight hepatomegaly, patchy uptake, or focal defects, findings that may persist for more than a year.

Abnormalities in urine and renal function were reported in about 10% of GCA patients (Truong et al. 1985). The most common of these have been microscopic hematuria and minimal proteinuria, with normal renal function. Nephrotic syndrome and renal failure have been reported a few times. The histopathological findings were intrarenal arteritis, and focal or membranous glomerulonephritis. Renal amyloidosis is very rare (Escriba et al. 2000).

The association between GCA-PMR and thyroid abnormalities remains controversial. While some studies reported increased prevalence of hypothyroidism (Bowness et al. 1991; Wiseman et al. 1989), others found no difference in prevalence compared with controls (Dasgupta et al. 1990; Duhaut et al. 1999b). Thyroid antibodies were observed in many GCA cases, but their prevalence was similar to that of the control group (Duhaut et al. 1999b).

Elevated levels of anticardiolipin antibodies have been found in 30–80% of GCA patients, and 5–30% of PMR patients (Chakravarty et al. 1995; Duhaut et al. 1998; Espinoza et al. 1991). Some studies found correlation between the presence of anticardiolipin antibodies and ischemic episodes, but this was not corroborated by others (Duhaut et al. 1998; Espinosa et al. 2001; Espinoza et al. 1991).

Elevated levels of von Willebrand factor, a marker of endothelial injury or activation, have been observed in GCA and PMR patients. The mean levels in GCA tend to be higher than in PMR patients, but there was no correlation between increased levels and ischemic complications. Levels did not decrease following the initiation of glucocorticoid therapy, and persisted for about 2 years (Cid et al. 1996).

Diagnostic approach

The diagnosis of PMR and GCA is made primarily on clinical grounds and is bolstered by laboratory evidence of an acute phase reaction. Various conditions can mimic GCA and PMR

(González-Gay *et al.* 2000b), and should be considered in the differential diagnosis (Table 24.4) (see Chapter 45).

Giant cell arteritis

The only test that confirms the diagnosis of GCA is a positive temporal (or occipital) artery biopsy. However, since the disease may affect the vessels focally, histologic examination is normal in some patients with GCA. The frequency of false-negative biopsies is about 15% (González-Gay *et al.* 2001b), and is influenced by the length of the arterial segment taken, the number of sections in the specimen, and time elapsed from the start of glucocorticoid treatment (Achkar *et al.* 1994; Allison and Gallagher 1984; Nordborg and Nordborg 1995).

A threshold size of 1 cm of artery specimen is associated with increased diagnostic yield (Taylor-Gjevre *et al.* 2005). Careful attention should be paid to processing the tissue sample. The arterial segment is cut into numerous short pieces which are embedded in one or more tissue blocks and then sectioned at multiple levels (see Figure 9.4 in Chapter 9). Obtaining biopsies from both temporal arteries increases the chance of a positive result by 1–14% (Danesh-Meyer *et al.* 2000; Hall and Hunder 1984; Pless *et al.* 2000). It is desirable to perform the biopsy as soon as possible, but there may be signs of arteritis even after 2–4 weeks of treatment (Achkar *et al.* 1994; Ray-Chaudhuri *et al.* 2002).

The necessity of obtaining a temporal artery biopsy in all cases suspected of having GCA is still debated, since a classic presentation may make this investigation seem unnecessary. Nevertheless, a positive biopsy gives the treating physician confidence in continuing glucocorticoid therapy, despite the potential for side-effects.

There are no independent validating criteria to determine whether GCA is present in individuals whose biopsy is negative. The American College of Rheumatology 1990 criteria for the classification of GCA (Hunder *et al.* 1990) may assist in diagnosis. These criteria include: (1) age at onset more than 50 years; (2) a new headache; (3) temporal artery abnormality such as tenderness to palpation or decreased pulsation; (4) ESR >50 mm/h; and (5) abnormal artery biopsy showing vasculitis with mononuclear cell or granulomatous inflammation usually with giant cells. At least three of the criteria must be present, which yields a sensitivity of 93% and a specificity of 91% among subjects with vasculitis.

Table 24.4 Conditions that should be considered in the differential diagnosis of polymyalgia rheumatica and giant cell arteritis

Polymyalgia rheumatica	Giant cell arteritis
Elderly-onset rheumatoid arthritis	Sinusitis
Fibromyalgia	Dental problems
Cervical spondylosis	Non-arteritic AION or CRAO
Hypothyroidism	Subacute thyroiditis
Viral infections, chronic infections	Chronic infections (infective endocarditis, etc.)
Polymyositis	Trigeminal neuralgia
Malignancy	Malignancy
Amyloidosis	Atherosclerotic cardiovascular disease

AION, anterior ischemic optic neuropathy; CRAO, central retinal artery occlusion.

Nevertheless, since physicians often misuse classification criteria as diagnostic criteria, it should be remembered that the GCA classification criteria were meant to distinguish patients with this disease from those with other vasculitides, and not from patients without vasculitis (Hunder 1998; Rao *et al.* 1998). Classification criteria work best in the study of groups of patients, and less well when used for the diagnosis of individual patients. Thus, meeting classification criteria is not equivalent to a diagnosis in an individual patient, and the final diagnosis should be based on all clinical features and laboratory findings.

In addition to temporal artery biopsy, various imaging modalities with relatively high sensitivity and specificity may aid in GCA diagnosis. Color duplex ultrasonography of the temporal arteries discloses a hypoechoic halo around the artery in many cases (Schmidt *et al.* 1997). This halo probably represents swelling of the vessel wall due to inflammation. Several studies have been conducted to assess the performance of this test in diagnosing GCA (LeSar *et al.* 2002; Nesher *et al.* 2002; Romera-Villegas *et al.* 2004; Salvarani *et al.* 2002). Most found a high negative predictive value (>95%), but the positive predictive value was lower. A recent meta-analysis concluded that when the pretest probability of GCA is low, negative results of ultrasonography practically exclude GCA (Karassa *et al.* 2005). Thus it appears that ultrasonography better serves to rule out GCA, while a positive test needs to be confirmed by a biopsy.

High-resolution contrast-enhanced magnetic resonance imaging (MRI) of the temporal arteries also enables evaluation of possible inflammation of the vessel wall, and preliminary results suggest high sensitivity (Bley *et al.* 2005). Gallium-67 scintigraphy may show increased uptake over the temporal region in GCA (Reitblat *et al.* 2003). Angiography of the aortic arch and its branches may diagnose large-vessel involvement (Brack *et al.* 1999). Non-invasive modalities, such as MRI and PET scanning, have been employed (Blockmans *et al.* 2000; Navarez *et al.* 2005).

Polymyalgia rheumatica

There is no single diagnostic test for PMR, but sets of diagnostic criteria have been suggested by different groups of investigators (Bird *et al.* 1979; Chuang *et al.* 1982; Healey 1984; Jones and Hazleman 1981) (Table 24.5). Bilateral shoulder or hip bursitis or synovitis found by ultrasonography or MRI has been reported in the majority of PMR patients and may support a diagnosis of PMR (Cantini *et al.* 2001, 2005; Salvarani *et al.* 1997b). Such findings, however, may also occur in elderly-onset RA (Lange *et al.* 1998). It is difficult at times to distinguish between PMR patients and those with elderly-onset RA and PMR-like presentation (Healey and Sheets 1988). A case–control study of shoulder MRI in patients with PMR or RA found signs of shoulder bursitis in all PMR patients, but in only 22% of the RA patients (Salvarani *et al.* 1997b); however, another study found no significant differences between PMR and RA, except for the presence of signs of extracapsular inflammation in PMR (McGonagle *et al.* 2001). In one-quarter of older-onset RA patients, PMR symptoms are the principal initial manifestation, and about 10% of patients with PMR presentation will eventually develop the characteristic features of RA (Caporali *et al.* 2001; Gran and Mykelbust 2000). The absence of anticyclic citrullinated peptide (anti-CCP) antibodies in PMR patients may help to differentiate them from patients with elderly-onset RA (Lopez-Hoyos *et al.* 2004). Differentiation of

Table 24.5 Criteria for the diagnosis of PMR suggested by various authors

	Healey 1984	Jones and Hazleman 1981	Bird *et al.* 1979	Chuang *et al.* 1982
Age (years)	>50		>65	>50
Onset			<2 weeks	
Duration		>2 months		>1 month
Area of pain	Neck, shoulder, or pelvic girdle	Shoulder and pelvic girdle	Bilateral shoulder pain and stiffness	Neck or torso, or proximal arms, shoulders hips or proximal thighs (at least 2 of 3)
Morning stiffness	>1 hour	Present	>1 hour	>30 min
Tenderness Systemic symptoms			Upper arms Depression, weight loss	
ESR	Elevated	>30 mm/h, or CRP >6 mg/l	>40 mm/h	>40 mm/h[1]
Response to glucocorticoids	Rapid, to 20 mg or less	Prompt and dramatic		
Requirements for diagnosis	Age must be >50, plus 3 of the other 4 criteria	All criteria	If any 3 criteria are present, sensitivity is 92% and specificity 80%	All criteria

[1] If ESR is borderline, look instead for other evidence to support the diagnosis: change in ESR compared to pre-illness period, rapid response to low-dose steroids, history of GCA, fever, weight loss or anemia).

PMR and rheumatoid arthritis may require several months of surveillance.

Giant cell arteritis in polymyalgia rheumatica

There is a wide range in the reported frequency of PMR in GCA patients (17–66%), and of GCA in PMR patients (4–31%). The two syndromes may appear together, but they may also be separated by long intervals and either one may appear first. No significant differences in PMR symptoms have been noted between patients who have been shown to have GCA and those whose temporal artery biopsies were negative (González-Gay *et al.* 1998b).

The approach for detecting GCA in PMR patients is a matter of controversy. One diagnostic option is to routinely biopsy the temporal arteries in all PMR patients. In this approach, the chance of missing GCA is negligible. Temporal artery biopsy may detect arteritis in persons with what was thought to be isolated PMR, but the frequency of positive biopsies is rather low (Healey 1991; Schmidt and Gromnica-Ihle 2002). Another strategy is to biopsy only those patients who have symptoms suggestive of GCA. The results are likely to vary according to the expertise of the examining physician (Hunder 1997).

There have been some attempts to develop guidelines for performing temporal artery biopsy for suspected GCA in PMR patients

(Gabriel *et al.* 1995; Rodriguez-Valverde *et al.* 1997). Patients who were younger than 70 years of age, and with no features of cranial vasculitis (such as a new headache, jaw claudication, abnormalities of the temporal arteries on examination, and amaurosis fugax) were unlikely to have a positive biopsy. Older patients with cranial vasculitis findings were more likely to have a positive biopsy. PMR patients with GCA tended to have higher ESR and platelet counts, and lower hemoglobin levels compared with patients with isolated PMR (González-Gay *et al.* 1998b). They also tend to have poor clinical response to low-dose glucocorticoid therapy, with persistent abnormalities in laboratory parameters of inflammation. GCA was unlikely in PMR patients with peripheral synovitis (Myklebust and Gran 1996).

Some patients with pure PMR may show signs of large-vessel inflammation when imaging modalities such as PET scanning are employed (Blockmans *et al.* 1999, 2000; Moosig *et al.* 2004). The significance of such involvement for the individual patient is yet unclear.

Management

Glucocorticoids are the mainstay of treatment for PMR and GCA. Symptoms typically begin to abate within 1–3 days of commencing therapy. This dramatic improvement is characteristic of both conditions. Prompt treatment is crucial in order to prevent the irreversible complications of stroke and visual loss. Therapy should not be delayed pending temporal artery biopsy, which should be performed as soon as possible. In GCA, most physicians begin treatment with a dose of 40–60 mg/day of prednisone, while in PMR the starting dose is 15–20 mg/day (Table 24.6). Patients with vascular complications such as visual loss or stroke are often treated initially with higher doses, such as 80–120 mg/day of prednisone, or 500–1000 mg/day of intravenous methyprednisolone for 3 consecutive days, followed by 60 mg/day of prednisone, in an attempt to prevent additional ischemic complications.

After 2–4 weeks, following improvement of the clinical features of the disease together with normalization of the acute phase reactants (ESR and CRP), the dose of glucocorticoids can be tapered (Table 24.6), with close monitoring for recurrence of symptoms. Levels of ESR and CRP do not always correlate with disease activity. Nevertheless, some researchers advocate that monitoring should be guided by the ESR and CRP levels only (Hayreh and Zimmerman 2003). Unfortunately, this approach may result in prolonged course of therapy: at an average of 2.5 years only 7% of those patients discontinued glucocorticoid therapy.

Elevation of CRP and ESR levels while the patient is asymptomatic is not an absolute indication to increase the dose of prednisone. In such cases, it is preferable to slow the rate of dosage tapering, and continue to watch closely for recurrence of symptoms. On the other hand, the dose should be increased if symptoms recur, even when ESR or CRP remains unchanged or within the normal range.

The duration of treatment varies. The average time is 2–3 years (Nesher *et al.* 1997; Proven *et al.* 2003), but in some patients it is necessary to continue low doses of prednisone (5–10 mg/day) for longer periods of time. One or more relapses are experienced by 25–65% of patients, mostly during the first year of treatment or the first year after discontinuation of glucocorticoids (Ayoub *et al.* 1985; Hachula *et al.* 2001; Nesher *et al.* 1997; Proven *et al.* 2003).

Table 24.6 Suggested guidelines for glucocorticoid therapy in giant cell arteritis and polymyalgia rheumatica[1]

	Giant cell arteritis	Polymyalgia rheumatica
Starting daily dose (prednisone)	40–60 mg for 2–4 weeks	15–20 mg for 2–4 weeks
Tapering and maintenance	Reduce by 5–10 mg every 2–4 weeks until dose is 20 mg, then reduce by 2.5–5 mg every 2–4 weeks until the dose is 10 mg, and then by 1–2.5 mg every 1–2 months thereafter	Reduce by 2.5–5 mg every 2–4 weeks until the dose is 10 mg, and then by 1–2.5 mg every 1–2 months thereafter

[1] See text for conditions where higher starting doses are recommended and for monitoring of disease activity during therapy. These dosages of steroids are suggestions only and are not to be interpreted rigidly, as individual cases vary greatly. The exact doses and the duration of treatment should be adjusted to the needs of the individual patient. It is advisable to add low-dose aspirin, and also calcium, vitamin D and bisphosphonates (see text)

During relapses, the dose of prednisone should be increased to the dose given before the relapse or even higher, depending on the nature and severity of the symptoms. In some PMR patients, symptoms of GCA develop while the glucocorticoid dose is tapered, and they will require a diagnostic and therapeutic approach appropriate for GCA.

The adverse effects of glucocorticoids are dose-related, so they are more frequent and severe in GCA patients than in PMR patients. The majority of the patients experience at least one adverse event (Nesher *et al.* 1994; Proven *et al.* 2003). The most common of these are weight gain, fluid retention, exacerbation of diabetes, hypertension and osteoporosis, recurrent infections, and changes in mood or affect. Treatment-related adverse effects may become a source of greater morbidity and mortality than the disease (Nesher *et al.* 1994).

Several approaches have been used to lower the cumulative doses of glucocorticoids. Treatment of GCA patients with alternate-day prednisone has not proved effective (Hunder *et al.* 1975). Initial treatment with intravenous pulses of 240 mg methylprednisolone had no long-term glucocorticoid-sparing effect (Chevalet *et al.* 2000). Another approach was to treat with a depot glucocorticoid preparation at varying intervals. One study in PMR patients, comparing the use of initial doses of 120 mg methylprednisolone given intramuscularly every 3 weeks, to 15 mg oral prednisolone given daily, reported similar efficacy; toxicity was far less with the depot preparation (Dasgupta *et al.* 1998).

A different approach to minimize side-effects is to define patients who are expected to have a mild course, so they can be treated with lower doses. It has been suggested that PMR patients with initial ESR of less than 50 mm/h and initial IL-6 levels less than 10 pg/ml have a short uncomplicated course, and that initial treatment with 10 mg/day of prednisone would be sufficient in this subgroup (Weyand *et al.* 1999).

Attempts have been made to find effective glucocorticoid-sparing agents (Nesher and Sonnenblick 1994). Unfortunately, the agents that have been tried (methotrexate, azathioprine, antimalarials such as hydroxychloroquine, cyclosporine, cyclophosphamide, dapsone, non-steroidal anti-inflammatory drugs, and statins) had no sparing effect or only marginal effect, and some had substantial rates of adverse effects. Although a modest glucocorticoid-sparing effect was reported with methotrexate (Jover *et al.* 2001), this finding was not corroborated by others (Hoffman *et al.* 2002). There have been several anecdotal reports on efficacy of antitumor necrosis factor (TNF) agents, but a recent prospective study did not find any significant glucocorticoid-sparing effect (Hoffman *et al.* 2005). Thus, the preferred approach to limit side-effects remains the use of the lowest dose possible for the shortest period of time, while avoiding disease relapse.

In a large-scale retrospective study, low-dose aspirin (100 mg/day) has been shown to significantly decrease the rate of vision loss and CVA (both at GCA presentation and during the course of glucocorticoid therapy), probably mediated by its antiplatelet effect (Nesher *et al.* 2004b). In an animal study, higher doses of aspirin (>20 mg/kg) had anti-inflammatory effects, probably mediated by suppression of IFN-γ production (Weyand *et al.* 2002). It seems advisable to add low-dose aspirin to glucocorticoid therapy in order to prevent cranial ischemic complications in GCA.

Glucocorticoid-induced osteoporosis occurs even at low doses (Pearce *et al.* 1998) and is preventable to some extent. Adequate intake of calcium and vitamin D should be ensured for all patients and the addition of bisphosphonates or other antiresortive agents should be considered (Hochberg *et al.* 1996).

Some GCA patients with thoracic vascular involvement may benefit from surgical interventions such as aortic valve replacement, resection of aortic aneurysms, and percutaneous balloon angioplasty of stenoses in subclavian or axillary arteries (Amann-Vesti *et al.* 2003; Evans *et al.* 1994). Aortic complications may occur late in the course of GCA, sometimes after the completion of drug treatment. It is advisable that all GCA patients have evaluation of the thoracic aorta during the follow-up period and after medication has been discontinued.

Prognosis

There is no objective way of determining the prognosis in an individual with GCA or PMR. The initial doses of glucocorticoids, the rate of tapering, and the duration of therapy should be adjusted to the needs of the individual patient. PMR, when not associated with GCA, is thought to have a benign course, with a variable degree of treatment-related morbidity. In contrast, GCA may cause serious irreversible complications, such as visual loss and stroke, and can be fatal (Lie 1995; Save-Soderberg *et al.* 1986). The major causes of mortality are vascular: stroke, coronary artery events, rupture of thoracic aortic aneurysms, and aortic dissection. Glucocorticoid-related toxicity may also increase mortality (Nesher *et al.* 1994).

It is clear that GCA can lead to potentially fatal complications, but their impact on the overall prognosis is controversial (Andersson *et al.* 1986; Bisgard *et al.* 1991; Boesen and Sorensen 1987; González-Gay *et al.* 1997; Graham *et al.* 1981; Gran *et al.* 2001; Matteson *et al.* 1996; Nesher *et al.* 1994; Nordborg and Bengtsson 1989; Schaufelberger *et al.* 1995; Uddhammar *et al.* 2002). Some of these epidemiologic studies reported increased mortality, mostly during the first year after diagnosis, while others found that the overall life expectancy among GCA patients was essentially identical to that of the general population.

References

Achkar, A. A., Lie, J. T., Hunder, G. G., O'Fallon, W. M. and Gabriel, S. E. (1994). How does previous corticosteroid treatment affect the biopsy findings in giant cell (temporal) arteritis? *Annals of Internal Medicine*, **120**, 987–92.

Aiello, P. D., Trautmann, J. C., McPhee, T. J., Kunselman, A. R. and Hunder, G. G. (1993). Visual prognosis in giant cell arteritis. *Ophthalmology*, **100**, 550–55.

Allison, M. C. and Gallagher, P. J. (1984). Temporal artery biopsy and corticosteroid treatment. *Annals of the Rheumatic Diseases*, **43**, 416–7.

Alvarez-Lafuente, R., Fernandez-Gutierrez, B., Jover, J. A., *et al.* (2005). Human parvovirus B19, varicella zoster virus, and human herpes virus 6 in temporal artery biopsy specimens of patients with giant cell arteritis. *Annals of Rheumatic Diseases*, **64**, 780–2.

Amann-Vesti, B. R., Koppensteiner, R., Rainoni, L., Pfamatter, T. and Schneider, E. (2003). Immediate and long-term outcome of upper extremity balloon angioplasty in giant cell arteritis. *Journal of Endovascular Therapy*, **10**, 371–5.

Amoli, M. M., Garcia-Porrua, C., Llorca, J., Ollier, W. E. and González-Gay, M. A. (2003). Endothelial nitric oxide synthase haplotype associations in biopsy-proven giant cell arteritis. *Journal of Rheumatology*, **30**, 2019–22.

Amor-dorado, J. C., Llorca, J., Garcia-porrua, C., Costa, C., Perez-Fernandez, N. and González-Gay, M. A. (2003). Audiovestibular manifestations in giant cell arteritis: a prospective study. *Medicine*, **82**, 13–26.

Andersson, R., Malmvall, B. O. and Bengtsson, B. A. (1986). Long-term survival in giant cell arteritis including temporal arteritis and polymyalgia rheumatica. *Acta Medica Scandinavica*, **220**, 361–4.

Ashton-Key, M. and Gallagher, P. H. (1991). Surgical pathology of cranial arteritis and polymyalgia rheumatica. *Bailliere's Clinical Rheumatology*, **5**, 387–404.

Ayoub, W. T., Franklin, C. M. and Torretti, D. (1985). Polymyalgia rheumatica. Duration of therapy and long-term outcome. *American Journal of Medicine*, **79**, 309–15.

Baldursson, O., Steinsson, K., Bjornsson, J. and Lie, J. T. (1994). Giant cell arteritis in Iceland. *Arthritis and Rheumatism*, **37**, 1007–12.

Bird, H. A., Esselinckx, W., Dison, A. S.J., Mowat, A. G. and Wood, P. H.N. (1979). An evaluation of criteria for polymyalgia rheumatica. *Annals of the Rheumatic Diseases*, **38**, 434–9.

Bisgard, C., Sloth, H., Keiding, N. and Juel, K. (1991). Excess mortality in giant cell arteritis. *Journal of Internal Medicine*, **230**, 119–23.

Bley, T. A., Weiben, O., Uhl, M., *et al.* (2005). Assessment of the cranial involvement pattern of giant cell arteritis with 3T magnetic resonance imaging. *Arthritis and Rheumatism*, **52**, 2470–7.

Blockmans, D., Maes, A., Stroobants, S., *et al.* (1999). New arguments for a vasculitic nature of polymyalgia rheumatica using positron emission tomography. *Rheumatology*, **38**, 444–7.

Blockmans, D., Stroobants, S., Maes, A. and Mortelmans, L. (2000). Positron emission tomography in giant cell arteritis and polymyalgia rheumatica: evidence for inflammation of the aortic arch. *American Journal of Medicine*, **108**, 246–9.

Boesen, P. and Sorensen, S. F. (1987). Giant cell arteritis, temporal arteritis, and polymyalgia rheumatica in a Danish county. *Arthritis and Rheumatism*, **30**, 294–9.

Boiardi, L., Casali, B., Nicoli, D., *et al.* (2003). Vascular endothelial growth factor gene polymorphisms in giant cell arteritis. *Journal of Rheumatology*, **30**, 2160–4.

Bowness, P., Shotliff, K., Middlemiss, A. and Myles, A. B. (1991). Prevalence of hypothyroidism in patients with polymyalgia rheumatica and giant cells arteritis. *British Journal of Rheumatology*, **30**, 349–51.

Brack, A., Martinez-Taboada, V., Stanson, A., Goronzy, J. J. and Weyand, C. M. (1999). Disease pattern in cranial and large-vessel giant-cell arteritis. *Arthritis and Rheumatism*, **42**, 311–17.

Cantini, F., Salvarani, C., Olivieri, I., *et al.* (2000). Erythrocyte sedimentation rate and C-reactive protein in the evaluation of disease activity and severity in polymyalgia rheumatica: a prospective follow-up study. *Seminars in Arthritis and Rheumatism*, **30**, 17–24.

Cantini, F., Salvarani, C., Olivieri, I., *et al.* (2001). Shoulder ultrasonography in the diagnosis of polymyalgia rheumatica: a case-control study. *Journal of Rheumatology*, **28**, 1049–55.

Cantini, F., Nicoli, L., Mannini, C., *et al.* (2005). Inflammatory changes of the hip synovial structures in polymyalgia rheumatica. *Clinical and Experimental Rheumatology*, **23**, 462–8.

Caporali, R., Montecucco, C., Epis, O., Bobbio-Pallavicini, F., Maio, T. and Cimmino, M. A. (2001). Presenting features of polymyalgia rheumatica (PMR) and rheumatoid arthritis with PMR-like onset: a prospective study. *Annals of the Rheumatic Diseases*, **60**, 1021–4.

Caporali, R., Cimmino, M. A., Feraccioli, G., *et al.* (2004). Prednisone plus methotrexate for polymyalgia rheumatica: a randomized, double-blind, placebo-controlled trial. *Annals of Internal Medicine*, **141**, 493–500.

Caselli, R. J. (1990). Giant cell (temporal) arteritis: a treatable cause of multi-infarct dementia. *Neurology*, **40**, 753–5.

Caselli, R. J., Hunder, G. G. and Whisnant, J. P. (1988a). Neurologic disease in biopsy-proven giant cell (temporal) arteritis. *Neurology*, **38**, 352–9.

Caselli, R. J., Daube, J. R., Hunder, G. G. and Whisnant, J. P. (1988b). Peripheral neuropathic syndromes in Giant cell (temporal) arteritis. *Neurology*, **38**, 685–9.

Chan, C. C., Paine, M. and O'day, J. (2005). Predictors of recurrent ischemic optic neuropathy in giant cell arteritis. *Journal of Neuroophthalmology*, **25**, 14–17.

Chakrabarty, A. and Franks, A. J. (2000). Temporal artery biopsy: is there any value in examining biopsies at multiple levels? *Journal of Clinical Pathology*, **53**, 131–6.

Chakravarty, K., Pountain, G., Merry, P., Byron, M., Hazleman, B. and Scott, D. G.I. (1995). A longitudinal study of anticardiolipin antibody in polymyalgia rheumatica and giant cell arteritis. *Journal of Rheumatology*, **22**, 1694–7.

Chevalet, P., Barrier, J. H., Pottier, P., *et al.* (2000). A randomized, multicenter, controlled trial using intravenous pulses of methylprednisolone in the initial treatment of simple forms of giant cell arteritis: a one-year followup study of 164 patients. *Journal of Rheumatology*, **27**, 1484–91.

Chou, C. T. and Schumacher, H. R., Jr (1984). Clinical and pathological studies of synovitis in polymyalgia rheumatica. *Arthritis and Rheumatism*, **27**, 1107–17.

Chuang, T. Y., Hunder, G. G., Ilstrup, D. M. and Kurland, L. T. (1982). Polymyalgia rheumatica: a 10-year epidemiologic and clinical study. *Annals of Internal Medicine*, **97**, 672–80.

Cid, M. C., Campo, E., Ercilla, G., *et al.* (1989). Immunohistochemical analysis of lymphoid and macrophage cell subsets and their immunologic activation markers in temporal arteritis. *Arthritis and Rheumatism*, **32**, 884–93.

Cid, M. C., Monteagudo, J., Oristrell, J., *et al.* (1996). Von Willebrand factor in the outcome of temporal arteritis. *Annals of the Rheumatic Diseases*, **55**, 927–30.

Cid, M. C., Font, C., Oristrell, J., *et al.* (1998). Association between strong inflammatory response and low risk of developing visual loss and other cranial ischemic complications in giant cell (temporal) arteritis. *Arthritis and Rheumatism*, **41**, 26–32.

Cid, M. C., Cebrian, M., Font, C., *et al.* (2000). Cell adhesion molecules in the development of inflammatory infiltrates in giant cell arteritis: inflammation-induced angiogenesis as the preferential site of leukocyte-endothelial cell interactions. *Arthritis and Rheumatism*, **43**, 184–94.

Combe, B., Sany, J., Le Quellec, A., Clot, J. and Eliaou, J. F. (1998). Distribution of HLA-DRB1 allels of patients with polymyalgia rheumatica and giant cell arteritis in a Mediterranean population. *Journal of Rheumatology*, **25**, 94–8.

Cornblath, W. T. and Eggenberger, E. R. (1997). Progressive visual loss from giant cell arteritis despite high-dose intravenous methylprednisolone. *Ophthalmology*, **104**, 854–8.

Corcoran, G. M., Prayson, R. A. and Herzog, K. M. (2001). The significance of perivascular inflammation in the absence of arteritis in temporal artery biopsy specimens. *American Journal of Clinical Pathology*, **115**, 342–7.

Dababneh, A., González-Gay, M. A., García-Porrua, C., Hajeer, A., Thomson, W. and Ollier, W. (1998). Giant cell arteritis and polymyalgia rheumatica can be differentiated by distinct patterns of HLA class II association. *Journal of Rheumatology*, **25**, 2140–5.

Danesh-Meyer, H. V., Savino, P. J., Eagle, R. C. Jr, Kubis, K. C. and Sergott, R. C. (2000). Low diagnostic yield with second biopsies in suspected giant cell arteritis. *Journal of Neuroophthalmology*, **20**, 213–5.

Danesh-Meyer, H. V., Savino, P. J. and Sergott, R. C. (2001). The prevalence of cupping in end-stage arteritic and nonarteritic anterior ischemic optic neuropathy. *Ophthalmology*, **108**, 593–8.

Danesh-Meyer, H., Savino, P. J. and Gamble, G. D. (2005a). Poor prognosis of visual outcome after visual loss from giant cell arteritis. *Ophthalmology*, **112**, 1098–103.

Danesh-Meyer, H., Savino, P. J., Spaeth, G. L. and Gamble, G. D. (2005b). Comparison of arteritis and nonarteritic anterior ischemic optic neuropathies with the Heidelberg Retina Tomograph. *Ophthalmology*, **112**, 1104–12.

Dasgupta, B., Grundy, F. and Stainer, E. (1990). Hypothyroidism in polymyalgia rheumatica and giant cell arteritis: lack of any association. *British Medical Journal*, **301**, 96–7.

Dasgupta, B., Dolan, A. L., Panayi, G. S. and Fernandes, L. (1998). An initially double-blind controlled 96 week trial of depot methylprednisolone against oral prednisolone in the treatment of polymyalgia rheumatica. *British Journal of Rheumatology*, **37**, 189–95.

Doran, M. F., Crowson, C. S., O'Fallon, W. M., Hunder, G. G. and Gabriel, S. E. (2002). Trends in the incidence of polymyalgia rheumatica over a 30 year period in Olmsted County, Minnesota, USA. *Journal of Rheumatology*, **29**, 1694–7.

Dudenhoefer, E. J., Cornblath, W. T. and Schatz, M. P. (1998). Scalp necrosis with giant cell arteritis. *Ophthalmology*, **105**, 1875–8.

Duhaut, P., Berruyer, M., Pinede, L., *et al.* (1998). Anticardiolipin antibodies and giant cell arteritis: a prospective, multicenter case-control study. *Arthritis and Rheumatism*, **41**, 701–9.

Duhaut, P., Bosshard, S., Calvet, A., *et al.* (1999a). Giant cell arteritis, polymyalgia rheumatica, and viral hypotheses: a multicenter, prospective case-control study. *Journal of Rheumatology*, **26**, 361–9.

Duhaut, P., Bornet, H., Pinedel, L., *et al.* (1999b). Giant cell arteritis and thyroid dysfunction: multicentre case-control study. *British Medical Journal*, **318**, 434–5.

Elling, P., Olsson, A. T. and Elling, H. (1996). Synchronous variations of the incidence of temporal arteritis and polymyalgia rheumatica in different regions of Denmark; association with epidemics of Mycoplasma pneumoniae infection. *Journal of Rheumatology*, **23**, 112–19.

Ely, G. M. (1998). Giant cells arteritis complicated by multiinfarct dimentia. *Journal of Clinical Rheumatology*, **4**, 209–15.

Escriba, A., Morales, E., Albizua, E., *et al.* (2000). Secondary (AA-type) amyloidosis in patients with polymyalgia rheumatica. *American Journal of Kidney Diseases*, **35**, 137–40.

Espinosa, G., Tassies, D., Font, J., *et al.* (2001). Antiphospholipid antibodies and thrombophilic factors in giant cell arteritis. *Seminars in Arthritis and Rheumatism*, **31**, 12–20.

Espinoza, L. R., Jara, L. J., Silveira, L. H., *et al.* (1991). Anticardiolipin antibodies in polymyalgia rheumatica-giant cell arteritis: association with severe vascular complications. *American Journal of Medicine*, **90**, 474–8.

Esteban, M. J., Font, C., Hernandez-Rodriguez, J., *et al.* (2001). Small-vessel vasculitis surrounding a spared temporal artery. *Arthritis and Rheumatism*, **44**, 1387–95.

Evans, J. M., Bowles, C. A., Bjornsson, J., Mullany, C. J. and Hunder, G. G. (1994). Thoracic aortic aneurysm and rupture in giant cell arteritis. *Arthritis and Rheumatism*, **37**, 1539–47.

Evans, J. M., O'Fallon, W. M. and Hunder, G. G. (1995). Increased incidence of aortic aneurysm and dissection in giant cell (temporal) arteritis. A population-based study. *Annals of Internal Medicine*, **122**, 502–7.

Font, C., Cid, M. C., Coll-Vinent, B., Lopez-Soto, A. and Grau, J. M. (1997). Clinical features in patients with permanent visual loss due to biopsy-proven giant cell arteritis. *British Journal of Rheumatology*, **36**, 251–4.

Franzen, P., Sutinien, S. and von Knorring, J. (1991). Giant cell arteritis and polymyalgia rheumatica in a region of Finland: an epidemiologic, clinical and pathologic study, 1984–1988. *Journal of Rheumatology*, **19**, 273–6.

Gabriel, S. E., O'Fallon, W. M., Achkar, A. A., Lie, J. T. and Hunder, G. G. (1995). The use of clinical characteristics to predict the results of temporal artery biopsy among patients with suspected giant cell arteritis. *Journal of Rheumatology*, **22**, 93–6.

Gabriel, S. E., Espy, M., Erdman, D. D., Bjornsson, J., Smith, T. F. and Hunder, G. G. (1999). The role of parvovirus B19 in the pathogenesis of giant cell arteritis: a preliminary evaluation. *Arthritis and Rheumatism*, **42**, 1255–8.

Gentric, A., Baccino, E., Mottier, D., Islam, S. and Cledes, J. (1988). Temporal arteritis revealed by a syndrome of inappropriate secretion of antidiuretic hormone. *American Journal of Medicine*, **85**, 559–60.

Ghanchi, F. D., Williamson, T. H., Lim, C. S., *et al.* (1996). Color Doppler imaging in giant cell (temporal) arteritis: serial examination and comparison with non-arteritic anterior ischaemic optic neuropathy. *Eye*, **10**, 459–64.

Gilbert, J. L., Coe, M. D., Nam, M. H., Kolsky, M. P. and Barth, W. F. (1999). Giant cell arteritis in African Americans. *Journal of Clinical Rheumatology*, **5**, 116–20.

Gillot, J. M., Masy, E., Davril, M., *et al.* (1997). Elastase derived elastin peptides: putative autoimmune targets in giant cell arteritis. *Journal of Rheumatology*, **24**, 677–82.

González-Gay, M. A. and Garciá-Porrua, C. (1998). Carotid tenderness: an ominous sign of giant cell arteritis? *Scandinavian Journal of Rheumatology*, **27**, 154–6.

González-Gay, M. A., Blanco, R., Abraira, V., *et al.* (1997). Giant cell arteritis in Lugo, Spain, is associated with low longterm mortality. *Journal of Rheumatology*, **24**, 2171–6.

González-Gay, M. A., Blanco, R., Rodriguez-Valverde, V., Martinez-Taboada, V. M., Delgado-Rodriguez, M. and Figueroa, M. (1998a). Permanent visual loss and cerebrovascular accidents in giant cell arteritis: predictors and response to treatment. *Arthritis and Rheumatism*, **41**, 1497–504.

González-Gay, M. A., García-Porrua, C. and Vazquez-Caruncho, M. (1998b). Polymyalgia rheumatica in biopsy proven giant cell arteritis does not constitute a different subset but differs from isolated polymyalgia rheumatica. *Journal of Rheumatology*, **25**, 1750–5.

González-Gay, M. A., García-Porrua, C., Vazquez-Caruncho, M., Dababneh, A., Hajeer, A. and Ollier, W. E. R. (1999). The spectrum of polymyalgia rheumatica in northwestern Spain: incidence and analysis of variables associated with relapse in a 10 year study. *Journal of Rheumatology*, **26**, 1326–32.

González-Gay, M. A., García-Porrua, C., Liorca J, *et al.* (2000a). Visual manifestations of giant cell arteritis. *Medicine*, **79**, 283–92.

González-Gay, M. A., García-Porrua, C., Salvarani, C., Olivieri, I. and Hunder, G. G. (2000b). Polymyalgia manifestations in different conditions mimicking polymyalgia rheumatica. *Clinical and Experimental Rheumatology*, **18**, 755–9.

González-Gay, M. A., García-Porrua, C., Rivas M. J., Rodriguez-Ledo, P. and Liorca, J. (2001a). Epidemiology of biopsy proven giant cell arteritis in northwestern Spain: trend over an 18 year period. *Annals of Rheumatic Diseases*, **60**, 367–71.

González-Gay, M. A., García-Porrua, C., Liorca, J., et al. (2001b). Biopsy-negative giant cell arteritis: clinical spectrum and predictive factors for positive temporal artery biopsy. Seminars in Arthritis and Rheumatism, 30, 249–56.

González-Gay, M. A., Amoli, M. M., García-Porrua, C. and Ollier, W. E. (2003), Genetic markers of disease susceptibility and severity in giant cell arteritis and polymyalgia rheumatica. Seminars in Arthritis and Rheumatism, 33, 38–48.

González-Gay, M. A., Hajeer, A. H., Dababneh, A., et al. (2004a). Interferon-gamma gene microsatellite polymorphisms in patients with biopsy-proven giant cell arteritis and isolated polymyalgia rheumatica. Clinical and Experimental Rheumatology, 22 (Suppl. 36), S18–20.

González-Gay, M. A., Pineiro, A., Gomez-Gigirey, A., et al. (2004b). Influence of traditional risk factors of atherosclerosis in the development of severe ischemic complications in giant cell arteritis. Medicine, 83, 342–7.

González-Gay, M. A., García-Porrua, C., Pineiro, A., Pego-Reigosa, R., Liorca, J. and Hunder, G. G. (2004c). Aortic aneurysm and dissection in patients with biopsy-proven giant cell arteritis from northwestern Spain: a population-based study. Medicine, 83, 335–41.

Graham, E., Holland, A., Avery, A. and Russell, R. W.R. (1981). Prognosis in giant cell arteritis. British Medical Journal, 282, 269–71.

Gran, J. T. and Myklebust, G. (1997). The Incidence of polymyalgia rheumatica and temporal arteritis in the country of Aust Agder, South Norway: a prospective study 1987–94. Journal of Rheumatology, 24, 1739–43.

Gran, J. T. and Myklebust, G. (2000). The incidence and clinical characteristics of peripheral arthritis in polymyalgia rheumatica and temporal arteritis: a prospective study of 231 cases. Rheumatology, 39, 283–7.

Gran, J. T., Mykelbust, G., Wilsgaard, T. and Jacobsen, B. K. (2001). Survival in polymyalgia rheumatica and temporal arteritis: a study of 398 cases and matched population controls. Rheumatology, 40, 1238–42.

Hachula, E., Boivin, V., Pasturel-Michon, U., et al. (2001). Prognostic factors and long-term evolution in a cohort of 133 patients with giant cell arteritis. Clinical and Experimental Rheumatology, 19, 171–6.

Hall, S. and Hunder, G. G. (1984). Is temporal artery biopsy prudent? Mayo Clinic Proceedings, 59, 793–6.

Haugberg, G., Paulsen, P. Q. and Bie, R. B. (2000). Temporal arteritis in Vest Augder County in southern Norway: incidence and clinical findings. Journal of Rheumatology, 27, 2624–7.

Hausch, R. C. and Harrington, T. (1998). Temporal arteritis and sensorineural hearing loss. Seminars in Arthritis and Rheumatism, 28, 206–9.

Hayreh, S. S. (1991). Ophthalmic features of giant cell arteritis. Bailliere's Clinical Rheumatology, 5, 431–55.

Hayreh, S. S., and Zimmerman, B. (2003). Management of giant cell arteritis. Our 27-year clinical study: new light on old controversies. Ophthalmologica, 217, 239–59.

Hayreh, S. S., Podhajsky, P. A., Raman, R. and Zimmerman, B. (1997). Giant cell arteritis: validity and reliability of various diagnosis criteria. American Journal of Ophthalmology, 123, 285–96.

Hayreh, S. S., Podhajsky, P. A. and Zimmerman, B. (1998). Ocular manifestation of giant cell arteritis. American Journal of Ophthalmology, 125, 509–20.

Hayreh, S. S., Zimmerman, B., and Kardon, R. H. (2002). Visual improvement with corticosteroid therapy in giant cell arteritis. Report of a large study and review of the literature. Acta Ophthalmologica Scandinavica, 80, 355–67.

Healey, L. A. (1984). Long-term follow-up of polymyalgia rheumatica: evidence for synovitis. Seminars in Arthritis and Rheumatism, 13, 322–8.

Healey, L. A. (1991). Relation of giant cell arteritis to polymyalgia rheumatica. Bailliere's Clinical Rheumatology, 5, 371–8.

Healey, L. A. and Sheets, P. K. (1988). The relation of polymyalgia rheumatica to rheumatoid arthritis. Journal of Rheumatology, 15, 750–52.

Healey, L. A., Parker, F. and Wilske, K. R. (1971). Polymyalgia rheumatica and giant cell arteritis. Arthritis and Rheumatism, 14, 138–41.

Hellmann, D. B. (2002). Temporal arteritis: a cough, toothache, and tongue infarction. Journal of the American Medical Association, 287, 2996–3000.

Hernandez-Rodriguez, J., Garcia-Martinez, A., Casademont, J., et al. (2002). A strong initial systemic inflammatory response is associated with higher corticosteroid requirements and longer duration of therapy in patients with giant-cell arteritis. Arthritis and Rheumatism, 47, 29–35.

Hernandez-Rodriguez, J., Segarra, M., Vilardell, C., et al. (2003). Elevated production of interleukin-6 is associated with lower incidence of disease-related ischemic events in patients with giant-cell arteritis. Angiogenic activity if interleukin 6 as a potential protective mechanism. Circulation, 107, 2428–34.

Hernandez-Rodriguez, J., Segarra, M., Vilardell, C., et al. (2004). Tissue production of pro-inflammatory cytokines (IL-1 beta, TNF-alpha and IL-6) correlates with the intensity of the systemic inflammatory response and with corticosteroid requirements in giant-cell arteritis. Rheumatology, 43, 294–301.

Hochberg, M. C., Prashker, M. J., Greenwald, M., et al. (1996). Recommendations for the prevention and treatment of glucocorticoid – induced osteoporosis. American college of rheumatology task force on osteoporosis guidelines. Arthritis and Rheumatism, 39, 1791–801.

Hoffman, G. S., Cid, M. C., Hellman, D. B., et al. (2002). A multicenter, randomized, double-blind, placebo-controlled trial of adjuvant methotrexate treatment for giant cell arteritis. Arthritis and Rheumatism, 46, 1309–18.

Hoffman, G. S., Cid, M. C., Weyand, C. M., et al. (2005). Phase II study of the safety and efficacy of infliximab in giant cell arteritis (GCA): 22 week interim analysis. Rheumatology, 44 (Suppl. 3), 18.

Hunder, G. G. (1998). The use and misuse of classification and diagnostic criteria for complex disease. Annals of Internal Medicine, 129, 417–8.

Hunder, G. G. (1997). Giant cell arteritis in polymyalgia rheumatica. American Journal of Medicine, 102, 514–6.

Hunder, G. G., Sheps, S. G., Allen, G. L. and Joyce, J. W. (1975). Daily and alternate-day corticosteroid regiments in treatment of giant cell arteritis. Comparison in a prospective study. Annals of Internal Medicine, 82, 613–8.

Hunder, G. G., Bloch, D. A., Michel, B. A., et al. (1990). The American College of Rheumatology 1990 criteria for the classification of giant cell arteritis. Arthritis and Rheumatism, 33, 1122–8.

Huston, K. A., Hunder, G. G., Lie, J. T., Kennedy, R. H., Elveback, L. R. (1978). Temporal arteritis: a 25-year epidemiologic, clinical, and pathologic study. Annals of Internal Medicine, 88, 162–7.

Johnson, H., Bouman, W. and Pinner, G. (1997). Psychiatric aspects of temporal arteritis: a case report and review of the literature. Journal of Geriatric Psychiatry and Neurology, 10, 142–5.

Jones, J. G. and Hazleman, B. L. (1981). Prognosis and management of polymyalgia rheumatica. Annals of the Rheumatic Diseases, 40, 1–5.

Jover, J. A., Hernandez-Garcia, C., Morado, I. C., et al. (2001). Combined treatment of giant-cell arteritis with methotrexate and prednisone. A randomized, double-blind, placebo-controlled trial. Annals of Internal Medicine, 134, 106–14.

Kaiser, M., Weyand, C. M., Bjornsson, J. and Goronzy, J. J. (1998). Platelet-derived growth factor, intimal hyperplasia, and ischemic complications in giant cell arteritis. Arthritis and Rheumatism, 41, 623–33.

Karassa, F. B., Matsagas, M. I., Schmidt, W. A. and Iannidis, J. P. (2005). Meta-analysis: test performance of ultrasonography for giant cell arteritis. Annals of Internal Medicine, 142, 359–69.

Kobayashi, S., Yano, T., Matsumoto, Y., et al. (2003). Clinical and epidemiologic analysis of giant cell (temporal) arteritis from a nationwide survey in 1998 in Japan: the first government-supported nationwide survey. Arthritis and Rheumatism, 49, 594–8.

Kramer, M. R., Melzer, E., Nesher, G. and Sonnenblick, M. (1987). Pulmonary manifestations of temporal arteritis. European Journal of Respiratory Diseases, 7, 430–3.

Kyle, V. (1991). Laboratory investigations including liver in polymyalgia rheumatica / giant cell arteritis. *Bailliere's Clinical Rheumatology*, **5**, 475–84.

Kyle, V., Silverman, B., Silman, A., *et al.* (1985). Polymyalgia rheumatica/ giant cell arteritis in a Cambridge general practice. *British Medical Journal*, **291**, 385–7.

Kyle, V., Cawston, T. E. and Hazleman, B. L. (1989). ESR and C-reactive protein in the assessment of polymyalgia rheumatica/giant cell arteritis on presentation and during follow-up. *Annals of the Rheumatic Diseases*, **48**, 667–71.

Lange, U., Teichmann, J., Stracke, H., Bretzel, R. G. and Neeck, G. (1998). Elderly onset rheumatoid arthritis and polymyalgia rheumatica: ultrasonographic study of the glenohumeral joints. *Rheumatology International*, **17**, 229–32.

Larson, T. S., Halls, S., Hepper, N. G.G. and Hunder, G. G. (1984). Resporatory tract symptoms as a clue to giant cell arteritis. *Annals of Internal Medicine*, **101**, 594–7.

Le Hello, C., Levesque, H., Jeanton, M., *et al.* (2001). Lower limb giant cell arteritis and temporal arteritis: followup of 8 cases. *Journal of Rheumatology*, **28**, 1407–12.

LeSar, C. J., Meier, G. H., DeMasi, R. J., *et al.* (2002). The utility of color duplex ultrasonography in the diagnosis of temporal arteritis. *Journal of Vascular Surgery*, **36**, 1154–60.

Lie, J. T. (1995). Aortic and extracranial large vessel giant cell arteritis: a review of 72 cases with histopathologic documentation. *Seminars in Arthritis and Rheumatism*, **24**, 422–31.

Lie, J. T., Brown, A. L. and Carter, E. T. (1970). Spectrum of aging changes in temporal arteries: its significance in interpretation biopsy of temporal artery. *Archives of Pathology and Laboratory Medicine*, **90**, 278–85.

Liozon, E., Herrmann, F., Ly, K., *et al.* (2001). Risk factors for visual loss in giant cell (temporal) arteritis: a prospective study of 174 patients. *American Journal of Medicine*, **111**, 211–7.

Liu, G. T., Glaser, J. S., Schatz, N. J. and Smith, J. L. (1994). Visual morbidity in giant cell arteritis, clinical characteristics and prognosis for vision. *Ophthalmology*, **100**, 1779–85.

Lopez-Hoyos, M., Ruis de Alegria, C., Blanco, R., *et al.* (2004). Clinical utility of anti-CCP antibodies in the differential diagtnosis of elderly0onset rheumatoid arthritis and polymyalgia rheumatica. *Rheumatology*, **43**, 655–7.

Ma-Krupa, W., Dewan, M., Jeon, M. S., *et al.* (2002). Trapping of misdirected dendritic cells in the granulomatous lesions of giant cell arteritis. *American Journal of Pathology*, **161**, 1815–23.

Ma-Krupa, W., Jeon, M. S., Spoerl, S., Tedder, T. F., Goronzy, J. J. and Weyand, C. M. (2004). Activation of arterial wall dendritic cells and breakdown of self-tolerance in giant cell arteritis. *Journal of Experimental Medicine*, **199**, 173–83.

Ma-Krupa, W., Kwan, M., Goronzy, J. J. and Weyand, C. M. (2005). Toll-like receptors in giant cell arteritis. *Clinical Immunology*, **115**, 38–46.

Macchioni, P., Boiardi, L., Salvarani, C., *et al.* (1993). Lymphocyte subpopulation analysis in peripheral blood in polymyalgia rheumatica/ giant cell arteritis. *British Journal of Rheumatology*, **32**, 666–70.

McGonagle, D., Pease, C., Marzo-Ortega, H., O'Connor, P., Gibbon, W. and Emery, P. (2001). Comparison of extracapsular changes by magnetic resonance imaging in patients with rheumatoid arthritis and polymyalgia rheumatica. *Journal of Rheumatology*, **28**, 1837–41.

Mallya, R. K., Hind,, C. R.K., Berry, H. and Pepys, M. B. (1985). Serum C-reactive protein in polymyalgia rheumatica: prospective serial study. *Arthritis and Rheumatism*, **28**, 383–7.

Martinez-Taboada, V., Hunder, N. N., Hunder, G. G., Weyand, C. M., Goronzy, J. J. (1996). Recognition of tissue residing antigen by T Cells in vasculitic lesions of giant cell arteritis. *Journal of Molecular Medicine*, **74**, 695–703.

Martinez-Taboada, V. M., Blanco, R., Armona, J., *et al.* (2000). Giant cell arteritis with an erythrocyte sedimantation rate lower than 50. *Clinical Rheumatology*, **19**, 73–5.

Martinez-Taboada, V. M., Blanco, R., Fito, C., Pacheco, M. J., Delgado-Rodriguez, M. and Rodriguez-Valverde, V. (2001). Circulating CD8+ T cells in polymyalgia rheumatica and giant cell arteritis: a review. *Seminars in Arthritis and Rheumatism*, **30**, 257–71.

Martinez-Taboada, V. M., Bartolome, M. J., Lopez-Hoyos, M., *et al.* (2004). HLA-DRB1 allele distribution in polymyalgia rheumatica and giant cell arteritis: influence on clinical subgroups and prognosis. *Seminars in Arthritis and Rheumatism*, **34**, 454–64.

Matteson, E. L., Gold, K. N., Bloch, D. A. and Hunder, G. G. (1996). Long-term survival of patients with giant cell arteritis in the American College of Rheumatology giant cell arteritis classification criteria cohort. *American Journal of Medicine*, **100**, 193–6.

Miller, N. R. (2001). Visual manifestations of temporal arteritis. *Rheumatic Disease Clinics of North America*, **27**, 781–97.

Moosig, F., Czech, N., Mehl, C., *et al.* (2004). Correlation between 18-fluorodeoxyglucose accumulation in large vessels and serological markers of inflammation in polymyalgia rheumatica: a quantitative PET study. *Annals of the Rheumatic Diseases*, **63**, 870–3.

Myklebust, G. and Gran, J. T. (1996). A prospective study of 287 patients with polymyalgia rheumatica and temporal arteritis: clinical and laboratory manifestations at onset of disease and at the time of diagnosis. *British Journal of Rheumatology*, **35**, 1161–8.

Navarez, J., Nolla-Sole, J. M., Navarez, J. A., Clavaguera, M. T., Valverde-Garcia, J., and Roig-Escofet, D. (2001). Musculoskeletal manifestations in polymyalgia rheumatica and temporal arteritis. *Annals of the Rheumatic Diseases*, **60**, 1060–3.

Navarez, J., Navarez, J. A., Nolla, J. M., Sirvent, E., Reina, D. and Valverde, J. (2005). Giant cell arteritis and polymyalgia rheumatica: usefulness of vascular magnetic resonance imaging studies in the diagnosis of aortitis. *Rheumatology*, **44**, 479–83.

Nesher, G. and Sonnenblick, M. (1994). Steroid-sparing medications and temporal arteritis: report of three cases and review of 174 reported patients. *Clinical Rheumatology*, **13**, 289–92.

Nesher, G., Rosenberg, P., Shorer, Z., Gilai, A., Solomonovich, A. and Sonnenblick, M. (1987). Involvement of the peripheral nervous system in temporal arteritis–polymyalgia rheumatica. Report of 3 cases and review of the literature. *Journal of Rheumatology*, **14**, 358–60.

Nesher, G., Sonnenblick, M. and Friedlander, Y. (1994). Analysis of steroid related complications and mortality in temporal arteritis: a 15-year survey of 43 patients. *Journal of Rheumatology*, **21**, 1283–6.

Nesher, G., Rubinow, A. and Sonnenblick, M. (1996). Trends in the clinical presentation of temporal arteritis in Israel: reflection of increased physician awareness. *Clinical Rheumatology*, **15**, 483–5.

Nesher, G., Rubinow, A. and Sonnenblick, M. (1997). Efficacy and adverse effects of different corticosteroid dose regimens in temporal arteritis: a retrospective study. *Clinical and Experimental Rheumatology*, **15**, 303–6.

Nesher, G., Nesher, R., Rozenman, Y. and Sonnenblick, M. (2001). Visual hallucinations in giant cell arteritis: association with visual loss. *Journal of Rheumatology*, **28**, 2046–8.

Nesher, G., Shemesh, D., Mates, M., Sonnenblick, M. and Abramowitz, H. B. (2002). The predictive value of the halo sign in color Doppler ultrasonography of the temporal arteries for diagnosing giant cell arteritis. *Journal of Rheumatology*, **29**, 1224–6.

Nesher, G., Berkun, Y., Mates, M., *et al.* (2004a). Risk factors for cranial ischemic complications in giant cell arteritis. *Medicine*, **83**, 114–22.

Nesher, G., Berkun, Y., Mates, M., Baras, M., Rubinow, A. and Sonnenblick, M. (2004b). Low-dose aspirin and prevention of cranial ischemic complications in giant cell arteritis. *Arthritis and Rheumatism*, **50**, 1332–7.

Neunninghof, D. M., Hunder, G. G., Christianson, T. J., McClelland, R. L. and Matteson, E. L. Incidence and predictors of large-artery complication (aortic aneurysm, aortic dissection, and/or large-artery stenosis) in patients with giant cell arteritis: a population-based study over 50 years. *Arthritis and Rheumatism*, **48**, 3522–31.

Nir-Paz, R., Gross, A. and Chajek-Shaul, T. (2002). Reduction of jaw opening (trismus) in giant cell arteritis. *Annals of Rheumatic Diseases*, **61**, 832–3.

Nordborg, E. and Bengtsson, B. A. (1989). Death rates and causes of death in 284 consecutive patients with giant cell arteritis confirmed by biopsy. *British Medical Journal*, **299**, 549–50.

Nordborg, E. and Nordborg, C. (1995). The influence of sectional interval on the reliability of temporal arterial biopsies in polymalgia rheumatica. *Clinical Rheumatology*, **14**, 330–4.

Nordborg, E. and Nordborg, C. (1998). The inflammatory reaction in giant cell arteritis: an immunohistochemical investigation. *Clinical and Experimental Rheumatology*, **16**, 165–8.

Nordborg, E., Bengtsson, B. A. and Nordborg, C. (1991). Temporal artery morphology and morphometry in giant cell arteritis. *Acta Pathologica et Microbiologica Scandinavica*, **99**, 1013–23.

Nordborg, E., Schaufelberger, C. and Bosaeus, I. (1998). The effect of glucocorticoids on fat and lean tissue masses in giant cell arteritis. *Scandinavian Journal of Rheumatology*, **27**, 106–11.

Olivieri, I., Salvarani, C. and Cantini, F. (1997). Remitting distal extremity swelling with pitting edema: a distinct syndrome or a clinical feature of different inflammatory rheumatic disease? *Journal of Rheumatology*, **24**, 249–52.

Ostberg, G. (1972). Morphological changes in the large arteries in polymyalgia arteritica. *Acta Medica Scandinavica*, **533** (Suppl.), 135–64.

Ostberg, G. (1973). On arteritis with special reference to polymyalgia arteritica. *Acta Pathologica et Microbiologica Scandinavica*, **237** (Suppl.), 1–59.

Pascuzzi, R. M., Roos, K. A. and Davis, T. E. (1989). Mental status abnormalities in temporal arteritis: a treatable cause of dementia in the elderly. *Arthritis and Rheumatism*, **32**, 1308–11.

Pearce, G., Ryan, P. F.J., Delmas, P. D., Tabensky, D. A. and Seeman, E. (1998). The deleterious effects of low-dose corticosteroids on bone density in patients with polymyalgia rheumatica. *British Journal of Rheumatology*, **37**, 292–9.

Pease, C. T., Haugeberg, G., Morgan, A. W., Montague, B., Hensor, E. M. and Bhakta, B. B. (2005). Diagnosing late-onset rheumatoid arthritis, polymyalgia rheumatica, and temporal arteritis in patients presenting with polymyalgic symptoms. A prospective longterm study. *Journal of Rheumatology*, **32**, 1043–6.

Petursdottir, V., Johansson, H., Nordborg, E. and Nordborg, C. (1999). The epidemiology of biopsy-positive giant cell arteritis: special reference to cyclic fluctuations. *Rheumatology*, **38**, 1208–12.

Pless, M., Rizzo, J. F. 3rd, Lamkin, J. C. and Lessell, S. (2000). Concordance of bilateral temporal artery biopsy in giant cell arteritis. *Journal of Neuroophthalmology*, **20**, 216–8

Pountain, G. and Hazleman, B. (1997). Erythrocyte sedimentation rate (ESR) at presentation is a prognostic indicator for duration of treatment in polymyalgia rheumatica (PMR). *British Journal of Rheumatology*, **36**, 508–9.

Proven, A., Gabriel, S. E., O'Fallon, W. M. and Hunder, G. G. (1999). Polymyalgia rheumatica with low erythrocyte sedimentation rate at diagnosis. *Journal of Rheumatology*, **26**, 1333–7.

Proven, A., Gabriel, S. E., Orces C, O'Fallon, W. M. and Hunder, G. G. (2003). Glucocorticoid therapy in giant cell arteritis: duration and adverse outcomes. *Arthritis and Rheumatism*, **49**, 703–8

Quillen, D. A., Cantore, W. A., Schwartz, S. R., Brod, R. D. and Sassani, J. W. (1993). Choroidal nonperfusion in giant cell arteritis. *American Journal of Ophthalmology*, **116**, 171–5.

Rao, J. K., Allen, N. B. and Pincus, T. (1998). Limitations of the 1990 American College of Rheumatology classification criteria in the diagnosis of vasculitis. *Annals of Internal Medicine*, **129**, 345–52.

Ray-Chaudhuri, N., Kine, D. A., Tijani, S. O., *et al.* (2002). Effect of prior steroid treatment on temporal artery biopsy findings in giant cell arteritis. *British Journal of Ophthalmology*, **86**, 530–2.

Reitblat, T., Ben-Horin, C. L. and Reitblat, A. (2003). Gallium-67 SPECT scintigraphy may be useful in diagnosis of temporal arteritis. *Annals of the Rheumatic Diseases*, **62**, 257–60.

Roche, N. E., Fulbright, J. W., Wagner, A. D., Hunder, G. G., Goronzy, J. J. and Weyand, C. M. (1993). Correlation of interleukin-6 production and disease activity in polymyalgia rheumatica and giant cell arteritis. *Arthritis and Rheumatism*, **36**, 1286–94.

Rodriguez-Pla, A., Bosch-Gil, J. A., Echevarria-Mayo, J. E., *et al.* (2004). No detection of parvovirus B19 or herpesvirus DNA in giant cell arteritis. *Journal of Clinical Virology*, **31**, 11–15.

Rodriguez-Valverde, V., Sarabia, J. M., González-Gay, M. A., Figueroa, M., Armona, J. and Blanco, R. (1997). Risk factors and predictive models of giant cell arteritis in polymyalgia rheumatica. *American Journal of Medicine*, **102**, 331–6.

Romera-Villegas, A., Villa-Coll, R., Poca-Dias, V. and Cairols-Castellote, M. A. (2004). The rople of color duplex sonography in the diagnosis of giant cell arteritis. *Journal of Ultrasound Medicine*, **23**, 1493–8.

Ruegg, S., Engelter, S., Jeanneret, C., *et al.* (2003). Bilateral vertebral artery occlusion resulting from giant cell arteritis: report of 3 cases and review of the literature. *Medicine*, **82**, 1–12.

Saldanha, G., Hongo, J., Plant, G., Acheson, J., Lavi, I. and Anand, P. (1999). Decreased CGRP, but preserved Trk immunoreactivity in nerve fibres in inflamed human superficial temporal arteries. *Journal of Neurology Neurosurgery and Psychiatry*, **66**, 390–92.

Salvarani, C. and Hunder, G. G. (2001). Giant cell arteritis with low erythrocyte sedimentation rate: frequency of occurrence in a population-based study. *Arthritis Care and Research*, **45**, 140–5.

Salvarani, C., Macchioni, P., Zizzi, F., *et al.* (1991). Epidemiologic and immuno-genetic aspects of polymyalgia rheumatica and giant cell arteritis in northern Italy. *Arthritis and Rheumatism*, **34**, 351–5.

Salvarani, C., Gabriel, S. and Hunder, G. G. (1996). Distal extremity swelling with pitting edema in polymyalgia rheumatica. *Arthritis and Rheumatism*, **39**, 73–80.

Salvarani, C., Macchioni, P. and Boiardi, L. (1997a). Polymyalgia rheumatica. *Lancet*, **350**, 43–7.

Salvarani, C., Cantini, F., Olivieri, I. *et al.* (1997b). Proximal bursitis in active polymyalgia rheumatica. *Annals of Internal Medicine*, **39**, 1199–207.

Salvarani, C., Cantini, F., Macchioni, P., *et al.* (1998). Distal musculoskeletal manifestations in polymyalgia rheumatica. *Arthritis and Rheumatism*, **41**, 1221–6.

Salvarani, C., Cantini, F., Olivieri, I. and Hunder, G. G. (1999). Polymyalgia rheumatica: a disorder of extraarticular synovial structures? *Journal of Rheumatology*, **26**, 517–21.

Salvarani, C., Silingardi, M., Ghirarduzzi, A., *et al.* (2002). Is Duplex ultrasonography useful for the diagnosis of giant-cell arteritis? *Annals of Internal Medicine*, **137**, 232–8.

Salvarani, C., Casali, B., Nicoli, D., *et al.* (2003). Endothelial nitric oxide synthase gene polymorphisms in giant cell arteritis. *Arthritis and Rheumatism*, **48**, 3219–23.

Salvarani, C., Crowson, C. S., O'Fallon, W. M., Hunder, G. G. and Gabriel, S. E. (2004). Reappraisal of the epidemiology of giant cell arteritis in Olmsted County, Minnesota, over fifty-year period. *Arthritis and Rheumatism*, **51**, 264–8.

Salvarani, C., Cimino L., Macchioni, P., *et al.* (2005a). Risk factors for visual loss in an Italian population-based cohort of patients with giant cell arteritis. *Arthritis and Rheumatism*, **53**, 293–7.

Salvarani, C., Cantini, F., Nicoli, L., *et al.* (2005b). Acute-phase reactants and the risk of relapse/recurrence in polymyalgia rheumatica: a prospective followup study. *Arthritis and Rheumatism*, **53**, 33–8.

Save-Soderbergh, J., Malmvall, B. E., Andersson, R. and Bengtsson, B. A. (1986). Giant cell arteritis as a cause of death. *Journal of the American Medical Association*, **255**, 493–6.

Schaufelberger, C., Bengtsson, B. A. and Andersson, R. (1995). Epidemiology and mortality in 220 patients with polymyalgia rheumatica. *British Journal of Rheumatology*, **34**, 261–4.

Schmidt, W. A., Kraft, H. E., Vorpahl, K., Volker, L. and Gromnica-Ihle, E. J. (1997). Color duplex ultrasonography in the diagnosis of temporal arteritis. *New England Journal of Medicine*, **337,** 1336–42.

Schmidt, W.A and Gromnica-Ihle, E. J. (2002). Incidence of temporal arteritis in patients with polymyalgia rheumatica: a prospective study using color Doppler ultrasonography of the temporal arteries. *Rheumatology*, **20,** 309–18.

Schmidt, W. A., Natusch, A., Moller, D. E., Vorpahl, K. and Gromnica-Ihle, E. J. (2002). Involvement of peripheral arteries in giant cell arteritis: a color Doppler sonography study. *Clinical and Experimental Rheumatology*, **41,** 46–52.

Siatkowski, M. R., Gass, J. D.M., Glaser, J. S., Smith, J. L., Schatz, N. J. and Schiffman, J. (1993). Fluorescein angiography in the diagnosis of giant cell arteritis. *American Journal of Ophthalmology*, **115,** 57–63.

Smith, A. J., Kyle, V., Cawston, T. E. and Hazleman, B. L. (1987). Isolation and analysis of immune complexes from sera of patients with polymyalgia rheumatica and giant cell arteritis. *Annals of the Rheumatic Diseases*, **46,** 468–74.

Smith, C. A., Fidler, W. J. and Pinals, R. (1983). The epidemiology of giant cell arteritis. Report of a ten-year study in Shelby county, Tennessee. *Arthritis and Rheumatism*, **26,** 1214–9.

Sonnenblick, M., Nesher, G., Friedlander, Y. and Rubinow, A. (1994). Giant cell arteritis in Jerusalem: a 12-year epidemiological study. *British Journal of Rheumatology*, **33,** 938–41.

Spiera, R. F., Mitnick, H. J., Kupersmith, M., *et al.* (2001). A prospective, double-blind, randomized, placebo controlled trial of methotrexate in the treatment of giant cell arteritis (GCA). *Clinical and Experimental Rheumatology*, **19,** 495–501.

Srigley, J. R. and Gardiner, G. W. (1980). Giant cell arteritis with small bowel infarction. *American Journal of Gastroenterology*, **73,** 157–61.

Staunton, H., Stafford, F., Leader, M. and O'Riordain, D. (2000). Deterioration of giant cell arteritis with corticosteroid therapy. *Archives of Neurology*, **57,** 581–4.

Straub, R. H., Herfarth, H. H., Rinkes, B., *et al.* (1999). Favorable role of interleukin-10 in patients with polymyalgia rheumatica. *Journal of Rheumatology*, **26,** 1318–25.

Taylor-Gjevre, R., Vo, M., Shukla, D. and Resch, L. (2005). Temporal artery biopsy for giant cell arteritis. *Journal of Rheumatology*, **32,** 1279–82.

Truong, L., Kopelman, R. G., Williams, G. S. and Pirani, C. L. (1985). Temporal arteritis and renal disease. *American Journal of Medicine*, **78,** 171–5.

Uddhammar, A., Boman, J., Juto, P. and Rantapaa-Dahlqvist, S. (1997). Antibodies against Chlamydia pneumoniae, cytomegalovirus, enteroviruses and respiratory syncytial virus in patients with polymyalgia rheumatica. *Clinical and Experimental Rheumatology*, **15,** 299–302.

Uddhammar, A., Rantapaa-Dahlqvist, S., Hedberg, B. and Thornell, L. E. (1998a). Deltoid muscle in patients with polymyalgia rheumatica. *Journal of Rheumatology*, **25,** 1344–51.

Uddhammar, A., Sundqvist, K. G., Ellis, B. and Rantapaa-Dahlqvist, S. (1998b). Cytokines and adhesion molecules in patients with polymyalgia rheumatica. *British Journal of Rheumatology*, **37,** 766–9.

Uddhammar, A., Eriksson, A. L., Nystrom, L., Stenling, R. and Rantapaa-Dahlqvist, S. (2002). Increased mortality due to cardiovascular disease in patients with giant cell arteritis in northern Sweden. *Journal of Rheumatology*, **29,** 737–42.

Wagner, A. D., Goronzy, J. J. and Weyand, C. M. (1994). Functional profile of tissue-infiltrating and circulating CD68+ cells in giant cell arteritis. *Journal of Clinical Investigation*, **94,** 1134–40.

Wagner, A. D., Bjornsson, J., Bartley, G. B., Goronzy, J. J. and Weyand, C. M. (1996). Inteferon-gamma-producing T cells in giant cell vasculitis represent a minority of tissue-infiltrating cells and are located distant from the site of pathology. *American Journal of Pathology*, **148,** 1925–33.

Wagner, A. D., Wittkop, U., Prahst, A., *et al.* (2003). Dendritic cells co-localize with activated CD4+ T cells in giant cell arteritis. *Clinical and Experimental Rheumatology*, **21,** 185–92.

Weyand, C. M. and Goronzy, J. J. (2003). Medium and large vessel vasculitis. *New England Journal of Medicine*, **349,** 160–9.

Weyand, C. M., Hicok, K. C., Hunder, G. G. and Goronzy, J. J. (1992). The HLA-DRB1 locus as a genetic component in giant cell arteritis. *Journal of Clinical Investigation*, **90,** 2355–61.

Weyand, C. M., Hicok, K. C., Hunder G. G. and Goronzy, J. J. (1994a). Tissue cytokine patterns in patients with polymyalgia rheumatica and giant cell arteritis. *Annals of Internal Medicine*, **121,** 484–91.

Weyand, C. M., Schonberger, J., Oppitz, U., Hunder, N. H.N., Hicok, K. C. and Goronzy, J. J. (1994b). Distinct vascular lesions in giant cell arteritis share identical T cell clonotypes. *Journal of Experimental Medicine*, **179,** 951–60.

Weyand, C. M., Wagner, A. D., Bjornsson, J. and Goronzy, J. J. (1996). Correlation of the topographical arrangement and the functional pattern of tissue-infiltrating macrophages in giant cell arteritis. *Journal of Clinical Investigation*, **98,** 1642–9.

Weyand, C. M., Tetzlaff, N., Bjornsson, J., Brack, A., Younge, B. and Goronzy, J. J. (1997). Disease patterns and tissue cytokine profiles in giant cell arteritis. *Arthritis and Rheumatism*, **40,** 19–26.

Weyand, C. M., Fulbright, J. W., Evans, J. M., Hunder, G. G. and Goronzy, J. J. (1999). Corticosteroid requirements in polymyalgia rheumatica. *Archives of Internal Medicine*, **159,** 577–84.

Weyand, C. M., Fulbright, J. W., Hunder, G. G., Evans, J. M. and Goronzy, J. J. (2000). Treatment of giant cell arteritis: interleukin-6 as a biologic marker of disease activity. *Arthritis and Rheumatism*, **43,** 1041–8.

Weyand, C. M., Kaiser, M., Yang, H., Younge, B. and Goronzy, J. J. (2002). Therapeutic effects of acetylsalicylic acid in giant cell arteritis. *Arthritis and Rheumatism*, **46,** 457–66.

Wilkinson, I. M.S. and Russell, R. W.R. (1972). Arteries of the head and neck in giant cell arteritis. *Archives of Neurology*, **27,** 378–91.

Wiseman, P., Stewart, K. and Rai, G. S. (1989). Hypothyroidism in polymyalgia rheumatica and giant cell arteritis. *British Medical Journal*, **298,** 647–8.

CHAPTER 25

Takayasu's arteritis

Yasushi Kobayashi

Introduction

Takayasu's arteritis (TA) is a chronic granulomatous vasculitis characterized by stenosis, occlusion, and sometimes aneurysm of large elastic arteries, mainly the aorta and its main branches including pulmonary and coronary arteries (Jennette *et al.* 1994; Kerr *et al.* 1994; Numano *et al.* 2000; Sharma *et al.* 1996) (Figure 25.1). TA generally affects young women during their reproductive period (Cipriano *et al.* 1977; Numano 2000).

TA was described by Mikito Takayasu, Professor of Ophthalmology of Kanazawa University, Japan, at the 12th Annual Meeting of the Japanese Ophthalmology Society held in 1905 (Takayasu 1908; Numano and Kakuta 1996). Takayasu described a 21-year old woman who had a peculiar wreath-like arteriovenous anastomosis (described as coronary anastomosis) around the papilla due to ischemia. The term Takayasu's arteritis was first used in 1942 (Shinmi 1942) and subsequently by many other researchers (Caccamise and Okuda 1954; Azizi and Rafat 1956; Jacobsen and Rasch 1956; Roedenbeck and Bauer 1956; Lobato 1956; Jimenez Casado and Moncada Moneu 1956). Morgagni had earlier reported a 40-year-old woman in Italy in 1761, whose radial pulses were not palpable for many years (Altschuler and Wheat 2000). In 1856, Savoy described a young woman in whom the main arteries of both upper extremities and of the left side of the neck were completely obliterated (Savoy 1856). Both these cases were likely to have been TA. TA has been called various names including pulseless disease (Jimenez Casado and Moncada Moneu 1956), aortitis syndrome (Kawai *et al.* 1975), aortic arch syndrome (Ross and Mc 1953), long-segment atypical coarctation of the aorta (Hatano *et al.* 1975), Martorell's syndrome (Planas 1978), and occlusive thromboaortopathy (Ishikawa 1978).

Epidemiology

Although TA has been reported all over the world, there is a wide variation in its prevalence in different geographical regions. TA is believed to be predominantly found in Asia (Koide 1992; Park *et al.* 1992; Zheng *et al.* 1992; Sharma *et al.* 1992; Piyachon and Suwanwela 1992), the Middle East (Rosenthal *et al.* 1992; Turkoglu *et al.* 1996; Ureten *et al.* 2004; el-Reshaid *et al.* 1995), and South America (Canas *et al.* 1998; Robles and Reyes 1994; Sato *et al.* 1998). Patients with TA have been increasingly recognized in Africa (Mwipatayi

et al. 2005), Europe (Vanoli *et al.* 2005), and North America (Kerr *et al.* 1994). The incidence of TA in Japan in 2005 was 4.2 per 100,000 persons. In Sweden and the USA, the prevalence was reported to be between 0.26 and 0.64 persons per 100,000 population (Hall *et al.* 1985; Waern *et al.* 1983).

TA causes different aortic lesions in different countries. TA in the Far East such as Japan, Korea, and China affects mainly the aortic arch. In contrast, TA in south Asian countries such as India, Thailand, and Turkey, Israel, and Middle Eastern countries frequently affects the abdominal aorta (Yajima *et al.* 1994).

Moreover, the female to male ratio of TA appears to decline from the Far East toward the West (Yajima *et al.* 1994). The apparent variation in prevalence and phenotype of TA in different geographical areas may reflect genetic factors as in giant cell arteritis, which is frequently found in Caucasian populations but not in others.

TA rarely affects very young children (Sharma *et al.* 1991; Millar *et al.* 1996; Mitchell and Parisi 1997; Hari *et al.* 2000; Stanley *et al.* 2003; Ladhani *et al.* 2001; D'Souza *et al.* 1998; Martini 1995; Cloux Blasco *et al.* 1991; Rose *et al.* 1990; Chiasson *et al.* 1990; Hong *et al.* 1992; Morales *et al.* 1991). Juvenile-onset type TA may differ from adult TA in its pathogenesis.

Etiology and pathogenesis

The etiology of TA still remains unknown; however, three major putative factors in its pathogenesis are: (1) external stress as a trigger; (2) inflammatory mechanisms; and (3) genetic factors. Unknown external stresses may trigger TA; among these, infection may be important. Tuberculosis was suspected for a long time as an etiologic factor of TA in India and Mexico (Lupi-Herrera *et al.* 1977; Sen *et al.* 1972). Tubercle bacilli injected into rabbits induced inflammatory changes resembling those of TA, and the presence of giant cell granulomata resembling tuberculosis follicles in the arterial wall suggested concomitant tuberculosis (Sen *et al.* 1972). Sharma and colleagues did not find an association between TA and tuberculosis and reported that the incidence of tuberculosis in TA was not higher than that in the general population (Jain *et al.* 1996; Sharma *et al.* 1992; Kothari, 1995). Tuberculosis may be a trigger of TA, but tuberculosis itself is now considered not to be a causative agent of TA. Cases of TA after hepatitis B vaccination have been

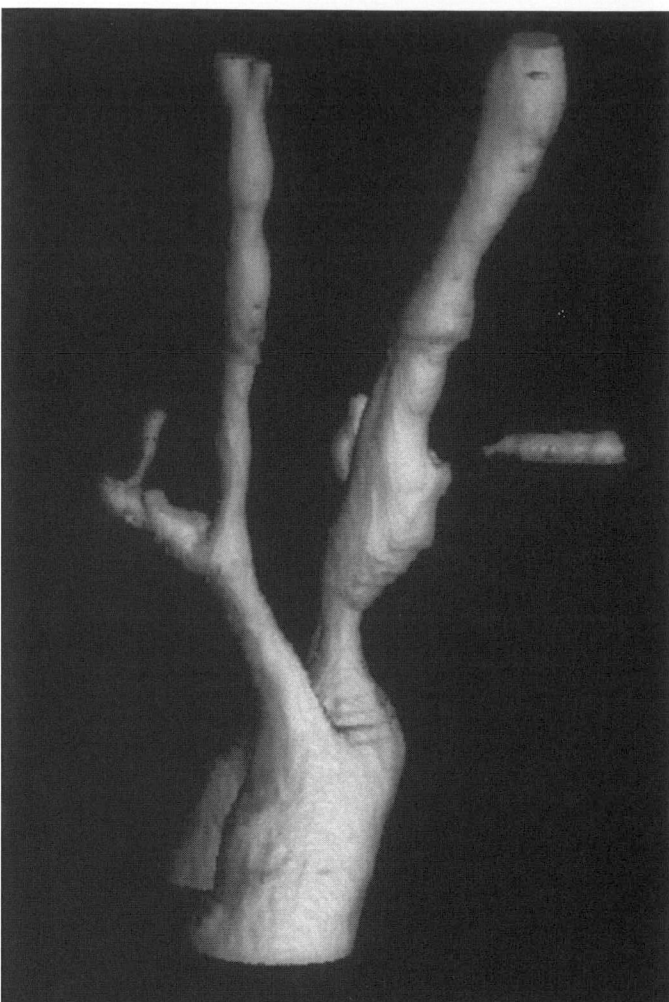

Figure 25.1 Three-dimensional reconstituted enhanced CT shows aneurysm formation in the left common carotid artery and obstruction in the left subclavian artery.

Seko *et al.* (2004) also observed that the expression of costimulatory molecule 4–1BBL, Fas, and the stress-induced molecule MICA were induced in the affected aortic tissue. These data suggested γδT cells infiltrated aortic tissue recognizing MICA, resulting in the induction of MHC antigens and costimulatory molecules, and infiltrating αβ T-cells recognized autoantigens presented by MHC antigens leading to chronic inflammation (Seko *et al.* 2004). The formation of granulomata may ensue under the control of proinflammatory cytokines such as INF-γ produced by T cells and TNF-α, a product of T cells and macrophages (Weyand and Goronzy 2003). The serum proinflammatory cytokines, IL-12, TNF-α, IL-6, and IL-1, are elevated in the serum of patients with active TA. These proinflammatory cytokines may promote granulomatous vascular lesion formation in TA (Park *et al.* 2005b; Tripathy *et al.* 2004; Verma *et al.* 2005).

Antiendothelial cell antibodies (AECA) have been reported in the serum of TA patients (Eichhorn *et al.* 1996). AECA may activate endothelial cells and be involved in the pathogenesis of TA (Blank *et al.* 1999; Kornberg *et al.* 2000; Tripathy *et al.* 2001). Antineutrophil cytoplasmic antibodies (ANCA), often found in many primary vasculitis syndromes, were reported to be associated with TA, but these data have not been confirmed (Hoffman and Ahmed 1998).

Nicklin and Iwakura have independently studied an Interleukin-1 receptor antagonist (IL-1ra) knockout mouse, in which IL-1 signaling is enhanced. IL-1ra-deficient mice developed transmural inflammation in elastic arteries at the site of turbulent flow, which is usually only observed in a mouse model of atherosclerosis (Nicklin *et al.* 2000; Shepherd and Nicklin 2005; Matsuki *et al.* 2005). In mildly affected mice, infiltrating cells were mainly observed in the adventitia. In severely affected mice, infiltrating cells consisted predominantly of monocytes, Th1 cells, and dendritic cells. Interestingly, Iwakura reported inflammation at the root of the aorta with massive infiltration of macrophages and monocytes and loss of lamellae in the aortic media (Matsuki *et al.* 2005). Moreover, left ventricular hypertrophy and aortic stenosis were also observed in these mice. Using adoptive transfer, they showed that T cells from IL-1ra knockout mice induced aortitis in nu/nu mice. These findings suggest that T cells may play an important role in the pathogenesis of TA. Iwakura also reported that abrogation of TNF-α, but not of IL-6, suppresses the development of aortitis, suggesting that IL-1 and TNF-α are key regulators in the development of inflammation in the aorta. TA may be caused by a spontaneous overproduction of IL-1α/β in response to stimuli that are usually tightly regulated in healthy individuals. Mutations resulting in constitutive elevation of IL-1α/β in mice may be a useful model of early-onset TA.

The higher incidence of TA in Asian, Middle Eastern, and South American populations, and some monozygotic twins imply a possible role of genetic factors in TA (Numano *et al.* 1978; Sasazuki *et al.* 1979), however, only about 1% of Japanese TA patients have relatives affected with TA (Kobayashi and Numano 2002), suggesting TA is not a monoallelic hereditary disease.

HLA studies of TA population in Japan revealed positive associations between TA and MHC class II alleles HLA-DRB1*1502 and DPB1* 0901 and MHC class I alleles HLA-B*5201 and HLA-B*3902 (Isohisa *et al.* 1978; Naito *et al.* 1978; Yoshida *et al.* 1993; Kimura *et al.* 2000). DRB1*1502 and DPB1*0901 were shown to be in strong linkage disequilibrium with HLA-B*5201 in the Japanese population (Kimura *et al.* 2000). Numano *et al.* reported TA patients

reported (Castresana-Isla *et al.* 1993; Zaas *et al.* 2001). The host response to infection may itself be a trigger of TA.

In a mouse model of infection, Virgin and colleagues reported a γ-herpes virus induced aortitis in IFN-γ signaling abrogated mice (Weck *et al.* 1997; Dal Canto *et al.* 2000). A γ-herpes virus, γHV68, causes inflammation in the elastic arteries in mice. Interestingly, younger mice were more susceptibility to γ-herpes virus-induced arteritis. (Dal Canto *et al.* 2000). α-herpes virus caused large-vessel inflammation in chickens (Fabricant 1985), and β-herpes virus and murine CMV can also cause aortic inflammation. The media of the aorta is often a target of aortitis in these mouse models.

The mechanism whereby inflammation damages aortic tissue in TA has been described. Seko showed perforin-secreting killer cells, γδ T cells, cytotoxic T lymphocytes, and natural killer cells infiltrated diseased aortic tissue from TA patients. A 65-kD heat shock protein (HSP-65), which may be one of the targets of γδT cells, was expressed at high levels in the media and along the vasa vasorum in the adventitia (Seko *et al.* 1994). αβT cells in the affected aortic tissue of TA had limited repertoires of TCR Vα and Vβ gene transcripts compared with atherosclerosis, which may indicate that a specific antigen in aortic tissue is targeted (Seko *et al.* 1996).

with HLA-Bw52 (HLA-B*5201) exhibited more severe inflammatory conditions and a higher degree of aortic insufficiency than those without Bw52 (Moriwaki and Numano 1992). In addition, HLA-B*3902 may be associated with renal vascular lesions in the Japanese TA population (Kitamura *et al.* 1998). The association of HLA with TA was also reported in North and South America: TA in Mexico with HLA-DRB1*1301 (Girona *et al.* 1996) and HLA-DRB1*1602 and DRB1*1001 with TA in Colombia (Salazar *et al.* 2000). A haplotype defined by several polymorphisms in the NFKBIL1 gene, which encodes a putative ankyrin repeat protein, may correlate with higher promoter activity of NFKBIL1 *in vitro* and appears to associate with TA (Shibata *et al.* 2006). Although the function of NFKBIL1 is unknown, it may confer the proinflammatory environment necessary for the development of TA.

TA has been reported to be associated with inflammatory bowel disease, including Crohn's disease (Lenhoff and Mee 1982; Owyang *et al.* 1979; Friedman and Tegtmeyer 1979; Yassinger *et al.* 1976; Baqir *et al.* 2006) and ulcerative colitis (Numano *et al.* 1996; Sakhuja *et al.* 1990; Achar and Al-Nakib 1986; Miwa *et al.* 1979; Chapman *et al.* 1978; Morita *et al.* 1996). These reports have fueled speculation that TA may share a developmental mechanism with Crohn's disease.

Autoinflammatory diseases, such as Crohn's disease, are characterized by attacks of seemingly unprovoked inflammation without significant levels of autoantibodies and autoreactive T cells (McDermott and Aksentijevich, 2002). Minor inflammatory injuries that would be unnoticed under normal circumstances may trigger unregulated inflammation in such disease states (Galeazzi *et al.* 2006). These disorders are presumably caused by primary dysfunction of the innate immune system, without evidence of adaptive immune dysregulation. To date, no causative autoantibodies or autoreactive T cells have been identified in TA, suggesting that TA may have a similar mechanism to that of other of autoinflammatory diseases.

One particular autoinflammatory disease, Blau syndrome, is a rare condition typically defined by granulomatous arthritis, skin eruption, and uveitis in the absence of lung or other visceral involvement, occurring in very young children (Blau 1985). Some variants of Blau syndrome cause large-vessel arteritis (Wang *et al.* 2002). A gain-of-function mutation in the Nod2 gene has been reported to activate NF-κB constitutively and cause Blau syndrome (Miceli-Richard *et al.* 2001). Early-onset TA may partially overlap with Blau syndrome (Rose *et al.* 1990; Schapiro *et al.* 1994; Fernandes *et al.* 2000; Hilario *et al.* 1998). Constitutive activation of IL-1 and NF-κB may cause early-onset TA, particularly in children.

Histopathological findings

Takayasu's arteritis is defined as an inflammatory vasculopathy that involves mainly large and middle-size vessels. The aorta is thick and often rigid, secondary to fibrosis of all three arterial layers, particularly the adventitia and intima (see Figures 9.1, 9.2, and 9.3 in Chapter 9). Extension of adventitial fibrosis and inflammatory cell infiltration to the adjacent structures is sometimes observed. Characteristic of TA is finding that the aortic lumen is narrowed in a "fusion that has skipped" area. These areas of narrowing may alternate with aneurysmal dilatations of the aortic wall. Ascending aortitis almost always results in dilatation of the aorta but not narrowing, perhaps due to hemodynamic influences. The gross appearance of the intima may be "cobblestoned" with round, well-circumscribed, variably-sized, white, gelatinous, smooth patches with intervening normal intima. The thick intima may have the gross appearance of tree bark due to longitudinal wrinkling and ridges. The affected aorta in end-stage TA may have a lead pipe appearance.

TA may be divided into an acute, florid inflammatory phase, and a chronic healed fibrotic phase. Both types may be seen simultaneously, suggesting recurrent inflammation in TA (Gravanis 2000). In the acute phase, the inflammatory lesions originate in the vasa vasorum and are characterized by perivascular cuffing mainly composed of γδT lymphocytes, cytotoxic T lymphocytes, and T helper cells (Figure 25.2). Luminal stenosis of adventitial small arteries due to intimal thickening is relatively common. An increase in adventitial thickness due to fibrosis is a histopathologic feature found in the chronic phase of TA. Inflammatory infiltrates in the arterial wall are typically arranged in granulomas that are dependent on T cells regulating the activity and integrity of macrophages. Neovascularization, often accompanied by infiltrates of lymphocytes, plasma cells, and occasional Langerhans-type giant cells, is seen in the media. Giant cells of the foreign body type are occasionally strewn around degraded elastic tissue. Patches of medial coagulation necrosis surrounded by a fence-like arrangement of epithelioid cells are occasionally noted at the periphery (Gravanis 2000). The inflammation caused by TA does not damage the aorta all at once but creates random lesions; usually the prominent lesion appears and disappears randomly (Nasu 1982; Gravanis 2000).

In the chronic stage of TA, intimal fibrosis is often accompanied by well-formed fibrous atherosclerotic plaques and calcification. Extension of the adventitial fibrosis and round cell infiltration to adjacent structures may result in retroperitoneal fibrosis, and extension of similar fibrotic processes to the pericardium may induce a fibrosing pericarditis. Inflammation may extend to the heart and cause myocarditis (Takeda *et al.* 2005). Active inflammation may be present in the arterial circuit even when the disease appears to be clinically silent. The activity of the disease often persists and new lesions in the arteries continue to appear (Bali *et al.* 1998).

Significant numbers of patients with TA have pulmonary artery involvement (approximately 50%). The morphologic changes in the pulmonary arterial wall such as inflammation and fibrosis of the adventitia and media and thickening of the intima secondary to fibrosis are similar to those in the aorta (Yamada *et al.* 1992).

Natural course

Paralleling the histopathologic changes, the clinical course of TA typically progresses through two basic stages, an acute stage and a chronic stage. Early in the acute stage, symptoms are non-specific features of aortic inflammation, including fever, fatigability, weight loss, arthralgias, hemoptysis, and tachycardia. After weeks, months, and years in some cases, vascular lesions appear and cause ischemic symptoms due to stenotic lesions or thrombus formation. Almost all patients will have ischemic disorders of the involved vessels, which can present as dizziness, syncope, visual disturbances, faint or absent pulses, or differences in systolic blood pressure between arms (Ishikawa and Maetani 1994; Iwai *et al.* 2000). Twenty percent of patients have a self-limited, monophasic inflammatory episode; however, a progressive and relapsing course is the rule. Serial angiographic studies show that new lesions can be found in 61% of

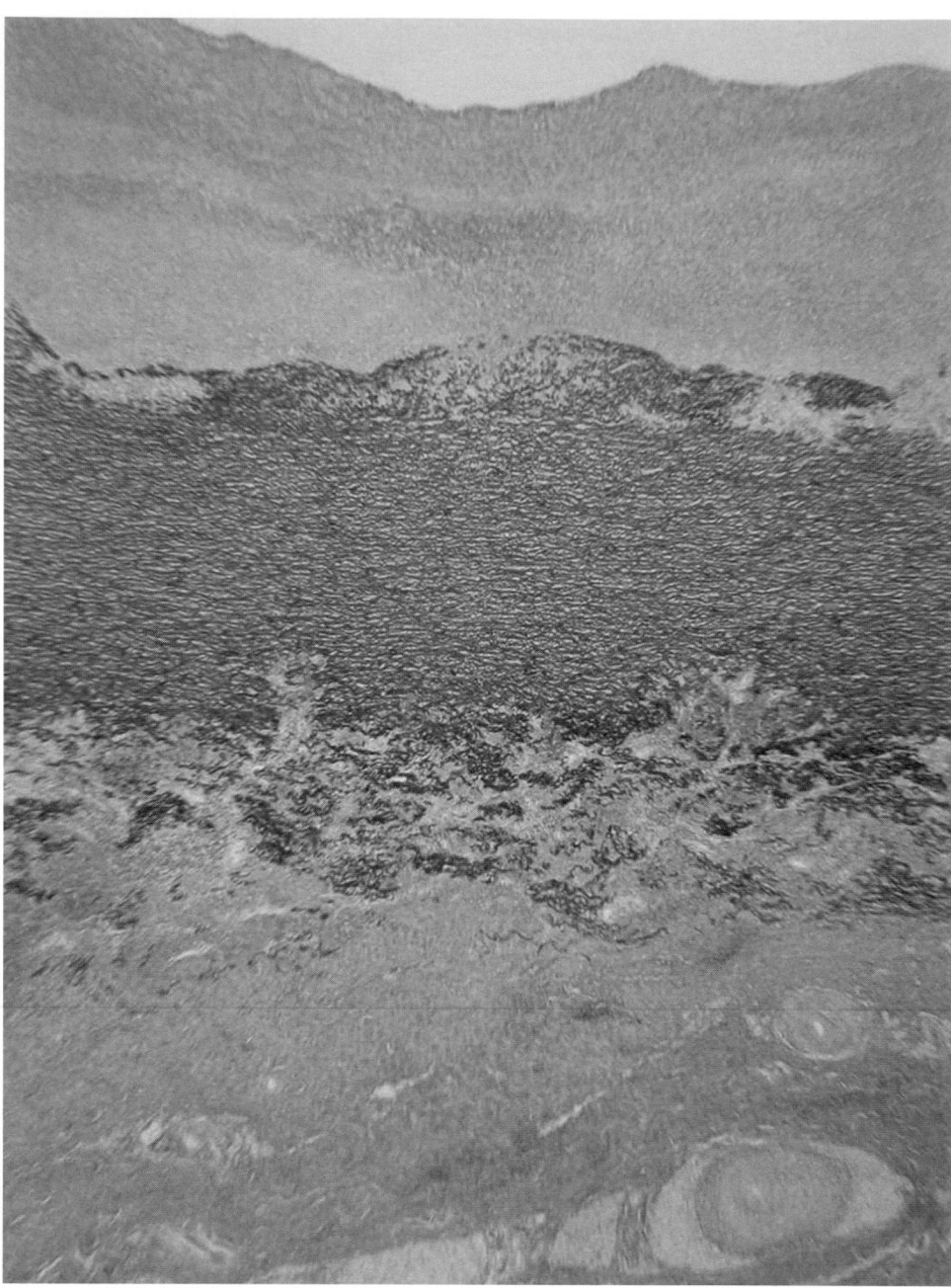

Figure 25.2 A section of the aorta showing intimal thickening, piecemeal necrosis in the outer media, and cellular infiltrate around the vasa vasorum. (See Color Plate 74).

patients even when the disease is thought to be in the chronic phase (Hoffman *et al.* 1994). Subsequent recurrence of TA is found in 20% of Japanese TA patients in remission. Among the complications of TA, aortic insufficiency and hypertension are highly associated with a poor prognosis.

TA patients have a high rate of atherosclerotic plaques, at least as frequent as those observed among autoimmune diseases (Seyahi *et al.* 2006). Activated immune mechanisms in TA may exacerbate the development of atherosclerosis.

Clinical features

In the acute stage, the symptoms of TA are usually non-specific, generalized inflammatory symptoms, as mentioned above. Early diagnosis is not easy because symptoms are not specific and

unique disease markers do not exist. The disease is characterized by a specific predilection for women, though the female-to-male ratio varies as follows: Japan 9:1, Korea 6.6:1, China 2.9:1, India 1.6:1, USA 29.1:1, Mexico 5.3:1 (Zheng *et al.* 1992; Hoffman *et al.* 1994; Koide 1992; Lupi-Herrera *et al.* 1977; Park and Park 1992; Bali *et al.* 1998). The average age of onset in Japanese and Indian patients is 15–35 years. The majority of TA patients present with symptoms due to vascular lesions. TA in far eastern countries affects the aortic arch most frequently, so decreased or absent pulses in upper limbs and difference of blood pressure in upper limbs is often observed. Decreased pulses in the left upper limb are more frequent due to the vascular anatomy. In contrast, TA in south Asian countries affects abdominal arteries; therefore hypertension may be the first clue to diagnosis. Easy fatigability of upper limbs, pain, and intermittent claudication may also be noticed.

Stroke (cerebral vascular accident/transient ischemic attack) and sudden blindness may be caused by thrombosis of cerebral arteries. Asthenia or dizziness are sometimes noticed, particularly in the acute stage. These symptoms may be due to stroke and in part to overstimulation of the baro-receptor in the aortic arch leading to hypotension (Takeshita *et al.* 1977). Hypertension may be caused from atypical coarctation of the aorta, loss of vascular compliance, aortic insufficiency, or renal artery stenosis (Abe *et al.* 1976; Ask-Upmark 1961; Sharma *et al.* 1985).

Aortic insufficiency is present in almost one-third of TA patients in the Japanese population; it may be caused by annuloaortic ectasia. Left ventricular hypertrophy is observed in the presence of aortic insufficiency. Aortic insufficiency and left ventricular hypertrophy may eventually result in heart failure, and carry a poor prognosis.

The inflammation of TA may involve the ostium of coronary arteries and thus lead to acute myocardial infarction or exertional angina (Matsubara *et al.* 1992). Pulmonary lesions were found in 15% of TA patients by angiography; however, clinical symptoms such as hemoptysis are rare (Frankel *et al.* 2006). Isolated pulmonary arteritis has also been reported (Nakabayashi *et al.* 1996; Lie 1996).

Crohn's disease, ulcerative colitis, and non-specific inflammatory colitis have been reported with TA (Baqir *et al.* 2006), and sometimes gastorointestinal bleeding is the first symptom in TA. The eyes can also be involved in TA; however, ocular complications due to TA are decreasing due to advances in early diagnosis and therapy. Emboli may cause sudden blindness in the acute stage. Ischemic retinopathy is often classified into three stages: Stage I – venous dilatation, Stage II – microaneurysm formation, and Stage III – arteriovenous anastomosis (Ishikawa *et al.* 1983; Vedantham *et al.* 2005). Hypertensive retinopathy is more commonly seen with TA. Other ocular complications of TA include cataracts, optic atrophy, loss of eye reflexes, iris atrophy, and rubeosis iris.

Dermatological lesions have been described with TA (Baqir *et al.* 2006). Erythema nodosum is reported as the most common skin lesion in TA in Caucasian populations, and ulcerative, subacute, nodular lesions have been described in Mexico and Japan. Pyoderma gangrenosum, papulonecrotic eruptions, nodular erythematous lesions, facial lupus-like rashes, and panniculitis have been also been reported. Skin lesions tend to occur without any relationship to the sites of vascular lesions; however, pathological findings include granulomatous features suggesting the same pathological mechanisms as those of the vasculitis.

Laboratory findings

The most frequent laboratory abnormality is an elevated erythrocyte sedimentation rate, which is considered a good index of disease activity. C-reactive protein is also used as a surrogate marker of the disease. White blood cell counts and γ-globulin levels are also elevated. Mild anemia and elevation of complement components are also observed, as are coagulopathies and platelet activation in the acute stage. These laboratory data reflect inflammation in general. ECG may show signs of left ventricular hypertrophy (Hashimoto *et al.* 1992).

Radiological findings

A comprehensive angiogram is usually performed to diagnose TA and evaluate the extent of disease and guide therapy.

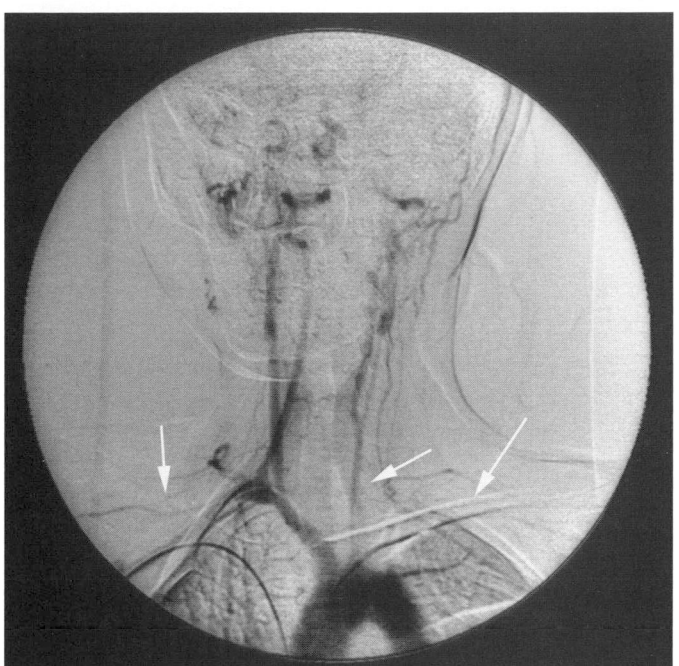

Figure 25.3 Angiogram shows obstruction of right and left subclavian arteries and marked narrowing in left common carotid artery (arrows).

Digital subtraction angiography (DSA), computed tomography (CT), and magnetic resonance angiography (MRA) may also provide valuable information (Sider *et al.* 1985) (Figures 25.3 and 25.4). The angiographic findings of segmental, fine dystrophic calcification with abrupt termination are very suggestive of TA. Similarly, calcification outlining a long stenotic segment of the aorta may be seen in young TA patients (Figure 25.5). Rib notching

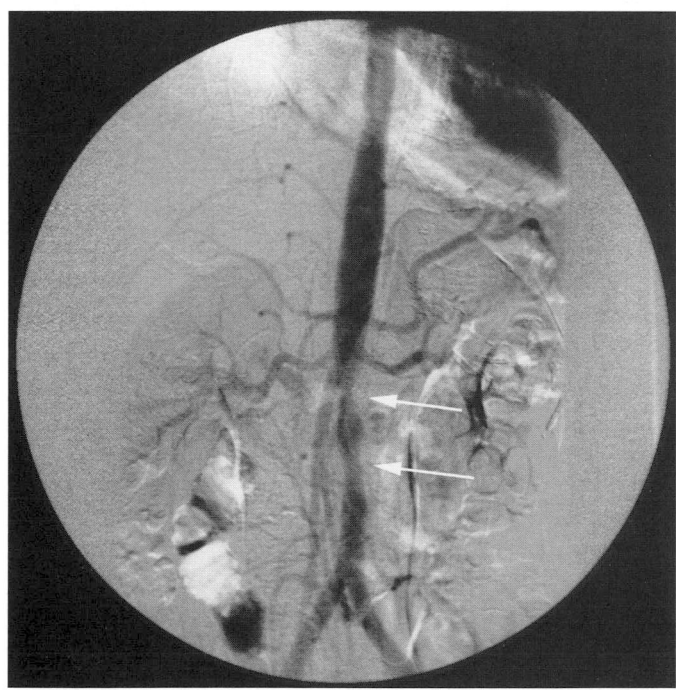

Figure 25.4 Angiogram demonstrating narrowing of the aorta (arrows).

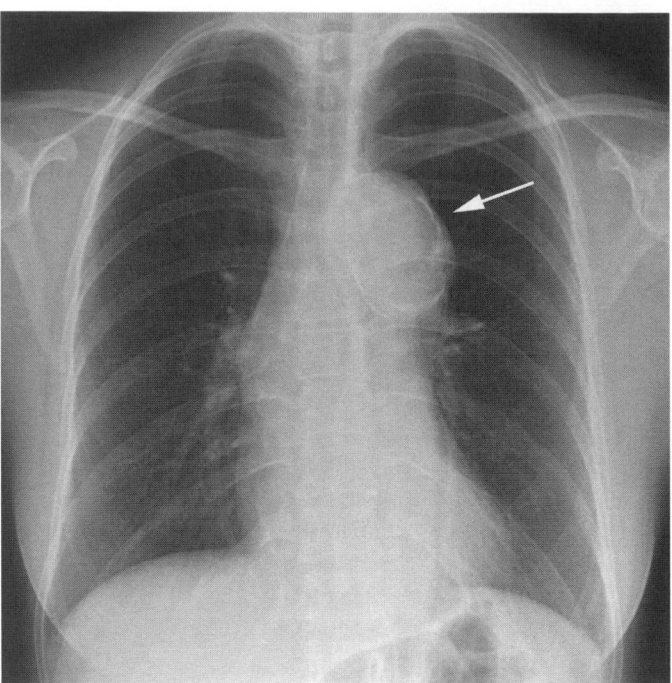

Figure 25.5 Chest radiograph showing calcification of the aortic arch and the descending aorta (arrow) in a 30-year-old TA patient.

due to aortic aneurysm or dilatation of the ascending aorta may also be found. Based on arteriographic involvement in a cohort of Japanese TA patients, Nasu (1975) classified the disease into four types, depending on which segments of the aorta and its branches were involved. A new classification proposed by an international co-operative study on Takayasu arteritis has been introduced to compare TA internationally, based on the location of vascular lesions (Hata *et al.* 1996).

Classification of the types of TA according to site of involvement is shown in Table 25.1. Involvement of the coronary or pulmonary artery is designated as C(+) or P(+) with any of the types (Hata *et al.* 1996; Moriwaki *et al.* 1997; Park *et al.* 2005a). Early angiographic changes include localized narrowing or irregularity of the aortic wall. Obliterative vascular lesions include narrowing and stenosis to complete occlusion. The vessel may be dilated or aneurysmal, and there may be a combination of obstruction and aneurysmal dilatation. Segments of narrowing are commonly found in angiogram.

The disease involves branches of the aorta at or near the point of origin and extends into the branch arteries for a variable distance. In India and other South Asian countries, the renal arteries are affected in the majority of the patients; bilateral disease can result

Table 25.1 Classification of Takayasu's arteritis

Type	Site of involvement
I	Branches of aortic arch
II	Ascending aorta, aortic arch and its branches
III	Ascending aorta, aortic arch and its branches, and thoracic descending aorta
IV	Abdominal aorta and/or renal arteries
V	Combination of Type IIb and IV

in severe renovascular hypertension. The pulmonary arteries are involved in half of TA patients and there is a predilection for involvement of the right pulmonary artery. Coronary artery lesions are usually ostial or limited to the proximal segment.

Aortic insufficiency and cardiac function can be assessed by echocardiography (Hashimoto *et al.* 1992; Hashimoto *et al.* 1993; Hashimoto *et al.* 1996). Ultrasonography may show carotid artery lesions and intimal thickness that may reflect disease activity (Park *et al.* 2001; Schmidt *et al.* 2001; Seth *et al.* 2006). MRI has been reported to detect vessel wall edema and can be used to monitor the disease activity of TA (Flamm *et al.* 1998).

Recently, ^{18}F-fluorodeoxyglucose positron emission tomography (^{18}F-FDG PET), has been introduced to diagnose TA (Hara *et al.* 1999; Belhocine 2004; Wenger *et al.* 2003; Webb *et al.* 2004; Meller *et al.* 2003a, 2003b; Kissin and Merkel 2004; Kobayashi *et al.* 2005) (see Chapter 20). ^{18}F-FDG is an analogue of glucose and accumulates in metabolically active cells such as tumor cells and inflammatory cells. The ^{18}F-FDG PET can show signs of inflammation and its location in the aorta directly, therefore early diagnosis of TA and exact estimation of the inflammatory activity can be made. Correlation using CT or MRI can help determine the exact location of inflammation in the aorta (Kobayashi *et al.* 2005) (Figure 25.6). To date, the diagnosis of TA has been made based on the vascular deformity shown by angiogram, CT, and MRI and early diagnosis of TA has been difficult. ^{18}F-FDG PET may facilitate early diagnosis before formation of vascular lesions. ^{18}F-FDG PET analyses showed that inflammatory activity did not always correlate with CRP and ESR level during treatment (Kobayashi *et al.* 2005). Because ^{18}F-FDG can accumulate in atherosclerotic lesions or other vascular diseases, FDG-PET data should be carefully interpreted along with other clinical findings (see Chapter 20).

Diagnosis

The diagnosis of TA is based on findings of vascular lesion formation in large and middle-size vessel by angiogram, CT, or MRI. Age of onset of vascular lesion formation should also be considered in making the diagnosis of TA. Usually in the early stages of TA, nonspecific inflammatory symptoms are common and a work up for fever of unknown origin may be performed (Wagner *et al.* 2005). The American College of Rheumatology proposed classification criteria (Arend *et al.* 1990), consisting of: (1) age of onset <40 years old; (2) claudication of an extremity; (3) decreased brachial artery pulse; (4) a difference of more than 10 mmHg systolic pressure between two limbs; (5) a bruit over subclavian arteries or the aorta; and (6) angiographic evidence of narrowing or occlusion of the aorta, its primary branches, or large arteries in the proximal upper or lower extremities. The presence of three of the six criteria is required for diagnosis among a set of subjects with systemic vasculitis.

The Japanese Research Committee on Vasculitis Syndromes proposed another set of diagnostic criteria: (1) angiographic evidence of narrowing or occlusion of the aorta, its primary branches, or large arteries in the proximal upper or lower extremities by angiogram, CT, or MRI; (2) early age of onset; (3) presence of markers of inflammation; and (4) exclusion of patients with atherosclerosis, inflammatory abdominal aortic aneurysm, vascular Behçet's syndrome, syphilitic aortitis, giant cell arteritis, congenital vascular abnormality, and mycotic aneurysm.

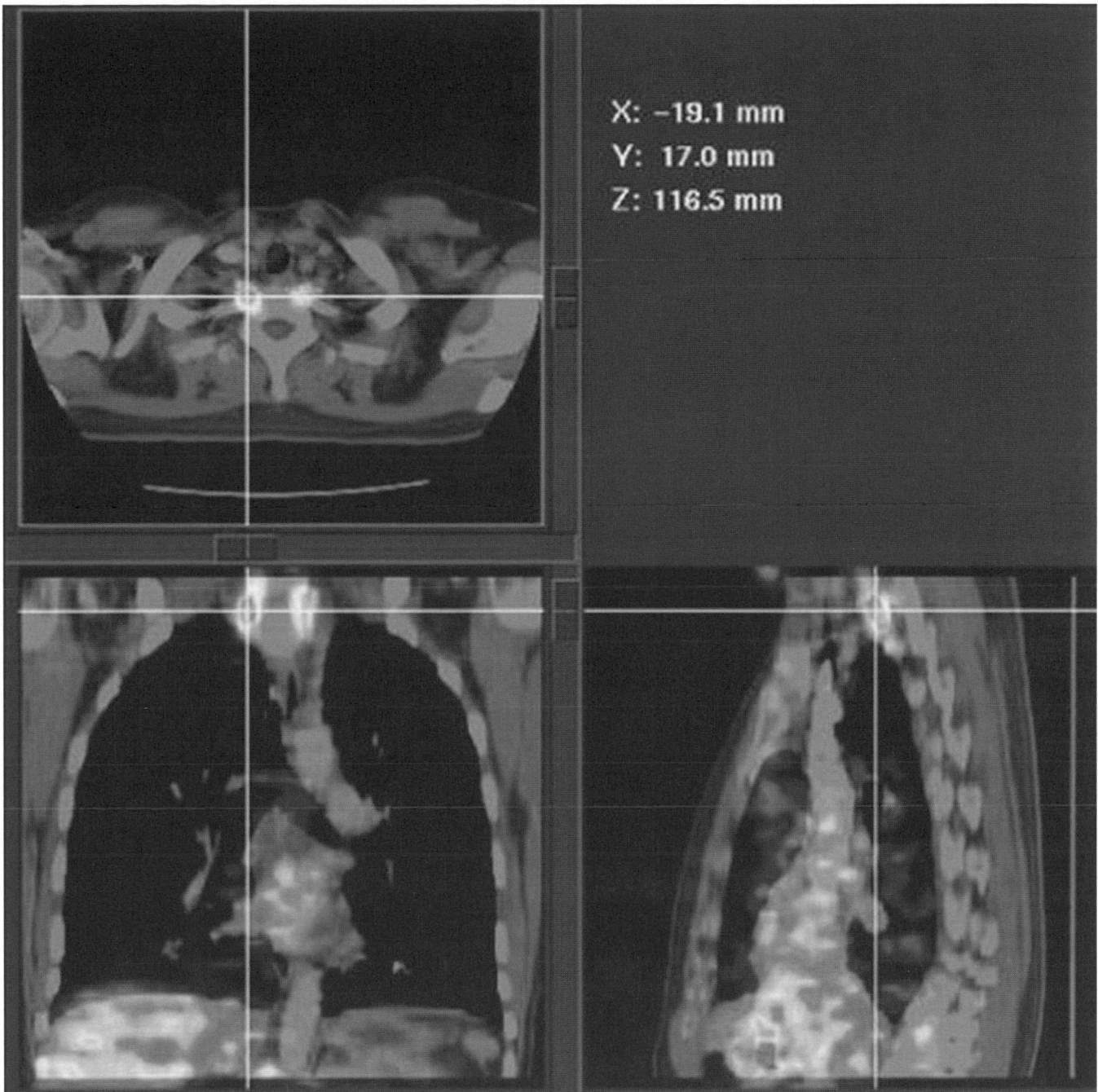

X: −19.1 mm
Y: 17.0 mm
Z: 116.5 mm

Figure 25.6 ¹⁸F-FDG PET image coimaged with enhanced CT showed active inflammation in both vertebral arteries. (See Color Plate 75).

Management

Medical management of TA in the acute stage consists of gluco-corticoids, particularly prednisone or prednisolone, as a first line therapy. Patients with active disease are initially treated with oral prednisolone at a dose of 0.5–1 mg/kg per day (Kerr *et al*. 1994) or an equivalent dose of prednisone. About 60 to 80% of TA patients will go into remission but relapse during taper occurs in more than 50% of patients. In Japan, HLA-B*5201-positive TA patients tend to need more prednisolone than HLA-B*5201-negative TA patients (Moriwaki and Numano 1992).

If patients cannot be tapered to an alternate-day regimen with-out disease exacerbation, a cytotoxic agent such as cyclosporine, cyclophosphamide, azathioprine, or methotrexate can be used. Cyclosporine is administered as a daily oral dose of 1 to 3 mg/kg per day in conjunction with daily glucocorticoids (Fullerton *et al*. 1991; Ujiie *et al*. 2004). Cyclophosphamide may be added to gluco-corticoids in severe refractory TA patients, but should be used with caution due to its cytotoxicity (Shelhamer *et al*. 1985). Azathioprine is administered as a daily oral dose of 1 to 2 mg/kg per day in con-junction with daily glucocorticoids (Valsakumar *et al*. 2003). Methotrexate can promote remission, given once weekly; the usual starting dose for methotrexate is about 15 mg/wk, with 2.5-mg increments every 1 to 2 weeks to achieve a maximum tolerated weekly dose of ~25 mg.

Excellent results have been reported with anti-TNF therapy in refractory TA (Hoffman *et al.* 2004) (Tato *et al.* 2005). Granulomatous inflammation in TA is dependent in part on macrophage secreted TNF-α. In addition to macrophages, T cells and natural killer cells also produce TNF-α. In a study by Hoffman *et al.*, the addition of anti-TNF-α therapy resulted in improvement in 14 out of 15 TA patients, and sustained remission in 10 of 15 patients who were able to discontinue glucocorticoids. Autologous stem cell transplantation has been performed in one refractory TA patient (Kotter *et al.* 2005). Further analyses will be needed to evaluate whether this approach is feasible (Kotter *et al.* 2005). Low-dose aspirin in addition to glucocorticoids treatment reduces the number of ischemic complications (Numano *et al.* 1985).

If severe ischemic organ dysfunction is present, surgical intervention may be needed because established vascular lesions are usually not reversible with medical treatment alone. Surgical treatment is common in patients with severe complications of TA, particularly: cerebrovascular disease due to cervicocranial vessel stenosis; coronary artery disease; severe to moderate aortic insufficiency; severe coarctation of the aorta; renovascular hypertension; limb claudication; and progressive aneurysm enlargement. For correction of vascular lesions, bypass graft procedures are often performed and good long-term outcomes have been reported (Kerr *et al.* 1994; Weaver *et al.* 1990; Lagneau *et al.* 1987).

There have been several retrospective reviews of surgical treatment of TA. Miyata *et al* reported 40 years of experience with vascular operations and found that patients with severe complications have a better prognosis with surgical intervention than with medication alone. The overall survival rate for surgical intervention at 20 years was 73.5%. The number of vascular lesions, age, and presence of aneurysm formation seemed to influence the prognosis. Matsuura *et al.* described their 20 years' experience of surgical treatment of aortic insufficiency in TA patients. They performed aortic valve replacement and composite graft repair. The overall 15-year survival rate was 76.1%. Matsuura reported that a major concern in aortic arch surgery was late dilatation of the residual segment of aorta (Matsuura *et al.* 2006). Matsuura also reported a retrospective analysis of long-term outcomes of surgical treatment for aortic valve regurgitation due to TA. Among 69 procedures performed over 25 years, the overall 15-year survival rate was 76.1%. Detachment of the valve and late dilation of the residual ascending aorta were reported as complications. Late dilation may have been due to active inflammation of TA leading to valve or graft dehiscence after surgery. Control of inflammation is important to improve the prognosis of surgical treatment (Miyata *et al.* 1998; Miyata *et al.* 2003). Taketani reported surgical treatment of atypical coarctation of the aorta. The overall survival rate and event-free survival rate over 20 years were 62.3% and 58.4% respectively. Serious long-term complications were anastomotic aneurysms, congestive heart failure, cerebrovascular accident, graft deterioration, abdominal aortic aneurysms, and renal failure. Control of hypertension was important in reducing complications (Taketani *et al.* 2005). Weaver reported renal revascularization in TA-induced renal artery stenosis. The authors stressed the importance of finding, for anastomosis, an anatomic site without apparent inflammation (Weaver *et al.* 2004).

Percutaneous transluminal angioplasty, with or without a stent, has been reported to have good to excellent short-term outcomes in TA by some authors (Sakaida *et al.* 2001; Sharma *et al.* 2000; Tyagi *et al.* 1998; Tyagi *et al.* 1993), however, other reports have been to the contrary (Fava *et al.* 1993; Weaver *et al.* 1990; Kerr *et al.* 1994), suggesting that TA vascular lesions may be less amenable to successful dilatation. Persistent inflammation in the TA vessel at the time of dilatation and stenting could also lead to enhanced myointimal proliferation. Still, for short focal lesions, excellent results have been reported.

Takayasu arteritis and pregnancy

TA is a disease that affects women of child-bearing age and sometimes presents during pregnancy and around the time of delivery. TA recurrences may also occur during these times. Numano and Shimamoto (1971) found continuous high level urinary excretion of total estrogens in TA patients. The exact mechanism is unknown, but hormonal change or other stress related to pregnancy or delivery may serve as a trigger.

Fertility is apparently not affected by the disease; however, severe complications due to TA may hamper pregnancy and delivery. Management of labor and the decision for caesarian section are based on the assessment of maternal risk factors. Inflammation during pregnancy may be managed by small amounts of glucocorticoids.

Prognosis

The prognosis of TA has much improved because of advances in imaging and early diagnosis. Major factors contributing to a poor prognosis of TA are complications such as aortic insufficiency, hypertension, and multiorgan failure. Therefore, it is important to diagnose TA early before formation of serious vascular lesions and appearance of complications.

Acknowledgement

I thank Professor Richard A. Flavell of Yale University for his support and Dr Fayazz Sutterwala of Yale University for critical reading and useful discussion. I also thank the late Emeritus Professor Fujio Numano for his long-time guidance with regard to basic and clinical studies of Takayasu's arteritis.

References

Abe, K., Miyazaki, S., Kusaka, T., Irokawa, N. and Aoyagi, H. (1976). Elevated plasma renin activity in aortitis syndrome. *Japanese Heart Journal*, **17**, 1–11.

Achar, K. N. and Al-Nakib, B. (1986). Takayasu's arteritis and ulcerative colitis. *American Journal of Gastroenterology*, **81**, 1215–7.

Altschuler, E. L. and Wheat, J. (2000). Morgagni-Takayasu arteritis. *Lancet*, **356**, 2013.

Arend, W. P., Michel, B. A., Bloch, D. A., Hunder, G. G., Calabrese, L. H., Edworthy, S. M., *et al.* (1990). The American College of Rheumatology 1990 criteria for the classification of Takayasu arteritis. *Arthritis and Rheumatism*, **33**, 1129–34.

Ask-Upmark, E. (1961). On the pathogenesis of the hypertension in Takayashu's syndrome. *Acta Medica Scandinavica*, **169**, 467–77.

Azizi, S. P. and Rafat, A. (1956). [Observation of a patient with Takayasu's disease; pulseless disease.]. *Acta Medica Iran*, **1**, 43–52.

Bali, H. K., Jain, S., Jain, A. and Sharma, B. K. (1998). Stent supported angioplasty in Takayasu arteritis. *International Journal of Cardiology*, **66** (Suppl. 1), S213–7; discussion S219–20.

Baqir, M., Usman, M. H., Adenwalla, H. N., Aziz, S., Noor, F., Islam, T. U., Ahmed, M. and Hotiana, M. (2006). Takayasu's arteritis with skin manifestations in a patient with inflammatory bowel disease: coincidence or concurrence? *Clinical Rheumatology*, **26**, 996–8.

Belhocine, T. (2004). 18FDG imaging of giant cell arteritis: usefulness of whole-body plus brain PET. *European Journal of Nuclear Medicine and Molecular Imaging*, **31**, 1055–6.

Blank, M., Krause, I., Goldkorn, T., Praprotnik, S., Livneh, A., Langevitz, P., Kaganovsky, E., Morgenstern, S., Cohen, S., Barak, V., Eldor, A., Weksler, B. and Shoenfeld, Y. (1999). Monoclonal anti-endothelial cell antibodies from a patient with Takayasu arteritis activate endothelial cells from large vessels. *Arthritis and Rheumatism*, **42**, 1421–32.

Blau, E. B. (1985). Familial granulomatous arthritis, iritis, and rash. *Journal of Pediatrics*, **107**, 689–93.

Caccamise, W. C. and Okuda, K. (1954). Takayasu's or pulseless disease: an unusual syndrome with ocular manifestations. *American Journal of Ophthalmology*, **37**, 784–6.

Canas, C. A., Jimenez, C. A., Ramirez, L. A., Uribe, O., Tobon, I., Torrenegra, A., Cortina, A., Munoz, M., Gutierrez, O., Restrepo, J. F., Pena, M. and Iglesias, A. (1998). Takayasu arteritis in Colombia. *International Journal of Cardiology*, **66** (Suppl. 1), S73–9.

Castresana-Isla, C. J., Herrera-Martinez, G. and Vega-Molina, J. (1993). Erythema nodosum and Takayasu's arteritis after immunization with plasma derived hepatitis B vaccine. *Journal of Rheumatology*, **20**, 1417–8.

Chapman, R., Dawe, C., Whorwell, P. J. and Wright, R. (1978). Ulcerative colitis in association with Takayasu's disease. *American Journal of Digestive Diseases*, **23**, 660–2.

Chiasson, D. A., Ipp, M., Benson, L. and Silver, M. M. (1990). Acute heart failure in an 8-year-old diabetic girl. *Journal of Pediatrics*, **116**, 472–7.

Cipriano, P. R., Silverman, J. F., Perlroth, M. G., Griepp, R. B. and Wexler, L. (1977). Coronary arterial narrowing in Takayasu's aortitis. *American Journal of Cardiology*, **39**, 744–50.

Cloux Blasco, J., Lozano de la Torre, M. J., Alvarez Granda, J. L., Vidal Sampedro, J. and Garcia Fuentes, M. (1991). [Takayasu arteritis in a 5-year-old girl]. *Anales Españoles de pediatría*, **35**, 134–6.

D'Souza, S. J., Tsai, W. S., Silver, M. M., Chait, P., Benson, L. N., Silverman, E., Hebert, D. and Balfe, J. W. (1998). Diagnosis and management of stenotic aorto-arteriopathy in childhood. *Journal of Pediatrics*, **132**, 1016–22.

Dal Canto, A. J., Virgin, H. W. T. and Speck, S. H. (2000). Ongoing viral replication is required for gammaherpesvirus 68-induced vascular damage. *Journal of Virology*, **74**, 11304–10.

Eichhorn, J., Sima, D., Thiele, B., Lindschau, C., Turowski, A., Schmidt, H., Schneider, W., Haller, H. and Luft, F. C. (1996). Anti-endothelial cell antibodies in Takayasu arteritis. *Circulation*, **94**, 2396–401.

El-Reshaid, K., Varro, J., Al-Duwairi, Q. and Anim, J. T. (1995). Takayasu's arteritis in Kuwait. *Journal of Tropical Medicine and Hygiene*, **98**, 299–305.

Fabricant, C. G. (1985). Atherosclerosis: the consequence of infection with a herpesvirus. *Advances in Veterinary Science and Comparative Medicine*, **30**, 39–66.

Fava, M. P., Foradori, G. B., Garcia, C. B., Cruz, F. O., Aguilar, J. G., Kramer, A. S. and Valdes, F. E. (1993). Percutaneous transluminal angioplasty in patients with Takayasu arteritis: five-year experience. *Journal of Vascular and Interventional Radiology*, **4**, 649–52.

Fernandes, S. R., Singsen, B. H. and Hoffman, G. S. (2000). Sarcoidosis and systemic vasculitis. *Seminars in Arthritis and Rheumatism*, **30**, 33–46.

Flamm, S. D., White, R. D. and Hoffman, G. S. (1998). The clinical application of 'edema-weighted' magnetic resonance imaging in the assessment of Takayasu's arteritis. *International Journal of Cardiology*, **66** (Suppl. 1), S151–9; discussion S161.

Frankel, S. K., Cosgrove, G. P., Fischer, A., Meehan, R. T. and Brown, K. K. (2006). Update in the diagnosis and management of pulmonary vasculitis. *Chest*, **129**, 452–65.

Friedman, C. J. and Tegtmeyer, C. J. (1979). Crohn's disease associated with Takayasu's arteritis. *Digestive Diseases and Sciences*, **24**, 954–8.

Fullerton, S. H., Abel, E. A., Getz, K. and El-Ramahi, K. (1991). Cyclosporine treatment of severe recalcitrant pyoderma gangrenosum in a patient with Takayasu's arteritis. *Archives of Dermatology*, **127**, 1731–2.

Galeazzi, M., Gasbarrini, G., Ghirardello, A., Grandemange, S., Hoffman, H. M., Manna, R., Podswiadek, M., Punzi, L., Sebastiani, G. D., Touitou, I. and Doria, A. (2006). Autoinflammatory syndromes. *Clinical and Experimental Rheumatology*, **24**, S79–85.

Girona, E., Yamamoto-Furusho, J. K., Cutino, T., Reyes, P., Vargas-Alarcon, G., Granados, J. and Alarcon-Segovia, D. (1996). HLA-DR6 (possibly DRB1*1301) is associated with susceptibility to Takayasu arteritis in Mexicans. *Heart Vessels*, **11**, 277–80.

Gravanis, M. B. (2000). Giant cell arteritis and Takayasu aortitis: morphologic, pathogenetic and etiologic factors. *International Journal of Cardiology*, **75** (Suppl. 1), S21–33; discussion S35–6.

Hall, S., Barr, W., Lie, J. T., Stanson, A. W., Kazmier, F. J. and Hunder, G. G. (1985). Takayasu arteritis. A study of 32 North American patients. *Medicine* (Baltimore), **64**, 89–99.

Hara, M., Goodman, P. C. and Leder, R. A. (1999). FDG-PET finding in early-phase Takayasu arteritis. *Journal of Computer Assisted Tomography*, **23**, 16–8.

Hari, P., Bagga, A. and Srivastava, R. N. (2000). Sustained hypertension in children. *Indian Pediatrics*, **37**, 268–74.

Hashimoto, Y., Oniki, T., Aerbajinai, W. and Numano, F. (1992). Aortic regurgitation in patients with Takayasu arteritis: assessment by color Doppler echocardiography. *Heart Vessels*, **7** (Suppl.), 111–5.

Hashimoto, Y., Oniki, T., Kaneko, E., Hata, A., Matsumura, A., Kobayashi, T. and Numano, F. (1993). Concentric left ventricular hypertrophy in patients with Takayasu arteritis. *Angiology*, **44**, 883–8.

Hashimoto, Y., Tanaka, M., Hata, A., Kakuta, T., Maruyama, Y. and Numano, F. (1996). Four years follow-up study in patients with Takayasu arteritis and severe aortic regurgitation; assessment by echocardiography. *International Journal of Cardiology*, **54** (Suppl.), S173–6.

Hata, A., Noda, M., Moriwaki, R. and Numano, F. (1996). Angiographic findings of Takayasu arteritis: new classification. *International Journal of Cardiology*, **54** (Suppl.), S155–63.

Hatano, R., Yamada, T., Sunamori, M., Tsukuura, T. and Sakamoto, T. (1975). Simplified operative technique for the long-segment atypical coarctation of the aorta. *Japanese Journal of Surgery*, **5**, 246–54.

Hilario, M. O., Terreri, M. T., Prismich, G., Len, C., Kihara, E. N., Goldenberg, J. and Sole, D. (1998). Association of ankylosing spondylitis, Crohn's disease and Takayasu's arteritis in a child. *Clinical and Experimental Rheumatology*, **16**, 92–4.

Hoffman, G. S. and Ahmed, A. E. (1998). Surrogate markers of disease activity in patients with Takayasu arteritis. A preliminary report from The International Network for the Study of the Systemic Vasculitides (INSSYS). *International Journal of Cardiology*, **66** (Suppl. 1), S191–4; discussion S195.

Hoffman, G. S., Leavitt, R. Y., Kerr, G. S., Rottem, M., Sneller, M. C. and Fauci, A. S. (1994). Treatment of glucocorticoid-resistant or relapsing Takayasu arteritis with methotrexate. *Arthritis and Rheumatism*, **37**, 578–82.

Hoffman, G. S., Merkel, P. A., Brasington, R. D., Lenschow, D. J. and Liang, P. (2004). Anti-tumor necrosis factor therapy in patients with difficult to treat Takayasu arteritis. *Arthritis and Rheumatism*, **50**, 2296–304.

Hong, C. Y., Yun, Y. S., Choi, J. Y., Sul, J. H., Lee, K. S., Cha, S. H., Hong, Y. M., Lee, H. J., Hong, Y. J. and Sohn, K. C. (1992). Takayasu arteritis in Korean children: clinical report of seventy cases. *Heart Vessels*, **7**(Suppl.), 91–6.

Ishikawa, K. (1978). Natural history and classification of occlusive thromboaortopathy (Takayasu's disease). *Circulation*, **57**, 27–35.

Ishikawa, K. and Maetani, S. (1994). Long-term outcome for 120 Japanese patients with Takayasu's disease. Clinical and statistical analyses of related prognostic factors. *Circulation*, **90**, 1855–60.

Ishikawa, K., Uyama, M. and Asayama, K. (1983). Occlusive thromboaortopathy (Takayasu's disease): cervical arterial stenoses, retinal arterial pressure, retinal microaneurysms and prognosis. *Stroke*, **14**, 730–5.

Isohisa, I., Numano, F., Maezawa, H. and Sasazuki, T. (1978). HLA-Bw52 in Takayasu disease. *Tissue Antigens*, **12**, 246–8.

Iwai, T., Inoue, Y., Matsukura, I., Sugano, N. and Numano, F. (2000). Surgical technique for management of Takayasu's arteritis. *International Journal of Cardiology*, **75** (Suppl. 1), S135–40.

Jacobsen, H. H. and Rasch, P. J. (1956). [Takayasu's syndrome, pulseless disease, or brachiocephalic arteritis.]. *Nordisk medicin*, **56**, 1328–31.

Jain, S., Kumari, S., Ganguly, N. K. and Sharma, B. K. (1996). Current status of Takayasu arteritis in India. *International Journal of Cardiology*, **54** (Suppl.), S111–6.

Jennette, J. C., Falk, R. J., Andrassy, K., Bacon, P. A., Churg, J., Gross, W. L., Hagen, E. C., Hoffman, G. S., Hunder, G. G., Kallenberg, C. G. and et al. (1994). Nomenclature of systemic vasculitides. Proposal of an international consensus conference. *Arthritis and Rheumatism*, **37**, 187–92.

Jimenez Casado, M. and Moncada Moneu, A. (1956). [Pulseless disease; Takayasu disease.]. *Revista clínica española*, **63**, 166–8.

Kawai, T., Yamada, Y., Tsuneda, J., Aoyagi, T. and Mikata, A. (1975). Pleural effusion associated with aortitis syndrome. *Chest*, **68**, 826–8.

Kerr, G. S., Hallahan, C. W., Giordano, J., Leavitt, R. Y., Fauci, A. S., Rottem, M. and Hoffman, G. S. (1994). Takayasu arteritis. *Annals of Internal Medicine*, **120**, 919–29.

Kimura, A., Ota, M., Katsuyama, Y., Ohbuchi, N., Takahashi, M., Kobayashi, Y., Inoko, H. and Numano, F. (2000). Mapping of the HLA-linked genes controlling the susceptibility to Takayasu's arteritis. *International Journal of Cardiology*, **75** (Suppl. 1), S105–10; discussion S111–2.

Kissin, E. Y. and Merkel, P. A. (2004). Diagnostic imaging in Takayasu arteritis. *Current Opinion in Rheumatology*, **16**, 31–7.

Kitamura, H., Kobayashi, Y., Kimura, A. and Numano, F. (1998). Association of clinical manifestations with HLA-B alleles in Takayasu arteritis. *International Journal of Cardiology*, **66** (Suppl. 1), S121–6.

Kobayashi, Y., Ishii, K., Oda, K., Nariai, T., Tanaka, Y., Ishiwata, K. and Numano, F. (2005). Aortic wall inflammation due to Takayasu arteritis imaged with 18F-FDG PET coregistered with enhanced CT. *Journal of Nuclear Medicine*, **46**, 917–22.

Kobayashi, Y. and Numano, F. (2002). 3. Takayasu arteritis. *Internal Medicine*, **41**, 44–6.

Koide, K. (1992). Takayasu arteritis in Japan. *Heart Vessels*, **7** (Suppl.), 48–54.

Kornberg, A., Renaudineau, Y., Blank, M., Youinou, P. and Shoenfeld, Y. (2000). Anti-beta 2-glycoprotein I antibodies and anti-endothelial cell antibodies induce tissue factor in endothelial cells. *Israel Medical Association Journal*, **2** (Suppl.), 27–31.

Kothari, S. S. (1995). Aetiopathogenesis of Takayasu's arteritis and BCG vaccination: the missing link? *Medical Hypotheses*, **45**, 227–30.

Kotter, I., Daikeler, T., Amberger, C., Tyndall, A. and Kanz, L. (2005). Autologous stem cell transplantation of treatment-resistant systemic vasculitis–a single center experience and review of the literature. *Clinical Nephrology*, **64**, 485–9.

Ladhani, S., Tulloh, R. and Anderson, D. (2001). Takayasu disease masquarading as interruption of the aortic arch in a 2-year-old child. *Cardiology in the Young*, **11**, 244–6.

Lagneau, P., Michel, J. B. and Vuong, P. N. (1987). Surgical treatment of Takayasu's disease. *Annals of Surgery*, **205**, 157–66.

Lenhoff, S. J. and Mee, A. S. (1982). Crohn's disease of the colon with takayasu's arteritis. *Postgraduate Medical Journal*, **58**, 386–9.

Lie, J. T. (1996). Isolated pulmonary Takayasu arteritis: clinicopathologic characteristics. *Modern Pathology*, **9**, 469–74.

Lobato, O. (1956). [Takayasu disease; case report.]. *Arquivos brasileiros de cardiologia*, **9**, 277–88.

Lupi-Herrera, E., Sanchez-Torres, G., Marcushamer, J., Mispireta, J., Horwitz, S. and Vela, J. E. (1977). Takayasu's arteritis. Clinical study of 107 cases. *American Heart Journal*, **93**, 94–103.

Marks, D. J., Harbord, M. W., Macallister, R., Rahman, F. Z., Young, J., Al-Lazikani, B., Lees, W., Novelli, M., Bloom, S. and Segal, A. W. (2006). Defective acute inflammation in Crohn's disease: a clinical investigation. *Lancet*, **367**, 668–78.

Martini, A. (1995). Behcet's disease and Takayasu's disease in children. *Current Opinion in Rheumatology*, **7**, 449–54.

Matsubara, O., Kuwata, T., Nemoto, T., Kasuga, T. and Numano, F. (1992). Coronary artery lesions in Takayasu arteritis: pathological considerations. *Heart Vessels*, **7** (Suppl.), 26–31.

Matsuki, T., Isoda, K., Horai, R., Nakajima, A., Aizawa, Y., Suzuki, K., Ohsuzu, F. and Iwakura, Y. (2005). Involvement of tumor necrosis factor-alpha in the development of T cell-dependent aortitis in interleukin-1 receptor antagonist-deficient mice. *Circulation*, **112**, 1323–31.

Matsuura, K., Ogino, H., Matsuda, H., Minatoya, K., Sasaki, H., Yagihara, T. and Kitamura, S. (2006). Surgical outcome of aortic arch repair for patients with Takayasu arteritis. *Annals of Thoracic Surgery*, **81**, 178–82.

McDermott, M. F. and Aksentijevich, I. (2002). The autoinflammatory syndromes. *Current Opinion in Allergy and Clinical Immunology*, **2**, 511–6.

Meller, J., Grabbe, E., Becker, W. and Vosshenrich, R. (2003a). Value of F-18 FDG hybrid camera PET and MRI in early takayasu aortitis. *European Radiology*, **13**, 400–5.

Meller, J., Strutz, F., Siefker, U., Scheel, A., Sahlmann, C. O., Lehmann, K., Conrad, M. and Vosshenrich, R. (2003b). Early diagnosis and follow-up of aortitis with [(18)F]FDG PET and MRI. *European Journal of Nuclear Medicine and Molecular Imaging*, **30**, 730–6.

Miceli-Richard, C., Lesage, S., Rybojad, M., Prieur, A. M., Manouvrier-Hanu, S., Hafner, R., Chamaillard, M., Zouali, H., Thomas, G. and Hugot, J. P. (2001). CARD15 mutations in Blau syndrome. *Nature Genetics*, **29**, 19–20.

Millar, A. J., Gilbert, R. D., Brown, R. A., Immelman, E. J., Burkimsher, D. A. and Cywes, S. (1996). Abdominal aortic aneurysms in children. *Journal of Pediatric Surgery*, **31**, 1624–8.

Mitchell, C. S. and Parisi, M. T. (1997). Magnetic resonance imaging of Takayasu's aortitis in an infant. *Journal of the American Osteopathic Association*, **97**, 607–9.

Miwa, Y., Nagasako, K., Sasaki, H., Ichikawa, K., Yaguchi, T., Hasegawa, K. and Kubokura, T. (1979). Aortitis syndrome associated with ulcerative colitis: report of a case. *Gastroenterologia Japonica*, **14**, 492–5.

Miyata, T., Sato, O., Deguchi, J., Kimura, H., Namba, T., Kondo, K., Makuuchi, M., Hamada, C., Takagi, A. and Tada, Y. (1998). Anastomotic aneurysms after surgical treatment of Takayasu's arteritis: a 40-year experience. *Journal of Vascular Surgery*, **27**, 438–45.

Miyata, T., Sato, O., Koyama, H., Shigematsu, H. and Tada, Y. (2003). Long-term survival after surgical treatment of patients with Takayasu's arteritis. *Circulation*, **108**, 1474–80.

Morales, E., Pineda, C. and Martinez-Lavin, M. (1991). Takayasu's arteritis in children. *Journal of Rheumatology*, **18**, 1081–4.

Morita, Y., Yamamura, M., Suwaki, K., Mima, A., Ishizu, T., Hirohata, M., Kashihara, N., Makino, H. and Ota, Z. (1996). Takayasu's arteritis associated with ulcerative colitis; genetic factors in this association. *Internal Medicine*, **35**, 574–8.

Moriwaki, R., Noda, M., Yajima, M., Sharma, B. K. and Numano, F. (1997). Clinical manifestations of Takayasu arteritis in India and Japan–new classification of angiographic findings. *Angiology*, **48**, 369–79.

Moriwaki, R. and Numano, F. (1992). Takayasu arteritis: follow-up studies for 20 years. *Heart Vessels*, **7** (Suppl.), 138–45.

Mwipatayi, B. P., Jeffery, P. C., Beningfield, S. J., Matley, P. J., Naidoo, N. G., Kalla, A. A. and Kahn, D. (2005). Takayasu arteritis: clinical features and management: report of 272 cases. *Australian and New Zealand Journal of Surgery*, **75**, 110–7.

Naito, S., Arakawa, K., Saito, S., Toyoda, K. and Takeshita, A. (1978). Takayasu's disease: association with HLA-B5. *Tissue Antigens*, **12**, 143–5.

Nakabayashi, K., Kurata, N., Nangi, N., Miyake, H. and Nagasawa, T. (1996). Pulmonary artery involvement as first manifestation in three cases of Takayasu arteritis. *International Journal of Cardiology*, **54** (Suppl.), S177–83.

Nasu, T. (1975). Takayasu's truncoarteritis in Japan. A statistical observation of 76 autopsy cases. *Patholgy and Microbiology*, **43**, 140–6.

Nasu, T. (1982). Takayasu's truncoarteritis. Pulseless disease or aortitis syndrome. *Acta Pathologica Japonica*, **32** (Suppl. 1), 117–31.

Nicklin, M. J., Hughes, D. E., Barton, J. L., Ure, J. M. and Duff, G. W. (2000). Arterial inflammation in mice lacking the interleukin 1 receptor antagonist gene. *Journal of Experimental Medicine*, **191**, 303–12.

Numano, F. (2000). Vasa vasoritis, vasculitis and atherosclerosis. *International Journal of Cardiology*, **75** (Suppl. 1), S1–8; discussion S17–9.

Numano, F., Isohisa, I., Kishi, U., Arita, M. and Maezawa, H. (1978). Takayasu's disease in twin sisters. Possible genetic factors. *Circulation*, **58**, 173–7.

Numano, F. and Kakuta, T. (1996). Takayasu arteritis–five doctors in the history of Takayasu arteritis. *International Journal of Cardiology*, **54** (Suppl.), S1–10.

Numano, F., Miyata, T. and Nakajima, T. (1996). Ulcerative colitis, Takayasu arteritis and HLA. *Internal Medicine*, **35**, 521–2.

Numano, F., Okawara, M., Inomata, H. and Kobayashi, Y. (2000). Takayasu's arteritis. *Lancet*, **356**, 1023–5.

Numano, F. and Shimamoto, T. (1971). Hypersecretion of estrogen in Takayasu's disease. *American Heart Journal*, **81**, 591–6.

Numano, F., Yajima, M., Shimokado, K. and Maruyama, Y. (1985). Aspirin treatment for patients with cardiovascular disease. *Advances in Prostaglandin Thromboxane and Leukotriene Research*, **15**, 543–6.

Owyang, C., Miller, L. J., Lie, J. T. and Fleming, C. R. (1979). Takayasu's arteritis in Crohn's disease. *Gastroenterology*, **76**, 825–8.

Park, M. C., Lee, S. W., Park, Y. B., Chung, N. S. and Lee, S. K. (2005a). Clinical characteristics and outcomes of Takayasu's arteritis: analysis of 108 patients using standardized criteria for diagnosis, activity assessment, and angiographic classification. *Scandinavian Journal of Rheumatology*, **34**, 284–92.

Park, M. C., Lee, S. W., Park, Y. B. and Lee, S. K. (2005b). Serum cytokine profiles and their correlations with disease activity in Takayasu's arteritis. *Rheumatology* (Oxford).

Park, M. H. and Park, Y. B. (1992). HLA typing of Takayasu arteritis in Korea. *Heart Vessels*, **7** (Suppl), 81–4.

Park, S. H., Chung, J. W., Lee, J. W., Han, M. H. and Park, J. H. (2001). Carotid artery involvement in Takayasu's arteritis: evaluation of the activity by ultrasonography. *Journal of Ultrasound Medicine*, **20**, 371–8.

Park, Y. B., Hong, S. K., Choi, K. J., Sohn, D. W., Oh, B. H., Lee, M. M., Choi, Y. S., Seo, J. D., Lee, Y. W. and Park, J. H. (1992). Takayasu arteritis in Korea: clinical and angiographic features. *Heart Vessels*, **7** (Suppl.), 55–9.

Piyachon, C. and Suwanwela, N. (1992). Takayasu arteritis in Thailand. *Heart Vessels*, **7** (Suppl.), 60–7.

Planas, E. (1978). [Martorell's syndrome and Takayasu arteritis]. *Angiologia*, **30**, 134–6.

Robles, M. and Reyes, P. A. (1994). Takayasu's arteritis in Mexico: a clinical review of 44 consecutive cases. *Clinical and Experimental Rheumatology*, **12**, 381–8.

Roedenbeck, S. D. and Bauer, J. (1956). [Takayasu's disease; neurological aspect of a case of pulseless disease.]. *Anales. Universidad Nacional Mayor de San Marcos. Facuttad de Medicina*, **39**, 1407–16.

Rose, C. D., Eichenfield, A. H., Goldsmith, D. P. and Athreya, B. H. (1990). Early onset sarcoidosis with aortitis– "juvenile systemic granulomatosis?" *Journal of Rheumatology*, **17**, 102–6.

Rosenthal, T., Morag, B. and Itzchak, Y. (1992). Takayasu arteritis in Israel. *Heart Vessels*, **7** (Suppl.), 44–7.

Ross, R. S. and Mc, K. V. (1953). Aortic arch syndromes; diminished or absent pulses in arteries arising from arch of aorta. *Archives of Internal Medicine*, **92**, 701–40.

Sakaida, H., Sakai, N., Nagata, I., Sakai, H., Iihara, K., Higashi, T., Kogure, S., Takahashi, J., Ohta, H., Nagamine, T., Anei, R., Soeda, A., Taniguchi, A., Shindo, A. and Kikuchi, H. (2001). [Stenting for the occlusive carotid and subclavian arteries in Takayasu arteritis]. *No Shinkei Geka*, **29**, 1033–41.

Sakhuja, V., Gupta, K. L., Bhasin, D. K., Malik, N. and Chugh, K. S. (1990). Takayasu's arteritis associated with idiopathic ulcerative colitis. *Gut*, **31**, 831–3.

Salazar, M., Varela, A., Ramirez, I. A., Uribe, O., Vasquez, G., Egea, F., Yunis, E. J. and Iglesias-Gamarra, A. (2000). Association of HLA-DRB1*1602 and DRB1*1001 with Takayasu arteritis in Colombian mestizos as markers of Amerindian ancestry. *International Journal of Cardiology*, **75** (Suppl. 1), S113–6.

Sasazuki, T., Kaneoka, H., Ohta, N., Hayase, R. and Iwamoto, I. (1979). Four common HLA haplotypes and their association with diseases in the Japanese population. *Transplantation Proceedings*, **11**, 1871–3.

Sato, E. I., Hatta, F. S., Levy-Neto, M. and Fernandes, S. (1998). Demographic, clinical, and angiographic data of patients with Takayasu arteritis in Brazil. *International Journal of Cardiology*, **66** (Suppl. 1), S67–70; discussion S71.

Savoy, W. (1856). Royal Medical and Chirurgical Society on a case of young woman in whom the main arteries of both upper extremities and of the left side of the neck were throughout completely obliterated. *Lancet*, **5**, 373.

Schapiro, J. M., Shpitzer, S., Pinkhas, J., Sidi, Y. and Arber, N. (1994). Sarcoidosis as the initial manifestation of Takayasu's arteritis. *Journal of Medicine*, **25**, 121–8.

Schmidt, W. A., Seipelt, E., Molsen, H. P., Poehls, C. and Gromnica-Ihle, E. J. (2001). Vasculitis of the internal carotid artery in Wegener's granulomatosis: comparison of ultrasonography, angiography, and MRI. *Scandinavian Journal of Rheumatology*, **30**, 48–50.

Seko, Y., Minota, S., Kawasaki, A., Shinkai, Y., Maeda, K., Yagita, H., Okumura, K., Sato, O., Takagi, A., Tada, Y. and et al. (1994). Perforin-secreting killer cell infiltration and expression of a 65-kD heat-shock protein in aortic tissue of patients with Takayasu's arteritis. *Journal of Clinical Investigation*, **93**, 750–8.

Seko, Y., Sato, O., Takagi, A., Tada, Y., Matsuo, H., Yagita, H., Okumura, K. and Yazaki, Y. (1996). Restricted usage of T-cell receptor Valpha-Vbeta genes in infiltrating cells in aortic tissue of patients with Takayasu's arteritis. *Circulation*, **93**, 1788–90.

Seko, Y., Sugishita, K., Sato, O., Takagi, A., Tada, Y., Matsuo, H., Yagita, H., Okumura, K. and Nagai, R. (2004). Expression of costimulatory molecules (4–1BBL and Fas) and major histocompatibility class I chain-related A (MICA) in aortic tissue with Takayasu's arteritis. *Journal of Vascular Research*, **41**, 84–90.

Sen, P. K., Kinare, S. G., Kelkar, M. D. and Parulkar, G. B. (1972). *Non-specific aortoarteritis*. Bombay, Tata McGraw Hill.

Seth, S., Goyal, N. K., Jagia, P., Gulati, G., Karthikeyan, G., Sharma, S. and Talwar, K. K. (2006). Carotid intima-medial thickness as a marker of disease activity in Takayasu's arteritis. *International Journal of Cardiology*, **108**, 385–90.

Seyahi, E., Ugurlu, S., Cumali, R., Balci, H., Seyahi, N., Yurdakul, S. and Yazici, H. (2006). Atherosclerosis in takayasu arteritis. *Annals of the Rheumatic Diseases*.

Sharma, B. K., Jain, S., Bali, H. K., Jain, A. and Kumari, S. (2000). A follow-up study of balloon angioplasty and de-novo stenting in Takayasu arteritis. *International Journal of Cardiology*, **75** (Suppl. 1), S147–52.

Sharma, B. K., Jain, S., Suri, S. and Numano, F. (1996). Diagnostic criteria for Takayasu arteritis. *International Journal of Cardiology*, **54** (Suppl.), S141–7.

Sharma, B. K., Sagar, S., Chugh, K. S., Sakhuja, V., Rajachandran, A. and Malik, N. (1985). Spectrum of renovascular hypertension in the young in north India: a hospital based study on occurrence and clinical features. *Angiology*, **36**, 370–8.

Sharma, B. K., Sagar, S., Singh, A. P. and Suri, S. (1992). Takayasu arteritis in India. *Heart Vessels*, **7** (Suppl.), 37–43.

Sharma, S., Rajani, M., Shrivastava, S., Kaul, U., Kamalakar, T., Talwar, K. K. and Saxena, A. (1991). Non-specific aorto-arteritis (Takayasu's disease) in children. *British Journal of Radiology*, **64**, 690–8.

Shelhamer, J. H., Volkman, D. J., Parrillo, J. E., Lawley, T. J., Johnston, M. R. and Fauci, A. S. (1985). Takayasu's arteritis and its therapy. *Annals of Internal Medicine* **103**, 121–6.

Shepherd, J. and Nicklin, M. J. (2005). Elastic-vessel arteritis in interleukin-1 receptor antagonist-deficient mice involves effector Th1 cells and requires interleukin-1 receptor. *Circulation*, **111**, 3135–40.

Shibata, H., Yasunami, M., Obuchi, N., Takahashi, M., Kobayashi, Y., Numano, F. and Kimura, A. (2006). Direct determination of SNP haplotype of NFKBIL1 promoter polymorphism by DNA conformation analysis and its application to association study of chronic inflammatory disease. *Human Immunology*, **67**, 363–73.

Shinmi, Y. (1942). A case of Takayasu's arteritis. *Sogo Gannka (Tokyo)*, **36**, 1404–10.

Sider, L., Mintzer, R. A., Vrla, R. F. and Mendelson, E. B. (1985). Use of DSA for diagnosis of Takayasu's arteritis. *Illinois Medical Journal*, **167**, 53–5.

Stanley, P., Roebuck, D. and Barboza, A. (2003). Takayusu's arteritis in children. *Tech Vasc Interv Radiol*, **6**, 158–68.

Takayasu, M. (1908). A case with peculiar changes of the retinal central vessels. *Acta Society of Ophtalmology of Japan*, **2**, 554–5.

Takeda, N., Takahashi, T., Seko, Y., Maemura, K., Nakasone, H., Sakamoto, K., Hirata, Y. and Nagai, R. (2005). Takayasu myocarditis mediated by cytotoxic T lymphocytes. *Internal Medicine*, **44**, 256–60.

Takeshita, A., Tanaka, S., Orita, Y., Kanaide, H. and Nakamura, M. (1977). Baroreflex sensitivity in patients with Takayasu's aortitis. *Circulation*, **55**, 803–6.

Taketani, T., Miyata, T., Morota, T. and Takamoto, S. (2005). Surgical treatment of atypical aortic coarctation complicating Takayasu's arteritis–experience with 33 cases over 44 years. *Journal of Vascular Surgery*, **41**, 597–601.

Tato, F., Rieger, J. and Hoffmann, U. (2005). Refractory Takayasu's arteritis successfully treated with the human, monoclonal anti-tumor necrosis factor antibody adalimumab. *International Angiology*, **24**, 304–7.

Tripathy, N. K., Chauhan, S. K. and Nityanand, S. (2004). Cytokine mRNA repertoire of peripheral blood mononuclear cells in Takayasu's arteritis. *Clinical and Experimental Immunology*, **138**, 369–74.

Tripathy, N. K., Upadhyaya, S., Sinha, N. and Nityanand, S. (2001). Complement and cell mediated cytotoxicity by antiendothelial cell antibodies in Takayasu's arteritis. *Journal of Rheumatology*, **28**, 805–8.

Turkoglu, C., Memis, A., Payzin, S., Akin, M., Kultusay, H., Akilli, A., Can, L. and Altintig, A. (1996). Takayasu arteritis in Turkey. *International Journal of Cardiology*, **54** (Suppl.), S135–6.

Tyagi, S., Singh, B., Kaul, U. A., Sethi, K. K., Arora, R. and Khalilullah, M. (1993). Balloon angioplasty for renovascular hypertension in Takayasu's arteritis. *American Heart Journal*, **125**, 1386–93.

Tyagi, S., Verma, P. K., Gambhir, D. S., Kaul, U. A., Saha, R. and Arora, R. (1998). Early and long-term results of subclavian angioplasty in aortoarteritis (Takayasu disease): comparison with atherosclerosis. *Cardiovascular and Interventional Radiology*, **21**, 219–24.

Ujiie, H., Sawamura, D., Yokota, K., Nishie, W., Shichinohe, R. and Shimizu, H. (2004). Pyoderma gangrenosum associated with Takayasu's arteritis. *Clinical and Experimental Dermatology*, **29**, 357–9.

Ureten, K., Ozturk, M. A., Onat, A. M., Ozturk, M. H., Ozbalkan, Z., Guvener, M., Kiraz, S., Ertenli, I. and Calguneri, M. (2004). Takayasu's arteritis: results of a university hospital of 45 patients in Turkey. *International Journal of Cardiology*, **96**, 259–64.

Valsakumar, A. K., Valappil, U. C., Jorapur, V., Garg, N., Nityanand, S. and Sinha, N. (2003). Role of immunosuppressive therapy on clinical, immunological, and angiographic outcome in active Takayasu's arteritis. *Journal of Rheumatology*, **30**, 1793–8.

Vanoli, M., Daina, E., Salvarani, C., Sabbadini, M. G., Rossi, C., Bacchiani, G., Schieppati, A., Baldissera, E. and Bertolini, G. (2005). Takayasu's arteritis: A study of 104 Italian patients. *Arthritis and Rheumatism*, **53**, 100–7.

Vedantham, V., Ratnagiri, P. K. and Ramasamy, K. (2005). Hypotensive retinopathy in Takayasu's arteritis. *Ophthalmic Surgery, Lasers and Imaging*, **36**, 240–4.

Verma, D. K., Tripathy, N. K., Verma, N. S. and Tiwari, S. (2005). Interleukin 12 in Takayasu's arteritis: plasma concentrations and relationship with disease activity. *Journal of Rheumatology*, **32**, 2361–3.

Waern, A. U., Andersson, P. and Hemmingsson, A. (1983). Takayasu's arteritis: a hospital-region based study on occurrence, treatment and prognosis. *Angiology*, **34**, 311–20.

Wagner, A. D., Andresen, J., Raum, E., Lotz, J., Zeidler, H., Kuipers, J. G. and Jendro, M. C. (2005). Standardised work-up programme for fever of unknown origin and contribution of magnetic resonance imaging for the diagnosis of hidden systemic vasculitis. *Annals of the Rheumatic Diseases*, **64**, 105–10.

Wang, X., Kuivaniemi, H., Bonavita, G., Mutkus, L., Mau, U., Blau, E., Inohara, N., Nunez, G., Tromp, G. and Williams, C. J. (2002). CARD15 mutations in familial granulomatosis syndromes: a study of the original Blau syndrome kindred and other families with large-vessel arteritis and cranial neuropathy. *Arthritis and Rheumatism*, **46**, 3041–5.

Weaver, F. A., Kumar, S. R., Yellin, A. E., Anderson, S., Hood, D. B., Rowe, V. L., Kitridou, R. C., Kohl, R. D. and Alexander, J. (2004). Renal revascularization in Takayasu arteritis-induced renal artery stenosis. *Journal of Vascular Surgery*, **39**, 749–57.

Weaver, F. A., Yellin, A. E., Campen, D. H., Oberg, J., Foran, J., Kitridou, R. C., Lee, S. E. and Kohl, R. D. (1990). Surgical procedures in the management of Takayasu's arteritis. *Journal of Vascular Surgery*, **12**, 429–37; discussion 438–9.

Webb, M., Chambers, A. A. A. L.-N., Mason, J. C., Maudlin, L., Rahman, L. and Frank, J. (2004). The role of 18F-FDG PET in characterising disease activity in Takayasu arteritis. *European Journal of Nuclear Medicine and Molecular Imaging*, **31**, 627–34.

Weck, K. E., Dal Canto, A. J., Gould, J. D., O'Guin, A. K., Roth, K. A., Saffitz, J. E., Speck, S. H. and Virgin, H. W. (1997). Murine gamma-herpesvirus 68 causes severe large-vessel arteritis in mice lacking interferon-gamma responsiveness: a new model for virus-induced vascular disease. *Nature Medicine*, **3**, 1346–53.

Wenger, M., Gasser, R., Donnemiller, E., Erler, H., Glossmann, H., Patsch, J. R., Moncayo, R. and Schirmer, M. (2003). Images in cardiovascular medicine. Generalized large vessel arteritis visualized by 18fluorodeoxyglucose-positron emission tomography. *Circulation*, **107**, 923.

Weyand, C. M. and Goronzy, J. J. (2003). Medium- and large-vessel vasculitis. *New England Journal of Medicine*, **349**, 160–9.

Yajima, M., Numano, F., Park, Y. B. and Sagar, S. (1994). Comparative studies of patients with Takayasu arteritis in Japan, Korea and India–comparison of clinical manifestations, angiography and HLA-B antigen. *Japanese Circulation Journal*, **58**, 9–14.

Yamada, I., Shibuya, H., Matsubara, O., Umehara, I., Makino, T., Numano, F. and Suzuki, S. (1992). Pulmonary artery disease in Takayasu's arteritis: angiographic findings. *American Journal of Roentgenology*, **159**, 263–9.

Yassinger, S., Adelman, R., Cantor, D., Halsted, C. H. and Bolt, R. J. (1976). Association of inflammatory bowel disease and large vascular lesions. *Gastroenterology*, **71**, 844–6.

Yoshida, M., Kimura, A., Katsuragi, K., Numano, F. and Sasazuki, T. (1993). DNA typing of HLA-B gene in Takayasu's arteritis. *Tissue Antigens*, **42**, 87–90.

Zaas, A., Scheel, P., Venbrux, A. and Hellmann, D. B. (2001). Large artery vasculitis following recombinant hepatitis B vaccination: 2 cases. *Journal of Rheumatology*, **28**, 1116–20.

Zheng, D., Fan, D. and Liu, L. (1992). Takayasu arteritis in China: a report of 530 cases. *Heart Vessels*, **7** (Suppl.), 32–6.

CHAPTER 26

Polyarteritis nodosa

Loïc Guillevin, Christian Pagnoux, and Luis Teixeira

Introduction

Polyarteritis nodosa (PAN) was first described by Küssmaul and Maier (1866). This necrotizing angiitis predominantly involves medium-sized arteries and can affect the majority of the organs in the body. Primary and secondary PAN can be distinguished, since PAN can be the consequence of hepatitis B virus (HBV) infection (Prince and Trépo 1971; Trépo and Thivolet 1970a) and sometimes other etiological agents (Corman and Dolson 1992; Calabrese 1991; Mader and Keystone 1992). Among vasculitides, PAN is now less frequent than in the past for reasons that will be discussed below. In this chapter, we review the classification criteria for PAN, the main characteristics of the disease, and its pathogenesis, outcome, and treatment.

Classification criteria

The first attempt to classify vasculitides was published in 1952, when P. Zeek (1952) proposed the generic term 'necrotizing vasculitis' to identify five distinct types of systemic vasculitides defined by their clinical and histological signs: hypersensitivity angiitis; allergic granulomatous angiitis; rheumatic arteritis; PAN; and temporal arteritis. All the subsequent classifications of vasculitides have been more or less derived from Zeek's endeavor. In Fauci's classification (Fauci *et al.* 1978), systemic vasculitides comprised PAN, Churg–Strauss syndrome (CSS), and overlap angiitis. In 1990, the American College of Rheumatology (ACR) (Table 26.1) established criteria for PAN classification (Lightfoot *et al.* 1990) but did not distinguish between PAN and microscopic polyangiitis (MPA). In the past, PAN and MPA have been considered unitarily because their main clinical manifestations are very similar, thereby explaining why the two were grouped together in the ACR classification criteria.

Nevertheless, major differences exist between these two entities, as clarified and clearly established in the Chapel Hill Nomenclature (Jennette *et al.* 1994) (Table 26.2). PAN predominantly affects medium-sized vessels and MPA small-sized vessels, especially arterioles, capillaries and venules. MPA is responsible for glomerulonephritis and lung capillaritis, while PAN is characterized by vascular nephropathy and never affects the lungs. The major differences between these two diseases are summarized in Table 26.3 (see also Chapter 27). These criteria are only satisfied in the patients presenting with the most severe forms of MPA or PAN, including nephropathy with or without lung involvement. Patients may not be classified so easily when clinical manifestations do not include kidney or lung involvement. In that setting, the Chapel Hill Nomenclature, like the ACR classification of PAN, does not contain enough items to clarify the distinction. Even biopsies are sometimes unable to contribute to the diagnosis because vessel type and size are not easy to describe.

Diagnostic criteria based on clinical manifestations and biological or immunological signs could be helpful to clinicians. Because antineutrophil cytoplasm antibodies (ANCA) are present in the majority of MPA patients, they can be a major indicator for classification and their presence should exclude the diagnosis of PAN. Diagnostic criteria are needed but have not yet been established and we propose herein a list of clinical items to help diagnose PAN (Table 26.4 and Figure 26.1) (Henegar *et al.* 2005).

Epidemiology

PAN is a rare disease that affects all racial/ethnic groups. Estimates of the annual incidence of PAN-type systemic vasculitides in the general population vary from 4.6 per 1,000,000 in England (Scott *et al.* 1982), and 9.0 per 1,000,000 in Olmsted County, Minnesota, to 77 per 1,000,000 in a hepatitis B-hyperendemic Alaskan Eskimo population (McMahon *et al.* 1989). In a German study (Reinhold-Keller *et al.* 2002), the incidence of PAN was extremely low (0.3–0.4/1,000,000 according to the year and part of the country). A comparison of the PAN incidence in two areas of Europe, Lugo, Spain and Norwich, United Kingdom (Watts *et al.* 2001), did not show significant differences: they were respectively, 6.2 and 9.7/1,000,000. In France, the prevalence of PAN was 34 per 1,000,000 in Seine–Saint-Denis, a northern suburb of the Paris (Mahr *et al.* 2004). Its prevalence was the highest among the vasculitides that were studied (MPA, PAN, CSS, and Wegener's granulomatosis [WG]) but its incidence has declined in parallel with that of HBV infection (Guillevin *et al.* 2005).

Pathogenesis

The immunopathogenic mechanisms leading to vascular injury in PAN are probably heterogeneous. The mechanism of vascular inflammation implicated most often, based on animal models,

Table 26.1 1990 ACR criteria for the classification of polyarteritis nodosa (Lightfoot *et al.* 1990)

Criterion	Definition
1. Weight loss > 4 kg	Loss of 4 kg or more of body weight since illness began, not due to dieting or other factors
2. Livedo reticularis	Mottled reticular pattern over the skin of portions of the extremities or torso
3. Testicular pain or tenderness	Pain or tenderness of the testicles, not due to infection, trauma, or other causes
4. Myalgias, weakness, or polyneuropathy	Diffuse myalgias (excluding shoulder and hip girdles), or weakness of muscles or tenderness of leg muscles
5. Mononeuropathy or polyneuropathy	Development of mononeuropathy, multiple mononeuropathies, or polyneuropathy
6. Diastolic BP >90 mmHg	Development of hypertension with the diastolic BP higher than 90 mmHg
7. Elevated BUN or creatinine	Elevation of BUN >40 mg/dl (14.3 μmol/l) or creatinine >1.5 mg/dl (132 μmol/l), not due to dehydration or obstruction
8. Hepatitis B virus	Presence of hepatitis B surface antigen or antibody in serum
9. Arteriographic abnormality	Arteriogram showing aneurysms or occlusions of the visceral arteries, not due to arteriosclerosis, fibromuscular dysplasia, or non-inflammatory causes
10. Biopsy of small- or medium-sized artery containing neutrophils	Histological changes showing the presence of granulocytes or granulocytes and mononuclear leukocytes in the artery wall

For classification purposes, a patient with vasculitis shall be said to have PAN if at least 3 of these 10 criteria are present. The presence of any 3 or more criteria yields a sensitivity of 82.2% and a specificity of 86.6%. BP: blood pressure; BUN: blood urea nitrogen.

is induction by immune-complexes (Trépo *et al.* 1974; Fye *et al.* 1977; Guillevin *et al.* 1990). In some cases, PAN is the consequence of HBV infection for which there is evidence of immune-complex disease, with hepatitis B surface antigen (HBsAg) being the triggering factor (Trépo and Thivolet 1970b; Guillevin *et al.* 1995b; Prince and Trépo 1971). Almost all cases of HBV-related PAN are associated with wild-type HBV, HBe antigenemia, and high HBV replication, supporting the concept that lesions could result from the deposition of soluble viral antigen–antibody (Ag–Ab) complexes in Ag excess, possibly involving HBeAg. According to this hypothesis, immune complexes would activate the complement cascade, whose activated products would, in turn, attract and activate neutrophils; however, the recent observation of PAN associated with a precore mutation, which abrogates the formation of HBeAg, counters that postulate. It might suggest that other, still undefined, circulating HBV-related Ag(s) distinct from HBeAg could be involved. Another mechanism could be direct injury of endothelial cells caused by viral replication. (Mason *et al.* 2005). No recent study has

Table 26.2 Names and definitions adopted by the Chapel Hill Consensus Conference on the nomenclature for systemic vasculitides (Jennette *et al.* 1994)

Large-vessel vasculitis[1]	
Giant-cell (temporal) arteritis	Granulomatous arteritis of the aorta and its major branches, with a predilection for the extracranial branches of the carotid artery. *Often involves the temporal artery. Usually occurs in patients older than 50 and is often associated with polymyalgia rheumatica.*
Takayasu's arteritis	Granulomatous arteritis of the aorta and its major branches. *Usually occurs in patients younger than 50.*
Medium-sized vessel vasculitis	
Polyarteritis nodosa (classic polyarteritis nodosa)	Necrotizing inflammation of medium-sized or small arteries without glomerulonephritis, or vasculitis in arterioles, capillaries or venules.
Kawasaki disease	Arteritis involving large, medium-sized, and small arteries, and associated with mucocutaneous lymph-node syndrome. *Coronary arteries are often involved. Aorta and veins may be involved. Usually occurs in children.*
Small-vessel vasculitis	
Wegener's granulomatosis[2]	Granulomatous inflammation involving the respiratory tract and necrotizing vasculitis affecting small- to medium-sized vessels (e.g. capillaries, venules, arterioles, and arteries). *Necrotizing glomerulonephritis is common.*
Churg–Strauss syndrome[2]	Eosinophil-rich and granulomatous inflammation involving the respiratory tract, and necrotizing vasculitis affecting small- to medium-sized vessels, associated with asthma and eosinophilia.
Microscopic polyangiitis[2] (microscopic polyarteritis)	Necrotizing vasculitis, with few or no immune deposits, affecting small vessels (i.e. capillaries, venules or arterioles). *Necrotizing arteritis involving small- and medium-sized vessels may be present. Necrotizing glomerulonephritis is very common. Pulmonary capillaritis often occurs.*
Henoch–Schönlein purpura	Vasculitis, with IgA-dominant immune deposits, affecting small vessels (i.e. capillaries, venules, or arterioles). *Typically involves skin, gut, and glomeruli, and is associated with arthralgias or arthritis.*
Essential cryoglobulinemia vasculitis	Vasculitis, with cryoglobulin immune deposits, affecting small vessels (i.e. capillaries, venules, or arterioles), and associated with cryoglobulins in serum. *Skin and glomeruli are often involved.*
Cutaneous leukocytoclastic angiitis	Isolated cutaneous leukocytoclastic angiitis without systemic vasculitis or glomerulonephritis.

[1] Large vessels refers to the aorta and the largest branches directed toward major body regions (e.g. to the extremities and the head and neck); medium-sized vessels refers to the main visceral arteries (e.g. renal, hepatic, coronary, and mesenteric arteries); small vessel refers to venules, capillaries, arterioles, and the intraparenchymal distal arteries that connect with arterioles. Some small- and large-vessel vasculitides may involve medium-sized arteries, but large and medium-sized vessel vasculitides do not involve vessels smaller than arteries. Essential components are represented by normal type; italics represent usual, but not essential, components.

[2] Strongly associated with antineutrophil cytoplasmic autoantibodies.

Table 26.3 Differential diagnosis of PAN and MPA

Criterion	PAN	MPA
Histology		
Type of vasculitis	Necrotizing with mixed cells, rarely granulomatous	Necrotizing with mixed cells, not granulomatous
Type(s) of vessels involved	Medium- and small-sized muscle arteries, sometimes arterioles	Small vessels (i.e. capillaries, venules, or arterioles); small- and medium-sized arteries may be also affected
Distribution and localization		
Kidney		
Renal vasculitis with renovascular hypertension, renal infarcts, and microaneurysms	Yes	No
Rapidly progressive glomerulonephritis	No	Very common
Lung		
Pulmonary hemorrhage	No	Yes
Peripheral neuropathy	50–80%	10–58%
Relapses	Rare	Frequent
Laboratory data		
ANCA	Rare (<10%)	Yes (50–75%)
HBV infection	Yes (uncommon)	No
Abnormal angiography (microaneurysms, stenoses)	Yes (variable)	No

Table 26.4 Proposed diagnostic criteria of polyarterits nodosa (Henegar *et al.* 2005)

Criteria	Odds ratio	95% CI	R^2
Positive for PAN			
HBV infection	16.85	6.30–45.08	0.320
Myalgias	1.93	1.06–3.53	0.517
Mononeuropathy or polyneuropathy	3.36	1.93–5.86	0.619
Arteriographic abnormalities	20.40	7.30–56.99	0.640
Testicular pain or tenderness	5.27	1.98–28.26	0.661
Negative (exclusion) for PAN			
ANCA positivity	0.11	0.05–0.23	0.668
Glomerulonephritis	0.07	0.02–0.29	0.674
Recent asthma onset	0.01	0.01–0.06	0.433

Based on the analysis of 582 systemic vasculitis patients with all data available in the French Vasculitis Study Group's database: 194 PAN (among whom 117 had HBV-related PAN) and 388 other systemic vasculitides (Wegener's granulomatosis, n = 144; Churg–Strauss syndrome n = 115; MPA, n = 101; cryoglobulinemia n = 28).

Dugué *et al.* 2004). Some authors (Chanseaud *et al.* 2005; Tamby *et al.* 2005) found that IgM and IgG from PAN patients reacted specifically with tissue antigens in artery and kidney extracts.

Cytokines are potentially involved in the pathogenesis of vasculitis. Marked increases of serum interferon-α and interleukin-2 levels, and moderately elevated levels of tumor necrosis factor-α and interleukin-1β have been detected in PAN and CSS patients (Grau *et al.* 1989). Immunohistochemical studies performed on biopsied perineurial and muscle vessels from homogeneous populations of PAN patients showed that inflammatory infiltrates consist mainly of macrophages and T lymphocytes, particularly of the CD8+ subset (Panegyres *et al.* 1990). A homogeneous immunofluorescent-labeling pattern of nerve and muscle vasculitic lesions suggests that some circulating factor, such as an antibody or complement component, binding to a common determinant expressed by muscle and nerve, may accumulate around epineurial and muscle endothelial cells (Panegyres *et al.* 1990). These observations

explored the pathogenic mechanisms of PAN which therefore remain largely unexplained.

ANCA were rarely found in earlier studies (Guillevin *et al.* 1993b), and re-examination of those data showed that the majority of ANCA-positive patients would now be thought to have MPA (Guillevin *et al.* 1995a). Our current opinion is that ANCA positivity should be considered a criterion for excluding the diagnosis of PAN.

Antiendothelial cell autoantibodies (AECA) are directed against antigens expressed on the surface of those cells and have been implicated as a participating pathogenic factor in vasculitis (Cid 1996), by causing direct endothelial damage, but little is known about the target autoantigens in vasculitis or whether AECA are really of pathogenic significance. Indeed, AECA are not disease specific, since they are detectable in both primary autoimmune vasculitides and vasculitides secondary to systemic autoimmune diseases, such as WG, MPA, and Kawasaki disease, as well as in PAN (Salojin *et al.* 1996; Le Tonqueze *et al.* 1996; Chanseaud *et al.* 2005; Tamby *et al.* 2005). The 60-kD heat-shock protein (Hsp60) was shown to be targeted by some AECA in sera from PAN patients (Salojin *et al.* 1996; Le Tonqueze *et al.* 1996; Jamin *et al.* 2005;

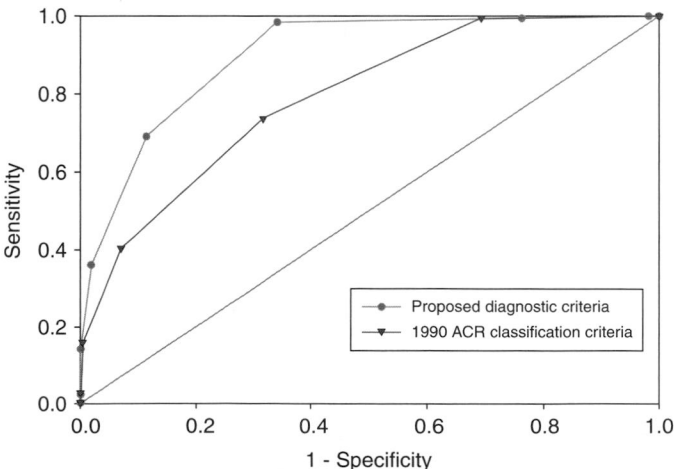

Figure 26.1 ROC curve analyses illustrating performances of the proposed clinical diagnostic set of criteria for PAN (see Table 26.4) compared to the 1990 ACR classification criteria (see Table 26.1).

suggest that T cell-mediated immune mechanisms may play a role in the development and perpetuation of PAN lesions.

To date, there is no reliable animal model of the disease (see Chapter 8). In fact, the PAN-like disease in synomolgus macaques (Porter *et al.* 2003; Colmegna and Maldonado-Cocco 2005), which is very similar to the human disease, occurs only sporadically.

Etiology and precipitating factors

For the majority of patients, the search for an etiology remains elusive. Nevertheless, in a few cases, infections, mainly viral, have been recognized as responsible for PAN, as in the case of HBV infection.

HBV-related PAN

Although viral antigens or immune complexes have rarely been found in the vessel walls of patients affected with PAN, a close relationship has been demonstrated between PAN and HBV infection (Trépo and Thivolet 1970a). In France, we observed that HBV infection transmitted by contaminated blood transfusion has now disappeared; the last proven case occurred in 1987 (Guillevin *et al.* 2005), but intravenous drug abuse has rapidly become a major cause of HBV-related PAN (Guillevin *et al.* 2005), as are cases due to sexual transmission of HBV in high-risk, unvaccinated individuals. The development of vaccines against HBV and their administration to people at risk also explain the dramatic decrease of the number of new cases observed since 1989. Over the past few years, the frequency of HBV-related PAN has declined by 20% (Guillevin *et al.* 2005). For the last 3 years, fewer than 10 patients a year have been diagnosed throughout France. Moreover, the frequency of PAN, due to HBV infection or not, has decreased in parallel.

Other etiologies

Some other viruses have also been associated with PAN but can explain few cases. The prevalence of HCV in our patients was anecdotal and some of the patients were coinfected (HBV–HCV). HCV does not seem to be an important etiological factor for PAN. GB virus-C, a virus searching for a disease, has been sought in patients with PAN, but has not been considered to be a cause of PAN (Servant *et al.* 1998). A few cases associated with parvovirus B19 infections have been described (Corman and Dolson 1992; Leruez *et al.* 1994) but systematic testing of PAN patients did not find them to have a higher frequency of parvovirus B19 infection than the control population (Leruez *et al.* 1994). Other viruses have been incriminated in PAN such as human immunodeficiency virus (anecdotal) (Calabrese 1991; Gherardi *et al.* 1993; Gisselbrecht *et al.* 1998). Herpes zoster could be responsible for vasculitis (Rodríguez Pereira *et al.* 1997), and some members of the *Herpes viridae* family, such as herpesvirus 68, have been possibly involved in the pathogenesis of large-vessel vasculitis in experimental models (Weck *et al.* 1997).

In addition to infectious causes, PAN has been described in association with cancers and blood diseases (mainly hematologic malignancies). The closest relationship has been with hairy-cell leukemia (Elkon *et al.* 1979; Krol *et al.* 1983; Hasler *et al.* 1995). Malignancies are, for the most part, associated with small-sized vessel vasculitides and very few cases of PAN have been reported. In a retrospective study from the Cleveland Clinic Foundation (Hutson and Hoffman 2000), there were only 69 patients who had both malignancies and systemic vasculitis over an 18-year period.

Of these 69 patients, only 12 had both vasculitis and cancer occurring within the same 12 month period, and only two of those 12 patients had PAN.

Pathology

The histological lesion defining PAN is focal segmental necrotizing vasculitis of medium-sized arteries, less commonly arterioles, and only rarely capillaries and venules. The lesion may occur in any artery of the body, but involvement of the aorta or other large elastic arteries or pulmonary arteries has been described only rarely. The acute phase of arterial wall inflammation is characterized by fibrinoid necrosis of the media and an intense pleomorphic cellular infiltration, with predominantly neutrophils and variable numbers of lymphocytes and eosinophils. The normal architecture of the vessel wall, including the elastic laminae, appears to be completely destroyed and replaced by a band of amorphous eosinophilic material, resembling fibrin when stained. Arterial aneurysms and thromboses can occur at the site of the lesion. Arterial healing is characterized by fibrotic endarteritis that may lead to regression of aneurysms or, when abundant, to vessel occlusion. One of the characteristic histological features of PAN is the coexistence of necrotizing vasculitis and a healed lesion or normal arteries in different tissues, or in different parts of the same tissues.

Biopsies from several sites can be diagnostic for PAN. The usefulness of muscle biopsy is discussed extensively in Chapter 14. In general, muscle biopsy should be performed at the site of myalgias or in the gastrocnemius or peroneal muscles. The diagnostic sensitivity of biopsies performed in proximal muscles (deltoid or quadriceps) is lower than in those performed in distal muscles. Nerve biopsy in a sensory branch of the sciatic or peroneal nerve can also be taken when the patient suffers from distal mononeuropathy multiplex in its sensory or sensorimotor form. When patients do not have sensory signs in a candidate region for biopsy, the results have low sensitivity. Nerve biopsy can often prove the presence of vasculitis but cannot easily give the diagnosis of PAN because arteries supplying nerves are usually small. Furthermore, the biopsy itself can cause a permanent sensory deficit. A deep skin biopsy is easy to obtain and can show medium-sized vessel involvement in patients with infiltrated necrotic purpura. In patients with visceral involvement, surgical specimens, such as small intestine for instance, can also provide the diagnosis. Because renal involvement results from ischemia and the risk of hematoma due to rupture of microaneurysm, renal biopsy is not recommended. Temporal artery biopsy can show necrotizing vasculitis of the main artery or one of its branches, even in the absence of clinical symptoms (Généreau *et al.* 1999; Hamidou *et al.* 2003; Haugeberg *et al.* 1997).

Clinical features

Age and sex

PAN can be observed in patients of all ages, including children and the elderly, but predominates between 40 and 60 years. There is no predilection for either sex. In our patients, the mean age was 47.5 years (range 4–92 years) (Table 26.5) (Gunal *et al.* 1997; Travers *et al.* 1979; Schrader *et al.* 1985; Fortin *et al.* 1995; Cohen *et al.* 1980; Leib *et al.* 1979; Frohnert and Sheps 1967; Guillevin *et al.* 1988; Mowrey and Lundberg 1954).

Table 26.5 Percentages of organ/system involvement in or manifestation of PAN according to larger published series

Reference	Organ/system involved ormanifestation (%)								
	Patients (n)	Mean age	Heart	Hypertension	Skin	CNS	PNS	Kidney	GI
Gunal et al. 1997	15 (children)	10	67	20	20	0	0	13	47
Travers et al. 1979[1]	17	41	89	29 (mild) 41 (severe)	65	41	59	77	65
Schrader et al. 1985[1]	36	–	61	72	–	–	–	76	–
Fortin et al. 1995	45	54	18	–	44	24	51	44	53
Cohen et al. 1980[1]	53	54	4	14	58	–	60	66	25
Leib et al. 1979[1]	64	47	30	25	28	25	72	63	42
Frohnert et al. 1967[1]	130	–	10	–	58	3	52	8	14
Guillevin et al. 1988	165	48	23	31	46	17	67	29	31
Mowrey et al. 1954[1]	607	–	–	58	25	–	66	83	48

[1] older populations may have included PAN patients who would now be diagnosed with MPA. CNS = central nervous system; GI = gastrointestinal; PNS = peripheral nervous system.

General (constitutional) symptoms

Poor general condition is common among patients presenting with PAN. Weight loss and fever are present in two-thirds of the patients. Non-specific symptoms occur early in the course of the disease, may be present at its onset, and isolated. The diagnosis of PAN is made only when other systemic manifestations occur. The characteristics of fever vary from one patient to another: high, remittent, with chills, or intermittent.

Myalgias and arthralgias

Half the patients suffer from myalgias. They may be intense, diffuse and occur spontaneously, or only after applying pressure on the muscle. The diagnosis of an inflammatory myopathy can be considered, but muscle enzymes are usually normal or only slightly elevated. Conversely, amyotrophy can be marked, but mostly reflects weight loss, sometimes of more than 20 kg. Some patients are bedridden due to the intensity of pain and amyotrophy. Magnetic resonance imaging (MRI) of painful muscles may show some inflammation, with hyperintensity on T2-weighted sequences (Figure 26.2),

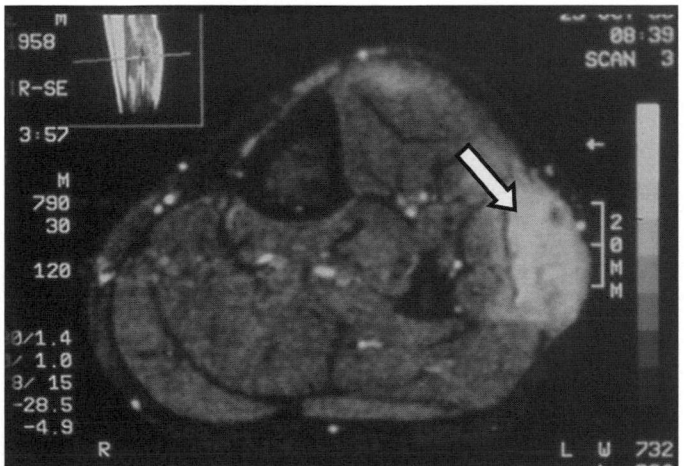

Figure 26.2 Peroneal muscle hypersignal (arrow) on T2-weighted MR images in a PAN patient with muscle involvement.

usually enhanced after gadolinium injection. Muscle biopsy can contribute decisively to the diagnosis of PAN when performed at this stage of illness. Forms of necrotizing vasculitis limited to one muscle or group of muscles with histological features of PAN but no other organ involvement are being described with an increasing frequency (Nakamura et al. 2003; Lupoli et al. 2004).

Arthralgias predominate in knees, ankles, elbows, and wrists, rather than shoulders or hips. Synovitis is rarely observed and joints are usually not deformed. Symptoms differ from those of rheumatoid arthritis, a disease that can also be associated with vasculitis as a secondary phenomenon (see Chapter 34).

Neurological manifestations

Peripheral neurological symptoms are frequent; central nervous system (CNS) involvement has been reported, but is rare.

Peripheral neuropathy

Peripheral neuropathy is the most frequent finding in PAN patients (50–75%) (Frohnert and Sheps 1967; Moore and Fauci 1981; Guillevin et al. 1992b) and is the earliest symptom of the disease in 23–33% (Frohnert and Sheps 1967; Guillevin et al. 1988). Indeed, there is a major variant of PAN that exclusively involves peripheral nerve and muscle (Abgrall et al. 2001). Onset is usually acute, but may be more indolent, particularly in the elderly. Sensory signs are responsible for hypo- or hyperesthesia, dysesthesia, or frank pain as the prominent and earliest features (Moore and Calabrese 1994). Usually, motor deficits start later, also with sudden onset, but may sometimes precede the sensory sign(s). The first manifestations often affect the lower limbs, with one particular nerve involved. Later, other nerves become affected in a pattern referred to as mononeuritis (or mononeuropathy) multiplex (see Chapter 14). Indeed, mononeuropathy multiplex affects 56.5–61.5% of PAN patients (Said and Lacroix 2005; Moore and Fauci 1981). Distal nerves are predominantly affected, and findings are often asymmetric. The following nerves are preferentially involved: superficial peroneal, sural, radial, cubital, and median. In its late stage, so many nerves can be involved that mononeuritis multiplex is mistaken for a symmetric process. Segmental edema may precede the development of palsies, reflecting capillary permeability dysfunction, which regresses either spontaneously or with treatment. Amyotrophy quickly ensues. Cerebrospinal fluid (CSF), when analyzed, is generally normal. Electromyography typically shows axonal neuropathy. Motor and sensory nerve action-potential amplitudes are markedly decreased, or may even be absent in the most severely affected nerves, while motor nerve-conduction velocities are normal or only slightly diminished. The extent of the neuropathy on electromyography may be greater than expected based on clinical manifestations (Said 1997; Bouche *et al.* 1986). Muscle and nerve biopsies may contain characteristic muscle and epineurial artery lesions.

Mononeuritis (simplex) is less frequently observed, in 16.5% of the patients, and distal symmetrical sensory, often patchy, or sensorimotor neuropathy in 25%. Very few cases of brachial plexus neuropathy have been reported (Jamieson *et al.* 1991). Conduction block, suggestive of demyelination, as in Guillain–Barré syndrome, nerve entrapment, or other acquired demyelinating neuropathies, has been described in rare cases (Ropert and Metral 1990; Allan *et al.* 1982).

Under treatment, mononeuropathy multiplex in PAN improves slowly and patients may recover without sequelae although 12 to 18 months are often necessary to evaluate maximal recovery. The degree of recovery is variable and unpredictable. In some patients, severe neuropathy with extensive palsies may regress completely, whereas in others, minor palsies or sensory symptoms may never totally disappear. Sensory symptoms, usually paresthesias, persist longer and sometimes indefinitely, and flares of peripheral neuropathy cannot be predicted. Electromyography can be used during follow-up to evaluate the regression or progression of neuropathy. Physical rehabilitation is indicated to prevent deformities and accelerate clinical improvement.

Central nervous system involvement

CNS involvement, much less common than peripheral neuropathy, is noted in 3–38% of PAN patients (Frohnert and Sheps 1967; Sack *et al.* 1975). It is usually a late manifestation and indicates a poor prognosis (Guillevin *et al.* 1996; Castaigne *et al.* 1970). Its common presentations include encephalopathy affecting cognitive function in 8–20% of patients (Moore and Fauci 1981; Scott *et al.* 1982). CNS involvement of PAN may be characterized by disorientation, psychosis and hallucinations, and delusion or diminished consciousness. Focal or multifocal disturbances of the brain and spinal cord, with seizures, strokes, and subarachnoid hemorrhages (Moore and Calabrese 1994) may result from vasculitis of a cerebral artery, rupture of cerebral artery aneurysm and hematoma, or as a consequence of malignant hypertension. A case of extrapyramidal syndrome has also been described (Mayo *et al.* 1986). Distal occlusion of spinal vessels can be responsible for spinal cord and cauda equina involvement (Castaigne *et al.* 1970), which in turn engenders sphincter dysfunction (Amarenco *et al.* 1988).

Computed tomography scans of the brain are usually normal but MRI may show T2-weighed hyperintensity localized to the white matter in various parts of the brain. These are suggestive although not specific. MR angiography and conventional cerebral angiography (which is performed less frequently than in the past) are often normal, but non-specific focal or diffuse segmental narrowing of the intracranial vessels may be seen.

Cranial nerve involvement

Cranial nerve palsies are found in approximately 1% of PAN patients (Guillevin *et al.* 1988). Oculomotor (III), trochlear (IV), abducens (VI), facial (VII), and acoustic (VIII) nerves (Ford and Sieckert 1965) are most often affected. Partial or full recovery can often be achieved with treatment, but is unlikely to be complete for the VIIIth vestibulocochlear nerve(s) (Vathenen *et al.* 1988). Vasculitis of the optic nerve, optic chiasm, and occipital cortex have been described (Kinyoun *et al.* 1987). Blurred vision or visual loss may also occur as a result of choroiditis (see below), retinitis, or brain parenchymal arteritis (Moore and Calabrese 1994). The CSF is usually normal but in a few cases an elevated protein concentration, without increased cellularity, is present (Hirohata *et al.* 1993).

Skin manifestations

Cutaneous lesions have been reported in 20–60% of patients with systemic PAN, but less frequently in those older than 65 years (Cohen *et al.* 1980; Puisieux *et al.* 1997). It must be remembered that in the majority of series, PAN and MPA were not differentiated and that today, most cutaneous manifestations would probably be attributed to MPA. Theoretically, cutaneous or subcutaneous nodules are hallmarks of PAN, occurring in 8–27% of patients. They occur in clusters along the trajectories of superficial arteries and often disappear spontaneously within a few days, before new ones develop. They measure 5–20 mm in diameter and are dermal and hypodermal, and mainly localized to the lower legs, especially the knees and feet. The most common cutaneous finding is palpable purpura, often necrotic (Figure 26.3), and corresponding to subcutaneous small vessel vasculitis, associated with the inflammation of medium-sized vessels. Although the Chapel Hill Nomenclature distinguishes large, medium-sized, and small-vessel vasculitides, it also recognizes some overlap forms such as PAN with some, but not predominant, involvement of small vessels, especially in skin biopsies (ANCA Workshop, Birmingham, UK, 1998, unpublished revised version of the Nomenclature). A convenient threshold for defining small-vessel vasculitis has been set, primarily for nerve biopsies, at around 50–70 μm in diameter for affected epineurial arteries and vasa nervorum (Gherardi *et al.* 1993; Moore 1995).

Ulcerations and livedo are less frequent (Leib *et al.* 1979). Livedo reticularis may precede, follow, or occur concomitantly with the onset of nodules. Livedo reticularis in PAN is typically localized on

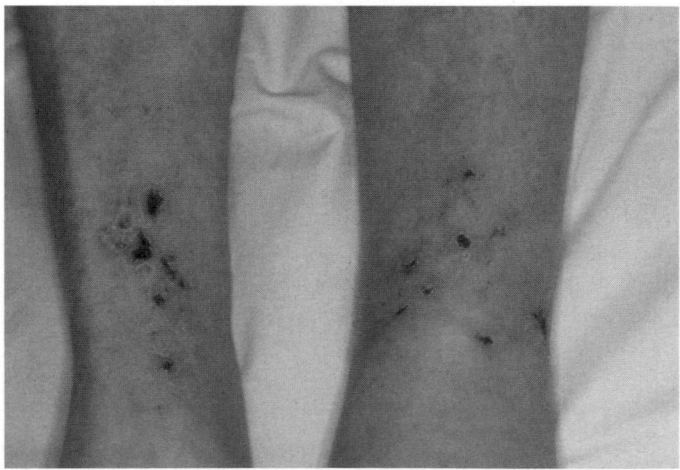

Figure 26.3 Necrotic purpura of the legs and ankles in a PAN patient. (See Color Plate 76).

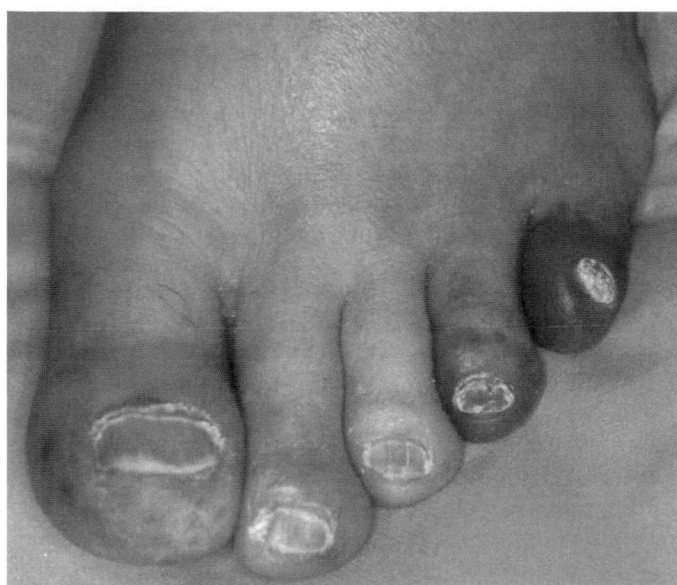

Figure 26.4 Toe ischemia in a PAN patient. (See Color Plate 77).

the lower limbs, the extensor surfaces of the arms and occasionally the trunk. It has a fishnet reticular pattern, with discontinuous circles, and often has infiltrated areas.

Local rupture of superficial arteries may lead to cutaneous hematoma or ecchymosis. A biopsy of infiltrated or central lesion zones can show changes of vasculitis. Painful ulcerations are frequently associated with indurated plaques resulting from the coalescence of nodules. Peripheral embolization of thrombi may cause infarction of the extremities (toes, fingers) (Figure 26.4) or skin, often in proximal areas, similar to the syndrome of cholesterol or atheromatous embolization.

Other reported manifestations include: bullous purpura and vesicles that may result in necrosis; urticaria; transient erythema or erythema annulare fugax; superficial phlebitis; Raynaud's phenomenon; and splinter hemorrhage. In most patients, cutaneous signs are associated with other PAN-related symptoms, such as arthralgias, hypertension, gastrointestinal manifestations, and peripheral neuropathy. Nevertheless, PAN may at first be limited to the skin in a few patients, with systemic PAN developing from 1 to 20 years after the first cutaneous signs (Diaz-Perez and Winkelmann 1974). Conversely, PAN may remain strictly confined to the skin, as a chronic disease, often associated with multiple cutaneous relapses (see Chapter 28).

Renal manifestations

Renal artery involvement can be responsible for mild to severe and malignant arterial hypertension and vascular ischemic nephropathy with renal insufficiency (Cohen *et al.* 1986), which has been identified as a poor prognosis factor (Guillevin *et al.* 1996). Angiography (when performed in spite of renal involvement) may show renal parenchymal infarcts and characteristic multiple stenoses and microaneurysms of branches of celiac-mesenteric and renal arteries (Figure 26.5) (in 90% and 40–62% of the cases with or without GI symptoms, respectively) (Ha *et al.* 2000; Camilleri *et al.* 1983; Miller 2000). Microaneurysms can occasionally rupture, spontaneously or after renal biopsy, which is strongly contraindicated

in the presence of microaneurysms (Akcicek *et al.* 1994; Cornfield *et al.* 1988; Tasdemir *et al.* 1988). Renal hematoma can be extensive and requires embolization (Hachulla *et al.* 1993) or even nephrectomy (San *et al.* 1990).

Acute renal insufficiency usually occurs early during the disease course or during a flare. Plasma exchanges might be required initially, but renal function outcome remains unpredictable. Some patients may come off dialysis but end-stage renal failure, resulting from chronic renal ischemia, may develop even years after the first manifestations of PAN.

Arterial hypertension

Hypertension is present in a mean of 40% of PAN patients and is usually mild; however, it can be triggered or exacerbated by glucocorticoids. Severe or malignant hypertension was detected in 7/165 (4%) of our patients (Guillevin *et al.* 1988) and 15% of those with HBV-related PAN (Guillevin *et al.* 1993a). Hypertension can be attenuated with angiotensin-converting enzyme inhibitors, which have been proven beneficial in this context.

Cardiac manifestations

Cardiac involvement was mentioned in the first publication on PAN (Kussmaul and Maier 1866), which described a case of "nodular coronaritis". It was subsequently reported with frequencies of 10% in clinical investigations of PAN patients (Frohnert and Sheps 1967), 40% when considering radiological and electrocardiographic anomalies,

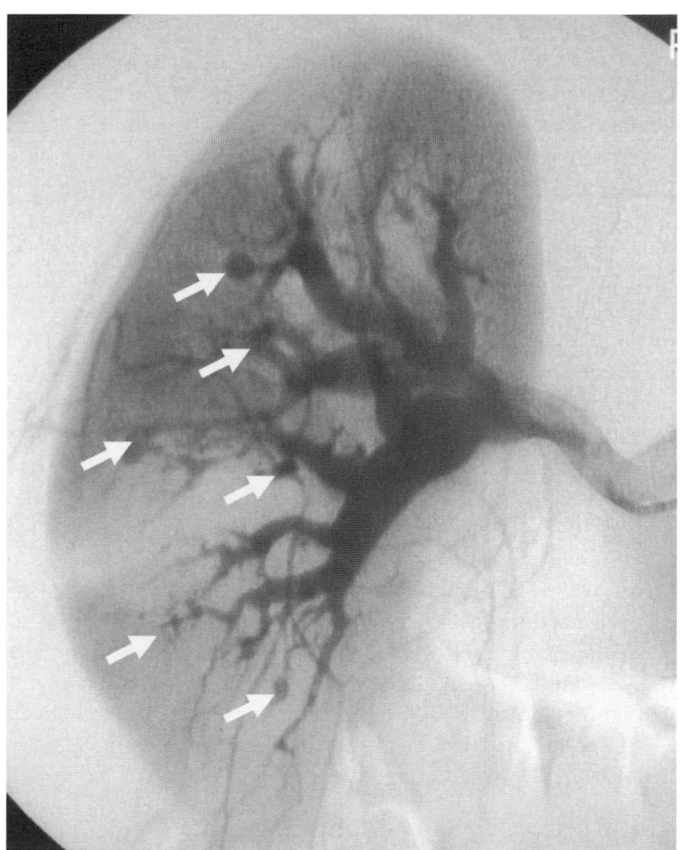

Figure 26.5 Multiple renal artery stenoses and microaneurysms (arrow) with an inferior kidney pole infarction on arteriography (paler, less well irrigated pyramidal corticoparenchymal area) in a PAN patient.

and 78% in a histopathological study (Holsinger *et al.* 1962). Congestive heart failure (CHF) is the main clinical feature, occurring in 6–57% of PAN patients, but usually less frequently than in Churg–Strauss syndrome. CHF in PAN is due to vasculitis of the coronary arteries, or their branches, with myocardial arteriolar infarcts, or from other vasculitis-related organ involvement or disorders, mainly hypertension and renal involvement (Blétry *et al.* 1980). Cardiomyopathy can occur as soon as 3 months after PAN onset. Despite coronary artery vasculitis, angina is rare, being reported in 2–18% of patients (Frohnert and Sheps 1967; Blétry *et al.* 1980). Myocardial infarctions are diagnosed in 1–12% of patients, but are commonly found at autopsy (Frohnert and Sheps 1967). Among 66 autopsied patients, 41 had features of myocardial infarction, but only three had clinical symptoms and only three had coronary atherosclerosis (Holsinger *et al.* 1962). Schrader *et al.* (1985) autopsied 36 PAN patients, 50% of whom had evidence of coronary arteritis, with severe lesions involving small subepicardial vessels as they entered the myocardium and 8% had large infarcts.

Angiography can prove coronary involvement in 85% of the patients with clinical signs of infarction. In the remaining 15%, infarction may be due to arteritis in small coronary vessels or vasospasm (Rajani *et al.* 1991). Coronary aneurysms were found in 9% of children with PAN (Takahashi 1993). Their rupture is rare but serious, as it can cause hemopericardium. Most cases have been described in infants (Holt and Jackson 1975; Tang and Segal 1971), some of whom might have had Kawasaki's disease rather than PAN. There are no guidelines for evaluation of coronary artery involvement in PAN patients without cardiac symptoms. Cardiac MRI seems to be promising but needs further evaluation.

The right ventricle may be involved, as reported in a small series (six of eight patients with heart involvement) (Blétry *et al.* 1980). Finally, interstitial myocarditis was seen in 14% of autopsied patients (Schrader *et al.* 1985).

Murmurs are relatively frequent, having been noted in 39% (Holsinger *et al.* 1962) of vasculitis patients. In most cases, they are innocuous, underlining the rarity of valve involvement in PAN. Indeed, endocarditis is rare in PAN, so other diagnoses should be sought in patients with findings to suggest endocarditis. Patients with mitral and tricuspid regurgitation supposedly specific to PAN have been reported, however (Gunal *et al.* 1997; Blétry *et al.* 1980).

The pericardium is affected clinically in less than 5% of PAN patients (Hu *et al.* 1997). The prevalence is higher (19% to 33%) (Gunal *et al.* 1997; Holsinger *et al.* 1962) in autopsy series. When not attributable to other causes, pericarditis is non-specific and may be secondary to myocardial involvement. About half of the initially reported cases of pericardial effusion were secondary to uremia, which is much less frequent now that diagnosis and management have improved.

In patients with cardiac involvement, sinus tachycardia is common, non-specific, and often precedes other cardiac symptoms. Arrhythmias and conduction disorders, mainly supraventricular, occur in 2–19% of PAN patients (Holsinger *et al.* 1962; Blétry *et al.* 1980) because of arteritis of the sinus node or neighboring nerve fibers.

Aortic dissection and peripheral vascular manifestations

Aortic dissection is a rare complication ignited by diffuse vasculitis of the aorta vasa vasorum. It has been reported to evolve to fatal tamponade (Iino *et al.* 1992). Dissections of proximal aortic branches have also been reported, with some attributed to other causes, such as atherosclerotic aneurysms (Hachulla *et al.* 1993; Bookman *et al.* 1983; Hautekeete *et al.* 1990; Lomeo *et al.* 1989); syphilis; cystic media necrosis; trauma; sepsis or hypertension.

Peripheral arterial occlusions may be responsible for distal gangrene of the toes or fingers. Angiography can demonstrate the presence of stenoses and microaneurysms (Figure 26.6) (Héron *et al.* 2003). Raynaud's phenomenon can remain isolated or be complicated by necrosis. In some patients, type II or III cryoglobulinemia can be found. It is not known whether cryoglobulinemia may accompany PAN, or if its detection should rather exclude the diagnosis of PAN. The latter position is more rigorous, and probably should be advocated, at least for clinical trials.

Gastrointestinal manifestations

GI tract involvement represents one of the most severe manifestations of PAN, reported with a frequency of 40–60% of the patients, more often in HBV-related PAN. GI manifestations are usually associated with other systemic manifestations of PAN, but they can be its first presenting signs in 2–16%, especially in HBV-related PAN (Zizic *et al.* 1982; Camilleri *et al.* 1983; Le Thi Huong *et al.* 1985). They are the major cause of deaths within the first year after PAN onset, and thereafter rank behind infections and heart disease with regard to causes of mortality (Bourgarit *et al.* 2005).

The spectrum of GI symptoms is wide and usually non-specific, with abdominal pain most frequent (30–40% of all patients, and 97% of those with GI involvement). It is difficult to establish the

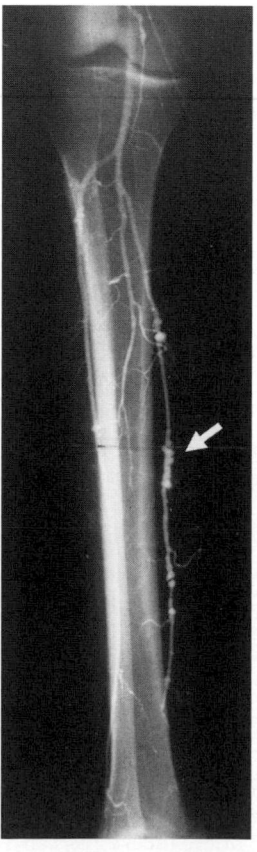

Figure 26.6 Tibial artery stenoses and microaneurysms in a PAN patient.

exact origin of this pain but it can be the symptom signaling more severe and life-threatening GI vasculitis, so should always be thoroughly investigated.

GI hemorrhage and small intestine perforation are its most feared manifestations (Guillevin *et al.* 1995c), with reported frequencies in PAN of 20–50% and 2–40% (mean 5%) respectively. Ischemic vasculitis mainly affects the small bowel and less often the colon or stomach. Esophageal perforations are rare (Lee and Kay 1958; Gourgoutis *et al.* 1971). Vasculitis of the gallbladder (2–17% of PAN patients) or the appendix (Parangi *et al.* 1991; Chen 1989; Ito *et al.* 1991; Nohr *et al.* 1989; Blidi *et al.* 1996) can be the first sign of PAN, and are sometimes isolated, hence possibly representing a localized form of PAN. Twenty-five percent of patients with isolated and histologically proven vasculitic appendicitis evolve to systemic PAN within 5 years (Godeau *et al.* 1979). Except for isolated appendicitis, whose vasculitic etiology might be perceived as a pathological curiosity (see Figure 9.36 in Chapter 9), medical therapy should not be used alone. The prognosis of limited forms remains good, owing to prompt combined medical and surgical treatment. Acute necrotizing or, less commonly, chronic pancreatitis, sometimes with pseudocysts, is diagnosed in 2–3% of patients (Cacoub *et al.* 1988). In these cases, the prognosis is dismal because of the frequent association with severe small intestine ischemia and perforations.

Digestive malabsorption and exudative enteropathy have also been reported on rare occasions. The liver and spleen can be involved, even in the absence of HBV infection, with infarcts (Figure 26.7) and hematomas (Li *et al.* 1979; Nakazawa *et al.* 1992) that are usually clinically silent. One case of fibrinoid necrosis of the splenic artery with subsequent splenic rupture has been described (Fortin *et al.* 1995).

In dealing with abdominal pain, abdominal computed tomography (CT) can be useful in detecting organ infarcts or pancreatitis, but its diagnostic sensitivity is only about 75%. GI vasculitis has no specific features, even though bowel-wall inflammation and thickening may be suggestive. Gastric and colon endoscopy can detect ischemic areas and ulcers that may precede perforation, but can also easily cause iatrogenic perforations in patients with fragile and inflamed GI mucosa. Furthermore, GI biopsies rarely contribute

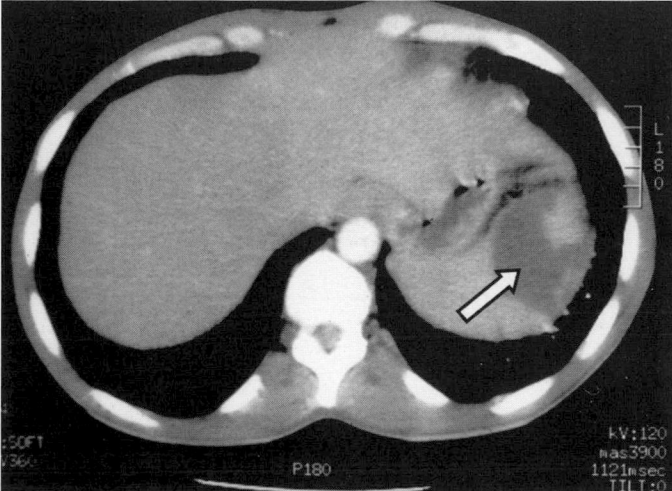

Figure 26.7 Splenic infarct (arrow) seen on a PAN patient's abdominal computed tomography scan.

to the diagnosis because they are usually not deep enough to reveal vasculitis.

In 90% of the patients with GI symptoms, angiography may detect infarcts, hematomas or more diagnostically useful arterial stenoses and microaneurysms. Microaneurysms (1–5 mm in diameter or more) appear mainly in renal (54%), celiac (24%), mesenteric (14%), hepatic, or, more rarely, splenic arteries (Camilleri *et al.* 1983; Miller 2000; Ewald *et al.* 1987), but have little or no prognostic value. When not rapidly fatal, intraperitoneal ruptures might be treatable with selective arterial embolization (Hachulla *et al.* 1993; Bookman *et al.* 1983).

Severe GI manifestations, such as bowel perforations and ischemia, peritonitis, intestinal occlusion, and pancreatitis (because of its frequent association with bowel perforations), imply a poor prognostic value. Treatment should combine prompt surgical intervention and medical therapy with glucocorticoids and immunosuppressants. The 5-year survival rate of patients with these severe GI manifestations is only 56%, compared to 82% for those with less severe GI involvement (Pagnoux *et al.* 2005; Levine *et al.* 2002).

Orchitis

Orchitis is one of the most characteristic manifestations of PAN (Warfield *et al.* 1994; Teichman *et al.* 1993; Guillevin *et al.* 1995b), and it was retained as one of the classification criteria established by the ACR (Lightfoot *et al.* 1990). It is rarely the first manifestation of the disease and is usually unilateral. It is the consequence of testicular artery ischemia, which may regress if treated immediately. No infectious etiology has been found. Fever and poor general condition are usually found in patients with orchitis. In isolated testicular involvement, a tumor or testicular torsion comes to mind and histological examination can provide the diagnosis (Warfield *et al.* 1994). We and others have observed that orchitis is often present in HBV-related PAN (Guillevin *et al.* 1995b) but no close relationship could be demonstrated between the viral infection and testicular manifestations.

Ureteral and urogenital manifestations

Ureteral manifestations are rare, and not specific to PAN. They most often have been considered characteristic of small vessel vasculitides. Unilateral or bilateral ureteral stricture (Gargollo *et al.* 2004), extrinsic compression of the ureter by retroperitoneal involvement (Lie 1992), and hydronephrosis due to ureteral myoneuropathy (Casserly *et al.* 1999) have been observed in PAN.

In patients with difficulty urinating, urodynamic and electrophysiological examinations can demonstrate hypoactivity of the detrusor, with increased compliance and loss of the urge to urinate. This often reflects hypoesthesia of the bladder due to vasculitis of the vaso vasorum of the vessels supplying the bladder rather than mucosal involvement. Spinal cord involvement or cauda equina syndrome should be considered, but are extremely rare.

Involvement of the glans penis resembling cancer has been described (Casserly *et al.* 1999). Cervical (Ganesan *et al.* 2000; Abu-Farsakh *et al.* 1994), ovarian (Kaya *et al.* 1994), and uterine arteries (Piette *et al.* 1987; Grasland *et al.* 1996) have been involved.

Pulmonary manifestations

In contrast to MPA, CSS, and WG, the lungs are spared in PAN. Autopsy studies, however, have shown asymptomatic vasculitis of bronchial arteries. When pulmonary symptoms occur, infection should be looked for first, and is usually found (Godeau *et al.* 1994).

Bone manifestations

Periosteal modifications can be seen (Short and Webley 1984; MacDonald and Blake 2004; Esteva-Lorenzo *et al.* 1994) particularly in the bones of the legs. Localized edema and pain are common, and biopsies reveal necrotizing vasculitis. A few cases of bone necrosis have also been reported (Wang *et al.* 1988).

Ophthalmological manifestations

The eye can be affected in PAN, sometimes severely, as with uni- or bilateral choroiditis (Kinyoun *et al.* 1987), iritis, iridocyclitis, retinal detachment, and retinal vasculitis (Akova *et al.* 1993; Horgan *et al.* 1986; Malan *et al.* 1986) (see Chapter 12).

Miscellaneous

Rare anecdotal descriptions of specific gingival (Cowpe and Hislop 1983; Thone 1988) and breast (Levy *et al.* 1986; Yamashina and Wilson 1985) lesions have been published.

Specific manifestations of HBV-PAN

The immunological process responsible for PAN occurs early in HBV infection, in most cases within 6 months after infection. PAN can be the first manifestation of HBV infection, preceding clinical evidence of hepatitis. Liver biopsies have frequently exhibited histologic evidence of chronic hepatitis, even in PAN occurring months after HBV infection. Hepatic cytolysis is usually moderate and cholestasis is minor or absent. In the group of patients with HBV-related PAN, clinical data were similar to those observed in PAN as a whole (Table 26.6) (Guillevin *et al.* 2005), but with some differences. Patients with HBV-associated PAN were usually under 40 years of age, and malignant hypertension (5%), renal infarction, and orchiepididymitis (25%) were more frequent than in non-HBV PAN (Guillevin *et al.* 2005; Guillevin *et al.* 1995b). Abdominal manifestations (53%) and surgical emergencies were frequently observed. In the study by Sergent *et al.* (1976), two of the three deaths (among nine patients), were attributed to vasculitis of the colon. Among Eskimo patients described by McMahon *et al.* (1989), 31% died and one of the four early deaths was due to small bowel perforation. GI and renal manifestations resulted from ischemia; angiography demonstrated the presence of microaneurysms and infarctions. Subsequent angiograms showed that the aneurysms had disappeared after PAN was effectively treated (Darras-Joly *et al.* 1995). Disappearance might reflect thrombosis of aneurysms and evolution to fibrosis.

HBV-related PAN is acute and initially severe but the outcome is excellent if adequate treatment is prescribed. Seroconversion of hepatitis serologies usually correlates with recovery. Sequelae are the consequence of vascular nephropathy but it is possible to obtain recovery of renal function with little residual impairment.

Localized forms of PAN

Localized PAN is rare except for the limited cutaneous forms that represent 10% of all PAN cases (Moreland and Ball 1990). Isolated involvement of one skeletal muscle or a muscle group, and isolated neuropathy (mononeuropathy multiplex or simplex) without systemic symptoms have been described (Dyck *et al.* 1987;

Table 26.6 Relevant clinical and biological symptoms in 115 patients with HBV-related PAN (Guillevin *et al.* 2005)

Clinical symptoms	Values[1]
Age, mean ± SD (years)	51.1 ± 17
Sex ratio	74 M/41 F
General symptoms	97
Fever	69
Weight loss	87
Arthralgias	56
Myalgias	47
Mononeuritis multiplex	84
GI-tract involvement	53
Abdominal pain	51
Bleeding	3
Appendicitis	2
Small intestine perforation	6
Cholecystitis	5
Pancreatitis	6
Renal and/or urogenital involvement	38
Creatininemia, mean ± SD (mg/dl)	1.52 ± 1.39
Orchitis	25
Microaneurysms[2]	69
Renal infarcts[2,3]	28
Skin involvement	31
Purpura	17
Infiltrated purpura	11
Livedo	10
Nodules	9
Edema (ankles)	16
Vascular manifestations	18
Hypertension	31
Malignant hypertension	5
Cardiac insufficiency	12
Raynaud's phenomenon	3
Pericarditis	5
Digital ischemia	4
Myocardial infarction	1
CNS involvement	10
Retinal vasculitis	2
Erythrocyte sedimentation rate >30 mm/h	78
ANCA[4]	0

[1] Values are %, unless otherwise indicated.

[2] 66 angiographies.

[3] Not related to vasculitis.

[4] ANCA assays were performed in sera of 66 patients.

Gallien *et al.* 2002). Occasional cases involve only the appendix, gallbladder (Pagnoux *et al.* 2005; Blidi *et al.* 1996), or uterus (Piette *et al.* 1987), in order of decreasing frequency. These forms usually carry good prognoses, often remitting spontaneously with local therapy (topical glucocorticoids for skin lesions) or after surgery (cholecystectomy or appendectomy). In PAN limited to the skin or muscle, however, relapses are frequent. Of the patients with appendicitis in whom PAN was found during histological examination, ~25% may subsequently develop systemic PAN (Godeau *et al.* 1979; Le Thi Huong *et al.* 1985).

PAN in childhood

After Kawasaki disease and Henoch–Schönlein purpura, PAN is the most common systemic necrotizing vasculitis in childhood (Ozen *et al.* 2004) (see Chapter 22). Neither the ACR nor the Chapel Hill Nomenclature for PAN is validated for children. European EULAR/PRES pediatricians have recently proposed specific classification criteria for juvenile vasculitides (Table 26.7) (Ozen *et al.* 2006). Among children, the mean age at diagnosis of PAN is 9 ± 4 years old, with an equal number of boys and girls. Clinical manifestations fall within the spectrum of disease seen in adults, but with more frequent skin disease. Indeed, 80% of affected children have skin involvement, and limited cutaneous forms may represent up to one-third of the cases (see Chapter 22).

Prognosis appears to be better in children than in adults, with overall mortality rate of 1–16%. Relapses are more frequent, may occur years after diagnosis, and are sometimes preceded by ENT infections. Evolution from a limited cutaneous disease to a systemic form is rare. Antistreptolysin antibodies should be systematically sought, with serial determinations when initially positive, because penicillin may help to cure the disease and has been shown to lower the relapse rate. The optimal antibiotic regimen is unknown, however, because relapses have been described up to 20 years after the first episode (Till and Amos 1997). HBV-related PAN is rare in children (<5%), especially after large campaigns to vaccinate children for HBV. Conversely, a link between PAN and streptococcal

infections has been identified, which may be relevant for as many as 75% of pediatric cases (Till and Amos 1997).

Laboratory tests

Indicators of inflammation are found in the majority of patients. An erythrocyte sedimentation rate >60 mm/hour (78–89% of patients); elevated C-reactive protein; high alpha-2 globulin level; elevated white blood cell count (45–75% of the patients) sometimes with eosinophilia >1500/mm^3; and normochromic anemia (34–79% of patients) are common laboratory findings. The presence of HBsAg should be systematically sought. The frequency of HBV infection in PAN patients was 38.5% during the period 1972–1976, peaked at 48.8% between 1982 and 1986, then fell to 17.4% in the period 1997–2002. HBV is now rarely found because of vaccination campaigns and increased safety of blood transfusions. Most recently, the majority of HBV-infected patients come from northern or sub-Saharan African countries that have no vaccination policy, or they are intravenous drug addicts, or are patients at risk for sexually transmitted infections. We have also observed that PAN without HBV infection has also become rarer than in the past for reasons which are unclear. We hypothesize that all PAN is the consequence of infection, even if a micro-organism has not been isolated in all patients.

ANCA are less common in PAN than in MPA, WG, and CSS. In the context of systemic vasculitides, the presence of ANCA giving a perinuclear labeling pattern (P-), primarily directed against myeloperoxidase (anti-MPO) in ELISA, should be considered exclusionary for PAN and be taken as an argument in favor of MPA. In some patients it is difficult, even when biopsies have been examined, to distinguish between PAN and MPA, especially in patients without renal involvement. This most likely explains why pANCA with MPO reactivity has been found in a small number of patients diagnosed with PAN (Gaskin *et al.* 1991). Hauschild *et al.* (1994) reported ANCA positivity in 7 of 36 patients (19.4%) with PAN (pANCA in three, cANCA in four).

Angiography

In 1965, Bron *et al.* (1965) showed that angiography could depict microaneurysms and stenoses in medium-sized vessels. Although microaneurysms are not pathognomonic, they are commonly present in PAN and rare in ANCA-associated vasculitides. Arterial saccular or fusiform aneurysms range in size from 1 to 5 mm and predominate in kidneys, mesentery, and liver. The lesions may disappear under effective vasculitis therapy (Darras-Joly *et al.* 1995). Angiography is a useful diagnostic tool when other diagnostic examinations are negative, especially when abdominal pain and nephropathy are present. Although the Chapel Hill Consensus Conference (Jennette *et al.* 1994) did not consider microaneurysms, we think their presence should be taken into consideration for the classification of PAN, representing an exclusionary criterion for MPA.

Outcome and prognosis of PAN

In its systemic form, PAN is an acute disease which can be severe and cause death if not treated adequately. In historical series, only about 12% (Leib *et al.* 1979) or 13% (Frohnert and Sheps 1967) of untreated patients survived. Since the introduction of glucocorticoids,

Table 26.7 EULAR/PRES proposed classification criteria for childhood PAN[1] (Ozen *et al.* 2006)

A systemic illness characterized by the presence of at least 2 of the following 7 criteria:
1. Skin involvement (livedo reticularis, tender subcutaneous nodules, other vasculitic lesions)
2. Myalgia or muscle tenderness
3. Systemic hypertension, relative to normal childhood values
4. Mononeuropathy or polyneuropathy
5. Abnormal urine analysis and/or impaired renal function
6. Testicular pain or tenderness
7. Signs or symptoms suggesting vasculitis of any other major organ system (GI, cardiac, respiratory, or CNS)
In the presence of (one, at least, of the below as a mandatory criterion)
1. Biopsy showing small and medium-sized artery necrotizing vasculitis
2. Angiographic abnormalities[2] (aneurysms or occlusions)

[1] Proposed criteria are currently being reviewed by the ACR.

[2] Should include angiography if MR angiography is negative.

and their later combination with immunosuppressants, antiviral therapy for HBV-related PAN, and plasma exchanges when appropriate, the prognosis of PAN improved and overall survival rates increased to 76–89% for PAN (Gayraud *et al*. 2001) and 64–70% for HBV-related PAN (Guillevin *et al*. 2005). Although treatment is now able to ensure a favorable outcome for the majority of patients, some relapse or die of disease- or treatment-related causes.

Relapses

Once remission has been obtained, PAN tends not to recur, unlike other systemic vasculitides such as WG or MPA. In an early study of 278 patients, 8% of HBV-related PAN and 19% of non-HBV–related PAN patients relapsed, with a mean time to first relapse of 37 and 29 months, respectively (Gayraud *et al*. 2001). In a more recent investigation, 10% of patients with HBV-related PAN relapsed (Guillevin *et al*. 2005). At present, it is not possible to identify the subgroup of non-HBV PAN patients who will relapse. In HBV-PAN, relapses occur in those patients who have persistent, active virus replication after treatment. The clinical pattern of

relapse does not necessarily repeat the original presentation, in that entirely new organs can be involved at relapse. Although the severity of relapses cannot be predicted, the clinical features at relapse are rash and arthralgias in most patients, and are generally less severe than during the initial presentation.

Deaths

Although the causes of death vary from one form of vasculitis to the other, they can be divided into two categories: deaths attributable to the vasculitic process and those due to treatment side-effects.

Deaths attributable to the vasculitis

Lethal complications may occur in any form of vasculitis that involves major organs. A few patients die during the first months of the disease from multivisceral involvement unresponsive to treatment (Bourgarit *et al*. 2005). Death most often occurs accompanied by fever, rapid weight loss, diffuse pain, and one or several major organ involvements. For PAN, deaths are often the consequence of GI disease. The major causes of death of PAN patients are summarized in Table 26.8 (Cohen *et al*. 1980; Gayraud *et al*. 2001;

Table 26.8 Causes of death in patients with PAN, including HBV-related PAN

	Gayraud *et al.* 2001	Cruz *et al.* 2003	Cacoub *et al.* 1988	Leib *et al.* 1979	Cohen *et al.* 1980	Guillevin *et al.* 2005
Number of patients	278	26	165	64	53	115
Type of vasculitis (n)	HBV-PAN (63)	Patients admitted to ICU[1]	PAN	PAN	PAN	HBV-related PAN
	PAN (93)	PAN (5)				
	MPA (58)	MPA (4)				
	and CSS (64)	CSS (7) and other (10)				
Deaths (%)	85 (31)	2 of the 5 PAN (20)	61 (37)†	32 (50)	22 (42)	41 (36)
Cause of death (%)						
Progressive vasculitis	22 (26)	0	21 (43)[2]	20 (63)	-	11 (27)
Bowel infarction	10	-	8	-	6 (27)	7
Cardiac failure	5	-	4	-	-	1
Multivisceral involvement	3	-	2	-	-	
Renal failure	3	-	5	-	6 (27)	
Stroke	1	-	2	-	-	
Infectious side-effects of treatment	11 (13)	2 (100)	13 (27)	2 (6)	-	4 (10)
Bacterial pneumonia	5	1	11	-	-	-
Septicemia	6	1	6 of 11	-	-	3 of the 4
Sudden deaths	9 (11)	0	3 (6)	-	-	1 (2)
Heart disease	8 (9)	0	6 (12)[2]	5 (16)	8 (36)[3]	5 (12)[3]
Cancer	13 (15)	0	5 (10)	1 (3)	1 (5)	3 (7)
Pulmonary embolism	3 (3.5)	0	2 (4)	-	-	
Chronic respiratory disease	3 (3.5)	0	-	-	-	
End-stage renal insufficiency	-	-	-	3 (9)	-	
Fulminant viral hepatitis	2 (2)	0	-	-	-	1 (2)
Miscellaneous	14 (17)	0	2 (4)	1 (3)	1 (5)	16 (39)

[1] ICU - intensive care unit.

[2] Patients died from heart disease due to vasculitis or other co-morbid diseases. The total of listed causes of death exceeds 100% because multiple causes were included. There were 61 deaths, with 49 having sufficient data for analyses.

[3] Includes cerebrovascular and cardiovascular complications.

Cruz *et al.* 2003; Cacoub *et al.* 1988; Leib *et al.* 1979; Guillevin *et al.* 2005).

Deaths due to treatment side-effects

While the deaths occurring during the first few months of the disease are often caused by uncontrolled vasculitis, those occurring during the following years may be the consequence of treatment side-effects and are not rare. These adverse events emphasize the importance of tailoring the therapeutic regimen after careful analysis of parameters available to predict the outcome (see below). Infections represent the primary cause of death. Septicemia occurs during the first months of treatment and is the consequence of the intense initial therapy with glucocorticoids and cytotoxic agents. Viral infections usually occur later and are the result of profound immunosuppression induced by drugs prescribed to control the vasculitis. Rare cases of *Pneumocystis jiroveci* pneumonia, which have mainly been described in WG (Jarrousse *et al.* 1993; Godeau *et al.* 1995), can also occur in PAN and MPA. Lowering doses and shortening treatment duration will probably lead to fewer infectious complications, but treatment intensity and duration needs to be further refined, based on prospective studies.

Early deaths in PAN

As in other vasculitides, a small number of patients die within weeks or months after the diagnosis of PAN, despite institution of adequate treatment. In a recent study (Bourgarit *et al.* 2005), it was shown that 38 of 309 patients died during the first year, predominantly from vasculitis (58%), with treatment side-effects as another cause. The primary cause of early death in PAN is severe GI involvement (perforations or hemorrhage), which is the rationale for including it in the Five-Factor Score (FFS) (see Chapter 23) (Guillevin *et al.* 1996).

When patients were hospitalized in intensive care units, the main prognostic factor for early deaths was the APACHE (Acute Physiology and Chronic Health Evaluation) score, which was not specifically devised for vasculitis. Scores specific for vasculitides, such as Birmingham Vasculitis Activity Score (BVAS) and FFS (see Chapter 23), were not associated with death in intensive care units (Cruz *et al.* 2003).

Treatment of PAN

Severity of vasculitis

The FFS has significant prognostic value and can be used to guide the physicians' choice of therapeutic agents and avoid overtreatment (Guillevin *et al.* 1996). The following parameters are associated with higher mortality: proteinuria (>1 g/day); renal insufficiency (serum creatinine >140 μmol/l [1.58 mg/dl]); cardiomyopathy due to PAN; GI manifestations; and CNS involvement. In a study of 342 patients with PAN and CSS, we found that when FFS = 0, mortality at 5 years was 12%; when FFS = 1, mortality was 26%; and when FFS >2, mortality was 46% (Guillevin *et al.* 1996). Although it has not yet been demonstrated that treatment should be chosen as a function of these criteria, they should probably be considered in deciding the therapeutic strategy. For PAN without poor prognostic factors (FFS = 0), we treat patients with glucocorticoids alone to lower the number of side-effects. This strategy is effective, with few minor relapses necessitating transient intensification of the glucocorticoid regimen or addition of an immunosuppressant agent (personal observations). Other criteria to determine the intensity of treatment, such as the BVAS (Luqmani *et al.* 1994), are being

tested in prospective trials proposed by the European Vasculitis Study Group (EUVAS).

Recommendations for specific conditions

Supportive care represents an important part of the treatment of patients with potentially fatal disease. Since maximal immunosuppression is given at the beginning of treatment, prevention of opportunistic infections, such as *Pneumocystis* pneumonia should be strongly considered (Jarrousse *et al.* 1993; Godeau *et al.* 1995). Pain control, prevention of pressure sores, and physical therapy are needed for mononeuropathy multiplex. Angiotensin-converting enzyme inhibitors are effective against severe hypertension due to renal vasculitis and have a beneficial effect on renal function. Fulminating vasculitis usually presents with GI involvement, renal failure, pulmonary hemorrhage, and rarely cerebral involvement.

In cases of GI involvement with persistent abdominal pain despite medical treatment, an exploratory laparotomy should be performed to identify and treat possible bowel perforations. For these patients, it seems reasonable to administer drugs intravenously to circumvent impaired drug absorption. Rapid and severe weight loss due to severe GI involvement must be countered with parenteral nutrition. Despite the fact that weight loss has not been demonstrated to be a factor of poor prognosis (Guillevin *et al.* 1996), good nutritional status may help to reduce the infection rate.

In angina or cardiac failure, echocardiography, cardiac catheterization, and coronary angiography can document involvement of PAN and detect comorbid conditions, for example atherosclerosis, which can be treated.

A Vasculitis Damage Index (VDI) (Exley *et al.* 1997) has been devised to measure the cumulative impact of scars and other sequelae of the disease and its therapy (see Chapter 23).

How should PAN be treated?

Nearly all the reported series of treatment and outcome of PAN included patients with MPA (Cohen *et al.* 1980; Leib *et al.* 1979; Frohnert and Sheps 1967), and sometimes with CSS (Guillevin *et al.* 1999). Today, treatments for MPA and WG are considered together (Rasmussen *et al.* 1995), based on their shared pathogenic mechanisms, such as the presence of ANCA, and it seems more reasonable to consider the therapeutic strategy for PAN independently from that of MPA.

Since the initial use of glucocorticoids in 1950 to treat PAN (Bagenstoss *et al.* 1950), their use has increased the 5-year survival rate from 10% for untreated patients to about 55% in the mid-to-late 1970s (Cohen *et al.* 1980; Leib *et al.* 1979; Frohnert and Sheps 1967). Survival was further prolonged by adding either azathioprine or cyclophosphamide (CYC) (Fauci *et al.* 1979a; Leib *et al.* 1979), to the treatment regimen, attaining a 5-year survival rate of 82% for patients given glucocorticoids and CYC (Leib *et al.* 1979). These results were obtained from retrospective studies and have not always been confirmed in prospective studies (Cohen *et al.* 1980). Fauci *et al.* (1979b), who advocated the use of CYC, found that the mean duration of glucocorticoid treatment at the time of entry into the study was 22 months (range 2–48 months). Studies that include such patients with longstanding vasculitis may introduce some biases in that most deaths directly attributable to uncontrolled vasculitis (Fauci *et al.* 1979b) usually occur within the first 6 months of treatment.

Glucocorticoids

Glucocorticoids are given to all patients with PAN. In the case of HBV-related PAN, glucocorticoids should be administered for only a few days. In the others, the treatment is prolonged, lasting around 12 months. High doses may be useful at the time of diagnosis. The administration of methylprednisolone pulses (usually 7.5–15 mg/kg IV over 60 minutes repeated at 24-hour intervals for 1 to 3 days) has become widely used at the initiation of therapy for severe systemic vasculitis, especially in the presence of life-threatening organ involvement or the extension phase of mononeuropathy multiplex. This regimen has a rapid onset of action and is relatively safe. The dose of pulse methylprednisolone is empiric and doses under 1000 mg may be as effective. Side-effects of pulse methylprednisolone are usually mild and transient and include a bitter taste; facial flushing; headache; asthenia; marked rise of blood pressure; and temporary glucose intolerance. The severe side-effects, fortunately rare, include sudden death, cardiac arrhythmia, myocardial infarction, digestive tract bleeding, and seizure. Oral glucocorticoids are given at a dose of 1 mg/kg/day of prednisone or its equivalent of methylprednisolone. Therapy should be consolidated into a single morning dose. As the patient's clinical status improves and the biological markers of inflammation (C-reactive protein, erythrocyte sedimentation rate) return to normal, usually within 3 weeks to 1 month, tapering of the prednisone dose can begin.

In the therapeutic trials conducted by the French Vasculitis Study Group (Guillevin et al. 1992b), the timetable for the tapering of prednisone was long and drawn out. The daily dose was decreased by 2.5 mg every 10 days for 1 month, and then by 2.5 mg every week until a level equivalent to half the initial dose was reached. This dose was maintained for 3 weeks and then further decreased by 2.5 mg every week, to approximately 20 mg/day. A more careful tapering schedule was followed for doses below 20 mg/day. The daily dose was decreased by 1 mg every 1 to 2 weeks, to a dose of 10 mg/day. This level was maintained for 3 weeks and was then further decreased by 1 mg every month until the treatment was completely withdrawn. This regimen is effective and may control the disease without the adjunction of cytotoxic agents. When concomitant CYC is used, the prednisone dose should be tapered more rapidly to avoid complications.

Cyclophosphamide

CYC is conventionally prescribed at a dose of 2 mg/kg/day or less for 1 year and, in combination with glucocorticoids, represents the traditional treatment of systemic necrotizing vasculitides. Although this regimen is effective, it has a low therapeutic/toxic index. Side-effects have been extensively described in WG patients, but are not disease-specific. Major side-effects associated with daily CYC administration include hemorrhagic cystitis, bladder fibrosis, bone marrow suppression, ovarian failure, and cancer (bladder cancer and hematological malignancies) (Hoffman et al. 1992; Stillwell et al. 1988; Sneller 2000). Severe infections represent a major cause of mortality of patients with systemic necrotizing vasculitis, especially while they are receiving high glucocorticoid doses with adjunctive immunosuppressive drugs (Bourgarit et al. 2005; Gayraud et al. 2001; Gayraud et al. 1997).

In an attempt to limit the morbidity associated with daily CYC administration, protocols using intermittent treatment with higher doses have been developed (Gayraud et al. 1997; Guillevin et al. 2003). Pulse CYC is now being used increasingly to treat systemic necrotizing vasculitides and might be preferred to daily oral CYC. The CYC content of each pulse, and both the total number and the frequency of the pulses, should be adjusted according to the patient's condition, renal function, hematological data, and response to previous therapies, including previous CYC pulses. High-dose IV CYC may be dangerous in patients with renal insufficiency, so dose reduction according to renal function is prudent. During pulse therapy, as with oral daily CYC, intense hydration and the use of sodium 2-mercaptoethanesulfonate (mesna) is recommended. Pulse CYC therapy allows a lower cumulative dose to be given and exposes the patient to less potential toxicity for shorter periods than oral CYC. In the protocols of the French Vasculitis Study Group, the CYC pulse dose was $0.6 \, g/m^2$ given once monthly. We have recently reviewed the results of 6 pulses versus 12 pulses of CYC administered every 2 weeks for the three first pulses, then every 4 weeks until reaching the number of pulses scheduled, with no subsequent maintenance treatment for PAN patients with FFS ≥1 (Guillevin et al. 2003). The event-free survival rate was much higher in the 12-pulse group than in the 6-pulse group (68% versus 19%, respectively). It may be feasible to treat severe PAN patients with CYC until remission has been achieved and then to maintain remission with another immunosuppressant (such as azathioprine) for 12 months, as has been reported for systemic WG (Jayne et al. 2003), but this approach has not been validated in a prospective trial of PAN.

In our opinion, CYC should not be prescribed systematically as first-line treatment for all PAN patients and the management decision must consider the anatomical location of the involvement and its severity. When patients fail to respond to pulse CYC, oral CYC has been successfully used to control disease activity or relapse within the first 6 months of treatment (Généreau et al. 1994).

Other cytotoxic agents

Azathioprine, methotrexate and several other cytotoxic agents have been tested in PAN. They are reserved for PAN patients with contraindications to CYC, or as maintenance therapy for patients with the more severe forms after stopping CYC, and the recommended treatment duration is 12–18 months.

Plasma exchanges

To date, no cogent argument supports the systematic prescription of plasma exchanges at the time of diagnosis of PAN without HBV infection (Guillevin et al. 1992a), even for patients with poor prognostic factors (Guillevin et al. 1995d). Plasma exchanges might be useful as second-line treatment in PAN refractory to conventional therapy and might be able to limit disease sequelae, as has been seen in severe renal disease in ANCA-associated vasculitides.

Treatment duration

Because PAN has a low relapse rate, PAN may be treated for a shorter time than other systemic necrotizing vasculitides. In PAN patients, treatment often cures the disease and no maintenance regimen is needed. For PAN patients with poor prognosis factors, therapy with both glucocorticoids and CYC is given for about 12 months. Alternatively, glucocorticoids and CYC may be used together for 6 months, followed by glucocorticoids plus a less toxic drug such as azathioprine or methotrexate. Ongoing protocols are comparing doses and intensities of treatment with conventional drugs, as well as evaluating the efficacy of autologous bone-marrow transplantation (Bacon et al. 1998).

Therapeutic specificities

HBV-related PAN

For HBV-related PAN, conventional treatment with glucocorticoids and CYC allows the virus to replicate, thus facilitating evolution towards chronic hepatitis and liver cirrhosis. Thus, CYC and prolonged glucocorticoid treatment are contraindicated. The preferred initial treatment approach is to combine plasma exchanges and antiviral treatment with glucocorticoids to rapidly control the most severe life-threatening manifestations which are common during the first weeks of the disease. Glucocorticoids are then abruptly discontinued to enhance immunological clearance of HBV-infected hepatocytes and favor seroconversion from a positive HBeAg to a positive anti-HBeAb.

In HBV-related PAN, the combination of antiviral agents (vidarabine or interferon alpha-2b) provides excellent therapeutic results (Guillevin *et al.* 1993a; Guillevin *et al.* 1994). The efficacy of this strategy was confirmed in a series of 41 patients: 23 (56.1%) patients no longer exhibited serological evidence of HBV replication and 80.5% were cured (Guillevin *et al.* 1995b). New antiviral agents, such as lamivudine, have been shown to increase the seroconversion rate up to 60% (Guillevin *et al.* 2005; Guillevin *et al.* 2004). They have not been shown to improve the survival rate at 18 months when compared to conventional glucocorticoids (with or without CYC) (mortality rate at 18 months, 27.5% without antiviral therapy vs. 17.5% with combined antiviral therapy, p = 0.46). The benefits of adjunctive antiviral therapy probably appear after prolonged follow-up, since these drugs lower the risk of cirrhosis or liver failure.

Localized forms

As with PAN without poor prognosis factors, localized forms of PAN can be initially treated without immunosuppressant drugs, but these drugs can be held in reserve for refractory or relapsing disease. It should be noted that isolated appendix or gallbladder involvement has a good prognosis only after surgical removal. Cutaneous polyarteritis, particularly in children, may be successfully treated with colchicine or disulone (dapsone), often in combination with topical glucocorticoids. Similarly, colchicine or dapsone may be efficacious in PAN restricted to skeletal muscles.

References

Abgrall, S., Mouthon, L., Cohen, P., *et al.* (2001). Localized neurological necrotizing vasculitides. Three cases with isolated mononeuritis multiplex. *Journal of Rheumatology*, **28**, 631–3.

Abu-Farsakh, H., Mody, D., Brown, R. W. and Truong, L. D. (1994). Isolated vasculitis involving the female genital tract: clinicopathologic spectrum and phenotyping of inflammatory cells. *Modern Pathology*, **7**, 610–5.

Akcicek, F., Dilber, S., Ozgen, G. *et al.* (1994). Spontaneous perirenal hematoma due to periarteritis nodosa. *Nephron*, **68**, 396.

Akova, Y. A., Jabbur, N. S. and Foster, C. S. (1993). Ocular presentation of polyarteritis nodosa. Clinical course and management with steroid and cytotoxic therapy. *Ophthalmology*, **100**, 1775–81.

Allan, S., Towla, H., Smith, C., *et al.* (1982). Painful brachial plexopathy: an unusual presentation of polyarteritis nodosa. *Postgraduate Medical Journal*, **58**, 311–3.

Amarenco, P., Amarenco, G., Guillevin, L., *et al.* (1988). Neuropathie vésicale au cours des vascularites systémiques [in French]. *Annales de Médecine Interne*, **139**, 183–5.

Bacon, P., Exley, A., Carruthers, D. *et al.* (1998). Immune ablation with peripheral stem cell rescue in Wegener's: systemic vasculitis. *Clinical and Experimental Immunology*, **112**, S156.

Bagenstoss, A., Shick, R. and Polley, H. (1950). The effect of cortisone on the lesions of periarteritis nodosa. *American Journal of Pathology*, **26**, 709.

Blétry, O., Godeau, P., Charpentier, G. *et al.*(1980). Manifestations cardiaques de la périartérite noueuse. Fréquence de la cardiomyopathie non hypertensive [in Frenc]. *Archives des Maladies du Coeur et des Vaisseaux*, **73**, 1027–35.

Blidi, M., Quang, T. N., Cassan, P. and Guillevin, L. (1996). Cholécystites aigues de la périartérite noueuse. Huit observations [in French]. *Annales de Médecine Interne* (Paris), **147**, 304–12.

Bookman, A., Goode, E., McLoughlin, M. and Cohen, Z. (1983). Polyarteritis nodosa complicated by a ruptured intrahepatic aneurysm. *Arthritis and Rheumatism*, **26**, 106–8.

Bouche, P., Léger, J. M., Travers, M. A., Cathala, H. P. and Castaigne, P. (1986). Peripheral neuropathy in systemic vasculitis: clinical and electrophysiologic study of 22 patients. *Neurology*, **36**, 1598–602.

Bourgarit, A., Le Toumelin, P., Pagnoux, C. *et al.* (2005). Deaths Occurring during the First Year after Treatment Onset for Polyarteritis Nodosa, Microscopic Polyangiitis or Churg–Strauss Syndrome. A Retrospective Analysis of Causes and Factors Predictive of Mortality Based on 595 Patients. *Medicine* (Baltimore), **84**, 323–30.

Bron, K., Strott, C. and Shapiro, A. (1965). The diagnostic value of angiographic observations in polyarteritis nodosa. A case of multiple aneurysms in the visceral organs. *Archives of Internal Medicine*, **116**, 454–9.

Cacoub, P., Le Thi Huong, D., Guillevin, L. and Godeau, P. (1988). Causes of death in systemic vasculitis of polyarteritis nodosa. Analysis of a series of 165 patients [in French]. *Annales de Médecine Interne* (Paris), **139**, 381–90.

Calabrese, L. H. (1991). Vasculitis and infection with the human immunodeficiency virus. *Rheumatic Diseases Clinics of North America*, **17**, 131–47.

Camilleri, M., Pusey, C., Chadwick, V. and Rees, A. (1983). Gastrointestinal manifestations of systemic vasculitis. *Quarterly Journal of Medicine*, **52**, 141–9.

Casserly, L. F., Reddy, S. M., Rennke, H. G., Carpinito, G. A. and Levine, J. S. (1999). Reversible bilateral hydronephrosis without obstruction in hepatitis B-associated polyarteritis nodosa. *American Journal of Kidney Disease*, **34**, e11.

Castaigne, P., Cambier, J., Escourolle, R. *et al.* (1970). Les manifestations nerveuses centrales de la périartérite noueuse. A propos d'une observation anatomo-clinique [in French]. *Annales de Médecine Interne* (Paris), **121**, 375–6.

Chanseaud, Y., Tamby, M. C., Guilpain, P. *et al.* (2005). Analysis of autoantibody repertoires in small- and medium-sized vessels vasculitides. Evidence for specific perturbations in polyarteritis nodosa, microscopic polyangiitis, Churg–Strauss syndrome and Wegener's granulomatosis. *Journal of Autoimmunity*, **24**, 169–79.

Chen, K. T. (1989). Gallbladder vasculitis. *Journal of Clinical Gastroenterology*, **11**, 537–40.

Cid, M. (1996). New developments in the pathogenesis of systemic vasculitis. *Current Opinion in Rheumatology*, **9**, 1–11.

Cohen, L., Guillevin, L., Meyrier, A., Bironne, P., Blétry, O. and Godeau, P. (1986). Malignant arterial hypertension in periarteritis nodosa. Incidence, clinicobiologic parameters and prognosis based on a series of 165 cases [in French]. *Archives des Maladies du Coeur et des Vaisseaux*, **79**, 773–8.

Cohen, R. D., Conn, D. L. and Ilstrup, D. M. (1980). Clinical features, prognosis, and response to treatment in polyarteritis. *Mayo Clinic Proceedings*, **55**, 146–55.

Colmegna, I. and Maldonado-Cocco, J. A. (2005). Polyarteritis nodosa revisited. *Current Rheumatology Reports*, **7**, 288–96.

Corman, L. C. and Dolson, D. J. (1992). Polyarteritis nodosa and parvovirus B19 infection. *Lancet*, **339**, 491.

Cornfield, J. Z., Johnson, M. L., Dolehide, J. and Fowler, J. J. (1988). Massive renal hemorrhage owing to polyarteritis nodosa. *Journal of Urology*, **140**, 808–9.

Cowpe, J. and Hislop, W. (1983). Oral presentation of polyarteritis nodosa. *Oral Surgery*, **56**, 597.

Cruz, B. A., Ramanoelina, J., Mahr, A. *et al.* (2003). Prognosis and outcome of 26 patients with systemic necrotizing vasculitis admitted to the intensive care unit. *Rheumatology* (Oxford), **42**, 1183–8.

Darras-Joly, C., Lortholary, O., Cohen, P., Brauner, M. and Guillevin, L. (1995). Regressing microaneurysms in 5 cases of hepatitis B virus-related polyarteritis nodosa. *Journal of Rheumatology*, **22**, 876–80.

Diaz-Perez, J. L. and Winkelmann, R. K. (1974). Cutaneous periarteritis nodosa. *Archives of Dermatology*, **110**, 407–14.

Dugué, C., Renaudineau, Y., Jamin, C. and Youinou, P. (2004). Diagnostic and pathogenic implications of the heterogeneity of antiendothelial cell antibodies. *Autoimmunity Reviews*, **3** (Suppl.1), 11–3.

Dyck, P., Benstead, T., Conn, D., Stevens, J. and Windebandk, A. (1987). Non systemic vasculitic neuropathy. *Brain*, **110**, 843–54.

Elkon, K. B., Hughes, G. R., Catovsky, D. *et al.* (1979). Hairy-cell leukaemia with polyarteritis nodosa. *Lancet*, **2**, 280–2.

Esteva-Lorenzo, F. J., Ferreiro, J. L., Tardaguila, F., de la Fuente, A., Falasca, G. and Reginato, A. J. (1994). Case report 866. Pseudotumor of the muscle associated with necrotizing vasculitis of medium- and small-sized arteries and chronic myositis. *Skeletal Radiology*, **23**, 572–6.

Ewald, E. A., Griffin, D. and McCune, W. J. (1987). Correlation of angiographic abnormalities with disease manifestations and disease severity in polyarteritis nodosa. *Journal of Rheumatology*, **14**, 952–6.

Exley, A., Carruthers, D., Luqmani, R. *et al.* (1997). Damage occurs early in systemic vasculitis and is an index of outcome. *Quarterly Journal of Medicine*, **90**, 391–9.

Fauci, A. S., Haynes, B. and Katz, P. (1978). The spectrum of vasculitis: clinical, pathologic, immunologic and therapeutic considerations. *Annals of Internal Medicine*, **89**, 660–76.

Fauci, A. S., Katz, P., Haynes, B. F. and Wolff, S. M. (1979a). Cyclophosphamide therapy of severe systemic necrotizing vasculitis. *New England Journal of Medicine*, **301**, 235–8.

Ford, R. and Sieckert, R. (1965). Central nervous system manifestations of periarteritis nodosa. *Neurology*, **15**, 114–22.

Fortin, P. R., Larson, M. G., Watters, A. K., Yeadon, C. A., Choquette, D. and Esdaile, J. M. (1995). Prognostic factors in systemic necrotizing vasculitis of the polyarteritis nodosa group–a review of 45 cases. *Journal of Rheumatology*, **22**, 78–84.

Frohnert, P. and Sheps, S. (1967). Long term follow-up study of periarteritis nodosa. *American Journal of Medicine*, **43**, 8–14.

Fye, K., Becker, M., Theofilopoulos, A., Moutsopoulos, H., Feldman, J. and Talal, N. (1977). Immune complexes in hepatitis B antigen-associated periarteritis nodosa: detection by antibody independent cell-mediated cytotoxicity and the Raji cell assay. *American Journal of Medicine*, **62**, 783–91.

Gallien, S., Mahr, A., Réty, F. *et al.* (2002). Magnetic resonance imaging of skeletal muscle involvement in limb restricted vasculitis. *Annals of the Rheumatic Diseases*, **61**, 1107–9.

Ganesan, R., Ferryman, S. R., Meier, L. and Rollason, T. P. (2000). Vasculitis of the female genital tract with clinicopathologic correlation: a study of 46 cases with follow-up. *International Journal of Gynecological Pathology*, **19**, 258–65.

Gargollo, P. C., Barnewolt, C. E. and Diamond, D. A. (2004). Calcified ureteral stricture in a child with polyarteritis nodosa. *Journal of Urology*, **171**, 1254–5.

Gaskin, G., Savage, C., Ryan, J. *et al.* (1991). Antineutrophil cytoplasmic antibodies and disease activity during long-term follow-up of 70 patients with systemic vasculitis. *Nephrology, Dialysis, Transplantation*, **6**, 689–94.

Gayraud, M., Guillevin, L., Cohen, P. *et al.* (1997). Treatment of good-prognosis polyarteritis nodosa and Churg–Strauss syndrome: comparison of steroids and oral or pulse cyclophosphamide in 25 patients. French Cooperative Study Group for Vasculitides. *British Journal of Rheumatology*, **36**, 1290–7.

Gayraud, M., Guillevin, L., le Toumelin, P. *et al.* (2001). Long-term followup of polyarteritis nodosa, microscopic polyangiitis, and Churg–Strauss syndrome: analysis of four prospective trials including 278 patients. *Arthritis and Rheumatism*, **44**, 666–75.

Généreau, T., Lortholary, O., Leclerq, P. *et al.* (1994). Treatment of systemic vasculitis with cyclophosphamide and steroids: daily oral low-dose cyclophosphamide administration after failure of a pulse intravenous high-dose regimen in four patients. *British Journal of Rheumatology*, **33**, 959–62.

Généreau, T., Lortholary, O., Pottier, M. A. *et al.* (1999). Temporal artery biopsy: a diagnostic tool for systemic necrotizing vasculitis. French Vasculitis Study Group. *Arthritis and Rheumatism*, **42**, 2674–81.

Ghérardi, R., Belec, L., Mhiri, C. *et al.* (1993). The spectrum of vasculitis in human immunodeficiency virus-infected patients. A clinicopathologic evaluation. *Arthritis and Rheumatism*, **36**, 1164–74.

Gisselbrecht, M., Cohen, P., Lortholary, O. *et al.* (1998). Human immunodeficiency virus-related vasculitis. Clinical presentation of and therapeutic approach to eight cases [in French]. *Annales de Médecine Interne* (Paris), **149**, 398–405.

Godeau, B., Coutant-Perronne, V., Le Thi Huong, D. *et al.* (1994). *Pneumocystis carinii* pneumonia in the course of connective tissue disease: report of 34 cases. *Journal of Rheumatology*, **21**, 246–51.

Godeau, B., Mainardi, J. L., Roudot, T. F. *et al.* (1995). Factors associated with *Pneumocystis carinii* pneumonia in Wegener's granulomatosis. *Annals of the Rheumatic Diseases*, **54**, 991–4.

Godeau, P., Guillevin, L., Tucat, G. *et al.* (1979). Périartérite noueuse avec pancréatite aiguë. Deux nouvelles observations [in French]. *Lyon Médical*, **242**, 279–81.

Gourgoutis, G. D., Paguirigan, A. A. and Berzins, T. (1971). Gastric perforation in polyarteritis nodosa. Report of a patient. *American Journal of Digestive Diseases*, **16**, 171–7.

Grasland, A., Pouchot, J., Damade, R. and Vinceneux, P. (1996). Uterine localization of periarteritis nodosa disclosed by fever of long duration [in French]. *Revue de Médecine Interne*, **17**, 58–60.

Grau, G. E., Roux, L. P., Gysler, C. *et al.* (1989). Serum cytokine changes in systemic vasculitis. *Immunology*, **68**, 196–8.

Guillevin, L., Cohen, P., Gayraud, M., Lhote, F., Jarrousse, B. and Casassus, P. (1999). Churg–Strauss syndrome. Clinical study and long-term follow-up of 96 patients. *Medicine* (Baltimore), **78**, 26–37.

Guillevin, L., Cohen, P., Mahr, A. *et al.* (2003). Treatment of polyarteritis nodosa and microscopic polyangiitis with poor prognosis factors: a prospective trial comparing glucocorticoids and six or twelve cyclophosphamide pulses in sixty-five patients. *Arthritis and Rheumatism*, **49**, 93–100.

Guillevin, L., Fain, O., Lhote, F. *et al.* (1992a). Lack of superiority of steroids plus plasma exchange to steroids alone in the treatment of polyarteritis nodosa and Churg–Strauss syndrome. A prospective, randomized trial in 78 patients. *Arthritis and Rheumatism*, **35**, 208–15.

Guillevin, L., Le Thi Huong, D., Godeau, P., Jais, P. and Wechsler, B. (1988). Clinical findings and prognosis of polyarteritis nodosa and Churg–Strauss angiitis: a study in 165 patients. *British Journal of Rheumatology*, **27**, 258–64.

Guillevin, L., Lhote, F., Jarrousse, B. and Fain, O. (1992b). Treatment of polyarteritis nodosa and Churg–Strauss syndrome. A meta-analysis of 3 prospective controlled trials including 182 patients over 12 years. *Annales de Medecine Interne*, **143**, 405–16.

Guillevin, L., Lhote, F., Leon, A., Fauvelle, F., Vivitski, L. and Trépo, C. (1993a). Treatment of polyarteritis nodosa related to hepatitis B virus with short term steroid therapy associated with antiviral agents and plasma exchanges. A prospective trial in 33 patients. *Journal of Rheumatology*, **20**, 289–98.

Guillevin, L., Lhote, F., Sauvaget, F. *et al.* (1994). Treatment of polyarteritis nodosa related to hepatitis B virus with interferon-alpha and plasma exchanges. *Annals of Rheumatic Diseases*, **53**, 334–7.

Guillevin, L., Lhote, F., Brauner, M. and Casassus, P. (1995a). Antineutrophil cytoplasmic antibodies (ANCA) and abnormal angiograms in polyarteritis nodosa and Churg–Strauss syndrome: indications for the diagnosis of microscopic polyangiitis. *Annales de Medecine Interne* (Paris), **146**, 548–50.

Guillevin, L., Lhote, F., Cohen, P. *et al.* (1995b). Polyarteritis nodosa related to hepatitis B virus. A prospective study with long-term observation of 41 patients. *Medicine* (Baltimore), **74**, 238–53.

Guillevin, L., Lhote, F., Gallais, V. *et al.* (1995c). Gastrointestinal tract involvement in polyarteritis nodosa and Churg- Strauss syndrome. *Annales de Medecine Interne*, **146**, 260–7.

Guillevin, L., Lhote, F., Cohen, P. *et al.* (1995d). Corticosteroids plus pulse cyclophosphamide and plasma exchanges versus corticosteroids plus pulse cyclophosphamide alone in the treatment of polyarteritis nodosa and Churg–Strauss syndrome patients with factors predicting poor prognosis. A prospective, randomized trial in sixty-two patients. *Arthritis and Rheumatism*, **38**, 1638–45.

Guillevin, L., Lhote, F., Gayraud, M. *et al.* (1996). Prognostic factors in polyarteritis nodosa and Churg–Strauss syndrome. A prospective study in 342 patients. *Medicine* (Baltimore), **75**, 17–28.

Guillevin, L., Mahr, A., Cohen, P. *et al.* (2004). Short-term corticosteroids then lamivudine and plasma exchanges to treat hepatitis B virus-related polyarteritis nodosa. *Arthritis and Rheumatism*, **51**, 482–7.

Guillevin, L., Mahr, A., Callard, P. *et al.* (2005). Hepatitis B virus-associated polyarteritis nodosa: clinical characteristics, outcome, and impact of treatment in 115 patients. *Medicine* (Baltimore), **84**, 313–22.

Guillevin, L., Ronco, P. and Verroust, P. (1990). Circulating immune complexes in systemic necrotizing vasculitis of the polyarteritis nodosa group. Comparison of HBV-related polyarteritis nodosa and Churg Strauss Angiitis. *Journal of Autoimmunology*, **3**, 789–92.

Guillevin, L., Visser, H., Noël, L. H. *et al.* (1993b). Antineutrophil cytoplasm antibodies in systemic polyarteritis nodosa with and without hepatitis B virus infection and Churg–Strauss syndrome- -62 patients. *Journal of Rheumatology*, **20**, 1345–9.

Gunal, N., Kara, N., Cakar, N., Kocak, H., Kahramanyol, O. and Cetinkaya, E. (1997). Cardiac involvement in childhood polyarteritis nodosa. *International Journal of Cardiology*, **60**, 257–62.

Ha, H. K., Lee, S. H., Rha, S. E. *et al.* (2000). Radiologic features of vasculitis involving the gastrointestinal tract. *Radiographics*, **20**, 779–94.

Hachulla, E., Bourdon, F., Taieb, S. *et al.* (1993). Embolization of two bleeding aneurysms with platinum coils in a patient with polyarteritis nodosa. *Journal of Rheumatology*, **20**, 158–61.

Hamidou, M. A., Moreau, A., Toquet, C., El Kouri, D., de Faucal, P. and Grolleau, J. Y. (2003). Temporal arteritis associated with systemic necrotizing vasculitis. *Journal of Rheumatology*, **30**, 2165–9.

Hasler, P., Kistler, H. and Gerber, H. (1995). Vasculitides in hairy cell leukemia. *Seminars in Arthritis and Rheumatism*, **25**, 134–42.

Haugeberg, G., Bie, R. and Johnsen, V. (1997). Vasculitic changes in the temporal artery in polyarteritis nodosa. *Scandinavian Journal of Rheumatology*, **26**, 383–5.

Hauschild, S., Csernok, E., Schmitt, W. H. and Gross, W. L. (1994). Antineutrophil cytoplasmic antibodies in systemic polyarteritis nodosa with and without hepatitis B virus infection and Churg–Strauss syndrome – 62 patients. *Journal of Rheumatology*, **21**, 1173–4.

Hautekeete, M. L., Babany, G., Marcellin, P. *et al.* (1990). Retroperitoneal fibrosis after surgery for aortic aneurysm in a patient with periarteritis nodosa: successful treatment with corticosteroids. *Journal of Internal Medicine*, **228**, 533–6.

Henegar, C., Puéchal, X., Pagnoux, C. *et al.* (2005). Development of a set of potential diagnostic criteria for polyarteritis nodosa by retrospective analysis of the French Vasculitis Study Group's patient database. *Arthritis and Rheumatism*, **52** (Supp.), S225.

Héron, E., Fiessinger, J. N. and Guillevin, L. (2003). Polyarteritis nodosa presenting as acute leg ischemia. *Journal of Rheumatology*, **30**, 1344–6.

Hirohata, S., Tanimoto, K. and Ito, K. (1993). Elevation of cerebrospinal fluid interleukin-6 activity in patients with vasculitides and central nervous system involvement. *Clinical Immunology and Immunopathology*, **66**, 225–9.

Hoffman, G. S., Kerr, G. S., Leavitt, R. Y. *et al.* (1992). Wegener granulomatosis: an analysis of 158 patients. *Annals of Internal Medicine*, **116**, 488–98.

Holsinger, D., Osmundson, P. and Edward, J. (1962). The heart in polyarteritis nodosa. *Circulation*, **25**, 610–8.

Holt, S. and Jackson, P. (1975). Ruptured coronary aneurysm and valvulitis in an infant with polyarteritis nodosa. *Journal of Pathology*, **117**, 83–7.

Horgan, C., Foster, C., D'Amico, D. *et al.*(1986). Retinal vasculitis in polyarteritis nodosa. *Retina*, **6**, 205.

Hu, P. J., Shih, I. M., Hutchins, G. M. and Hellmann, D. B. (1997). Polyarteritis nodosa of the pericardium: antemortem diagnosis in a pericardiectomy specimen. *Journal of Rheumatology*, **24**, 2042–4.

Hutson, T. E. and Hoffman, G. S. (2000). Temporal concurrence of vasculitis and cancer: a report of 12 cases. *Arthritis Care and Research*, **13**, 417–23.

Iino, T., Eguchi, K., Sakai, M., Nagataki, S., Ishijima, M. and Toriyama, K. (1992). Polyarteritis nodosa with aortic dissection: necrotizing vasculitis of the vasa vasorum. *Journal of Rheumatology*, **19**, 1632–6.

Ito, M., Sano, K., Inaba, H. and Hotchi, M. (1991). Localized necrotizing arteritis. A report of two cases involving the gallbladder and pancreas. *Archives of Pathology and Laboratory Medicine*, **115**, 780–3.

Jamieson, P., Giuliani, M. and Martinez, A. (1991). Necrotizing angiopathy presenting with multifocal conduction blocks. *Neurology*, **41**, 442–4.

Jamin, C., Dugué, C., Alard, J. E. *et al.* (2005). Induction of endothelial cell apoptosis by the binding of anti-endothelial cell antibodies to Hsp60 in vasculitis-associated systemic autoimmune diseases. *Arthritis and Rheumatism*, **52**, 4028–38.

Jarrousse, B., Guillevin, L., Bindi, P. *et al.* (1993). Increased risk of *Pneumocystis carinii* pneumonia in patients with Wegener's granulomatosis. *Clinical and Experimental Rheumatology*, **11**, 615–21.

Jayne, D., Rasmussen, N., Andrassy, K., Bacon, P. *et al.* (2003). A randomized trial of maintenance therapy for vasculitis-associated with antineutrophil cytoplasmic antibodies. *New England Journal of Medicine*, **349**, 36–44.

Jennette, J. C., Falk, R. J., Andrassy, K. *et al.* (1994). Nomenclature of systemic vasculitides. Proposal of an international consensus conference. *Arthritis and Rheumatism*, **37**, 187–92.

Kaya, E., Utas, C., Balkanli, S., Basbug, M. and Onursever, A. (1994). Isolated ovarian polyarteritis nodosa. *Acta Obstetricia et Gynecologica Scandinavica*, **73**, 736–8.

Kinyoun, J., Kalina, R. and Klein, M. (1987). Choroidal involvement in systemic necrotizing vasculitis. *Archives of Ophthalmology*, **105**, 939.

Krol, T., Robinson, J., Bekeris, L. and Messmore, H. (1983). Hairy cell leukemia and a fatal periarteritis nodosa-like syndrome. *Archives of Pathology and Laboratory Medicine*, **107**, 583–5.

Kussmaul, A. and Maier, R. (1866). Ueber eine bisher nicht beschriebene eigenthümliche Arterienerkrankung (Periarteritis nodosa), die mit Morbus Brightii und rapid fortschreitender allgemeiner Muskellähmung einhergeht. *Deutsches Archiv für Klinische Medizin*, **1**, 484–518.

Le Thi Huong, D., Wechsler, B., Guillevin, L. *et al.* (1985). Digestive manifestations of periarteritis nodosa in a series of 120 cases. [in French]. *Gastroentérologie Clinique et Biologique*, **9**, 697–703.

Le Tonqueze, M., Jamin, C., Bohme, M., Le Corre, R., Dueymes, M. and Youinou, P. (1996). Establishment and characterization of permanent human endothelial cell clones. *Lupus*, **5**, 103–12.

Lee, C. and Kay, S. (1958). Primary polyarteritis nodosa of the stomach and small intestine as a cause of gastro-intestinal hemorrhage. *Annals of Surgery*, **147**, 714–25.

Leib, E. S., Restivo, C. and Paulus, H. E. (1979). Immunosuppressive and corticosteroid therapy of polyarteritis nodosa. *American Journal of Medicine*, **67**, 941–7.

Leruez, V. M., Lauge, A., Morinet, F., Guillevin, L. and Dény, P. (1994). Polyarteritis nodosa and parvovirus B19. *Lancet*, **344**, 263–4.

Levine, S. M., Hellmann, D. B. and Stone, J. H. (2002). Gastrointestinal involvement in polyarteritis nodosa (1986–2000): presentation and outcomes in 24 patients. *American Journal of Medicine*, **112**, 386–91.

Levy, A., Weinberger, A., Mor, C. and Pinkhas, J. (1986). Localized polyarteritis nodosa: cases involving the lower extremities and the breast. *Rheumatology International*, **6**, 43–4.

Li, A., Rhodes, J. and Valentine, A. (1979). Spontaneous liver rupture in polyarteritis nodosa. *British Journal of Surgery*, **66**, 251–2.

Lie, J. T. (1992). Retroperitoneal polyarteritis nodosa presenting as ureteral obstruction. *Journal of Rheumatology*, **19**, 1628–31.

Lightfoot, Jr. R. W., Michel, B. A., Bloch, D. A. *et al.* (1990). The American College of Rheumatology 1990 criteria for the classification of polyarteritis nodosa. *Arthritis and Rheumatism*, **33**, 1088–93.

Lomeo, R. M., Silver, R. M. and Brothers, M. (1989). Spontaneous dissection of the internal carotid artery in a patient with polyarteritis nodosa. *Arthritis and Rheumatism*, **32**, 1625–6.

Lupoli, S., Gargiulo, A., Rossi, R. and Ames, P. R. (2004). Myositis as a presenting feature of polyarteritis nodosa. *Clinical and Experimental Rheumatology*, **22**, 507–8.

Luqmani, R., Bacon, P., Moots, R. *et al.* (1994). Birmingham Vasculitis Activity Score (BVAS) in systemic necrotizing vasculitis. *Quaterly Journal of Medicine*, **87**, 671–8.

MacDonald, W. B. and Blake, M. P. (2004). Periostitis and localized myositis in polyarteritis nodosa. *Clinical Nuclear Medicine*, **29**, 703–5.

Mader, R. and Keystone, E. C. (1992). Infections that cause vasculitis. *Current Opinion in Rheumatology*, **4**, 35–8.

Mahr, A., Guillevin, L., Poissonnet, M. and Ayme, S. (2004). Prevalences of polyarteritis nodosa, microscopic polyangiitis, Wegener's granulomatosis, and Churg–Strauss syndrome in a French urban multiethnic population in 2000: a capture-recapture estimate. *Arthritis and Rheumatism*, **51**, 92–9.

Malan, P., Ciurana, A. and Boudet, C. (1986). Artérite rétinienne bilatérale avec dilatations anévrysmales multiples [in French]. *Journal Français d'Ophtalmologie*, **9**, 23–8.

Mason, A., Theal, J., Bain, V., Adams, E. and Perrillo. R. (2005). Hepatitis B virus replication in damaged endothelial tissues of patients with extrahepatic disease. *American Journal of Gastroenterology*, **100**, 972–6.

Mayo, J., Arias, M., Leno, C. and Berciano, J. (1986). Vascular parkinsonism and periarteritis nodosa. *Neurology*, **36**, 874–5.

McMahon, B. J., Heyward, W. L., Templin, D. W., Clement, D. and Lanier, A. P. (1989). Hepatitis B-associated polyarteritis nodosa in Alaskan Eskimos: clinical and epidemiologic features and long-term follow-up. *Hepatology*, **9**, 97–101.

Miller, D. L. (2000). Angiography in polyarteritis nodosa. *American Journal of Roentgenology*, **175**, 1747–8.

Moore, P. and Fauci, A. (1981). Neurologic manifestations of systemic vasculitis: a retrospective and prospective study of the clinico-pathologic features and responses to therapy in 25 patients. *American Journal of Medicine*, **71**, 517–24.

Moore, P. M. and Calabrese, L. H. (1994). Neurologic manifestations of systemic vasculitides. *Seminars in Neurology*, **14**, 300–6.

Moore, P. M. (1995). Neurological manifestation of vasculitis: update on immunopathogenic mechanisms and clinical features. *Annals of Neurology*, **37** (Suppl. 1), 131–41.

Moreland, L. W. and Ball, G. V. (1990). Cutaneous polyarteritis nodosa. *American Journal of Medicine*, **88**, 426–30.

Mowrey, F. H. and Lundberg, E. A. (1954). The clinical manifestations of essential polyangiitis (periarteritis nodosa), with emphasis on the hepatic manifestations. *Annals of Internal Medicine*, **40**, 1145–64.

Nakamura, T., Tomoda, K., Yamamura, Y., Tsukano, M., Honda, I. and Iyama, K. (2003). Polyarteritis nodosa limited to calf muscles: a case report and review of the literature. *Clinical Rheumatology*, **22**, 149–53.

Nakazawa, K., Itoh, N., Duan, H. J., Komiyama, Y. and Shigematsu, H. (1992). Polyarteritis nodosa with atrophy of the left hepatic lobe. *Acta Pathologica Japonica*, **42**, 662–6.

Nohr, M., Laustsen, J. and Falk, E. (1989). Isolated necrotizing panarteritis of the gallbladder. Case report. *Acta Chirurgica Scandinvica*, **155**, 485–7.

Ozen, S., Anton, J., Arisoy, N. *et al.* (2004). Juvenile polyarteritis: results of a multicenter survey of 110 children. *Journal of Pediatrics*, **145**, 517–22.

Ozen, S., Ruperto, N., Dillon, M. J., *et al.* (2006) EULAR/PReS endorsed consensus criteria for the classification of childhood vasculitides. *Annals of the Rheumatic Diseases*, **65**, 936–41.

Pagnoux, C., Mahr, A., Cohen, P. and Guillevin, L. (2005). Presentation and outcome of gastrointestinal involvement in systemic necrotizing vasculitides: analysis of 62 patients with polyarteritis nodosa, microscopic polyangiitis, Wegener granulomatosis, Churg–Strauss syndrome, or rheumatoid arthritis-associated vasculitis. *Medicine* (Baltimore), **84**, 115–28.

Panegyres, P., Blumberg, P., Leong, A. and Bourne, A. (1990). Vasculitis of peripheral nerve and skeletal muscle: clinicopathological correlation and immunopathic mechanisms. *Journal of Neurological Sciences*, **100**, 193–202.

Parangi, S., Oz, M. C., Blume, R. S. *et al.* (1991). Hepatobiliary complications of polyarteritis nodosa. *Archives of Surgery*, **126**, 909–12.

Piette, J. C., Bourgault, I., Legrain, S. *et al.* (1987). Systemic polyarteritis nodosa diagnosed at hysterectomy. *American Journal of Medicine*, **82**, 836–8.

Porter, B. F., Frost, P. and Hubbard, G. B. (2003). Polyarteritis nodosa in a cynomolgus macaque (Macaca fascicularis). *Veterinary Pathology*, **40**, 570–3.

Prince, A. M. and Trépo, C. (1971). Role of immune complexes involving SH antigen in pathogenesis of chronic active hepatitis and polyarteritis nodosa. *Lancet*, **1**, 1309–12.

Puisieux, F., Woesteland, H., Hachulla, E., Hatron, P. Y., Dewailly, P. and Devulder, B. (1997). Clinical symptomatology and prognosis of periarteritis nodosa in the elderly. Retrospective study of 25 periarteritis nodosa cases in young adults and 22 cases in aged patients [in French]. *Revue de Médecine Interne*, **18**, 195–200.

Rajani, R. M., Dalvi, B. V., D'Silva, S. A., Lokhandwala, Y. Y. and Kale, P. A. (1991). Acute myocardial infarction with normal coronary arteries in a case of polyarteritis nodosa: possible role of coronary artery spasm. *Postgraduate Medical Journal*, **67**, 78–80.

Rasmussen, N., Jayne, D., Abramowicz, D. *et al.* (1995). European therapeutic trials in ANCA-associated systemic vasculitis: disease scoring, consensus regimens and proposed clinical trials. *Clininical and Experimental Immunology*, **101**, 29–34.

Reinhold-Keller, E., Herlyn, K., Wagner-Bastmeyer, R. *et al.* (2002). No difference in the incidences of vasculitides between north and south Germany: first results of the German vasculitis register. *Rheumatology* (Oxford), **41**, 540–9.

Rodríguez Pereira, C., Suárez Peñaranda, J. M., del Río, E. and Forteza Vila, J. (1997). Cutaneous granulomatous vasculitis after herpes zoster infection showing polyarteritis nodosa-like features. *Clinical and Experimental Dermatology*, **22**, 274–6.

Ropert, A. and Metral, S. (1990). Conduction block in neuropathies with necrotizing vasculitis. *Muscle and Nerve*, **13**, 102–5.

Sack, M., Cassidy, J. T. and Bole, G. G. (1975). Prognostic factors in polyarteritis. *Journal of Rheumatology*, **2**, 411–20.

Said, G. (1997). Necrotizing peripheral nerve vasculitis. *Neurologic Clinics*, **15**, 835–48.

Said, G. and Lacroix, C. (2005). Primary and secondary vasculitic neuropathy. *Journal of Neurology*, **252**, 633–41.

Salojin, K. V., Le Tonqueze, M., Nassovov, E. L. *et al.* (1996). Anti-endothelial cell antibodies in patients with various forms of vasculitis. *Clinical and Experimental Rheumatology*, **14**, 163–9.

San, A., Aydin, N. E., Akcay, G., Selcuk, Y. and Okyar, G. (1990). Spontaneous bilateral rupture of kidneys in a patient with polyarteritis nodosa. A case report. *Scandinavian Journal of Urology and Nephrology*, **24**, 319–21.

Schrader, M. L., Hochman, J. S. and Bulkley, B. H. (1985). The heart in polyarteritis nodosa: a clinicopathologic study. *American Heart Journal*, **109**, 1353–9.

Scott, D., Bacon, P., Elliott, P., Tribe, C. and Wallington, T. (1982). Systemic vasculitis in a district general hospital 1972–1980: clinical and laboratory features, classification and prognosis in 80 cases. *Quarterly Journal of Medicine*, **51**, 292–311.

Sergent, J., Lockshin, M., Christian, C. and Gocke, D. (1976). Vasculitis with hepatitis B antigenemia: long term observations in nine patients. *Medicine*, **55**, 1–18.

Servant, A., Bogard, M., Delaugerre, C., Cohen, P., Dény, P. and Guillevin, L. (1998). GB virus C in systemic medium- and small-vessel necrotizing vasculitides. *British Journal of Rheumatology*, **37**, 1292–4.

Short, D. J. and Webley, M. (1984). Periosteal new bone formation complicating juvenile polyarteritis nodosa. *Journal of the Royal Society of Medicine*, **77**, 325–7.

Sneller, M. C. (2000). Cystitis, bladder cancer, and myelodysplasia in patients with Wegener's granulomatosis: comment on the article by Reinhold-Keller et al. *Arthritis and Rheumatism*, **43**, 2853–5.

Stillwell, T., Benson, R., DeRemee, R. *et al.* (1988). Cyclophosphamide'induced bladder toxicity in Wegener's granulomatosis. *Arthritis and Rheumatism*, **31**, 465–70.

Takahashi, M. (1993). Inflammatory diseases of the coronary artery in children. *Coronary Artery Disease*, **4**, 133–8.

Tamby, M. C., Chanseaud, Y., Humbert, M. *et al.* (2005). Anti-endothelial cell antibodies in idiopathic and systemic sclerosis associated pulmonary arterial hypertension. *Thorax*, **60**, 765–72.

Tang, P. H. and Segal, A. J. (1971). Polyarteritis nodosa of infancy. Fatal late complication. *Journal of the American Medical Association*, **217**, 1666–70.

Tasdemir, I., Turgan, C., Emri, S. *et al.* (1988). Spontaneous perirenal haematoma secondary to polyarteritis nodosa. *British Journal of Urology*, **62**, 219–22.

Teichman, J. M., Mattrey, R. F., Demby, A. M. and Schmidt, J. D. (1993). Polyarteritis nodosa presenting as acute orchitis: a case report and review of the literature. *Journal of Urology*, **149**, 1139–40.

Thone, M. (1988). Buccal ulceration in a case of periarteritis nodosa [in French]. *Acta Stomatologica Belgica*, **85**, 69–75.

Till, S. H. and Amos, R. S. (1997). Long-term follow-up of juvenile-onset cutaneous polyarteritis nodosa associated with streptococcal infection. *British Journal of Rheumatology*, **36**, 909–11.

Travers, R. L., Allison, D. J., Brettle, R. P. and Hughes, G. R. (1979). Polyarteritis nodosa: a clinical and angiographic analysis of 17 cases. *Seminars in Arthritis and Rheumatism*, **8**, 184–99.

Trépo, C. and Thivolet, J. (1970a). Hepatitis associated antigen and periarteritis nodosa. *Vox Sanguinis*, **19**, 410–1.

Trépo, C. and Thivolet, J. (1970b). Antigène Australia, virus de l'hépatite et périartérite noueuse. *Presse Médicale*, **78**, 1575.

Trépo, C., Zuckerman, A., Bird, R. and Prince, A. (1974). The role of circulating hepatitis B antigen/antibody immune complexes in the pathogenesis of vascular and hepatic manifestations in polyarteritis nodosa. *Journal of Clinical Pathology*, **27**, 863–8.

Vathenen, A., Skinner, D. and Shale, D. (1988). Treatment response with bilateral mixed deafness and facial palsy in polyarteritis nodosa. *American Journal of Medicine*, **84**, 1081–2.

Wang, T., Avlonitis, E. and Relkin, R. (1988). Systemic necrotizing vasculitis causing bone necrosis. *American Journal of Medicine*, **84**, 1085–6.

Warfield, A. T., Lee, S. J., Phillips, S. M. and Pall, A. A. (1994). Isolated testicular vasculitis mimicking a testicular neoplasm. *Journal of Clinical Pathology*, **47**, 1121–3.

Watts, R., Gonzalez-Gay, M., Lane, S. *et al.* (2001). Geoepidemiology of systemic vasculitis: comparison of the incidence in two regions of Europe. *Annals of the Rheumatic Diseases*, **60**, 170–2.

Weck, K. E., Dal Canto, A. J., Gould, J. D. *et al.* (1997). Murine gamma-herpesvirus 68 causes severe large-vessel arteritis in mice lacking interferon-gamma responsiveness: a new model for virus-induced vascular disease. *Nature Medicine*, **3**, 1346–53.

Yamashina, M. and Wilson, T. K. (1985). A mammographic finding in focal polyarteritis nodosa. *British Journal of Radiology*, **58**, 91–2.

Zeek, P. (1952). Periarteritis nodosa. A critical review. *American Journal of Pathology*, **22**, 277–90.

Zizic, T. M., Classen, J. N. and Stevens, M. B. (1982). Acute abdominal complications of systemic lupus erythematosus and polyarteritis nodosa. *American Journal of Medicine*, **73**, 525–31.

CHAPTER 27

Microscopic polyangiitis

Loïc Guillevin, Christian Pagnoux, and Luis Teixeira

Introduction

Initially considered a 'microscopic' form of polyarteritis nodosa (PAN), microscopic polyangiitis (MPA) was viewed as distinct from PAN by Wohlwill (1923), and then redefined by Davson *et al.* (1948). Its unanimous recognition as a clearly different entity among systemic vasculitides occurred only years later (Jennette *et al.* 1994). MPA is a small-sized vessel systemic necrotizing vasculitis whose typical clinical manifestations are similar to those encountered in PAN, thereby explaining decades of confusion. In further contrast to PAN, MPA belongs to the group of vasculitides associated with antineutrophil cytoplasmic antibodies (ANCA), such as Wegener's granulomatosis (WG) and Churg–Strauss syndrome (CSS). Recognition of MPA as a separate entity also implied different therapeutic strategies than those adopted for PAN and closer to the treatment of WG; however, MPA has some unique features which are detailed below.

Classification criteria

MPA did not appear in the classification criteria established in 1990 by the American College of Rheumatology (ACR) (Bloch *et al.* 1990; Lightfoot *et al.* 1990). In the past, PAN and MPA were thought to be different forms of the same disease because their main clinical manifestations (constitutional symptoms, neurological, gastrointestinal manifestations, etc.) are very similar, thereby explaining why they were considered together in the ACR classification criteria. However, major differences exist between these two entities, and this divergence needed to be clarified. MPA is a small-sized vessel vasculitis, which explains some of its clinical characteristics, such as glomerular involvement, with frequent presence of rapidly progressive glomerulonephritis (RPGN), and sometimes pulmonary capillaritis, manifesting as alveolar hemorrhage, signs of which are not found in PAN (Savage *et al.* 1985). Since the discovery of ANCA (van der Woude *et al.* 1985), which are only present in patients with some small-sized vessel vasculitides and not in those with PAN, MPA has been further differentiated from PAN.

The Chapel Hill international consensus conference established a new nomenclature for the classification of systemic vasculitides that defines and clearly separates MPA and PAN (Jennette *et al.* 1994) (see Table 26.2 in Chapter 26). In this nomenclature, which is intended for classification and not for diagnosis, MPA is defined as a necrotizing vasculitis, with few or no immune deposits, that affects small-sized vessels, especially arterioles, capillaries, and venules, and is often responsible for glomerulonephritis and lung capillaritis. However, it recognizes that MPA may also, but not predominantly, affect medium-sized vessels. This may raise a real diagnostic dilemma for clinicians and pathologists confronted with such an overlapping clinical picture.

Epidemiology

Like all other vasculitides, MPA is a rare disease. Furthermore, as stated above, PAN and MPA have long been grouped together in published studies. Hence, valid epidemiological data are sparse, and only the more recent studies can be considered reliable for MPA incidence and prevalence. MPA has been reported world-wide and affects all racial/ethnic groups, but with a probable predominance in Caucasians (Falk *et al.* 1990b; Handa *et al.* 2001). Males are affected slightly more frequently with a male:female ratio ranging from 1.1 to 1.8 (Adu *et al.* 1987; Savage *et al.* 1985). The average age at onset is about 50 years old. Soon after the introduction of ANCA testing and the Chapel Hill Consensus Conference, total annual incidence was estimated at 3.6 per 1,000,000 in England (Watts *et al.* 1996). As for WG, some authors reported a possible North–South gradient, with the highest annual incidence being observed in Northern European countries, at 16 per 1,000,000 in Sweden, for example (Tidman *et al.* 1998). In France, MPA prevalence was 25.1 per 1,000,000 in Seine-Saint-Denis, a northern suburb of Paris (Mahr *et al.* 2004), suggesting a possible increasing frequency of MPA within the last few decades. The recognition of MPA as a distinct clinical entity and the use of ANCA testing might also explain (at least in part) these results, which must be confirmed by additional studies.

Pathogenesis

MPA is an ANCA-related vasculitis. Perinuclear-labeling (pANCA) with antimyeloperoxidase (MPO) specificity (Jennette *et al.* 1989) has been found in nearly 75% of MPA patients (Guillevin *et al.* 1999). MPO is a 140-kDa protein composed of two identical heterodimers encoded by a single gene, located in chromosome 17q21.3. MPO constitutes about 5% of all neutrophil proteins and is present in the cytoplasmic granules at very high concentrations.

Investigators have thought that this enzyme catalyzes the H_2O_2-dependent oxidation of halides that can react with and kill microbes. Another possible MPO function is to protect the digestive enzymes from oxidative denaturation by removing H_2O_2 from the phagocytic vacuole. In fact, MPO-knockout mice are abnormally susceptible to bacterial (Hirche *et al.* 2005) and mainly fungal infections (Aratani *et al.* 2000).

A few MPA patients have cytoplasm-labeling cANCA with antiproteinase 3 (PR3) specificity. PR3 is a 29-kDa neutrophil serine protease, encoded by a single gene, located in chromosome 19p13.3. This protein is stored in granules of human neutrophils and monocytes. PR3 is mostly involved in the pathogenesis of WG.

ANCA are now considered a useful immunological marker for the diagnosis of vasculitis (see Chapter 6). Over the last decade, numerous *in vitro* data and two animal models (Heeringa *et al.* 1998; Pfister *et al.* 2004; Xiao *et al.* 2002) have supported a direct pathogenic role of ANCA in systemic vasculitis (see Chapters 7 and 8). Falk *et al.* (1990a) showed that IgG-ANCA can activate tumor necrosis factor (TNF)-α primed neutrophils, thereby inducing the production of reactive oxygen metabolites and the release of lysosomal proteolytic enzymes, including ANCA-target antigens. It has been demonstrated that ANCA promote neutrophil adhesion to endothelial cells and their lysis. The mechanisms involved in ANCA-mediated neutrophil activation are not clearly understood. Following TNF-α priming, neutrophils express the ANCA-target antigen on their cell membrane, making it accessible for interaction with ANCA (Csernok *et al.* 1999). These target antigens are also expressed on the surface membranes of apoptotic non-primed neutrophils and recognized by ANCA (Gilligan 1996; Falk *et al.* 1990a).

It has been shown that ANCA-induced activation is dependent on the cross-linking of surface molecules; for example IgG-ANCA and F(ab)$_2$ fragments, but not Fab fragments, were able to stimulate the production of oxygen radicals by primed neutrophils (Kettritz *et al.* 1997). Because neither PR3 nor MPO contains a transmembrane domain and a cytoplasmic tail for signal transduction, other molecules or receptors, such as FcγRIIa receptors, which are extensively involved in neutrophil activation, must perform this function (Mulder *et al.* 1994). In addition, β_2-integrins have been shown to bind MPO (Reumaux *et al.* 1995) and are a third factor required for ANCA activation of neutrophils. Indeed, ANCA-mediated neutrophil activation does not occur when neutrophil adhesion is prevented either by continuous stirring of the cell suspension or by the addition of antibodies directed against CD18, a subunit of β_2-integrins.

The signal-transduction pathways involved after ANCA activation of neutrophils have only been investigated recently (see Chapter 7). Importantly, ANCA can also activate monocytes, which results in enhanced production of reactive oxygen species (Weidner *et al.* 2001), interleukin (IL)-8, and monocyte chemoattractant protein-1 (MCP-1) (Casselman *et al.* 1995; Ralston *et al.* 1997).

Animal models of ANCA-associated vasculitis with glomerulonephritis have failed to implicate ANCA as an independent cause of the disease (reviewed in Heeringa *et al.* 1998). Convincing evidence came from MPO-deficient mice developed by Xiao *et al.* (2002). Their experimental model is based on immunization of MPO-deficient mice to circumvent tolerance of MPO. First, the immunization with murine MPO generated antimurine MPO antibodies. Second, another immune-deficient mouse, lacking T and B cells, was created by inactivating the recombinase-activating gene-2 deficient (*rag2*) to obtain rag2-deficient animals to study the effect of adoptive transfer of foreign antibodies or graft immunity. When splenocytes from MPO$^{-/-}$ immunized mice were transferred into *rag2$^{-/-}$* mice, anti-MPO antibodies were detected a few days later and all mice developed severe necrotizing crescentic glomerulonephritis, closely resembling human disease. Other *rag2$^{-/-}$* mice developed systemic vasculitis with lung, spleen, and lymph-node involvement. These diseases were reproduced by passive transfer of purified IgG-anti-MPO from MPO$^{-/-}$ mice into *rag2$^{-/-}$* and wild-type mice, thereby demonstrating their pathogenicity. Subsequent studies using this experimental model have focused on the crucial role of neutrophils in glomerulonephritis (Xiao *et al.* 2005). The Chapel Hill group showed that selective neutrophil depletion in these mice with a monoclonal antibody protected them against vasculitis. These data raised the question of whether a therapeutic strategy should, or even could, be devised to target neutrophils. The same group demonstrated the role of TNF-α in this experimental MPA model. They showed that pretreatment with anti-TNF-α antibodies attenuated glomerulonephritis induced by MPO-ANCA and bacterial lipopolysaccharides (Huugen *et al.* 2005).

Little *et al.* (2006) used an experimental rat model to demonstrate that MPO-ANCA are pathogenic. Immunization of this rat strain with human MPO led to the synthesis of antibodies recognizing murine MPO, and to the development of systemic vasculitis with pauci-immune glomerulonephritis, closely resembling human disease. In addition, passive transfer of purified IgG anti-MPO from immunized rat into non-immunized rats also induced systemic vasculitis. Intravital microscopy of these rats showed dynamic leukocyte interaction with vessel walls after injection of purified MPO-ANCA. Furthermore, these modifications of leukocyte adhesion and vessel walls interactions were confirmed *in vitro* for this animal model. Recently, transplacental transfer of MPO-ANCA resulting in neonatal MPA was reported, supporting MPO-ANCA pathogenicity in humans (Bansal and Tobin 2004; Schlieben *et al.* 2005).

The general concept derived from all these studies is that ANCA-induced vasculitis may be a two-hit process, in which ANCA together with proinflammatory stimuli, most likely infectious, are required for the development of full-blown disease.

Antiendothelial cell antibodies (AECA) constitute a heterogeneous group of autoantibodies distinct from ANCA (see Chapter 7). AECA have been detected in systemic lupus erythematosus, systemic sclerosis, and primary and secondary systemic vasculitides (Chan and Cheng 1996; Praprotnik *et al.* 2000; Salojin *et al.* 1997). The presence of AECA has also been well-documented in idiopathic retinal vasculitis, WG, MPA, and Kawasaki disease, and their titers paralleled disease activity. A growing body of evidence suggests that AECA might be pathogenic, inducing systemic vasculitis by enhancing leukocyte adhesion to endothelial cells. AECA targets comprise a wide range of extracellular matrix proteins, DNA, or phospholipids, but their precise nature in patients with small- and medium-sized vessel systemic vasculitides remains unknown. Using a quantitative immunoblotting technique, Chanseaud *et al.* (2003) showed that IgM and, to a lesser degree, IgG from MPA patients recognize multiple endothelial cell antigens, but their precise identity remains unknown.

The role of T cells in MPA, as opposed to WG, is poorly established; however, T-cell responses to MPO have been observed

(King *et al.* 1998; Popa *et al.* 2002). The lack of substantial lymphocyte participation in the early stages of MPA is consistent with the observation that, in the mouse model of Xiao *et al.* (2002), glomerulonephritis can be induced by injecting IgG anti-MPO into *rag2*$^{-/-}$ mice that lack functional T cells.

Clinical features

Clinical features of MPA are summarized in Table 27.1. It should be kept in mind that, in addition to failure to distinguish between PAN and MPA in earlier series, the first reported studies on patients who satisfied MPA classification criteria were primarily from departments of nephrology and only later from internal medicine departments as well. Hence, the reported frequencies of involvement of each organ in MPA should always be interpreted after considering the patient's demographic characteristics.

General symptoms and clinical presentation at disease onset

Systemic symptoms (for example myalgias, arthralgias, or arthritis) are present in 56–76% of patients before MPA is diagnosed. There can be an indolent course of several months or even years before diagnosis, with general symptoms or even episodic, mildly bloody sputum which is ignored by the patient.

Renal and urogenital involvement

Renal involvement, predominantly RPGN, is a major feature of MPA. Renal involvement appeared to be nearly constant in the first series of MPA patients, but they were reported by nephrologists, leading to referral bias in the incidence of renal disease. Most of the patients have renal impairment at diagnosis and renal function that rapidly deteriorates if not treated. Eight of the 34 patients reported by Savage *et al.* (1985) required dialysis for oliguric or anuric renal disease, as did 20 of the 43 patients described by Adu *et al.* (1987). Initial renal manifestations are often silent, but detection of microscopic hematuria with or without proteinuria usually precedes deterioration in renal function. Several MPA flares with very few clinical symptoms may occur before renal manifestations become evident, as shown by the results of renal biopsies, which can reveal the coexistence of acute glomerular lesions and glomerular scars.

Ureteral involvement, which is much more suggestive of WG, is rare in MPA. It has been described rarely in PAN, but some of those cases might have been MPA rather than PAN. Uni- or bilateral ureteral stenoses may occur, and are usually localized to the lower part of ureters or more rarely at the ureteropelvic junction. Abdominal pain and anuria are the most common, but non-specific, symptoms of this complication. Indeed, some patients have no clinical urinary warning symptoms and renal destruction may progress silently. Diagnosis of ureteral stenoses can be confirmed by intravenous urography (when renal impairment does not preclude iodinated contrast-medium injection). Alternatively, ultrasonography or magnetic resonance imaging can be used, as both these techniques are safer. Vasculitis may be detected in the ureteral wall or in the periureteral fat. Retroperitoneal involvement might also be responsible for ureteral obstruction, as has been described for PAN (Lie 1992; van Bommel *et al.* 2002).

Table 27.1 Microscopic polyangiitis: clinical features and organ or system involvement, expressed as percentages of the studied population (n = 235)

	Serra *et al.* 1984	Savage *et al.* 1985	D'Agati *et al.* 1986	Adu *et al.* 1987	Guillevin *et al.* 1999
No. of patients	53	34	20	43	85
Mean age (yr)	53	50	50	–	57
Sex ratio (M/F)	1.5	1.8	1	1.7	1.2
General signs (fever, asthenia, myalgias, arthralgias)	79	76	–	–	73
Hypertension	26	29	35	21	34
Kidney	100	100	100	100	79
Skin	60	–	35	53	62
Purpura	40	44	–	–	41
Lung	55	–	55	34	25
Hemoptysis	23	32	–	–	–
Infiltrates	30	–	–	–	10
Pleural effusion	19	15	–	–	6
Gastrointestinal tract	51	–	–	56	30
Ear, nose, throat	30	–	–	20	–
Sinusitis	6	9	–	–	11
Eyes	30	–	–	28	–
Nervous system	28	–	–	–	–
Peripheral	19	18	15	14	58
Central	15	18	40	0	12
Heart	15	–	–	9	–

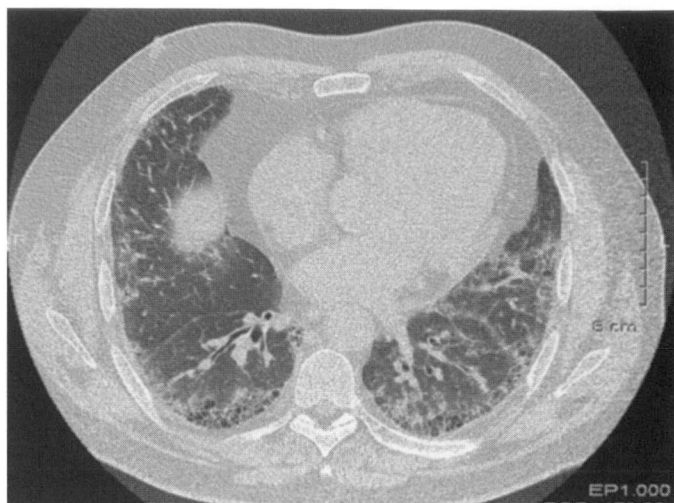

Figure 27.1 Computed tomography scan showing microcystic fibrosis of the lung in a patient with anti-MPO ANCA.

Pulmonary involvement

Pulmonary alveolar hemorrhage occurs in MPA. Moreover, as in WG or Goodpasture's syndrome, MPA can also be responsible for a pulmonary–renal syndrome. Hemoptysis, or even moderately bloody expectorations, may precede severe pulmonary hemorrhage, which is characterized by dyspnea and anemia, and may progress to diffuse alveolar damage and respiratory distress due, at least in part, to capillaritis (Savage *et al.* 1985). Bronchial arteritis with intimal thickening and focal destruction of the internal elastic lamina associated with subintimal fibrous scarring in the media may be found on histological examination of lung biopsy material.

Diffuse alveolar damage and interstitial lung fibrosis (Figure 27.1) are also complications, mainly in patients with anti-MPO pANCA; fibrosis and vasculitis can evolve independently (Souid *et al.* 2001). Lung fibrosis has also been described as an isolated process in some patients with anti-MPO pANCA, but no other clinical evidence of systemic vasculitis. Hence, lung fibrosis with anti-MPO ANCA may possibly be a separate entity from MPA (Hiromura *et al.* 2000; Homma *et al.* 2004). Chest CT scans usually show honeycombing fibrosis in the bases of the lungs, with histological features compatible with the usual interstitial pneumonia pattern and vasculitis, in less than half the patients. The mortality rate of patients with lung fibrosis and anti-MPO pANCA was found to be similar to that of that of idiopathic alveolar fibrosis, but worse than for fibrosis associated with other collagen vascular diseases in which anti-MPO pANCA is not found (Homma *et al.* 2004).

Cutaneous manifestations

Skin lesions are found in 30–60% of patients with MPA (Lhote *et al.* 1998; Penas *et al.* 1996). Maculopapular purpuric lesions of the lower limbs are the most frequent skin manifestations. Other lesions have been described, such as mouth ulcers, vesicles, necrosis, ulcerations, nodules, splinter hemorrhages, livedo reticularis, hand and finger erythema, and facial edema (Homas *et al.* 1992; Seishima *et al.* 2004). Leukocytoclastic vasculitis of the small vessels of the dermis is usually observed. Sometimes, arterioles or smaller vessels of the deep dermis and subcutis are also involved, thereby explaining the nodular appearance of some skin lesions.

In one patient, vasculitis was associated with eosinophilic panniculitis (Penas *et al.* 1996). All these cutaneous lesions usually disappear rapidly under treatment, but relapses may occur.

Other clinical manifestations

Not surprisingly, clinical features are similar to those of PAN. Peripheral neuropathy is found in 10–58% of patients, much less frequently than in PAN (Guillevin *et al.* 1999; Rodgers *et al.* 1989; Savage *et al.* 1985). Mononeuropathy multiplex is, as in all other vasculitides, the main clinical feature, and is sometimes isolated. Of patients with peripheral nervous system involvement, ~69% have mononeuropathy multiplex, ~12% have symmetric polyneuropathy, and ~19% have asymmetric polyneuropathy (Hattori *et al.* 2002). Necrotizing vasculitis has been reported in up to 81% of sural nerve biopsies. Central nervous system involvement (mostly encephalopathy and stroke) and cranial neuropathies have been reported in 12–18% of patients (Généreau *et al.* 1999; Savage *et al.* 1985), reflecting small vessel vasculitis. Pachymeningitis thought to possibly result from dural necrotizing vasculitis has also been described (Kono *et al.* 2000).

Gastrointestinal symptoms, seen in 30–60% of patients, include abdominal pain (32–58%) and GI bleeding (29%). Severe small intestine or large bowel ischemia, ulcerations, and perforations occur as in PAN, but published case reports indicate it is clearly less frequent in MPA (Tsai *et al.* 2004; Ueda *et al.* 2001).

Reports of cardiovascular complications in MPA are rare. Among the 85 MPA patients described by Guillevin *et al.* (1999), heart failure and pericarditis occurred at respective frequencies of 17.6% and 10%. Severe acute congestive heart failure has been reported, but rarely with documented myocardial infarction due to myocardial or coronary small vessel arteritis (Wang *et al.* 2002); however, subclinical myocardial infarctions may be more frequent, as in PAN and other small-vessel vasculitides. MPA lung and kidney disease appear to be associated with pANCA, whereas heart involvement may be more frequent in ANCA-negative patients, as in those with CSS (Sablé-Fourtassou *et al.* 2005; Sinico *et al.* 2005).

Ocular manifestations, including eyelid inflammation, iridocyclitis, scleritis, retinal cotton-wool spots, retinal vasculitis, and choroiditis are seen in MPA. Although these manifestations are more frequent than in PAN, they occur in less than 30% of the patients, and they often remain clinically silent (Caster *et al.* 1996; Mihara *et al.* 2005).

There is some controversy regarding ear, nose, and throat involvement, which is more characteristic of WG and is sometimes considered by some authors to be an exclusion for the diagnosis of MPA, which is probably too dogmatic a point of view. Mild non-granulomatous, non-erosive sinus inflammation may be noted in up to 29% of MPA patients (Lane *et al.* 2005; Serra *et al.* 1984).

Laboratory findings

Non-specific tests reflect the systemic inflammatory nature of MPA. The major abnormalities are elevated erythrocyte sedimentation rate, serum C-reactive protein and albumin concentrations, platelet and white blood cell counts, and low hemoglobin (normochromic normocytic anemia). All patients reported by Savage *et al.* (1985) had impaired renal function with serum creatinine >120 µmol/l (1.4 mg/dl) and only 15% of those described by Serra *et al.* (1984) had normal plasma creatinine levels. The mean plasma creatinine was 574 µmol/l (6.5 mg/dl) (range: 147–1405 µmol/l, 1.7–15.9 mg/dl) in the Hammersmith series (Savage *et al.* 1985). Microscopic hematuria is constant and proteinuria, often >3 g/24 hours, is found in more than 90% of patients.

ANCA are frequently detected in MPA patients. For example, 75% of the 33 MPA patients reported by Hauschild *et al.* (1994) had ANCA: 60% (20/33) pANCA and 15% cANCA. Most ANCA detected in MPA are pANCA anti-MPO, although anti-PR3 can also be found. Among our 85 patients selected according to the Chapel Hill nomenclature, 74.5% were ANCA-positive (Guillevin *et al.* 1999). The usefulness of anti-MPO ANCA to diagnose MPA is now well established (Jennette *et al.* 1989). However, despite the close connection between those autoantibodies and MPA, the immunodiagnostic potency of this anti-MPO ANCA subspecificity is not as high as that for anti-PR3 ANCA in WG because pANCA are found in a variety of different inflammatory disorders and are not specific to vasculitis or glomerulonephritis.

Visceral angiography is usually normal, without stenoses or microaneurysms characteristic of PAN. ANCA-positivity and concomitant abnormal angiograms are exceptional. Therefore, it does not seem informative to perform angiography before renal biopsy in ANCA-positive patients (Guillevin *et al.* 1996a).

Renal histology is characterized by focal segmental thrombosing and necrotizing glomerulonephritis. Extracapillary crescents are present in nearly all renal biopsies and often involve more than 60% of the glomeruli. The severity of renal impairment is related to the presence of glomerular sclerosis and frequent severe tubular damage, more than to active glomerular disease and crescents (Hogan *et al.* 1996; Kapitsinou *et al.* 2003; Zauner *et al.* 2002).

Outcome and prognosis

Relapses

Relapses are frequent in MPA. Savage *et al.* (1985) reported that 12 of 33 (36.4%) MPA patients had relapses. In the study by Gordon *et al.* (1993), relapses occurred less frequently (25.3%); median time to relapse was 24 months. In our MPA population, 34.1% relapsed (Guillevin *et al.* 1999). At present, it is not be possible to identify the subgroup of patients who will relapse, or to predict the severity of the relapses. The clinical pattern of relapse does not necessarily repeat the original presentation and organs that were not previously affected can be involved. Nevertheless, relapses are usually less severe than initial manifestations, most often consisting of rash and arthralgias.

Deaths

Deaths attributed to vasculitis

When vital organs are involved, lethal complications may occur. A few patients die during the first months of the disease from multivisceral involvement because treatment is unable to control the disease, which is characterized by fever, rapid weight loss, diffuse pain, and one or multiple major organ involvements. The remaining deaths are mainly attributed to renal failure and lung hemorrhage.

Deaths due to treatment side-effects

Iatrogenic deaths are not rare. Those occurring during the first few months of the disease are often caused by uncontrolled vasculitis, while deaths during the following years may be the consequence of treatment side-effects. These adverse events emphasize the importance of an individually tailored regimen, established after careful analysis of parameters which might predict outcome. Infections are the primary cause of such deaths, influenced by glucocorticoids and cytotoxic agents. Minimizing doses and shortening the duration of treatment can limit these complications, but optimal treatment intensity and duration need to be refined based on prospective studies. Septicemia can develop during the first months of treatment as a consequence of intense initial therapy. Viral infections usually arise later and result from the profound immunosuppression induced by the drugs prescribed to control the vasculitis. We want to emphasize that rare cases of *Pneumocystis jiroveci* pneumonia, which have mainly been described in WG (Godeau *et al.* 1994; Jarrousse *et al.* 1993), also occur in MPA.

Treatment

Disease severity

To help the clinician choose the most effective therapy and avoid overly aggressive treatment, we have devised a prognostic score, the Five Factor Score (FFS) (Guillevin *et al.* 1996b) (Table 27.2) (see Chapter 23). Parameters correlated with higher mortality include: proteinuria >1 g/day, renal insufficiency (serum creatinine >140 µmol/l [1.58 mg/dl]), cardiomyopathy attributable to MPA, gastrointestinal manifestations, and central nervous system involvement. Treatment should be chosen as a function of these criteria. Other criteria, such as those included in the Birmingham Vasculitis Activity Score (BVAS) (Luqmani *et al.* 1994; 1997) (see Chapter 23), are also used to determine the intensity of treatment to be prescribed, but BVAS has not yet been validated for that purpose (Bacon *et al.* 1995).

Recommendations for specific manifestations

Supportive care, prevention of opportunistic infections, including *Pneumocystis carinii* and *jiroveci* pneumonia, and physical therapy are all important parts of the treatment of patients with MPA, as is the case for those with PAN (see Chapter 26). The clinical presentation of fulminating MPA is usually that of pulmonary–renal failure and, more rarely, cerebral or gastrointestinal involvement. Deterioration of renal function often necessitates hemodialysis.

Table 27.2 The five-factor score (FFS), as established based on 342 patients with PAN or CSS (Guillevin *et al.* 1996) and further validated for patients with MPA (Gayraud *et al.* 2001)

Five Factor Score
Proteinuria >1 g/24 hours
Serum creatinine >140 µmol/l
Specific gastrointestinal involvement
Specific cardiomyopathy
Specific central nervous system involvement

1 point for each of these 5 items when present

FFS	5 year survival rate (%)	Relative risk
0	88.1	0.62
1	74.1*	1.35
≥ 2	54.1**	2.40

*p <0.005 and **p <0.0001 as compared to patients with FFS = 0.

Treatment of massive alveolar hemorrhage requires immediate fluid resuscitation, with hemodynamic and respiratory support. In the case of gastrointestinal involvement with constant abdominal pain despite medical treatment, an exploratory surgical procedure should be performed to identify and treat possible bowel perforation. For the same groups of patients, it seems reasonable to administer drugs parenterally to circumvent impaired drug absorption. The prognosis of fulminating MPA is poor. Savage *et al.* (1985) reported on 34 MPA patients, whose actuarial survival and kidney survival at 5-year follow-up were, respectively, 65 and 55%. Two-thirds of the deaths were due to active vasculitis complicated by renal failure, lung hemorrhage or treatment side effects. Age over 50 and plasma creatinine >500 μmol/l (5.7 mg/dl) portend a poor prognosis (Gordon *et al.* 1993).

Treatment principles

There is a tendency to consider the treatment of MPA with poor prognosis factors in a manner similar to that of treatment of WG, based on their shared pathogenic mechanisms (association with the presence of ANCA) and their risk of relapses. In contrast, when no such factors of poor prognosis are present, there is a tendency to relate MPA therapy to that of PAN (Gayraud *et al.* 1997; Hoffman *et al.* 1992). Indeed, it has become obvious that MPA without poor prognostic criteria does not require the systematic use of cyclophosphamide or other cytotoxic agents in addition to glucocorticoids. Most MPA patients who relapse do so when treatment is discontinued (33%), although relapses while tapering the glucocorticoid dose are frequent (Gordon *et al.* 1993). Gaskin *et al.* (1991) analyzed the relationship between ANCA detection by immunofluorescence and clinical evidence of relapse in 70 patients with WG or MPA. They found that patients who relapsed invariably had detectable ANCA, that some relapses were preceded by the reappearance of ANCA, but that many ANCA-positive patients did not relapse during the study. Relapses during long-term follow-up were generally associated with high or rising ANCA titers, although the temporal relationship between clinical relapse and ANCA changes was not constant. Relapses were rare in patients with low or undetectable ANCA.

Glucocorticoids

These drugs are prescribed to all patients with MPA, and high doses may be useful at onset. Because of their rapid action and relative safety, methylprednisolone pulses (usually 15 mg/kg IV over 60 min repeated at 24-hour intervals for 1–3 days), have become widely used at the initiation of therapy for severe disease, especially in the presence of life-threatening organ involvement or the extension phase of mononeuropathy multiplex (Guillevin *et al.* 1990). The dose of pulse methylprednisolone is empiric and doses less than 1000 mg may be as effective. Oral glucocorticoids are given at the dose of 1 mg/kg/day of prednisone or its equivalent of methylprednisolone, with dose tapering according to the European vasculitis study group EUVAS (Table 27.3). This regimen is effective and may control MPA, without the addition of cytotoxic agents, in patients without factors of poor prognosis.

Cyclophosphamide

Cyclophosphamide (CYC) should not be systematically prescribed as the first-line treatment to all MPA patients. Factors influencing the decision to use this drug include the anatomical location of the

Table 27.3 EUVAS oral glucocorticoid dosing regimen for ANCA-associated vasculitides (in this setting, combined with an immunosuppressant drug)

Time of treatment	Prednisone dose
Onset	1 mg/kg/day
1st week	0.75 mg/kg/day
2nd week	0.5 mg/kg/day
4th week	0.4 mg/kg/day
7th week	0.3 mg/kg/day
10th week	0.28 mg/kg/day[1]
13th week	0.25 mg/kg/day[1]
3rd month	15 mg/day[1]
4th month	12.5 mg/day[1]
5th month	10 mg/day
6th month	7.5 mg/day
12th month	5 mg/day
18th month	2.5 mg/day
24th month	0

[1] for thinner patients, the minimum dose for the first 3 months is 10 mg/day, which should then be maintained until the 5th month.

involvement, its severity and the intensity of disease activity, as outlined above. Although oral CYC (2 mg/kg/day or less), in combination with glucocorticoids is effective for the treatment of vasculitis, it has a low therapeutic/toxic index. Major side-effects associated with CYC, such as infections, and attempts to decrease their related morbidity, such as protocols using intermittent IV pulses, are detailed in the chapter on PAN (see Chapter 26).

The current recommended regimen is based on initial CYC doses varying from 0.5 to 2.5 g (0.5–0.7 g/m^2) at 2-week intervals initially (days 1, 15, and 30) then every 3 weeks, as for WG, or monthly (depending on the patient's general condition), until remission is obtained, followed by maintenance therapy (Jayne *et al.* 2003, 2005; Nachman *et al.* 1996). The inability of CYC to prevent relapse has been disappointing. The duration of CYC treatment and the total amount received did not differ between patients with vasculitis who relapsed and those who did not. Serra *et al.* (1984) reported 18 MPA patients who had chronically active disease that they described as a smoldering vasculitis. Those patients had poorer outcomes than long-term survivors with stable, inactive vasculitis.

When patients fail to respond to pulse CYC, oral CYC has been successfully introduced to control disease activity or treat relapses within the first 6 months of treatment (Généreau *et al.* 1994); however, combined glucocorticoid and CYC therapy should not exceed 1 year.

Maintenance therapy for MPA with poor prognosis factor(s)

Azathioprine (2 mg/kg/day) (Jayne *et al.* 2003), methotrexate (0.3 mg/kg/week) (de Groot *et al.* 2005) and several other cytotoxic agents, such as mycophenolate mofetil, have been used in MPA (Nowack *et al.* 1999). They are now recommended for maintenance therapy, after remission has been achieved in MPA patients with factors of poor prognosis, as for WG. This maintenance therapy must be continued for more than 6 months, but its optimal duration remains undefined, but is currently being evaluated in a prospective EUVAS trial. Use of these cytotoxic agents is not recommended as first-line therapy for MPA with poor-prognosis factors, for which CYC is mandatory.

Plasma exchanges

Plasma exchanges can improve renal outcome, but not patient survival, when kidney involvement is severe (defined as oliguria (<400 ml/24 hours) or requiring dialysis or with serum creatinine >500 μmol/l (5.7 mg/dl). A typical regimen includes exchanges of 60 ml/kg of body weight with 4% albumin replacement fluid three times/week for 2–3 weeks, then twice/week for 3 weeks, then once/week for 1–3 weeks. The effectiveness of this regimen is demonstrated by the definitive results of the EUVAS MEPEX (methylprednisolone or plasma exchange for severe renal vasculitis) trial, presented as an abstract at the 2005 EUVAS Workshop, in Heidelberg, Germany (Jayne et al. 2006, submitted for publication; Rahman and Harper 2006). Plasma exchanges may also be beneficial for patients with intra-alveolar hemorrhage, as for Goodpasture's syndrome, which is also due to pulmonary capillaritis (Guillevin and Pagnoux 2003; Levy et al. 2001; Simpson et al. 1982; Tesar et al. 2003).

Other treatments

The use of IV immunoglobulins (IVIg) to treat systemic vasculitis has been stimulated by its success in Kawasaki disease, in which IVIg prevented the development of coronary artery aneurysms (Newburger et al. 1991). IVIg has been used to treat WG and MPA, often with sustained benefit and reduced requirement for immunosuppression (Jayne et al. 1991; Jayne and Lockwood 1996); however, there are some discrepancies in published studies. IVIg was administered to 15 patients with ANCA-associated systemic vasculitis who were poor responders to conventional therapy (Jayne and Lockwood 1996) and their outcomes were less promising: only 40% of them benefited from IVIg treatment and complete remission of disease activity was not obtained. In contrast, IVIg was highly effective in our recent prospective trial on relapsing ANCA-associated vasculitis patients. All 20 patients achieved remission after six IVIg infusions, but eight of them relapsed after its cessation (Martinez et al. 2005).

Monoclonal antibodies that target proinflammatory cytokine(s), such as anti-TNF a (infliximab, etanercept) (Bartolucci et al. 2002; Booth et al. 2002), T cells (Lockwood et al. 1993), or B cells (anti-CD20 (rituximab) (Keogh et al. 2005), offer alternatives to conventional immunosuppressive drugs and have been used to the treat systemic vasculitis patients, who obtained substantial and sustained benefit. Prospective studies are ongoing to define their roles in treating MPA. At present, these biological agents are mostly prescribed for refractory forms of the disease or to patients who suffer multiple relapses despite conventional therapies.

References

Adu, D., Howie, A. J., Scott, D. G., Bacon, P. A., McGonigle, R. J. and Micheal, J. (1987). Polyarteritis and the kidney. *Quarterly Journal of Medicine*, **62**, 221–37.

Aratani, Y., Kura, F., Watanabe, H., Akagawa, H., Takano, Y., Suzuki, K., Maeda, N. and Koyama, H. (2000). Differential host susceptibility to pulmonary infections with bacteria and fungi in mice deficient in myeloperoxidase. *Journal of Infectious Diseases*, **182**, 1276–9.

Bacon, P. A., Moots, R. J., Exley, A., Luqmani, R. and Rasmussen, N. (1995). VITAL (Vasculitis integrated Assessment Log) assessment of vasculitis. *Clinical and Experimental Rheumatology*, **13**, 275–8.

Bansal, P. J. and Tobin, M. C. (2004). Neonatal microscopic polyangiitis secondary to transfer of maternal myeloperoxidase-antineutrophil cytoplasmic antibody resulting in neonatal pulmonary hemorrhage and renal involvement. *Annals of Allergy Asthma and Immunology*, **93**, 398–401.

Bartolucci, P., Ramanoelina, J., Cohen, P., et al. (2002). Efficacy of the anti-TNF-alpha antibody infliximab against refractory systemic vasculitides: an open pilot study on 10 patients. *Rheumatology* (Oxford), **41**, 1126–32.

Bloch, D. A., Michel, B. A., Hunder, G. G., et al. (1990). The American College of Rheumatology 1990 criteria for the classification of vasculitis. Patients and methods. *Arthritis and Rheumatism*, **33**, 1068–73.

Booth, A. D., Jefferson, H. J., Ayliffe, W., Andrews, P. A. and Jayne, D. R. (2002). Safety and efficacy of TNFalpha blockade in relapsing vasculitis. *Annals of the Rheumatic Diseases*, **61**, 559.

Casselman, B. L., Kilgore, K. S., Miller, B. F. and Warren, J. S. (1995). Antibodies to neutrophil cytoplasmic antigens induce monocyte chemoattractant protein-1 secretion from human monocytes. *Journal of Laboratory and Clinical Medicine*, **126**, 495–502.

Caster, J. C., Shetlar, D. J., Pappolla, M. A. and Yee, R. W. (1996). Microscopic polyangiitis with ocular involvement. *Archives of Ophthalmology*, **114**, 346–8.

Chan, T. M. and Cheng, I. K. (1996). A prospective study on anti-endothelial cell antibodies in patients with systemic lupus erythematosus. *Clinical Immunology and Immunopathology*, **78**, 41–6.

Chanseaud, Y., Pena-Lefebvre, P. G., Guilpain, P., et al. (2003). IgM and IgG autoantibodies from microscopic polyangiitis patients but not those with other small- and medium-sized vessel vasculitides recognize multiple endothelial cell antigens. *Clinical Immunology*, **109**, 165–78.

Csernok, E., Muller, A. and Gross, W. L. (1999). Immunopathology of ANCA-associated vasculitis. *Internal Medicine*, **38**, 759–65.

D'Agati, V., Chander, P., Nash, M. and Mancilla-Jimenez, R. (1986). Idiopathic microscopic polyarteritis nodosa: ultrastructural observations on the renal vascular and glomerular lesions. *American Journal of Kidney Diseases*, **7**, 95–110.

Davson, J., Ball, J. and Platt, R. (1948). Kidney in periarteritis nodosa. *Quarterly Journal of Medicine*, **17**, 175–202.

de Groot, K., Rasmussen, N., Bacon, P. A., et al. (2005). Randomized trial of cyclophosphamide versus methotrexate for induction of remission in early systemic antineutrophil cytoplasmic antibody-associated vasculitis. *Arthritis and Rheumatism*, **52**, 2461–9.

Falk, R. J., Terrell, R. S., Charles, L. A. and Jennette, J. C. (1990a). Anti-neutrophil cytoplasmic autoantibodies induce neutrophils to degranulate and produce oxygen radicals *in vitro*. *Proceedings of the National Academy of Sciences USA*, **87**, 4115–9.

Falk, R. J., Hogan, S., Carey, T. S. and Jennette, J. C. (1990b). Clinical course of anti-neutrophil cytoplasmic autoantibody-associated glomerulonephritis and systemic vasculitis. The Glomerular Disease Collaborative Network. *Annals of Internal Medicine*, **113**, 656–63.

Gaskin, G., Clutterbuck, E. J. and Pusey, C. D. (1991). Renal disease in the Churg–Strauss syndrome. Diagnosis, management and outcome. *Contributions to Nephrology*, **94**, 58–65.

Gayraud, M., Guillevin, L., Cohen, P., et al. (1997). Treatment of good-prognosis polyarteritis nodosa and Churg–Strauss syndrome: comparison of steroids and oral or pulse cyclophosphamide in 25 patients. French Cooperative Study Group for Vasculitides. *British Journal of Rheumatology*, **36**, 1290–7.

Généreau, T., Lortholary, O., Leclerq, P., et al. (1994). Treatment of systemic vasculitis with cyclophosphamide and steroids: daily oral low-dose cyclophosphamide administration after failure of a pulse intravenous high-dose regimen in four patients. *British Journal of Rheumatology*, **33**, 959–62.

Généreau, T., Lortholary, O., Pottier, M. A., et al. (1999). Temporal artery biopsy: a diagnostic tool for systemic necrotizing vasculitis. French Vasculitis Study Group. *Arthritis and Rheumatism*, **42**, 2674–81.

Gilligan, H. M., Bredy, B., Brady, H. R., *et al* (1996). Antineutrophil cytoplasmic autoantibodies interact with primary granule constituents on the surface of apoptotic neutrophils in the absence of neutrophil priming. *Journal of Experimental Medicine*, **184**, 2231–41.

Godeau, B., Coutant-Perronne, V., Lê Thi Huong, D., *et al.* (1994). Pneumocystis carinii pneumonia in the course of connective tissue disease: report of 34 cases. *Journal of Rheumatology*, **21**, 246–51.

Gordon, M., Luqmani, R. A., Adu, D., *et al.* (1993). Relapses in patients with a systemic vasculitis. *Quarterly Journal of Medicine*, **86**, 779–89.

Guillevin, L., Durand-Gasselin, B., Cevallos, R., *et al.* (1999). Microscopic polyangiitis: clinical and laboratory findings in eighty-five patients. *Arthritis and Rheumatism*, **42**, 421–30.

Guillevin, L., Fain, O., Lhote, F., *et al.* (1992b). Lack of superiority of steroids plus plasma exchange to steroids alone in the treatment of polyarteritis nodosa and Churg–Strauss syndrome. A prospective, randomized trial in 78 patients. *Arthritis and Rheumatism*, **35**, 208–15.

Guillevin, L., Lhote, F., Jarrousse, B. and Fain, O. (1992a). Treatment of polyarteritis nodosa and Churg–Strauss syndrome. A meta-analysis of 3 prospective controlled trials including 182 patients over 12 years. *Annales de Médecine Interne*, **143**, 405–16.

Guillevin, L., Lhote, F., Amouroux, J., Ghérardi, R., Callard, P. and Casassus, P. (1996a). Antineutrophil cytoplasmic antibodies, abnormal angiograms and pathological findings in polyarteritis nodosa and Churg–Strauss syndrome: indications for the classification of vasculitides of the polyarteritis Nodosa Group. *British Journal of Rheumatology*, **35**, 958–64.

Guillevin, L., Lhote, F., Gayraud, M., *et al.* (1996b). Prognostic factors in polyarteritis nodosa and Churg–Strauss syndrome. A prospective study in 342 patients. *Medicine* (Baltimore), **75**, 17–28.

Guillevin, L. and Pagnoux, C. (2003). Indications of plasma exchanges for systemic vasculitides. *Therapeutic Apheresis and Dialysis*, **7**, 155–60.

Guillevin, L., Rosser, J., Cacoub, P., Mousson, C. and Jarrousse, B. (1990). Methylprednisolone in the treatment of Wegener's granulomatosis, polyarteritis nodosa and Churg-Strauss angiitis. *APMIS*, **19** (Suppl.), 52–3.

Handa, R., Wali, J. P., Gupta, S. D., *et al.* (2001). Classical polyarteritis nodosa and microscopic polyangiitis – a clinicopathologic study. *The Journal of the Association of Physicians of India*, **49**, 314–9.

Hattori, N., Mori, K., Misu, K., Koike, H., Ichimura, M. and Sobue, G. (2002). Mortality and morbidity in peripheral neuropathy associated Churg–Strauss syndrome and microscopic polyangiitis. *Journal of Rheumatology*, **29**, 1408–14.

Hauschild, S., Csernok, E., Schmitt, W. H. and Gross, W. L. (1994). Antineutrophil cytoplasmic antibodies in systemic polyarteritis nodosa with and without hepatitis B virus infection and Churg–Strauss syndrome – 62 patients. *Journal of Rheumatology*, **21**, 1173–4.

Heeringa, P., Brouwer, E., Tervaert, J. W., Weening, J. J. and Kallenberg, C. G. (1998). Animal models of anti-neutrophil cytoplasmic antibody associated vasculitis. *Kidney International*, **53**, 253–63.

Hiromura, K., Nojima, Y., Kitahara, T., *et al.* (2000). Four cases of anti-myeloperoxidase antibody-related rapidly progressive glomerulonephritis during the course of idiopathic pulmonary fibrosis. *Clinical Nephrology*, **53**, 384–9.

Hirche, T. O., Gaut, J. P., Heinecke, J. W. and Belaaouaj, A. (2005). Myeloperoxidase plays critical roles in killing Klebsiella pneumoniae and inactivating neutrophil elastase: effects on host defense. *Journal of Immunology*, **174**, 1557–65.

Hoffman, G. S., Kerr, G. S., Leavitt, R. Y., *et al.* (1992). Wegener granulomatosis: an analysis of 158 patients. *Annals of Internal Medicine*, **116**, 488–98.

Hogan, S. L., Nachman, P. H., Wilkman, A. S., Jennette, J. C. and Falk, R. J. (1996). Prognostic markers in patients with antineutrophil cytoplasmic autoantibody-associated microscopic polyangiitis and glomerulonephritis. *Journal of the American Society for Nephrology*, **7**, 23–32.

Homas, P. B., David-Bajar, K. M., Fitzpatrick, J. E., West, S. G. and Tribelhorn, D. R. (1992). Microscopic polyarteritis. Report of a case with cutaneous involvement and antimyeloperoxidase antibodies. *Archives of Dermatology*, **128**, 1223–8.

Homma, S., Matsushita, H. and Nakata, K. (2004). Pulmonary fibrosis in myeloperoxidase antineutrophil cytoplasmic antibody-associated vasculitides. *Respirology*, **9**, 190–6.

Huugen, D., Xiao, H., van Esch, A., *et al.* (2005). Aggravation of anti-myeloperoxidase antibody-induced glomerulonephritis by bacterial lipopolysaccharide: role of tumor necrosis factor-alpha. *American Journal of Pathology*, **167**, 47–58.

Jarrousse, B., Guillevin, L., Bindi, P., *et al.* (1993). Increased risk of Pneumocystis carinii pneumonia in patients with Wegener's granulomatosis. *Clinical and Experimental Rheumatology*, **11**, 615–21.

Jayne, D. (2005). How to induce remission in primary systemic vasculitis. *Best Practice and Research in Clinical Gastroenterology*, **19**, 293–305.

Jayne, D. R., Davies, M. J., Fox, C. J., Black, C. M. and Lockwood, C. M. (1991). Treatment of systemic vasculitis with pooled intravenous immunoglobulin. *Lancet*, **337**, 1137–9.

Jayne, D. R. and Lockwood, C. M. (1996). Intravenous immunoglobulin as sole therapy for systemic vasculitis. *British Journal of Rheumatology*, **35**, 1150–3.

Jayne, D., Rasmussen, N., Andrassy, K., *et al.* (2003). A randomized trial of maintenance therapy for vasculitis associated with antineutrophil cytoplasmic autoantibodies. *New England Journal of Medicine*, **349**, 36–44.

Jennette, J. C., Falk, R. J., Andrassy, K., *et al.* (1994). Nomenclature of systemic vasculitides. Proposal of an international consensus conference. *Arthritis and Rheumatism*, **37**, 187–92.

Jennette, J. C., Wilkman, A. S. and Falk, R. J. (1989). Anti-neutrophil cytoplasmic autoantibody-associated glomerulonephritis and vasculitis. *American Journal of Pathology*, **135**, 921–30.

Kapitsinou, P. P., Ioannidis, J. P., Boletis, J. N., *et al.* (2003). Clinicopathologic predictors of death and ESRD in patients with pauci-immune necrotizing glomerulonephritis. *American Journal of Kidney Diseases*, **41**, 29–37.

Keogh, K. A., Wylam, M. E., Stone, J. H. and Specks, U. (2005). Induction of remission by B lymphocyte depletion in eleven patients with refractory antineutrophil cytoplasmic antibody-associated vasculitis. *Arthritis and Rheumatism*, **52**, 262–8.

Kettritz, R., Jennette, J. C. and Falk, R. J. (1997). Crosslinking of ANCA-antigens stimulates superoxide release by human neutrophils. *Journal of the American Society for Nephrology*, **8**, 386–94.

King, W. J., Brooks, C. J., Holder, R., Hughes, P., Adu, D. and Savage, C. O. (1998). T lymphocyte responses to anti-neutrophil cytoplasmic autoantibody (ANCA) antigens are present in patients with ANCA-associated systemic vasculitis and persist during disease remission. *Clinical and Experimental Immunology*, **112**, 539–46.

Kono, H., Inokuma, S., Nakayama, H. and Yamazaki, J. (2000). Pachymeningitis in microscopic polyangiitis (MPA): a case report and a review of central nervous system involvement in MPA. *Clinical and Experimental Rheumatology*, **18**, 397–400.

Lane, S. E., Watts, R. A., Shepstone, L. and Scott, D. G. (2005). Primary systemic vasculitis: clinical features and mortality. *Quarterly Journal of Medicine*, **98**, 97–111.

Levy, J. B., Turner, A. N., Rees, A. J. and Pusey, C. D. (2001). Long-term outcome of anti-glomerular basement membrane antibody disease treated with plasma exchange and immunosuppression. *Annals of Internal Medicine*, **134**, 1033–42.

Lhote, F., Cohen, P. and Guillevin, L. (1998). Polyarteritis nodosa, microscopic polyangiitis and Churg–Strauss syndrome. *Lupus*, **7**, 238–58.

Lie, J. T. (1992). Retroperitoneal polyarteritis nodosa presenting as ureteral obstruction. *Journal of Rheumatology*, **19**, 1628–31.

Lightfoot, R. W. Jr, Michel, B. A., Bloch, D. A., *et al.* (1990). The American College of Rheumatology 1990 criteria for the classification of polyarteritis nodosa. *Arthritis and Rheumatism*, **33**, 1088–93.

Little, M. A., Bhangal, G., Smyth, C. L., *et al.* (2006). Therapeutic effect of anti-TNF-alpha antibodies in an experimental model of anti-neutrophil cytoplasm antibody-associated systemic vasculitis. *Journal of the American Society for Nephrology*, **17**, 160–9.

Lockwood, C. M., Thiru, S., Isaacs, J. D., Hale, G. and Waldmann, H. (1993). Long-term remission of intractable systemic vasculitis with monoclonal antibody therapy. *Lancet*, **341**, 1620–2.

Luqmani, R. A., Bacon, P. A., Moots, R. J., *et al.* (1994). Birmingham Vasculitis Activity Score (BVAS) in systemic necrotizing vasculitis. *Quarterly Journal of Medicine*, **87**, 671–8.

Luqmani, R. A., Exley, A. R., Kitas, G. D. and Bacon, P. A. (1997). Disease assessment and management of the vasculitides. *Baillieres Clinical Rheumatology*, **11**, 423–46.

Mahr, A., Guillevin, L., Poissonnet, M. and Aymé, S. (2004). Prevalences of polyarteritis nodosa, microscopic polyangiitis, Wegener's granulomatosis, and Churg-Strauss syndrome in a French urban multiethnic population in 2000: a capture-recapture estimate. *Arthritis and Rheumatism*, **51**, 92–9.

Martinez, V., Cohen, P., Mouthon, L., Guillevin, L. for the FVSG (2005). Intravenous immunoglobulins for relapses of ANCA-associated systemic vasculitides: final analysis of a prospective, open and multicenter trial [abstract]. *Arthritis and Rheumatism*, **52**, S649.

Mihara, M., Hayasaka, S., Watanabe, K., Kitagawa, K. and Hayasaka, Y. (2005). Ocular manifestations in patients with microscopic polyangiitis. *European Journal of Ophthalmology*, **15**, 138–42.

Mulder, A. H., Broekroelofs, J., Horst, G., Limburg, P. C., Nelis, G. F. and Kallenberg, C. G. (1994). Anti-neutrophil cytoplasmic antibodies (ANCA) in inflammatory bowel disease: characterization and clinical correlates. *Clinical and Experimental Immunology*, **95**, 490–7.

Nachman, P. H., Hogan, S. L., Jennette, J. C. and Falk, R. J. (1996). Treatment response and relapse in antineutrophil cytoplasmic autoantibody-associated microscopic polyangiitis and glomerulonephritis. *Journal of the American Society for Nephrology*, **7**, 33–9.

Newburger, J. W., Takahashi, M., Beiser, A. S., *et al.* (1991). A single intravenous infusion of gamma globulin as compared with four infusions in the treatment of acute Kawasaki syndrome. *New England Journal of Medicine*, **324**, 1633–9.

Nowack, R., Gobel, U., Klooker, P., Hergesell, O., Andrassy, K. and van der Woude, F. J. (1999). Mycophenolate mofetil for maintenance therapy of Wegener's granulomatosis and microscopic polyangiitis: a pilot study in 11 patients with renal involvement. *Journal of the American Society for Nephrology*, **10**, 1965–71.

Penas, P. F., Porras, J. I., Fraga, J., Bernis, C., Sarria, C. and Dauden, E. (1996). Microscopic polyangiitis. A systemic vasculitis with a positive P-ANCA. *British Journal of Dermatology*, **134**, 542–7.

Pfister, H., Ollert, M., Frohlich, L. F., *et al.* (2004). Antineutrophil cytoplasmic autoantibodies against the murine homolog of proteinase 3 (Wegener autoantigen) are pathogenic in vivo. *Blood*, **104**, 1411–8.

Popa, E. R., Franssen, C. F., Limburg, P. C., Huitema, M. G., Kallenberg, C. G. and Tervaert, J. W. (2002). In vitro cytokine production and proliferation of T cells from patients with antiproteinase 3- and antimyeloperoxidase-associated vasculitis, in response to proteinase 3 and myeloperoxidase. *Arthritis and Rheumatism*, **46**, 1894–904.

Praprotnik, S., Rozman, B., Blank, M. and Shoenfeld, Y. (2000). Pathogenic role of anti-endothelial cell antibodies in systemic vasculitis. *Wiener Klinische Wochenschrift*, **112**, 660–4.

Rahman, T. and Harper, L. (2006). Plasmapheresis in nephrology: an update. *Current Opinion in Nephrology and Hypertension*, **15**, 603–9.

Ralston, D. R., Marsh, C. B., Lowe, M. P. and Wewers, M. D. (1997). Antineutrophil cytoplasmic antibodies induce monocyte IL-8 release. Role of surface proteinase-3, alpha1-antitrypsin, and Fcgamma receptors. *Journal of Clinical Investigation*, **100**, 1416–24.

Reumaux, D., Vossebeld, P. J., Roos, D. and Verhoeven, A. J. (1995). Effect of tumor necrosis factor-induced integrin activation on Fc gamma receptor II-mediated signal transduction: relevance for activation of neutrophils by anti-proteinase 3 or anti-myeloperoxidase antibodies. *Blood*, **86**, 3189–95.

Rodgers, H., Guthrie, J. A., Brownjohn, A. M. and Turney, J. H. (1989). Microscopic polyarteritis: clinical features and treatment. *Postgraduate Medical Journal*, **65**, 515–8.

Sablé-Fourtassou, R., Cohen, P., Mahr, A., *et al.* (2005). Antineutrophil cytoplasmic antibodies and the Churg–Strauss syndrome. *Annals of Internal Medicine*, **143**, 632–8.

Salojin, K. V., Le Tonqueze, M., Saraux, A., *et al.* (1997). Antiendothelial cell antibodies: useful markers of systemic sclerosis. *American Journal of Medicine*, **102**, 178–85.

Savage, C. O., Winearls, C. G., Evans, D. J., Rees, A. J. and Lockwood, C. M. (1985). Microscopic polyarteritis: presentation, pathology and prognosis. *Quarterly Journal of Medicine*, **56**, 467–83.

Schlieben, D. J., Korbet, S. M., Kimura, R. E., Schwartz, M. M. and Lewis, E. J. (2005). Pulmonary-renal syndrome in a newborn with placental transmission of ANCAs. *American Journal of Kidney Diseases*, **45**, 758–61.

Seishima, M., Oyama, Z. and Oda, M. (2004). Skin eruptions associated with microscopic polyangiitis. *European Journal of Dermatology*, **14**, 255–8.

Serra, A., Cameron, J. S., Turner, D. R., *et al.* (1984). Vasculitis affecting the kidney: presentation, histopathology and long-term outcome. *Quarterly Journal of Medicine*, **53**, 181–207.

Simpson, I. J., Doak, P. B., Williams, L. C., *et al.* (1982). Plasma exchange in Goodpasture's syndrome. *American Journal of Nephrology*, **2**, 301–11.

Sinico, R. A., Di Toma, L., Maggiore, U., *et al.* (2005). Prevalence and clinical significance of antineutrophil cytoplasmic antibodies in Churg–Strauss syndrome. *Arthritis and Rheumatism*, **52**, 2926–35.

Souid, M., Terki, N. H., Nochy, D. and Hillion, D. (2001). Myeloperoxidase anti-neutrophil cytoplasmic autoantibodies (MPO-ANCA)-related rapidly progressive glomerulonephritis (RPGN) and pulmonary fibrosis (PF) with dissociated evolution. *Clinical Nephrology*, **55**, 337–8.

Tesar, V., Rihova, Z., Jancova, E., Rysava, R. and Merta, M. (2003). Current treatment strategies in ANCA-positive renal vasculitis-lessons from European randomized trials. *Nephrology Dialysis Transplantation*, **18** (Suppl. 5), 2–4.

Tidman, M., Olander, R., Svalander, C. and Danielsson, D. (1998). Patients hospitalized because of small vessel vasculitides with renal involvement in the period 1975–95: organ involvement, anti-neutrophil cytoplasmic antibodies patterns, seasonal attack rates and fluctuation of annual frequencies. *Journal of Internal Medicine*, **244**, 133–41.

Tsai, C. N., Chang, C. M., Chuang, C. H., Jin, Y. T., Liu, M. F. and Wang, C. R. (2004). Extended colonic ulcerations in a patient with microscopic polyangiitis. *Annals of the Rheumatic Diseases*, **63**, 1521–2.

Ueda, S., Matsumoto, M., Ahn, T., *et al.* (2001). Microscopic polyangiitis complicated with massive intestinal bleeding. *Journal of Gastroenterology*, **36**, 264–70.

van Bommel, E., Brouwers, A., Makkus, A. and van Vliet, A. (2002). Retroperitoneal fibrosis and p-ANCA-associated polyarteritis nodosa: coincidental or common etiology? *European Journal of Internal Medicine*, **13**, 392.

van der Woude, F. J., Rasmussen, N., Lobatto, S., *et al.* (1985). Autoantibodies against neutrophils and monocytes: tool for diagnosis and marker of disease activity in Wegener's granulomatosis. *Lancet*, **1**, 425–9.

Wang, L., Thelmo, W. L. and Axiotis, C. A. (2002). Microscopic polyangiitis with massive myocardial necrosis and diffuse pulmonary hemorrhage. *Virchows Archiv*, **441**, 202–4.

Watts, R. A., Jolliffe, V. A., Carruthers, D. M., Lockwood, M. and Scott, D. G. (1996). Effect of classification on the incidence of polyarteritis nodosa and microscopic polyangiitis. *Arthritis and Rheumatism*, **39**, 1208–12.

Weidner, S., Neupert, W., Goppelt-Struebe, M. and Rupprecht, H. D. (2001). Antineutrophil cytoplasmic antibodies induce human monocytes to produce oxygen radicals *in vitro*. *Arthritis and Rheumatism*, **44,** 1698–706.

Wohlwill, F. (1923). Ueber die nur mikroskopisch erkennbare Form der Periarteritis nodosa. *Virchows Archiv A-Pathological Anatomy and Histopathology*, **246,** 377–411.

Xiao, H., Heeringa, P., Hu, P., *et al.* (2002). Antineutrophil cytoplasmic autoantibodies specific for myeloperoxidase cause glomerulonephritis and vasculitis in mice. *Journal of Clinical Investigation*, **110,** 955–63.

Xiao, H., Heeringa, P., Liu, Z., *et al.* (2005). The role of neutrophils in the induction of glomerulonephritis by anti-myeloperoxidase antibodies. *American Journal of Pathology*, **167,** 39–45.

Zauner, I., Bach, D., Braun, N., *et al.* (2002). Predictive value of initial histology and effect of plasmapheresis on long-term prognosis of rapidly progressive glomerulonephritis. *American Journal of Kidney Diseases*, **39,** 28–35.

CHAPTER 28

Cutaneous polyarteritis

Holly M. Bastian

Introduction

Cutaneous polyarteritis nodosa (CPAN) is a chronic, relapsing arteritis of subcutaneous, and deep dermal, small and medium-sized vessels. It spares visceral organs, and only rarely evolves into a systemic disease (David *et al.* 1993; Dewar and Bellamy 1992; Dyk 1973). The hallmark of CPAN is painful nodules, which may ulcerate, and which usually arise on the lower extremities (see Figure 10.11 in Chapter 10), often with a starburst of livedo reticularis or racemose livedo (Figure 28.1). Regional neurological and musculoskeletal symptoms are not uncommon.

CPAN was first recognized as a distinct entity, separate from polyarteritis nodosa (PAN), with the description by Lindberg in 1931 of two patients whose skin lesions were due to necrotizing arteritis, but without signs of visceral involvement. Reports by Carol and Prakken (1937), Miescher (1946), Lindgren and Lundmark (1956), Borrie (1972), Diaz-Perez and Winkelmann (1974), and others more recently (Chen 1989; Daoud *et al.* 1997; Khoo and Ng 1998), have reinforced the classification of CPAN as a distinctive disease. Numerous authors have emphasized the view that the microscopic anatomy warrants its classification as a form of polyarteritis, and in the absence of clinical or laboratory evidence of systemic lesions, as CPAN (Fisher and Orkin 1964; Ketron and Bernstein 1939; Rawlinson and Ball 1981; Slinger and Starck 1951; Thomas and Black 1983). This view embraces the fact that as many as one-quarter of patients with classical PAN have skin lesions, though not usually arteritic, which could be a major source of nosologic confusion. It also emphasizes that CPAN should not be diagnosed until a reasonable search is made for visceral disease; skin biopsies showing arteritis should be the sole basis for a diagnosis of CPAN only when systemic disease has been excluded. A large number of patients with CPAN have died from unrelated causes, and systemic arteritis was not found at autopsy. Furthermore, large numbers of patients have been followed who did not display signs of progression to systemic disease. Diaz-Perez and Winkelmann (1974) followed 23 such patients a mean of 6.9 years, and Daoud *et al.* (1997) followed 24 for a minimum of 10 years, observing no conversion to PAN. Finally, in this regard, Borrie (1972) followed 15 CPAN patients for as long as 23 years, and a mean of 11.5, finding no evidence of systemic spread. Because strict histologic criteria have not always been followed, some cases that were defined as CPAN were, in retrospect, examples of systemic polyarteritis (Minkowitz *et al.* 1991) and other forms of vasculitis (Chen 1989; Dewar and Bellamy 1992; Dyk 1973; Miescher 1946).

Histopathology

Microscopically, the vascular lesions of CPAN can be very similar to those of systemic PAN (Figure 28.2) (Kleeman *et al.* 1998). In both conditions the lesions usually consist of necrotizing inflammation, in various stages of healing, which involve small and medium-sized arteries; however, in CPAN only the deep dermal and subcutaneous vessels are compromised (Albornoz *et al.* 1998). Systemic polyarteritis rarely presents as a nodular arteritis of the skin, and the histopathology is usually of small-vessel leukocytoclastic vasculitis involving postcapillary venules of the superficial vessels (Minkowitz *et al.* 1991). Early lesions of CPAN are panarteritic, with degeneration of the arterial wall, varying amounts of destruction of the external and internal elastic lamina, and fibrinoid necrosis. A neutrophilic infiltrate with leukocytoclasis is found in and around the vessel wall, with or without eosinophils. During later stages, complete occlusion of the lumina may occur due to thrombosis and proliferation of the endothelium, and lead to ischemia and epidermal ulceration. Healing is characterized by mononuclear cells and proliferation of fibroblasts. Focal lobular panniculitis may be found near the affected vessels (Chiu and Rajapakse 1991; Goodless *et al.* 1990; Lever and Shaumberg-Lever 1990; Malaviya *et al.* 1999).

Pathogenesis

The pathogenesis of both CPAN and systemic PAN is poorly understood. Support for hypersensitivity as a possible cause for CPAN includes examples of cases that have developed following exposure to minocycline (Pelletier *et al.* 2003; Schaffer *et al.* 2001; Schrodt and Callen 2006); sulfonamide; streptomycin; penicillin (Borrie 1972); metolazone (Weinrauch *et al.* 1982); estrogens (Keyloun *et al.* 1967); and antituberculous (Swarc and Kaminski *et al.* 1971) and chemotherapeutic drugs. It has also been described following treatment with 2-chlorodeoxyadenosine (Rosen *et al.* 1995).

CPAN has been diagnosed in newborn infants of three mothers with the disease, invoking a potential role for transfer of antigens

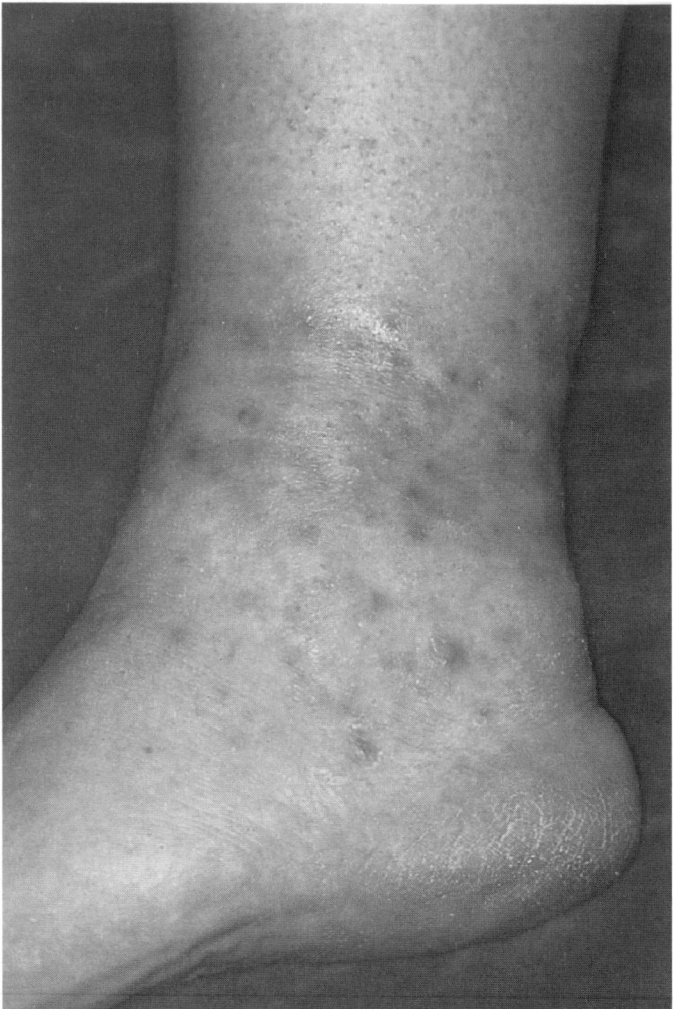

Figure 28.1 Tender nodules and livedo reticularis about the left ankle of a woman with cutaneous polyarteritis. (See Color Plate 78).

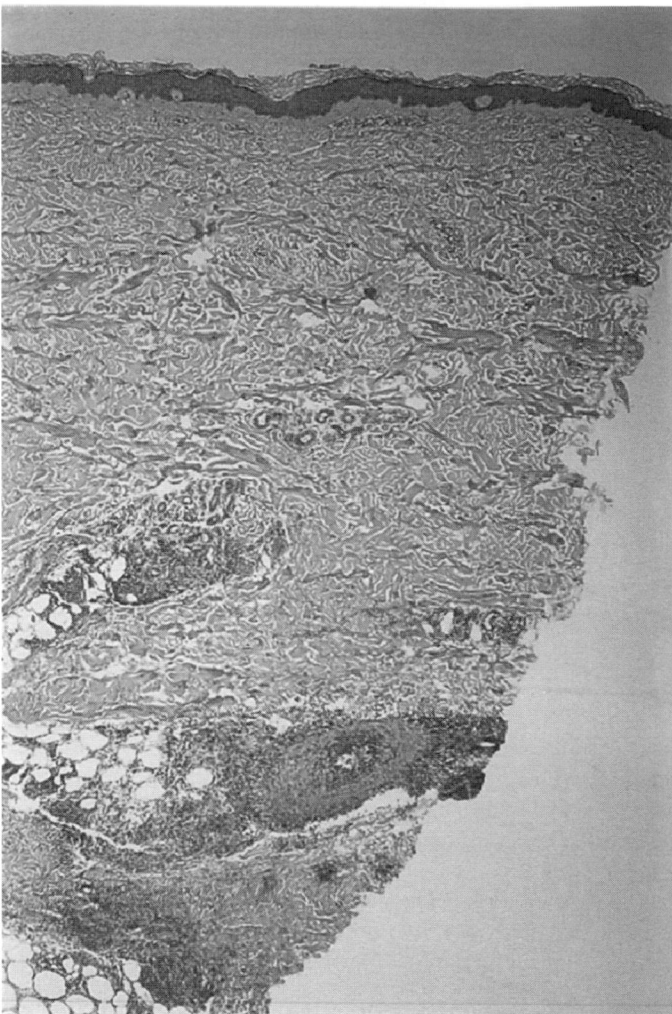

Figure 28.2 Skin punch biopsy. Inflammatory cells infiltrating the medium sized arteries of the deep reticular dermis. (H and E stain.) (See Color Plate 79).

(Boren and Everett 1965; Miller, III and Fries 1975; Stone *et al.* 1993). There have also been a few cases of CPAN following hepatitis B vaccination (Bourgeais *et al.* 2003; Whittaker *et al.* 1986), suggesting an immunological cause. Although systemic PAN has been reported to follow streptococcal pharyngitis (David *et al.* 1993; Fink 1991; Fordham, III *et al.* 1964; Friedberg and Gross 1934; Rose and Spencer 1957), CPAN has been less frequently associated with streptococcal pharyngitis in adults (Stein *et al.* 2001; Albornoz *et al.* 1998) than in children (Albornoz *et al.* 1998; Daoud *et al.* 1997; Orkin and Winkelmann 1970).

The presence of IgM, IgG, and complement (Kiraly *et al.* 1978) supports an immunological etiology for the lesions. In addition, deposition of IgM in the vessel walls has been found in six of 10 cases, and C3 in four of 10 cases described by Diaz-Perez *et al.* (1980), and elevated C1q levels have been found in a group of patients with cutaneous vasculitis (Sano *et al.* 1979).

Clinical features

Unlike systemic PAN, CPAN seems to occur slightly more often in women (1.7:1) according to one large case series (Daoud *et al.* 1997);

however, it had been previously reported as occurring with equal frequency in men and women (Diaz-Perez *et al.* 1980). It has been found in persons ranging from infancy to age 72. The age of onset does not seem to influence severity of the disease (Avedisian and Adelizzi 1985; Daoud *et al.* 1997). Three classes of CPAN have been described (Table 28.1) (Chen 1989; Daoud *et al.* 1997). Class I (mild cutaneous) consists primarily of nodular skin lesions and livedo reticularis. Class II (severe cutaneous) involves prominent livedo lesions, ulceration and pain. Class III is defined by the presence of necrotizing livedo and acral gangrene.

The typical nodules of CPAN are tender and sometimes painful; they tend to be red early on and blue later. They range in size from 0.5 to 3 cm in diameter, and tend to occur in clusters of up to several hundred nodules. Common sites of involvement are the lower legs, ankles, and feet, but they may occur on the arms, trunk, head, or face and, rarely, on mucosal surfaces (Borrie 1972). The nodules tend to occur in different stages and may last for a few days or a few weeks. Lower limb ulcerations have been seen in as many as 50% of patients with CPAN (Daoud *et al.* 1997; Diaz-Perez *et al.* 1980).

The musculoskeletal and peripheral nervous systems are also affected in CPAN. One of the most common presenting features is

Table 28.1 Cutaneous PAN: classes of severity

Class	Cutaneous manifestations	Extracutaneous manifestations
I – Mild cutaneous	Nodular skin lesions Livedo reticularis	Mild polyneuropathy may be present
II – Severe cutaneous	Livedo more prominent Ulceration Pain	Mild polyneuropathy frequently present Fever, malaise, arthralgias (acute phase)
III – Progressive systemic	Necrotizing livedo Acral gangrene	Progressive musculoskeletal involvement Foot drop Visceral involvement (eventually) Autoimmune tests positive

Adapted from: Chen K.R. Cutaneous polyarteritis nodosa: a clinical and histopathological study of 20 cases. *Journal of Dermatology*, **16**(6), 429–42, 1989. Daoud, M.S., Hutton, K.P. and Gibson L.E. Cutaneous periarteritis nodosa: a clinicopathological study of 79 cases. *British Journal of Dermatology*, **136**, 706–13, 1997.

arthralgias; however, a few patients may present with arthritis manifested by stiffness and recurrent inflammatory effusions with a predominance of polymorphonuclear leukocytes. The arthritis is usually non-destructive and non-erosive (Gottlieb 1978; Mekori *et al.* 1984), but it may be rapidly progressive (Mekori *et al.* 1984) and require aggressive treatment (Gottlieb 1978). Radiographic findings have included cystic changes, and joint space narrowing of the carpus and ankles (Quintana *et al.* 2004). CPAN has been described with periosteal new bone formation (Flanagan *et al.* 1999; Peron *et al.* 1999). Synovial biopsies typically reveal non-specific synovitis without evidence of vasculitis (Mekori *et al.* 1984; Smukler and Schumacher 1977).

Myalgias and myositis occur less frequently than arthralgias and arthritis. The former usually occur in the calves (Soubrier *et al.* 1997), but may be widespread. Myositis may occur in proximity to nodules. Muscle biopsy features are usually those of PAN, and inflammation may persist for months or years (Borrie 1972). Peripheral sensorimotor neuropathy, most often expressed as mononeuropathy multiplex, is of varying severity, and involves feet and lower legs more often than hands and forearms. This has been reported in as many as 50% of patients (Daoud *et al.* 1997; Diaz-Perez *et al.* 1980). The course may unfold to complete recovery or permanent damage with wasting and contractures of the limbs.

Unusual presentations of CPAN have been reported, for example nail lesions with classic histologic changes of CPAN (Kassis *et al.* 1985). The nail plates were thin, excessively ridged, and split longitudinally. The abnormalities slowly resolved with glucocorticoid therapy. Ocular inflammation (Grinbaum *et al.* 1994) and Raynaud's phenomena (Andreu-Sanchez *et al.* 1991) have been reported as initial presenting features of CPAN. Single case reports of myasthenia gravis (Sayed *et al.* 2006), collagenous colitis (Procopiou *et al.* 2004),

necrotizing fasciitis (Stein *et al.* 2001), morphea associated with ANCA positivity (Reddy *et al.* 2005), and necrosis of the fingers (Chiu and Rajapakse 1991; Schanz and Ulmer 2006; Stussi *et al.* 2001) in association with CPAN have been documented. Even though serious debilitation is uncommon and perhaps unheard of until recently in association with CPAN, a case of CPAN complicated by anterior tibial artery occlusion leading to amputation of a limb has been reported (Kuriya *et al.* 2006). Other vascular occlusions and abnormalities have been documented in CPAN, including thrombosis of the superior and inferior vena cavae without documented coagulation abnormalities (Lightman *et al.* 1988), and the finding of multiple aneurysms of small and medium sized renal vessels in a patient with no other evidence of systemic involvement. The latter has supported the notion that differentiation between CPAN and systemic polyarteritis nodosa is an oversimplification (Orton and Whittaker 2000).

Diagnostic features

As in systemic PAN, there are no serologic tests that are diagnostic for CPAN. However, investigations of basic fibroblast growth factor (bFGF) and vascular endothelial growth factor (VEGF) have revealed that these angiogenic cytokines are significantly elevated in patients with CPAN and systemic PAN in comparison to healthy controls. In addition, the levels of both cytokines seem to be significantly higher in patients with the systemic form of the disease (Kikuchi *et al.* 2005) than in CPAN. Irrespective of these findings, the diagnosis of CPAN is dependent on the clinical history and biopsy of the cutaneous lesions. An elevated sedimentation rate is the most frequently occurring laboratory abnormality. Serum rheumatoid factor, antinuclear antibodies, antineutrophil cytoplasmic antibodies, serum complement levels, cryoglobulins, and hepatitis B and C serologies are usually absent or normal (Daoud *et al.* 1997; Moreland and Ball 1990; Verbov and Stansfeld 1972). Similarly, routine serum chemistry panels, blood counts, and urinalyses are normal (Table 28.2).

In persons with CPAN, systemic symptoms should be evaluated to determine the presence of visceral polyarteritis. Abdominal pain, gastrointestinal blood loss, hypertension, and elevated creatinine may warrant evaluation with imaging studies to exclude generalized

Table 28.2 Comparison between systemic and cutaneous polyarteritis nodosa

	Systemic	Cutaneous
Blood pressure	Frequently elevated	Normal
Leukocytosis	Frequent; at times very high	Normal to moderate increase
Eosinophilia	Frequent	None
Visceral involvement: heart, GI tract, liver	Present	None
Neuromuscular changes	Diffuse	Localized to areas of skin lesions
Prognosis	Frequently fatal in first 2 years	Chronic; relapsing, benign disease

Adapted from: Diaz-Perez and Winkelmann (1974).

vasculitis. Central nervous system symptoms may mandate complete evaluations of the brain. Extracutaneous manifestations including constitutional symptoms, local neurological and musculoskeletal manifestations may be associated with CPAN (Bauza *et al.* 2002). Myalgias and muscle weakness should be evaluated as indicated. Nerve conduction velocity tests and sural nerve biopsy may be useful.

Differential diagnosis

In addition to systemic PAN, multiple conditions may resemble or mimic CPAN, as shown in Table 28.3. Of these conditions, only PAN exhibits panarteritis histologically. Furthermore, nodules are uncommon in PAN as the majority of skin lesions present as hemorrhagic purpura (Pak *et al.* 1998). CPAN has also been mimicked by or found in association with a number of other diseases, including bacterial and atypical infections. Meliodosis, an infectious disease caused by the bacterium *Burkholderia pseudomallei*, was documented in a Thai woman presenting with high fever, leukocytosis, splenomegaly, splenic abscesses, arthralgias, and erythematous painful nodules which were histologically consistent with CPAN (Choonhakarn and Jirarattanapochai 1998). A patient with CPAN and leukocytoclastic vasculitis related to *Mycobacterium fortuitum* has also been described (Chen *et al.* 2004), and a man with CPAN, a strongly positive purified protein derivative skin test for tuberculosis, and exposure to active tuberculosis (Antony and Sidhu 1977) was reported to have resolution of his painful lesions with antituberculous therapy. Finally, CPAN has been reported after necrotizing fasciitis associated with Group A streptococcal infection (Stein *et al.* 2001). CPAN-like lesions may be associated with certain autoimmune diseases including relapsing polychondritis (Rauh *et al.* 1993) and rheumatoid arthritis (Chen *et al.* 2002; Magro and Crowson 2003). Behçet's syndrome with CPAN-like lesions on biopsy has been described (Chen 1989; Liao *et al.* 1999; Vikas *et al.* 2003). Leukocytoclastic vasculitis has been reported in association with two cases of CPAN (deShazo *et al.* 1977; Pischel and Zvaifler 1984). A few reports have described patients with CPAN by biopsy who were later diagnosed with Takayasu's arteritis (Mousa *et al.* 1985; Nikolic *et al.* 1993). In addition, patients with

Table 28.3 Conditions that may mimic cutaneous polyarteritis

Cellulitis
Recurrent thrombophlebitis
Rheumatoid arthritis with nodulosis
Erythema nodosum
Chronic cutaneous leukocytoclastic vasculitis
Weber Christian disease
Angiocentric T cell lymphoma (Thomas *et al.* 1994)
Aortic angiosarcoma (Sparsa *et al.* 2006)
Atrophie blanche (Mimouni *et al.* 2003)
Papulonecrotic tuberculids (Borrie 1972)
Bazin's erythema induratum (Ruiter 1958)
Nodular vasculitis (Kint and Van Herpe 1979)
Necrotizing vasculitis (Goodless *et al.* 1990)
Pyoderma gangrenosum (Nguyen *et al.* 2003)

Takayasu's arteritis, with typical stenosing lesions involving the aorta and its branches, as well as biopsy-proven CPAN have been described (Cajigas *et al.* 1987; Mousa *et al.* 1985). CPAN has also been observed in persons with Crohn's disease and ulcerative colitis (Chiu and Rajapakse 1991; Goslen *et al.* 1983; Grana *et al.* 1991; Kahn *et al.* 1980; Matsumura *et al.* 2000; Solley *et al.* 1975; Volk and Owen 1986; Voulgarelis *et al.* 1998). Although inflammatory bowel disease usually precedes CPAN, the reverse has been documented (Gudbjornsson and Hallgren 1990; Solley *et al.* 1975). In addition, there appears to be little correlation between the occurrence of flares of CPAN and those of ulcerative colitis. Further, resection of the colon does not appear to prevent the recurrence of CPAN (Paller 1986; Volk and Owen 1986).

In general, viral infections have been described infrequently in the setting of CPAN. Despite the fact that several reports have described an association of parvovirus B19 with necrotizing vasculitis and systemic PAN (Corman and Staud 1992; Nikkari *et al.* 1994; Viguier *et al.* 2001), this pathogen has been described in association with necrotizing CPAN only rarely (Dusunsel *et al.* 2002). Although human immunodeficiency virus (HIV) is not usually associated with PAN, at least two cases of HIV and CPAN have been reported. In one, the patient was HIV-positive, and had a fever, rash, and lesions consistent with CPAN, which responded to therapy with glucocorticoids (Pereira *et al.* 1995). The other was of a patient with CPAN having HIV which was documented in a retrospective study of the occurrence of hepatitis C in 16 patients with CPAN (Soufir *et al.* 1999). In this same study, five of the 16 patients with CPAN also tested positive for hepatitis C by ELISA, which was confirmed by immunoblot assay. This finding could suggest that CPAN may also have an association with hepatitis C infection (Soufir *et al.* 1999); however, only one case of CPAN was reported in a review of the dermatological manifestations of 35 patients with hepatitis C infection (Crowson *et al.* 2003).

Hepatitis B surface antigen in systemic PAN is a well-recognized association. Prior to 1986 only two cases of hepatitis B in association with CPAN had been published (Van de Pette *et al.* 1984; Whittaker *et al.* 1986); however, in 1991 Minkowitz noted that four out of nine (44%) of patients initially diagnosed with CPAN had serologic evidence of hepatitis B infection and that seven of nine patients (78%) went on to have organ manifestations other than skin (Minkowitz *et al.* 1991). This finding serves to remind us that the distinction between CPAN and the systemic form of polyarteritis nodosa may lack certainty.

Therapy

Remissions may occur spontaneously or the disease may require treatment. Non-steroidal anti-inflammatory drugs have been effective in some cases; however, successful treatment usually involves moderate dosages of glucocorticoids, which sometime induce a remission of the disease or a reduction in pain within 3–6 months. Some cases are unresponsive to such treatment and other drugs such as sulfapyridine, dapsone, pentoxifylline (Calderon *et al.* 1993), or stanazol (Thomas and Black 1983) have been used. In patients with tissue loss, mononeuropathy multiplex, and myositis, disease modifying antirheumatic drugs (DMARDs) have been tried. Successful treatment with low-dose weekly methotrexate has been reported in about seven persons (Jorizzo *et al.* 1991; Queiro *et al.* 2002; Schartz *et al.* 2001). Other DMARDS, including azathioprine (Fitzgerald and Verbov 1996; Thomas and Black 1983), intravenous cyclophosphamide (Fort and Abruzzo 1988), and intravenous gamma globulin (Gedalia *et al.* 1995; Gedalia and Sorensen 1998) have been used with some success. In 2003, successful response to infliximab was also reported in a patient with polyarteritis nodosa-like cutaneous vasculitis and undifferentiated spondyloarthropathy (Garcia-Porrua and Gonsales-Gay 2003).

The effect of exogenous estrogens on CPAN activity is uncertain. One woman experienced clinical remission with each of her three pregnancies (Cherubin 1966), but another developed active CPAN during pregnancy (Janin-Mercier *et al.* 1982). CPAN has been reported in a presumed postmenopausal woman who was still producing detectable levels of estrogens (Cvancara *et al.* 1998), but who responded to treatment with tamoxifen (a non-steroidal antiestrogen and partial estrogen agonist). The response was attributed to an antiestrogen effect.

Cutaneous polyarteritis nodosa in children

CPAN rarely occurs in children. The first case reported was in 1980 by Verbov. Non-recurring CPAN has been observed in neonates (Boren and Everett 1965; Miller, III and Fries 1975; Stone *et al.* 1993) who were born to mothers with the chronic form of CPAN. The recurring form has been reported in children as young as 1 or 2 years of age (Kumar *et al.* 1995; Siberry *et al.* 1994); however, the usual age of occurrence is somewhat older. CPAN of childhood is very similar to that of adults (Ginarte *et al.* 1998; Siberry *et al.* 1994). The clinical course is one of periods of remissions and exacerbations. Fever and tender, subcutaneous, dermal nodules, occurring predominantly in the lower extremities, characterize the disease. Neonates and small children may experience gangrene and autoamputation of fingers or toes (Boki *et al.* 1997; Boren and Everett 1965; Kumar *et al.* 1995; Miller, III and Fries 1975). Acral necrosis has been attributed to the small caliber of acral arteries in the newborn (Stone *et al.* 1993). As in adults, arthritis and myositis are not unusual occurrences. Diagnosis is based on biopsy findings. Putative initiating events are similar to those seen in adults and include streptococcal infections (which may be a more common precipitant in children), rheumatic fever, Crohn's disease, and ulcerative colitis. Other possible triggers include: diphtheria–pertussis–tetanus immunization; insect bites; *Plasmodium falciparum* malaria; treatment with minocycline or tetracycline; and other childhood immunizations (Schrodt and Callen 2006; Calderon *et al.* 1993; Daoud *et al.* 1997; Mekori *et al.* 1984; Sheth *et al.* 1994; Till and Amos 1997). In contrast to adults, no cases have been reported in children in association with HIV, hepatitis B virus infection, or familial Mediterranean fever (Ginarte *et al.* 1998; Siberry *et al.* 1994). The differential diagnosis of CPAN in children includes: superficial thrombophlebitis; systemic PAN; Kawasaki's disease; Henoch–Schönlein purpura; Churg–Strauss syndrome; juvenile inflammatory arthritis; erythema multiforme; rheumatic fever; and panniculitis (Sheth *et al.* 1994; Siberry *et al.* 1994).

As in adulthood, CPAN in childhood rarely progresses to PAN, and the effects of treatment can be difficult to evaluate. An international survey of pediatricians from 21 pediatric centers identified 110 children with PAN, 33 of whom had cutaneous lesions (Ozen *et al.* 2004). Of the 33 children with CPAN, 40% had an upper respiratory infection at the start of their disease. Eleven of the patients received prophylactic penicillin, and about 25 received

glucocorticoids at some point during their illness. In addition, three were treated with azathioprine and five with cyclophosphamide because they had constitutional symptoms and a high level of acute phase reactants. There were only four relapses and overall the prognosis was good.

In general, most children are treated with acetylsalicylic acid, other non-steroidal anti-inflammatory drugs, or glucocorticoids (prednisone equivalent 1–2 mg/kg/day) or 30 mg/kg methylprednisolone injection per month during flares of the disease (Mocan *et al.* 1998; Sheth *et al.* 1994; Siberry *et al.* 1994). Because CPAN tends to be a benign, chronic condition, a more conservative approach has been suggested with a goal of relieving pain rather than resolution of the lesions (Draaisma *et al.* 1992). Intravenous immunoglobulin therapy proved to be efficacious in a child where there was concern for long-term treatment with glucocorticoids (Uziel and Silverman 1998). Some authors have advocated penicillin prophylaxis and treatment of streptococcal infections with penicillin to prevent recurrences of CPAN (Falcini 2004; Fink 1991), but treatment with penicillin under these circumstances has not always been helpful (Fathalla *et al.* 2005; Sheth *et al.* 1994; Till and Amos 1997). Some patients appear to have responded well to pentoxifylline (Calderon *et al.* 1993) or chloroquine (Goodless *et al.* 1990). Patients in whom there is a significant threat of tissue loss may require treatment with cytotoxic agents such as methotrexate (Jorizzo *et al.* 1991), or cyclophosphamide (Kumar *et al.* 1995).

In conclusion, many, if not most, patients experience persistence of cutaneous lesions for as long as 20 years, but it is important to recognize the uncommon progression to systemic arteritis after years of confinement to the skin. Long-term surveillance of this disease is therefore essential.

References

Albornoz, M. A., Benedetto, A. V., Korman, M., McFall, S., Tourtellotte, C. D., and Myers, A. R. (1998). Relapsing cutaneous polyarteritis nodosa associated with streptococcal infections. *International Journal of Dermatology*, **37**, 664–6.

Andreu-Sanchez, J. L., Martin-Santos, J. M., Isasi-Zaragoza, C., Trujillo-Castellanos, A., Cuende-Quintana, E., and Mulero, J. (1991). Raynaud's phenomenon as initial manifestation of cutaneous polyarteritis nodosa. *Annals of the Rheumatic Diseases*, **50**, 48–50.

Antony, L. and Sidhu, G. S. (1977). Cutaneous polyarteritis nodosa. *Archives of Dermatology*, **113**, 518–9.

Avedisian, R. and Adelizzi, R. A. (1985). Cutaneous polyarteritis nodosa: report of case and literature review. *Journal of the American Osteopathic Association*, **85**, 93–6.

Bauza, A., Espana, A., and Idoate, M. (2002). Cutaneous polyarteritis nodosa. *British Journal of Dermatology*, **146**, 694–9.

Boki, K. A., Dafni, U., Karpouzas, G. A., Papasteriades, C., Drosos, A. A., and Moutsopoulos, H. M. (1997). Necrotizing vasculitis in Greece: clinical, immunological and immunogenetic aspects. A study of 66 patients. *British Journal of Rheumatology*, **36**, 1059–66.

Boren, R. J. and Everett, M. A. (1965). Cutaneous vasculitis in mother and infant. *Archives of Dermatology*, **92**, 568–70.

Borrie, P. (1972). Cutaneous polyarteritis nodosa. *British Journal of Dermatology*, **87**, 87–95.

Bourgeais, A. M., Dore, M. X., Croue, A., Leclech, C., and Verret, J. L. (2003). Cutaneous polyarteritis nodosa following hepatitis B vaccination. *Annales de Dermatologie et de Venereologie*, **130**, 205–7.

Cajigas, J. C., Amigo, M. C., Pineda, C., Herrera, R., Sanchez-Torres, G., and Martinez-Lavin, M. (1987). Association between Takayasu's arteritis and cutaneous polyarteritis nodosa. *American Journal of Medicine*, **82**, 382–4.

Calderon, M. J., Landa, N., Aguirre, A. and Diaz-Perez, J. L. (1993). Successful treatment of cutaneous PAN with pentoxifylline. *British Journal Dermatology*, **128**, 706–8.

Carol, W. L. L. and Prakken, J. R. (1937). Die kutane form de periarteritis nodosa. *Acta Dermato-Venereologica*, **18**, 102–18.

Chen, H. H., Hsaio, C. H. and Chui, H. C. (2004). Successive development of cutaneous polyarteritis nodosa, leucocytoclastic vasculitis and Sweet's syndrome in a patient with cervical lymphadenitis caused by *Mycobacterium fortuitum. British Journal of Dermatology*, **151**, 1096–100.

Chen, K. R. (1989). Cutaneous polyarteritis nodosa: a clinical and histopathological study of 20 cases. *Journal of Dermatology*, **16**, 429–42.

Chen, K. R., Toyohara, A., Suzuki, A. and Mizuno, M. (2002). Clinical and histopathological spectrum of cutaneous vasculitis in rheumatoid arthritis. *British Journal of Dermatology*, **147**, 905–13.

Cherubin, C. E. (1966). So-called cutaneous polyarteritis nodosa. *New York State Journal of Medicine*, **66**, 1673–8.

Chiu, G. and Rajapakse, C. N. (1991). Cutaneous polyarteritis nodosa and ulcerative colitis. *Journal of Rheumatology*, **18**, 769–70.

Choonhakarn, C. and Jirarattanapochai, K. (1998). Cutaneous polyarteritis nodosa: a report of a case associated with melioidosis (Burkholderia pseudomallei). *International Journal of Dermatology*, **37**, 433–53.

Corman, L. and Staud, R. (1992). Polyarteritis nodosa and parvovirus B19 infection. *Lancet*, **343**, 339–491.

Crowson, A. N., Nuovo, G., Ferri, C. and Magro, C. M. (2003). The dermatopathologic manifestations of hepatitis C infection: a clinical, histological, and molecular assessment of 35 cases. *Human Pathology*, **34**, 573–9.

Cvancara, J. L., Meffert, J. J. and Elston, D. M. (1998). Estrogen-sensitive cutaneous polyarteritis nodosa: response to tamoxifen. *Journal American Academy of Dermatology*, **39**, 643–6.

Daoud, M. S., Hutton, K. P. and Gibson, L. E. (1997). Cutaneous periarteritis nodosa: a clinicopathological study of 79 cases. *British Journal of Dermatology*, **136**, 706–13.

David, J., Ansell, B. M., and Woo, P. (1993). Polyarteritis nodosa associated with streptococcus. *Archives of Disease in Childhood*, **69**, 685–8.

deShazo, R. D., Levinson, A. I., Lawless, O. J., and Weisbaum, G. (1977). Systemic vasculitis with coexistent large and small vessel involvement. A classification dilemma. *Journal of the American Medical Association*, **238**, 1940–2.

Dewar, C. L. and Bellamy, N. (1992). Necrotizing mesenteric vasculitis after longstanding cutaneous polyarteritis nodosa. *Journal of Rheumatology*, **19**, 1308–11.

Diaz-Perez, J. L., Schroeter, A. L., and Winkelmann, R. K. (1980). Cutaneous periarteritis nodosa: Immunofluorescence studies. *Archives of Dermatology*, **116**, 56–8.

Diaz-Perez, J. L. and Winkelmann, R. K. (1974). Cutaneous periarteritis nodosa. *Archives of Dermatology*, **110**, 407–14.

Draaisma, J. M., Fiselier, T. J., and Mullaart, R. A. (1992). Mononeuritis multiplex in a child with cutaneous polyarteritis. *Neuropediatrics*, **23**, 28–9.

Dusunsel, R., Goldsmith, A., and Yehuda, B. (2002). Parvovirus B19 infection associated with myelosuppression and cutaneous polyarteritis nodosa. *British Society for Rheumatology*, **41**, 1210–2.

Dyk, T. (1973). Cutaneous polyarteritis. *British Medical Journal*, **1**, 551.

Falcini, F. (2004). Vascular and connective tissue diseases in the paediatric world. *Lupus*, **13**, 77–84.

Fathalla, B., Miller, L., Brady, S., and Schaller, J. (2005). Cutaneous polyarteritis nodosa in children. *Journal of the American Academy of Dermatology*, **53**, 724–8.

Fink, C. W. (1991). The role of the streptococcus in poststreptococcal reactive arthritis and childhood polyarteritis nodosa. *Journal of Rheumatology*, **29** (Suppl.), 14–20.

Fisher, I. and Orkin, M. (1964). Cutaneous form of periarteritis nodosa – an entity? *Archives of Dermatology*, **89**, 180–9.

Fitzgerald, D. A. and Verbov, J. L. (1996). Cutaneous polyarteritis nodosa. *Archives of Disease in Childhood*, **74**, 367.

Flanagan, N., Casey, E. B., Watson, R., and Barnes, L. (1999). Cutaneous polyarteritis nodosa with seronegative arthritis. *Rheumatology* (Oxford), **38**, 1161–2.

Fordham, C. C., III, Epstein, F. H., Huffiness, W. D., and Harrington, J. T. (1964). Polyarteritis and acute post-streptococcal glomerulonephritis. *Annals of Internal Medicine*, **61**, 89–97.

Fort, J. G. and Abruzzo, J. L. (1988). Reversal of progressive necrotizing vasculitis with intravenous pulse cyclophosphamide and methylprednisolone. *Arthritis and Rheumatism*, **31**, 1194–8.

Friedberg, C. K. and Gross, L. (1934). Periarteritis nodosa (necrotizing arteritis) associated with, rheumatic heart disease with a note on abdominal rheumatism. *Archives in Internal Medicine*, **54**, 170–98.

Garcia-Porrua, C and Gonzales-Gay, M. (2003). Successful response to infliximab in a patient with undifferentiated spondyloarthropathy coexisting with polyarteritis nodosa-like cutaneous vasculitis. *Clinical and Experimental Rheumatology*, **21** (Suppl. 32), S138.

Gedalia, A., Correa, H., Kaiser, M., and Sorensen, R. (1995). Case report: steroid sparing effect of intravenous gamma globulin in a child with necrotizing vasculitis. *American Journal of Medical Science*, **309**, 226–8.

Gedalia, A. and Sorensen, R. (1998). Intravenous immunoglobulin in childhood cutaneous polyarteritis nodosa. *Clinical and Experimental Rheumatology*, **16**, 767.

Ginarte, M., Pereiro, M., and Toribio, J. (1998). Cutaneous polyarteritis nodosa in a child. *Pediatric Dermatology*, **15**, 103–7.

Goodless, D. R., Dhawan, S. S., Alexis, J. M.B., and Wiszniak, J. (1990). Cutaneous periarteritis nodosa. *International Journal of Dermatology*, **29**, 611–5.

Goslen, J. B., Graham, W., and Lazarus, G. S. (1983). Cutaneous polyarteritis nodosa. Report of a case associated with Crohn's disease. *Archives of Dermatology*, **119**, 326–9.

Gottlieb, N. L. (1978). Arthropathy associated with cutaneous polyarteritis. *Arthritis and Rheumatism*, **21**, 281–2.

Grana, G. J., Alonso, A. P., Yebra Pimental, M. T., Sanchez, B. J., Vasquez Iglesias, J. L., and Galdo, F. F. (1991). Cutaneous polyarteritis nodosa and Crohn's disease. *Clinical Rheumatology*, **10**, 196–200.

Grinbaum, A., Ashkenazi, A., Avni, I., and Treister, G. (1994). Ocular inflammation as an initial manifestation of cutaneous polyarteritis nodosa. *British Journal of Dermatology*, **131**, 451–2.

Gudbjornsson, B. and Hallgren, R. (1990). Cutaneous polyarteritis nodosa associated with Crohn's disease. Report and review of the literature. *Journal of Rheumatology*, **17**, 386–90.

Janin-Mercier, A., Beyvin, A J., Pablo, M., and Jacquetin, B. (1982). Cutaneous periarteritis nodosa occurring during pregnancy. *Acta Dermato-Venereologica*, **62**, 256–8.

Jorizzo, J. L., White, W. L., Wise, C. M., Zanolli, M. D., and Sherertz, E. F. (1991). Low-dose weekly methotrexate for unusual neutrophilic vascular reactions: Cutaneous polyarteritis nodosa and Behcet's disease. *Journal of American Academy of Dermatology*, **24**, 973–8.

Jorizzo, J. L., White, W. L., Wise, C. M., Zanolli, M. D., and Sherertz, E. F. (1991). Low-dose weekly methotrexate for unusual neutrophilic vascular reactions: cutaneous polyarteritis nodosa and Behcet's disease. *Journal of American Academy of Dermatology*, **24**, 973–8.

Kahn, E. I., Daum, F., Aiges, H. W., and Silverberg, M. (1980). Cutaneous polyarteritis nodosa associated with Crohn's disease. *Diseases of the Colon and Rectum*, **23**, 258–62.

Kassis, V., Kassis, E., and Thomsen, H. K. (1985). Benign cutaneous periarteritis nodosa with nail defects. *Journal of the American Academy of Dermatology*, **13**, 661–3.

Ketron, L. W. and Bernstein, J. C. (1939). Cutaneous manifestations of periarteritis nodosa. *Archives of Dermatology and Syphilology*, **40**, 929–44.

Keyloun, V., Halperin, I., and Grace, W. J. (1967). Periarteritis nodosa caused by hypersensitivity to estrogens. *Vascular Disease*, **4**, 21–6.

Khoo, B. P. and Ng, S. K. (1998). Cutaneous polyarteritis nodosa: a case report and literature review. *Annals of the Academy of Medicine*, **27**, 868–72.

Kikuchi, K., Hoashi, T., Kanazawa, S., and Tamaki, K. (2005). Angiogenic cytokines in serum and cutaneous lesions of patients with polyarteritis nodosa. *Journal of American Academy of Dermatology*, **1**, 57–61.

Kint, A. and Van Herpe, L. (1979). Cutaneous periarteritis nodosa. *Dermatologica*, **158**, 85–189.

Kiraly, K., Fulop, E., and Vajda, T. (1978). [Immunofluorescence in cutaneous vasculitis. Immunological tests]. *Minerva Medica*, **69**, 2177–90.

Kleeman, D., Kempf, W., Burg, G., and Hafner, J. (1998). Cutaneous polyarteritis nodosa. *Zeitschrift fur Gefasskrankheiten. Journal for Vascular Diseases*, **27**, 54–7.

Kumar, L., Thapa, B. R., Sarkar, B., and Walia, B. N. (1995). Benign cutaneous polyarteritis nodosa in children below 10 years of age–a clinical experience. *Annals of Rheumatology Diseases*, **54**, 134–6.

Kuriya, G., Izumi, Y., Satou, T., Tanaka, F., Miyashita, T., Kamachi, M., Ida, H., Kawakami, A., Hayashi, T., and Eguchi, K. (2006). [Cutaneous polyarteritis nodosa complicated with anterior tibial artery occlusion, leading to the amputation of the left leg]. *Nippon Naika Gakkai Zasshi*, **95**, 739–41.

Lever, W. and Shaumberg-Lever, G. (1990). Vascular diseases. In *Histopathy of the skin* (G. Shaumberg-Lever, ed.)., 7th edn. J. B. Lippincott, Philadelphia.

Levy, A., Weinberger, A., Mor, C., and Pinkhas, J. (1986). Localized polyarteritis nodosa: cases involving the lower extremities and the breast. *Rheumatology International*, **6**, 43–4.

Liao, Y. H., Hsiao, G. H., and Hsiao, C. H. (1999). Behcet's disease with cutaneous changes resembling polyarteritis nodosa. *British Journal of Dermatology*, **140**, 358–77.

Lightman, H. I., Valderrama, E., and Ilowite, N. T. (1988). Cutaneous polyarteritis nodosa and thromboses of the superior and inferior venae cavae. *Journal of Rheumatology*, **15**, 113–6.

Lindgren, I. and Lundmark, C. (1956). Periarteritis nodosa as a skin disease. *Acta Dermato-Venereogical*, **36**, 343–54.

Magro, C. M. and Crowson, A. N. (2003). The spectrum of cutaneous lesions in rheumatoid arthritis: a clinical and pathological study of 43 patients. *Journal of Cutaneous Pathology*, **30**, 10.

Malaviya, A. N., Francis, I. M., Kashia, P., and Ayahs, E. H. (1999). Musculoskeletal manifestations with panniculitis–a hospital based study on 62 patients in Kuwait. *Rheumatology International*, **19**, 51–7.

Matsumura Y, Mizuno K, Oath K, Okamoto H, and Imamura S (2000). A case of cutaneous polyarteritis nodosa associated with ulcerative colitis. *British Journal of Dermatology*, **142**, 561–2.

Mekori, Y. A., Awai, L. E., Widely, J. D., and Kohler, P. F. (1984). Cutaneous polyarteritis nodosa associated with rapidly progressive arthritis. *Arthritis and Rheumatism*, **27**, 574–88.

Miescher, V. G. (1946). Uber kutane formen der Periarteritis Nodosa. *Dermatologica*, **92**, 225–45.

Miller, J. J., III and Fries, J. F. (1975). Simultaneous vasculitis in a mother and newborn infant. *Journal of Pediatrics*, **87**, 443–5.

Mimouni, D., Ng, P. P., Rencic, A., Nikolskaia, O. V., Bernstein, B. D., and Nousari, H. C. (2003). Cutaneous polyarteritis nodosa in patients presenting with atrophie blanche. *British Journal of Dermatology*, **148**, 789–94.

Minkowitz, G., Smoller, B. R., and McNutt, N. S. (1991). Benign cutaneous polyarteritis nodosa. Relationship to systemic polyarteritis nodosa and to hepatitis B infection. *Archives of Dermatology*, **127**, 1520–3.

Mocan, H., Mocan, M. C., Peru, H., and Ozoran, Y. (1998). Cutaneous polyarteritis nodosa in a child and a review of the literature. *Acta Paediatrica*, **87**, 351–3.

Moreland, L. W. and Ball, G. V. (1990). Cutaneous polyarteritis nodosa. *American Journal of Medicine*, **88**, 426–30.

Mousa, A. R., Marafie, A. A., and Dajani, A. I. (1985). Cutaneous necrotizing vasculitis complicating Takayasu's Arteritis with a review of cutaneous manifestants. *Journal of Rheumatology*, **12**, 607–10.

Nguyen, K. H., Miller, J. J., and Helm, K. F. (2003). Case reports and a review of the literature on ulcers mimicking pyoderma gangrenosum. *International Journal of Dermatology*, **42**, 84–94.

Nikkari, S., Mertsola, J., Kovernata, H., Vainiopaa, R., and Toinavanen, P. (1994). Wegener's granulomatosus and parvovirus B19 infection. *Arthritis and Rheumatism*, **37**, 1707–8.

Nikolic, J., Peclard, N., Deleamont, P., Chavaz, P., Schifferli, J., and Bounameaux, H. (1993). Takayasu arteritis preceded by cardiac and cutaneous lesions. A case report. *Zeitschrift fur Gefasskrankheiten. Journal for Vascular Diseases*, **22**, 347–51.

Orkin, M. and Winkelmann, R. K. (1970). Cutaneous manifestations. *Archives of Dermatology*, **102**, 571–2.

Orton, D. I. and Whittaker, S. J. (2000). Renal angiogram abnormalities in a case of cutaneous polyarteritis nodosa. *Clinical and Experimental Dermatology*, **25**, 33–5.

Ozen, S., Anton, J., Arisoy, N., Bakkaloglu, A., Besbas, N., Brogan, P., *et al.* (2004). Juvenile polyarteritis: results of a multicenter survey of 110 children. *Journal of Pediatrics*, **145**, 517–22.

Pak, H., Montemarano, A. D., and Berger, T. (1998). Purpuric nodules and macules on the extremities of a young woman. Cutaneous polyarteritis nodosa. *Archives of Dermatology*, **134**, 231–5.

Paller, A. S. (1986). Cutaneous changes associated with inflammatory bowel disease. *Pediatrics of Dermatology*, **3**, 439–45.

Pelletier, F., Puzenat, E., Blanc, D., Faivre, B., Humbert, P., and Aubin, F. (2003). Minocycline-induced cutaneous polyarteritis nodosa with antineutrophil cytoplasmic antibodies. *European Journal of Dermatology*, **4**, 396–8.

Pereira, B. A., Silva, N. A., Ximenes, A. C., Alvarenga, S. L., and Barbosa, V. S. (1995). Cutaneous polyarteritis nodosa in a child with positive antiphospholipid and P-ANCA. *Scandinavian Journal of Rheumatology*, **24**, 386–8.

Peron, S., Tilly-Gentric, A., Hutin, P., Le Ninivin, P., Le Goff, P., and Pennec, Y. L. (1999). [Localized periarteritis nodosa with periostal new bone formation]. *LaRevue De Medicine Interne*, **12**, 132–4.

Pischel, K. D. and Zvaifler, N. J. (1984). Simultaneous occurrence of polyarteritis nodosa and leukocytoclastic vasculitis. *Journal of Rheumatology*, **11**, 542–4.

Procopiou, M., Egger, J. F., and De Torrente, A. (2004). Collagenous colitis and cutaneous polyarteritis nodosa in the same patient. *Scandinavian Journal of Gastroenterology*, **39**, 89–92.

Queiro, R. and De Dios, J. R. (2002). Successful treatment with low-dose weekly methotrexate in a case of undifferentiated spondyloarthropathy coexisting with cutaneous polyarteritis nodosa. *Clinical Rheumatology*, **4**, 304–5.

Quintana, G., Matteson, E. L., Fernandez, A., Restrepo, J. F., and Iglesias, A. (2004). Localized nodular vasculitis: a new variant of localized cutaneous polyarteritis nodosa. *Clinical and Experimental Rheumatology*, **22**, 31–4.

Rauh, G., Kamilli, I., Gresser, U., and Landthaler, M. (1993). Relapsing polychondritis presenting as cutaneous polyarteritis nodosa. *Clinical and Investigative*, **71**, 305–9.

Rawlinson, T. and Ball, G. V. (1981). Chronic cutaneous polyarteritis nodosa: a distinct subset of polyarteritis nodosa. *Archives of Internal Medicine*, **141**, 961.

Reddy, S. M., Pui, J. C., Gold, L. I., Mitnick, H. J. (2005). Postirradiation morphea and subcutaneous polyarteritis nodosa: case report and literature review. *Seminars in Arthritis and Rheumatism*, **34**(5): 728–34.

Rose, G. A. and Spencer, H. (1957). Polyarteritis nodosa. *Quarterly Journal of Medicine*, **26**, 43–81.

Rosen, A. M., Haines, K., III, Tallman, M. S., Hakimian, D., and Ramsey-Goldman, R. (1995). Rapidly progressive cutaneous vasculitis in a patient with chronic myelomonocytic leukemia. *American Journal of Hematology*, **50**, 310–2.

Ruiter, M. (1958). The so-called cutaneous type of periarteritis nodosa. *British Journal of Dermatology*, **70**, 102–6.

Sano, S., Shinkai, H., and Yonemasu, K. (1979). Immunobiological aspects of Clq in sera of patients with cutaneous vasculitis and collagen diseases. *Acta Dermato-venereologica*, **59**, 33–8.

Sayed, F., Dhaybi, R., Ammoury, A., Chababit, M., and Bazex, J. (2006). Myasthenia gravis with cutaneous polyarteritis nodosa. *Clinical Dermatology*, **31**, 215–7.

Schaffer, J., Davidson, D., McNiff, J., and Bolognia, J. (2001). Perinuclear antineutrophilic cytoplasmic antibody-positive cutaneous polyarteritis nodosa associated with minocycline therapy for acne vulgaris. *Journal of the American Academy of Dermatology*, **44**, 198–206.

Schanz, S. and Ulmer, A. (2006). Medical mystery: gangrene and cutaneous nodules–the answer. *New England Journal of Medicine*, **354**, 2393–4.

Schartz, N., Alaoui, S., Vignon-Pennamen, M. D., Cordoliani, F., Fermand, J., Morel, P., *et al.* (2001). Successful treatment in two cases of steroid-department cutaneous polyarteritis nodosa with low-dose methotrexate. *Dermatology*, **203**, 336–8.

Schrodt, B. J. and Callen, J. P. (2006). Polyarteritis nodosa attributable to minocycline treatment for acne vulgaris. *Pediatrics*, **103**, 503–4.

Sheth, A. P., Olson, J. C., and Esterly, N. B. (1994). Cutaneous polyarteritis nodosa of childhood. *Journal American Academy Dermatology*, **31**, 561–6.

Siberry, G. K., Cohen, B. A., and Johnson, B. (1994). Cutaneous polyarteritis nodosa. Reports of two cases in children and review of the literature. *Archives Dermatology*, **130**, 884–9.

Slinger, W. and Starck, V. (1951). Cutaneous form of polyarteritis nodosa; report of a case. *Archives of Dermatology and Syphilology*, **63**, 461–8.

Smukler, N. M. and Schumacher, H. R., Jr. (1977). Chronic nondestructive arthritis associated with cutaneous polyarteritis. *Arthritis and Rheumatism*, **20**, 1114–20.

Solley, G. O., Winklemann, R. K., and Rovelstad, R. A. (1975). Correlation between regional enterocolitis and cutaneous polyarteritis nodosa. Two case reports and review of the literature. *Gastroenterology*, **69**, 235–9.

Soubrier, M., Bangil, M., Franc, S., Dubost, J. J., Ristori, J. M., Kemeny, J. L., and Bussiere, J. L. (1997). Vasculitis confined to the calves. Report of a case. *Revue Du Rhumatisme. English Edition*, **64**, 414–6.

Soufir, N., Descamps, V., Crickx, B., Thibault, V., Cosnes, A., Becherel, P. A. *et al.* (1999). Hepatitis C virus infection in cutaneous polyarteritis nodosa: a retrospective study of 16 cases. *Archives of Dermatology*, **135**, 1001–2.

Sparsa, A., Liozon, E., Wechsler, J., Soria, P., Delage-Core, M., Loustaud, V. (2006). Aortic angiosarcoma clinically mimicking polyarteritis nodosa. *Scandanavian Journal of Rheumatology*, **35**, 237–40.

Stein, R., Phelps, R., and Sapadin, A. (2001). Cutaneous polyarteritis nodosa after streptococcal necrotizing fasciitis. *Mount Sinai Journal of Medicine*, **68**, 336–8.

Stone, M. S., Olson, R. R., Weismann, D. N., Giller, R. H., and Goeken, J. A. (1993). Cutaneous vasculitis in the newborn of a mother with cutaneous polyarteritis nodosa. *Journal of American Academy Dermatology*, **28**, 101–5.

Stussi, G., Schneider, E., Trueb, R., and Seebach, J. (2001). Acral necrosis of the fingers as initial manifestation of cutaneous polyarteritis nodosa. *Angiology*, **52**, 63–7.

Swarc, M. and Kaminski, Z. (1971). Polyarteritis nodosa probably caused by hypersensitivity to antitubercular drugs. *Gruzlica*, **39**, 135–42.

Thomas, R., Vuitch, F., and Lakhanpal, S. (1994). Angiocentric T cell lymphoma masquerading as cutaneous vasculitis. *Journal Rheumatology*, **21**, 760–2.

Thomas, R. H. and Black, M. M. (1983). The wide clinical spectrum of polyarteritis nodosa with cutaneous involvement. *Clinical and Experimental Dermatology*, **8**, 47–59.

Till, S. and Amos, R. (1997). Long-term follow-up of juvenile-onset cutaneous polyarteritis nodosa associated with streptococcal infection. *British Journal of Rheumatology*, **36**, 909–11.

Trueb, R., Scheidegger, E., Pericin, M., Singh, A., Hoffmann, U., Sauvant, G., *et al.* (1999). Periarteritis nodosa presenting as a breast lesion: report of a case and review of the literature. *British Journal of Dermatology*, **141**, 1117–21.

Uziel, Y. and Silverman, E. D. (1998). Intravenous immunoglobulin therapy in a child with cutaneous polyarteritis nodosa. *Clinical and Experimental Rheumatology*, **16**, 187–9.

Van de Pette, J. E., Jarvis, J. M., Wilton, J. M., and MacDonald, D. M. (1984). Cutaneous periarteritis nodosa. Hepatitis B surface antigen-containing immunocomplexes and polymorphonuclear-leukocyte lysosomal enzyme release. *Archives of Dermatology*, **120**, 109–11.

Verbov, J. and Stansfeld, A. G. (1972). Cutaneous polyarteritis nodosa and Crohn's disease. *Transactions of the St. Johns Hospital Dermatological Society*, **58**, 261–8.

Viguier, M., Guillevin, L., and Laroche, L. (2001). Treatment of parvovirus B19-associated polyarteritis nodosa with intravenous immune globulin. *New England Journal of Medicine*, **344**, 1481–2.

Vikas, A., Atul, S., Singh, R., Sarbmeet, L., and Mohan, H. (2003). Behcet disease with relapsing cutaneous polyarteritis nodosa-like lesions, responsive to oral cyclosporine therapy. *Dermatology Online Journal*, **9**, 9.

Volk, D. M. and Owen, L. G. (1986). Cutaneous polyarteritis nodosa in a patient with ulcerative colitis. *Journal of Pediatrics Gastroenterology and Nutrition*, **5**, 970–2.

Voulgarelis, M., Chorti, M., Kittas, C., Karachristos, A., Ikonomopoulos, G., and Skopouli, F. (1998). Fever and abdominal pain in a 45-year old woman with cutaneous necrotising vasculitis. *Clinical and Experimental Rheumatology*, **16**, 72–6.

Weinrauch, L. A., Belok, S. S., Gauvin, G. P., and D'Elia, J. A. (1982). Palpable acute necrotizing arteritis secondary to metolazone. *Cutis*, **30**, 83–4.

Whittaker, S. J., Dover, J. S., and Greaves, M. W. (1986). Cutaneous polyarteritis nodosa associated with hepatitis B surface antigen. *Journal of the American Academy of Dermatology*, **15**, 1142–5.

CHAPTER 29

Kawasaki's disease

Hirohisa Kato and Kei Takahashi

Kawasaki's disease (KD) is an acute vasculitis in small and medium-sized arteries, particularly the coronary arteries (Kawasaki *et al*.1974), in which lesions develop aneurysms, thrombotic occlusion, and progress to coronary artery disease and premature atherosclerosis (Kato *et al*. 1995). This coronary artery vasculitis may cause myocardial infarction or sudden death in the young.

This disease was first described by Dr Tomisaku Kawasaki in Japan, who recognized his first case in 1961 (Kawasaki 1967). At first, it was thought to be benign with a good prognosis, because all acute symptoms disappear within 2 or 3 weeks. Yamamoto reported a case complicated with myocarditis (Yamamoto *et al*. 1968); however, he did not recognize the presence of coronary artery involvement. In 1970 the first nationwide survey in Japan reported that 1.7% of the patients died from acute myocardial infarction, and all four autopsies performed showed coronary arteritis accompanied by aneurysms and thrombotic occlusion. At that time most pediatricians thought that Kawasaki's disease was complicated by vasculitis in only a small number of cases, because of the great contrast in prognosis between these rare fatalities and the large number of examples without obvious heart disease.

In 1973, Kato performed coronary angiography in 20 infants and children when their acute symptoms had disappeared. Twelve had multiple coronary aneurysms in both the right and left coronary arteries, which was the first recognition that coronary aneurysms are present not only in fatal cases, but also in survivors free from cardiac symptoms (Kato *et al*.1975). Through pathological study and coronary angiographic findings, KD is now recognized as a systemic vasculitis syndrome in small and medium-sized arteries in infants and young children.

In the past KD may have been misdiagnosed as scarlet fever, measles, rheumatic fever, juvenile rheumatoid arthritis, Stevens–Johnson syndrome, and infantile polyarteritis, which are included in its differential diagnosis (Shibuya *et al*. 2002). Landing reported that pathological findings are identical between fatal KD and infantile polyarteritis, which was described through autopsy (Landing and Larson 1977), thus unifying the two.

Epidemiology

The epidemiology of KD in Japan, where it is most prevalent, has been well documented by the Research Committee organized by the Health and Welfare Department of the Japanese Government (Yanagawa *et al*. 1995), and can be summarized as follows. The number of patients has increased since 1968 and now totals over 190,000. KD affects over 9000 children each year in Japan and the incidence has been increasing yearly to 150 per 100,000 children less than 4 years of age. Onset may be as early as 1 month of age and peaks at 1 year of age. Fifty percent of children with DK are less than 2 years of age; those over 10 years of age are quite rare. Boys are affected more than girls with a male:female ratio of 1.5:1. KD is more prevalent in Japanese and other Asians than in Caucasians. No urban–rural or geographical differences exist within Japan. Seasonal variation is not distinct, but there are small peaks during the winter and spring. The recurrence rate is about 3.3%, and 1–2% of cases are familial. Time–space clustering and outbreaks in communities are recognized; however, there is no evidence of person-to-person transmission. In 1979, 1982, and 1986 there were large outbreaks in Japan, but the last 25 years have not seen a large epidemic.

KD is now widely recognized all over the world but is most prevalent in Japan and eastern Asia (Nakamura *et al*. 2004). In the US, an estimated 4248 children were hospitalized with KD in 2000. The incidence in children <5 years old is 32.5/100,000 among those of Asian and Pacific Island descent, 16.9 in non-Hispanic African-Americans, 11.1 in Hispanics, and is lowest in Caucasians at only 9.1.

The fatality rate was approximately 2% in the 1970s and had declined to 0.1% in the 1990s in Japan. In the US, the in-hospital mortality rate is 0.17%, with peak mortality occurring 15 to 45 days after the onset of illness (Chang *et al*. 2002).

Pathology

Kawasaki's disease is classified among the systemic vasculitides involving the small or medium-sized arteries, particularly the coronary arteries (Jennette *et al*. 1994). The rare "ischemic heart disease in infants" can be caused by formation of a thrombus in an aneurysm arising due to vasculitis (Figure 29.1). At autopsy, myocarditis (interstitial myocarditis with mild necrosis), pericarditis, endocarditis, cholecystitis, cholangitis, pancreatic ductitis, sialoadenitis, meningitis, and lymphadenitis are also frequently seen.

Coronary artery lesions in the acute stage

Coronary arteritis begins as edematous dissociation of the media 6 to 8 days after the disease onset. On about the 10th day of disease, lymphocyte and macrophage infiltration into the arterial wall from

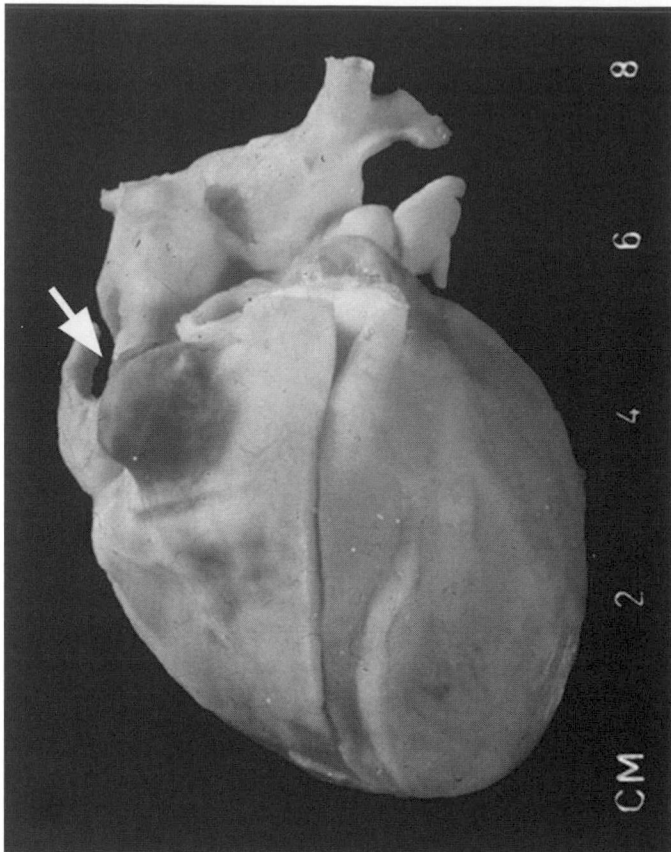

Figure 29.1 Gross appearance of the heart with spherical coronary aneurysm (arrow). (Courtesy of Dr A.E. Becker, Amsterdam, The Netherlands).

the luminal side and adventitial sides begins, leading immediately to inflammation of all layers of the artery, that is panarteritis (Figure 29.2). The inflammation spreads around the artery. The internal elastic lamina, smooth muscle cells of the media, and other structural components of the artery are subjected to intense damage; the artery then begins to dilate. When the damage is severe, aneurysms may develop on about the 12th day after disease onset of the disease. Blood moves in a vortex in the aneurysm, permitting the formation of thrombi, and thrombotic occlusion is found in the coronary artery aneurysm of many autopsy cases of acute-stage KD (Amano *et al.* 1980; Masuda *et al.* 1981) (Figure 29.3).

Arteritis in KD is characterized by proliferative and granulomatous inflammation with marked accumulation of macrophages. Aberrant activation of those macrophages is thought to be involved in the formation of vascular lesions (Naoe *et al.* 1991a; 1991b). Histopathological studies from our group have revealed that lesions in the initial stage of inflammation contain not only macrophages and lymphocytes but also many neutrophils (Takahashi *et al.* 2005). This finding suggests that the proteases, etc. that are produced and released by neutrophils are integrally involved in damage to the arterial walls.

Inflammatory cell infiltration continues until about 3–4 weeks of disease duration, after which the cells gradually decrease in number and are almost completely gone by about 6 weeks. A scar from the inflammation remains.

Coronary artery lesions in convalescent or long-term stage

Most deaths in the remote stage of KD are unexpected, occurring during or immediately after physical or emotional stress (Tanaka *et al.* 1986; Takahashi *et al.* 2001). It is thought that death occurs due to cardiac ischemia or arrhythmia. Coronary artery lesions in the remote-stage can be divided into two histological types: severe dilatory changes such as aneurysms, and mild dilatation, which can be thought of as transient.

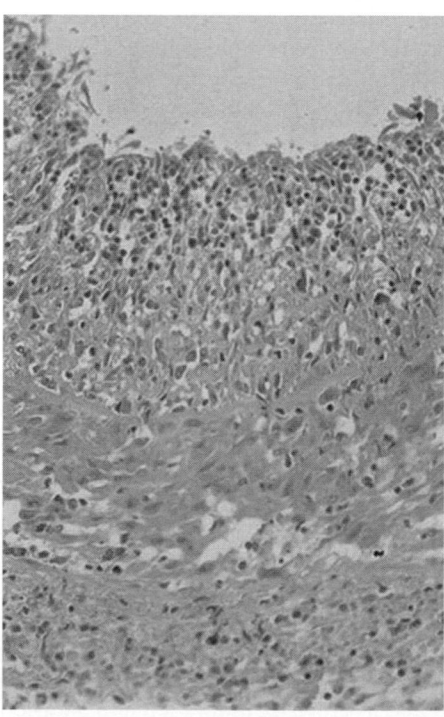
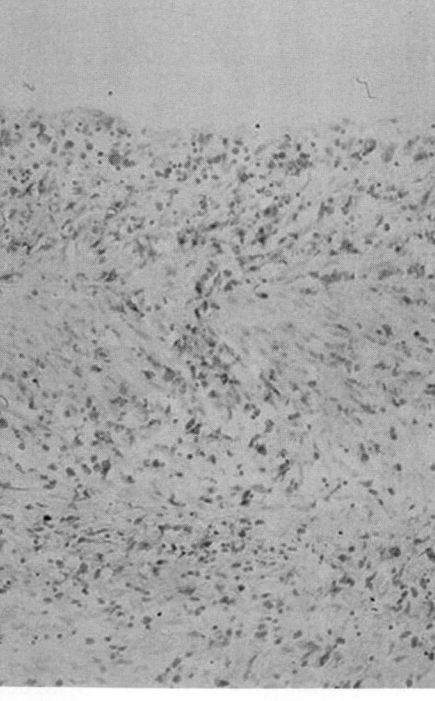

Figure 29.2 Panarteritis, inflammation of all layers of the artery, of a coronary artery in a patient who died 10 days after the onset of Kawasaki's disease. (a) Hematoxylin and eosin stain; (b) immunohistochemical study using anti-CD68 antibody. (See Color Plate 80).

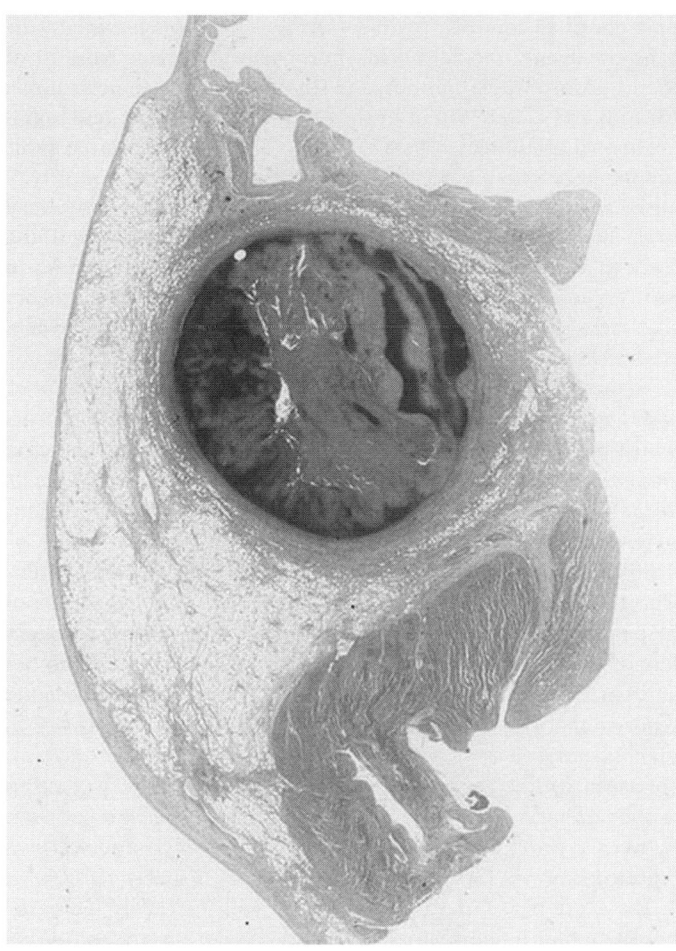

Figure 29.3 Coronary artery aneurysm filled in with a fresh thrombus in patient who died 18 days after the onset of KD.

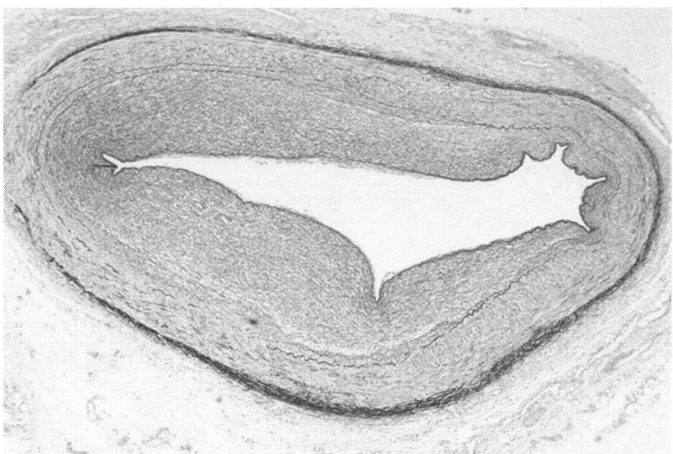

Figure 29.4 Coronary artery of a patient who died of meningitis 14 years after the onset of Kawasaki's disease. This patient had no coronary aneurysms but coronary arteries showed circumferential intimal thickening.

Patients with residual aneurysms

As noted earlier, blood in an aneurysm may thrombose. It is common for the wall of an aneurysm to be accompanied by laminar calcification surrounding it, with an organized thrombus on the inner side; plugging of the lumen by a fresh thrombus may then be lethal. In addition, portions of the artery on both the proximal and distal sides of the coronary aneurysm have centripetal intimal thickening, and in some cases it can be surmised that death occurred because of luminal stenosis due to intimal thickening.

On the other hand, some lesions suggest that the vessel has been recanalized due to partial thrombolysis (Fujiwara *et al.* 1986). Ordinarily, multiple channels are opened within the aneurysm, and smooth muscle cells migrate to surround the blood vessels. In patients who die a number of years after contracting KD, the recanalized vessels can have a structure that closely resembles that of normal arteries. One central artery may bifurcate into multiple new vessels within the aneurysm, which then rejoin on the opposite side to form a coronary artery (Naoe and Takahashi 1993). There are also cases in which a recanalized vessel becomes reoccluded due to new intimal thickening.

Patients with no residual aneurysm

In our studies, no patients without an aneurysm had severe cardiac sequelae. That is, all fatalities were due to causes unrelated to KD.

In most of the patients, the coronary arteries showed a mild tendency to dilation with circumferential thickening of the intima (Figure 29.4), but in many there were no changes suggestive of scars from previous arteritis. It is thought that these changes represent dilation during the acute inflammatory stage which underwent regression during the convalescent stage (Sasaguri and Kato 1982). Thus, the finding of intimal thickening in patients with no residual aneurysm in the remote stages, suggests that coronary arteritis was present in the past (Naoe *et al.* 1987).

Relationship between sequelae of coronary arteritis and atherosclerosis

Histological findings in autopsy cases with coronary aneurysms were compared with pathological reports with regard to atherosclerosis of the coronary arteries in age-matched Japanese not having aneurysms. Those confirmed that there were clearly more severe atherosclerotic lesions in the coronary aneurysms of subjects in their 30s compared with the control subjects having no aneurysms (Figure 29.5). Therefore, it appears that a past history of KD with residual coronary artery aneurysm represents a risk factor for atherosclerosis (Takahashi *et al.* 2001). Much is unknown about the long-term prognosis of patients who have comparatively mild scarring due to vasculitis; further study of these subjects is warranted.

Relationships between Kawasaki's disease arteritis vs. classical polyarteritis nodosa (PAN) and infantile polyarteritis nodosa

Kussmaul–Maier-type classical polyarteritis nodosa (PAN) is characterized by changes in the medium- and small-sized arteries similar to those seen in KD. One of the histological characteristics of PAN is the simultaneous presence of arterial lesions in the acute inflammatory stages (stages I and II) with neutrophil infiltration and fibrinoid necrosis, and lesions in the scarring stages (stages III and IV). As a rule, KD arteritis does not show fibrinoid necrosis, and the arterial lesions are in the acute inflammatory stage or the scarring stage, but not both.

It is difficult to make a simple comparison of KD and infantile polyarteritis nodosa (IPN), since the former is a clinical entity

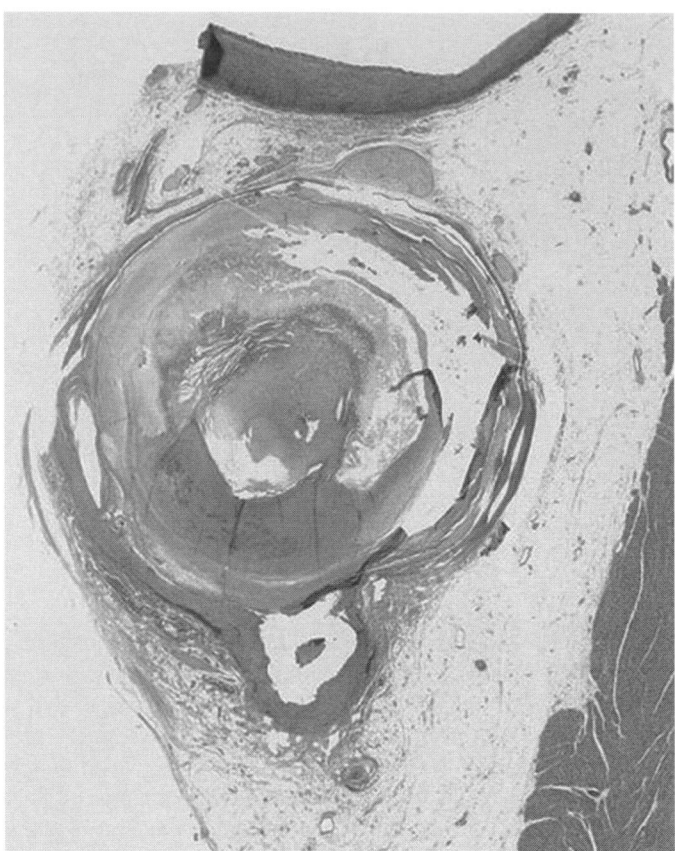

Figure 29.5 Coronary artery aneurysm of 39-year-old male with severe atherosclerotic lesion with thrombus formation in the aneurysm.

whereas IPN is a pathological entity. Many patients diagnosed with IPN cannot be histologically differentiated from those with KD, and illnesses that should be diagnosed as "PAN in infants" are also classified as IPN (Tanaka 1975; Landing and Larson 1987). That is, there is a possibility that patients who are pathologically diagnosed as IPN include patients with KD or other similar diseases.

Pathogenesis and etiology

The etiology of KD remains unknown despite extensive investigation. Based on clinical features and epidemiologic data, KD is now considered to be an infection due to unknown agent(s) or an infection-triggered immune disorder with concomitant activation of proinflammatory cytokines. A variety of possible causative agents has been proposed, including bacteria, spirochetes, fungi, mycoplasma, rickettsiae, and viruses.

KD has clinical similarities to scarlet fever and toxic shock syndrome, both of which are caused by toxin-producing bacteria. These toxins have superantigen activity which allows them to stimulate T cells expressing particular variable regions of the T cell receptor beta chain. A study on peripheral blood T cells in KD has shown that T cells expressing T cell receptor variable regions Vbeta2 and Vbeta8 were selectively expanded (Abe *et al*. 1992). These observations suggest that KD may be caused by a micro-organism that produces a toxin with superantigen properties. Leung *et al*. cultured bacteria from the throat, rectum, axilla, and groin of 16 patients with untreated acute KD and 15 controls. Bacteria producing toxins were isolated from 13 of 16 KD patients but from only one of 15 controls. Toxin-secreting *Staphylococcus aureus* (the causative agent in toxic shock syndrome) was isolated from 11 of the 13 toxin-positive cultures, and streptococcal pyogenic exotoxin (SPE) B and C were found in the other two cultures. These toxins are known to stimulate Vbeta2+ T cells. These data suggested a role for *Staphylococcus aureus* group A streptococci (Leung *et al*. 1993). Yoshioka *et al*. reported that SPEC induces activation and polyclonal expansion of Vbeta2- and Vbeta6.5-positive T cells, and that SPEC-induced activation of T cells may contribute to the pathogenesis of KD (Yoshioka *et al*. 2003). Other studies have not supported the theory that these bacterial species contribute to KD, however (Sakaguchi *et al*. 1995).

Yersinia pseudotuberculosis may be an etiologic agent (Sato *et al*. 1983) in a small group of KD patients. *Propionibacterium acnes* which produced a cytotoxic protein similar to bacterial exotoxin was isolated from the cervical lymph nodes of patients (Kato *et al*. 1983; Tomita *et al*. 1987), but a causal relationship to KD remains to be determined.

Epstein–Barr virus (EBV) may rarely induce a clinical picture mimicking that of KD (Kikuta *et al*. 1984), as one study found that three of 37 patients with chronic active EBV infection developed coronary lesions, but epidemiologic, serologic, and virological studies do not support EBV as a causative agent of KD. Rowley and colleagues reported that IgA plasma cells infiltrate the vascular wall as well as other tissues such as myocardium, respiratory tract, kidney, and pancreas in acute KD. They suggested a mucosal portal of entry of a conventional antigen (Rowley *et al*. 2001). Recently a possible association between a novel human Corona virus (HcoV-NH) and KD was reported; however, further studies are necessary (Esper *et al*. 2005).

The acute phase of KD is associated with markedly increased production of inflammatory cytokines. TNF-α, IL-1β, and γ-IFN induce activation antigens and adhesion molecules such as endothelial leukocyte adhesion molecule 1 and intercellular adhesion molecule 1 (ICAM-1) on endothelial cells, and TNF-α and γ-IFN cause endothelial injury *in vitro* (Furukawa *et al*. 1988). Leung and associates have proposed that antiendothelial cell antibodies (AECA) cause endothelial injury in KD, based on the findings that these autoantibodies were cytotoxic against human umbilical vein endothelial cells treated with TNF-α, IL-1β, or γ-IFN (Leung *et al*. 1986). Coronary artery endothelial cells in KD were found to express activation antigens in a necropsy study (Terai *et al*. 1990). Vascular endothelial growth factor (VEGF) and monocyte chemotactic and activating factor (MCAF or MCP-1), may also have important roles in the pathogenesis of KD vasculitis (Yasukawa *et al*. 2002; Furukawa *et al*. 1994; Lin *et al*. 1992).

Many hypotheses on the etiology and pathogenesis of KD have appeared, but no host–microbial relationship specific to KD has been identified. KD is widely scattered in the community, self-limiting, characterized by multiorgan involvement with possible recurrences, and has a tendency toward occurring in epidemics. These traits suggest that this disease may be caused in susceptible children by ubiquitous infectious agents.

Clinical presentations

Symptoms and diagnosis of Kawasaki's disease

Common clinical findings in KD are shown in Figure 29.6. In the absence of a specific laboratory test, the diagnosis of KD is made according to diagnostic guidelines such as those shown in

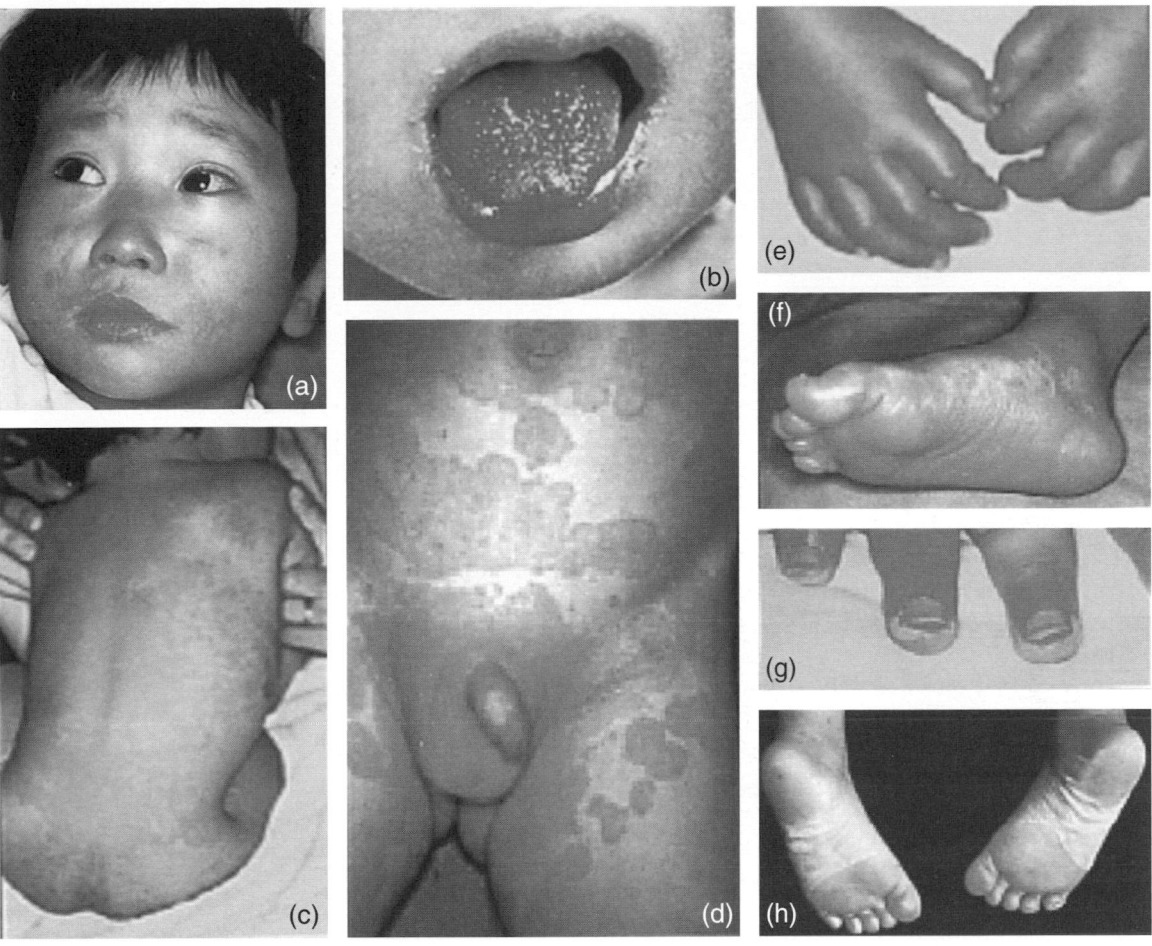

Figure 29.6 Clinical manifestations of KD. (a) Typical appearance of Kawasaki face, bilateral conjunctival congestion, and reddening and fissuring of lips. (b) Strawberry tongue. (c and d) Polymorphous exanthema. (e) Indurative edema of the hands. (f) Redness and swelling of the sole. (g and h) Desquamation of fingers and foot. (See Color Plate 81).

Table 29.1 (5th Revised Edition, Japanese Kawasaki Disease Research Committee, 2002). The principal diagnostic criteria of KD are: persistent fever; conjunctival injection; changes in the mucosa of the oropharynx (erythema of the lips, strawberry tongue, diffuse injection); changes in the peripheral extremities (erythema of the palms and soles, indurative edema in the acute stage, desquamation of the skin on the fingertips in the convalescent stage); erythematous rash; and cervical lymphadenopathy. At least five of six principal symptoms should be met for diagnosis of KD. Some patients who have only four of the six symptoms are thought to have incomplete KD. The duration of fever may be less than 5 days, particularly in those treated with intravenous gamma globulin (IVIg). Patients with four findings can be diagnosed with KD when coronary abnormalities such as dilatation or non-uniformity of arterial lumen, or enhanced brightness of the arterial wall, are recognized on two-dimensional echocardiography. Patients less than 6 months of age or those over 7 years of age may present with atypical symptoms. Incomplete KD should be considered in children with unexplained fever for more than 4 days and three other principal symptoms. High CRP (>3 mg/dL), elevated ESR (more than 40 mm/h), thrombocytosis (>400,000/mm³), high white blood cell count (>15,000/mm³), and erythema and induration at the site of previous vaccination with BCG (Bacille Calmette–Guérin) are helpful in diagnosing incomplete KD. In older children (>7 years old), high fever and cervical lymphadenopathy are initial symptoms. Other significant symptoms and laboratory findings are listed in Table 29.1.

Spectrum of cardiovascular disease

The spectrum of cardiovascular disease among 2180 patients with acute KD during the last 31 years in our hospital is shown in Table 29.2. Of all patients, 14.9% were diagnosed with coronary aneurysms. After 1992 (when treatment with IVIg was commonly used), the incidence of coronary aneurysms declined to 8.7%. The coronary arteries are the most common sites of aneurysms in KD; however, aneurysms in other arteries such as in the axillary, iliac, or renal arteries may occur (see below). Valvular heart disease appeared in about 1.5% of the patients. Myocardial infarction occurred in 24 cases, 10 of whom died. It is important to note that approximately half of the fatal cases did not have any symptoms of coronary artery disease before the onset of myocardial infarction.

The main cause of death in KD is acute myocardial infarction (MI). In one study of 104 fatal cases in KD in Japan, 56.7% died of acute myocardial infarction, 18% died of congestive heart failure,

Table 29.1 Diagnostic guidelines for Kawasaki's disease (5th Revised Edition, February 2002, Japanese Kawasaki Disease Research Committee)

KD is a disease of unknown etiology affecting most frequently infants and young children under 5 years of age.	2. GI tract: Diarrhea Vomiting Abdominal pain Hydrops of gall bladder Paralytic ileus Mild jaundice Slight increase of serum transaminases
The symptoms can be classified into two categories: principal symptoms and other significant symptoms or findings.	
A. Principal symptoms	
1. Fever persisting 5 days or more (inclusive of those cases in whom the fever has subsided before the 5th day in response to therapy)	3. Blood test abnormalities: Leukocytosis with shift to the left Mild anemia Thrombocytosis Increased ESR or CRP Hypoalbuminemia Increased alpha 2-globulin
2. Bilateral conjunctival congestion	
3. Changes of lips and oral cavity: Reddening of lips Strawberry tongue Diffuse injection of oral and pharyngeal mucosa	
4. Polymorphous exanthema	4. Urine abnormalities: Proteinuria Pyuria
5. Changes of peripheral extremities: Initial stage: Reddening of palms and soles Indurative edema Convalescent stage: Membranous desquamation from fingertips	5. Skin: Erythema and crusting at the site of BCG inoculation Pustules Transverse furrows of the finger nails
6. Acute non-purulent cervical lymphadenopathy	6. Respiratory: Cough Rhinorrhea Abnormal chest X-ray film
At least five items of 1–6 should be satisfied for diagnosis of KD. However, patients with four of the principal symptoms can be diagnosed as KD when coronary aneurysm is noted on two-dimensional echocardiography or coronary angiography.	
B. Other significant symptoms or findings	7. Joint pain or swelling
1. Cardiovascular: Auscultation abnormalities (heart murmur, gallop rhythm, distant heart sounds) ECG changes (prolonged PR/QT intervals, abnormal Q wave, low voltage, ST-T wave changes, dysrhythmias) Chest radiograph abnormalities (cardiomegaly) 2-D echocardiographic abnormalities (pericardial effusion, coronary aneurysms) Aneurysm of peripheral arteries Angina pectoris or myocardial infarction	8. Neurological: Pleocytosis of mononuclear cells in CSF Seizures Loss of consciousness Facial nerve palsy Paralysis

For item 5 in principal symptoms, the convalescent stage is considered important. Non-purulent cervical lymphadenopathy is less frequently encountered (approximately 65%) than other principal symptoms during the acute phase. Male: Female ratio: 1.3–1.5: 1, patients under 5 years of age: 80–85%, fatality rate: 0.1%. Recurrence rate: 2–3%. Proportion of siblings cases: 1–2%. Approximately 10% of the total cases do not fulfill five of the six principal symptoms, in which other diseases can be excluded and Kawasaki's disease is suspected. In some of these patients coronary artery aneurysms (including so-called coronary artery ectasia) have been confirmed.

and five persons died from rupture of coronary aneurysms. In the 1970s, the fatality rate was about 2%; however, in the 1990s it declined to 0.2% in Japan. From a nation-wide survey in Japan, 195 KD patients with MI were analyzed (Kato *et al.* 1986): MI mostly occurred within 1 year of illness, however, deaths several years after acute KD have increased recently; 37% of patients with MI were asymptomatic; 22% of patients suffering MI died in the first attack; 16% of survivors from the first attack had subsequent MIs, with increasing mortality. Not surprisingly, coronary angiographic studies showed that most patients who died had obstructions in the left main coronary artery or in both the right main coronary artery and the anterior descending artery while survivors tended to have one-vessel obstruction, particularly in the right coronary artery (see Figure 29.7).

The early recognition and treatment for acute MI are critical. Since the mortality of subsequent MI is high, careful management is needed. Patients with complications, such as ventricular aneurysm, papillary muscle dysfunction, heart failure, severe arrhythmias, and postinfarction angina, should be meticulously managed by medical or surgical approaches.

Systemic artery involvement

Aneurysms in non-coronary arteries were observed in 1.0% of the patients (Kato *et al.* 1996). Our angiographic study of 22 patients with systemic artery aneurysms demonstrated that axillary arteries were affected in 18 cases; common iliac arteries in 16; internal iliac arteries in 12; renal arteries in six; mesenteric arteries in two; and internal thoracic arteries in two. One patient had a large common

Table 29.2 Spectrum of cardiovascular manifestations in Kawasaki disease, Kurume University 1973–2003

Manifestation	No. of patients affected total no. of patients (% affected)
Coronary artery involvement	
Transient dilatation in acute stage	282/1558 (18.1%)
Coronary aneurysm	325/2180 (14.9%)
1973–1990 (aspirin treatment era)	253/1355 (18.6%)
1991–2001 (IVIg plus aspirin treatment era)	72/825 (8.7%)
Systemic artery aneurysms (axillary, iliac, renal, etc.)	22/2180 (1.0%)
Mitral regurgitation	28/2180 (1.3%)
Aortic regurgitation	5/2180 (0.2%)
Pericarditis or pericardial effusion	241/1871 (12.9%)
Myocarditis	617/2180 (28.3%)
Myocardial infarction	24/2180 (1.1%)
Fatal cases	10/2180 (0.45%)

iliac artery aneurysm associated with aortic dilatation. Although the prognosis of systemic artery aneurysms is generally favorable, renovascular hypertension may develop in a patient having a renal artery lesion, and lesions in intrathoracic arteries may complicate coronary bypass surgery. Digital gangrene has been reported (Tomita *et al.* 1992).

Valvular heart disease, myocarditis, and pericarditis

Valvular heart disease appears in about 1% of patients, mostly in the mitral valve and rarely the aortic valve. We demonstrated acute mitral regurgitation in 28 of 2180 cases (1.3%), which resolved in one-half of patients after a few months to several years. The etiology may be valvulitis or papillary muscle dysfunction caused by ischemia (Akagi *et al.* 1990). We had five patients with aortic regurgitation (0.2%). It is noteworthy that aortic regurgitation appeared after the acute or subacute stage of illness and slowly progressed to severe regurgitation in some patients (Gidding *et al.* 1986). Subclinical pericarditis or pericardial effusion appeared in 12.9% of the patients in the acute phase, which typically resolved within 1 or 2 weeks. Massive pericardial effusion or cardiac tamponade was rare. There have been no reports on its progression to chronic or constrictive pericarditis. Relatively mild myocarditis was observed

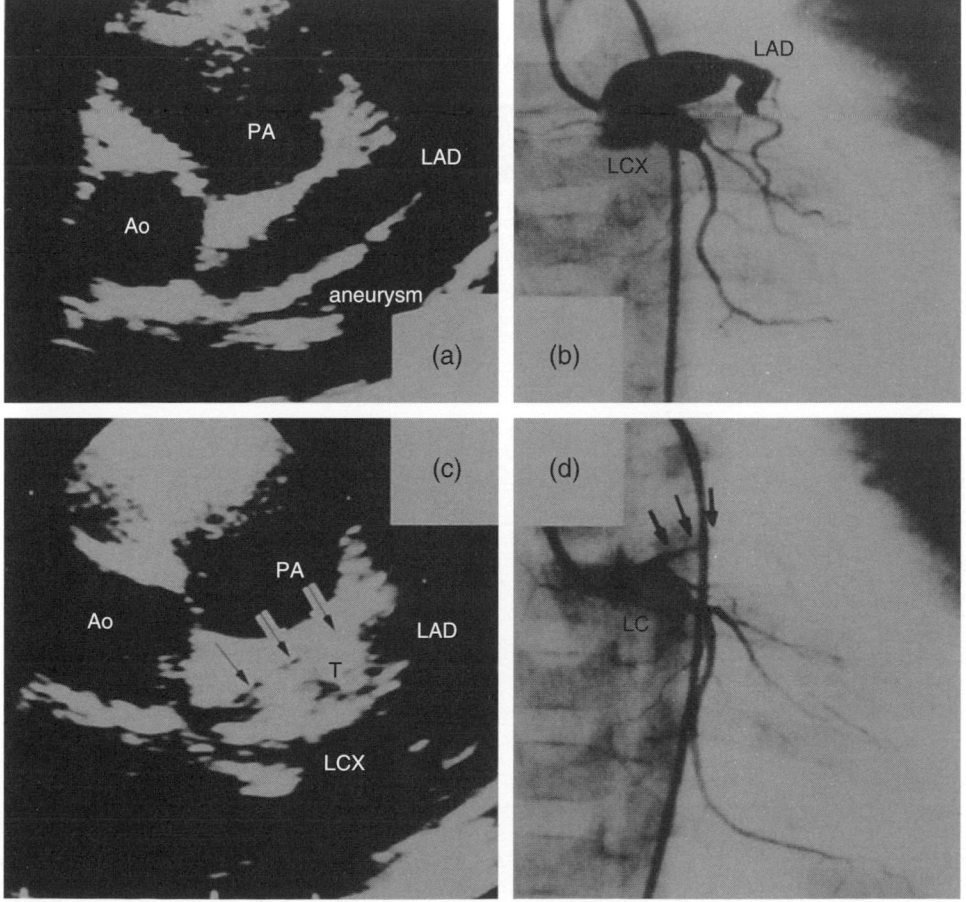

Figure 29.7 Myocardial infarction caused by acute thrombotic occlusion in a 3-year-old boy with KD. (a) Giant aneurysms in both the right and left coronary arteries shown by two-dimensional echocardiography. (b) Coronary angiography demonstrated large aneurysm in left main coronary artery and circumflex artery and stenosis in the left anterior descending artery. No ischemic findings were recognized at that time. (c) Three months later, he complained of frequent chest pain and vomiting. Echocardiogram during the acute myocardial infarction demonstrated complete occlusion in the left main coronary artery and the anterior descending artery. (d) The follow-up coronary angiography just after myocardial infarction demonstrated complete obstruction of the left anterior descending artery.

in about 28.3% of the patients in the acute phase, especially in the first and second weeks of illness, regardless of the presence of coronary aneurysms. The presence of a cardiac gallop, distant heart sounds, ST-T segment changes and decreased voltage of R waves on EKG may suggest the presence of myocarditis. In many instances, cardiac enzyme levels did not change significantly. Acute myocarditis may cause cardiomegaly or decreased ejection fraction of the left ventricle, but seldom develops into a chronic condition or causes cardiomyopathy.

Cardiac evaluation

The evaluation of the coronary artery lesions in KD in the acute stage of illness is essential, and is usually done by two-dimensional echocardiography (2DE) and coronary angiography.

Echocardiography

Serial 2DE studies are the most useful method to evaluate coronary aneurysms. The importance of 2DE in KD is stressed in the Japan Kawasaki Disease Research Committee on standardization of diagnostic criteria and reporting of coronary artery lesions (Kamiya *et al.* 1984) and the Committee Report of the American Heart Association (Dajani *et al.* 1994). Recent reports suggest that these criteria may underestimate the true incidence of coronary artery dilatation (de Zorzi *et al.* 1998; Kurotobi *et al.* 2002). If a patient has abnormal findings on serial 2DE studies, coronary angiography is indicated (Kato *et al.* 1982a).

The evaluation of coronary artery morphology is particularly important in KD. The technical method for evaluation by echocardiography is well described in the American Heart Association

Scientific Statement on KD (Newburger *et al.* 2004). The precordial short axis segment is the standard approach for evaluation of the left main coronary artery, left anterior descending artery, and right main coronary artery. The posterior descending artery can be evaluated by the apical four-chamber view, as is the middle segment of the right coronary artery. Our experience with 2DE has found that it can be used to diagnose left main coronary artery aneurysms with 98% sensitivity and 95% specificity compared to angiography. Echocardiographic evaluation for right coronary artery lesions is less sensitive. False-negative results were mainly due to the rare presence of isolated small peripheral coronary artery aneurysms. From echocardiographic studies, it is evident that coronary artery dilatation appears at around 10 days of illness in about 40% of patients. Transient dilatation is seen in two-thirds of these, with regression within 3–5 weeks from the onset of illness. This means that Kawasaki's vasculitis may cause various degrees of coronary artery dilatation from mild transient dilatation, and small or moderate-sized aneurysms to giant aneurysms in more than half of the patients in acute phase of the disease (Kato 2004). Aneurysms are classified as saccular or as fusiform. If the coronary artery diameter looks larger than normal without segmental dilatation, the coronary artery is considered ectatic. Follow-up echocardiography is essential to assess changes. We perform 2DE at the time of diagnosis, after 8–10 days of illness (when coronary dilatation may appear), at 2 weeks, and 8 weeks after the onset of the disease. Coronary aneurysms are classified as small (<5 mm internal diameter), medium (5–8 mm), and giant or large (>8 mm) (Figure 29.8).

Acute coronary thrombosis may also be diagnosed by outpatient 2DE, and can be treated with thrombolytic agents such as urokinase or tissue plasminogen activator (tPA) (Kato *et al.* 1991).

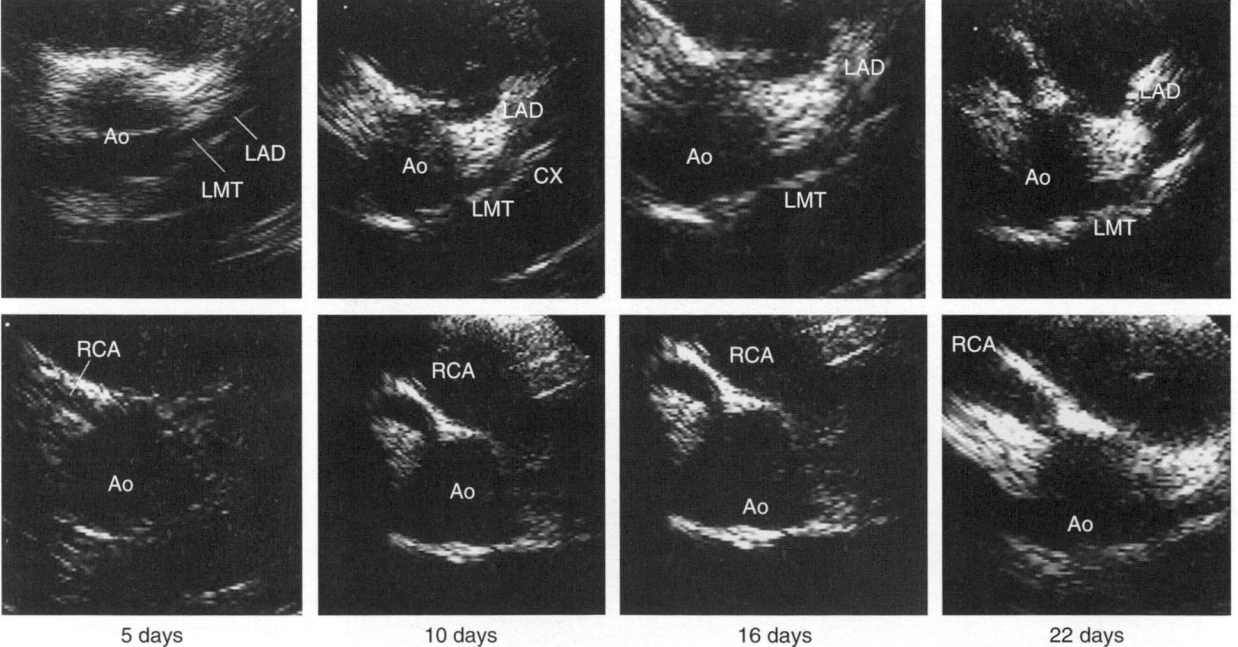

| 5 days | 10 days | 16 days | 22 days |

Figure 29.8 Serial two-dimensional echocardiography of the coronary artery in acute Kawasaki's disease. Upper panel: Left main coronary artery. At 5 days of illness, the size of left main coronary artery looked to be normal. At 10 days of illness it demonstrated mild dilatation and enhanced echocardiographic density in the arterial wall, and subsequently underwent gradually dilatation and developed a coronary aneurysm. Lower panel: Right main coronary artery. At 5 days of illness, the size of main right coronary artery appeared normal, but the arterial wall demonstrated increased echogenicity. At 10 days of illness, it demonstrated mild dilatation and an aneurysm had developed.

Evaluation of stenotic coronary artery lesions is sometimes difficult by 2DE; however, a careful examination with a high frequency transducer may identify such lesions. Echocardiographic features sought on the 2DE exam include loss of the uniformity of the arterial lumen, and irregularities or increased echogenicity in the arterial walls.

Other non-invasive techniques

Magnetic resonance imaging (MRI) may evaluate aneurysms in the proximal coronary artery as well as the coronary flow profile (Greil et al. 2002). Ultrafast CT is also available to evaluate coronary aneurysms (Frey et al. 1988); however, further studies on larger patient groups will be necessary.

Coronary angiography and heart catheterization

Selective coronary artery angiography is the most accurate method to define the presence and severity of coronary arterial abnormalities in KD. We have used specially designed catheters (three types) for selective coronary angiography for infants, toddler, and school children, by which coronary angiography can be performed safely and successfully (Kato et al. 1982a; 1982b). The indications for CAG include the presence of abnormal 2DE findings; the presence of symptoms or signs of ischemia; audible valve regurgitation during auscultation; evidence of cardiac dysfunction; and the use of intracoronary thrombolytic treatment. In patients with severe coronary lesions, evaluation for other systemic vascular involvement (such as aneurysms in the axillary, iliac, renal, or intrathoracic arteries) should be considered based on clinical findings. Because regression of coronary artery aneurysms or progression to stenotic lesions mostly occur within 2 years of the onset of illness, follow-up coronary angiography is essential in patients with coronary aneurysms (Kato et al. 1996). The definition of regression of coronary aneurysms is that the follow-up coronary angiography demonstrates completely normal findings (disappearance of aneurysms and no irregularities in the walls of any arteries in the coronary artery system). 2DE may miss some mild abnormal findings, which subsequently progress to coronary artery disease. Coronary angiography is essential for the evaluation of stenotic or obstructive lesions of the coronary artery and for assessment of collateral circulation (Figure 29.9).

Intravascular ultrasound imaging of the coronary arteries in patients with KD may show mild or marked intimal thickening at the site of aneurysms that have resolved (Sugimura et al. 1994). Remodeling may contribute to maintenance of the normal lumen diameter despite mild intimal thickening (Glagov et al. 1987). Intravascular ultrasound is a useful technique for long-term follow-up of arteries affected by KD.

Evaluation for myocardial ischemia

Because the morbidity and mortality of KD mostly depend on the extent of associated coronary artery disease, it is particularly

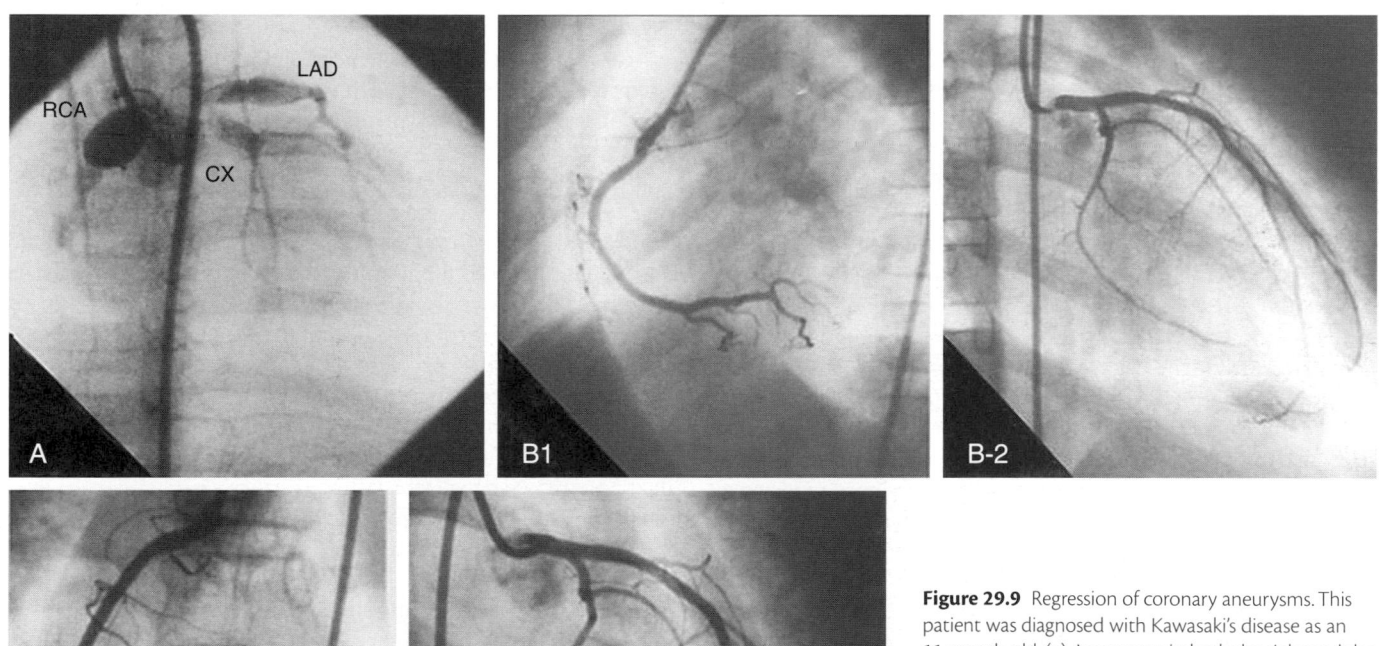

Figure 29.9 Regression of coronary aneurysms. This patient was diagnosed with Kawasaki's disease as an 11-month-old. (a) Aneurysms in both the right and the left coronary arteries. (b-1, b-2) One year and 2 months later the follow-up coronary angiography demonstrated disappearance of the coronary aneurysms. There were no stenoses or irregularities of the arterial lumen. (c-1,c-2). The follow-up coronary angiography 12 years later demonstrated no aneurysms, stenosis, or irregularities of the arterial lumen in either the left or right coronary arteries.

important to identify myocardial ischemia during follow-up, but current diagnostic methods have limitations. 2DE can detect coronary aneurysms, but is not satisfactory in the evaluation of stenotic lesions. Coronary angiography is an accurate method to assess coronary artery involvement, but repeated evaluations are difficult because of the invasiveness and cost of the procedure. The exercise stress test can detect myocardial ischemia and is non-invasive, but its sensitivity is suboptimal, even in patients with significant coronary stenosis. Furthermore, it is difficult to perform on young children. Myocardial single-photon emission computed tomography (SPECT) using pharmacological stress (dipyridamole infusion) is considered as the most accurate diagnostic method for identifying myocardial ischemia in children for whom the exercise stress test cannot be performed. Because the SPECT stress test provides quantitative analysis, the severity of myocardial ischemia can be assessed serially.

Kamiya and colleagues reported the sensitivities of various methods in detecting myocardial ischemia in patients with significant coronary stenosis (over 75% occlusion) (Kamiya 1995). The most sensitive method was dipyridamole stress SPECT (85% sensitivity). In contrast, the sensitivity of standard treadmill exercise test is less than 50% (Fukuda *et al.* 1998). Many types of stress tests have recently been reported in children with KD, including nuclear perfusion scans with exercise (Kondo *et al.* 1989), exercise echocardiography (Pahl *et al.* 1995), stress echocardiography using dobutamine (Noto *et al.* 1996), and contrast echocardiography with dipyridamole stress (Ishii *et al.* 2002b).

Management

Treatment of acute Kawasaki's disease

The major therapeutic approach to acute KD is a combination of aspirin (100 mg/kg body weight per day, through the 14th day of illness, then 3 to 5 mg/kg/day) and high-dose IVIg (Newburger *et al.* 2002). In 1984, high dose gamma globulin treatment was reported to be effective by Furusho in Japan (Furusho *et al.* 1984); this was confirmed by a randomized, multicenter trial in the US (Newburger *et al.* 1986). These two studies indicate that 400 mg/kg of body weight of IVIg should be given daily for 4 days for prevention of coronary aneurysms. Although IVIg treatment is now accepted as standard treatment, the optimal dose and selection of patients for this treatment are controversial. Some reports demonstrated a dose-dependent effect, with higher doses in single infusion being more effective (Terai and Shulman 1997). One dose of 2 g/kg has been reported to be effective (Newburger *et al.* 1991; Sato *et al.* 1999). This treatment should be started no later than 10 days after the onset of illness, and, if possible, within 7 days. It is uncertain whether earlier treatment (within 4 days of illness) is more effective (Muta *et al.* 2004).

Coronary aneurysms develop in less than 20% of KD patients, so the optimal strategy would be to identify patients at high risk for developing coronary aneurysms and treat them with IVIg. This would avoid the cost and morbidity of treating patients who would not have developed aneursysms even without treatment. Harada's scoring system (Harada 1991) may be useful to identify high-risk patients for IVIg treatment. Criteria used in this system include: (1) white blood cell count >12,000/mm³; (2) platelet count <350,000/mm³; (3) serum CRP >3 mg/dL; (4) hematocrit <35%; (5) serum albumin <3.5 mg/dL; (6) age <12 months; and (7) male sex. In their

analysis, the presence of more than four of these seven criteria indicates the need for IVIg treatment. It should be noted that coronary artery aneurysms may develop in up to 13% of patients treated with high-dose IVIg. Repeat doses of IVIg (2 g/kg) or pulse high-dose methylprednisolone (30 mg/kg for 3 days) may be indicated (Wright *et al.* 1996).

The mechanisms of action of IVIg are uncertain. Possibilities include: Fc-mediated down-regulation of inflammatory cytokines; modulation of T/B-cell functions through binding to lymphocyte Fc receptors; and inhibition of activated complement binding to targets such as endothelium. Potential Fab-mediated mechanisms include neutralization of microbial toxins, cytokines, and anti-idiotypic reactions against autoantibodies.

Aspirin is an important drug in KD for its antipyretic, anti-inflammatory, and antiplatelet effects, but the optimal dosage is still controversial (Kato *et al.* 1979; Akagi *et al.* 1991). The American Heart Association recommended high-dose aspirin (80 to 100 mg/kg) initially, with reduction of the dose to 3 to 5 mg/kg/day after the child has been afebrile for 48 to 72 hours. High-dose aspirin and IVIg appear to possess additive anti-inflammatory effects. In Japan, a lower dose of aspirin is generally used, such as 30 mg/kg/day in two doses for 2 weeks followed by 5 mg/kg/day thereafter (Kato *et al.* 1979).

Liver dysfunction is seen more often in high-dose aspirin groups; in such cases flurbiprofen may be substituted. Giving several lower doses of aspirin during the day may reduce aspirin intoxication, liver dysfunction, gastrointestinal irritation, and lower the risk of Reye syndrome. For these reasons, we recommend 30 mg/kg/day of aspirin in the acute stage and 5 mg/kg/day in the convalescent stage (Newburger *et al.* 2004).

Is glucocorticoid therapy beneficial? In the in 1970s, 2 mg/kg prednisone for 2 weeks was used frequently for KD vasculitis. The presence of coronary aneurysms, lack of regression of lesions, and frequent rupture in glucocorticoid-treated KD patients (Suzuki *et al.* 1999) suggested a lack of efficacy for coronary artery aneurysms. Short courses of glucocorticoid pulse therapy with or without IVIg has been reported to shorten the duration of fever (Sundel *et al.* 2003); however, the use of prednisone for 2 weeks may have adverse effects on coronary aneurysms in KD, underscoring the importance of frequent assessment by echocardiography and long-term follow-up.

Other treatments for acute KD include pentoxifylline, which has been shown to inhibit TNF transcription (Furukawa *et al.* 1994); ulinastatin (an inhibitor of neutrophil elastase) (Zaitsu *et al.* 2000); plasma exchange (for IVIg-refractory cases) (Imanaga *et al.* 2004); the anti-TNF antibody infliximab (Weiss *et al.* 2004; Burns *et al.* 2005); and cytotoxic agents such as cyclophosphamide and cyclosporin (Wallace *et al.* 2000). The antiplatelet agent abciximab (platelet glycoprotein IIb/IIIa receptor inhibitor) may enhance regression of coronary aneurysms (Williams *et al.* 2002). All these drugs may have some efficacy for treatment of KD; however, there are no results from randomized, controlled trials.

Long-term management

Long-term management of patients with KD depends on the degree of coronary arterial involvement. Low-dose aspirin (3 to 5 mg/kg/day single dose) is basic treatment in the convalescent phase and should be continued for up to 6–8 weeks in patients without coronary abnormalities. If coronary arterial abnormalities are detected, low-dose aspirin should be continued until these have been documented to have resolved. Coronary angiography is recommended in children in whom cardiovascular abnormalities have been found by 2DE. Since the risk of progression to ischemic heart disease is high, particularly in those with giant aneurysms, these patients should be managed by pediatric cardiologists. We recommend the combination of aspirin and warfarin for patients with giant coronary aneurysms. Beta-blockade may be indicated for patients with ischemic symptoms. Table 29.3 summarizes recommendations for long-term management.

When symptoms of acute MI are noted, the patient should be immediately hospitalized and treated with supportive measures as is current practice for patients with suspected MI due to atherosclerotic coronary artery disease. Since the main cause of acute MI in KD is acute thrombotic occlusion in stenotic coronary aneurysms, thrombolytic and anticoagulation therapy including intravenous tPA, intracoronary infusion of urokinase, and heparin are needed. Intracoronary infusion of urokinase within 6 hours after the onset of MI is the most effective treatment of thrombolysis (Kato et al. 1991);

however, tPA can be given by intravenous infusion. Therefore, when acute MI is recognized, pediatricians should use it immediately intravenously and refer the patient to a cardiac center. Vasodilators, nitroglycerin, and diuretics are useful; cardiogenic shock, heart failure, and arrhythmias should be treated promptly.

Long-term results of interventional techniques for treating coronary artery disease in KD are unknown. Balloon angioplasty is effective in some patients within 6–8 years from disease onset; however, it is less effective than in adult atherosclerotic coronary lesions because of the elastic recoil and stiffness of the coronary artery (Ino et al. 1996). We have successfully performed coronary rotational ablation for late severe coronary artery stenosis associated with severe calcification (Sugimura et al. 1997). Stent implantation may be useful in some patients (Ishii et al. 2001), and intervention procedures may postpone or supplant coronary artery bypass surgery (Kato et al. 1998; Akagi et al. 2000; Ishii et al. 2002a) (Figure 29.10).

Coronary artery bypass surgery may be indicated for patients with serious coronary artery lesions; the results are generally favorable

Table 29.3 Therapeutic recommendations for KD

Acute phase:	Patients with regressed coronary aneurysms
Aspirin	discontinue aspirin
80 to 100 mg/kg (4 divided daily doses) for 48 to 72 hours until afebrile, then 3 to 5 mg/kg for 6 to 8 weeks	follow-up every several years
or	no restriction of physical activity
30 mg/kg (2 divided daily doses) for 2 weeks then 5 mg/kg for 8 weeks	Patients with giant coronary aneurysms
IVIg (in addition to aspirin)	aspirin with warfarin
2 g/kg as a single dose infusion over 12 hours	follow-up every 3–6 months
For cases refractory to initial IVIg	consider coronary angiography
additional 2 g/kg as a single dose infusion over 12 hours	For acute thrombosis
or	thrombolytic treatment with:
glucocorticoid pulse therapy (IV methylprednisolone 30 mg/kg once daily for 3 days)	tissue plasminogen activator (bolus 1.25 mg/kg, infuse 0.1–0.5 mg/kg/hour for 6 hours)
Optional treatments for refractory cases	*or*
pentoxifylline, ulinastatin, plasma exchange, infliximab, cyclophosphamide, cyclosporine	urokinase (bolus 4400 U/kg, infuse 4400 U/kg/hour)
Convalescence phase:	Patients with coronary stenosis with or without aneurysms
Aspirin	aspirin with warfarin (for giant aneurysms)
3 to 5 mg/kg/day as a single dose for patients with coronary aneurysm	follow-up every 3–6 months
Optimal	physical activity restricted depending on stress test
consider adding dipyridamole 2–5 mg/kg, ticlopidine 5–7 mg/kg	assess the need for percutaneous intervention or bypass surgery
For patients with giant coronary aneurysms	screen for risk factors for atherosclerotic at school age
warfarin (0.05–0.12 mg/kg/day to keep INR 1.5–2.5) in combination with aspirin	**Indications for percutaneous interventions:**
Long-term management:	Ischemic symptoms or findings
Patients with no coronary lesions	Localized stenosis
stop aspirin, follow at 1 and 2 years later and at school age	PTCA is preferable in younger patients without severe calcification
no restriction of physical activity	Stent is indicated in older children over 10 years of age
Patients with small or moderate-sized aneurysms	Rotational ablation is indicated for patients with severe calcification
continue aspirin (3–5 mg/kg/day)	**Indications for coronary bypass surgery:**
follow-up coronary angiography 1–2 years after onset to check for regression of coronary	Ischemic symptoms or findings
aneurysms or progression to stenotic lesions	Severe multivessel obstruction
no restriction of physical activity	Obstruction in the left main trunk, stenosis in the left anterior descending artery and right main coronary artery
	Severe valvular disease
	Indication for heart transplantation:
	Severe ischemic cardiomyopathy (intractable)

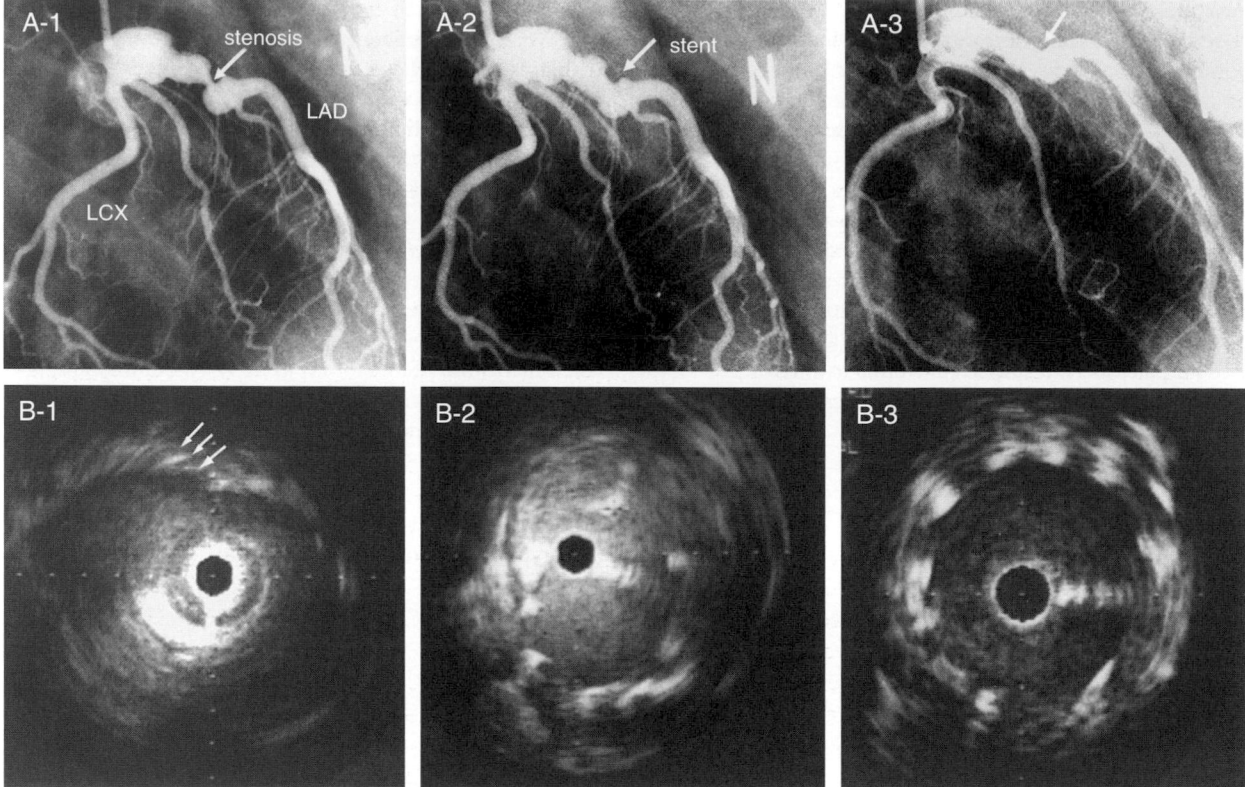

Figure 29.10 Percutaneous interventions for stenotic lesions. Left coronary artery angiography and intravascular ultrasound imaging in a 13-year-old boy with severe stenosis of the left anterior descending artery (LAD). (a-1) 95% localized stenosis of the LAD (arrow) before stent implantation. (a-2, b-2) Coronary stenosis improved after stent placement. (b-2, b-3) Intravascular ultrasound imaging image at the site of the coronary artery stenosis after stent placement showing the stent and improved coronary artery lumen diameter. (a-3, b-3). Follow-up coronary angiography and intravascular ultrasound imaging images 1 year later showed maintenance of the successfully dilated coronary artery lumen.

(Kitamura *et al.* 1994; Tsuda and Kitamura 2004). Surgical indications include: (1) three-vessel occlusion; (2) severe occlusion of the left main coronary artery; and (3) severe occlusion in both the left anterior descending artery and right coronary artery. A native, intrathoracic arterial graft is preferable, since it can grow with the child as he or she matures (Yoshikawa *et al.* 2000). Infants and small children under 3 years of age present technical difficulties for bypass surgery. Viability of the myocardium should be evaluated by thallium myocardial scintigraphy. Several patients have undergone cardiac transplantation in the US or UK (Checchia *et al.* 1997). Transplantation may be indicated in the rare instances of severe diffuse myocardial fibrosis due to ischemia or previous multivessel bypass surgery with difficult revascularization.

Prognosis and long-term issues

Long-term consequences of coronary aneurysms

The natural history or fate of coronary aneurysms is an important issue in KD (Kato 1996). We studied 594 consecutive patients with acute KD between 1973 and 1983, with follow-up ranging from 10 to 21 years (Kato *et al.* 1996). In all patients, we evaluated the coronary lesions by coronary angiography just after the acute stage. One hundred and forty-six patients (24.6%) were diagnosed as having coronary aneurysms. A second angiogram obtained 1 to 2 years later

in all 146 cases who previously had coronary aneurysms, demonstrated that 72 (49.3%) of these 146 had regression in coronary aneurysms. None of the patients with regression of coronary aneurysms had cardiac symptoms in the long-term follow-up periods; results of EKGs, exercise stress tests, thallium myocardial scintigraphy, and left ventricular function assessments were all within normal limits. Of the 594 patients, stenosis in the coronary aneurysms had developed in 28 cases. Myocardial infarction occurred in 11 patients, five of whom died. From this study, it is estimated that about 4% of patients with KD may develop ischemic heart disease.

We studied the timing and the incidence of regression or progression to obstructive lesions from the onset of KD using the Kaplan–Meyer life table method. Regression of coronary aneurysms mostly occurred within 2 years from the onset of illness, whereas obstructive lesions developed in 2 years and gradually increased thereafter.

We investigated various factors that could affect the prognosis of coronary aneurysms (Ichinose *et al.* 1986). The risk factors for coronary aneurysms to develop into ischemic heart disease are: (1) aneurysms with diameter >8 mm; (2) large diffuse aneurysms or saccular morphology; (3) prolonged fever (more than 21 days); and (4) age at onset >2 years. In the 26 patients with giant coronary aneurysms, stenotic lesions developed in 12, and no regression occurred in our follow-up study. Thus, the presence of giant coronary aneurysms is a critical problem because it has a high likelihood to progress to ischemic heart disease. In our series, the incidence of giant coronary aneurysms was 17.8% among patients with coronary aneurysms and 4.4% among all KD patients.

The mechanism of regression of aneurysms is marked intimal proliferation, with abundant smooth muscle cells, well-regenerated endothelium, and no thrombus formation (Sasaguri and Kato 1982). Hemodynamic forces may influence such arteries to maintain adequate luminal diameter. It is uncertain whether intimal thickening eventually develops into obstructive lesions; however, from our long-term follow-up study, none of the patients whose aneurysms regressed developed subsequent ischemic heart disease. Our experience suggests that stenotic lesions do not develop, at least within 10–20 years, in the patients with complete regression of coronary aneurysms (Figure 29.11).

Kawasaki's vasculitis may be a risk factor for atherosclerosis

The histologic picture of the coronary artery in KD several years after its onset is that of marked intimal proliferation. In some patients, calcified deposits of protein-like material and hyalinized degeneration in the thickened intima are seen. These findings are quite similar to atherosclerotic lesions. Suzuki reported that active expression of various growth factors were observed in the coronary artery in the late phase of KD, which suggests that active vascular remodeling continues years after disease onset (Suzuki et al. 2000, 2004). An important issue is whether these coronary artery lesions develop into atherosclerotic coronary artery disease in adulthood.

We have studied the distensibility of the coronary arterial wall by intracoronary infusion of isosorbide dinitrate (Sugimura et al. 1992)

and endothelial function by intracoronary infusion of acetylcholine (Yamakawa et al. 1998; Iemura et al. 2000). Mitani and Dhillon reported that endothelial dysfunction was observed even in the normal arteries of patients with KD (Dhillon et al. 1996; Mitani et al. 1997; Silva et al. 2001). Mitani found that the persistence of coronary artery lesions late after KD was independently associated with levels of CRP and serum amyloid A, suggesting that inflammation may contribute to coronary artery disease in patients with a remote history of KD (Mitani et al. 2005) (Figure 29.12).

Adult coronary artery disease due to childhood Kawasaki's disease

It has now been more than 35 years since the first description of KD as a new clinical entity, and a number of the early KD children are now adults. We surveyed these adults to look for coronary sequelae that might have been due to their earlier KD, and reported 21 such cases and their cardiac conditions (Kato et al. 1992). Most of these 21 patients were diagnosed originally with fever of unknown origin, sepsis, or pneumonia; their illnesses antedated Dr Kawasaki's first description in 1968. Most of the 21 patients had experienced ischemic symptoms, such as MI or angina pectoris two or three decade after the onset of suspected KD. Some patients had mitral regurgitation or arrhythmias. Almost all patients had multiple coronary aneurysms with obstruction or stenosis and severe calcification of the arteries.

Suggested criteria for recognition of coronary artery sequelae of KD are as follows: (1) history of KD in infancy or childhood; (2) abnormal Q waves or mitral regurgitation of unknown origin in younger adults; and most importantly (3) angiographic evidence of multiple aneurysms, frequently associated with calcification.

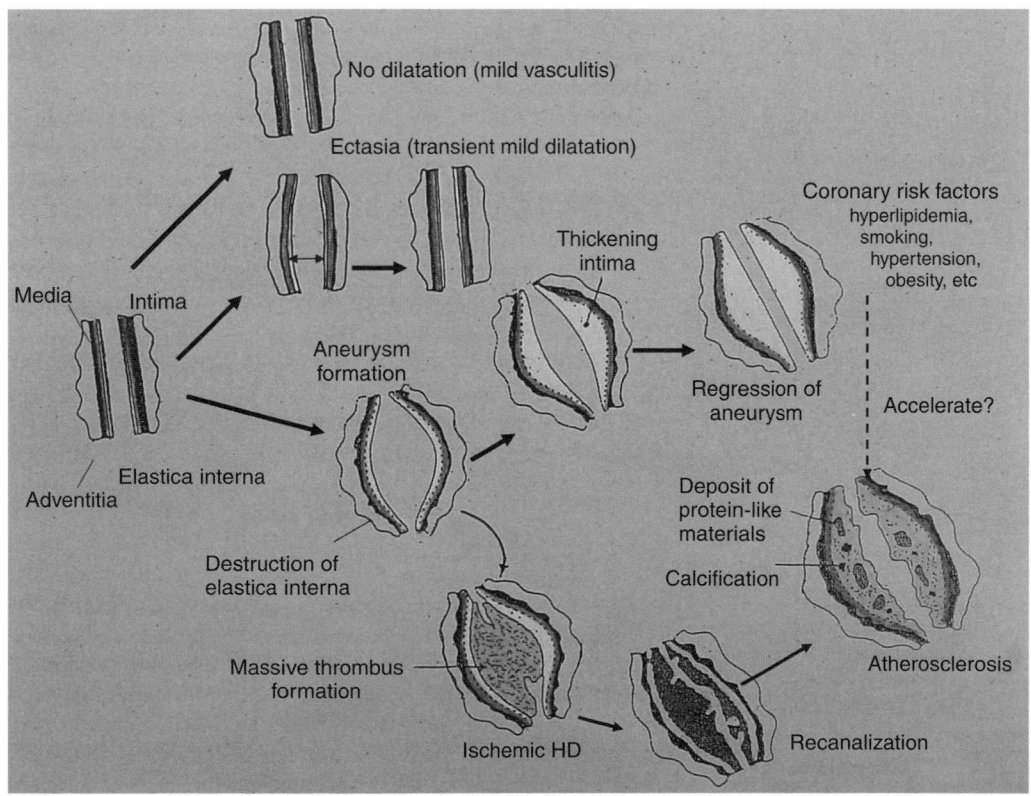

Figure 29.11 Pathological sequences of coronary aneurysms. (See Color Plate 82).

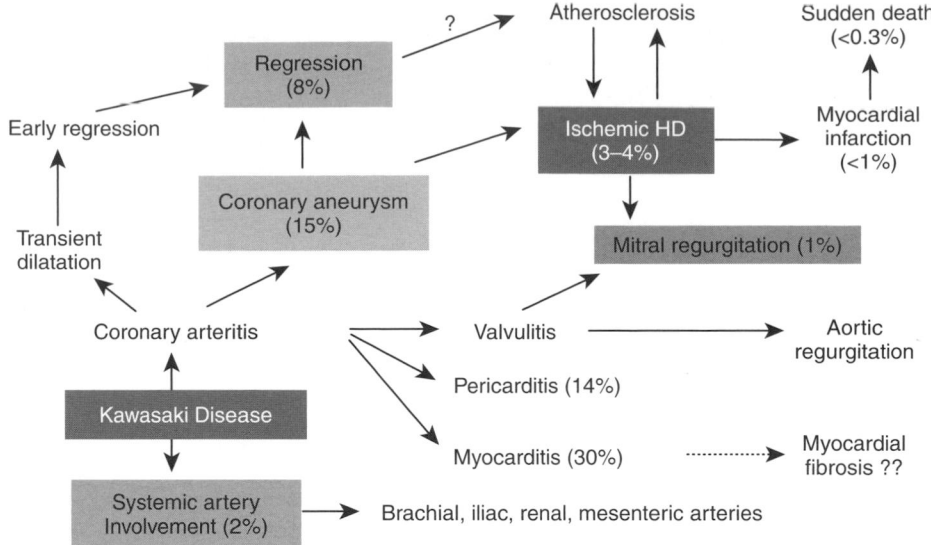

Figure 29.12 The cardiovascular spectrum and natural history.

Dyslipidemia should be excluded. Subsequent to our article, there were many case reports of adult coronary artery disease probably due to childhood KD (reviewed in Burns *et al.* 1996). The coronary artery sequelae of KD may be a significant cause of ischemic heart disease in adults under 40 years of age, and adult cardiologists should incorporate this condition into the differential diagnosis of early-onset coronary artery disease in adults.

Summary

KD is a common, acute febrile illness with mucocutaneous involvement that affects infants and young children. It is a vasculitis syndrome mostly affecting small and medium-sized arteries, particularly coronary arteries. Coronary aneurysms occur in 10–20% of the patients and may cause MI, sudden death, or coronary artery disease. In Japan, North America, and Western Europe, KD has replaced rheumatic fever as the leading cause of acquired heart disease in children. Long-term follow-up study is needed to clarify the prognosis from childhood through adult life.

References

Abe, J., Kotzin, B. L., Jujo, K., Melish, M. E., Glode, M. P., Kohsaki, T. and Leung, D. Y. M. (1992). Selective expansion of T cells expressing T-cell receptor variable regions Vbeta2 and Vbeta8 in Kawasaki disease. *Proceedings of the National Academy of Sciences of the USA*, **89**, 4066–70.

Akagi, T., Kato, H., Inoue, O. and Sato, N. (1990). Valvular heart disease in Kawasaki syndrome: Incidence and natural history. *American Heart Journal*, **120**, 366–72.

Akagi, T., Kato, H., Inoue, O. and Sato, N. (1991). Salicylate treatment in Kawasaki disease: high dose or low dose? *European Journal Pediatrics*, **150**, 642–6.

Akagi, T., Ogawa, S., Ino, T., Iwasa, M., Echigo, S., Kishida, K., Baba, K., Matsushima, M., Hamaoka, K., Tomita, H., Ishii, M. and Kato, H. (2000). Catheter interventional treatment in Kawasaki disease: A report from the Japanese Pediatric Interventional Cardiology Investigation group. *Journal of Pediatrics*, **137**, 181–6.

Amano, S., Hazawa, F., Kubagawa, H., *et al.* (1980) General pathology of Kawasaki disease on the morphological alterations corresponding to the clinical manifestations. *Acta Pathologica Japonica*, **30**, 681–94.

Burns, J. C., Shike, H., Gordon, J. B., Malhotra, A., Schoenwetter, M. and Kawasaki, T. (1996). Sequelae of Kawasaki disease in adolescents and young adults. *Journal of the American College of Cardiology*, **28**, 253–7.

Burns, J. C., Mason, W. H., Hauger, S. B., Janai, H., Bastian, J., Wohrely, J. D., Balpour, I., Shen, C. A., Michel, E. D., Shulman, S. T. and Melish, M. E. (2005). Infliximab treatment for refractory Kawasaki syndrome. *Journal of Pediatrics*, **146**, 662–7.

Chang, R. K. (2002). Hospitalization for Kawasaki disease among children in the United States, 1988–1997. *Pediatrics*, **109**, e87.

Checchia, P. A., Pahl, E., Shaddy, R. E. and Shulman, S. T. (1997). Cardiac transplantation for Kawasaki disease. *Pediatrics*, **100**, 695–9.

Dajani, A. S., Taubert, K. A., Takahashi, M., Bierman, F. Z., Freed, M. D., Ferrieri, P., Gerber, M., Shulman, S. T., Karchmer, A. W., Wilson, W., Peter, G., Durack, D. T. and Rahimtoola, S. H. (1994). Guidelines for long-term management of patients with Kawasaki disease, Committee Report of Council on Cardiovascular Disease in the Young, American Heart Association. *Circulation*, **89**, 916–22.

de Zorzi, A., Colan, S. D., Gauvreau, K. and Newbuirger, J. (1998). Coronary artery dimensions may be misclassified as normal in Kawasaki disease. *Journal of Pediatrics*, **133**, 254–8.

Dhillon, R., Clarkson, P., Donald, A. E., Powe, A. J., Nash, M., Novelli, V., Dillon, M. J. and Deanfield, J. E. (1996). Endothelial dysfunction late after Kawasaki disease. *Circulation*, **94**, 2103–6.

Esper, F., Shapiro, E. D., Welbel, C., Ferguson, D., Landry, M. L. and Kahn, J. S. (2005). Association between a novel human Coronavirus and Kawasaki disease. *Journal of Infectious Diseases*, **191**, 499–502.

Frey, E. E., Matherne, G. P., Mahony, L. T., Sato, Y., Stanford, W. and Smith, W. L. (1988). Coronary artery aneurysms due to Kawasaki disease: diagnosis with ultrafast CT. *Radiology*, **167**, 725–6.

Fujiwara, H. and Hamashima, Y. (1978). Pathology of the heart in Kawasaki disease. *Pediatrics*, **61**, 100–7.

Fujiwara, H., Fujiwara, T., Kao, T. C., Ohshio, G. and Hamashima, Y. (1986) Pathology of Kawasaki disease in the healed stage; relationship between typical and atypical cases of Kawasaki disease. *Acta Pathologica Japonica*, **36**, 857–67.

Fukuda, T., Akagi, T., Ishibashi, M., Inoue, O., Sugimura, T. and Kato, H. (1998). Noninvasive evaluation of myocardial ischemia in Kawasaki disease: Comparison between dipyridamole stress thallium imaging and exercise stress testing. *American Heart Journal*, **135**, 482–7.

Furukawa, S., Matsubara, T., Jujoh, K., Yone, K., Sugawara, T., Sasai, K., Kato, H. and Yabuta, K. (1988). Peripheral blood monocyte / macrophages and serum tumor necrosis factor in Kawasaki disease. *Clinical Immunology and Immunopathology*, **48**, 247–51.

Furukawa, S., Matsubara, T., Umezawa, Y., Okamura, K. and Yabuta, K. (1994). Serum levels of p60 soluble tumor necrosis factor receptor during acute Kawasaki disease. *Journal of Pediatrics*, **124**, 721–5.

Furukawa, S., Matsubara, T., Umezawa, Y., Motohashi, T., Ino, T. and Yabuta, K. (1994). Pentoxifylline and intravenous gamma globulin combination therapy for acute Kawasaki disease. *European Journal of Pediatrics*, **153**, 663–7.

Furusho, K., Kamiya, T., Nakano, H., Kiyosawa, N., Shinamiya, K., Hayashidera, T., Tamura, T., Hirose, O., Manabe, Y. and Yokoyama, T. (1984). High-dose intravenous gammaglobulin for Kawasaki disease. *Lancet*, **2**, 1055–8.

Gidding, S. S., Shulman, S. T., Ilbawi, M., Crussi, F. and Duffy, C. E. (1986). Mucocutaneous lymph node syndrome (Kawasaki disease): delayed aortic and mitral insufficiency secondary to valvulitis. *Journal of American College of Cardiology*, **7**, 894–7.

Glagov, S., Weinsenberg, E. and Kolettis, G. (1987). Compensatory enlargement of human coronary arteries. *New England Journal of Medicine*, **316**, 1371–5.

Greil, G. F., Stuber, M., Botnar, R. M., Kissinger, K. V., Geva, T., Newburger, J. W., Manning, W. J. and Powell, A. J. (2002). Coronary magnetic resonance angiography in adolescent and young adults due to Kawasaki disease. *Circulation*, **105**, 908–11.

Harada, K. (1991). Intravenous gammaglobulin treatment in Kawasaki disease. *Acta Paediatrica Japonica*, **33**, 805–10.

Hayakawa, S., Nakamura, Y., Yashiro, M., Uehara, R., Oki, I., Tajimi, M., Ojima, T., Terai, M. and Yanagawa, H. (2003). Analyses of fatal cases of Kawasaki disease in Japan using vital statistical data over 27 years. *Journal of Epidemiology*, **13**, 246–50.

Ichinose, E., Inoue, O., Hiyoshi, Y. and Kato, H. (1986). Fate of coronary aneurysms in Kawasaki disease: Analysis of prognostic factors. In *Pediatric cardiology* (Doyle, E. F., Engle, M. A. and Gersony, W., eds), pp. 1099–101. Saunders, New York.

Iemura, M., Ishii, M., Sugimura, T., Akagi, T. and Kato, H. (2000). Long term consequences of regressed coronary aneurysms after Kawasaki disease: vascular wall morphology and function. *Heart*, **83**, 307–11.

Imanaga, T., Mori, M., Miyamae, T., Ito, S., Nakamura, T., Tasui, K., Kimura, H. and Yokota, S. (2004). Plasma exchange for refractory Kawasaki disease. *European Journal of Pediatrics*, **163**, 263–4.

Ino, T., Akimoto, K., Ohkubo, M., Nishimoto, K., Yabuta, K., Takaya, J. and Yamaguchi, H. (1996). Application of percutaneous transluminal coronary angioplasty to coronary arterial stenosis in Kawasaki disease. *Circulation*, **93**, 1709–15.

Ishii, M., Ueno, T., Akagi, T., Baba, K., Harada, K., Hamaoka, K., Kato, H., Tsuda, E., Uemura, S., Saji, T., Ogawa, S., Echigo, S., Yamaguchi, T. and Kato, H. (2001).Guidelines for catheter intervention in coronary artery lesion in Kawasaki disease. *Pediatrics International*, **43**, 558–62.

Ishii, M., Ueno, T., Ikeda, H., Iemura, M., Sugimura, T., Furui, J., Sugahara, Y., Muta, H., Akagi, T., Nomura, Y., Homma, T., Yokoi, H., Nobuyoshi, M., Matsuishi, T. and Kato, H. (2002a). Sequential follow-up results of catheter intervention for coronary artery lesions after Kawasaki disease: quantitative coronary artery angiography and intravascular ultrasound imaging study. *Circulation*, **105**, 3004–10.

Ishii, M., Himeno, W., Sawa, M., Iemura, M., Furui, J., Muta, H., Sugawara, Y., Egami, K., Akagi, T., Ishibashi, M. and Kato, H. (2002b). Assessment of the ability of myocardial contrast echocardiography with harmonic power Doppler imaging to identify perfusion abnormalities in patients with Kawasaki disease at rest and during dipyridamole stress. *Pediatric Cardiology*, **23**, 192–9.

Jennette, J. C., Falk, R. J., Andrassy, K., Bacon, P. A., Churg, J., Gross, W. L., Hagen, E. C., Hoffman, G. S., Hunder, G. G. and Kallenberg, C. G. (1994). Nomenclature of systemic vasculitides. Proposal of an international consensus conference. *Arthritis and Rheumatism*, **37**, 187–92.

Kamiya, T. (1984). *Research Committee on Kawasaki disease. Report of subcommittee on standardization of diagnostic criteria and reporting of coronary artery lesions in Kawasaki disease.* Tokyo, Japan: Ministry of Health and Welfare.

Kamiya, T. (1995). How to evaluate the myocardial ischemic in Kawasaki disease. In *Kawasaki disease* (Kato, H., ed.), pp. 447–50. Elsevier, Amsterdam.

Kato, H., Koike, S., Yamamoto, M., Ito, Y. and Yano, E. (1975). Coronary aneurysms in infants and young children with acute febrile mucocutaneous lymph node syndrome. *Journal of Pediatrics*, **86**, 892–8.

Kato, H., Koike, S. and Yokoyama, T. (1979). Kawasaki disease: effect of treatment on coronary artery involvement. *Pediatrics*, **63**, 175–9.

Kato, H., Ichinose, E., Yoshioka, F., Takechi, T., Matsunaga, S., Suzuki, K. and Rikitake, N. (1982a). Fate of coronary aneurysms in Kawasaki disease: serial coronary angiography and long-term follow-up study. *American Journal of Cardiology*, **49**, 1758–66.

Kato, H., Inoue, O., Ichinose, E., Akagi, T. and Sato, N. (1982b). Intracoronary urokinase in Kawasaki disease: treatment and prevention of myocardial infarction. *Acta Paediatrica Japonica*, **33**, 27–35.

Kato, H., Fujimato, T., Inoue, O., Kondo, M., Koga, Y., Yamamoto, S., Shingu, M., Tominaga, K. and Sasaguri, Y. (1983). Variant strain of Propionibacterium acnes: a clue to the aetiology of Kawasaki disease. *Lancet*, **2**,1383–8.

Kato, H., Ichinose, E. and Kawasaki, T. (1986). Myocardial infarction in Kawasaki disease: clinical analyses in 195 cases. *Journal of Pediatrics*, **108**, 923–7.

Kato, H. and Kitamura, S. (1987). Guideline for treatment and management of cardiovascular sequelae in Kawasaki disease. Subcommittee of Cardiovascular Sequelae, Subcommittee of Surgical Treatment, Kawasaki Disease Research Committee. *Heart and Vessels*, **3**, 50–4

Kato, H., Inoue, O., Ichinose, E., Akagi, T. and Sato, N. (1991). Intracoronary urokinase in Kawasaki disease: treatment and prevention of myocardial infarction. *Acta Paediatrica Japonica*, **33**, 27–35.

Kato, H., Inoue, O., Kawasaki, T., Fujiwara, H., Watanabe, T. and Toshima, H. (1992). Adult coronary artery disease probable due to childhood Kawasaki disease. *Lancet*, **340**, 1127–9.

Kato, H., Akagi, T., Sugimura, T., Sato, N., Kazue, T., Hashino, K., Nishiyori, A. and Sakaguchi, M. (1995). Kawasaki disease. *Coronary Artery Disease*, **6**, 94–206.

Kato, H., Sugimura, T., Akagi, T., Sato, N., Hashino, K., Maeno, Y., Kazue, T., Eto, G. and Yamakawa, R. (1996). Long-term consequences of Kawasaki disease: A 10-to-21-year follow-up study of 594 patients. *Circulation*, **94**, 1379–85.

Kato, H. (1997). Long-term consequences of Kawasaki disease: pediatrics to adults. In *Kawasaki disease* (Kato, H., ed.), pp. 557–66. Elsevier, Amsterdam.

Kato, H., Ishii, M., Akagi, T., Eto, G., Iemura, M., Tsutsumi, T. and Ueno, T. (1998). Interventional catheterization in Kawasaki disease. *Journal of Interventional Cardiology*, **11**, 355–61.

Kato, H. (2004). Cardiovascular complications in Kawasaki disease: coronary artery lumen and long-term consequences. *Progress of Pediatric Cardiology*, **19**, 137–45.

Kawasaki, T. (1967). Acute febrile mucocutaneous syndrome with lymphoid involvement with specific desquamation of the fingers and toes in children. *Japanese Journal of Allergy*, **16**, 178–222.

Kawasaki, T., Kosaki, F., Okawa, S., Shigematsu, I. and Yanagawa, H. (1974). A new infantile acute febrile mucocutaneous lymph node syndrome prevailing in Japan. *Pediatrics*, **54**, 271–6.

Kikuta, H., Mizuno, F. and Osato, T. (1984). Kawasaki disease and an unusual primary infection with Epstein-Barr virus. *Pediatrics*, **73**, 413–4.

Kitamura, S., Kameda, Y., Seki, T., Kawachi, K., Endo, M., Takeuchi, Y., Kawasaki, T. and Kawashima, Y. (1994). Long-term outcome of myocardial revascularization in patients with Kawasaki coronary artery disease, A multicenter cooperative study. *Journal of Thoracic and Cardiovascular Surgery*,**107**, 663–73.

Kondo, C., Hiroe, M., Nakanishi, T. and Takao, A. (1987). Detection of coronary artery stenosis in children with Kawasaki disease. *Circulation*, **80**, 615–24.

Kurotobi, S., Nagai, T. and Kawakami, N. (2002). Coronary diameter in normal infants, children and patients with Kawasaki disease. *Pediatrics International*, **44**, 1–4.

Landing, B. H. and Larson, E. J. (1977). Are infantile periarteritis nodosa with coronary artery involvement and fetal mucocutaneous lymph node syndrome the same? comparison of 20 patients from North America with patients from Hawaii and Japan. *Pediatrics*, **59**, 651–62.

Landing, H. L. and Larson, E. (1987) Pathological features of Kawasaki disease (mucocutaneous lymph node syndrome). *American Journal of Cardiovascular Pathology*, **1**, 215–29.

Leung, D. Y.M., Collins, T., LaPierre, L. A., Geha, R. S. and Pober, J. S. (1986). Immunoglobulin M antibodies present in the acute phase of Kawasaki syndrome lyse cultured vascular endothelial cells stimulated by gamma interferon. *Journal of Clinical Investigation*, **77**, 1428–35.

Leung, D. Y.M., Meissner, H. C., Fulton, D. R., Murray, D., Kotzin, B. L. and Schllevert, P. M. (1993). Toxic shock syndrome toxin-secreting staphylococcus aureus in Kawasaki syndrome. *Lancet*, **342**, 1385–8.

Lin, C. Y., Lin, C. C., Hwang, B. and Chiang, B. (1992). Serial changes of serum interleukin-6, interleukin-8, and tumor necrosis factor alpha among patients with Kawasaki disease. *Journal of Pediatrics*, **121**, 924–6.

Masuda, H., Naoe, S. and Tanaka, N. (1981) A pathological study of coronary artery in Kawasaki disease (MCLS) – with special reference to morphogenesis of aneurysm. *Journal of the Japanese College of Angiology*, **21**, 899–912.

Mitani, Y., Okuda, Y., Shimpo, H., Uchida, F., Hamanaka, K., Aoki, K. and Sajurai, M. (1997). Impaired endothelial function in epicardial coronary arteries after Kawasaki disease. *Circulation*, **96**, 454–61.

Mitani, Y., Sawada, H., Hayakawa, H., Aoki, K., Ohashi, H., Matsumura, M., Kuroe, K., Shimpo, H., Nakano, M. and Kodama, Y. (2005). Elevated levels of high-sensitivity C-reactive protein and serum amyloid-A late after Kawasaki disease: association between inflammation and late coronary sequelae in Kawasaki disease. *Circulation*, **111**, 38–43.

Muta, H., Ishii, M., Egami, K., Furui, J., Sugawara, Y., Akagi, T., Nakamura, Y., Yanagawa, H. and Matsuishi, T. (2004). Early intravenous gamma globulin treatment for Kawasaki disease: the nationwide survey in Japan. *Journal of Pediatrics*, **144**, 496–9.

Nakamura, Y., Yanagawa, H., Harada, K. and Kawasaki, T. (2002). Mortality among persons with a history of Kawasaki disease in Japan. The fifth look. *Archives of Pediatric and Adolescent Medicine*, **156**, 162–5.

Nakamura, Y. and Yanagawa, H. (2004). The worldwide epidemiology of Kawasaki disease. *Progress of Pediatric Cardiology*, **19**, 99–108.

Naoe, S., Takahashi, K., Masuda, H. and Tanaka, N. (1987). Coronary findings post Kawasaki disease in children who died of other causes. In *Kawasaki disease* (Schulman ST, ed.), pp. 341–6. Liss, New York.

Naoe, S., Takahashi, K., Masuda, H. and Tanaka, N. (1991a) Kawasaki disease with particular emphasis on arterial lesions. *Acta Pathologica Japonica*, **41**, 785–97.

Naoe, S., Shibuya, K., Takahashi, K., Wakayama, M., Masuda, H. and Tanaka, M. (1991b). Pathological observations concerning the cardiovascular lesions in Kawasaki disease. *Cardiology in the Young*, **3**, 212–20.

Naoe, S. and Takahashi, K. (1993). Kawasaki disease with the focus on sequelae. In *Intractable vasculitis syndromes* (Tanabe, T. ed.) pp. 93–103. Hokkaido University Press, Sapporo.

Newburger, J. W., Takahashi, M., Burns, J. C., Beiser, A. S., Chung, K. J., Duffy, C. E., Glode, M. P., Mason, W. H., Reddy, V. and Sanders, S. P. (1986). The treatment of Kawasaki syndrome with intravenous gamma globulin. *New England Journal of Medicine*, **315**, 341–7.

Newburger, J. W., Takahashi, M., Beiser, A. S., Burns, J. C., Bastian, J., Chung, K. J., Colan, S. D., Duffy, E., Fulton, D. R. and Glode, M. P. (1991). A single intravenous infusion of gamma globulin as compared with four infusions in the treatment of acute Kawasaki syndrome. *New England Journal of Medicine*, **324**, 1633–9.

Newburger, J. W., Takahashi, M., Gerber, M. A., Gewitz, M. H., Tani, L. Y. and Burns, J. C., *et al.* (2004). Diagnosis, treatment, and long-term management of Kawasaki disease. American Heart Association Scientific Statement. *Circulation*, **110**, 2747–71.

Noto, N., Ayusawa, M., Karasawa, K., Yamaguchi, H., Sumitomo, N., Okada, T. and Harada, K. (1996). Dobutamine stress echocardiography for detection of coronary artery stenosis in children with Kawasaki disease. *Journal of the American College of Cardiology*, **27**, 1251–6.

Pahl, E., Sehgal, R., Chrystof, D., Neches, W. H., Webb, C. L., Duffy, E., Shulman, S. T. and Chanudhy, F. A. (1995). Feasibility of exercise stress echocardiography for the follow-up of children with coronary involvement secondary to Kawasaki disease. *Circulation*, **91**, 122–8.

Rowley, A. H., Shulman, S. T., Spike, B. T., Mask, C. A. and Baker, S. C. (2001). Oligoclonal IgA response in the vascular wall in acute Kawasaki disease. *Journal of Immunology*, **166**, 1334–43.

Sakaguchi, M., Kato, H., Nishiyori, A., Sagawa, K. and Itoh, K. (1995). Characterization of CD4+ T helper cells in patients with Kawasaki disease: Preferential production of TNF- alph by Vbeta2 and Vbeta8 CD4+ T helper cells. *Clinical and Experimental Immunology*, **99**, 276–82.

Sasaguri, Y. and Kato, H. (1982). Regression of aneurysms in Kawasaki disease: A pathologic study. *Journal of Pediatrics*, **100**, 225–31.

Sato, K., Ouichi, K. and Taki, M. (1983). Yersinia pseudotuberculosis infection in children, resembling Izumi fever and Kawasaki syndrome. *Pediatric Infectious Disease Journal*, **2**, 123–6.

Sato, N., Sugimura, T., Akagi, T., Yamakawa, R., Hashino, K., Eto, G., Iemura, M., Ishii, M. and Kato, H. (1999). Selective high dose gamma-globulin treatment in Kawasaki disease: Assessment of clinical aspects and cost effectiveness. *Pediatrics International*, **41**, 1–7.

Shibuya, N., Shibuya, K., Kato, H. and Yanagisawa, M. (2002). Kawasaki disease before Kawasaki at Tokyo University Hospital. *Pediatrics*, **110**, e17.

Silva, A. A., Maeno, Y., Hashmi, A., Smallhorn, J. F., Silverman, E. D. and McCrindle, B. W. (2001). Cardiovascular risk factors after Kawasaki disease: A case-control study. *Journal of Pediatrics*, **138**, 400–5.

Sugimura, T., Kato, H., Inoue, O., Takagi, J., Fukuda, T. and Sato, N. (1992). Vasodilatory response of the coronary arteries after Kawasaki disease: evaluation by intracoronary injection of isosorbide dinitrate. *Journal of Pediatrics*, **121**, 684–8.

Sugimura, T., Kato, H., Inoue, O., Fukuda, T., Sato, N., Ishii, M., Takagi, J., Akagi, T., Maeno, Y., Kawano, T., Takagishi, T. and Sasaguri, Y. (1994). Intravascular ultrasound of coronary arteries in children: Assessment of the wall morphology and the lumen after Kawasaki disease. *Circulation*, **89**, 258–65.

Sugimura, T., Yokoi, H., Sato, N., Akagi, T., Kimura, T., Iemura, M., Nobuyoshi, M. and Kato, H. (1997). Interventional treatment for children with severe coronary artery stenosis with calcification after long-term Kawasaki disease. *Circulation*, **96**, 3928–33.

Sundel, R. P., Baker, A. L., Fulton, D. R. and Newburger, J. W. (2003). Corticosteroids in the initial treatment of Kawasaki disease:report of a randomized trial. *Journal of Pediatrics*, **142**, 611–6.

Suzuki, A., Miyagawa-Tomita, S., Komatsu, K., Nishikawa, T., Sakomura, Y., Horie, T. and Nakazawa, M. (2000). Active remodeling of the coronary arterial lesions in the late phase of Kawasaki disease: immunohistochemical study. *Circulation*, **101**, 2935–41.

Suzuki, A., Miyagawa-Tomita, S., Komatsu, K., Nakazawa, M., Fukaya, T., Baba, K. and Yutani, C. (2004). Immunohistochemical study of apparently intact coronary artery in a child after Kawasaki disease. *Pediatrics International*, **46**, 590–6.

Suzuki, N., Seguchi, M., Kouno, C., Inukai, K., Kito, H. and Kobayashi, H. (1999). Rupture of coronary aneurysm in Kawasaki disease. *Pediatrics International*, **41**, 318–20.

Takahashi, K., Oharaseki, T. and Naoe, S. (2001) Pathological study of postcoronary arteritis in adolescents and young adults, with reference to the relationship between sequelae of Kawasaki disease and atherosclerosis *Pediatric Cardiology*, **22**, 138–42.

Takahashi, K., Oharaseki, T., Naoe, S., Wakayama, M. and Yokouchi, Y. (2005) Neutrophilic involvement in the damage to coronary arteries in acute stage of Kawasaki disease. *Pediatrics International*, **47**, 305–10.

Tanaka, N. (1975) Kawasaki disease (acute febrile infantile mucocutaneous lymph node syndrome) in Japan: relationship with infantile periarteritis nodosa. *Pathology and Microbiology*, **43**, 204–18.

Tanaka, N., Naoe, S., Masuda, H. and Ueno, T. (1986) Pathological study of sequelae of Kawasaki disease (MCLS) with special reference to heart and coronary arterial lesions. *Acta Pathologica Japonica*, **36**, 1513–27.

Terai, M., Kohno, Y., Nanba, M., Uemiya, T., Niwa, K., Nakajima, H. and Mikata, A. K. (1990). Class II antigen expression in the coronary artery endothelium in Kawasaki disease. *Human Pathology*, **21**, 231–4.

Terai, M. and Shulman, S. (1997). Prevalence of coronary artery abnormalities in Kawasaki disease is highly dependent on gamma globulin dose but independent of salycilate dose. *Journal of Pediatrics*, **131**, 888–93.

Tomita, S., Kato, H., Fujimoto, T., Inoue, O., Kondo, M., Koga, Y. and Kuriya, N. (1987). Cytopathogenic protein in filtrates from cultures of Propionibacterium acnes isolated from patients with Kawasaki disease. *British Medical Journal*, **295**, 1229–32.

Tomita, S., Chung, K., Mas, M., Gidding, S. and Shulman, S. T. (1992). Peripheral gangrene associated with Kawasaki disease. *Clinical Infectious Disease*, **14**, 121–6.

Tsuda, E. and Kitamura, S. (2004). Cooperative study group of Japan: National survey of coronary artery bypass grafting for coronary stenosis caused by Kawasaki disease in Japan. *Circulation*, **110** (Suppl. 1), II 61–6.

Wallace, C. A., French, J. W., Kahn, S. J. and Sherry, D. D. (2000). Initial intravenous gamma globulin treatment failure in Kawasaki disease. *Pediatrics*, **24**, 145–8.

Weiss, J. E., Eberhard, B. A., Chowdhury, D. and Gottlieb, B. S. (2004). Infliximab as a novel therapy for refractory Kawasaki disease. *Journal of Rheumatology*, **31**, 808–10.

Williams, R. V., Wilke, V. M., Tani, L. Y. and Minch, L. L. (2002). Does abcixmab enchance regression of coronary aneurysms resulting from Kawasaki disease? *Pediatrics*, **109**, E4.

Wright, D. A., Newburger, J. W., Baker, A. and Sundel, R. P. (1996). Treatment of immune globulin-resistant Kawasaki disease with pulsed doses of corticosteroids. *Journal of Pediatrics*, **128**, 146–9.

Yamakawa, R., Ishii, M., Sugimura, T., Akagi, T., Eto, G., Iemura, M., Tsutsumi, T. and Kato, H. (1998). Coronary endothelial dysfunction after Kawasaki disease: Evaluation by intracoronary injection of acetylcholine. *Journal of American College of Cardiology*, **31**, 1074–80.

Yamamoto, T. and Kimura, J. (1968). A case report of acute febrile MCLS complicated with myocarditis (in Japanese). *Shonika Rinsho*, **21**, 336–9.

Yanagawa, H., Yashiro, M., Nakamura, T., Kawasaki, T. and Kato, H. (1995). Results of twelve nationwide epidemiological incidence surveys of Kawasaki disease in Japan. *Archives of Pediatric and Adolescent Medicine*, **149**, 779–83.

Yasukawa, K., Terai, M., Shulman, S. T., Toyozaki, T., Yajima, S., Kohno, Y. and Rowley, A. H. (2002). Systemic production of vascular endothelial growth factor in fms-like tyrosine kinase-1 receptor in acute Kawasaki disease. *Circulation*, **105**, 766–9.

Yokoyama, T., Ichinose, E. and Kato, H. (1980). Aspirin treatment and platelet function in Kawasaki disease. *Kurume Medial Journal*, **27**, 57–60.

Yoshikawa, Y., Yagihara, T., Kameda, Y., Taniguchi, S., Tsuda, E., Kawahira, Y., Uemura, H. and Kitamura, S. (2000). Result of surgical treatments in patients with coronary-arterial obstructive disease after Kawasaki disease. *European Journal of Cardiothoracic Surgery*, **17**, 515–9.

Yoshioka, T., Matsutani, T., Toyosaki-Maeda, T., Suzuki, H., Uemura, S., Suzuki, R., Koike, M. and Hinuma, Y. (2003). Relation of streptococcal pyrogenic exotoxin C as a causative superantigen for Kawasaki disease. *Pediatric Research*, **53**, 403–10.

Yutani, C., Okano, K., Kamiya, T., Oguchi, K., Kozuka, T., Ota, M. and Onishi, S. (1980). Histopathological study on right endomyocardial biopsy of Kawasaki disease. *British Heart Journal*, **43**, 589–92.

Zaitsu, M., Hamasaki, Y., Tashiro, K., Matsuo, M., Ichimura, T., Fujita, I., Tasaki, H. and Miyazaki, S. (2000). Ulinastatin, an elastase inhibitor, inhibits the increased mRNA expression of prostaglandin H2 synthase-type 2 in Kawasaki disease. *Journal of Infectious Disease*, **181**, 1101–9.

CHAPTER 30

Wegener's granulomatosis: pathogenesis

Peter Lamprecht, Konstanze Holl-Ulrich, and Wolfgang L. Gross

Wegener's granulomatosis (WG) is a chronic, inflammatory, autoimmune disease of unknown cause characterized by granulomatous lesions and necrotizing vasculitis. Full-blown WG is an organ- or life-threatening disorder in which pulmonary–renal syndrome is common. Antineutrophil cytoplasmic autoantibodies specific for "Wegener's autoantigen" proteinase 3 (PR3-ANCA) are detected in more than 95% of the patients with generalized WG, whereas PR3-ANCA are present in less than half of the patients with very early, initial-phase WG (so-called localized WG). Data from *in vitro* and *in vivo* studies suggest that PR3-ANCA play an important role in the pathogenesis of the autoimmune vasculitis in WG. It is unclear how pathogenic granulomatous inflammation, a defining feature of WG, is related to the presence of PR3-ANCA. There is evidence, however, from animal models of autoimmune disease and recent *ex vivo* studies in humans to support the concept of ectopic autoantigen presentation in inflammatory lesions such as granulomatous lesions, ultimately resulting in autoimmune disease (Zinkernagel and Hengartner 1999; Weyand *et al.* 2001). These data refuel Wegener's and Fienberg's proposition of WG starting as a granulomatous disease in which vasculitis evolves subsequently (Wegener 1939; Fienberg 1981).

Genetic factors

Association with HLA

Cases of siblings with WG have been reported (Knudson *et al.* 1988), but are uncommon (Reinhold-Keller *et al.* 2000). WG affects predominantly Caucasians, but the genetic factors involved in this predilection are unknown (Hoffman *et al.* 1992). A hypothetical consideration suggests that there is an inverse relationship between the intensity of genetic predisposition and the time necessary to develop an autoimmune disease. The delayed onset of an autoimmune disease such as WG (which has a mean age at diagnosis of about 50 years) could indicate that the underlying genetic abnormality might be quite subtle (Lipsky 2001).

MHC class I and II molecules present peptide fragments from foreign antigens and potential autoantigens to CD8+ and CD4+ T-cells bearing the appropriate T-cell receptor for antigen recognition. Polymorphism of MHC molecules determines which amino acid sequences are preferentially bound to the peptide binding groove through specific anchor residues. In this way the MHC restricts the ability of T-cells to recognize antigens, but could also support responses to autoantigens in predisposed individuals. In a study from south Germany, HLA-DRB1*04 alleles were over-represented in WG-patients with end-stage renal disease and HLA-DRB1*13 and HLA-DQB1*0603 alleles were under-represented. A protective role of HLA-DRB1*13 alleles was postulated, but these results could have been biased by over- and under-representation of HLA alleles within the general population of that particular region of Germany (Gencik *et al.* 1999). Earlier studies suggested an association of WG with HLA-DR1 or HLA-DR2 alleles (Elkon *et al.* 1983; Paphiha *et al.* 1992), whereas later studies failed to establish an association between HLA alleles and WG (Zhang *et al.* 1995). The fact that approximately half of normal Caucasian individuals are HLA-DR2 positive might explain why no particular HLA gene appears to convey susceptibility to WG (Peen and Williams 2000). More recently, a strong association of the HLA-DPB1*0401 allele with WG has been reported (Jagiello *et al.* 2004). Intriguingly, susceptibility to another granulomatous disease – chronic beryllium disease – is also conveyed by HLA-DPB1 alleles (Richeldi *et al.* 1993).

Cytokine and signal transducer genes

Tumor necrosis factor (TNF)-α primes neutrophil granulocytes before they interact with PR3-ANCA and is known to promote granuloma formation (reviewed in Lamprecht and Gross 2004). In this context, the role of polymorphisms in the TNF gene has been analyzed. Although the prevalence of homozygosity for the minor allele (A) of the TNF −308 single nucleotide polymorphism (SNP) was slightly higher among WG patients than healthy controls (6% vs. 2%), no statistically significant differences in TNF gene polymorphisms, or high and low producers of TNFα could be demonstrated (Marscher *et al.* 1998). The TNF −308 SNP was recently excluded as a risk factor for WG in a larger cohort (Gencik *et al.* 1999).

The AA genotype of the SNP at position −1082 in the promoter region of the interleukin 10 (IL-10) gene favors Th1-type reactions, because this genotype is associated with reduced IL-10 secretion from activated macrophages and certain T-cell subsets. Analysis of this SNP showed a significant shift towards the AA genotype in WG (Muraközy *et al.* 2001).

Cytotoxic T-lymphocyte associated antigen (CTLA)-4 (CD152) is an inducible negative regulator of T-cell activation. A SNP at position −318 of the promoter region of CTLA-4 is associated with WG (Giscombe *et al.* 2002). In contrast to familial Crohn's disease (another granulomatous disease), no association with NOD2 gene mutations have yet been found in WG (Newman *et al.* 2003). Two studies suggest a role for signaling abnormalities as predisposing factors for WG. One study reported on the association of the retinoid X receptor b gene (RXRB03) with WG. The RXRB protein forms heterodimers with a variety of nuclear receptors, such as the vitamin D receptor (Jagiello *et al.* 2004). Another study disclosed a significant increase in the frequency of the lymphoid protein tyrosine phosphatase non-receptor 22 (PTPN22) 620W allele in PR3-ANCA+ WG (Jagiello *et al.* 2005).

PR3 expression and ANCA

It has been suggested that free PR3 might mediate vasculitic lesions in the context of an acquired or genetically determined protease/antiprotease imbalance. An association has been found between ANCA activity and distinct alleles (Z and S) of alpha$_1$-antitrypsin (α1-AT) in ANCA-associated systemic vasculitis (Esnault *et al.* 1993). α1-AT interacts with both of the major ANCA antigens. It is the main inhibitor of polymorphonuclear neutrophil (PMN), neutral serine proteases (PR3), and neutrophil elastase, and is inactivated by myeloperoxidase (MPO). Lack of PR3 inhibitor could induce exposure of cryptic antigenic PR3-epitopes. Furthermore, decreased neutralization of PR3 and HLE could favor damage at the sites of inflammation. The interaction of PR3 with α1-AT is inhibited by ANCA (Dolman *et al.* 1993). Secretory leukocyte proteinase inhibitor mRNA expression is upregulated in circulating leukocytes and nasal biopsies in WG and could indicate an altered protease/antiprotease balance inducing its upregulation (Ohlsson *et al.* 2003).

High constitutive expression of PR3 on the surface of neutrophil granulocytes is genetically determined and correlates with disease activity in WG (Csernok *et al.* 1994; Muller Kobold *et al.* 1998; Schreiber *et al.* 2005). Furthermore, there is an association of WG with the A-564G polymorphism in the PR3 promoter region, which affects a putative transcription factor-binding site. Over-expression of PR3 could predispose individuals to the development of WG (Gencik *et al.* 2000). Since PR3-ANCA interacts with Fcg receptors, several investigators have focused on analysis of FcgR polymorphisms. PMN express a normal representation of the alleles FcgRIIa-H131 and R131 in WG (Edberg *et al.* 1997). Another neutrophil receptor, FcgRIIIb, has two common allelic forms originally defined serologically as NA1 and NA2. FcgRIIIb-NA1 alleles are associated with severe renal disease in WG (Wainstein *et al.* 1996); however, another group of investigators showed that FcgRIIIb receptor polymorphism is not a major factor predisposing to development of ANCA+ vasculitis or nephritis (Tse *et al.* 2000).

Rare patients with cANCA-negative and PR3-ANCA-negative WG-like syndrome (TAP-deficiency syndrome) have been identified (Moins-Teisserenc *et al.* 1997; Schultz *et al.* 2003). The syndrome resembles WG both clinically and histologically. Patients present with necrotizing granulomatous lesions in the upper respiratory tract and skin associated with recurrent bacterial respiratory infections and skin vasculitis. Although only two of six patients had detectable ANCA by immunofluorescence, bactericidal/permeability-increasing protein (BPI)-ANCA were detected by ELISA in five out of six patients. The disease is caused by mutations

of transporter associated with antigen presentation (TAP) genes resulting in defective TAP complex expression and severely reduced MHC class I molecule expression. In contrast to WG, granulomatous lesions of TAP-deficiency patients contain predominantly NK-cells. This finding suggests a failure to downregulate NK-cell activity as a result of lacking MHC class I molecule expression ("missing self" hypothesis for NK-cell activation).

Environmental factors

The cause of WG is still unknown, but hypersensitivity mechanisms have long been implicated (Fienberg 1981). The clinical course of WG with initial respiratory tract involvement (so-called localized WG) followed by vasculitis suggests a chain of events in which a pathogenic agent gains entry to the respiratory tract and elicits an inflammatory response with subsequent self-perpetuation of the process and extension to other tissues. The nasal and bronchial mucosa is the first site of contact with inhaled antigens. Nasal and bronchial associated lymphoid tissue (NALT/BALT) orchestrates immune responses to antigens. A recently published animal model suggests that pathogens can also induce BALT (Moyron-Quiroz *et al.* 2004). Environmental factors thought to be associated with WG include exposure to inhaled substances (fumes or particulate matter), infections by airborne or opportunistic pathogens (viruses, bacteria), and medications.

Infections in WG

To date, the most convincing evidence of an etiological association of bacterial infections with WG comes from studies dealing with *Staphylococcus aureus*. Nasal carriage of *Staphylococcus aureus* is approximately three times higher in WG compared to healthy individuals and disease controls, and constitutes a risk factor for disease exacerbation of WG (Stegeman *et al.* 1994; Gadola *et al.* 1997). Prophylactic treatment with trimethoprim–sulfamethoxazole reduces respiratory and non-respiratory tract infections and the risk of WG relapses (Stegeman *et al.* 1996). An earlier case series had indicated that trimethoprim–sulfamethoxazole induces remissions in localized WG (DeRemee 1985). A later study confirmed that induction of remission with trimethoprim–sulfamethoxazole is efficacious in localized WG (Reinhold-Keller *et al.* 1996). Whereas clonal T-cell expansions in WG are not related to the presence of *Staphylococcus aureus* or its superantigen, there are data indicating that *Staphylococcus aureus* B-cell superantigens such as staphylococcal protein A might play a role in stimulating autoreactive PR3-producing B-cells within granulomatous lesions of the respiratory tract (Popa *et al.* 2003; Voswinkel *et al.* 2005). Moreover, sera from patients with WG recognize endothelial-bound *Staphylococcus aureus* acid phosphatase. It has been hypothesized that staphylococcal acid phosphatase could act as a planted antigen to induce vasculitis (Brons *et al.* 2000). Intriguingly, transient rises of PR3- or MPO-ANCA and vasculitic manifestations have been reported in subacute bacterial endocarditis. Treatment of endocarditis resulted in declining ANCA-titers, indicating transient induction of humoral autoimmunity (Choi *et al.* 2000).

A number of studies suggest an association of viral infections with WG. A case–control study excluded an association between parvovirus B19 infection and WG (Nikkari *et al.* 1995). Few anecdotal reports on cytomegalovirus infection or reactivation associated with WG exacerbation have been published, but relevance and interdependency of CMV infection and WG activity and immunosuppressive treatment has remained as yet unclear (Meyer *et al.* 2000).

Silica

Silica (inorganic mineral form of silicone) and silicone (synthetic polymers with a SiO backbone) have been implicated in the pathogenesis of ANCA-associated rapidly progressive glomerulonephritis and WG (Gregorini *et al.* 1993; Nuyts *et al.* 1995). Silicates activate T-cells by a superantigen-like mechanism via T-cell receptor (TCR) Vb chain stimulation. Silica can induce rupture of macrophage phagosomes with subsequent release of lysosomal enzymes such as PR3. Furthermore, macrophages are activated by silicates *in vitro*. Other occupational exposures have not consistently been shown to be associated with WG (Cohen Tervaert *et al.* 1998).

Drug-induced WG and ANCA+ vasculitis

Intranasal cocaine abuse induces inflammatory destructive lesions resulting in nasal perforation. Drug-induced granulomatous inflammation and autoimmunity has been reported in patients with cocaine-induced midline destructive lesions (CIMDL) (Wiesner *et al.* 2004). Moreover, ANCA with human neutrophil elastase specificity (HNE-ANCA) or PR3-ANCA are induced in these patients. Although severe ANCA-induced vasculitis is unusual in such patients, their disease course with exogenous induction of nasal lesions and ANCA might mimic early pathological events in WG (Wiesner *et al.* 2004).

Cases of drug-induced WG and ANCA-positive vasculitis have been described in a number of anecdotal reports. Antithyroid drugs, especially propylthiouracil, but also methimazole and carbimazole, are a rare cause of ANCA+ cutaneous vasculitis and glomerulonephritis (Pillinger and Staud 1998; Bonaci-Nikolic *et al.* 2005). MPO-ANCA is more frequently induced than PR3-ANCA (Bonaci-Nikolic *et al.* 2005). Another case report described a superimposed episode of propylthiouracil-induced MPO-ANCA+ vasculitis in a patient with PR3-ANCA+ WG (Choi *et al.* 1999). A MPO-ANCA+ lupus-like syndrome is induced in a cat model; modification of MPO ("altered self") by reactive metabolites of propylthiouracil is thought to be the key initiating event resulting in MPO-ANCA production and lupus-like disease in this model (Waldhauser and Uetrecht 1996). Presence of neutrophil granulocytes and MPO is essential in drug-induced lupus-like reactions (Jiang *et al.* 1994). Other drugs, such as hydralazine, minocycline, and penicillamine, may also induce ANCA+ vasculitis. Again, MPO-ANCA is usually detected in such cases, but sometimes PR3-ANCA is seen (reviewed in Merkel 1998).

WG and malignancy

WG patients have an increased risk of preceding or concurrent malignancy. There is a two-fold overall increased risk for cancer, with the most pronounced increases for bladder cancer, skin cancer, leukemia, and malignant lymphoma (Tatsis *et al.* 1998; Westman *et al.* 1998; Knight *et al.* 2002; Pankhurst *et al.* 2004). Hemorrhagic cystitis induced by chemotherapy is a risk factor for the development of bladder cancer; cyclophosphamide treatment

results in a nine to 45-fold increased risk for this cancer. The relative risk for bladder cancer is increased for cumulative cyclophosphamide doses over 25 g or an exposure ≥12 months and is particularly high with doses over 100 g and exposure ≥30 months. Use of mesna (2-mercapto-ethane sulphonate sodium) reduces the risk of bladder cancer (Reviewed in Hellmich *et al.* 2004). There seems to be an association of WG with malignancy independent of the known risk associated with drugs used to treat the disease. One study found renal cell carcinoma in 7 of 23 WG-patients with malignant disease: in five out of these seven patients the carcinoma was diagnosed before or simultaneously with WG (Tatsis *et al.* 1999). The cause for this association remains unclear, but PR3 mRNA has been reported to be expressed in renal epithelial and glomerular cell lines. ANCA induces signaling in renal epithelial cells by binding to PR3 and PR3 stimulates the growth of tubular epithelial cells (Relle *et al.* 2003; reviewed in Hellmich *et al.* 2004).

Granulomatous lesions

Granulomatous lesions – pathology

Granulomatous inflammation, "geographic" necrosis, and small-vessel vasculitis have been established as classical morphological features of WG. The full triad of morphological criteria is found only in about one-third of respiratory tract biopsies. In two-thirds of such biopsies, only one of these three features is displayed (Holl-Ulrich *et al.* 2002). Granulomatous lesions may be found in virtually any organ, such as retroorbital tissues or meninges, but renal granulomas have been reported to be rare (Kradin and Mark 2002; Bajema *et al.* 1998).

In WG, the granulomatous inflammation displays several different morphologies (Table 30.1). Therefore, it is usually referred to as "granulomatous lesion" rather than "granuloma". Within a surrounding inflammatory background, poorly formed epitheloid cell granulomas, scattered histiocytic giant cells of Langhans type, or palisading histiocytes around central necrosis may be seen. Well-defined sarcoid-type granulomas are rare (Travis *et al.* 2002). Parenchymal necrosis in WG can take the form of either neutrophilic microabscesses (Figures 30.1 and 30.2) or large zones

Table 30.1 Major pathologic manifestations (diagnostic criteria) of WG in respiratory tract lesions (adapted from Travis *et al.* 2002)

I.	**Vasculitis**
	A. Arteritis, venulitis, capillaritis
	B. Six types: acute, chronic, necrotizing granulomatous, non-necrotizing granulomatous, fibrinoid necrosis, cicatricial changes
II.	**Parenchymal necrosis**
	A. Microabscess
	B. Geographic necrosis
III.	**Granulomatous inflammation (mixed inflammatory infiltrate)**
	A. Microabscess surrounded by granulomatous inflammation
	B. Palisading histiocytes
	C. Scattered giant cells
	D. Poorly formed granulomas
	E. Sarcoid-like granulomas (rare)

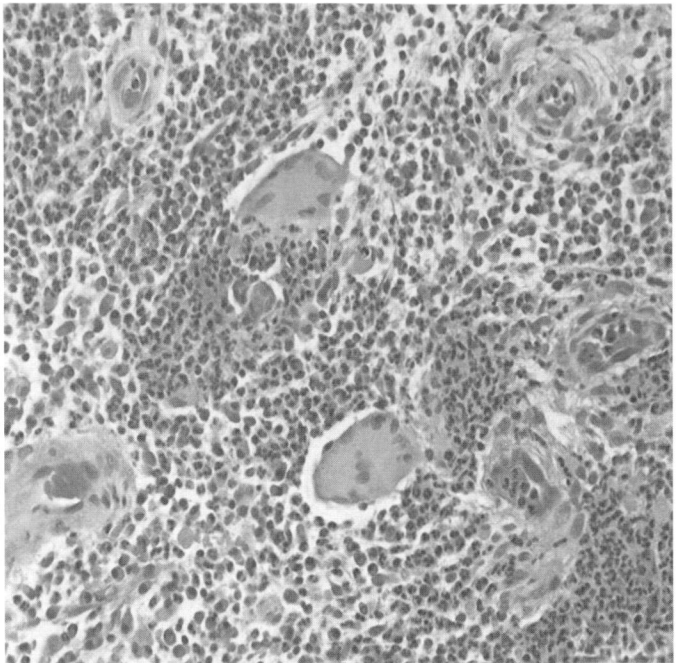

Figure 30.1 Wegener's granulomatosis—granulomatous and vasculitic lesions in nasal biopsy: diffuse granulomatous tissue, several dispersed multinucleated giant cells, and neutrophilic microabscesses. Vasculitis of small venule (upper right) with onion-skin appearance of vessel wall and intramural inflammatory infiltrates. (See Color Plate 83).

of "geographic" necrosis with irregular serpinginous margins (Figure 30.3) bounded by palisading histiocytes and giant cells (Travis *et al.* 2002). The mixed inflammatory infiltrate in WG is composed of lymphocytes, plasma cells, neutrophils, eosinophils, monocytes, macrophages, histiocytes, and giant cells (Fienberg 1981, 1989; Travis 1996; Kradin and Mark 2002). Eosinophils are scanty in the cellular parts of the lesion outside the edges of the necrotic tissue; however, an eosinophilic variant of WG has been described. These cases are similar to classic WG, except for the marked infiltration by eosinophils (Yousem and Lombard 1988). Tissue damage such as destruction of nasal cartilage or bone (Figure 30.4) leading to the characteristic saddle nose of WG, may be a direct consequence of the destructive necrotizing inflammation.

Granulomatous lesions – pathophysiology

Studies by Fienberg disclosed that the earliest lesions in the lung are foci of swollen collagen fibers apparently representing tissue injury and necrosis. Thereafter, mononuclear histiocytes migrate to the vicinity of the necrosis. Neutrophil granulocytes, lymphocytes, epitheloid cells, and multinucleated giant cells appear subsequently. Finally, the histiocytes become oriented in a palisading manner around the central area of necrosis. In the lung, granulomatous lesions can be found in proximity to inflamed vessels and at extravascular sites (Fienberg 1981, 1989; Kradin and Mark 2002). Fienberg suggested that WG starts as granulomatous disease in the respiratory tract, and systemic vasculitis develops subsequently (Fienberg 1989). It has been argued, however, that early foci of fibrinoid necrosis could also be a consequence of initial necrotizing

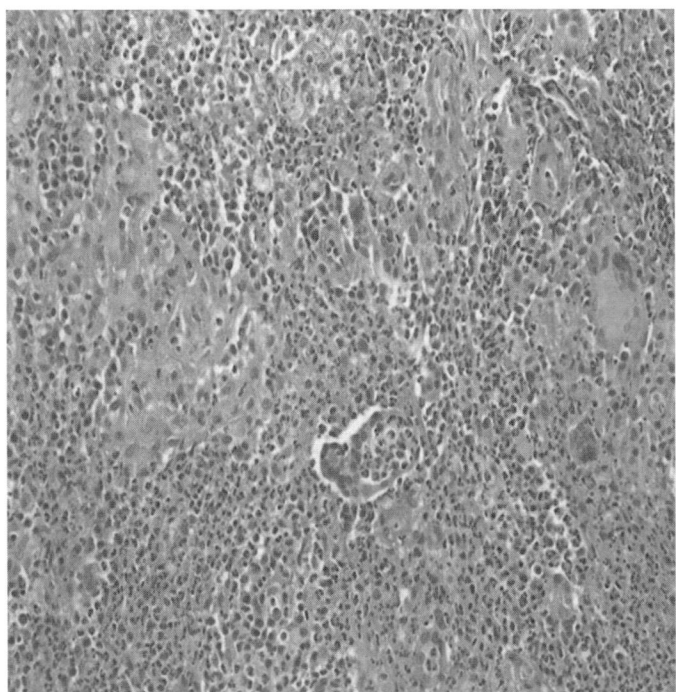

Figure 30.2 Wegener's granulomatosis—granulomatous lesions in nasal biopsy: typical ill-defined epitheloid cell granulomas with several multinucleated giant cells and neutrophilic microabscesses. (See Color Plate 84).

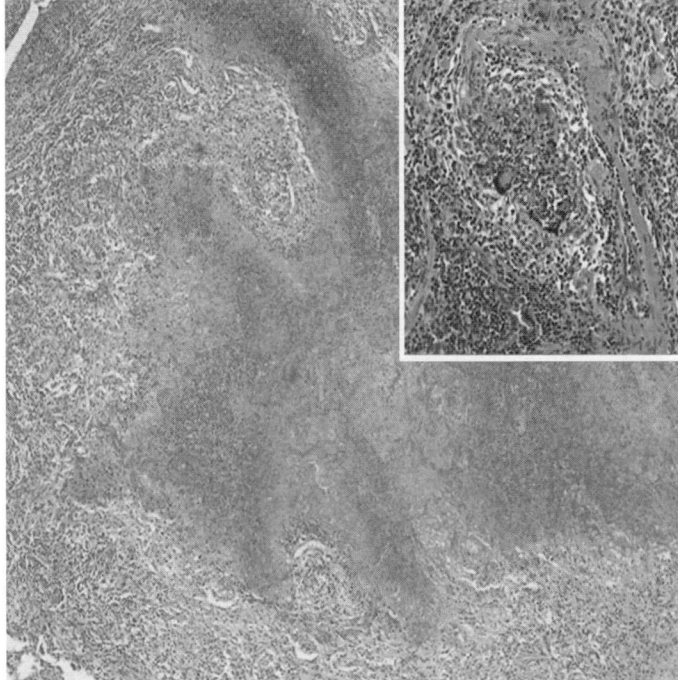

Figure 30.3 Wegener's granulomatosis—granulomatous lesions in lung biopsy: large necrotizing granuloma with palisading histiocytes and large central geographical necrosis. Inset: granulomatous vasculitis of lung (medium-sized vessel) with obliteration of vessel lumen and dense intramural inflammatory infiltrates, including numerous multinucleated giant cells. (See Color Plate 85).

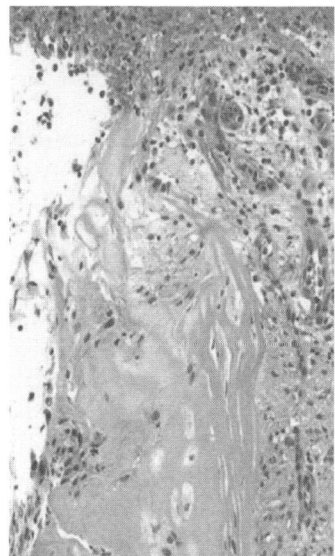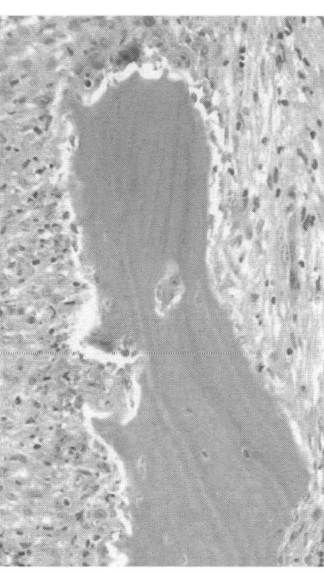

Figure 30.4 Wegener's granulomatosis—granulomatous lesions in nasal biopsy: Destruction of nasal cartilage (a) and bone (b) by inflammatory granulomatous tissue. (See Color Plate 86).

capillaritis. A different scenario would envision initial formation of extravascular granulomata followed by granulomatous lesions in the vicinity of inflamed vessels once autoimmunity with PR3-ANCA is established.

Formation of lymphoid-like structures within chronically inflamed tissue rich in T-cells is seen in many autoimmune diseases such as Hashimoto's thyroiditis and rheumatoid arthritis, and it is hypothesized that autoimmune responses could be maintained in such lesions (Zinkernagel and Hengartner 1999; Zinkernagel 2004). Greater abundance of neutrophils and monocytes as a potential source of PR3 has been demonstrated in granulomatous lesions in WG compared to other granulomatous diseases (Braun *et al.* 1990). PR3 is present in inflammatory lesions of lung and kidney sections in WG (Gross *et al.* 1995; Brockmann *et al.* 2002). Macrophages, histiocytes, and giant cells, all of which could function as (auto)antigen presenting cells, surround necrotic areas and interspersed PR3. In WG, there is *in vitro* evidence that inactivation and processing of PR3 from apoptotic neutrophils via antigen presenting cells is aberrant (Moosig *et al.* 2000). In WG, neutrophil granulocytes acquire characteristics of antigen presenting cells such as HLA-DR expression (Iking-Konert *et al.* 2001). PR3 induces protease-activated receptor (PAR)-2-mediated maturation of dendritic cells, which subsequently drive Th1-type responses of PR3-specific CD4+ T-cells favoring granuloma formation in WG. The induced Th1-type response is stronger in WG compared to healthy and disease (Crohn's disease) controls (Csernok *et al.* 2006). This study indicates that "gate-way" receptors might determine how a particular autoantigen, such as PR3, becomes a target of adaptive immunity.

Clusters of CD20+ B-cells are present in granulomatous lesions in WG (Müller *et al.* 2000; Voswinkel *et al.* 2005). There is evidence of immunoglobulin heavy chain usage and affinity maturation in these lesions is similar to that found in circulating PR3-ANCA-producing B-cells (Voswinkel *et al.* 2006). It is unclear, however, whether follicular structures are formed and plasma cells or their

precursors are generated in granulomatous lesions. Moreover, *de novo* formation of ectopic lymphoid tissue could be incomplete in the presence of a strong proinflammatory cytokine response.

Since interferon-gamma (IFNγ) and T-cells play pivotal roles in granuloma formation, alterations of the T-cell and cytokine response could contribute to anomalous autoantigen-presentation in ectopic lymphoid-like structures and sustain autoimmunity to PR3 (Ehlers *et al.* 2001; Aries *et al.* 2005; Lamprecht 2005). Skewing of the T-cell phenotype with expansion of CD4+ and CD8+ T-cells lacking CD28 expression is seen in WG. CD28– T-cells are reminiscent of so-called late differentiated or effector memory T-cells. Expansion of CD28– T-cells is already evident in localized WG and further increases in generalized WG. The expansion is independent of age and immunosuppressive treatment and correlates with organ involvement (Moosig *et al.* 1998; Komocsi *et al.* 2002; Lamprecht *et al.* 2003a). CD28– T-cells are enriched in bronchoalveolar fluid and are a major source of T-cell TNFα and IFNγ production in granulomatous lesions (Lamprecht *et al.* 2001; Komocsi *et al.* 2002). Abundant IFNγ, CD26 (Th1-type marker), and Th1-type CC chemokine receptor CCR5 expression are seen in granulomatous lesions of the respiratory tract in localized WG, but appears less strong in generalized WG (Müller *et al.* 2000; Lamprecht *et al.* 2003b). Moreover, a fraction of Th2-type IL-4 producing CCR3+ T cells is present in the circulation and tissue lesions in generalized, but not in localized, WG (Ludviksson *et al.* 1998; Csernok *et al.* 1999; Balding *et al.* 2001; Lamprecht *et al.* 2003b). The CC chemokine RANTES (regulated on activation normal T cell expressed and secreted/CCL5), a ligand for both Th1-type CCR5 and Th2-type CCR3, is expressed in granulomatous lesions of the respiratory tract and could favor migration of T-cell subsets into granulomatous lesions (Coulomb-L'Hermine *et al.* 2001).

These data suggest that an aberrant Th1-type response favoring granuloma formation might play a role in initiation of WG (Sneller 2002). Ectopic presentation of the "Wegener's autoantigen" PR3 and autoimmunity to PR3 might be sustained within inflammatory lesions and by skewed T-cell and cytokine responses (Aries *et al.* 2005; Lamprecht 2005). Progression from localized to generalized WG is associated with the appearance of another subset of Th2-type cells, which could be a consequence of B-cell expansion and T-cell dependent PR3-ANCA production during disease progression (Popa *et al.* 2002; Aries *et al.* 2005; Lamprecht 2005).

Vasculitis

Vasculitis – pathology

Generalized WG is characterized by a necrotizing vasculitis affecting predominantly small vessels and medium-sized vessels, that is capillaries, venules, arterioles, and arteries (Jennette and Falk 1997). The vasculitis is termed "pauci-immune" because few or no immunoglobulin or complement deposits are detected in glomerular lesions and at other sites.

The histological picture of vasculitis in WG shows an extremely wide morphologic spectrum (Table 30.1) (see Chapter 9). Classical locations of necrotizing small vessel vasculitis in WG are the kidney (necrotizing crescentic glomerulonephritis) and lung (acute pulmonary capillaritis), which may lead to life-threatening pulmonary hemorrhage (Lieberman and Churg 1991; Harper and Savage 2000). Within the lung, however, several other patterns of vasculitis can be detected (Table 30.1). Necrotizing granulomatous arteritis involving medium-sized vessels is commonly found close to large necrotizing granulomatous foci in the lung, whereas outside the lung granulomatous vasculitis is rare. Non-granulomatous fibrinoid necrosis of vessel walls is rare in the lung, but may affect bronchial arteries.

Cutaneous manifestations of WG most often show a leukocytoclastic vasculitis. As a systemic disease, WG may evoke vasculitic lesions in virtually any other organ. Moreover, vasculitis morphologically identical to that seen in classical polyarteritis and microscopic polyangiitis, both in size of the vessels involved and the presence of fibrinoid necrosis, may be seen in WG (Lieberman and Churg 1991; Kradin and Mark 2002).

Endothelial cells are the target of the initial vessel injury. The earliest changes affect the vascular endothelium with swelling, necrosis, and de-adherence. Lysed neutrophil granulocytes are found within affected vessels. In the kidney, rupture of the basement membrane subsequent to neutrophil degranulation gives rise to glomerular capillary thrombosis followed by segmental necrosis of the tuft. Necrotic material, blood, and fibrin spill into Bowman's space. As a consequence, there is accumulation and proliferation of monocytes and parietal (Bowman's) epithelial cells with the formation of crescents. The growing crescent compresses the capillary tuft, leading to segmental and global loss of circulation through the glomerulus. In the lung, capillaries, venules, and arterioles are infiltrated by polymorphonuclear leukocytes.

Vasculitis – pathophysiology

The vasculitis of WG is "pauci-immune" because few or no immunoglobulin or complement deposits are detected in glomerular lesions and at other sites. In the early 1980s, the crucial role of ANCA in the pathophysiology of WG became evident. ANCA were first described in the early 1980s as a cause of diffuse granular cytoplasmic immunofluorescence staining on ethanol-fixed neutrophils (cANCA pattern). PR3 is the principal target antigen for cANCA (Csernok et al. 1990; Jenne et al. 1990; Lüdemann et al. 1990). The serological hallmark of WG is the presence of circulating ANCA to proteinase 3 (PR3-ANCA) in about 95% of the patients. Nevertheless, PR3-ANCA are detected infrequently during initial-phase WG (granulomatous disease localized only in the respiratory tract). In contrast, PR3-ANCA are nearly always

Table 30.2 Results of *in vitro* studies supporting the concept of ANCA-induced vascular damage and vasculitis in WG

Key result of study	Reference
ANCA induce the release of primary granule contents from neutrophil granulocytes in a dose-dependent manner. Priming with TNFα results in translocation of MPO on the cell surface and enhance degranulation.	Falk et al. 1990
TNFα and IL-8 induce translocation of PR3 from azurophilic granules to the cell surface of neutrophil granulocytes where PR3 becomes accessible for PR3-ANCA.	Csernok et al. 1994
TNFα primed neutrophil granulocytes stimulated with PR3-ANCA and arachidonic acid secrete superoxide and leukotriene 4. PR3-ANCA also activate endothelial cells.	Grimminger et al. 1996, Sibelius et al. 1998
PR3 is also constitutively expressed on the cell surface of neutrophil granulocytes and high expression is associated with relapses in WG.	Muller Kobald et al. 1998
Production of IL-8 by ANCA-stimulated neutrophil granulocytes with the intravascular compartment inhibits neutrophil transmigration and, thus, may contribute to endothelial damage by premature neutrophil degranulation.	Cockwell et al. 1999
ANCA stabilize adhesion and promote migration of flowing neutrophil granulocytes on endothelial cells activated with TNFα.	Radford et al. 2001
PR3 enhances endothelial MCP-1 production and induces increased adhesion of neutrophil granulocytes to endothelial cells by upregulating ICAM-1.	Taekema-Roelvink et al. 2001
Release of neutrophilic PR3 results in its uptake in endothelial cells and activation of distinct signaling proapoptotic events.	Preston et al. 2002

Table 30.3 Results of studies in animal models supporting the concept of ANCA-induced vascular damage and vasculitis in WG

Key result of study	Reference
Brown Norway rats treated with mercuric chloride (HgC1₂) develop MPO-ANCA and a necrotizing vasculitis including leukocytoclastic vasculitis of the gut.	Esnault et al. 1992 Qasim et al. 1995
Brown Norway rats immunized with MPO develop MPO-ANCA.	Brouwer et al. 1993
Subsequent perfusion of a kidney or lung with a lysosomal enzyme extract results in crescentic glomerulonephritis, vasculitis, and pulmonary tissue injury. Immune deposits are seen in early glomerular lesions.	Foucher et al. 1999
Similar approach to Brouwer et al. 1993. In contrast, immune complex-mediated glomerulonephritis was found.	Yang et al. 1994
Mice immunized with human ANCA develop anti-human ANCA and anti-anti-human ANCA (mouse ANCA) as well as perivascular mononuclear cell infiltrates in the lungs and glomerular pathology.	Blank et al. 1995 Tomer et al. 1995
Crescentic glomerulonephritis and systemic necrotizing vasculitis is induced in Rag2 (−/−) mice lacking T- and B-cells after transfer of splenocytes from MPO (−/−) knockout mice immunized with MPO. Similar lesions are induced in Rag2 (−/−) mice and wild-type C57BL/6J (intact immune system) mice receiving anti-MPO IgG (MPO-ANCA).	Xiao et al. 2002
SCG/Kj mice spontaneously develop crescentic glomerulonephritis, systemic vasculitis, and pANCA. Presence of glomerular immune deposits differs from the pauci-immune pattern found in human WG and MPA	Neumann et al. 2003.
ANCA against murine PR3 generated in PR3/elastase-deficient mice induce panniculitis upon passive transfer into mice challenged with intradermal TNF-α injection. Stronger pulmonary and renal inflammation in LPS primed mice in the presence of PR3-ANCA	Pfister et al. 2004
MPO-ANCA induce vasculitis in a rat experimental autoimmune vasculitis model.	Little et al. 2005

detected in generalized WG (95% of patients). ANCA directed against myeloperoxidase (MPO-ANCA) are seldom detected in WG (about 3% of patients). Of note, a few cases of persistently ANCA-negative disease courses have been described (Nölle *et al.* 1989; Bacon 2005). Changes in ANCA titers seem to reflect changes in disease activity and predict impending relapse (Boomsma *et al.* 2000; Slot *et al.* 2004).

Several *in vitro* studies and animal models using different approaches support the concept of a pathogenic role of PR3-ANCA in the induction of vasculitis in WG (Tables 30.2 and 30.3) (see Chapter 8). So far, most animal models have provided evidence that vasculitis is induced by MPO-ANCA, which is the principal ANCA in microscopic polyangiitis. In contrast, it has been more difficult to demonstrate direct evidence of PR3-ANCA-induced vasculitis in animal models. One of the reasons is that murine PR3 shows little sequence homology to human PR3 and is not recognized by human PR3-ANCA. None of the models has been able to mimic granulomatous disease and vasculitis typical of WG (Table 30.3). The interaction of PR3-ANCA with neutrophils primed with cytokines such as TNFα or IL-1 results in their premature degranulation, subsequent endothelial cell damage, and leukocyte recruitment (Figure 30.5). Priming of neutrophils with TNFα or IL-1 results in translocation of ANCA target antigens such

as PR3 from intracellular granules to the cell surface of neutrophils, where they can interact with ANCA (Lüdemann *et al.* 1990; Falk *et al.* 1990; Csernok *et al.* 1994). Moreover, high constitutive membrane expression of PR3 correlates with disease activity (Csernok *et al.* 1994; Muller Kobold *et al.* 1998; Schreiber *et al.* 2005).

Cockwell *et al.* (1999) analyzed the intraglomerular expression of IL-8 in ANCA-associated glomerulonephritis. The production of IL-8 by ANCA-stimulated neutrophils within the intravascular compartment may facilitate neutrophil transmigration, encourage intravascular stasis, and contribute to bystander damage to glomerular endothelial cells (Cockwell *et al.* 1999). Binding of the ANCA-Fc-chain or F(ab′)$_2$-fragments induces production of oxygen radicals and degranulation of primed neutrophils (Csernok *et al.* 1994; Muller Kobold *et al.* 1998; Schreiber *et al.* 2005). Simultaneous binding of the F(ab′)$_2$ to membrane expressed PR3 and the Fc-chain to Fcg receptors FcgRIIa and Fcg-RIIIb on neutrophils seems to be important for the full activation of primed neutrophils by ANCA (Csernok *et al.* 1994; Porges *et al.* 1994; Kocher *et al.* 1998). Furthermore, involvement of both F(ab′)$_2$ and the Fc-chain of ANCA in the activation of primed neutrophils could account for apparent differences compared to the activation solely by Fcg receptors. ANCA activate the (p101/p110g) isoform of phosphatidylinositol 3-kinase. In contrast, Fcg receptor ligation

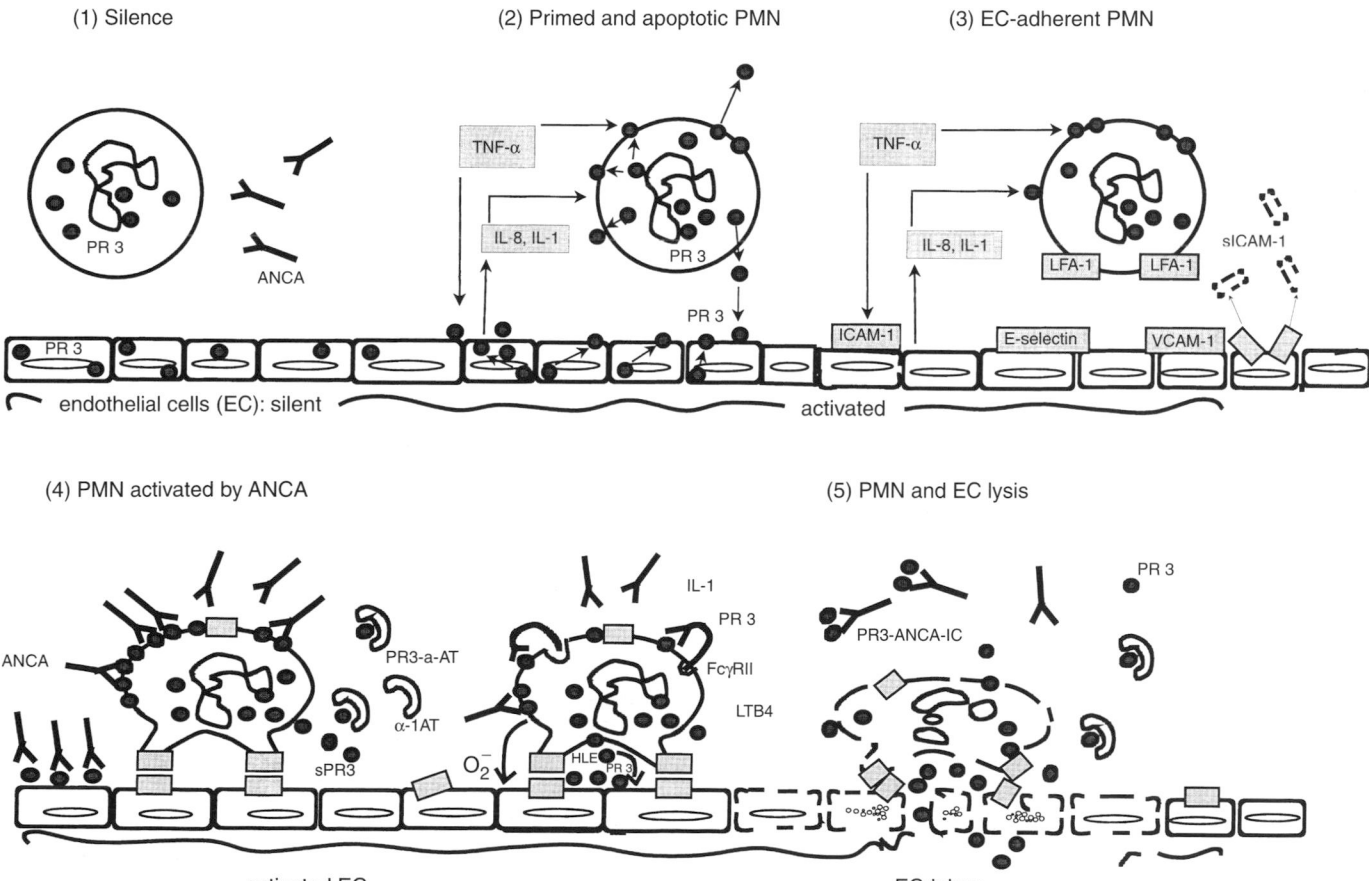

Figure 30.5 Antineutrophil cytoplasmic antibody (ANCA)-cytokine sequence theory. (1) Resting neutrophil-proteinase 3 (PR3) mostly sequestered in azurophil granules. (2) Primed (such as by cytokines) and apoptotic PMN intracytoplasmic PR3 is translocated to the cell surface and becomes accessible to ANCA: Expression of adhesion molecules. (3) Adhesion of PMN to endothelial cells. (4) Interaction between ANCA and PR3 leads to activation of neutrophils with degranulation, generation of oxygen radicals and endothelial cell injury. (5) This finally results in intravascular lysis of PMN and necrotizing vasculitis.

activates the (p85/p110) isoform of phosphatidylinositol 3-kinase (Ben-Smith *et al.* 2001; Kettritz *et al.* 2002). Moreover, ANCA and ANCA-F(ab')$_2$ fragments activate the G$_{i/o}$ GTPase (Williams *et al.* 2003). A number of other kinases such as ERK (extracellular receptor-activated kinase) and p38 MAPK (mitogen-activated protein kinase) have been reported to play a role in ANCA-mediated neutrophil activation (Kettritz *et al.* 2001). Several leukocyte genes are activated upon stimulation with ANCA, such as DIF-2, COX-2, and IL-8. Gene expression and protein levels of monocyte differentiation factor DIF-2 correlate with disease activity and ANCA titers (Yang *et al.* 2002).

Because PR3 is also a constituent of granules from monocytes, these cells are likely to be targets for ANCA as well. Activated monocytes are detected in renal biopsies (Rastaldi *et al.* 1996) and in nasal biopsies from patients with WG (Müller *et al.* 2000). ANCA binding to PR3 expressed on the surface of monocytes may result in FcgR crosslinking and subsequent IL-8 release (Ralston *et al.* 1997). Furthermore, monocytes can be activated to produce reactive oxygen intermediates by ANCA enhanced by priming with TNF. ANCA stimulate monocytes to produce monocyte chemoattractant protein-1 (MCP-1) *in vitro* thereby amplifying local monocyte recruitment (Casselman *et al.* 1995).

Differential diagnosis of pathologic findings

For granulomatous lesions, especially of the respiratory tract, granulomatous infection is the most important differential diagnosis. Both fungal and tuberculous infections share many histologic features with WG, including vasculitic changes. This may also be true for pulmonary manifestations of rheumatoid arthritis and necrotizing sarcoid granulomatosis. Pulmonary capillaritis in WG can be clinically indistinguishable from other forms of alveolar hemorrhage syndromes. In the kidney, morphology alone may not discriminate between WG and other types of pauci-immune ANCA-associated glomerulonephritis. As noted above, vasculitis morphologically identical to that seen in classical polyarteritis nodosa and microscopic polyangiitis may be seen in WG (Lieberman and Churg 1991; Kradin and Mark 2002).

References

Aries, P. M., Lamprecht, P. and Gross, W. L. (2005). Wegener's granulomatosis: A view from the granulomatous side of the disease. *Israel Medical Association Journal*, 7, 768–73.

Bacon, P. A. (2005). The spectrum of Wegener's granulomatosis and disease relapse. *New England Journal of Medicine*, 352, 330–2.

Bajema, I. M., Hagen, E. C., Ferrario, F., *et al.* (1998). Renal granulomas in systemic vasculitis. EC/BCR project for ANCA-assay standardization. *Clinical Nephrology*, 48, 16–20.

Balding, C. E., Howie, A. J., Drake-Lee, A. B. and Savage, C. O. (2001). Th2 dominance in nasal mucosa in patients with Wegener's granulomatosis. *Clinical and Experimental Immunology*, 125, 332–9.

Ben-Smith, A., Dove, S. K., Martin, A., Wakelam, M. J. and Savage, C. O. (2001). Antineutrophil cytoplasm autoantibodies from patients with systemic vasculitis activate neutrophils through distinct signaling cascades: comparison with conventional Fc-gamma receptor ligation. *Blood*, 98, 1448–55.

Blank, M., Tomer, Y., Stein, M., *et al.* (1995). Immunization with anti-neutrophil cytoplasmic antibody (ANCA) induces the production of mouse ANCA and perivascular lymphocyte infiltration. *Clinical and Experimental Immunology*, 102, 120–30.

Bonaci-Nikolic, B., Nikoloc, M. M., Andrejevic, S., Zoric, S. and Bukilica, M. (2005). Antineutrophil cytoplasmic antibody (ANCA)-associated autoimmune diseases induced by antithyroid drugs: comparison with idiopathic ANCA vasculitides. *Arthritis Research and Therapy*, 7, R1072–81.

Boomsma, M. M., Stegeman, C. A., van der Leij, *et al.* (2000). Prediction of relapses in Wegener's granulomatosis by measurement of antineutrophil cytoplasmic antibody levels: a prospective study. *Arthritis and Rheumatism*, 43, 2025–33.

Braun, M. G., Csernok, E., Gross, W. L. and Muller-Hermelink, H. K. (1990). Proteinase 3, the target antigen of anticytoplasmic antibodies circulating in Wegener's granulomatosis. Immunolocalization in normal and pathologic tissues. *American Journal of Pathology*, 139, 831–8.

Brockmann, H., Schwarting, A., Kriegsmann, J., *et al.* (2002). Proteinase-3 as the major autoantigen of c-ANCA is strongly expressed in lung tissue of patients with Wegener's granulomatosis. *Arthritis Research*, 4, 220–5.

Brons, R. H., Bakker, H. I., van Wijk, R. T., *et al.* (2000). Staphylococcal acid phosphatase binds to endothelial cells via charge interaction; a pathogenic role in Wegener's granulomatosis. *Clinical and Experimental Immunology*, 119, 566–73.

Brouwer, E., Huitema, M. G., Klok, P. A., *et al.* (1993). Antimyeloperoxidase-associated proliferative glomerulonephritis: an animal model. *Journal of Experimental Medicine*, 177, 905–14.

Casselman, B. L., Kilgore, K. S., Miller, B. F. and Warren, J. S. (1995). Antibodies to neutrophil cytoplasmic antigens induce monocyte chemoattractant protein-1 secretion from human monocytes. *Journal of Laboratory and Clinical Medicine*, 126, 495–502.

Choi, H. K., Merkel, P. A., Tervaert, J. W., Black, R. M., McCluskey, R. T. and Niles, J. L. (1999). Alternating antineutrophil cytoplasmic antibody specificity: drug-induced vasculitis in a patient with Wegener's granulomatosis. *Arthritis and Rheumatism*, 42, 384–8.

Choi, H. K., Lamprecht, P., Niles, J. L., Gross, W. L. and Merkel, P. A. (2000). Subacute bacterial endocarditis with positive cytoplasmic antineutrophil cytoplasmic antibodies and anti-proteinase 3 antibodies. *Arthritis and Rheumatism*, 43, 226–31.

Cockwell, P., Brooks, C. J., Adu, D. and Savage, C. O.S. (1999). Interleukin-8: A pathogenic role in antineutrophil cytoplasmic autoantibody-associated glomerulonephritis. *Kidney International*, 55, 852–63.

Cohen Tervaert, J. W., Stegeman, C. A. and Kallenberg, C. G.M. (1998). Silicon exposure and vasculitis. *Current Opinion in Rheumatology*, 10, 12–7.

Coulomb-L'Hermine, A., Capron, F., Zhou, W., *et al.* (2001). Expression of the chemokine RANTES in pulmonary Wegener's granulomatosis. *Human Pathology*, 32, 320–6.

Csernok, E., Lüdemann, J., Gross, W. L. and Bainton, D. (1990). Ultrastructural localization of proteinase 3, the target antigen of anti-cytoplasmic antibodies circulating in Wegener's granulomatosis. *American Journal of Pathology*, 137, 1113–20.

Csernok, E., Ernst, M., Schmitt, W. H., Bainton, D. F. and Gross, W. L. (1994). Activated neutrophils express proteinase 3 on their plasma membrane in vitro and in vivo. *Clinical and Experimental Immunology*, 95, 244–50.

Csernok, E., Trabandt, A., Müller, A., *et al.* (1999). Cytokine profiles in Wegener's granulomatosis: predominance of type 1 (Th1) in the granulomatous inflammation. *Arthritis and Rheumatism*, 42, 742–50.

Csernok, E., Ai, M., Gross, W. L., *et al.* (2006). Wegener's autoantigen induces maturation of dendritic cells and licences them for Th1 priming via the protease-activated receptor-2 pathway. *Blood*, In press.

DeRemee, R. A., McDonald, T. J. and Weiland, L. H. (1985). Wegener's granulomatosis: observations on treatment with antimicrobial agents. *Mayo Clinical Proceedings*, 60, 27–32.

Dolman, K. M., Stegemann, C. A., van de Wiel, B. A., *et al.* (1993). Relevance of classic anti-neutrophil cytoplasmic autoantibody (cANCA)-mediated inhibition of proteinase 3-alpha1-antitrypsin complexation to disease activity in Wegener's granulomatosis. *Clinical and Experimental Immunology*, **93**, 405–10.

Edberg, J. C., Wainstein, E., Csernok, E., *et al.* (1997). Analysis of Fcg II gene polymorphisms in Wegener's granulomatosis. *Experimental and Clinical Immunogenetics*, **14**, 183–95.

Ehlers, S., Benini, J., Held, H. D., Rock, C., Alber, G. and Uhlig, S. (2001). ab TCR+ cells and IFNg, but not iNOS are critical for granuloma necrosis in a mouse model for mycobacteria-induced pulmonary immunopathology. *Journal of Experimental Medicine*, **194**, 1847–59.

Elkon, K. B., Sutherland, D. C., Rees, A. J., Hughes, G. R.V. and Batchelor, J. R. (1983). HLA frequencies in systemic vasculitis. Increase in HLA-DR2 in Wegener's granulomatosis. *Arthritis and Rheumatism*, **26**, 102–5.

Esnault, V. L., Mathieson, P. W., Thiru, S., Oliveira, D. B. and Lockwood, M. C. (1992). Autoantibodies to myeloperoxidase in brown Norway rats treated with mercuric chloride. *Laboratory and Investigation*, **67**, 114–20.

Esnault, V. L.M., Testa, A., Aucrain, M., *et al.* (1993). Alpha$_1$-antitrypsin genetic polymorphism in ANCA positive systemic vasculitis. *Kidney International*, **43**, 1329–32.

Falk, R. J., Terrell, R. S., Charles, L. A. and Jennette, J. C. (1990). Anti-neutrophil cytoplasmic autoantibodies induce neutrophils to degranulate and produce oxygen radicals in vitro. *Proceedings of the National Academy of Science USA*, **87**, 4115–19.

Fienberg, R. (1981). The protracted superficial phenomenon in pathergic (Wegener's) granulomatosis. *Human Pathology*, **12**, 458–67.

Fienberg, R. (1989). A morphologic and immunohistologic study of the evolution of the necrotizing palisading granuloma of pathergic (Wegener's) Granulomatosis. *Seminars in Respiratory Medicine*, **10**, 126–32.

Foucher, P., Heeringa, P., Petersen, A. H., *et al.* (1999). Antimyeloperoxidase-associated lung disease. An experimental model. *American Journal of Respiratory Critical Care Medicine*, **160**, 987–94.

Gadola, S., Sahly, H., Reinhold-Keller, E., Hellmich, B., Paulsen, J. and Gross, W. L. (1997). Nasal carriage of staphylococcus aureus in patients with Wegener's granulomatosis (WG), rheumatoid arthritis (RA), and polyposis nasi (PN) (Abstract). *Sarcoidosis Vasculitis and Diffuse Lung Diseases*, **14** (Suppl.1), 29.

Gencik, M., Borgmann, S., Zahn, R., *et al.* (1999). Immunogenetic risk factors for anti-neutrophil cytoplasmic antibody (ANCA) associated systemic vasculitis. *Clinical and Experimental Immunology*, **117**, 412–17.

Gencik, M., Mueller, S., Borgmann, S. and Fricke, H. (2000). Proteinase 3 gene polymorphisms and Wegener's granulomatosis. *Kidney International*, **58**, 2473–7.

Giscombe, R., Wang, X., Huang, D. and Lefvert, A. K. (2002). Coding sequence 1 and promoter single nucleotide polymorphisms in the CTLA-4 gene in Wegener's granulomatosis. *Journal of Rheumatology*, **29**, 950–3.

Gregorini, G., Ferioli, A., Donato, F., *et al.* (1993). Association between silica exposure and necrotizing crescentic glomerulonephritis with p-ANCA and anti-MPO antibodies: a hospital based case-control study. *Advances in Experimental Medicine and Biology*, **336**, 435–40.

Grimminger, F., Hattar, K., Papavassilis, C., *et al.* (1996). Neutrophil activation by anti-proteinase 3 antibodies in Wegener's granulomatosis: role of exogenous arachidonic acid and leukotriene B4 generation. *Journal of Experimental Medicine*, **184**, 1567–72.

Gross, W. L., Csernok, E. and Hellmchen, U. (1995). Antineutrophil cytoplasmic autoantibodies, autoantigens, and systemic vasculitis. *Acta Pathologica Microbiologica et Immunologica Scandinavica*, **103**, 81–97.

Harper, L. and Savage, C. O.S. (2000). Pathogenesis of ANCA-associated systemic vasculitis. *Journal of Pathology*, **190**, 349–359.

Hellmich, B., Kausch, I., Doehn, C., Jocham, D., Holl-Ulrich, K. and Gross, W. L. (2004). Urinary bladder cancer in Wegener's granulomatosis: Is it more than cyclophosphamide? *Annals of the Rheumatic Diseases*, **63**, 1183–5.

Hoffman, G. S., Kerr, G. S., Leavitt, R. Y., *et al.* (1992). Wegener's granulomatosis: an analysis of 158 patients. *Annals of Internal Medicine*, **116**, 488–98.

Holl-Ulrich, K., Reinhold-Keller, E., Müller, A. and Feller, A. C. (2002). Pathology of vasculitis: Differential diagnosis and selected disorders. *Verhandlungen der Deutsche Gesellschaft für Pathologie*, **86**, 83–90.

Iking-Konert, C., Vogt, S., Radsak, M., Wagner, C., Hänsch, G. M. and Andrassy, K. (2001). Polymorphonuclear neutrophils in Wegener's granulomatosis acquire characteristics of antigen presenting cells. *Kidney International*, **60**, 2247–62.

Jagiello, P., Gencik, M., Arning, L., *et al.* (2004). New genomic region for Wegener's granulomatosis as revealed by an extended association screen with 202 apoptosis-related genes. *Human Genetics*, **114**, 468–77.

Jagiello, P., Aries, P., Arning, L., *et al.* (2005). The PTPN22 620W polymorphism is associated with the occurrence of autoantibodies to proteinase 3 in Wegener's granulomatosis. *Arthritis and Rheumatism*, **52**, 4039–43.

Jenne, D., Tschopp, J., Lüdemann, J., Utccht, B. and Gross, W. L. (1990). Wegener's autoantigen decoded. *Nature*, **346**, 520.

Jennette, J. C. and Falk, R. (1997). Small vessel vasculitis. *New England Journal of Medicine*, **337**, 1512–23.

Jiang, X., Khursigara, G. and Rubin, R. L. (1994). Transformation of lupus-inducing drugs to cytotoxic products by activated neutrophils. *Science*, **266**, 810–3.

Kettritz, R., Schreiber, A., Luft, F. C. and Haller, H. (2001). Role of mitogen-activated protein kinases in activation of human neutrophils by antineutrophil cytoplasm antibodies. *Journal of the American Society of Nephrology*, **12**, 37–46.

Kettritz, R., Choi, M., Butt, W., *et al.* (2002). Phosphatidylinositol 3-kinase controls antineutrophil cytoplasm antibodies-induced resprriratory burst in human neutrophils. *Journal of the American Society of Nephrology*, **13**, 1740–9.

Knight, A., Askling, J. and Ekbom, A. (2002). Cancer incidence in a population-based cohort of patients with Wegener's granulomatosis. *International Journal of Cancer*, **100**, 82–5.

Knudson, B. B., Joergensen, T. and Munch-Jensen, B. (1988). Wegener's granulomatosis in a family. *Scandinavian Journal of Rheumatology*, **17**, 225–7.

Kocher, M., Edberg, J. C., Fleit, H. B. and Kimberly, R. P. (1998). Antineutrophil cytoplasm antibodies preferentially engage Fc gammaRIIIb on human neutrophils. *Journal of Immunology*, **161**, 6909–14.

Komocsi, A., Lamprecht, P., Csernok, E., *et al.* (2002). Peripheral blood and granuloma CD4+CD28− T-cells are a major source of IFN-g and TNF-a in Wegerner's granulomatosis. *American Journal of Pathology*, **160**, 1717–24.

Kradin, R. L. and Mark, E. J. (2002). Case records of the Massachusetts General Hospital: Weekly clnicopathological exercises. Case 18–2002, A 48-year-old man with a cough and bloody sputum. *New England Journal of Medicine*, **346**, 1892–9.

Lamprecht, P., Moosig, F., Csernok, E., *et al.* (2001). CD28 negative T cells are enriched in granulomatous lesions of the respiratory tract in Wegener's granulomatosis. *Thorax*, **56**, 751–7.

Lamprecht, P., Erdmann, A., Müller, A., *et al.* (2003a). Heterogeneity of CD4+ and CD8+ memory T cells in localized and generalized Wegener's granulomatosis. *Arthritis Research and Therapy*, **5**, R25–31.

Lamprecht, P., Brühl, H., Erdmann, A., *et al.* (2003b). Differences in CCR5 expression on peripheral blood CD4+CD28− T-cells and in granulomatous lesions between localized and generalized Wegener's granulomatosis. *Clinical Immunology*, **108**, 1–7.

Lamprecht, P. and Gross, W. L. (2004). Wegener's granulomatosis. *Herz*, **29**, 47–56.

Lamprecht, P. (2005). Off balance: T-cells in antineutrophil cytoplasmic antibody (ANCA)-associated vasculitides. *Clinical and Experimental Immunology*, **141**, 201–10.

Lieberman, K. and Churg, A. (1991). Wegener's granulomatosis. In *Systemic vasculitis* (Churg, A. and Churg, J., eds), pp. 79–99. Igaku Shoin Medical Publishers, Inc. Tokyo.

Lipsky, P. (2001). Systemic lupus erthematosus: an autoimmune disease of B cell hyperactivity. *Nature Immunology*, **2**, 764–6.

Little, M. A., Smyth, L., Yadav, R., *et al.* (2005). Antineutrophil cytoplasm antibodies directed against myeloperoxidase augment leukocyte-microvascular interactions in vivo. *Blood*, **106**, 2050–8.

Lüdemann, J., Utecht, B. and Gross, W. L. (1990). Anti-neutrophil cytoplasm antibodies in Wegener's granulomatosis recognize an elastinolytic enzyme. *Journal of Experimental Medicine*, **171**, 357–62.

Ludviksson, B. R., Sneller, M. C., Chua, T. S., *et al.* (1998). Active Wegener's granulomatosis is associated with HLA-DR+ CD4+ T cells exhibiting an unbalanced Th1-type T cell cytokine pattern: reversal with IL-10. *Journal of Immunology*, **160**, 3602–9.

Marscher, B., Schmitt, W. H., Csernok, E., *et al.* (1998). Polymorphisms in the tumor necrosis factor genes in Wegener's granulomatosis. *Experimental and Clinical Immunogenetics*, **14**, 226–33.

Merkel, P. A. (1998). Drugs associated with vasculitis. *Current Opinion in Rheumatology*, **10**, 45–50.

Meyer, M. F., Hellmich, B., Kotterba, S. and Schatz, H. (2000). Cytomegalovirus infection in systemic necrotizing vasculitis: causative agent or opportunistic infection? *Rheumatology International*, **20**, 35–8.

Moins-Teisserenc, H. T., Gadola, S. D., Cella, M., *et al.* (1999). Association of a syndrome resembling Wegener's granulomatosis with low surface expression of HLA class-I molecules. *Lancet*, **354**, 1596–603.

Moosig, F., Csernok, E., Wang, G. and Gross, W. L. (1998). Costimulatory molecules in Wegener's granulomatosis (WG): lack of expression of CD28 and preferential up-regulation of its ligands B7–1 (CD80) and B7–2 (CD86) on T cells. *Clinical and Experimental Immunology*, **114**, 113–8.

Moosig, F., Csernok, E., Kumanovics, G., and Gross, W. L. (2000). Opsonization of apoptotic neutrophils by anti-neutrophil cytoplasmic antibodies (ANCA) leads to enhanced uptake by macrophages and increased release of tumour necrosis factor-alpha (TNF-alpha). *Clinical and Experimental Immunology*, **122**, 499–503.

Moyron-Quiroz, J. E., Rangel-Moreno, R., Kusser, K., *et al.* (2004). Role of inducible bronchus associated lymphoid tissue (iBALT) in respiratory immunity. *Nature Medicine*, **10**, 927–34.

Muller-Kobold, A. C., Kallenberg, C. G. and Tervaert, J. W. (1998). Leukocyte membrane expression of proteinase 3 correlates with disease activity in patients with Wegener's granulomatosis. *British Journal of Rheumatology*, **37**, 901–7.

Müller, A., Trabandt, A., Glöckner-Hofmann, K., *et al.* (2000). Localized Wegener's granulomatosis: predominance of CD26 and IFN-g expression. *Journal of Pathology*, **192**, 113–20.

Muraközy, G., Gäde, K. I., Ruprecht, B., *et al.* (2001). Gene polymorphism of immunoregulatory cytokines and angiotensin-converting enzyme in Wegener's granulokatosis. *Journal of Molecular Medicine*, **79**, 665–70.

Neumann, I., Birck, R., Newman, M., *et al.* (2003). SCG/Kinjoh mice: a model of ANCA-associated crescentic glomerulonephritis with immune deposits. *Kidney International*, **64**, 140–8.

Newman, B., Rubin, L. A. and Siminovitch, K. A. (2003). NOD2/CARD15 gene mutation is not associated with susceptibility to Wegener's granulomatosis. *Journal of Rheumatology*, **30**, 305–7.

Nikkari, S., Vainionpää, R., Toivanen, P., *et al.* (1995). Wegener's granulomatosis and parvovirus B19 infection. *Arthritis and Rheumatism*, **38**, 1175–6.

Nölle, B., Specks, U., Lüdemann, J., Rohrbach, M. S., DeRemee, R. A. and Gross, W. L. (1989). Anticytoplasmic autoantibodies: Their immundiagnostic value in Wegener's granulomatosis. *Annals of Internal Medicine*, **111**, 28–40.

Nuyts, G. D., van Vlem, E., de Vos, A., *et al.* (1995). Wegener's granulomatosis is associated to exposure to silicon compounds: a case-control study. *Nephrology Dialysis and Transplantation*, **10**, 1162–5.

Ohlsson, S., Falk, R., Yang, J. J., Ohlsson, K., Segelmark, M. and Wieslander, J. (2003). Increased expression of the secretory leukocyte proteinase inhibitor in Wegener's granulomatosis. *Clinical and Experimental Immunology*, **131**, 190–6.

Pankhurst, T., Savage, C. O., Gordon, C. and Harper, L. (2004). Malignancy is increased in ANCA-associated vasculitis. *Rheumatology*, **43**, 1532–5.

Papiha, S. S., Murty, G. E., Ad'Hia, A., Mains, B. T. and Venning, M. (1992). Association of Wegener's granulomatosis with HLA antigens and other genetic markers. *Annals of Rheumatic Diseases*, **51**, 246–8.

Peen, E. and Williams, Jr R. C. (2000). What you should know about PR3-ANCA, structural aspects of antibodies to proteinase 3 (PR3). *Arthritis Research*, **2**, 255–9.

Pfister, H., Ollert, M., Fröhlich, L. F., *et al.* (2004). Antineutrophil cytoplasmic autoantibodies (ANCA) against the murine homolog of proteinase 3 (Wegener's autoantigen) are pathogenic in vivo. *Blood*, **104**, 1411–8.

Popa, E. R., Stegeman, C. A., Kallenberg, C. G.M. and Cohen Tervaert, J. W. (2002). Staphylococcus aureus and Wegener's granulomatosis. *Arthritis Research*, **4**, 77–9.

Popa, E. R., Stegeman, C. A., Bos, N. A., Kallenberg, C. A. and Terwaert, J. W. (2003). Staphylococcal superantigens and T cell expansions in Wegener's granulomatosis. *Clinical and Experimental Immunology*, **132**, 496–504.

Porges, A. J., Redecha, P. B., Kimberly, W. T., Csernok, E., Gross, W. L. and Kimberly, R. P. (1994). Antineutrophil cytoplasmic antibodies engage and activate human neutrophils via Fc gamma RIIa. *Journal of Immunology*, **153**, 1271–80.

Pillinger, M. and Staud, R. (1998). Wegener's granulomatosis in a patient receiving propylthiouracil for Graves' disease. *Seminars in Arthritis and Rheumatism*, **28**, 124–9.

Preston, G. A., Zarella, C. S., Pendergraft, W. F., *et al.* (2002). Novel effects of neutrophil-derived proteinase 3 and elastase on the endothelium involve in vivo cleavage of NF-kB and proapoptotic changes in JNK, ERK, and p38 MAPK signaling pathways. *Journal of the American Society of Nephrology*, **13**, 2840–9.

Qasim, F. J., Thiru, S., Mathieson, P. W. and Oliveira, D. B. (1995). The time course and characterization of mercuric chloride-induced immunopathology in the brown Norway rat. *Journal of Autoimmunity*, **8**, 193–208.

Radford, D. J., Luu, N. T., Hewins, P., Nash, G. and Savage, C. O.S. (2001). Antineutrophil antibodies stabilize adhesion and promote migration of flowing neutrophils on endothelial cells. *Arthritis and Rheumatism*, **44**, 2851–61.

Ralston, D. R., Marsh, C. B., Lowe, M. P. and Wewers, M. D. (1997). Antineutrophil cytoplasmic antibodies induce monocyte IL-8 release. *Journal of Clinical Investigation*, **100**, 1416–26.

Rastaldi, M. P., Ferrario, F., Yang, L., Tunesi, S., Ludaco, A., Zou, H. and D'Amico, G. (1996). Adhesion molecules expression in non-crescentic acute post-streptococcal glomerulonephritis. *Journal of the American Society of Nephrology*, **11**, 2419–27.

Reinhold-Keller, E., Beuge, N., Latza, U., *et al.* (2000). An interdisciplinary approach to the care of patients with Wegener's granulomatosis: Long term outcome in 155 patients. *Arthritis and Rheumatism*, **43**, 1021–32.

Reinhold-Keller, E., De Groot, K., Rudert, H., Nölle, B., Heller, M. and Gross, W. L. (1996). Response to trimethoprim/sulfamethoxazole in Wegener's granulomatosis depends on the phase of disease. *Quarterly Journal of Medicine*, **89**, 15–23.

Relle, M., Mayet, W. J., Strand, D., Brenner, W., Galle, P. R. and Schwarting, A. (2003). Proteinase 3/myeloblastin as a growth factor in human kidney cells. *Journal of Nephrology*, **16**, 831–40.

Richeldi, L., Sorrentino, R. and Saltini, C. (1993). HLA-DPB1 glutamate 69: a genetic marker of beryllium disease. *Science*, **262**, 242–4.

Schreiber, A., Otto, B., Ju, X., *et al.* (2005). Membrane proteinase 3 expression in patients with Wegener's granulomatosis and in human hematopoietic stem cell-derived neutrophils. *Journal of the American Society of Nephrology*, **16**, 2216–24.

Schultz, H., Schinke, S., Weiss, J., Cerundolo, V., Gross, W. L., and Gadola, S. (2003). BPI-ANCA in transporter associated with antigen presentation (TAP) deficiency: possible role in susceptibility to gram-negative bacterial infections. *Clinical and Experimental Immunology*, **133**, 252–9.

Sibelius, U., Hattar, K., Schenkel, A., *et al.* (1998). Wegener's granulomatosis: anti-proteinase 3 antibodies are potent inductors of human endothelial cell signaling and leakage response. *Journal of Experimental Medicine*, **187**, 497–503.

Slot, M. C., Tervaert, J. W., Boomsma, M. M. and Stegeman, C. A. (2004). Positive classic antineutrophil cytoplasmic antibody (C-ANCA) titer at switch to azathioprine therapy associated with relapse in proteinase 3-related vasculitis. *Arthritis and Rheumatism*, **51**, 269–73.

Sneller, M. C. (2002). Granuloma formation, implications for the pathogensis of vasculitis. *Cleveland Clinical Journal of Medicine*, **69** (Suppl. 2), SII-40–2.

Stegeman, C. A., Tervaert, J. W., Sluiter, W. J., Manson, W. L., de Jong, P. E. and Kallenberg, C. G.M. (1994). Association of chronic nasal carriage of Staphylococcus aureus and higher relapse rates in Wegener's granulomatosis. *Annals of Internal Medicine*, **120**, 12–7.

Stegeman, C. A., Tervaert, J. W., de Jong, P. E. and Kallenberg, C. G.M. (1996). Trimethoprim-sulfmethoxazole (co-trimoxazole) for the prevention of relapses of Wegener's granulomatosis. Dutch Co-Trimoxazole Wegener Study Group. *New England Journal of Medicine*, **335**, 16–20.

Taekema-Roelvink, M. E., Kooten, C., Kooij, S. V., Heemskerk, E. and Daha, M. R. (2001). Proteinase 3 enhances endothelial monocyte chemoattractant protein-1 production and induces increased adhesion of neutrophils to endothelial cells by upregulating intercellular cell adhesion molecule-1. *Journal of the American Society of Nephrology*, **12**, 932

Tatsis, E., Reinhold-Keller, E., Steindorf, K., Feller, A. C. and Gross, W. L. (1999). Wegener's granulomatosis associated with renal cell carcinoma. *Arthritis and Rheumatism*, **42**, 751–6.

Tomer, Y., Gilburd, B., Blank, M., *et al.* (1995). Characterization of biologically active antineutrophil cytoplasmic antibodies induced in mice. Pathogenetic role in experimental vasculitis. *Arthritis and Rheumatism*, **38**, 1375–81.

Travis, W. D. (1996). Pathology of pulmonary granulomatous vasculitis. *Sarcoidosis Vasculitis and Diffuse Lung Diseases*, **13**, 14–27.

Travis, W. D., Colby, T. V., and Koss, M. N. (2002). *Non-Neoplastic Disorders of the Lower Respiratory Tract. Atlas of Nontumor Pathology*, 1st Series, Fasc. 2. American Registry of Pathology/Armed Foreces Institute of Pathology, Washington, DC.

Tse, W. Y., Abadeh, S., Jefferis, R., Savage, C. O. and Adu, D. (2000). Neutrophil FcgammaRIIIb allelic polymorphism in anti-neutrophil cytoplasmic antibody (ANCA)-positive systemic vasculitis. *Clinical and Experimental Immunology*, **119**, 574–7.

Voswinkel, J., Muller, A. and Lamprecht, P. (2005). Is PR3-ANCA formation initiated in Wegener's granulomatosis lesions? Granulomas as potential lymphoid tissue maintaining autoantibody production. *Annals of the New York Academy of Science*, **1051**, 12–9.

Voswinkel, J., Mueller, A., Krämer, J. A., *et al.* (2006). B lymphocyte maturation in Wegener's granulomatosis: a comparative analysis of VH genes from endonasal lesions. *Annals of the Rheumatic Diseases*, **65**, 859–64.

Wainstein, E., Edberg, J. C., Csernok, E., *et al.* (1996). FcgRIIIB alleles predict renal dysfunction in Wegener's granulomatosis. *Arthritis and Rheumatism*, **39**, (Suppl.) S210 (Abstract).

Waldhauser, L. and Uetrecht, J. (1996). Antibodies to myeloperoxidase in propylthiouracil-induced autoimmune disease in the cat. *Toxicology*, **114**, 155–62.

Wegener, F. (1937). Über generalisierte, septische Gefässerkrankungen. *Verhandlungen der Deutschen Gesellschaft für Pathologie*, **29**, 202–8.

Wegener, F. (1939). Über eine eigenartige rhinogene Granulomatose mit besonderer Beteiligung des Arteriensystems und der Nieren. *Beiträge zur Pathologischen Anatomie*, **102**, 36–68.

Westman, K. W., Bygren, P. G., Olsson, H., Ranstam, J. and Wieslander, J. (1998). Relapse rate, renal survival, and cancer morbidity in patients with Wegener's granulomatosis or microscopic polyangiitis with renal involvement. *Journal of the American Society for Nephrology*, **9**, 842–52.

Weyand, C. M., Kurtin, P. J. and Goronzy, J. J. (2001). Ectopic lymphoid organogenesis – a fast track for autoimmunity. *American Journal of Pathology*, **159**, 787–93.

Wiesner, O., Russell, K. A., Lee, A. S., *et al.* (2004). Antineutrophil cytoplasmic antibodies reacting with human neutrophil elastase as a diagnostic marker for cocaine-induced midline destructive lesions but not autoimmune vasculitis. *Arthritis and Rheumatism*, **50**, 2954–65.

Williams, J. M., Ben-Smith, A., Hewins, P., *et al.* (2003). Activation of the G(i) heterotrimeric G protein by ANCA IgG F(ab')(2) fragments is necessary but not sufficient to stimulate the recruitment of those downstream mediators used by intact ANCA IgG. *Journal of the American Society of Nephrology*, **14**, 661–9.

Xiao, H., Heeringa, P., Hu, P., *et al.* (2002). Antineutrophil cytoplasmic autoantibodies specific for myeloperoxidase cause glomerulonephritis and vasculitis in mice. *Journal of Clinical Investigation*, **110**, 955–63.

Yang, J. J., Jennette, J. C. and Falk, R. J. (1994). Immune complex glomerulonephritis is induced in rats immunized with heterologous myeloperoxidase. *Clinical and Experimental Immunology*, **97**, 466–73.

Yang, J. J., Preston Gical, A., Alcorta, D. A., *et al.* (2002). Expression profile of leukocyte genes activated by anti-neutrophil cytoplasmic autoantibodies (ANCA). *Kidney International*, **62**, 1638–49.

Yousem, S. A. and Lombard, C. M. (1988). The eosinophilic variant of Wegener's granulomatosis. *Human Pathology*, **19**, 682–8.

Zhang, L., Jayne, D., Zhao, M., Lockwood, C. and Oliveira, D. (1995). Distribution of MHC class II allels in primary systemic vasculitis. *Kidney International*, **47**, 294–8.

Zinkernagel, R. M. and Hengartner, H. (2001). Regulation of the immune response by antigen. *Science*, **293**, 251–3.

Zinkernagel, R. M. (2004). On reactivity versus tolerance. *Immunology and Cell Biology*, **82**, 343–52.

CHAPTER 31

Wegener's granulomatosis: clinical and immunodiagnostic aspects

Wolfgang L. Gross and Elena Csernok

Wegener's granulomatosis (WG) is a systemic, inflammatory disease with a broad clinical spectrum. The disease was first described in 1931 by a medical student at the Charité in Berlin, Heinz Klinger, who mistakenly believed it to be an atypical form of polyarteritis nodosa (Klinger 1932). At the 29th Meeting of the German Society of Pathology in Breslau, Friedrich Wegener, a good friend of Klinger's, reported on the post-mortem findings in three of his patients. He was able to convince famous German pathologists, including Ludwig Aschoff (Freiburg), that the findings represented a new disease entity (reviewed in Socias and James 1987; Wegener 1990). At that time Wegener was, like his friend Klinger, fascinated by the vascular lesions that dominate the final stage of the disease, entitling his report "About generalized septic vessel diseases" (Wegener 1935), although, in its complete form the disease is characterized by necrotizing granulomatous inflammation of the upper and lower respiratory tracts, vasculitis, and glomerulonephritis (the so-called WG triad). A second report by Wegener in 1939 further detailed the clinical course of the three patients, with special emphasis on the granulomatous lesions: "About a peculiar rhinogenic granulomatosis with particular involvement of the arteries and kidneys" (Wegener 1939). He noted that symptoms began with severe upper respiratory infections followed by a fulminant vasculitic course. This sequence of events (spreading of granulomatous inflammation and, secondarily, the development of systemic vasculitis) has been confirmed both by clinical means and histological studies (reviewed in Gross et al. 2000). The term pathergic granulomatosis was introduced in 1955 in order to include a localized form of WG in the lung, an absolutely new concept at the time (Fienberg 1955), but later confirmed by Carrington and Liebow (1966). In the 1990s, this concept was revived with the growing recognition of WG subsets. Today, the pathological hallmark of WG is the coexistence of granulomas and vasculitis.

Definition and classification

According to the definitions of the vasculitides adopted by the Chapel Hill Consensus Conference (CHCC) on the nomenclature of systemic vasculitides (Jennette et al. 1994) (see Table 26.2 in Chapter 26), WG is characterized by granulomatous inflammation of the respiratory tract and a necrotizing vasculitis affecting small to medium-sized vessels, for example capillaries, venules, arterioles, and arteries, with necrotizing glomerulonephritis being a common manifestation. WG is associated with antineutrophil cytoplasmic antibodies (ANCA). Immunohistochemistry reveals no (or only few) immune deposits in the kidney lesion; hence the term pauci-immune glomerulonephritis (Jennette et al. 1994).

Classification criteria have been developed by the American College of Rheumatology (ACR) for seven forms of vasculitis (Hunder et al. 1990) including WG (Leavitt et al. 1990). In the presence of vasculitis, at least two of the following four criteria should additionally be met for the purpose of the classification of WG: (1) nasal or oral inflammation (defined as the development of painful or painless oral ulcers or purulent or bloody nasal discharge); (2) abnormal chest radiograph (the presence of cavitating or noncavitating nodules, or fixed infiltrates); (3) an abnormal urinary sediment (microscopic hematuria with >5 red blood cells/high power field or red cell casts in urine sediment); and (4) granulomatous inflammation (histological changes showing granulomatous inflammation within the wall of an artery or arteriole or in the perivascular or extravascular area) on a biopsy specimen (Leavitt et al. 1990). The presence of any two or more criteria yields a sensitivity of 88.2% and a specificity of 92.0%.

Epidemiology

Estimates of disease prevalence vary between 30 (US) and 60 (Germany) cases per million (Cotch et al. 1996; Reinhold-Keller et al. 1998). There may be a simple explanation for the difference between the two countries: in contrast to the population-based German study, Cotch et al. (1996) analyzed only hospitalized or deceased patients with WG. Furthermore, the US study covered the years 1979–1988 and thus included a long period prior to the introduction of ANCA testing in the mid-1980s; the German rate was for the year 1994. The incidence rose from 0.7 per million per year between 1980 and 1986 (Andrews et al. 1990) to 8.5 between 1988 and 1994 (Watts et al. 1995). This increase in reported incidence reflects both greater awareness of the disease and improved detection due to ANCA testing (Andrews et al. 1990). A comparative study between groups in Norway, England, and Spain, in which care was taken to classify patients in a consistent fashion, showed that WG was more common in north Norway compared with Spain (Watts et al. 2001). There is a lack of reliable data from other parts

Table 31.1 Incidence rates for primary systemic vasculitides (PSV) in Schleswig-Holstein from 1998 to 2002: new cases per year and per one million (95% CI)

	1998	1999	2000	2001	2002
All PSV	54 (39;68)	48 (34;61)	45 (34;61)	40 (31;50)	42 (31;52)
GCA	17 (8;24)	9 (3;15)	9 (3;15)	10 (4;16)	13 (6;20)
>50 years[1]	46 (33;59)	25 (14;36)	31 (18;44)	27 (16;38)	37 (23;50)
ANCA-associated PSV	11 (5;18)	9.5 (4;16)	12 (5;19)	12 (5;19)	16 (8;24)
WG	8 (2;14)	6 (1;11)	8 (2;13)	9 (3;15)	12 (5;19)
MPA	3 (0;6)	2.5 (0;6)	3 (0;6)	2 (0;4)	3 (0;6)
CSS	0 (0)	1 (0;3)	1.5 (0;3)	1 (0;3)	2 (0;4)
PAN	1 (0;3)	2 (0;4)	1 (0;2)	0.4 (0;2)	0.4 (0;2)
HSP	7 (2;12)	10 (4;16)	6 (3;9)	7 (4;11)	3 (0;6)
CLA	9 (3;15)	8 (2;14)	9 (3;15)	6 (3;9)	4 (1;7)
TA	1 (0;3)	1 (0;3)	0.5 (0;2)	0.4 (0;2)	0.4 (0;2)
KD	0	1 (0;3)	1 (0;2)	1 (0;3)	0
UV	9 (3;15)	8 (2;14)	6 (3;9)	3 (0;6)	5 (2;8)

[1] In the population 50 years and older. GCA, giant cell arteritis; WG, Wegener's granulomatosis; MPA, microscopic polyangiitis; CSS, Churg–Strauss syndrome; PAN, polyarteritis nodosa; HSP, Henoch–Schönlein purpura; CLA, cutaneous (isolated) leukocytoclastic angiitis; TA, Takayasu's arteritis; KD, Kawasaki's disease; UV, unclassified vasculitis. (From Reinhold-Keller *et al.* with permission).

of the world. Results of a population-based vasculitis register over 5 years for the incidence of primary systemic vasculitides among 2.78 million habitants in northern Germany revealed a stable incidence for all primary systemic vasculitides (PSV) (Table 31.1) (Reinhold-Keller *et al.* 2005). WG may present at any age, the mean age at presentation being 40 years; WG occurs in the elderly (Chakravarty *et al.* 1994; Weiner *et al.* 1986), and in children (Dillon 1998; Hall *et al.* 1985; McHugh *et al.* 1991; Rottem *et al.* 1993).

Pathological features

WG is a necrotizing granulomatous disease rather than a primary vasculitic disorder (Lie 1990). The classic triad of WG consists of necrotizing granulomas in the upper or lower respiratory tract or both; necrotizing or granulomatous vasculitis, usually of small arteries and veins, almost always in the lung, and more selectively in other organs; and focal, segmental, necrotizing glomerulitis (see Chapter 9).

The typical pulmonary lesions of WG are necrotizing granulomas combined with necrotizing granulomatous vasculitis. The granulomas may be discrete or confluent, forming an irregular geographic pattern of lung parenchymal necrosis. Eosinophils may be present in the inflammatory infiltrate but seldom in excessive numbers. The vasculitis is more often necrotizing than granulomatous and diffuse lung hemorrhage from capillaritis has been documented in 5–45% of biopsied or autopsied cases. Focal, segmental necrotizing glomerulonephritis is the predominant type of renal lesion in WG. Renal vasculitis occurs in less than 50% of patients and when present it may be of the polyarteritis type of necrotizing vasculitis or a granulomatous vasculitis (Lie 1990).

The lesions of glomerulonephritis range from a focal and segmental process to a diffuse necrotizing process with crescent formation. Characteristically no immunodeposits are seen by immunohistochemistry (pauci-immune glomerulonephritis) in contrast to the immune complex diseases, such as Henoch–Schönlein purpura or antiglomerular basement membrane disease (Goodpasture's syndrome).

The nasal mucosa is frequently involved in WG and is easily accessible for biopsy although it is typically of limited diagnostic value (Del Buono and Flint 1991; Devaney *et al.* 1990; Lombard *et al.* 1990). Applying the proposed criteria for the diagnosis of WG to findings on biopsy specimens from the head and neck region can usually render open lung biopsy unnecessary. The presence of all three major pathological criteria (granulomatous inflammation, necrosis, and vasculitis) in a biopsy specimen may be considered diagnostic of WG if the patients have the classic triad of involvement or evidence of typical disease in the lung or kidney. The concept that persistent granulomata can be at the root of relapses of WG underscores the need to understand their pathogenesis; much more needs to be learned about the mechanisms of the granulomatous component of WG. New data indicate that different subgroups of T cells predominate in localized WG and vasculitic lesions: in nasal tissues derived from patients with untreated localized WG a predominance of CD4+/CD26+ T cells as well as INFγ-positive cells support a polarized Th1-like immune response (Figure 31.1) (Müller *et al.* 2000). A shift from a type 1 helper T-cell response to a type 2 helper T cell-response has been associated with the abrupt development of systemic disease in patients with WG.

Clinical features

Presentation

In many cases the disease is localized at first, with granulomatous lesions mostly in the upper respiratory tract, before systemic vasculitis occurs. The presenting features are therefore protean, ranging from indolent ENT findings with asymptomatic lesions on chest radiograph to progressive multiorgan failure. The presenting signs and symptoms in 155 patients from the Medical University Lübeck are compared with those of three other WG cohorts in Table 31.2.

The presenting features cross the barriers of the various medical disciplines, and so an interdisciplinary assessment of disease activity and extent should be performed by a team of rheumatologists, ENT surgeons, ophthalmologists, pulmonologists, and sometimes neurologists or dermatologists. The spectrum of WG manifestations in each of these specialties has been reviewed in detail elsewhere (Frances *et al.* 1994; Harman and Margo 1998; Kempf 1989; Nadeau 1997; Nishino *et al.* 1993).

The most common presenting symptoms (Figure 31.2) are related to the upper respiratory tract ("E region" according to the ELK classification) (DeRemee *et al.* 1976). These include symptoms induced by granulomatous inflammation in the nose (nasal obstruction, serosanguineous discharge, epistaxis, progressive saddle nose deformity); the oral cavity and oropharynx (ulcerative stomatitis, hyperplastic gingivitis); the upper trachea (subglottic stenosis); the external ear (chondritis); the middle ear (otitis media, mastoiditis); and the orbits (protrusio bulbi). All these manifestations can occur initially without symptoms of a systemic inflammatory disease such as fever, malaise, arthralgia, and weight loss, and without clinical signs of systemic vasculitis. In this stage,

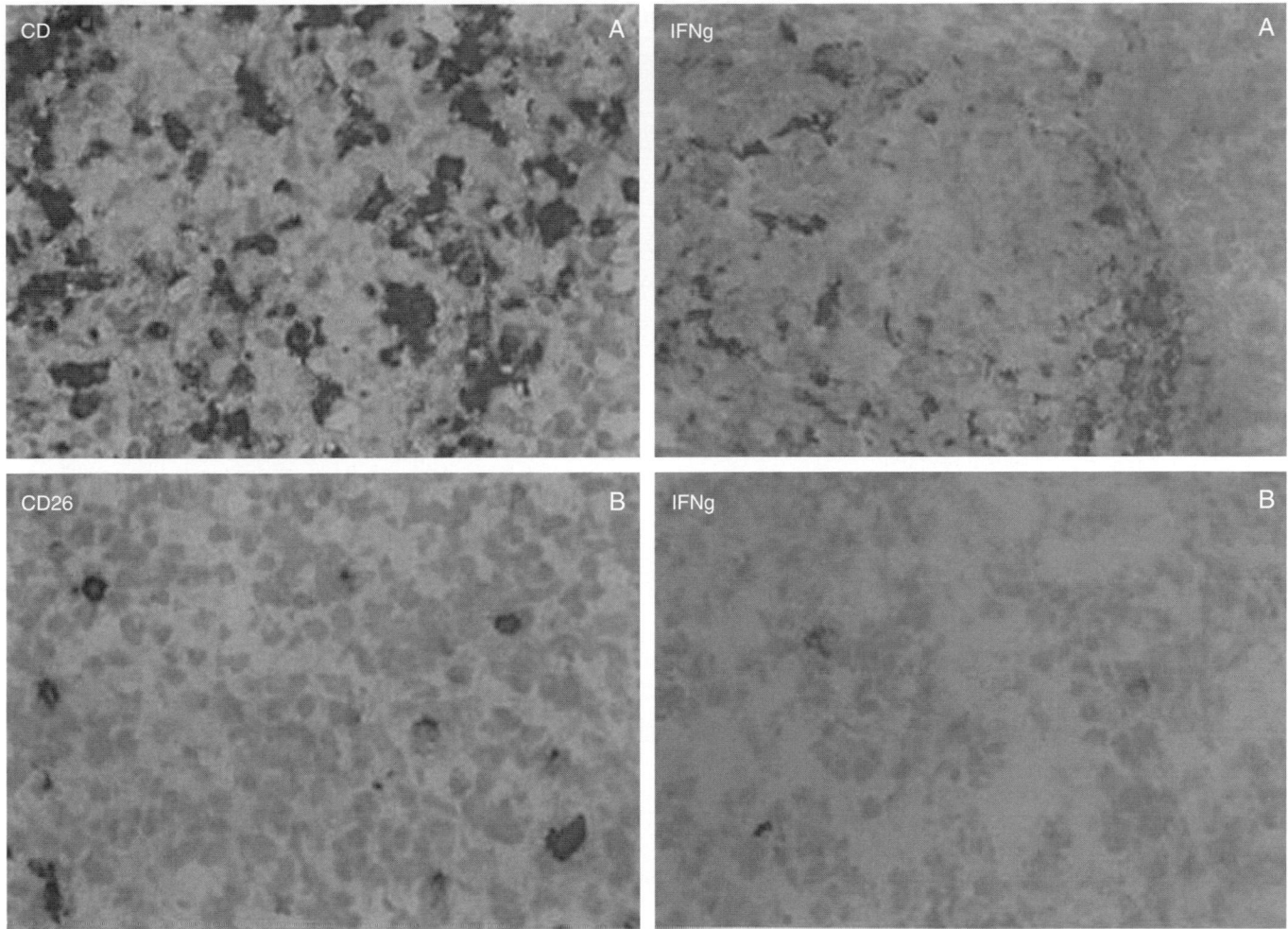

Figure 31.1 Immunohistological assessment of CD26-positive cells (MIB DS2/7) and IFNγ-positive cells (GZ-4) in clinically and histologically representative cases of nasal mucosal biopsies derived from a patient with untreated localized WG (a, two upper images) and a patient with untreated generalized WG (b, two lower images). Staining was performed with APAAP method. × 300. (From Müller *et al.* (2000). *Journal of Pathology,* 192, 113–120, with permission)..

the disease has many names, including localized WG and initial-phase WG.

Arthralgias are frequent symptoms at the presentation of the generalized phase of WG, together with other symptoms of systemic inflammation, such as fatigue, malaise, and weight loss (constitutional symptoms; "B-symptoms"). Fever often occurs and may be related to the underlying inflammatory disease although it can be associated with secondary bacterial infection of the involved paranasal sinuses. The transition from the initial stage to the active generalized phase with its frequent fulminant course is heralded by these indirect constitutional symptoms. Clinically, the combination of constitutional symptoms together with rheumatic complaints and the striking laboratory abnormalities typical of this phase of disease (markedly elevated ESR and CRP, leukocytosis, thrombocytosis) warrants close scrutiny of the patient. Early recognition of complications (rapidly progressive glomerulonephritis; alveolar hemorrhage) is important because, if untreated, they can lead to the life-threatening situations inherent in this disease.

Signs of small vessel vasculitis in generalized WG are red eye (due to episcleritis, scleritis); cutaneous vasculitis manifested as palpable purpura or necrotic nodules, usually on the lower extremities; and peripheral neuropathy. The most ominous manifestations of small-vessel WG involve the kidney (K) or lung (L). Rapidly progressive glomerulonephritis together with pulmonary capillaritis lead to a pulmonary–renal syndrome, which cannot be differentiated clinically from other such syndromes (for example Goodpasture's syndrome). Only rapid diagnosis and immediate immunosuppressive treatment can control this life-threatening condition. In some instances the vasculitis can lead to sensorineural deafness, vertigo, or pericarditis or myocarditis.

Laboratory tests

There is no single laboratory finding that is diagnostic for WG. Besides the clinical picture, disease activity must be assessed with the help of serological acute phase reactants such as ESR and CRP. Leukocytosis, which is usually associated with moderate eosinophilia, thrombocytosis, and normochromic normocytic anemia, is also common. All these parameters are only slightly abnormal or even sometimes normal in the initial phase of WG and, by contrast, maximally elevated in the fulminant generalized stage of WG,

Table 31.2 Comparison of 155 Wegener's granulomatosis (WG) patients with three other WG cohorts

	Hoffman *et al.* 1992	Anderson *et al.* 1992	Matteson *et al.* 1996	Reinhold-Keller *et al.* 2000
Total no. of patients	158 (Single center)	265 (Multicenter)	77 (Multicenter)	155 (Single center)
Male/female (%)	50/50	55/45	64/36	49/51
Age at diagnosis (mean)	41	50	45	48
Calendar year of diagnosis	1966–90	1975–85	1978–87	1966–93
Mean follow-up (years)	8	ni	7.1	7
Total patient-years	1229	ni	ni	2144
Follow-up more than 5 years (%)	63	ni	ni	78
Date of end of follow-up	ni	January, 1986	June, 1993	March, 1997
cANCA positive (%)[1]	88	ni	ni	84
Involved organ systems at diagnosis/ over the whole course (%)[2,3]				
E	73/92	75/ni	ni/ni	93/99
K	18/77	60/ni	ni/73	54/70
L	45/85	63/ni	ni/53	55/66
EY	15/52	14/ni	ni/ni	40/61
H	ni/8	ni/ni	ni/14	13/25
P	ni/15	ni/ni	ni/[4]	21/40
C	ni/8	ni/ni	ni/[4]	6/11
GI	ni/ni	ni/ni	ni/19	3/6
S	13/46	25/ni	ni/ni	21/33
A	32/67	20/ni	ni/ni	61/77
Initial phase at diagnosis (%)	ni	22	ni	15
Cyclophosphamide therapy (%)	89	29[5]	60	92
Prednisone therapy (mg/day)[6]				
Initial	70	ni	ni	70
After 3 months	30	ni	ni	10
Infections (%)	46	ni	ni	26
Median survival (years)	ni	8.5	ni	21.7
Mortality (%)	20	56	36	14
Death due to WG and/ or its therapy (%)	13	ni	ni	12
Death due to infections (%)	3	12	10	3

[1] Classic antineutrophil cytoplasmic antibodies in the present study proved to be directed against proteinase 3.

[2] In the study of Hoffmann *et al.* information only on onset of disease; in that of Anderson *et al.* information at presentation.

[3] For abbreviations see Table 31.3.

[4] Involvement of both peripheral and central nervous systems 31%.

[5] Initial therapy within the first 3 months (information about further treatment not available).

[6] Based on a body weight of 70 kg.

ni = no information.

which sometimes is associated with leukemoid reactions. These tests do not allow a distinction between vasculitic disease activity and a concomitant infection or other source of inflammation. The extent of organ lesions can be monitored by other tests, such as serum creatinine and urinary sediment for renal involvement.

In contrast to the group of collagen vascular diseases, for example SLE, generalized WG is associated with no or only mild hypergammaglobulinemia, negative or low titer antinuclear antibody (ANA), no evidence of complement consumption and no serum cryoglobulins. Rheumatoid factor may be present in up to 50% of patients.

Antineutrophil cytoplasmic antibodies (ANCA)

ANCA represent a class of autoantibodies that are specifically directed to multiple intracellular antigens in neutrophils and monocytes (see Chapter 7). ANCA are routinely detected by indirect immunofluorescence (IIF) on ethanol-fixed neutrophils (Hagen *et al.* 1993a). At least three different patterns of fluorescence can be distinguished: the cytoplasmic granular fluorescence with central interlobular accentuation (cANCA); the perinuclear with nuclear extension pattern (pANCA); and the combination of cytoplasmic and perinuclear staining (atypical ANCA) (see Chapter 6).

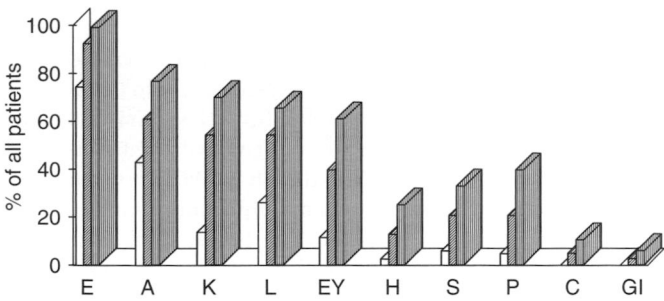

Figure 31.2 Disease extent at the onset of symptoms (open bars), at the time of diagnosis (shadowed bars), and over the whole course of disease (striped bars) in 155 patients with Wegener's granulomatosis. E, upper respiratory tract; A, rheumatic complaints; K, kidney; L, lung; EY, inflammatory eye involvement; H, heart; S, skin; P, peripheral nervous system; C, central nervous system; GI, gastrointestinal tract.

In vasculitis, cANCA is a seromarker for WG and pANCA is a marker for microscopic polyangitis (MPA); the cytoplasmic pattern associated with WG is characteristically induced by proteinase 3 (PR3)-ANCA, the perinuclear pattern seen in MPA by myeloperoxidase (MPO)-ANCA. These associations are not absolute and PR3-ANCA are sometimes seen in MPA and MPO-ANCA in WG (reviewed in Hoffman and Specks 1998).

The early literature on the clinical utility of ANCA as a diagnostic marker for WG has been evaluated in a meta-analysis by Rao and colleagues (Rao *et al.* 1995). The sensitivities of cANCA testing for WG ranged from 34% to 92%, and the specificities range from 88% to 100%. The pooled sensitivity was 66%, and the pooled specificity was 98%. Over the past few years, several new studies have been conducted, most of them being retrospective, and the reported sensitivities and specificities of ANCA tests range widely, depending not only on the test characteristics of the assays used but also on the population under study. Between 60% and 95% of all ANCA found in WG are cANCA and PR3-ANCA. Hagen *et al.* (1993b) showed that the value of the immunofluorescence test for ANCA detection can be greatly increased by the addition of a well-standardized antigen-specific ELISA. When the results of IIF were combined with those of the ELISA (cANCA /PR3-ANCA and pANCA /MPO-ANCA), the diagnostic specificity increased to 99%. The sensitivity of the combination of cANCA /PR3-ANCA and pANCA /MPO-ANCA for WG, MPA, or primary pauci-immune crescentic glomerulonephritis was 73%, 67%, and 82%, respectively (Hagen *et al.* 1998). The sensitivity of cANCA /PR3-ANCA for WG is related to the extent, severity, and activity of disease at the time of sampling. The association of MPA with pANCA /MPO-ANCA is reported to be in the range of 40–80% (Hagen *et al.* 1998). Few patients with WG are pANCA /MPO-ANCA positive and few patients with MPA are cANCA /PR3-ANCA positive. ANCA have been detected with variable frequency (10–70%) in Churg–Strauss syndrome (CSS). Both PR3 and MPO have been described as target antigens. In general, ANCA levels are usually high at presentation and ANCA testing can been used to monitor disease activity and to differentiate disease flares from intercurrent illness. PR3-ANCA has also been observed in other disorders such as cryoglobulinemic vasculitis, ulcerative colitis, infectious diseases (tuberculosis, leprosy, subacute bacterial endocarditis, etc.), and drug-induced syndromes (cocaine-induced midline destructive lesions). However, the clinical value of PR3-ANCA testing in these conditions is very limited.

Although the diagnostic value of ANCA is well established, the usefulness of measuring ANCA titers in assessing disease activity and guiding therapy is somewhat controversial (Langford 2005). Generally, since rises in ANCA occur in most patients prior to a relapse, serial measurements of ANCA titers in patients with ANCA-associated vasculitis (AAV) during remission can help predict relapses; however, ANCA levels should not be used by themselves to guide treatment. A significant increase in ANCA titers, or reappearance of ANCA, should alert the clinicians and lead to a more vigilant patient care.

The internationally accepted gold standard for ANCA detection remains IIF on human neutrophils fixed with ethanol. As mentioned above, the value of IIF for ANCA detection is increased by the addition of standardized antigen-specific ELISA (Hagen *et al.* 1998). Recently, an international group of ANCA researchers published a consensus statement on ANCA testing (Savige *et al.* 1999). These guidelines mandate that in cases of positive IIF-testing for ANCA an ELISA test is obligatory; however, many hospital and referral laboratories only use commercially available ELISA kits to detect ANCA. The performances of commercial direct ANCA ELISA vary significantly from each other and, in some cases, from that of IIF ANCA assays; there are significant differences in sensitivity, specificity, and predictive value among available commercial ELISA kits (Holle *et al.* 2005). Another method for quantifying PR3-ANCA may prove to be superior to direct ELISA, namely capture ELISA. The first results obtained in a new European Vasculitis Study Group (EUVAS) study demonstrated that capture ELISA seems to be the superior method of PR3-ANCA detection in WG (Csernok *et al.* 2004).

Among all the described ANCA target antigens, only ANCA against the PR3 and MPO antigens are closely associated with small-vessel vasculitis; the reason for this is unclear. Several studies have compared the clinical and histopathological associations between patients with PR3-ANCA and MPO-ANCA. A direct comparison of clinical features of patients categorized by their ANCA-status revealed that extrarenal manifestations, granuloma formation, and relapse were more frequent in patients with PR3-ANCA than in those with MPO-ANCA (Fransen *et al.* 1998; Schönermarck *et al.* 2001). Analysis of renal biopsy specimens from 173 patients obtained at the time of diagnosis suggested that active and chronic renal lesions are more common in MPO-ANCA-positive patients than in PR3-ANCA-positive patients (Hauer *et al.* 2002). Thus, despite substantial overlap there appear to be clinical and pathologic differences between patients with PR3-ANCA and patients with MPO-ANCA that may reflect different pathogenic molecular interactions between ANCA, their target antigens, and organ involvement. About 10% of patients with WG do not have ANCA that can be demonstrated by IIF or in antigen-specific assays (ELISA, immunoblotting). Patients with ANCA-negative WG are likely to have localized disease. ANCA-negative patients with generalized WG are younger, more likely to be female, have less lung and kidney involvement, a lower rate of relapse, and a better outcome than ANCA-positive patients.

Within the last 20 years ANCA have been the subject of intensive studies and a growing body of evidence has arisen for a specific role of ANCA in the pathogenesis of the ANCA-associated vasculitis. Recently, a direct causal link between ANCA and the development of glomerulonephritis and vasculitis has been demonstrated in animal models (Pfister *et al.* 2004; Xiao *et al.* 2002).

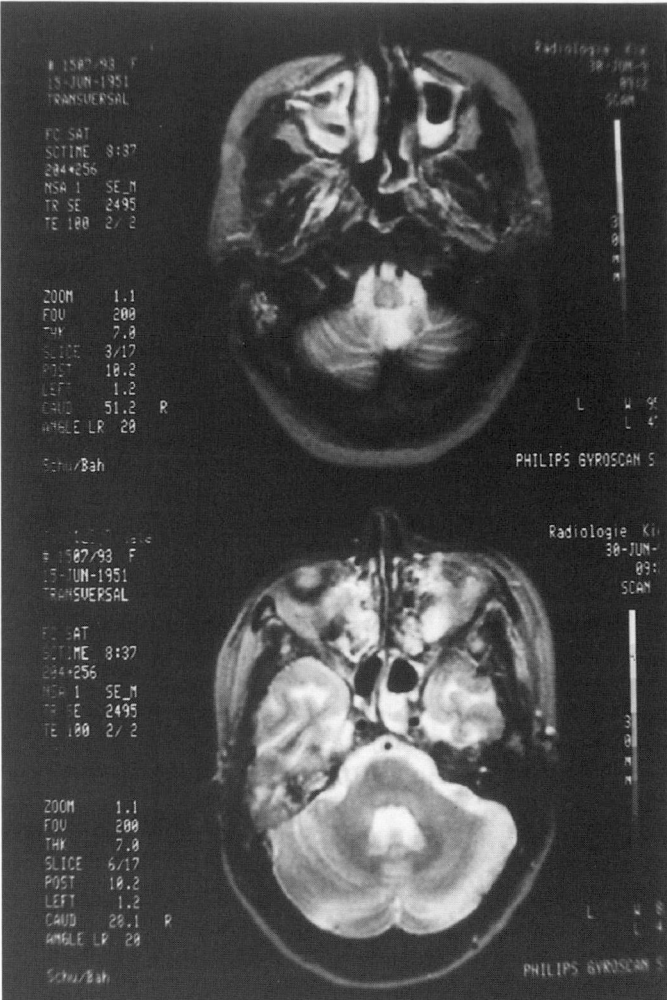

Figure 31.3 Cranial MRI of a patient with WG. T2-weighted images show increased soft tissues in the maxillary and sphenoid sinuses, with high signal intensity, indicating active sinusitis.

Surrogate markers

Cytokines, cytokine receptor molecules, and adhesion molecules in serum or plasma of WG patients have been shown to be associated with clinical disease activity. Soluble IL-2 receptor (sIL2-R) levels were found to be higher in sera of patients with generalized WG than in sera from patients with initial-phase WG. Persistent elevation of sIL2-R during remission may indicate a higher risk of relapse in these patients (Schmitt *et al.* 1992). Soluble CD30 has recently been shown to correlate with disease activity in the generalized vasculitic phase of WG (Wang *et al.* 1997). Elevated procalcitonin levels are a useful variable in the differential diagnosis of flares and bacterial infection in WG patients (Eberhard *et al.* 1997; Moosig *et al.* 1998).

The diagnostic value of endothelial cell markers such as von Willebrand factor and thrombomodulin is being investigated. Soluble thrombomodulin reflects the course of clinical disease activity more closely than the cANCA titer (Boehme *et al.* 1996). Antiendothelial cell antibodies (AECA) have been detected in WG but do not seem to be useful in diagnosis.

Imaging

Cranial MRI is a helpful clinical technique for the visualization of nasal, sinusoidal, orbital (retrobulbar), and mastoidal lesions in WG (Figure 31.3). Not only can it help in locating biopsy sites but characteristic patterns have been delineated for highly active mucosal disease, subacute granulomatous disease, and cicatricial changes (Muhle 1997). Moreover, MRI is vastly superior to computed tomography in detecting vascular cerebral lesions.

The imaging of pulmonary WG was greatly improved by the introduction of high-resolution computed tomography of the chest (see Chapters 13 and 19). The diffuse infiltrates characteristic of florid vasculitic lung disease are adequately depicted by conventional radiography (Cordier 1990), but high-resolution computed tomography (HRCT) proved to be superior to conventional radiography in detecting the more subtle changes of subacute pulmonary WG (Reuter 1998). The most common abnormalities among the latter are small nodules, septal and non-septal linear opacities, and low-attenuation (ground-glass) opacities (Figure 31.4a and b). A large study comparing HRCT with conventional radiography

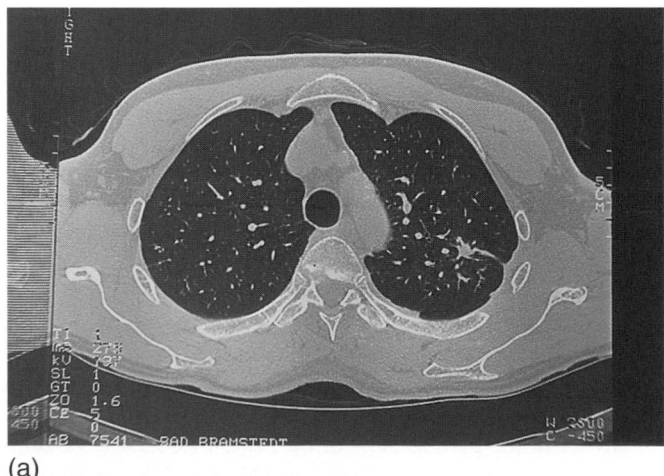

(a)

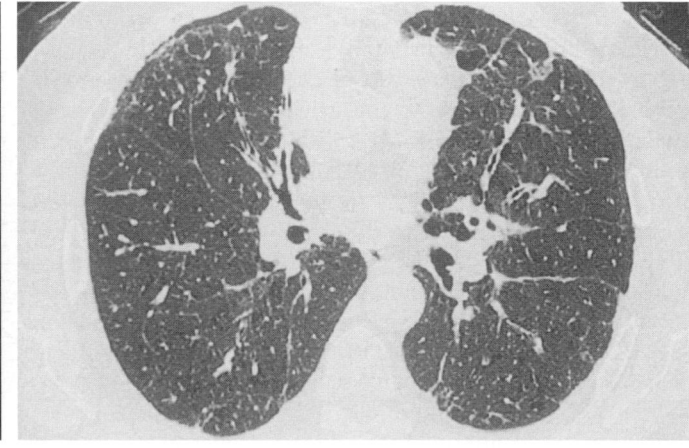

(b)

Figure 31.4 (a and b) High resolution CT scan in WG, showing small nodules, septal and non-septal lines.

found the former to be three times more sensitive in detecting nodules and masses and 1.7 times more sensitive in detecting linear opacities than the latter (Reuter 1998). Focal low-attenuation infiltrates, which evade detection in the conventional radiograph, were found in 10% of patients. Longitudinal observation suggests that nodules and low-attenuation opacities are ordinarily a reflection of active disease, whereas linear opacities can be either active or cicatricial lesions.

Angiography (including non-invasive techniques such as MR angiography) is a valuable technique for detecting abnormalities in large and intermediate vessels (see Chapter 18). Since vasculitic involvement of intermediate vessels is not uncommon in WG, angiography can be helpful for the discrimination between vasculitic and atherosclerotic disease, such as in a patient with active WG and concomitant angina, intestinal ischemia, or hypoperfusion of an extremity. Digital gangrene has been reported in WG (Frances *et al.* 1994; Karjalainen and Hakala 1996) (Figure 31.5a and b). Documentation of small-vessel disease, the most common feature in WG, is beyond the capability of standard angiography.

Bronchoscopy, bronchoalveolar lavage

Subglottic tracheal stenosis is a characteristic lesion in WG that can be visualized by laryngoscopy, conventional radiography, and spiral computed tomography (Daum *et al.* 1995). The introduction of bronchoscopy led to the realization that WG airway lesions are much more common than one might expect from chest radiographs. Bronchoscopy studies found tracheobronchial lesions in 26–59% of WG patients (Cordier *et al.* 1990; Daum *et al.* 1995; Schnabel *et al.* 1997). The abnormalities comprise ulcerative bronchitis, inflammatory pseudotumors, inflammatory and cicatricial bronchial stenoses, diffuse inflammation, and focal bleeding. A fixed extrathoracic major airway stricture may be detected by pulmonary function studies, in which there is attenuation of both the inspiratory and expiratory limbs of the flow volume loop. Active inflammatory tracheobronchial lesions produce a high yield of positive biopsies (Daum *et al.* 1995; Schnabel *et al.* 1997).

The cell profile in fluid obtained from bronchoalveolar lavage (BAL) depends on the underlying lesion (Schnabel *et al.* 1999). In highly active vasculitic disease associated with diffuse opacities on the chest radiograph, the BAL cell profile is dominated by neutrophils (Figure 31.6). In lung disease of low or moderate disease activity characterized by nodular or linear opacities, lymphocytes prevail. For the most part these are CD4+ T cells; functional studies have disclosed a predominant Th1 cytokine profile (Csernok *et al.* 1999; Schnabel *et al.* 1999). It is of foremost importance to examine all BAL materials microbiologically to rule out infection; this is probably the main purpose for performing BAL in WG patients with pulmonary disease.

Measurement of disease activity and extent

The assessment of therapy in WG is hampered by the absence of well-defined end-points of disease activity. The critical factors for determining therapeutic options are the location, extent and severity of the disease, and its response to current or previous treatment. For an in-depth discussion of assessment of disease activity and damage in vasculitis, see Chapter 23.

With recent recognition of the diversity of disease courses in WG, treatment needs to be more individualized. Therefore, a uniform patient assessment seems indispensable. Clinical symptoms need to be evaluated on a regular and standardized basis by an interdisciplinary team of physicians. Ideally, these results should yield an objective and reproducible measure of at least two parameters: disease extent and disease activity (differentiated from irreversible damage) that allow a comparison between patients on a semiquantitative basis. As there is no laboratory test (besides the cANCA titer) that is both specific for WG and correlates closely with disease activity and extent in all disease stages, scoring systems are mainly confined to clinical symptoms attributable to vasculitic activity.

Disease activity of WG is quantified by disease assessment tools which record disease activity in different organ systems in specified item lists. Most frequently used are the Birmingham vasculitis activity score (BVAS) (Luqmani *et al.* 1994) and some of its variations (see Chapter 23). The BVAS/WG incorporates several items specific for WG (Stone *et al.* 2001) (see Table 23.1 in Chapter 23) while the BVAS 2003 is a further development of the initial BVAS (see Chapter 32 for further details). On the basis of the extended ELK classification (DeRemee *et al.* 1976) a disease extent index (DEI) (Table 31.3) was developed (de Groot *et al.* 2001; Reinhold-Keller *et al.* 1994). This instrument assigns two points to every

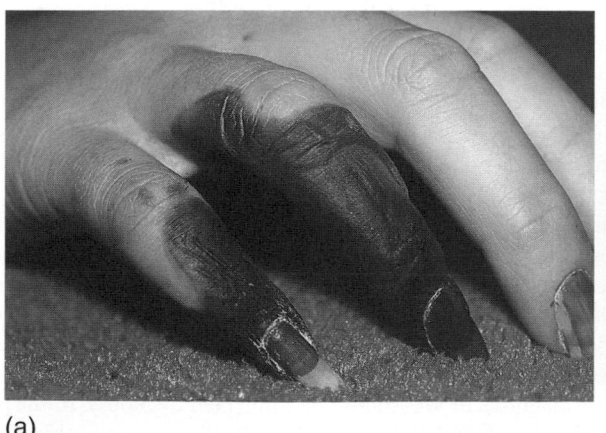
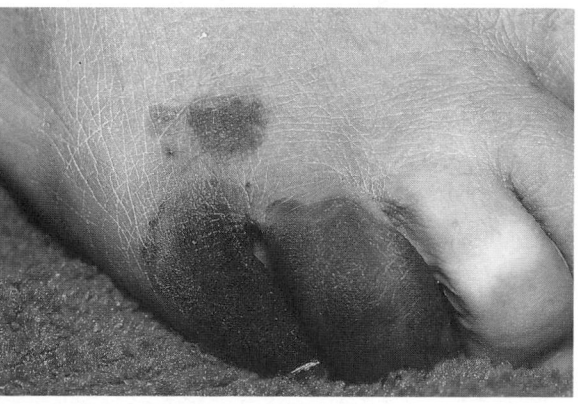

(a)   (b)

Figure 31.5 Hand (a) and foot (b) of an 18-year-old woman with digital necrosis due to WG. (Courtesy of Dr Gene Ball.) (See Color Plate 87).

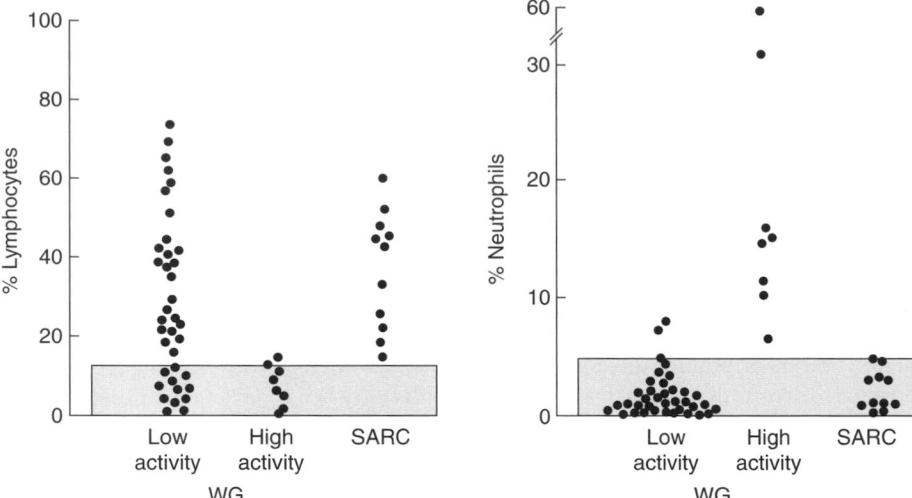

Figure 31.6 The cell profile of bronchoalveolar lavage (BAL) fluid from highly active WG is dominated by neutrophils, while lymphocytes predominate in less active WG.

organ system affected by active WG with the exception of constitutional symptoms (B) which are allocated only one point because they are largely subjective. The maximum attainable score is 21 points. The DEI has proven to be easy and quick to apply, can be used prospectively or retrospectively, and shows a very low inter- and intraobserver variability. It has become part of the every

day clinical practice in some centers, as it indicates at a glance the actual disease extent.

Diagnosis

Although the ACR vasculitis classification criteria were never intended for diagnosis of individual patients, clinicians often use them for that purpose. Recently, Rao *et al.* (1998) examined the operating characteristics of the ACR classification criteria in the diagnosis of four vasculitides including WG. In this prospective cohort study (198 consecutive patients referred to rheumatologists for evaluation of possible vasculitis), the positive predictive values for the four vasculitides according to ACR criteria ranged from 17% to 29% for the entire cohort and from 29% to 75% for only the patients with a final diagnosis of vasculitis. The authors therefore concluded that the ACR classification criteria work poorly in the diagnosis of specific vasculitides.

In everyday practice, WG should be suspected in patients who report unexplained symptoms of systemic inflammatory disease (fever, malaise, arthralgias, weight loss), direct signs of vasculitis (cutaneous vasculitis, etc.), and airway complaints (upper and lower airway symptoms), with or without signs of glomerulonephritis (such as active urine sediment or elevated creatinine). If WG is suspected, the patient should be questioned about symptoms of nasal, sinus, tracheal, and ear abnormalities, which are responsible for initial symptoms in nearly 90% of patients. It is important to look for pulmonary infiltrates and nodules, and for active urine sediment, since at least one-third of patients have asymptomatic pulmonary and renal involvement first.

If the cANCA test is positive in a patient with the appropriate clinical findings, WG is likely. ELISA must be used to define the subspecificity of PR3 antibodies (PR3-ANCA). The specificity of cANCA /PR3-ANCA for WG has been found to be as high as 98%. It is noteworthy that ANCA are found in only about 50% of WG patients without obvious clinical vasculitis (initial-phase WG).

The diagnosis of WG should be confirmed by biopsy. In the past, the majority of patients with pulmonary disease were subjected to open lung biopsy to establish a pathological diagnosis because biopsies of other organs such as kidney or other airways were often non-specific. Today, the diagnosis is often made by the typical

Table 31.3 The extended ELK classification leading to the Disease Extent Index (DEI)

	Involved organ	Score	Standard diagnostic procedure
E	ENT/upper respiratory tract	2	Clinical assessment by ENT specialist, cranial MRI, sinoscopy
L	Lung	2	Chest radiograph, HRCT, bronchoscopy, bronchoalveolar lavage
EY	Eye	2	Ophthalmological referral, cranial MRI
K	Kidney	2	Urinalysis, serum creatinine, abdominal ultrasound
H	heart	2	ECG, chest radiograph, echocardiogram, myocardial scintigram, coronary angiogram
GI	Gastrointestinal tract	2	Abdominal ultrasound, endoscopy, (mesenteric angiogram, laparotomy)
S	Skin	2	Clinical assessment, biopsy
P	Peripheral nervous system	2	Neurological referral, ENG, EMG (nerve biopsy)
C	Central nervous system	2	Neurological referral, lumbar puncture, cranial MRI
A	Rheumatic complaints	2	Radiographs, ultrasound, diagnostic arthrocentesis, bone scan, serum-CK, EMG, MRI, muscle biopsy
B	Constitutional symptoms	1	
	Maximum DEI score	21 points	

From de Groot *et al.* (2001). Abbreviations: MRI, magnetic resonance imaging; HRCT, high resolution computed tomography; ECG, electrocardiogram; ENG, electroneurography; EMG, electromyography.

clinical findings, ANCA serology, and minor biopsies, mostly from the ENT region.

Natural history and prognosis

WG usually progresses without therapy, but the tempo varies greatly among individual patients. Up to the mid-1980s, before the institution of effective therapy, the prognosis for WG was extremely grave. The mean survival of untreated WG was thought to be 5 months, with 82% of patients dying within 1 year and more than 90% within 2 years (Fauci *et al.* 1983). Walton (1958) reported, in a retrospective study of 10 of his own patients and of 46 others selected from the literature, that although a few cases lived for up to 4 years, most died rapidly (average of 5 months) from renal or respiratory failure. He further reported that the natural history of WG clearly involved two phases and that "the initial lesion in WG is not polyarteritis nodosa, but the ulceration in the respiratory tract."

In addition to full-blown forms with possible fatal outcome, indolent or less extensive, and non-life-threatening variants of WG have been shown to be more frequent than previously thought (Gross 1989; Gross *et al.* 1986). In an updated analysis of 158 patients with WG, investigators at the National Institutes of Health (NIH) emphasized the variability of the disease prior to diagnosis: WG followed a confusing and indolent course in many cases (particularly in patients without renal manifestation) for up to 16 years before a definitive diagnosis was established. The median and mean periods from the onset of symptoms to a diagnosis of WG were 4.7 and 15 months, respectively. Diagnosis of WG was made within 3 months after onset of symptoms in only 42% of patients. In a British study of 265 WG patients observed between 1975 and 1985 (Anderson *et al.* 1992), the mean time from onset of symptoms to presentation and from presentation to diagnosis were each approximately 7 months; correct diagnosis was often missed for many years (range 1–188 months). The mean survival of 4.2 years in patients receiving no drug treatment (10%) during the first 3 months indicates that some variants must have been very mild. Furthermore, it is striking that the median survival of 72 patients treated with glucocorticoids alone within the first 3 months exceeded 12 years.

More recently, long-term survival of WG patients from the cohort of subjects used for development of the ACR classification criteria was determined. Not surprisingly, the life expectancy of WG patients was lower than that of the general population. Although the disease manifestations in these patients were heterogeneous, the overall mortality rate was 4.7 times higher than expected. Causes of death among 28 patients in this cohort were infection in eight (28.6%); cardiac disease in five (17.9%); renal failure in five (17.9%); and malignancy in four (14.2%) (Matteson *et al.* 1996).

Prognosis varies considerably depending on the clinical status of the patient, and thus affects management decisions. It is a difficult question whether to treat a symptomatic patient with only minor lesions in the upper respiratory tract in the initial phase of WG with trimethoprim/ sulfamethoxazole, low-dose prednisone, both medications, or not at all. On the other hand, in fulminant WG one should not hesitate to immediately use the standard treatment regimen. For a full discussion of treatment of WG, see Chapter 32.

References

Anderson, G., Crane, M., Douglas, A. C., Gibbs, A. R., Coles, E. T., Geddes, D. M., Peel, E. T. and Wood, J. B. (1992). Wegener's granuloma. A series of 265 British cases seen between 1975 and 1985. A report by a sub-committee of the British Thoracic Society Research Committee. *Quarterly Journal of Medicine*, **302**, 427–38.

Andrews, M., Edmunds, M., Campbell, A., Walls, J. and Feehally, J. (1990). Systemic vasculitis in the 1980s – Is there an increasing incidence of Wegener's granulomatosis and microscopic polyarteritis? *Journal of the Royal College of Physicians of London*, **24**, 284–8.

Boehme, M. W., Schmitt, W. H., Youinou, P., Stremmel, W. R. and Gross, W. L. (1996). Clinical relevance of elevated serum thrombomodulin and soluble E-selectin in patients with Wegener's granulomatosis and other systemic vasculitides. *American Journal of Medicine*, **101**, 387–94.

Carrington, C. B. and Liebow, A. A. (1966). Limited forms of angiitis and granulomatosis of Wegener's type. *American Journal of Medicine*, **41**, 497–502.

Chakravarty, K., Scott, D. G. I., Blyth, J. and Courteney- Harris, R. G. (1994). Wegener's granulomatosis in the elderly – unusual presentations and misdiagnosis. *Journal of Rheumatology*, **21**, 1157–9.

Cordier, J.-F., Valeyre, D., Guillevin, L., Loire, R. and Brechot, J.-M. (1990). Pulmonary Wegener's granulomatosis. A clinical imaging study of 77 cases. *Chest*, **97**, 906–12.

Cotch, M. F., Hoffman, G. S., Yerg, D. E., Kaufman, G. I., Targonski, P. and Kaslow, R. A. (1996). The epidemiology of Wegener's granulomatosis. *Arthritis and Rheumatism*, **39**, 87–92.

Csernok, E., Trabandt, A., Müller, A., Wang, G., Moosig, F., Paulsen, J., Schnabel, A. and Gross, W. L. (1999). Cytokine profiles in Wegener's granulomatosis: predominance of type 1 (Th1) in the granulomatous inflammation. *Arthritis and Rheumatism*, **42**, 742–50.

Csernok, E., Holle, J., Hellmich, B., Willem, J., Tervaert, C., Kallenberg, C. G., *et al.* (2004). Evaluation of capture ELISA for detection of neutrophil cytoplasmatic antibodies directed against proteinase 3 in Wegener's granulomatosis: first results from a multicenter study. *Rheumatology* (Oxford), **43**, 174–80.

Daum, T. E., Specks, U., Colby, T. V., Edell, E. S., Brutinel, M. W., Prakash, U. B. and DeRemee, R. A. (1995). Transbronchial involvement in Wegener's granulomatosis. *American Journal of Respiratory and Critical Care Medicine*, **151**, 522–6.

de Groot, K., Gross, W. L., Herlyn, K. and Reinhold-Keller, E. (2001). Development and validation of a disease extent index for Wegener's granulomatosis. *Clinical Nephrology*, **55**, 31–8.

Del Buono, E. A. and Flint, A. (1991). Diagnostic usefulness of nasal biopsy in Wegener's granulomatosis. *Human Pathology*, **22**, 107–10.

DeRemee, R. A., McDonald, T. J., Harrison, E. G.J. R. and Coles, D. T. (1976). Wegener's granulomatosis. Anantomic correlates, a proposed classification. *Mayo Clinic Proceedings*, **51**, 777–81.

Devaney, K. O., Travis, W. D., Hoffman, G., Leavitt, R., Lebovics, R. and Fauci, A. S. (1990). Interpretation of head and neck biopsies in Wegener's granulomatosis. *American Journal of Surgical Pathology*, **14**, 555–64.

Dillon, M. J. (1998). Childhood vasculitis. *Lupus*, **7**, 259–65.

Eberhard, O. K., Haubitz, M., Brunkhorst, F. M., Kliem, V., Koch, K. M. and Brunkhorst, R. (1997). Usefulness of procalcitonin for differentiation between activity of systemic autoimmune disease (systemic lupus erythematosus/systemic antineutrophil cytoplasmic antibody-associated vasculitis) and invasive bacterial infection. *Arthritis and Rheumatism*, **40**, 1250–6.

Fauci, A. S., Haynes, B. F., Katz, P. and Wolff, S. M. (1983). Wegener's granulomatosis: Prospective clinical and therapeutic experience with 85 patients for 21 years. *Annals of Internal Medicine*, **98**, 76–85.

Fienberg, R. (1955). Pathergic granulomatosis. *American Journal of Medicine*, **19**, 829.

Frances, C., Huong Du, L. T., Piette, J. C., Saada, V., Boisnic, S., Wechsler, B., Bletry, O. and Godeau, P. (1994). Wegener's granulomatosis: dermatological manifestations in 75 cases with clinicopathologic correlation. *Archives of Dermatology*, **130**, 861.

Franssen, C., Gans, R., Kallenberg, C., Hageluken, C. and Hoorntje, S. (1998). Disease spectrum of patients with antineutrophil cytoplasmic autoantibodies of defined specificity: distinct differences between patients with anti-proteinase 3 and anti-myeloperoxidase autoantibodies. *Journal of Internal Medicine*, **244**, 209–16.

Gross, W. L. (1989). Wegener's granulomatosis. New aspects of the disease course, immunodiagnostic procedures and stage-adapted treatment. *Sarcoidosis*, **6**, 15–29.

Gross, W. L. and Csernok, E. (1995). Immunodiagnostic and pathophysiologic aspects of antineutrophil cytoplasmic antibodies in vasculitis. *Current Opinion in Rheumatology*, **7**, 11–19.

Gross, W. L., Lüdemann, G., Kiefer, G. and Lehmann, H. (1986). Anticytoplasmic antibodies in Wegener's granulomatosis. *Lancet*, **1**, 806.

Gross, W. L., Schnabel, A. and Trabandt, A. (2000). New perspectives in pulmonary angiitis. *Sarcoidosis*, **17**, 33–52.

Hagen, E. C., Andrassy, K., Csernok, E., Daha, M. R., Gaskin, G., Gross, W. L., Lesavre, P., Ludemann, J., Pusey, C. D., Rasmussen, N., Savage, C. O., Sinico, R. A., Wiik, A. and van der Woude, F. J. (1993a). The value of indirect immunofluorescence and solid phase techniques for ANCA detection. A report on the first phase of an international cooperative study on the standardization of ANCA assays. *Journal of Immunological Methods*, **159**, 1–16.

Hagen, E. C., Ballieux, B. E., van Es, L. A., Daham, M. R. and van der Woude, F. J. (1993b). Antineutrophil cytoplasmic autoantibodies: a review of the antigens involved, the assays, and the clinical and possible pathogenetic consequences. *Blood*, **81**, 1996–2002.

Hagen, E. C., Daha, M. R., Hermans, J., Andrassy, K., Csernok, E., Gaskin, G., *et al.*(1998). Diagnostic value of standardized assays for anti-neutrophil cytoplasmic antibodies in idiopathic systemic vasculitis. EC/BCR Project for ANCA Assay Standardization. *Kidney International*, **53**, 743–53.

Hall, S. L., Miller, L. C., Duggan, E., Mauer, S. M., Beatty, E. C. and Hellerstein, S. (1985). Wegener granulomatosis in pediatric patients. *Journal of Pediatrics*, **106**, 739–44.

Harman, L. E. and Margo, C. E. (1998). Wegener's granulomatosis. *Survey of Ophthalmology*, **42**, 458–80.

Hauer, H. A., Bajema, I. M., van Houwelingen, H. C., Ferrario, F., Noel, L. H., Waldherr, R., Jayne, D. R., Rasmussen, N., Bruijn, J. A. and Hagen, E. C. (2002). Renal histology in ANCA-associated vasculitis: differences between diagnostic and serologic subgroups. *Kidney International*, **61**, 80–9.

Hoffman, G. S. and Specks, U. (1998). Antineutrophil cytoplasmic antibodies. *Arthritis and Rheumatism*, **41**, 1521–37.

Holle, J. U., Hellmich, B., Backes, M., Gross, W. L. and Csernok, E. (2005). Variations in performance characteristics of commercial enzyme immunoassay kits of the detection of antineutrophil cytoplasmatic antibodies: What is the optimal cut-off? *Annals of the Rheumatic Diseases*, **64**, 1773–9.

Hunder, G. G., Arend, W. P., Bloch, D. A., Calabrese, L. H., Fauci, A. S., Fries, J. F., Leavitt, R. Y., Lie, J. T., Lightfoot, R. W., Jr. and Masi, A. T. (1990). The American College of Rheumatology 1990 criteria for the classification of vasculitis. Introduction. *Arthritis and Rheumatism*, **33**, 1065–7.

Jennette, J. C., Falk, R. J., Andrassy, K., Bacon, P. A., Churg, J., Gross, W. L., Hagen, E. C., Hoffman, G. S., Hunder, G. G., Kallenberg, C. G.M., McCluskey, R. T., Sinico, R. A., Rees, A. J., Van Es, L. A., Waldherr, R. and Wiik, A. (1994). Nomenclature of systemic vasculitides. Proposal of an International Consensus Conference. *Arthritis and Rheumatism*, **37**, 187–92.

Karjalainen, A. and Hakala, M. (1996). Still another case of Wegener's granulomatosis with a digital gangrene [letter]. *Scandinavian Journal of Rheumatology*, **25**, 339.

Kempf, H.-G. (1989). Ear involvement in Wegener's granulomatosis. *Clinical Otolaryngology*, **14**, 451–6.

Klinger, H. (1932). Grenzformen der Periarteritis nodosa. *Frankfurter Zeitschrift für Pathologie*, **42**, 455–80.

Langford, C. A. (2005). How can relapses be detected and prevented in primary systemic small-vessel vasculitides? *Best Practice and Research Clinical Rheumatology*, **19**, 307–20.

Leavitt, R. Y., Fauci, A. S., Bloch, D. A., Michel, B. A., Hunder, G. G., Arend, W. P., Calabrese, L. H., Fries, J. F., Lie, J. T., Lightfoot, R. W., Masi, A. T., McShane, D. J., Mills, J. A., Stevens, M. B., Wallace, S. L. and Zvaifler, N. J. (1990). The American College of Rheumatology 1990 criteria for the classification of Wegener's granulomatosis. *Arthritis and Rheumatism*, **33**, 1101–7.

Lie, J. T. (1990). Illustrated histopathologic classification criteria for selected vasculitis syndromes. *Arthritis and Rheumatism*, **33**, 1074–87.

Lombard, C. M., Duncan, S. R., Rizk, N. W. and Colby, T. V. (1990). The diagnosis of Wegener's granulomatosis from transbronchial biopsy specimens. *Human Pathology*, **21**, 838–42.

Luqmani, R. A., Bacon, P. A., Moots, R. J., Janssen, B. A., Pall, A., Emery, P., Savage, C. and Adu, D. (1994). Birmingham Vasculitis Activity Score (BVAS) in systemic necrotizing vasculitis. *Quarterly Journal of Medicine*, **87**, 671–8.

Matteson, E. L., Gold, K. N., Bloch, D. A. and Hunder, G. A. (1996). Long-term survival of patients with Wegener's granulomatosis from the American College of Rheumatology Wegener's granulomatosis classification criteria cohort. *American Journal of Medicine*, **101**, 129–34.

McHugh, K., Manson, D., Eberhard, B. A., Shore, A. and Laxer, R. M. (1991). Wegener's granulomatosis in childhood. *Pediatric Radiology*, **21**, 552–5.

Moosig, F., Csernok, E., Reinhold-Keller, E., Schmitt, W. H. and Gross, W. L. (1998). Elevated procalcitonin levels in active Wegener's granulomatosis. *Journal of Rheumatology*, **25**, 1531–3.

Muhle, C., Reinhold-Keller, E., Richter, C., Duncker, G., Beigel, A., Brinkmann, G., Gross, W. L. and Heller, M. (1997). MRI of the nasal cavity, the paranasal sinuses and orbits in Wegener's granulomatosis. *European Radiology*, **7**, 566–70.

Müller, A., Trabandt, A., Glöckner-Hofmann, K., Seitzer, U. and Csernok, E. (2000). Localized Wegener's granulomatosis: predominance of CD26 and IFN-g expression. *Journal of Pathology*, **192**, 113–20.

Nadeau, S. E. (1997). Diagnostic approach to central and peripheral nervous system vasculitis. *Neurologic Clinics*, **15**, 759–77.

Nishino, H., Rubino, F. A., DeRemee, A., Swanson, J. W. and Parisi, J. E. (1993). Neurological involvement in Wegener's granulomatosis: An analysis of 324 consecutive patients at the Mayo Clinic. *Annals of Neurology*, **33**, 4–9.

Pfister, H., Ollert, M., Frohlich, L. F., *et al.* (2004). Antineutrophil cytoplasmic autoantibodies against the murine homolog of proteinase 3 (Wegener autoantigen) are pathogenic in vivo. *Blood*, **104**, 1411–18.

Rao, J. K., Weinberger, M., Oddone, E. Z., Allen, N. B., Landsman, P., Feussner, J. R. (1995). The role of antineutrophil cytoplasmatic antibody (C-ANCA) testing in the diagnosis of Wegener granulomatosis. *Annals of Internal Medicine*, **123**, 925–32.

Rao, J. K., Allen, N. B. and Pincus, T. (1998). Limitations of the 1990 American College of Rheumatology classification criteria in the diagnosis of vasculitis. *Annals of Internal Medicine*, **129**, 345–52.

Reinhold-Keller, E., Kekow, J., Schnabel, A., Schmitt, W. H., Heller, M., Beigel, A., Duncker, G. and Gross, W. L. (1994). Influence of disease manifestation and antineutrophil cytoplasmic antibody titer in the response to pulse cyclophosphamide therapy in patients with Wegener's granulomatosis. *Arthritis and Rheumatism*, **37**, 919–24.

Reinhold-Keller, E., de Groot, K., Rudert, H., Nölle, B., Heller, M. and Gross, W. L. (1996). Response to trimethoprim/sulfamethoxazole in Wegener's granulomatosis depends on the phase of disease. *Quarterly Journal of Medicine*, **89**, 15–23.

Reinhold-Keller, E., Beuge, N., Latza, U., de Groot, K., Rudert, H., Nölle, B., Heller, M., Gross, W. L. (2000). An interdisciplinary approach to the care of patients with Wegener's granulomatosis. *Arthritis and Rheumatism*, **43**, 1021–32.

Reinhold-Keller, E., Herlyn, K., Wagner-Bastmeyer, R., Gross, W. L. (2005). Stable incidence of primary systemic vasculitides over five years: results from the German vasculitis register. *Arthritis and Rheumatism*, **53**, 93–9.

Reuter, M., Schnabel, A., Wesner, F., Tetzlaff, K., Rishcng, Y., Gross, W. L. and Heller, M. (1998). Pulmonary Wegener's granulomatosis: correlation between high-resolution CT findings and clinical scoring of disease activity. *Chest*, **114**, 500–6.

Rottem, M., Fauci, A. S., Hallahan, C. W., Kerr, G. S., Lebovics, R., Leavitt, R. Y. and Hoffman, G. S. (1993). Wegener granulomatosis in children and adolescents: Clinical presentation and outcome. *Journal of Pediatrics*, **122**, 26–31.

Savige, J., Gillis, D., Benson, E., Davies, D., Esnault, V., Falk, R. J., *et al.* (1999). international consensus statement on testing and reporting of antineutrophil cytoplasmic antibodies (ANCA). *American Journal of Clinical Pathology*, **111**, 507–13.

Schmitt, W. H., Heesen, C., Csernok, E., Rautmann, A. and Gross, W. L. (1992). Elevated serum levels of soluble inter- leukin-2 receptor in patients with Wegener's granulomatosis. *Arthritis and Rheumatism*, **35**, 1088–96.

Schnabel, A., Holl-Ullrich, K., Dalhoff, K., Reuter, M. and Gross, W. L. (1997). Efficacy of transbronchial biopsy in pulmonary vasculitides. *European Respiratory Journal*, **10**, 2738–43.

Schnabel, A., Reuter, M., Gloeckner, K., Müller-Querheim, J. and Gross, W. L. (1999). Bronchoalveolar lavage cell profiles in Wegener's granulomatosis. *Respiratory Medicine*, **93**, 498–506.

Schönermarck, U., Lamprecht, P., Csernok, E. and Gross, W. L. (2001). Prevalence and spectrum of rheumatic diseases associated with proteinase 3-antineutrophil cytoplasmic antibodies (ANCA) and myeloperoxidase-ANCA. *Rheumatology* (Oxford) **40**, 178–84.

Socias, R. and James, D. G. (1987). Wegener and Wegener's granulomatosis. *Thorax*, **42**, 920–21.

Stone, J. H., Hoffman, C. S., Merkel, P. A. *et al.* (2001). A disease-specific activity index for Wegener's granulomatosis: modification of the Birmingham Vasculitis Activity Score. International Network for the Study of the Systematic Vasculitides (INSSYS). *Arthritis and Rheumatism* **44**, 912–20.

Walton, E. W. (1958). Giant-cell granuloma of the respiratory tract (Wegener's granulomatosis). *British Medical Journal*, 265–9.

Wang, G., Hansen, H., Tatsis, E., Csernok, E. and Gross, W. L. (1997). High plasma levels of the soluble form of CD30 activation molecule reflect disease activity in patients with Wegener's granulomatosis. *American Journal of Medicine*, **101**, 517–23.

Watts, R. A., Carruthers, D. M. and Scott, D. G. I. (1995). Epidemiology of systemic vasculitis: Changing incidence or definition? *Seminars in Arthritis and Rheumatism*, **1**, 28–34. [Abstract]

Watts, R. A., Lane, S. E., Scott, D. G., *et al.* (2001). Epidemiology of vasculitis in Europe. *Annals of the Rheumatic Diseases*, **60**: 1156–7.

Watts, R. A., Lane, S. and Scott, D. G. I. (2005). What is known about the epidemiology of the vasculitides? Best Practice and Research. *Clinical Rheumatology*, **19**, 191–207.

Wegener, F. (1935). Über generalisierte, septische Gefässerkrankungen. *Verhandlungen der Deutschen Pathologischen Gesellschaft*, **29**, 202–10.

Wegener, F. (1939). Über eine eigenartige rhinogene Granulomatose mit besonderer Beteiligung des Arteriensystems und der Nieren. *Beiträge zur Pathologischen Anatomie und zur Allgemeinen pathologie*, **102**, 36–8.

Wegener, F. (1990). 50 years of Wegener's granulomatosis. *Immunität und Infektion*, **18**, 11–19.

Weiner, S. R., Paulus, H. E. and Weisbart, R. H. (1986). Wegener's granulomatosis in the elderly. *Arthritis and Rheumatism*, **29**, 1157–9.

Xiao, H., Heeringa, P., Hu, P., Liu, Z., Zhao, M., Aratani, Y., Maeda, N., Falk, R. J. and Jennette, J. C. (2002). Antineutrophil cytoplasmic autoantibodies specific for myeloperoxidase cause glomerulonephritis and vasculitis in mice. *Journal of Clinical Investigation*, **110**, 955–63.

CHAPTER 32

Wegener's granulomatosis: treatment

Bernhard Hellmich and Wolfgang L. Gross

Introduction

Wegener's granulomatosis (WG) is characterized by granulomatous inflammation primarily affecting the upper and lower respiratory tract, necrotizing vasculitis, and rapidly progressive glomerulonephritis (see Chapter 30). WG is a disease that can affect multiple organ systems at one time and has a variable clinical presentation (see Chapter 31), which can range from isolated granulomatous inflammation to generalized vasculitis. A treatment plan for an individual patient should be based primarily on the stage of disease (Table 32.1) and the current activity state (Table 32.2). Therefore, a thorough evaluation of the activity and extent of the clinical picture at the time of presentation and a basic understanding of the underlying immunopathogenetic processes are important requirements for formulating a treatment plan that is tailored to the needs of the individual patient (see Chapter 23).

Friedrich Wegener's first description of the disease was based on autopsy cases (Wegener 1939), reflecting the fact that WG generally had a fatal outcome prior to the advent of immunosuppressive therapy (Walton 1958). Although glucocorticoids are an integral part of any treatment regimen for WG, they are usually not sufficient for disease control when given alone. A comparison of historic cohorts shows that treatment with glucocorticoids alone prolongs the median 5-months survival of untreated patients (Walton 1958) by not more than half a year (Hollander et al. 1967). However, a retrospective chart review of 265 WG cases from the UK between 1975 and 1985 revealed that some patients can survive for several years without any treatment (Anderson et al. 1992). Walton recognized the variable course of the disease (Walton 1958).

Only the combination of glucocorticoids with cyclophosphamide (CYC), as first introduced by Fauci and Wolf in the early 1970s,

Table 32.1 Definitions for disease stages used for subclassification of patients with WG in clinical trials (D Jayne 2001, The WGET Research Group 2002)

Study group	Clinical subgroup	Systemic vasculitis outside ENT tract and lung	Threatened vital organ function	Other definitions	Serum creatinine (μmol/l)	Clinical trials using definition
EUVAS	Localized	no	no	No constitutional symptoms, ANCA typically negative	<120	
	Early systemic	yes	no	Constitutional symptoms present, ANCA positive or negative	<120	NORAM
	Generalized	yes	yes	ANCA positive	<500	CYCAZAREM
	Severe	yes	Organ failure	ANCA positive	>500	MEPEX
	Refractory	yes	yes	Refractory to standard therapy	any	SOLUTION
WGET Research Group/VCRC	Limited	allowed	no	No red blood cell casts, nor rise of creatinine >25 of baseline	≤124, if hematuria, but no red blood cell casts present	WEGET
	Severe	yes	yes	Any patient not classifiable as limited	any	WEGET

EUVAS, European Vasculitis Study Group; WGET, Wegener's granulomatosis etanercept trial; VCRC, vasculitis clinical research consortium

Table 32.2 Definitions for disease states used for assessment of outcome in WG (Jayne 2001, The WGET Research Group 2002)

Study group	Disease state	Definitions
EUVAS	Complete remission	Absence of any disease activity,[1] BVAS = 0
	Partial remission	Significant decrease of disease activity with persisting low grade activity believed to regress by continued treatment
	Minor relapse	Recurrent or new disease activity *not* threatening vital organs which is controllable by an increase of glucocorticoid dosage only
	Major relapse	Recurrent or new disease activity threatening vital organs or leading to functional impairment which usually requires reinstitution of cyclophospharide
WEGET Research Group/VCRC	Sustained remission	BVAS/WG of 0 for 6 months
	Low level of disease activity flare	BVAS/WG <3 for 6 months
		Increase of at least one point in BVAS/WG

[1] Clinical features, serology, and imaging. EUVAS, European Vasculitis Study Group; WGET, Wegener's granulomatosis etanercept trial; VCRC, vasculitis clinical research consortium; BVAS, Birmingham Vasculitis Activity Score; BVAS/WG, Birmingham Vasculitis Activity Score for Wegener's Granulomatosis.

has clearly prolonged survival, with median survival times of more than 20 years (Hoffman *et al.* 1992; Reinhold-Keller *et al.* 2000b). As the therapeutic efficacy of CYC is documented for any disease stage and activity state, daily oral CYC together with glucocorticoids is still the standard of care (so-called "NIH-standard" or "Fauci protocol") for severe generalized WG, although the substantial, long-term toxicity of this protocol limits its use. Therefore, alternative treatment strategies for less severe disease and maintenance of remission have been sought, including less toxic drugs such as methotrexate, azathioprine, or leflunomide. In recent years, efficacy of numerous alternative treatment approaches has been documented in clinical trials. New treatment modalities such as B cell blockade and neutralization of tumor necrosis factor-α (TNFα) have been used, based on a better understanding of the immunopathogenesis of WG.

Design and interpretation of therapeutic trials in WG: points to consider

Classification and definitions of disease stages

Only a few of the clinical trials in WG published to date have had a randomized, controlled design and have been sufficiently powered in size to allow a direct head-to-head comparison of two or more drugs. Therefore, recommendations for the treatment of WG are largely based on the evaluation of treatments across different clinical trials (such as evaluation of methotrexate or azathioprine for maintenance of remission). One basic requirement for such comparisons across clinical trials is a comparable trial methodology in the respective studies. This, however, was not the case in many recent studies.

Although in most studies both the vasculitis classification criteria of the American College of Rheumatology (ACR) and the definition of the Chapel Hill Consensus Conference (CHCC) for vasculitides were applied, investigators from both sides of the Atlantic have used divergent definitions for disease stages to classify patients with WG into clinical subgroups (Table 32.1). Furthermore, in some studies, patients with microscopic polyangiitis (MPA) or polyarteritis nodosa (PAN) were included. This can be problematic since outcome can be different between patients with WG and other ANCA-associated vasculitis, as shown for relapse rates in the CYCAZAREM trial (Jayne *et al.* 2003).

Outcome parameters and end points

Definitions of outcome parameters have not been uniform across clinical trials. Outcome is usually defined in terms of disease states such as remission or relapse (Table 32.1) and is quantified by the use of disease assessment instruments (see Chapter 23). In the past, complete remission was defined as the absence of any disease activity related to active WG. American investigators designing the WGET trial (see below) felt that, in addition, the disease should be inactive in the absence of glucocorticoid treatment for a specified period before a patient should be considered in complete remission (Table 32.2). Other investigators (EUVAS) allow the use of low-dose glucocorticoids in their definition of remission. Although a complete withdrawal of glucocorticoids is desirable, it seems questionable whether this is a realistic goal for all patients and whether it should be a common end point for clinical studies in WG, given the relatively high relapse rates during maintenance therapy without glucocorticoids.

Disease assessment tools

Disease activity of WG is quantified by disease assessment tools which record disease activity in different organ systems in specified item lists. Most frequently used are the Birmingham vasculitis activity score (BVAS) (Luqmani *et al.* 1994) and some of its variations (see Chapter 23). The BVAS/WG incorporates several items specific for WG (Stone *et al.* 2001a) while the BVAS 2003 is a further refinement of the initial BVAS. BVAS2, which documents persistent disease, is a modification of the original BVAS1 in which only new disease activity is captured. In contrast to the BVAS and its derivatives, the disease extent index (DEI) incorporates no subjective weighting by severity of manifestations, but is easier to use in trials and in everyday practice (de Groot *et al.* 2001b). Although differing in some items, preliminary results of a comparative multicenter case exercise by experienced investigators indicate that BVAS, BVAS 2003, BVAS WG, and the DEI are highly correlated (Merkel *et al.* 2004), suggesting that comparison of these assessment tools across clinical trials is possible to some extent. However, differences in disease assessment tools may still account for different findings across studies. Thus, a uniform and internationally accepted disease assessment tool in WG or ANCA-associated vasculitis is highly desirable and initiatives towards such consensus instruments involving the OMERACT process are in progress.

Differences in the frequency and intensity of clinical evaluations of patients during a clinical study may influence the reported outcomes. For example, a study in which there is close surveillance with frequent evaluation for subclinical disease using sensitive imaging procedures such as magnetic resonance imaging (MRI) or high resolution CT (HRCT) is likely to detect more disease flares in a specified period than a study in which such measures are not used. Furthermore, the assessment of certain symptoms is likely to vary among investigators. For example, the evaluation of granulomatous manifestations such as nasal crusting or retro-orbital granuloma is particularly challenging as it is often difficult to distinguish between damage ("scar tissue") and persistent low-grade activity (grumbling disease). In addition, the length of follow-up is crucial for the interpretation of relapse rates. Finally, concomitant treatments and glucocorticoids doses often contribute significantly to outcome, especially in uncontrolled observational studies. In summary, variations in trial design and particularly disease assessment are likely to have a major impact on reported outcomes in therapeutic trials in WG.

Approaches to therapy of WG

Current management of WG has been strongly influenced by the principles of study design in WG developed by the EUVAS study group and NIH investigators in the last century. The first aim is induction of remission, the next goal is maintenance of remission, and the final challenge lies in the treatment of refractory disease states.

Treatment for induction of remission during active disease (Table 32.3) is usually followed by less aggressive therapy for maintenance of remission (Table 32.4). Note that the categories of evidence and grades of recommendations for Tables 32.3, 32.4, and 32.5 are based on the study or studies with the highest level of evidence or grade of recommendations according to Shekelle et al. (1999) (See Table 32.6 for definitions). As detailed below, CYC is the treatment of choice for patients with active WG, but methotrexate (MTX)

may be substituted in less severe disease. However, preliminary results of the NORAM trial (de Groot et al. 2005b, see below) show that after withdrawal of treatment at 12 months, relapse rates at 18 months were 70% in the MTX arm and 45% in the CYC arm, suggesting that continued treatment for maintenance of remission is advisable. Given the high cumulative toxicity of CYC, treatment should be switched to less toxic agents such as MTX, azathioprine (AZA), or mycophenolate mofetil (MMF) as soon as remission is accomplished. In about 10% of cases, administration of CYC and glucocorticoids alone is insufficient to control disease activity completely. In these cases, additional therapy with biologic agents, plasmapheresis, or alternative treatments such as deoxyspergualin may be needed (Table 32.5).

Standard therapeutic regimes in WG

Glucocorticoids

It is generally accepted that glucocorticoids alone are insufficient to control active, generalized WG. In historic cohorts, glucocorticoid monotherapy prolonged median survival by only a few months (Hollander et al. 1967) compared to a median survival time of 5 months in the era prior to glucocorticoids (Walton 1958). Nevertheless, glucocorticoids given as an adjunct to other immunosuppressive agents (CYC, MTX, etc.) are a cornerstone in the treatment of active WG and for maintenance of remission. For induction of remission, 1 mg/kg prednisolone is given as a starting dose, together with CYC or MTX. In case of life- or organ-threatening disease, for example alveolar hemorrhage, rapidly progressive glomerulonephritis, etc., high-dose intravenous methylprednisolone (250–1000 mg/day on 3 consecutive days) should be added. The dosage is then tapered in increments of 5 to 10 mg/day according to the activity of the disease. In view of the predictable, long-term side effects of high-dose glucocorticoids, they should be tapered to as low a dose as possible. Therefore, a prednisolone dose near or below the Cushing threshold of 7.5 mg/day is desirable. Many patients report symptoms of active disease such as arthralgias when

Table 32.3 Recommendations for induction of remission in Wegener's granulomatosis

Protocol	Disease stage[3]	Dose	Category of evidence[4]	Grade of recommendations[4]	References
Cyclophosphamide (daily oral)[1]	Generalized	2 mg/kg/day p.o.	I-b	A	Fauci et al. 1983, Guillevin et al. 1997, Hoffman et al. 1992, Jayne et al. 2003, Reinhold-Keller et al. 2000b
Cyclophosphamide (pulse)[1]	Generalized	15-20 mg/kg i.v. every 3rd week	I-a	A	Adu et al. 1997, de Groot et al. 2001a, de Groot et al. 2005a,
Methotrexate[1]	Early systemic	0,3 mg/kg/week i.v., s.c. or p.o	I-b	A	de Groot et al. 1998, de Groot et al. 2005b, Sneller et al. 1995 Guillevin et al. 1997
Trimethoprim/ sulfamethoxazole	Localized	2 × 960 mg/day p.o.	II-a	A	Reinhold-Keller et al. 1996
Plasma exchange[2]	Severe	40–60 ml/kg (4-7×)	I-b	A	Gaskin et al. 2002

[1] Plus prednisone (starting dose 1mg/kg).

[2] Plus Cyclophosphamide (daily oral) and prednisone (starting dose 1mg/kg).

[3] For definitions of disease stages see Table 32.4.

[4] Based on the study(-ies) with the highest level of evidence or grade of recommendations according to Shekelle et al. (1999), see Table 32.6 for definitions.

Table 32.4 Recommendations for maintenance of remission in Wegener's granulomatosis

Protocol	Dose	Category of evidence[2]	Grade of recommendations[2]	References
Azathioprine[1]	2 mg/kg/day p.o.	I-b	A	Jayne et al. 2003
Methotrexate[1]	0.3 mg/kg/week. i.v./p.o.	I-b	A	de Groot et al. 1996, Langford et al. 1999, Metzler et al. 2005, Reinhold-Keller et al. 2002)
Leflunomide[1]	30–40 mg/day	I-b	A	Metzler et al. 2004, Metzler et al. 2005
Trimethoprim/ Sulfamethoxazole[1]	2 × 960 mg/day p.o.	I-b[3]	A[3]	Reinhold-Keller et al. 1996, Stegeman et al. 1996
Mycophenolate mofetil[1]	2 g/day	II-c	B	Haubitz et al. 2002, Langford et al. 2004, Nowack et al. 1999
Desoxyspergualin	0.5 mg/kg/day	III	C	Schmitt et al. 2005

[1]prednisone should have been tapered to ≤ 7.5 mg/d.

[2]based on the study(-ies) with the highest level of evidence or grade of recommendations according to Shekelle et al. (1999), see Table 32.6 for definitions.

[3]significantly reduced incidence of relapses for upper airway disease only.

glucocorticoids are completely withdrawn. Thus, it is often necessary to continue a low dose (5 mg or below) during the maintenance phase. In studies where glucocorticoids were rapidly withdrawn (as in the WGET study), relapse rates were surprisingly high (Wegener's Granulomatosis Etanercept (WGET) Research Group 2005).

Cyclophosphamide

Oral cyclophosphamide

Investigators at the NIH were the first to formally study the effects of CYC in combination with glucocorticoids in patients with WG (Fauci et al. 1983, 1973). They used CYC, 2 mg/kg/day orally, together with prednisone at an initial dose of 1 mg/kg/day to induce and maintain remission. In a cohort of 133 patients treated with this regimen at the NIH, 91% responded, with 75% of patients achieving complete remission (Hoffman et al. 1992). In a series of 155 patients treated at our institution, of which 92% received CYC as daily oral therapy (Modified NIH standard) and 4% as pulse therapy, 54% went into complete remission while in the

remaining 46% partial remission was accomplished (Reinhold-Keller et al. 2000b). Mortality related to WG or its therapy was 13% in the NIH study and 12% in our cohort during a mean follow-up of approximately 8 and 7 years, respectively. The relapse rate in patients followed for at least 5 years was somewhat higher in our cohort (71%) than in the NIH cohort (50%) (Hoffman et al. 1992; Reinhold-Keller et al. 2000b). This may be a consequence of extended administration of CYC for maintenance of remission in the NIH cohort. Due to the lack of alternative treatments at that time, combination therapy was used in many cases, resulting in a high cumulative dose of both CYC and glucocorticoids and a resultant high degree of treatment-related morbidity and mortality.

The extended use of CYC is often limited by serious morbidity including infections, leukopenia related to bone marrow failure, infertility, and hemorrhagic cystitis. Beside the risk of hemorrhagic cystitis, a large body of evidence suggests that administration of cyclophosphamide is linked to a 9- to 45-fold increased risk for bladder cancer in WG patients (Hellmich et al. 2004; Hoffman et al. 1992; Knight et al. 2002; Reinhold-Keller et al. 2000a; Talar-Williams

Table 32.5 Recommendations for treatment of refractory disease in Wegener's granulomatosis

Protocol	Dose	Category of evidence[2]	Grade of recommendations[2]	References
Intravenous immunoglobulin	5 × 400 mg/kg i.v.	I-b	A	Jayne et al. 2000
Etanercept[1]	25 mg twice weekly	II-c	B	Stone et al. 2001b
Infliximab[1]	5 mg/kg twice monthly	II-c	B	Booth et al. 2004, Lamprecht et al. 2002b
Rituximab[1]	375 mg/m[2]/week for 4 weeks	III	B	Keogh et al. 2005a
Desoxyspergualin	0.5 mg/kg/day	II-c	B	Birck et al. 2003
Azathioprine (pulse)	1200 mg i.v. monthly, 2 mg/kg in weeks 2 and 3	III	B	Aries et al. 2004
Antithymocyte globulin (ATG)	5 mg/kg i.v. for 10 days	III	C	Schmitt et al. 2004

[1]plus standard therapy (cyclophosphamide and prednisone).

[2]based on the study or studies with the highest level of evidence or grade of recommendations according to Shekelle et al. (1999), see Table 32.6 for definitions.

Table 32.6 Categorization of evidence and recommendations according to Shekelle *et al.* 1999

Category of evidence	Strength of recommendations
Ia Evidence from metaanalysis of randomized controlled trials	**A** Directly based on category I evidence
Ib Evidence from at least one randomized controlled trial	
IIa Evidence from at least one controlled study without randomisation	**B** Directly based on category II evidence or extrapolated recommendation form category I evidence
IIb Evidence from at least one other type of quasi-experimental study	
III Evidence form non-experimental descriptive studies, and case–control studies	**C** Directly based on category III evidence or extrapolated recommendation from category I or II evidence
IV Evidence form expert committee reports or opinions or clinical experience of respected authorities, or both	**D** Directly based on category IV evidence or extrapolated recommendation from category I, II or III evidence

et al. 1996). In a large cohort of 1065 patients with WG from Sweden, Knight and coworkers reported a 31-fold relative risk and a cumulative risk of 3% at 10 years and 10% at 15 years after treatment with cyclophosphamide (Knight *et al.* 2002). Interestingly, eight patients in this cohort had a diagnosis of bladder cancer *before* WG was diagnosed, resulting in a relative risk of 2.1 (95% CI 0.6–3.6) compared to the expected prevalence of bladder cancer in Sweden (Knight *et al.* 2004). This finding further substantiates earlier observations of our group suggesting that WG is associated with cancer (such as renal cell carcinoma) (Tatsis *et al.* 1999). Although epidemiologic studies have not yet shown a clear cut-off, the risk of cyclophosphamide-associated malignancies appears to increase substantially at cumulative cyclophosphamide doses above 100 g.

In view of the fact that long-term toxicity of CYC is correlated with the cumulative doses, approaches to limit the total exposure to CYC have been studied. Cumulative CYC doses can be limited by either shortening the period of oral CYC therapy or alternatively by using pulse therapy. The former strategy was the subject of study in the CYCAZAREM trial conducted by the EUVAS (Jayne *et al.* 2003). Patients with a diagnosis of ANCA-associated vasculitis (N = 155), of which 61% had WG, and who went into remission after treatment with CYC, 2 mg/kg, and glucocorticoids for 3 to 6 months were randomized to either continue CYC therapy for a total of 12 months or to receive azathioprine as a substitute for CYC. After 12 months, the CYC group was also switched to AZA and followed for an additional 6 months. Relapse rates during the 18-month period were similar for the long-term (13.7%) compared to the short-term CYC group (15.5%). Given the increased risk of toxicity with prolonged CYC administration, results of the CYCAZAREM trial suggest that CYC exposure should be limited to phases of active disease and should be replaced by a less toxic therapy as soon as remission is accomplished.

Pulse cyclophosphamide

The intermittent application of intravenous pulses is an alternative strategy to reduce the cumulative CYC dose. To date, results of five prospective trials on the efficacy of pulse CYC therapy in WG have been published, of which three had a randomized design (Adu *et al.* 1997; Guillevin *et al.* 1997; Haubitz *et al.* 1998). None of these trials was sufficiently sized to permit confident conclusions regarding the efficacy of pulse versus oral CYC. Furthermore, the inclusion of patients with MPA and PAN in two of the three randomized trials represents an important confounding factor for the efficacy analysis, as it has been shown in the CYCAZAREM that patients with WG relapsed more frequently (18%) than patients with MPA (8%) (Jayne *et al.* 2003). A meta-analysis of the above-mentioned three randomized trials indicated that compared to daily oral CYC, pulse CYC appeared to be similarly effective in inducing remission with less adverse events (de Groot *et al.* 2001a); however, relapse rates tended to be higher with intermittent pulse therapy.

In view of the methodological limitations of the above mentioned studies, results from a sufficiently large randomized, controlled trial (CYCLOPS) conducted by the EUVAS are highly anticipated. In the CYCLOPS trial, 160 patients with previously untreated "generalized" but not life-threatening ANCA-associated vasculitis (AAV) were randomized to either continuous oral or intermittent pulse CYC, each combined with equivalent doses of glucocorticoids (de Groot *et al.* 2005a). Three months after successful induction of remission, therapy was switched to AZA and glucocorticoids. The primary end point was the time from remission until the first relapse (disease-free period). According to the recently presented preliminary survival analysis of CYCLOPS, disease-free periods did not differ significantly between the two treatment arms (de Groot *et al.* 2005a). On an intention-to-treat basis, the cumulative CYC doses were twice as high in the oral as they were in the pulse group (de Groot *et al.* 2005a). Although these preliminary data sound promising, it seems premature to conclude that pulse CYC can safely replace oral daily CYC until a complete data report from CYCLOPS, including subgroup analyses for patients with WG, is published.

Practice points: cyclophosphamide

Taken together, these data and the daily experience in vasculitis centers suggest that CYC and glucocorticoids according to the protocol used by investigators at the US National Institutes of Health (NIH), the so-called NIH protocol, is still the standard therapy to induce remission in WG. This treatment schedule is mostly used only for 3 to 6 months and will then be switched to AZA (according to CYCAZAREM) in order to maintain remission for an additional 18 to 24 months. If there is no renal insufficiency or if there are contraindications to AZA, for example intolerance, drug fever, etc., then MTX or LEF can be used instead of AZA.

Methotrexate

Two open label studies and one randomized trial evaluated the efficacy of MTX as a potentially less toxic alternative for induction treatment in WG (de Groot *et al.* 1998, 2005b; Sneller *et al.* 1995). In the two prospective, open-label studies, MTX was given at doses of ~0.3 mg/kg/week, in combination with glucocorticoids, to patients with WG who did not have life-threatening disease and who had normal or nearly normal renal function. Successful induction of remission was seen in 10 of 17 (59%) and 33 of 42 patients (79%), respectively.

In a prospective, unblinded and controlled trial (NORAM), 100 patients with AAV, of which 89 (94%) had WG, and who did not have life- or organ-threatening disease, were randomized to treatment with either MTX at a target dose of 20–25 mg/week or daily oral CYC (2 mg/kg). After 12 months from study entry therapy was stopped in both treatment arms and no maintenance treatment was given. Results of the NORAM trial show that MTX can be nearly as effective as CYC, with remission rates of 89.8% for MTX and 93.5% for CYC (de Groot *et al.* 2005b). Time to remission was also similar in the MTX and CYC groups; however, relapse rates at 6 months after discontinuation of therapy were high for both the MTX (69.5%) and CYC (46.5%) groups. Thus, a major lesson of the NORAM trial is that some form of immunosuppressive treatment should be continued beyond 12 months for maintenance of remission. MTX did not have fewer serious adverse events during the 18-months study period, but a favorable toxicity profile of MTX compared to CYC is likely to emerge at a later time point, as long-term CYC toxicity is observed after years of treatment. A long-term follow-up study by the EUVAS to address the important issue of late adverse events and long-term outcome is in progress.

The unfavorable relapse rates observed in the NORAM trial highlights the need for maintenance therapy in WG. Two standardised, randomized open-label trials have investigated the efficacy of MTX for maintenance of remission in WG after successful induction of remission with oral CYC (Langford *et al.* 1999, 2003; Reinhold-Keller *et al.* 2002). In a series of 71 patients followed for a mean period of 24 months at our center, 26 relapses (36%) were seen after a mean of 19 months when prednisolone was tapered to a very low dose (<5 mg/d) (Reinhold-Keller *et al.* 2002). Of note, an unexpectedly high rate of kidney involvement (in a few cases with organ-threatening rapidly progressive glomerulonephritis (RPGN) was seen in 16 of 26 relapses (61%) (Reinhold-Keller *et al.* 2002). In a study conducted by Langford and coworkers, 22 relapses were seen in 42 patients (52%) studied during a median follow-up period of 32 months (Langford *et al.* 2003). No reliable parameters to predict relapse in MTX-treated patients emerged from either study. Compared to CYC, adverse events from MTX were rare in both studies. The administration of folic acid during MTX therapy has been shown to reduce the frequency of adverse events in patients with rheumatoid arthritis and is thus recommended in WG patients.

Practice points: methotrexate

MTX and glucocorticoids can be used in early systemic WG to induce remission (according to NORAM) when there is no kidney involvement or renal insufficiency. MTX should be used for maintenance of remission and doses of glucocorticoids lowered (<7.5 mg/day). Close follow-up is mandatory to detect relapses as early as possible.

Azathioprine

Results of the CYCAZAREM trial have convincingly demonstrated the potency of AZA to prevent relapses in patients with WG (Jayne *et al.* 2003), as outlined above. The French vasculitis study group recently presented preliminary data from a prospective, multicenter, randomized trial comparing AZA (2 mg/kg/day) versus MTX (0.3 mg/kg/week) for maintenance of remission in 114 patients with WG or MPA following successful induction of remission with CYC pulses (Mahr *et al.* 2005). Relapse rates 36 months after diagnosis were reported to be 33% for MTX and 41% for AZA,

suggesting that these agents are similarly effective in maintenance of remission (Mahr *et al.* 2005). A trend towards a higher frequency of treatment-related adverse events in the MTX arm was reported (Mahr *et al.* 2005).

Recent data show that AZA induces apoptosis of T cells via modulation of RAC-1 activation upon CD28 stimulation (Tiede *et al.* 2003). These experimental data raise interest in whether AZA might be a valuable drug not only for maintenance therapy but also for active WG, where activated T cells play a central role. Controlled studies investigating AZA as induction therapy for WG have not been reported. Retrospective observation in a small number of subjects did not indicate that oral AZA (2 mg/kg) was effective in inducing remission (Fauci *et al.* 1983). Interestingly, recent observations suggest that intermittent administration of high doses of AZA may be effective for refractory cases of WG. We treated two patients with WG and refractory granulomatous manifestations, particularly retro-orbital disease, who had not responded to therapy with CYC, infliximab, and rituximab. AZA was given in intravenous pulses (1200 mg/day) once per month and at a daily oral dose of 100 mg in weeks 2 and 3 between each i.v. pulse (Aries *et al.* 2004). Regression of granulomatous disease was seen in both patients after the second AZA pulse with additional improvement seen later (Aries *et al.* 2004). Two additional patients with refractory WG were treated with pulse AZA at our center, with clear clinical benefit seen in one and lack of efficacy in the other. Benenson and colleagues treated four patients with active WG with a similar regimen of pulse AZA (1200–1800 mg/month) (Benenson *et al.* 2005). Successful induction of remission was reported in two patients, while AZA had to be withdrawn in the remaining two patients due to persistent disease (Benenson *et al.* 2005). No severe adverse events were reported in either of the two small cohorts.

Practice points: azathioprine

AZA is the only agent to date that has been shown in a randomized, controlled trial (CYCAZAREM) to maintain remission following induction treatment with CYC in generalized WG. A role of AZA for the induction of remission has not yet been established.

Leflunomide

Leflunomide (LEF) inhibits *de novo* pyrimidine synthesis and inhibits responses of activated T and B cells. In a phase II, open-label clinical trial, LEF (30 mg/day) was given to 20 patients with WG for maintenance of remission following CYC induction therapy (Metzler *et al.* 2004). During a median follow-up of 21 months only one major relapse requiring reinstitution of CYC was recorded (Metzler *et al.* 2004). Eight minor flares were successfully treated by increasing the LEF dose to 40 mg/day. In a multicenter, randomised, controlled clinical trial (the LEM trial) by the German rheumatology network the potency of LEF (30 mg/day) to prevent relapses in patients with WG after successful induction of remission with CYC was compared to MTX (20 mg weekly). The first results of that trial were recently reported and show a significantly higher rate of severe relapses in the MTX limb (n = 7) compared to the LEF limb (n = 1) (Metzler *et al.* 2005). The study was therefore prematurely terminated. Adverse events (hypertension, neuropathy, leukopenia) necessitated withdrawal of LEF in four of 26 patients (Metzler *et al.* 2005). The dose escalation scheme used for MTX may partially account for the higher relapse rate in the MTX arm.

Practice points: leflunomide

The available preliminary results of the LEM trial suggest that LEF warrants further investigation as a drug for maintenance therapy of WG. In clinical practice, LEF can be used as an alternative treatment for maintenance of remission if AZA or MTX are contraindicated or have previously failed to maintain remission.

Mycophenolate mofetil

The safety and efficacy of MMF for maintenance of remission has been evaluated in three small, open-label clinical trials including five to 14 patients with AAV (Haubitz et al. 2002; Langford et al. 2004; Nowack et al. 1999). In the study by Nowak and coworkers only one relapse in 11 patients was seen during a follow up time of 15 months. In contrast, in the study by Langford and coworkers, six of 14 patients relapsed during a median 18 month of follow-up. Dosage and duration of CYC therapy for induction of remission as well as MMF dosage (2 g/day) was similar in both studies. However, differences in glucocorticoid therapy may account for the divergent outcome, as in the study by Langford and colleagues glucocorticoid were completely discontinued after a median of 8 months while in the study by Nowak et al. a median dose of 5 mg prednisolone was maintained. Tolerability of MMF was reported to be good in both studies. However, in a small series of five patients with AAV and end-stage renal disease, MMF doses of >1 g were not well tolerated, with anemia, leukopenia, and gastrointestinal symptoms being the most frequently reported adverse events (Haubitz et al. 2002).

Practice points: mycophenolate mofetil

Overall, as published data on MMF in AAV are limited and derived from non-randomized trials, MMF can be regarded as an agent of second choice for maintenance of remission only if other better established treatments (MTX, AZA, LEF) fail, are not tolerated, or are contraindicated. Given the promising results of the open-label studies mentioned above, the first results of a recently completed, randomized, controlled trial by the EUVAS comparing MMF and AZA for maintenance of remission in AAV (IMPROVE) are greatly anticipated (Jayne 2001).

Trimethoprim/sulfamethoxazole

The use of trimethoprim/sulfamethoxazole (T/S) in WG was first introduced by DeRemee in 1985 (DeRemee et al. 1985) and has since been studied for its potential to induce and maintain remission. In a prospective, open-label clinical trial, T/S was given to 72 patients with WG and different disease stages (Reinhold-Keller et al. 1996). Treatment with T/S induced partial or complete remission, which lasted for a median of 43 months, in 11 of 19 patients (58%) with localized WG (Reinhold-Keller et al. 1996). Of the remaining eight patients, five showed local disease progression, and three progressed to generalized disease. In contrast, neither T/S alone nor in combination with glucocorticoids induced sustained remissions among patients with generalized WG.

The efficacy of T/S for maintenance of remission following standard therapy has been evaluated in a prospective, randomized, placebo-controlled clinical trial (Stegeman et al. 1996). After 24 months, relapse rates in the T/S group were lower (18%) than the placebo group (40%). Subgroup analyses revealed that only relapses in the ENT region were significantly reduced by T/S while relapses in all major organ systems were not prevented.

Practice Points: T/S

T/S can only be recommended in patients with localized disease restricted to the upper respiratory tract who do not show signs of rapid disease progression or destructive disease.

Treatment of refractory WG

Standard CYC therapy fails to induce remission in up to 25% of patients with WG. In refractory patients on pulse CYC, a switch to the daily oral dose (2 mg/kg) is sometimes successful, possibly related to the higher cumulative doses applied. Until recently, the use of an intensified CYC protocol (3–4 mg/kg/day for a few days) was recommended for patients refractory to daily oral CYC (2 mg/kg) (Fauci et al. 1983). However, as Fauci and Wolf emphasized in their first report in 1973, the induction of neutropenia is not necessary for a favorable response to CYC (Fauci et al. 1973), but is associated with a high risk for infections (Bradley et al. 1989). In fact, the use of this intensified CYC protocol is associated with a substantially higher incidence of severe adverse events, particularly bone marrow suppression and infections. Therefore, the use of alternative regimens such as biologic agents or plasmapheresis, which are outlined below, should be considered in cases of refractory WG.

TNF blockade

In contrast to RA or ankylosing spondylitis, TNFα has not been convincingly demonstrated to be a key player in the pathogenesis of WG. Nonetheless, in view of its central role in the mediation of systemic inflammatory responses in general, several recent studies have evaluated the efficacy of TNF blockade in AAV. Etanercept, a soluble TNFα inhibitor consisting of two extracellular p75 TNFα receptor domains linked to the Fc portion of human IgG1, was found to be effective in an open-label, prospective trial involving patients with refractory WG (Stone et al. 2001b). Based on these positive data, a randomized, placebo-controlled trial (WGET) to evaluate etanercept for maintenance of remission in 180 patients was conducted (WGET Research Group 2002). Etanercept was given in addition to standard therapy, which was tapered and finally discontinued with only etanercept remaining as the sole maintenance therapy (WGET Research Group 2002). Overall, results of the WGET trial were disappointing. The rate of sustained remissions, the primary end point of WGET, was similar in etanercept-treated patients and controls (WGET Research Group 2005). Furthermore, the risk of disease flares, the periods of low disease activity (BVAS/WG <3 for 6 months) and the number of adverse events were similar in both groups. Given the large number of well-defined patients of WG and the strength of the randomized, placebo-controlled design, the results of WGET suggest that etanercept is of little value for maintenance of remission with concomitant immunosuppressive therapy.

However, based on the WGET data alone, it seems premature and inappropriate to exclude the possibility that etanercept or other TNF-blocking agents may be useful in the treatment of WG, based on the following reasons. First, a TNF-blocking agent can only work in situations where TNFα production is increased. This is the case during active disease rather than during remission, making a beneficial effect of etanercept for maintenance therapy less likely. Second, cyclophosphamide and glucocorticoids can effectively abolish TNFα secretion in patients with WG within 2 weeks (Lamprecht et al. 2002a). Thus, in patients responding to

CYC and glucocorticoids, addition of a TNF-blocking agent has little chance of additional benefit. Given the fact that 75–100% of patients with WG respond to standard therapy with CYC or MTX (de Groot *et al.* 2005a; Hoffman *et al.* 1992; Jayne *et al.* 2003; Reinhold-Keller *et al.* 2000b), at best only 20 out of the 89 patients in the etanercept arm of WGET might have had benefit from addition of etanercept (with regard to induction of remission). Twenty evaluable patients seems too small a group to observe a potential therapeutic effect. As noted above, experimental data (Lamprecht *et al.* 2002a) suggest that TNF blockade might have a positive effect in refractory patients with active disease, and presumably continuously elevated TNFα production, despite standard therapy. This finding might explain the divergent outcomes of the initial pilot trial, which included patients with refractory disease; the randomized trial included only previously untreated patients. Third, data obtained on the efficacy of etanercept may not be applicable to other TNF-blocking agents. For example, infliximab, a monoclonal chimeric anti-TNFα antibody, was shown to effectively induce remission in Crohn's disease, but etanercept has little efficacy (Akobeng *et al.* 2004). Although both agents neutralize TNFα effectively, differential effects on the immune system have been demonstrated, which may account for divergent clinical effects. For example, infliximab is more potent than etanercept at binding to peripheral and lamina propria T cells and inducing apoptosis (Van den Brande *et al.* 2003). It has been suggested that these data may provide a biological basis for the difference in clinical efficacy of the two TNFα-neutralizing drugs.

In three open-label clinical trials involving six, eight, and 32 patients with AAV who were refractory to standard therapy, infliximab, given at doses of 3–5 mg/kg in 2 to 8-week intervals, was found to be effective (Bartolucci *et al.* 2002; Booth *et al.* 2004; Lamprecht *et al.* 2002b). In the largest of these trials, however, two deaths and seven serious infections were noted (Booth *et al.* 2004), highlighting the importance of close monitoring and cautious use of such intensive immunosuppression. Due to the difficulties in controlling for potential effects of concomitant immunosuppressive therapies in open-label trials, a well-designed, randomized, controlled clinical trial to evaluate the efficacy of infliximab in patients with WG would be highly desirable.

Practice points: TNF-blockade

Available data indicate a differential role of etanercept and infliximab on granulomatous inflammation as in WG. While the WGET study did not confirm a role for etanercept in the treatment of non-refractory WG, open-label studies suggest an effect of infliximab in refractory WG. Therefore, in clinical practice the administration of three pulses of infliximab (5 mg/kg) given at 2-week intervals may be given to patients with WG who are unresponsive to CYC and glucocorticoids alone. If there is a good response, infliximab may be continued until prednisolone is tapered to a dose below 10 mg/day. The high risk of infectious and other serious complications associated with this intensive immunosuppression warrants close clinical monitoring.

Rituximab

Several lines of evidence suggest a pathogenetic role of ANCA in the pathogenesis of WG (see Chapters 7 and 30). Preliminary data suggest that B cells are present in early granulomatous lesions in nasal tissue in WG. Therefore, B cells, the precursors of ANCA-producing plasma cells, are an interesting target of therapy in WG (see Chapter 43). Rituximab is a chimeric monoclonal antibody directed against the CD20 molecule on the surface of B lymphocytes. In an open-label study evaluating the efficacy of rituximab in patients with AAV (10 of whom had WG) refractory to CYC or with contraindications for its use, remission was induced in all 11 patients after 4 doses of rituximab (375 mg/m^2) given weekly (Keogh *et al.* 2005a). This was accompanied by a decrease in ANCA titers and depletion of peripheral blood B cells (Keogh *et al.* 2005a). Since all patients received concomitant high-dose glucocorticoids and three patients were also treated with plasma exchange, it is difficult to determine the extent of contribution of rituximab. In three patients with an asymptomatic rise in ANCA titers, a second course of rituximab failed to induce a significant decline in ANCA titers (Keogh *et al.* 2005a). It has thus been speculated that ANCA in WG may be produced by long-lived plasma cells which do not express CD20 and thus would be unaffected by rituximab therapy (Sneller 2005). The group at the Mayo Clinic reported a second series of 10 patients with WG refractory to CYC and glucocorticoids treated with four infusions of rituximab (375 mg/m^2) given weekly and oral prednisone (1 mg/kg/d) in a prospective, open-label study (Keogh *et al.* 2005b). All patients achieved complete remission at 3 months and glucocorticoids were tapered at 6 months. In seven patients with WG and two patients with MPA, rituximab was given together with various conventional immunosuppressive drugs and successful induction of remission was reported in all cases (Eriksson 2005); however, in another eight patients with refractory WG and predominantly granulomatous disease, administration of rituximab in addition to standard therapy failed to induce clinical improvement in the majority of patients (Aries *et al.* 2005). Efficacy in vasculitis, but not granulomatous retro-orbital disease or sinusitis was confirmed in another report on two patients (Omdal *et al.* 2005).

Practice points: rituximab

Since treatment options for patients with refractory WG are limited, four infusions of rituximab (375 mg/m^2) given weekly can be used as an alternative to a rescue treatment with infliximab. There are not sufficient data to conclude which of the two alternatives is the better. In view of the limited and partially conflicting data, results of an ongoing randomized, controlled trial evaluating rituximab therapy in patients with AAV (RAVE) will be needed in order to define a potential role of this drug in the therapy of WG.

Intravenous immunoglobulin

Although early case reports and case series suggested that intravenous immunoglobulin (IVIg) might be effective in patients with refractory WG, there are few data from clinical trials confirming this impression. In an open-label study in 15 patients with WG who were refractory to CYC and glucocorticoids, a clinical response to IVIg was seen in 40% of cases, but no patient reached complete remission (Richter *et al.* 1995). In a series of six previously untreated patients with AAV, of whom three had WG without severe organ involvement, clinical improvement was seen in all and complete remission in two patients following administration of IVIg at a dose of 500 mg/kg/day for 4 consecutive days. Results from a small, randomized, double-blind, placebo-controlled study in 34 patients with AAV, including 24 patients with WG, suggest that IVIg (400 mg/kg/day for 4 consecutive days) had a significant but modest effect on disease persisting despite conventional immunosuppressive therapy (Jayne *et al.* 2000). Clinical improvement defined as a reduction of BVAS scores of 50% or more was seen in 14 of 17 patients in the IVIg arm and six of 17 in the placebo arm. Arthritis/arthralgias, ENT, and pulmonary symptoms as well as peripheral neuropathy were the manifestations that primarily responded to IVIg therapy. Overall, results of this study suggest that IVIg can be a reasonable adjunct to standard therapy in patients with persistent disease but without severe organ dysfunction. Because patients with glomerulonephritis and severe lung disease were not included (Jayne *et al.* 2000), the efficacy of IVIg in such patients remains uncertain.

15-Deoxyspergualin

15-Deoxyspergualin (DSG) is a synthetic analogue of spergualin, a natural product of the bacterium *Bacillus lactosporus*. Although its exact mechanism of action remains obscure, DSG has immunosuppressive properties and is licensed in Japan for treatment of recurrent kidney transplant rejection. In an open-label, pilot study up to six cycles of DSG were given to 20 patients with AAV, 19 of whom had WG unresponsive to, or with contraindications to, conventional immunosuppressive drugs (Birck *et al.* 2003). A clinical response to DSG was seen in 70% of patients, with six of 20 patients attaining complete remission (Birck *et al.* 2003). In four of these patients and three additional patients with WG, DSG was given on a long-term basis for an average of 26 months and a relapse-free disease course was reported in all seven patients (Schmitt *et al.* 2005). Currently, a larger multicenter phase II trial evaluating the efficacy and safety of DSG in refractory WG is in progress.

Specific therapies for organ failure

Plasmapheresis for renal failure and alveolar hemorrhage

Preliminary results of a multicenter randomized controlled study (MEPEX) indicate that plasmapheresis, compared to methylprednisolone pulses, may lead to higher rates of renal recovery and dialysis independence in patients with AAV (Gaskin and Jayne 2002). The overall mortality reported in that study was still high, possibly reflecting the severe disease in this patient subgroup with severely impaired renal function. Final results of the MEPEX trial are expected to be available soon. A retrospective review of 20 patients with diffuse alveolar hemorrhage who received plasmapheresis as an adjunct to intensive immunosuppressive therapy reported good recovery from alveolar bleeding in all patients (Klemmer *et al.* 2003).

Renal transplantation

Retrospective studies from several centers indicate that the survival and graft function of patients with WG after renal transplantation is comparable to other non-diabetic patients (Deegens *et al.* 2003; Elmedhem *et al.* 2003; Schmitt *et al.* 1993). Immunosuppressive therapy after transplantation was not uniform in the different cohorts and consisted of cyclosporine A, AZA, glucocorticoids, or combinations of these drugs. Extrarenal flares can occur despite immunosuppression, but recurrence of WG in the kidney allografts is rare and mild. Therefore, renal transplantation should be offered to patients with WG who progress to end-stage renal disease.

Subglottic stenosis

Subglottic stenosis occurs in about 20% of patients with WG. In a series of 43, seen at the NIH, the diagnosis of subglottic stenosis was made when no disease activity of WG was seen at other sites (Langford *et al.* 1996). Systemic immunosuppressive therapy often has little or no effect on subglottic stenosis, suggesting that scarring contributes to the progressive narrowing. Ten of 18 patients in the NIH cohort who were receiving immunosuppressive agents subsequently required tracheostomy (Langford *et al.* 1996). Intralesional injection of methylprednisolone into the stenotic segment, followed by microsurgical lysis of the stenotic ring and serial dilatation was reported to prevent tracheostomy in a series of 21 patients with WG (Hoffman *et al.* 2003). This therapeutic approach is therefore recommended before surgical tracheostomy is performed. In the rare event of severe bronchial narrowing with atelectasis, endobronchial placement of stents can prevent respiratory failure (Hellmich *et al.* 2003).

Prophylaxis and treatment of complications

The high rate and severity of adverse effects of drugs commonly used in the treatment of WG warrants close monitoring and, for certain drugs, specific prophylaxis (Table 32.7). Although prophylactic therapies reduce the incidence of complications, patient education is also important. Specific educational courses can help patients to learn about the symptoms and prophylaxis of the most frequent adverse events of drugs used in the treatment of WG. In addition to patient education the following measures are recommended:

Pneumocystis carinii prophylaxis

Patients with WG are at a particularly high risk to acquire *Pneumocystis carinii* pneumonia (PCP); mortality rates over 35% have been reported (Ognibene *et al.* 1995; Sneller 1998). The largest retrospective review of PCP cases in patients with autoimmune disease revealed that 8.9 of 1000 hospitalizations of patients with WG are caused by PCP (Ward *et al.* 1999). Lymphopenia (<1000 cells/mm^3) caused by CYC therapy and high glucocorticoid doses have been identified as the two major risk factors for PCP (Sowden *et al.* 2004). Patients with a CD4+ T cell count of <200 cells/mm^3 and a glucocorticoid dose of >15 mg prednisolone equivalent or duration of treatment greater than 3 months are at particularly high risk for PCP (Sowden *et al.* 2004). Although there are no prospective studies on the use of PCP prophylaxis in patients with WG, we recommend the administration of cotrimoxazole three times weekly during induction therapy with CYC, a regimen for prophylaxis that it is in common use in many centers. Furthermore, it has been suggested that PCP prophylaxis be continued independent of current treatment in patients with CD4+ counts of <200 cells/mm^3 (Sowden *et al.* 2004). Although full doses of cotrimoxazole increase the risk of adverse events in MTX-treated patients, the recommended trice-weekly dose can be administered safely (Sneller *et al.* 1995). In sulfa allergic patients, inhaled pentamidine 300 mg every 3 to 4 weeks may be used (Table 32.7).

Osteoporosis prophylaxis

In view of the often extended need for glucocorticoid, a risk assessment for the development of glucocorticoid-induced osteoporosis is advisable, which ideally should include bone density

Table 32.7 Frequently used drugs for treatment of WG: adverse effects, monitoring, prophylaxis

Medication	Common adverse effects (expected frequency)	Monitoring	Prophylaxis
Glucocorticoids (GC)	Osteoporosis[1]	Dual-X-ray absorptiometry (in case of other risk factors and/or high cumulative GC exposure)	Calcium 1000–1500 mg, Vitamin D 400–800 IU, consider bisphosphonate if T-score is <1.5mg and/or are present fractures
	Diabetes mellitus (<2%)	Blood glucose 3-monthly	Patient education: diet
	Infections[1]	Clinical	Patient education: avoid contact to infected people, recognize early symptoms
	Cushing's syndrome[1]	Clinical	Early tapering of GC
	Skin atrophy[1]	Clinical	Early tapering of GC
Cyclophosphamide (CYC)	Hemorrhagic cystitis (1–50%), transitional bladder cancer (1–5%)	Urinalysis, cystoscopy in case of non-renal hematuria	Give CYC only in the morning
			Advise patients to drink sufficient fluids (2–3 liters/day)
			Give Mesna (dosage in mg = CYC dosage, oral CYC: divide on two doses in morning and afternoon, pulse CYC divide into three doses at 0, 4 and 8 hours)
			Limit cumulative CYC exposure
	Hematological: Leukopenia (50–100%), anemia, thrombocytopenia	Blood cell counts, 2–3 times weekly during daily oral therapy, at days 8, 10 and 12 during pulse therapy	Frequent monitoring
	Severe infections (20–30 %)	Clinical	Patient education: avoid contact to infected people, recognize early symptoms
	Pneumocystis carinii pneumonia	Clinical	Trice weekly doses of co-trimoxazole.
		Lymphocyte counts	In sulfa-allergic patients, inhaled pentamidine 300 mg every 3 to 4 weeks
	Nausea, vomiting (>50%)	Clinical	Ondansetrone 4–8 mg
	Myelodysplasia (1–8%)	Blood cell counts, MCV	Limit cumulative CYC exposure
Methotrexate (MTX)	Stomatitis (5–30%), alopecia	Clinical	Folate 15–20 mg 24 h after MTX
	Hematological (5–30%): Leukopenia anemia, thrombopenia	Blood cell counts, weekly at first 4 weeks, then 2- to 4-weekly	Stop when renal function declines
		Serum creatinine	Folate 15–20 mg 24 h after MTX
	Elevation of liver enzymes (10–15 %)[1]	ALT, AST, weekly at first 4 weeks, then 2- to 4-weekly	Folate 15–20 mg 24 h after MTX
	Infections (>10%)	Clinical	Patient education: avoid contact to infected people, recognize early symptoms
	Pneumocystis carinii pneumonia[1]	Clinical	Trice weekly doses of co-trimoxazole
		Lymphocyte counts	In sulfa-allergic patients, inhaled pentamidine 300 mg every 3 to 4 weeks
	Pneumonitis (1–10%)	Clinical, consider bronchoalveolar lavage in case of unexplained pneumonitis	Patient education: symptoms (cough, fever)
	Nausea, vomiting (2–50%)	Clinical	Give MTX parenterally
			In severe cases, theophylline on day of MTX

Drug	Adverse events	Monitoring	Recommendations
Azathioprine (AZA)	Hematological (5–30%): Leukopenia anemia, thrombopenia	Blood cell counts, weekly at first 4 weeks, then 2- to 4-weekly; Serum creatinine	Avoid comedication with allopurinol; Patient education: regular lab checks; Check thiopurinemethyltransferase (TPMT) in case of frequent leukopenia
	Elevation of liver enzymes (1–10%)	ALT, AST, weekly at first 4 weeks, then 2- to 4-weekly	Patient education: regular lab checks
	Infections (> 20%)	Clinical	Patient education: avoid contact to infected people, recognize early symptoms
	Drug fever (1%)	Clinical	Patient education: consult physician in case of unexplained fever
	Nausea, vomiting, abdominal pain (5–20%)	Clinical	Check TPMT
Leflunomide	Hematological (5–30%): Leukopenia anemia, thrombocytopenia	Blood cell counts, weekly at first 4 weeks, then 2- to 4-weekly; Serum creatinine	Patient education: regular lab checks
	Elevation of liver enzymes (1–10%)	ALT, AST, weekly at first 4 weeks, then 2- to 4-weekly	Patient education: regular lab checks
	Infections (general)	Clinical	Patient education: avoid contact to infected people, recognize early symptoms
	Diarrhea (>20 %)	Clinical	Patient education: report symptoms
	Hypertension	Blood pressure 2-weekly	Avoid in patients with pre-existing severe hypertension
Mycophenolate mofetil	Hematological[1]: Leukopenia anemia, thrombopenia	Blood cell counts, weekly at first 4 weeks, then 2- to 4-weekly; Serum creatinine	Patient education: regular lab checks
	Elevation of liver enzymes[1]	ALT, AST, weekly at first 4 weeks, then 2- to 4-weekly	Patient education: regular lab checks
	Infections (general)[1]	Clinical	Patient education: avoid contact to infected people, recognize early symptoms
	Diarrhea[1]	Clinical	Patient education: report symptoms
	Nausea, vomiting, abdominal pain[1]	Clinical	Check TPMT
	Hypertension[1]	Blood pressure 2-weekly	Avoid in patients with pre-existing severe hypertension

The frequencies of adverse events were obtained form different randomized trials and cohort studies involving patients with WG with different times of observation and therefore only represent rough estimates.

[1] Insufficient data on frequency in WG.

measurements. In patients with a bone mineral density (T-score) of <−1 standard deviations, evidence based guidelines recommend the prophylactic use of bisphosphonates in patients treated with >7.5 mg/day of prednisone for more than 3 months. Prophylaxis with vitamin D (400–800 IU daily) and calcium (500–1000 mg of elemental calcium daily) should be given to each patient on glucocorticoid therapy.

Prophylaxis of transitional bladder cancer

Comparison of the two largest cohorts of WG patients yet suggests that the use of mesna during CYC therapy limits the risk of developing bladder cancer (Hellmich *et al.* 2004; Hoffman *et al.* 1992; Reinhold-Keller *et al.* 2000a, 2000b). Patients in the large cohort of WG patients observed at the NIH did not receive mesna along with cyclophosphamide treatment (Hoffman *et al.* 1992; Talar-Williams *et al.* 1996). In that cohort, 68 of 158 patients (43%) and, after extended follow-up, 42 of 145 patients (29%) developed hemorrhagic cystitis due to cyclophosphamide treatment (Hoffman *et al.* 1992; Talar-Williams *et al.* 1996). In contrast, in patients receiving mesna together with cyclophosphamide in the German WG cohort reported by Reinhold-Keller and coworkers, only 17 of 142 patients (12%) had cyclophosphamide-induced cystitis (Reinhold-Keller *et al.* 2000a). Comparison of both cohorts shows a relative risk for the occurrence of hemorrhagic cystitis of 0.41 (95% CI 0.25–0.69) without administration of mesna compared to only 0.28 (95% CI 0.17–0.45) with administration of mesna (Reinhold Keller *et al.* 2000). The incidence of hemorrhagic cystitis in the cohort given mesna was significantly lower than that reported in the two NIH studies, in which no mesna was administered ($P = 0.00001$, and $P = 0.0004$, respectively) (Reinhold Keller *et al.* 2000a). Furthermore, the incidence of bladder cancer was significantly lower in the mesna-treated cohort (1 of 155 patients) compared to the non-mesna treated NIH cohort (7 of 158 patients; $P = 0.034$) (Reinhold Keller *et al.* 2000b). We therefore recommend the use of mesna in patients receiving CYC. Mesna can be given orally in three divided daily doses of 50 mg during oral CYC therapy or in three doses during the day of intravenous CYC pulses. Urine cytology should be checked every 6 months. Allergic reactions, which may sometimes be difficult to distinguish from cutaneous vasculitis, and elevation of serum liver enzymes are the most frequently adverse events of mesna. CYC should be given at a single dose in the morning and patients should be advised to drink water frequently. Patients who have previously experienced hemorrhagic cystitis should have cystoscopy every year to look for evidence of early transitional cell carcinoma.

Treatment of drug-induced myelosuppression

Bone marrow suppression is frequently observed in patients with WG who have been treated with CYC (Bradley *et al.* 1989). In most cases, neutropenia is modest and resolves with cessation of CYC therapy for a few days; however, sometimes neutropenia can be severe and may last for a week or even longer. Such patients are at a particularly high risk of developing opportunistic infections (Bradley *et al.* 1989). In patients with WG and agranulocytosis due to CYC therapy lasting more than 3 days, recombinant human granulocyte-colony stimulating factor (rhG-CSF) was shown to induce a significantly faster rise in neutrophil counts compared to historic controls with a similar degree of neutropenia (Hellmich *et al.* 1999a). In addition, the use of rhG-CSF was associated with a lower incidence of infections (Hellmich *et al.* 1999a).

A particular concern of administration of recombinant cytokines to patients with autoimmune diseases is the potential of these cytokines to trigger the activity of the underlying inflammatory disease. Clinical observations suggest that the administration of rhG-CSF to patients with CYC-induced agranulocytosis does not cause flares of WG unless rhG-CSF is not stopped when neutrophil counts are at 1000/µl or above (Hellmich *et al.* 1999a). However, flares of other autoimmune disease such as Felty's syndrome were observed when neutrophilia developed as a result of growth factor treatment (Hellmich *et al.* 1999b; Starkebaum 1997). Thus, we recommend the rhG-CSF treatment only in patients with agranulocytosis lasting more than 3 days and its discontinuation when neutrophil counts recover (above 1000/µl). In contrast to rhG-CSF, granulocyte-macrophage colony-stimulating factor (GM-CSF) has the potential to increase the surface expression of the ANCA target antigen PR3 on neutrophils *in vitro*, and thus theoretically confers an additional risk of triggering a flare of WG (Hellmich *et al.* 2000).

Summary

Data from randomized, controlled clinical trials and accumulated experience in vasculitis centers indicate that CYC and glucocorticoid according to the "NIH-protocol" are still the standard therapy to induce remission in generalized and severe WG. In early systemic WG without renal involvement, MTX can be used instead of CYC, but treatment to maintain remission and close monitoring are mandatory. Efficacy as maintenance therapy in WG is documented in randomized controlled trials for azathioprine, leflunomide, and methotrexate (Table 32.4). Given the above mentioned limitations in trial methodology, currently available data do not suggest a superiority of one of these agents. Thus, the patient's individual history needs to be weighed against the toxicity profile of the respective compounds. Previous intolerability, treatment failure of certain medications, and impaired organ function (for example of the kidney, liver, or bone marrow) are important factors to be considered in the choice of a maintenance treatment for an individual patient with WG.

References

Adu, D., Pall, A., Luqmani, R. A., *et al.* (1997). Controlled trial of pulse versus continuous prednisolone and cyclophosphamide in the treatment of systemic vasculitis. *Quarterly Journal of Medicine*, **90**, 401–9.

Akobeng, A. K. and Zachos, M. (2004). Tumor necrosis factor-alpha antibody for induction of remission in Crohn's disease. *Cochrane Database Syst Rev*, CD003574.

Anderson, G., Coles, E., Crane, M., *et al.* (1992). Wegener's granuloma: A series of 265 British cases seen between 1975 and 1985. A report by the sub-committee of the British Thoracic Society. *Quarterly Journal of Medicine*, **83**, 427–438.

Aries, P. M., Hellmich, B., Both, M., *et al.* (2005). Lack of efficacy of Rituximab in Wegener's Granulomatosis with refractory granulomatous manifestations. *Annals of the Rheumatic Diseases*, **3**, 3.

Aries, P. M., Hellmich, B., Reinhold-Keller, E. and Gross, W. L. (2004). High-dose intravenous azathioprine pulse treatment in refractory Wegener's granulomatosis. *Rheumatology (Oxford)*, **43**, 1307–8.

Bartolucci, P., Ramanoelina, J., Cohen, P., *et al.* (2002). Efficacy of the anti-TNF-alpha antibody infliximab against refractory systemic vasculitides: an open pilot study on 10 patients. *Rheumatology (Oxford)*, **41**, 1126–32.

Benenson, E., Fries, J. W., Heilig, B., Pollok, M. and Rubbert, A. (2005). High-dose azathioprine pulse therapy as a new treatment option in patients with active Wegener's granulomatosis and lupus nephritis refractory or intolerant to cyclophosphamide. *Clinical Rheumatology*, **24**, 251–7.

Birck, R., Warnatz, K., Lorenz, H. M., *et al.* (2003). 15-Deoxyspergualin in patients with refractory ANCA-associated systemic vasculitis: a six-month open-label trial to evaluate safety and efficacy. *Journal of the American Society for Nephrology*, **14**, 440–7.

Booth, A., Harper, L., Hammad, T., *et al.* (2004). Prospective study of TNFalpha blockade with infliximab in anti-neutrophil cytoplasmic antibody-associated systemic vasculitis. *Journal of the American Society for Nephrology*, **15**, 717–21.

Bradley, J., Brandt, K. and Katz, B. (1989). Infectious complications of cyclophosphamide-induced severe neutropenia in Wegener's granulomatosis. *Arthritis and Rheumatism*, **32**, 45–53.

de Groot, K., Reinhold-Keller, E., Tatsis, E., *et al.* (1996). Therapy for the maintenance of remission in sixty-five patients with generalized Wegener's granulomatosis. Methotrexate versus trimethoprim/ sulfamethoxazole. *Arthritis and Rheumatism*, **39**, 2052–61.

de Groot, K., Muhler, M., Reinhold-Keller, E., Paulsen, J. and Gross, W. L. (1998). Induction of remission in Wegener's granulomatosis with low dose methotrexate. *Journal of Rheumatology*, **25**, 492–5.

de Groot, K., Adu, D. and Savage, C. (2001a). The value of pulse cyclophosphamide in ANCA-associated vasculitis: meta-analysis and critical review. *Nephrology Dialysis Transplantation*, **16**, 2018–27.

de Groot, K., Gross, W. L., Herlyn, K. and Reinhold-Keller, E. (2001b). Development and validation of a disease extent index for Wegener's granulomatosis. *Clinical Nephrology*, **55**, 31–8.

de Groot, K., Jayne, D., Tesar, V. and Savage, C. (2005a). Randomised controlled trial of daily oral versus pulse cyclophosphamide for induction of remission in ANCA-associated systemic vasculitis. *Kidney and Blood Pressure Research*, **28**, 195 [Abstract].

de Groot, K., Rasmussen, N., Bacon, P., *et al.* (2005b). Randomized trial of cyclophosphamide versus methotrexate for induction of remission in early systemic antineutrophil cytoplasmic antibody-associated vasculitis. *Arthritis and Rheumatism*, **52**.

Deegens, J., Artz, M., Hoitsma, A. and Wetzels, J. (2003). Outcome of renal transplantation in patients with pauci-immune small vessel vasculitis and anti-GBM disease. *Clinical Nephrology*, **59**, 1–9.

DeReeme, R., McDonald, T. J. and Wiland, L. (1985). Wegener's granulomatosis: observations on treatment with observational agents. *Mayo Clinic Proceedings*, **60**, 27–32.

Elmedhem, A., Adu, D. and Savage, C. (2003). Relapse rate and outcome of ANCA-associated small vessel vasculitis after transplantation. *Nephrology Dialysis Transplantation*, **18**, 1001–4.

Eriksson, P. (2005). Nine patients with anti-neutrophil cytoplasmic antibody-positive vasculitis successfully treated with rituximab. *Journal of Internal Medicine*, **257**, 540–8.

Fauci, A., Haynes, B., Katz, P. and Wolff, S. (1983). Wegener's granulomatosis: prospective clinical and therapeutic experience with 85 patients for 21 years. *Annals of Internal Medicine*, **98**, 76–85.

Fauci, A. and Wolff, S. (1973). Wegener's granulomatosis: studies in eigtheen patients and review of the literature. *Medicine*, **52**, 535–61.

Gaskin, G. and Jayne, D. (2002). Adjuctive Plasmaexchange is superior to methylprednisolone in acute renale failure due to ANCA-associated glomerulonephritis. *Journal of the American Society for Nephrology*, **13**, F-FC010.

Guillevin, L., Cordier, J., Lhote, F., *et al.* (1997). A prospective, multicenter, randomized trial comparing steroids and pulse cyclophosphamide versus steroids and oral cyclophosphamide in the treatment of generalized Wegener's granulomatosis. *Arthritis and Rheumatism*, **40**, 2187–98.

Haubitz, M. and de Groot, K. (2002). Tolerance of mycophenolate mofetil in end-stage renal disease patients with ANCA-assocaited vasculitis. *Clinical Nephrology*, **57**, 421–4.

Haubitz, M., Schellong, S., Gobel, U., *et al.* (1998). Intravenous pulse administration of cyclophosphamide versus daily oral treatment in patients with antineutrophil cytoplasmic antibody-associated vasculitis and renal involvement: a prospective, randomized study. *Arthritis and Rheumatism*, **41**, 1835–44.

Hellmich, B., Csernok, E., Trabandt, A., Gross, W. and Ernst, M. (2000). Granulocyte-macrophage colony-stimulating factor (GM-CSF), but not granulocyte-colony stimulating factor (G-CSF) induces surface expression of proteinase 3(PR3) on neutrophils in vitro. *Clinical and Experimental Immunology*, **120**, 392–8.

Hellmich, B., Hering, S., Duchna, H. W., *et al.* (2003). Airway manifestations of relapsing polychondritis: treatment with cyclophosphamide and placement of bronchial stents. *Zeitschrift fur Rheumatologie*, **62**, 73–9.

Hellmich, B., Kausch, I., Doehn, C., Jocham, D., Holl-Ulrich, K. and Gross, W. L. (2004). Urinary bladder cancer in Wegener's granulomatosis: is it more than cyclophosphamide? *Annals of the Rheumatic Diseases*, **63**, 1183–5.

Hellmich, B., Schnabel, A. and Gross, W. (1999a). Granulocyte colony-stimulating factor treatment for cyclophosphamide-induced severe neutropenia in Wegener's granulomatosis. *Arthritis and Rheumatism*, **42**, 1752–62.

Hellmich, B., Schnabel, A. and Gross, W. L. (1999b). Treatment of severe neutropenia due to Felty's syndrome or systemic lupus erythematosus with granulocyte colony-stimulating factor. *Seminars in Arthritis and Rheumatism*, **29**, 82–99.

Hoffman, G., Kerr, G., Leavitt, R., *et al.* (1992). Wegener's granulomatosis: an analysis of 158 patients. *Archives of Internal Medicine*, **116**, 488–99.

Hoffman, G., Thomas-Golbanov, C., Chan, J., Akst, L. and Eliachar, I. (2003). Treatment of subglottic stenosis, due to Wegener's granulomatosis, with intralesional corticosteroids and dilation. *Journal of Rheumatology*, **30**, 1017–21.

Hollander, D. and Manning, R. (1967). The use of alcylating agents in the treatment of Wegener's granulomatosis. *Annals of Internal Medicine*, **67**, 393–8.

Jayne, D., Chapel, H., Adu, D., *et al.* (2000). Intravenous immunoglobulin for ANCA-associated systemic vasculitis with persistent disease activity. *Quarterly Journal of Medicine*, **93**, 433–9.

Jayne, D. (2001). Update on the European Vasculitis Study Group (EUVAS). *Current Opinion in Rheumatology*, **13**, 48–55.

Jayne, D., Rasmussen, N., Andrassy, K., *et al.* (2003). A randomized trial of maintenance therapy for vasculitis associated with antineutrophil cytoplasmic autoantibodies. *New England Journal of Medicine*, **349**, 36–44.

Keogh, K., Wylam, M., Stone, J. and Specks, U. (2005a). Induction of remission by B lymphocyte depletion in eleven patients with refractory antineutrophil cytoplasmic antibody-associated vasculitis. *Arthritis and Rheumatism*, **52**, 262–8.

Keogh, K. A., Ytterberg, S. R., Fervenza, F. C., Carlson, K. A., Schroeder, D. R. and Specks, U. (2005b). Rituximab for refractory Wegener's granulomatosis: report of a prospective, open-label pilot trial. *American Journal of Respiratory and Critical Care Medicine*, **13**, 13.

Klemmer, P. J., Chalermskulrat, W., Reif, M. S., Hogan, S. L., Henke, D. C. and Falk, R. J. (2003). Plasmapheresis therapy for diffuse alveolar hemorrhage in patients with small-vessel vasculitis. *American Journal of Kidney Diseases*, **42**, 1149–53.

Knight, A., Askling, J. and Ekbom, A. (2002). Cancer incidence in a population-based cohort of patients with Wegener's granulomatosis. *International Journal of Cancer*, **100**, 82–5.

Knight, A., Askling, J., Granath, F., Sparen, P. and Ekborn, A. (2004). Urinary bladder cancer in Wegener's granulomatosis, risks and relation to cyclophosphamide. *Annals of the Rheumatic Diseases*, **63**, 1307–11.

Lamprecht, P., Kumanovics, G., Mueller, A., *et al.* (2002a). Elevated monocytic IL-12 and TNF-alpha production in Wegener's granulomatosis is normalized by cyclophosphamide and corticosteroid therapy. *Clinical and Experimental Immunology*, **128**, 181–6.

Lamprecht, P., Voswinkel, J., Lilienthal, T., *et al.* (2002b). Effectiveness of TNF-alpha blockade with infliximab in refractory Wegener's granulomatosis. *Rheumatology* (Oxford), **41**, 1303–7.

Langford, C. A., Sneller, M. C., Hallahan, C. W., *et al.* (1996). Clinical features and therapeutic management of subglottic stenosis in patients with Wegener's granulomatosis. *Arthritis and Rheumatism*, **39**, 1754–60.

Langford, C. A., Talar-Williams, C., Barron, K. S. and Sneller, M. C. (1999). A staged approach to the treatment of Wegener's granulomatosis:

induction of remission with glucocorticoids and daily cyclophosphamide switching to methotrexate for remission maintenance. *Arthritis and Rheumatism*, **42**, 2666–73.

Langford, C. A., Talar-Williams, C., Barron, K. S. and Sneller, M. C. (2003). Use of a cyclophosphamide-induction methotrexate-maintenance regimen for the treatment of Wegener's granulomatosis: extended follow-up and rate of relapse. *American Journal of Medicine*, **114**, 463–9.

Langford, C. A., Talar-Williams, C. and Sneller, M. C. (2004). Mycophenolate mofetil for remission maintenance in the treatment of Wegener's granulomatosis. *Arthritis and Rheumatism*, **51**, 278–83.

Luqmani, R. A., Bacon, P. A., Moots, R. J., *et al.* (1994). Birmingham Vasculitis Activity Score (BVAS) in systemic necrotizing vasculitis. *Quarterly Journal of Medicine*, **87**, 671–8.

Mahr, A., Pagnoux, C., Cohen, P., *et al.* (2005). Treatment of ANCA-associated vasculitides: corticosteroids and pulse cyclophosphamide followed by maintenance therapy with methotrexate or azathioprine: a prospective multicenter randomized trial (Wegent). *Kidney and Blood Pressure Research*, **28**, 194 [Abstract].

Merkel, P. A., Cuthbertson, D., Hellmich, B., *et al.* (2004). Comparison of disease activity measures for ANCA-associated vasculitis. *Arthritis and Rheumatism*, **50**, S229–30.

Metzler, C., Fink, C., Lamprecht, P., Gross, W. L. and Reinhold-Keller, E. (2004). Maintenance of remission with leflunomide in Wegener's granulomatosis. *Rheumatology*, **63**, 339–40.

Metzler, C., Wagner-Bastmeyer, R., Gross, W. and Reinhold Keller, E. (2005). Leflunomide versus methotrexate for maintenance of remission in Wegener's granulomatosis – unexpected high relapse rate under oral methotrexate. *Annals of the Rheumatic Diseases*, **64** (Suppl. 3), 85.

Nowack, R., Gobel, U., Klooker, P., Hergesell, O., Andrassy, K. and van der Woude, F. J. (1999). Mycophenolate mofetil for maintenance therapy of Wegener's granulomatosis and microscopic polyangiitis: a pilot study in 11 patients with renal involvement. *Journal of the American Society for Nephrology*, **10**, 1965–71.

Ognibene, F. P., Shelhamer, J. H., Hoffman, G., *et al.* (1995). Pneumocystis carinii pneumonia: a major complication of immunosuppressive therapy in patients with Wegener's granulomatosis. *American Journal of Respiratory and Critical Care Medicine*, **151**, 795–99.

Omdal, R., Wildhagen, K., Hansen, T., Gunnarsson, R. and Kristoffersen, G. (2005). Anti-CD20 therapy of treatment-resistant Wegener's granulomatosis: favourable but temporary response. *Scandinavian Journal of Rheumatology*, **34**, 229–32.

Reinhold Keller, E., de Groot, K. and Gross, W. (2000). Reply to: Cystitis, bladder cancer, and myelodysplasia in patients with Wegener's granulomatosis [Letter]. *Arthritis and Rheumatism*, **43**, 2854.

Reinhold-Keller, E., Beuge, N., Latza, U., *et al.* (2000). An interdisciplinary approach to the care of patients with Wegener's granulomatosis: long-term outcome in 155 patients. *Arthritis and Rheumatism*, **43**, 1021–32.

Reinhold-Keller, E., De Groot, K., Rudert, H., Noelle, B., Heller, M. and Gross, W. (1996). Response to trimethoprim/ sulfamethoxazole in Wegener's granulomatosis depends on the phase of disease. *Quarterly Journal of Medicine*, **89**, 15–23.

Reinhold-Keller, E., Fink, C., Herlyn, K., Gross, W. L. and de Groot, K. (2002). High rate of renal relapse in 71 patients with Wegener's granulomatosis under maintenance of remission with low-dose methotrexate. *Arthritis Care Research*, **47**, 326–32.

Richter, C., Schnabel, A., Csernok, E., De Groot, K., Reinhold-Keller, E. and Gross, W. L. (1995). Treatment of anti-neutrophil cytoplasmic antibody (ANCA)-associated systemic vasculitis with high-dose intravenous immunoglobulin. *Clinical and Experimental Immunology*, **101**, 2–7.

Schmitt, W., Hagen, E., Neumann, I., Nowack, R., Flores-Suarez, L. F. and van der Woude, F. (2004). Treatment of refractory Wegener's granulomatosis with antithymocyte globulin (ATG): an open study in 15 patients. *Kidney International*, **65**, 1440–8.

Schmitt, W., Haubitz, M., Mistry, N., Brunkhorst, R., Erbslöh-Möller, B. and Gross, W. (1993). Renal transplantation in Wegener's granulomatosis. *Lancet*, **342**, 860 [Letter].

Schmitt, W. H., Birck, R., Heinzel, P., *et al.* (2005). Prolonged treatment of refractory Wegener's granulomatosis with 15-deoxyspergualin: an open study in seven patients. *Nephrology Dialysis Transplantation*, **20**, 1083–92.

Shekelle, P. G., Woolf, S. H., Eccles, M. and Grimshaw, J. (1999). Clinical guidelines: developing guidelines. *British Medical Journal*, **318**, 593–6.

Sneller, M. C. (1998). Evaluation, treatment, and prophylaxis of infections complicating systemic vasculitis. *Current Opinion in Rheumatology*, **10**, 38–44.

Sneller, M. C. (2005). Rituximab and Wegener's granulomatosis: Are B cells a target in vasculitis treatment? *Arthritis and Rheumatism*, **52**, 1–5.

Sneller, M. C., Hoffman, G. S., Talar-Williams, C., Kerr, G. S., Hallahan, C. W. and Fauci, A. S. (1995). An analysis of forty-two Wegener's granulomatosis patients treated with methotrexate and prednisone. *Arthritis and Rheumatism*, **38**, 608–13.

Sowden, E. and Carmichael, A. (2004). Autoimmune inflammatory disorders, systemic corticosteroids and pneumocystis pneumonia: a strategy for prevention. *BMC Infectious Diseases*, **4**, 42.

Starkebaum, G. (1997). Use of colony-stimulating factors in the treatment of neutropenia associated with collagen vascular disease. *Current Opinion in Hematology*, **4**, 196–9.

Stegeman, C. A., Tervaert, J. W., de Jong, P. E. and Kallenberg, C. G. (1996). Trimethoprim-sulfamethoxazole (co-trimoxazole) for the prevention of relapses of Wegener's granulomatosis. Dutch Co-Trimoxazole Wegener Study Group. *New England Journal of Medicine*, **335**, 16–20.

Stone, J. H., Hoffman, G. S., Merkel, P. A., *et al.* (2001a). A disease-specific activity index for Wegener's granulomatosis: modification of the Birmingham Vasculitis Activity Score. International Network for the Study of the Systemic Vasculitides (INSSYS). *Arthritis and Rheumatism*, **44**, 912–20.

Stone, J. H., Uhlfelder, M. L., Hellmann, D. B., Crook, S., Bedocs, N. M. and Hoffman, G. S. (2001b). Etanercept combined with conventional treatment in Wegener's granulomatosis: a six-month open-label trial to evaluate safety. *Arthritis and Rheumatism*, **44**, 1149–54.

Talar-Williams, C., Hijazi, Y. M., Walther, M. M., *et al.* (1996). Cyclophosphamide-induced cystitis and bladder cancer in patients with Wegener granulomatosis. *Annals of Internal Medicine*, **124**, 477–84.

Tatsis, E., Reinhold-Keller, E., Steindorf, K., Feller, A. C. and Gross, W. L. (1999). Wegener's granulomatosis associated with renal cell carcinoma. *Arthritis and Rheumatism*, **42**, 751–6.

Tiede, I., Fritz, G., Strand, S., *et al.* (2003). CD28-dependent Rac1 activation is the molecular target of azathioprine in primary human CD4+ T lymphocytes. *Journal of Clinical Investigation*, **111**, 1133–45.

Van den Brande, J. M., Braat, H., van den Brink, G. R., *et al.* (2003). Infliximab but not etanercept induces apoptosis in lamina propria T-lymphocytes from patients with Crohn's disease. *Gastroenterology*, **124**, 1774–85.

Walton, E. (1958). Giant cell granuloma of the respiratory tract (Wegener's granulomatosis). *British Medical Journal*, **2**, 265–70.

Ward, M. and Donald, F. (1999). Pneumocystis carinii pneumnia in patients with connective tissue diseases: the role of hospital experience in diagnosis and mortality. *Arthritis and Rheumatism*, **42**, 780–9 [Abstract].

Wegener, F. (1939). Über eine eigenartige rhinogene Granulomatose mit besonderer Beteiligung des Arteriensystems und der Nieren. *Beitrage zur Pathologischen Anatomie und zur Allgemeinen Pathologie*, **102**, 36–68.

Wegener's Granulomatosis Etanercept (WGET) Research Group (2005). Etanercept plus standard therapy for Wegener's granulomatosis. *New England Journal of Medicine*, **352**, 351–61.

WGET Research Group (2002). Design of the Wegener's granulomatosis etanercept trial (WGET). *Controlled Clinical Trials*, **23**, 450–68.

CHAPTER 33

Churg–Strauss syndrome

Ulrich Specks

Original description, disease definitions, and classification

Churg–Strauss syndrome (CSS) was first described as "allergic granulomatosis and angiitis" in patients with asthma who had three pathological features: necrotizing vasculitis, eosinophilic inflammation, and extravascular granulomas (Churg and Strauss 1951). It is now recognized as a small-vessel vasculitis, which preferentially affects the capillaries, arterioles, and venules, even though the disease process occasionally extends to larger vessels (Jennette *et al.* 1994). Because of the frequent occurrence of antineutrophil cytoplasmic antibodies (ANCA) and clinical and histopathologic similarities, CSS has been classified along with Wegener's granulomatosis and microscopic polyangiitis as one of the ANCA-associated vasculitides (Cohen Tervaert *et al.* 1991; Cohen Tervaert and Kallenberg 1993; Guillevin *et al.* 1993, 1999; Jennette *et al.* 1994; Reid *et al.* 1998; Solans *et al.* 2001; Keogh and Specks 2003).

The original description of the disease was based on autopsy observations. All three pathologic features of the syndrome defined by Churg and Strauss in 1951 (necrotizing vasculitis, eosinophilic inflammation, and extravascular granulomas) (Figures 33.1, 33.2, and 33.3) are rarely present in patients at the time of original presentation.

Three schemes of clinical criteria and definitions have subsequently been proposed for the disease. Lanham's criteria emphasize the clinical presentation: a patient is said to have CSS if asthma, peripheral blood eosinophilia, and systemic vasculitis in two or more organs are detected (Lanham *et al.* 1984). The Chapel Hill Consensus Conference definition (see Table 26.2 in Chapter 26) is based on the combination of clinical and histopathologic features: a patient fulfills the definition if asthma, peripheral eosinophilia, eosinophil-rich granulomatous inflammation involving the respiratory tract, and necrotizing vasculitis affecting small to medium-sized vessels are found; radiographic or clinical surrogates for vasculitis are accepted (Jennette *et al.* 1994). Finally, the American College of Rheumatology criteria were designed to differentiate patients with CSS from those with other forms of vasculitis. According to these criteria, a patient with vasculitis is said to have CSS if four of the following six features are present: asthma; peripheral eosinophilia; peripheral neuropathy attributed to vasculitis; transient pulmonary infiltrates; paranasal sinus disease; and a

biopsy containing a blood vessel with extravascular eosinophils (Masi *et al.* 1990). Even though these three schemes are not meant to serve as stand-alone diagnostic criteria, they are frequently used in that capacity. None of the three schemes captures all patients (Keogh and Specks 2003).

Diagnosing patients with CSS is further complicated because the various clinical manifestations of the syndrome rarely coincide. Lanham and colleagues distinguished three clinical phases (Lanham *et al.* 1984). The first prodromal phase consists of asthma, with or without allergic rhinitis and nasal polyposis. It may precede other manifestations of the disease, particularly vasculitis, by a number of years (Lanham *et al.* 1984). The second phase is characterized by peripheral blood eosinophilia and eosinophilic tissue infiltration. Eosinophilic manifestations may also remit and recur over a number of years. The third and most severe phase of CSS consists of systemic vasculitis, and may be life-threatening. However, these three phases do not always occur sequentially, and in a minority of cases the onset of asthma may follow the onset of vasculitis (Chumbley *et al.* 1977; Keogh and Specks 2003). Occasionally

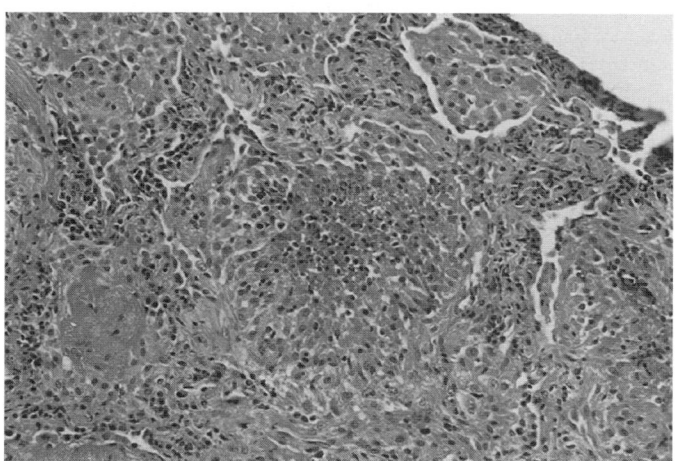

Figure 33.1 Extravascular granuloma in the lung, also referred to as the Churg–Strauss or allergic granuloma. (Courtesy of Dr Jeffrey L. Myers). From: R.A. DeRemee. Chapter 27: Churg–Strauss Syndrome. In: *Vasculitis*, 1st edn, G. V. Ball and S. L. Bridges, Jr, eds. Oxford University Press, 2002. (See Color Plate 88).

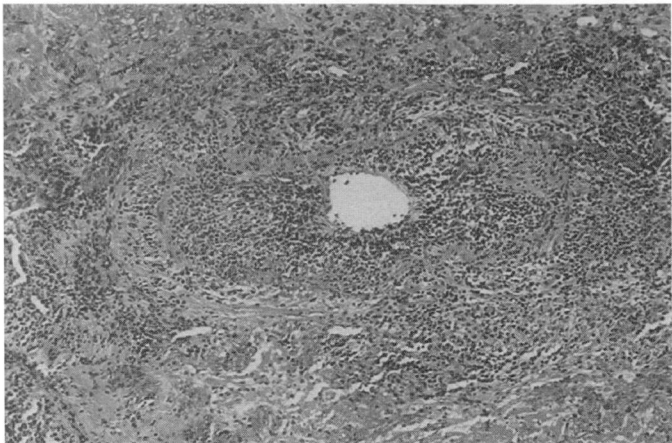

Figure 33.2 Necrotizing vasculitis of a small pulmonary artery with prominent eosinophilic infiltration. (Courtesy of Dr Jeffrey L. Myers). From: R.A. DeRemee. Churg–Strauss Syndrome. In: *Vasculitis*, 1st edn, G. V. Ball and S. L. Bridges, Jr, eds. Oxford University Press, 2002. (See Color Plate 89).

eosinophilic vasculitis or eosinophilic granulomatous inflammation is limited to one organ in asthmatic patients who lack other signs of systemic disease. Moreover, overt manifestations of vasculitis may be suppressed by oral glucocorticoid therapy of asthma, only to emerge when the glucocorticoids are withdrawn. Such conditions have been referred to as "limited forms" or as "formes frustes" of CSS (Lie 1993; Churg *et al.* 1995; Churg 2001).

Pathogenesis

The pathogenesis of CSS remains poorly understood. An allergic background seems to be common to all patients. Direct tissue injury is attributed to toxic eosinophil and neutrophil degranulation products. Activation of T-lymphocytes seems to be a significant force maintaining the eosinophilic inflammation. Most recent reports of successful treatment of CSS with B-lymphocyte depletion suggest that B-lymphocytes may also play an, as yet

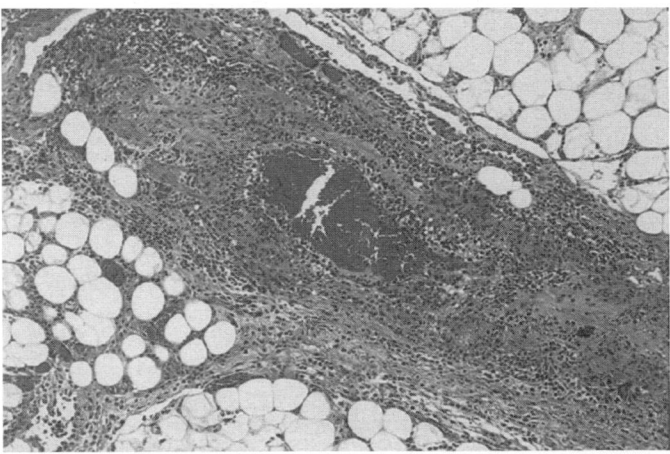

Figure 33.3 Necrotizing vasculitis of a small extrapulmonary artery. (Courtesy of Dr Jeffrey L. Myers). From: R.A. DeRemee. Churg–Strauss Syndrome. In: *Vasculitis*, 1st edn, G. V. Ball and S. L. Bridges, Jr, eds. Oxford University Press, 2002. (See Color Plate 90).

unrecognized, important role in the pathogenesis of the disease. Finally, there is evidence in support of a pathogenic role of ANCA, which seems to modulate the disease phenotype.

Peripheral blood and tissue eosinophilia are hallmarks of CSS. These eosinophils are activated, and markers of eosinophil activation parallel disease activity and predict relapses (Cottin *et al.* 1995; Schmitt *et al.* 1998; Hurst *et al.* 2000; Kurosawa *et al.* 2000). Both eosinophil and neutrophil degranulation products are found in areas of prominent inflammation and tissue necrosis in affected organs (Schnabel *et al.* 1999; Peen *et al.* 2000; Ramakrishna *et al.* 2000; Drage *et al.* 2002). It has been suggested that the eosinophilic inflammation and possibly the allergic background in CSS are the result of abnormally activated T-lymphocytes. Markers of T-lymphocyte activation (soluble interleukin-2 receptor) are elevated in patients with active CSS and correlate with markers of endothelial cell damage (soluble thrombomodulin) (Schmitt *et al.* 1998). T-lymphocytes of patients with CSS release predominantly Th-2-type cytokines, such as interleukin-4 (IL-4), interleukin-5 (IL-5), and interleukin-13 (IL-13), and are thought to be responsible for the recruitment, activation, and delayed apoptosis of eosinophils (Schonermarck *et al.* 2000; Kiene *et al.* 2001).

Abnormalities in the CD95/CD95-ligand system have also been observed in CSS (Muschen *et al.* 1999). This mechanism may contribute to delayed lymphocyte and eosinophil apoptosis, as well as to the clonal expansion of autoreactive T-cells (Muschen *et al.* 1999). It has been documented that clonally expanded T-cells from CSS patients exhibit preferential V-gene usage for a gene from the Vβ21 family, and that they display similar T-cell receptor specificities. This suggests recognition of a limited number of shared antigens among the patients studied (Muschen *et al.* 1999). These findings also support a previous clinical observation, which implicated inhaled antigen(s) as triggers of CSS (Guillevin *et al.* 1991; Muschen *et al.* 1999).

Two types of ANCA are associated with small-vessel vasculitis (see Chapter 6). Those reacting with proteinase 3 (PR3) predominate in Wegener's granulomatosis (WG), whereas ANCA reacting with myeloperoxidase (MPO) are more commonly found in microscopic polyangiitis (MPA) and CSS. The reported frequency of ANCA in active CSS varies between 40 and 75% (Cohen Tervaert and Kallenberg 1993; Schmitt *et al.* 1998; Guillevin *et al.* 1999; Solans *et al.* 2001; Keogh and Specks 2003; Sinico *et al.* 2005), and the frequency as well as the levels of detected ANCA seem to correlate with disease activity (Keogh and Specks 2003).

In vitro and animal model studies have documented a variety of proinflammatory effects of ANCA, suggesting that ANCA are important for the leukocyte activation and endothelial cell injury observed in ANCA-associated vasculitis (Savage *et al.* 2002; Xiao *et al.* 2002; Pfister *et al.* 2004; Specks 2004) (see Chapter 7). For MPO-ANCA, which are the predominant type of ANCA encountered in CSS, the evidence from rodent models is particularly strong (Xiao *et al.* 2002) (see Chapters 8 and 30). The clinical observations made in a cohort of 93 patients further support a potentially pathogenic and disease-modifying role of ANCA in CSS (Sinico *et al.* 2005). Manifestations of small-vessel vasculitis, including purpura, alveolar hemorrhage, mononeuritis multiplex, and glomerulonephritis, were found to be significantly more common in ANCA-positive patients than in those who lacked these autoantibodies (Sinico *et al.* 2005).

Leukotriene receptor antagonists and other drugs

There has been much discussion about a possible pathogenic link between leukotriene receptor antagonists (LRA) and the onset of CSS. The introduction of LRA for the treatment of asthma was followed by anecdotal reports of CSS in patients exposed to agents of this class (Knoell *et al.* 1998; Wechsler *et al.* 1998; Tuggey and Hosker 2000; Wechsler *et al.* 2000; Hashimoto *et al.* 2001; Guilpain *et al.* 2002; Solans *et al.* 2002). The most significant argument put forth in favor of a pathogenic role was an observed two to three-fold increase in incidence of CSS coinciding with the wide-spread use of LRA (Watts *et al.* 1995, 2000); however, many arguments speak against a pathogenic role of LRA. The observed increased incidence of CSS over the last decade can easily be attributed to improved physician awareness (Watts *et al.* 1995, 2000), possibly compounded by the original case reports of LRA-associated CSS, themselves. The estimated annual incidence of CSS cases per million asthma patients (0–67) overlaps with the estimated incidence of about 60 cases per million LRA users (Wechsler *et al.* 2000; Loughlin *et al.* 2002; Harrold *et al.* 2005). The clinical disease manifestations, including time from onset of asthma to onset of vasculitis symptoms, do not differ between CSS patients exposed to these drugs and those never exposed (Keogh and Specks 2003). One-hundred sixty-five patients who developed CSS while receiving LRA were analyzed at a workshop sponsored by the National Institutes of Health and the US Food and Drug Administration, and in 88% of these cases, the onset of vasculitis was associated with a dose reduction of oral glucocorticoids (Weller *et al.* 2001). Finally, there is little chemical similarity between the different agents in this class or other drugs reported in association with CSS, including acetaminophen, macrolides, carbamazepine, cocaine, and other asthma treatments used to reduce the use of oral glucocorticoids (such as inhaled glucocorticoids, cromolyn sodium, and beta-agonists) (Sheffer *et al.* 1975; Churg *et al.* 1995; Orriols *et al.* 1996; Hübner *et al.* 1997; Bili *et al.* 1999; Le Gall *et al.* 2000; Lilly *et al.* 2002; Masuzawa *et al.* 2005). All of these arguments suggest that LRA unmask a smoldering vasculitis by allowing a dose reduction of systemic glucocorticoids used for asthma management, rather than causing CSS.

Epidemiology

Given the described diagnostic uncertainties and the rare nature of the disease, it is difficult to interpret the reported incidence and prevalence numbers for CSS; however, it is the rarest of the three ANCA-associated vasculitides. The estimated annual incidence is 1–3 cases per million (Watts *et al.* 1995, 2000; Gonzalez-Gay *et al.* 2003; Reinhold-Keller *et al.* 2005) (see Chapter 2). Among asthma patients, the incidence of CSS is as high as 67 per million (Loughlin *et al.* 2002; Harrold *et al.* 2005). CSS affects men slightly more often than women. The disease is typically diagnosed in middle-age patients, but it has been reported in children (Chumbley *et al.* 1977; Lanham *et al.* 1984; Reid *et al.* 1998; Guillevin *et al.* 1999; Solans *et al.* 2001; Keogh and Specks 2003; Hernandez-Bautista *et al.* 2006).

Specific organ manifestations

The reported frequencies of organ manifestations and clinical features of CSS are summarized in Table 33.1.

Table 33.1 Frequency of clinical manifestations in Churg–Strauss syndrome

Organ involvement	
Upper respiratory tract	50–60%
Lungs	
Asthma	90–100%
Lung nodules	<10%
Eosinophilic infiltrates	30–50%
Alveolar hemorrhage/capillaritis	0–20%
Skin	51–70%
Nervous system	
Central nervous system	6–39%
Peripheral neuropathy, multiple mononeuropathies	66–76%
Gastrointestinal tract	13–59%
Kidneys	25–58%
Heart	
Endomyocardial	13–47%
Pericardial	8–32%
Eyes	<5%
Laboratory abnormalities	
Peripheral blood eosinophilia	90–100%
ANCA	40–75%

Based on Chumbley *et al.* 1977; Lanham *et al.* 1984; Guillevin *et al.* 1999; Solans *et al.* 2001; Keogh and Specks, 2003; Sinico *et al.* 2005.

Respiratory tract

Asthma is the disease-defining feature of CSS, which is central to all three classification schemes. It occurs in almost all patients (~99%) (Guillevin *et al.* 1999; Keogh and Specks 2003). In 83% of patients, it precedes the onset of vasculitis, with a median time between onset of asthma and a diagnosis of CSS of 4 years (inter-quartile range 2–11.5 years) (Keogh and Specks 2003). In 14% of patients the diagnosis of asthma coincided with that of vasculitis, and in rare cases vasculitis precedes the asthma by over a decade (Keogh and Specks 2003).

The paranasal sinuses are affected in ~75% of patients (Keogh and Specks 2003). It usually takes the form of nasal polyposis and allergic or granulomatous inflammation. Severe necrotizing inflammation is much less common in CSS than in Wegener's granulomatosis.

Radiographic imaging studies reveal pulmonary parenchymal abnormalities in up to two-thirds of patients. Mostly, these are caused by eosinophilic or granulomatous inflammation with or without vasculitis (Guillevin *et al.* 1999; Keogh and Specks 2003). Fleeting, patchy, pulmonary infiltrates with a peripheral predominance occur in half of the patients with CSS at some stage of the disease (Figure 33.4) (Worthy *et al.* 1998). They are radiographically and histopathologically indistinguishable from chronic eosinophilic pneumonitis (Silva *et al.* 2005). Poorly defined, small, centrilobular nodules are occasionally identified on high-resolution computed tomography, and larger nodules with a diameter of 1–3 cm or granulomatous mass lesions are rare (Worthy *et al.* 1998; Choi *et al.* 2000; Keogh and Specks 2003; Silva *et al.* 2005).

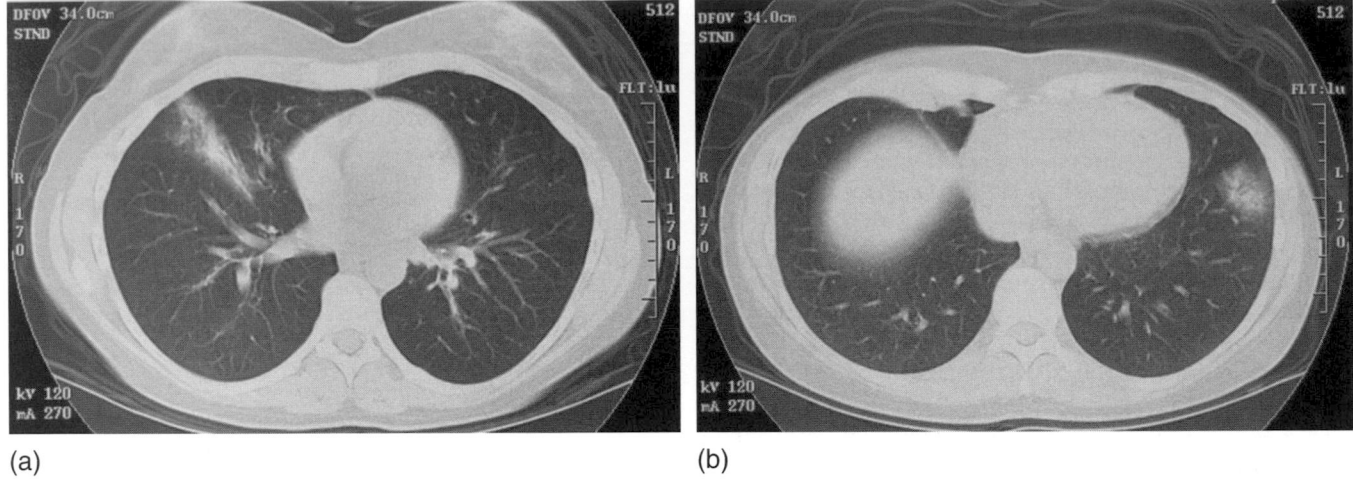

Figure 33.4 Computed tomography of the chest showing peripheral infiltrates in the right middle lobe (a) and left lower lobe (b) caused by eosinophilic inflammation of Churg–Strauss syndrome.

Pleural effusions occurring in up to 10% of patients can be caused by eosinophilic pleuritis or by congestive heart failure resulting from cardiac involvement. The former is typically associated with eosinophils found in the pleural fluid. Mediastinal adenopathy caused by either reactive hyperplasia or eosinophilic infiltration is also rare (Choi *et al.* 2000; Lesens *et al.* 2002). Alveolar hemorrhage has been reported in CSS patients (Clutterbuck and Pusey, 1987; Lai *et al.* 1998). Three large case series have reported a frequency ranging from 0 to 25% (Guillevin *et al.* 1999; Keogh and Specks, 2003; Sinico *et al.* 2005).

The differential diagnosis of eosinophilic lung disease includes: acute and chronic eosinophilic pneumonia; allergic bronchopulmonary aspergillosis; parasitic infections; drug reactions; and idiopathic hypereosinophilic syndrome. Of these, only idiopathic hypereosinophilic syndrome, a myeloproliferative disorder, affects extrapulmonary organs as does CSS.

Skin

About half of the patients with CSS have skin involvement resembling that of the other systemic small-vessel vasculitic disorders (Davis *et al.* 1997; Guillevin *et al.* 1999; Keogh and Specks, 2003). Nodules and papules on extensor surfaces of joints are called "Churg–Strauss granuloma" and represent cutaneous extravascular granulomas. The term refers to the histological pattern of palisading granulomas with central necrosis. Despite its name, this is a non-specific finding, which may occur in isolation or in the setting of other systemic diseases including WG, systemic lupus erythematosus, and rheumatoid arthritis (Finan and Winkelmann 1983). Vasculitic cutaneous involvement of CSS may also present as a petechial rash, palpable purpura, or an erythematous maculopapular rash, typically developing on the lower extremities and expanding proximally. The histopathologic correlate is leukocytoclastic vasculitis with or without prominent eosinophilic infiltration (Davis *et al.* 1997).

Central and peripheral nervous system

Neurological manifestations are common in patients with CSS. They are similar to those found in MPA and WG and are a consequence of vasculitis affecting epineural vessels or the central nervous system (Vital *et al.* 2006). Up to 76% of patients have peripheral nerve involvement, typically in the form of multiple mononeuropathies (Sehgal *et al.* 1995; Guillevin *et al.* 1999; Keogh and Specks 2003). Distal symmetrical polyneuropathy (24%) and less commonly asymmetric polyneuropathy (3%) and lumbar radiculopathy (3%) are also seen (Sehgal *et al.* 1995). Central nervous system involvement presents as confusion, seizures, or coma, with or without cranial nerve palsies or evidence of cerebral infarction. It is less common than peripheral nerve involvement, but causes significant morbidity and mortality in affected patients.

Gastrointestinal manifestations

Gastrointestinal tract involvement occurs in one-third of patients (Guillevin *et al.* 1999; Keogh and Specks 2003) (see Chapter 15). Symptoms may range from abdominal pain, nausea, vomiting, diarrhea, and gastrointestinal bleeding to an acute abdomen (Pagnoux *et al.* 2005). Eosinophilic gastroenteritis or colitis and small-vessel vasculitis affecting the small or large bowel can cause bowel ischemia and may lead to mucosal ulcerations and possibly perforation (Peen *et al.* 2000; Memain *et al.* 2002).

Heart

Reports of cardiac involvement vary widely (10–49%) (Chumbley *et al.* 1977; Lanham *et al.* 1984; Guillevin *et al.* 1999; Keogh and Specks, 2003; Sable-Fourtassou *et al.* 2005; Sinico *et al.* 2005). Clinical manifestations range from cardiac arrest, congestive heart failure and myocardial infarction, to valvular and pericardial disease, and the predominant finding is eosinophilic myocarditis (Morgan *et al.* 1989; Ramakrishna *et al.* 2000; Val-Bernal *et al.* 2003; Stollberger *et al.* 2005) (see Chapter 13). Like other forms of eosinophilic infiltration of the myocardium, CSS typically affects the ventricles and the diagnosis is best made by echocardiography (Morgan *et al.* 1989). Endomyocardial fibrosis, restrictive cardiomyopathy, and superimposed intracavitary thrombus can cause life-threatening complications (Ramakrishna *et al.* 2000). Contiguous valvular involvement, most commonly of the atrioventricular valves, may lead to valve destruction (Ramakrishna *et al.* 2000).

Acute or chronic constrictive pericarditis, and pericardial effusion with or without cardiac tamponade, can result from eosinophilic pericardial disease (Ramakrishna *et al.* 2000; Stollberger *et al.* 2005). Whereas the original autopsy studies found small-vessel coronary vasculitis in the majority of patients (Churg and Strauss 1951), and ischemia is thought to contribute to myocardial dysfunction, angiographically detectable involvement of the major coronary vessels is rare (Hasley *et al.* 1990; Kozak *et al.* 1995; Hellemans *et al.* 1997).

Kidneys

Renal involvement occurs in one-quarter of patients with CSS (Guillevin *et al.* 1999; Keogh and Specks 2003; Sinico *et al.* 2006) (see Chapter 16), far less commonly than in WG or MPA, where renal involvement affects up to 80% of patients. Furthermore, renal disease is usually mild and rarely causes renal failure. Investigators from the United Kingdom have reported higher frequencies of renal involvement in CSS (50–80%), and in the report from the Hammersmith Hospital nephrology group, renal outcome seemed similar to that of microscopic polyangiitis (Clutterbuck *et al.* 1990; Reid *et al.* 1998). The most common histopathologic abnormality on renal biopsy is that of a pauci-immune focal segmental necrotizing glomerulonephritis with crescent formation, indistinguishable from the other ANCA-associated vasculitides (Clutterbuck *et al.* 1990; Sinico *et al.* 2006). Eosinophilic or granulomatous inflammation of the kidney are rare findings in CSS (Clutterbuck *et al.* 1990; Kikuchi *et al.* 2001; Sinico *et al.* 2006).

Other clinical manifestations

In addition to these most frequent clinical manifestations, any organ system may be affected in CSS. Eye, ear, and salivary gland involvement have been reported (Robin *et al.* 1985; Vitali *et al.* 1996; Granata *et al.* 2001; Ishiyama and Canalis 2001; Takanashi *et al.* 2001; Cackett and Singh 2006; Hoffman *et al.* 2005; Boin *et al.* 2006). Myositis, and even breast involvement may occur (De Vlam *et al.* 1995). Patients with CSS also seem to have a propensity for thromboembolic events, similar to that seen in patients with WG (Ames *et al.* 1996; Garcia *et al.* 2005; Merkel *et al.* 2005).

Differential diagnosis

The diagnostic approach to patients suspected of CSS is governed by the predominant symptom. If symptoms are centered on the respiratory tract, the differential diagnosis needs to exclude other pulmonary eosinophilic syndromes. Once parasitic infections and drug reactions are excluded, CSS needs to be differentiated from acute and chronic eosinophilic pneumonia, from allergic bronchopulmonary aspergillosis, and from idiopathic hypereosinophilic syndrome. As mentioned above, only the last affects extrapulmonary organs as does CSS. If the clinical presentation features prominent peripheral eosinophilia and multiorgan involvement, but vasculitic features and asthma are not obvious, idiopathic hypereosinophilic syndrome is the more likely diagnosis, and additional evaluations should focus on identification of specific subsets, such as clonal abnormalities in the eosinophil lineage, atypical myeloproliferative variants, and T-lymphocytic variants. If multisystem disease and vasculitis are apparent, CSS also needs to be

differentiated from WG and MPA, particularly if the patient is ANCA-positive.

Diagnostic procedures and laboratory testing

Laboratory tests and diagnostic procedures should be performed to firmly establish the diagnosis and differentiate it from other eosinophilic and vasculitic disorders, to establish the extent and severity of organ involvement, and to provide baseline markers of disease activity for the future assessments of treatment response.

Peripheral blood eosinophilia detected on complete blood count is an important component of the diagnosis and a marker of disease activity. Immunoglobulin E levels, erythrocyte sedimentation rate, and C-reactive protein levels are other markers of inflammatory activity that should be followed. Serum chemistries and urine microscopy are critical for detecting evidence of renal involvement and following its severity. A variety of other surrogate markers of disease activity have been proposed, including serum markers of endothelial damage, lymphocyte and eosinophil activation such as soluble thrombomodulin, vascular endothelial growth factor, soluble interleukin-2 receptor, and eosinophil cationic protein. But routine measurements of these parameters are currently not practical in clinical practice (Schmitt *et al.* 1998; Mitsuyama *et al.* 2006).

Chest radiographs or computed tomography of the chest are indicated to detect pulmonary parenchymal involvement (Figure 33.4). Flexible bronchoscopy with bronchoalveolar lavage can help to establish the presence of eosinophilic inflammation in patients with radiographically detected infiltrates. This may obviate the need for more invasive lung biopsy procedures. The differential cell count of the bronchoalveolar lavage fluid usually confirms the presence of eosinophils in patients with lung infiltrates caused by CSS (Wallaert *et al.* 1993; Schnabel *et al.* 1999).

Pulmonary function testing and peak flow measurements are integral components of the management of asthma. Pulmonary function testing should go beyond simple spirometry. Abnormalities of the shape of the flow-volume curve may suggest large airway involvement, and a reduction in diffusion capacity can be a clue to the presence of venous thromboembolic complications (Matsushima *et al.* 2006). If there is any concern for cardiac involvement, patients with suspected or confirmed CSS should also undergo echocardiography. A histopathologic diagnosis should be sought whenever possible, with biopsy of the most accessible affected tissue.

Therapy

The management of CSS remains challenging, and there are no conclusive clinical trial results in well-defined patient populations that would provide guidance. For practical management reasons it may be helpful to conceptually separate the asthma component of the disease from the eosinophilic tissue inflammation and vasculitis. Systemic glucocorticoids remain the mainstay of therapy and data about the use of additional immunosuppressive agents are scarce (Langford *et al.* 1998). Most vasculitis experts seem to apply the same principles of treatment used for the other

ANCA-associated vasculitides to the management of CSS. Patients are separated into those who have severe disease, and those who are not so classified. Having severe disease indicates that the patient's life or a vital organ (heart, nervous system, kidney) are at risk of irreversible damage. In such patients cyclophosphamide should be added to glucocorticoids for remission induction. Patients who are not thought to have severe disease by that definition are primarily treated with glucocorticoids. Methotrexate, azathioprine, mycophenolate mofetil, or hydroxyurea can be added if glucocorticoids cannot be tapered to acceptably low doses (Della Rossa *et al.* 2002; Assaf *et al.* 2004; Metzler *et al.* 2004).

For patients who are resistant to standard immunosuppressive agents, particularly if eosinophilic inflammation dominates the clinical presentation, interferon-alpha has been proposed as an alternative (Tatsis *et al.* 1998; Termeer *et al.* 2001; Lesens *et al.* 2002). However, interferon-alpha therapy may need to be continued long-term, in order to prevent relapses, and there is evidence for potentially serious treatment toxicity (Gordon *et al.* 1998; Metzler *et al.* 2005). B-cell depletion with rituximab has recently been reported to be beneficial in several patients with refractory CSS (Koukoulaki *et al.* 2006).

Prognosis

The long-term outcome and prognosis of CSS is not entirely clear. Before therapy with glucocorticoids, the disease appeared universally fatal (Churg and Strauss, 1951); however, this perception may have been confounded by selection bias towards the most severe cases. Guillevin and colleagues developed the prognostic Five-Factor Score based on 260 patients with polyarteritis nodosa and 82 patients with CSS who were followed prospectively (Guillevin *et al.* 1996). The five factors (see Table 23.2 in Chapter 23) are elevation of serum creatinine (>1.58 mg/dl); proteinuria due to vasculitis or glomerulonephritis (>1 g/24hours); gastrointestinal involvement; cardiomyopathy; and central nervous system involvement. Two or more of these manifestations present at diagnosis were associated with increased mortality (Guillevin *et al.* 1996).

In the 1970s, CSS was estimated to carry a mortality of about 40% (Chumbley *et al.* 1977). A subsequent analysis of patients evaluated at the same center during the 1990s did not detect a significantly increased mortality for CSS (n = 91) (Keogh and Specks 2003). This improvement in prognosis may be the result of earlier diagnosis and optimized use of immunosuppressive therapy, and it may also reflect a referral bias, favoring patients with less life-threatening disease manifestations. A population-based study conducted in a cohort of 18 CSS patients treated at the Norwich University Hospital, UK, between 1988 and 2000, revealed 1- and 5-year survival rates of 83.2% and 68.1%, respectively (Lane *et al.* 2005). These patients were relatively old, and a significant increase in mortality with age was observed (Lane *et al.* 2005).

In addition to mortality, the long-term morbidity associated with the disease and drugs used to treat it are frequently major concerns of patients with CSS. The vasculitic manifestations of the disease usually respond promptly to appropriate therapy; however, asthma usually persists and is often difficult to manage. This may be the major factor responsible for the cumulative glucocorticoid toxicity observed in so many patients with CSS. Neuropathic sequelae of the disease are another long-term management challenge which persists long after the acute inflammation has subsided.

References

Ames, P. R. J., Roes, L., Lupoli, S. M. P., Brancaccio, V., Khamashta, M. A. and Hughes, G. R.V. (1996). Thrombosis in Churg-Strauss syndrome. Beyond vasculitis? *British Journal of Rheumatology*, **35**, 1181–1183.

Assaf, C., Mewis, G., Orfanos, C. E. and Geilen, C. C. (2004). Churg-Strauss syndrome: successful treatment with mycophenolate mofetil. *British Journal of Dermatology*, **150**, 598–600.

Bili, A., Condemi, J. J., Bottone, S. M. and Ryan, C. K. (1999). Seven cases of complete and incomplete forms of Churg-Strauss syndrome not related to leukotriene receptor antagonists. *Journal of Allergy and Clinical Immunology*, **104**, 1060–5.

Boin, F., Sciubba, J. J. and Stone, J. H. (2006). Churg-Strauss syndrome presenting with salivary gland enlargement and respiratory distress. *Arthritis and Rheumatism*, **55**, 167–70.

Cackett, P. and Singh, J. (2006). Churg-Strauss syndrome in association with proliferative retinopathy. *Eye*, **20**: 394–6.

Choi, Y. H., Im, J. G., Han, B. K., Kim, J. H., Lee, K. Y. and Myoung, N. H. (2000). Thoracic manifestation of Churg-Strauss syndrome: radiologic and clinical findings. *Chest*, **117**, 117–24.

Chumbley, L. C., Harrison, E. G. and DeRemee, R. A. (1977). Allergic granulomatosis and angiitis (Churg-Strauss syndrome). *Mayo Clinic Proceedings*, **52**, 477–84.

Churg, A. (2001). Recent Advances in the Diagnosis of Churg-Strauss Syndrome. *Modern Pathology*, **14**, 1284–93.

Churg, A., Brallas, M., Cronin, S. R. and Churg, J. (1995). Formes frustes of Churg-Strauss syndrome. *Chest*, **108**, 320–3.

Churg, J. C. and Strauss, L. (1951). Allergic granulomatosis, allergic angiitis and periarteritis nodosa. *American Journal of Pathology*, **27**, 277–301.

Clutterbuck, E. J., Evans, D. J. and Pusey, C. D. (1990). Renal involvement in Churg-Strauss syndrome. *Nephrology Dialysis Transplantation*, **5**, 161–7.

Clutterbuck, E. J. and Pusey, C. D. (1987). Severe alveolar haemorrhage in Churg-Strauss syndrome. *European Journal of Respiratory Diseases*, **71**, 158–63.

Cohen Tervaert, J. W. and Kallenberg, C. G. M. (1993). Anti-myeloperoxidase antibodies in Churg-Strauss syndrome. *Journal of Neurology*, **240**, 449–52.

Cohen Tervaert, J. W., Limburg, P. C., Elema, J. D., Huitema, M. G., Horst, G., The, T. H. and Kallenberg, C. G. M. (1991). Detection of autoantibodies against myeloid lysosomal enzymes: a useful adjunct to classification of patients with biopsy-proven necrotizing arteritis. *American Journal of Medicine*, **91**, 59–66.

Cottin, V., Tardy, F., Gindre, D., Vernet, G., Deviller, P. and Cordier, J. F. (1995). Urinary eosinophil-derived neurotoxin in Churg-Strauss syndrome. *Journal of Allergy and Clinical Immunology*, **96**, 261–4.

Davis, M. D., Daoud, M. S., McEvoy, M. T. and Su, W. P. (1997). Cutaneous manifestations of Churg-Strauss syndrome: a clinicopathologic correlation. *Journal of the American Academy of Dermatology*, **37**, 199–203.

De Vlam, K., De Keyser, F., Goemaere, S., Praet, M. and Veys, E. M. (1995). Churg-Strauss syndrome presenting as polymyositis. *Clinical and Experimental Rheumatology*, **13**, 505–7.

Della Rossa, A., Baldini, C., Tavoni, A., Tognetti, A., Neglia, D., Sambuceti, G., Puccini, R., Colangelo, C. and Bombardieri, S. (2002). Churg-Strauss syndrome: clinical and serological features of 19 patients from a single Italian centre. *Rheumatology* (Oxford), **41**, 1286–94.

Drage, L. A., Davis, M. D., De Castro, F., Van Keulen, V., Weiss, E. A., Gleich, G. J. and Leiferman, K. M. (2002). Evidence for pathogenic involvement of eosinophils and neutrophilsin Churg-Strauss syndrome. *Journal of the American Academy of Dermatology*, **47**, 209–16.

Finan, M. C. and Winkelmann, R. K. (1983). The cutaneous extravascular necrotizing granuloma (Churg-Strauss granuloma) and systemic disease: a review of 27 cases. *Medicine* (Baltimore), **62**, 142–58.

Garcia, G., Achouh, L., Cobarzan, D., Fichet, D. and Humbert, M. (2005). Severe venous thromboembolic disease in Churg-Strauss syndrome. *Allergy*, **60**, 409–10.

Gonzalez-Gay, M. A., Garcia-Porrua, C., Guerrero, J., Rodriguez-Ledo, P. and Llorca, J. (2003). The epidemiology of the primary systemic vasculitides in northwest Spain: implications of the Chapel Hill Consensus Conference definitions. *Arthritis and Rheumatism*, **49**, 388–93.

Gordon, A. C., Edgar, J. D. and Finch, R. G. (1998). Acute exacerbation of vasculitis during interferon-alpha therapy for hepatitis C-associated cryoglobulinaemia. *Journal of Infection*, **36**, 229–30.

Granata, M., Ammendolea, C., Trudu, R., Spimpolo, N. and Martelletti, P. (2001). Thrombosis of the retinal artery in a patient with Churg-Strauss syndrome. *Clinical and Experimental Rheumatology*, **19**, 234.

Guillevin, L., Amouroux, J., Arbeille, B. and Boura, R. (1991). Churg-Strauss angiitis. Arguments favoring the responsibility of inhaled antigens. *Chest*, **100**, 1472–3.

Guillevin, L., Cohen, P., Gayraud, M., Lhote, F., Jarrousse, B. and Casassus, P. (1999). Churg-Strauss syndrome. Clinical study and long-term follow-up of 96 patients. *Medicine*, **78**, 26–37.

Guillevin, L., Lhote, F., Gayraud, M., Cohen, P., Jarrousse, B., Lortholary, O., Thibult, N. and Casassus, P. (1996). Prognostic factors in polyarteritis nodosa and Churg-Strauss syndrome. *Medicine*, **75**, 17–28.

Guillevin, L., Visser, H., Noel, L. H., Pourrat, J., Vernier, I., Gayraud, M., Oksman, F. and Lesavre, P. (1993). Antineutrophil cytoplasm antibodies in systemic polyarteritis nodosa with and without hepatitis B virus infection and Churg-Strauss syndrome – 62 patients. *Journal of Rheumatology*, **20**, 1345–9.

Guilpain, P., Viallard, J. F., Lagarde, P., Cohen, P., Kambouchner, M., Pellegrin, J. L. and Guillevin, L. (2002). Churg-Strauss syndrome in two patients receiving montelukast. *Rheumatology* (Oxford), **41**, 535–9.

Harrold, L. R., Andrade, S. E., Go, A. S., Buist, A. S., Eisner, M., Vollmer, W. M., Chan, K. A., Frazier, E. A., Weller, P. F., Wechsler, M. E., Yood, R. A., Davis, K. J. and Platt, R. (2005). Incidence of Churg-Strauss syndrome in asthma drug users: a population-based perspective. *Journal of Rheumatology*, **32**, 1076–80.

Hashimoto, M., Fujishima, T., Tanaka, H., Kon, H., Saikai, T., Suzuki, A., Nakatsugawa, M. and Abe, S. (2001). Churg-Strauss syndrome after reduction of inhaled corticosteroid in a patient treated with pranlukast for asthma. *Internal Medicine*, **40**, 432–4.

Hasley, P. B., Follansbee, W. P. and Coulehan, J. L. (1990). Cardiac manifestations of Churg-Strauss syndrome: report of a case and review of the literature. *American Heart Journal*, **120**, 996–9.

Hellemans, S., Dens, J. and Knockaert, D. (1997). Coronary involvement in the Churg-Strauss syndrome. *Heart*, **77**, 576–8.

Hernandez-Bautista, V. M., Espinosa-Padilla, S. E., Yamazaki-Nakashimada, M. A., Lopez-Lara, D., Gonzalez-Serrano, E., Staines-Boone, T. and Espinosa-Rosales, F. (2006). Pediatric Churg-Strauss syndrome in Mexico. *Pediatric Pulmonology*, **41**, 379–82.

Hoffman, P. M., Godfrey, T. and Stawell, R. J. (2005). A case of Churg-Strauss syndrome with visual loss following central retinal artery occlusion. *Lupus*, **14**, 174–5.

Hübner, C., Dietz, A., Stremmel, W., Stiehl, A. and Andrassy, K. (1997). Macrolide-induced Churg-Strauss syndrome in a patient with atopy. *Lancet*, **350**, 563.

Hurst, S., Chizzolini, C., Dayer, J. M., Olivieri, J. and Roux-Lombard, P. (2000). Usefulness of serum eosinophil cationic protein (ECP) in predicting relapse of Churg and Strauss vasculitis. *Clinical and Experimental Rheumatology*, **18**, 784–5.

Ishiyama, A. and Canalis, R. F. (2001). Otological manifestations of Churg-Strauss syndrome. *Laryngoscope*, **111**, 1619–24.

Jennette, J. C., Falk, R. J., Andrassy, K., Bacon, B. A., Churg, J., Gross, W. L., Hagen, E. C., Hoffmann, G. S., Hunder, G. G., Kallenberg, C. G. M., McCluskey, R. T., Sinico, R. A., Rees, A. J., Van Es, L. A., Waldherr, R. and Wiik, A. (1994). Nomenclature of systemic vasculitides: The proposal of an international consensus conference. *Arthritis and Rheumatism*, **37**, 187–92.

Keogh, K. A. and Specks, U. (2003). Churg-Strauss syndrome. clinical presentation, antineutrophil cytoplasmic antibodies, and leukotriene receptor antagonists. *American Journal of Medicine*, **115**, 284–90.

Kiene, M., Csernok, E., Muller, A., Metzler, C., Trabandt, A. and Gross, W. L. (2001). Elevated interleukin-4 and interleukin-13 production by T cell lines from patients with Churg-Strauss syndrome. *Arthritis and Rheumatism*, **44**, 469–73.

Kikuchi, Y., Ikehata, N., Tajima, O., Yoshizawa, N. and Miura, S. (2001). Glomerular lesions in patients with Churg-Strauss syndrome and the anti- myeloperoxidase antibody. *Clinical Nephrology*, **55**, 429–35.

Knoell, D. L., Lucas, J. and Allen, J. N. (1998). Churg-Strauss Syndrome associated with Zafirlukast. *Chest*, **114**, 332–4.

Koukoulaki, M., Smith, K. G. and Jayne, D. R. (2006). Rituximab in Churg-Strauss syndrome. *Annals of the Rheumatic Diseases*, **65**, 557–9.

Kozak, M., Gill, E. A. and Green, L. S. (1995). The Churg-Strauss syndrome. A case report with angiographically documented coronary involvement and a review of the literature. *Chest*, **107**, 578–80.

Kurosawa, M., Nakagami, R., Morioka, J., Inamura, H., Mizushima, Y., Sugawara, N., Yamashita, T., Yokoseki, T., Kitamura, S., Omura, Y., Shibata, M. and Chihara, J. (2000). Interleukins in Churg-Strauss syndrome. *Allergy*, **55**, 785–7.

Lai, R. S., Lin, S. L., Lai, N. S. and Lee, P. C. (1998). Churg-Strauss syndrome presenting with pulmonary capillaritis and diffuse alveolar hemorrhage. *Scandinavian Journal of Rheumatology*, **27**, 230–2.

Lane, S. E., Watts, R. A., Shepstone, L. and Scott, D. G. (2005). Primary systemic vasculitis: clinical features and mortality. *Quarterly Journal of Medicine*, **98**, 97–111.

Langford, C. A., Klippel, J. H., Balow, J. E., James, S. P. and Sneller, M. C. (1998). Use of cytotoxic agents and cyclosporine in the treatment of autoimmune disease. Part 2: Inflammatory bowel disease, systemic vasculitis, and therapeutic toxicity. *Annals of Internal Medicine*, **129**, 49–58.

Lanham, J. G., Elkon, K. B., Pusey, C. D. and Hughes, G. R. (1984). Systemic vasculitis with asthma and eosinophilia: a clinical approach to the Churg-Strauss syndrome. *Medicine*, **63**, 65–81.

Le Gall, C., Pham, S., Vignes, S., Garcia, G., Nunes, H., Fichet, D., Simonneau, G., Duroux, P. and Humbert, M. (2000). Inhaled corticosteroids and Churg-Strauss syndrome: a report of five cases. *European Respiratory Journal*, **15**, 978–81.

Lesens, O., Hansmann, Y., Nerson, J., Pasquali, J., Gasser, B., Wihlm, J. and Christmann, D. (2002). Severe Churg-Strauss syndrome with mediastinal lymphadenopathy treated with interferon therapy. *European Journal of Internal Medicine*, **13**, 458.

Lie, J. T. (1993). Limited forms of Churg-Strauss syndrome. *Pathology Annual*, **28**, 199–220.

Lilly, C. M., Churg, A., Lazarovich, M., Pauwels, R., Hendeles, L., Rosenwasser, L. J., Ledford, D. and Wechsler, M. E. (2002). Asthma therapies and Churg-Strauss syndrome. *Journal of Allergy and Clinical Immunology*, **109**, S1–19.

Loughlin, J. E., Cole, J. A., Rothman, K. J. and Johnson, E. S. (2002). Prevalence of serious eosinophilia and incidence of Churg-Strauss syndrome in a cohort of asthma patients. *Annals of Allergy Asthma and Immunology*, **88**, 319–25.

Masi, A. T., Hunder, G. G., Lie, J. T., Michel, B. A., Bloch, D. A., Arend, W. P., Calabrese, L. H., Edworthy, S. M., Fauci, A. S., Leavitt, R. Y., Lightfoot, R. W., McShane, D. J., Mills, J. A., Stevens, M. B., Wallace, S. L. and Zvaifler, N. J. (1990). The American College of Rheumatology 1990 criteria for the classification of Churg-Strauss syndrome (allergic granulomatosis and angiitis). *Arthritis and Rheumatism*, **33**, 1094–100.

Masuzawa, A., Moriguchi, M., Tsuda, T., Sugawara, H., Otsuka, M., Yamada, S., Tabei, K. and Kawakami, M. (2005). Churg-Strauss syndrome associated with hypersensitivity to acetaminophen. *Internal Medicin*, **44**, 496–8.

Matsushima, H., Takayanagi, N., Kurashima, K., Tokunaga, D., Ubukata, M., Kawabata, Y. and Sugita, Y. (2006). Multiple tracheobronchial mucosal lesions in two cases of Churg-Strauss syndrome. *Respirology*, **11**, 109–12.

Memain, N., De, B. M., Guillevin, L., Wechsler, B. and Meyer, O. (2002). Delayed relapse of Churg-Strauss syndrome manifesting as colon ulcers with mucosal granulomas: 3 cases. *Journal of Rheumatology*, **29**, 388–91.

Merkel, P. A., Lo, G. H., Holbrook, J. T., Tibbs, A. K., Allen, N. B., Davis, J. C., Jr., Hoffman, G. S., McCune, W. J., St Clair, E. W., Specks, U., Spiera, R., Petri, M. and Stone, J. H. (2005). High incidence of venous thrombotic events among patients with Wegener granulomatosis: the Wegener's Clinical Occurrence of Thrombosis (WeCLOT) Study. *Annals of Internal Medicine*, **142**, 620–6.

Metzler, C., Hellmich, B., Gause, A., Gross, W. L. and de Groot, K. (2004). Churg Strauss syndrome – successful induction of remission with methotrexate and unexpected high cardiac and pulmonary relapse ratio during maintenance treatment. *Clinical and Experimental Rheumatology*, **22**, S52–61.

Metzler, C., Lamprecht, P., Hellmich, B., Reuter, M., Arlt, A. C. and Gross, W. L. (2005). Leucoencephalopathy after treatment of Churg-Strauss syndrome with interferon α. *Annals of the Rheumatic Diseases*, **64**, 1242–3.

Mitsuyama, H., Matsuyama, W., Iwakawa, J., Higashimoto, I., Watanabe, M., Osame, M. and Arimura, K. (2006). Increased serum vascular endothelial growth factor level in Churg-Strauss syndrome. *Chest*, **129**, 407–11.

Morgan, J. M., Raposo, L. and Gibson, D. G. (1989). Cardiac involvement in Churg-Strauss syndrome shown by echocardiography. *British Heart Journa*, **62**, 462–6.

Muschen, M., Warskulat, U., Perniok, A., Even, J., Moers, C., Kismet, B., Temizkan, N., Simon, D., Schneider, M. and Haussinger, D. (1999). Involvement of soluble CD95 in Churg-Strauss syndrome. *American Journal of Pathology*, **155**, 915–25.

Orriols, R., Munoz, X., Ferrer, J., Huget, P. and Morell, F. (1996). Cocaine-induced Churg-Strauss vasculitis. *European Respiratory Journal*, **9**, 175–7.

Pagnoux, C., Mahr, A., Cohen, P. and Guillevin, L. (2005). Presentation and outcome of gastrointestinal involvement in systemic necrotizing vasculitides: analysis of 62 patients with polyarteritis nodosa, microscopic polyangiitis, Wegener granulomatosis, Churg-Strauss syndrome, or rheumatoid arthritis-associated vasculitis. *Medicine* (Baltimore), **84**, 115–28.

Peen, E., Hahn, P., Lauwers, G., Williams, R. C., Jr., Gleich, G. and Kephart, G. M. (2000). Churg-Strauss syndrome: localization of eosinophil major basic protein in damaged tissues. *Arthritis and Rheumatism*, **43**, 1897–900.

Pfister, H., Ollert, M., Frohlich, L. F., Quintanilla-Martinez, L., Colby, T. V., Specks, U. and Jenne, D. E. (2004). Antineutrophil cytoplasmic autoantibodies against the murine homolog of proteinase 3 (Wegener autoantigen) are pathogenic in vivo. *Blood*, **104**, 1411–8.

Ramakrishna, G., Connolly, H. M., Tazelaar, H. D., Mullany, C. J. and Midthun, D. E. (2000). Churg-Strauss syndrome complicated by eosinophilic endomyocarditis. *Mayo Clinic Proceedings*, **75**, 631–5.

Reid, A. J.C., Harrison, B. D.W., Watts, R. A., Watkin, S. W., McCann, B. G. and Scott, D. G.I. (1998). Churg-Strauss syndrome in a district hospital. *Quarterly Journal of Medicine*, **91**, 219–29.

Reinhold-Keller, E., Herlyn, K., Wagner-Bastmeyer, R. and Gross, W. L. (2005). Stable incidence of primary systemic vasculitides over five years: results from the German vasculitis register. *Arthritis and Rheumatism*, **53**, 93–9.

Robin, J. B., Schanzlin, D. J., Meisler, D. M., de Luise, V. P. and Clough, J. D. (1985). Ocular involvement in the respiratory vasculitides. *Survey of Opthalmology*, **30**, 127–140.

Sable-Fourtassou, R., Cohen, P., Mahr, A., Pagnoux, C., Mouthon, L., Jayne, D., Blockmans, D., Cordier, J. F., Delaval, P., Puechal, X., Lauque, D., Viallard, J. F., Zoulim, A. and Guillevin, L. (2005). Antineutrophil cytoplasmic antibodies and the Churg-Strauss syndrome. *Annals of Internal Medicine*, **143**, 632–8.

Savage, C. O., Harper, L. and Holland, M. (2002). New findings in pathogenesis of antineutrophil cytoplasm antibody- associated vasculitis. *Current Opinion in Rheumatology*, **14**, 15–22.

Schmitt, W. H., Csernok, E., Kobayashi, S., Klinkenborg, A., Reinhold-Keller, E. and Gross, W. L. (1998). Churg-Strauss syndrome. Serum markers of lymphocyte activation and endothelial damage. *Arthritis and Rheumatism*, **41**, 445–52.

Schnabel, A., Csernok, E., Braun, J. and Gross, W. L. (1999). Inflammatory cells and cellular activation in the lower respiratory tract in Churg-Strauss syndrome. *Thorax*, **54**, 771–8.

Schonermarck, U., Csernok, E., Trabandt, A., Hansen, H. and Gross, W. L. (2000). Circulating cytokines and soluble CD23, CD26 and CD30 in ANCA- associated vasculitides. *Clinical and Experimental Rheumatology*, **18**, 457–63.

Sehgal, M., Swanson, J. W., DeRemee, R. A. and Colby, T. V. (1995). Neurologic manifestations of Churg-Strauss syndrome. *Mayo Clinic Proceedings*, **70**, 337–41.

Sheffer, A. L., Rocklin, R. E. and Goetzl, E. J. (1975). Immunologic components of hypersensitivity reactions to cromolyn sodium. *New England Journal of Medicine*, **293**, 1220–4.

Silva, C. I., Muller, N. L., Fujimoto, K., Johkoh, T., Ajzen, S. A. and Churg, A. (2005). Churg-Strauss syndrome: high resolution CT and pathologic findings. *Journal of Thoracic Imaging*, **20**, 74–80.

Sinico, R. A., Di Toma, L., Maggiore, U., Bottero, P., Radice, A., Tosoni, C., Grasselli, C., Pavone, L., Gregorini, G., Monti, S., Frassi, M., Vecchio, F., Corace, C., Venegoni, E. and Buzio, C. (2005). Prevalence and clinical significance of antineutrophil cytoplasmic antibodies in Churg-Strauss syndrome. *Arthritis and Rheumatism*, **52**, 2926–35.

Sinico, R. A., Di Toma, L., Maggiore, U., Tosoni, C., Bottero, P., Sabadini, E., Giammarresi, G., Tumiati, B., Gregorini, G., Pesci, A., Monti, S., Balestrieri, G., Garini, G., Vecchio, F. and Buzio, C. (2006). Renal involvement in Churg-Strauss syndrome. *American Journal of Kidney Diseases*, **47**, 770–9.

Solans, R., Bosch, J. A., Perez-Bocanegra, C., Selva, A., Huguet, P., Alijotas, J., Orriols, R., Armadans, L. and Vilardell, M. (2001). Churg-Strauss syndrome: outcome and long-term follow-up of 32 patients. *Rheumatology* (Oxford), **40**, 763–71.

Solans, R., Bosch, J. A., Selva, A., Orriols, R. and Vilardell, M. (2002). Montelukast and Churg-Strauss syndrome. *Thorax*, **57**, 183–5.

Specks, U. (2004). Antineutrophil cytoplasmic antibodies: are they pathogenic? *Clinical and Experimental Rheumatology*, **22**, S7–12.

Stollberger, C., Finsterer, J. and Winkler, W. B. (2005). Eosinophilic pericardial effusion in Churg-Strauss syndrome. *Respiratory Medicine*, **99**, 377–9.

Takanashi, T., Uchida, S., Arita, M., Okada, M. and Kashii, S. (2001). Orbital inflammatory pseudotumor and ischemic vasculitis in Churg-Strauss syndrome: report of two cases and review of the literature. *Ophthalmology*, **108**, 1129–33.

Tatsis, E., Schnabel, A. and Gross, W. L. (1998). Interferon-a treatment of four patients with the Churg-Strauss syndrome. *Annals of Internal Medicine*, **129**, 370–4.

Termeer, C. C., Simon, J. C. and Schopf, E. (2001). Low-dose interferon alfa-2b for the treatment of Churg-Strauss syndrome with prominent skin involvement. *Archives of Dermatology*, **137**, 136–8.

Tuggey, J. M. and Hosker, H. S. (2000). Churg-Strauss syndrome associated with montelukast therapy. *Thorax*, **55**, 805–6.

Val-Bernal, J. F., Mayorga, M., Garcia-Alberdi, E. and Pozueta, J. A. (2003). Churg-Strauss syndrome and sudden cardiac death. *Cardiovascular Pathology*, **12**, 94–7.

Vital, A., Vital, C., Viallard, J. F., Ragnaud, J. M., Canron, M. H. and Lagueny, A. (2006). Neuro-muscular biopsy in Churg-Strauss syndrome: 24 cases. *Journal of Neuropathology and Experimental Neurology*, **65**, 187–92.

Vitali, C., Genovesi-Ebert, F., Romani, A., Jeracitano, G. and Nardi, M. (1996). Ophthalmological and neuro-ophthalmological involvement in Churg-Strauss syndrome: a case report. *Graefe's Archives of Clinical and Experimental Ophthalmology*, **234**, 404–8.

Wallaert, B., Gosset, P., Prin, L., Bart, F., Marquette, C. H. and Tonnel, A. B. (1993). Bronchoalveolar lavage in allergic granulomatosis and angiitis. *European Respiratory Journal*, **6**, 413–7.

Watts, R. A., Carruthers, D. M. and Scott, D. G.I. (1995). Epidemiology of systemic vasculitis: changing incidence or definition? *Seminars in Arthritis and Rheumatism*, **25**, 28–34.

Watts, R. A., Lane, S. E., Bentham, G. and Scott, D. G. (2000). Epidemiology of systemic vasculitis: a ten-year study in the United Kingdom. *Arthritis and Rheumatism*, **43**, 414–9.

Wechsler, M. E., Finn, D., Gunawardena, D., Westlake, R., Barker, A., Haranath, S. P., Pauwels, R. A., Kips, J. C. and Drazen, J. M. (2000). Churg-Strauss syndrome in patients receiving montelukast as treatment for asthma. *Chest*, **117**, 708–13.

Wechsler, M. E., Garpestad, E., Flier, S. R., Kocher, O., Weiland, D. A., Polito, A. J., Klinek, M. M., Bigby, T. D., Wong, G. A., Helmers, R. A. and Drazen, J. M. (1998). Pulmonary infiltrates, eosinophilia, and cardiomyopathy following corticosteroid withdrawal in patients with asthma receiving zafirlukast. *Journal of the American Medical Association*, **279**, 455–7.

Weller, P. F., Plaut, M., Taggart, V. and Trontell, A. (2001). The relationship of asthma therapy and Churg-Strauss syndrome: NIH workshop summary report. *Journal of Allergy and Clinical Immunology*, **108**, 175–83.

Worthy, S. A., Muller, N. L., Hansell, D. M. and Flower, C. D. (1998). Churg-Strauss syndrome: the spectrum of pulmonary CT findings in 17 patients. *American Journal of Roentgenology*, **170**, 297–300.

Xiao, H., Heeringa, P., Hu, P., Liu, Z., Zhao, M., Aratani, Y., Maeda, N., Falk, R. J. and Jennette, J. C. (2002). Antineutrophil cytoplasmic autoantibodies specific for myeloperoxidase cause glomerulonephritis and vasculitis in mice. *Journal of Clinical Investigation*, **110**, 955–63.

CHAPTER 34

Vasculitis in primary connective tissue diseases

Laura B. Hughes

Introduction

In 1957, Bywaters suggested that vasculitis was an inherent component of all connective tissue diseases (Bywaters 1957). While vasculitis arising in the context of a pre-existing connective tissue disease (CTD) is well documented, its presence varies widely among such diseases. Characterized as multisystem inflammatory processes, CTDs such as rheumatoid arthritis (RA) and systemic lupus erythematosus (SLE) may have vascular involvement as a major clinical manifestation. Vasculitis in these cases often shares characteristics: (1) it may affect vessels of any caliber, concurrently or sequentially; (2) it can vary from mild protean symptoms to severe, life-threatening disease; and (3) it rarely precedes other manifestations of the particular CTD (Danning et al. 1998). In general, vasculitis in connective tissue disease is often found in patients with more severe disease activity and with longer disease duration. The clinical manifestations of vasculitis associated with CTDs, along with therapeutic considerations, are described in this chapter. Key clinical features of vasculitis in these conditions are summarized in Table 34.1.

Rheumatoid vasculitis

Epidemiology

The occurrence of vasculitis in RA underscores the systemic, inflammatory nature of the disease. RA is primarily manifested by symmetric inflammation in the synovial lining of diarthrodial joints. Extra-articular disease, particularly involving the skin (rheumatoid nodules), lungs (for example, pleuritis, interstitial lung disease (ILD) with pulmonary fibrosis), and heart (pericarditis, myocarditis), is also well recognized. Vasculitis in RA can lead to a variety of extra-articular conditions ranging from mild to severe. The overall annual incidence of RV is <1%, with a lifetime risk of 1 in 9 for males and 1 in 38 for females with RA (Panush et al. 1983; Watts et al. 1994). Post-mortem studies place the incidence of RV closer to 25% of RA patients, perhaps consistent with the view that RV is associated with more severe RA (Bacon and Carruthers 1995). The severe form of RV (threatening end-organ damage) is estimated to occur in less than 1 per 100,000 of the general population (Goronzy and Weyand 1994). Although the prevalence of RV is low, it has been more common than other primary vasculitides such as Wegener's granulomatosis (WG) or polyarteritis nodosa

(PAN) (Watts et al. 1994). Examples of clinical and angiographic manifestations of rheumatoid vasculitis (RV) are shown in Figure 34.1 and Figure 18.16.

RV appears to affect patients with more aggressive RA. It occurs on average 10–14 years after the onset of RA; however, it can occur before or at the time of RA diagnosis (Chen et al. 2002; Gray and Poppo 1983; Vollertsen et al. 1986). There are many patient factors that have been associated with an increased risk for the development of RV. Some of these factors include: a high titer rheumatoid factor (RF); ANA positivity; male gender; smoking; presence of joint erosions; or subcutaneous nodules or other extra-articular manifestations; increased number of disease-modifying antirheumatic drugs (DMARDs); and longer disease duration when compared with age-matched RA patients without RV (Struthers et al. 1981;Voskuyl et al. 1996a). Similarly, RV is reported in as many as 30% of persons with Felty's syndrome (Campion et al. 1990). Of the factors associated with RV, RF positivity has the strongest association (Voskuyl et al. 1996a). The association with smoking may be due to its immunomodulatory effects or to endothelial damage that predisposes to vascular inflammation (Struthers et al. 1981; Turesson et al. 2004).

Significant morbidity and mortality can occur in patients with RV. The mortality has been reported to be as high as 43%, most notably within the first 6 months after onset of vasculitis (Scott et al. 1981c). A more recent study, however, found only a trend toward a excess mortality (Hazard Ratio (HR) 1.26, 95% CI 0.79–2.01) in RV patients compared to RA controls, after controlling for the effects of age and sex (Voskuyl et al. 1996b). Predictors of decreased survival include: younger age at diagnosis of RV; delayed diagnosis; abnormal urinary sediment; high titer RF; and hypergammaglobulinemia (Geirsson et al. 1986). Cardiac involvement, gangrene, mononeuropathy multiplex, and bowel infarctions portend lethality (Chen et al. 2002; Geirsson et al. 1987).

Pathogenesis

In 1959, the dominant paradigm for RV attributed its pathogenesis to the effect of RF on the vessel wall. Several clinical and experimental studies support this theory in describing circulating immune complexes containing IgG and IgA rheumatoid factor, deposition of complement, and the presence of autoantibodies (such as antiendothelial cell antibodies) which form deposits in

Table 34.1 Characteristic of vasculitis associated with primary connective tissue diseases

	Disease vessel size	**Comments**
Rheumatoid arthritis	Small vessel, typically leukocytoclastic vasculitis. Necrotizing vasculitis of larger arteries occurs.	Vasculitis is a complication of RA in 10–15% of patients, usually those with more severe disease.
SLE	Usually small vessel/leukocytoclastic. Can rarely involve the great vessels.	Diseases resulting in pseudovasculitis (atherosclerosis; thromboembolism with or without APLs) are common in SLE.
Sjögren's syndrome	Usually small vessel/leukocytoclastic.	Mixed cryoglobulinemia may occur and concurrent infection with Hepatitis C has been reported. Latent HIV infection should also be considered. Hyperviscosity can also produce 'vasculitis.'
Systemic sclerosis	Cases reported involve small vessels.	Vasculitis is decidedly rare in primary, diffuse SSc. Most instances of vasculitis occur with limited variant (with anticentromere antibodies) or Sjögren's overlap.
SNSA	Vasculitis reported in anecdotal cases.	Clinical suspicion should be raised for underlying HIV infection when vasculitis complicates the SNSAs.
Relapsing polychondritis	Valvular (aortic) disease is most common but necrotizing vasculitis of medium to large arteries has been reported.	RP may also occur in other rheumatic conditions where vasculitis is common as well as in certain malignancies.
Inflammatory myopathies	Rare and involves small vessels/capillaries when present.	Vasculitis is more common in pediatric cases.
Retroperitoneal fibrosis	10% of cases have true vasculitis of the aorta.	Treatment requires long-term immunosuppression.

RA, rheumatoid arthritis; SLE, systemic lupus erythematosus; APLs, antiphospholipid antibodies; HIV, human immunodeficiency virus; SSc, systemic sclerosis; SNSA, seronegative spondyloarthropathies; RP, relapsing polychondritis.

vessel walls and trigger an inflammatory reaction (Breedveld *et al.* 1988; Jans *et al.* 1983; Scott *et al.* 1981a). Indeed, patients with RV typically have polyclonal hypergammaglobulinemia with high titer rheumatoid factor, detectable serum immune complexes (IC), and often diminished levels of serum complement (Bacons and

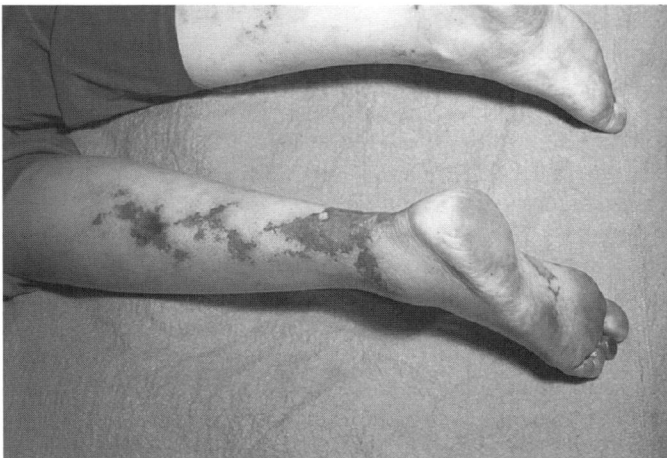

Figure 34.1 Extensive, rapidly developing, necrosis due to rheumatoid vasculitis in a 60-year-old woman, who subsequently died with inflammation in the coronary arteries as well. (Courtesy of Dr Gene Ball.) From: R. Jones and L. Moreland. Vasculitis in Primary Connective Tissue Diseases. In: *Vasculitis*, 1st edn. G. V. Ball and S. L. Bridges, Jr., eds. Oxford University Press, 2002. (See Color Plate 91).

Kitas 1994). Rappaport *et al.* reported an association between cutaneous immune complex deposition, detected via direct immunofluorescence, and cutaneous RV (Rapoport *et al.* 1980).

More recently T cell-mediated processes have been postulated. Because ICs cannot always be detected, vasculitis mediated by direct cell–cell contacts has been postulated by Goronzy *et al* (Goronzy and Weyand 1994). T cell abnormalities observed in patients with RV (and extra-articular RA) include expansion of CD8+ large granular lymphocytes, and immunosenescent CD4+CD28– cells (Goronzy and Weyand 2003; Martens *et al.* 1997). Flipo *et al.* (1994) recently proposed a TH-1-mediated process leading to an increase in ICAM-1, E-selectin, and TNF-α expression in endothelial and perivascular infiltrative cells in active RV lesions. In their study, labial salivary gland biopsies were obtained from RV patients before and after treatment, RA patients without vasculitis, and patients with primary Sjögren's syndrome. Expression of adhesions factors and TNF-α was found only in RV patients before treatment. This study introduces a possible diagnostic role for labial salivary gland biopsy in patients with suspected RV who are without other accessible affected tissue (Flipo *et al.* 1994). Finally, there is evidence to suggest a role for both B and T cells in RV, which possibly includes dysregulated B cell–T cell interaction (Turesson *et al.* 2005).

Increased levels of circulating fibronectin have been detected in patients with RV (versus other CTDs), perhaps indicating activation of vascular endothelium (Voskuyl *et al.* 1998a). Autoantibodies reportedly associated with RV include antiendothelial cell antibodies (AECA), which were detected in 87% of patients with RV in one series (van der Zee *et al.* 1991). It is not clear whether these represent pathogenically active molecules or are simply indicators of the ongoing inflammatory process (see Chapter 7). AECAs have been detected in vasculitis seen with other CTDs as well as in primary vasculitis. The role they play in the pathogenesis of vasculitic processes remains unclear.

To date, the relationship of ANCA to RV remains equivocal (Bosch *et al.* 1995; Braun *et al.* 1996; Coremans *et al.* 1992; De Bandt *et al.* 1996). Perinuclear ANCAs (pANCA) were most often found; however, no pANCA that recognized myeloperoxidase or cathepsin G, the usual targets for pANCA, were found in these large studies of RV (Bosch *et al.* 1995; Braun *et al.* 1996; Coremans *et al.* 1992; De Bandt *et al.* 1996). These, as well as other, investigators found pANCA in patients with RA (typically long-standing) but without RV, therefore attenuating diagnostic significance of ANCA (De Bandt *et al.* 1996).

There is increasing evidence to support a role for particular genes in RV. An association of RV with the MHC class II HLA-DR4 genes containing the RA-associated shared epitope (SE) alleles has been described in several studies (Gonzalez *et al.* 1997; Hillarby *et al.* 1991; Jaraquemada *et al.* 1986; Toussirot *et al.* 1999; Turesson *et al.* 2005; Voskuyl *et al.* 1997; Weyand *et al.* 1992). These associations tend to be stronger in studies of northern European and Caucasian American RA populations. The presence of two HLA-DRB1*04 SE alleles was associated with RV (OR2.44, 95%CI 1.22–4.89) in a multicenter study of patients from Minnesota and Sweden (Turesson *et al.* 2005). Other studies have found an association between mild cutaneous RV and the *0401 and *0404 alleles (Voskuyl *et al.* 1997). In a recent meta-analysis RV was found to be associated with three specific genotypes containing a double dose of the SE, HLE-DRB1*0401/*0401, *0401/*0404, and *0401/*0101 (Gorman *et al.* 2004). Other genes, such as the MHC class I alleles HLA-C*03 and HLA-C*05 and the *KIR2DS2* gene, encoding a stimulatory killer-immunoglobulin-like receptor (KIR) on natural killer (NK) cells, have also been associated with vasculitis in RA (Yen *et al.* 2001).

RV can affect vessels of varying size with varying degrees of inflammation, which may occur concurrently in the same patient. Milder forms of RV typically involve smaller vessels (such as digital arteries and postcapillary venules) of the skin characterized by intimal proliferation, immune complex deposition, and intravascular thrombosis (Chen *et al.* 2002; Turesson and Jacobsson 2004). Medium and large artery involvement, manifest as necrotizing granulomatous vasculitis and abdominal microaneurysms, may be seen in more severe forms of RV (Chen *et al.* 2002). Mild cutaneous vasculitis may coexist with, or be followed by, more severe, systemic necrotizing vasculitis creating difficulties in the diagnosis and treatment of the patients with RV (Chen *et al.* 2002; Lindsay *et al.* 1973).

Cutaneous

Cutaneous RV is most common and is seen in 75–89% of RV patients (Chen *et al.* 2002; Geirsson *et al.* 1987; Scott *et al.* 1981c; Voskuyl *et al.* 1996a; Watts *et al.* 1994). The most common cutaneous findings include cutaneous ulcers (up to 63%), petechiae or palpable purpura (up to 56%), digital infarcts including innocuous nail-fold infarcts (up to 41%), and gangrene (up to 38%) (reviewed in Sayah and English 2005). Ulcers of the lower extremities have been described in up to 38% of subjects with RV and are typically acute in onset, painful, punched-out lesions occurring along the lateral malleolus or pretibial region. Other less common, cutaneous manifestations include: non-specific maculopapular or nodular erythema; hemorrhagic blisters; livedo reticularis; erythema elevatum diutinum; and atrophie blanche (Sayah and English 2005). Among a study of 11 subjects with RV, all but one had coexistence of different forms of cutaneous vasculitis (Chen *et al.* 2002).

Neurological

The most common extracutaneous manifestation of RV is a peripheral, non-compressive neuropathy. Mononeuritis multiplex and distal symmetric sensory or sensorimotor neuropathy occur in up to 50% of subjects with RV (see Chapter 14) (Bacon and Carruthers 1995; Puechal *et al.* 1995; Schneider *et al.* 1985). In a recent study of 32 subjects with biopsy confirmed RV of the peripheral nerves, morphologic analysis revealed epi- or perineural necrotizing vasculitis, with axonal degeneration in the majority of the nerve fibers (Puechal *et al.* 1995). In this study, the coexistence of cutaneous vasculitis, a multifocal neuropathy, or a depressed C4 level were associated with increased mortality. At a mean follow-up of 7.2 years, prolonged remission of the vasculitis was observed in 53% of the patients while 25% showed signs of relapse. A severe inflammatory myositis with small-vessel vasculitis has been found on muscle biopsy in a patient with mononeuritis multiplex with severe muscle weakness (Chatterjee and Kupsky 2005). Involvement is less common, but can lead to significant morbidity and mortality unless recognized and properly treated (Kim *et al.* 1982). Rheumatoid nodules and meningitis may occur independently or along with CNS vasculitis (Bathon *et al.* 1989).

Pulmonary

Pulmonary involvement in RA is common and can be due to the disease itself as well as to the therapies used to treat it. Lung disease has been reported to affect between 1 and 40% of patients with RA (Horton 2004). RA-associated interstitial lung disease (ILD) is often subtle in onset, slowly progressive, and of unclear etiology (Horton 2004). A case of diffuse alveolar hemorrhage (DAH) due to pulmonary capillaritis has been documented in a patient with RA and mixed connective tissue disease (MCTD) (Schwarz *et al.* 1998).

Cardiac and peripheral vascular

Cardiac vasculitis affecting medium and small intramyocardial arteries has been described in up to 20% of autopsy cases (Bonfiglio and Atwater 1969). This may lead to patchy myocardial necrosis due to microinfarction or ischemia (Bonfiglio and Atwater 1969; Cathcart and Spodick 1962; Sokoloff 1953). A non-occlusive vasculitis of the epicardial vessels has also been described (Morris *et al.* 1986; Voyles *et al.* 1980).

Aortitis of the thoracic and abdominal aorta or both has been described in a series of 10 RV patients (Gravallese *et al.* 1989). Mesenteric vasculitis is rare but is associated with significant mortality (Chen *et al.* 2002; Pagnoux *et al.* 2005). This should be suspected in RV patients with skin or peripheral nerve involvement who develop acute abdominal pain, colonic ulcerations, or appendicitis (Chen *et al.* 2002; Nagahama *et al.* 2000; Pagnoux *et al.* 2005; Scott and Bacon 1983; van Laar *et al.* 1998). Necrotizing vasculitis of renal vessels is rare (Bacons and Kitas 1994).

Ocular

Scleritis/keratitis has been reported to occur in up to 20% of patients with other manifestations of RV and has been described as a herald of diffuse vasculitis (Jifi-Bahlool *et al.* 1995).

Diagnosis and treatment

Ideally, the diagnosis of RV is made by histological examination of a biopsy specimen of an affected organ or by angiogram. Biopsy of clinically unaffected muscle, rectum, and labial salivary glands have also shown potential for diagnosing RV (Flipo *et al.* 1994; Tribe *et al.* 1981; Voskuyl *et al.* 1998b; Voskuyl *et al.* 2003). The diagnosis of RV can be inferred from classic clinical signs alone. This is demonstrated by the 1984 Scott and Bacon criteria for the diagnosis of RV which includes the presence of one or more of the following in a patient with RA: (1) mononeuritis multiplex or peripheral neuropathy; (2) peripheral gangrene; (3) biopsy evidence of acute necrotizing arteritis plus systemic illness, for example fever, weight loss; and (4) deep cutaneous ulcers or extra-articular disease, for example pleurisy, pericarditis, scleritis, if associated with typical digital infarcts or biopsy evidence of vasculitis (Scott and Bacon 1984). More recently, Voskuyl and others sought to determine the optimal diagnostic strategy for RA patients suspected of having RV (Voskuyl *et al.* 2003). In their cohort of 81 subjects with suspected RV they found peripheral neuropathy or purpura/petechiae were the most important clinical features to discriminate RA patients with and without histological proven RV. The presence of a high number of recent onset (≤6 months) extra-articular RA manifestations, an elevated IgA RF level, and decreased C3 also were associated with increased probability of RV.

There are no randomized, controlled trials of the treatment of RV. The treatment of RV varies according to clinical severity. Several diseases may mimic RV and should be considered prior to initiation of RV treatment. These include cholesterol embolization syndrome (cutaneous lesions and infarcts), peripheral vascular disease or venous insufficiency (leg ulcers), diabetes mellitus (mononeuritis multiplex), other forms of primary vasculitis such as polyarteritis nodosa and cryoglobulinemia.

In its mildest form, simple nail-fold infarcts may be treated either by adjustment of DMARD therapy as one would for routine synovitis, or by close observation (Vollertsen and Conn 1990). Leg ulcerations and leukocytoclastic vasculitis are typically managed with aggressive topical therapy, moderate dose glucocorticoids, and DMARD therapy such as methotrexate (MTX) (McRorie *et al.* 1998). Other unvalidated therapies for treatment of vasculitic leg ulcers include topical nerve growth factor (not available in the US), and pinch skin grafting (Oien *et al.* 2001; Tuveri *et al.* 2000).

More severe forms of RV, such as mononeuropathy multiplex, digital infarction, mesenteric vasculitis, or cutaneous vasculitis that fails to respond to more conservative measures, require more aggressive therapy. Standard treatment includes high-dose pulse or continuous cyclophosphamide along with glucocorticoids (Scott and Bacon 1984). Pulse-dose regimens consist of IV prednisolone at 6.6–10 mg/kg and IV cyclophosphamide at 10–15 mg/kg at 2–4 week intervals, with dose adjustment for associated cytopenias (Luqmani *et al.* 1994, 2005). Oral regimens include prednisone at 1 mg/kg/day with a slow taper to 10 mg/day or less over several months with oral daily cyclophosphamide at 2 mg/kg/day which is continued as the glucocorticoid dose is tapered to 7.5 mg/day or less (Sundy *et al.* 2004). If remission is maintained for 9–12 months then cyclophosphamide can be slowly tapered over 2 to 3 months (Sundy *et al.* 2004).

Methotrexate (MTX) by intrathecal administration has been reported to be effective in CNS vasculitis complicating RA (Bathon *et al.* 1989). Success using MTX by the oral route has been reported in one case (Ohno *et al.* 1994). MTX has been implicated as a possible causative agent of drug-induced vasculitis, however, a review of patients from the Mayo Clinic over 20 years failed to detect an increased incidence of RV from MTX (Goronzy and Weyand 1994). Other therapies used for RV, either alone or in combination with glucocorticoids, include D-penicillamine, cyclosporin, azathioprine, leflunomide, and plasma exchange (Axson 1979; Heurkens *et al.* 1991; Jaffe and Smith 1968; Knab *et al.* 2005; Nicholls *et al.* 1973; Schneider *et al.* 1985; Scott *et al.* 1981b).

The efficacy of anti-TNF therapy for RV is limited but encouraging. There have been approximately 10 case reports in the literature and the clinical response was good in all patients treated with infliximab (n = 8), as well as in two patients receiving the TNF-α-binding fusion proteins etanercept and lenercept (Armstrong *et al.* 2005; den Broeder *et al.* 2001; Garcia-Porrua *et al.* 2006; Richter *et al.* 2000; van der Bijl *et al.* 2005). In six of these patients, initial treatment with cyclophosphamide was ineffective and in four patients anti-TNF agents were added to maintenance therapy. In contrast, one report describes a patient with progression of pre-existing mononeuritis during infliximab therapy after initial therapy with glucocorticoids and cyclophosphamide (Richette *et al.* 2004). While some are now advocating anti-TNF agents as first-line therapy for RV it certainly can be considered in patients who do not respond to immunosuppressive drugs or in those with a contraindication for such treatment (Garcia-Porrua *et al.* 2006; van der Bijl *et al.* 2005).

Infection and cardiovascular disease have been reported as the two most common causes of death in RV in a large series (Voskuyl *et al.* 1996b). Frequent and careful surveillance for treatment-related adverse events are an essential aspect of treatment for RV. There is also the evolving concept that such local vascular inflammation in RV has important effects on distant vascular endothelium (Buckley *et al.* 2005). This systemic endothelial dysfunction may further contribute to the increased cardiovascular disease described in patients with RV.

Systemic lupus erythematosus and vasculitis

Systemic lupus erythematosus (SLE) is a chronic, immune-mediated, inflammatory multisystem disorder (Mills 1994). Involvement of blood vessels may be a manifestation of SLE itself or the clinical presentation of a syndrome more compatible with other types of vasculopathy. Thus, vascular disease in SLE occurs through a variety of lesions (and combinations thereof), including atherosclerosis, thrombosis due to aggregates of leukocytes or platelets with or without antiphospholipid (APL) antibodies or inflammation (Danning *et al.* 1998; McDonald *et al.* 1992; Rocca *et al.* 1994). Evaluating the contributions made by these potential etiologies of vascular injury is important, as optimal treatment should be based on the operative mechanisms (Greisman *et al.* 1991; Somer 1993).

Epidemiology

Vasculitis as a manifestation of SLE is not rare. In a largely Caucasian population, the reported incidence of SLE vasculitis was 3.6 per million persons, nearly the same as one estimate of vasculitis due to infection (Watts *et al.* 1995). When patients with SLE are examined as a group most studies report a prevalence of vasculitis ranging between 11% and 36% (Cardinali *et al.* 2000; Drenkard *et al.* 1997; Gonzalez-Gay and Garcia-Porrua 1999; Ramos-Casals *et al.* 2006; Vitali *et al.* 1992; Vlachoyiannopoulos *et al.* 1993). Cutaneous vasculitis involving small arteries and venules of the skin is most common, accounting for between 82% and 90% of cases. Medium vessel involvement is less frequent, accounting for less than 15% of cases, and is manifest as mononeuritis multiplex in the majority of cases, followed by abdominal vasculitis (Drenkard *et al.* 1997; Ramos-Casals *et al.* 2006). Lupus-associated, large-vessel vasculitis is rare with a few reported cases of lower extremity large-artery vasculitis and coronary vasculitis (Drenkard *et al.* 1997). Visceral involvement portends increased morbidity and mortality. Between 10% and 40% of lupus vasculitis patients have both cutaneous and visceral involvement.

In a large cohort of SLE subjects (n = 667) described by Drenkard *et al.* (1997), patients with vasculitis were more commonly male (odds ratio 2.2), had onset of disease at an earlier age (mean age 26 years), and had longer duration of disease than those without vasculitis. Clinical features associated with the presence of vasculitis included documented Raynaud's phenomenon, APL syndrome, neuropsychiatric lupus, myocarditis, serositis, and lymphopenia. In another large cohort of SLE subjects (n = 670), from Spain, those with vasculitis had a significantly greater prevalence of livedo reticularis, greater SLE disease activity, more frequent anemia, higher ESR, and greater prevalence of anti-La/SS-B antibodies, compared to those without vasculitis (Ramos-Casals *et al.* 2006). In this study, APL antibodies were more common in patients with vasculitis on univariate analysis (52% vs. 23%; p = 0.002); however, this did not remain significant in the multivariate analysis.

Pathogenesis

Vascular injury in SLE is thought to be primarily mediated by IC deposition in vessel walls, leading to an inflammatory cascade through complement activation (Ansari *et al.* 1986; Fauci *et al.* 1978). Most biopsy specimens of vasculitic lesions from SLE patients demonstrate deposits of IgG, components of complement, and fibrin deposition, indicating an IC-mediated process. However, the presence of IC cannot always be demonstrated. There is anecdotal evidence that vasculitis in a given patient with SLE may involve different organ systems by distinct mechanisms, such as cell–cell interactions (Feriozzi *et al.* 1997). CD40 ligand is expressed on a higher number of T and B cells in SLE patients than in controls, and *in vitro* evidence suggests that interaction with CD40 on endothelial cells produces activation of B cells and increased expression of adhesion molecules (Koshy *et al.* 1996). In addition to cell–cell interactions, cytokine 'priming' and autoantibody stimulation of the endothelium in SLE may also play roles in vascular activation (Alexander *et al.* 1985; Belmont *et al.* 1996). By these mechanisms, the final common pathways in SLE vasculitis are increased expression of adhesion molecules by activated endothelium along with production of complement split products, which promote inflammatory cell recruitment and migration (see below).

Serum levels of soluble adhesion molecules are elevated in a variety of inflammatory conditions that involve vascular injury, both with and without vasculitis (Carson *et al.* 1993). Several investigators have attempted to correlate expression of vascular adhesion signals with disease activity in SLE patients with vasculitis. Lymphocytes from SLE patients with active vasculitis are known to have increased surface density of the integrin Very Late Antigen-4 (VLA-4) (Takeuchi *et al.* 1995). Soluble ICAM-1 and E-selectin levels have not been shown to correlate with disease activity in either SLE or other forms of vasculitis (Janssen *et al.* 1994).

AECAs have been proposed as "endothelial activators" and several investigators have noted an increased occurrence of AECAs in SLE patients with vasculitis (Alarcon-Segovia *et al.* 1992; d'Cruz 1998; d'Cruz *et al.* 1997; Li *et al.* 1996). Two groups have noted that APLs tend to occur along with AECAs in SLE patients with vasculitis and therefore a causal role for AECAs in vasculitis remains speculative (Drenkard *et al.* 1997; Navarro *et al.* 1997).

A considerable literature exists regarding the existence and clinical significance of ANCA in SLE (reviewed in Sen and Isenberg 2003). Approximately 15–20% of SLE patients have pANCA antibodies (Sen and Isenberg 2003). Several attempts have been made to correlate activity of vasculitis in SLE with the presence of ANCA (Pedrollo *et al.* 1993; Waldendorf and Schneider 1993). There appears to be a link between pANCA levels and disease activity in some patients; however, there is no consensus regarding a correlation between ANCA levels and the presence of vasculitis (Chin *et al.* 2000; Lee and Lawton 1992; Nishiya *et al.* 1997; Schnabel *et al.* 1995; Sen and Isenberg 2003).

There is a well-established correlation between cutaneous vasculitis (as well as subacute cutaneous lupus) and the presence of anti-SSA/Ro antibodies (Lee and Norris 1989; Simmons-O'Brien *et al.* 1995). Others have reported associations between cutaneous vasculitis and anti-Smith, anti-SSB-La and anti-dsDNA antibodies (Beaufils *et al.* 1983; Ramos-Casals *et al.* 2006; Tikly *et al.* 1996). A study involving a cohort of more than 300 patients with SLE found a particular association between the presence of anti-dsDNA antibodies of the IgA subclass with clinical vasculitis (Witte *et al.* 1998).

Cutaneous

The most common organ affected by vasculitis in SLE is the skin (Belmont *et al.* 1996) (see Figure 34.2). Cutaneous vasculitis is more common in children with SLE than adults (Carreno *et al.* 1999). Cutaneous vasculitis has diverse manifestations, perhaps due primarily to variation in skin depth and intensity of vessel involvement. Although morphologic features usually suggest vasculitis, punch biopsy is the standard diagnostic method employed to confirm the diagnosis. This is particularly important in SLE where mimickers of vasculitis (atherosclerotic disease, thrombosis, etc., see Chapter 45) are prevalent and the treatments pursued are sharply divergent from that of vasculitis.

Erythematous punctuate lesions on the fingertips and palms are the most common cutaneous finding, occurring in up to two-thirds of patients (Drenkard *et al.* 1997; Ramos-Casals *et al.* 2006). Palpable purpura is also common (~25%) followed by ischemic lesions or ulcers (~14%), urticarial lesions (~5–10%), and nodular lesions (~5%); a combination of lesions is found in approximately 30% of patients. The most frequent location of the lesions were: the lower

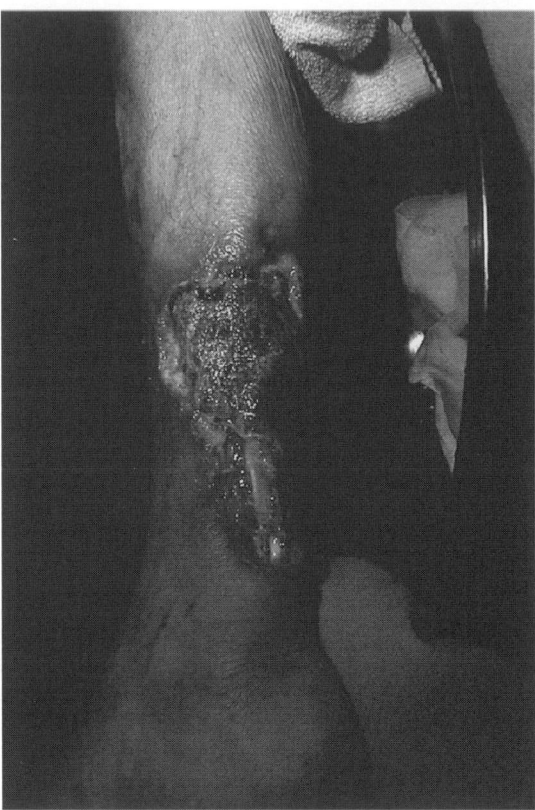

Figure 34.2 Vasculitis in a young woman with systemic lupus erythematosus. (Courtesy of Dr Gene Ball.) From: R. Jones and L. Moreland. Vasculitis in Primary Connective Tissue Diseases. In: *Vasculitis*, 1st edn. G. V. Ball and S. L. Bridges, Jr, eds. Oxford University Press, 2002. (See Color Plate 92).

extremities (42%); hands (40%); upper extremities (20%); trunk (5%); and face (3%); 3% were generalized.

Leukocytoclastic vasculitis is the most common pattern reported on biopsy with classic findings of fibrinoid changes in the vessel walls composed of immunoglobulin, especially IgM, and complement (Calamia and Balabanova 2004). Diffuse neutrophilic and mononuclear/lymphocytic perivascular infiltrates have also been described, possibly associated with the age of the lesion (Calamia and Balabanova 2004). Lesions of small arterioles or venules high in the dermal layer produce a petechial morphology but necrosis can occur if the vasculitis is particularly robust (Lee and Norris 1989). Not all petechial lesions represent vasculitis, as thrombocytopenia can also produce such lesions. Palpable purpura or urticaria result from vascular involvement deeper in the dermis. Extensive damage at this level may result in bullous-type lesions. Such lesions almost always are due to leukocytoclastic vasculitis (Laman and Provost 1994; Tsuchida *et al.* 1994). Subcutaneous nodules akin to polyarteritis nodosa are the consequence of vasculitis at the dermal–epidermal junction. Ulcerations from these lesions may result if collateral circulation is impaired, for example from coexistent atherosclerotic or thrombotic disease (Martens *et al.* 1999; Sanchez *et al.* 1981).

Urticarial lesions that persist for more than 24 hours may be a vasculitis manifestation of SLE (Calamia and Balabanova 2004). Urticarial lesions in SLE have been shown to be commonly associated with hypocomplementemia (d'Cruz 1998). Hypocomplementemic urticarial vasculitis (HUV) is associated with anti-C1q antibodies (Trendelenburg *et al.* 1999). Anti-C1q antibodies are also present in SLE; therefore, the distinction between these two disease entities can sometimes be blurred.

Treatment of cutaneous vasculitis in SLE is tailored to the underlying disease process. Antimalarials such as hydroxychloroquine may be effective in mild cases. Dapsone (100–200 mg/day) has also been utilized (Holtman *et al.* 1990). Reported side-effects of dapsone (hemolytic anemia, agranulocytosis, and neuropathy) are not trivial and all patients should have a documented normal complete blood count and G6PD level prior to starting dapsone. Thalidomide may also be considered for use in carefully selected patients (Godfrey *et al.* 1998). Glucocorticoids are often used as "bridge" therapy to control moderate to severe disease while waiting for a more potent cytotoxic agent such as azathioprine to produce clinical benefit (Callen *et al.* 1991). Cyclophosphamide is effective, but should be reserved for severe, refractory cases of cutaneous vasculitis (Nishijima *et al.* 1999). Mycophenolate mofetil (MMF) has recently been reported to show promise for several dermatologic conditions, and for other manifestations of SLE, but a role in SLE cutaneous vasculitis remains to be defined (Goyal and Nousari 2001; Liu and Mackool 2003; Pisoni *et al.* 2005). Similarly, rituximab may be a promising treatment for SLE and may have utility in the treatment of severe or treatment resistant, cutaneous, lupus vasculitis (Van den *et al.* 2005; Weide *et al.* 2003).

Visceral

Extracutaneous involvement is observed in 12% to 20% of subjects with lupus vasculitis (Drenkard *et al.* 1997; Ramos-Casals *et al.* 2006). Mononeuropathy multiplex accounts for over one half of the cases described (see below). The second most common is abdominal vasculitis (see Chapter 15). Intestinal vasculitis is most commonly described, primarily located in the ileum or colon. In a report by Medina *et al.* (1997), of 13 SLE subjects with ileal or colonic vasculitis, the mortality approached 50%, particularly if the patient presented with an acute abdomen or if surgery were delayed. Other less frequent sites of visceral vasculitic involvement include the pancreas, gallbladder, urinary bladder, liver, and uterus (Alarcon-Segovia *et al.* 1984; Bando *et al.* 2003; Feriozzi *et al.* 1997; Karrar *et al.* 2001; Matsumoto *et al.* 1992; Medina *et al.* 1997; Newbold *et al.* 1987).

Abdominal pain is common in SLE patients (~20%) and differentiating benign from life-threatening causes can be difficult (Lee *et al.* 2002; Medina *et al.* 1997). In a recent study of 175 subjects admitted to the hospital with SLE, 22% presented with acute abdominal pain and of those 45% were due to gastrointestinal vasculitis (Lee *et al.* 2002). A similar percentage was found by Medina *et al.* (1997), and this percentage increased to over 50% in those patients with active disease. In patients with inactive SLE the overall incidence of mesenteric vasculitis is reportedly low (<1%) (Sultan *et al.* 1999). Postprandial timing of pain, vomiting, fever, guiac-positive stool, or overt hematochezia suggest mesenteric vasculitis as a cause of abdominal pain (Wallace and Metzger 1997). Antiphospholipid antibody syndrome may also cause vessel obstruction from thrombosis and it can be difficult to distinguish from vasculitis (Asherson *et al.* 1985; Asherson *et al.* 1986; Provenzale and Ortel 1995).

Arteriography is the gold standard diagnostic test (Zizic *et al.* 1982), although computed tomography has advantages in terms of wide availability and promptness of result (Ko *et al.* 1997;

Zizic *et al.* 1982). The successful use of CT to detect mesenteric vasculitis in 11 of 15 patients with SLE has been reported (Ko *et al.* 1997). Characteristic findings included pallisading vessels in areas adjacent to ischemic bowel as well as thickening of the affected bowel wall with enhancement (Lee *et al.* Moon 2002). High-dose intravenous methylprednisolone and cyclophosphamide are the usual treatments (Grimbacher *et al.* 1998; Laing 1988).

Pulmonary

Pulmonary involvement occurs in approximately 60% of patients with SLE during the course of the disease (Paran *et al.* 2004). Pulmonary vasculitis, however, is rare, occurring in less than 2% patients according to an autopsy study (Haupt *et al.* 1981). Pulmonary vasculitis can occur with or without diffuse alveolar hemorrhage (DAH) (Zamora *et al.* 1997). Pulmonary hemorrhage was the initial clinical event in SLE in 10–20% of the few cases where DAH was secondary to SLE (Schwab *et al.* 1993; Zamora *et al.* 1997) (see Chapter 13). Most patients with this syndrome have associated nephritis (perhaps unrecognized) and a diagnosis of SLE of less than 5 years (Calamia and Balabanova 2004; Liu *et al.* 1998). DAH may have an occult presentation but most patients initially report abrupt onset of dyspnea (Blanche *et al.* 1996). Hemoptysis is a presenting complaint in less than 50%. Fever, hypoxemia, patchy infiltrates on chest radiographs, and decreasing hematocrit should prompt clinical suspicion (Zamora *et al.* 1997). The last of these features distinguishes DAH from the otherwise similar presentation of acute lupus pneumonitis. An increased single breath carbon monoxide diffusion determination further suggests DAH (Greening and Hughes 1981). Bloody fluid on bronchoalveolar lavage in these circumstances strongly supports DAH (Leatherman *et al.* 1984). Radiographic features of DAH are indistinguishable from pneumonia and pulmonary edema; therefore, aggressive procurement of material for culture as well as broad antibiotic/antifungal/antiviral coverage should be considered (Zamora *et al.* 1997). The histological lesions seen in DAH due to vasculitis are those of capillaritis. An associated lesion is "microangiitis," where capillaries as well as arterioles and small muscular arteries are involved (Myers and Katzenstein 1986; Santos-Ocampo *et al.* 2000; Zamora *et al.* 1997). This lesion has been purported to be pathognomonic for SLE (Myers and Katzenstein 1986).

Pulmonary manifestations of antiphospholipid antibody syndrome (APS) can be strikingly similar to SLE related pulmonary vasculitis and DAH (Nguyen *et al.* 2005). Apart from pulmonary embolism and pulmonary hypertension, catastrophic APS can cause diffuse pulmonary infiltrates, capillaritis, and diffuse alveolar hemorrhage (Nguyen *et al.* 2005). Fortunately, pulmonary APS and SLE vasculitis are reported to exhibit a similar clinical course and response to treatment.

The mortality in SLE patients with DAH is greater than 50% in most studies (Zamora *et al.* 1997). Early diagnosis and aggressive therapy has been shown to improve survival considerably (Santos-Ocampo *et al.* 2000; Schwab *et al.* 1993). Although multiple interventions have been utilized, pulse-dose glucocorticoids are a mainstay of therapy with or without concurrent cyclophosphamide (Santos-Ocampo *et al.* 2000). Utilization of plasmapheresis in synchrony with cyclophosphamide pulses has been reported, with variable success (Erickson *et al.* 1994; Schroeder and Euler 1989). The use of mycophenolate mofetil (MMF) has been shown to be effective for SLE nephritis and other lupus disease manifestations

indicating its potential for treatment of pulmonary vasculitis and DAH (Bijl *et al.* 2003). SLE patients with DAH who survive are at increased risk of future episodes of DAH as well as other severe manifestations of SLE; therefore, they have diminished life-expectancy compared with SLE patients without DAH (Zamora *et al.* 1997).

Vasculitis in SLE may also involve the upper airway, albeit rarely. Ulcerations of the larynx as well as overt necrotizing vasculitis of the larynx, tracheal structures, and large bronchi have been reported (Boumpas *et al.* 1995; Teitel *et al.* 1992).

Cardiac and peripheral vascular

Pericarditis is the most common cardiac manifestation of SLE, found in up to 60% of cases examined post-mortem (Doherty *et al.* 1988). Echocardiographic studies show pericardial abnormalities in 11% to 54% of patients with SLE (Doria *et al.* 2005). Pericardial disease appears more frequently at disease onset or during relapses (Doria *et al.* 2005). Immune complex deposition in small vessels of the pericardium is the underlying cause (Bidani *et al.* 1980). Pericardial effusions vary in size, but complications such as tamponade, constrictive pericarditis, or purulent pericarditis are rare. Non-steroidal anti-inflammatory drugs or low-dose glucocorticoids are effective in mild, symptomatic pericarditis; a moderate dose of oral glucocorticoids (prednisone 1 mg/kg/day) is usually effective for more severe cases. In patients with refractory or recurring pericarditis, chronic immunosuppression with methotrexate, azathioprine, MMF, or IVIg may be beneficial. Invasive procedures such as pericardiocentesis or pericardial window are rarely required (Doria *et al.* 2005).

Valvular abnormalities in SLE are common. Libman–Sachs (verrucous) endocarditis is the most characteristic lesion; however, valvular thickening and regurgitation are more common than verrucous endocarditis (Doria *et al.* 2005). Anatomic valvular lesions are observed in 18–74% of all patients with SLE and tend to occur in the mitral and aortic valves. Actual valvulitis with vasculitis and resultant fibrinoid necrosis may be seen on histological examination in the rare instances of severe valvular disease. Fortunately, lesions of such severity probably occur in only 1–2% of all cases (Straaton *et al.* 1988). Severe valvulitis is managed by valve replacement when clinically indicated.

Clinical myocarditis occurs in 7% to 10% of SLE patients (Bidani *et al.* 1980; Bulkley and Roberts 1975; Doria *et al.* 2005; Roberts and High 1999). When severe, the condition presents as congestive heart failure and the diagnosis is confirmed by the clinical context and endomyocardial biopsy (Fairfax *et al.* 1988). Biopsy material shows intravascular IC deposition with vasculitis and adjacent myocarditis. Treatment with moderate to high doses of glucocorticoids has been effective in some cases (Fairfax *et al.* 1988). Importantly, myocardial dysfunction in SLE may be secondary to other causes such as coronary artery disease due to premature atherosclerosis, hypertension, valvular disease, or toxicity to medications, for example cyclophosphamide or chloroquine (Doria *et al.* 2005; Kao and Manzi 2002).

Coronary artery disease occurs in 6% to 10% of SLE patients and is most often due to atherosclerosis (Petri *et al.* 1992; Toloza *et al.* 2004). The risk of developing coronary artery disease is four to eight times higher than controls and the risk of myocardial infarction is increased 50-fold in young women with SLE (Manzi *et al.* 1997). Current knowledge indicates that atherosclerosis is an active inflammatory and immune-mediated process. Therefore, the processes characteristic of SLE can undoubtedly contribute to the accelerated vascular disease seen in these patients (Kao *et al.* 2003). Coronary arteritis is rare and may be exacerbated by coexistent atherosclerosis (Moder *et al.* 1999). Differentiating coronary arteritis from lesions due to atherosclerosis may be difficult but important for therapeutic decisions. The presence of aneurysmal dilatation and rapid progression of lesions on arteriography support vasculitis (Heibel *et al.* 1976; Nobrega *et al.* 1996). Active SLE and a short duration of symptoms should also heighten clinical suspicion for coronary arteritis (Badui *et al.* 1985; Doria *et al.* 2005). In case of coronary vasculitis, glucocorticoids at high doses are recommended. When atherosclerotic coronary artery disease is suspected, diagnosis and treatment should follow current recommended guidelines. Additionally, a concerted effort to modify both traditional risk factors and immune and inflammatory processes in SLE patients is critical in preventing premature cardiovascular disease (Kao *et al.* 2003).

Large-vessel vasculitis, indistinguishable from that of Takayasu's arteritis, has been reported in SLE. Due to the lack of common pathologic and serologic features between SLE vasculitis and Takayasu's arteritis, it has been suggested that these 'overlap' cases represent random occurrences of two different autoimmune diseases in one individual (Lorber *et al.* 1994). Most reported cases of large-vessel vasculitis have responded to moderate doses of oral prednisone (1 mg/kg/day), while others have required the addition of cyclophosphamide (Saxe and Altman 1992). Azathioprine and MMF are other therapeutic options (Daina *et al.* 1999; Kao *et al.* 2003).

Renal

Renal vessels, including the specialized vascular bed of the glomeruli, are at particular risk for immune complex binding or deposition (Calamia and Balabanova 2004; Hricik *et al.* 1998). Histologically, the pattern of glomerular injury may vary to include capillary proliferation, fibrinoid necrosis, or hyaline thrombi. The most common form of renal vasculitis is capillaritis and is the underlying vascular lesion in the proliferative forms of lupus nephritis (WHO classes III and IV). Less commonly, lesions reminiscent of necrotizing vasculitis may involve larger renal arteries which is associated with severe renal disease (Bacon and Carruthers 1995). Glucocorticoids with cyclophosphamide have been the cornerstones of therapy for renal vasculitis. Recent, short-term studies have indicated the therapeutic equivalence of mycophenolate mofetil and cyclophosphamide for in induction of remission, but results are still far from ideal (Boumpas *et al.* 1995; Ginzler *et al.* 2005).

Neurological

Neuropsychiatric SLE (NPSLE) affects 17% to 72% of patients and is manifested by a wide variety of symptoms (Eber *et al.* 2005; West 1994). In 1999, the ACR produced a standard nomenclature and diagnostic criteria for 19 neuropsychiatric syndromes known to occur in SLE (American College of Rheumatology 1999). The most frequent NPSLE symptoms include cognitive dysfunction, headache, mood disorder, cerebrovascular disease, seizures, polyneuropathy, anxiety, and psychosis (Hanly and Harrison 2005). Three primary immunopathogenic mechanisms are most often implicated in NPSLE: vasculopathy of primarily small intracranial vessels; autoantibody production, for example antineuronal, antiribosomal, antiphospholipid; and the generation of inflammatory

mediators, for example IL-6, IL-10, IL-2, IL-8, and MMP-9 (Hanly 2005). Vasculitis is an uncommon cause of NPSLE, accounting for less than 10% of cases (Drenkard *et al.* 1997); however, small-vessel involvement and occlusions may cause signs and symptoms of NPSLE (Boumpas *et al.* 1995). Large-vessel occlusive disease is rare and typically presents as a stroke or intracerebral hemorrhage and carries a relatively poor prognosis (Mitsias and Levine 1994; Weiner and Allen 1991). Arterial thrombus, dissection, fibromuscular dysplasia, and vasculitis should be considered with large vessel involvement.

In diagnosing NPSLE, cerebrospinal fluid studies are important to exclude infection; although cell count, total protein, and oligoclonal band determination are not reliable indicators of NPSLE (West 1994). Studies have demonstrated an association of antiribosomal-P antibodies and psychiatric manifestations of NPSLE; however, others have disputed it (reviewed in Eber *et al.* 2005). Imaging studies are more likely to be revealing in patients with focal neurological deficits rather than diffuse encephalopathy (Boumpas *et al.* 1995). MRI is more likely to show small-vessel vasculopathy, but asymptomatic periventricular white matter changes are found in a large number of patients with SLE (Kent *et al.* 1994; Rovaris *et al.* 2000). MR arteriography (MRA), computed tomography (CT), and radiocontrast arteriography are useful only in detecting the rare instances of larger-vessel vasculitis (see Chapters 18 and 19). Positron emission tomography (PET) spectroscopy (see Chapter 20) has reportedly proven useful in demonstrating diminished CNS blood flow in SLE vasculitis, but this finding awaits confirmation in larger series (Hanly 1998).

Management of NPSLE needs to be tailored according to the individual patient and the manifestation of the disease. Initial attention should be focused on treating non-SLE-related factors including infection, hypertension, or metabolic abnormalities. Symptomatic therapy with anticonvulsants, antidepressants, or antipsychotic medications should be considered (Hanly and Harrison 2005). Immunosuppressive therapy with moderate-dose oral prednisone (1 mg/kg daily) or methylprednisolone pulse therapy can be used. Administration of cyclophosphamide should be considered for refractory or life-threatening disease (Boumpas *et al.* 1995). Azathioprine, MMF, and intravenous immunoglobulin (IVIg) are other therapeutic options.

Transverse myelitis consists of segmental spinal cord compromise due to vascular occlusion and occurs in SLE due to either thrombosis or vasculitis. A strong association between transverse myelitis and APLs exists in patients with SLE (Lavalle *et al.* 1990). Patients present with hemiparesis, often complicated by urinary sphincter dysfunction. The diagnosis is confirmed by MRI, which shows increased cord diameter as well as increased T1 and T2-weighted signal in the affected cord segments (Provenzale *et al.* 1994). When recognized early, myelitis has been successfully treated with high-dose methylprednisolone and cyclophosphamide (Barile and Lavalle 1992; Harisdangkul *et al*, 1995). Treatment should not be abandoned early, as there are reports of response after months of treatment. A single case report described the successful use of combination methylprednisolone/azathioprine for transverse myelitis (Schantz *et al.* 1998).

Peripheral neuropathy has been reported in up to 28% of SLE patients (Ainiala *et al.* 2001; Brey *et al.* 2002; Hanly *et al.* 2004; Hanly and Harrison 2005). It is usually a sensorimotor neuropathy which is mild, persistent, and frequently occurs independently of other disease characteristics (Hanly and Harrison 2005; Omdal *et al.* 2001). Other, less frequent forms of peripheral neuropathy include mononeuritis multiplex, autonomic neuropathies, cranial neuropathies, plexopathy, and Guillain–Barré syndrome (Bloch *et al.* 1979; Hanly and Harrison 2005; Liote and Osterland 1994; Martinez-Taboada *et al.* 1996; Straub *et al.* 1996; van Laarhoven *et al.* 2001). The diagnosis should be established by nerve conduction velocity assessment followed by nerve biopsy (usually the sural nerve) for histologic confirmation. Non-specific axonal degeneration with demyelination is the most common finding, but necrotizing vasculitis of perineural vessels has been reported (Griffin 2001). The distinction may be important in terms of therapeutic approach; IVIg may be the preferred treatment for the former, while combination prednisone/cytotoxic agent therapy is indicated for the latter (Enevoldson and Wiles 1991; Lesprit *et al.* 1996).

Ophthalmologic

SLE can affect every structure in the eye and ocular inflammation can antedate the diagnosis of the disease. The most common ocular manifestation is keratoconjunctivitis sicca (Peponis *et al.* 2006). Recurrent episcleritis has been reported in up to 28% of SLE patients and has a clinically benign course (Frith *et al.* 1990). Less frequently scleritis occurs in SLE and causes severe ocular morbidity (Peponis *et al.* 2006). SLE retinopathy has been reported in up to 25% of patients and in most cases is due to an immune complex mediated vasculopathy. Abnormalities in the retinal vasculature include vascular sheathing, arterial narrowing, capillary and venous dilation, tortuosity, and microaneurysms. Severe vasoocclusive retinopathy due to vasculitis or associated with antiphospholipid antibodies is rare; however, unlike the immune complex mediated retinopathy, it carries a high risk of ensuing visual loss (Au and O'Day 2004; Klinkhoff *et al.* 1986). This form of retinal disease is also reported to be associated with similar changes in the CNS vasculature (Jabs *et al.* 1986; Klinkhoff *et al.* 1986). Treatment of retinal vasculitis is with glucocorticoids, but ischemic retinal vasculopathy due to APLs may require anticoagulation. Several reports indicate SLE retinopathy (1) parallels systemic disease activity and (2) is a marker of poor prognosis for survival (Klinkhoff *et al.* 1986; Stafford-Brady *et al.* 1988). SLE patients should, therefore, have regular ophthalmologic examinations, even if they are not on antimalarial therapy.

In summary, vasculitis has widespread and diverse manifestations in SLE. It is most commonly recognized in the skin but may be present as capillarities in all organs and as larger vessel disease in a number of organs and its presence is associated with increased morbidity and mortality. Causes of pseudovasculitis, including APS, are also common in SLE and should be considered in the evaluation of ischemic events. The degree of disease severity dictates therapy ranging from careful observation, to high-dose glucocorticoids and cytotoxic agents. The increased availability and research utilizing targeted immunotherapy holds promise for improved treatment and understanding of disease pathogenesis (Calamia and Balabanova 2004).

Sjögren's syndrome and vasculitis

Epidemiology

Primary Sjögren's syndrome (SS) is an autoimmune disorder characterized by lymphocytic infiltration of lacrimal and salivary glands leading to xerostomia and keratoconjunctivitis sicca, and systemic production of antibodies (Fox 2005). Systemic (extraglandular) manifestations occur in one-third of patients with SS. Vasculitis is one of the most characteristic extraglandular manifestations with biopsy-proven vasculitis occurring in approximately 13% of patients (Tsokos *et al.* 1987). Vasculitis in SS can affect arteries of different sizes, veins, and capillaries in various organs with cutaneous small-vessel vasculitis being the most common (Ramos-Casals *et al.* 2006). Several studies have described an association with the presence of anti-SSA/Ro antibodies and vasculitis while another group found no differences in autoantibodies between SS patients with and without vasculitis (Alexander and Provost 1983).

Cutaneous

Cutaneous vasculitis has been reported in 9%–32% of patients with SS with a predominance of small-vessel vasculitis (SVV) (Garcia-Carrasco *et al.* 2002; Ramos-Casals *et al.* 2002). Cutaneous SVV can be further categorized, in order of frequency, as: (1) non-cryoglobulinemic, non-urticarial vasculitis presenting as palpable purpura in the lower extremities; (2) cryoglobulinemic vasculitis manifesting as palpable purpura primarily affecting the lower extremities; and (3) urticarial vasculitis with erythematosus, urticariform macules on the lower or upper extremities (Ramos-Casals *et al.* 2006). Cutaneous medium-vessel, necrotizing vasculitis is rare and typically presents as ischemic/ulcerative lesions (Ramos-Casals *et al.* Font 2006). Venous and arterial thrombotic lesions can also occur. SS patients with cutaneous vasculitis typically have a higher prevalence of anemia, an elevated ESR, hypergammaglobulinemia, and a higher frequency of immunologic markers (ANA, RF, antiRo/SSA antibodies) compared to those SS patients without cutaneous vasculitis (Alexander *et al.* 1983; Garcia-Carrasco *et al.* 2002; Ramos-Casals *et al.* 2002; Tsokos *et al.* 1987). Treatment of cutaneous vasculitis typically involves glucocorticoids in low to moderate doses. Other drugs such as hydroxychloroquine, dapsone, IVIg, methotrexate, azathioprine, and cyclophosphamide can be used alone or in combination with glucocorticoids depending on disease severity (Fox 2005; Price *et al.* 1998; Skopouli *et al.* 1996).

Neurological

The nervous system can be globally involved in SS, observed in approximately 20%–25% of cases (Delalande *et al.* 2004). Peripheral nervous system involvement is most common, affecting 10%–20% of cases (Garcia-Carrasco *et al.* 2002; Govoni *et al.* 1999; Ramos-Casals *et al.* 2002). Peripheral sensory or sensory–motor neuropathies are most common, followed by cranial neuropathies affecting trigeminal, facial, and cochlear nerves (Delalande *et al.* 2004; Grant *et al.* 1997). Multiple mononeuropathy, although far less common, frequently occurs in patients with more severe systemic disease and can be associated with small to medium-vessel vasculitis (Delalande *et al.* 2004; Fox 2005). Central nervous system (CNS) involvement is well documented in SS although the frequency varies widely across studies. In a recent study of 82 patients with neurologic manifestations associated with SS, CNS involvement was described in 68% of patients and preceded the diagnosis of SS in 45 patients (Delalande *et al.* 2004). Almost one-half of the patients had brain involvement, either focal mimicking stroke or relapsing–remitting multiple sclerosis, or diffuse manifesting as cognitive impairment. Optic neuritis and rare cases of aseptic menigoencephilitis and recurrent encephalitis are also described (Delalande *et al.* 2004;

Rogers *et al.* 2004). Spinal cord involvement was found in 29% of patients and is well reported in the literature (Delalande *et al.* 2004; Rogers *et al.* 2004; Williams *et al.* 2001). Acute transverse myelitis is a frequent spinal cord manifestation which carries a high mortality (Delalande *et al.* 2004; Rogers *et al.* 2004). Chronic or progressive myelitis has also been reported presenting as a progressive paraparesia, often mimicking primary progressive multiple sclerosis. Less common spinal cord manifestations include lower motor neuron disease, neurogenic bladder, and Brown–Sequard syndrome.

Diagnosis of suspected CNS SS begins with a high index of suspicion and typically an MRI of the brain or spinal cord. Spinal cord MRI typically reveals T2-weighted hyperintensities which can be extended to involve large parts of the spinal cord in cases of acute myelopathy (Delalande *et al.* 2004). In the brain, white matter lesions, which can be similar to MS lesions, are commonly found. Some differences can help distinguish CNS SS from MS and include: (1) the localization of MRI lesions (rare corpus callosum lesions, involvement of the basal ganglia); (2) associated peripheral nerve involvement (common in SS); (3) lower prevalence of oligocloncal bands in the spinal fluid; and (4) the presence of sicca symptoms or extraglandular features of SS. Cutaneous vasculitis is frequently found patients with neurologic SS, as are laboratory abnormalities such as lymphopenia, hypergammaglobulinemia, ANA, anti-SSA/Ro antibodies, and cryoglobulins.

Severe disability can result rapidly from CNS SS, therefore, intensive and early treatment is recommended. In patients with myelopathy, IV glucocorticoids plus IV cyclophosphamide is effective (Alexander 1992; Williams *et al.* 2001). Other immunosuppressive treatments have been tried with variable efficacy, including azathioprine, chlorambucil, and plasmapheresis (Alexander 1992; Hermisson *et al.* 2002; Konttinen *et al.* 1987; Williams *et al.* 2001; Wright *et al.* 1999).

Cardiac and pulmonary

Cardiopulmonary involvement occurs in SS. The most common pulmonary symptom is cough, observed in up to 41% of patients which is often a symptom of tracheobronchial sicca (Papiris *et al.* 1999). In a recent study of 61 patients with SS, mild interstitial-like changes on chest X-ray were found in approximately one-half of subjects (Papiris *et al.* 1999). High resolution chest CT revealed predominantly segmental bronchial wall thickening. Transbronchial biopsy specimens demonstrated peribronchial and/or peribronchiolar mononuclear inflammation in all samples, and interstitial inflammation coexisted in only two patients. Other SS-related pulmonary disorders include hypersensitivity of the lung, toxic effects of drugs such as methotrexate, and opportunistic infections in patients on immunosuppressive drugs (Fox 2005; Kim *et al.* 2002). Pericarditis, pulmonary hypertension, and cardiovascular tests consistent with an autonomic neuropathy can also occur in SS (Fox 2005; Gyongyosi *et al.* 1996).

Renal

Renal involvement in SS occurs in approximately 30% of subjects; however, most often it is unrecognized (Bossini *et al.* 2001). The majority of patients have subclinical renal tubular dysfunction, due to tubulointerstitial nephritis. A frank distal tubular acidosis can be found in approximately 5% of subjects who present with hypokalemia, hyperchloremic acidosis, nephrolitiasis, and rarely hypokalemic paralysis (Bossini *et al.* 2001). Histological examination

typically reveals a focal or diffuse lymphocytic infiltrate in the interstitial tissue. Interstitial fibrosis and tubular atrophy are associated with chronic disease. Immune-mediate glomerulonephritis is rare in SS occurring in less than 5% of patients. The most frequent types of glomerular involvement include membranoproliferative, membranous, or mesangioproliferative glomerlulonephropathies. Subclinical tubular abnormalities require no treatment. Mild to moderate renal tubular acidosis requires potassium replacement and alkalinization with potassium citrate. For cases resistant to replacement therapy or those with renal insufficiency, glucocorticoids are the treatment of choice (Carsons 2001).

Gastrointestinal

Vasculitis of the gastrointestinal tract is rare in SS and is associated with a high mortality. Case reports document polyarteritis nodosa-like vasculitis localized to the bowel, gallbladder, spleen, and pancreas (Carsons 2001; Sato *et al.* 1987; Tsokos *et al.* 1987).

In summary, vasculitis can be one many extraglandular manifestation of SS, with the skin and nervous systems most commonly affected. Treatment depends on the severity of vasculitis and the site of involvement. CNS vasculitis may be more common than previously reported and carries a high risk of morbidity if not recognized and treated aggressively.

Systemic sclerosis and vasculitis

Systemic sclerosis (SSc) is a disease characterized by immunologic abnormalities, microangiopathy, and excessive deposition of collagen in unregulated fashion. Organ systems affected include skin, GI tract, lungs, heart, and kidneys. The pathology of SSc has three major facets, the first being a structural and functional vasculopathy characterized by endothelial cell injury and activation. This is followed by inflammation caused by a perivascular monocytic/macrophage infiltrate, and finally varying degrees of tissue fibrosis (Denton and Black 2004). Despite the systemic vasculopathy associated with SSc, true vasculitis is rare.

Vasculitis in SSc usually occurs in one of two clinical circumstances: (1) SSc in association with Sjögren's syndrome; or (2) in the limited cutaneous form of SSc, which is seropositive for anticentromere antibody (Oddis *et al.* 1987). Histologically, the vasculitis is typically cutaneous and leukocytoclastic. Occurence of pleuropericarditis secondary to leukocytoclastic vasculitis has been reported in a patient with diffuse SSc (Abu-Shakra *et al.* 1995). Rarely, necrotizing vasculitis of larger arteries may occur in the limited form and has been reported as digital gangrene and CNS disease (Herrick *et al.* 1994a, 1994b). There are several case reports of MPO-ANCA-positive microscopic polyangiitis in patients with SSc presenting with crescentic glomerulonephritisor, a pulmonary renal syndrome (Anders *et al.* 1999; Carvajal *et al.* 1997; Maes *et al.* 2000; Mizutani *et al.* 2000; Omote *et al.* 1997; Yamashita *et al.* 2000). Others, however, have found no clinical significance of ANCA antibodies in patients with SSc (Locke *et al.* 1997; Ruffatti *et al.* 2002). Treatment with prednisone or other immunosuppressives should be dictated by the severity of disease.

Polychondritis and vasculitis

Relapsing polychondritis (RP) is a rare systemic disorder characterized by episodic inflammation of cartilaginous structures, including the elastic cartilage of the ear and nose, and cartilage of the tracheobronchial tree. Inflammation can involve other non-cartilagenous structures including the eyes, heart, blood vessels, inner ear, and kidneys (Letko *et al.* 2002). Approximately one-third of patients with RP have an associated hematological disorder, connective tissue disease, systemic inflammatory arthritis, or other autoimmune disease (Letko *et al.* 2002).

Vasculitis is an accepted feature of RP, occurring in as many as 56% of patients with the disease (McAdam *et al.* 1976). The spectrum varies from leukocytoclastic vasculitis of small cutaneous vessels to necrotizing vasculitis of the great vessels (Letko *et al.* 2002; Michet 1990). Dermatologic manifestations of RP are found in up to 35% of patients, with the majority of lesions associated with leukocytoclastic vasculitis (Frances *et al.* 2001). These skin lesions include purpura, livedo reticularis, urticarial papules, erythema nodosum-like lesions, erythema elevatum diutinum, and distal ulceration of the limbs. Other non-vasculitic RP-related skin lesions include oral apthosis (common), neutrophilic dermatosis, superficial phlebitis, and septal panniculitis.

Ocular manifestations occur in up to 60% of RP patients (Isaak *et al.* 1986). Episclcritis and scleritis is most common, followed by conjunctivitis sicca, iritis, retinopathy, keratitis, optic neuritis, and corneal melt. Orbital pseudotumor, extraocular muscle palsy, and lid edema can also occur.

Renal lesions occur in approximately 10%–20% of RP patients and are usually associated with extrarenal vasculitis and a worse prognosis (Chang-Miller *et al.* 1987; Kent *et al.* 2004). Kidney involvement is caused by RP itself, or with an associated underlying vasculitis, or SLE (Isaak *et al.* 1986). Mild mesangial proliferation is the most common histological finding. Other findings include IgA nephropathy, tubulointerstitial nephritis, and segmental necrotizing crescentic glomerulonephritis (Chang-Miller *et al.* 1987; Letko *et al.* 2002).

Peripheral neuropathies (mononeuritis multiplex and mixed motor-sensory types) can occur in RP due to vasculitis of small, epineurial vessels (Michet 1990). Cerebral vasculitis affecting both small and medium vessels has also been reported (Stewart *et al.* 1988).

Cardiovascular disease manifestations in RP are well documented (Michet 1990). The spectrum of involvement includes aortitis, thoracic and abdominal aortic aneurysms, Takayasu's-like aortic arch syndrome, conduction system abnormalities, pericarditis, coronary vasculitis, and valvulitis. The aortic valve is most commonly involved followed by the mitral valve, which can cause catastrophic heart failure even if other features of RP are clinically quiet (Pappas and Johnson 1972). Baseline echocardiography has been advocated to screen for aortic valve disease, but no evidence supports its routine use (Buckley and Ades 1992).

Glucocorticoids are used in therapy of vasculitis associated with RP; azathioprine, cyclophosphamide, chlorambucil, cyclosporin, and methotrexate have been used for glucocorticoid-resistant cases (Kent *et al.* 2004; Michet 1990). There are no controlled studies documenting the effectiveness of any of these agents. One recent report describes a child successfully treated with oral type II collagen as a toleragen (Navarro *et al.* 2002). Several biologics have been used as salvage therapy in RP including anti-CD4 chimeric monoclonal antibody and infliximab, with generally good results, however, there was one death from severe septicemia with infliximab (Cazabon *et al.* 2005; Choy *et al.* 1991; Matzkies *et al.* 2003;

Mpofu *et al.* 2003; Richez *et al.* 2004; Saadoun *et al.* 2003). Although in its infancy, autologous stem cell transplantation for the use of refractory connective tissue diseases including RP may be a viable option (Rosen *et al.* 2000). Finally, valve replacement or aneurysm grafting should be performed when indicated, although the inflammatory process may continue in proximity to installed devices resulting in therapeutic failures (Lang-Lazdunski *et al.* 1995; Michet 1990).

Seronegative spondyloarthropathies

The seronegative spondyloarthropathies (SNSAs) consist of a cluster of interrelated, overlapping inflammatory rheumatic diseases that includes ankylosing spondylitis (AS), reactive arthritis, psoriatic arthritis, arthritis associated with Crohn's disease and ulcerative colitis, and undifferentiated spondyloarthropathies (Khan 2002). These diseases share several characteristics including: (1) an asymmetric erosive inflammatory arthropathy; (2) inflammation at the site of ligament-to-bone insertion (enthesopathy); and (3) inflammation in the axial skeleton and sacroiliac joints (Kerr and Sturrock 1999). Extra-articular features of the spondyloarthropathies include anterior uveitis, colitis, aortitis, and apical lung fibrosis (especially in the case of AS) (Kerr and Sturrock 1999).

Acute anterior uveitis occurs in 20%–40% of patients with AS, but is less common in the other spondyloarthropathies (Gran and Skomsvoll 1997). The uveitis is characterized by recurrent, alternating, unilateral attacks of a painful, inflamed eye which is typically confined to those who are HLA-B27 positive (Monnet *et al.* 2004; Rothova *et al.* 1992). Musculoskeletal symptoms precede the first attack of anterior uveitis in more than 80% of cases (Monnet *et al.* 2004). Glucocorticoids are the treatment of choice in topical, periocular or systemic formulations. Sulfasalazine and methotrexate are recommended for those who fail to respond to systemic glucocorticoids or who have frequent recurrences (Munoz-Fernandez *et al.* 2003; Munoz-Fernandez and Martin-Mola 2006). The use of anti-TNF agents to treat patients with AS with has also demonstrated a significant decrease in the number of anterior uveitis flares (Braun *et al.* 2005).

Cardiovascular manifestations of AS include aortic root thickening and dilation, aortic valve thickening and insufficiency, mitral valve insufficiency and conduction system abnormalities. Vasculitis or a vasculopathy affecting the small arteries of the cardiac and aortic tissues result in intimal proliferation (obliterative endarteritis) and fibrosis (Bergfeldt 1997). Overall, aortic regurgitation has been described in 2% to 40% of patients with AS and in 2.8% of patients with reactive arthritis (Bachmann *et al.* 1976; Bergfeldt 1997; Kinsella *et al.* 1974; Roldan *et al.* 1998). Atrioventricular conduction blocks have been described in up to one-third of patients with AS (Bergfeldt *et al.* 1982; O'Neill and Bresnihan 1992). Myocarditis and pericarditis are rare features of SNSA (Bergfeldt 1997). Medium and large-vessel vasculitis has been described in patients with SNSA including polyarteritis nodosa, Takayasu's arteritis, and aneurysms with arteritis of the ascending, thoracic, and abdominal aorta (Duvernoy and Schatz 1966; Kawasuji *et al.* 1982; Paloheimo *et al.* 1966; Somer and Siltanen 1970; Stamp *et al.* 2000; Takagi *et al.* 2003).

IgA nephropathy has been reported to occur in association with all types of SNSAs. Patients typically present with microscopic or gross hematuria and proteinuria (Satko *et al.* 2000). Other glomer-ulopathies reported include mesangial proliferative glomerulone-phritis, amyloid nephropathy, and membranous nephropathy (Botey *et al.* 1981; Malaviya *et al.* 1981; Satko *et al.* 2000; Shu *et al.* 1986). A recent report describes a significantly increased frequency of renal stones in patients with AS (25%) compared to healthy con-trols (3.3%), especially those with longer disease duration (Korkmaz *et al.* 2005). An important note of caution is that patients with SNSA may develop renal insufficiency unrelated to their primary disease, but rather as a consequence of treatment with NSAIDs (Satko *et al.* 2000; Shu *et al* 1986).

Vasculitic skin lesions are rarely described in the SNSAs. There are cases of leukocytoclastic vasculitis which have occurred in asso-ciation with reactive arthritis, psoriatic arthritis, and in those with IgA nephropathy (Jennette *et al.* 1982; Magro *et al.* 1995; Wong and Marks 1994). When vasculitis is seen in the context SNSA, latent HIV infection should be excluded as a cause (Kaye 1989).

Nervous system involvement in SNSA is limited to case reports describing transverse myelitis and cauda equina syndrome (Bilgen *et al.* 1999; Gabay *et al.* 1978; Haddad *et al.* 1990; Koenigsberg *et al.* 1995; Kushwaha and Steinberg 1992; Oh *et al.* 2001; Sant and O'Connell 1995; Schroder *et al.* 1994; Travis and Byrne 1987).

Idiopathic inflammatory myopathies and vasculitis

Polymyositis (PM) and dermatomyositis (DM) are members of a group of inflammatory myopathies that have in common the pres-ence of muscle weakness and inflammation in the muscle (Dalakas and Hohlfeld 2003). Dermatomyositis is distinguished by charac-teristic skin findings (heliotrope rash, erythema on the face, neck and anterior chest, and Gottron's papules) associated with the muscle disease. Pathologically, DM is a humorally mediated micro-angiopathy with activation and deposition of complement in the endomysial capillaries resulting in muscle ischemia in a perivascu-lar and perifasicular distribution (Arahata and Engel 1988; Dalakas and Hohlfeld 2003; Engel and Arahata 1984). In polymyositis there is no rash and the inflammation is due to invasion of CD8-positive cytotoxic T-cells which invade muscle fibers that express MHC class I antigens (Arahata and Engel 1988; Engel and Arahata 1984; Engel *et al.* 1990). Vasculitis is not a common component of either DM or PM.

Small-vessel cutaneous vasculitis characterized by periungual infarcts and digital ulcerations has been reported and is more fre-quent in child-onset DM compared to adult-onset DM (Feldman *et al.* 1983; Kadoya *et al.* 1994). In some, but not all studies, leuko-cytoclastic vasculitis in adult DM has been a marker of an underly-ing malignancy (Feldman *et al.* 1983; Hunger *et al.* 2001).

Interstitial lung disease is well described in PM/DM, frequently in association with the antibodies to antihistidyl transfer RNA syn-thetase (Anti-Jo-l) or mucin like glycoprotein (KL-6) (Hirakata and Nagai 2000). In a recent study of 70 subjects with PM or DM and diffuse interstitial lung disease, the majority (~81%) of lung biopsies revealed non-specific interstitial pneumonia (NSIP), while there were isolated cases of diffuse alveolar damage (DAD), bron-chiolitis obliterans organizing pneumonia (BOOP), and usual interstitial pneumonia (UIP) (Douglas *et al.* 2001). In a separate report, pulmonary capillaritis with DAH is described in two patients with PM (Schwarz *et al.* 1995).

Renal involvement is uncommon in DM/PM and glomerulone-phritis is rare. In a recent review of the literature, Takizawa *et al.* (2007), found 15 cases of biopsy proven cases of glomerulo-nephritis in patients with PM and six cases in DM patients. Mesangioproliferative GN is the primary lesion found in PM while membranous GN was more common in DM. The GN responds like the muscle disease to glucocorticoids or immunosuppressive agents.

Large-vessel vasculitis although rare, is reportedly more common in children than adults; however, one survey of 43 adult cases found evidence of large-vessel vasculitis in five patients (Kalovidouris *et al.* 1988; Pachman 1995). Mesenteric vasculitis has rarely been described in adult-onset DM, but is a known complication of pediatric DM (Eshraghi *et al.* 1998; Pachman *et al.* 1998; See *et al.* 1997). A peripheral polyneuropathy due to microangiopathic changes is reported in two cases of child-onset DM (Vogelgesang *et al.* 1995).

Idiopathic retroperitoneal fibrosis

Seen mostly in middle-aged to older men, retroperitoneal fibrosis is a rare disease characterized by inflammation in the retroperito-neum with associated fibrosis (Gilkeson and Allen 1996). Retroperitoneal fibrosis can be characterized as idiopathic (IRP), which accounts for more than two-thirds of cases, and secondary IP which is associated with certain drugs (such as ergot alkaloids); neoplasms (carcinoid tumors, lymphomas, sarcomas, carcinomas); infections (tuberculosis, histoplasmosis, actinomycosis); trauma; radiotherapy; and surgery (Koep and Zuidema 1977; Vaglio *et al.* 2006b). The pathogenesis of IPF is unclear and likely multifacto-rial. A prominent theory has suggested that IPF is a form of chronic periaortitis which is secondary to a local inflammatory reaction to oxidized low-density lipoproteins (LDL) from atherosclerotic plaques in the abdominal aorta (Mitchinson 1984; Parums *et al.* 1990a, 1990b). More recently, IPF is considered a systemic autoim-mune disease due to the frequent findings of constitutional symp-toms, elevated acute phase reactants, and autoantibodies in IPF patients (Vaglio *et al.* 2006b).

Due to the anatomic location of the inflammation, patients often complain early of vague lower back or abdominal pain. Hydronephrosis due to ureteral compression is a common compli-cation (Rhee *et al.* 1994). Constitutional symptoms including fatigue, low grade fever, nausea, anorexia, weight loss, and myalgias are also common (Vaglio *et al.* 2006b). CT or MRI scans are used to diagnose and follow the course of IRP which typically demon-strates a soft tissue mass, surrounding the aorta and iliac arteries with the possible encasement of neighboring structures such as the ureters and inferior vena cava. The presence of an elevated ESR and CRP can help to substantiate the diagnosis. A biopsy of the tissue is recommended if the mass shows an atypical presentation, or if the presence of a malignancy or infection is suspected.

Histologically, there are similarities in cases of IPF and large-vessel vasculitis. There is often: (1) pronounced aortic adventitial inflammation; (2) vasculitis of the vasa vasorum and periaortic small vessels; and (3) infiltrates of lymphocytes, macrophages, plasma cells, and eosinophils (Gilkeson and Allen 1996; Vaglio *et al.* 2006b). Additionally in 10% of cases, frank vasculitis with fibri-noid necrosis is found in the small and medium retroperitoneal vessels of the inflammatory mass. It is unknown whether the vasculitis plays an initiating role or represents sequelae of the fibrotic inflammatory mass.

The goals of treatment of IPF are to stop the progression of the disease, relieve or prevent ureteral obstruction, normalize acute phase reactants, and prevent disease relapse (Vaglio *et al.* 2006b). Glucocorticoids are most often used with initial doses of prednisone of 40 mg to 60 mg per day (Kardar *et al.* 2002; Marcolongo *et al.* 2004). Other immunosuppressive agents (cyclophosphamide, azathioprine, and methotrexate) have been used both as steroid-sparing agents as well as rescue therapy for steroid-resistant cases (Harreby *et al.* 1994). The successful use of cyclosporin and MMF has also been reported (Grotz *et al.* 1998; Marzano *et al.* 2001). Case reports support the use of tamoxifen in IPF due to the ability of the drug to inhibit transforming growth factor-beta, a putative mediator of the inflammatory changes in the disorder (Al Salman and Makhdomi 2002; Bourouma *et al.* 1997; Clark *et al.* 1991; Dedeoglu *et al.* 2001; Loffeld and van Weel 1993; Vaglio *et al.* 2006a). Although encouraging, tamoxifen is generally viewed as second line therapy in IPF. The treatment of IPF may be prolonged up to 2 years in some cases to prevent disease relapse (Harreby *et al.* 2002).

Summary

Vasculitis occurring in the context of connective tissue diseases presents difficult diagnostic challenges due to the variety of vessels and organ systems that can become involved. Fortunately, most are responsive to currently available therapies, especially when the diagnosis is made and appropriate therapy instituted in a timely fashion. The most important factors in successfully making these diagnoses are familiarity with common patterns of vasculitis within a given disease process and appropriate consideration of vasculitis in the differential diagnosis.

References

Abu-Shakra, M., Koh, E. T., Treger, T., and Lee, P. (1995). Pericardial effusion and vasculitis in a patient with systemic sclerosis. *Journal of Rheumatology*, **22**, 1386–8.

Ainiala, H., Hietaharju, A., Loukkola, J., Peltola, J., Korpela, M., Metsanoja, R., and Auvinen, A. (2001). Validity of the new American College of Rheumatology criteria for neuropsychiatric lupus syndromes: a population-based evaluation. *Arthritis and Rheumatism*, **45**, 419–23.

Al Salman, J. and Makhdomi, A. R. (2002). Treatment of retroperitoneal fibrosis with tamoxifen. *Southern Medical Journal*, **95**, 947.

Alarcon-Segovia, D., Abud-Mendoza, C., Reyes-Gutierrez, E., Iglesias-Gamarra, A., and Diaz-Jouanen, E. (1984). Involvement of the urinary bladder in systemic lupus erythematosus. A pathologic study. *Journal of Rheumatology*, **11**, 208–10.

Alarcon-Segovia, D., Perez-Vazquez, M. E., Villa, A. R., Drenkard, C., and Cabiedes, J. (1992). Preliminary classification criteria for the antiphospholipid syndrome within systemic lupus erythematosus. *Seminars in Arthritis and Rheumatism*, **21**, 275–86.

Alexander, E. (1992). Central nervous system disease in Sjögren's syndrome. New insights into immunopathogenesis. *Rheumatic Disease Clinics of North America*, **18**, 637–72.

Alexander, E. L., Arnett, F. C., Provost, T. T., and Stevens, M. B. (1983). Sjögren's syndrome: association of anti-Ro(SS-A) antibodies with vasculitis, hematologic abnormalities, and serologic hyperreactivity. *Annals of Internal Medicine*, **98**, 155–9.

Alexander, E. L., Moyer, C., Travlos, G. S., Roths, J. B., and Murphy, E. D. (1985). Two histopathologic types of inflammatory vascular disease in MRL/Mp autoimmune mice. Model for human vasculitis in connective tissue disease. *Arthritis and Rheumatism*, **28**, 1146–55.

Alexander, E. L. and Provost, T. T. (1983). Cutaneous manifestations of primary Sjögren's syndrome: a reflection of vasculitis and association with anti-Ro(SSA) antibodies. *Journal of Investigative Dermatology*, **80**, 386–91.

American College of Rheumatology (ACR) (1999). The American College of Rheumatology nomenclature and case definitions for neuropsychiatric lupus syndromes. *Arthritis and Rheumatism*, **42**, 599–608.

Anders, H. J., Wiebecke, B., Haedecke, C., Sanden, S., Combe, C., and Schlondorff, D. (1999). MPO-ANCA-Positive crescentic glomerulonephritis: a distinct entity of scleroderma renal disease? *American Journal of Kidney Diseases*, **33**, e3.

Ansari, A., Larson, P. H., and Bates, H. D. (1986). Vascular manifestations of systemic lupus erythematosus. *Angiology*, **37**, 423–32.

Arahata, K. and Engel, A. G. (1988). Monoclonal antibody analysis of mononuclear cells in myopathies. V: Identification and quantitation of T8+ cytotoxic and T8+ suppressor cells. *Annals of Neurology*, **23**, 493–9.

Armstrong, D. J., McCarron, M. T., and Wright, G. D. (2005). Successful treatment of rheumatoid vasculitis-associated foot-drop with infliximab. *Journal of Rheumatology*, **32**, 759–60.

Asherson, R. A., Mackworth-Young, C. G., Harris, E. N., Gharavi, A. E., and Hughes, G. R. (1985). Multiple venous and arterial thromboses associated with the lupus anticoagulant and antibodies to cardiolipin in the absence of SLE. *Rheumatology International*, **5**, 91–3.

Asherson, R. A., Morgan, S. H., Harris, E. N., Gharavi, A. E., Krausz, T., and Hughes, G. R. (1986). Arterial occlusion causing large bowel infarction–a reflection of clotting diathesis in SLE. *Clinical Rheumatology*, **5**, 102–6.

Au, A. and O'Day, J. (2004). Review of severe vaso-occlusive retinopathy in systemic lupus erythematosus and the antiphospholipid syndrome: associations, visual outcomes, complications and treatment. *Clinical and Experimental Ophthalmology*, **32**, 87–100.

Axson, F. A. (1979). D-penicillamine in the treatment of rheumatoid vasculitis. *Journal of the South Carolina Medical Association*, **75**, 211–5.

Bachmann, F., Hartl, W., Veress, M., and Frind, W. (1976). [Cardiovascular complications of ankylosing spondylitis (Bechterew's disease)]. *Medizinische Welt*, **27**, 2149–50.

Bacon, P. A. and Carruthers, D. M. (1995). Vasculitis associated with connective tissue disorders. *Rheumatic Disease Clinics of North America*, **21**, 1077–96.

Bacons, P. A. and Kitas, G. D. (1994). The significance of vascular inflammation in rheumatoid arthritis. *Annals of the Rheumatic Diseases*, **53**, 621–3.

Badui, E., Garcia-Rubi, D., Robles, E., Jimenez, J., Juan, L., Deleze, M., Diaz, A., and Mintz, G. (1985). Cardiovascular manifestations in systemic lupus erythematosus. Prospective study of 100 patients. *Angiology*, **36**, 431–41.

Bando, H., Kobayashi, S., Matsumoto, T., Tamura, N., Yamanaka, K., Yamaji, C., Takasaki, C., Takasaki, Y., and Hashimoto, H. (2003). Acute acalculous cholecystitis induced by mesenteric inflammatory veno-occlusive disease (MIVOD) in systemic lupus erythematosus. *Clinical Rheumatology*, **22**, 447–9.

Barile, L. and Lavalle, C. (1992). Transverse myelitis in systemic lupus erythematosus – the effect of IV pulse methylprednisolone and cyclophosphamide. *Journal of Rheumatology*, **19**, 370–2.

Bathon, J. M., Moreland, L. W., and DiBartolomeo, A. G. (1989). Inflammatory central nervous system involvement in rheumatoid arthritis. *Seminars in Arthritis and Rheumatism*, **18**, 258–66.

Beaufils, M., Kouki, F., Mignon, F., Camus, J. P., Morel-Maroger, L., and Richet, G. (1983). Clinical significance of anti-Sm antibodies in systemic lupus erythematosus. *American Journal of Medicine*, **74**, 201–5.

Belmont, H. M., Abramson, S. B., and Lie, J. T. (1996). Pathology and pathogenesis of vascular injury in systemic lupus erythematosus.

Interactions of inflammatory cells and activated endothelium. *Arthritis and Rheumatism*, **39**, 9–22.

Bergfeldt, L. (1997). HLA-B27-associated cardiac disease. *Annals of Internal Medicine*, **127**, 621–9.

Bergfeldt, L., Edhag, O., and Vallin, H. (1982). Cardiac conduction disturbances, an underestimated manifestation in ankylosing spondylitis. A 25-year follow-up study of 68 patients. *Acta Medica Scandinavica*, **212**, 217–23.

Bidani, A. K., Roberts, J. L., Schwartz, M. M., and Lewis, E. J. (1980). Immunopathology of cardiac lesions in fatal systemic lupus erythematosus. *American Journal of Medicine*, **69**, 849–58.

Bijl, M., Horst, G., Bootsma, H., Limburg, P. C., and Kallenberg, C. G. (2003). Mycophenolate mofetil prevents a clinical relapse in patients with systemic lupus erythematosus at risk. *Annals of the Rheumatic Diseases*, **62**, 534–9.

Bilgen, I. G., Yunten, N., Ustun, E. E., Oksel, F., and Gumusdis, G. (1999). Adhesive arachnoiditis causing cauda equina syndrome in ankylosing spondylitis: CT and MRI demonstration of dural calcification and a dorsal dural diverticulum. *Neuroradiology*, **41**, 508–11.

Blanche, P., Krebs, S., Renaud, B., Dusser, D., and Sicard, D. (1996). Systemic lupus erythematosus presenting as iron deficiency anemia due to pulmonary alveolar hemorrhage. *Clinical and Experimental Rheumatology*, **14**, 228.

Bloch, S. L., Jarrett, M. P., Swerdlow, M., and Grayzel, A. I. (1979). Brachial plexus neuropathy as the initial presentation of systemic lupus erythematosus. *Neurology*, **29**, 1633–4.

Bonfiglio, T. and Atwater, E. C. (1969). Heart disease in patients with seropositive rheumatoid arthritis; a controlled autopsy study and review. *Archives of Internal Medicine*, **124**, 714–9.

Bosch, X., Llena, J., Collado, A., Font, J., Mirapeix, E., Ingelmo, M., Munoz-Gomez, J., and Urbano-Marquez, A. (1995). Occurrence of antineutrophil cytoplasmic and antineutrophil (peri)nuclear antibodies in rheumatoid arthritis. *Journal of Rheumatology*, **22**, 2038–45.

Bossini, N., Savoldi, S., Franceschini, F., Mombelloni, S., Baronio, M., Cavazzana, I., Viola, B. F., Valzorio, B., Mazzucchelli, C., Cattaneo, R., Scolari, F., and Maiorca, R. (2001). Clinical and morphological features of kidney involvement in primary Sjögren's syndrome. *Nephrology Dialysis Transplantation*, **16**, 2328–36.

Botey, A., Torras, A., and Revert, L. (1981). Membranous nephropathy in ankylosing spondylitis. *Nephron*, **29**, 203.

Boumpas, D. T., Austin, H. A., III, Fessler, B. J., Balow, J. E., Klippel, J. H., and Lockshin, M. D. (1995). Systemic lupus erythematosus: emerging concepts. Part 1: Renal, neuropsychiatric, cardiovascular, pulmonary, and hematologic disease. *Annals of Internal Medicine*, **122**, 940–50.

Bourouma, R., Chevet, D., Michel, F., Cercueil, J. P., Arnould, L., and Rifle, G. (1997). Treatment of idiopathic retroperitoneal fibrosis with tamoxifen. *Nephrology Dialysis Transplantation*, **12**, 2407–10.

Braun, J., Baraliakos, X., Listing, J., and Sieper, J. (2005). Decreased incidence of anterior uveitis in patients with ankylosing spondylitis treated with the anti-tumor necrosis factor agents infliximab and etanercept. *Arthritis and Rheumatism*, **52**, 2447–51.

Braun, M. G., Csernok, E., Schmitt, W. H., and Gross, W. L. (1996). Incidence, target antigens, and clinical implications of antineutrophil cytoplasmic antibodies in rheumatoid arthritis. *Journal of Rheumatology*, **23**, 826–30.

Breedveld, F. C., Heurkens, A. H., Lafeber, G. J., van Hinsbergh, V. W., and Cats, A. (1988). Immune complexes in sera from patients with rheumatoid vasculitis induce polymorphonuclear cell-mediated injury to endothelial cells. *Clinical Immunology and Immunopathology*, **48**, 202–13.

Brey, R. L., Holliday, S. L., Saklad, A. R., Navarrete, M. G., Hermosillo-Romo, D., Stallworth, C. L., Valdez, C. R., Escalante, A., del, R., I, Gronseth, G., Rhine, C. B., Padilla, P., and McGlasson, D. (2002). Neuropsychiatric syndromes in lupus: prevalence using standardized definitions. *Neurology*, **58**, 1214–20.

Buckley, C. D., Ed, R. G., Nash, G. B., and Raza, K. (2005). Endothelial cells, fibroblasts and vasculitis. *Rheumatology* (Oxford), **44**, 860–3.

Buckley, L. M. and Ades, P. A. (1992). Progressive aortic valve inflammation occurring despite apparent remission of relapsing polychondritis. *Arthritis and Rheumatism*, **35**, 812–4.

Bulkley, B. H. and Roberts, W. C. (1975). The heart in systemic lupus erythematosus and the changes induced in it by glucocorticoid therapy. A study of 36 necropsy patients. *American Journal of Medicine*, **58**, 243–64.

Bywaters, E. G. L. (1957). Peripheral vascular obstruction in rheumatoid arthritis and its relationship to other vascular lesions. *Annals of the Rheumatic Diseases*, **16**, 84–103.

Calamia, K. T. and Balabanova, M. (2004). Vasculitis in systemic lupus erythematosis. *Clinical Dermatology*, **22**, 148–56.

Callen, J. P., Spencer, L. V., Burruss, J. B., and Holtman, J. (1991). Azathioprine. An effective, glucocorticoid-sparing therapy for patients with recalcitrant cutaneous lupus erythematosus or with recalcitrant cutaneous leukocytoclastic vasculitis. *Archives of Dermatology*, **127**, 515–22.

Campion, G., Maddison, P. J., Goulding, N., James, I., Ahern, M. J., Watt, I., and Sansom, D. (1990). The Felty syndrome: a case-matched study of clinical manifestations and outcome, serologic features, and immunogenetic associations. *Medicine* (Baltimore), **69**, 69–80.

Cardinali, C., Caproni, M., Bernacchi, E., Amato, L., and Fabbri, P. (2000). The spectrum of cutaneous manifestations in lupus erythematosus–the Italian experience. *Lupus*, **9**, 417–23.

Carreno, L., Lopez-Longo, F. J., Monteagudo, I., Rodriguez-Mahou, M., Bascones, M., Gonzalez, C. M., Saint-Cyr, C., and Lapointe, N. (1999). Immunological and clinical differences between juvenile and adult onset of systemic lupus erythematosus. *Lupus*, **8**, 287–92.

Carson, C. W., Beall, L. D., Hunder, G. G., Johnson, C. M., and Newman, W. (1993). Serum ELAM-1 is increased in vasculitis, scleroderma, and systemic lupus erythematosus. *Journal of Rheumatology*, **20**, 809–14.

Carsons, S. (2001). A review and update of Sjogren's syndrome: manifestations, diagnosis, and treatment. *American Journal of Managed Care*, **7** (Suppl.), S433–43.

Carvajal, I., Bernis, C., Sanz, P., Garcia, A., Garcia-Vadillo, A., and Traver, J. A. (1997). Antineutrophil cytoplasmic autoantibodies (ANCA) and systemic sclerosis. *Nephrology Dialysis Transplantation*, **12**, 576–7.

Cathcart, E. S. and Spodick, D. H. (1962). Rheumatoid heart disease. A study of the incidence and nature of cardiac lesions in rheumatoid arthritis. *New England Journal of Medicine*, **266**, 959–64.

Cazabon, S., Over, K., and Butcher, J. (2005). The successful use of infliximab in resistant relapsing polychondritis and associated scleritis. *Eye*, **19**, 222–4.

Chang-Miller, A., Okamura, M., Torres, V. E., Michet, C. J., Wagoner, R. D., Donadio, J. V., Jr., Offord, K. P., and Holley, K. E. (1987). Renal involvement in relapsing polychondritis. *Medicine* (Baltimore), **66**, 202–17.

Chatterjee, S. and Kupsky, W. J. (2005). Severe proximal myopathy and mononeuritis multiplex in rheumatoid arthritis: manifestations of rheumatoid vasculitis. *Journal of Clinical Rheumatology*, **11**, 50–5.

Chen, K. R., Toyohara, A., Suzuki, A., and Miyakawa, S. (2002). Clinical and histopathological spectrum of cutaneous vasculitis in rheumatoid arthritis. *British Journal of Dermatology*, **147**, 905–13.

Chin, H. J., Ahn, C., Lim, C. S., Chung, H. K., Lee, J. G., Song, Y. W., Lee, H. S., Han, J. S., Kim, S., and Lee, J. S. (2000). Clinical implications of antineutrophil cytoplasmic antibody test in lupus nephritis. *American Journal of Nephrology*, **20**, 57–63.

Choy, E. H., Chikanza, I. C., Kingsley, G. H., and Panayi, G. S. (1991). Chimaeric anti-CD4 monoclonal antibody for relapsing polychondritis. *Lancet*, **338**, 450.

Clark, C. P., Vanderpool, D., and Preskitt, J. T. (1991). The response of retroperitoneal fibrosis to tamoxifen. *Surgery*, **109**, 502–6.

Coremans, I. E., Hagen, E. C., Daha, M. R., van der Woude, F. J., van der Voort, E. A., Kleijburg-van der Keur, C., and Breedveld, F. C. (1992).

Antilactoferrin antibodies in patients with rheumatoid arthritis are associated with vasculitis. *Arthritis and Rheumatism*, **35**, 12, 1466–75.

d'Cruz, D. (1998). Vasculitis in systemic lupus erythematosus. *Lupus*, **7**, 270–4.

d'Cruz, D., Khamashta, M., and Hughes, G. (1997). Antiendothelial cell antibodies (AECA) in systemic lupus erythematosus (SLE). *Clinical Reviews in Allergy and Immunology*, **15**, 53–63.

Daina, E., Schieppati, A., and Remuzzi, G. (1999). Mycophenolate mofetil for the treatment of Takayasu arteritis: report of three cases. *Annals of Internal Medicine*, **130**, 422–6.

Dalakas, M. C. and Hohlfeld, R. (2003). Polymyositis and dermatomyositis. *Lancet*, **362**, 9388, 971–82.

Danning, C. L., Illei, G. G., and Boumpas, D. T. (1998). Vasculitis associated with primary rheumatologic diseases. *Current Opinion in Rheumatology*., **10**, 58–65.

De Bandt, M., Meyer, O., Haim, T., and Kahn, M. F. (1996). Antineutrophil cytoplasmic antibodies in rheumatoid arthritis patients. *British Journal of Rheumatology*, **35**, 38–43.

Dedeoglu, F., Rose, C. D., Athreya, B. H., Conard, K., Grissom, L., and Magnusson, M. (2001). Successful treatment of retroperitoneal fibrosis with tamoxifen in a child. *Journal of Rheumatology*, **28**, 1693–5.

Delalande, S., de Seze, J., Fauchais, A. L., Hachulla, E., Stojkovic, T., Ferriby, D., Dubucquoi, S., Pruvo, J. P., Vermersch, P., and Hatron, P. Y. (2004). Neurologic manifestations in primary Sjogren syndrome: a study of 82 patients. *Medicine* (Baltimore), **83**, 280–91.

den Broeder, A. A., van den Hoogen, F. H., and van de Putte, L. B. (2001). Isolated digital vasculitis in a patient with rheumatoid arthritis: good response to tumour necrosis factor alpha blocking treatment. *Annals of the Rheumatic Diseases*, **60**, 538–9.

Denton, C. P. and Black, C. M. (2004). Scleroderma–clinical and pathological advances. *Best Practice and Research in Clinical Rheumatology*, **18**, 271–90.

Doherty, N. E., III, Feldman, G., Maurer, G., and Siegel, R. J. (1988). Echocardiographic findings in systemic lupus erythematosus. *American Journal of Cardiology*, **61**, 1144.

Doria, A., Iaccarino, L., Sarzi-Puttini, P., Atzeni, F., Turriel, M., and Petri, M. (2005). Cardiac involvement in systemic lupus erythematosus. *Lupus*, **14**, 683–6.

Douglas, W. W., Tazelaar, H. D., Hartman, T. E., Hartman, R. P., Decker, P. A., Schroeder, D. R., and Ryu, J. H. (2001). Polymyositis-dermatomyositis-associated interstitial lung disease. *American Journal of Respiratory and Critical Care Medicine*, **164**, 1182–5.

Drenkard, C., Villa, A. R., Reyes, E., Abello, M., and Alarcon-Segovia, D. (1997). Vasculitis in systemic lupus erythematosus. *Lupus*, **6**, 235–42.

Duvernoy, W. F. and Schatz, I. J. (1966). Rheumatoid spondylitis associated with aneurysmal dilatation of the entire thoracic aorta. *Henry Ford Hospital Medical Journal*, **14**, 309–12.

Eber, T., Chapman, J., and Shoenfeld, Y. (2005). Anti-ribosomal P-protein and its role in psychiatric manifestations of systemic lupus erythematosus: myth or reality?. *Lupus*, **14**, 571–5.

Enevoldson, T. P. and Wiles, C. M. (1991). Severe vasculitic neuropathy in systemic lupus erythematosus and response to cyclophosphamide. *Journal of Neurology Neurosurgery and Psychiatry*, **54**, 468–9.

Engel, A. G. and Arahata, K. (1984). Monoclonal antibody analysis of mononuclear cells in myopathies. II: Phenotypes of autoinvasive cells in polymyositis and inclusion body myositis. *Annals of Neurology*, **16**, 209–15.

Engel, A. G., Arahata, K., and Emslie-Smith, A. (1990). Immune effector mechanisms in inflammatory myopathies. *Research Publications-Association for Research in Nervous and Mental Disease*, **68**, 141–57.

Erickson, R. W., Franklin, W. A., and Emlen, W. (1994). Treatment of hemorrhagic lupus pneumonitis with plasmapheresis. *Seminars in Arthritis and Rheumatism*, **24**, 114–23.

Eshraghi, N., Farahmand, M., Maerz, L. L., Campbell, S. M., Deveney, C. W., and Sheppard, B. C. (1998). Adult-onset dermatomyositis with severe gastrointestinal manifestations: case report and review of the literature. *Surgery*, **123**, 356–8.

Fairfax, M. J., Osborn, T. G., Williams, G. A., Tsai, C. C., and Moore, T. L. (1988). Endomyocardial biopsy in patients with systemic lupus erythematosus. *Journal of Rheumatology*, **15**, 593–6.

Fauci, A. S., Steinberg, A. D., Haynes, B. F., and Whalen, G. (1978). Immunoregulatory aberrations in systemic lupus erythematosus. *Journal of Immunology*, **121**, 1473–9.

Feldman, D., Hochberg, M. C., Zizic, T. M., and Stevens, M. B. (1983). Cutaneous vasculitis in adult polymyositis/dermatomyositis. *Journal of Rheumatology*, **10**, 85–9.

Feriozzi, S., Muda, A. O., Amini, M., Faraggiana, T., and Ancarani, E. (1997). Systemic lupus erythematosus with membranous glomerulonephritis and uterine vasculitis. *American Journal of Kidney Diseases*, **29**, 277–9.

Flipo, R. M., Janin, A., Hachulla, E., Houvenagel, E., Foulet, A., Cardon, T., Desbonnet, A., Grardel, B., Duquesnoy, B., and Delcambre, B. (1994). Labial salivary gland biopsy assessment in rheumatoid vasculitis. *Annals of the Rheumatic Diseases*, **53**, 648–52.

Fox, R. I. (2005). Sjogren's syndrome. *Lancet*, **366**, 321–31.

Frances, C., el Rassi, R., Laporte, J. L., Rybojad, M., Papo, T., and Piette, J. C. (2001). Dermatologic manifestations of relapsing polychondritis. A study of 200 cases at a single center. *Medicine* (Baltimore), **80**, 173–9.

Frith, P., Burge, S. M., Millard, P. R., and Wojnarowska, F. (1990). External ocular findings in lupus erythematosus: a clinical and immunopathological study. *British Journal of Ophthalmology*, **74**, 163–7.

Gabay, R., Guignard, D., and Chantraine, A. (1978). A rare extra-articular manifestation of ankylosing spondylitis: cauda equina syndrome. *Journal of Rheumatology*, **5**, 234–5.

Garcia-Carrasco, M., Ramos-Casals, M., Rosas, J., Pallares, L., Calvo-Alen, J., Cervera, R., Font, J., and Ingelmo, M. (2002). Primary Sjogren syndrome: clinical and immunologic disease patterns in a cohort of 400 patients. *Medicine* (Baltimore), **81**, 270–80.

Garcia-Porrua, C., Gonzalez-Gay, M. A., and Quevedo, V. (2006). Should anti-tumor necrosis factor-alpha be the first therapy for rheumatoid vasculitis?. *Journal of Rheumatology*, **33**, 433–4.

Geirsson, A. J., Sturfelt, G., and Truedsson, L. (1987). Clinical and serological features of severe vasculitis in rheumatoid arthritis: prognostic implications. *Annals of the Rheumatic Diseases*, **46**, 727–33.

Gilkeson, G. S. and Allen, N. B. (1996). Retroperitoneal fibrosis. A true connective tissue disease. *Rheumatic Disease Clinics of North America*, **22**, 23–38.

Ginzler, E. M., Dooley, M. A., Aranow, C., Kim, M. Y., Buyon, J., Merrill, J. T., Petri, M., Gilkeson, G. S., Wallace, D. J., Weisman, M. H., and Appel, G. B. (2005). Mycophenolate mofetil or intravenous cyclophosphamide for lupus nephritis. *New England Journal of Medicine*, **353**, 2219–28.

Godfrey, T., Khamashta, M. A., and Hughes, G. R. (1998). Therapeutic advances in systemic lupus erythematosus. *Current Opinion in Rheumatology*, **10**, 435–41.

Gonzalez, A., Nicovani, S., Massardo, L., Aguirre, V., Cervilla, V., Lanchbury, J. S., and Jacobelli, S. (1997). Influence of the HLA-DR beta shared epitope on susceptibility to and clinical expression of rheumatoid arthritis in Chilean patients. *Annals of the Rheumatic Diseases*, **56**, 191–3.

Gonzalez-Gay, M. A. and Garcia-Porrua, C. (1999). Systemic vasculitis in adults in northwestern Spain, 1988–1997. Clinical and epidemiologic aspects. *Medicine* (Baltimore), **78**, 292–308.

Gorman, J. D., David-Vaudey, E., Pai, M., Lum, R. F., and Criswell, L. A. (2004). Particular HLA-DRB1 shared epitope genotypes are strongly associated with rheumatoid vasculitis. *Arthritis and Rheumatism*, **50**, 3476–84.

Goronzy, J. J. and Weyand, C. M. (1994). Vasculitis in rheumatoid arthritis. *Current Opinion in Rheumatology*, **6**, 290–4.

Goronzy, J. J. and Weyand, C. M. (2003). Aging, autoimmunity and arthritis: T-cell senescence and contraction of T-cell repertoire diversity – catalysts of autoimmunity and chronic inflammation. *Arthritis Research and Theory*, **5**, 225–34.

Goules, A., Masouridi, S., Tzioufas, A. G., Ioannidis, J. P., Skopouli, F. N., and Moutsopoulos, H. M. (2000). Clinically significant and biopsy-documented renal involvement in primary Sjogren syndrome. *Medicine* (Baltimore), **79**, 241–9.

Govoni, M., Bajocchi, G., Rizzo, N., Tola, M. R., Caniatti, L., Tugnoli, V., Colamussi, P., and Trotta, F. (1999). Neurological involvement in primary Sjögren's syndrome: clinical and instrumental evaluation in a cohort of Italian patients. *Clinical Rheumatology*, **18**, 299–303.

Goyal, S. and Nousari, H. C. (2001). Treatment of resistant discoid lupus erythematosus of the palms and soles with mycophenolate mofetil. *Journal of the American Academy of Dermatology*, **45**, 142–4.

Gran, J. T. and Skomsvoll, J. F. (1997). The outcome of ankylosing spondylitis: a study of 100 patients. *British Journal of Rheumatology*, **36**, 766–71.

Grant, I. A., Hunder, G. G., Homburger, H. A., and Dyck, P. J. (1997). Peripheral neuropathy associated with sicca complex. *Neurology*, **48**, 855–62.

Gravallese, E. M., Corson, J. M., Coblyn, J. S., Pinkus, G. S., and Weinblatt, M. E. (1989). Rheumatoid aortitis: a rarely recognized but clinically significant entity. *Medicine* (Baltimore), **68**, 95–106.

Gray, R. G. and Poppo, M. J. (1983). Necrotizing vasculitis as the initial manifestation of rheumatoid arthritis. *Journal of Rheumatology*, **10**, 326–8.

Greening, A. P. and Hughes, J. M. (1981). Serial estimations of carbon monoxide diffusing capacity in intrapulmonary haemorrhage. *Clinical Science*, **60**, 507–12.

Greisman, S. G., Thayaparan, R. S., Godwin, T. A., and Lockshin, M. D. (1991). Occlusive vasculopathy in systemic lupus erythematosus. Association with anticardiolipin antibody. *Archives of Internal Medicine*, **151**, 389–92.

Griffin, J. W. (2001). Vasculitic neuropathies. *Rheumatic Disease Clinics of North America*, **27**, 751–60, vi.

Grimbacher, B., Huber, M., von Kempis, J., Kalden, P., Uhl, M., Kohler, G., Blum, H. E., and Peter, H. H. (1998). Successful treatment of gastrointestinal vasculitis due to systemic lupus erythematosus with intravenous pulse cyclophosphamide: a clinical case report and review of the literature. *British Journal of Rheumatology*, **37**, 1023–8.

Grotz, W., von, Z., I, Andre, M., and Schollmeyer, P. (1998). Treatment of retroperitoneal fibrosis by mycophenolate mofetil and glucocorticoids. *Lancet*, **352**, 1195.

Gyongyosi, M., Pokorny, G., Jambrik, Z., Kovacs, L., Kovacs, A., Makula, E., and Csanady, M. (1996). Cardiac manifestations in primary Sjögren's syndrome. *Annals of the Rheumatic Diseases*, **55**, 450–4.

Haddad, F. S., Sachdev, J. S., and Bellapravalu, M. (1990). Neuropathic bladder in ankylosing spondylitis with spinal diverticula. *Urology*, **35**, 313–16.

Hanly, J. G. (1998). Evaluation of patients with CNS involvement in SLE. *Baillieres Clinical Rheumatology*, **12**, 415–31.

Hanly, J. G. (2005). Neuropsychiatric lupus. *Rheumatic Disease Clinics of North America*, **31**, 273–98, vi.

Hanly, J. G. and Harrison, M. J. (2005). Management of neuropsychiatric lupus. *Best Practice and Research in Clinical Rheumatology*, **19**, 799–821.

Hanly, J. G., McCurdy, G., Fougere, L., Douglas, J. A., and Thompson, K. (2004). Neuropsychiatric events in systemic lupus erythematosus: attribution and clinical significance. *Journal of Rheumatology*, **31**, 2156–62.

Harisdangkul, V., Doorenbos, D., and Subramony, S. H. (1995). Lupus transverse myelopathy: better outcome with early recognition and aggressive high-dose intravenous glucocorticoid pulse treatment. *Journal of Neurology*, **242**, 326–31.

Harreby, M., Bilde, T., Helin, P., Meyhoff, H. H., Vinterberg, H., and Nielsen, V. A. (1994). Retroperitoneal fibrosis treated with methylprednisolon pulse and disease-modifying antirheumatic drugs. *Scandinavian Journal of Urology and Nephrology*, **28**, 237–42.

Haupt, H. M., Moore, G. W., and Hutchins, G. M. (1981). The lung in systemic lupus erythematosus. Analysis of the pathologic changes in 120 patients. *American Journal of Medicine*, **71**, 791–8.

Heibel, R. H., O'Toole, J. D., Curtiss, E. I., Medsger, T. A., Jr., Reddy, S. P., and Shaver, J. A. (1976). Coronary arteritis in systemic lupus erythematosus. *Chest*, **69**, 700–3.

Hermisson, M., Klein, R., Schmidt, F., Weller, M., and Kuker, W. (2002). Myelopathy in primary Sjogren's syndrome: diagnostic and therapeutic aspects. *Acta Neurologica Scandinavica*, **105**, 450–3.

Herrick, A. L., Oogarah, P., Brammah, T. B., Freemont, A. J., and Jayson, M. I. (1994a). Nervous system involvement in association with vasculitis and anticardiolipin antibodies in a patient with systemic sclerosis. *Annals of the Rheumatic Diseases*, **53**, 349–50.

Herrick, A. L., Oogarah, P. K., Freemont, A. J., Marcuson, R., Haeney, M., and Jayson, M. I. (1994b). Vasculitis in patients with systemic sclerosis and severe digital ischaemia requiring amputation. *Annals of the Rheumatic Diseases*, **53**, 323–6.

Heurkens, A. H., Westedt, M. L., and Breedveld, F. C. (1991). Prednisone plus azathioprine treatment in patients with rheumatoid arthritis complicated by vasculitis. *Archives of Internal Medicine*, **151**, 2249–54.

Hillarby, M. C., Clarkson, R., Grennan, D. M., Bate, A. S., Ollier, W., Sanders, P. A., Chattophadhyay, C., Davis, M., O'Sullivan, M. M., and Williams, B. (1991). Immunogenetic heterogeneity in rheumatoid disease as illustrated by different MHC associations (DQ, Dw and C4) in articular and extra-articular subsets. *British Journal of Rheumatology*, **30**, 5–9.

Hirakata, M. and Nagai, S. (2000). Interstitial lung disease in polymyositis and dermatomyositis. *Current Opinion in Rheumatology*, **12**, 501–8.

Holtman, J. H., Neustadt, D. H., Klein, J., and Callen, J. P. (1990). Dapsone is an effective therapy for the skin lesions of subacute cutaneous lupus erythematosus and urticarial vasculitis in a patient with C2 deficiency. *Journal of Rheumatology*, **17**, 1222–5.

Horton, M. R. (2004). Rheumatoid arthritis associated interstitial lung disease. *Critical Reviews in Computed Tomography*, **45**, 429–40.

Hricik, D. E., Chung-Park, M., and Sedor, J. R. (1998). Glomerulonephritis. *New England Journal of Medicine*, **339**, 888–99.

Hunger, R. E., Durr, C., and Brand, C. U. (2001). Cutaneous leukocytoclastic vasculitis in dermatomyositis suggests malignancy. *Dermatology*, **202**, 123–6.

Isaak, B. L., Liesegang, T. J., and Michet, C. J., Jr. (1986). Ocular and systemic findings in relapsing polychondritis. *Ophthalmology*, **93**, 681–9.

Jabs, D. A., Fine, S. L., Hochberg, M. C., Newman, S. A., Heiner, G. G., and Stevens, M. B. (1986). Severe retinal vaso-occlusive disease in systemic lupus erythematous. *Archives of Ophthalmology*, **104**, 558–63.

Jaffe, I. A. and Smith, R. W. (1968). Rheumatoid vasculitis. Report of a second case treated with penicillamine. *Arthritis and Rheumatism*, **11**, 585–92.

Jans, H., Halberg, P., and Lorenzen, I. (1983). Circulating immune complexes in rheumatoid arthritis with extra-articular manifestations. *Scandinavian Journal of Rheumatology*, **12**, 215–18.

Janssen, B. A., Luqmani, R. A., Gordon, C., Hemingway, I. H., Bacon, P. A., Gearing, A. J., and Emery, P. (1994). Correlation of blood levels of soluble vascular cell adhesion molecule-1 with disease activity in systemic lupus erythematosus and vasculitis. *British Journal of Rheumatology*, **33**, 1112–16.

Jaraquemada, D., Ollier, W., Awad, J., Young, A., Silman, A., Roitt, I. M., Corbett, M., Hay, F., Cosh, J. A., and Maini, R. N. (1986). HLA and rheumatoid arthritis: a combined analysis of 440 British patients. *Annals of the Rheumatic Diseases*, **45**, 627–36.

Jennette, J. C., Ferguson, A. L., Moore, M. A., and Freeman, D. G. (1982). IgA nephropathy associated with seronegative spondylarthropathies. *Arthritis and Rheumatism*, **25**, 144–9.

Jifi-Bahlool, H., Saadeh, C., and O'Connor, J. (1995). Peripheral ulcerative keratitis in the setting of rheumatoid arthritis: treatment with immunosuppressive therapy. *Seminars in Arthritis and Rheumatism*, **25**, 67–73.

Kadoya, A., Akahoshi, T., Sekiyama, N., Hosaka, S., and Kondo, H. (1994). Cutaneous vasculitis in a patient with dermatomyositis without muscle involvement. *Internal Medicine*, **33**, 809–12.

Kalovidouris, A. E., Stoesz, E., Muller, J., Kimes, T., and Brandt, K. D. (1988). Relationships between clinical features and distribution of mononuclear cells in muscle of patients with polymyositis. *Journal of Rheumatology*, **15**, 1401–6.

Kao, A. H. and Manzi, S. (2002). How to manage patients with cardiopulmonary disease? *Best Practice and Research in Clinical Rheumatology*, **16**, 211–27.

Kao, A. H., Sabatine, J. M., and Manzi, S. (2003). Update on vascular disease in systemic lupus erythematosus. *Current Opinion in Rheumatology*, **15**, 519–27.

Kardar, A. H., Kattan, S., Lindstedt, E., and Hanash, K. (2002). Steroid therapy for idiopathic retroperitoneal fibrosis: dose and duration. *Journal of Urology*, **168**, 550–5.

Karrar, A., Sequeira, W., and Block, J. A. (2001). Coronary artery disease in systemic lupus erythematosus: A review of the literature. *Seminars in Arthritis and Rheumatism*, **30**, 436–43.

Kawasuji, M., Hetzer, R., Oelert, H., Stauch, G., and Borst, H. G. (1982). Aortic valve replacement and ascending aorta replacement in ankylosing spondylitis: report of three surgical cases and review of the literature. *Thoracic and Cardiovascular Surgery*, **30**, 310–14.

Kaye, B. R. (1989). Rheumatologic manifestations of infection with human immunodeficiency virus (HIV). *Annals of Internal Medicine*, **111**, 158–67.

Kent, D. L., Haynor, D. R., Longstreth, W. T., Jr., and Larson, E. B. (1994). The clinical efficacy of magnetic resonance imaging in neuroimaging. *Annals of Internal Medicine*, **120**, 856–71.

Kent, P. D., Michet, C. J., Jr., and Luthra, H. S. (2004). Relapsing polychondritis. *Current Opinion in Rheumatology*, **16**, 56–61.

Kerr, H. E. and Sturrock, R. D. (1999). Clinical aspects, outcome assessment, disease course, and extra-articular features of spondyloarthropathies. *Current Opinion in Rheumatology*, **11**, 235–7.

Khan, M. A. (2002). Update on spondyloarthropathies. *Annals of Internal Medicine*, **136**, 896–907.

Kim, E. A., Lee, K. S., Johkoh, T., Kim, T. S., Suh, G. Y., Kwon, O. J., and Han, J. (2002). Interstitial lung diseases associated with collagen vascular diseases: radiologic and histopathologic findings. *Radiographics*, **22**, S151–65.

Kim, R. C., Collins, G. H., and Parisi, J. E. (1982). Rheumatoid nodule formation within the choroid plexus. Report of a second case. *Archives of Pathology and Laboratory Medicine*, **106**, 83–4.

Kinsella, T. D., Johnson, L. G., and Ian, R. (1974). Cardiovascular manifestations of ankylosing spondylitis. *Canadian Medical Association Journal*, **111**, 1309–11.

Klinkhoff, A. V., Beattie, C. W., and Chalmers, A. (1986). Retinopathy in systemic lupus erythematosus: relationship to disease activity. *Arthritis and Rheumatism*, **29**, 1152–6.

Knab, J., Goos, M., and Dissemond, J. (2005). Successful treatment of a leg ulcer occurring in a rheumatoid arthritis patient under leflunomide therapy. *Journal of the European Academy of Dermatology and Venereology*, **19**, 243–46.

Ko, S. F., Lee, T. Y., Cheng, T. T., Ng, S. H., Lai, H. M., Cheng, Y. F., and Tsai, C. C. (1997). CT findings at lupus mesenteric vasculitis. *Acta Radiologica*, **38**, 115–20.

Koenigsberg, R. A., Klahr, J., Zito, J. L., Patel, M., and Carsons, S. (1995). Magnetic resonance imaging of cauda equina syndrome in ankylosing spondylitis: a case report. *Journal of Neuroimaging*, **5**, 46–8.

Koep, L. and Zuidema, G. D. (1977). The clinical significance of retroperitoneal fibrosis. *Surgery*, **81**, 250–7.

Konttinen, Y. T., Kinnunen, E., von Bonsdorff, M., Lillqvist, P., Immonen, I., Bergroth, V., Segerberg-Konttinen, M., and Friman, C. (1987). Acute transverse myelopathy successfully treated with plasmapheresis and prednisone in a patient with primary Sjogren's syndrome. *Arthritis and Rheumatism*, **30**, 339–44.

Korkmaz, C., Ozcan, A., and Akcar, N. (2005). Increased frequency of ultrasonographic findings suggestive of renal stones in patients with ankylosing spondylitis. *Clinical and Experimental Rheumatology*, **23**, 389–92.

Koshy, M., Berger, D., and Crow, M. K. (1996). Increased expression of CD40 ligand on systemic lupus erythematosus lymphocytes. *Journal of Clinical Investigation*, **98**, 826–37.

Kushwaha, S. S. and Steinberg, V. L. (1992). Cauda equina syndrome associated with ankylosing spondylitis in a female. *Postgraduate Medical Journal*, **68**, 485–6.

Laing, T. J. (1988). Gastrointestinal vasculitis and pneumatosis intestinalis due to systemic lupus erythematosus: successful treatment with pulse intravenous cyclophosphamide. *American Journal of Medicine*, **85**, 555–8.

Laman, S. D. and Provost, T. T. (1994). Cutaneous manifestations of lupus erythematosus. *Rheumatic Disease Clinics of North America*, **20**, 195–212.

Lang-Lazdunski, L., Hvass, U., Paillole, C., Pansard, Y., and Langlois, J. (1995). Cardiac valve replacement in relapsing polychondritis. A review. *Journal of Heart Valve Diseases*, **3**, 227–35.

Lavalle, C., Pizarro, S., Drenkard, C., Sanchez-Guerrero, J., and Alarcon-Segovia, D. (1990). Transverse myelitis: a manifestation of systemic lupus erythematosus strongly associated with antiphospholipid antibodies. *Journal of Rheumatology*, **17**, 34–7.

Leatherman, J. W., Davies, S. F., and Hoidal, J. R. (1984). Alveolar hemorrhage syndromes: diffuse microvascular lung hemorrhage in immune and idiopathic disorders. *Medicine* (Baltimore), **63**, 343–61.

Lee, C. K., Ahn, M. S., Lee, E. Y., Shin, J. H., Cho, Y. S., Ha, H. K., Yoo, B., and Moon, H. B. (2002). Acute abdominal pain in systemic lupus erythematosus: focus on lupus enteritis (gastrointestinal vasculitis). *Annals of the Rheumatic Diseases*, **61**, 547–50.

Lee, L. A. and Norris, D. A. (1989). Mechanisms of cutaneous tissue damage in lupus erythematosus. *Immunology Series*, **46**, 359–86.

Lee, S. S. and Lawton, J. M. (1992). Antimyeloperoxidase antibody in systemic lupus erythematosus. *Journal of Internal Medicine*, **232**, 283–4.

Lesprit, P., Mouloud, F., Bierling, P., Schaeffer, A., Cesaro, P., Brun-Buisson, C., and Godeau, B. (1996). Prolonged remission of SLE-associated polyradiculoneuropathy after a single course of intravenous immunoglobulin. *Scandinavian Journal of Rheumatology*, **25**, 177–9.

Letko, E., Zafirakis, P., Baltatzis, S., Voudouri, A., Livir-Rallatos, C., and Foster, C. S. (2002). Relapsing polychondritis: a clinical review. *Seminars in Arthritis and Rheumatism*, **31**, 384–95.

Li, J. S., Liu, M. F., and Lei, H. Y. (1996). Characterization of anti-endothelial cell antibodies in the patients with systemic lupus erythematosus: a potential marker for disease activity. *Clinical Immunology and Immunopathology*, **79**, 211–6.

Lindsay, M. K., Tavadia, H. B., Whyte, A. S., Lee, P., and Webb, J. (1973). Acute abdomen in rheumatoid arthritis due to necrotizing arteritis. *British Medical Journal*, **2**, 592–3.

Liote, F. and Osterland, C. K. (1994). Autonomic neuropathy in systemic lupus erythematosus: cardiovascular autonomic function assessment. *Annals of the Rheumatic Diseases*, **53**, 671–4.

Liu, M. F., Lee, J. H., Weng, T. H., and Lee, Y. Y. (1998). Clinical experience of 13 cases with severe pulmonary hemorrhage in systemic lupus erythematosus with active nephritis. *Scandinavian Journal of Rheumatology*, **27**, 291–5.

Liu, V. and Mackool, B. T. (2003). Mycophenolate in dermatology. *Journal of Dermatological Treatment*, **14**, 203–11.

Locke, I. C., Worrall, J. G., Leaker, B., Black, C. M., and Cambridge, G. (1997). Autoantibodies to myeloperoxidase in systemic sclerosis. *Journal of Rheumatology*, **24**, 86–9.

Loffeld, R. J. and van Weel, T. F. (1993). Tamoxifen for retroperitoneal fibrosis. *Lancet*, **341**, 382.

Lorber, M., Gershwin, M. E., and Shoenfeld, Y. (1994). The coexistence of systemic lupus erythematosus with other autoimmune diseases: the kaleidoscope of autoimmunity. *Seminars in Arthritis and Rheumatism*, **24**, 105–13.

Luqmani, R. A., Pathare, S., and Kwok-Fai, T. L. (2005). How to diagnose and treat secondary forms of vasculitis. *Best Practice and Research in Clinical Rheumatology*, **19**, 321–36.

Luqmani, R. A., Watts, R. A., Scott, D. G., and Bacon, P. A. (1994). Treatment of vasculitis in rheumatoid arthritis. *Annales de Médecine Interne* (Paris), **145**, 566–76.

Maes, B., Van Mieghem, A., Messiaen, T., Kuypers, D., Van Damme, B., and Vanrenterghem, Y. (2000). Limited cutaneous systemic sclerosis associated with MPO-ANCA positive renal small vessel vasculitis of the microscopic polyangiitis type. *American Journal of Kidney Diseases*, **36**, E16.

Magro, C. M., Crowson, A. N., and Peeling, R. (1995). Vasculitis as the basis of cutaneous lesions in Reiter's disease. *Human Pathology*, **26**, 633–8.

Malaviya, A. N., Raina, V., Mittal, V., Narayanan, K., Malhotra, K. K., Bhuyan, U. N., and Mehra, N. K. (1981). Glomerulonephritis in seronegative spondylarthritis syndrome. *Arthritis and Rheumatism*, **24**, 751–2.

Manzi, S., Meilahn, E. N., Rairie, J. E., Conte, C. G., Medsger, T. A., Jr., Jansen-McWilliams, L., D'Agostino, R. B., and Kuller, L. H. (1997). Age-specific incidence rates of myocardial infarction and angina in women with systemic lupus erythematosus: comparison with the Framingham Study. *American Journal of Epidemiology*, **145**, 408–15.

Marcolongo, R., Tavolini, I. M., Laveder, F., Busa, M., Noventa, F., Bassi, P., and Semenzato, G. (2004). Immunosuppressive therapy for idiopathic retroperitoneal fibrosis: a retrospective analysis of 26 cases. *American Journal of Medicine*, **116**, 194–7.

Martens, P. B., Goronzy, J. J., Schaid, D., and Weyand, C. M. (1997). Expansion of unusual CD4+ T cells in severe rheumatoid arthritis. *Arthritis and Rheumatism*, **40**, 1106–14.

Martens, P. B., Moder, K. G., and Ahmed, I. (1999). Lupus panniculitis: clinical perspectives from a case series. *Journal of Rheumatology*, **26**, 68–72.

Martinez-Taboada, V. M., Alonso, R. B., Armona, J., Fernandez-Sueiro, J. L., Gonzalez, V. C., and Rodriguez-Valverde, V. (1996). Mononeuritis multiplex in systemic lupus erythematosus: response to pulse intravenous cyclophosphamide. *Lupus*, **5**, 74–6.

Marzano, A., Trapani, A., Leone, N., Actis, G. C., and Rizzetto, M. (2001). Treatment of idiopathic retroperitoneal fibrosis using cyclosporin. *Annals of the Rheumatic Diseases*, **60**, 427–8.

Matsumoto, T., Yoshimine, T., Shimouchi, K., Shiotu, H., Kuwabara, N., Fukuda, Y., and Hoshi, T. (1992). The liver in systemic lupus erythematosus: pathologic analysis of 52 cases and review of Japanese Autopsy Registry Data. *Human Pathology*, **23**, 1151–8.

Matzkies, F. G., Manger, B., Schmitt-Haendle, M., Nagel, T., Kraetsch, H. G., Kalden, J. R., and Schulze-Koops, H. (2003). Severe septicaemia in a patient with polychondritis and Sweet's syndrome after initiation of treatment with infliximab. *Annals of the Rheumatic Diseases*, **62**, 81–2.

McAdam, L. P., O'Hanlan, M. A., Bluestone, R., and Pearson, C. M. (1976). Relapsing polychondritis: prospective study of 23 patients and a review of the literature. *Medicine* (Baltimore), **55**, 193–215.

McDonald, J., Stewart, J., Urowitz, M. B., and Gladman, D. D. (1992). Peripheral vascular disease in patients with systemic lupus erythematosus. *Annals of the Rheumatic Diseases*, **51**, 56–60.

McRorie, E. R., Ruckley, C. V., and Nuki, G. (1998). The relevance of large-vessel vascular disease and restricted ankle movement to the aetiology of leg ulceration in rheumatoid arthritis. *British Journal of Rheumatology*, **37**, 1295–8.

Medina, F., Ayala, A., Jara, L. J., Becerra, M., Miranda, J. M., and Fraga, A. (1997). Acute abdomen in systemic lupus erythematosus: the importance of early laparotomy. *American Journal of Medicine*, **103**, 100–05.

Michet, C. J. (1990). Vasculitis and relapsing polychondritis. *Rheumatic Disease Clinics of North America*, **16**, 441–4.

Mills, J. A. (1994). Systemic lupus erythematosus. *New England Journal of Medicine*, **330**, 1871–9.

Mitchinson, M. J. (1984). Chronic periaortitis and periarteritis. *Histopathology*, **8**, 589–600.

Mitsias, P. and Levine, S. R. (1994). Large cerebral vessel occlusive disease in systemic lupus erythematosus. *Neurology*, **44**, 385–93.

Mizutani, A., Tanaka, I., Katayama, M., Oshima, H., Komatsu, Y., Asano, S., Kato, K., Matsumura, H., Ishii, K., Miyama, H., Nagai, T., Kato, K., Fukaya, S., Yoshida, S., Hasegawa, M., Kawashima, S., and Torikai, K. (2000). [A case of myeloperoxidase-antineutrophil cytoplasmic antibody (MPO-ANCA) related glomerulonephritis associated with systemic sclerosis treated by steroid pulse therapy: a case report]. *Ryumachi*, **40**, 828–32.

Moder, K. G., Miller, T. D., and Tazelaar, H. D. (1999). Cardiac involvement in systemic lupus erythematosus. *Mayo Clinic Proceedings*, **74**, 275–84.

Monnet, D., Breban, M., Hudry, C., Dougados, M., and Brezin, A. P. (2004). Ophthalmic findings and frequency of extraocular manifestations in patients with HLA-B27 uveitis: a study of 175 cases. *Ophthalmology*, **111**, 802–9.

Morris, P. B., Imber, M. J., Heinsimer, J. A., Hlatky, M. A., and Reimer, K. A. (1986). Rheumatoid arthritis and coronary arteritis. *American Journal of Cardiology*, **57**, 689–90.

Moutsopoulos, H. M., Balow, J. E., Lawley, T. J., Stahl, N. I., Antonovych, T. T., and Chused, T. M. (1978). Immune complex glomerulonephritis in sicca syndrome. *American Journal of Medicine*, **64**, 955–60.

Mpofu, S., Estrach, C., Curtis, J., and Moots, R. J. (2003). Treatment of respiratory complications in recalcitrant relapsing polychondritis with infliximab. *Rheumatology* (Oxford), **42**, 1117–18.

Munoz-Fernandez, S., Hidalgo, V., Fernandez-Melon, J., Schlincker, A., Bonilla, G., Ruiz-Sancho, D., Fonseca, A., Gijon-Banos, J., and Martin-Mola, E. (2003). Sulfasalazine reduces the number of flares of acute anterior uveitis over a one-year period. *Journal of Rheumatology*, **30**, 1277–9.

Munoz-Fernandez, S. and Martin-Mola, E. (2006). Uveitis. *Best Practice and Research in Clinical Rheumatology*, **20**, 487–505.

Myers, J. L. and Katzenstein, A. A. (1986). Microangiitis in lupus-induced pulmonary hemorrhage. *American Journal of Clinical Pathology*, **85**, 552–6.

Nagahama, T., Matsui, T., Matsumura, M., Matake, H., Tsuda, S., Sakurai, T., Yao, T., and Schlemper, R. (2000). Rheumatoid arthritis accompanied by colonic lesions. *Internal Medicine*, **39**, 235–8.

Navarro, M., Cervera, R., Font, J., Reverter, J. C., Monteagudo, J., Escolar, G., Lopez-Soto, A., Ordinas, A., and Ingelmo, M. (1997). Anti-endothelial cell antibodies in systemic autoimmune diseases: prevalence and clinical significance. *Lupus*, **6**, 521–6.

Navarro, M. J., Higgins, G. C., Lohr, K. M., and Myers, L. K. (2002). Amelioration of relapsing polychondritis in a child treated with oral collagen. *American Journal of Medical Science*, **324**, 101–3.

Newbold, K. M., Allum, W. H., Downing, R., Symmons, D. P., and Oates, G. D. (1987). Vasculitis of the gall bladder in rheumatoid arthritis and systemic lupus erythematosus. *Clinical Rheumatology*, **6**, 287–9.

Nguyen, V. A., Gotwald, T., Prior, C., Oberrnoser, G., and Sepp, N. (2005). Acute pulmonary edema, capillaritis and alveolar hemorrhage: pulmonary manifestations coexistent in antiphospholipid syndrome and systemic lupus erythematosus?. *Lupus*, **14**, 557–60.

Nicholls, A., Snaith, M. L., Maini, R. N., and Scott, J. T. (1973). Proceedings: Controlled trial of azathioprine in rheumatoid vasculitis. *Annals of the Rheumatic Diseases*, **32**, 589–91.

Nishijima, C., Hatta, N., Inaoki, M., Sakai, H., and Takehara, K. (1999). Urticarial vasculitis in systemic lupus erythematosus: fair response to prednisolone/dapsone and persistent hypocomplementemia. *European Journal of Dermatology*, **9**, 54–6.

Nishiya, K., Chikazawa, H., Nishimura, S., Hisakawa, N., and Hashimoto, K. (1997). Anti-neutrophil cytoplasmic antibody in patients with systemic lupus erythematosus is unrelated to clinical features. *Clinical Rheumatology*, **16**, 70–5.

Nobrega, T. P., Klodas, E., Breen, J. F., Liggett, S. P., Higano, S. T., and Reeder, G. S. (1996). Giant coronary artery aneurysms and myocardial infarction in a patient with systemic lupus erythematosus. *Catheterization and Cardiovascular Interventions*, **39**, 75–9.

O'Neill, T. W. and Bresnihan, B. (1992). The heart in ankylosing spondylitis. *Annals of the Rheumatic Diseases*, **51**, 705–6.

Oddis, C. V., Eisenbeis, C. H., Jr., Reidbord, H. E., Steen, V. D., and Medsger, T. A., Jr. (1987). Vasculitis in systemic sclerosis: association with Sjögren's syndrome and the CREST syndrome variant. *Journal of Rheumatology*, **14**, 942–8.

Oh, D. H., Jun, J. B., Kim, H. T., Lee, S. W., Jung, S. S., Lee, I. H., and Kim, S. Y. (2001). Transverse myelitis in a patient with long-standing ankylosing spondylitis. *Clinical and Experimental Rheumatology*, **19**, 195–6.

Ohno, T., Matsuda, I., Furukawa, H., and Kanoh, T. (1994). Recovery from rheumatoid cerebral vasculitis by low-dose methotrexate. *Internal Medicine*, **33**, 615–20.

Oien, R. F., Hakansson, A., and Hansen, B. U. (2001). Leg ulcers in patients with rheumatoid arthritis–a prospective study of aetiology, wound healing and pain reduction after pinch grafting. *Rheumatology* (Oxford), **40**, 816–20.

Omdal, R., Loseth, S., Torbergsen, T., Koldingsnes, W., Husby, G., and Mellgren, S. I. (2001). Peripheral neuropathy in systemic lupus erythematosus–a longitudinal study. *Acta Neurologica Scandinavica*, **103**, 386–91.

Omote, A., Muramatsu, M., Sugimoto, Y., Hosono, S., Murakami, R., Tanaka, H., Watanabe, Y., Sano, H., and Kato, K. (1997). Myeloperoxidase-specific anti-neutrophil cytoplasmic autoantibodies – related scleroderma renal crisis treated with double-filtration plasmapheresis. *Internal Medicine*, **36**, 508–13.

Pachman, L. M. (1995). An update on juvenile dermatomyositis. *Current Opinion in Rheumatology*, **7**, 437–41.

Pachman, L. M., Hayford, J. R., Chung, A., Daugherty, C. A., Pallansch, M. A., Fink, C. W., Gewanter, H. L., Jerath, R., Lang, B. A., Sinacore, J., Szer, I. S., Dyer, A. R., and Hochberg, M. C. (1998). Juvenile dermatomyositis at diagnosis: clinical characteristics of 79 children. *Journal of Rheumatology*, **25**, 1198–204.

Pagnoux, C., Mahr, A., Cohen, P., and Guillevin, L. (2005). Presentation and outcome of gastrointestinal involvement in systemic necrotizing vasculitides: analysis of 62 patients with polyarteritis nodosa, microscopic polyangiitis, Wegener granulomatosis, Churg-Strauss syndrome, or rheumatoid arthritis-associated vasculitis. *Medicine* (Baltimore), **84**, 115–28.

Paloheimo, J. A., Julkunen, H., Siltanen, P., and Kajander, A. (1966). Takayasu's arteritis and ankylosing spondylitis. Report of four cases. *Acta Medica Scandinavica*, **179**, 77–85.

Panush, R. S., Katz, P., Longley, S., CarterR, Love, J., and Stanley, H. (1983). Rheumatoid vasculitis: diagnostic and therapeutic decisions. *Clinical Rheumatology*, **2**, 321–30.

Papiris, S. A., Maniati, M., Constantopoulos, S. H., Roussos, C., Moutsopoulos, H. M., and Skopouli, F. N. (1999). Lung involvement in primary Sjögren's syndrome is mainly related to the small airway disease. *Annals of the Rheumatic Diseases*, **58**, 61–4.

Pappas, G. and Johnson, M. (1972). Mitral and aortic valvular insufficiency in chronic relapsing polychondritis. *Archives of Surgery*, **104**, 712–4.

Paran, D., Fireman, E., and Elkayam, O. (2004). Pulmonary disease in systemic lupus erythematosus and the antiphospholpid syndrome. *Autoimmunity Reviews*, **3**, 70–5.

Parums, D. V., Brown, D. L., and Mitchinson, M. J. (1990a). Serum antibodies to oxidized low-density lipoprotein and ceroid in chronic periaortitis. *Archives of Pathology and Laboratory Medicine*, **114**, 383–7.

Parums, D. V., Dunn, D. C., Dixon, A. K., and Mitchinson, M. J. (1990b). Characterization of inflammatory cells in a patient with chronic periaortitis. *American Journal of Cardiovascular Pathology*, **3**, 121–9.

Pedrollo, E., Bleil, L., Bautz, F. A., Kalden, J. R., and Bautz, E. K. (1993). Antineutrophil cytoplasmic autoantibodies (ANCA) recognizing a recombinant myeloperoxidase subunit. *Advances in Experimental Medicine and Biology*, **336**, 87–92.

Peponis, V., Kyttaris, V. C., Tyradellis, C., Vergados, I., and Sitaras, N. M. (2006). Ocular manifestations of systemic lupus erythematosus: a clinical review. *Lupus*, **15**, 3–12.

Petri, M., Perez-Gutthann, S., Spence, D., and Hochberg, M. C. (1992). Risk factors for coronary artery disease in patients with systemic lupus erythematosus. *American Journal of Medicine*, **93**, 513–19.

Pisoni, C. N., Obermoser, G., Cuadrado, M. J., Sanchez, F. J., Karim, Y., Sepp, N. T., Khamashta, M. A., and Hughes, G. R. (2005). Skin manifestations of systemic lupus erythematosus refractory to multiple treatment modalities: poor results with mycophenolate mofetil. *Clinical and Experimental Rheumatology*, **23**, 393–6.

Price, E. J., Rigby, S. P., Clancy, U., and Venables, P. J. (1998). A double blind placebo controlled trial of azathioprine in the treatment of primary Sjögren's syndrome. *Journal of Rheumatology*, **25**, 896–9.

Provenzale, J. M., Barboriak, D. P., Gaensler, E. H., Robertson, R. L., and Mercer, B. (1994). Lupus-related myelitis: serial MR findings. *American Journal of Neuroradiology*, **15**, 1911–17.

Provenzale, J. M. and Ortel, T. L. (1995). Anatomic distribution of venous thrombosis in patients with antiphospholipid antibody: imaging findings. *American Journal of Roentgenology*, **165**, 365–8.

Puechal, X., Said, G., Hilliquin, P., Coste, J., Job-Deslandre, C., Lacroix, C., and Menkes, C. J. (1995). Peripheral neuropathy with necrotizing vasculitis in rheumatoid arthritis. A clinicopathologic and prognostic study of thirty-two patients. *Arthritis and Rheumatism*, **38**, 1618–29.

Ramos-Casals, M., Font, J., Garcia-Carrasco, M., Brito, M. P., Rosas, J., Calvo-Alen, J., Pallares, L., Cervera, R., and Ingelmo, M. (2002). Primary Sjögren's syndrome: hematologic patterns of disease expression. *Medicine* (Baltimore), **81**, 281–92.

Ramos-Casals, M., Nardi, N., Lagrutta, M., Brito-Zeron, P., Bove, A., Delgado, G., Cervera, R., Ingelmo, M., and Font, J. (2006). Vasculitis in systemic lupus erythematosus: prevalence and clinical characteristics in 670 patients. *Medicine* (Baltimore), **85**, 95–104.

Rapoport, R. J., Kozin, F., Mackel, S. E., and Jordon, R. E. (1980). Cutaneous vascular immunofluorescence in rheumatoid arthritis. Correlation with circulating immune complexes and vasculitis. *American Journal of Medicine*, **68**, 325–31.

Rhee, R. Y., Gloviczki, P., Luthra, H. S., Stanson, A. W., Bower, T. C., and Cherry, K. J., Jr. (1994). Iliocaval complications of retroperitoneal fibrosis. *American Journal of Surgery*, **168**, 179–83.

Richette, P., Dieude, P., Damiano, J., Liote, F., Orcel, P., and Bardin, T. (2004). Sensory neuropathy revealing necrotizing vasculitis during infliximab therapy for rheumatoid arthritis. *Journal of Rheumatology*, **31**, 2079–81.

Richez, C., Dumoulin, C., Coutouly, X., and Schaeverbeke, T. (2004). Successful treatment of relapsing polychondritis with infliximab. *Clinical and Experimental Rheumatology*, **22**, 629–31.

Richter, C., Wanke, L., Steinmetz, J., Reinhold-Keller, E., and Gross, W. L. (2000). Mononeuritis secondary to rheumatoid arthritis responds to etanercept. *Rheumatology* (Oxford), **39**, 1436–7.

Roberts, W. C. and High, S. T. (1999). The heart in systemic lupus erythematosus. *Current Problems in Cardiology*, **24**, 1–56.

Rocca, P. V., Siegel, L. B., and Cupps, T. R. (1994). The concomitant expression of vasculitis and coagulopathy: synergy for marked tissue ischemia. *Journal of Rheumatology*, **21**, 556–60.

Rogers, S. J., Williams, C. S., and Roman, G. C. (2004). Myelopathy in Sjögren's syndrome: role of nonsteroidal immunosuppressants. *Drugs*, **64**, 123–32.

Roldan, C. A., Chavez, J., Wiest, P. W., Qualls, C. R., and Crawford, M. H. (1998). Aortic root disease and valve disease associated with ankylosing spondylitis. *Journal of the American College of Cardiology*, **32**, 1397–404.

Rosen, O., Thiel, A., Massenkeil, G., Hiepe, F., Haupl, T., Radtke, H., Burmester, G. R., Gromnica-Ihle, E., Radbruch, A., and Arnold, R. (2000). Autologous stem-cell transplantation in refractory autoimmune diseases after in vivo immunoablation and ex vivo depletion of mononuclear cells. *Arthritis Research*, **2**, 327–36.

Rothova, A., Buitenhuis, H. J., Meenken, C., Brinkman, C. J., Linssen, A., Alberts, C., Luyendijk, L., and Kijlstra, A. (1992). Uveitis and systemic disease. *British Journal of Ophthalmology*, **76**, 137–41.

Rovaris, M., Viti, B., Ciboddo, G., Gerevini, S., Capra, R., Iannucci, G., Comi, G., and Filippi, M. (2000). Brain involvement in systemic immune mediated diseases: magnetic resonance and magnetisation transfer imaging study. *Journal of Neurology Neurosurgery and Psychiatry*, **68**, 170–7.

Ruffatti, A., Sinico, R. A., Radice, A., Ossi, E., Cozzi, F., Tonello, M., Grypiotis, P., and Todesco, S. (2002). Autoantibodies to proteinase 3 and myeloperoxidase in systemic sclerosis. *Journal of Rheumatology*, **29**, 918–23.

Saadoun, D., Deslandre, C. J., Allanore, Y., Pham, X. V., and Kahan, A. (2003). Sustained response to infliximab in 2 patients with refractory relapsing polychondritis. *Journal of Rheumatology*, **30**, 1394–5.

Sanchez, N. P., Peters, M. S., and Winkelmann, R. K. (1981). The histopathology of lupus erythematosus panniculitis. *Journal of the American Academy of Dermatology*, **5**, 673–80.

Sant, S. M. and O'Connell, D. (1995). Cauda equina syndrome in ankylosing spondylitis: a case report and review of the literature. *Clinical Rheumatology*, **14**, 224–6.

Santos-Ocampo, A. S., Mandell, B. F., and Fessler, B. J. (2000). Alveolar hemorrhage in systemic lupus erythematosus: presentation and management. *Chest*, **118**, 1083–90.

Satko, S. G., Iskandar, S. S., and Appel, R. G. (2000). IgA nephropathy and Reiter's syndrome. Report of two cases and review of the literature. *Nephron*, **84**, 177–82.

Sato, K., Miyasaka, N., Nishioka, K., Yamaoka, K., Okuda, M., Nishido, T., and Uchima, H. (1987). Primary Sjögren's syndrome associated with systemic necrotizing vasculitis: a fatal case. *Arthritis and Rheumatism*, **30**, 717–18.

Saxe, P. A. and Altman, R. D. (1992). Takayasu's arteritis syndrome associated with systemic lupus erythematosus. *Seminars in Arthritis and Rheumatism*, **21**, 295–305.

Sayah, A. and English, J. C., III (2005). Rheumatoid arthritis: a review of the cutaneous manifestations. *Journal of the American Academy of Dermatology*, **53**, 191–209.

Schantz, V., Oestergaard, L. L., and Junker, P. (1998). Shrinking spinal cord following transverse myelopathy in a patient with systemic lupus erythematosus and the phospholipid antibody syndrome. *Journal of Rheumatology*, **25**, 1425–8.

Schnabel, A., Csernok, E., Isenberg, D. A., Mrowka, C., and Gross, W. L. (1995). Antineutrophil cytoplasmic antibodies in systemic lupus erythematosus. Prevalence, specificities, and clinical significance. *Arthritis and Rheumatism*, **38**, 633–7.

Schneider, H. A., Yonker, R. A., Katz, P., Longley, S., and Panush, R. S. (1985). Rheumatoid vasculitis: experience with 13 patients and review of the literature. *Seminars in Arthritis and Rheumatism*, **14**, 280–6.

Schroder, R., Urbach, H., and Zierz, S. (1994). Cauda equina syndrome with multiple lumbar diverticula complicating long-standing ankylosing spondylitis. *Clinical Investigation*, **72**, 1056–9.

Schroeder, J. O. and Euler, H. H. (1989). Treatment combining plasmapheresis and pulse cyclophosphamide in severe systemic lupus erythematosus. *Advances in Experimental Medicine and Biology*, **260**, 203–13.

Schwab, E. P., Schumacher, H. R., Jr., Freundlich, B., and Callegari, P. E. (1993). Pulmonary alveolar hemorrhage in systemic lupus erythematosus. *Seminars in Arthritis and Rheumatism*, **23**, 8–15.

Schwarz, M. I., Sutarik, J. M., Nick, J. A., Leff, J. A., Emlen, J. W., and Tuder, R. M. (1995). Pulmonary capillaritis and diffuse alveolar hemorrhage. A primary manifestation of polymyositis. *American Journal of Respiratory and Critical Care Medicine*, **151**, 2037–40.

Schwarz, M. I., Zamora, M. R., Hodges, T. N., Chan, E. D., Bowler, R. P., and Tuder, R. M. (1998). Isolated pulmonary capillaritis and diffuse alveolar hemorrhage in rheumatoid arthritis and mixed connective tissue disease. *Chest*, **113**, 1609–15.

Scott, D. G. and Bacon, P. A. (1983). Rheumatoid vasculitis. *Clinical Rheumatology*, **2**, 311–14.

Scott, D. G. and Bacon, P. A. (1984). Intravenous cyclophosphamide plus methylprednisolone in treatment of systemic rheumatoid vasculitis. *American Journal of Medicine*, **76**, 377–84.

Scott, D. G., Bacon, P. A., Allen, C., Elson, C. J., and Wallington, T. (1981a). IgG rheumatoid factor, complement and immune complexes in rheumatoid synovitis and vasculitis: comparative and serial studies during cytotoxic therapy. *Clinical and Experimental Rheumatology*, **43**, 54–63.

Scott, D. G., Bacon, P. A., Bothamley, J. E., Allen, C., Elson, C. J., and Wallington, T. B. (1981b). Plasma exchange in rheumatoid vasculitis. *Journal of Rheumatology*, **8**, 433–9.

Scott, D. G., Bacon, P. A., and Tribe, C. R. (1981c). Systemic rheumatoid vasculitis: a clinical and laboratory study of 50 cases. *Medicine* (Baltimore), **60**, 288–97.

See, Y., Martin, K., Rooney, M., and Woo, P. (1997). Severe juvenile dermatomyositis complicated by pancreatitis. *British Journal of Rheumatology*, **36**, 912–16.

Sen, D. and Isenberg, D. A. (2003). Antineutrophil cytoplasmic autoantibodies in systemic lupus erythematosus. *Lupus*, **12**, 651–8.

Shu, K. H., Lian, J. D., Yang, Y. F., Lu, Y. S., Wang, J. Y., Lan, J. L., and Chou, G. (1986). Glomerulonephritis in ankylosing spondylitis. *Clinical Nephrology*, **25**, 169–74.

Simmons-O'Brien, E., Chen, S., Watson, R., Antoni, C., Petri, M., Hochberg, M., Stevens, M. B., and Provost, T. T. (1995). One hundred anti-Ro (SS-A) antibody positive patients: a 10-year follow-up. *Medicine* (Baltimore), **74**, 109–30.

Skopouli, F. N., Jagiello, P., Tsifetaki, N., and Moutsopoulos, H. M. (1996). Methotrexate in primary Sjogren's syndrome. *Clinical and Experimental Rheumatology*, **14**, 555–8.

Sokoloff, L. (1953). The heart in rheumatoid arthritis. *American Heart Journal*, **45**, 635–43.

Somer, T. (1993). Thrombo-embolic and vascular complications in vasculitis syndromes. *European Heart Journal*, **14** (Suppl. K), 24–9.

Somer, T. and Siltanen, P. (1970). Aneurysm of the descending thoracic aorta, amyloidosis and renal carcinoma in a patient with ankylosing spondylitis. *American Journal of Medicine*, **49**, 408–15.

Stafford-Brady, F. J., Urowitz, M. B., Gladman, D. D., and Easterbrook, M. (1988). Lupus retinopathy. Patterns, associations, and prognosis. *Arthritis and Rheumatism*, **31**, 1105–10.

Stamp, L., Lambie, N., and O'Donnell, J. (2000). HLA-B27 associated spondyloarthropathy and severe ascending aortitis. *Journal of Rheumatology*, **27**, 2038–40.

Stewart, S. S., Ashizawa, T., Dudley, A. W., Jr., Goldberg, J. W., and Lidsky, M. D. (1988). Cerebral vasculitis in relapsing polychondritis. *Neurology*, **38**, 150–2.

Straaton, K. V., Chatham, W. W., Reveille, J. D., Koopman, W. J., and Smith, S. H. (1988). Clinically significant valvular heart disease in systemic lupus erythematosus. *American Journal of Medicine*, **85**, 645–50.

Straub, R. H., Zeuner, M., Lock, G., Rath, H., Hein, R., Scholmerich, J., and Lang, B. (1996). Autonomic and sensorimotor neuropathy in patients with systemic lupus erythematosus and systemic sclerosis. *Journal of Rheumatology*, **23**, 87–92.

Struthers, G. R., Scott, D. L., Delamere, J. P., Sheppeard, H., and Kitt, M. (1981). Smoking and rheumatoid vasculitis. *Rheumatology International*, **1**, 145–6.

Sultan, S. M., Ioannou, Y., and Isenberg, D. A. (1999). A review of gastrointestinal manifestations of systemic lupus erythematosus. *Rheumatology* (Oxford), **38**, 917–32.

Sundy, J. S., Jaffe, G. J., and McCallum, R. M. (2004). Extraarticular disease. In *Rheumatoid Arthritis* (St Clair, E. W., Pisetsky, D. S. and Haynes, B. F., eds), pp. 483–95. Lippincott Williams and Wilkins, Philadelphia, PA.

Takagi, H., Mori, Y., Umeda, Y., Fukumoto, Y., Kato, Y., Shimokawa, K., and Hirose, H. (2003). Abdominal aortic aneurysm with arteritis in ankylosing spondylitis. *Journal of Vascular Surgery*, **38**, 613–16.

Takeuchi, T., Aoki, K., Koide, J., Sekine, H., and Abe, T. (1995). Systemic lupus erythematosus with necrotizing vasculitis and upregulated expression of VLA-4 antigen. *Clinical Rheumatology*, **14**, 370–4.

Takizawa, Y., Kanda, H., Sato, K., Kawahata, K., Yamaguchi, A., Uozaki, H., Shimizu, J., Tsuji, S., Misaki, Y., and Yamamoto, K. (2007). Polymyositis associated with focal mesangial proliferative glomerulonephritis with depositions of immune complexes. *Clinical Rheumatology*, **26**, 792–6.

Teitel, A. D., MacKenzie, C. R., Stern, R., and Paget, S. A. (1992). Laryngeal involvement in systemic lupus erythematosus. *Seminars in Arthritis and Rheumatism*, **22**, 203–14.

Tikly, M., Burgin, S., Mohanlal, P., Bellingan, A., and George, J. (1996). Autoantibodies in black South Africans with systemic lupus erythematosus: spectrum and clinical associations. *Clinical Rheumatology*, **15**, 143–7.

Toloza, S. M., Uribe, A. G., McGwin, G., Jr., Alarcon, G. S., Fessler, B. J., Bastian, H. M., Vila, L. M., Wu, R., Shoenfeld, Y., Roseman, J. M., and Reveille, J. D. (2004). Systemic lupus erythematosus in a multiethnic US cohort (LUMINA). XXIII. Baseline predictors of vascular events. *Arthritis and Rheumatism*, **50**, 3947–57.

Toussirot, E., Auge, B., Tiberghien, P., Chabod, J., Cedoz, J. P., and Wendling, D. (1999). HLA-DRB1 alleles and shared amino acid sequences in disease susceptibility and severity in patients from eastern France with rheumatoid arthritis. *Journal of Rheumatology*, **26**, 1446–51.

Travis, R. C. and Byrne, P. (1987). The cauda equina syndrome: a rare extra-articular manifestation of ankylosing spondylitis – a case report. *Australian Radiology*, **31**, 395–6.

Trendelenburg, M., Courvoisier, S., Spath, P. J., Moll, S., Mihatsch, M., Itin, P., and Schifferli, J. A. (1999). Hypocomplementemic urticarial vasculitis or systemic lupus erythematosus?. *American Journal of Kidney Diseases*, **34**, 745–51.

Tribe, C. R., Scott, D. G., and Bacon, P. A. (1981). Rectal biopsy in the diagnosis of systemic vasculitis. *Journal of Clinical Pathology*, **34**, 843–50.

Tsokos, M., Lazarou, S. A., and Moutsopoulos, H. M. (1987). Vasculitis in primary Sjogren's syndrome. Histologic classification and clinical presentation. *American Journal of Clinical Pathology*, **88**, 26–31.

Tsuchida, T., Furue, M., Kashiwado, T., and Ishibashi, Y. (1994). Bullous systemic lupus erythematosus with cutaneous mucinosis and leukocytoclastic vasculitis. *Journal of the American Academy of Dermatology*, **31**, 387–90.

Turesson, C. and Jacobsson, L. T. (2004). Epidemiology of extra-articular manifestations in rheumatoid arthritis. *Scandinavian Journal of Rheumatology*, **33**, 65–72.

Turesson, C., Schaid, D. J., Weyand, C. M., Jacobsson, L. T., Goronzy, J. J., Petersson, I. F., Sturfelt, G., Nyhall-Wahlin, B. M., Truedsson, L., Dechant, S. A., and Matteson, E. L. (2005). The impact of HLA-DRB1 genes on extra-articular disease manifestations in rheumatoid arthritis. *Arthritis Research and Theory*, **7**, R1386–93.

Turesson, C., Weyand, C. M., and Matteson, E. L. (2004). Genetics of rheumatoid arthritis: Is there a pattern predicting extraarticular manifestations?. *Arthritis and Rheumatism*, **51**, 853–63.

Tuveri, M., Generini, S., Matucci-Cerinic, M., and Aloe, L. (2000). NGF, a useful tool in the treatment of chronic vasculitic ulcers in rheumatoid arthritis. *Lancet*, **356**, 1739–40.

Vaglio, A., Greco, P., and Buzio, C. (2006a). Tamoxifen therapy for retroperitoneal fibrosis. *Annals of Internal Medicine*, **144**, 619–20.

Vaglio, A., Salvarani, C., and Buzio, C. (2006b). Retroperitoneal fibrosis. *Lancet*, **367**, 241–51.

Van den, B. B., Selleslag, D., Boelaert, J. R., Matthys, E. G., Schurgers, M., Vandecasteele, S., and De Vriese, A. (2005). Management of therapy-resistant systemic lupus erythematosus with rituximab: report of a case and review of the literature. *Acta Clinica Belgica*, **60**, 102–5.

van der Bijl, A. E., Allaart, C. F., Van Vugt, J., Van Duinen, S., and Breedveld, F. C. (2005). Rheumatoid vasculitis treated with infliximab. *Journal of Rheumatology*, **32**, 1607–9.

van der Zee, J. M., Heurkens, A. H., van der Voort, E. A., Daha, M. R., and Breedveld, F. C. (1991). Characterization of anti-endothelial antibodies in patients with rheumatoid arthritis complicated by vasculitis. *Clinical and Experimental Rheumatology*, **9**, 589–94.

van Laar, J. M., Smit, V. T., de Beus, W. M., Collee, G., Jansen, E. H., and Breedveld, F. C. (1998). Rheumatoid vasculitis presenting as appendicitis. *Clinical and Experimental Rheumatology*, **16**, 736–8.

van Laarhoven, H. W., Rooyer, F. A., van Engelen, B. G., van Dalen, R., and Berden, J. H. (2001). Guillain-Barre syndrome as presenting feature in a patient with lupus nephritis, with complete resolution after cyclophosphamide treatment. *Nephrology Dialysis Transplantation*, **16**, 840–2.

Vitali, C., Bencivelli, W., Isenberg, D. A., Smolen, J. S., Snaith, M. L., Sciuto, M., d'Ascanio, A., and Bombardieri, S. (1992). Disease activity in systemic lupus erythematosus: report of the Consensus Study Group of the European Workshop for Rheumatology Research. I. A descriptive analysis of 704 European lupus patients. European Consensus Study Group for Disease Activity in SLE. *Clinical and Experimental Rheumatology*, **10**, 527–39.

Vlachoyiannopoulos, P. G., Karassa, F. B., Karakostas, K. X., Drosos, A. A., and Moutsopoulos, H. M. (1993). Systemic lupus erythematosus in Greece. Clinical features, evolution and outcome: a descriptive analysis of 292 patients. *Lupus*, **2**, 303–12.

Vogelgesang, S. A., Gutierrez, J., Klipple, G. L., and Katona, I. M. (1995). Polyneuropathy in juvenile dermatomyositis. *Journal of Rheumatology*, **22**, 1369–72.

Vollertsen, R. S. and Conn, D. L. (1990). Vasculitis associated with rheumatoid arthritis. *Rheumatic Disease Clinics of North America*, **16**, 445–61.

Vollertsen, R. S., Conn, D. L., Ballard, D. J., Ilstrup, D. M., Kazmar, R. E., and Silverfield, J. C. (1986). Rheumatoid vasculitis: survival and associated risk factors. *Medicine* (Baltimore), **65**, 365–75.

Voskuyl, A. E., Emeis, J. J., Hazes, J. M., van Hogezand, R. A., Biemond, I., and Breedveld, F. C. (1998a). Levels of circulating cellular fibronectin are increased in patients with rheumatoid vasculitis. *Clinical and Experimental Rheumatology*, **16**, 429–34.

Voskuyl, A. E., Hazes, J. M., Schreuder, G. M., Schipper, R. F., de Vries, R. R., and Breedveld, F. C. (1997). HLA-DRB1, DQA1, and DQB1 genotypes and risk of vasculitis in patients with rheumatoid arthritis. *Journal of Rheumatology*, **24**, 852–5.

Voskuyl, A. E., Hazes, J. M., Zwinderman, A. H., Paleolog, E. M., van der Meer, F. J., Daha, M. R., and Breedveld, F. C. (2003). Diagnostic strategy for the assessment of rheumatoid vasculitis. *Annals of the Rheumatic Diseases*, **62**, 407–13.

Voskuyl, A. E., van Duinen, S. G., Zwinderman, A. H., Breedveld, F. C., and Hazes, J. M. (1998b). The diagnostic value of perivascular infiltrates in muscle biopsy specimens for the assessment of rheumatoid vasculitis. *Annals of the Rheumatic Diseases*, **57**, 114–17.

Voskuyl, A. E., Zwinderman, A. H., Westedt, M. L., Vandenbroucke, J. P., Breedveld, F. C., and Hazes, J. M. (1996a). Factors associated with the development of vasculitis in rheumatoid arthritis: results of a case-control study. *Annals of the Rheumatic Diseases*, **55,** 190–2.

Voskuyl, A. E., Zwinderman, A. H., Westedt, M. L., Vandenbroucke, J. P., Breedveld, F. C., and Hazes, J. M. (1996b). The mortality of rheumatoid vasculitis compared with rheumatoid arthritis. *Arthritis and Rheumatism*, **39,** 266–71.

Voyles, W. F., Searles, R. P., and Bankhurst, A. D. (1980). Myocardial infarction caused by rheumatoid vasculitis. *Arthritis and Rheumatism*, **23,** 860–3.

Waldendorf, M. and Schneider, M. (1993). Anti-neutrophil cytoplasmic antibodies in patients with systemic lupus erythematosus. *Advances in Experimental Medicine and Biology*, **336,** 381–4.

Watts, R. A., Carruthers, D. M., and Scott, D. G. (1995). Epidemiology of systemic vasculitis: changing incidence or definition?. *Seminars in Arthritis and Rheumatism*, **25,** 28–34.

Watts, R. A., Carruthers, D. M., Symmons, D. P., and Scott, D. G. (1994). The incidence of rheumatoid vasculitis in the Norwich Health Authority. *British Journal of Rheumatology*, **33,** 832–3.

Weide, R., Heymanns, J., Pandorf, A., and Koppler, H. (2003). Successful long-term treatment of systemic lupus erythematosus with rituximab maintenance therapy. *Lupus*, **12,** 779–82.

Weiner, D. K. and Allen, N. B. (1991). Large vessel vasculitis of the central nervous system in systemic lupus erythematosus: report and review of the literature. *Journal of Rheumatology*, **18,** 748–51.

West, S. G. (1994). Neuropsychiatric lupus. *Rheumatic Disease Clinics of North America*, **20,** 129–58.

Weyand, C. M., Hicok, K. C., Conn, D. L., and Goronzy, J. J. (1992). The influence of HLA-DRB1 genes on disease severity in rheumatoid arthritis. *Annals of Internal Medicine*, **117,** 801–6.

Williams, C. S., Butler, E., and Roman, G. C. (2001). Treatment of myelopathy in Sjogren syndrome with a combination of prednisone and cyclophosphamide. *Archives of Neurology*, **58,** 815–19.

Witte, T., Hartung, K., Matthias, T., Sachse, C., Fricke, M., Deicher, H., Kalden, J. R., Lakomek, H. J., Peter, H. H., and Schmidt, R. E. (1998). Association of IgA anti-dsDNA antibodies with vasculitis and disease activity in systemic lupus erythematosus. SLE Study Group. *Rheumatology International*, **18,** 63–9.

Wong, S. S. and Marks, R. (1994). Cutaneous vasculitis in psoriasis. *Acta Dermato-venereologica*, **74,** 57–60.

Wright, R. A., O'Duffy, J. D., and Rodriguez, M. (1999). Improvement of myelopathy in Sjogren's syndrome with chlorambucil and prednisone therapy. *Neurology*, **52,** 386–8.

Yamashita, K., Yorioka, N., Kyuden, Y., Naito, T., Tanji, C., Ueda, C., Usui, K., Shigemoto, K., Harada, S., and Yamakido, M. (2000). A case of CREST syndrome and myeloperoxidase-specific anti-neutrophil cytoplasmic autoantibody-associated glomerulonephritis. *Clinical Nephrology*, **53,** 296–300.

Yen, J. H., Moore, B. E., Nakajima, T., Scholl, D., Schaid, D. J., Weyand, C. M., and Goronzy, J. J. (2001). Major histocompatibility complex class I-recognizing receptors are disease risk genes in rheumatoid arthritis. *Journal of Experimental Medicine*, **193,** 1159–67.

Zamora, M. R., Warner, M. L., Tuder, R., and Schwarz, M. I. (1997). Diffuse alveolar hemorrhage and systemic lupus erythematosus. Clinical presentation, histology, survival, and outcome. *Medicine* (Baltimore), **76,** 192–202.

Zizic, T. M., Classen, J. N., and Stevens, M. B. (1982). Acute abdominal complications of systemic lupus erythematosus and polyarteritis nodosa. *American Journal of Medicine*, **73,** 525–31.

CHAPTER 35

Behçet's syndrome: pathogenesis, clinical manifestations, and treatment

Izzet Fresko, Melike Melikoglu,
Emire Kural-Seyahi, and Hasan Yazici

Introduction

There is little doubt that elements of Behçet's syndrome (BS) were discussed in the medical literature before Behçet first proposed it as a distinct entity (Behçet 1937). Hippocrates described something akin to BS but it was not mentioned in the medical literature until the early part of the last century.

In his original paper Hulusi Behçet, a professor of dermatovenereology at the University of Istanbul, described three patients, two men and a woman, with aphthous and genital ulceration along with hypopyon uveitis (Saylan 1997). It is interesting to note that these three patients were studied over a course of 17 years. Starting with skin disease, it soon became apparent that many other organ systems were involved in addition to the initial "trisymptom disease" as originally proposed.

Recent years have seen a global interest in BS reflected in a large number of scientific publications each year. In 2004, the 11th International Conference on Behçet's Disease was held in Turkey with 275 participants from many disciplines. BS is the leading cause of acquired blindness in Japan and the Japanese government has been supporting a National Behçet's Disease Research Committee since 1972. Also, there are dedicated, university-based units in Turkey and Iran. The wide interest in BS is not simply due to the obvious concerns of clinical medicine and health services. There are many physicians and scientists interested in BS from the standpoints of endothelial injury, genetics, and relations between inflammatory and immunologic insult and tissue localization and inflammation, to name but a few.

There is debate whether the entity described by Behçet is better designated as a disease or a syndrome. We prefer the latter as we do not know the pathogenesis of the illness, nor is there a definitive diagnostic test.

Epidemiology

BS has a distinct geographical distribution (see Chapter 2). As shown in Figure 35.1, most of the reported cases are from the countries around the Mediterranean basin and Japan. There is a paucity of patients, for unknown reasons, in Northern Europe, Northern Asia, most of continental Africa, Australia, and the Americas. Travel along the Silk Route has been repeatedly implicated as the means through which a putative etiological agent was spread. Perhaps the reason Pakistan and India are mostly spared from BS is that the Silk Route ran north of these regions.

BS has been reported in patients from every race; however, there is a definite under-representation of black patients from Africa and elsewhere (Poon *et al.* 2003). Even though it can affect every age group, onset before puberty or after the sixth decade is relatively rare. There has been a recent awareness of pediatric BS (Kone-Paut *et al.* 1998; Uziel Y *et al.* 1998); however, a survey of 47,000 children in Turkey (Ozen *et al.* 1998) did not identify a single patient with BS.

The usual onset is in the third decade. No socioeconomic class seems to be spared and no environmental agent has been identified as causative. Most prevalence data on BS is based on outpatient records. In addition to the survey of children cited above, there have been three other field surveys of BS in Turkey. In the first, involving 5000 persons aged 10 years or older who were living near Istanbul, there were four cases, giving a prevalence of 80 per 100,000 (Demirhindi *et al.* 1981). In the second study (Yurdakul *et al.* 1988), conducted again among 5000 individuals aged 10 years or older in Camas (Northern Turkey), the prevalence was 380 per 100,000. In the third survey conducted in Istanbul, the reported prevalence was 420 per 100,000 (Azizlerli *et al.* 2003). Table 35.1 summarizes the reported prevalence of BS in various geographic regions (Al Dalaan *et al.* 1996; Gonzalez-Gay *et al.* 2000; Kaklamani *et al.* 1998; O'Duffy 1994; Shimizu *et al.* 1979; Zoubulis *et al.* 1996).

Apart from the unexplained differences in disease prevalence between different geographical areas, some of the manifestations of BS show regional differences as well. Gastrointestinal (GI) manifestations are common in Japanese patients (Shimizu *et al.* 1979); however, these are rather infrequent in Turkey (Yurdakul *et al.* 1996) and the Middle East. The same is true for the prevalence of pathergy, the non-specific hypersensitivity of the skin to a needle

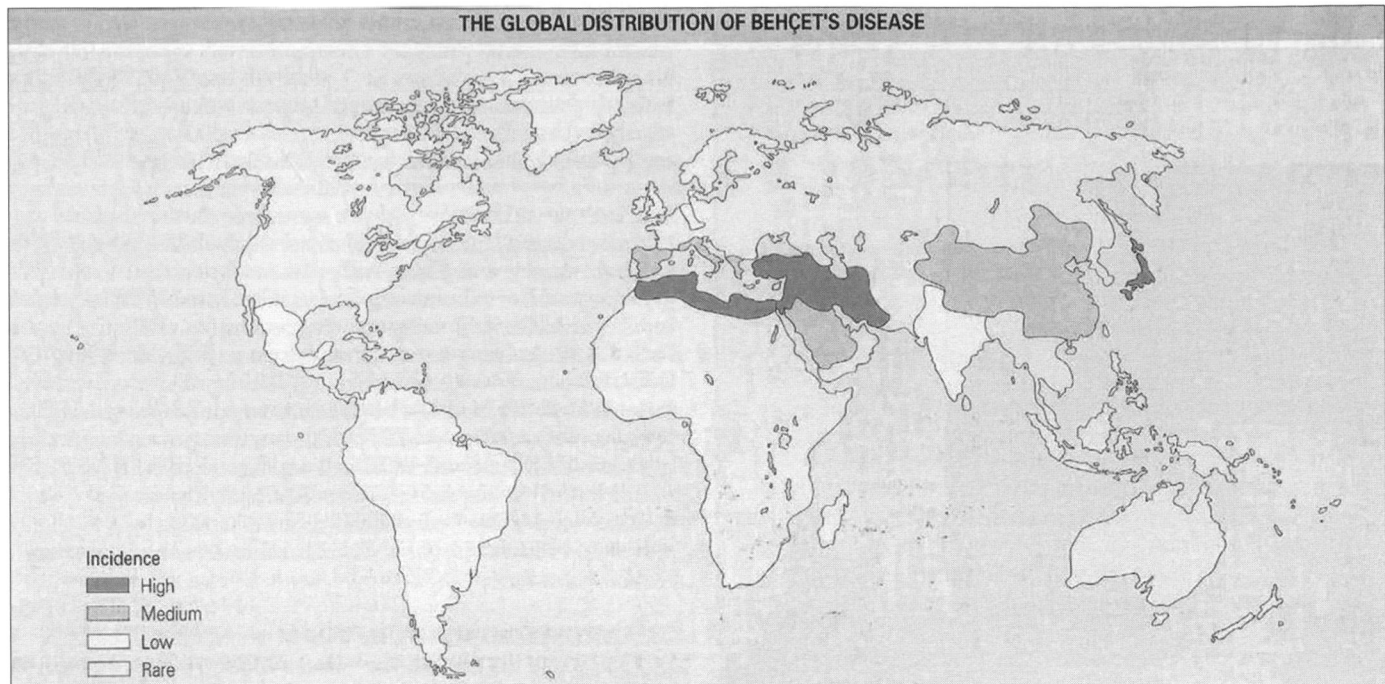

Figure 35.1 Geographical distribution of Behçet's syndrome. From: Yazici, H. (1994). Behçet's syndrome. In *Rheumatology* (eds J. H. Klippel and P. A. Dieppe). Mosby, pp. 20, 1–6 and H. Yazici, I. Fresko, R. Tunç, and M. Melikoglu (2002). Behçet's Syndrome: Pathogenesis, Clinical Manifestations and Treatment. In: *Vasculitis*. 1st edn. G. V. Ball and S. L. Bridges, Jr, eds. Oxford University Press.

prick, which is less common in North European and United States patients (Yazici *et al*. 1984b). Finally the HLA B51 association is most pronounced among patients from the Middle and the Far East.

Clinical findings

BS is a systemic vasculitis that affects many organs. The clinical manifestations include a variety of skin and mucosa lesions; uveitis that may result in blindness; a wide range of central nervous system (CNS) abnormalities; major-vessel disease; musculoskeletal problems; and GI problems. The diagnosis is based on clinical findings. Initial manifestations typically include one or more of the following: oral and genital ulcers; ocular lesions; papulopustular skin lesions; erythema nodosum; and arthritis. Table 35.2 shows the frequency of clinical manifestations of BS. The course is characterized by remissions and exacerbations that generally abate in intensity with the passage of time.

Table 35.1 Prevalence of BS in various countries

Region	Prevalence per 100,000
Turkey	80–420 (aged 10 or over)
Japan	100
Iran	16–100
Germany (West Berlin)	1.6
USA (Olmstead County, Minn.)	10–30
Northwestern Spain	0.7
Saudi Arabia	20

Mucocutaneous findings

Oral ulcers

Oral ulcers occur in virtually all patients and are frequently the first disease manifestation (Figure 35.2); however, 1–3% of patients can have several of the other features of the disease without ever having oral ulcers. It is not uncommon for some patients to have only oral

Table 35.2 Frequency of clinical manifestations of BS

Manifestation	Frequency
Oral ulcers	97–99%
Genital ulcers	~85%
Scar	~50% (likely more prevalent in males)
Skin lesions	
Papulopustular lesions	~85%
Erythema nodosum	~50%
Pathergy reaction	~60% (Mediterranean countries and Japan)
Uveitis	~50%
Arthritis	30–50%
Subcutaneous thrombophlebitis	25%
Deep vein thrombosis	~5%
Arterial occlusion/ aneurysm	~4%
CNS involvement	~5%
Epididymitis	~5%
Gastrointestinal lesions	1–30% (more prevalent in Japan)

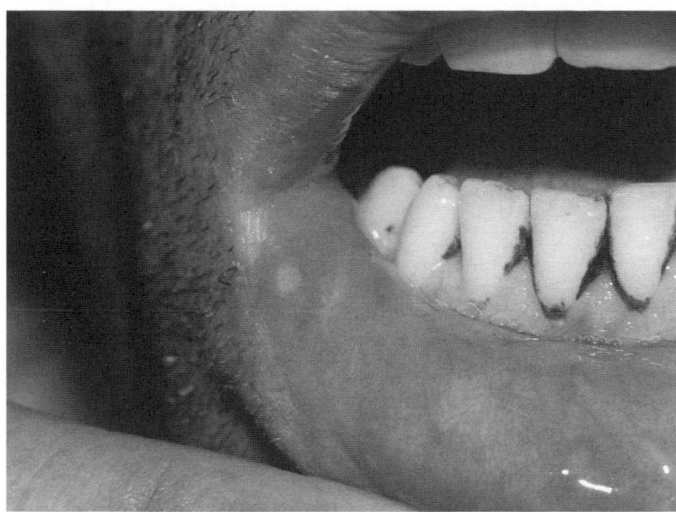

Figure 35.2 Oral ulcers. (See Color Plate 93).

ulcers for many years before other stigmata appear. It is sometimes difficult or impossible to tell when the disease actually started. The majority of the oral ulcers are indistinguishable from ordinary canker sores (see Chapter 11); however, they are more frequent and multiple. They frequently appear as erythematous, circular, and slightly raised areas evolving into oval or round ulcers within 48 hours.

The oral ulcerations in BS are classified as minor, major, or herpetiform (Grattan and Scully 1986). Minor aphthous ulcers are the most common clinical form and are round or oval, shallow ulcers, usually multiple, less than 10 mm in diameter, with a grey-white pseudomembrane surrounded by a thin erythematous inflammatory halo. The involved sites are usually the mucous membranes of the lips, gingiva, cheeks, and tongue. The palate, tonsils, and pharynx are less commonly involved; in contrast to herpetic lesions, the skin-covered portions of the lips are spared. The ulcers of BS usually have regular borders, unlike the lesions of Stevens–Johnson syndrome and Reiter's syndrome. Minor ulcers constitute around 90% of all oral ulcers in BS and usually heal in about 15 days without scarring. Like ordinary canker sores, they cause varying amounts of discomfort and occasionally make eating difficult.

Major aphthous ulcers are seen less often. These lesions range from 1–3 cm in diameter, have a grey-white ulcer base and may involve any region of the oral mucosa. They are usually more painful than minor ulcers and have a tendency to heal with a scar. They may cause dysphagia and lead to pharyngeal stenosis, resulting in malnutrition or even death (Kobayashi et al. 1982). Herpetiform aphthous ulcers are rather uncommon. They consist of crops of ulcers, 2–3 mm in diameter, distributed throughout the oral cavity. They heal in a short time without scarring.

The frequency and type of oral ulcers in BS patients were recently evaluated at a single time point in a hospital-based population in Istanbul. Minor aphthous ulcers were the most common type of aphthae in BS (85%); the frequency of major oral ulcerations, more common in females, was 14% (Coskun et al. 2004).

In the general population, the prevalence of recurrent aphthous stomatitis (RAS) is roughly 10 to 20% (Crivelli et al. 1988; Azizlerli et al. 2003) (see Chapter 11). We found that the prevalence of RAS was 16% (Yurdakul et al. 1988), noted that the prevalence of BS

was 2.8% among patients with RAS, and suggested that BS and RAS represent two ends of a clinical spectrum (Lehner and Batchelor 1979). This view has been challenged from the clinical standpoint, in that few patients present with aphthous ulcers plus one other symptom, and from the genetic point of view, in that there is not an increased frequency of the HLA B51 gene among patients with RAS (Ozbakir et al. 1987). A study from Israel, however, did report an association of HLA B51 with RAS (Shohat-Zabarski et al. 1992). There is preliminary evidence for a negative correlation between oral ulcers and tobacco use; cessation of smoking exacerbated mucocutaneous lesions and oral ulcers (Soy et al. 2000; Kaklamani et al. 2003).

Histopathologic examination of oral ulcers in BS shows lymphocytic and monocytic inflammatory infiltrates in the basal layer and dermis with an eroded epidermis. In the early stages, plasma cells are usually absent; as the ulcer ages, neutrophils become the dominant cell (Muller and Lehner 1982) and there is vascular proliferation along with endothelial swelling. Leukocytoclastic vasculitis is also occasionally observed (Chun et al. 1990). There is no difference between the findings on macroscopic examination of the aphthae in patients with BS and those with RAS.

Genital ulcers

Genital ulcers of BS usually begin as papules or pustules that ulcerate in a short time period. They are usually round or oval with a punched-out appearance (Figure 35.3). The base is covered with grey-white fibrin, and at times with surrounding edema with induration. They tend to be more readily infected than oral ulcers. In males they are usually localized on the scrotum and commonly leave scars. They are less frequent on the shaft and the glans penis, inguinal area, pubis, and perineum. Compared with oral ulcers, perianal ulcers are larger, deeper, less recurrent, and more resistant to healing.

In females, ulcers are commonly found on both major and minor labiae; vaginal and cervical lesions are less frequent and may go unnoticed unless complicated by infection and associated discharge. Therefore, gynecologic examination should be carried out in all female patients with suspected BS. Genital scarring is usually good evidence of BS in a patient suspected of having this syndrome.

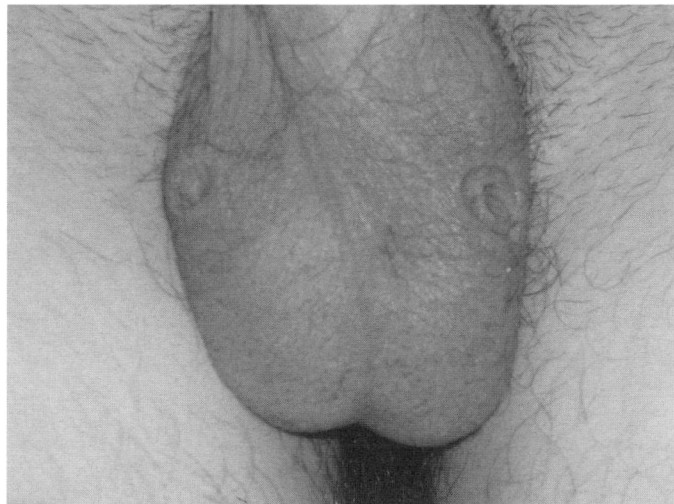

Figure 35.3 Genital ulcers. (See Color Plate 94).

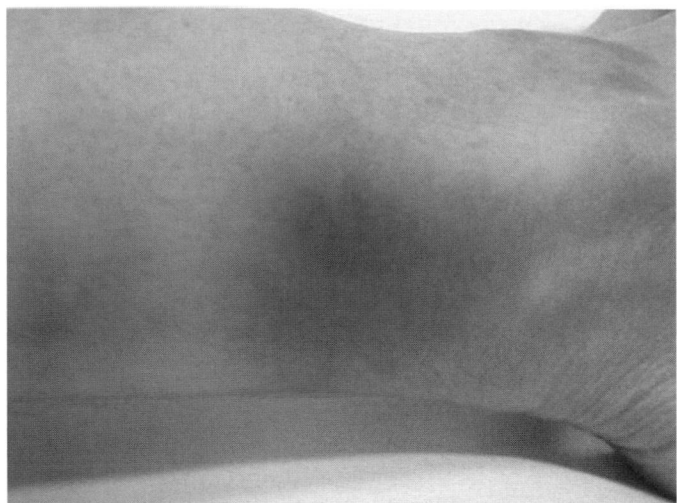

Figure 35.4 Erythema nodosum like lesion. (See Color Plate 95).

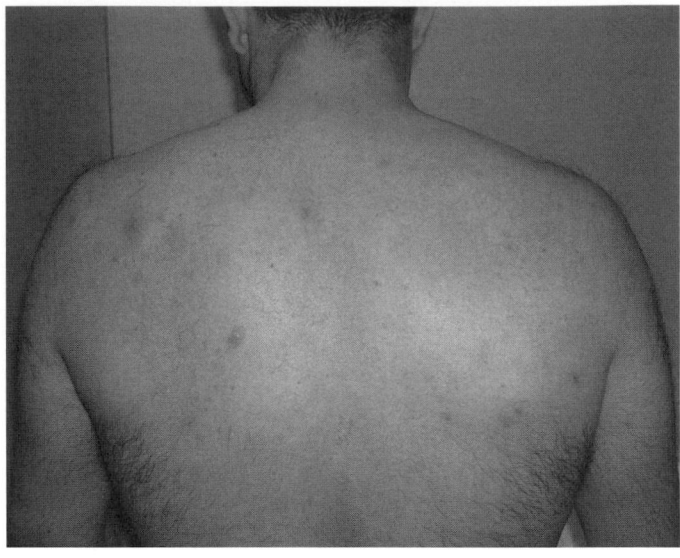

Figure 35.5 Osteofollicular (acne) like lesions. (See Color Plate 96)

The fate of genital ulcers was recently analyzed. They usually heal in 10–30 days if they are not secondarily infected. Not surprisingly, large ulcers have a higher rate of scarring compared to small ulcers both in males and females (Mat *et al.* 2006). The histopathologic features of genital ulcers are similar to that of the oral ulcers.

Other skin lesions

There are three broad categories of other types of skin lesions in BS: (1) erythema nodosum-like lesions and superficial thrombophlebitis; (2) papulopustular lesions; and (3) other lesions, including ulcers, Sweet's syndrome, and pyoderma gangrenosum. Erythema nodosum-like lesions are observed in 50% of patients. They may be indistinguishable clinically from idiopathic or other disease-associated erythema nodosum (Figure 35.4), but they tend to be deeper and less well demarcated. Erythema nodosum lesions related to BS have more histopathologic features of vasculitis than erythema nodosum due to other causes (Demirkesen *et al.* 2001). Superficial thrombophlebitis lesions morphologically look very much like erythema nodosum, which might explain the negative association described between the two (Krause *et al.* 1999). On biopsy, superficial thrombophlebitis lesions have a central thrombosed vein. We have preliminary evidence to suggest that ultrasonography can differentiate between erythema nodosum-like lesions and superficial thrombophlebitis.

The acne-like lesions of BS (papulopustular lesions) were once considered to represent dermal vasculitis and thus to be different from ordinary acne; however, the two can hardly be differentiated. Acne-like lesions of BS are frequently seen at the usual sites of acne vulgaris, such as the face, upper chest, and upper back, and it is not uncommon for them to appear on the legs and arms (Figure 35.5). Histologically, the acne-like lesions of BS are indistinguishable from those of acne vulgaris (Ergun *et al.* 1998). Sebum production is increased in BS, as it is in acne vulgaris (Yazici *et al.* 1987). Acne lesions of BS are mainly of cosmetic concern.

It is curious why BS patients, usually in their late 20s or mid-30s, suddenly begin having acne lesions which are more characteristic of adolescence. It is well known that acne is an androgen-dependent lesion and in view of the more severe disease in BS among males, one could speculate that acne lesions represent androgen

hypersensitivity but data do not consistently support this hypothesis. Androgen levels are normal in BS (Yazici *et al.* 1986) with no evidence for increased androgen receptors on the skin (Mat *et al.* 1998a); however, increased androgen receptor activity has been demonstrated in specimens of skin pathergy reactions from men (Alpsoy *et al.* 2005). Although papulopustular lesions in BS were thought to be sterile, it has recently been shown that these lesions are colonized with bacteria, most commonly *Staphylococcus aureus* and less frequently by *Prevotella* species (Hatemi *et al.* 2004). One recent, interesting observation is the association of acne lesions with the presence of arthritis in BS (Diri *et al.* 2001; Tunc *et al.* 2002).

Skin ulcers may also be observed rarely in the axillary and interdigital areas (Azizlerli *et al.* 1992) and an occasional patient might have dermal punched-out lesions similar to those of polyarteritis nodosa (PAN). The association of BS with neutrophilic dermatitis (Sweet's syndrome) can be confusing. Typical lesions of Sweet's syndrome, slightly elevated and somewhat shiny, can be seen in 2.4 to 4% of patients with BS (Shi Hui-Li 1993). On the other hand, some clinical features of BS, such as oral ulceration and arthritis, can be seen during the course of primary Sweet's syndrome (Oğuz *et al.* 1992). Thus the differential diagnosis between the two may occasionally be a semantic exercise.

Pathergy

The pathergy phenomenon is a non-specific hyper-reactivity in response to minor trauma. It is rarely observed in normal individuals or those with other diseases except for pyoderma gangrenosum and chronic myeloid leukemia treated with interferon-alpha (Tüzün *et al.* 1980; Budak Alpdogan *et al.* 1998). It is one of the characteristic manifestations of BS and is usually elicited for diagnostic purposes by inserting a 20 gauge needle into the dermis of the forearm. A positive response is defined by a papule or pustule that forms 48 hours later (Figure 35.6). It has been claimed that surgical procedures might also lead to pathergic-type reactions, which may influence the outcome of the procedures, but such findings have not been consistent. It is worth noting that wound healing appears to be normal BS patients (Mat *et al.* 1998).

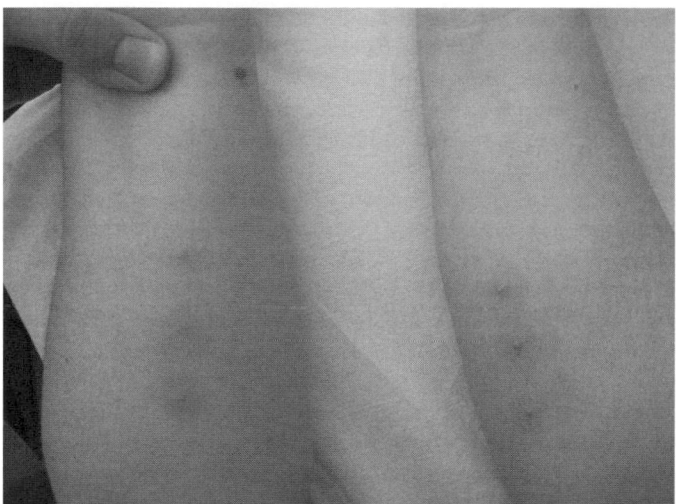

Figure 35.6 Positive pathergy reaction. (See Color Plate 97).

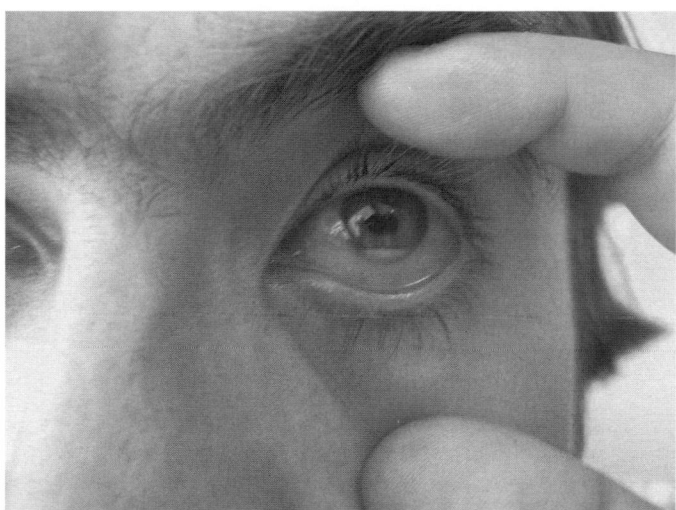

Figure 35.7 Hypopyon uveitis. (See Color Plate 98).

It is thought by some groups that pathergy occurs during the active phases of the disease and disappears when the disease remits, but others find no such correlation (Krause *et al.* 2000). Male patients have stronger pathergy reactions (Yazici *et al.* 1985).

A positive pathergy test is an important parameter in the diagnosis of BS in Middle Eastern countries. The specificity of the pathergy test is high (Tüzün *et al.* 1980) but sensitivity varies in different studies. The frequency of a positive reaction decreases sharply in countries outside the Middle East, Far East, and the Mediterranean regions (Yazici *et al.* 1984b). Furthermore, analysis of case series suggests that the rate of pathergy has decreased steadily since 1968 (Saylan *et al.* 1999). It has been hypothesized that the use of less traumatic disposable needles may account for this decrease (Ozarmağan *et al.* 1991). The pathergy test has limited reproducibility due to intra- and interobserver variation in its assessment, and the reaction may vary in intensity in the same patient over time (Altaç *et al.* 1982).

Ocular involvement

Eye involvement is the most serious manifestation of BS when one takes into consideration both its frequency and morbidity. It is a common cause of blindness in the Mediterranean basin, Middle East, and Far East. Eye disease in BS is a non-granulomatous panuveitis and retinal vasculitis with exacerbations and remissions of the inflammatory process (Pazarli *et al.* 1986; Shimizu *et al.* 1979) (see Chapter 12). While the overall prevalence is about 50%, it occurs in close to 70% of males aged less than 25 years (Yazici *et al.* 1984a). Eye disease is frequently present at the onset of the disease or within the first 2 years and it is quite rare for this to develop after the initial 5 years of disease (Kural-Seyahi *et al.* 2003).

Eye involvement is bilateral in 70–80% of patients (Tugal-Tutkun *et al.* 2004; Kural-Seyahi *et al.* 2003). It affects the posterior uvea more often and more severely than the anterior uvea. Patients usually complain of ocular discomfort and visual blurring. Anterior uveitis appears as a solitary finding in 10% of those with ocular involvement. It is not associated with a poor visual outcome. Hypopyon formation, which represents a profuse accumulation of inflammatory cells forming a visible layering of pus anterior to the iris (Figure 35.7), occurs in about 20% of patients with

eye involvement. As a rule, patients with hypopyon suffer from associated severe retinal vasculitis and thereby have a grave visual prognosis. It has been shown that optic atrophy ensues within a few months in about half of those with hypopyon uveitis (Pazarli *et al.* 1986).

Gross pathologic changes include vitreous deposits, choroiditis, and retinitis. Retinitis involves capillaries at the disc, macula, and the periphery. Early retinal vasculitis can be seen as patches of fluorescein leaks along vessels in otherwise asymptomatic patients with a normal ophthalmoscopic examination. In well-established disease, fundoscopic examination reveals vitreal deposits; choroidal or retinal exudates with sheathing of the blood vessels; hemorrhages; cytoid bodies or white patches; venous thrombosis; papilledema; and macular disease. It is sometimes difficult to differentiate papilledema due to primary eye disease from that due to increased intracranial pressure.

Recurrent inflammatory activity in the anterior chamber may lead to anterior and posterior synechiae, secondary glaucoma, optic atrophy, and macular degeneration. Cataracts may form with or without the additional insult of glucocorticoid therapy. Even with treatment, total loss of vision occurs in up to 20% of those affected. Ocular inflammation can persist among patients with complete loss of vision and total global atrophy. Enucleation might be the only way to control the pain of ongoing inflammation in these patients. Histological examination of the enucleated blind eye reveals atrophy and marked lymphocyte infiltration (predominantly T cells) of all intraocular tissues (Shimizu *et al.* 1979; George *et al.* 1997). Episcleritis, conjunctivitis, corneal ulcerations, and lid lesions are not characteristic features of eye disease in BS, but are noted occasionally.

Central nervous system disease

Neurological disease, of acute and chronic onset, is one of the most serious features of BS. Although the prevalence of neurological involvement has been reported to be between 5% and 59% (Farah *et al.* 1998), a prevalence of 5.3% was found in a prospective survey of Turkish patients (Serdaroglu *et al.* 1989). Japanese autopsy registry data (Lakhanpal *et al.* 1985) suggest that cerebrospinal tract demyelination is the most common pathologic finding, followed

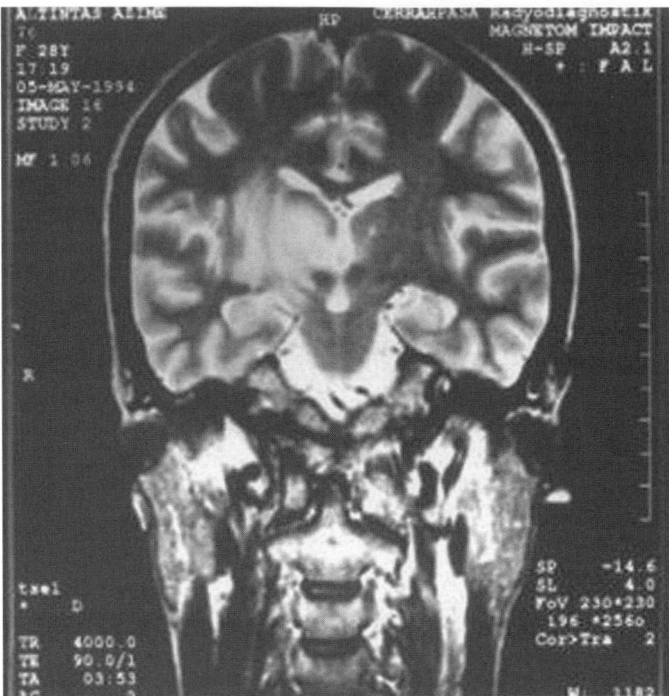

Figure 35.8 CT scan of parenchymal central nervous system involvement. Note the hyperintense lesion in the brain stem.

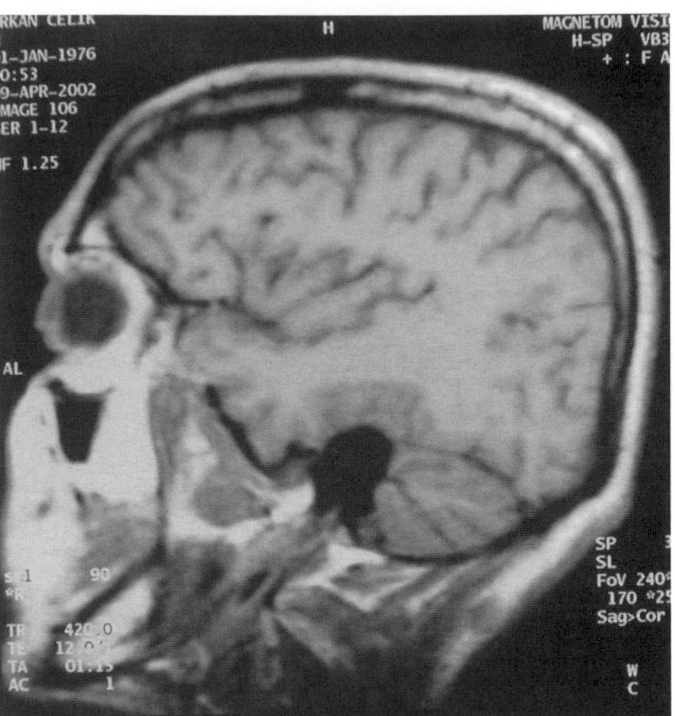

Figure 35.9 CT scan of dural sinus thrombosis.

by encephalomalacia, perivascular cellular infiltration, and cerebral atrophy. The role, if any, of vasculitis *per se* in the pathogenesis of CNS involvement is not certain. A histopathological study showed that active neurological involvement was associated with perivascular infiltration of CD45RO+ T lymphocytes, and CD68+ monocytes with few CD20+ B lymphocytes. Most of the neurons were undergoing apoptosis. Clinically inactive lesions were characterized by atrophy and isomorphic gliosis (Hirohata *et al.* 2003).

There are mainly two types of CNS involvement in BS (Serdaroglu 1998). About 75% of patients with CNS disease have parenchymal lesions (Figure 35.8) and the remainder have dural sinus thrombi (Figure 35.9). Venous thrombosis in the CNS typically causes headaches with or without bilateral papilledema and increased cerebrospinal fluid pressure. It is rare to have both lesions in the same patient (Siva *et al.* 2004). Table 35.3 summarizes the clinical symptoms and findings of CNS involvement in BS.

The brain stem is the most commonly afflicted site, followed by the spinal cord, cerebrum, and cerebellum (Lakhanpal *et al.* 1985). Pyramidal motor signs are the most common clinical features, followed by cerebellar and sensory signs and symptoms. Isolated cerebellar involvement, however, is most unusual (Serdaroglu 1998). Signs and symptoms of meningeal irritation and increased intracranial pressure also occur.

Headaches are ascribed to CNS lesions only if other associated neurologic signs and symptoms are present (Serdaroglu *et al.* 1989), but one should keep in mind that a non-structural migraine type headache unrelated to neurological involvement is also common among patients with BS (Saip *et al.* 2005). Hearing loss and vertigo may also occur (Kulahli *et al.* 2005). Lesions of the nervous system may progress to produce fatal bulbar paralysis. As with almost all other manifestations, neurological involvement runs a more severe course among males.

Table 35.3 Features of neurologic involvement in BS

Symptoms and signs	%
Pyramidal signs	82
Headache	65
Cerebellar signs	24
Sensory symptoms and/or signs	24
Pseudobulbar signs	12
Intracranial hypertension	12
Meningeal irritation signs	12
Hemianopsia	6
Dementia	6
Personality changes	6
Tremor	6
Myoclonic jerks	6

Problems related to higher cortical function, such as character disorders, impairment of memory and dementia, and other psychiatric symptoms, are sometimes noted (Oktem-Tanor *et al.* 1999; Monastero *et al.* 2004). Some of these disturbances are related to the situational response to a chronic disease or possibly to glucocorticoid use. Peripheral nervous system involvement is distinctly unusual in BS.

Cerebrospinal fluid analysis usually reveals non-specific findings such as mild pleocytosis and slightly elevated protein concentration. Glucose levels are usually normal but occasionally they can be low. Despite the lack of specificity of these findings, patients with abnormal CSF had the worst prognosis in a study in which 7-year follow-up was reported (Akman-Demir *et al.* 1996).

If there is a localized neurologic disease, CT scans and magnetic resonance imaging can correlate anatomic findings with clinical features. Lesions include hypodense areas on CT scans and hyperdense areas on MRI, similar to those seen in vasculitis. The brain stem and basal ganglia are the sites most frequently abnormal on MRI of patients with acute BS. Seventy-five percent of these lesions were large and confluent, mainly extending from the brain stem to the diencephalon and basal ganglia. The brain stem or basal ganglia were involved in one-third of patients with chronic BS. Brain stem atrophy was seen in 21% of the patients with a specificity of 100% in the absence of cortical atrophy (Coban *et al.* 1999). MRI findings in BS indicate the presence of a small-vessel vasculitis with mainly venular involvement (Kocer *et al.* 1999). There are reports that single photon emission computed tomography (SPECT) may be more sensitive in detecting early CNS lesions than MRI but controlled studies are lacking (Avci *et al.* 1998; Nobili *et al.* 2002; Siva and Yazici 2004).

Major vessel involvement

The spectrum of vascular disease is broad and unique in BS. It is one of the few vasculitides that can involve large vessels, both arterial and venous. It is virtually the only disorder that leads to the formation of pulmonary artery aneurysms (Figure 35.10). Close scrutiny suggests that the Hughes–Stovin syndrome (pulmonary arterial aneurysms with systemic thrombosis) is indeed BS (Erkan *et al.* 2004). As many as 50% of BS patients have large-vessel involvement; this, too, is more common in men. Vascular disease most often occurs late in the course of the disease, usually 5 to 10 years after the diagnosis (Koc *et al.* 1992; Kural-Seyahi *et al.* 2003). Deep veins of the lower extremity are the most common sites of venous thrombosis, which constitute 60–80% of vascular lesions. The veins affected in descending order of frequency are: inferior and superior vena cavae, dural sinuses; axillary; brachial; hepatic; and portal veins. Superficial thrombophlebitis tends to be associated with deep vein thrombosis in the lower extremity and inferior vena cava. Furthermore, chronic relapsing deep vein thromboses in the legs tend to precede the other sites

of major vessel involvement. One should also note that major vessel involvement is closely associated with dural sinus thrombi, suggesting that this is also part of the vascular spectrum (Tunc *et al.* 2004).

The pattern of vascular inflammation in BS is diffuse rather than patchy, and large segments of the vessel wall are involved, with superimposed inflammatory thrombi. Sometimes the entire length of the inferior vena cava is affected. Clinical signs of venous lesions vary according to their site. Chronic recurrent thrombosis of the lower extremities leads to erythema, dermatitis, hyperpigmentation, and subsequently to crural ulcers (Figure 35.11). Chronic obliteration of the caval systems leads to the appearance of prominent venous collaterals on the thoracic and abdominal walls, forming caput medusae. Obstruction of superior vena cava may also cause esophageal varices, chylothorax and chylous pericardial effusions, but pericardial involvement is rare.

Budd–Chiari syndrome from hepatic vein occlusion presents with ascites or liver failure. It is a rare complication of BS, but carries a high mortality rate. In one large series from Turkey, BS was the single most frequent cause of Budd–Chiari syndrome, accounting for roughly half of such patients. It carried a mortality of 60% (Saatci *et al.* 1993).

Inflammation of the aorta, pulmonary, and peripheral arteries is one of the most serious complications of BS and is responsible for the majority of deaths (Hamza 1987; Lie 1992). Its prevalence is about 1.5–7.5% (Kural-Seyahi *et al.* 2003), so it is less common than venous disease. There is a marked male dominance. Arterial lesions can cause aneurysms which can be complicated by *in situ* thrombosis, leading to variable degrees of occlusion. Any part of the arterial tree can be diseased, but the abdominal aorta is the most frequent site. Arteritis can also be localized to the iliac, femoral, popliteal, carotid, and subclavian vessels, where it is usually of the occlusive type. Renal, cerebral, and coronary arteritis have been reported rarely. Abdominal visceral ischemia is uncommon. Arterial disease is mostly unilateral and in a single vessel, but multiple, mainly false, aneurysms are possible. Abdominal aortic aneurysms sometimes produce abdominal pain. Bruits can be heard over the affected large arteries and a pulsating mass may be found.

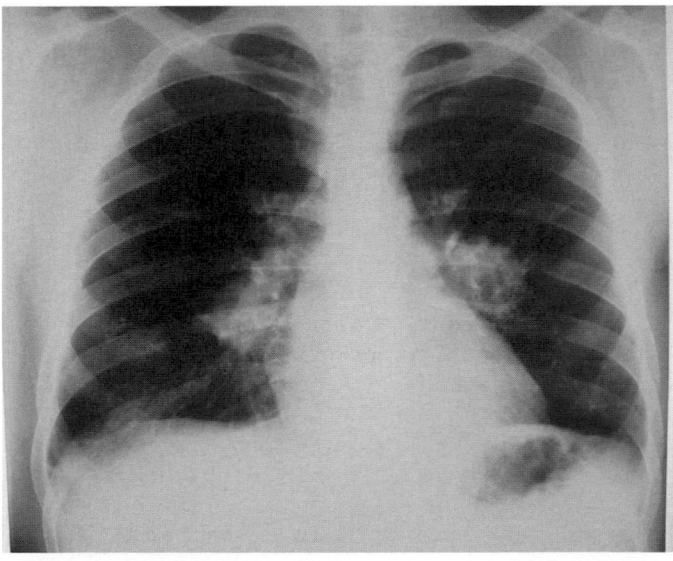

Figure 35.10 Radiographic appearance of pulmonary arterial aneurysms.

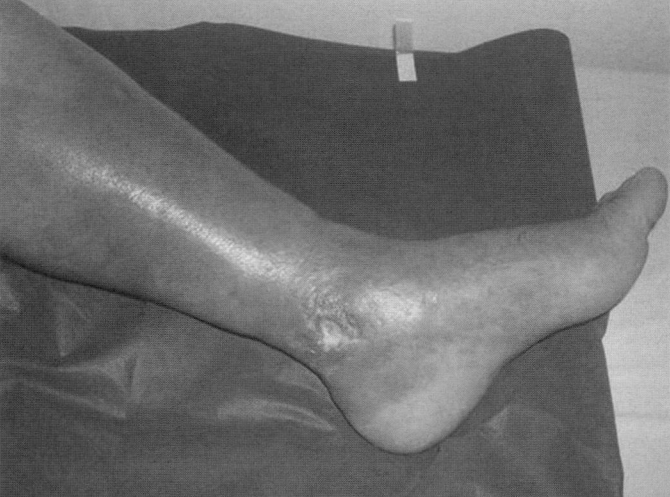

Figure 35.11 Chronic thrombosis of the leg veins with hyperpigmentation and a skin ulcer. (See Color Plate 99).

Most patients with arterial lesions have constitutional signs and symptoms, such as fever and weight loss. Peripheral arterial involvement causes reduced or absent pulses with intermittent claudication, cold extremities, or even gangrene.

A histopathologic study of six resected peripheral arterial aneurysms reported a predominantly neutrophilic vascular injury of the vasa vasorum, with a significantly increased number of vasa vasorum. The internal elastic membrane was intact, and there was increased expression of HLA-DR-positive cells in the endothelium (Kobayashi *et al.* 2000). Chronic aneurysmal lesions are characterized by periadventitial fibrosis with the entire vessel being encased in fibrous tissue. Large segments of thrombi are observed, and as a rule there are no free-floating thrombus tails. Reactive lymph nodes have also been reported in the immediate vicinity of peripheral arterial aneurysms (Tuzun *et al.* 1997).

Pulmonary arterial involvement is rare, but it leads to the most life-threatening complication of the disease: aneurysms, thrombosis, pulmonary infarction, and pulmonary hemorrhage (Efthimiou *et al.* 1986; Hamuryudan *et al.* 1994). Aneurysm formation is frequently complicated by rupture with a mortality rate as high as 50%. Early detection and use of immunosuppressive drugs have decreased the mortality to as low as 20% (Hamuryudan *et al.* 2004a). Histopathologically, the inflammatory process is located primarily in the vasa vasorum. Necrosis of the vessel wall occurs with the formation of true or false aneurysms (Hamuryudan *et al.* 2004b). They in turn erode into the bronchial tree and cause hemoptysis, the most frequent symptom. Thrombophlebitis of leg veins and inferior vena cava coexist with pulmonary vascular disease in 90% of cases (Hamuryudan *et al.* 1994).

The clinical picture of recurrent hemoptysis accompanied by pleuritic chest pain and dyspnea closely resembles that of pulmonary embolism. Ventilation perfusion lung scans may be misleading in that they reveal segmental perfusion defects compatible with pulmonary thromboembolism. In reality, this appearance is due to multiple pulmonary arterial thromboses secondary to vasculitis. No association between pulmonary embolism and deep vein thrombosis is found in BS, perhaps because thrombi are tightly adherent to inflamed veins. It follows that anticoagulant therapy is not only unhelpful but is dangerous in this situation (Efthimiou *et al.* 1986).

Pulmonary aneurysms are seen as perihilar or peripheral non-cavitating nodular opacities on chest radiographs, and pulmonary angiography reveals single or multiple arterial aneurysms or occlusions. There is a small risk of pseudoaneurysm formation at the puncture site after pulmonary angiography (Kingston *et al.* 1979). CT scans and magnetic resonance angiography (MRA) are noninvasive and preferred alternative approaches for documentation of arterial involvement (Tunaci *et al.* 1995).

Cardiac disease

Cardiac involvement is infrequent in BS (Ozkan *et al.* 1992), but may on occasion cause complex problems. Many types of conduction problems, valvular disease, and aortitis have been documented, as have ventricular aneurysms and coronary vasculitis. One bizarre development is endomyocardial fibrosis with intracardiac thrombi. This usually involves the right side of the heart and carries a high mortality (Houng *et al.* 1997; Mogulkoc *et al.* 2000).

Musculoskeletal manifestations

Arthritis or arthralgias have been noted at some point in the disease in as many as 50% of patients (Yurdakul *et al.* 1983). It is usually monoarticular or oligoarticular and may occasionally precede the diagnosis of BS by months or years. Arthritis most often involves large joints: knees, ankles, elbows, and wrists, in more or less that order. The arthritis is usually non-destructive and typically resolves in several days or weeks, but synovitis lasting months to years with deformity and erosions, has been encountered. It is accompanied by a moderately elevated erythrocyte sedimentation rate. The issue of sacroiliitis as a component of BS and the inclusion of BS among the seronegative spondylarthritides is controversial, but the consensus is that BS should not be included in this group (Chamberlain and Robertson 1993; Olivieri *et al.* 1997; Yazici *et al.* 1981a).

Synovial fluid in BS-associated arthritis is inflammatory, with a predominance of polymorphonuclear leucocytes. The histological changes of synovium in BS are not disease-specific. Ulceration and replacement of the superficial layer by heavily inflamed granulation tissue, and paucity of plasma cells are the salient features. Articular symptoms may also arise from aseptic osteonecrosis, where it is taken as evidence of vasculitis, and not necessarily the result of glucocorticoid use (Sugioka *et al.* 1966).

Inflammatory myositis is usually local and confined to the leg, but generalized forms have been described (Arkin *et al.* 1980; Yazici *et al.* 1981b). Serum levels of muscle enzymes are not elevated in localized forms. The histologic picture of these lesions is similar to that observed in polymyositis. The prevalence of "fibromyalgia" is around 10%, and is mainly in female patients with mild to moderate disease activity (Yavuz *et al.* 1998).

Gastrointestinal involvement

Lesions of BS occur throughout the GI tract (Yurdakul *et al.* 1996) (see Chapter 15). Mucosal ulcers dominate and are histologically indistinguishable from those found in inflammatory bowel disease. These are multiple, deep, round, and not specific, sometimes granulomatous, ulcers associated with chronic inflammation. Normal intervening mucosa is also characteristic (Fukuda and Watanabe 1979). Three-quarters of the mucosal ulcers in BS are found in the terminal ileum and cecum and less often in the stomach and duodenum (Mori *et al.* 1983). In contrast to ulcerative colitis, rectal involvement in BS is rare. Esophageal lesions include esophagitis and ulcers in various stages of healing and stenosis (Griffin *et al.* 1982).

GI complaints include dysphagia, vomiting, colicky abdominal pain, and diarrhea, which can be bloody. They are characterized by exacerbations and remissions. During exacerbations, a mass is often palpable in the abdomen. Ileocecal lesions are quite prone to perforation (Kasahara *et al.* 1981; Shimizu *et al.* 1979). GI involvement in BS is sometimes difficult to distinguish from Crohn's disease in which oral ulcers, erythema nodosum, and intermittent arthritis are also features. A study of enteroclysis findings has shown that GI involvement in BS is milder than that of Crohn's disease. Scalloping, ulceronodular patterns, and abscess and fistula formation are not part of BS (Iida *et al.* 1993; Korman *et al.* 2003).

As noted above, Budd–Chiari syndrome occurs in BS patients, but primary involvement of the liver without occlusion of the hepatic vein is uncommon. Splenomegaly is noted in 20% of patients, even without portal hypertension secondary to venous thrombosis (Soysal *et al.* 1990).

Amyloidosis and renal involvement

As in other chronic inflammatory states, there may be secondary amyloidosis of the AA type. Widely different frequencies ranging from 400/100,000 to 2000/100,000 have been reported (Dilsen *et al.* 1988; Yurdakul *et al.* 1990). In BS, amyloidosis predominantly occurs in males, and nephrotic syndrome is the typical clinical presentation. The onset of amyloidosis is about a decade after the disease begins; however, it can be seen as early as the third year. There seems to be a close association with large-vessel disease and arthritis. The nephrotic syndrome due to amyloidosis has a mortality rate of over 50% within 3.5 years of its onset (Melikoglu *et al.* 2001).

Glomerulonephritis attributable to BS has been increasingly reported (Akpolat *et al.* 2003; Altiparmak *et al.* 2002), with lesions varying from IgA nephropathy to rapidly progressive glomerulonephritis. Immune complexes are not a constant feature. We have had a successful kidney transplant with 4-year follow-up, in a patient with renal failure (Apaydın *et al.* 1999).

Urological problems

Urethritis and urogenital infections are rare in BS. An occasional patient may present with a meatal ulcer. Apart from the genital ulcerations there are three primary problems related to the genitourinary system in BS: epididymitis, cystitis, and erectile dysfunction. In a recent prospective survey based on a standard urological history questionnaire, the prevalence of epididymitis was found to be as high as 19% (Cetinel *et al.* 1998). In the same survey, the frequency of lower urinary tract symptoms was also significantly higher in BS than in controls. Clinicians have noted voiding disturbances due to neurologic involvement, as well as primary bladder dysfunction due to mucosal ulcers or what resembles interstitial cystitis, without demonstrable neurological defects (Cetinel *et al.* 1999). Erectile dysfunction has been reported recently to have a frequency of 63% among patients with neurologic involvement (Erdogru *et al.* 1999).

Pathogenesis

The pathogenesis of BS remains unclear. The scope and the specificity of immunological alterations suggests that immunologically mediated mechanisms are the main trigger of the vasculitis of BS. The arguments against a primary autoimmune process are as follows:

1 Clinical and laboratory findings usually found in autoimmune diseases (Raynaud's phenomenon, serosal involvement, photosensitivity, thrombocytopenia, hemolytic anemia) are not usually seen in BS. Most importantly there is no association with Sjögren's syndrome.

2 There is no increased prevalence of autoimmune diseases among BS patients or their families.

3 The HLA gene associated with BS, HLA B51, is not found in autoimmune diseases and the HLA alleles associated with other autoimmune diseases are not frequent in BS.

4 Although there is evidence of polyclonal B cell activation, there is no specific association autoantibody (Gunaydin *et al.* 1994; Yazici 1997).

The absence of the classical features of autoimmunity along with the paucity of specific autoantibodies has led to the suggestion that BS is an autoinflammatory disorder (Gul 2005). On the other hand there is no association of BS with mutations in genes implicated in autoinflammatory disorders such as familial Mediterranean fever or TNF-receptor associated periodic syndrome (MEVF and TNFR2, respectively). Furthermore, BS is more frequent than the classical autoinflammatory conditions and tends to abate with time, which also argues against its inclusion as an autoinflammatory disease (Yazici and Fresko 2005).

Lymphocytes and cytokines

Increasing evidence suggests that Th1-type T cells are the main cells responsible for tissue destruction (Frassanito *et al.* 1999; Ben-Ahmed *et al.* 2004); the possibility of specific or non-specific T-cell activation is still a matter of debate. The former is supported by increased susceptibility to infectious triggers (Kaneko *et al.* 2003); the upregulation of heat-shock protein (HSP60) expression in mucosal lesions of BS (Ergun *et al.* 2001; Lehner *et al.* 1997); and a strong oligoclonal T-cell response to human hsp60 and to other strains of streptoccocci or various microbial agents (Direskeneli *et al.* 1999; Esin *et al.* 1997; Pervin *et al.* 1993). In this context, one attractive hypothesis is the involvement of heat-shock proteins in a Th1-type immune response without TCR engagement, linking the innate immune system to T-cell immunity (Direskeneli and Saruhan-Direskeneli 2003). On the other hand, the overproduction of proinflammatory cytokines by innate immune cells of BS (Mege *et al.* 1993; Zierhut *et al.* 2003) may result in a non-specific T-cell response. An interesting, preliminary observation is the production of oral tolerization in BS patients with uveitis, by the uveitogenic BS specific peptide of the human 60 kD heat shock protein (Stanford *et al.* 2004).

Another potential connection between the innate and adaptive immune systems involves the interaction of MHC class I molecules with the killer cell immunoglobulin-like receptors (KIRs) which are expressed by natural killer cells and T cells. A particular association between HLA B51 and KIR3DL1 or KIR3DS1 receptors on inflammatory cells has been reported in BS (Saruhan-Direskeneli *et al.* 2004).

Neutrophils

For many years it was thought that neutrophil hyper-reactivity in BS was central to its pathogenesis (Takeuchi *et al.* 1981), which explained the usefulness of colchicine. Closer scrutiny indicates that the data are, in fact, somewhat contradictory. In a well-controlled study, there was no evidence of increased PMN activity in BS (Tüzün *et al.* 1999). Carletto and colleagues found increased activity of PMNs only during active BS (Carletto *et al.* 1997); under basal conditions, no evidence for increased superoxide production or adhesion was noted. Another study found an increased oxidative burst response in neutrophils and monocytes in patients with BS although the reaction was not specific to this condition (Gogus *et al.* 2005).

Immune complexes and hypercoagulability

It is controversial whether immune complexes or B cells play a role in the pathogenesis of BS. Antineutrophil cytoplasmic antibodies (ANCA) (Ben Hmida *et al.* 1997) and anticardiolipin antibodies

(Tokay *et al.* 2001) are absent. Antibodies to *Saccharomyces cerevisiae* (Fresko *et al.* 2005; Krause *et al.* 2002), to α-tropomysin (Mahesh *et al.* 2005) and to α-enolase (Lee *et al.* 2003) have been described, but their role in the pathogenesis of BS is not clear. A detailed analysis has revealed that no procoagulant factors are definitely associated with the tendency to thrombosis observed in BS (Espinosa *et al.* 2002; Leiba *et al.* 2004). It has been suggested; however, that there is a defect in fibrinolysis related to a deficiency of tissue plasminogen activator (tPA) production in acute thrombosis of BS (Yurdakul *et al.* 2005).

Endothelial cells

Several findings suggest endothelial dysfunction in BS: increased levels of von Willebrand factor; increased endothelin I production; decreased prostaglandin I_2 (PGI$_2$) synthesis; decreased nitrous oxide (NO) production; and enhanced E-selectin expression in endothelium (see Chapter 4). Von Willebrand factor and endothelin are synthesized and stored in the endothelium and both are elevated in BS (Direskeneli *et al.* 1995; Ural *et al.* 1994). Elevated levels of these proteins in the peripheral blood might be due to increased synthesis, perhaps secondary to an inflammatory insult. There is also decreased production of PGI$_2$ (Kansu *et al.* 1986) and nitric oxide synthetase (NOS). Both molecules are potent vasodilators and are strong inhibitors of platelet aggregation and thrombosis. There are two lines of evidence for decreased NOS production from the endothelium in BS. NOS levels in the peripheral blood are decreased (Orem *et al.* 1999), and flow-mediated vasodilation, a well established function of the endothelium, is impaired (Chambers *et al.* 1998; Oflaz H *et al.* 2005). The VNTR polymorphism in the endothelial NOS gene has been associated with BS, suggesting the role of genetic factors in endothelial dysfunction (Karasneh *et al.* 2005a). The presence of antiendothelial antibodies in BS is controversial. One study suggested that their quantity is related to disease activity (Direskeneli *et al.* 1995) while another study did not find increased levels (Dinc *et al.* 2003).

Genetics

Family studies have provided evidence of a genetic predisposition to BS. The sibling relative risk ratio (l_s) in Turkey has been estimated to be between 11 and 53, implying a strong genetic influence on disease expression (Gul *et al.* 2000). Although multicase family studies have suggested a multifactorial mode of inheritance, an autosomal recessive pattern of inheritance has been implicated in childhood BS (Molinari *et al.* 2003). HLA B51 has been the most consistently reported HLA association in BS in spite of various associations with the MICA gene (Mizuki *et al.* 2000). The mechanism whereby HLA B51 confers susceptibility to BS is not known. A HLA B51-related peptide might function as a cross-reactive antigen, such as in the proposed role played by the retinal S antigen and HLA B27 in the pathogenesis of ankylosing spondylitis (Kurhan-Yavuz *et al.* 2000). HLA B51 may account for no more than 20% of the sibling relative risk (Gul *et al.* 2001b), which supports the view that susceptibility is dependent on other genetic loci in addition to environmental triggers. Evidence suggestive of linkage has been reported on chromosome 6p22–23 (Gul *et al.* 2001c). A preliminary whole-genome screening also provided evidence of non-major histocompatibility complex (MHC) genetic-susceptibility loci in BS (Karasneh *et al.* 2005b).

The following genetic polymorphisms have been implicated in the pathogenesis of BS: the *CTLA4* +49 A allele (Sallakci *et al.* 2005); an insertion/deletion polymorphism characterized by the presence or absence of a 287-base pair Alu repeat within intron 16 of the angiotensin converting enzyme (*ACE*) gene (Ozturk *et al.* 2005); an HYPA haplotype in the mannose binding lectin 2 (*MBL2*) gene defined by –550G (H)/–221G (Y)/ +4C (P)/ +54Gly (A) SNP alleles (Park *et al.* 2005); an IL-1 beta (*IL1B*) +3953 T allele and TT genotype (Coskun *et al.* 2005); N-acyltransferase 2 (*NAT2*) *5A and *6A genotypes (Tamer *et al.* 2005); vascular endothelial growth factor (*VEGF*) 634C and I alleles (Salvarani *et al.* 2005; Nam *et al.* 2005), and gluthathione S transferase (*GSTM1*) null genotypes (Tursen *et al.* 2004a; Uzunoglu *et al.* 2006). The statistical power of these studies, however, does not allow definitive conclusions. Polymorphisms in the *CARD15/NOD2* (Ahmad *et al.* 2005; Uyar *et al.* 2004) and apolipoprotein E (apoE) genes (Tursen *et al.* 2004b) have been reported not to be associated with BS. Similarly, SNPs in the IL-8 gene (–353 A/G, +1530 T/C, +3331 A/G), and the CXCR2 gene (+785 C/T and +1208 T/C) have been found to have no role in the increased expression of IL-8 in BS (Duymaz-Tozkir *et al.* 2005).

Pathogenesis of pathergy

The pathergy reaction is related to the increased inflammatory state that characterizes BS but the exact pathogenesis of the phenomenon is unknown. Pathogenetically, it shows features in common with T-cell-mediated immune response (Gul *et al.* 1995). A recent study suggested that injury to the skin of BS patients elicits a T helper 1 (TH1)-cell response due to interleukin (IL)-12-mediated production of interferon (IFN)-gamma by CD4+ T cells (Melikoglu *et al.* 2002). The intradermal inoculation of monosodium urate (MSU) crystals also produces a longer lasting erythema in BS patients than healthy or diseased controls (Çakır *et al.* 1991). An interesting observation is the induction of the pathergy reaction with interferon α (Budak-Alpdoğan *et al.* 1997). In these patients the symptoms of BS subsided on withdrawal of interferon-α therapy. The same group (Budak-Alpdoğan *et al.* 1998) reported a positive pathergy test in 25% of chronic myelogenous leukemia (CML) patients using interferon-α. A number of patients with BS and coexistent myelodysplastic syndrome have been reported (Ohno *et al.* 1997). The majority of these patients had trisomy 8. The association of BS with the myelodysplastic syndrome and the induction of the pathergy reaction among patients with CML brings us back to the argument of whether the neutrophil is central to the pathogenesis of BS.

In summary, several points are worth emphasizing regarding the pathogenesis of BS. Most immunological data have been based either on healthy controls alone or patients with other autoimmune diseases. Data from patients with other vasculitides, infectious diseases such as tuberculosis, and those with other inflammatory diseases such as gout and FMF, are clearly needed. Second, some of the observations related to the etiopathogenesis might be more relevant to the severity of disease expression than to susceptibility. The data related to HLA-B51, as discussed above, are a case in point. Finally, perhaps not all the clinical findings of BS are explained by the same pathogenetic mechanism. The previously mentioned clinical association between acne-like lesions and arthritis certainly brings to mind reactive arthritis. On the other hand, eye and genital lesions in BS do not resemble the findings seen in reactive arthritis such as Reiter's syndrome.

Laboratory findings and differential diagnosis

The laboratory features of BS are non-specific. Mild anemia of chronic disease and neutrophilic leucocytosis are observed in 15% of the patients, but they do not correlate with clinical activity of the disease. The erythrocyte sedimentation (ESR) rate and the C-reactive protein (CRP) may be moderately elevated; the latter may correlate with erythema nodosum and acute thrombophlebitis (Muftuoglu *et al.* 1986). Elevated serum alkaline phosphatase levels have been noted in ~10% of patients; the levels were correlated with ESR and CRP (Takeuchi *et al.* 1989).

Serum immunoglobulins (especially IgA) may be increased, but rheumatoid factor and antinuclear antibody are absent. Tests for antineutrophil cytoplasmic antibodies (ANCA) are usually negative. Patients with BS who have gastrointestinal involvement seem to have high levels of anti-*Saccharomyces cerevisiae* antibodies (ASCA), but larger numbers of patients are needed to confirm this finding (Fresko *et al.* 2005).

A group of physicians involved in the care of large numbers of patients with BS formed an International Study Group (ISG) and in 1990 published the ISG Criteria of Diagnosis of Behçet's Disease (International Study Group for Behçet's Disease 1990). After determining the sensitivity and specificity of the various findings, a set of criteria that seemed to perform better than all the previously proposed criteria emerged (International Study Group for Behçet's Disease 1992). Oral ulceration was the *sine qua non*, as its presence was almost universal.

In the original control groups, the representation of Reiter's syndrome and inflammatory bowel disease was deficient. The performance of the criteria remained robust when a group of patients with inflammatory bowel disease was included in the control group (Tunc *et al.* 2001). In the differential diagnosis of the individual patient it is important to remember that BS very rarely occurs without recurrent oral ulceration, which is also rather common in otherwise healthy people. On the other hand, oral ulcers of BS tend to occur more frequently.

The so-called MAGIC syndrome (oral and genital ulcers with cartilage inflammation), which is relevant to the differential diagnosis of BS (Firestein *et al.* 1985), is probably nothing other than BS with secondary relapsing polychondritis. RAS in AIDS patients can also be confusing. The absence of dysuria or urethritis and the usual sparing of glans penis are helpful in diagnosis. It must be stressed that in females secondary infection is very common.

Finally, there remains a group of patients in whom it is not possible to make a firm diagnosis of BS. Particularly bothersome are those patients with no recurrent oral ulceration but with other manifestations, patients with isolated CNS or major vascular disease, and those patients with inflammatory bowel disease. Among these patients the presence of scar-forming genital disease is most helpful in diagnosis.

As discussed above, there has been a recent debate concerning the inclusion of BS among the so called autoinflammatory diseases (Gul 2005). These diseases, TRAPS (tumor necrosis factor receptor-associated periodic syndrome), MWS (Muckle–Wells syndrome), HIDS (hyperimmunoglobulinemia D with periodic fever syndrome), FMF, and to a lesser extent Crohn's disease, are characterized by the absence of specific high-titer antibodies, and specific mutations that are related to the syndromes (CARD, NOD, and various pyrin mutations). Aphthae, genital ulcers, acneiform skin lesions, pathergy like skin reactions, uveitis, arthritis, and orchioepididimitis are occasionally seen during their course. However, apart from FMF, all of these are very rare. Most of these entities begin in infancy, but pediatric BS is infrequent. Paroxysmal attacks that last from a few hours to a couple of weeks with frequent serosal involvement and fever characterize the former whereas they are not typical of BS. Arthritis and skin involvement are non-specific findings that are also observed in SLE, a prototype autoimmune disease. Extensive vasculitis, hypercoagulability, increased severity among males and less severe disease after age 40 are findings that are peculiar to BS (Yazici and Fresko 2005). It should also be kept in mind that the presence of one of these conditions may lead to an increased awareness and diagnosis of a second disease, the so-called Berkson's bias (Ben-Chetrit and Yazici 2002). Important considerations in the differential diagnosis are summarized in Table 35.4 (Barnes and Yazici 1999).

Prognosis and management

In a survey of the 20-year outcome of a cohort of patients with BS, mortality was specifically increased among young males, among whom morbidity was also the highest (Kural-Seyahi *et al.* 2003). The main cause of mortality in this age group was major-vessel disease (especially pulmonary arterial aneurysms) and neurological involvement. The mortality rate decreased with the passage of time, as did all mucocutaneous and articular manifestations. Both the onset of eye disease and its greatest damage were also usually within the first few years of disease. These suggest that BS "burns out" after approximately 40 years of age, with the exception of central nervous system involvement and major-vessel disease. They can have late onset (5–10 years after the disease starts). The disease was less severe among females for almost all of its manifestations. There were no female patients with arterial aneurysms in this cohort.

More than two decades ago, BenEzra and Cohen (1986) noted the eventual loss of vision in three-quarters of their patients. We are certainly doing better today – loss of useful vision ensues in one-fifth of our BS patients. Severely impaired vision does not always mean an eventual loss of useful vision, and those patients with late onset of eye disease have a better visual prognosis (Kural-Seyahi *et al.* 2003; Tugal-Tutkun *et al.* 2004).

A recent study of pulmonary arterial aneurysms has shown that the mortality has decreased from 50% to around 20% in the last decade due to earlier recognition or more rational use of immunosuppressives (Hamuryudan *et al.* 2004a).

Therapeutic options range from simple reassurance to aggressive immunosuppression, depending on the signs and symptoms and the individual needs of the patient. There is no widely accepted way of assessing disease activity, although a disease activity scheme has been prepared by international effort (Hamuryudan *et al.* 1999). The approach to the management of the systemic manifestations of the disease can be summarized as below.

Table 35.4 Highlights of the clinical manifestations of BS and differential diagnosis (Barnes and Yazici 1999)

Area affected	Clinical features
Mouth ulcers	Majority similar to common aphthous ulcers regarding appearance, localization and discomfort/pain More frequent and frequently multiple May scar
Genital ulcers	Most commonly scrotal or vulval, painful, recurrent and usually with scarring Urethral discharge and penile lesions very rare
Skin	Acneiform lesions as common acne in appearance and histology but also at uncommon sites such as the extremities Erythema nodosum-like lesions leaving pigmentation Not psoriasis
Eyes	Panuveitis and retinal vasculitis, usually bilateral occurring within about 2 years of the onset of the disease Conjunctivitis and sicca syndrome most unusual
Joints	Monarthritis in 50%, otherwise oligoarticular or polyarticular involving relatively few joints May be symmetrical; knees most frequently Intermittent resolving in 2–4 weeks or chronic and continuous Not involving sacroiliac joints or spine Deformity and erosions rare Synovial fluid usually inflammatory with good mucin clot
Peripheral arterial and venous disease	Subclinical peripheral large vein disease uncommon Usually involves large segments with skip areas without embolization Arteritis with occlusion and/or pseudo-aneurysms Microaneurysms of the polyarteritic type very uncommon
Neurological involvement	Peripheral neuropathy and isolated cerebellar involvement very unusual Headaches with dural sinus thrombosis Vascular CNS lesions including transverse myelitis-type manifestation Multiple sclerosis with aphthous ulcers a problem but no plaques on MRI
Pulmonary involvement	Hemoptysis associated with pulmonary arterial aneurysm Pulmonary artery occlusion Pleural involvement uncommon Interstitial involvement very rare
Gastrointestinal involvement	Severe abdominal pain Ulcerative lesions at any level but mainly in the ileocaecal region Mild GI symptoms should not be associated with BS
Cardiac disease	Pericarditis, valve lesions and coronary artery involvement uncommon Rarely intracardiac thrombi

Mucocutaneous manifestations

Oral and genital ulcers cause pain and interfere with the quality of life and they may lead to difficulty in swallowing and walking. Most of them can be managed by topical glucocorticoids and reassurance but systemic therapy may be required in a substantial number. Colchicine has been used by many for this problem. A 2-year, double-blind study revealed that the drug was equally effective in both sexes for arthritis, but it appeared to be effective for genital ulcers and erythema nodosum only in women (Yurdakul et al. 1998). This was probably due to the more severe course of the disease in men. The usual maximum tolerated dose of colchicine is 1.5 mg/day.

A 24-week, double-blind trial compared 100 mg/day and 300 mg/day of thalidomide with placebo (Hamuryudan et al. 1998). All mucocutaneous symptoms responded to both doses of thalidomide, but they recurred after the drug was stopped. There was also a paradoxical increase in the frequency of erythema nodosum

during the first 8 weeks of the trial. Peripheral neuropathy, the principal side-effect of the drug, usually occurred in elderly females and was not a major problem (Ochonisky et al. 1994). Thalidomide seems to be an effective drug but its use is limited because of its potential teratogenicity. Patients resistant to conventional therapy may be managed by brief courses of glucocorticoids or azathioprine (2.5 mg/kg/day).

A recent study evaluated the effect of depot glucocorticoids (40 mg methyprednisolone acetate every 3 weeks for 27 weeks) on mucocutaneous lesions. They were useful only in controlling erythema nodosum among the females, but were not effective in males (Mat et al. 2005).

A trial of topical interferon (Hamuryudan et al. 1991) and of topical cyclosporine A (Ergun et al. 1997) did not produce improvement in the number, size, and healing time of oral ulcers. Intralesional injection of recombinant human granulocyte-macrophage colony stimulating factor (Alli et al. 1997) and the topical use of sucralfate (Alpsoy *et al.* 1999) may be of some value. Dapsone may also be beneficial (Sharquie *et al.* 2002).

Various antibiotics have also been claimed to be effective in suppressing mucocutaneous lesions and arthritis with the rationale of eradicating streptococci implicated in the pathogenesis. A prospective study reported favorable results with penicillin (Calgüneri *et al.* 1996). The combination of benzathine penicillin with colchicine has been reported to be superior to colchicine alone in managing mucocutaneous and arthritic episodes of BS (Al-Waiz *et al.* 2005). Minocycline was also claimed to be effective in treating mucocutaneous symptoms based on an uncontrolled study (Kaneko *et al.* 1997). Controlled trials with antibiotics are required before their use can be recommended.

TNF-α inhibitors have increasingly been used in the treatment of BS. A controlled, 4-week trial with etanercept among male patients showed that it was effective in controlling most of the mucocutaneous manifestations of BS while it did not suppress the pathergy phenomenon (Melikoglu *et al.* 2005).

Joint involvement

The arthritis of BS is usually self-limited (Yurdakul *et al.* 1983). Non-steroidal anti-inflammatory drugs and local glucocorticoid injections are not very beneficial, but colchicine seems to be helpful in both men and women (Yurdakul *et al.* 2001). Brief courses of oral glucocorticoids may be given in patients who have protracted symptoms. Interferon-α seems to be effective but the cost of the drug, the absence of a standardized dose, and toxicity limit its use.

Ocular involvement

Azathioprine was one of the first drugs extensively evaluated for ophthalmitis of BS. One group showed that it was effective in controlling eye disease at a dose of 2.5 mg/kg/day (Yazici *et al.* 1990). It was also superior to placebo in preventing progression from unilateral to bilateral eye disease and in decreasing the use of glucocorticoids in patients who had established eye disease. Patients enrolled in the initial study with azathioprine were reanalyzed with the aim of determining the long-term effects of the drug (Hamuryudan *et al.* 1997). After 8 years, patients who were on azathioprine were still doing better (in terms of emergence of blindness, drop in visual acuity, and extraocular complications) than patients who had received placebo. The outcome was even better for patients allocated to azathioprine within the first 2 years of eye involvement. This raises the question whether young male patients without eye disease should be treated with this drug without waiting for its emergence.

Cyclosporin A (CSA) has been utilized consistently since the 1980s and was found to be superior to monthly pulses of cyclophosphamide in a single blinded study conducted in a limited number of patients (Ozyazgan *et al.* 1992). In doses of 2–5 mg/kg/day, it induces a rapid decrease in inflammation, but care is required to monitor its toxic effects such as increased serum creatinine, hypertension, occasional episodes of neuropathy, and hearing loss. Based on evidence from transplantation studies and a retrospective study in BS, its use is not recommended in CNS disease (Kötter *et al.* 2005).

Some clinicians combine azathioprine and CSA in cases of severe uveitis. Although visual acuity improved with this combination, baseline visual acuity determined during quiescent disease, which is a more precise measure of visual function, remained stable. The toxicity of the combination was low (Ozyazgan *et al.* 1996).

Tacrolimus (FK506), a potent immunosuppressive macrolide antibiotic, has been evaluated in patients with posterior uveitis resistant to CsA. There is no controlled study of its efficacy but open studies claim that it is effective in preserving visual acuity in cases of refractory posterior uveitis (Sloper *et al.* 1999). Mild increases in serum creatinine, hyperglycemia, and neurological symptoms constitute its side-effects but they can usually be managed by lowering the dose of the drug.

Alpha interferon has also been used in the uveitis of BS. A retrospective survey of this drug showed that 94% of the patients with uveitis who used the drug exhibited a partial or complete response. The drug was beneficial even in resistant posterior uveitis. Side-effects were dose dependent (Kotter *et al.* 2004). These results should be interpreted with caution, because the data are mainly uncontrolled and there is no consensus on the dose of interferon.

Emerging data suggest that TNF-α blockade, either with monoclonal antibodies to TNF-α or with soluble TNF-α receptors, are effective in BS. The anti-TNF monoclonal antibody infliximab at 5 mg/kg exerts rapid control of severe and resistant uveitis but relapses necessitate continuous treatment (Ohno *et al.* 2004; Sfikakis *et al.* 2004; Tugal-Tutkun *et al.* 2005).

Many ophthalmologists use glucocorticoids but there are no controlled trials evaluating their efficacy in eye disease. Glucocorticoids should be used as briefly as possible and should be tapered as soon as an immunosuppressive is added to the regimen. Local corticoid eye drops combined with mydriatics are also used during acute attacks with the aim of preventing synechiae.

Vitrectomy and cataract surgery do not seem to add much to the maintenance of vision in BS. Reports on the beneficial effects of photocoagulation (Atmaca *et al.* 1996) certainly need further evaluation.

Major vessel disease

An important clinical point concerning vascular disease is the relative absence of embolic phenomena in spite of the thrombotic episodes. The role of anticoagulation in deep vein thrombosis has not been evaluated in a controlled study, but one group does not use routine anticoagulation other than low-dose aspirin in the elderly patient. Azathioprine is given to young patients based on the results of the long-term follow-up of patients in an azathioprine trial (Hamuryudan *et al.* 1997) and the association of life-threatening pulmonary arterial aneurysms with deep vein thrombosis in this age group (Hamuryudan *et al.* 1994, 2004a).

Limited experience with fibrinolytic therapy has been mostly disappointing. A recent study evaluated the role of side-to-side portocaval shunts in the treatment of the dreaded Budd–Chiari syndrome, which has a reported mortality rate of 61% (Orloff and Orloff 1999). The procedure resulted in a substantial increase in survival (80% at a mean of 10.6 years of follow-up), coupled with a decrease in ascites and diuretic use.

Arterial disease in BS causes substantial morbidity and mortality. Aneurysms of peripheral arteries should be corrected surgically although there is a recurrence rate of about 30% (Tüzün *et al.* 1996; Kalko *et al.* 2005). The recommended adjunctive medical treatment consists of monthly pulses of cyclophosphamide combined with 1 mg/kg of prednisolone with tapering in the course of a few months to a dose below 30 mg/day. Medical management of pulmonary arterial aneurysms should follow the same regimen. Anticoagulation is contraindicated because of the risk of bleeding and surgical repair should not usually be performed because of the high risk of mortality. Intra-arterial embolization has been attempted (Cantasdemir *et al.* 2002; Mouas *et al.* 1996) but the value of this procedure is not clear. There are various reports that suggest that endovascular surgery may be beneficial in major arterial and venous disease (Castelli *et al.* 2005).

Occasionally, patients present with cardiac disease such as mitral and aortic insufficiency and intracavitary thrombi. Surgical thrombectomy (Kirali *et al.* 1998) and valve replacement (Zakaria *et al.* 1998) have been reported with variable success.

Central nervous system disease

There are no controlled studies evaluating the management of CNS disease in BS. Thrombosis of the dural sinuses and increased intracranial pressure is empirically treated with 1 g of methylprednisolone administration intravenously daily for 3–5 days, followed by oral maintenance doses. Parenchymal involvement, which manifests itself as varying degrees of cognitive, pyramidal, and cerebellar symptoms, is usually treated with cyclophosphamide or azathioprine combined with glucocorticoids. The use of CSA should be avoided in CNS disease because of its potential neurotoxicity (Kotter *et al.* 2005). Chlorambucil, claimed beneficial by some (O'Duffy *et al.* 1984), has not found wide use mainly due to its myelotoxicity. An open trial in a small number of patients suggests that low-dose, oral methotrexate (7.5–12.5 mg/week) stops the progression of chronic neurological involvement (Hirohata *et al.* 1998), but larger studies are needed to confirm this finding.

A few case reports suggest that the TNF-α blocker infliximab is beneficial in treating parenchymal neurological disease refractory to other medications (Licata *et al.* 2003).

Gastrointestinal disease

Gastrointestinal manifestations in BS resemble those of inflammatory bowel disease or less frequently, ileocecal perforation. Thalidomide seems to be effective in healing the ulcers of some patients (Postema *et al.* 1996). Sulfasalazine at a dose of 2–4 g/day has not been efficacious. Surgical repair should be instituted in case of resistant ulcerations and perforations. Recurrences after gastrointestinal surgery have been reported and inspection of the entire bowel during the operation is highly recommended (Lee *et al.* 1997). Small case series suggest that the TNF-α blocker infliximab is beneficial in treating refractory cases of gastrointestinal BS (Travis *et al.* 2001).

In summary, clinicians generally have some degree of success in treating the eye and mucocutanous manifestations of BS. Management of CNS disease, and the major vascular complications, including thrombotic events, is still difficult, with suboptimal success.

References

Ahmad, T., Zhang, L., Gogus, F., *et al.* (2005). CARD15 polymorphisms in Behçet's disease. *Scandinavian Journal of Rheumatology*, **34**, 233–7.

Akman-Demir, G., Baykan-Kurt, B., Serdaroglu, P., *et al.* (1996). Seven-year follow-up of neurologic involvement in Behçet's syndrome. *Archives of Neurology*, **53**, 691–4.

Akpolat, T., Diri, B., Oguz, Y., Yilmaz, E., Yavuz, M. and Dilek, M. (2003). Behçet's disease and renal failure. *Nephrology Dialysis Transplantation*, **18**, 888–91.

Al Dalaan, A., AlBalla, S., Alsukait, M., *et al.* (1996). The prevalence of Behçet's disease in al. Quassim region of Saudi Arabia. *Revue de Rhumatisme* (English Edition) (abs.), **63**, 538.

Alli, N., Karakayalı, G., Kahraman, I. and Artuz, F. (1997). Local intralesional therapy with rhGM-CSF for a large genital ulcer in Behçet's disease. *British Journal of Dermatology*, **136**, 639–40.

Alpsoy, E., Elpek, G. O., Yilmaz, F., *et al.* (2005). Androgen receptor levels of oral and genital ulcers and skin pathergy test in patients with Behçet's disease. *Dermatology*, **210**, 31–5.

Alpsoy, E., Er, H., Durusoy, C. and Yılmaz, E. (1999). The use of sucralfate suspension in the treatment of oral and genital ulceration of Behçet disease: a randomized, placebo-controlled, double-blind study. *Archives of Dermatology*, **135**, 529–32.

Altac, M., Tuzun, Y., Yurdakul, S., Binyildiz, P. and Yazici, H. (1982). The validity of pathergy test (non-specific skin hyperreactivity) in Behçet's disease: A double blind study by independent observers. *Acta Dermato-Venereologica*, **62**, 158–9.

Altiparmak, M. R., Tanverdi, M., Pamuk, O. N., Tunc, R. and Hamuryudan, V. (2002). Glomerulonephritis in Behçet's disease: report of seven cases and review of the literature. *Clinical Rheumatology*, **21**, 14–8.

Al-Waiz, M. M., Sharquie, K. E., A-Qaissi, M. H. and Hayani, R. K. (2005). Colchicine and benzathine penicillin in the treatment of Behçet disease: a case comparative study. *Dermatology Online Journal*, **11**, 3.

Apaydin, S., Erek, E., Ulku, U., Hamuryudan, V., Yazici, H. and Sariyar, M. (1999). A successful renal transplantation in Behçet's syndrome. *Annals of the Rheumatic Diseases*, **58**, 719.

Arkin, C. R., Rothschild, B. M., Florendo, N. T. and Popoff, N. (1980). Behçet's syndrome with myositis. A case report with pathologic findings. *Arthritis and Rheumatism*, **23**, 600–4.

Atmaca, L. S., Batioglu, F. and Idil, A. (1996). Retinal and disc neovascularization in Behçet's disease and efficacy of laser photocoagulation. *Graefes Archives of Clinical and Experimental Ophtalmology*, **234**, 94–9.

Avci, O., Kutluay, E., Argon, N., Erdem, S. and Tahsin, G. A. (1998). Subclinical cerebral involvement in Behçet's disease: A SPECT study. *European Journal of Neurology*, **5**, 49–53.

Azizlerli, G., Kose, A. A., Sarica, R., *et al.* (2003). Prevalence of Behçet's disease in Istanbul, Turkey. *International Journal of Dermatology*, **42**, 803–6.

Azizlerli, G., Ozarmagan, G., Ovul, C., Sarica, R. and Mustafa, S. O. (1992). A new kind of skin lesion in Behçet's disease: extragenital ulcers. *Acta Dermato-Venereologica*, **72**, 286.

Barnes, C. G. and Yazici, H. (1999). Behçet's syndrome. *Rheumatology* (Oxford), **38**, 1171–4.

Behçet, H. (1937). Ueber rezidivierende aphtose durch ein virus verursachte geschwuere am mund, am auge und an den genitalien. *Dermatologische Woschenschrift*, **105**, 1152–7.

Ben Ahmed, M., Houman, H., Miled, M., Dellagi, K. and Louzir, H. (2004). Involvement of chemokines and Th1 cytokines in the pathogenesis of mucocutaneous lesions of Behçet's disease. *Arthritis and Rheumatism*, **50**, 2291–5.

Ben-Chetrit, E. and Yazici, H. (2002). Thoughts on the proposed links between Behçet's disease and familial Mediterranean fever. *Clinical and Experimental Rheumatology*, **20** (Suppl. 26), S1–2.

Benezra, D. and Cohen, E. (1986). Treatment and visual prognosis in Behçet's disease. *British Journal of Ophthalmology*, **70**, 589–92.

Ben Hmida, M., Hachicha, J., Kaddour, N., *et al.* (1997). ANCA in Behçet's disease. *Nephrology, Dialysis, Transplantation*, **12**, 2465–6.

Budak-Alpdogan, T., Demircay, Z., Alpdogan, O., *et al.* (1997). Behçet's disease in patients with chronic myelogenous leukemia: possible role of interferon-alpha treatment in the occurrence of Behçet's symptoms. *Annals of Haematology*, **74**, 45–8.

Budak-Alpdogan, T., Demircay, Z., Alpdogan, O., *et al.* (1998). Skin hyperreactivity of Behçet's patients (pathergy reaction) is also positive in interferon alpha-treated chronic myeloid leukaemia patients, indicating similarly altered neutrophil functions in both disorders. *British Journal of Rheumatology*, **37**, 1148–51.

Cakir, N., Yazici, H., Chamberlain, M. A., *et al.* (1991). Response to intradermal injection of monosodium urate crystals in Behçet's syndrome. *Annals of the Rheumatic Diseases*, **50**, 634–6.

Calguneri, M., Kiraz, S., Ertenli, I., Benekli, M., Karaarslan, Y. and Celik, I. (1996). The effect of prophylactic penicillin treatment on the course of arthritis episodes in patients with Behçet's disease. A randomized clinical trial. *Arthritis and Rheumatism*, **39**, 2062–5.

Cantasdemir, M., Kantarci, F., Mihmanli, I., *et al.* (2002). Emergency endovascular management of pulmonary artery aneurysms in Behçet's disease: report of two cases and a review of the literature. *Cardiovascular and Interventional Radiology*, **25**, 533–7.

Carletto, A., Pacor, M. L., Biasi, D., *et al.* (1997). Changes of neutrophil migration without modification of in vitro metabolism and adhesion in Behçet's disease. *Journal of Rheumatology*, **24**, 1332–6.

Castelli, P., Caronno, R., Piffaretti, G., *et al.* (2005). Endovascular treatment for superior vena cava obstruction in Behçet disease. *Journal of Vascular Surgery*, **41**, 548–51.

Cetinel, B., Obek, C., Solok, V., Yaycioglu, O. and Yazici, H. (1998). Urologic screening for men with Behçet's syndrome. *Urology*, **52**, 863–5.

Cetinel, B., Akpinar, H., Tufek, I., Uygun, N., Solok, V. and Yazici, H. (1999). Bladder involvement in Behçet's syndrome. *Journal of Urology*, **161**, 52–6.

Chamberlain, M. A. and Robertson, R. J. (1993). A controlled study of sacroiliitis in Behçet's disease. *British Journal of Rheumatology*, **32**, 693–8.

Chambers, J. C., Haskard, D. O. and Kooner, J. S. (2001). Vascular endothelial function and oxidative stress mechanisms in patients with Behçet's syndrome. *Journal of the American College of Cardiology*, **37**, 517–20.

Chun, S. I., Su, W. P. and Lee, S. (1990). Histopathologic study of cutaneous lesions in Behçet's syndrome. *Journal of Dermatology*, **17**, 333–41.

Coban, O., Bahar, S., Akman-Demir, G., *et al.* (1999). Masked assessment of MRI findings: is it possible to differentiate neuro-Behçet's disease from other central nervous system. *Neuroradiology*, **41**, 255–60.

Coskun, M., Bacanli, A., Sallakci, N., Alpsoy, E., Yavuzer, U. and Yegin, O. (2005). Specific interleukin-1 gene polymorphisms in Turkish patients with Behçet's disease. *Experimental Dermatology*, **14**, 124–9.

Coskun, S., Seyahi, E., Mat, C. and Yazici, H. (2004). Female Behçet's syndrome patients have more severe oral ulcerations. *Clinical and Experimental Rheumatology*, **22**, S-86, abs A 16.

Crivelli, M. R., Aguas, S., Adler, I., Quarracino, C. and Berque, P. (1988). Influence of socioeconomic status on oral mucosa lesion prevalence in schoolchildren. *Community Dentistry and Oral Epidemiology*, **16**, 58–60.

Demirhindi, O., Yazici, H., Binyildiz, P., *et al.* (1981). Silivri Fener koyu ve yoresinde Behçet hastaligi sikligi ve bu hastaligin toplum icinde taranabilmesinde kullanabilecek bir yontem. *Cerrahpasa Tip Dergisi*, **12**, 509–14.

Demirkesen, C., Tuzuner, N., Mat, C., *et al.* (2001). Clinicopathologic evaluation of nodular cutaneous lesions of Behçet syndrome. *American Journal of Clinical Pathology*, **116**, 341–6.

Dilsen, E., Konice, M., Aral, O., *et al.* (1988). Behçet's disease associated with amyloidosis in Turkey and in the world. *Annals of the Rheumatic Diseases*, **47**, 157–63.

Dinc, A., Takafuta, T., Jiang, D., Melikoglu, M., Saruhan-Direskeneli, G. and Shapiro, S. S. (2003). Anti-endothelial cell antibodies in Behçet's disease. *Clinical and Experimental Rheumatology*, **21** (Suppl. 30), S27–30.

Direskeneli, H. and Saruhan-Direskeneli, G. (2003). The role of heat shock proteins in Behçet's disease. *Clinical and Experimental Rheumatology*, **21**, S44–8.

Direskeneli, H., Keser, G., D'Cruz, D., *et al.* (1995). Anti-endothelial cell antibodies, endothelial proliferation and von Willebrand factor antigen in Behçet's disease. *Clinical Rheumatology*, **14**, 55–61.

Direskeneli, H., Eksioglu-Demiralp, E., Kibaroglu, A., Yavuz, S., Ergun, T. and Akoglu, T. (1999). Oligoclonal T cell expansions in patients with Behçet's disease. *Clinical and Experimental Immunology*, **117**, 166–70.

Diri, E., Mat, C., Hamuryudan, V., Yurdakul, S., Hizli, N. and Yazici, H. (2001). Papulopustular skin lesions are seen more frequently in patients with Behçet's syndrome who have arthritis: a controlled and masked study. *Annals of the Rheumatic Diseases*, **60**, 1074–6.

Duymaz-Tozkir, J., Yilmaz, V., Uyar, F. A., Hajeer, A. H., Saruhan-Direskeneli, G. and Gul, A. (2005). Polymorphisms of the IL-8 and CXCR2 genes are not associated with Behçet's disease. *Journal of Rheumatology*, **32**, 93–7.

Efthimiou, J., Johnston, C., Spiro, S. G. and Turner-Warwick, M. (1986). Pulmonary disease in Behçet's syndrome. *Quarterly Journal of Medicine*, **227**, 259–80.

Erdogru, T., Kocak, T., Serdaroglu, P., Kadioglu, A. and Tellaloglu, S. (1999). Evaluation and therapeutic approaches of voiding and erectile dysfunction in neurological Behçet's syndrome. *Journal of Urology*, **162**, 147–53.

Ergun, T., Gurbuz, O., Yurdakul, S., Hamuryudan, V., Bekiroglu, N. and Yazici, H. (1997). Topical cylosporine-A for treatment of oral ulcers of Behçet's syndrome. *International Journal of Dermatology*, **36**, 720.

Ergun, T., Gürbüz, O., Dogusoy, G., Mat, C. and Yazici, H. (1998). Histopathologic features of the spontaneous pustular lesions of Behçet's syndrome. *International Journal of Dermatology*, **37**, 194–6.

Ergun, T., Ince, U., Eksioglu-Demiralp, E., *et al.* (2001). HSP 60 expression in mucocutaneous lesions of Behçet's disease. *Journal of the American Academy of Dermatology*, **45**, 904–9.

Erkan, D., Yazici, Y., Sanders, A., Trost, D. and Yazici, H. (2004). Is Hughes-Stovin syndrome Behçet's disease? *Clinical and Experimental Rheumatology*, **22**, S64–8.

Esin, S., Gül, A., Hodara, V., *et al.* (1997). Peripheral blood T cell expansions in patients with Behçet's disease. *Clinical and Experimental Immunology*, **107**, 520–7.

Espinosa, G., Font, J., Tassies, D., *et al.* (2002). Vascular involvement in Behçet's disease: relation with thrombophilic factors, coagulation activation and thrombomodulin. *American Journal of Medicine*, **112**, 37–43.

Farah, S., Al-shubaili, A., Montaser, A., *et al.* (1998). Behçet's syndrome: a report of 41 patients with emphasis on neurological manifestations. *Journal of Neurology Neurosurgery and Psychiatry*, **64**, 382–4.

Firestein, G. S., Gruber, H. E., Weisman, M. H., Zvaifler, N. J., Barber, J. and O'Duffy, J. D. (1985). Mouth and genital ulcers with inflamed cartilage: MAGIC syndrome. Five patients with features of relapsing polychondritis and Behçet's disease. *American Journal of Medicine*, **79**, 65–72.

Frassanito, M. A., Dammacco, R., Cafforio, P. and Dammacco, F. (1999). Th1 polarization of the immune response in Behçet's disease: a putative pathogenetic role of interleukin-12. *Arthritis and Rheumatism*, **42**, 1967–74.

Fresko, I., Ugurlu, S., Ozbakir, F., *et al.* (2005). Anti-Saccharomyces cerevisiae antibodies (ASCA) in Behçet's syndrome. *Clinical and Experimental Rheumatology*, **23** (Suppl. 38), S67–70.

Fukuda, Y. and Watanabe, I. (1979). Pathological studies on intestinal Behçet's (entero-Behçet's) disease. In *Behçet's disease*. Proceedings of an International Symposium on Behçet's Disease (eds Dilsen, N., Konice, M. and Ovul, C.), pp. 90–5. Excerpta Medica, Amsterdam.

George, R. K., Chan, C. C., Whitcup, S. M. and Nussenblatt, R. B. (1997). Ocular immunopathology of Behçet's disease. *Survey of Ophthalmology*, **42**, 157–62.

Gogus, F., Fresko, I., Elbir, Y., Eksioglu-Demiralp, E. and Direskeneli, H. (2005). Oxidative burst response to monosodium urate crystals in patients with Behçet's syndrome. *Clinical and Experimental Rheumatology*, **23** (Suppl. 38), S81–5.

Gonzalez-Gay, M. A., Garcia-Porrua, C., Branas, F., Lopez-Lazaro, L. and Olivieri, I. (2000). Epidemiologic and clinical aspects of Behçet's disease in a defined area of Northwestern Spain, 1988–1997. *Journal of Rheumatology, 27,* 703–7.

Grattan, C. E. and Scully, G. (1986). Oral ulceration: a diagnostic problem. *British Medical Journal, 292,* 1093–4.

Griffin, J. W. Jr, Harrison, H. B., Tedesco, F. J. and Mills, L. R. 4th (1982). Behçet's disease with multiple sites of gastrointestinal involvement. *Southern Medical Journal, 75,* 1405–8.

Gul, A. (2001). Behçet's disease: an update on the pathogenesis. *Clinical and Experimental Rheumatology, 19* (Suppl. 24), S6–12.

Gul, A. (2005). Behçet's disease as an autoinflammatory disorder. *Current Drug Targets. Inflammation and Allergy, 4,* 81–3.

Gul, A., Esin, S., Dilsen, N., Konice, M., Wigzell, H. and Biberfeld, P. (1995). Immunohistology of skin pathergy reaction in Behçet's disease. *British Journal of Dermatology, 132,* 901–7.

Gul, A., Inanc, M., Ocal, L., Aral, O. and Konice, M. (2000). Familial aggregation of Behçet's disease in Turkey. *Annals of the Rheumatic Diseases, 59,* 622–5.

Gul, A., Hajeer, A. H., Worthington, J., Ollier, W. E. and Silman, A. J. (2001). Linkage mapping of a novel susceptibility locus for Behçet's disease to chromosome 6p22–23. *Arthritis and Rheumatism, 44,* 2693–6.

Gunaydin, I., Ustundag, C., Kaner, G., *et al.* (1994). The prevalence of Sjögren's syndrome in Behçet's syndrome. *Journal of Rheumatology, 21,* 1662–4.

Hamuryudan, V., Yurdakul, S., Rosenkaimer, F. and Yazici, H. (1991). Inefficacy of topical alpha interferon in the treatment of oral ulcers in Behçet's syndrome: a randomized, double blind trial. *British Journal of Rheumatology, 30,* 395–6.

Hamuryudan, V., Yurdakul, S., Moral, F., *et al.* (1994). Pulmonary arterial aneurysms in Behçet's syndrome: A report of 24 cases. *British Journal of Rheumatology, 33,* 48–51.

Hamuryudan, V., Ozyazgan, Y., Hizli, N., *et al.* (1997). Azathioprine in Behçet's syndrome: Effects on long term prognosis. *Arthritis and Rheumatism, 40,* 769–74.

Hamuryudan, V., Mat, C., Saip, S., *et al.* (1998). Thalidomide in the treatment of mucocutaneous lesions of the Behçet's syndrome. A randomized, double-blind, placebo-controlled trial. *Annals of Internal Medicine, 128,* 443–50.

Hamuryudan, V., Fresko, I., Direskeneli, H., *et al.* (1999). Evaluation of the Turkish translation of a disease activity form for Behçet's syndrome. *Rheumatology* (Oxford), *38,* 734–6.

Hamuryudan, V., Er, T., Seyahi, E., *et al.* (2004a). Pulmonary artery aneurysms in Behçet syndrome. *American Journal of Medicine, 117,* 867–70.

Hamuryudan, V., Oz, B., Tuzun, H. and Yazici, H. (2004b). The menacing pulmonary artery aneurysms of Behçet's syndrome. *Clinical and Experimental Rheumatology, 22,* S1–3.

Hamza, M. (1987). Large artery involvement in Behçet's disease. *Journal of Rheumatology, 14,* 554–9.

Hatemi, G., Bahar, H., Uysal, S., *et al.* (2004). The pustular skin lesions in Behçet's syndrome are not sterile. *Annals of the Rheumatic Diseases, 63,* 1450–2.

Hirohata, S., Suda, H. and Hashimoto, T. (1998). Low-dose methotrexate for progressive neuropsychiatric manifestations in Behçet's disease. *Journal of the Neurological Sciences, 159,* 181–5.

Hirohata, S., Arai, H. and Matsumoto, T. (2003). Immunohistological studies in neuro-Behçet's disease. *Advances in Experimental Medicine and Biology, 528,* 385–7.

Houng, D. I., Wechsler, B., Papo, T., *et al.* (1997). Endomyocardial fibrosis in Behçet's disease. *Annals of the Rheumatic Diseases, 56,* 205–8.

Iida, M., Kobayashi, H., Matsumoto, T., *et al.* (1993). Intestinal Behçet's disease: serial changes at radiography. *Radiology, 188,* 65–9.

International Study Group for Behçet's Disease (1990). Criteria for diagnosis of Behçet's disease. *Lancet, 335,* 1078–80.

International Study Group for Behçet's Disease (1992). Evaluation of diagnostic (classification) criteria in Behçet's disease – towards internationally agreed criteria. *British Journal of Rheumatology, 31,* 299–308.

Kaklamani, G., Vaiopoulos, G. and Kaklamanis, P. G. (1998). Behçet's Disease. *Seminars in Arthritis and Rheumatism, 27,* 197–217.

Kaklamani, V. G., Tzonou, A., Markomichelakis, N., Papazoglou, S. and Kaklamanis, P. G. (2003). The effect of smoking on the clinical features of Adamantiades-Behçet's disease. *Advances in Experimental Medicine and Biology, 528,* 323–7.

Kalko, Y., Basaran, M., Aydin, U., Kafa, U., Basaranoglu, G. and Yasar, T. (2005). The surgical treatment of arterial aneurysms in Behçet disease: a report of 16 patients. *Journal of Vascular Surgery, 42,* 673–7.

Kaneko, F., Oyama, N. and Nishibu, A. (1997). Streptococcal infection in the pathogenesis of Behçet's disease and clinical effects of minocycline on the disease symptoms. *Yonsei Medical Journal, 38,* 444–54.

Kaneko, F., Tojo, M., Sato, M. and Isogai, E. (2003). The role of infectious agents in the pathogenesis of Behçet's disease. *Advances in Experimental Medicine and Biology, 528,* 181–3.

Kansu, E., Sahin, G., Sahin, F., Sivri, B., Sayek, I. and Batman, F. (1986). Impaired prostacyclin synthesis by vessel walls in Behçet's disease. *Lancet, 2,* 1154.

Karasneh, J. A., Hajeer, A. H., Silman, A., Worthington, J., Ollier, W. E. and Gul, A. (2005a). Polymorphisms in the endothelial nitric oxide synthase gene are associated with Behçet's disease. *Rheumatology* (Oxford), *44,* 614–7.

Karasneh, J., Gul, A., Ollier, W. E., Silman, A. J. and Worthington, J. (2005b). Whole-genome screening for susceptibility genes in multicase families with Behçet's disease. *Arthritis and Rheumatism, 52,* 1836–42.

Kasahara, Y., Tanaka, S., Nishino, M., Umemura, H., Shiraha, S. and Kuyama, T. (1981). Intestinal involvement in Behçet's disease: Review of 136 surgical cases in Japanese literature. *Diseases of the Colon and Rectum, 24,* 103–6.

Kingston, M., Ratcliffe, J. R., Alltree, M. and Merendino, K. A. (1979). Aneurysm after arterial puncture in Behçet's disease. *British Medical Journal, 11,* 1766–7.

Kirali, K., Civelek, A., Daglar, B., *et al.* (1998). An uncommon complication of Behçet's disease: intracardiac thrombosis needing surgical treatment. *Thoracic and Cardiovascular Surgeon, 46,* 102–5.

Kobayashi, M., Ito, M., Nakagawa, A., *et al.* (2000). Neutrophil and endothelial cell activation in the vasa vasorum in vasculo-Behçet disease. *Histopathology, 36,* 362–71.

Kobayashi, T., Kikawada, T., Shima, K. and Fukuda, O. (1982). Ulceration and stenosis of the hypopharynx and its surgical management. *Head and Neck Surgery, 5,* 66–9.

Koc, Y., Gullu, I., Akpek, G., *et al.* (1992). Vascular involvement in Behçet's disease. *Journal of Rheumatology, 19,* 402–10.

Kocer, N., Islak, C., Siva, A., *et al.* (1999). CNS involvement in neuro-Behçet syndrome: an MR study. *American Journal of Neuroradiolgy, 20,* 1015–24.

Kone-Paut, I., Yurdakul, S., Bahabri, S. A., *et al.* (1998). Clinical features of Behçet's disease in children: an international colloborative study of 86 cases. *Journal of Pediatrics, 132,* 721–5.

Korman, U., Cantasdemir, M., Kurugoglu, S., *et al.* (2003). Enteroclysis findings of intestinal Behçet disease: a comparative study with Crohn disease. *Abdominal Imaging, 28,* 308–12.

Kotter, I., Gunaydin, I., Zierhut, M. and Stubiger, N. (2004). The use of interferon alpha in Behçet disease: review of the literature. *Seminars in Arthritis and Rheumatism, 33,* 320–35.

Kotter, I., Gunaydin, I., Batra, M., *et al.* (2005). CNS involvement occurs more frequently in patients with Behçet's disease under cyclosporin A (CSA) than under other medications-results of a retrospective analysis of 117 cases. *Clinical Rheumatology, 25,* 482–6.

Krause, I., Leibovici, L., Guedj, D., Molad, Y., Uziel, Y. and Weinberger, A. (1999). Disease patterns of patients with Behçet's disease demonstrated by factor analysis. *Clinical and Experimental Rheumatology*, **17**, 347–50.

Krause, I., Molad, Y., Mitrani, M., Weinberger, A. (2000). Pathergy reaction in Behçet's disease: lack of correlation with mucocutaneous manifestations and systemic disease expression. *Clinical and Experimental Rheumatology*, **18**, 71–4.

Krause, I., Monselise, Y., Milo, G. and Weinberger, A. (2002). Anti-Saccharomyces cerevisiae antibodies–a novel serologic marker for Behçet's disease. *Clinical and Experimental Rheumatology*, **20** (Suppl. 26), S21–4.

Kulahli, I., Balci, K., Koseoglu, E., Yucc, I., Cagli, S. and Senturk, M.(2005). Audio-vestibular disturbances in Behçet's patients: report of 62 cases. *Hearing Research*, **203**, 28–31.

Kural-Seyahi, E., Fresko, I. and Seyahi, N. (2003). The long-term mortality and morbidity of Behçet syndrome: a 2-decade outcome survey of 387 patients followed at a dedicated center. *Medicine* (Baltimore), **82**, 60–76.

Kurhan-Yavuz, S., Direskeneli, H., Bozkurt, N., *et al.* (2000). Anti-MHC autoimmunity in Behçet's disease: T cell responses to an HLA-B-derived peptide cross-reactive with retinal-S antigen in patients with uveitis. *Clinical and Experimental Immunology*, **120**, 162–6.

Lakhanpal, S., Tani, K., Lie, J. T., Katoh, K., Ishigatsubo, Y. and Ohokubo, T. (1985). Pathologic features of Behçet's syndrome. A review of Japanese autopsy registry data. *Human Pathology*, **16**, 790–5.

Lee, K. H., Chung, H. S., Kim, H. S., *et al.* (2003). Human alpha-enolase from endothelial cells as a target antigen of anti-endothelial cell antibody in Behçet's disease. *Arthritis and Rheumatism*, **48**, 2025–35.

Lee, K. S., Kim, S. J., Lee, B. C., Yoon, D. S., Lee, W. J. and Chi, H. S. (1997). Surgical treatment of intestinal Behçet's disease. *Yonsei Medical Journal*, **38**, 455–60.

Lehner, T. and Batchelor, J. R. (1979). Classification and an immunogenetic basis of Behçet's syndrome. In *Behçet's Disease* (eds Lehner, T. and Barnes, C. G.), pp. 13–32. Excerpta Medica, London.

Lehner, T. (1997). The role of heat shock protein, microbial and autoimmune agents in the etiology of Behçet's disease. *International Review of Immunology*, **14**, 21–32.

Leiba, M., Seligsohn, U., Sidi, Y., *et al.* (2004). Thrombophilic factors are not the leading cause of thrombosis in Behçet's disease. *Annals of the Rheumatic Diseases*, **63**, 1445–9.

Licata, G., Pinto, A. and Tuttolomondo, A. (2003). Anti-tumour necrosis factor alpha monoclonal antibody therapy for recalcitrant cerebral vasculitis in a patient with Behçet's syndrome. *Annals of the Rheumatic Diseases*, **62**, 280–1.

Lie, J. T. (1992). Vascular involvement in Behçet's disease: Arterial and venous and vessels of all sizes. *Journal of Rheumatology*, **19**, 341–3.

Mahesh, S. P., Li, Z., Buggage, R., *et al.* (2005). Alpha tropomyosin as a self-antigen in patients with Behçet's disease. *Clinical and Experimental Immunology*, **140**, 368–75.

Mat, C., Nazarbaghi, M., Tuzun, Y., *et al.* (1998). Wound healing in Behçet's syndrome. *International Journal of Dermatology*, **37**, 120–3.

Mat, C., Demirkesen, C., Cokerler, O., *et al.* (2001). Androgen receptor density in scrotal skin of Behçet's disease. In *Behçet's disease*. Proceeding of the 8th International Congress of Behçet's Disease (eds Bang, D., Lee, E.-S. and Lee, S). pp. 646–8. Design Mecca Publishing, Seoul.

Mat, C., Yurdakul, S., Uysal, S., *et al.* (2005). A double-blind trial of depot glucocorticoids in Behçet's syndrome. *Rheumatology* (Oxford) **45**, 245–7.

Mat, C., Goksugur, N., Engin, B., Yurdakul, S. and Yazici, H. (2006). The frequency of scarring after genital ulcers in Behçet's Syndrome: A prospective study. *International Journal of Dermatology*, **45**, 554–6.

Mege, J. L., Dilsen, N., Sanguedolce, V., *et al.* (1993). Overproduction of monocyte derived tumor necrosis factor alpha, interleukin (IL) **6**, IL-8 and increased neutrophil superoxide generation in Behçet's disease.

A comparative study with familial Mediterranean fever and healthy subjects. *Journal of Rheumatology*, **20**, 1544–9.

Melikoglu, M., Altiparmak, M. R., Fresko, I., *et al.* (2001). A reappraisal of amyloidosis in Behçet's syndrome. *Rheumatology* (Oxford), **40**, 212–5.

Melikoglu, M., Uysal, S., Kaplan, G., *et al.* (2002). Leukocyte phenotype and cytokine expression at the skin pathergy reaction in Behçet's disease: evidence for a type I immune response (abstract). *Arthritis and Rheumatism*, **46**, S191.

Melikoglu, M., Fresko, I., Mat, C., *et al.* (2005). Short-term trial of etanercept in Behçet's disease: a double blind, placebo controlled study. *Journal of Rheumatology*, **32**, 98–105.

Mizuki, N., Ota, M., Yabuki, K., *et al.* (2000). Localization of the pathogenic gene of Behçet's disease by microsatellite analysis of three different populations. *Investigative Ophthalmology and Visual Science*, **41**, 3702–8.

Mogulkoc, N., Burgess, M. I. and Bishop, P. W. (2000). Intracardiac thrombus in Behçet's disease: a systematic review. *Chest*, **118**, 479–87.

Molinari, N., Kone Paut, I., Manna, R., Demaille, J., Daures, J. P. and Touitou, I. (2003). Identification of an autosomal recessive mode of inheritance in paediatric Behçet's families by segregation analysis. *American Journal of Medical Genetics. Part A*, **122**, 115–8.

Monastero, R., Camarda, C., Pipia, C., *et al.* (2004). Cognitive impairment in Behçet's disease patients without overt neurological involvement. *Journal of the Neurological Sciences*, **220**, 99–104.

Mori, S., Yoshihara, A., Kavamura, H., Takeuchi, A., Hashimoto, T. and Inaba, G. (1983). Esophageal involvement in Behçet's disease. *American Journal of Gastroenterology*, **78**, 548–53.

Mouas, H., Lorthorary, O., Lacombe, P., *et al.* (1996). Embolization of multiple pulmonary arterial aneurysms in Behçet's disease. *Scandinavian Journal of Rheumatology*, **25**, 58–60.

Muftuoglu, A. U., Yazici, H., Yurdakul, S., *et al.* (1986). Behçet's disease. Relation of serum C-reactive protein and erythrocyte sedimentation rates to disease activity. *International Journal of Dermatology*, **25**, 235–9.

Muller, W. and Lehner, T. (1982). Quantitative electron microscopical analysis of leucocyte infiltration in oral ulcers of Behçet's syndrome. *British Journal of Dermatology*, **106**, 535–44.

Nobili, F., Cutolo, M., Sulli, A., Vitali, P., Vignola, S. and Rodriguez, G. (2002). Brain functional involvement by perfusion SPECT in systemic sclerosis and Behçet's disease. *Annals of the New York Academy of Sciences*, **966**, 409–14.

Nam, E. J., Han, S. W., Kim, S. U., Cho, J. H., Sa, K. H., Lee, W. K., Park, J. Y. and Kang, Y. M. (2005). Association of vascular endothelial growth factor gene polymorphisms with Behçet disease in a Korean population. *Human Immunology*, **66**, 1068–73.

Ochonisky, S., Verroust, J., Bastuji-Garin, S., Gherardi, R. and Revuz, J. (1994). Thalidomide neuropathy incidence and clinico-electrophysiologic findings in 42 patients. *Archives of Dermatology*, **130**, 66–9.

O'Duffy, J. D. (1994). Behçet's disease. *Current Opinion in Rheumatology*, **6**, 39–43.

O'Duffy, J. D., Robertson, D. M. and Goldstein, N. P. (1984). Chlorambucil in the treatment of uveitis and maningoencephalitis of Behçet's disease. *American Journal of Medicine*, **76**, 75–84.

Oflaz, H., Mercanoglu, F., Karaman, O., *et al.* (2005). Impaired endothelium-dependent flow-mediated dilation in Behçet's disease: more prominent endothelial dysfunction in patients with vascular involvement. *International Journal of Clinical Practice*, **59**, 777–81.

Oguz, A., Serdaroglu, S., Tuzun, Y., Erdogan, N., Yazici, H. and Savaskan, H. (1992). Acute febrile neutrophilic dermatosis associated with Behçet's syndrome. *International Journal of Dermatology*, **31**, 645–6.

Ohno, E., Ohtsuka, E., Watanabe, K., *et al.* (1997). Behçet's disease associated with myelodysplastic syndromes. A case report and a review of the literature. *Cancer*, **79**, 262–8.

Ohno, S., Nakamura, S., Hori, S., *et al.* (2004). Efficacy, safety, and pharmacokinetics of multiple administration of infliximab in Behçet's disease with refractory uveoretinitis. *Journal of Rheumatology*, **31,** 1362–8.

Oktem-Tanor, O., Baykan-Kurt, B., Gurvit, I. H., Akman-Demir, G. and Serdaroglu, P. (1999). Neuropsychological follow up of 12 patients with neuro-Behçet's disease. *Journal of Neurology*, **246,** 113–19.

Olivieri, I., Salvarini, C. and Cantini, F. (1997). Is Behçet's disease part of the spondyloartritis complex? *Journal of Rheumatology*, **34,** 1870–1.

Orem, A., Vanizor, B., Cimsir, G., Kiran, E., Deger, O. and Malkoc, M. (1999). Decreased nitric oxide production in patients with Behçet's disease. *Dermatology*, **198,** 33–6.

Orloff, L. A. and Orloff, M. J. (1999). Budd-Chiari syndrome caused by Behçet's disease: treatment by side-to-side portocaval shunt. *Journal of the American College of Surgeons*, **188,** 396–407.

Ozarmagan, G., Saylan, T., Azizlerli, G., Ovul, C. and Aksungur, V. L. (1991). Re-evaluation of the pathergy test in Behçet's disease. *Acta Dermato-Venereologica*, **71,** 75–6.

Ozbakir, F., Yazici, H., Mat, C., Tuzun, Y., Yurdakul, S. and Yilmazer, S. (1987). HLA antigens in reccurrent oral ulcer: evidence against a common disease spectrum with Behçet's syndrome. *Clinical and Experimental Rheumatology*, **5,** 263–5.

Ozen, S., Karaaslan, Y., Ozdemir, O., *et al.*(1998). Prevalence of juvenile chronic arthritis and familial Mediterranean fever in Turkey: a field study. *Journal of Rheumatology*, **25,** 2445 –9.

Ozkan, M., Emel, O., Ozdemir, M., *et al.* (1992). M-mode, 2-D and Doppler echocardiographic study in 65 patients with Behçet's syndrome. *European Heart Journal*, **13,** 638–41.

Ozturk, M. A., Calguneri, M. and Kiraz, S. (2004), Angiotensin-converting enzyme gene polymorphism in Behçet's disease. *Clinical Rheumatology*, **23,** 142–6.

Ozyazgan, Y., Hamuryudan, V., Fresko, I., Yurdakul, S., Mat, C. and Yazici, H. (1996). Maintenance of visual acuity with combined cyclosporine A and azathioprine treatment among 141 Behçet syndrome patients with uveitis. In *4th International Symposium on Ocular Inflammation*, p. 150. Abstract Book, London, UK.

Ozyazgan, Y., Yurdakul, S., Yazici, H., *et al.* (1992). Low dose cylosporin A versus pulsed cyclophosphamide in Behçet's syndrome: a single masked trial. *British Journal of Ophthalmology*, **4,** 241–3.

Park, K. S., Min, K., Nam, J. H., Bang, D., Lee, E. S. and Lee, S. (2005). Association of HYPA haplotype in the mannose-binding lectin gene-2 with Behçet's disease. *Tissue Antigens*, **65,** 260–5.

Pazarli, H., Ozyazgan, Y., Bahcecioglu, H., *et al.* (1986). Ocular involvement in Behçet's syndrome in Turkey. In *Behçet's Disease,* vol. 103 (eds Lehner, T. and Barnes, C. G.), pp. 267–8. Royal Society of Medicine Services, London.

Poon, W., Verity, D. H., Larkin, G. L., Graham, E. M. and Stanford, M. R. (2003). Behçet's disease in patients of west African and Afro-Caribbean origin. *British Journal of Ophthalmology*, **87,** 876–8.

Postema, P. T., den Haan, P., van Hagen, P. M. and van Blankenstein, M. (1996). Treatment of colitis in Behçet's disease with thalidomide. *European Journal of Gastroenterology and Hepatology*, **8,** 929–31.

Saatci, I., Ozmen, M., Balkanci, F., Akhan, O. and Senaati, S. (1993). Behçet's disease in the etiology of Budd-Chiari disease. *Angiology*, **44,** 392–8.

Saip, S., Siva, A., Altintas, A., *et al.* (2005). Headache in Behçet's syndrome. *Headache*, **45,** 911–9.

Sallakci, N., Bacanli, A., Coskun, M., Yavuzer, U., Alpsoy, E. and Yegin, O. (2005). CTLA-4 gene 49A/G polymorphism in Turkish patients with Behçet's disease. *Clinical and Experimental Dermatology*, **30,** 546–50.

Salvarani, C., Boiardi, L., Casali, B., *et al.* (2004). Vascular endothelial growth factor gene polymorphisms in Behçet's disease. *Journal of Rheumatology*, **31,** 1785–9.

Saruhan-Direskeneli, G., Uyar, F. A., Cefle, A., *et al.* (2004). Expression of KIR and C-type lectin receptors in Behçet's disease. *Rheumatology* (Oxford), **43,** 423–7.

Saylan, T. (1997). Life story of Dr. Hulusi Behçet. *Yonsei Medical Journal*, **38,** 327–32.

Saylan, T., Mat, C., Fresko, I. and Melikoglu, M. (1999). Behçet's Disease in the Middle East. *Clinics in Dermatology*, **17,** 209–23.

Serdaroglu, P. (1998). Behçet's disease and nervous system. *Journal of Neurology*, **245,** 197–205.

Serdaroglu, P., Yazici, H., Ozdemir, C., Yurdakul, S., Bahar, S. and Aktin, E. (1989). Neurologic involvement in Behçet's syndrome. A prospective study. *Archives of Neurology*, **46,** 265–69.

Sfikakis, P. P., Theodossiadis, P. G., Katsiari, C. G., Kaklamanis, P. and Markomichelakis, N. N. (2001). Effect of infliximab on sight-threatening panuveitis in Behçet's disease. *Lancet*, **358,** 295–6.

Sharquie, K. E., Najim, R. A. and Abu-Raghif, A. R. (2002). Dapsone in Behçet's disease: a double-blind, placebo-controlled, cross-over study. *Journal of Dermatology*, **29,** 267–79.

Shi Hui-li and Huang-Zheng-ji (1993). Study on cutaneous lesions in Behçet's disease and meanings of relative laboratory parameters. In *Behçet's Disease. Proceedings of the 6th International Conference on Behçet's Disease* (eds Godeau, F. and Weschler, B.), p. 325. Excerpta Medica, Amsterdam.

Shimizu, T., Ehrlich, G. E., Inaba, G. and Hayashi, K. (1979). Behçet's disease. *Seminars in Arthritis and Rheumatism*, **8,** 223–60.

Shohat-Zabarski, R., Kalderon, S., Klein, T. and Weinberger, A. (1992). Close association of HLA–B5a in persons with recurrent aphtous stomatitis. *Oral Surgery, Oral Medicine and Oral Pathology*, **74,** 455–8.

Siva, A. and Yazici, H. (2004). Behçet's syndrome. In *Handbook of Systemic Autoimmune Diseases, Neurologic Involvement in Systemic Autoimmune Diseases* (eds Erkan, D. and Levine, S. R.), vol. 3, pp. 193–216. Elsevier, New York.

Siva, A., Altintas, A. and Saip, S. (2004). Behçet's syndrome and the nervous system. *Current Opinion in Neurology*, **17,** 347–57.

Sloper, C. M., Powell, R. J. and Dua, H. S. (1999). Tacrolimus (FK 506) in the treatment of posterior uveitis refractory to cylosporine. *Opthalmology*, **106,** 723–8.

Soy, M., Erken, E., Konca, K. and Ozbek, S. (2000). Smoking and Behçet's disease. *Clinical Rheumatology*, **19,** 508–9.

Soysal, M., Denizci, U., Alhan, S., *et al.* (1990). Splenic size in Behçet's syndrome. *British Journal of Rheumatology*, **29,** 497–8.

Stanford, M., Whittall, T., Bergmeier, L. A., *et al.* (2004). Oral tolerization with peptide 336–351 linked to cholera toxin B subunit in preventing relapses of uveitis in Behçet's disease. *Clinical and Experimental Immunology*, **137,** 201–8.

Sugioka, Y., Ohe, H. and Tanaka, T. (1966). Two cases of hip joint deformation associated with Behçet's syndrome. *Orthopedic Surgery and Traumatology*, **15,** 131.

Takeuchi, A., Kobayashi, K., Mori, M. and Mizushima, Y. (1981).The mechanism of hyperchemotaxis in Behçet's disease. *Journal of Rheumatology*, **8,** 40–4.

Takeuchi, A., Haraoka, H. and Hashimoto, T. (1989). Increased serum alkaline phosphatase activity in Behçet's disease. *Clinical and Experimental Rheumatology*, **7,** 19–21.

Tamer, L., Tursen, U. and Eskandari, G. (2005). N-acetyltransferase 2 polymorphisms in patients with Behçet's disease. *Clinical and Experimental Dermatology*, **30,** 56–60.

Tokay, S., Direskeneli, H., Yurdakul, S. and Akoglu, T. (2001). Anticardiolipin antibodies in Behçet's disease: a reassessment. *Rheumatology* (Oxford), **40,** 192–5.

Travis, S. P., Czajkowski, M., McGovern, D. P., Watson, R. G. and Bell, A. L. (2001). Treatment of intestinal Behçet's syndrome with chimeric tumour necrosis factor alpha antibody. *Gut*, **49,** 725–8.

Tugal-Tutkun, I., Onal, S., Altan-Yaycioglu, R., Huseyin Altunbas, H. and Urgancioglu, M. (2004). Uveitis in Behçet disease: an analysis of 880 patients. *American Journal of Ophthalmology*. **138,** 373–80.

Tugal-Tutkun, I., Mudun, A., Urgancioglu, M., *et al.* (2005). Efficacy of infliximab in the treatment of uveitis that is resistant to treatment with the combination of azathioprine, cyclosporine, and glucocorticoids in Behçet's disease: an open-label trial. *Arthritis and Rheumatism,* **52,** 2478–84.

Tunaci, A., Berkmen, Y. M. and Gokmen, E. (1995). Thoracic involvement in Behçet's disease: pathologic, clinical, and imaging features. *American Journal of Roentgenology,* **164,** 51–6.

Tunc, R., Keyman, E., Melikoglu, M., Fresko, I. and Yazici, H. (2002). Target organ associations in Turkish patients with Behçet's disease: a cross sectional study by exploratory factor analysis. *Journal of Rheumatology,* **29,** 2393–6.

Tunc, R., Uluhan, A., Melikoglu, M., Ozyazgan, Y., Ozdogan, H. and Yazici, H. (2001). A reassessment of the International Study Group criteria for the diagnosis (classification) of Behçet's syndrome. *Clinical and Experimental Rheumatology,* **19** (Suppl. 24), S45–7.

Tunc, R., Saip, S., Siva, A. and Yazici, H. (2004). Cerebral venous thrombosis is associated with major vessel disease in Behçet's syndrome. *Annals of the Rheumatic Diseases,* **63,** 1693–4.

Tursen, U., Tamer, L., Eskandari, G., *et al.* (2004a). Glutathione S-transferase polymorphisms in patients with Behçet's disease. *Archives for Dermatological Research,* **296,** 185–7.

Tursen, U., Eskandari, G., Kaya, T. I., Tamer, L., Ikizoglu, G. and Atik, U. (2004b). Apolipoprotein E polymorphism and lipoprotein compositions in patients with Behçet's disease. *International Journal of Dermatology,* **43,** 900–3.

Tuzun, B., Tuzun, Y., Yurdakul, S., Hamuryudan, V., Yazici, H. and Ozyazgan, Y. (1999). Neutrophil chemotaxis in Behçet's syndrome. *Annals of the Rheumatic Diseases,* **58,** 658.

Tuzun, H., Hamuryudan, V., Yildirim, S., *et al.* (1996). Surgical therapy of pulmonary arterial aneurysms in Behçet's syndrome. *Annals of Thoracic Surgery,* **61,** 733–5.

Tuzun, H., Besirli, K. and Sayin, A. (1997). Management of aneurysms in Behçet's syndrome: an analysis of 24 patients. *Surgery,* **121,** 150–6.

Tuzun, Y., Altac, M., Yazici, H., *et al.* (1980). Nonspecific skin hyperreactivity in Behçet's disease. *Haematologica,* **65,** 395–8.

Ural, A. U., Yalcin, A., Beyan, C., Isimer, A. and Bayhan, H. (1994). Plasma endothelin-1 concentrations in patients with Behçet's disease. *Scandinavian Journal of Rheumatology,* **23,** 322–5.

Uyar, F. A., Saruhan-Direskeneli, G. and Gul, A. (2004). Common Crohn's disease-predisposing variants of the CARD15/NOD2 gene are not associated with Behçet's disease in Turkey. *Clinical and Experimental Rheumatology,* **22** (Suppl. 34), S50–2.

Uziel, Y., Brik, R., Padeh, S., *et al.* (1998). Juvenile Behçet's disease in Israel. The Pediatric Rheumatology Study Group of Israel. *Clinical and Experimental Rheumatology,* **16,** 502–5.

Uzunoglu, S., Acar, H., Okudan, N., Gokbel, H., Mevlitoglu, I. and Sari, F. (2006). Evaluation of the association between null genotypes of glutathione-S-transferases and Behçet's disease. *Archives of Dermatology Research,* **297,** 289–93.

Yavuz, S., Fresko, I., Hamuryudan, V., Yurdakul, S. and Yazici, H. (1998). Fibromyalgia in Behçet's syndrome. *Journal of Rheumatology,* **25,** 2219–20.

Yazici, H. (1997). The place of Behçet's syndrome among the autoimmune diseases. *International Review of Immunology,* **14,** 1–10.

Yazici, H. and Fresko, I. (2005). Behçet's disease and other autoinflammatory conditions: what's in a name? *Clinical and Experimental Rheumatology,* **23** (Suppl. 38), S1–2.

Yazici, H., Tuzlaci, M. and Yurdakul, S. (1981a). A controlled survey of sacroiliitis in Behçet's disease. *Annals of the Rheumatic Disease,* **40,** 558–9.

Yazici, H., Tuzuner, N., Tuzun, Y. and Yurdakul, S. (1981b). Localized myositis in Behçet's disease. *Arthritis and Rheumatism,* **24,** 636.

Yazici, H., Tuzun, Y., Pazarli, H., *et al.* (1984a). Influence of age of onset and patient's sex on prevalence and severity of manifestations of Behçet's syndrome. *Annals of the Rheumatic Disease,* **43,** 783–9.

Yazici, H., Chamberlain, M. A., Tuzun, Y., Yurdakul, S. and Muftuoglu, A. (1984b). A comparative study of the pathergy among Turkish and British patients with Behçet's disease. *Annals of the Rheumatic Diseases,* **43,** 74–5.

Yazici, H., Tuzun, Y., Tanman, A. B., *et al.* (1985). Male patients with Behçet's syndrome have stronger pathergy reactions. *Clinical and Experimental Rheumatology,* **3,** 137–41.

Yazici, H., Tuzun, Y., Pazarli, H., *et al.* (1986). Sex factor and Behçet's syndrome. In *Recent Advances in Behcet's Disease* (eds Lehner, T., Barnes, C. G.), vol. 013, pp. 205–6. Royal Society of Medicine Services, London.

Yazici, H., Mat, C., Deniz, S., *et al.* (1987). Sebum production is increased in Behçet's syndrome and even more so in rheumatoid arthritis. *Clinical and Experimental Rheumatology,* **5,** 371–4.

Yazici, H., Pazarli, H., Barnes, C. G., *et al.* (1990). A controlled trial of azathioprine in Behçet's syndrome. *New England Journal of Medicine,* **322,** 281–5.

Yurdakul, S., Yazici, H., Tuzun, Y., *et al.* (1983). The arthritis of Behçet's disease: a prospective study. *Annals of the Rheumatic Disease,* **42,** 505–15.

Yurdakul, S., Gunaydin, I., Tuzun, Y., *et al.* (1988). The prevalence of Behçet's syndrome in a rural area in northern Turkey. *Journal of Rheumatology,* **15,** 820–2.

Yurdakul, S., Tuzuner, N., Yurdakul, I., Hamuryudan, V. and Yazici, H. (1990). Amyloidosis in Behçet's syndrome. *Arthritis and Rheumatism,* **33,** 1586–9.

Yurdakul, S., Tuzuner, N., Yurdakul, I., Hamuryudan, V. and Yazici, H. (1996). Gastrointestinal involvement in Behçet's syndrome: a controlled study. *Annals of the Rheumatic Diseases,* **55,** 208–10.

Yurdakul, S., Mat, C., Tuzun, Y., *et al.* (2001). A double blind trial of colchicine in Behçet's syndrome. *Arthritis and Rheumatism,* **44,** 2686–92.

Yurdakul, S., Hekim, N., Soysal, T., *et al.* (2005). Fibrinolytic activity and d-dimer levels in Behçet's syndrome. *Clinical and Experimental Rheumatology,* **23** (Suppl. 38), S53–8.

Zakaria, M., Sasaki, S., Matsui, Y., Shiiya, N., Murashita, T. and Yasuda, K. (1998). Successful repair of cardio-Behçet's disease with aortic and mitral regurgitation. *Journal of Cardiovascular Surgery,* **39,** 803–5.

Zierhut, M., Mizuki, N., Ohno, S., *et al.* (2003). Immunology and functional genomics of Behçet's disease. *Cellular and Molecular Life Sciences,* **60,** 1903–22.

Zouboulis, C. C., Djawari, D., Kirch, D., *et al.* (1996). Adamantiades-Behçet's disease in Germany: Data of the German Registry in 1996. *Revue de Rheumatism,* English Edition (abs.), **63,** 538.

CHAPTER 36

Juvenile Behçet's syndrome

Gülsevim Azizlerli

Introduction

Behçet's syndrome (BS) is a chronic, relapsing, multisystemic inflammatory disease of unknown etiology. It was first described in 1937 by Hulusi Behçet as a trisymptom complex comprised of oral and genital ulcerations and iridocyclitis with hypopyon (Behçet 1937). BS has been reported all over the world but has a distinct geographic distribution (Chapters 2 and 35). The prevalence of BS is much higher in countries along the ancient Silk Road, extending from Japan to the Mediterranean and Middle Eastern countries, including Turkey, than in northern Europe and the USA (Sakane et al. 1999; Verity et al. 1999). Field surveys in Turkey have found prevalence rates in the range of 8–42 /10,000 which ranks it as the country with the highest rate of BS in the world (Demirhindi et al. 1981; Yurdakul et al. 1988; Idil et al. 2002; Azizlerli et al. 2003) (see Chapter 35).

The prevalence of BS varies both between countries and between different regions of the same country. These regional differences are probably due to ethnic as well as geographical factors. The disease is rare in children. The term juvenile Behçet's syndrome (JBS) is applicable to those persons who fulfill the criteria for diagnosis before the age of 16. Of the 2334 Behçet's syndrome patients diagnosed according to International Study Group Criteria, and followed at the Behçet's Disease Outpatient Clinic in the Department of Dermatology of the University of Istanbul Medical Faculty, 62 had JBS (International Study Group for Behçet's Disease 1990). The prevalence of JBS in the Turkish series is 2.6% (62/2334), 1.6% in the Japanese report (42/2519) (Meada and Nakae 1977), and 3% in Iran (67/2175) (Shafaie et al. 1993). In another series from Turkey it was found to be 2% (44/1921) (Özdoğan 1996; Yurdakul et al. 1993). Kone-Paut and Bernard, in 1993, detected 17 JBS patients in an overall survey of 239 departments in France. Based on these reports, the prevalence of JBS is around 1.6–3% of BS patients. In the adult type, sex and age influence the course of the disease (Lang et al. 1990). The finding that the course is more aggressive in young males who develop the disease before age 25 has led to increased interest in the juvenile form of BS (Sarica et al. 1996; Yazici et al. 1984).

The clinical manifestations of the 62 JBS patients who are followed at the Turkish outpatient clinic are given in Table 36.1. The initial symptom encountered in 95.1% of patients is aphthous ulceration. Within a mean interval of 2.8 years, the second lesion appears, most commonly as genital ulceration. Systemic involvement ensues with a mean of 7.4 ± 6.2 (0–22) years after the detection of the initial symptom.

Compared with the clinical features of the adult BS, no difference was observed in oral–genital ulcerations, but erythema nodosum and pseudofolliculitis were more frequent in JBS. While extragenital ulceration occurred in 3% of adult BS patients, it is noteworthy that there was none in the JBS group. Arthritis and eye involvement was slightly more common in the JBS patients compared with the adult, but the difference was not significant. Epididymitis, neurologic signs, and deep vein thrombosis were more frequent in the JBS group than in the adult group. To evaluate the factors affecting the course of the disease, the patients were divided into two groups, one showing severe disease with systemic involvement, and the other with mild disease, mostly with mucocutaneous lesions. In the severe disease group, which comprised 21 patients, 13 were male and eight were female. In the mild disease group of 41 patients, 17 were male and 24 were female. In adult BS, male preponderance in systemic involvement is statistically significant; however, in the JBS group, there was no significant sex difference. In our 62 JBS patients, a mild course was observed in 66%, as it was in our adult patient group of 1127 individuals (Sarica et al. 1996). Although it has been reported that the disease begins within a wide age range, namely between age 2 and 16, most frequently the onset is around age 10–14. Twenty-six of our 62 JBS patients have been followed for 5–25 years. Results of evaluation with respect to mucocutaneous, ocular, arthritic, vascular, and CNS manifestations at consecutive 5-year intervals are shown in Table 36.2.

In the first 5-year period, JBS was observed to follow a predominantly mucocutaneous course (61.5%) similar to the adult type. Most ocular involvement, however, was observed within the first 5 years of the disease and was more common in males (36.3%) than in females (13.3%). Only one of the 26 patients had new ocular disease after the first 5-year period. In JBS patients with eye involvement, amaurosis developed within 2–3 years after onset in two of six patients. In the second 5-year period, 88.4% of the patients had only mucocutaneous lesions. Organ involvement was observed in 11.5% of patients (all of whom were male), including vascular and neurological involvement in one patient and arthritis in two patients. In the third 5-year follow-up period, 85.7% of the patients continued having a mild course with only mucocutaneous lesions,

Table 36.1 Clinical features of JBS and adult Behçet's syndrome in University of Istanbul, Faculty of Medicine, Dermatology Clinic 'Behçet's Disease Study Group'

Clinical feature	Adult BS (n = 1127) % of patients M = 610, F = 517	Juvenile BS (n = 62) % of patients M = 30, F = 32
Aphthous ulceration	100	100
Genital ulceration	87.4	85.4
Pseudofolliculitis	58.1	69.3
Erythema nodosum	45.9	69.3
Extragenital ulceration	3.1	0
Eye involvement	29.1	32.2
Arthritis	28.9	35.4
Superficial thrombophlebitis	15.8	12.9
Deep vein thrombosis	3.9	4.9
Epididymitis	2.5	4.8
Neurological involvement	3.0	6.4
Pulmonary involvement	2.1	1
GI symptoms	0.8	3.2
Pathergy positivity	74.6	82.3
HLA B5 positivity	82.4	73.3
Family history	6.1	11.0
Age of onset	27.2 ± 7.5 years (range 17–60)	11.3 ± 3.1 years (range 4–16)
Interval between first and second symptom	2.2 ± 3.8 years	2.8 ± 2.9 years

and 14% had organ involvement: eye and deep vein thrombosis (DVT) in one male and arthritis and DVT in one female. In the fourth 5-year period, there are data on only four males: three had only mucocutaneous involvement and one had pulmonary arteritis. In the fifth 5-year period, DVT developed in both male patients for whom there were data. In conclusion, vascular lesions in JBS, most frequently DVT, appear primarily in males after their transition from childhood to early adulthood, which is similar to adult BS. Arterial disease occurs in later years, and then only rarely. Thus, long-term surveillance indicates that JBS follows a clinical course with exacerbations and remissions, and with predominantly mucocutaneous involvement just as in the adult type.

Clinical manifestations

Mucocutaneous findings

As in the adult, the initial lesion in JBS is oral aphthae (see also Chapter 11). Minor aphthae are more frequent than major or herpetiform types. The mean interval between the first and second lesion is 2–3 years. Genital ulcerations, which reportedly have a predilection in females, are next in frequency. Reports from Iran assert that aphthae and genital ulcerations are infrequent in the JBS group compared with the adult group (Shafaie *et al.* 1993). Yurdakul *et al.* (1993) found that the frequency of genital ulceration is low in the prepubertal age group, increasing after puberty. Our data show no difference between JBS and adult BS in the frequency of genital ulcers. These commonly leave scars after healing (see Chapter 35). Others report that the most common signs of disease were mucocutaneous, with nearly the same frequency as in adults (Kone-Paut *et al.* 1998).

Other skin lesions

Pseudofolliculitis is encountered more in the JBS group and acneiform lesions develop mostly with puberty. Erythema nodosum occurs more often in the JBS group than in the adults. Extragenital aphthous-like ulcerations, which are seen in 3% of BS patients, develop in sites other than the genital region and also heal with scars (Azizlerli *et al.* 1992). In the JBS group no such lesion was

Table 36.2 Classification of 26 JBS cases in long-term follow-up according to clinical features and years

	Year 0–5		Year 5–10		Year 10–15		Year 15–20		Year 20–25	
	F=15	M=11	F=15	M=11	F=5	M=9	F=0	M=4	F=0	M=2
Mucocutaneous findings (genital ulceration and other skin findings)	11	5	15	8	4	8	–	3	–	–
Eye involvement	2	4	–	–	–	1[1]	–	–	–	–
Lose of useful visual acuity	1[1]	1[1]	–	–	–	–	–	–	–	–
Arthritis	2	2	–	2	1[1]	–	–	–	–	–
Vascular involvement										
Veins	–	–	–	1[1]	1[1]	1[1]	–	–	–	2
Arteries	–	–	–	–	–	–	–	Pulmonary	–	–
CNS involvement	–	–	–	1[1]	–	–	–	–	–	–
	15	11	15	11	5	9	0	4	0	2
Total number of patients	26		26		14		4		2	

[1] Indicates two different sites of involvement in the same patient.

encountered, so extragenital ulceration seems to be a specific feature of adult BS.

Eye involvement

Eye disease is one of the most serious afflictions of BS. In adult BS it is more frequent in males (Sarica *et al.* 1996), with a predominant onset in the first 5 years of disease. Its frequency is slightly higher in the JBS group than in adults, but the difference is not statistically significant. The frequency of uveitis in JBS is 14% in Tunisia, 47% in France, 31% in Iran, and 32.2% in our clinics (Table 36.3). Childhood-onset Behçet uveitis is more common among males. Bilateral panuveitis with retinal vasculitis and retinitis is reported to be the most common form of ocular involvement in the adult patient (Tugal-Tutkun *et al.* 2003).

Arthritis

Small joints of the hands and feet, knees, and elbows are the most common sites of arthritis. Arthritis is usually monoarticular, and articular destruction is seldom seen. There is no gender predilection. Arthritis is slightly more common in the JBS group than in adults: 35.4% versus 28.9%, respectively (Table 36.1). The proportion of patients with arthritis differs according to geographical region. It was reported to be 21% in Tunisia, 69% in France, and 13% in Iran (Hamza 1993; Kone-Paut and Bernard 1993; Shafaie *et al.* 1993).

Vascular involvement

Vasculitis involving veins, arteries, or both, is a serious prognostic sign and one of the main causes of death. Peripheral veins of the calf, superior and inferior vena cava, and hepatic veins may be involved, and more than one region may be diseased in the same patient. In one series, DVT was found in 4.9% of the patients, all of whom were male. In these patients, as well as in those from another group in Turkey and one in Tunisia, vascular involvement in JBS appears to be largely confined to males (Hamza 1993;

Yurdakul *et al.* 1993). There is no difference between JBS and adult BS with regard to frequency of superficial thrombophlebitis. DVT may sometimes be the first manifestation of this disease but is rare in children (Leiba *et al.* 2004). Moreover, arterial lesions typically seen as late-stage complications of adult BS have been observed in our JBS patients (Table 36.3). Overall, vascular complications are less frequent in children than in adults (Kone-Paut *et al.* 1998).

Gastrointestinal involvement

Gastrointestinal (GI) symptoms in JBS are abdominal pain and non-specific "gastric upset". Kone-Paut *et al.* reported in 1998 that GI involvement in children is rare and minor because severe iliocolitis has not been reported.

Central nervous system involvement

Central nervous system (CNS) disease is another leading cause of mortality in BS. Headache and symptoms attributable to raised intracranial pressure are typical. Two major forms of neurological disease seen in BS are CNS parenchymal involvement and cerebral venous sinus thrombosis. The frequency of neurological involvement in adult BS differs in different geographical regions (O'Neill *et al.* 1993): in northern America and Europe it is reported to be 10–25%, but in Turkey it is 3–5%. This differing prevalence in adult BS parallels the differences in JBS: it is 18% in France, and 6–7% in Turkey and Tunisia (Table 36.3). There was no difference in CNS involvement between the sexes in JBS, but frequency is 6.4% in JBS, compared with 3% of adult BS.

Other clinical manifestations

Another clinical feature which is more frequent in JBS than in the adult type is epididymitis (Table 36.1). Neither sex nor age seems to influence the frequency of pathergy. With the aforementioned exceptions, JBS and adult BS are similar in clinical features and clinical course; prepubertal onset of the disease has no deleterious effect on the course of the disease.

Table 36.3 Clinical features and systemic involvement of juvenile BS patients from five different centers

	France (n = 17)	Tunisia (n = 14)	Iran (n = 67)	Turkey (1st Med. Fac.) (n = 62)	Turkey (Cerrahpasa Med. Fac.) (n = 44)
Oral ulcers	94	100	77	100	100
Genital ulcers	53	60	26	85.4	70
Skin lesions	92	86	61	–	–
Pseudofolliculitis	–	71	–	69.3	77
Erythema nodosum	–	14	–	69.3	59
Eye involvement	47	14	31	32.2	48
Arthritis	69	21	13	35.4	34
CNS involvement	18	7	–	6.4	6
Vascular involvement	6	33	–	4.8	12
Pathergy	60	65	–	82.3	68
HLA B5	54	30	–	73.3	52

Numbers shown are percentages of patients. Dashes indicate findings that were not identified.

Immunogenetics

Familial aggregation has been well documented in Behçet's syndrome, and the sibling recurrence risk ratio for BS was found to be between 11.4 and 52.5 in Turkey (Gul et al. 2000). Analysis of a small group of multicase families did not show any particular Mendelian inheritance pattern (Bird 1986). HLA-B51 has been the strongest genetic association described so far with BS; however, genetic analysis of multicase families suggested that the contribution of the HLA–B locus to the overall genetic susceptibility to BS (λ_{HLA}) is less than 20% (Gul et al. 2001). In 30 patients, HLA-B5 was found in 22 (73.3%); the majority were in the mild disease group (18/22).

Management

Colchicine is effective in the treatment of erythema nodosum, arthritis, and genital ulcerations. Local application of antiseptic solutions and topical glucocorticoids, combined with periodontal care, reduces the frequency of aphthous lesions. Systemic glucocorticoids alone or combined with immunosuppressive drugs can be used (see Chapter 35).

References

Azizlerli, G., Özarmagan, G., Övül, C., et al. (1992). A new kind of skin lesion in Behçet's disease. Extragenital ulcerations. *Acta Dermatologica Venerologica*, **72**, 286.

Azizlerli, G., Akdag Köse, A., Sarica, R., et al. (2003). Prevalence of Behçet's disease in Istanbul, Turkey. *International Journal of Dermatology*, **42**, 803–6.

Behçet, H. (1937). Über rezidivierende apthöse, durch ein Virus verursachte Geschwüre am Mund, am Auge, und an dem Genitalien. *Dermatologische Wochenschrift*, **105**, 1152–7.

Bird, S. J. A.(1986). Genetic analysis of families of patients with Behçet's syndrome: Data incompatible with autosomal recessive inheritance. *Annals of the Rheumatic Diseases*, **45**, 265–8.

Demirhindi, O., Yazıcı, H., Binyildiz, P., et al. (1981). Silivri Fener Köyü ve yöresinde Behçet Hastalığı sıklığı ve bu hastalığın toplum içinde taranmasında kullanılabilecek bir yöntem. *Cerrahpaşa Tıp Dergisi*, **12**, 509–14.

Gul, A., Inanc, M., Ocal, L., Aral, O. and Konice, M. (2000). Familial aggregation of Behçet's disease in Turkey. *Annals of the Rheumatic Diseases*, **59**, 622–5.

Gul, A., Hajeer, A. H., Worthington, J., Barrett, J. H., Ollier, W. E. and Silman, A. J. (2001). Evidence for linkage of the HLA–B locus in Behçet's disease, obtained using the transmission disequilibrium test. *Arthritis and Rheumatism*, **44**, 239–40.

Hamza, M. (1993). Juvenile Behçet's disease. In *Behçet's disease* (eds Godeau, P. and Wechsler, B.), pp. 337–80. Elsevier, Amsterdam.

Idil, A., Gurler, A., Boyvat, A., et al. (2002). The prevalence of Behçet's disease above the age of 10 years. The results of a pilot study conducted at the Park Primary Health Care Center in Ankara, Turkey. *Opthalmic Epidemiology*, **9**, 325–31.

International Study Group for Behçet's Disease (1990). Criteria for diagnosis of Behçet's disease. *Lancet*, **335**, 1078–80.

Kone-Paut, I. and Bernard, J. L. (1993). Behçet's disease in children. A French nation wide survey. In *Behçet's disease* (eds Godeau, P. and Wechsler, B.), pp. 385–9. Elsevier, Amsterdam.

Kone-Paut, I., Yurdakul, S., Bahabri, S. A., et al. (1998). Clinical features of Behçet's disease in children: An international collaborative study of 86 cases. *Journal of Pediatrics*, **132**, 721–5.

Lang, B. A., Laxer, R. M., Thorner, P., Greenberg, M. and Silverman, E. D. (1990). Pediatric onset of Behçet's syndrome with myositis. Case report and literature review illustrating unusual features. *Arthritis and Rheumatism*, **33**, 418–25.

Leiba, M., Seligsohn, U., Sidi, Y., et al. (2004). Thrombophilic factors are not the leading cause of thrombosis in Behçet's disease. *Annals of the Rheumatic Diseases*, **63**, 1445–9.

Maeda, K. and Nakae, K. (1977). Recent epidemiological review on Behçet's disease in Japan. *Asian Medical Journal*, **20**, 568–82.

O' Neill, T. W., Rigby, A. S., McHugh, S., Silman, A. J. and Barnes, C. on behalf of the International Study Group for Behçet's Disease (1993). Regional differences in clinical manifestations of Behçet's disease. In *Behçet's disease* (eds Godeau, P. and Wechsler, B.), pp. 159–63. Elsevier, Amsterdam.

Özdoğan, H. (1996). Behçet's syndrome in children. In *Vasculitides* (eds Ansell, B. M., Bacon, P. A., Lie, J. T. and Yazici, H.), pp. 419–24. Chapman and Hall, London.

Sakane, T., Takeno, M., Suzuki, N. and Inaba, G. (1999). Behçet's disease. *New England Journal of Medicine*, **341**, 1284–91.

Sarica, R., Azizlerli, G., Akdag Köse, A., et al. (1996). The course of disease activity among 1127 Turkish adult Behçet's patient. In *Behçet's disease 7th Congress on Behçet's Disease Proceedings* (ed. Haniza, M.), pp. 157–9. Adhoua, Tunis.

Shafaie, N., Shahram, F., Davatchi, F., et al. (1993). Behçet's disease in children. In *Behçet's disease* (eds Godeau, P. and Wechsler, B.), pp. 385–9. Elsevier, Amsterdam.

Tugal-Tutkun, I. and Urgancıogu, M., (2003). Childhood-onset uveitis in Behçet's disease: a descriptive study of 36 cases. *American Journal of Ophthalmology*, **136**, 1114–9.

Verity, D. H., Marr, J. E., Ohno, S., Wallace, G. R., Stanford, M. R.(1999). Behçet's disease, the Silk Road and HLA-B51: historical and geographical perspectives. *Tissue Antigens*, **54**, 213–20.

Yazici, H., Tüzün, Y., Pazarli, H., et al. (1984). Influence of age of onset and patient's sex on the prevalence and severity of manifestations of Behçet's syndrome. *Annals of the Rheumatic Diseases*, **83**, 783–9.

Yurdakul, S., Günaydın, I., Tüzün, Y., et al. (1988). The prevalence of Behçet's syndrome in a rural area in northern Turkey. *Journal of Rheumatology*, **15**, 820–2.

Yurdakul, S., Özdogan, H., Kasapçopur, Ö., et al. (1993). Behçet's syndrome with juvenile onset: Report of 44 patients. *Clinical and Experimental Rheumatology*, **11**, 71.

CHAPTER 37

Vasculitis of the central nervous system

Leonard H. Calabrese and George F. Duna

Introduction

Vasculitis affecting the central nervous system (CNS) remains one of the most elusive forms of vascular inflammatory disease. Factors contributing to our relative lack of understanding of CNS vasculitis include its rarity, the lack of an efficient, non-invasive test, a paucity of pathologic material to study, and the absence of animal models simulating the disease. Despite these limitations, the past 15 years have witnessed significant progress in our understanding of the clinical heterogeneity of these disorders and their subclassification into clinical subsets.

Vasculitis affecting the CNS can be classified into primary and secondary forms. Primary angiitis of the CNS (PACNS) is vasculitis confined to the CNS, including brain and spinal cord and their coverings. Secondary vasculitis of the CNS implies vascular inflammation of CNS as part of a larger process such as an infection, connective tissue disease, drug reaction, or other systemic disorder. This chapter will outline the epidemiologic, clinical, diagnostic, and therapeutic aspects of both primary and secondary forms of CNS vasculitis.

Primary angiitis of the CNS (PACNS)

Classification and diagnostic criteria

The modern era of PACNS began in the late 1950s with the elegant descriptive report of a few patients with an isolated, progressive, fatal form of vasculitis affecting the CNS (Cravioto and Feigin 1959). Upon pathologic examination of these cases all were found to be granulomatous in nature, leading to the alternative term granulomatous angiitis of the CNS (GACNS). Following this early description, others were slow to be reported, with less than 40 total cases by the mid 1980s (Calabrese and Mallek 1988). With the advent of cerebral angiography as a diagnostic tool for vasculitis, combined with its spreading clinical application, a flurry of new case reports was published in the mid to late 1980s; many of these lacked pathologic confirmation. Cases diagnosed solely on angiographic grounds were considered clinically equivalent to those documented on the basis of ante-mortem biopsy, with both representing examples of a progressive, fatal form of granulomatous arteritis. In the early 1980s, a small series of PACNS, successfully treated with a combination of cyclophosphamide and glucocorticoids, increased the enthusiasm for diagnosing PACNS. It became standard practice to treat all cases aggressively with this combination of drugs regardless of the method of diagnosis or clinical picture (Cupps et al. 1983). In the mid 1990s, several investigators noted that not all cases of PACNS appeared to have the inexorable and fatal course of those reported earlier and they proposed that benign variants may exist (Hankey 1991; Calabrese et al. 1993). Many of these benign variants have recently been demonstrated to be secondary to a reversible cerebral angiopathy and not vasculitis (Singhal 2004a). Finally, variants of PACNS have been described including those associated with cerebral amyloid, lymphoproliferative diseases, and unusual or novel infections (Calabrese et al. 1997).

In 1988, Calabrese and Mallek proposed three working criteria for the diagnosis of PACNS (Calabrese and Mallek 1988). Despite changes in our view of PACNS, particularly with the appreciation of its broadening clinical spectrum and the increasing number of mimics, these criteria still serve as a useful starting place for classification. The criteria are:

1. a history of a clinical finding of an acquired neurologic deficit that remains unexplained after a thorough, initial basic evaluation;

2. either classic (high probability) angiographic evidence or histopathologic demonstration of angiitis within the CNS;

3. no evidence of systemic vasculitis or any other condition to which the angiographic or pathologic condition could be attributed (see Table 37.1).

While these criteria can be used to secure a diagnosis of PACNS, further categorization into one of several currently recognizable, clinical subsets is essential to determine prognosis and prescribe optimal therapy. Among the clinical forms of PACNS, a few may represent distinct nosologic entities, for example granulomatous angiitis of the CNS (GACNS) and amyloidosis, with distinct histology and possibly unique pathobiology. Other subsets may merely represent alternative but clinically important clinical presentations (spinal cord, mass lesion), warranting specialized clinical approaches to diagnosis or treatment which justifies their distinction. Finally, as our knowledge increases, new forms, such as that sharing the complex relationship with varicella zoster virus (VZV) infection, may in the future more appropriately be viewed as secondary disease.

Table 37.1 Conditions resembling PACNS excluded by the preliminary diagnostic criteria (adapted from Calabrese 1995)

Systemic vasculitides
 Polyarteritis nodosa
 Allergic granulomatosis
 Hypersensitivity vasculitis (cutaneous leukocytoclastic vasculitis) and
  related disorders
 Vasculitis of connective tissue diseases
 Wegener's granulomatosis
 Giant cell arteritis
 Takayasu's arteritis
 Behçet's syndrome
 Lymphomatoid granulomatosis
 Cogan's syndrome

Infections
 Viral
 Bacterial
 Fungal
 Rickettsial

Neoplasms
 Angioimmunoproliferative disorders
 Carcinomatous meningitis
 Infiltrating glioma
 Malignant angioendotheliomatosis

Drug use
 Amphetamines
 Ephedrine
 Phenylpropanolamine
 Cocaine
 Ergotamine

Vasospastic disorders
 Postpartum angiopathy
 Eclampsia
 Pheochromocytoma
 Subarachnoid hemorrhage
 Migraine and exertional headache

Other vasculopathies and mimicking conditions
 Fibromuscular dysplasia
 Moyamoya disease
 Thrombotic thrombocytopenic purpura
 Sickle cell anemia
 Neurofibromatosis
 Cerebrovascular atherosclerosis
 Demyelinating disease
 Sarcoidosis
 Emboli (subacute bacterial endocarditis, cardiac myxoma,
  paradoxical emboli)
 Acute posterior placoid pigment epitheliopathy and cerebral vasculitis
 Antiphospholipid antibody syndrome
 Susac's syndrome (encephalopathy, branch retinal artery occlusions and
  sensorineural hearing loss)
 MELAS (mitochondrial myopathy, encephalopathy, lactic acidosis and
  stroke-like episodes)
 CADASIL (cerebral autosomal dominant arteriopathy with subcortical
  infarcts and leukoencephalopathy)

Clinical subsets

Granulomatous angiitis of the CNS (GACNS)

Clinical manifestations

While there are no formal diagnostic criteria established for GACNS, the essential features of this syndrome are outlined in Table 37.2. Within the spectrum of PACNS, it is difficult to estimate the percentage of patients who fulfill these criteria since they have not been applied prospectively to any large series of patients. We estimate that no more than one-third of patients diagnosed would fulfill such criteria.

The epidemiology of the disease is poorly understood, but it does appear to be a male-predominant disorder occurring at virtually any age (Calabrese *et al.* 1997; Calabrese and Duna 1995; Younger *et al.* 1997). In 1997, Younger and colleagues (Younger *et al.* 1997) reviewed the cumulative literature on GACNS and analyzed 136 reported cases and one new case. Fifty-one of these patients had associated conditions including lymphoproliferative diseases, VZV infection, amyloidosis, sarcoidosis, or one of several other conditions. Whether such cases are equivalent to GACNS occurring *de novo* is unknown, but this analysis remains the basis of much of the clinical appreciation for this relatively rare disorder.

The most common clinical manifestations in GACNS are headache and mental changes. These features generally evolve over weeks to months and are followed by focal cerebral signs including seizure, aphasia, hemiparesis, or tetraparesis in the vast majority of patients. Thus, the combination of focal and non-focal neurologic dysfunction remains the hallmark of GACNS.

The onset of GACNS may occasionally be acute, but is more commonly subacute. While fulminant presentations have been reported, an insidious onset is much more common. Neurologic signs and symptoms may predate the diagnosis by months or even years. Curiously, headache, the most common symptom, may be extraordinarily severe or relatively mild. The headache may wax and wane, with periods of prolonged symptom-free remission unassociated with therapy (Calabrese 1995). A variety of less common clinical manifestations of GACNS have also been reported, including cranial neuropathies, visual changes, ataxia, and coma. Patients with GACNS may rarely present with cerebral hemorrhage. As noted, non-focal neurologic deficits are characteristic of this

Table 37.2 Key features of GACNS

Clinical
 Variable onset but most frequently a prolonged prodrome of 3–6 or
  more months
 Mixture of focal and non-focal neurologic signs
 CSF analysis abnormal in 90% (aseptic meningitis findings)

Radiographic
 Neuroimaging reveals signs of multifocal ischemia of varying ages
 Variable presence of leptomeningeal enhancement
 Angiography normal in approximately 40%; high probability in 40%

Pathology
 Vasculitis of small and medium vessels of leptomeninges and underlying
  cortex with variable degrees of granulomatous changes
 Giant cells may or may not be present

Exclusions
 Diseases and conditions in Table 37.1

disorder and include an acute or subacute encephalopathy (Scolding *et al.* 1997) which rarely may manifest as dementia alone. A decreasing or fluctuating level of consciousness is more common, however. A pseudo-multiple sclerosis like presentation has also been described (Scolding *et al.* 1997). The signs and symptoms of systemic vasculitis such as fever, weight loss, peripheral neuropathy, and visceral end-organ dysfunction are only rarely part of GACNS. Wasting and low grade fever may be observed following prolonged neurologic dysfunction, but these are not part of the primary disorder.

Diagnostic studies

Diagnostic studies for GACNS include routine laboratory testing, cerebral spinal fluid analysis (CSF), neuroimaging studies, cerebral angiography, and biopsy of CNS tissues. Screening laboratory studies performed on blood have little positive predictive value since there are no tests of sufficient specificity to secure a diagnosis but various tests for chemistries, autoantibodies, and cultures, and other investigations are useful for ruling out the conditions listed in Table 37.1.

Examination of the cerebral spinal fluid (CSF) is extremely important. It is essential to help exclude other conditions such as malignancy and infection, and it is abnormal in 80–90% of patients with GACNS. The characteristic CSF findings are those of elevated protein and pleocytosis. The white count is rarely over 250 cells/mm³ and protein rarely exceeds 500 mg % (Calabrese *et al.* 1992a; Younger *et al.* 1997). Neuroimaging studies are important in the diagnostic process, but CT, MRI, and MRA are insufficiently specific to establish the diagnosis of GACNS. MRI is more sensitive than CT and is the preferred diagnostic imaging technique when acute cerebral hemorrhage is suspected. The most common MRI findings in GACNS as well as other forms of PACNS are those of multifocal cerebral ischemia. These include multiple bilateral infarcts with lesions in the cortex, deep white matter, and leptomeninges (Greenan *et al.* 1992; Pierot *et al.* 1991; Hurst and Grossman 1994). Enhancement, particularly of the leptomeninges, may be variably observed and serves to increase the sensitivity of a biopsy guided to this region (Cheng *et al.* 1994). Occasionally, GACNS may appear as diffuse white matter disease mimicking primary demyelinating diseases (Finelli *et al.* 1997). Collectively, abnormalities of CSF or MRI are noted in close to 100% of patients. Thus, when normal, these studies generate a high negative predictive value, making the diagnosis of GACNS, but not other forms of PACNS, unlikely (Stone *et al.* 1994).

Angiography has a limited role in the diagnosis of GACNS. The angiogram may be normal in up to 40% of patients with GACNS and non-specific in another 20% (Calabrese *et al.* 1992b). A high probability angiogram, defined as multiple areas of stenosis and ectasia in multiple vascular beds, may be seen in up to 40% of cases, although the specificity of this finding has been clearly demonstrated to be low for the diagnosis of any form of PACNS (Duna and Calabrese 1995; Kadkhodayan *et al.* 2004; Chu *et al.* 1998).

The gold standard for the diagnosis of GACNS is biopsy of CNS affected tissue. GACNS is defined in large part by its histopathology (Lie 1992). The gross neuropathologic findings in GACNS consist of multiple small foci of infarction or hemorrhage, but occasionally larger areas have been involved. Microscopically, GACNS is a segmental necrotizing and granulomatous vasculitis of the small- and medium-sized arteries, predominantly in the leptomeninges and cortex. Veins are affected in about half of the cases. The predominant inflammatory cell is the small lymphocyte with an admixture of epithelioid cells, plasma cells, macrophages, and giant cells of both the Langhans and foreign body types. Not all of these features are present in all patients, and the abnormalities have a patchy distribution throughout the CNS. Frank, well-formed granulomas may be seen, but are relatively rare (Figure 37.1). More commonly, there is loose granuloma formation with giant cells (Figure 37.2). Lastly, up to 20% of cases are lymphocytic forms without prominent granulomatous features. Whether these represent true GACNS is unknown, but most patients have other clinical and demographic features of the subset and thus should be considered to have a GACNS variant.

When biopsy is performed, it should include both brain and leptomeninges. The preferred site for brain biopsy is the temporal tip of the non-dominant hemisphere in an area with a longitudinally oriented surface vessel (Parisi and Moore 1994). An infratentorial approach should be strongly considered in patients suspected of having conditions such as tuberculosis or sarcoidosis, which preferentially involve the basilar meninges (Gripshover and Ellner 1998). A normal or non-diagnostic biopsy may be encountered in up to one-fourth of the patients (Younger *et al.* 1997), limiting the diagnostic accuracy of this test. Reasons for a non-diagnostic biopsy include failure to sample both cortex and leptomeninges and the patchy distribution of lesions. Most importantly, it must be realized that the biopsy serves not only to establish the diagnosis of GACNS, but also to rule out other forms of inflammatory infiltrative, infective, and neoplastic diseases which may mimic PACNS in clinical presentation (see Chapter 45). Biopsy can be performed with minimal morbidity and should be urged in all cases where combined glucocorticoid and cytotoxic therapy is being considered.

Diagnosis and differential diagnosis

The diagnosis of GACNS is most commonly considered in a patient with an unexplained neurologic event and CSF findings consistent with chronic meningitis. The differential diagnosis of this problem is lengthy and complex. Many of the conditions that need to be considered are found in Table 37.1 and include infectious,

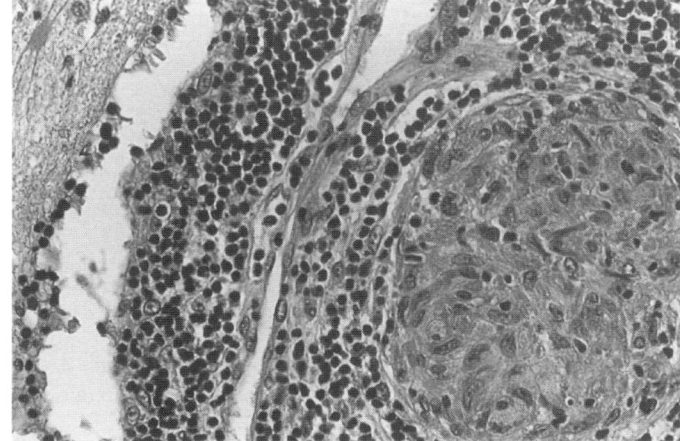

Figure 37.1 Marked mononuclear inflammatory infiltrates in cortical vessel with a well formed paravascular granuloma (Hematoxylin and eosin stain, magnification × 200). (Reprinted with permission from Calabrese 1995.)

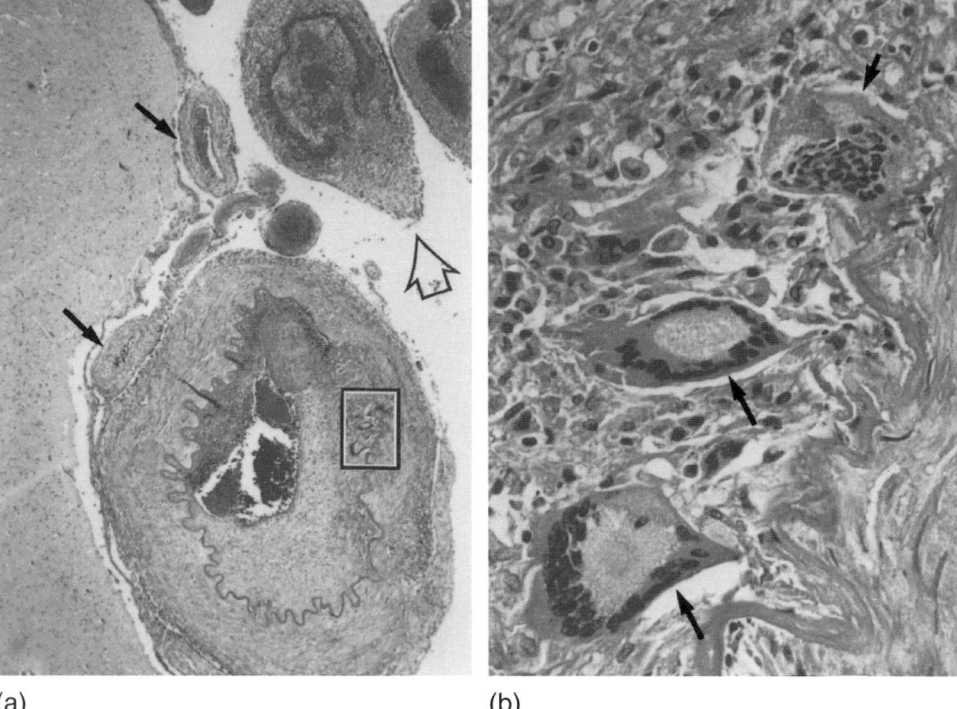

Figure 37.2 (a) Brain biopsy findings of granulomatous vasculitis in PACNS side by side with a polyarteritis nodosa-type necrotizing vasculitis (open arrow) and two normal arterioles (short arrows). (b) Close-up showing foreign body (short arrows) and Langhans' (long arrow) giant cells in the granulomatous inflammation. (Hematoxylin and eosin stain, magnification × 64 and × 400). (Reprinted with permission from Calabrese *et al.* 1997.)

(a)   (b)

neoplastic, and inflammatory diseases. In general we have found that even in a highly biased referral practice, the majority of patients suspected of having some form of PACNS who actually come to angiography or brain biopsy are found eventually to have another condition (Villa-Forte *et al.* 1998). Thus, a team approach including experts in both inflammatory and non-inflammatory vascular diseases, infectious diseases, neuroradiology, neuropathology, and neurosurgery is desirable.

Evaluations for suspected GACNS should be individualized, but several underlying principles deserve emphasis. Infections are the most important category of illness to exclude. Infections occasionally associated with PACNS, and of particular importance since they may be overlooked, are those due to HIV, *Borrelia burgdorferi*, and varicella zoster viruses (VZV). As discussed below, VZV may confound the diagnosis of GACNS since it may co-occur with histologically documented vasculitis in the absence of preceding or concurrent clinical infection (Gilden *et al.* 1996, 2000). If after a careful exclusionary process the diagnosis of GACNS is still a serious consideration, we favor CNS biopsy over angiography as the next step, given the non-specificity and low positive predictive value of the latter (Gilden *et al.* 1996, 2000). The importance of the biopsy is not only to secure the diagnosis of GACNS, but also to rule out the many mimicking conditions noted in Table 37.1 (Kadkhodayan *et al.* 2004; West 2003).

Treatment and prognosis

There are no controlled clinical trials in GACNS. Therapeutic guidelines are informal and have been based upon a collective experience suggesting that GACNS is progressive and uniformly fatal if untreated (Calabrese *et al.* 1997). More recent reviews of this topic have questioned whether this observation is accurate. These indicate that the reported mortality reflect historical bias, with the majority of untreated cases discovered at post-mortem

examination (Calabrese *et al.* 1997; Younger *et al.* 1997). Younger and colleagues (Younger *et al.* 1997) analyzed outcome in 50 reported cases and noted that 70% of patients treated with glucocorticoids with or without cyclophosphamide survived, although often with significant sequelae. We believe that the majority of patients with documented GACNS should be treated with combined therapy, at least initially, until the disease has been controlled. Attempts should then be made to limit exposure to the alkylating agent by either discontinuation or switching to an antimetabolite such as methotrexate or azathioprine (Calabrese *et al.* 1997). A total treatment period of 6–12 months is usual. All patients should receive prophylaxis for *Pneumocystis carinii* infection (see Table 32.7 in Chapter 32) (Calabrese 1997b).

Following disease activity in GACNS can be problematic. Clinical symptoms and signs may be slow to change as in any ischemic insult to the brain. MRI changes should improve, but are likely to leave residual scar. In our experience, improvement in CSF abnormalities is a useful indication of decreased activity, and should be documented after 8–12 weeks. Following clinical stability, serial MRI examinations at 3–6 month intervals should be performed during the tapering phase of immunosuppressive therapy. Relapses do occur and may appear after many years of clinical stability. As with long-term treatment of any vasculitis with immunosuppressive drugs, vigilance to reduce treatment-related morbidity from infections, osteoporosis, and other complications is of paramount importance (Calabrese *et al.* 1997).

Reversible cerebral vasoconstrictive syndromes (RCVS) (formerly benign angiopathy of the CNS)
Clinical manifestations

Perhaps the greatest single advance in CNS vasculitis has been recognition that the most common clinical mimic (angiographic mimic) of PACNS is reversible cerebral segmental vasoconstriction or vasospasm, now referred to under the heading of reversible cerebral vasoconstrictive syndromes (RCVS) (Calabrese *et al.* 2007). These include a group of conditions all sharing similar reversible vasoconstriction and each presenting with angiographic findings indistinguishable from CNS arteritis.

The evolution of our current understanding of RCVS has been impeded by: (1) a lack of a clear underlying pathologic basis; (2) a diagnosis reliant on non-specific clinical and radiographic abnormalities; and (3) a lack of a consensus definition. Furthermore, patients with RCVS have historically presented to different specialists such as neurologists, headache specialists, obstetricians, and rheumatologists, depending on their symptoms. These investigators have imparted their own biases in nomenclature, theories of pathogenesis, and clinical approaches. Only in recent years have investigators (Singhal 2004a; Calabrese *et al.* 2007) begun to define the unifying features of those disorders that we now consider under the umbrella of RCVS.

In the field of neurology the concept of cerebral vasospasm has long been understood in the setting of delayed vasoconstriction following subarachnoid hemorrhage, and in rare patients described with what was once thought of as migranous vasospasm (Solomon *et al.* 1990). In 1988, Call and colleagues reported 19 patients with "reversible cerebral arterial segmental vasoconstriction syndrome" (Call *et al.* 1988). These patients were predominantly women who had acute headaches with or without focal neurologic deficits, occurring either spontaneously or in association with a variety of conditions, such as vasoactive drug exposure, trauma, and others. CSF analysis was largely benign. While the pathophysiology was unknown, migranous vasospasm (vasospasm secondary to migraine headache) was considered likely. The eponym Call–Fleming syndrome has endured in neurology and is still applied to patients with reversible cerebral vasoconstriction (Nowak *et al.* 2003).

In rheumatology, the 1970s witnessed an increasing use of cerebral angiography for the diagnosis of PACNS in the absence of confirming histopathology (Calabrese *et al.* 1997). It is of interest that many of these patients with RCVS documented by angiography were women who had benign outcomes and normal or near normal CSF. In 1993, Calabrese and co-workers (Calabrese *et al.* 1993) reviewed these cases and proposed the term "benign angiopathy of the central nervous system (BACNS)" to define a subset of patients with PACNS defined on the basis of their acute presentation, angiographic abnormalities, normal spinal fluid examinations, and monophasic course. While patients fitting this picture often had favorable outcomes and thus were benign (Snyder and McClelland 1978; Serdaru *et al.* 1984; Bettoni *et al.* 1984) compared to those PACNS patients with the granulomatous variant, BACNS patients could also have more severe outcomes such as stroke. The term "angiopathy" was employed to emphasize that in the absence of histopathologic confirmation there was considerable uncertainty with regards to vessel wall status. When PACNS was last reviewed in *Arthritis and Rheumatism* (Calabrese *et al.* 1997), BACNS was thought to be an angiographically diagnosed variant of PACNS; its pathophysiology was unknown and it was presumed to be due possibly to a reversible vasoconstrictive process among others. It is now clear that BACNS and Call–Fleming syndrome are indistinguishable and likely represent the same disorder.

Hajj-Ali *et al.* (2002) reported that, in a series of 16 similar patients studied serially by neurovascular imaging, there was dramatic resolution of angiographic abnormalities in 4 to 12 weeks without intensive immunosuppressive therapy. Several of these patients received either calcium channel blockers alone or were merely observed. In two patients biopsies were obtained, revealing no evidence of vasculitis. Based upon these data it became increasingly apparent that for most patients presenting with what was recognized as BACNS the underlying vascular lesion was reversible vasoconstriction rather than arteritis.

Similar cases of RCVS have been described in the obstetrical literature under the labels postpartum angiopathy (Bogousslavsky *et al.* 1989; Janssens *et al.* 1995; Kubo *et al.* 2002; Ihara *et al.* 2000; Geocadin *et al.* 2002; Konstantinopoulos *et al.* 2004; Song *et al.* 2004; Calado *et al.* 2004; Singhal 2004b), postpartum angiitis (Farine *et al.* 1984), benign isolated angiitis of the CNS (Sugiyama *et al.* 1997), puerperal vasospasm (Geraghty *et al.* 1991), and PACNS (Calabrese and Mallek 1988). More recently, a similar disorder has also been described in the setting of idiopathic "thunderclap headache", an intense, rapidly progressive headache which generally leads to a negative evaluation for subarachnoid hemorrhage. RCVS can be seen as a consequence of exposure to vasoactive agents such as cocaine, amphetamines, ephedrine, pseudoephedrine, phenylpropanolamine, or other drugs (Henry *et al.* 1984; Janssens *et al.* 1995; Levine *et al.* 1987; Merkel *et al.* 1995; Singhal *et al.* 2002, 2004a). Finally, a syndrome resembling RCVS has also been described in various other settings, such as: the presence of catecholamine-secreting tumors (Nighoghossian *et al.* 1998; Razavi *et al.* 1999); the period after trauma; after vascular manipulation or neurosurgical procedures (Chang *et al.* 1999; Hyde-Rowan *et al.* 1983; LeRoux *et al.* 1991; Schaafsma *et al.* 2002; Singhal 2004a); the presence of hypercalcemia (where activation of vascular smooth muscle has been documented) (Kaplan 1998; Yamamoto *et al.* 1999); acute porphyria (Hinchey *et al.* 1996); and following therapy with intravenous immunoglobulin (Sztajzel *et al.* 1999; Voltz *et al.* 1996). In several of these conditions, the pathophysiologic link to reversible vasoconstriction remains unclear. Diagnostic criteria for RCVS have recently been proposed (Calabrese *et al.* 2007) (Table 37.3).

Differentiating RCVS from GACNS

The differentiation of RCVS from GACNS is of vital clinical importance since their therapies differ greatly; patients with RCVS can be spared immunosuppression. The differentiation of these disorders

Table 37.3 Key features of reversible cerebral vasoconstrictive syndromes (RCVS)

A diagnosis of RCA requires all of following criteria:

1. A severe and acute headache with or without other associated neurologic signs and symptoms
2. No evidence of aneurismal subarachnoid hemorrhage
3. Normal or near normal cerebrospinal fluid analysis
   a. Protein <70 mg%
   b. White blood cell count <20 cells per/mm^3
   c. Normal glucose
   d. No evidence of subarachnoid hemorrhage
4. Reversible cerebral segmental vasoconstriction involving arteries of Circle of Willis (see Figure 37.3)
   a. Documented by serial angiography, CT, or MR angiography or flow-related vascular technique (transcranial Doppler) within 12 weeks after onset

Table 37.4 Comparison of GACNS and RCVS

	GACNS	RCVS
Sex predominance	Male 3:2	Female 2:1
Onset	Long prodrome; 3–6 months	Acute; hours to days
Symptoms and signs	Chronic headache, focal, and non-focal	Headache and/or focal event
CSF analysis	Chronic meningitis findings	Normal
Angiogram	Normal in 40%, high probability in 50%	High probability >95%
Biopsy	Arteritis in leptomeninges and/or cortex in 75–80%	

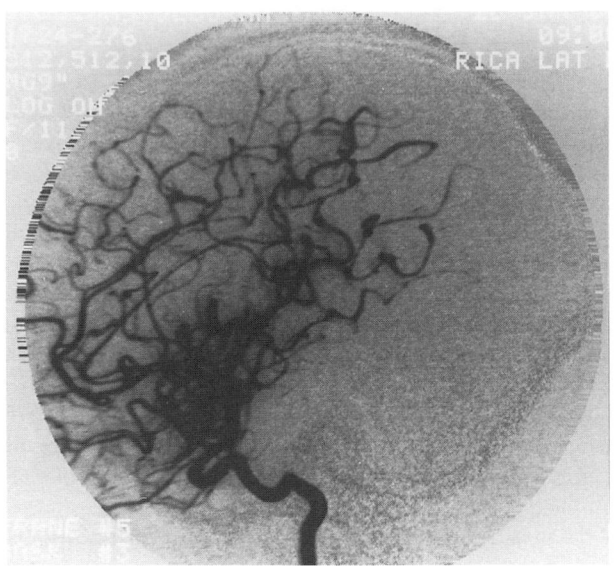

Figure 37.3 A high probability angiogram demonstrating numerous areas of focal stenosis and ectasia from a patient with RCVS.

generally is straightforward but it can be complex. Despite similar angiographic findings in RCVS and GACNS, the diagnosis may be secured by the clinical presentation, CSF analysis, and the presence of other clinical factors (see Table 37.4). Patients with RCVS generally have a background of excellent health, though a history of migraine is not uncommon. The most common presentation is that of a severe, acute headache with or without other neurologic signs and symptoms. Headache is the most common symptom in patients with GACNS as well but it is not of the thunderclap variety, and the history reveals a more prolonged and recurrent problem (Younger *et al.* 1997). CSF analysis is normal or near normal in RCVS while it is almost always abnormal in GACNS (Calabrese *et al.* 1997; Younger *et al.* 1997). Furthermore, in patients with RCVS there is frequently a history of associated cofactors providing clues to the diagnosis, such as a recent pregnancy, typical history of "thunderclap" headache often precipitated by exercise, sexual activity, or exposure to vasoactive drugs. Occasional patients with PACNS, who do not display granulomatous features and who have been referred to as "atypical" (Calabrese *et al.* 1997), may at times be difficult to differentiate; however, the clinical picture is often more subacute, CSF more frequently abnormal, and findings on neuroimaging studies more suggestive of true arteritis.

MR imaging is frequently normal in RCVS but can reveal evidence of infarction (particularly in watershed areas), edema, or bleeding in up to 60% of patients (Singhal 2002). Changes consistent with posterior reversible leukoencephalopthy have also been reported (Dodick *et al.* 2003). The MRI is abnormal in the vast majority of patients with GACNS though rare examples of normal MRI in the presence of typical angiographic features have been described (Wasserman *et al.* 2001). There is no specific MRI finding indicative of GACNS though multifocal areas of ischemia, infarction, or both of different ages involving grey and white matter are most common.

Diagnostic studies
By definition all patients have a high probability angiogram. The angiographic features are illustrated in Figure 37.3 and include alternating areas of stenosis or ectasia in multiple vessels in multiple vascular beds. At times the vessels may display long areas of smooth tapering or areas of cut-off. A clinical point of great importance in regards to CNS vasculitis and RCVS is that angiography, even in cases with high probability findings, lacks specificity and it is insufficient to secure a diagnosis of cerebral vasculitis on purely

radiographic grounds. Duna and Calabrese (1995) demonstrated that in the evaluation of suspected GACNS, a high probability angiogram is likely to represent a false-positive test. Differentiating vasoconstriction from vasculitis and either of these forms of vascular abnormalities from other forms of non-inflammatory vascular disease is not possible in the majority of cases. Careful clinical correlation is essential to allow proper interpretation.

Routine blood tests, acute phase reactants, and autoantibody assays are not revealing in RCVS and serve primarily to rule out mimicking conditions. As noted in Table 37.4, CSF examination is essential and findings of chronic meningitis should greatly dissuade one from the diagnosis of RCVS.

Diagnosis and differential diagnosis
In patients presenting with a history of complex headaches, and an acute onset of unexplained severe headache or focal neurologic event, RCVS should be considered. Examination of CSF is an essential study in suspected RCVS and should be normal or nearly so. As noted above, a detailed search must be made for exposure to sympathomimetic drugs, including over-the-counter agents and those that may be found in herbal preparations and other complementary and alternative medicines. An assessment for conditions such as pheochromocytoma is also important. In our experience there is often a strong history of cigarette smoking, though this is anecdotal. Other conditions in the differential diagnosis include embolization and hypercoaguable states.

Treatment and prognosis
There are no controlled studies of the treatment of RCVS and thus we are guided by observational data and our experience. A therapeutic view of RCVS must reconcile two conflicting observations. On the one hand, successful outcomes, including alleviation of symptoms and rapid reversibility of vascular abnormalities, have been reported with a variety of approaches including treatment with calcium channel blockers (Dodick 2003; Lu *et al.* 2004), brief courses of glucocorticoids (Hajj-Ali *et al.* 2002), magnesium sulfate (Singhal 2004b), and, most importantly, observation without treatment

(Hajj-Ali *et al.* 2002; Singhal *et al.* 2002). The clinical course may also be pernicious, as it is not uncommon for symptoms to initially clear, and return repeatedly, culminating in stroke (Hajj-Ali *et al.* 2002; Lu *et al.* 2004; Sturm and Macdonell 2000). Stroke as an outcome was noted in up to 54% of patients in one systematic review (Singhal 2002). At present, the absence of clear predictors of benign versus progressive disease confounds clinical decision making.

Simple observation, without treatment, is acceptable for patients presenting with self-limited headache syndrome without stroke. For patients presenting with severe and recurrent headache with or without stroke, oral or intravenous calcium channel blockers such as verapamil or nimodipine have been used successfully (Lu *et al.* 2004; Dodick 2003; Hajj-Ali *et al.* 2002).

Regression of angiographic lesions can be followed using MRA in the majority of patients. Alternatively, vascular flow rates can be followed serially by transcranial Doppler analysis. Improvement can be observed within days to weeks. In general, regression of symptoms such as headache is prompt, and failure to improve should be viewed with alarm. For patients whose symptoms and angiographic findings worsen, there are no clear treatment options, but short-term, high-dose glucocorticoids have been reported to be effective (Hajj-Ali *et al.* 2002). The rationale for this approach is based on the efficacy of high-dose glucocorticoids in reversing experimentally-induced vasoconstriction (Chen *et al.* 2002). For patients presenting with massive stroke or a prolonged clinical course, the diagnosis should always be viewed with caution. In these settings, clinicians should consider a diagnosis such as true cerebral arteritis, or progression to a stage of vascular necrosis. In these settings biopsy of central nervous system tissues may have a role.

Clinical variants

Spinal cord and mass lesion presentations

Several other distinctive clinical presentations deserve comment for they often pose diagnostic difficulties. Spinal cord involvement is well-documented, but uncommon in PACNS (Ropper *et al.* 2003; Campi *et al.* 2001; Younger *et al.* 1997). Spinal cord involvement may or may not coincide with cortical involvement. When isolated it may pose a formidable diagnostic challenge. Most cases reported in the literature were diagnosed post-mortem and only recently has ante-mortem diagnosis become more common. The symptoms and signs of spinal cord involvement are non-specific and are similar to any other vascular or inflammatory myelopathy. Treatment is similar to that of GACNS.

Less well-appreciated is the presentation of PACNS as a mass lesion in about 15% of reported cases (Duna *et al.* 1995). The clinical findings in this setting are non-specific, but headache and a variety of focal and diffuse abnormalities are common. Angiography is generally abnormal, with a "mass effect". Frank beading as seen in RCVS is rare (Duna *et al.* 1995). Mass lesions are generally defined by CT or MRI, and enhancement has been reported variably (Calabrese *et al.* 1997; Greenan *et al.* 1992; Pierot *et al.* 1991). These vasculitic mass lesions have no distinctive features to differentiate them from other pathologic lesions, so they must all be approached as potentially neoplastic. This is the sole indication for stereotactic biopsy, which has been successful in diagnosing PACNS (Whiting *et al.* 1992). In our experience a sizable percentage of these lesions are non-granulomatous, often with leukocytoclastic features. The optimal therapy for such patients is unknown, but rare instances of excisional cure have been documented (Berger *et al.* 1995).

GACNS and giant cell arteritis (GCA)

Central nervous system complications of GCA are distinctly uncommon. When they do occur, they appear to primarily result from arteritis of the large vessels at the base of the brain. Carotid artery involvement is usually extracranial, although proximal intracranial segments can be affected. Vertebral arteritis is extracranial, but it may extend intracranially for roughly 5 mm beyond dural penetration (Caselli and Hunder 1993). There are numerous well-documented cases summarized in two studies (Buttner *et al.* 1994; Rhodes *et al.* 1995). Bilateral vertebral artery involvement leading to catastrophic cerebral ischemia has also been reported (Ruegg *et al.* 2003). Virtually all autopsied cases of GCA with intracranial involvement involved a single branch of the circle of Willis with vasculitis in at least one extracranial site (Rhodes *et al.* 1995). In only a single patient was small-vessel involvement documented (Buttner *et al.* 1994), though in this patient extracranial disease was not well-documented.

It is our opinion that extensive small-vessel cerebral arteritis is not a complication of classical GCA. CNS involvement is likely due to either atherosclerosis in the elderly, or, rarely, large-vessel arteritis at the base of the brain. Furthermore, we believe that in suspected cases of GACNS, there is no indication for temporal artery biopsy if the suspected pathology involves small intracranial vessels. Much of the confusion regarding intracranial GCA arises from the fact that the lesions of GCA and GACNS are similar and that confusing terminology was used in the older literature.

GACNS and sarcoidosis

A small number of cases of GACNS concomitant with sarcoidosis have been reported (Younger *et al.* 1997). It was felt that the neurologic disease in these patients was essentially similar to those of patients with pure GACNS. Because well-formed perivascular granulomas may occasionally be seen in GACNS, the histologic features separating GACNS from sarcoidosis may at times be obscure. Most cases of GACNS do not have well-formed non-caseating granulomas, so histologic differentiation is somewhat easier. Since the presence of non-caseating granulomas is not a specific histopathologic marker for sarcoidosis, several clinical guidelines can help separate these conditions. First, we believe that any case of vascular granulomatous angiitis occurring in the setting of multisystemic sarcoidosis represents CNS sarcoidosis. Secondly, we believe that if well-formed granulomas are found within the CNS in a vascular distribution and there is no evidence of granulomatous disease outside the CNS, these cases should be viewed as GACNS. Lastly, a small group of cases will always remain difficult to classify, but the principles of treatment should be similar to those of GACNS (Ulrich 1977). The differentiation of these two disorders has recently been discussed (Calabrese 2003).

GACNS and amyloidosis

There have been 34 persons with cerebral amyloidosis reported to have features of GACNS (Scolding *et al.* 2005). The mean age of the group was 67 years, which is older than patients with GACNS. Alterations in mental status, headaches, seizures, and focal deficits were common. Hallucinations were the presenting manifestation in 12%. MRI findings consisting of extensive white matter changes were common and CSF revealed modest elevations of cells and protein.

There are several explanations for the relationship between amyloidosis and GACNS. One is that this represents the chance concurrence of two uncommon conditions. This seems unlikely on a purely probabilistic basis; furthermore, amyloidosis localizes to the leptomeninges with sparing of other regions of the brain. A more satisfying explanation is that GACNS is secondary to the amyloidosis or that amyloidosis is induced by GACNS.

A pathophysiologic study by Anders and colleagues (Anders *et al.* 1997) described six patients with GACNS and cerebral amyloid angiopathy. These authors point out that the inflammatory infiltrate in these cases is somewhat atypical for classical GACNS in that the mononuclear cells are found only in the outer portion of the vessels and surrounding brain parenchyma and are not transmural (Anders *et al.* 1997). In their study, they clearly demonstrated the presence of beta/A4 peptide deposition primarily in the thickened media of vessels damaged by amyloid and within the cytoplasm of multinucleated giant cells. They proposed that the granulomatous angiitis seen in these cases most likely represented a foreign body response to amyloid proteins causing secondary destruction of the vessel wall.

Therapy for this variant of PACNS in unsettled but some patients have responded to aggressive therapy (Propst *et al.* 1997; Shintaku *et al.* 1986; Ginsberg *et al.* 1988). Cyclophosphamide alone was reported to be efficacious in one person, implying that glucocorticoids may not be needed in all cases (Fountain and Eberhard 1996).

PACNS associated with varicella zoster infection (VZV)

While PACNS associated with infection is generally considered a secondary form of arteritis, the relationship between PACNS and VZV is perplexing enough to warrant a separate discussion. The association of VZV infection with CNS vascular disease is well known. Several syndromes have been well described, especially that of contralateral hemiplegia in the setting of herpes zoster ophthalmicus or VZV infection of the trigeminal nerve (Sigal 1987; Martin *et al.* 1990). The clinical features of this syndrome include an ischemic CNS event that occurs several weeks to months following VZV infection. The ischemia relates to vasculitis of the middle cerebral artery or several of its branches and occasionally the internal carotid artery. Vasculitis follows, from retrograde spread of VZV via anastomotic branches of the gasserian ganglion to the cerebral circulation (Doyle *et al.* 1983; Linnemann and Alvira 1980; MacKenzie *et al.* 1981). In general, the arteritis remains anatomically localized and monophasic in course, and we do not view this as true PACNS, from which it is readily differentiated on clinical and angiographic grounds.

A more complex VZV-associated syndrome of CNS vascular disease indistinguishable from classic GACNS has been described in patients who frequently have altered host defenses (Lie 1992; Martin *et al.* 1990). This disease may evolve in the setting of VZV infection of the trigeminal nerve or a somatic dermatome, or even in the absence of clinical VZV infection. For example, Gilden and colleagues (Gilden *et al.* 1996, 2000) have described GACNS where VZV was identified, via molecular techniques, in a patchy distribution throughout the inflamed cerebral vessels in an elderly patient with no clinical evidence of preceding VZV infection. Another investigation found that VZV infection of somatic dermatomes frequently extends into the CNS, producing a subclinical inflammatory response. This tends to corroborate a role for occult VZV infection in PACNS (Haanpaa *et al.* 1998). It is therefore possible that VZV may belie the "idiopathic" label of many cases of GACNS.

This may be particularly germane to immunocompromised patients developing GACNS, such as those with lymphoproliferative disease, HIV infection, organ transplantation on immunosuppressive drugs, or graft-versus-host disease (Younger *et al.* 1997; Ma *et al.* 2002). The treatment for such cases is problematic but probably requires a combination of antiviral and immunosuppressive drugs. There are no controlled trials on which to base therapy.

Secondary forms of CNS vasculitis

Treatment of secondary systemic vasculitis

Cerebral vasculitis may be associated with a variety of conditions including infections, drugs, lymphoproliferative diseases, systemic vasculitides, and connective tissue diseases (Calabrese 1997b) (Table 37.1). Although direct evidence is generally lacking, removal of the exogenous inciting agent or control of the associated systemic disease may ameliorate a secondary CNS vasculitis. A diligent search for associated conditions is thus essential in the approach to the patient with suspected cerebral arteritis.

Infections

In the evaluation of CNS vasculitis, it is imperative to search for infection through microbiologic analysis of CSF and biopsy material. This cannot be overemphasized since the clinical and angiographic presentations of infection-related cerebral arteritis mimic those of PACNS (Calabrese 1997a; Calabrese *et al.* 1997; Mandell and Calabrese 1998; Younger 2004). Furthermore, the underlying infection may be occult when the neurovascular complication occurs. Suspicion of specific pathogens should be guided by epidemiologic features and individual risk factors. Infection with human immunodeficiency virus (HIV-1), VZV, HCV, or syphilis should be considered (Table 37.1) (West 2003; Mandell and Calabrese 1998).

Evaluating patients with HIV infection for possible CNS vasculitis is particularly challenging. An array of CNS vascular diseases, both inflammatory and non-inflammatory, has been associated with HIV infection (Table 37.5). In an analysis of CNS specimens from 100 cases of acquired immunodeficiency syndrome (AIDS), pathologic changes were detected in 87 (Mossakowski and Zelman 1997). Encephalitis, leptomeningitis, or vasculitis were described in 35% of cases. Opportunistic CNS infections, however, accounted for the majority of brain lesions (59%). Of note, the coexistence of multiple pathologic processes in a brain was characteristic in this series (Table 37.5). A peculiar variant of isolated CNS vasculitis associated with microaneurysm has been reported in HIV-infected children (Calabrese 2004). This illustrates the complexities of the relationship between HIV infection and CNS vasculitis.

The clinical outcome of infection-associated CNS vasculitis is variable even when appropriate antimicrobial drugs are given. This reflects the diverse pathophysiologic mechanisms involved, which include a direct cytopathic effect of the pathogen invading the blood vessel, injury to endothelial cells via induction of neoantigen formation, and immune complex-mediated damage (Jennette and Falk 1997). Adjunctive anti-inflammatory or immunosuppressive therapy may be beneficial in patients who do not respond to antimicrobial therapy although such an approach has not been tested.

Table 37.5 HIV-associated CNS disease

Pathologic findings
Encephalitis
Leptomeningitis
Vasculitis
Vacuolar myelopathy
Leukoencephalopathy
Etiologies
HIV
Opportunistic infections
Lymphoproliferative diseases
Drug-associated vasculopathy

Table 37.6 Differential diagnosis of CNS disease in patients with systemic vasculitis

Vasculitis
Infections
CNS
Systemic
Drug toxicities
Glucocorticoid-induced CNS effects
Cyclophosphamide-induced hyponatremia
Extracranial end-organ damage
Hypoxic encephalopathy due to pulmonary or cardiac disease
Uremic encephalopthy
Accelerated hypertension
Thromboembolic disease

Drugs

As noted in the section on RCVS, a variety of drugs, particularly those with sympathomimetic properties, have been associated with neurologic complications, including cerebral infarcts, intracerebral bleeding, and subarachnoid hemorrhage. The most commonly implicated drugs are oral and intravenous amphetamines, cocaine, heroin, ephedrine, and phenylpropanolamine (Table 37.1).

Recognizing and withdrawing the offending drug is obviously the cornerstone of treatment. For drugs of abuse, the risk profile dictates the need to look for associated infections. When present, hypertension should be controlled and for most angiographically defined cases, we recommend the use of calcium channel blockers and a limited course of glucocorticoids. The use of long-term glucocorticoid therapy and the addition of cytotoxic drugs should be reserved for pathologically documented cases of CNS arteritis.

Lymphoproliferative diseases

Vasculitis of the CNS has been reported in association with Hodgkin's lymphoma, non-Hodgkin's lymphoma, and angioimmunolymphoproliferative lesions (AIL) (Calabrese *et al.* 1997). Of note, the anatomic location of the lymphoproliferative disease is not necessarily within the CNS. Although the clinical presentation is generally similar to that of PACNS, mass lesions, spinal cord involvement, and CNS hemorrhage should raise suspicion for an underlying lymphoproliferative disease (Calabrese *et al.* 1997). It is important to realize that a biopsy of the CNS lesion may only reveal the angiitis without evidence of malignancy. On the other hand, a lymphocytic angiitis may itself be the malignant lesion of AIL, a diagnosis established by detailed immunohistochemistry, T-cell receptor analysis, and B-cell immunoglobulin studies. Finally, one should also look for concomitant infections, particularly VZV.

Treatment is generally directed at the underlying lymphoproliferative disease, be it within or outside the CNS. This generally consists of combination chemotherapy and irradiation. Favorable neurologic outcomes have been reported (Greco *et al.* 1976; Kleinschmidt-DeMasters *et al.* 1992).

Systemic vasculitides

Vasculitis of the CNS may occur with any of the systemic vasculitides, but is most commonly reported in polyarteritis nodosa (PAN), microscopic polyangiitis (MPA), Behçet's syndrome (BS), Wegener's granulomatosis (WG), and Churg–Strauss syndrome (CSS) (Calabrese *et al.* 1997; West 2003; Younger 2004). The true prevalence of CNS arteritis in systemic vasculitides is difficult to estimate since the diagnosis is most often presumed on clinical grounds when neurologic events occur in the setting of systemic disease (angiographic premortem pathologic evidence of CNS vasculitis is rarely sought). Alternative explanations should be considered in patients with systemic vasculitis presenting with symptoms or signs of CNS dysfunction (Table 37.6) (Calabrese *et al.* 1997; West 2003).

Treatment of CNS disease is directed at the underlying systemic vasculitis and generally consists of high-dose glucocorticoids. Cytotoxic drugs are added in MPA and WG as well as in other serious systemic vasculitides in which permanent CNS damage may occur.

Connective tissue diseases

CNS involvement is not uncommon in connective tissue diseases, mainly systemic lupus erythematosus (SLE) and Sjögren's syndrome (SS) (see Chapter 34) (Younger 2004; West 2003). In SLE, brain lesions most often represent vasculopathy, with small-vessel hyalinization, thickening, intramural platelet deposition, and thrombus formation (Jennekens and Kater 2002a, 2002b). Frank CNS vasculitis occurs in less than 7% of cases of SLE (Ellis and Verity 1979). When SLE patients present with CNS symptoms and signs, it is important to consider causes other than CNS vasculitis (Table 37.1). Treatment of CNS vasculitis in SLE generally consists of high-dose intravenous glucocorticoids plus cyclophosphamide in critically ill or progressively deteriorating patients. The use of intravenous immunoglobulin (IVIg) remains anecdotal, but may be considered as adjunctive therapy.

In Sjögren's syndrome, CNS manifestations may be caused by a mononuclear inflammatory vasculopathy involving the small vessels of the cortex and meninges (Alexander 1993; Soliotis *et al.* 2004; Morgen *et al.* 2004). Angiographic abnormalities consistent with vasculitis are seen uncommonly. Treatment issues remain unresolved.

Miscellaneous conditions

A variety of other disorders are capable of mimicking the clinical and angiographic picture of CNS vasculitis, while others are associated with true CNS arteritis (Table 37.1) (Calabrese 1995). The antiphospholipid antibody (APL) syndrome (see Chapter 44) is of particular interest since it is clearly associated with CNS ischemic events related to thrombosis. In one study, 74% of patients with the APL syndrome and ischemic cerebrovascular events had angiographic abnormalities, the majority of which were arterial (Provenzale *et al.* 1994). The abnormalities were solely intracranial in 59%, solely extracranial in 35%, and mixed in 6%. Of patients with intracranial abnormalities, 60% were solitary stem or branch occlusions of the cerebral or basilar arteries while 40% were "suggestive of" vasculitis. This is potentially misleading since the occurrence of true histologic vasculitis in the APL syndrome is distinctly unusual. Treatment consists of anticoagulation rather than immunosuppression.

Radiation and, in particular, over-irradiation, has been associated with CNS vasculitis (Alfonso *et al.* 1997). In eight patients with over-irradiation myelopathy due to a malfunctioning linear electron accelerator, an obliterative vasculitis of the spinal cord was present in all four in whom autopsies were performed (Alfonso *et al.* 1997). Of note, MRI of the spine was normal in the acute phase in all patients. In a rat pial window model, single high doses of radiation caused an increase in leukocyte–endothelial cell interactions and a decrease or loss of arteriolar flow in the cerebral vasculature, perhaps explaining the radiation vasculitis described in humans (Acker *et al.* 1998). Finally, PACNS has been increasingly described in the setting of graft-versus-host disease (Ma *et al.* 2002).

References

Acker, J. C., Marks, L. B., Spencer, D. P., Yang, W., Avery, M. A., Dodge, R. K., *et al.* (1998). Serial in vivo observations of cerebral vasculature after treatment with a large single fraction of radiation. *Radiation Research*, **149**, 350–9.

Alexander, E. L. (1993). Neurologic disease in Sjögren's syndrome: mononuclear inflammatory vasculopathy affecting central/peripheral nervous system and muscle. A clinical review and update of immunopathogenesis. *Rheumatic Diseases Clinics of North America*, **19**, 869–908.

Alfonso, E. R., De Gregorio, M. A., Mateo, P., Esco, R., Bascon, N., Morales, F., *et al.* (1997). Radiation myelopathy in over-irradiated patients: MR imaging findings. *European Radiology*, **7**, 400–4.

Anders, K. H., Wang, Z. Z., Kornfeld, M., Gray, F., Soontornniyomkij, K., Reed, L., *et al.* (1997). Giant cell arteritis with cerebral amyloid angiopathy: immunohistochemical and molecular studies. *Human Pathology*, **28**, 1237–46.

Berger, J. R., Romano, J., Menkin, M. and Norenberg, M. (1995). Benign focal cerebral vasculitis: case report. *Neurology*, **45**, 1731–4.

Bettoni, L., Juvarra, G., Bortone, E. and Lechi, A. (1984). Isolated benign cerebral vasculitis. Case report and review. *Acta Neurologica Belgica*, **84**, 161–73.

Bogousslavsky, J., Despland, P. A., Regli, F. and Dubuis, P. Y. (1989). Postpartum cerebral angiopathy: reversible vasoconstriction assessed by transcranial Doppler ultrasounds. *European Neurology*, **29**, 102–5.

Buttner, T., Heye, N. and Przuntek, H. (1994). Temporal arteritis with cerebral complications: report of four cases. *European Neurology*, **34**, 162–7.

Calabrese, L. H. (1995). Vasculitis of the central nervous system. *Rheumatic Diseases Clinics of North America*, **21**, 1059–76.

Calabrese, L. H. (1997a). Human immunodeficiency virus infection and rheumatic disease. *Bulletin on the Rheumatic Diseases*, **46**, 2–5.

Calabrese, L. H. (1997b). Therapy of systemic vasculitis.[Erratum appears in *Neurologic Clinics* (1998),16, x]. *Neurologic Clinics*, **15**, 973–91.

Calabrese, L. H. (2003). A headache and a mass lesion: vasculitis or CNS sarcoid? *Clinical and Experimental Rheumatology*, **21**, S131–2.

Calabrese, L. H. (2004). Infection with the human immunodeficiency virus type 1 and vascular inflammatory disease. *Clinical and Experimental Rheumatology*, **22**, S87–93.

Calabrese, L. H., Dodick, D. W., Schwedt, T. J. and Singhal, A. B. (2007). Narrative review: reversible cerebral vasoconstriction syndromes. *Annals of Internal Medicine*, **146**, 34–44.

Calabrese, L. H. and Duna, G. F. (1995). Evaluation and treatment of central nervous system vasculitis. *Current Opinion in Rheumatology*, **7**, 37–44.

Calabrese, L. H., Duna, G. F. and Lie, J. T. (1997). Vasculitis in the central nervous system. *Arthritis and Rheumatism*, **40**, 1189–201.

Calabrese, L. H., Furlan, A. and Gragg, L. A. (1992a). Primary angiitis of the central nervous system: Diagnostic criteria and clinical approach. *Cleveland Clinic Journal of Medicine*, **59**, 293–306.

Calabrese, L. H., Furlan, A. J., Gragg, L. A. and Ropos, T. J. (1992b). Primary angiitis of the central nervous system: diagnostic criteria and clinical approach. *Cleveland Clinic Journal of Medicine*, **59**, 293–306.

Calabrese, L. H., Gragg, L. A. and Furlan, A. J. (1993). Benign angiopathy: a distinct subset of angiographically defined primary angiitis of the central nervous system. *Journal of Rheumatology*, **20**, 2046–50.

Calabrese, L. H. and Mallek, J. A. (1988). Primary angiitis of the central nervous system. Report of 8 new cases, review of the literature, and proposal for diagnostic criteria. *Medicine*, **67**, 20–39.

Calado, S., Vale-Santos, J., Lima, C. and Viana-Baptista, M. (2004). Postpartum cerebral angiopathy: vasospasm, vasculitis or both? *Cerebrovascular Diseases*, **18**, 340–1.

Call, G. K., Fleming, M. C., Sealfon, S., Levine, H., Kistler, J. P. and Fisher, C. M. (1988). Reversible cerebral segmental vasoconstriction. *Stroke*, **19**, 1159–70.

Campi, A., Benndorf, G., Martinelli, V., Terreni, M. R. and Scotti, G. (2001). Spinal cord involvement in primary angiitis of the central nervous system: a report of two cases. *American Journal of Neuroradiology*, **22**, 577–82.

Caselli, R. J. and Hunder, G. G. (1993). Neurologic aspects of giant cell (temporal) arteritis. *Rheumatic Diseases Clinics of North America*, **19**, 941–53.

Chang, S. D., Yap, O. W. and Adler, J. R., Jr. (1999). Symptomatic vasospasm after resection of a suprasellar pilocytic astrocytoma: case report and possible pathogenesis. *Surgical Neurology*, **51**, 521–6; discussion 526–7.

Chen, D., Nishizawa, S., Yokota, N., Ohta, S., Yokoyama, T. and Namba, H. (2002). High-dose methylprednisolone prevents vasospasm after subarachnoid hemorrhage through inhibition of protein kinase C activation. *Neurological Research*, **24**, 215–22.

Cheng, T. M., O'Neill, B. P., Scheithauer, B. W. and Piepgras, D. G. (1994). Chronic meningitis: the role of meningeal or cortical biopsy. *Neurosurgery*, **34**, 590–5; discussion 596.

Chu, C. T., Gray, L., Goldstein, L. B. and Hulette, C. M. (1998). Diagnosis of intracranial vasculitis: a multi-disciplinary approach. *Journal of Neuropathology and Experimental Neurology*, **57**, 30–8.

Cravioto, M. and Feigin, I. (1959). Noninfectious granulomatous angiitis with a predilection for the nervous system. *Neurology*, **9**, 599.

Cupps, T. R., Moore, P. M. and Fauci, A. S. (1983). Isolated angiitis of the central nervous system. Prospective diagnostic and therapeutic experience. *American Journal of Medicine*, **74**, 97–105.

Dodick, D. W. (2003). Reversible segmental cerebral vasoconstriction (Call-Fleming syndrome): the role of calcium antagonists.[comment]. *Cephalalgia*, **23**, 163–5.

Dodick, D. W., Eross, E. J., Drazkowski, J. F. and Ingall, T. J. (2003). Thunderclap headache associated with reversible vasospasm and posterior leukoencephalopathy syndrome. *Cephalalgia*, **23**, 994–7.

Doyle, P. W., Gibson, G. and Dolman, C. L. (1983). Herpes zoster ophthalmicus with contralateral hemiplegia: identification of cause. *Annals of Neurology*, **14**, 84–5.

Duna, G. F. and Calabrese, L. H. (1995). Limitations of invasive modalities in the diagnosis of primary angiitis of the central nervous system. *Journal of Rheumatology*, **22**, 662–7.

Duna, G. F., George, T., Rybicki, L. and Calabrese, L. H. (1995). Primary angiitis of the central nervous system: An analysis of unusual presentations. *Arthritis and Rheumatism*, **38**, S340.

Ellis, S. G. and Verity, M. A. (1979). Central nervous system involvement in systemic lupus erythematosus: A review of neuropathologic findings in 57 cases. *Seminars in Arthritis and Rheumatism*, **8**, 212.

Farine, D., Andreyko, J., Lysikiewicz, A., Simha, S. and Addison, A. (1984). Isolated angiitis of brain in pregnancy and puerperium. *Obstetrics and Gynecology*, **63**, 586–8.

Finelli, P. F., Onyiuke, H. C. and Uphoff, D. F. (1997). Idiopathic granulomatous angiitis of the CNS manifesting as diffuse white matter disease. *Neurology*, **49**, 1696–9.

Fountain, N. B. and Eberhard, D. A. (1996). Primary angiitis of the central nervous system associated with cerebral amyloid angiopathy: report of two cases and review of the literature. *Neurology*, **46**, 190–7.

Geocadin, R. G., Razumovsky, A. Y., Wityk, R. J., Bhardwaj, A. and Ulatowski, J. A. (2002). Intracerebral hemorrhage and postpartum cerebral vasculopathy. *Journal of the Neurological Sciences*, **205**, 29–34.

Geraghty, J. J., Hoch, D. B., Robert, M. E. and Vinters, H. V. (1991). Fatal puerperal cerebral vasospasm and stroke in a young woman. *Neurology*, **41**, 1145–7.

Gilden, D. H., Kleinschmidt DeMasters, B. K., LaGuardia, J. J., Mahalingam, R. and Cohrs, R. J. (2000). Neurologic complications of the reactivation of varicella-zoster virus. *New England Journal of Medicine*, **342**, 635–45.

Gilden, D. H., Kleinschmidt-DeMasters, B. K., Wellish, M., Hedley-Whyte, E. T., Rentier, B. and Mahalingam, R. (1996). Varicella zoster virus, a cause of waxing and waning vasculitis: the New England Journal of Medicine case 5–1995 revisited. *Neurology*, **47**, 1441–6.

Ginsberg, L., Geddes, J. and Valentine, A. (1988). Amyloid angiopathy and granulomatous angiitis of the central nervous system: a case responding to corticosteroid treatment. *Journal of Neurology*, **235**, 438–40.

Greco, F. A., Kolins, J., Rajjoub, R. K. and Brereton, H. D. (1976). Hodgkin's disease and granulomatous angiitis of the central nervous system. *Cancer*, **38**, 2027–32.

Greenan, T. J., Grossman, R. I. and Goldberg, H. I. (1992). Cerebral vasculitis: MR imaging and angiographic correlation. *Radiology*, **182**, 65–72.

Gripshover, B. M. and Ellner, J. J. (1998). Chronic meningitis. In *Principles and practice of infectious diseases, 4th edition* (eds, Mandell, G. L., Bennett, J. E. and Dolin, R.). Churchill Livingstone, Philadelphia.

Haanpaa, M., Dastidar, P., Weinberg, A., Levin, M., Meittenin, A., Lapinlampli, A., Laippala, P. and Nurmikko, T. (1998). CSF and MRI findings in patients with acute herpes zozster arteritis. *Neurology*, **51**, 1405.

Hajj-Ali, R. A., Furlan, A., Abou-Chebel, A. and Calabrese, L. H. (2002). Benign angiopathy of the central nervous system: cohort of 16 patients with clinical course and long-term followup. *Arthritis and Rheumatism*, **47**, 662–9.

Hankey, G. J. (1991). Isolated angiitis/angiopathy of the central nervous system. *Cerebrovascular Diseases*, **1**, 2–15.

Henry, P. Y., Larre, P., Aupy, M., Lafforgue, J. L. and Orgogozo, J. M. (1984). Reversible cerebral arteriopathy associated with the administration of ergot derivatives. *Cephalalgia*, **4**, 171–8.

Hinchey, J., Chaves, C., Appignani, B., Breen, J., Pao, L., Wang, A., Pessin, M. S., Lamy, C., Mas, J. L. and Caplan, L. R. (1996). A reversible posterior leukoencephalopathy syndrome. *New England Journal of Medicine*, **334**, 494–500.

Hurst, R. W. and Grossman, R. I. (1994). Neuroradiology of central nervous system vasculitis. *Seminars in Neurology*, **14**, 320–40.

Hyde-Rowan, M. D., Roessmann, U. and Brodkey, J. S. (1983). Vasospasm following transsphenoidal tumor removal associated with the arterial changes of oral contraception. *Surgical Neurology*, **20**, 120–4.

Ihara, M., Yanagihara, C. and Nishimura, Y. (2000). Serial transcranial color-coded sonography in postpartum cerebral angiopathy. *Journal of Neuroimaging*, **10**, 230–3.

Janssens, E., Hommel, M., Mounier-Vehier, F., Leclerc, X., Guerin du Masgenet, B. and Leys, D. (1995). Postpartum cerebral angiopathy possibly due to bromocriptine therapy. *Stroke*, **26**, 128–30.

Jennekens, F. G. and Kater, L. (2002a). The central nervous system in systemic lupus erythematosus. Part 1. Clinical syndromes: a literature investigation. *Rheumatology*, **41**, 605–18.

Jennekens, F. G. and Kater, L. (2002b). The central nervous system in systemic lupus erythematosus. Part 2. Pathogenetic mechanisms of clinical syndromes: a literature investigation. *Rheumatology*, **41**, 619–30.

Jennette, J. C. and Falk, R. J. (1997). Small-vessel vasculitis. *New England Journal of Medicine*, **337**, 1512–23.

Kadkhodayan, Y., Alreshaid, A., Moran, C. J., Cross, D. T., Powers, W. J. and Derdeyn, C. P. (2004). Primary angiitis of the central nervous system at conventional angiography. *Radiology*, **233**, 878–82.

Kaplan, P. W. (1998). Reversible hypercalcemic cerebral vasoconstriction with seizures and blindness: a paradigm for eclampsia? *Clinical Electroencephalography*, **29**, 120–3.

Kleinschmidt-DeMasters, B. K., Filley, C. M. and Bitter, M. A. (1992). Central nervous system angiocentric, angiodestructive T-cell lymphoma (lymphomatoid granulomatosis). *Surgical Neurology*, **37**, 130–7.

Konstantinopoulos, P. A., Mousa, S., Khairallah, R. and Mtanos, G. (2004). Postpartum cerebral angiopathy: an important diagnostic consideration in the postpartum period. *American Journal of Obstetrics and Gynecology*, **191**, 375–7.

Kubo, S., Nakata, H., Tatsumi, T. and Yoshimine, T. (2002). Headache associated with postpartum cerebral angiopathy: monitoring with transcranial color-coded sonography. *Headache*, **42**, 297–300.

LeRoux, P. D., Haglund, M. M., Mayberg, M. R. and Winn, H. R. (1991). Symptomatic cerebral vasospasm following tumor resection: report of two cases. *Surgical Neurology*, **36**, 25–31.

Levine, S. R., Washington, J. M., Jefferson, M. F., Kieran, S. N., Moen, M., Feit, H. and Welch, K. M. (1987). "Crack" cocaine-associated stroke. *Neurology*, **37**, 1849–53.

Lie, J. T. (1992). Primary (granulomatous) angiitis of the central nervous system: a clinicopathologic analysis of 15 new cases and a review of the literature. *Human Pathology*, **23**, 164–71.

Linnemann, C. C., Jr. and Alvira, M. M. (1980). Pathogenesis of varicella-zoster angiitis in the CNS. *Archives of Neurology*, **37**, 239–40.

Lu, S. R., Liao, Y. C., Fuh, J. L., Lirng, J. F. and Wang, S. J. (2004). Nimodipine for treatment of primary thunderclap headache. *Neurology*, **62**, 1414–6.

Ma, M., Barnes, G., Pulliam, J., Jezek, D., Baumann, R. J. and Berger, J. R. (2002). CNS angiitis in graft vs host disease. *Neurology*, **59**, 1994–7.

MacKenzie, R. A., Forbes, G. S. and Karnes, W. E. (1981). Angiographic findings in herpes zoster arteritis. *Annals of Neurology*, **10**, 458–64.

Mandell, B. F. and Calabrese, L. H. (1998). Infections and systemic vasculitis. *Current Opinion in Rheumatology*, **10**, 51–7.

Martin, J. R., Mitchell, W. J. and Henken, D. B. (1990). Neurotropic herpesviruses, neural mechanisms and arteritis. *Brain Pathology*, **1**, 6–10.

Merkel, P. A., Koroshetz, W. J., Irizarry, M. C. and Cudkowicz, M. E. (1995). Cocaine-associated cerebral vasculitis. *Seminars in Arthritis and Rheumatism*, **25**, 172–83.

Morgen, K., McFarland, H. F. and Pillemer, S. R. (2004). Central nervous system disease in primary Sjogrens syndrome: the role of magnetic resonance imaging. *Seminars in Arthritis and Rheumatism*, **34**, 623–30.

Mossakowski, M. J. and Zelman, I. B. (1997). Neuropathological syndromes in the course of full blown acquired immune deficiency syndrome (AIDS) in adults in Poland (1987–1995). *Folia Neuropathologica*, **35**, 133–43.

Nighoghossian, N., Derex, L. and Trouillas, P. (1998). Multiple intracerebral hemorrhages and vasospasm following antimigrainous drug abuse. *Headache*, **38**, 478–80.

Nowak, D. A., Rodiek, S. O., Henneken, S., Zinner, J., Schreiner, R., Fuchs, H. H. and Topka, H. (2003). Reversible segmental cerebral vasoconstriction (Call-Fleming syndrome): are calcium channel inhibitors a potential treatment option? *Cephalalgia*, **23**, 218–22.

Parisi, J. E. and Moore, P. M. (1994). The role of biopsy in vasculitis of the central nervous system. *Seminars in Neurology*, **14**, 341–8.

Pierot, L., Chiras, J., Debussche-Depriester, C., Dormont, D. and Bories, J. (1991). Intracerebral stenosing arteriopathies. Contribution of three radiological techniques to the diagnosis. *Journal of Neuroradiology*, **18**, 32–48.

Propst, T., Propst, A., Nachbauer, K., Graziadei, I., Willeit, H., Margreiter, R. and Vogel, W. (1997). Papillitis and vasculitis of the arteria spinalis anterior as complications of hepatitis C reinfection after liver transplantation. *Transplant International*, **10**, 234–7.

Provenzale, J. M., Heinz, E. R., Ortel, T. L., Macik, B. G., Charles, L. A. and Alberts, M. J. (1994). Antiphospholipid antibodies in patients without systemic lupus erythematosus: neuroradiologic findings. *Radiology*, **192**, 531–7.

Razavi, M., Bendixen, B., Maley, J. E., Shoaib, M., Zargarian, M., Razavi, B. and Adams, H. P. (1999). CNS pseudovasculitis in a patient with pheochromocytoma. *Neurology*, **52**, 1088–90.

Rhodes, R. H., Madelaire, N. C., Petrelli, M., Cole, M. and Karaman, B. A. (1995). Primary angiitis and angiopathy of the central nervous system and their relationship to systemic giant cell arteritis. *Archives of Pathology and Laboratory Medicine*, **119**, 334–49.

Ropper, A. H., Ayata, C. and Adelman, L. (2003). Vasculitis of the spinal cord. *Archives of Neurology*, **60**, 1791–4.

Ruegg, S., Engelter, S., Jeanneret, C., Hetzel, A., Probst, A., Steck, A. J. and Lyrer, P. (2003). Bilateral vertebral artery occlusion resulting from giant cell arteritis: report of 3 cases and review of the literature. *Medicine*, **82**, 1–12.

Schaafsma, A., Veen, L. and Vos, J. P. (2002). Three cases of hyperperfusion syndrome identified by daily transcranial Doppler investigation after carotid surgery. *European Journal of Vascular and Endovascular Surgery*, **23**, 17–22.

Scolding, N. J., Jayne, D. R., Zajicek, J. P., Meyer, P. A., Wraight, E. P. and Lockwood, C. M. (1997). Cerebral vasculitis–recognition, diagnosis and management. *Quarterly Journal of Medicine*, **90**, 61–73.

Scolding, N. J., Joseph, F., Kirby, P. A., Mazanti, I., Gray, F., Mikol, J., Ellison, D., Hilton, D. A., Williams, T. L., MacKenzie, J. M., Xuereb, J. H. and Love, S. (2005). Abeta-related angiitis: primary angiitis of the central nervous system associated with cerebral amyloid angiopathy. *Brain*, **128**, 500–15.

Serdaru, M., Chiras, J., Cujas, M. and Lhermitte, F. (1984). Isolated benign cerebral vasculitis or migrainous vasospasm? *Journal of Neurology, Neurosurgery and Psychiatry*, **47**, 73–6.

Shintaku, M., Osawa, K., Toki, J., Maeda, R. and Nishiyama, T. (1986). A case of granulomatous angiitis of the central nervous system associated with amyloid angiopathy. *Acta Neuropathologica*, **70**, 340–2.

Sigal, L. H. (1987). The neurologic presentation of vasculitic and rheumatologic syndromes. A review. *Medicine*, **66**, 157–80.

Singhal, A. B. (2002). Cerebral vasoconstriction without subarachnoid blood: associated conditions, clinical and neuroimaging characteristics. *Annals of Neurology*, **52**, S59–S60. (abstract).

Singhal, A. B. (2004a). Cerebral vasoconstriction syndromes. *Topics in Stroke Rehabilitation*, **11**, 1–6.

Singhal, A. B. (2004b). Postpartum angiopathy with reversible posterior leukoencephalopathy. *Archives of Neurology*, **61**, 411–6.

Singhal, A. B., Caviness, V. S., Begleiter, A. F., Mark, E. J., Rordorf, G. and Koroshetz, W. J. (2002). Cerebral vasoconstriction and stroke after use of serotonergic drugs. *Neurology*, **58**, 130–3.

Snyder, B. D. and McClelland, R. R. (1978). Isolated benign cerebral vasculitis. *Archives of Neurology*, **35**, 612–4.

Soliotis, F. C., Mavragani, C. P. and Moutsopoulos, H. M. (2004). Central nervous system involvement in Sjogren's syndrome. *Annals of the Rheumatic Diseases*, **63**, 616–20.

Solomon, S., Lipton, R. B. and Harris, P. Y. (1990). Arterial stenosis in migraine: spasm or arteriopathy? *Headache*, **30**, 52–61.

Song, J. K., Fisher, S., Seifert, T. D., Cacayorin, E. D., Alexandrov, A. V., Malkoff, M. D., Grotta, J. C. and Campbell, M. S. (2004). Postpartum cerebral angiopathy: atypical features and treatment with intracranial balloon angioplasty. *Neuroradiology*, **46**, 1022–6.

Stone, J. H., Pomper, M. G., Roubenoff, R., Miller, T. J. and Hellmann, D. B. (1994). Sensitivities of noninvasive tests for central nervous system vasculitis: a comparison of lumbar puncture, computed tomography, and magnetic resonance imaging. *Journal of Rheumatology*, **21**, 1277–82.

Sturm, J. W. and Macdonell, R. A. (2000). Recurrent thunderclap headache associated with reversible intracerebral vasospasm causing stroke. *Cephalalgia*, **20**, 132–5.

Sugiyama, Y., Muroi, A., Ishikawa, M., Tsukamoto, T. and Yamamoto, T. (1997). A benign form of isolated angiitis of the central nervous system in puerperium: an identical disorder to postpartum cerebral angiopathy? *Internal Medicine*, **36**, 931–4.

Sztajzel, R., Le Floch-Rohr, J. and Eggimann, P. (1999). High-dose intravenous immunoglobulin treatment and cerebral vasospasm: A possible mechanism of ischemic encephalopathy? *European Neurology*, **41**, 153–8.

Ulrich, H. (1977). Neurosarcoidosis or granulomatous angiitis: a problem of definition. *Mount Sinai Journal of Medicine*, **44**, 718–25.

Villa-Forte, A., Vassilopoulos, D. and Calabrese, L. H. (1998) What is not primary angiitis of the CNS (PACNS). *Arthritis and Rheumatism*, **41** (Suppl.), S124 (Abstract).

Voltz, R., Rosen, F. V., Yousry, T., Beck, J. and Hohlfeld, R. (1996). Reversible encephalopathy with cerebral vasospasm in a Guillain-Barré syndrome patient treated with intravenous immunoglobulin, *Neurology*, **46**, 250–1.

Wasserman, B. A., Stone, J. H., Hellmann, D. B. and Pomper, M. G. (2001). Reliability of normal findings on MR imaging for excluding the diagnosis of vasculitis of the central nervous system. *American Journal of Roentgenology*, **177**, 455–9.

West, S. G. (2003). Central nervous system vasculitis. *Current Rheumatology Reports*, **5**, 116–27.

Whiting, D. M., Barnett, G. H., Estes, M. L., Sila, C. A., Rudick, R. A., Hassenbusch, S. J. and Lanzieri, C. F. (1992). Stereotactic biopsy of non-neoplastic lesions in adults. *Cleveland Clinic Journal of Medicine*, **59**, 48–55.

Yamamoto, Y., Georgiadis, A. L., Chang, H. M. and Caplan, L. R. (1999). Posterior cerebral artery territory infarcts in the New England Medical Center Posterior Circulation Registry. *Archives of Neurology*, **56**, 824–32.

Younger, D. S. (2004). Vasculitis of the nervous system. *Current Opinion in Neurology*, **17**, 317–36.

Younger, D. S., Calabrese, L. H. and Hays, A. P. (1997). Granulomatous angiitis of the nervous system. *Neurologic Clinics*, **15**, 821–34.

Thromboangiitis obliterans (Buerger's disease)

Kitti Totemchokchyakarn

Introduction

Humans have been fighting "diseases of civilization" since they began congregating in large numbers. One of these diseases is thrombo-angiitis obliterans (TAO), or Buerger's disease, which is a non-necrotizing vasculitis affecting primarily small and medium-sized arteries and veins, especially the distal arteries and veins of upper and lower extremities. It develops predominantly in young adults, usually men in the second through fourth decades of life, although the incidence in women is increasing. The active phase of the disease is almost always associated with use of tobacco, although the exact pathogenetic mechanisms are not yet well defined and most hypotheses are controversial.

In the past, several isolated case reports of obliterative athero-sclerosis of the extremities were described under a variety of diag-nostic terms. In 1879, Felix von Winiwater, an Austrian surgeon, described the cellular thrombus and adjacent wall pathology of a single patient. In 1908, Leo Buerger of New York published his observations on clinical and pathologic studies of a small group of patients. He introduced the term "thromboangiitis obliterans" to describe the disease (Buerger 1908). The eponym "von Winiwater–Buerger's disease" is commonly used in Europe. In Buerger's subse-quent reports, he described the histopathology of acute and healing arteries, the focal and segmental distribution of the lesions, and the clinical course of the disease, which includes gangrene, vaso-motor, and trophic disorders (Buerger 1924). He was unaware of the relationship of tobacco and the disease, and his differentia-tion of TAO from atherosclerotic gangrene caused confusion, lead-ing to overdiagnosis of TAO for many years. Many examples of atherosclerosis of the extremities, particularly in younger persons, were loosely diagnosed as TAO. After careful retrospective review of both clinical and pathologic changes, Wessler et al. (1960) con-cluded that the histopathology of what had been diagnosed as TAO was indistinguishable from atherosclerosis, systemic embolism, or idiopathic arterial or venous thrombosis, and they questioned the distinctiveness of TAO. McKusick et al. (1962) studied the clinical profile and histopathology of TAO, and noted that the interpreta-tion of tissue specimens was dependent on the site of the biopsy and the stage of the disease. McPherson, Juergens and Gifford (1963) found no difference between the survival of patients with TAO and normal, age-matched controls, whereas the survival of

patients with premature atherosclerosis was decreased because of cardiac and cerebral events. Szilagyi et al. (1964) correlated clinical and histologic features with angiography, and established criteria for angiographic diagnosis of TAO.

TAO accounts for 0.5–5% of occlusive vascular disease. Though TAO has a world-wide distribution, its prevalence is greatest in Eastern Europe, the Middle East, and southeastern Asia. In Europe, TAO represents 0.5 to 2% of all ischemic disease, while in Japan it reaches 20–30%. In Nepal, the incidence of TAO is stated to be 50 times higher than in North America (Fleshman 1998). The ratio of men to women with TAO has been given as 100:1 in the past, but at present women account for 10–20% of the patients, and 5–10% are more than 60 years old (Reny and Cabane 1998). This may indi-cate increased use of tobacco by women in recent decades and also their better access to health care. TAO in women is as severe as it is in men (Lie 1987).

Etiologic factors

The cause of TAO is unknown. It is observed universally that the disease and its exacerbations occur in active tobacco smokers, and that cessation of smoking brings remission. Many observers report that most TAO patients are, or have been, heavy smokers, often smoking more than 20 cigarettes daily. Rather surprisingly, a case–control study of tobacco dependence in TAO vis-à-vis coronary atherosclerosis concluded that there was no significant difference in the age at first tobacco exposure of the study cohorts, and in the degree of tobacco dependence (Cooper et al. 2006). The disease has been reported in pipe smokers and in persons using chewing tobacco only (Lie 1988a), but has been reported rarely in non-smokers. Disease progression is also moderately related to continued tobacco use. Nicotine and carboxyhemoglobin may cause functional distur-bances and structural damage to endothelial cells of the vessels, initiating atherosclerosis. Additional effects of smoking include hyperfibrinogenemia, lowering of HDL cholesterol, and increased oxidation of LDL cholesterol, which can also precipitate arterio-sclerosis. Passive exposure to smoke has minimal effects on TAO patients, yet it should probably be avoided (Matsushita et al. 1991). Only a small number of smokers develop TAO; however, heavy smokers frequently have atherosclerosis (coronary artery disease, peripheral vascular disease, etc.). This suggests that additional factors such as genetic predisposition and alterations of the immune response may contribute to development of TAO.

Laohapensang and colleagues have reported a significant seasonal variation in admissions for TAO to Chiang Mai University Hospital in northern Thailand. Among 121 admissions, 52% took place during winter, 34.6% during the rainy season, and only 11.6% in the summer. They did not comment on the extent of seasonal variations in temperatures, although winters can be cool in the mountainous areas of northern Thailand (Laohapensang *et al.* 2004). The disease was at first thought to occur exclusively in Jews, a misconception stemming from Buerger's work. It is now known to occur in all populations, with increased prevalence in Middle Easterners and Asians compared with Caucasians. In the vast majority of persons with TAO, no hereditary basis has been established, despite reports of familial occurrence of the disease and isolated kindreds (Goodman *et al.*1965). An association with certain histocompatibility leukocyte antigens (HLA) has been reported from several countries. For example, the HLA-B54-DRB1*0405-DQB1*0401-DQA1*03-DPB1*0501 haplotype has been reported to be associated with Buerger's disease in Japanese populations (Aerbajinai *et al.* 1996). This is inconclusive because HLA patterns vary with ethnic populations, not all patients have a given haplotype, and asymptomatic controls overlap with those having TAO. Further studies are needed to define the genetic influences on TAO. In regards to socioeconomic status, almost all patients in one study from the Orient were farmers from a low socioeconomic class (McKusick and Harris 1961). Farmers in Asia usually work in rice fields and have their feet immersed in water for long periods of time and smoke the cheapest type of strong, locally grown tobacco wrapped in nonporous leaf, both of which are believed to worsen their disease (Hill and Smith 1974; Hill *et al.* 1973).

Evidence supporting an immunologic pathogenesis for TAO includes the intense cellular infiltration of the thrombus and adjacent vessel, and the distribution of focal segmental lesions. Adar *et al.* (1983) have identified increased sensitivity of leukocytes from TAO patients to collagen types I and III and a modest increase in anti-collagen antibodies in their sera. Kobayashi *et al.* (1999) have shown that TAO is an endarteritis caused by T cell- and B cell-mediated immunity and activation of macrophages or dendritic cells in the intima. They also demonstrated the deposition of IgG, IgA, IgM, and complement factors 3d and 4c (C3d, C4c) along the internal elastic lamina. Antinuclear antibodies and rheumatoid factors are not found. Slavov *et al.* have found increased *in vitro* production of IL-6 and IL-12, and decreased IL-10 in PBMC harvested from TAO patients compared to controls. Spontaneous and induced apoptosis was also higher in TAO compared to controls (Slavov *et al.* 2005). Antiendothelial cell antibodies (AECA), whose titers are strikingly high in TAO patients with active disease compared with patients in remission and normal controls, may be useful in following disease activity and may play a role in the pathogenesis of TAO (Eichhorn *et al.* 1998). In one study, lymphocytes were challenged with tobacco glycoprotein antibody; those from smokers, but not those from non-smokers, responded, but there was no difference between smokers with and without TAO. The evidence favoring a hypercoagulable state in the blood of patients who have TAO is fragmentary and inconclusive. Glueck *et al.* (2006) hypothesized that genetic polymorphisms associated with arterial vasospasm (5A/6A in the stromelysin-1 gene and -786 T/C in the eNOS gene) and the 677 C/T and 1298 A/C polymorphisms in the methylene tetrahydrofolate reductase (MTHFR) gene interact with cigarette-cannabis smoking, causing reduction in vasodilatory nitric oxide, which would promote arterial spasm and thrombosis. Based on preliminary experimental evidence, they speculated that the development and severity of TAO were related to a gene–environment vasospastic interaction with reduced NO-mediated vasodilatation.

Preliminary data have identified putative roles for plasma endothelin-1 levels in exacerbation of clinical symptoms of TAO, and increased concentrations of selectin P in endothelial injury (Czarnacki *et al.* 2004). Investigators in Japan have examined the prevalence of oral (periodontal) bacteria found in periodontitis and in arterial lesions of TAO. Occluded arteries including the superficial femoral, popliteal, anterior tibial, and posterior tibial were removed and studied. DNA of *Treponema denticola* was found by polymerase chain reaction (PCR) amplification in 12 of 14 arterial and in all 14 oral samples. Other organisms were identified less frequently. No evidence of periodontal bacteria was found in control arterial samples. This study suggested a possible etiologic link between oral bacterial infections and TAO (Iwai *et al.* 2005).

Pathology

The gross pathologic features of TAO are distinct from those of other vascular lesions such as atherosclerosis or polyarteritis nodosa. TAO is primarily a disease of the blood vessels of the extremities; it involves the lower extremities more commonly, and usually more severely, than the upper extremities. It has also been found sometimes in various viscera, "spreading" from the extremities. The disease usually begins in medium-sized or small arteries, most commonly the posterior tibial, anterior tibial, radial, ulnar, plantar, palmar, and digital arteries. Larger arteries are affected only when the disease is severe and progressive. Involvement of veins is less common, and preferentially affects small and medium-sized vessels. The lesions are focal or segmental, and are separated by normal segments of vessels, with fairly distinct demarcations. The lesions can be classified as an inflammatory, non-suppurative panarteritis or panphlebitis with thrombosis.

Buerger classified pathological changes of TAO into acute, subacute, and chronic phases. He considered the acute lesion crucial for the diagnosis. In acute lesions, the artery or vein is modestly swollen, with moderate lymphocytic infiltration of the adventitia and media. The lumen is occluded by a highly cellular thrombus with the appearance of a microabscess, in which the number of lymphocytes usually exceeds the number of neutrophils, and giant cells or eosinophils may be seen. The occlusion may extend for variable lengths and then stop abruptly, and sometimes can occur at two different levels in the same vessel; between the sites of occlusions the lumen is patent. In the subacute phase, cellular infiltration has diminished; the microabscess has disappeared and recanalization has begun. Organized and recanalized thrombi in fibrotic small vessels are characteristic of the late-phase lesion. The structure of the vessel wall remains intact, without necrosis, and in general the lesions throughout a single affected segment seem to be of essentially the same age. Lie has shown a photomicrograph of acute phlebitis, without thrombus, made from a segment of an acutely inflamed superficial vein, which supports the hypothesis that TAO begins with a reaction of the vessel wall or endothelium (Lie 1988b). It is not certain that the initial lesions in veins are exactly the same as the early lesions in arteries.

The secondary pathologic changes seen in TAO result mainly from ischemia of the tissue of the limbs. The skeletal muscle may be atrophic and is occasionally replaced by fibrous tissue. Osteoporosis of the bones of the foot and lower part of the leg may occur. When gangrene is present, bone may become necrotic and its destruction, or osteomyelitis, may be evident. The nails may be distorted and their growth slows. Trauma to the tissue usually starts the development of ulceration and gangrene. Gangrene and ulcers, most commonly seen in the toes, frequently begin in the region of the nails where minor trauma is produced by the pressure of the shoe in ordinary walking. If infection and pus formation develop in ulcers and at the margin of gangrenous lesions, it may lead to diffuse cellulitis or ascending lymphangitis.

Clinical manifestations

The onset of TAO usually starts between 19 and 45 years of age, with a median age of 30–35 years (Wessler *et al.* 1960; McPherson *et al.* 1963). Clinical manifestations of TAO result mainly from impairment of arterial blood flow to tissues, and local venous insufficiency. These include: intermittent claudication; rest pain; coldness or cold sensitivity; impaired arterial pulsation; color changes; temperature changes; superficial thrombophlebitis; ulceration; and gangrene (Figure 38.1) (see also Figure 17.2B in Chapter 17). Some patients with TAO may have joint pain or, less commonly, inflammatory arthritis (Johnson and Enzenauer 2003). The patient may present with pain, which may be expressed as an ache, a sense of fatigue, a persistent cramp, or a squeezing pain occurring only after a certain amount of exercise of the affected limb and relieved by rest. This intermittent claudication can be found in other occlusive peripheral arterial diseases also, but claudication of the foot is almost pathognomonic of TAO. It is frequently the first symptom, but can occur at any stage of the disease and may persist for the remainder of the patient's life when all other symptoms have disappeared. Claudication severity ascends with disease progression and some patients will have intermittent claudication in one or both upper extremities. Resting pain, which is usually localized in the digits, may persist for hours at a time and become more severe at night. Cold sensitivity is sometimes severe, and associated with paresthesias and color changes. Other types of sensation such as tickling, prickling, or burning may be bothersome. In most persons with TAO, pulsations of the dorsalis pedis and posterior tibial arteries are impaired or absent, and radial and ulnar pulsations are affected in at least 40% of persons. Early on, the affected extremities may have a normal color but in advanced cases they are often abnormally red, or cyanotic. These color changes usually are unilateral or involve only certain digits or portions of feet or hands. Asymmetric postural color changes also occur in TAO, indicating the degree of ischemia. Raynaud's phenomenon is common, and usually asymmetric and irregular in distribution. Superficial thrombophlebitis, which occurs in 30–45% of patients with TAO, is frequently found in the area of arterial involvement. These lesions involve small and medium-sized superficial veins, causing red, raised, and tender indurated cords of 0.5–3.0 cm in length. Symptoms usually last for 1–3 weeks before the redness and tenderness disappear, but occlusion of the veins may persist. When superficial thrombophlebitis is seen with occlusive arterial disease, the diagnosis of TAO should be considered.

Digital ulceration or gangrene is found in 18–60% of patients. These may occur spontaneously, but most are induced by mechanical, chemical, or thermal trauma, such as nail trimming or pressure from footwear. Pressure from shoes on the nails during walking can cause necrosis of skin and underlying tissue when the blood supply is impaired. Nails may become loosened and slough, followed by ulceration of the nail bed. Ulcerations usually develop on the tips of the digits, in the fold at the base of the flexor surface of the toe, or between the toes. Contact ulcers may develop from pressure on the side of the toes. There may be swelling and redness around the margin of ulcers, but the base of the ischemic ulcers is usually yellowish-white, brown, or black in color. Secondary infection can precipitate further loss of necrotic tissue or gangrene. Cellulitis and abscess formation from ulceration or gangrenous lesions are common.

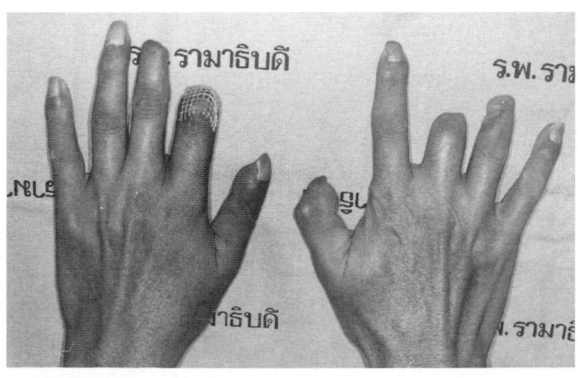

(a)

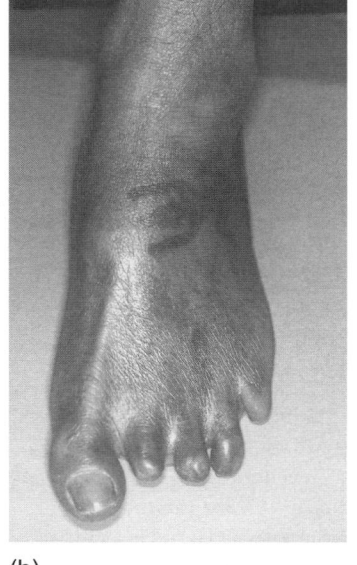

(b)

Figure 38.1 Hands (a) and feet (b) of a patient with TAO and healed amputations.

In moderate to severe ischemia, trophic changes such as slow nail growth, small scars, depression or pits on the tip of the digits are inevitable. Absorption of fat causes shrunken digits; and in advanced cases the whole foot may appear shrunken. The muscles of calf and thigh may also atrophy. In severe arterial insufficiency, osteoporosis of the foot and leg is not uncommon. Obstruction of venous blood flow by venous thrombosis, local lymphangitis, malnutrition of tissue, and prolonged dependency can contribute to lower extremity edema.

Despite a patient's complaints referable to only one limb, examination usually detects other limb involvement as well. Shionoya and colleagues analyzed 255 TAO patients and reported involvement of all four limbs in 40%, of three limbs in 43%, and of two limbs in 17% of the patients (Shionoya et al. 1982). Features that help distinguish TAO from premature atherosclerosis are foot claudication, involvement of upper extremities, bilateral or three or four limb involvement, superficial phlebitis, and Raynaud's phenomenon.

TAO is a significant cause of limb loss in youthful patients, but it is not lethal. The rate of leg amputation, mostly below the knee, is 3–30% of patients, of the toe and forefoot 19–23% of patients, and of the fingers, 3–15%. These amputation rates depend on the effectiveness of local care of the ischemic limbs, the duration of follow-up, and, most importantly, whether the patients have stopped smoking or not. Complete abstinence from tobacco use is crucial for stabilization of the process, but in advanced stage of the disease, despite cessation of smoking, recurrent episodes of ischemia or tissue loss are not rare.

Occlusive arterial disease of viscera may occur in patients with TAO, as demonstrated by Lie (Lie 1998c). It appears that the visceral arteries of TAO patients are somewhat more susceptible to thrombotic occlusion or atherosclerotic changes than normal, and abdominal pain in a TAO patient should alert the clinician to the possibility of mesenteric ischemia. Intestinal TAO is uncommon, there being some 50 or so reported examples, including some in women, but this should be considered in all patients with TAO and abdominal symptoms. Symptoms related to mesenteric artery lesions range from abdominal angina to acute pain due to intestinal perforation (Medlicott et al. 2003; Cho et al. 2005; Kobayashi et al. 2003).

Cerebral lesions are apparently rare. No et al. (2005) described a patient with TAO and repeated transient ischemic attacks. Angiography showed multiple areas of arterial occlusions in the distal segments of both middle cerebral arteries and collateral vessels around the occluded segment resembling the "corkscrew" vessels described peripherally in some patients. Few patients have been reported to have multisystem involvement, such as cerebral and bowel infarctions as well as cavernomatous transformation of the portal vein (Rai et al. 2004; Calguneri et al. 2004). Less common still is coronary artery disease (Hong et al. 2005).

Diagnosis

The diagnosis of TAO should be considered in tobacco users presenting with digital ischemia of the feet or hands. In a typical case of TAO, the diagnosis can be made on clinical basis alone and by excluding other diseases with selected laboratory testing. Special confirmatory investigations include Doppler flow-velocity, arteriography, and biopsy. The standard criterion for the diagnosis of TAO is typical histologic changes in the arteries of the extremities. Shionoya proposed clinical criteria for diagnosis of TAO consisting of: (1) smoking history; (2) onset before the age of 50 years; (3) infrapopliteal arterial occlusions; (4) either upper limb involvement or phlebitis migrans; and (5) absence of atherosclerotic risk factors other than smoking (Shionoya 1998).

Laboratory investigations

The diagnosis of TAO is made on a clinical basis. Laboratory tests are needed to exclude hyperlipidemia, diabetes mellitus, other rheumatic diseases, clotting disorders, and dysproteinemia. An appropriate workup should include lipid profile, fasting serum glucose, ANA, erythrocyte sedimentation rate, complement C_3, C_4, and CH_{50}, prothrombin time and partial thromboplastin time, hematocrit and platelet count, anticardiolipin antibody/lupus anticoagulant, serum protein electrophoresis, protein C, protein S, and antithrombin III levels.

The Doppler flow-velocity detector is used to demonstrate decreased or absent flow signals through arteries of digits or limbs. Laser flow velocities are useful in assessing occlusive disease of the fingers and their potential response to sympathetic block. In the presence of trophic changes, ulcerations, or gangrene, radiographs of the foot or hand are needed to determine whether necrosis of bone has occurred. They also help in determining the presence of osteoporosis, but this is seen only after substantial loss of bone mineral density has occurred.

Arteriography

The role of arteriography in TAO is controversial. Some consider it necessaary for diagnosis, some agree with its corroborative role, and others claim it is not crucial when the clinical features are typical. Arteriograms show multiple occluded segments in the small and medium-sized arteries of legs and arms, thus digital, pedal and calf vessel involvement is common (see Figure 18.10 in Chapter 18). Shionoya demonstrated bilateral infrapopliteal involvement in all limbs of his patients, with abnormal anterior tibial (90%), posterior tibial (80%), and peroneal arteries (50%) (Shionoya et al. 1982). He also observed toe ulceration in 57% of his patients with three-vessel obstruction, in contrast to only 7% when at least one vessel was patent. An extensive reticular network of collateral vessels is seen around the occlusive area. These collateral vessels sometimes have a "corkscrew" appearance (see Figure 18.9 in Chapter 18), which had been attributed by some to recanalization of the occluded arteries and by others to collateral flow through vasa vasorum that surround the thrombosed segment. Suzuki et al. (1996) found corkscrew-appearing collateral vessels in 27% of limbs affected by TAO and in 2% in limbs of patients with atherosclerotic disease. They also concluded that corkscrew-shaped vessels that extend from the sites of the arterial occlusion to the periphery of the feet without opacification of the main pedal arteries are a characteristic feature of TAO and also indicate a poor prognosis.

Arteriography is not recommended as a routine diagnostic procedure, but might be appropriate for identifying patients who might be candidates for bypass surgery, and to rule out a proximal site of atherosclerosis. The patterns of occlusion seen by arteriography can be correlated with both the distribution and severity of the disease.

Differential diagnosis

Bearing the typical clinical features in mind, the differential diagnosis of TAO is usually not difficult. Premature atherosclerosis is the most common occlusive disease of arteries causing leg claudication and ischemia in young men and women, which should be considered first in differential diagnosis. Patients with premature atherosclerosis usually have risk factors of diabetes mellitus or hyperlipidemia, and radiographic calcification in involved arterial segments, and they have more proximal symptoms. Pairolero *et al.* (1984) studied by arteriography 50 patients under the age of 35, who had lower limb ischemia. Twenty-four of the 50 had premature atherosclerosis, 14 had TAO, and the remaining 12 had other problems. In the premature atherosclerosis group, 10 had diabetes, eight had increased lipids or hypertension, and only one was a heavy smoker.

Vascular occlusion can occur in various rheumatic diseases and hematologic disorders. Raynaud's phenomenon, acrocyanosis, and acrolysis are major manifestations of scleroderma, as well as of TAO, but skin disease manifest as thickening, induration, and vitiligo, is not seen in TAO. Systemic lupus erythematosus, with or without antiphospholipid syndrome, or primary antiphospholipid syndrome itself, can present with thrombi in large digital arteries or veins, but these are usually accompanied by other manifestations which yield the diagnosis. Occlusion of arteries with impairment or absence of pulsation is rare in polyarteritis nodosa, although isolated areas of purpura, ischemia, or infarction of skin may be present. Thrombocytosis, polycythemia vera, dysproteinemia, and hypercoagulable states can cause microcirculatory occlusion. It is unclear whether use of cannabis can cause onset of TOA or whether it can provoke arterial disease resembling TAO (Karila *et al.* 2004). Occlusive arterial disease of the hand due to chronic occupational trauma is usually confined to the dominant hand, while TAO involves upper extremities bilaterally, often with one or both lower extremities. Reflex sympathetic dystrophy may be associated with coldness, sudomotor, and color changes in the hands due to arterial insufficiency, but skin temperature and pulsations become normal during vasodilation.

Embolic arterial occlusion can be differentiated from TAO on clinical grounds. Progressive claudication and distal emboli with ischemia are common findings in popliteal entrapment syndrome, cystic disease of the popliteal artery, and thoracic outlet syndrome. Other rare hereditary diseases of connective tissue such as Ehler–Danlos syndrome and pseudoxanthoma elasticum can cause occlusion of arteries with the formation of aneurysm or thrombosis with embolism. Combined arterial and venous occlusions are highly suggestive of TAO.

Treatment

Complete abstinence from tobacco is the first and most important step in stabilizing the process of the disease and preventing relapses. This must be clearly conveyed to the patient and family. Pain relief is another essential step in helping the patient. Intermittent claudication can be relieved by rest and oral analgesia, but patients with rest pain, ulceration, gangrene, or infection often require hospitalization, where they can be placed in a warm environment, with avoidance of weight bearing and other trauma to ischemic limbs. Continuous intravenous narcotics or epidural anesthesia are required in severe cases. Special wound care and infection control are essential for patients with ulceration, infection, or gangrene.

Vasodilating agents such as calcium channel blockers can be used, but their efficacy regarding ischemic pain and wound healing is controversial. There is preliminary evidence suggesting that prostacyclin (PGI_2) or its analogs, such as treprostinil, may be beneficial in the treatment of TAO that does not improve with smoking cessation. Regional sympathetic ganglionectomy may be of some value in TAO patients with extensive gangrene. Surgical sympathetic ganglionectomy is preferable to injection of alcohol into sympathetic ganglia, because interruption is more certain and permanent.

A Turkish clinic treated 344 TAO patients surgically between 1980 and 2004. The most common complaints were foot coldness in 90%; color changes in 84%: resting pin in 46%; claudication in 66%; and necrotic ulcers in 53%. Lumbar sympathectomy was done in 278 patients followed by thoracic and combined thoracic and lumbar sympathectomies; few bypass procedures were done. Sympathectomies appeared to be helpful in healing ulcers and decreasing symptoms (Ates *et al.* 2006). It may be advisable for the patients to avoid exposure to cold, as well as to drugs that may produce vasoconstriction.

It is logical to heparinize patients with acute severe exacerbations, or evidence of fresh cutoff sign on arteriography, with the goal of preventing further clot propagation. Long-term anticoagulant therapy would be of some value in chronic cases. Trials with glucocorticoids are needed to establish their efficacy (Gur'eva *et al.* 2003).

Arterial bypass surgery can be considered only in a small group of patients whose distal segments are suitable for grafting. Shionoya *et al.* reported patency rates of 90% at 1 year, 70% at 2 years, and 70% at 10 years for suprainguinal (aortofemoral or iliofemoral) grafts and patency rates of 56%, 48%, and 32% respectively for femoropopliteal or tibioperoneal grafts (Shionoya *et al.* 1994). The small size of the arteries involved and the multiplicity of occluded arterial segments make surgical approaches ineffective and potentially hazardous to the ischemic region. When rest pain, ulceration, or gangrene cannot be controlled by conventional measures within 4 weeks or when severe infection is superimposed, early amputation should be considered. It is useless to delay amputation of the leg when gangrene extends well into the foot. When amputation is necessary, an attempt should be made to keep the procedure below the knee. The success of the medical and surgical therapy of TAO usually depends on the severity of ischemia and the pattern of occlusion in a given patient.

Prognosis

TAO, although a significant cause of limb loss in youthful patients, is not a lethal disease. McPherson *et al.* (1963) reported a survivorship equal to a matched control group of non-smokers and distinctively different from the arteriosclerosis obliterans group. In both groups, coronary heart disease appeared to be the main cause of death, but it happened at an earlier age and with greater frequency in patients with arteriosclerosis obliterans than in TAO patients. The survival of digits or legs from amputation usually depends on the stage of the disease when treatment is first instituted, the abstinence of tobacco use, and avoidance of trauma to the ischemic tissue.

References

Adar, R., Papa, M. Z., Halpern, Z., Mozes, M., Shoshan, S., *et al.* (1983). Cellular sensitivity to collagen in thromboangiitis obliterans. *New England Journal of Medicine*, **308,** 1113–6.

Aerbajinai, W., Tsuchiya, T., Kimura, A., Yasukochi, Y. and Numano, F. (1996). HLA class II DNA typing in Buerger's disease. *International Journal of Cardiology*, **54** (Suppl.), 197–202.

Ates, A., Yekeler, I., Ceviz, M. *et al.* (2006). One of the most frequently vascular diseas in northeastern of Turkey: Thromboangiitis obliterans or Buerger's disease experience with 344 cases). *International Journal of Cardiology*, **111**, 147–53.

Buerger, L. (1908). Thrombo-angiitis obliterans: a study of the vascular lesions leading to presenile spontaneous gangrene. *American Journal of Medical Science*, **136**, 567.

Buerger, L. (1924). *The circulatory disturbances of the extremities: including gangrene, vasomotor, and trophic disorder*. Saunders, Philadelphia.

Calgüneri, M., Ozturk, M. A., Ay, H., Arsava, E. M., Altinok, D., Ertenli, I. and Kiraz, S. (2004). Buerger's disease with multisystem involvement, a case report and a review of literature. *Angiology*, **55**, 325–8.

Cho, Y. P., Kang, G. H., Han, M. S., Jang, H. J., *et al.* (2005). Mesenteric involvement of acute-stage Buerger's disease as the initial clinical manifestation: report of a case. *Surgery Today*, **35**, 499–501.

Cooper, L. T., Henderson, S. S., Ballman, K. V., Offord, K. P., *et al.* (2006). A prospective case-control study of tobacco dependence in thromboangiitis obliterans (Buerger's Disease). *Angiology*, **57**, 72–8.

Czarnacki, M., Gacka, M. and Adamiec, R. (2004). A role of endothelin 1 in the pathogenesis of thromboangiitis obliterans (initial news). *Przegl Lek*, **61**, 1346–50.

Eichhorn, J., Sima, D., Lindschau, C. and Turowski, A. (1998). Antiendothelial cell antibodies in thromboangiitis obliterans. *American Journal of Medical Science*, **315**, 17–23.

Fernandez, B. and Strootman, D. (2006). The prostacyclin analog, treprostinil sodium, provides symptom relief in severe Buerger's disease–a case report and review of literature. *Angiology*, **57**, 99–102.

Fleshman, K. (1998). Buerger's disease in Nepal. *Tropical Doctor*, **28**, 203–6.

Goodman, R. M., Elian, B., Mozes, M., *et al.* (1965). Buerger's disease in Israel. *American Journal of Medicine*, **39**, 601–15.

Glueck, C. J., Haque, M., Winarska, M., Dharashivkar, S., Fontaine, R. N., Zhu, B. and Wang, P. (2006). Stromelysin-1 5A/6A and eNOS T-786C polymorphisms, MTHFR C677T and A1298C mutations, and cigarette-cannabis smoking: a pilot, hypothesis-generating study of gene-environment pathophysiological associations with Buerger's disease. *Clinical and Applied Thrombosis-Hemostasis*, **12**, 427–39.

Gur'eva, M. S., Baranov, A. A., Bagrakova, S. V. and Kurdiukov, A. A. (2003). Pulse-therapy with glucocorticoids and cyclophosphamide in the treatment of thromboangiitis obliterans. *Klinicheskaya Meditsina* (Mosk), **81**, 53–7.

Hill, G. L. and Smith, A. H. (1974). Buerger's disease in Indonesia: clinical course and prognostic factors. *Journal of Chronic Disease*, **27**, 205–16.

Hill, G. L., Moeliono, J., Tumewu, F., Brataamadja, D. and Tohardi A. (1973). 'Asian cigarette' is an adverse prognostic factor in peripheral arterial disease. *Nature*, **246**, 492–3.

Hong, T. E. and Faxon, D. P. (2005). Coronary artery disease in patients with Buerger's disease. *Reviews in Cardiovascular Medicine*, **6**, 222–6.

Iwai, T., Inoue, Y., Umeda, M., *et al.* (2005). Oral bacteria in the occluded arteries of patients with Buerger disease. *Journal of Vascular Surgery*, **42**, 107–15.

Johnson, J. A. and Enzenauer, R. J. (2003). Inflammatory arthritis associated with thromboangiitis obliterans. *Journal of Clinical Rheumatology*, **9**, 37–40.

Karila, L., Daniel, T., Coscas, S., Chambon, J. P. and Reynaud, M. (2004). Progressive cannabis-induced arteritis: a clinical thromboangiitis obliterans sub-group? *Presse Medicale*, **33** (18 Suppl.), 21–3.

Kobayashi, M., Ito, M., Nakagawa, A., Nishikimi, N. and Nimura, Y. (1999). Immunohistochemical analysis of arterial wall cellular infiltration in Buerger's disease. *Journal of Vascular Surgery*, **29**, 451–8.

Kobayashi, M., Kurose, K., Kobata, T., Hida, K., Sakamoto, S. and Matsubara, J. (2003). Ischemic intestinal involvement in a patient with

Buerger disease: case report and literature review. *Journal of Vascular Surgery*, **38**, 170–4.

Laohapensang, K., Kerkasem, K. and Kattipattanapong, V. (2004). Seasonal variation of Buerger's disease in Northern part of Thailand. *European Journal of Vascular and Endovascular Surgery*, **28**, 418–20.

Lie, J. T. (1987). Thromboangiitis obliterans (Buerger's disease) in women. *Medicine* (Baltimore), **66**, 65–72.

Lie, J. T. (1988a). Thromboangiitis obliterans (Buerger's disease) and smokeless tobacco. *Arthritis and Rheumatism*, **31**, 812–3.

Lie, J. T. (1988b). Thromboangiitis obliterans (Buerger's disease) revisited. *Pathology Annual*, **23**, 257–91.

Lie, J. T. (1988c). Visceral intestinal Buerger's disease. *International Journal of Cardiology*, **66**, (Suppl. 1), S249–56.

Matsushita, M., Shionoya, S. and Matsumoto, T. (1991). Urinary cotinine measurements in patients with Buerger's disease-effect of active and passive smoking on the disease process. *Journal of Vascular Surgery*, **14**, 53–8.

McKusick, V. A., Harris, W. S., Oxtesen, O. E., Goodman, R. M., Shelley, W. M. and Bloodwell, R. D. (1962). Buerger's disease: a distinct clinical and pathologic entity. *Journal of the American Medical Association*, **181**, 5–12.

McKusick, V. A. and Harris, W. S. (1961). The Buerger syndrome in the Orient. *Bulletin of Johns Hopkins Hospital*, **109**, 241–91.

McPherson, J. R., Juergens, J. L. and Gifford, R. W. (1963). Thromboangiitis obliterans and arteriosclerosis obliteran: clinical and prognostic differences. *Annals of Internal Medicine*, **59**, 288–96.

Medlicott, S. A., Beaudry, P., Morris, G., Hollaar, G. and Sutherland, F. (2003). Intestinal thromboangiitis obliterans in a woman: a case report and discussion of chronic ischemic changes. *Canadian Journal of Gastroenterology*, **17**, 559–61.

No, Y. J., Lee, E. M., Lee, D. H. and Kim, J. S. (2005). Cerebral angiographic findings in thromboangiitis obliterans. *Neuroradiology*, **47**, 912–5.

Pairolero, P. C., Joyce, J. W., Skinner, C. R., Hollier, L. H. and Cherry, K. J. Jr. (1984). Lower limb ischemia in young adults: prognostic implications. *Journal of Vascular Surgery*, **1**, 459–64.

Rai, M., Miyashita, K., Oe, H., Nishigami, K. and Naritomi, H. (2004). Multiple brain infarctions in a young patient with Buerger's disease. A case report of cerebral thromboangiitis obliterans. *Rinsho Shinkeigaku*, **44**, 522–6.

Reny, J. L. and Cabane, J. (1998). Buerger's disease or thromboangiitis obliterans. *Review Medicine Interne*, **19**, 34–43.

Shionoya, S. (1994). Buerger's disease (thromboangiitis obliterans). In *Vascular surgery* (Rutherford, R. B., ed), 4th edn. Saunders, Philadelphia.

Shionoya, S. (1998). Diagnostic criteria of Buerger's Disease. *International Journal of Cardiology*, **66** (Suppl.), S243–5.

Shionoya, S., Hiari, M. and Kawai, S. (1982). Pattern of arterial occlusion in Buerger's disease. *Angiology*, **33**, 375–84.

Slavov, E. S., Stanilova, S. A., Petkov, D. P. and Dobreva, Z. G. (2005). Cytokine production in thromboangiitis obliterans patients: new evidence for an immune-mediated inflammatory disorder. *Clinical and Experimental Rheumatology*, **23**, 219–26.

Suzuki, S., Yamada, I. and Himeno, Y. (1996). Angiographic findings in Buerger disease. *International Journal of Cardiology*, **54** (Suppl.), S189–95.

Szilagyi, E. D., De Russo, F. J. and Elliot, J. P. (1964). Thromboangiitis obliterans: clinico-angiographic correlations. *Archives of Surgery*, **88**, 824.

Wessler, S., Ming, S.-C. and Gurewich, V. (1960). A critical evaluation of thromboangiitis obliterans: the case against Buerger's disease. *New England Journal of Medicine*, **262**, 1149–60.

CHAPTER 39

Cutaneous small-vessel vasculitis

Amy E. DeVore and Joseph L. Jorizzo

Cutaneous small-vessel vasculitis (CSVV), or as it is referred to elsewhere in this text, cutaneous leukocytoclastic vasculitis, is the most common form of vasculitis in the skin. There is a spectrum of clinical lesions, with palpable purpura on dependent sites being most common. Histopathologic examination of classic lesions reveals fibrinoid necrosis of vessel walls, endothelial cell swelling, and segmental neutrophilic inflammation with leukocytoclasia (Lotti *et al.* 1996; Soter and Austen 1978). This immune-complex driven vasculitis specifically affects postcapillary venules. Although the skin is often the only organ involved, systemic involvement must be ruled out in each presentation. The majority of cases are idiopathic, but medications, infections, malignancies, or other systemic disease can induce this form of vasculitis.

Classification

Due to the variability in both clinical and histologic features of the various types of vasculitis, establishment of a generally accepted classification scheme has been challenging. In the early 1950s, Zeek first attempted to classify the vasculitides (Zeek 1953) followed by many subsequent alternative classification systems (Fauci *et al.* 1978; Gilliam and Smiley 1976; Lie 1989). In 1990, the American College of Rheumatology (ACR) defined criteria for the diagnosis of hypersensitivity vasculitis, which corresponds to CSVV (Hunder *et al.* 1990) as outlined in Table 39.1. Some of the problems with this scheme are the histologic requirements, restrictions on age of onset, and the specification of a medication at onset as a criterion. Several working classifications of the various vasculitides have been described (see Chapter 1). Shown in Table 39.2 are cutaneous small-vessel vasculitides (Ghersetich *et al.* 1995; Jorizzo 1993). To date, a non-controversial classification that is clinically relevant, workable by various medical subspecialists throughout the world, and addresses the various features and causes of vasculitis has yet to be defined.

Epidemiology

CSVV affects 9% of all patients presenting to rheumatologists with the diagnosis of vasculitis (Hunder *et al.* 1990). It occurs equally in both males and females and at all ages of life (Comacchi *et al.* 1998; Lotti *et al.* 1996). Approximately 10% of those affected are children

(Lynch 1988; Resnick and Esterly 1985), thus highlighting a weakness of the ACR criteria for CSVV. Caucasians are predominantly affected (Ekenstam and Callen 1984).

Etiology

Factors known to contribute to the etiology of CSVV are limited, and the cause of disease remains undetermined in the majority

Table 39.1 American College of Rheumatology criteria for hypersensitivity vasculitis (Hunder *et al.* 1990)

1. Age at disease onset >16 years
2. Medication at disease onset
3. Palpable purpura
4. Maculopapular rash
5. Biopsy including arteriole and venule with histologic changes showing granulocytes in a perivascular or extravascular location

Hypersensitivity vasculitis is diagnosed if a patient meets 3 or more criteria.

Specificity of 83.9% and sensitivity of 71%.

Table 39.2 Cutaneous small-vessel vasculitides from a proposed working classification of vasculitis (Ghersetich *et al.* 1995)

Idiopathic cutaneous small-vessel vasculitis
Henoch–Schönlein purpura
Essential mixed cryoglobulinemia
Waldenström's hypergammaglobulinemic purpura
Collagen vascular disease associated
Urticarial vasculitis
Erythema elevatum diutinum
Rheumatoid nodules
Reactive leprosy
Septic vasculitis

Table 39.3 Associations with cutaneous small-vessel vasculitis (Sams and Sams 2001; Lotti *et al.* 1998)

Drugs	Allopurinol, aminosalicylic acid, beta-blockers, herbicides, hydantoins, insecticides, insulin, iodides, oral contraceptives, penicillin, petroleum products, phenacetin, phenothiazines, phenylbutazone, propylthiouracil, quinine, quinidine, serum, streptokinase, streptomycin, sulfonamides, tamoxifen, thiazides, vaccines(influenza), vitamins
Infections	*Candida albicans*, cytomegalovirus, Epstein barr virus, hepatitis A, B and C, herpes simplex, histoplasmosis, influenza, *Mycobacterium leprae*, *Mycobacterium tuberculosis*, *Onchocerca volvulus*, *Plasmodium malariae*, *Schistosoma haematobium*, *Schistosoma mansoni*, *Staphylococcus aureus*, *Streptococcus* group A
Malignancies	Adult T-cell leukemia, chronic lymphocytic leukemia, hairy cell leukemia, Hodgkin's disease, lymphosarcoma, multiple myeloma, mycosis fungoides, solid tumors (breast, colon colon, head and neck, lung, prostate, and renal)
Other conditions	Behçet's syndrome, bowel bypass syndrome, chronic active hepatitis, cryoglobulinemia, cystic fibrosis, hemolytic anemia, HIV/AIDS, hyperglobulinemic states, primary biliary cirrhosis, rheumatoid arthritis, Sjögren's syndrome, systemic lupus erythematosus, ulcerative colitis

of patients (Braun-Falco *et al.* 1991; Comacchi *et al.* 1998; Lotti *et al.* 1996; Ryan 1992). There are no recognized genetic factors (Soter and Wolff 1987). Infections, medications, chemicals, food proteins, malignancies, and systemic diseases such as the connective tissue diseases are potential causes (Table 39.3) (Braun-Falco *et al.* 1991; Comacchi *et al.* 1998; Lotti *et al.* 1996; Ryan 1992; Sams and Sams 2001; Soter and Wolff 1987). Many of the etiologic factors have been incriminated by association alone, without direct confirmatory evidence (Lotti *et al.* 1998). Only the streptococcal M protein, *Mycobacterium tuberculosis*, and hepatitis B surface antigen have been found in the same pattern in the same affected vessels as the corresponding antibodies (Gower *et al.* 1978; Parish 1971; Thorne *et al.* 1977). A practical approach is to evaluate drugs, infections, and diseases associated with immune complexes, such as connective tissue vascular diseases, inflammatory bowel disease, chronic active hepatitis, and myelodysplastic malignancy, as possible etiologies.

Pathogenesis

The deposition of circulating immune complexes initiates the vasculitic process in patients with CSVV and likely results in the classic histologic pattern (Mackel and Jordon 1982). Immunoglobulins (IgG, IgM, IgA), complement components (C1q, C3) and fibrin deposits have been documented in postcapillary venules using immunofluorescence and ultrastructural techniques (Braun-Falco *et al.* 1991; Braverman and Yen 1975; Comacchi *et al.* 1998; Lotti *et al.* 1996; Ryan 1992; Soter and Wolff 1987). Deposited immune complexes activate the classical and alternative complement pathways (Lynch 1988; Tosca and Stratigos 1988; Yancey and Lawley 1984) leading to mast cell degranulation, neutrophil migration, and neutrophil activation with release of tissue destructive enzymes (protease, collagenase,

elastase) (Braun-Falco *et al.* 1991; Jorizzo *et al.* 1988; Tosca and Stratigos 1988). These enzymes, along with oxygen free radicals produced by neutrophils, cause endothelial damage (Braun-Falco *et al.* 1991; Tosca and Stratigos 1988). Cytokines and other mediators of inflammation such as tumor necrosis factor, leukotriene B4, histamine, interleukin-1, interleukin-6, thrombin, and interferons accelerate neutrophil influx and induce the synthesis and expression of surface adhesion molecules on endothelium promoting neutrophil migration (Bevilacqua *et al.* 1985; Braun-Falco *et al.* RK 1991; Tosca and Stratigos 1988; Yancey and Lawley 1984; Zimmerman *et al.* 1992; Zimmerman and Hill 1984). Neutrophils phagocytose and degrade the deposited immune complexes, with the entire cycle of events from immune complex deposition to removal usually requiring 18–24 hours (Jorizzo *et al.* 1988; Tosca and Stratigos 1988; Yancey and Lawley 1984).

Multiple factors influence the deposition of immune complexes and amplify tissue destruction. These include the erythrocyte's ability to transport immune complexes to the fixed macrophage system; the functional state of the macrophage system, hydrostatic pressure and turbulent flow; serotonin and histamine release from platelets facilitating initial immune complex deposition; and the integrity of the fibrinolytic system (Lotti *et al.* 1998). Fibrinolytic activity is increased in the early stages of disease and reduced in later stages. Immune complexes, through interaction with the Fc receptor on the endothelium, cause release of tissue plasminogen activator (t-PA), inducing fibrinolytic activity and increased vascular permeability. Increased tissue deposition of immune complexes is an end result (Bianchini *et al.* 1983; Parish 1972; Teofoli and Lotti 1995).

Neuropeptides, such as substance P, neurokinin A, and calcitonin gene-related peptide, are hypothesized to play a role in the pathogenesis of vasculitis. Mechanisms include modulation of the fibrinolytic system and local immune system, activation of macrophages and mast cells, vasodilatation and increased vascular permeability, and expression of endothelial cell adhesion molecules (Lotti *et al.* 1998).

T lymphocytes that express γ and δ polypeptide chains in the T-cell receptor (γ/δ T cells) recognize human heat shock proteins (HSP) that may cross react with HSPs from infectious pathogens. γ/δ T cells and HSP-72 have been observed in lesional skin of patients with CSVV due to documented infectious causes (Comacchi *et al.* 1999). This suggests that the infectious agent led to selectively elevated tissue levels of HSPs preferentially recognized by this subpopulation of T cells. At this point, γ/δ T cells have only been implicated in the pathogenesis of infectious causes of CSVV, but their involvement has not been definitively proven.

Clinical features

The classic presentation of CSVV is petechial macules which progress to palpable purpura (Figure 39.1). Individual lesions are usually less than 1 cm diameter and demonstrate sharply demarcated margins (Figure 39.2). Adjacent lesions may coalesce to form large plaques (Figure 39.3). Dermal inflammation causes distension, resulting in palpability. Extravasation of red blood cells from involved vessels leads to the non-blanchable, purpuric nature of lesions. Other less common clinical signs include nodules, pustules (Figures 39.4), necrosis (Figures 39.5 and 39.6), ulcers (Figure 39.7), urticarial lesions, and retiform patterns.

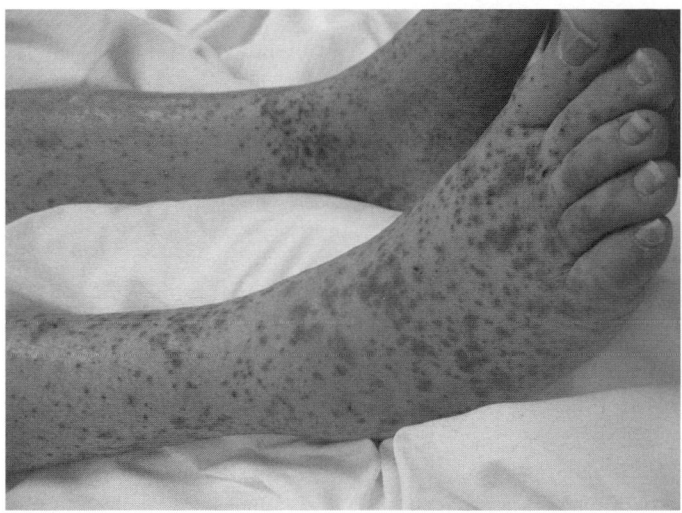

Fig. 39.1 Diffuse palpable purpura on the bilateral lower extremities representing CSVV. (See Color Plate 100).

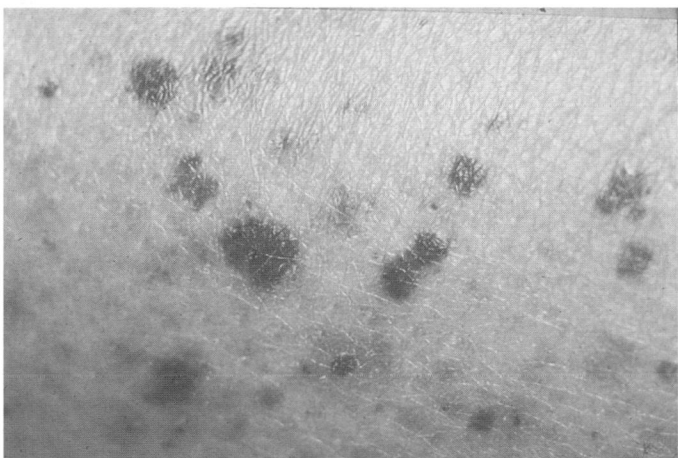

Fig. 39.2 Individual lesions are usually less than 1 cm diameter and demonstrate sharply demarcated margins. (From Sams, H. H. and Sams, W. M. Jr (2002). Cutaneous leukocytoplastic vasculitis. In *Vasculitis* (Ball, G. V. and Bridges, S. L. Jr, eds), 1st edn, pp. 467–75. Oxford University Press, New York.) (See Color Plate 101).

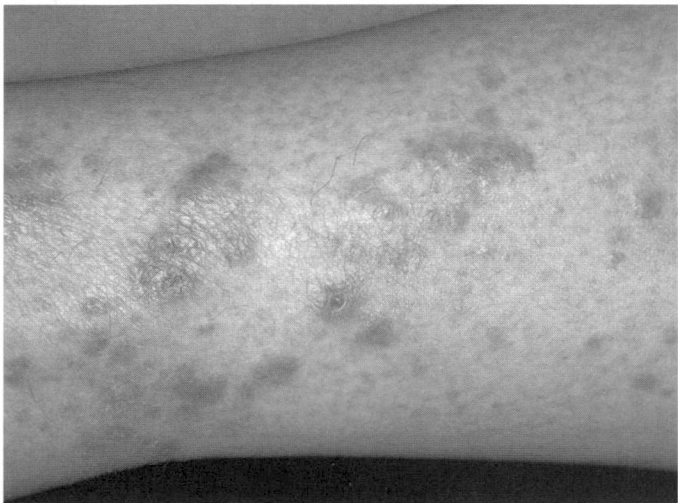

Fig. 39.3 Individual lesions may coalesce to larger plaques. (See Color Plate 102).

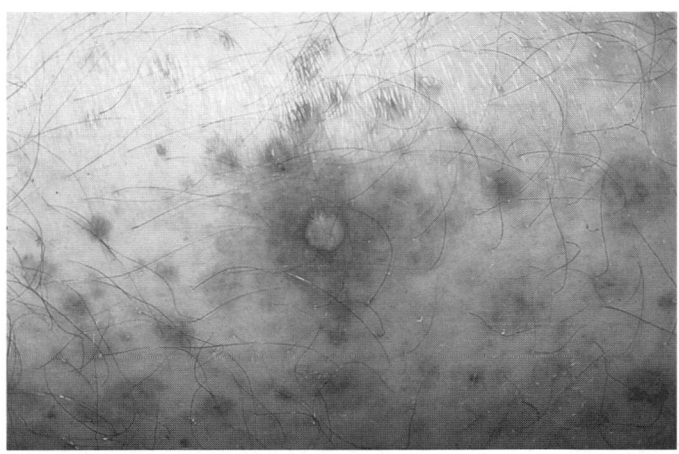

Fig. 39.4 Intense neutrophilic infiltrate may lead to pustule formation on a hemorrhagic base. (From Sams, H. H. and Sams, W. M. Jr (2002). Cutaneous leukocytoplastic vasculitis. In *Vasculitis* (Ball, G. V. and Bridges, S. L. Jr, eds), 1st edn, pp. 467–75. Oxford University Press, New York.) (See Color Plate 103).

Vascular lesions usually occur first and predominate on the ankles and legs. Other dependent areas may show involvement due to sludging of blood and decreased vascular flow. Areas of trauma, including cutaneous surfaces under tight-fitting clothing, may also be affected. These lesions are commonly asymptomatic, although pruritus and burning are often reported (Hautmann *et al.* 1999).

Given that CSVV is typically due to an inciting agent, these lesions typically occur as a single crop that resolves spontaneously after weeks or months (Swerlick and Lawley 1989). Postinflammatory hyperpigmentation is common after resolution, and scarring occurs after ulcerative or necrotic lesions (Figures 39.8, and 39.9). Ten percent of patients may progress to chronic recurrent disease with intervals ranging from months to years. Chronicity can be predicted by coexistent arthralgias and cryoglobulinemia without fever (Sais *et al.* 1998).

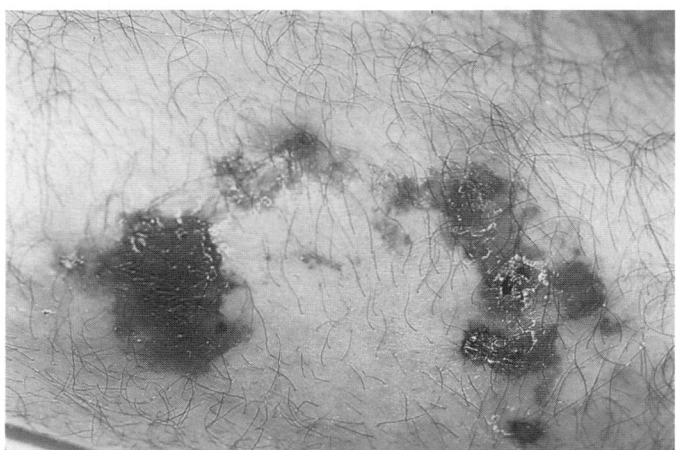

Fig. 39.5 With sufficient vascular destruction, necrosis ensues, often with irregular borders. (From Sams, H. H. and Sams, W. M. Jr (2002). Cutaneous leukocytoplastic vasculitis. In *Vasculitis* (Ball, G. V. and Bridges, S. L. Jr, eds), 1st edn, pp. 467–75. Oxford University Press, New York.) (See Color Plate 104).

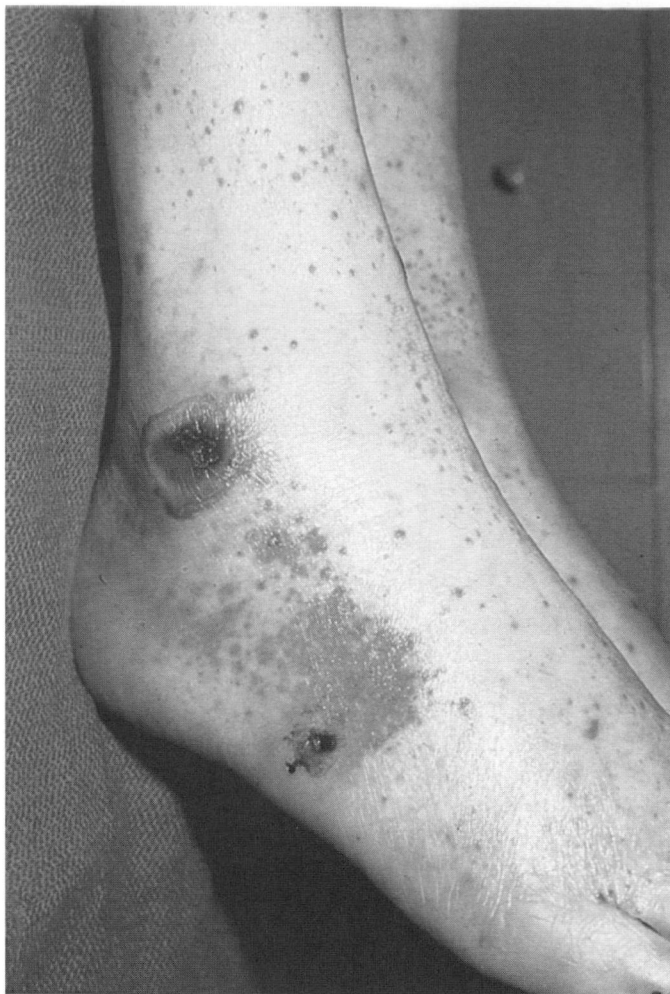

Fig. 39.6 Necrosis and blister formation may occur, as this example proximal to the lateral malleolus. (From Sams, H. H. and Sams, W. M. Jr (2002). Cutaneous leukocytoplastic vasculitis. In *Vasculitis* (Ball, G. V. and Bridges, S. L. Jr, eds), 1st edn, pp. 467–75. Oxford University Press, New York.) (See Color Plate 105).

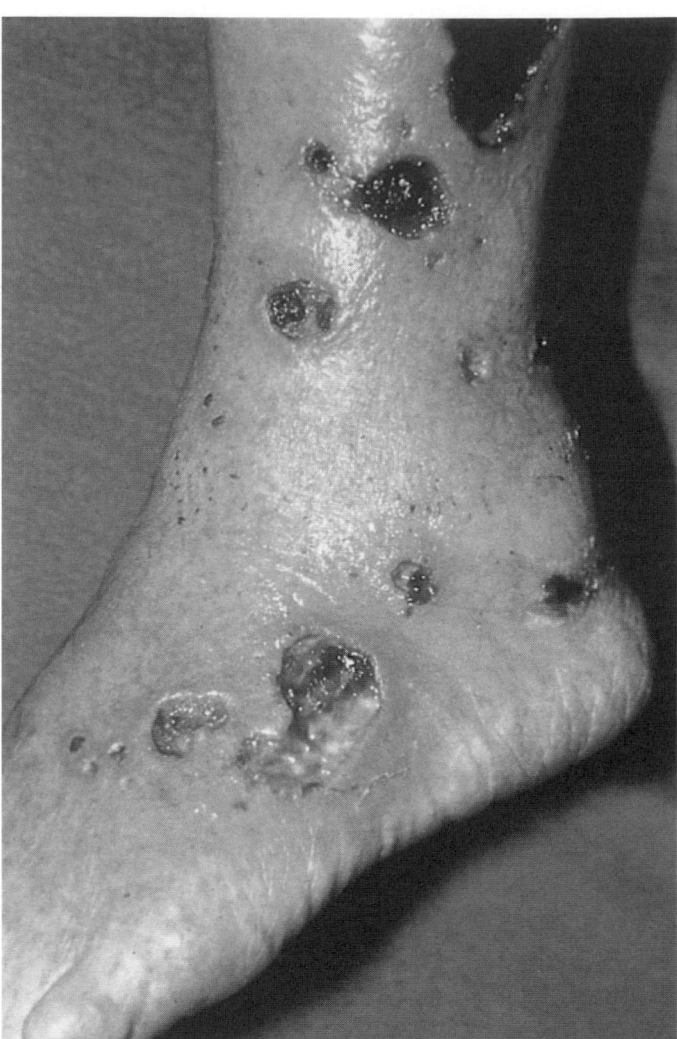

Fig. 39.8 Severe ulcers may form in CSVV. (From Sams, H. H. and Sams, W. M. Jr (2002). Cutaneous leukocytoplastic vasculitis. In *Vasculitis* (Ball, G. V. and Bridges, S. L. Jr, eds), 1st edn, pp. 467–75. Oxford University Press, New York.) (See Color Plate 107).

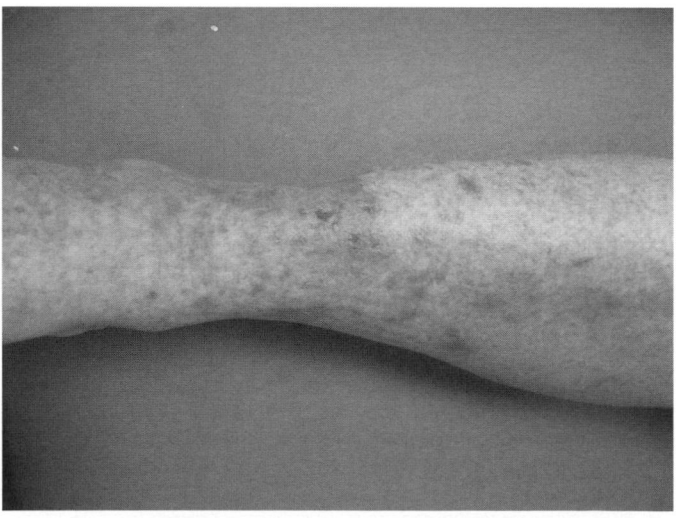

Fig. 39.7 This patient with CSVV had palpable purpura complicated by ulceration. (See Color Plate 106).

Systemic involvement

Systemic vasculitis often has cutaneous manifestations, but CSVV often occurs without any demonstrable systemic manifestations (Lotti *et al.* 1998). In any patient presenting with classic CSVV, a thorough history and physical examination as well as laboratory studies should be performed to exclude systemic involvement (Table 39.4). Synovium, pleura, pericardium, and gastrointestinal tract are frequently affected locations. The renal system and upper respiratory tract should also be evaluated. A practical approach to patient assessment would be to consider where circulating immune complexes could be filtered, other than the skin.

Laboratory evaluation

All patients with chronic disease or suspected systemic involvement should have laboratory evaluation to determine the etiology and extent of disease. Those tests evaluating etiology of disease need only be performed during the initial episode, whereas those tests determining extent of disease should be performed during each

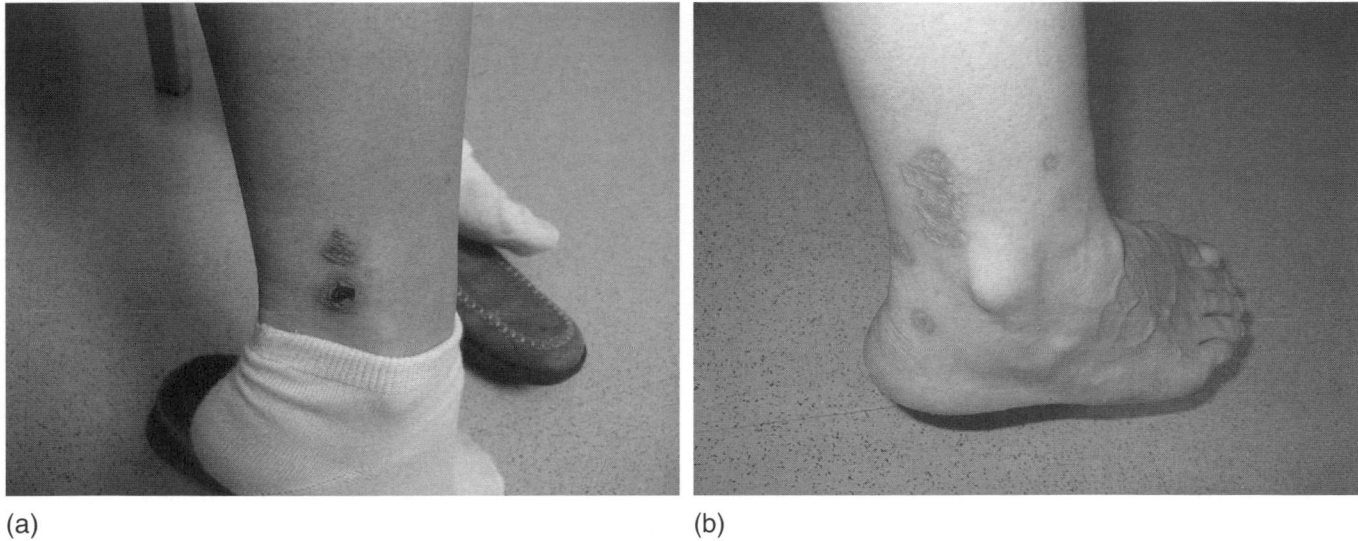

(a)

(b)

Figure 39.9 Ulcerations (a) may heal with scar formation (b), as seen in this 40-year-old woman who had resolution of CSVV. (Courtesy of Dr Lou Bridges.) (See Color Plate 108).

episode. Useful tests include: CBC with differential; hepatitis B and C serologies; serum cryoglobulins; complement levels; ANA; rheumatoid factor; and antistreptolysin titers. Positive ANCA tests must be evaluated with tests to further characterize reactivity to antigens such as MPO and PR3. In the absence of other specific systemic signs or symptoms, a chest radiograph and complete blood count are adequate screens for malignancy. In febrile patients with a new heart murmur, echocardiography and blood cultures should be ordered to rule out endocarditis (Fiorentino 2003). Laboratory tests to determine extent of disease include blood urea nitrogen, creatinine, liver function tests, urinalysis, and stool guaiac. ESR is elevated in up to 60% of patients, but is not useful for diagnostic purposes or prediction of disease progression (Ekenstam and Callen 1984).

Histopathology

The clinical diagnosis should be confirmed by biopsy, which needs to be performed in a timely fashion. A biopsy specimen taken too late (after 48 hours) may show more pathologic features of tissue repair and a monocytic infiltrate as opposed to the initial injury (Ryan 1999). Early lesions typically show the classic pathologic finding of leukocytoclastic vasculitis (Figures 39.10 and 39.11). This is characterized by angiocentric segmental inflammation, endothelial swelling, erythrocyte extravasation, fibrinoid necrosis of blood vessel walls, and an infiltrate around and within blood vessels composed primarily of neutrophils which show fragmentation of nuclei (Lotti *et al.* 1998). Thrombosis within affected vessels and hyalinization of vessel walls can be observed in the later phase (Soter *et al.* 1976). Direct immunofluorescence may show IgG, IgM, C1q, and C3 both within and around vessels in lesions as early as 8 hours after onset, while these immunoreactants disappear as the inflammatory sequence evolves.

Treatment

Identification and removal of any identifiable trigger factor such as medications or infection can be an effective first-line approach to

Table 39.4 Systemic manifestations of cutaneous small-vessel vasculitis (Lotti *et al* 1998)

Joints	Arthralgias and arthritis
Pulmonary	Cough and hemoptysis or asymptomatic
Cardiac	Myocardial angiitis and pericarditis
Gastrointestinal	Nausea, vomiting, diarrhea, colicky pain, melena, hematemesis, melena, and pancreatitis
Renal	Nephritis with microscopic hematuria and proteinuria, acute and chronic renal failure
Ophthalmologic	Retinal vasculitis, conjunctivitis, keratitis, and pseudotumor cerebri
Nervous system	Headache, diplopia, hypoesthesia, paresthesia
Constitutional	Fever

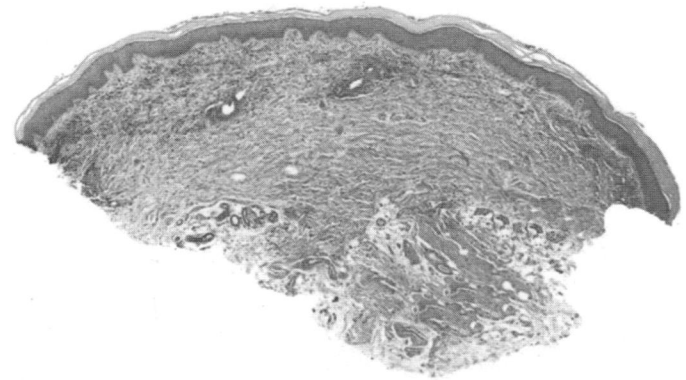

Fig. 39.10 Low power histopathologic skin specimen showing dense superficial perivascular inflammation. (Courtesy of Dr Omar Sangueza.) (See Color Plate 109).

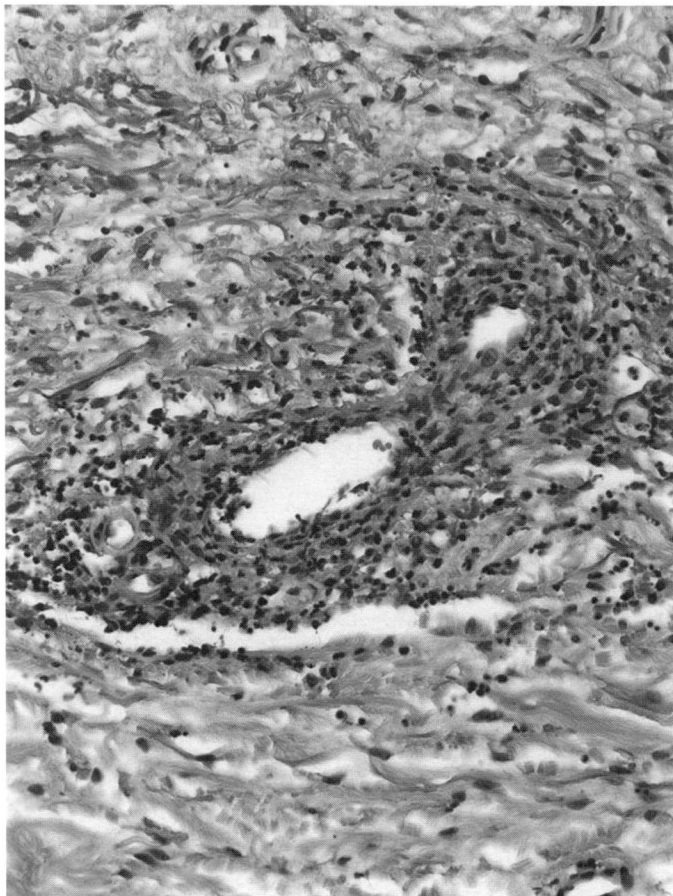

Figure 39.11 The affected small vessel demonstrates fibrinoid necrosis of the wall, neutrophilic infiltration with nuclear dust, and extravasation of red blood cells. (Courtesy of Dr Omar Sangueza.) (See Color Plate 110).

treatment of CSVV. Unfortunately, it has been estimated that only 50% of those with disease have a definable etiology (Fiorentino 2003). A watchful waiting approach may also be taken for asymptomatic disease, as in the majority of patients it will be self-limited and resolve spontaneously.

Gradient support stockings, by reducing edema, may be useful in lower extremity involvement of CSVV. In limited symptomatic disease, topical glucocorticoids may be helpful (Braun-Falco *et al.* 1991; Comacchi *et al.* 1998; Lotti *et al.* 1996). Small case series have also demonstrated some benefit from aspirin, NSAIDs, and oral antihistamines (Fiorentino 2003). Dapsone (50–200 mg daily) has been effective, typically in patients with only cutaneous involvement (Braun-Falco *et al.* 1991; Comacchi *et al.* 1998; Lotti 1991; Lotti *et al.* 1996; Ryan 1992).

For those with more diffuse, symptomatic, or systemic disease, more aggressive systemic therapy is warranted. Systemic glucocorticoids (prednisone 60–80 mg/day) are prescribed for those with systemic manifestations or those with significant cutaneous ulceration (Lotti, *et al.* 1998). Therapy should be continued until improvement is noted, and the dose should be tapered slowly (over 3–6 weeks) to avoid rebound (Braun-Falco *et al.* 1991; Comacchi *et al.* 1998; Jorizzo *et al.* 1988; Lotti *et al.* 1996; Ryan 1992). Colchicine (0.6 mg, two or three times daily) may be helpful in chronic disease by inhibiting neutrophil chemotaxis (Braun-Falco *et al.* 1991;

Comacchi *et al.* 1998; Jorizzo *et al.* 1988; Lotti *et al.* 1996; Ryan 1992; Soter and Wolff 1987). Fibrinolytic agents such as stanozolol (5 mg twice daily), have been effective in those patients with decreased cutaneous fibrinolytic activity (as defined by the maximum amount of plasminogen activator released in the skin after certain stimuli); aminocaproic acid has been used in those with increased fibrinolytic activity (Lotti 1991; Lotti *et al.* 1998).

In severe, rapidly progressive disease unresponsive to glucocorticoids, other systemic immunosuppressive agents such as cyclophosphamide (2 mg/kg/day or monthly intravenous therapy), methotrexate (10–25 mg/week), azathioprine (50–200 mg/day), or cyclosporine (3–5 mg/kg/day) may be used (Comacchi *et al.* 1998; Fiorentino 2003; Habif 1990; Jorizzo *et al.* 1988; Lotti *et al.* 1996; Lynch 1988). Appropriate laboratory testing to monitor for toxicity is indicated with all of the above-mentioned therapies. A therapeutic ladder is outlined in Table 39.5 (Barham *et al.* 2004). When approaching treatment of cutaneous small-vessel vasculitis, the physician must realize that almost no double-blind,

Table 39.5 Therapeutic ladder for the treatment of CSVV (Barham *et al.* 2004)

Skin lesions alone
Supportive therapy[3]
Antihistamines[3]
Non-steroidal anti-inflammatory drugs[2]
Pentoxiphylline[3]
Hydroxychloroquine[3]
Colchicine[1]
Dapsone[2]
Ulcerative skin lesions alone
Thalidomide[3]
Low-dose weekly methotrexate[3]
Prednisone[2]
Systemic disease
Prednisone[2]
Azathioprine 1–2.5 mg/kg/day PO as single dose or divided twice a day[2]
Cyclophosphamide pulsed dosing regimen, 40–50 mg/kg IV in divided doses over 2–5 days OR 10–15 mg/kg IV every 7–10 days OR 3–5 mg/kg IV twice weekly[2]
Mycophenolate mofetil 500 mg–2000 mg PO bid[3]
Methotrexate 7.5–15 mg once a week
Cyclosporine 2.5 mg/kg/day PO divided twice daily; after 4 weeks, dose may be increased 0.5 mg/kg/day at 2-week intervals; maximum of 4 mg/kg/day[3]
Interferon-α and ribavirin (if hepatitis C-associated) 3 million units, 3 times a week, and 1000 mg/day respectively[1]
Intravenous gammaglobulin[3]
Extracorporeal immunomodulation[3]
Biologic agents (TNF-α inhibitors) – infliximab, etanercept[3]

[1] Evidence from double-blind studies.

[2] Evidence from case series.

[3] Evidence from case reports.

placebo-controlled trials exist and current treatment recommendations are based on small clinical trials, case series, and anecdotal reports.

References

Barham, K. L, Jorizzo, J. L., Grattan, B., and Cox, N. H. (2004). Vasculitis and neutrophilic vascular reactions. In *Rook's Textbook of Dermatology* (Burns, T. *et al.* eds), 7th edn, p. 49.1–49.46. Blackwell Publishing, Oxford.

Bevilacqua, M. P., Pober, J. S., Wheeler, M. E., Cotran, R. S. and Gimbrone, M. A., Jr. (1985). Interleukin 1 acts on cultured human vascular endothelium to increase the adhesion of polymorphonuclear leukocytes, monocytes, and related leukocyte cell lines. *Journal of Clinical Investigation*, **76**, 2003–11.

Bianchini, G., Lotti, T. and Fabbri, P. (1983). Fibrin deposits and fibrinolytic activity in Schonlein-Henoch syndrome. *International Journal of Dermatology*, **22**, 103–6.

Braun-Falco, O., Plewing, G., Wolff, H. H. and Winkelmann, R. K. (1991). *Dermatology*. Springer-Verlag, Berlin.

Braverman, I. M. and Yen, A. (1975, Demonstration of immune complexes in spontaneous and histamine-induced lesions and in normal skin of patients with leukocytoclastic angiitis. *Journal of Investigative Dermatology*, **64**, 105–12.

Comacchi, C., Ghersetich, I., Katsambas, A. and Lotti, T. M. (1999). gamma/delta T lymphocytes and infection: pathogenesis of leukocytoclastic cutaneous necrotizing vasculitis. *Clinical Dermatology*, **17**, 603–7.

Comacchi, C., Ghersetich, I. and Lotti, T. (1998). Vasculite necrotizzante cutanea. *Giornale Italiano di dermatologia evenereologia*, **133**, 23–49.

Ekenstam, E. and Callen, J. P. (1984).Cutaneous leukocytoclastic vasculitis. Clinical and laboratory features of 82 patients seen in private practice. *Archives of Dermatology*, **120**, 484–9.

Fauci, A. S., Haynes, B. and Katz, P. (1978). The spectrum of vasculitis: clinical, pathologic, immunologic and therapeutic considerations. *Annals of Internal Medicine*, **89**, 660–76.

Fiorentino, D. F. (2003). Cutaneous vasculitis. *Journal of the American Academy of Dermatology*, **48**, 311–40.

Ghersetich, I., Jorizzo, J. L. and Lotti, T. (1995). Working classification of vasculitis. *International Angiology*, **14**, 101–6.

Gilliam, J. N. and Smiley, J. D. (1976). Cutaneous necrotizing vasculitis and related disorders. *Annals of Allergy*, **37**, 328–39.

Gower, R. G., Sausker, W. F., Kohler, P. F., Thorne, G. E. and McIntosh, R. M. (1978). Small vessel vasculitis caused by hepatitis B virus immune complexes. Small vessel vasculitis and HBsAG. *Journal of Allergy and Clinical Immunology*, **62**, 222–8.

Habif, T. P. (1990). *Clinical dermatology*. Mosby, St. Louis.

Hautmann, G., Campanile, G. and Lotti, T. M. (1999). The many faces of cutaneous vasculitis. *Clinical Dermatology*, **17**, 515–31.

Hunder, G. G., Arend, W. P., Bloch, D. A., Calabrese, L. H., Fauci, A. S., Fries, J. F., Leavitt, R. Y., Lie, J. T., Lightfoot, R. W., Jr., Masi, A. T., *et al.* (1990). The American College of Rheumatology 1990 criteria for the classification of vasculitis. Introduction. *Arthritis and Rheumatism*, **33**, 1065–7.

Jorizzo, J. L. (1993). Classification of vasculitis. *Journal of Investigative Dermatology*, **100**, 106S–10S.

Jorizzo, J. L., Solomon, A. R., Zanolli, M. D. and Leshin, B. (1988). Neutrophilic vascular reactions. *Journal of the American Academy of Dermatology*, **19**, 983–1005.

Lie, J. T. (1989). Systemic and isolated vasculitis. A rational approach to classification and pathologic diagnosis. *Pathology Annual*, **24**, 25–114.

Lotti, T. (1991). The management of systemic complications of vasculitis. In *Dermatology in Europe* (Panconesi, E, ed.), pp. 330–2. Blackwell Science Publications, Oxford.

Lotti, T., Comacchi, C. and Ghersetich, I. (1996). Cutaneous necrotizing vasculitis. *International Journal of Dermatology*, **35**, 457–74.

Lotti, T., Ghersetich, I., Comacchi, C. and Jorizzo, J. L. (1998). Cutaneous small-vessel vasculitis, *Journal of the American Academy of Dermatology*, **39**, 667–87.

Lynch, P. J. (1988). Vascular reactions. In *Pediatric dermatology* (Schachner, L. A. and Hansen, R. C., eds), pp. 959–1014. Churchill Livingstone, New York.

Mackel, S. E. and Jordon, R. E. (1982). Leukocytoclastic vasculitis. A cutaneous expression of immune complex disease. *Archives of Dermatology*, **118**, 296–301.

Parish, W. E. (1971). Studies on vasculitis. I. Immunoglobulins, 1C, C-reactive protein, and bacterial antigens in cutaneous vasculitis lesions. *Clinical Allergy*, **1**, 97–109.

Parish, W. E. (1972). Cutaneous vasculitis: antigen-antibody complexes and prolonged fibrinolysis. *Proceedings of the Royal Society of Medicine*, **65**, 276–8.

Resnick, A. H. and Esterly, N. B. (1985). Vasculitis in children. *International Journal of Dermatology*, **24**, 139–46.

Ryan, T. J. (1992). Cutaneous vasculitis. In *Textbook of dermatology* (Rook, A., Wilkinson, D. S. and Ebling, F. J.G., eds), pp. 1893–1961. Blackwell Scientific Publications, Oxford.

Ryan, T. J. (1999). Common mistakes in the clinical approach to vasculitis. *Clinical Dermatology*, **17**, 555–7.

Sais, G., Vidaller, A., Jucgla, A., Servitje, O., Condom, E. and Peyri, J. (1998). Prognostic factors in leukocytoclastic vasculitis: a clinicopathologic study of 160 patients. *Archives of Dermatology*, **134**, 309–15.

Sams, H. H. and Sams, W. M. (2001). Cutaneous leukocytoclastic vasculitis. In *Vasculitis* (Ball, G. V. and Bridges, S. L. eds), pp. 467–75. Oxford University Press.

Soter, N. A. and Austen, K. F. (1978). Cutaneous necrotizing angiitis. In *Immunological diseases* (Samter, M., ed.), p. 993. Little, Brown, Boston.

Soter, N. A. and Wolff, S. M. (1987). Necrotizing vasculitis. In *Dermatology in general medicine* (Fitzpatrick, T. B. *et al.* eds), pp. 1300–12. McGraw Hill, New York.

Soter, N. A., Mihm, M. C., Jr., Gigli, I., Dvorak, H. F. and Austen, K. F. (1976). Two distinct cellular patterns in cutaneous necrotizing angiitis. *Journal of Investigative Dermatology*, **66**, 344–50.

Swerlick, R. A. and Lawley, T. J. (1989). Cutaneous vasculitis: its relationship to systemic disease. *Medical Clinics of North America*, **73**, 1221–35.

Teofoli, P. and Lotti, T. (1995). Cytokines, fibrinolysis and vasculitis. *International Angiology*, **14**, 125–9.

Thorne, E. G., Gower, R. G. and Claman, H. N. (1977). Hepatitis B surface antigen and leukocytoclastic vasculitis. *Journal of Investigative Dermatology*, **68**, 243–7.

Tosca, N. and Stratigos, J. D. (1988). Possible pathogenetic mechanisms in allergic cutaneous vasculitis. *International Journal of Dermatology*, **27**, 291–6.

Yancey, K. B. and Lawley, T. J. (1984). Circulating immune complexes: their immunochemistry, biology, and detection in selected dermatologic and systemic diseases. *Journal of the American Academy of Dermatology*, **10**, 711–31.

Zeek, P. M. (1953). Periarteritis nodosa and other forms of necrotizing angiitis. *New England Journal of Medicine*, **248**, 764–72.

Zimmerman, B. J., Anderson, D. C. and Granger, D. N. (1992). Neuropeptides promote neutrophil adherence to endothelial cell monolayers. *American Journal of Physiology*, **263**, G678–82.

Zimmerman, G. A. and Hill, H. R. (1984). Inflammatory mediators stimulate granulocyte adherence to cultured human endothelial cells. *Thrombosis Research*, **35**, 203–17.

CHAPTER 40

Henoch–Schönlein purpura

Miguel A. González-Gay and Carlos Garcia-Porrúa

Introduction

In the first half of the nineteenth century, Schönlein (1837) named the association between arthralgia and purpuric cutaneous lesions in a child "purpura rheumatica". His pupil Edward-Heinrich Henoch (1874) described a syndrome of purpura, severe abdominal colic and melena. It was not until the end of the nineteenth century that this author referred to nephritis as a complication of this syndrome (1895). Although the term Schönlein–Henoch purpura is more appropriate historically, Henoch–Schönlein purpura (HSP) is used more commonly by rheumatologists in the USA, so this term will be used throughout this chapter. The first description of a child with the syndrome that we currently know as HSP was by Heberden (1801) in his treatise "On cutaneous disease". A child with joint pain and painful subcutaneous edema, abdominal pain, vomiting, bloody stools and urine, and "bloody points" over the skin of his legs was described. In 1915, Frank called this syndrome "anaphylactoid purpura" (Frank 1915). This term is not commonly used, however, because an allergic etiology has not been substantiated.

Definition

Henoch–Schönlein purpura is a systemic vasculitis characterized by purpuric skin lesions unrelated to any underlying coagulopathy, abdominal pain and bleeding, arthritis, and renal involvement (González-Gay et al. 2005; Saulsbury 2001). Although the classic clinical triad of HSP is palpable purpura, joint symptoms, and abdominal pain, the most serious complication is renal involvement. HSP is characterized histologically by infiltration of the small blood vessels with polymorphonuclear leukocytes and the presence of leukocytoclasia. Immunofluorescence staining usually reveals the presence of IgA-dominant immune deposits in the walls of the small vessels (capillaries, venules, or arterioles) and in the renal glomeruli (Giancomo and Tsai 1977; Jennette et al. 1994). Henoch–Schönlein purpura is essentially a childhood disease. The pediatric form of HSP has been widely described and it is generally considered a benign, self-limited disorder (Calviño et al. 2001; Cassidy and Petty 1995; Trapani et al. 2005). HSP in adults is less common and is generally associated with a worse outcome (Garcia-Porrúa and González-Gay 1999a; Garcia-Porrúa et al. 2002).

Epidemiology

Henoch–Schönlein purpura is the most common vasculitis in children (González-Gay and Garcia-Porrúa 2001) (see Chapter 2). Although it may occur from 6 months of age through adulthood, 50% of the cases occur in children less than 5 years of age, and 75% of patients are less than 10 years old. Indeed, the disease is observed predominantly in children between the ages of 2 and 10, and the median age of onset is 4 years. In some reports girls and boys were affected equally. A lower frequency of boys (46%) than girls was observed in pediatric HSP from the Lugo region of northwestern Spain (Calviño et al. 2001). In contrast, in Charlottesville, Virginia, USA, boys outnumbered girls (57 of 100) (Saulsbury 1999). Previous studies also found a higher incidence in boys than girls (Allen et al. 1960; Robson and Leung 1994; Sterky and Thilén 1960). In adults with HSP Garcia-Porrúa and González Gay reported a higher frequency in males (1999a).

Classic studies described an annual incidence rate of HSP in children between 135 and 180 per million (Nielsen 1988; Robson and Leung 1994; Stewart et al. 1988). Nielsen (1988) showed that while the average annual incidence rate in the county of Copenhagen was 180 per million for children aged 0–14, it was only 8 per million for the population 15 years and older. Two more recent European epidemiological studies yielded a slightly lower annual incidence rate of HSP in children. In the Czech Republic, the estimated annual incidence of HSP between 1997 and 1999 was 102 per million children (Dolezalova et al. 2004). In the Lugo region of northwestern Spain the annual incidence rate of pediatric HSP during the period was 126 per million children (Calviño et al. 2001).

The incidence of HSP is much lower in adults than in children. Previous reports described a similar incidence among men and women (Clauvel et al. 1972; Debray et al. 1971), but a recent epidemiological study from northwestern Spain disclosed a higher incidence in men than women (2:1 ratio) (Garcia-Porrúa and González-Gay 1999a).

Based on the American College of Rheumatology (ACR) classification criteria for HSP (Mills et al. 1990), the annual incidence of HSP in an English population of patients older than 16 years was 13.0 per million (Watts et al. 1998). In northwestern Spain, the annual incidence rate of biopsy-proven HSP in a population 21 years of age and older was 14.3 per million (Garcia-Porrúa and González-Gay 1999a).

Genetic factors

HSP seems to be a polygenic disease and it has been described in parents, offspring, and siblings of affected individuals. Environmental factors may explain these cases (Knight 1990; Cakir et al. 2004); however, the familial occurrence of HSP in different episodes separated by several years supports a genetic predisposition (Lofters et al. 1973). Genetic susceptibility to HSP may be conferred by the interaction of a number of loci, including the major histocompatibility complex (MHC). A weak genetic association of HSP with HLA B35 and DR4 has been reported (Knight 1990). Amoroso et al. (1997) analyzed 152 patients with HSP (105 with renal disease) and found that HLA-DRB1*01 and DRB1*11 were more common among HSP patients than controls, while HLA DRB1*07 was less common in HSP patients than in controls. These authors did not find significant differences in DRB, DQB, and DQA alleles between patients with or without renal disease.

HSP in a population from northwest Spain was significantly associated with HLA-DRB1*01; in Italians HLA-DRB1*07 was significantly reduced compared with controls (Amoli et al. 2001b). In individuals from northwestern Spain, the multiallelic (CCTTT)$_n$ polymorphism in the promoter region of the gene encoding inducible nitric oxide synthase (NOS2A) was associated with susceptibility to HSP (Martin et al. 2005).

Both HSP nephritis and IgA nephropathy have been associated with deficiencies in the second and fourth components of complement (C2 and C4), and with deletion of C4 genes (Ault et al. 1990; Jin et al. 1992; Sussman et al. 1973). Jin et al. (1996) showed that locus II deletion of C4 is a risk factor for these diseases, and the deleted gene can be either C4A or C4B. An increased frequency of DQA1*0301 was present among these patients, suggesting that this allele could also be a genetic risk factor for these diseases. More recently, Stefansson Thors et al. (2005) reported that C4 null alleles were found in 66% of 56 HSP patients from Iceland compared with only 41% of 98 blood donors used as controls. This difference was due to an increased frequency of C4B*Q0 allele in the group of HSP patients.

Recent genetic studies in the Lugo region of northwestern Spain have examined the role of ICAM-1, HLA-B35, IL1RN, Interleukin (IL)-8, IL-1beta, and VEGF in disease severity (Table 40.1).

Precipitating factors

The etiology of HSP remains unknown. Seasonal increases in the incidence of HSP, with peaks in the spring, fall, and winter, have been reported, but these findings are controversial. While in children from northwest Spain HSP appeared more commonly in fall and winter, summer and winter were the most common seasons of onset in adults from the same region (Garcia-Porrúa et al. 2002). This may be related to a higher frequency of upper respiratory tract infections (URI) in children, in particular during the coldest months of the year. The site of infection varies: pharyngitis; rhinopharyngitis, and tracheobronchitis are frequently observed. Other foci of infection, such as the skin, have been considered uncommon. In northwestern Spain, URIs in children with HSP were almost twice as frequent as in adults (Garcia-Porrúa et al. 2002). In some series, infection was a presumed precipitant in more than 50% of cases. A URI preceding the onset of the disease was reported to occur in 32 (41%) of 78 children with HSP in the Lugo region of northwestern Spain

Table 40.1 Genetic polymorphisms associated with disease severity in HSP patients from northwestern Spain

Authors	Gene polymorphism	Type of complication
Amoli et al. (2001a)	Codon 469 of ICAM-1	Gastrointestinal
Amoli et al. (2002a)	HLA-B35	Susceptibility to nephritis
Amoli et al. (2002b)	IL1RN	Nephrotic syndrome and/or renal insufficiency
Amoli et al. (2002c)	Interleukin-8	Susceptibility to nephritis
Amoli et al. (2004)	Interleukin-1beta	Nephrotic syndrome and/or renal insufficiency
Rueda et al. (2006)	VEGF	Susceptibility to nephritis

ICAM-1, Intercellular adhesion molecule-1 locus; IL1RN, Interleukin 1 receptor antagonist gene polymorphism; VEGF, Vascular endothelial growth factor.

(González-Gay et al. 2004). Among them, 15 children had tonsillitis, two tracheitis, and 15 a history of influenza with pharyngitis or rhinitis (González-Gay et al. 2004). In adults, Debray et al. (1971) reported an infectious precipitating event in 27% of patients. In northwestern Spain (Garcia-Porrúa and González-Gay 1999a), underlying URIs occurring within 7 days before the onset of the disease were observed in four of 27 adults (18.5%) with HSP. In a controlled study, Farley et al. (1989) observed throat infections in 52% of patients with HSP, but in only 22% of controls; almost 60% of the throat infections were streptococcal.

In general, an infection precedes the onset of the disease by several days to weeks. The organism most frequently isolated is the beta-hemolytic streptococcus group A (pyogenes) (Ballard et al. 1970; Farley et al. 1989). Other organisms implicated in HSP include: other streptococci; Staphylococcus aureus; Escherichia coli; Mycobacterium tuberculosis; yersinia species; legionella species; Mycoplasma pneumoniae; Epstein–Barr virus; hepatitis B virus; varicella; adenovirus; cytomegalovirus; and parvovirus B19 (Cimolai and Macnab 1991; Pacheco 1991; Szer 1994; Somer and Finegold 1995). Vaccinations against typhoid, paratyphoid A and B, measles, cholera, and yellow fever have also been implicated in the development of HSP (reviewed in Mormile et al. 2004).

Mesangial deposition of nephritis-associated plasmin receptor, a group A streptococcal antigen, has been detected in the glomeruli of children with HSP with nephritis (Masuda et al. 2003). In northwestern Spain, approximately 72% of children with HSP and URIs had renal involvement, manifested by hematuria with or without proteinuria, compared with only 39% of children without URI (González-Gay et al. 2004). Helicobacter pylori (H. pylori) has also been implicated in the gastrointestinal and extragastrointestinal manifestations of HSP. IgG antibodies to H. pylori were present, mostly in acute HSP compared with controls. Ratios of IgA/IgG antibodies to H. pylori were significantly higher in the remitting phase (Novak et al. 2003).

Some drugs, especially penicillin, ampicillin and erythromycin, paracetamol, and non-steroidal anti-inflammatory drugs have been thought to precipitate HSP (Blanco et al. 1997b; Calviño et al. 2001; Garcia-Porrúa and González-Gay 1999a; Garcia-Porrúa et al. 1999; González-Gay et al. 2004). A history of use of these drugs was reported to occur in 30% children. These drugs were generally prescribed because of the presence of URI. A history of medication use was not associated with worse outcome (González-Gay *et al.* 2004). Exposure to cold, insect bites, and food allergens have also been implicated as potential triggers. A recent report describes the potential role of pregnancy as a trigger for HSP or its recurrence (Cummins *et al.* 2003).

Clinical manifestations

Cutaneous

A rash of erythematous papules followed by non-thrombocytopenic palpable purpura constitutes the most common initial manifestation of HSP. The rash occurs in all cases, but it is not always the presenting sign (Szer 1994; Calviño *et al.* 2001). The rash is more commonly petechial or purpuric with contiguous erythematous plaques, often associated with macular, papular, or vesicular elements. In the series from Lugo (Calviño *et al.* 2001), besides the typical palpable purpura (Figure 40.1), other skin lesions, generally macular, papular, or more rarely urticarial or vesicular, were observed in 44% of children with HSP. In all cases, however, palpable purpura was the predominant cutaneous lesion. The purpuric eruption evolves from red to purple, then becomes rust-colored with a brownish hue

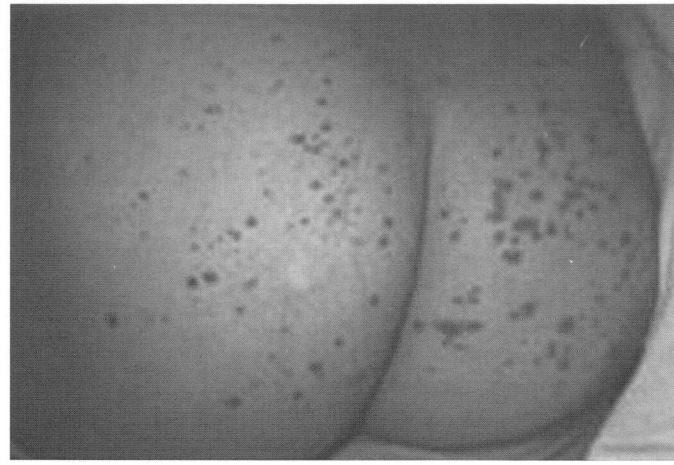

Figure 40.2 A bedridden boy with palpable purpura in a dependent and pressure-bearing area of the buttocks.

and then fades. The rash does not blanch with pressure. Purpura may be preceded by a pruritic, urticarial rash. Palpable purpura occurs in dependent and pressure-bearing areas such as the lower limbs and buttocks (Figure 40.2). The distribution is roughly symmetrical (Figure 40.3); it typically appears on the lower extremities and then spreads to the thighs and buttocks. The upper extremities and the abdomen are involved less frequently. The rash is usually intermittently progressive and is exacerbated by prolonged standing.

In young children, facial involvement and subcutaneous edema of the hands, feet, scalp, and ears are observed as early manifestations in up to 45% of cases (Dillon and Ansell 1995; Szer 1994). Adults may experience skin necrosis in areas of severe hemorrhage that are subjected to significant pressure, such as dependent areas (Cream *et al.* 1970).

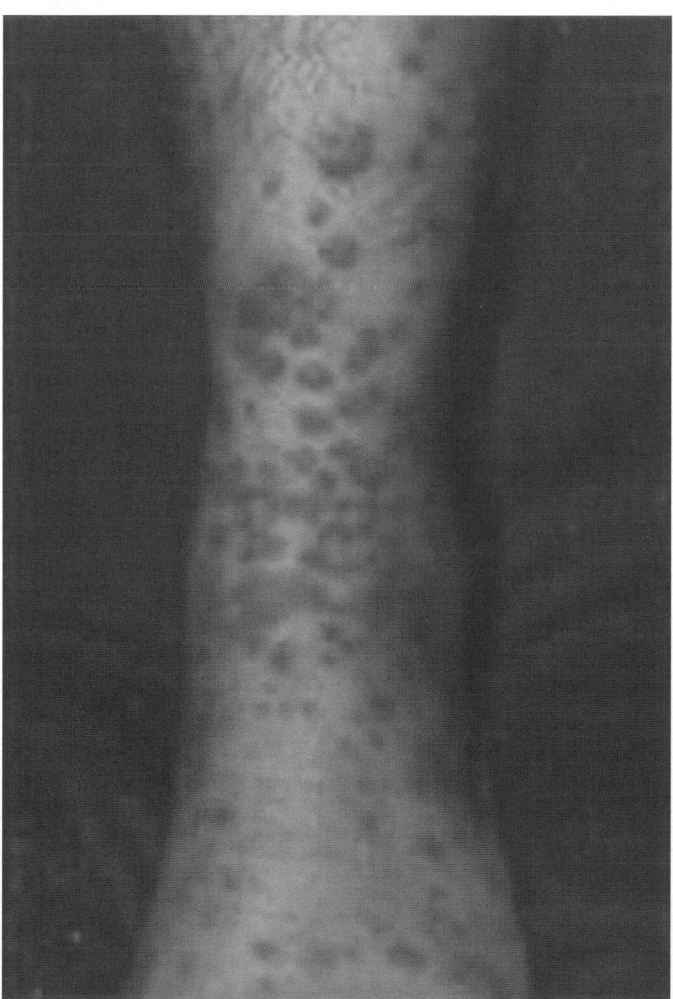

Figure 40.1 Typical palpable purpura in dependent areas of the lower extremities.

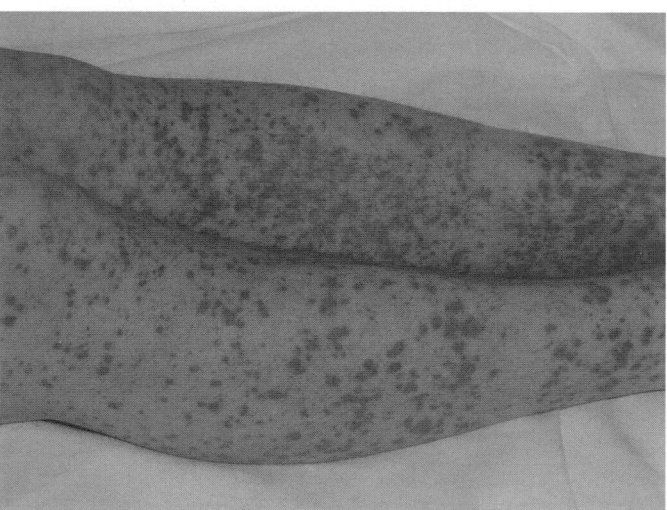

Figure 40.3 Symmetrical distribution of cutaneous lesions in legs.

Gastrointestinal

Gastrointestinal (GI) symptoms are common; the main gastrointestinal complications include abdominal pain, nausea and vomiting, and GI bleeding manifest as melena or hematemesis, sometimes with massive hemorrhage and shock. Children may suffer acute intussusception. Other GI manifestations include bowel infarction and perforation; duodenojejunal stenosis; malabsorption and exudative enteropathy; and intestinal serositis and hemorrhagic ascites.

Abdominal pain constitutes the second most frequent clinical manifestation of HSP, occurring in approximately 60–75% of patients (Bailey *et al.* 1998; Calviño *et al.* 2001; Kraft *et al.* 1998). In children from northwestern Spain, abdominal pain was often the initial manifestation, preceding the onset of purpura by 1 to 10 days (mean 3.3 days), in 17% of the cases (Calviño *et al.* 2001). Abdominal pain is frequently colicky, sometimes severe, and is associated with nausea and vomiting. It occurs in waves, returning as the purpuric skin lesions spread. The pain is commonly periumbilical; it may some-times mimic an acute abdomen. The pain is due to peritoneal or visceral purpura leading to submucosal and mucosal extravasation of blood and edema fluid, which may lead to ulceration of the bowel mucosa. There may eventually be bleeding into the lumen, with occult blood in the stool. Melena and hematemesis have been reported in up to 50% and 15% of patients, respectively (Allen *et al.* 1960). Interestingly, the frequency of GI bleeding in two epidemiological studies of unselected children with HSP from Lugo (Calviño *et al.* 2001) and Charlottesville Virginia, USA (Saulsbury 1999) was similar (31% in Lugo and 33% in Charlottesville). In patients with hematemesis or melena, upper GI endoscopy usually discloses erythema, petechiae, and mucosal ulcerations and erosions, especially in the second part of duodenum (Kato *et al.* 1992). Submucosal hemorrhages have been observed in the stomach, duodenum, and sigmoid colon (Goldman and Lindenberg 1981) (Figure 40.4). Colonoscopy may disclose petechial colonic lesions in the descending colon.

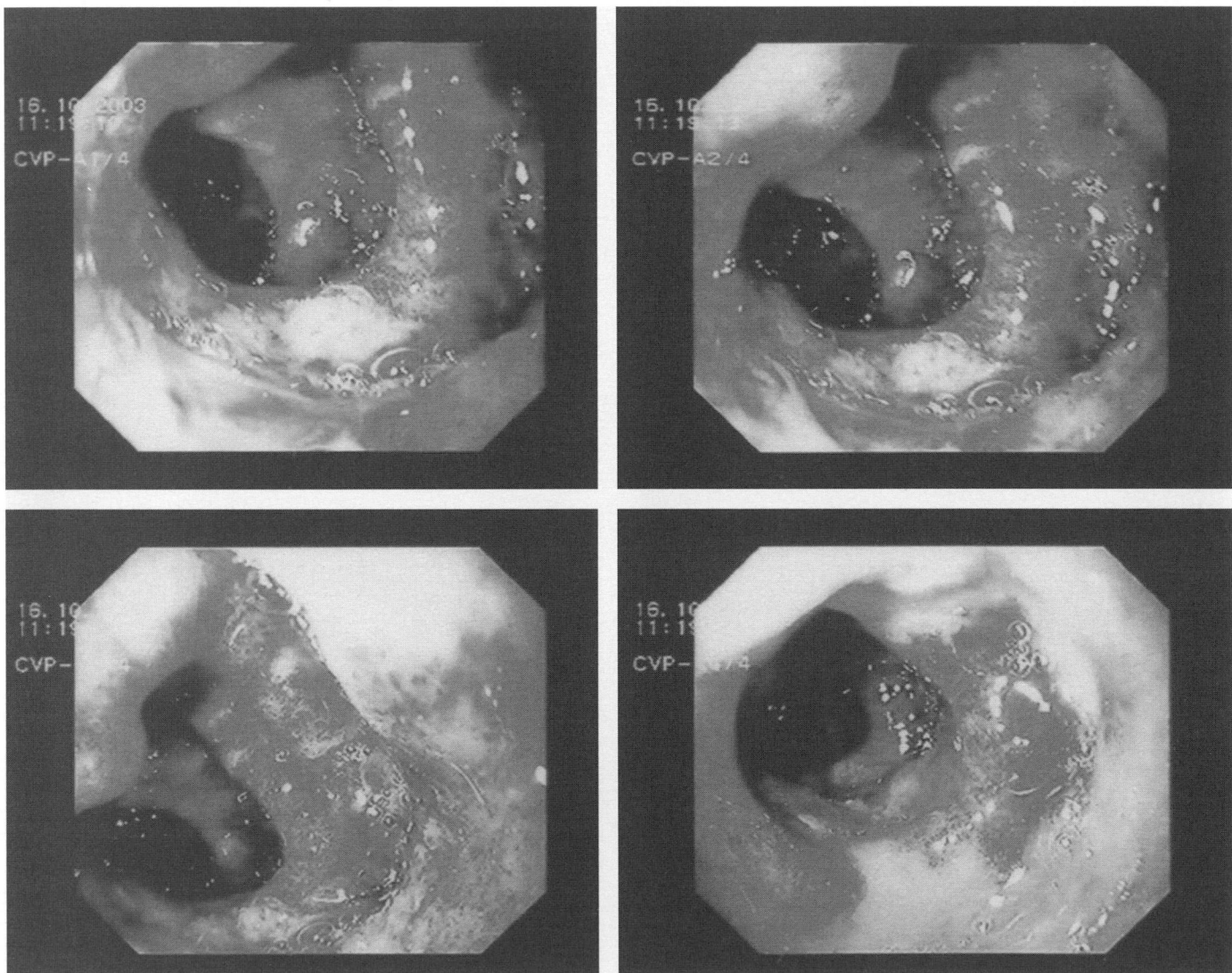

Figure 40.4 An adult with HSP manifested as erythema, edema, and hemorrhagic lesions involving the duodenal mucosa.

Acute intussusception may be observed in 1–5% of children (Allen *et al.* 1960; Cull *et al.* 1990; Robson and Leung 1994). This is usually ileoileal and less commonly ileocolic and jejunojejunal (Macpherson 1974). Perforation is a rare, but serious, complication. Severe cases may proceed to hemorrhage and shock or even to duodenojejunal stenosis (Allen *et al.* 1960; Boyer *et al.* 1978). Other uncommon complications such as malabsorption, exudative enteropathy, intestinal serositis, and hemorrhagic ascites have been reported (Archimandritis *et al.* 1994; Jones *et al.* 1966; Roy 1972; Santiago *et al.* 1996).

Radiologic changes include thickening of mucosal folds, prolongation of transit time, and increased distance between loops of small intestine. Abdominal ultrasonography may be the imaging modality of choice to investigate intestinal manifestations of HSP, such as thickening in the bowel wall, reduced peristalsis, intussusception, and free peritoneal fluid (Connolly and O'Halpin 1994). Ozdemir *et al.* (1995) reported the use of sonography in the diagnosis and follow-up of children with HSP. They observed dilatation of intestinal segments; hypomotility; eccentric thickening of the wall of the small intestine; centrally located intestinal contents; and intramural hemorrhage. Ultrasonography may also be useful in differentiating HSP from other non-hemorrhagic GI diseases (Ozdemir *et al.* 1995). Jeong *et al.* (1997) have emphasized the importance of computed tomography (CT) scan as another tool to delineate GI involvement in HSP. CT scans may disclose multifocal bowel wall thickening, mesenteric edema, and vascular engorgement. Hepatosplenomegaly has also been reported in patients with HSP (Kraft *et al.* 1998).

Joints

Joint manifestations have been reported to precede the development of palpable purpura by several days in up to 25% of cases (Piette 1994). Farley *et al.* (1989) observed in some cases a delay between the onset of joint manifestations and the occurrence of cutaneous lesions ranging from 1–75 days, with an average of 5 days. During the course of the disease, joint symptoms may occur in more than 50% of cases. Joint manifestations were observed in 78% of children with HSP (Calviño *et al.* 2001). Arthralgias, with or without arthritis, preceded purpura in 13% of cases (Calviño *et al.* 2001). In most cases, the pattern of joint involvement was oligoarthritis involving feet and ankles or knees and, less commonly, upper extremity joints (Calviño *et al.* 2001). Although Duquesnoy (1991) reported that joint manifestations were more common in adults than in children, we have observed arthritis more commonly in children (64%) than in adults (23%) (Garcia-Porrúa *et al.* 2002). Joint manifestations are generally transient; permanent deformities are rarely seen. Patients may present with arthralgias without objective signs of synovitis. In our series of adults with HSP, arthralgia without clinically evident synovitis was twice as common as joint inflammation (Garcia-Porrúa *et al.* 2002). In this region of Spain, arthralgias were reported in 42% of adults and in only 11% of children. Arthralgias or arthritis of the knees and ankles (Garcia-Porrúa and González-Gay 1999a) may be associated with edema; upper extremity joints such as elbows and wrists may also be involved (Garcia-Porrúa and González-Gay 1999a; Calviño *et al.* 2001).

Renal

Renal involvement constitutes the most serious feature of HSP, and occurs in 20–80% of patients (Chang *et al.* 2005; Garcia-Porrúa *et al.* 2002; Kaku *et al.* 1998), most commonly in older children and adults.

In unselected patients with HSP from northwestern Spain the incidence of nephritis, manifest as hematuria, with or without proteinuria, was similar in children (54%) (Calviño *et al.* 2001) and adults (~50%) (Garcia-Porrúa and González-Gay 1999a). Renal sequelae, characterized by nephrotic syndrome or renal insufficiency, were more common in adults (Garcia-Porrúa *et al.* 2002). Renal complications are infrequent in children younger than 2 years, where it occurs in no more than 25% of the cases. Renal disease may be more common than is clinically apparent, as minor degrees of focal mesangial proliferation have been reported in the absence of urinary abnormalities (White 1994).

Renal involvement generally occurs within the first 3 months after clinical onset of the disease (Calviño *et al.* 2001); however, it may be observed later, generally in the setting of relapses of palpable purpura. Nephropathy in patients with HSP usually presents with gross hematuria lasting a few days (although it may persist for several weeks), followed by microscopic hematuria that may persist for months or even years. Recurrences of gross hematuria may be observed in association with relapses of skin lesions. Recurrences of hematuria long after other manifestations of HSP have resolved are less common. Hematuria may be isolated or associated with proteinuria.

Persistent, severe proteinuria accompanied by microscopic hematuria suggests the presence of glomerulonephritis. Initial hematuria may be accompanied by hypertension and elevation of serum creatinine (Meadow *et al.* 1972). In addition to nephrotic syndrome (Niaudet and Habib 1989), the most severe clinical presentation is that of mixed nephritic and nephrotic syndromes, with hematuria, hypertension and renal insufficiency, severe proteinuria, and hypoalbuminemia. In HSP nephritis the glomerular filtration rate is moderately reduced early and is more impaired in patients with proteinuria and more advanced histopathologic changes on kidney biopsy (Halling *et al.* 2005).

The long-term morbidity and mortality of HSP are almost completely due to renal involvement. Many of early reports documented a relatively high frequency of chronic renal failure in children and adults, but these suffered from selection bias, in that patients were usually referred because of kidney dysfunction (Counahan *et al.* 1977; Fogazzi *et al.* 1989; Lee *et al.* 1986; Meadow *et al.* 1972; Roth *et al.* 1985). Garcia-Porrúa *et al.* (2002) observed that the frequency of severe renal manifestations or renal insufficiency during the course of the disease was significantly lower in children than adults. Other studies (Blanco *et al.* 1997b; Uthman *et al.* 1998) also found a higher frequency of severe renal involvement in adults. The final outcome in both age groups is good in most cases. After 6 years median follow-up, complete recovery was observed in 65 of 73 children; however, after 5 years median follow-up almost 40% of 31 adults had persistent hematuria and three of them (10%) had renal insufficiency, two of whom required hemodialysis (Garcia-Porrúa *et al.* 2002).

The urine should be routinely tested for blood and protein at onset and during the follow-up until systemic signs have resolved. Proteinuria, if present, should be quantified. Narchi (2005) reviewed 12 studies that included 1133 children with HSP to assess the risk of long-term renal impairment. Hematuria and proteinuria were found in 34% of the children, occurring in 85% of cases within 4 weeks of the diagnosis of HSP, in 91% within 6 weeks, and in 97% within 6 months. Thus, if there are no abnormalities on the urinalysis within the first 6 months of the disease, urinalysis testing need not be performed thereafter (Narchi 2005).

In most cases, the severity of disease at onset appears to predict outcome. The presence of both proteinuria and hematuria at the onset of the disease may be linked to progression to renal insufficiency (Kraft *et al.* 1998). In 69 children from Lugo, Spain, development of nephrotic syndrome within the first 3 months of disease was the best predictor of renal sequelae during the extended follow-up (Calviño *et al.* 2001). In a long-term study of 78 children with HSP with nephritis, Goldstein *et al.* (1992) observed that 44% of those with nephritic syndrome, nephrotic syndrome, or both at the onset of the disease had long-term impairment of renal function. In another study of 114 children with HSP nephritis the presence of nephrotic syndrome, decreased factor XIII activity, hypertension, and renal failure at onset were more frequently observed in those who had a bad outcome at last follow-up (Kawasaki *et al.* 2003).

Based on the morphological classification of HSP glomerulonephritis in the International Study for Kidney Disease in Children (ISKDC), in which renal biopsy findings may be graded from grade I to VI (Counahan *et al.* 1977), Goldstein *et al.* (1992) correlated outcomes with the severity of the lesions on initial renal biopsy. In this study, 58% of the children in whom more than half of the glomeruli were affected by crescent formation (corresponding to grades IV and V of the ISKDC classification) had a poor outcome. Of those with crescents in less than one-half of glomeruli (grade III) or with no crescents (grades I and II), the outcome was poor in only 17%. Other studies have confirmed that children with glomerular crescents have a high chance of developing end-stage renal disease (Lanzkowsky *et al.* 1992). Kaku *et al.* (1998) studied factors associated with the progression of renal involvement in children with HSP. Renal disease appeared in 63 of their 194 children between 3 days and 17 months after onset of HSP. The probability of renal involvement in HSP was influenced by the presence of severe abdominal symptoms, persistent purpura, and decreased activity of coagulation factor XIII. In contrast, treatment with glucocorticoids reduced the risk of nephritis. An increased risk of developing renal insufficiency was associated with age at onset of more than 7 years, the presence of persistent proteinuria, and decreased activity of coagulation factor XIII. In a series of 28 adults with long-term follow-up of HSP, hematuria at the onset of the disease, or renal manifestations during the course of the disease (frequently observed in patients with relapses), were the main risk factors for renal sequelae (Garcia-Porrúa *et al.* 2001). In adults with nephritis, Fogazzi *et al.* (1989) observed a high rate of renal function deterioration (11 of 16 adults with a mean follow-up of 90.5 months). Although patients who developed renal insufficiency had a higher percentage of crescents at the disease onset, no clinical features at presentation predicted the course of the disease (Fogazzi *et al.* 1989). In fact, in this series most adults with HSP who had normal renal function at onset subsequently developed renal insufficiency; however, this poor outcome and high frequency of renal insufficiency in adults has not been corroborated by more recent studies (Blanco *et al.* 1997b; Garcia-Porrúa and González-Gay 1999a; Garcia-Porrúa *et al.* 2002).

Other clinical manifestations

Other features of HSP, which are rare or under-reported, are summarized below. Extrarenal genitourinary problems sometimes precede the onset of purpuric lesions (Szer 1994). Acute scrotal swelling due to inflammation and hemorrhage was observed in 32% of the series of boys reported by Chamberlain and Greenberg (1992). These authors emphasized the need to differentiate this complication from testicular torsion of the spermatic cord, as it too may be the initial manifestation of HSP. In patients with testicular torsion, both Doppler flow and radionuclide scan are abnormal, while in children with scrotal swelling due to HSP, Doppler and radionuclide scan show normal or increased blood flow. Orchitis has also been reported in HSP (Gibson and Su 1995).

Neurologic complications are probably more common in HSP patients than are generally described. Central nervous system involvement usually causes headache, which Ostergaard and Storm (1991) reported in 31% of 26 cases. Other neurologic problems include: behavioral changes due to encephalopathy; changes in mental status; apathy; hyperactivity; mood swings; and seizures (Fielding *et al.* 1998; Woolfenden *et al.* 1998). Subdural hematomas, intracranial hemorrhage, intraparenchymal bleeding, and non-hemorrhagic vasculitis of the cerebral parenchyma have been documented less often (Chiaretti *et al.* 1995; Ha and Cha 1996; Misra *et al.* 2004). Peripheral nervous system lesions may appear as mononeuropathy involving the facial, ulnar, femoral, sciatic, or peroneal nerves; polyneuropathy such as Guillain–Barré syndrome, polyradiculoneuropathy, and brachial plexopathy have been reported (Robson and Leung 1994).

Interstitial pulmonary disease is common, but it is generally asymptomatic. Impairment of lung diffusion capacity has been reported in the majority of children during the active phase of the disease (Chaussain *et al.* 1992). A few cases of pulmonary hemorrhage consisting of diffuse alveolar hemorrhage, leading in some cases to death, or more rarely interstitial pneumonia, have been described (Olson *et al.* 1992; Paller *et al.* 1997; Nadrous *et al.* 2004). Other manifestations such as malaise and low-grade fever are observed in half of the patients with HSP (Robson and Leung 1994).

Laboratory investigation

Elevation of acute phase reactants, moderate leukocytosis, and thrombocytosis are common during the active phase of disease. The hemoglobin is generally normal unless severe GI or pulmonary bleeding occurs. A pathogenic role for IgA is supported by its presence in cryoprecipitate (see below), (Garcia Fuentes *et al.* 1977) and the finding of an increased number of circulating IgA-secreting cells in patients with active HSP (Casanueva *et al.* 1983; Levinsky and Barratt 1979; Trygstad and Stiehm 1971). IgA-dominant immune deposits are observed in many cases of HSP (Hené *et al.* 1986), and their presence has been included in the definition adopted by the Consensus Conference on the Nomenclature of Systemic Vasculitides (Jennette *et al.* 1994). Although IgA levels in the serum are reportedly increased in 50% of children in acute phases of disease (Dillon and Ansell 1995), they were increased in only 5.6% of the tested patients in the American College of Rheumatology (ACR) study database (Mills *et al.* 1990). In Spain, increased values of serum IgA were only observed in 10 of 27 (37%) adults and 20 of 37 (54%) children (Garcia-Porrúa *et al.* 2002).

Circulating IgA-containing immune complexes and cryoglobulins have also been found (Blockmans and Bobbaers 1998; Levinsky and Barratt 1979; Trygstad and Stiehm 1971). Serum C3, C4, and CH50 are generally normal; however, in a series of patients with HSP and IgA nephropathy the measurement of plasma anaphylatoxins C3a and C4a showed significant correlation with plasma creatinine and urea values (Abou-Ragheb *et al.* 1992). This suggests a role for plasma anaphylatoxin determination as a sensitive indicator of complement activation and a useful parameter in monitoring HSP activity. Complement activation through both the alternative and lectin pathways has been found in patients with HSP nephritis (Hisano *et al.* 2005).

Antineutrophil cytoplasmic antibodies (ANCA) have been identified in a wide variety of vasculitic disorders, but the presence of ANCA in sera of patients with HSP is controversial. Van den Wall Bake *et al.* (1987) suggested a role for ANCA in the pathogenesis of HSP, as they detected IgA ANCA in 55% of their patients. O'Donoghue *et al.* (1992) did not confirm that observation, as none of 30 children with early HSP were ANCA-positive. Coppo *et al.* (1997) suggested that the conflicting reports on IgA ANCA might be due to atypical characteristics of the reaction in some ELISA assays. More recently, Ozaltin *et al.* (2004) undertook a prospective study to establish the presence of ANCA IgA subclass in HSP. IgA ANCA in a cytoplasmic pattern was detected in a higher percentage of children diagnosed with HSP (82% of 35) in the acute phase compared to children with other vasculitides (38% of 13). In the resolution phase of HSP, IgA ANCA was negative in 88% of patients. No relationship was found between disease severity of HSP and IgA ANCA. Accordingly, IgA ANCA testing might be useful to confirm the diagnosis of HSP in children (Ozaltin *et al.* 2004).

As with other vasculitides, and as a consequence of vascular endothelial damage, high concentrations of von Willebrand factor have been observed (Ates *et al.* 1994; De Mattia *et al.* 1995), suggesting its possible use as a marker of disease severity. Elevated levels of serum thrombomodulin, derived from damaged endothelium, have also been observed in patients with HSP nephritis (Fujieda *et al.* 1998). The prothrombin time and partial thromboplastin time are typically normal. Reduced factor XIII activity has been found in patients with severe GI complications (De Mattia *et al.* 1995).

Pathophysiology

In HSP, IgA-dominant immune deposits are observed in the wall of the small vessels and in the renal glomeruli. IgA$_1$ accounts for 80–90% of serum IgA. Secretory IgA is composed of roughly equal proportions of IgA$_1$ and IgA$_2$ (Saulsbury 1999). Aberrant glycosylation of the hinge region of IgA$_1$ may be responsible for the clinical and histopathologic features of HSP (Saulsbury 1999; Saulsbury 2001). Although the pathogenic role of IgA is widely accepted, the diagnostic significance of IgA vascular immune deposits detected by direct immunofluorescence is not completely defined, as similar immune deposits have been observed in patients with other types of cutaneous vasculitis (Sams *et al.* 1975). Helander *et al.* (1995) found that the presence of vascular deposits of IgA was sensitive, but not specific for diagnosis. Nevertheless, the presence of IgA immune deposits, when combined with selected clinical data such as GI involvement, previous history of URI, or age less than 20 years, improved the diagnostic accuracy of HSP (Helander *et al.* 1995).

Increased IgA may be due to increased production or decreased clearance. An unknown antigen may stimulate IgA production, activating pathways leading to necrotizing vasculitis. In addition to elevations in serum IgA concentration, there may be IgA-containing immune complexes and IgA isotype autoantibodies (rheumatoid factor, ANCA, and antiendothelial cell antibodies) (Tizard 1999). IgA deposits are present in both skin and glomeruli. The IgA immune complexes are capable of activating complement, leading to the formation of chemotactic factors such as C5a, which in turn recruit polymorphonuclear leukocytes to the site of deposition. The release of lysosomal enzymes due to the ingestion of immune complexes by the polymorphonuclear leukocytes results in vessel damage. The membrane-attack complex (MAC) is also required for the endothelial damage; serum concentration of the C5b-9 complex has been found to be significantly elevated in many patients at the time of disease flare. The MAC has been found along with IgA and C3 on the vessel walls of the skin and on the capillary walls and mesangium of patients with HSP nephritis (Kawana and Nishiyama 1992). Measurement of the terminal complement complex is another possibly useful tool for monitoring disease activity in HSP patients. Although serum C3 and C4 levels are generally normal in most patients with HSP, anaphylatoxins C3a and C4a are sensitive indicators of complement activation and indicators of disease activity in some patients with HSP and IgA nephritis (Abou-Ragheb *et al.* 1992). Complement abnormalities such as C2 deficiency, the homozygous null C4 phenotype, and C4B deficiency have been detected in some patients (Tizard 1999). Although high C3d concentrations and glomerular C3 and properdin deposition in the acute phase of disease activity have suggested complement activation, a study of three multimolecular complement activation protein complexes failed to support complement activation in the disease (Smith *et al.* 1997). Hisano *et al.* (2005) confirmed complement activation through both the alternative and lectin pathways in patients with HSP nephritis and they showed that complement activation is promoted *in situ* in the glomerulus. In HSP patients with nephritis, complement activation through the lectin pathway may play a role in the development of advanced glomerular injuries and prolonged urinary abnormalities (Hisano *et al.* 2005). Finally, proinflammatory cytokines seems to be involved in the pathogenesis of nephritis in HSP. In the acute phase of the disease, serum TNF-α levels were significantly higher in HSP with proteinuria compared to those without renal involvement. These observations suggest that increased TNF-α levels in the serum are involved in the acute phase of glomerular disease, and may correlate with disease activity of HSP in patients with severe renal involvement (Ha 2005).

Histology

Skin

Consonant with other small-sized blood vessel vasculitides involving the skin (González-Gay *et al.* 2004, 2005), cutaneous lesions of patients with HSP generally involve capillaries, postcapillary venules, and non-muscular arterioles (less than 50 μm in diameter) found mainly within the superficial papillary dermis (Figure 40.5). Biopsy samples of the cutaneous lesions in patients with HSP show: a leukocytoclastic vasculitis of small blood vessels with infiltration of neutrophils within and around vessel walls; leukocytoclasia; fibrinoid necrosis of the damaged vessel walls; necrosis, swelling, and proliferation of the endothelial cells; and red cell extravasation (Figure 40.6). Eosinophils may also be present. Necrosis of small blood vessels and platelet thrombi in capillaries and venules are common findings. IgA, C3, and fibrin may deposit within the walls of the dermal vessels as well as in the connective tissue of the upper dermis of the purpuric skin lesions (Giancomo and Tsai 1977). IgA deposits have also been found, albeit less often, in biopsy specimens of non-purpuric skin (Giancomo and Tsai 1977).

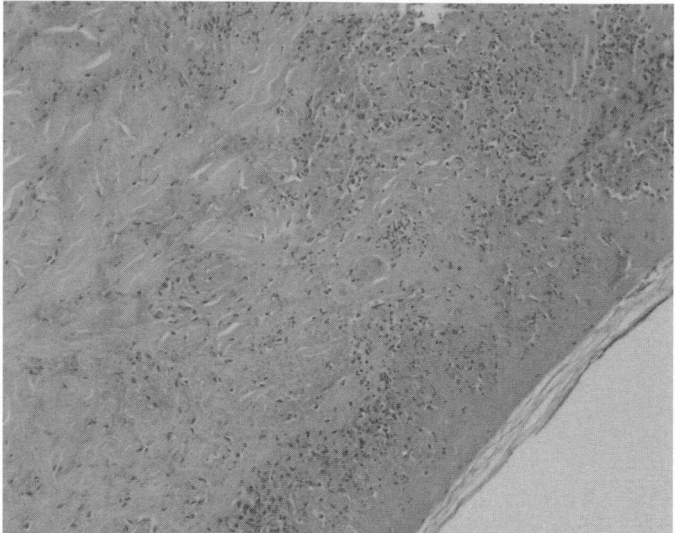

Figure 40.5 Skin biopsy of a patient with HSP showing dermal vascular neutrophilic inflammatory infiltration, leukocytoclasia, vessel wall fibrinoid necrosis, and hematic extravasation (Hematoxylin and eosin × 100.) (See Color Plate 111).

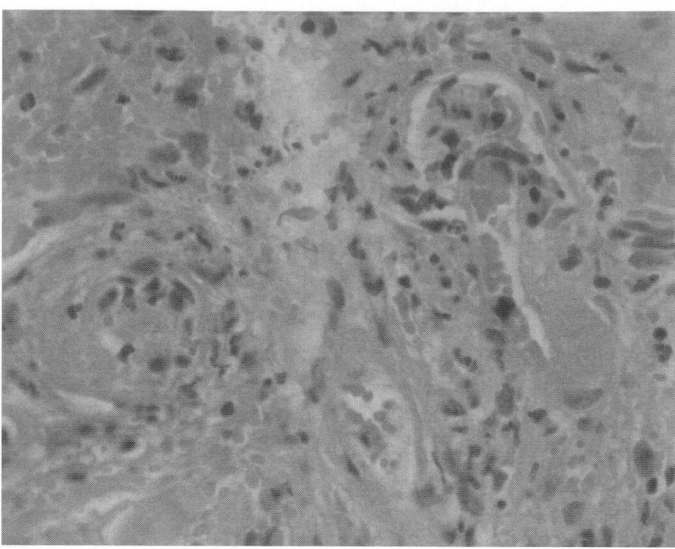

Figure 40.6 Skin biopsy disclosing small-sized blood vessel vasculitis with two vessels showing peripheral leukocytoclasia, fibrin thrombosis, fibrinoid necrosis, and red cell extravasation consistent with leukocytoclastic vasculitis. (Hematoxylin and eosin × 400.) (See Color Plate 112).

Gastrointestinal tract

Non-specific inflammatory infiltrates of lymphocytes and IgA deposits in the capillaries of the stomach and duodenal mucosa have been reported (Kato *et al.* 1992) and mild inflammation and endothelial cell proliferation have been observed in colonic biopsies (Cappell and Gupta 1990).

Kidney

The early lesion is an endocapillary, focal or diffuse, proliferative glomerulonephritis involving both endothelial and mesangial cells (Robson and Leung 1994). The glomeruli are infiltrated with polymorphonuclear and mononuclear cells. Proliferation of extracapillary cells, including epithelial cells and Bowman's capsule cells, may result in variable degrees of crescent formation, due to adhesion of

the proliferating cells to the glomerular tuft (Figure 40.7). Interstitial inflammation and tubular changes with atrophy and tubular casts are common. Disease of renal arterioles occurs infrequently; therefore the brunt of the disease is borne by the glomeruli, which characteristically show two basic lesions: mesangial proliferative and epithelial crescent formation (White 1994) (Figure 40.8).

Renal biopsy findings may be graded according to the classification of the ISKDC (see above), which is based on the percentage of glomeruli showing crescents and segmental lesions (Counahan *et al.* 1977). Renal biopsies may reveal minimal to severe glomerulonephritis indistinguishable from IgA nephropathy. When renal involvement is minimal, glomeruli appear normal on light microscopy (Yoshikawa *et al.* 1981). Mesangial proliferation may be either diffuse or focal and segmental. Associated features include

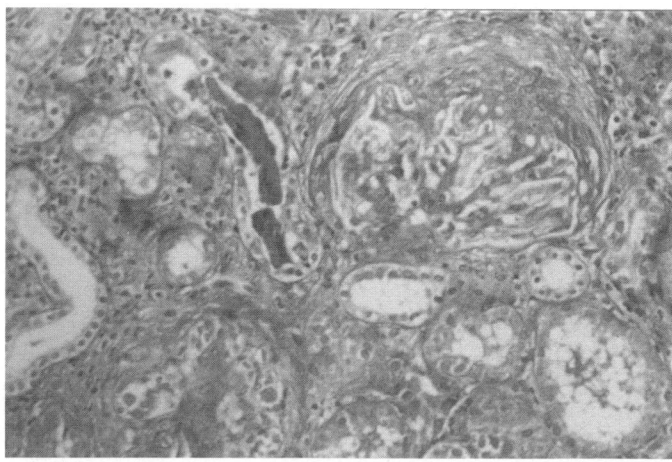

Figure 40.7 Kidney biopsy showing glomerular sclerosis and crescent formation. (Masson × 400.) (See Color Plate 113).

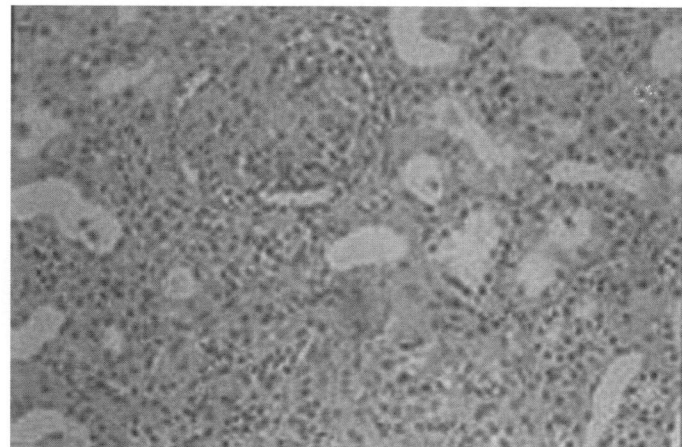

Figure 40.8 Renal biopsy showing two glomeruli. One of them has an extracapillary proliferative crescent that obliterates the glomerular tuft. The other glomerulus shows diffuse mesangial proliferative involvement. (Hematoxylin and eosin × 100.) (See Color Plate 114).

thrombosis and necrosis. Epithelial crescents vary in size from small segmental wedges, affecting one or two lobules, to circumferential forms. Large cellular crescents cause extensive obliteration of the urinary spaces. In the acute phase, crescents are predominantly cellular, but become fibrous after being infiltrated with collagen. Adherent glomerular capillaries become sclerotic. The extent of tubular atrophy and interstitial cellular infiltration and fibrosis is a measure of the severity of the glomerular lesions (White 1994).

Immunofluorescence microscopy almost invariably reveals diffuse distribution of mesangial deposits of IgA (Figure 40.9), which are generally associated with minimal amounts of IgG, IgM, C3, and properdin. In patients with more severe disease, IgA deposits may extend into the capillary walls; fibrin, which could have a role in crescent formation, may also be seen (Heaton 1977). Electron microscopy shows that some deposits are found in the mesangial regions, especially in the perimesangium. Smaller deposits are also observed in the subendothelial zone of the capillary walls adjacent to the mesangiocapillary junction, and to a minor extent in the subepithelial region (White 1994).

Lung

In pulmonary specimens obtained at autopsy, IgA deposits have been found along the alveolar septa (Kathuria and Cheifec 1982).

Diagnosis

The clinical diagnosis of HSP is supported by finding leukocytoclastic vasculitis on skin biopsy, with IgA immunofluorescence in small vessels of the skin and in the renal glomeruli. Elevation of serum IgA may suggest a diagnosis of HSP. Its histologic picture is

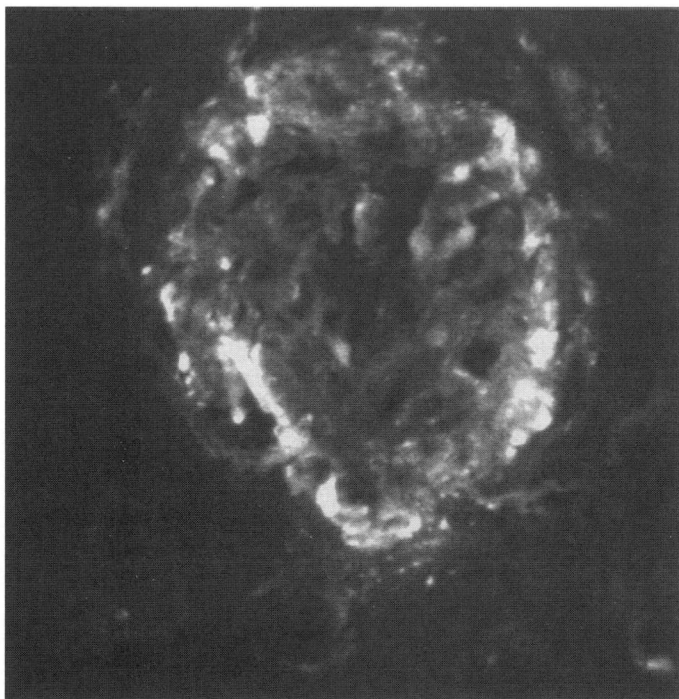

Figure 40.9 Glomerulus from a patient with HSP and proliferative mesangial glomerulonephritis with granular mesangial deposits of IgA. (IgA immunofluorescence × 400.) (See Color Plate 115).

not specific, since HSP is characterized by a leukocytoclastic vasculitis that is indistinguishable from leukocytoclastic (hypersensitivity) vasculitis and other systemic vasculitides involving small blood vessel of the skin (González-Gay et al. 2004, 2005).

As no absolute diagnostic test is available, classification criteria and definitions are commonly used. Classification of vasculitides is often confusing and controversial. In 1990, the American College of Rheumatology proposed classification criteria for HSP (Hunder et al. 1990). The criteria were presented in two forms, a traditional format and a tree format. The traditional format for the classification of HSP included the following four features: palpable purpura defined by the presence of slightly raised skin lesions unrelated to thrombocytopenia; age at the onset of the vasculitis younger than 20 years old; bowel angina consisting of diffuse abdominal pain or bowel ischemia, with or without bloody diarrhea; and histologic changes showing granulocytes in the walls of arterioles or venules on skin biopsy (Mills et al. 1990). For the classification of HSP at least two of these four criteria were required to be present. However, both HSP and hypersensitivity vasculitis (for which the preferred term is leukocytoclastic) are small-sized blood vessel vasculitides involving preferentially the skin, which share many clinical and pathologic features such as leukocytoclasia and palpable purpura. Furthermore, the overall sensitivity of the ACR criteria for classification of "hypersensitivity" vasculitis was low (Calabrese et al. 1990).

A considerable overlap between the ACR 1990 criteria for HSP and that for leukocytoclastic vasculitis was reported. In fact, in previous classifications such as that proposed by Fauci et al. (1978), HSP was classified as a subgroup of hypersensitivity vasculitis. Likewise, Gilliam and Smiley (1976) classified HSP within the group of leukocytoclastic, hypersensitivity, or allergic vasculitis.

In 1992, to compare the characteristics of leukocytoclastic vasculitis and HSP as separate and definable clinical syndromes, Michel et al. using the ACR database, investigated which clinical criteria best differentiated these two vasculitides. They reported that requiring the presence of three or more criteria, from a list of six, yielded correct classification of 87.1% of HSP cases. Two or fewer criteria from the same list of six criteria yielded a percentage of correctly classified leukocytoclastic vasculitis cases of 74.2%. In Table 40.2, the traditional format of criteria for differentiating HSP from "hypersensitivity" vasculitis is shown. In 1994, the Consensus Conference on the Nomenclature of Systemic Vasculitides required the presence of IgA-dominant immune deposits for the definition of HSP (Jennette et al. 1994). Immunofluorescence, however, was not routinely performed in the series of systemic vasculitis reported by Watts et al. (1998) and in that of González-Gay and García-Porrúa (1999). As expected, when Chapel Hill Consensus Conference definitions were applied to some series of systemic vasculitides (González-Gay and García-Porrúa 1999), many of the patients classified as HSP according to the ACR and Michel's classification criteria, fell into the category of microscopic polyangiitis. Furthermore, the requirement of immunofluorescence data would have underestimated the number of HSP patients reported in other series (Blanco et al. 1997b).

Conditions associated with HSP

Drugs (Calviño et al. 2001; Garcia-Porrúa et al. 1999), malignancies (Garcia-Porrúa and González-Gay 1998), and infections (Garcia-Porrúa and González-Gay 1999b; González-Gay and

Table 40.2 Criteria for differentiating Henöch–Schonlein purpura from hypersensitivity vasculitis (traditional format)

Criterion	Definition
1. Palpable purpura	Slightly elevated purpuric rash over one or more areas of the skin not related to thrombocytopenia.
2. Bowel angina	Diffuse abdominal pain worse after meals or bowel ischemia usually including bloody diarrhea.
3. Gastrointestinal bleeding	Gastrointestinal bleeding, including melena, hematochezia or positive test for occult blood in the stool.
4. Hematuria	Gross hematuria or microhematuria.
5. Age at onset <20 years	Development of first symptoms at age 20 or less.
6. No medications	Absence of any medications at onset of disease, which may have been a precipitating factor.

The presence of any three or more of the six criteria yields a correct classification of HSP cases of 87.1%. Two or fewer criteria yield a corrected classification of hypersensitivity vasculitis cases of 74.2%.

Data from Michael *et al.* (1992), with permission from *Journal of Rheumatology*.

Garcia-Porrúa 1999) have been associated with HSP. Cutaneous vasculitis, including HSP, may be associated with malignant disorders and behave as a paraneoplastic syndrome (González-Gay *et al.* 2000); however, there is no consensus about the actual proportion of patients with HSP and malignancy. Gibson and Su (1995) reported a frequency of 8% of cutaneous vasculitis associated with malignancy. Cutaneous vasculitis may antedate the discovery of the neoplasia, coincide, or appear after the malignancy has already been recognized; it may also indicate recurrence of cancer (Fortin 1996; García-Porrúa and González-Gay 1998; González-Gay *et al.* 2000; Mertz and Conn 1992; Sánchez-Guerrero *et al.* 1990). Hematologic disorders constituted the most common group of neoplasms associated with cutaneous vasculitis (Fortin 1996; García-Porrúa and González-Gay 1998; Mertz and Conn 1992). Cutaneous vasculitis associated with solid tumors often fulfills criteria for the diagnosis of HSP (Kurzrock *et al.* 1994; Sánchez-Guerrero *et al.* 1990; Garcia-Porrúa and González-Gay 1998; Weiler-Bisig *et al.* 2005).

There are several possible mechanisms accounting for either HSP or other cutaneous vasculitis in the setting of malignancy (González-Gay *et al.* 2000), such as impaired clearance of normally produced immune complexes. Alternatively, there may be abnormal production of immunoglobulins that react either with vascular antigens (causing formation of *in situ* immune complexes) or with a circulating antigen (forming circulating immune complexes that then deposit in the vessel walls). Finally, there may be production of immunoglobulins directed to the abnormal tumor cells as well as normal endothelium.

Drugs are often implicated in the development of cutaneous vasculitis. A history of drug exposure prior to the onset of the cutaneous vasculitis has traditionally been considered an important criterion for differentiating leukocytoclastic vasculitis (Michel *et al.* 1992) from HSP. A history of prior drug use is common in leukocytoclastic vasculitis; antecedent medication at disease onset was adopted by the ACR Subcommittee on Classification of Vasculitis as a classification criterion for "hypersensitivity" vasculitis (Calabrese *et al.* 1990). Although found at a lower frequency in HSP than in patients with "hypersensitivity" vasculitis, a history of recent drug intake has also been implicated in its pathogenesis (Blanco *et al.* 1997b; Garcia-Porrúa *et al.* 1999).

As with leukocytoclastic vasculitis and mixed cryoglobulinemia, HSP has been related to bacterial and viral infections (Somer and Finegold 1995). In the majority of series, Gram-positive cocci (staphylococcus and streptococcus species) (Saulsbury 1999; Calviño *et al.* 2001) and *Neisseria meningitidis* and *gonorrhoeae* were the most common bacteria implicated in this process; however, HSP has been reported in the context of infections with Gram-negative bacteria, anaerobes, mycobacteria, and brucella (Pacheco 1991). Parvovirus B19 has been related to HSP in anecdotal reports, but this association was uncommon in a case–control study (Ferguson *et al.* 1996). If some cases of HSP are caused by infection, responsible mechanisms might include immune complex formation and activation initiated by antigen products of the responsible organisms, or abnormal immunoregulation related to the infectious disease (Garcia-Porrúa and González-Gay 1999b).

Differences between HSP in children and adults

A few studies have discussed clinical and epidemiological differences of HSP according to the age of onset (Blanco *et al.* 1997b; Garcia-Porrúa *et al.* 2002; Ilan and Naparstek 1991; Lin *et al.* 1998; Uthman *et al.* 1998). Ilan and Naparstek (1991) did not find significant differences in clinical and laboratory findings between children and adult patients with HSP from Israel. In their series, renal failure was observed in two of the 15 adults and in five of the 46 children during the course of the disease, but none developed chronic renal failure (Ilan and Naparstek 1991). In contrast, other investigators reported a more severe disease in adults. In a retrospective study of patients with HSP classified according to the criteria proposed by Michel *et al.* (1992), Blanco *et al.* (1997b) observed more frequent and severe renal disease in patients older than 20 years than in those younger than 20. Similarly, Uthman *et al.* (1998) found a statistically significant difference in the incidence of nephropathy between adults and children, with two of 10 adults (age more than 20) developing renal failure compared with none of 35 children. A Chinese study also found that renal involvement was more common and severe in adults with HSP (Lin and Huang 1998). To establish clear differences in terms of age at disease onset in Spain, individuals older than 20 years (considered as adults) were compared with those younger than 14 years. In this series adults complained of arthralgias more often than children but swelling in the joints was observed more frequently in children. The frequency of GI manifestations was similar in both age groups. During the course of disease, six of the 31 adults (19%) from Spain had severe renal manifestations and another four (13%) renal insufficiency, whereas in 73 children from the same region the frequency of severe renal manifestations was 8% and of renal insufficiency 3%. After a median follow-up period of ~6 years, complete recovery was observed in 89% of the 73 children. None of the children developed chronic renal insufficiency and the few who developed renal insufficiency during the course of the disease had improved renal function at last follow-up. After 5 years median follow-up almost 40% of adults had persistent hematuria, three (10%) had renal insufficiency, of whom two required hemodialysis (Garcia-Porrúa *et al.* 2002). Relapses were also more common in adults but the difference was not statistically significant (Garcia-Porrúa *et al.* 2002). Complete recovery was reported in 107 of the 114 children and 33 of the 38 adults studied by Blanco *et al.* (1997b). Among these, persistent microscopic hematuria alone was observed in six children and mild renal insufficiency in four adults (Blanco *et al.* 1997).

Adults from the Lugo region of Spain developed the disease during the summer months more frequently than did children. The pediatric disease occurred more commonly in the coldest months of the year (Garcia-Porrúa *et al.* 2002). These observations were in keeping with the data reported in Israel by Ilan and Naparstek (1991).

Differential diagnosis

Diagnosis of HSP is straightforward in children presenting with the classic triad of palpable purpura, arthritis, and GI manifestations or hematuria. HSP is more common in children, and leukocytoclastic vasculitis is more common in adults (González-Gay *et al.* 2004, 2005). HSP in adults tends to involve organs more extensively, and the prognosis appears to be worse than in those with leukocytoclastic vasculitis (García-Porrúa and González-Gay 1999a). The clinical criteria proposed by Michel *et al.* are useful in differentiating HSP from leukocytoclastic vasculitis.

As in HSP, other systemic vasculitides such as microscopic polyangiitis (MPA) and Wegener's granulomatosis (WG) may present with skin lesions and crescentic glomerulonephritis. In addition to other clinical features, the presence of ANCA may be useful in differentiating these conditions. Perinuclear ANCA (pANCA) is found frequently in MPA while cytoplasmic (cANCA) is more commonly observed in WG (Gross *et al.* 1993; Guillevin *et al.* 1996; Rao *et al.* 1995; Specks and Homburger 1994).

Patients with mixed cryoglobulinemia and cryoglobulinemic vasculitis may present with recurrent episodes of purpuric skin lesions, frequently associated with visceral involvement, for example glomerulonephritis and neuropathy. Thus, patients should be tested for cryoglobulin, C4 and C3 complement serum levels, rheumatoid factor, and hepatitis C and B virus (González-Gay *et al.* 2004).

Connective tissue diseases, in particular systemic lupus erythematosus (SLE), may present with vasculitic skin lesions (González-Gay and Garcia-Porrúa 1999) and systemic symptoms. Although antinuclear antibodies (ANA) have been reported in some patients with HSP (Saulsbury 1986), ANA and anti-dsDNA antibodies, and low levels of serum C3 and C4, differentiate patients with SLE from those with HSP. Furthermore, leukocytoclastic cutaneous vasculitis in patients with SLE has been reported to occur more commonly in the setting of a flare of the disease (González-Gay and García-Porrúa 1999).

A careful clinical history in patients presenting with palpable purpura may be useful in differentiating vasculitic skin lesions from those produced by trauma, drug reactions, or physical trauma such as that seen in child abuse (González-Gay *et al.* 2004). Purpuric rash may also be due to sepsis, bacterial endocarditis, meningococcemia, Rocky Mountain spotted fever, or other infections (Stevens *et al.* 1995). Thrombotic disorders, such as the antiphospholipid antibody syndrome or thromboembolism, thrombocytopenia, pseudovasculitic lesions such as atheroembolic disease, neoplasms such as

the cardiac myxoma, or scurvy, may also cause purpuric cutaneous lesions and mimic vasculitis (González-Gay *et al.* 1999, 2004).

Abdominal pain, particularly in children, in which it often precedes cutaneous lesions, prompts the consideration of acute abdomen (Glasier *et al.* 1981). IgA glomerulonephritis is not pathognomonic of HSP; rheumatic diseases other than SLE (seronegative spondyloarthropathy), dermatologic diseases (psoriasis or dermatitis herpetiformis), neoplasms, and intestinal disorders (celiac sprue or hepatic cirrhosis) have been infrequently associated with this type of glomerulonephritis. These conditions can be clearly differentiated from IgA glomerulonephritis in the context of HSP, or from idiopathic IgA glomerulonephritis by clinical features (Galla 1995).

Finally, in infants younger than 2 years there is a syndrome called acute hemorrhagic edema that has been reported most often from Europe. It is characterized by a cutaneous leukocytoclastic vasculitis and edema, and ecchymotic, target-like purpura on the limbs and face. In many of the infants with this syndrome there is a history of recent illness, use of drugs or immunizations. Visceral involvement is the exception, and spontaneous recovery occurs generally within 1–3 weeks. It is not clear whether this syndrome should be considered a benign infantile form of HSP or an independent disease within the spectrum of conditions presenting with leukocytoclastic vasculitis (Athreya 1996; Ince *et al.* 1995).

Treatment

There is no specific treatment for HSP. Indeed, HSP in most cases is a self-limiting disease (Garcia-Porrúa *et al.* 2002). Treatment is largely supportive and, besides bed rest, includes adequate hydration and monitoring of vital signs. Non-steroidal anti-inflammatory drugs can improve joint pain, but they should be avoided in patients with renal insufficiency.

There is no consensus on the efficacy of glucocorticoid therapy to prevent severe complications in children with HSP and use of glucocorticoids in relapses is controversial (González-Gay and Llorca 2005). Glucocorticoids have been used, although not without controversy, in patients with severe GI manifestations, such as abdominal pain (Szer 1996). Abdominal pain improves in some children independent of glucocorticoids (Glasier *et al.* 1981; Rosenblum and Winter 1987). Rosenblum and Winter, however, described improvement of abdominal pain within the first 24 hours of glucocorticoid therapy in almost 50% of children, compared with a spontaneous resolution of only 14%. Many clinicians use glucocorticoids in all cases of HSP with abdominal pain. It appears that the risk of intussusception in children with abdominal pain is lower in those treated with glucocorticoids. Children and adults with HSP with severe abdominal pain, melena, and massive hemorrhage are routinely and, in general, successfully treated with these drugs (Blanco *et al.* 1997b; Calviño *et al.* 2002; García-Porrúa and González-Gay 1999a). Marked improvement of abdominal pain was observed in a patient immediately after the administration of factor XIII concentrate (Shimomura *et al.* 2005).

Another important point of contention is the role of glucocorticoids in the prevention of nephritis. Mollica *et al.* (1992) reported a prospective, randomized, controlled study on glucocorticoid prevention of renal disease in children with HSP. One hundred and sixty-eight children with HSP without nephritis were randomized to receive either prednisone (1 mg/kg per day orally for 2 weeks) or no glucocorticoids. None of the treated group (n = 84), but 10 of the control group (n = 84), developed nephropathy within 6 weeks. Two other controls developed nephropathy at 24 and 72 weeks. The results of this study suggested a role for prednisone in preventing HSP nephritis; however, a retrospective study based on 50 children with HSP without nephritis at the time of diagnosis, showed a similar frequency of nephritis in those patients treated or not treated with glucocorticoids (Saulsbury 1993). Kaku *et al.* (1998) reported results of a multivariate analysis and found that glucocorticoid treatment reduced the risk of nephritis and advocated its use in patients with risk factors for renal involvement. More recently, Huber *et al.* (2004) performed a randomized, placebo-controlled study of 40 children with HSP to assess whether glucocorticoid administration within 7 days of disease onset could reduce the rate of renal or GI complications. Twenty-one children were treated with oral prednisone, 2 mg/kg/day for 1 week, with weaning over a second week, while the remaining 19 received placebo. In this study, early prednisone therapy did not reduce the risk of renal involvement at 1 year, or the risk of acute GI complications (Huber *et al.* 2004).

The management of HSP nephritis is also highly controversial. Patients with severe nephritis have been treated with glucocorticoids (oral or pulse therapy) alone, or in combination with immunosuppressive agents such as cyclophosphamide, azathioprine, chlorambucil, or cyclosporine; plasmapheresis; high-dose intravenous immunoglobulin therapy; danazol; and fish oil (Kawasaki *et al.* 2004a, 2004b; Szer 1996; Shin *et al.* 2005a, 2005b; Tarshish *et al.* 2004; White 1994).

In most cases the absence of randomized, placebo-controlled studies makes valid conclusions difficult. Based on a series of 20 patients with HSP nephritis, Shin *et al.* (2005b) suggested that combined therapy of azathioprine and glucocorticoids might be beneficial in improving histopathological features and the clinical course of HSP patients with severe nephritis. An uncontrolled study of combined glucocorticoids, immunosuppressive drugs, and anticoagulants in patients with rapidly progressive glomerulonephritis due to various causes, including HSP, suggested that deterioration of renal function could be retarded if the patient was not severely oliguric (Brown *et al.* 1974). Niaudet and Habib (1998) evaluated the efficacy of methylprednisolone pulse therapy on the outcome of nephropathy in 38 children with severe forms of HSP. All patients were treated with high-dose methylprednisolone pulse therapy for 3 days, followed by oral prednisone for 3 months, and followed for a mean of 67 months. Based on clinical symptoms and histopathological changes, the investigators suggested that methylprednisolone pulse therapy should be limited to HSP patients with nephritis who are at risk of progressive renal disease, especially those with nephrotic syndrome or crescentic glomerulonephritis. They considered this therapy useful when it was started early in the disease, before crescents became fibrosed.

The prognosis is poor if patients present with rapidly progressive glomerulonephritis. Tarshish *el al.* (2004) found no differences in outcome between 56 patients with histopathologically severe HSP nephritis randomized to receive supportive therapy with or without cyclophosphamide, 90 mg/m^2/day for 42 days. In an uncontrolled study of 12 children with HSP and biopsy-proven rapidly progressive crescentic glomerulonephritis, Oner *et al.* (1995) suggested that a combination of methylprednisolone for 3 days (30 mg/kg/day) followed by oral prednisone at 45 mg/m^2/day tapered over 2 months, oral cyclophosphamide at 2 mg/kg/day

for 2 months, and dipyridamole at 5 mg/kg/day for 6 months, may be effective in normalizing glomerular filtration. Only one patient from this small series developed persistent nephropathy with nephrotic syndrome, gross hematuria, and renal failure. Another study with a longer follow-up (mean 7.5 years) of 14 children with severe nephritis and crescent formation corresponding to grades IV and V of the ISKDC iterated the benefit from intensive combination therapy (prednisolone, cyclophosphamide, heparin/warfarin, and dipyridamole) (Iijima *et al.* 1998). Kawasaki *el al.* (2004b) studied 37 patients with HSP who had been diagnosed with glomerulonephritis of at least grade IVb. Twenty of them were treated with methylprednisolone and urokinase pulse therapy (group A), and the remaining 17 (group B) were treated with methylprednisolone and urokinase pulse therapy combined with cyclophosphamide. After 6 months of treatment, the mean urinary protein excretion in group B was significantly lower than those in Group A, and on the second kidney biopsy, the chronicity index of Group B was lower than that of Group A. These observations support the use of methylprednisolone and urokinase pulse therapy combined with cyclophosphamide in HSP patients with severe nephritis.

In an uncontrolled, retrospective study, Shin *et al.* (2005a) reported a beneficial effect of cyclosporine in HSP children with nephrotic syndrome. High-dose intravenous immunoglobulin (IVIG) has proved to be effective in the treatment of several immune-mediated diseases, including systemic vasculitis (Dwyer 1992; Jayne *et al.* 1991). Rostoker *et al.* (1994, 1995) reported that both low-and high-dose IVIg may be effective in treating either moderate or severe nephritis in HSP and IgA nephropathy. There has been concern about renal deterioration following such treatment in cases of systemic vasculitis and SLE (Barron *et al.* 1992; Pasatiempo *et al.* 1994; Schifferlie *et al.* 1991). Although the occurrence of acute renal failure after high-dose IVIg seems to be rare, persistent deterioration was observed in renal function following this therapy in an adult with HSP and focal proliferative glomerulonephritis with mesangial IgA and C3 deposits (Blanco *et al.* 1997a).

Outcomes of treatment with plasma exchange combined with glucocorticoids, anticoagulants, cyclophosphamide, and azathioprine (in different combinations) in children with crescentic glomerulonephritis related to HSP (and various other conditions) were retrospectively examined by Jardim *et al.* (1992). In 30 patients, they observed a progression to end-stage renal failure in 50% of the children. The interval between disease onset and commencement of therapy was an important prognostic factor for the outcome. A retrospective study of plasma exchange in children with rapidly progressive nephritis or cerebral vasculitis associated with HSP was reported by Gianviti *et al.* (1996). These investigators described 17 HSP patients treated with plasma exchange and combinations of glucocorticoids, cyclophosphamide, and azathioprine. Fourteen of them had severe glomerulonephritis (30–100% of glomeruli with crescents) or were dialysis-dependent, and three had cerebral vasculitis. Recovery was observed in all three children with cerebral vasculitis. In those with severe nephritis, the time of onset of therapy was a determinant of outcome, as all nine with renal vasculitis who started plasma exchange within 1 month of disease onset had significant improvement in renal function. In contrast, five of six children with HSP nephritis treated later in the disease developed end-stage renal failure. No relapses of vasculitis were observed after treatment with plasma exchange. These results suggest that plasma exchange associated with immunosuppressive therapy may be useful in cases of severe renal or extrarenal HSP.

Renal transplantation may be considered for the few patients who progress to end-stage renal disease. Recurrences have been observed and when the graft function was seriously impaired, other systemic manifestations, including typical purpura, tended to recur. Recurrences of the disease appear to be strongly associated with living related donor transplants (Baliah *et al.* 1974; Hasegawa *et al.* 1989; Nast *et al.* 1987). The significance of this association is unknown, but it may suggest a genetic predisposition for the development of the disease.

Clinical course and outcome

Most patients with HSP have a self-limited disease (Garcia-Porrúa *et al.* 2002). On occasion, hormone therapy has been reported to be associated with remission in some patients (Lahita 1997). The average duration of the disease is 4 weeks (Allen *et al.* 1960); however, in both children and adults, relapses of the disease are common. They are characterized by flares of purpuric skin lesions which in some patients are associated with renal and GI complications.

Allen *et al.* (1960) reported relapses in 40% of children. Blanco *et al.* (1997b) described relapses in 43% of HSP patients younger than 20 years. In children from Spain, Calviño *et al.* (2001) reported relapses (defined as an HSP patient asymptomatic for at least 1 month presenting with a flare of skin lesions or other systemic complications) in 15% of 69 children followed for at least 12 months. In two studies of HSP in adults, relapses occurred in 36% (Blanco *et al.* 1997b) and 21% (García-Porrúa and González-Gay 1999a) of patients. Although the prognosis is not as good for adults as for children, the overall outcome in HSP is better than that observed in polyarteritis nodosa, WG, or Churg–Strauss syndrome (González-Gay and García-Porrúa 1999; Hunder 1996). Comparisons among different series are tenuous because most recent epidemiological studies (Blanco *et al.* 1997b; García-Porrúa and González-Gay 1999a; Garcia-Porrúa *et al.* 2002; Trapani *et al.* 2005) have been based on unselected patients classified according to the 1990 ACR classification criteria or those of Michel *et al.* (Michel *et al.* 1992; Mills *et al.* 1990), or on the basis of IgA deposits in the dermal vessel walls (Tancrede-Bohin *et al.* 1997). In contrast, some have been based on selected patient populations, usually those with kidney dysfunction (Fogazzi *et al.* 1989; Lee *et al.* 1986; Roth *et al.* 1985). Some studies have included patients with several different types of cutaneous vasculitis, and some patients with underlying diseases (Cream *et al.* 1970). Thus, different methods of selection of patients may explain a discrepancy in reported outcomes of the disease.

The long-term morbidity and mortality of HSP are predominantly attributable to renal involvement. HSP has been reported to account for between 5–15% of end-stage renal failure in children (Bunchman *et al.* 1988; Meadow 1978). Bunchman *et al.* (1988) observed that a failure to reach a creatinine clearance higher than 70 ml/min/1.73 m^2 by 3 years after the onset of HSP predicted progression to end-stage renal failure. In an unselected series of 141 children with HSP, Koskimies *et al.* (1981) reported persistence of abnormal urinary sediment for at least 1 month in 28% of their patients. After a mean follow-up of 7.2 years, only one child progressed to end-stage renal failure (0.7%) and two (1.4%) developed chronic glomerular disease. In another unselected series of 270 children, Stewart *et al.* (1988) observed evidence of renal involvement

in 55 (20%). Re-examination at an average of 8.3 years after the onset of the disease showed a good overall prognosis, with mortality less than 1% overall and long-term morbidity of only 1.1% (Stewart *et al.* 1988). Unlike adults, none of 73 unselected children with HSP from Spain who were followed at least 1 year developed end-stage renal failure (Garcia-Porrúa *et al.* 2002). All these studies (Garcia-Porrúa *et al.* 2002; Koskimies *et al.* 1981; Stewart *et al.* 1988) support a better prognosis for HSP nephritis in children than the majority of published estimates. In extensive surveillance for 23.4 years of 78 of 99 children with HSP nephritis (Goldstein *et al.* 1992), the severity of the clinical presentation and the initial findings on the renal biopsy correlated well with the outcome. In 16 of 44 girls, pregnancies were complicated by proteinuria and hypertension, even in the absence of active renal disease. Because of that, Goldstein *et al.* (1992) suggested that HSP nephritis in children should be followed long-term, and especially during pregnancy.

As discussed above, severe renal involvement is more common in adults than in children (Blanco *et al.* 1997b; Garcia-Porrúa *et al.* 2002; Uthman *et al.* 1998) but in the unselected series of Blanco *et al.* (1997b), the final outcome was equally good in both age groups. For patients older than 15 who were studied based on the presence of cutaneous IgA deposits and purpura, Tancrede-Bohin (1997) observed a good outcome. In an unselected series of 27 HSP adults (older than 20 years) with biopsy-proven leukocytoclastic vasculitis, García-Porrúa and González-Gay (1999a) observed the development of renal insufficiency in 8.3% of patients after a median follow-up of 3 years. These data suggest that the prognosis in adults with HSP is not as good as that reported in children.

Conclusions

HSP is an IgA-mediated disease affecting small blood vessels. It is the most common vasculitis in children and an infrequent condition in adults. It may follow an intercurrent illness, usually infection of the upper respiratory tract. Skin, joints, gut, and kidneys are the organs most commonly involved. It is a benign and self-limited condition in the vast majority of children and most adults, but a small percentage, especially adults, progress to renal insufficiency. For this reason, close follow-up with repeated urinalysis is advisable in those who present renal manifestations during the first 6 months after the onset of the disease. Pharmacological treatments are controversial and so far no management of HSP has been declared optimal in patients with renal disease or severe GI complications. Reports on prophylactic glucocorticoid therapy to prevent renal disease are contradictory. Long-term follow-up studies are required for a better understanding of this vasculitis.

References

Abou-Ragheb, H. H. A., Williams, A. J., Brown, C. B. and Milford-Ward, A. (1992). Plasma levels of the anaphylatoxins C3a and C4a in patients with IgA nephropathy/Henoch–Schönlein nephritis. *Nephron*, **62**, 22–6.

Allen, D., Diamond, L. K. and Howell, D. A. (1960). Anaphylactoid purpura in children (Schönlein-Henoch syndrome). *American Journal of Diseases of Children*, **99**, 833–54.

Amoli, M. M., Calviño, M. C., Garcia-Porrúa, C., Llorca, J., Ollier, W. E. and González-Gay, MA. (2004). Interleukin 1beta gene polymorphism association with severe renal manifestations and renal sequelae in Henoch–Schönlein purpura. *Journal of Rheumatology*, **31**, 295–8.

Amoli, M. M., Mattey, D. L., Calviño, M. C., *et al.* (2001a). Polymorphism at codon 469 of the intercellular adhesion molecule-1 locus is associated with protection against severe gastrointestinal complications in Henoch–Schönlein purpura. *Journal of Rheumatology*, **28**, 1014–8.

Amoli, M. M., Thomson, W., Hajeer, A. H., *et al.* (2001b). HLA-DRB1*01 association with Henoch–Schönlein purpura in patients from northwest Spain. *Journal of Rheumatology*, **28**, 1266–70.

Amoli, M. M., Thomson, W., Hajeer, A. H., *et al.* (2002a). HLA-B35 association with nephritis in Henoch–Schönlein purpura. *Journal of Rheumatology*, **29**, 948–9.

Amoli, M. M., Thomson, W., Hajeer, A. H., *et al.* (2002b). Interleukin 1 receptor antagonist gene polymorphism is associated with severe renal involvement and renal sequelae in Henoch–Schönlein purpura. *Journal of Rheumatology*, **29**, 1404–7.

Amoli, M. M., Thomson, W., Hajeer, A. H., *et al.* (2002c). Interleukin-8 gene polymorphism is associated with increased risk of nephritis in cutaneous vasculitis. *Journal of Rheumatology*, **29**, 2367–70.

Amoroso, A., Berrino, M., Canale, L., Coppo, R., Cornaglia, M., Guarrera, S., *et al.* (1997). Immunogenetics of Henoch–Schönlein disease. *European Journal of Immunogenetics*, **24**, 323–33.

Archimandritis, A., Kalos, A., Pantzos, A., Sakellariou, D., Malamas, N. and Fertakis, A. (1994). Hemorrhagic ascites in a patient with anaphylactoid purpura. *Journal of Clinical Gastroenterology*, **18**, 257–8.

Ates, E., Bakkaloglu, A., Saatci, U., Soylemezoglu, O. (1994). Von Willebrand factor antigen compared with other factors in vasculitic syndromes. *Archives of Disease in Childhood*, **70**, 40–3.

Athreya, B. H. (1996). Vasculitis in children. *Current Opinion in Rheumatology*, **8**, 477–84.

Ault, B. H., Stapleton, F. B., Rivas, M. L., Waldo, F. B., Roy, S., McLean, R. H., *et al.* (1990). Association of Henoch–Schönlein purpura glomerulonephritis with C4B deficiency. *Journal of Pediatrics*, **117**, 753–5.

Baliah, T., Kim, K., Anthone, S., Anthone, R., Montes, M. and Andres, G. (1974). Recurrence of Henoch–Schönlein purpura glomerulonephritis in transplanted kidneys. *Transplantation*, **18**, 343–6.

Bailey, M., Chapin, W., Licht, H. and Reynolds, J. C. (1998). The effects of vasculitis on the gastrointestinal tract and liver. *Gastroenterology Clinics of North America*, **27**, 747–82.

Ballard, H. S., Eisinger, R. P. and Gallo, G. (1970). Renal manifestations of the Henoch–Schönlein syndrome in adults. *American Journal of Medicine*, **79**, 328–35.

Barron, K. S., Sher, M. R. and Silverman, E. D. (1992). Intravenous immunoglobulin therapy: Magic or black magic. *Journal of Rheumatology*, **19** (Suppl. 33), 94–7.

Blanco, R., González-Gay, M. A., Ibañez, D., Sanchez-Andrade, A. and González-Vela, C. (1997a). Paradoxical and persistent renal impairment in Henoch–Schönlein purpura after high-dose immunoglobulin therapy. *Nephron*, **76**, 247–8.

Blanco, R., Martinez-Taboada, V. M., Rodriguez-Valverde, V., García-Fuentes, M. and González-Gay, M. A. (1997b). Henoch–Schönlein purpura in the adulthood and in the childhood: two different expressions of the same syndrome. *Arthritis and Rheumatism*, **40**, 859–64.

Blockmans, D. and Bobbaers, H. (1998). Inflammation phenomena in vasculitis: from immune complexes to less immune forms. *Acta Clinica Belgica*, **53**, 83–91.

Brown, C. B., Wilson, D., Turner, D., Cameron, J. S., Ogg, C. S., Chantler, C., *et al.* (1974). Combined immunosuppression and anticoagulation in rapidly progressive glomerulonephritis. *Lancet*, **2**, 1166–72.

Boyer, J., Baudet, P., Ben Bouali, A., Ronceray, J. and Joubaud, F. (1978). Unusual manifestations during rheumatoid purpura. Apropos of 2 cases. *La Semaine des Hôpitaux de Paris*, **54**, 298–302.

Bunchman, T. E., Mauer, S. M., Sibley, R. K. and Vernier, R. L. (1988). Anaphylactoid purpura: characteristics of 16 patients who progressed to renal failure. *Pediatric Nephrology*, **2**, 393–7.

Cakir, N., Pamuk, O. N. and Donmez, S. (2004). Henoch–Schönlein purpura in two brothers imprisoned in the same jail: presentation two months apart. *Clinical and Experimental Rheumatology*, **22**, 235–7.

Calabrese, L. H., Michel, B. A., Bloch, D. A., Arend, W. P., Edworthy, S. M., Fauci, A. S., *et al.* (1990). The ACR 1990 criteria for the classification of hypersensitivity vasculitis. *Arthritis and Rheumatism*, **33**, 1108–13.

Calvino, M. C., Llorca, J., Garcia-Porrúa, C., Fernandez-Iglesias, J. L., Rodriguez-Ledo, P and González-Gay, M. A. (2001). Henoch–Schönlein purpura in children from northwestern Spain: a 20-year epidemiologic and clinical study. *Medicine* (Baltimore), **80**, 279–90.

Cappell, M. S. and Gupta, A. M. (1990). Colonic lesions associated with Henoch–Schönlein purpura. *American Journal of Gastroenterology*, **85**, 1186–8.

Casanueva, B., Rodriguez-Valverde, Merino, J., Arias, M. and García-Fuentes, M. (1983). Increased IgA-producing cells in the blood of patients with active Henoch–Schönlein purpura. *Arthritis and Rheumatism*, **26**, 854–60.

Casanueva, B., Rodriguez-Valverde, V. and Luceño, A. (1988). Circulating IgA-producing cells in the differential diagnosis of Henoch–Schönlein purpura. *Journal of Rheumatology*, **15**, 1229–33.

Cassidy, J. T. and Petty, R. E. (1995). Henoch–Schönlein purpura. In *Textbook of pediatric rheumatology* (Cassidy, J. T. and Petty, R. E., eds), 3rd edn, pp. 384–8. W. B. Saunders Company, Philadelphia.

Chamberlain, R. S. and Greenberg, L. W. (1992). Scrotal involvement in Henoch–Schönlein purpura. A case report and review of literature. *Pediatric Emergency Care*, **8**, 213–5.

Chang, W. L., Yang, Y. H., Wang, L. C., Lin, Y. T., and Chiang, B. L. (2005). Renal manifestations in Henoch–Schönlein purpura: a 10-year clinical study. *Pediatric Nephrology*, **20**, 1269–72.

Chaussain, M., De Boissieu, D., Kalifa, G., Epelbaum, S., Niaudet, P., Badoual, J., *et al.* (1992). Impairment of lung diffusion capacity in Henoch–Schönlein purpura. *Journal of Pediatrics*, **121**, 12–6.

Clauvel, J. P., Touraine, R. and Bernard, J. (1972). Rheumatoid purpura in adults. Apropos of 22 cases. *Nouvelle Revue Française d'Hématologie*, **12**, 117–22.

Chiaretti, A., Scommegna, S., Castorina, M., Piastra, M., Tortorolo, L., Villali, A., *et al.* (1995). Intracranial hemorrhage in Henoch–Schönlein syndrome. *Pediatria Medica e Chirurgica*, **17**, 177–9.

Cimolai, N. and Macnab, A. (1991). Henoch–Schönlein purpura and *Streptococcus equisimilis*. *British Journal of Dermatology*, **125**, 403.

Connolly, B. and O'Halpin, D. (1994). Sonographic evaluation of the abdomen in Henoch–Schönlein purpura. *Clinical Radiology*, **49**, 320–3.

Coppo, R., Cirina, P., Amore, A., Sinico, R. A., Radice, A. and Rollino, C. (1997). Properties of circulating IgA molecules in Henoch–Schönlein purpura nephritis with focus on neutrophil cytoplasmic antigen IgA binding (IgA-ANCA): new insight into a debated issue. Italian Group of Renal Immunopathology Collaborative Study on Henoch–Schönlein purpura in adults and children. *Nephrology, Dialysis, Transplantation*, **12**, 2269–76.

Counahan, R., Winterborn, M. H., White, R. H.R., Heaton, J. M., Meadow, S. R., Bluett, N. H., *et al.* (1977). Prognosis of Henoch–Schönlein purpura in children. *British Medical Journal*, **2**, 11–14.

Cream, J. J., Gample, J. M. and Peachey, R. D.G. (1970). Schönlein-Henoch purpura in the adult. *Quarterly Journal of Medicine*, **39**, 461–82.

Cull, D. L., Rosario, V., Lally, K. P., Ratner, I. and Mahour, G. H. (1990). Surgical implications of Henoch–Schönlein purpura. *Journal of Pediatric Surgery*, **25**, 741–3.

Cummins, DL., Mimouni, D., Rencic, A., Kouba, D. J. and Nousari, C. H. (2003). Henoch–Schönlein purpura in pregnancy. *British Journal of Dermatology*, **149**, 1282–5.

Debray, J., Krulik, M. and Giorgi, H. (1971). Le purpura rhumatoide de l'adulte (syndrome de Schönlein-Henoch). A propos de 22 observations. *Semaine des Hopitaux de Paris*, **47**, 1805–19.

De Mattia, D., Penza, R., Giordano, P., Del Vecchio, G. C., Aceto, G., Altomare, M., *et al.* (1995). Von Willebrand factor and factor XIII in children with Henoch–Schönlein purpura. *Pediatric Nephrology*, **9**, 603–5.

Dillon, M. J. and Ansell, B. M. (1995). Vasculitis in children and adolescents. *Rheumatic Diseases Clinics of North America*, **21**, 1115–36.

Dolezalova, P., Telekesova, P., Nemcova, D. and Hoza, J. (2004). Incidence of vasculitis in children in the Czech Republic: 2-year prospective epidemiology survey. *Journal of Rheumatology*, **31**, 2295–9.

Duquesnoy, B. (1991). Henoch–Schönlein purpura. *Bailliere's Clinical Rheumatology*, **5**, 253–61.

Dwyer, J. M. (1992). Manipulating the immune system with immune globulin. *New England Journal of Medicine*, **326**, 107–16.

Farley, T. A., Gillespi, S., Rasoulpour, M., Tolentino, N., Hadler, J. L. and Hurwitz, E. (1989). Epidemiology of a cluster of Henoch–Schönlein purpura. *American Journal of Diseases of Children*, **143**, 798–803.

Fauci, A. S., Haynes, B. F. and Katz, P. (1978). The spectrum of vasculitis: clinical, pathologic, immunologic, and therapeutic considerations. *Annals of Internal Medicine*, **89**, 660–76.

Ferguson, P. J., Saulsbury, F. T., Dowell, S. F., Török, T. J., Erdman, D. A. and Anderson, L. A. (1996). Prevalence of human parvovirus B19 infection in children with Henoch–Schönlein purpura. *Arthritis and Rheumatism*, **39**, 880–2.

Fielding, R. E., Hawkins, C. P., Hand, M. F., Heath, P. D. and Davies, S. J. (1998). Seizure complicating Henoch–Schönlein purpura. *Nephrology, Dialysis, Transplantation*, **13**, 761–2.

Fogazzi, G. B., Pasquali, S., Moriggi, M., Casanova, S., Damilano, I., Mihatsch, M. J., *et al.* (1989). Long-term outcome of Schönlein–Henoch nephritis in the adult. *Clinical Nephrology*, **31**, 60–6.

Fortin, P. R. (1996). Vasculitides associated with malignancy. *Current Opinion in Rheumatology*, **8**, 30–3.

Frank, E. (1915). Die essentielle thrombopenie. *Berliner Klinische Wochenschrift*, **52**, 454.

Fujieda, M., Oishi, N., Naruse, K., Hashizume, M., Nishiya, K., Kurashige, T., *et al.* (1998). Soluble thrombomodulin and antibodies to bovine glomerular endothelial cells in patients with Henoch–Schönlein purpura. *Archives of Disease in Childhood*, **78**, 240–4.

Galla, J. H. (1995). IgA nephropathy. *Kidney International*, **47**, 377–87.

García Fuentes, M., Chantler, C. and Williams, D. G. (1977). Cryoglobulinaemia in Henoch–Schönlein purpura. *British Medical Journal*, **2**, 163–5.

Garcia-Porrúa, C., Calvino, M. C., Llorca, J., Couselo, J. M. and González-Gay, M. A. (2002). Henoch–Schönlein purpura in children and adults: clinical differences in a defined population. *Seminars Arthritis Rheumatism*, **32**, 149–56.

Garcia-Porrúa, C. and González-Gay, M. A. (1998). Cutaneous vasculitis as a paraneoplastic syndrome in adults. *Arthritis and Rheumatism*, **41**, 1133–5.

Garcia-Porrúa, C. and González-Gay, M. A. (1999a). Comparative clinical and epidemiologic study of hypersensitivity vasculitis versus Henoch–Schönlein purpura in adults. *Seminars in Arthritis and Rheumatism*, **28**, 404–12.

Garcia-Porrúa, C. and González-Gay, M. A. (1999b). Bacterial infection presenting as cutaneous vasculitis in adults. *Clinical and Experimental Rheumatology*, **17**, 471–3.

Garcia-Porrúa, C., González-Gay, M. A. and Lopez-Lazaro, L. (1999). Drug-associated cutaneous vasculitis in adulthood. Clinical and epidemiological associations in a defined population of Northwestern Spain. *Journal of Rheumatology*, **26**, 1942–4.

Garcia-Porrúa, C., González-Louzao, C., Llorca, J. and González-Gay, MA. (2001). Predictive factors for renal sequelae in adults with Henoch–Schönlein purpura. *journal of Rheumatology*, **28**, 1019–24.

Giancomo, J. and Tsai, C. C. (1977). Dermal and glomerular deposition of IgA in anaphylactoid purpura. *American Journal of Diseases of Children*, **131**, 981–3.

Gianviti, A., Trompeter, R. S., Barratt, T. M., Lythgoe, M. F. and Dillon, D. J. (1996). Retrospective study of plasma exchange in patients with idiopathic rapidly progressive glomerulonephritis and vasculitis. *Archives of Disease in Childhood*, **75**, 186–90.

Gibson, L. E. and Su, W. F. (1995). Cutaneous vasculitis. *Rheumatic Diseases Clinics of North America*, **21**, 1097–113.

Gilliam, J. N. and Smiley, J. D. (1976). Cutaneous necrotizing vasculitis and related disorders. *Annals of Allergy*, **37**, 328–39.

Glasier, C. M., Siegel, M. J., McAlister, W. H. and Shackelford, G. D. (1981). Henoch–Schönlein syndrome in children: gastrointestinal manifestations. *American Journal of Roentgenology*, **136**, 1081–5.

Goldman, L. P. and Lindenberg, R. L. (1981). Henoch–Schönlein purpura: gastrointestinal manifestations with endoscopic correlation. *American Journal of Gastroenterology*, **75**, 357–60.

Goldstein, A. R., White, R. H., Akuse, R. and Chantler, C. (1992). Long-term follow-up of childhood Henoch–Schönlein nephritis. *Lancet*, **339**, 280–2.

González-Gay, M. A., Calviño, M. C., Vazquez-Lopez, M. E., Garcia-Porrúa, C., Fernandez-Iglesias, J. L., Dierssen, T., *et al.* (2004). Implications of upper respiratory tract infections and drugs in the clinical spectrum of Henoch–Schönlein purpura in children. *Clinical and Experimental Rheumatology*, **22**, 781–4.

González-Gay, M. A. and García-Porrúa, C. (1999). Systemic vasculitis in adults in Northwestern Spain, 1988–1997: Clinical and epidemiologic aspects. *Medicine* (Baltimore), **78**, 292–308.

González-Gay, M. A. and Garcia-Porrúa, C. (2001). Epidemiology of the vasculitides. *Rheumatic Diseases Clinics of North America*, **27**, 729–49.

González-Gay, M. A., García-Porrúa, C., Afonso, E., Basanta, D. and Moreno-Lugris, C. (1999). Scurvy: a condition mimicking cutaneous vasculitis. Report of three cases. *Revue du Rhumatisme (English Edition)*, **66**, 360–1.

González-Gay, M. A., Garcia-Porrúa, C and Pujol, R. M. (2005). A clinical approach to cutaneous vasculitis. *Current Opinion in Rheumatology*, **17**, 56–61

González-Gay, M. A., Garcia-Porrúa, C., Salvarani, C. and Hunder, G.G (2000). Cutaneous vasculitis and cancer: a clinical approach. *Clinical and Experimental Rheumatology*, **18**, 305–7.

González-Gay, M. A., Garcia-Porrúa, C., Salvarani, C., Lo Scocco, G. and Pujol, R. M. (2003). Cutaneous vasculitis: a diagnostic approach. *Clinical and Experimental Rheumatology*, **21** (6 Suppl. 32), S85–8.

González-Gay, M. A. and Llorca, J. (2005). Controversies on the use of corticosteroid therapy in children with Henoch–Schönlein purpura. *Seminars in Arthritis and Rheumatism*, **35**, 135–7.

Gross, W. L., Schmitt, W. H. and Csernok, E. (1993). ANCA and associated diseases: immunodiagnostic and pathogenetic aspects. *Clinical and Experimental Immunology*, **91**, 1–12.

Guillevin, L., Lhote, F., Amouroux, J., Gherardi, R., Callard, P. and Casassu, P. (1996). Antineutrophil cytoplasmic antibodies, abnormal angiograms and pathological findings in polyarteritis nodosa and Churg-Strauss syndrome: indications for the classification of the vasculitides of the polyarteritis nodosa group. *British Journal of Rheumatology*, **35**, 958–64.

Ha, T. S. (2005). The role of tumor necrosis factor-alpha in Henoch–Schönlein purpura. *Pediatric Nephrology*, **20**, 149–53.

Ha, T. S. and Cha, S. H. (1996). Cerebral vasculitis in Henoch–Schönlein purpura: a case report with sequential magnetic resonance imaging. *Pediatric Nephrology*, **10**, 634–6.

Halling, S. F., Soderberg, M. P. and Berg, U. B. (2005). Henoch–Schönlein nephritis: clinical findings related to renal function and morphology. *Pediatric Nephrology*, **20**, 46–51.

Hasegawa, A., Kawamura, T., Ito, H., Hasegawa, O., Ogawa, O., Honda, M., *et al.* (1989). Fate of renal grafts with recurrent Henoch–Schönlein purpura nephritis in children. *Transplantation Proceedings*, **21**, 2130–3.

Heaton, J. M., Turner, D. R. and Cameron, J. S. (1977). Localization of glomerular deposits in Henoch–Schönlein nephritis. *Histopathology*, **1**, 93–104.

Heberden, W. (1801). *Commentarii de Marlbaun. Historia et curatione*. London, Payne.

Helander, S. D., de Castro, F. R. and Gibson, L. E. (1995). Henoch–Schönlein purpura: Clinicopathologic correlation of cutaneous vascular IgA deposits and the relationship to leukocytoclastic vasculitis. *Acta Dermato-Venereologica*, **75**, 125–9.

Hené, R. J., Velthuis, P., van de Wiel, A., Klepper, D., Mees, E. J.D. and Kater, L. (1986). The relevance of IgA deposits in vessel walls of clinically normal skin. *Archives of Internal Medicine*, **146**, 745–9.

Henoch, E. H.H. (1874). Über eine eigentümliche Form von Purpura. *Berliner Klinische Wochenschrift*, **2**, 641–3.

Henoch, E. H.H. (1895). *Vorlesungen über Kinderkrankheiten*. Berlin, Hirschwald.

Hisano, S., Matsushita, M., Fujita, T. and Iwasaki, H. (2005). Activation of the lectin complement pathway in Henoch–Schönlein purpura nephritis. *American Journal of Kidney Diseases*, **45**, 295–302.

Huber, A. M., King, J., McLaine, P., Klassen, T. and Pothos, M. (2004). A randomized, placebo-controlled trial of prednisone in early Henoch–Schönlein Purpura. *BioMed Central Medicine*, **2**, 7.

Hunder, G. (1996). Vasculitis: Diagnosis and therapy. *American Journal of Medicine*, **100** (Suppl. 2A), 37S–45S.

Hunder, G. G., Arend, W. P., Bloch, D. A., Calabrese, L. H., Fauci, A. S., Fries, J. F., *et al.* (1990). The ACR 1990 criteria for the classification of vasculitis. *Arthritis and Rheumatism*, **33**, 1065–7.

Iijima, K., Ito-Kariya, S., Nakamura, H. and Yoshikawa, N. (1998). Multiple combined therapy for severe Henoch–Schönlein nephritis in children. *Pediatric Nephrology*, **12**, 244–8.

Ilan, Y. and Naparstek, Y. (1991). Schönlein-Henoch syndrome in adults and children. *Seminars in Arthritis and Rheumatism*, **21**, 103–9.

Ince, E., Mumcu, Y., Suskan, E., Yalcincaya, F., Tumer, N. and Cin, S. (1995). Infantile acute hemorrhagic edema: a variant of leukocytoclastic vasculitis. *Pediatric Dermatology*, **12**, 224–7.

Jardim, H. M., Leake, J., Risdon, R. A., Barrat, T. M. and Dillon, M. J. (1992). Crescentic glomerulonephritis in children. *Pediatric Nephrology*, **6**, 231–5.

Jayne, D. R.W., Davies, M. J., Fox, C. J.V., Black, C. M. and Lockwood, C. M. (1991). Treatment of systemic vasculitis with pooled intravenous immunoglobulin. *Lancet*, **337**, 1137–9.

Jennette, J. C., Falk, R. J., Andrassy, K., Bacon, P. A., Churg, J., Gross, W. L., *et al.* (1994). Nomenclature of systemic vasculitides: proposal of an international consensus conference. *Arthritis and Rheumatism*, **37**, 187–92.

Jeong, Y. K., Hu, H. K., Yoon, C. H., *et al.* (1997). Gastrointestinal involvement in Henoch–Schönlein syndrome: CT findings. *American Journal of Roentgenology*, **168**, 965–8.

Jin, D. K., Kohsaka, T., Jun, A. and Kobayashi, N. (1992). Complement 4 gene deletion in patients with IgA nephropathy and Henoch–Schönlein nephritis. *Child Nephrology and Urology*, **12**, 208–11.

Jin, D. K., Kohsaka, T., Koo, J. W., Ha, I. S., Cheong, H. I. and Choi, Y. (1996). Complement 4 locus II gene deletion and DQA1*0301 gene: genetic risk factors for IgA nephropathy and Henoch–Schönlein nephritis. *Nephron*, **73**, 390–5.

Jones, N. F., Creamer, B. and Gimlette, T. M.D. (1966). Hypoproteinemia in anaphylactoid purpura. *British Medical Journal*, **2**, 1166–8.

Kaku, Y., Nohara, K. and Honda, S. (1998). Renal involvement in Henoch–Schönlein purpura: a multivariate analysis of prognostic factors. *Kidney International*, **53**, 1755–9.

Kato, S., Shibuya, H., Naganuma, H. and Nakagawa, H. (1992). Gastrointestinal endoscopy in Henoch–Schönlein purpura. *European Journal of Pediatrics*, **151**, 482–4.

Kathuria, S. and Cheifec, G. (1982). Fatal pulmonary Henoch–Schönlein syndrome. *Chest*, **82**, 654–6.

Kawana, S. and Nishiyama, S. (1992). Serum SC5b-9 (terminal complement complex) level, a sensitive indicator of disease activity in patients with Henoch–Schönlein purpura. *Dermatology*, **184**, 171–6.

Kawasaki, Y., Suzuki, J., Sakai, N., Nemoto, K., Nozawa, R., Suzuki, S., *et al.* (2003). Clinical and pathological features of children with Henoch–Schönlein purpura nephritis: risk factors associated with poor prognosis. *Clinical Nephrology*, **60**, 153–60.

Kawasaki, Y., Suzuki, J., Murai, M., Takahashi, A., Isome, M., Nozawa, R., *et al.* (2004a). Plasmapheresis therapy for rapidly progressive Henoch–Schönlein nephritis. *Pediatric Nephrology*, **19**, 920–3.

Kawasaki, Y., Suzuki, J. and Suzuki, H (2004b). Efficacy of methylprednisolone and urokinase pulse therapy combined with or without cyclophosphamide in severe Henoch–Schönlein nephritis: a clinical and histopathological study. *Nephrology Dialysis Transplantation*, **19**, 858–64.

Knight, J. F. (1990). The rheumatic poison: a survey of some published investigations of the immunopathogenesis of Henoch–Schönlein purpura. *Pediatric Nephrology*, **4**, 533–41.

Koskimies, O., Mir, S., Rapola, J. and Vilska, J. (1981). Henoch–Schönlein nephritis: long-term prognosis of unselected patients. *Archives of Disease in Childhood*, **56**, 482–4.

Kraft, D. A., Mckee, D. and Scott, C. (1998). Henoch–Schönlein purpura: A review. *American Family Physician*, **58**, 405–8.

Kurzrock, R., Cohen, P. and Markowitz, A. (1994). Clinical manifestations of vasculitis in patients with solid tumors. *Archives of Internal Medicine*, **154**, 334–40.

Lahita, R. G. (1997). Influence of age on Henoch–Schönlein purpura. *Lancet*, **350**, 1116–7.

Lanzkowsky, S., Lanzkowsky, L. and Lanzkowsky, P. (1992). Henoch–Schönlein purpura. *Pediatrics in Review*, **13**, 130–7.

Lee, H. S., Koh, H. I., Kim, M. J. and Rha, H. Y. (1986). Henoch–Schönlein nephritis in adults: a clinical and morphological study. *Clinical Nephrology*, **26**, 125–30.

Levinsky, R. J. and Barratt, T. M. (1979). IgA immune complexes in Henoch–Schönlein purpura. *Lancet*, **2**, 1100.

Lin, S. J., and Huang, J. L. (1998). Henoch–Schönlein purpura in Chinese children and adults. *Asian Pacific Journal of Allergy and Immunology*, **16**, 21–5.

Lofters, W. S., Pineo, G. F., Luke, K. H. and Yaworsky, R. G. (1973). Henoch–Schönlein purpura occurring in three members of a family. *Canadian Medical Association Journal*, **109**, 46–8.

Macpherson, R. I. (1974). The radiologic manifestations of Henoch–Schönlein purpura. *Journal of the Canadian Association of Radiologists*, **25**, 275–81.

Martin, J., Paco, L., Ruiz, M. P., *et al.* (2005). Inducible nitric oxide synthase polymorphism is associated with susceptibility to Henoch–Schönlein purpura in Northwestern Spain. *Journal of Rheumatology*, **32**, 1081–5.

Masuda, M., Nakanishi, K., Yoshizawa, N., Iijima, K. and Yoshikawa, N. (2003). Group A streptococcal antigen in the glomeruli of children with Henoch–Schönlein nephritis. *American Journal of Kidney Diseases*, **41**, 366–70.

Meadow, S. R. (1978). The prognosis of Henoch–Schönlein nephritis. *Clinical Nephrology*, **9**, 87–90.

Meadow, S. R., Glasgow, E. F., Whire, R. H.R., Moncrieff, M. W., Cameron, J. S. and Ogg, C. S. (1972). Schönlein-Henoch nephritis. *Quarterly Journal of Medicine*, **41**, 241–58.

Mertz, L. E. and Conn, D. L. (1992). Vasculitis associated with malignancy. *Current Opinion in Rheumatology*, **4**, 39–46.

Michel, B. A., Hunder, G. G., Bloch, D. A. and Calabrese, L. H. (1992). Hypersensitivity vasculitis and Henoch–Schönlein purpura: A comparison between the 2 disorders. *Journal of Rheumatology*, **19**, 721–8.

Mills, J. A., Michel, B. A., Bloch, D. A., Calabrese, L. H., Hunder, G. G., Arend, W. P., *et al.* (1990). The ACR 1990 criteria for the classification of Henoch–Schönlein purpura. *Arthritis and Rheumatism*, **33**, 1114–21.

Misra, A. K., Biswas, A., Das, S. K., Gharai, P. K. and Roy, T. (2004). Henoch–Schönlein purpura with intracerebral haemorrhage. *Journal of Association of Physicians India*, **52**, 833–4.

Mollica, F., Li Volti, S., Garozzo, R. and Russo, G. (1992). Effectiveness of early prednisone treatment in preventing the development of nephropathy in anaphylactoid purpura. *European Journal of Pediatrics*, **15**, 140–4.

Mormile R, D'Alterio V, Treccagnoli G, Sorrentino P. (2004). Henoch–Schönlein purpura with antiphospholipid antibodies after influenza vaccination: how fearful is it in children? *Vaccine*, **23**, 567–8.

Nadrous, H. F., Yu, A. C., Specks, U. and Ryu, J. H. (2004). Pulmonary involvement in Henoch–Schönlein purpura. *Mayo Clinic Proceeding*, **79**, 1151–7.

Narchi, H. (2005). Risk of long term renal impairment and duration of follow up recommended for Henoch–Schönlein purpura with normal or minimal urinary findings: a systematic review. *Archives of Disease in Childhood*, **90**, 916–20.

Nast, C. C., Ward, H. J., Kyole, M. A. and Cohen, A. H. (1987). Recurrent Henoch–Schönlein purpura following renal transplantation. *American Journal of Kidney Diseases*, **9**, 39–43.

Niaudet, P. and Habib, R. (1989). Nephropathie du purpura rhumatoïde. *Presse Medicale*, **18**, 99–101.

Niaudet, P. and Habib, R. (1998). Methylprednisolone pulse therapy in the treatment of severe forms of Schönlein-Henoch purpura nephritis. *Pediatric Nephrology*, **12**, 238–43.

Nielsen, H. E. (1988). Epidemiology of Schönlein–Henoch purpura. *Acta Paediatrica Scandinava*, **77**, 125–31.

Novak, J., Szekanecz, Z., Sebesi, J., *et al.* (2003). Elevated levels of anti-Helicobacter pylori antibodies in Henoch–Schönlein purpura. *Autoimmunity*, **36**, 307–11.

O'Donoghue, D. J., Nusbaum, P., Noel, L. H., Halbwachs-Mecarelli, L. and Lesavre, P. H. (1992). Antineutrophil cytoplasmic antibodies in IgA nephropathy and Henoch–Schönlein purpura. *Nephrology Dialysis Transplantation*, **7**, 534–8.

Olson, J. C., Kelly, K. J., Pan, C. G. and Wortmann, D. W. (1992). Pulmonary disease with hemorrhage in Henoch–Schönlein purpura. *Pediatrics*, **89**, 1177–81.

Oner, A., Tinaztepe, K. and Erdogan, O. (1995). The effect of triple therapy on rapidly progressive Henoch–Schönlein nephritis. *Pediatric Nephrology*, **9**, 6–10.

Ostergaard, J. R. and Storm, K. (1991). Neurologic manifestations of Schönlein-Henoch purpura. *Acta Paediatrica Scandinava*, **80**, 339–42.

Ozaltin, F., Bakkaloglu, A., Ozen, S., Topaloglu, R., Kavak, U., Kalyoncu, M. and Besbas, N. (2004). The significance of IgA class of antineutrophil cytoplasmic antibodies (ANCA) in childhood Henoch–Schönein purpura. *Clinical Rheumatology*, **23**, 426–9.

Ozdemir, H., Isik, S., Buyan, N. and Hasanoglu, E. (1995). Sonographic demonstration of intestinal involvement in Henoch–Schönlein syndrome. *European Journal of Radiology*, **20**, 32–4.

Pacheco, A. (1991). Henoch–Schönlein vasculitis and tuberculosis. *Chest*, **100**, 293–4.

Paller, A. S., Kelly, K. and Sethi, R. (1997). Pulmonary hemorrhage: an often fatal complication of Henoch–Schönlein purpura. *Pediatric Dermatology*, **14**, 299–302.

Pasatiempo, A. M.G., Kroser, J. A., Rudnick, M. and Hoffman, B. I. (1994). Acute renal failure after intravenous immunoglobulin therapy. *Journal of Rheumatology*, **21**, 347–9.

Piette, W. W. (1994). The differential diagnosis of purpura f rom a morphologic perspective. *Advances in Dermatology*, **9**, 3–23.

Rao, J. K., Weinberger, M., Oddone, E. Z., Allen, N. B., Landsman, P. and Feussner, J. R. (1995). The role of anti-neutrophil cytoplasmic antibody (c-ANCA) testing in the diagnosis of Wegener granulomatosis. A literature review and meta-analysis. *Annals of Internal Medicine*, **123**, 925–32.

Robson, W. L.M. and Leung, A. K.C. (1994). Henoch–Schönlein purpura. *Advances in Pediatrics*, **41**, 163–94.

Rosenblum, N. D. and Winter H. S. (1987). Steroid effects on the course of abdominal pain in children with HSP. *Pediatrics*, **79**, 1018–21.

Rostoker, G., Desvaux-Belghiti, D., Pilatte, Y., Petit-Phar, M., Philippon, C., Deforges, L., *et al.* (1994). Immunoglobulin therapy for severe IgA nephropathy and Henoch–Schönlein purpura. *Annals of Internal Medicine*, **120**, 476–84.

Rostoker, G., Desvaux-Belghiti, D., Pilatte, Y., Petit-Phar, M., Philippon, C., Deforges, L., *et al.* (1995). Immuno-modulation with low-dose immunoglobulins for moderate IgA nephropathy and Henoch–Schönlein purpura. *Nephron*, **69**, 327–34.

Roth, R., Wilz, D. R. and Theil, G. B. (1985). Schönlein–Henoch syndrome in adults. *Quarterly Journal of Medicine*, **55**, 145–59.

Roy, S. (1972). Steatorrhoea in Henoch's syndrome. *British Medical Journal*, **3**, 682.

Sams, W. M., Claman, H. N., Kholer, P. F., McIntosh, R. M., Small, P. and Mass, P. S. (1975). Human necrotizing vasculitis: immunoglobulins and complement in vessel walls of cutaneous lesions and normal skin. *Journal of Investigative Dermatology*, **64**, 441–5.

Rueda, B, Perez-Armengol, C, Lopez-Lopez, S, Garcia-Porrúa, C, Martin, J. and González-Gay, M. A. (2006). Association between functional haplotypes of vascular endothelial growth factor and renal complications in Henoch–Schönlein purpura. *Journal of Rheumatology* **33**, 69–73.

Sánchez-Guerrero, J., Gutiérrez-Ureña, S., Vidaller, A., Reyes, E., Iglesias, A. and Alarcón-Segovia, D. (1990). Vasculitis as a paraneoplastic syndrome. Report of 11 cases and review of the literature. *Journal of Rheumatology*, **17**, 1458–62.

Santiago, J., Blanco, R., González-Gay, M. A., Mateos, A., Roses, L., Andrade, A. S., *et al.* (1996). Henoch–Schönlein purpura with hemorrhagic ascites and intestinal serositis. *Gastrointestinal Endoscopy*, **44**, 624–5.

Saulsbury, F. T. (1986). Case report: antinuclear antibody in Henoch–Schönlein purpura. *American Journal of the Medical Science*, **291**, 180–2.

Saulsbury, F. T. (1993). Corticosteroid therapy does not prevent nephritis in Henoch–Schönlein purpura. *Pediatric Nephrology*, **7**, 69–71.

Saulsbury, F. T. (1999). Henoch–Schönlein purpura in children. Report of 100 patients and review of the literature. *Medicine (Baltimore)*, **78**, 395–409.

Saulsbury, F. T. (2001). Henoch–Schönlein purpura. *Current Opinion in Rheumatology*, **13**, 35–40.

Schifferli, J., Leski, M., Favre, H., Imbach, P., Nydegger, U. and Davies, K. (1991). High-dose intravenous IgG treatment and renal function. *Lancet*, **337**, 457–8.

Schönlein, J. L. (1837). *Allgemeine und specielle Pathologie und Therapie*, Vol. 2, 3rd edn. Wurzburg, Herisau.

Shimomura, N., Kawai, K., Watanabe, S., Katsuumi, K. and Ito, M. (2005). Henoch–Schönlein purpura with severe abdominal pain treated with dapsone and factor XIII concentrate. *Journal of Dermatology*, **32**, 124–7.

Shin, J. I., Park, J. M., Shin, Y. H., Kim, J. H., Kim, P. K., Lee, J. S., *et al.* (2005a). Cyclosporin A therapy for severe Henoch–Schönlein nephritis with nephrotic syndrome. *Pediatric Nephrology*, **20**, 1093–7.

Shin, J. I., Park, J. M., Shin, Y. H., Kim, J. H., Lee, J. S., Kim, P. K., *et al.* (2005b). Can azathioprine and steroids alter the progression of severe Henoch–Schönlein nephritis in children? *Pediatric Nephrology*, **20**, 1087–92.

Smith, G. C., Davidson, J. E., Hughes, D. A., Holme, E. and Beattie, T. J. (1997). Complement activation in Henoch–Schönlein purpura. *Pediatric Nephrology*, **11**, 477–80.

Somer, T. and Finegold, S. M. (1995). Vasculitides associated with infections, immunizations and antimicrobial drugs. *Clinical Infectious Diseases*, **20**, 1010–36.

Specks, U. and Homburger, H. A. (1994). Laboratory medicine and pathology. Anti-neutrophil cytoplasmic antibodies. *Mayo Clinic Proceedings*, **69**, 1197–8.

Stefansson Thors, V., Kolka, R., Sigurdardottir, S. L., Edvardsson, V. O., Arason, G. and Haraldsson, A. (2005). Increased frequency of C4B*Q0 alleles in patients with Henoch–Schönlein purpura. *Scandinavian Journal of Immunology*, **61**, 274–8.

Sterky, G. and Thilén, A. (1960). A study on the onset and prognosis of acute vascular purpura (the Schönlein-Henoch syndrome) in children. *Acta Paediatrica*, **49**, 217–29.

Stevens, G. L., Adelman, H. M. and Wallach, P. M. (1995). Palpable purpura: an algorithmic approach. *American Family Physician*, **52**, 1355–62.

Stewart, M., Savage, J. M., Bell, B. and McCord, B. (1988). Long term renal prognosis of Henoch–Schönlein purpura in an unselected childhood population. *European Journal of Pediatrics*, **147**, 113–5.

Sussman, M., Jones, J. H., Almeida, J. D. and Lachmann, P. J. (1973). Deficiency of second component of complement associated with anaphylactoid purpura and presence of mycoplasma in the serum. *Clinical and Experimental Immunology*, **14**, 531–9.

Szer, I. S. (1994). Henoch–Schönlein purpura. *Current Opinion in Rheumatology*, **6**, 25–31.

Szer, I. S. (1996). Henoch–Schönlein purpura: when and how to treat. *Journal of Rheumatology*, **23**, 1661–5.

Tancrede-Bohin, E., Ochonisky, S., Vignon-Pennamen, M. D., Flageul, B., Morel, P. and Rybojad, M. (1997). Schönlein-Henoch purpura in adult patients: predictive factors for IgA glomerulonephritis in a retrospective study of 57 cases. *Archives of Dermatology*, **133**, 438–42.

Tarshish, P., Bernstein, J. and Edelmann, C. M. Jr. (2004). Henoch–Schönlein purpura nephritis: course of disease and efficacy of cyclophosphamide. *Pediatric Nephrology*, **19**, 51–6.

Tizard, E. J. (1999). Henoch–Schönlein purpura. *Archives Diseases in Children*, **80**, 380–3.

Trapani, S., Micheli, A., Grisolia, F., Resti, M., Chiappini, E., Falcini, F., *et al.* (2005). Henoch Schönlein purpura in childhood: epidemiological and clinical analysis of 150 cases over a 5-year period and review of literature. *Seminars Arthritis Rheumatism*, **35**, 143–53.

Trygstad, C. W. and Stiehm, E. R. (1971). Elevated serum IgA globulin in anaphylactoid purpura. *Pediatrics*, **47**, 1023–8.

Uthman, I., Kassak, K. and Nasr, F. W. (1998). Henoch–Schönlein purpura in adulthood and childhood. *Arthritis and Rheumatism*, **41**, 1518.

Van den Wall Bake, A., Lobatto, S. and Jonges, L. (1987). IgA antibodies directed against cytoplasmic antigens of polymorphonuclear leukocytes in patients with Henoch–Schönlein purpura. *Nephrology Dialysis Transplantation*, **7**, 1238–41.

Watts, R. A., Jolliffe, V. A., Grattan, C. E.H., Elliot, J., Lockwood, M. and Scott, D. G.I. (1998). Cutaneous vasculitis in a defined population: clinical and epidemiological associations. *Journal of Rheumatology*, **25**, 920–4.

Weiler-Bisig, D., Ettlin, G., Brink, T., Arnold, W., Glatz-Krieger, K. and Fischer, A. (2005). Henoch–Schönlein purpura associated with esophagus carcinoma and adenocarcinoma of the lung. *Clinical Nephrology*, **63**, 302–4.

White, R. H.R. (1994). Henoch–Schönlein nephritis. A disease with significant late sequelae. *Nephron*, **68**, 1–9.

Woolfenden, A. R., Hukin, J., Poskitt, K. J. and Connolly, M. B. (1998). Encephalopathy complicating Henoch–Schönlein purpura: reversible MRI changes. *Pediatric Neurology*, **19**, 74–7.

Yoshikawa, N., White, R. H.R. and Cameron, A. H. (1981). Prognostic significance of the glomerular changes in Henoch–Schönlein nephritis. *Clinical Nephrology*, **16**, 223–9.

CHAPTER 41

Cryoglobulinemic vasculitis

Massimo Galli, Fulvio Invernizzi, and Giuseppe Monti

Professor Angelo Monteverde, MD, who participated with us in writing the first edition, died in 2001. We would like to dedicate this chapter to our memory of the exceptional contribution his ideas and enthusiastic assistance gave to our research and patient care.

Definition

Cryoglobulinemic vasculitis is a systemic vasculitis affecting small and medium-sized vessels that is caused by immune complexes of cryoprecipitating immunoglobulins and is sustained by benign B-cell clonal proliferation. The most frequent pathological trigger is an infection which, in the large majority of cases, is due to hepatitis C virus (HCV). Palpable purpura is the clinical hallmark of the disease.

Historical note

The formation of a cryoprecipitate (a sugar-like deposit at the bottom of a test tube of serum at temperatures of less than 37°C) (Figure 41.1) was first observed in 1933 in relation to a patient with multiple myeloma (Wintrobe and Buell 1933). The term "cryoglobulin" was introduced in 1947 by Lerner and Watson, who demonstrated the reversibility of the phenomenon when the sera were heated to 37°C. Steinhard and Fisher (1954) first described cryoglobulinemias apparently unassociated with lymphoproliferative diseases as "essential". In the same year, Petermann and Braunsteiener reported cryoprecipitates of immunoglobulins with different sedimentation rates, thus introducing the concept of "mixed cryoglobulinemia". The role of a rheumatoid factor (RF) in cryoprecipitation was first demonstrated by Lospalluto *et al.* in 1962.

The classic triad of symptoms (purpura, asthenia, and arthralgia) was first described by Meltzer and Franklin (1966), who applied the term "essential mixed cryoglobulinemia" (EMC) to the cases unassociated with lymphoproliferative or autoimmune diseases. Some years later, Brouet *et al.* (1974), proposed their immunochemical classification of monoclonal cryoglobulin (type I), mixed cryoglobulins with a monoclonal component (type II), and mixed polyclonal cryoglobulins (type III).

In 1977, Levo *et al.* suggested hepatitis B virus as the possible etiological agent in EMC. Although not confirmed (Dienstag *et al.* 1977; Galli *et al.* 1980; Popp *et al.* 1980), this hypothesis influenced research until, 13 years later, Pasqual *et al.* (1990) demonstrated an association between EMC and the newly discovered HCV, thus

opening up new research perspectives and suggesting new therapeutic opportunities.

Etiopathogenesis

Cryoglobulinemic vasculitis as an immune complex disease

As mentioned above, type I monoclonal cryoglobulins have a single monoclonal component that usually consists of IgM, IgG, IgA, or, very rarely, Bence–Jones proteins. Monoclonal cryoglobulins account for 6–15% of the total in the largest case series (Monti *et al.* 1995a; Dammacco *et al.* 2001), and are associated with lymphoproliferative cell disorders such as Waldenström's macroglobulinemia, multiple myeloma, or, less frequently, chronic lymphocytic leukemia. The large amount of circulating monoclonal immunoglobulins mainly causes a hyperviscosity syndrome that may rarely be accompanied by cutaneous manifestations such as purpura and ulcers.

A potential vasculitis-causing role of monoclonal immunoglobulin (Ig) was first suggested by the experiments of Spertini *et al.* (1988), who induced true vasculitis in mice after an intraperitoneal injection of an IgG_3-producing hybridoma. These monoclonal immunoglobulins showed a self-association due to non-immunological interactions, which generated cryoglobulins that caused skin lesions and severe acute glomerulonephritis. More recently, the same group (Kuroki *et al.* 2002) has demonstrated that the cryoglobulin activity is primarily determined by the galactose content of CH2 oligosaccharide chains, with the secondary involvement of VH chains.

The cryoprecipitation of single monoclonal paraproteins seems to be an intrinsic characteristic that is strictly linked to the quaternary structure of the immunoglobulins, because the separated Fc and Fab fragments usually lose their cold-induced precipitability. Wang (1988) found relatively lower amounts of serine, lysine, methionine, and isoleucine, and higher amounts of leucine and threonine, in the variable region of a monoclonal cryoprecipitable Bence–Jones protein than in non-cryoprecipitable immunoglobulins, thus suggesting that hydrophobicity may influence cryoprecipitation. It has been shown that a combination of weak non-ionic and hydrophobic interactions allows the association of IgG cryoglobulins (Hall and Abraham 1984), and polymerization may be enhanced by an increase in the ionic strength of the medium.

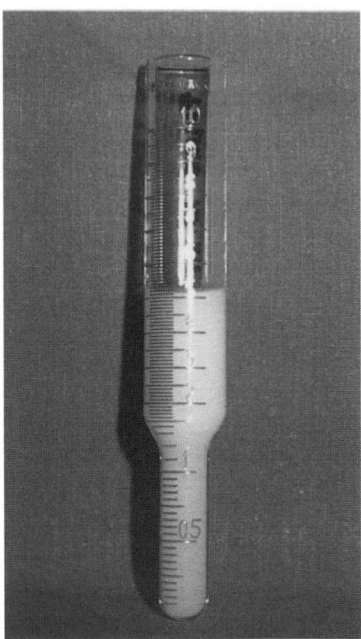

Figure 41.1 Cryoglobulin precipitation in a cryocrit tube.

The cryoprecipitability of IgG is also enhanced by a relative decrease in the number of the negatively charged carbohydrate moieties that contribute to the solubility of the molecule. For example, sialic acid is frequently absent in both monoclonal (Brouet *et al.* 1974) and mixed cryoglobulins (Levo 1980; Zinnemann *et al.* 1968).

The most frequent cause of cryoglobulinemic vasculitis is the presence of mixed cryoglobulins, which usually consist of monoclonal (type II mixed cryoglobulinemia) or polyclonal IgM (type III mixed cryoglobulinemia). The IgG component is always polyclonal: type II mixed cryoglobulinemias accounted for 62% of a large series of 694 cryoglobulinemic patients and type III for 31% (Monti *et al.* 1995a).

Distinguishing the different types of mixed cryoglobulins strictly depends on the accuracy and sensitivity of the methodology used. A new type of cryoglobulin consisting of polyclonal IgG associated with a mixture of polyclonal and monoclonal IgM was detected by Tissot *et al.* in 1994 using two-dimensional polyacrylamide gel electrophoresis, and was named type II-III cryoglobulin. This new type accounted for 26.8% of a series of 265 cases of cryoglobulinemia, whereas the traditional three types respectively accounted for 9% (type I), 26% (type II), and 43.8% (type III). Comparison with previous series suggests that the cases classified as the new type were previously considered type II cryoglobulins, and so it is likely that type II/III is an intermediate form. Moreover, the existence of this intermediate form suggests a progressive selection of the monoclonal components, with the evolution of cryoglobulins with multiple monoclonal IgM components to cryoglobulins with a single IgM rheumatoid factor.

Ever since the first studies of cryoglobulins, it has been hypothesized that the IgG component represents antibodies against bacterial or viral antigens. Weger *et al.* (1969) suggested that, "some unknown antigens first formed complexes with their proper IgG antibody. This complex in its turn gives rise to a rheumatoid factor-like IgM response ... The series of events might have a protective function". It has since been confirmed that the transient appearance of serum RF is a common feature of many acute infections. It has become evident that IgG monomers do not induce RF efficiently, whereas IgG-coated micro-organisms do. These low-affinity RFs correspond to the natural antibodies found in normal individuals, and the normal function of RF is to present the antigens contained in immune complexes to T cells (Newkirk 2002).

In mixed IgM–IgG cryoglobulins, it is the anti-IgG IgM component that determines the cryoprecipitation. Williams and Malone (1994) demonstrated that the RF is specific for multiple antigenic determinants in the second and third domains of the immunoglobulin gamma chain constant region, and on the basis of the crystallographic structure of the RF bound to IgG Fc, Sutton *et al.* (2000) proposed that some RFs simultaneously bind to an as yet unknown antigen via conventional antigen binding, and bind to the Fc region of IgG via an adjacent site. Cryoprecipitable IgM RF has a low affinity for IgG at 37°C, but its affinity increases when the temperature drops (Stone and Fedak 1974). After the interaction of IgM and IgG, the solubility of the immune complexes is significantly less than that of their individual components. The precipitation of mixed cryoglobulins is influenced more by the size of the complexes than by small increases in the binding constant of an IgM cryoglobulin at lower temperatures. Brandau *et al.* (1986) confirmed that lower temperatures increase the number of binding sites of the RF complexes, which are so large that the number of intermolecular contacts between their surfaces outweighs favorable solvent–complex interactions.

On the other hand, RFs may also react with greater affinity and precipitate circulating immune complexes (ICs) of IgG antibodies and their specific antigens, which should be found in the cryoprecipitates (Maid *et al.* 1991). This type of IgM RF reaction occurs with immune complexes or IgG aggregates deposited in tissues. Local complement activation might be insufficient to dissociate the aggregates in the presence of IgM RF. The release of the complement fragments responsible for inflammation may even be enhanced by the ternary complex formed by RF, antigen, and the Fc region of IgG (Sutton *et al.* 2000).

In emphasizing the role of complement in cryoglobulinemia secondary to HCV infection, Schifferly (1996) suggested three possible causes of the inefficient elimination of circulating ICs: (1) the presence of large ICs of HCV/anti-HCV antibodies and rheumatoid factor; (2) the depletion of complement due to these complexes; and (3) inefficient complement fixation by rheumatoid factor. In addition, the function of the splenic reticuloendothelial system in removing immune complexes has been found to be defective in clearing IgG-coated erythrocytes (Walport *et al.* 1985).

The view that IgM monoclonal or polyclonal RF and IgG circulate as immune complexes in cryoglobulinemic sera has been challenged by Agnello and Abel (1997), who found both IgM and IgG as dissociated components in serum at a temperature of 37°C, and suggested that cryoglobulinemic cutaneous vasculitis may be due to the colocalization of HCV, IgG, and IgM caused by the *in situ* formation of complexes of HCV, IgG, and monoclonal RF. On the other hand, circulating immune complexes containing hepatitis antigens and HBV-DNA or HCV-RNA have been reported in viral hepatitis patients with and without cryoglobulins (Hijicata Y *et al.* 1993; Nityanand *et al.* 1997).

Sansonno *et al.* (1996) have shown that in acute and chronic non-cryoglobulinemic HCV infection, hepatitis C virions are bound to anti-HCV-specific IgG, which in turn are linked to IgM; they subsequently confirmed these observations in cryoglobulinemic vasculitis by revealing the role of IgMRF high-affinity antibody (Sansonno and Dammacco 2005).

Multiple lines of evidence suggest that CD5+ B cells (also called B1 cells) spontaneously produce multispecific, low-affinity IgM autoantibodies with RF activity (Nakamura *et al.* 1988). In the majority of cases, monoclonal RFs with cryoglobulin activity express public cross-reactive idiotypes that are recognized by the same monoclonal antibodies (Mageed and Jefferis 1988). The most common public specificity in monoclonal cryoglobulins is the Wa cross-reactive idiotype (CRI) (Agnello *et al.* 1995), which correlates with, but is not restricted to, light chain variable regions of the VκIIIb subfamily. The VκIIIb determinants with Wa reactivity are encoded by the single gene, Hum VK325 (A27) (Kipps *et al.* 1989; Radoux *et al.* 1986), whose product is recognized by monoclonal antibody 17.109. Wa reactivity frequently correlates also with a product of the VH1 gene (Hum VH783, V_{1-69}), which is recognized by the G6 monoclonal antibody (Kunkel *et al.* 1973). Overall, G6 and 17.109 reactive idiotypes are present in 30–35% of subjects with type II cryoglobulinemia (Mageed and Jefferis 1988). More recently, Sansonno *et al.* (2003b) have found cryoprecipitates and purified cryoglobulins with IgM RF bearing the 17.109 cross idiotype that were linked to anti-HCV core protein IgGs.

Viral hypotheses and the role of hepatitis C virus

Circulating cryoglobulins have been found in more than 20 acute and chronic infections due to a variety of pathogens (reviewed in Galli *et al.* 1986) (Table 41.1). In the majority of cases, the cryoglobulins disappear from the circulation with the regression of the symptoms. Variable but generally small amounts of cryoglobulins have also been reported during HIV-1 infection (Galli *et al.* 1986; Matsuda *et al.* 1994; Taillan *et al.* 1993), but there is some doubt as to whether these are attributable to HIV-1 or co-infections with viruses such as EBV or HCV.

A number of authors (Florin-Christensen *et al.* 1974; Iori and Buonanno 1972; Levo 1980; Mcintosh *et al.* 1976; Realdi *et al.* 1974) have suggested that hepatotropic viruses play a role in evoking cryoglobulins. Evaluable cryoglobulin production is induced during the acute phase of hepatitis A (Galli *et al.* 1986; Shalit *et al.* 1982), and polyclonal IgM (including anti-HAV-specific IgM) have been found in the cryoprecipitates, which rapidly decrease with symptom remission (Galli *et al.* 1986; Galli *et al.* 1995). On the basis of serological data, Levo *et al.* (1977) claimed that the large majority of EMCs were caused by hepatitis B virus (HBV), but the real significance of these findings has been subsequently questioned and attributed to confounding variables such as age, geographical origin, socioeconomic status, and frequent hospitalizations (Dienstag *et al.* 1977; Galli *et al.* 1980; Popp *et al.* 1980). In particular, only a slight difference in the prevalence of serological markers of HBV was found when a large series of cryoglobulinemic patients was compared with hospitalized patients or blood donors resident in the same areas (Galli 1991; Galli *et al.* 1992a). Nevertheless, the primary role of HBV in causing cryoglobulinemia in some patients cannot be excluded (see below).

In the early 1990s, the discovery of active HCV infection in the vast majority of patients with mixed cryoglobulinemia clearly supported the major causative role of HCV and underlined the

Table 41.1 Infectious agents reported in association with, or as possible causes of, cryoglobulinemia

RNA viruses
HIV-1
HTLV-1
Hepatitis A virus
Hepatitis C virus
DNA viruses
Adenovirus
Epstein–Barr virus
Cytomegalovirus
Hepatitis B virus
Bacteria and Spirochetes
Streptococcus spp.
Proteus mirabilis
Brucella spp.
Leptospira icterohaemorrhagiae
Borrelia burgdorferi
Treponema pallidum
Chlamydia and Rickettsia
Chlamydia psittaci
Rickettsia conorii
Protozoa
Toxoplasma gondii
Leishmania donovani
Plasmodium falciparum
Helminths
Echinococcus granulosus
Schistosoma mansoni
Fungi
Coccidioides immitis

importance of other infectious agents as etiological factors in cryoglobulinemic syndrome (Agnello *et al.* 1992: Casato *et al.* 1991; Disdier *et al.* 1991; Durand *et al.* 1991; Ferri *et al.* 1991; Galli *et al.* 1992b; Pascual *et al.* 1990; Sansonno *et al.* 1997). Cryoglobulinemic vasculitis is therefore now considered to be the most common extrahepatic manifestation of HCV infection, and is the only one that has so far been definitely validated (Agnello and De Rosa 2004).

HCV is a single-stranded positive-sense RNA virus that belongs to the Flaviviridae family of RNA viruses and has a genome consisting of ~9500 nucleotides. Six major genotypes have been identified. The virus mutates rapidly and generates quasispecies, a series of related but immunologically distinct variants. HCV RNA has been detected by PCR in the peripheral blood mononuclear cells and bone marrow of patients with mixed cryoglobulinemia (Ferri *et al.* 1993; Galli *et al.* 1995; Zignego *et al.* 1992), and studies of fractioned subpopulations have detected it almost exclusively at B-cell level (Zehender *et al.* 1997). Moreover, immunohistochemical and *in situ* hybridization studies have revealed HCV proteins in the cytoplasm of lymphoid cells (Sansonno *et al.* 1996a, 1996b).

The E2 HCV envelope protein binds human CD81, a tetraspanin expressed by various cell types, including hepatocytes and B lymphocytes (Pileri *et al.* 1998). It is considered to be the receptor involved in the HCV-mediated activation of B cells that leads to their polyclonal proliferation and expansion (Rosa *et al.* 2005). The presence of HCV in immune complexes in the kidney, cutaneous vasculitis lesions, and vessel walls of cryoglobulinemic patients (Agnello 1997; Agnello and Abel 1997; Agnello *et al.* 1992; Sansonno *et al.* 1997) suggests that the virus may play a role in complex-mediated damage. Furthermore, HCV-containing monoclonal B cell infiltrates in bone marrow and liver may be the source of production of cryoglobulins (Gabrielli *et al.* 1994; Galli *et al.* 1995; Monteverde *et al.* 1997; Sansonno *et al.* 1996c, 1998). The presence of higher concentrations of HCV RNA and HCV-containing antigen/ antibody complexes in cryoprecipitates than in sera suggests that HCV plays a direct role in inducing the production of the monoclonal component of cryoglobulins (Agnello *et al.* 1992).

One of the most intriguing questions regarding HCV-associated cryoglobulinemic vasculitis is what factors lead some HCV-infected patients to produce cryoglobulins whereas others produce none or only small amounts. Studies of patients with chronic hepatitis C have shown that cryoglobulins are detectable in 15–54% of cases, but almost always in small amounts and classifiable as type III. The other important question is why the presence of circulating cryoglobulins is associated with clinical manifestations in only some cases. According to Meyers *et al.* (2003), symptomatic cryoglobulinemia occurs in no more than 1% of HCV-infected patients. In a case series of 1071 HCV-positive patients with chronic active hepatitis studied by some of us (Pioltelli *et al.* unpublished data), 821 (77%) were cryoglobulin negative and, of the 250 (23%) with cryoglobulins, 194 (78%) were completely symptom-free, and only 32 of the 56 patients with symptoms attributable to cryoglobulinemia showed signs of vasculitis. Lunel *et al.* (1994) found that the prevalence of mixed cryoglobulinemia increases with the progression of chronic hepatitis C, and reaches 34% in patients with cirrhosis (Kayali *et al.* 2002). Interestingly, even in these advanced HCV infections, vasculitis was absent in most cryoglobulinemic patients

In summary, it can be concluded that:

1 Cryoglobulins are a frequent finding in patients with chronic HCV infections, but do not have any clinical significance in the majority of cases.

2 The detection of cryoglobulins (particularly when they are produced in small amounts) depends on the accuracy of the method, the maintenance of a temperature of ≥37°C during sample handling, and the amount of blood processed.

3 In line with this, the percentage of chronically HCV-infected patients producing cryoglobulins is probably underestimated.

4 The patients developing a frank cryoglobulinemic syndrome represent a small minority of chronically HCV-infected patients, and a minority of the HCV-infected patients in whom cryoglobulin is at least occasionally isolated.

5 The origin of the investigated cases (rheumatology or hematology versus hepatology or gastroenterology units) may lead to

selection biases, and the reported variability in the prevalence of MC (Agnello and De Rosa 2004).

The cause of cryoglobulin overproduction in a minority of patients is generally attributed to the particular characteristics of the host, although it is also possible that there may be a strain of HCV that has a particular propensity to produce cryoglobulin. Like other RNA viruses, HCV is characterized by a high degree of genetic heterogeneity (Ogata *et al.* 1991; Okamoto *et al.* 1992). MC patients do not show any particular distribution of HCV genotypes (Zehender *et al.* 1995; Zignego *et al.* 1996); the high prevalence of genotype 2 in type II MC in one of these studies (Zehender *et al.* 1996) was probably due to its high frequency in elderly patients in Italy. A recent review of a large series of cases (Pioltelli *et al.* unpublished data) has confirmed that cryoglobulinemic vasculitis is not linked to a particular HCV genotype.

More recently, questions concerning a specific MC-associated mutation in HCV genome have been raised by the finding of a single amino acid insertion/deletion at codons 384–385 of the hypervariable region 1 (HVR 1) of HCV in one-third of a population of MC patients (Gerotto *et al.* 2001). We could not confirm the existence of an "MC-inducing quasispecies" after analyzing 360 clones from 10 MC patients and eight patients with non-cryoglobulinemic chronic hepatitis C (Zehender *et al.* 2005). Only one of our patients was infected by a virus showing a five amino acid insertion at codon 385–389 of the HVR, which was observed with minimal variations in all of the clones obtained from the plasma, cryoprecipitate, and lymphocyte samples. Nevertheless, in comparison with the controls, the HCV of the MC patients was less heterogeneous and more frequently compartmentalized (the plasma, cryoprecipitates, and PBMCs contained different quasispecies). Reduced HCV heterogeneity has been observed in patients with long-lasting infections (Allain *et al.* 2000) and in immunocompromised hosts (Toyoda *et al.* 1997; Booth *et al.* 1998), but the role of compartmentalization in the pathogenesis of MC syndrome is still unclear and needs to be defined by longitudinal studies. In brief, there are still no data to support the possibility that MC is due to infection with a particular HCV strain. The demonstration of cryoglobulins in only a percentage of patients with chronic hepatitis C also suggests that their formation, persistence and clinical effects need other factors in addition to HCV infection.

Patients with symptomatic cryoglobulinemia are mainly women more than 50 years of age, who often have no history of common risk factors for HCV infection. Moreover, changes in the epidemiological pattern of HCV infection in Western countries due to the epidemic of intravenous drug abuse, and the introduction of new HCV subtypes caused by international contacts and immigration, has not yet significantly affected this patient profile.

It has been postulated that a particular genetic background of the host may lead to an anomalous cryoglobulin-generating response to HCV, but the results of HLA studies are contradictory: Lenzi *et al.* (1998) observed a greater frequency of haplotype HLA-B8-DR3 in a small series of cryoglobulinemic patients, but this finding could not be confirmed (Amoroso *et al.* 1998). Cacoub *et al.* (2001) suggest that HLA-DR11 is more frequent in patients with type II MC than in those without it, but there was no correlation with the presence or absence of vasculitis.

Abnormalities in IC clearance have been observed in MC patients (Madi *et al.* 1991) and it has been shown that patients with active nephritis have impaired liver uptake of IC and cryoglobulin processing (Roccatello *et al.* 1997). Moreover, *in vitro* studies suggest that a high rate of spontaneous *in vitro* RF production due to an increase in the number of B-cell clones committed to RF synthesis is accompanied by a T-cell defect (Meroni *et al.* 1984). More recent studies have found a high concentration of soluble TNF-α receptors (sTNFR1 and sTNFR2) in patients with severe visceral vasculitis (Kaplanski *et al.* 2002), a defect in CD4+/CD25+ regulatory T cells (Boyer *et al.* 2004), and an increase in B lymphocytic stimulator (BLyS) (Fabris *et al.* 2005).

The prominent role of HCV as a probable etiological factor in the cryoglobulinemic syndrome questions not only the relevance, but also the existence, of HCV-negative vasculitic cryoglobulinemias. In a still ongoing study, we have reviewed the cases of symptomatic persistent cryoglobulinemia observed by 11 centers in the Italian Group for the Study of Cryoglobulinemias (GISC), and have so far identified 125 cases with repeatedly negative tests for antibodies to HCV. The majority of these patients were female (83%) and their median age at first cryoglobulin determination was 55 years. Palpable purpura was present in about 56% of cases. Cryocrit levels of >1% were found in 37% of patients, and type II cryoglobulins were found in 49% of patients (66% of the typed cases). In many respects, these patients are therefore not different from HCV-positive cryoglobulinemic subjects: 17% had systemic lupus erythematosus (SLE), 7% non-Hodgkin's lymphoma, and 15% Sjögren's syndrome. There were eight subjects whose sera were positive for HBsAg, three of whom also presented one of the aforementioned conditions. The remaining 60% did not show any signs of autoimmune, lymphoproliferative, or chronic infectious disease.

It can thus be provisionally concluded that patients with symptomatic HCV-negative cryoglobulinemias are not rare and probably account for at least 2–3% of the symptomatic cryoglobulinemic patients attending our centers. A possible role of latent HCV infection in causing at least some cases of apparently HCV-negative cryoglobulinemia has been suggested by Casato *et al.* (2003), who reported the appearance of HCV-RNA in the serum of three previously HCV-RNA negative and persistently anti-HCV-negative subjects with type II mixed cryoglobulinemia. It is difficult to explain the absence of any specific antibody response in the presence of latent/reactivating HCV infection in these patients. In our study cited above, we identified some sustained responders to anti-HCV therapy who maintained symptomatic cryoglobulinemia despite persistently negative HCV-RNA.

It may thus be concluded that HCV is the main etiological agent of cryoglobulinemic vasculitis, but the disorder may arise only in a subgroup of patients who lack particular mechanisms of controlling their humoral immune response against the virus. The same type of defects might be involved in cases of symptomatic cryoglobulinemia not triggered by HCV.

Lymphoproliferation in cryoglobulinemic vasculitis

The role of HCV in inducing lymphoproliferation and causing lymphomas has been widely debated. HCV lymphotropism was identified in the early 1990s with the demonstration of viral segments in peripheral blood mononuclear cells (Zignego *et al.* 1992), and has subsequently been confirmed in the PBMCs of patients with mixed cryoglobulinemias (Ferri *et al.* 1993), in CD34 hemopoietic progenitor cells (Sansonno *et al.* 1993), and in

B lymphocytes in peripheral blood (Zehender *et al.* 1997). Lymphoid aggregates with pseudofollicular features are detectable in the liver and bone marrow of cryoglobulinemic patients, and show monoclonal B cell restriction (Figure 41.2) (Monteverde *et al.* 1988, 1995, 1997; Sansonno *et al.* 1998).

A number of authors have reported an increased prevalence of HCV infection in patients with non-Hodgkin's lymphoma (NHL) (Ferri *et al.* 1994; Mazzaro *et al.* 1988; Pioltelli *et al.* 1996). Pioltelli *et al.* (2000) found HCV infection in 16% of 300 patients with B-cell NHL and 8.5% of 969 controls, including 247 with neoplasms other than lymphoma, 122 treated with immunosuppressive drugs, and 600 age- and sex-matched subjects without neoplasms. The prevalence of HCV was not significantly different among the different NHL histological subtypes, and the HCV subtype distribution was similar in the NHL patients and controls.

Similar prevalences of HCV infection (17.5%) were found by Mele *et al.* (2003) in a population of 400 B-cell NHL patients, and by investigators from Japan (Kuniyoshi *et al.* 2001). Epidemiological studies suggest that geographic and racial factors may influence the involvement of HCV in B-cell lymphoma. In Europe, prevalence seems to increase from north to south; in the United States, there is a high prevalence in southern California (22%) but no difference from the general population in other parts of the country (reviewed in Ferri *et al.* 2000).

A possible relationship between cryoglobulinemia and B-cell NHL was suggested many years before the discovery of HCV (Invernizzi *et al.* 1983). Monti *et al.* (2005) have recently analyzed a series of 1255 HCV-positive patients with symptomatic cryoglobulinemia followed up for 8928 person-years and found that the overall risk of developing aggressive NHL was about 12 times higher than the general population. The cumulative incidence (1.6%) was lower than that (7–11%) reported in previous, smaller Italian series (Monteverde *et al.* 1988; Invernizzi *et al.* 1990; La Civita *et al.* 1995); more than 90% of the patients who developed NHLs had type II cryoglobulins.

These observations are supported by laboratory findings. Monteverde *et al.* (1989) first reported lymphoid aggregates in the

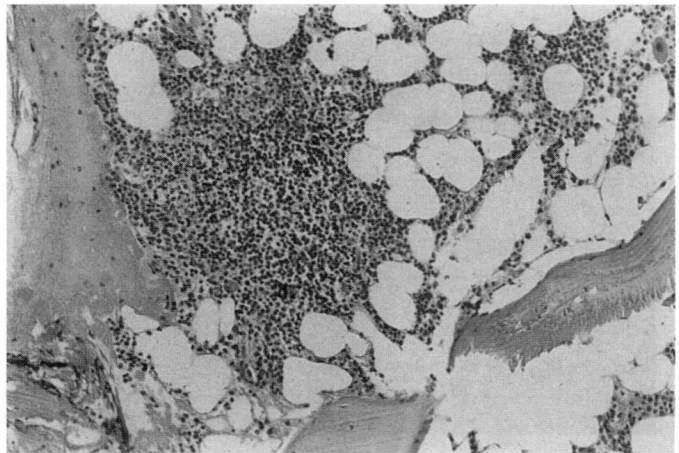

Figure 41.2 Bone marrow biopsy of a patient with type II HCV-related cryoglobulinemia showing a nodular infiltrate consisting of small lymphocytes, lymphoplasmacytoid elements, and plasma cells (Giemsa, 250 × magnification). (See Color Plate 116).

liver and bone marrow (Figure 41.2) of cryoglobulinemic patients showing Bcl-2 overexpression, monotype IgMκ restriction of cryoglobulin production, and a high rate of IgM rearrangements. Zignego *et al.* (1997, 2000), and Zuckerman (2001) confirmed the Bcl-2 overexpression in B cells with the t (14;18) translocation. Machida *et al.* (2004) suggested that HCV might cause mutations in immunoglobulin genes and proto-oncogenes and transform cells through a hit-and-run mechanism. According to Agnello and De Rosa (2004), the critical question is whether HCV is directly lymphomagenic or, as they suggest, whether lymphomagenesis is a stochastic process in the HCV-driven proliferation of B cells.

Vasculitis lesions

Many factors are involved in the failure to clear circulating ICs in cryoglobulinemic vasculitis. According to Madi *et al.* (1991), IgM-RF depletes complement proteins, enhances immune aggregation reactions, and inhibits the opsonization of IC. A failure in macrophage clearance also contributes to the deposition of immune aggregates. Sansonno and Dammacco (2005) has shown substantially enriched C1q protein and C1q binding activity in cryoprecipitates, contrasting with a reduction in C3 and C4 proteins. The large complexes containing HCV core protein can specifically bind the C1q receptor expressed by endothelial cells.

Sansonno *et al.* (1995) also demonstrated HCV-related proteins as intraluminal and perivascular deposits in the skin blood vessels of patients with cryoglobulinemic vasculitis. Agnello and Abel (1997) obtained the same results by means of an *in situ* hybridization technique in the purpuric lesions of patients with type II cryoglobulinemia, thus suggesting that immune complexes are formed *in situ* by HCV, monomeric IgM-RF, and IgG.

Capillary and postcapillary vasculitis represents the basic pathogenetic lesion of various organ systems. The histopathological picture of cutaneous purpura (the most common lesion) is that of leukocytoclastic vasculitis with endothelial swelling, perivascular leukocytic infiltration, varying degrees of leukocytoclasis, the extravasation of red blood cells, fibrinoid necrosis, and hyaline thrombi. These typical lesions are mainly observed in specimens obtained at the onset of the purpuric rash, whereas the later lesions show a perivascular infiltrate of mononuclear cells with a nonspecific inflammatory pattern. Deposits of immunoglobulins and complement factors can be detected by immunofluorescence, and HCV proteins can be revealed by immunochemistry.

In addition to cutaneous leukocytoclastic vasculitis, widespread vasculitis involving small and medium-size vessels in the heart, gastrointestinal tract, liver, nervous system, muscles, lung, and adrenal glands have been shown post mortem (Gorevic *et al.* 1980).

Clinical aspects of cryoglobulinemic vasculitis

The triad of symptoms first described by Meltzer and Franklin (1966), and considered to be the classical presentation of the disease (purpura, asthenia, and arthralgia) is reported in varying percentages of patients: for example, a large multicenter study found it in only 27.5% of the participants (Monti *et al.* 1995a). Asthenia and arthralgia are less specific symptoms than purpura, which is the typical clinical marker of the syndrome. Moreover, asthenia has been variably evaluated and reported in different studies, and

arthralgia is generally less frequent than purpura, which has been described in 80–100% of patients with mixed cryoglobulinemia. Almost all patients with symptomatic cryoglobulinemia and HCV infection experience purpura during the course of the disease.

Cryoglobulinemic vasculitis is a true syndrome resembling experimental serum sickness. The following set of criteria has been proposed: (1) cryocrit >1% for at least 6 months; (2) positive rheumatoid factor in serum and C4 <8 mg%; and (3) at least two of the following: purpura, weakness, and arthralgias (Invernizzi *et al.* 1995). The type of circulating cryoglobulin is highly relevant: compared to type III, patients with type II cryoglobulins have a more severe presentation and course, are more likely to have serum complement C4 <8 mg%, mean cryocrit level >3%, higher RF levels, and more severe cutaneous purpura and renal involvement. Finally, in our case series of 1255 HCV-positive patients followed up for a total of 8928 person-years, 93% of those developing NHL had type II cryoprecipitate.

Purpura

Purpura is the most evident manifestation of cryoglobulinemic vasculitis (Table 41.2), and is due to the precipitation of immune complexes in the small vessels of derma and (less frequently) subcutaneous tissue (Figure 41.3). The lesions are infiltrating, palpable, polymorphic, and mainly localized to the legs (Figure 41.4), although the thighs and less frequently the trunk may also be involved. Prolonging standing, exercise, and low temperatures facilitate the appearance of the purpuric manifestations, which are

Table 41.2 Signs and symptoms of cryoglobulinemic syndrome at clinical onset, as reported in the literature before and after the identification of HCV as an etiological agent of EMC (modified from Monteverde *et al.* 1996)

	Before HCV identification	After HCV identification
Female sex	59–66%	62–93%
Median age (years)	42–52	54–64
Meltzer's triad	nr	27.5%
Purpura	88–100%	73–95%
Weakness	60–67%	10–100%
Arthralgias	51–70%	33–90%
Leg ulcers	9–30%	4–8%
Urticaria	1–2%	2%
Raynaud's phenomenon	10–40%	7–31%
Peripheral neuropathy	2–31%	12–69%
Nephropathy	8–54%	8–33%
Liver involvement	9–88%	26–62%
Speen enlargement	4–50%	35%
Peripheral lymphadenopathy	16%	nr
Sicca syndrome	0–14%	10–40%
Hypertension	35%	nr
Pulmonary involvement	rare	nr

nr = not reported.

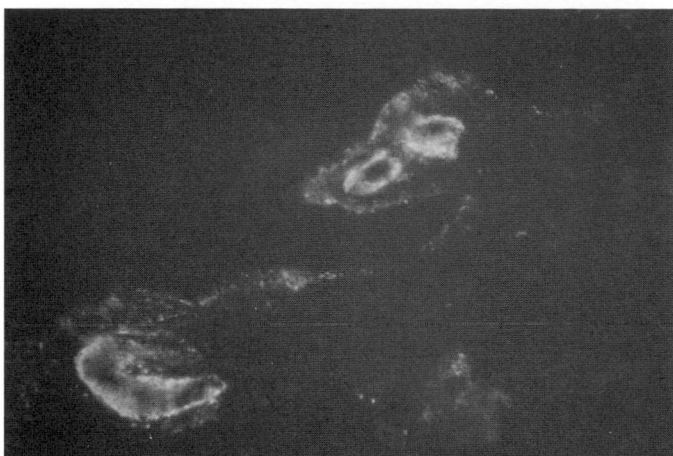

Figure 41.3 Immune complex deposits at the level of the basal membrane of dermal vessels. Immunofluorescence staining with anti-IgM antiserum of a cutaneous purpuric lesion (320 × magnification). (See Color Plate 117).

generally intermittent. The hallmark of long-lasting cryoglobulinemic purpura is an ocherous pigmentation of the involved areas.

Cutaneous ulcers

Skin ulcers are relatively frequent and often have a chronic, disabling course (Figure 41.5). They represent an important aspect of disease activity, and possibly serve as an indication for aggressive treatment with plasmapheresis and cytotoxic drugs. Their most frequent location is around the malleoli of the ankles, but the fingers and toes may be involved in some cases.

Raynaud's phenomenon

Raynaud's phenomenon (which is sometimes the first clinical manifestation of the syndrome) is more frequent in females, observed in about 20% of cryoglobulinemic patients, and is triggered by low temperatures. The endothelial damage caused by precipitating immune complexes is involved in its pathogenesis and facilitates relapses. Raynaud's phenomenon is particularly frequent in the type of cryoglobulinemia associated with connective tissue diseases (particularly scleroderma), in which its prevalence reaches 37% (Monti *et al.* 1995a).

Arthralgias/ arthritis

Arthralgias (with or without arthritis) are generally intermittent and migratory, without any typical pattern. The synovial membranes do not show any pathological changes even in individuals with long-standing arthralgia. Arthritis is present in about 10% of cases (Monti *et al.* 1995b), may have an acute or chronic course, and does not generally give rise to erosive lesions (Monteverde *et al.* 1996). Myalgias (mainly involving the shoulder girdle) or rheumatic polymyalgia-like patterns may be present in a minority of cases (Monteverde *et al.* 1996).

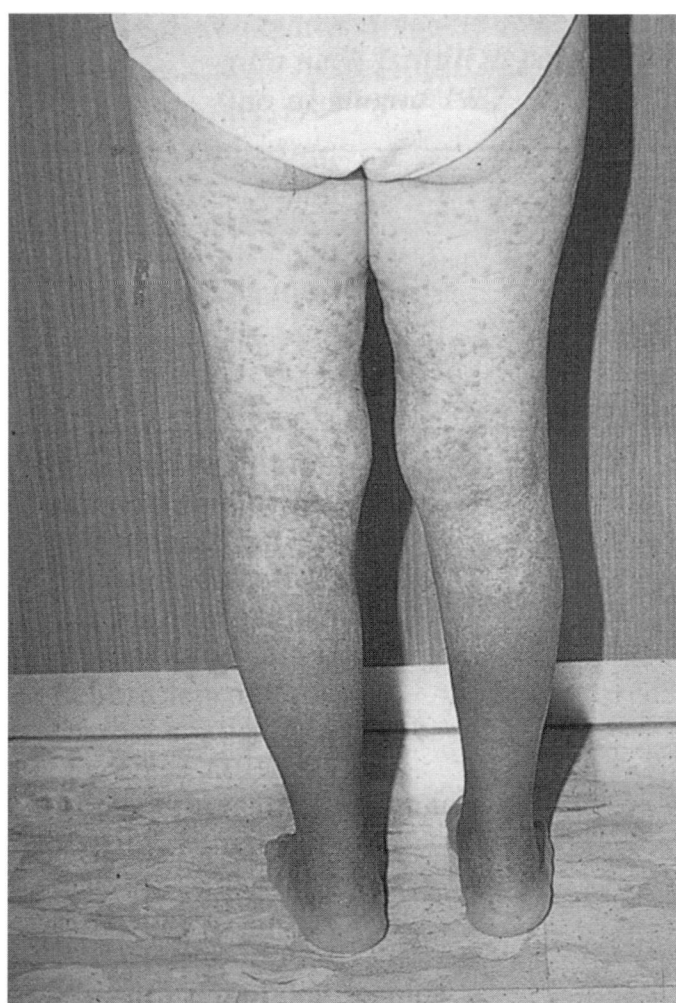

Figure 41.4 Typical presentation of lower-limb purpural lesions in a patient with type II HCV-related cryoglobulinemia.

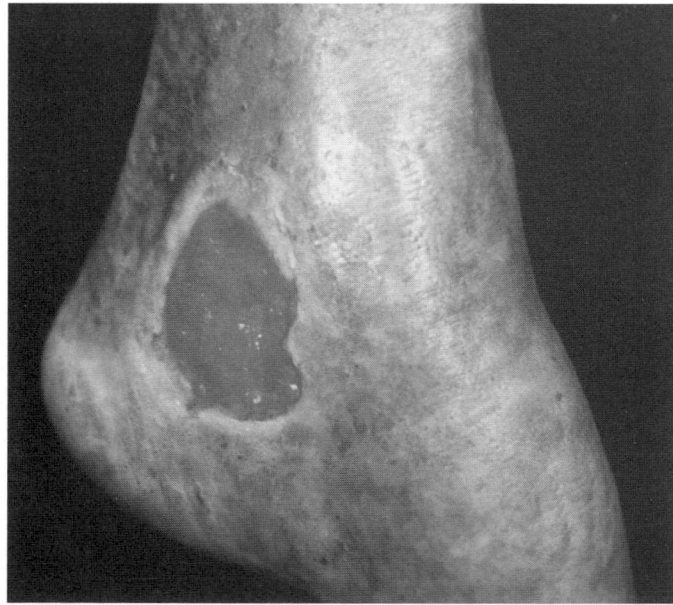

Figure 41.5 Malleolar ulcer in a patient with cutaneous type III HCV-related cryoglobulinemia. The surrounding skin shows areas of ocherous pigmentation due to longstanding cryoglobulinemic purpura. (See Color Plate 118).

Cryoglobulinemic neuropathy

The prevalence of neuropathic symptoms has been variously reported between 2% and 69%, a large difference that may be due to diagnostic criteria, study design, or case selection; the increasing number of recent reports (Pioltelli *et al.* 1995) may be due to improved diagnostic techniques and increasing awareness. Chronic or relapsing distal peripheral neuropathy has been reported at presentation and during the course of cryoglobulinemic syndrome. The most frequent symptoms are paresthesia, painful dysesthesia, and myalgias, associated with asthenia. The deep tendon reflexes are generally diminished. In the majority of cases, the electrophysiological picture confirms the presence of symmetrical distal sensorimotor polyneuropathy, which may sometimes have a severe course, with intense painful symptoms and functional importance. These conditions may respond to plasmapheresis. Cases of mononeuropathy are rare. Electrophysiological studies have revealed axonal damage attributable to epineural vasculitis caused by immune complexes, with subsequent ischemic damage and possible alterations in blood flow (Ferri *et al.* 1992).

Cell-mediated damage with monocytic infiltration has been suggested (Benetti *et al* 1997), and confirmed by the demonstration of Th1 cytokines and chemokines in the inflammatory vascular lesions (Saadoun 2005). No direct involvement of HCV has been demonstrated. The peripheral neuropathy may be associated with autonomic neuropathy, which is rarely found by conventional tests but relatively frequent if evaluated by means of cutaneous sympathetic responses (Migliaresi *et al.* 1999).

Nephropathy

The percentage of patients with renal involvement at the time of diagnosis varies from 8% to 54% in large series (Monteverde *et al.* 1996), and is greatly influenced by the patient selection criteria. In our experience, renal impairment is present at diagnosis in 12% of the patients with type III cryoglobulins and 35% of those with type II (Monti *et al.* 1995a). Agnello and De Rosa (2004) have also reported a prevalence of membranoproliferative glomerulonephritis (MPGN) of about 30% in HCV-positive type II MC. The clinical picture ranges from acute nephritic syndrome with hematuria, proteinuria, and altered renal function (often associated with arterial hypertension), to a mild and slowly-developing form with urinary abnormalities, but without progression towards renal insufficiency. However, when present at onset, acute nephritic or nephrotic syndromes may sometimes be rapidly progressive. Although partial or complete remission has been observed in 30% of such cases, these syndromes are a frequent cause of death (Invernizzi *et al.* 1990). Relapsing renal impairment has been described in about 20% of patients with symptomatic mixed cryoglobulinemia, and is generally associated with a poor prognosis (Tarantino *et al.* 1986).

The typical pathological form of cryoglobulinemic nephropathy is MPGN (see Figure 41.6), which is characterized by IC deposits in the mesangium and subendothelial space. Its particular features are: (1) abundant endocapillary proliferation with heavy mononuclear cell infiltration, mainly represented by monocytes that are thought to have the function of scavenger cells; (2) amorphous deposits within the glomerular capillaries that appear to consist of IgM, IgG, and C3; and (3) a split capillary basement membrane. Electron microscopy reveals subendothelial electron-dense deposits in the

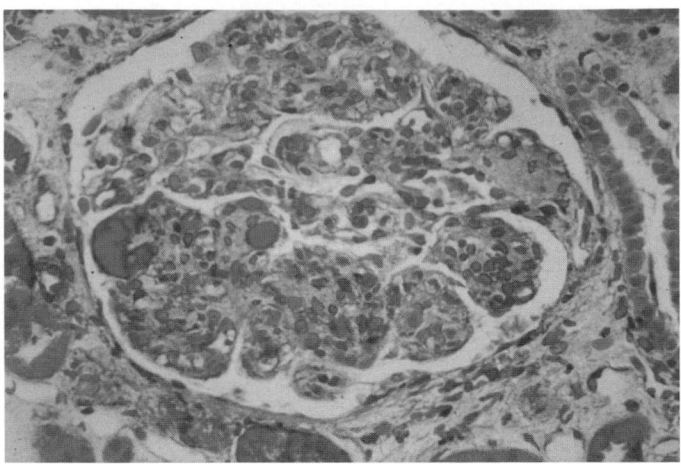

Figure 41.6 Kidney biopsy in a patient with type II HCV-related cryoglobulinemia showing membranoproliferative glomerulonephritis with mononuclear cell infiltration and intraluminal thrombi (PAS, 320 × magnification). (See Color Plate 119).

glomerular capillary walls, with a finely fibrillar pattern identical to that observed in precipitated cryoglobulins *in vitro* (Monga *et al.* 1986). More than one-third of the patients undergoing renal biopsy or pathologic examination of renal tissue at autopsy have evidence of vasculitis of the small and medium-sized arteries, with fibrinoid necrosis and monocyte infiltration.

A recent review of HCV-related renal diseases reports that 50–70% of the HCV-positive patients with MPGN have circulating cryoglobulins, with the majority of them also being RF positive and having low serum C4 levels (Meyers *et al.* 2003). These data suggest a large overlap of so-called HCV nephropathies and MC syndromes.

Liver disease in cryoglobulinemic syndrome

The influence of cryoglobulinemia on the course of HCV-related liver disease continues to be debated. Many authors suggest that patients with type II cryoglobulinemia show milder liver involvement than those with non-cryoglobulinemic chronic hepatitis C infection. In particular, Agnello (1997) hypothesized that IgMκ-RF bearing the Wa cross reactive idiotype plays a protective role by binding HCV lipoproteins to LDL, which may block the viral endocytosis in hepatocytes. In contrast, Lunel *et al.* (1994) have reported more severe liver damage in patients with cryoglobulinemia than in those without and, more recently, a meta-analysis of 19 studies (Kayali *et al.* 2002) concluded that the risk of liver cirrhosis was significantly higher in cryoglobulinemic patients. The findings in our clinical series (Monteverde *et al.* 1996) did not support either of the two positions as they did not show any significant differences in liver damage or disease progression between the patients with and without cryoglobulinemia over 6 years' follow-up. Possible major biases need to be taken into account when considering all of these studies. Although not supported by data, our experience and the opinions of other experts suggest that the onset of cryoglobulinemic syndrome is generally not preceded by clinical evidence of acute hepatitis.

Given the relatively late onset of cryoglobulinemic syndrome (the fifth decade of life or later), it is possible that the patients have sustained infection with HCV, and this should be considered when selecting control groups for clinical studies. Moreover, definitions vary among studies and the patients with cryoglobulinemic syndrome are not always distinguished from asymptomatic patients with detectable circulating cryoglobulins. Of the 19 studies considered in the meta-analysis, only 11 provided typing of cryoglobulins, seven of which reported type III cryoglobulin in the majority of cases (Kayali *et al.* 2002). This finding conflicts with the results of the largest series of patients with cryoglobulinemic syndrome.

The liver is clearly involved in the clonal B cell expansion observed in MC, as lymphocytic infiltrates with a pseudofollicular appearance are the site of the clonal B cell proliferation that produces IgMκ-RF bearing the Wa cross-reactive idiotype (Monteverde *et al.* 1997). These germinal center-like structures are found most often in type II cryoglobulinemias, and tend to decrease with the progression of liver disease. Although monoclonal IgMκ restriction is always detectable in type II cryoglobulinemia, the expression of immunoglobulin light chains is always polyclonal in the B cells of lymphoid aggregates found in the liver of patients with non-cryoglobulinemic chronic hepatitis or type III cryoglobulins (Monteverde *et al.* 1997) (Table 41.3).

Cardiovascular abnormalities

It has been reported that congestive heart failure is the most prevalent cardiovascular manifestation in cryoglobulinemic patients (Gorevic *et al.* 1990), and vasculitic lesions of the myocardium have been reported upon post-mortem examination in at least one patient who died of congestive heart disease (Saccardo *et al.* 1986). A recent report from Hong Kong (Au *et al.* 2005) has described structural aortic abnormalities, including multiple dissections, aneurysms, and congenital aortic arch abnormalities, in four cases of HCV-negative patients with cryoglobulinemia. Three patients had underlying malignancies, and the fourth was HBV positive. The authors suggest that cryoglobulins may cause a peculiar form of aortic intimal damage in Chinese patients. Monteverde *et al.* (1996) reported hypertension, often refractory to conventional therapy (particularly when associated with renal impairment) in 42% of 145 patients with type II MC.

The role of hyperviscosity syndrome in increasing cardiovascular risk of cryoglobulinemic patients still needs to be assessed. The syndrome is often reported in type I monoclonal HCV-unrelated cryoglobulinemias, and seems to be relatively infrequent in type II and type III MC. Measurements of serum viscosity in 43 unselected MC patients (Ferri *et al.* 1990) were altered in a small minority of cases, with some variations affected by temperature changes.

Gastrointestinal abnormalities

Abdominal pain, which is sometimes severe and requires surgical procedures, has been reported in about 5–20% of patients with cryoglobulinemic syndrome (Gorevic *et al.* 1980; Montagnino 1988; Ramos-Casals *et al.* 2005). The presence of vasculitic lesions in the GI tract was not confirmed by Gorevic *et al.* (1980), but has been subsequently reported by some authors (Robinson and Kirkhan 1984; Montagnino 1988; Monteverde *et al.* 1996). In a recent survey, Ramos-Casals *et al.* (2005) found vasculitic abdominal involvement in nine of 268 cryoglobulinemic patients.

Pulmonary involvement

Bombardieri *et al.* (1979) described pulmonary involvement in 60% of MC cases, with a pattern of interstitial lung disease. Ramon-Casals *et al.* (2005) have reported pulmonary alveolitis in six of 268 cryoglobulinemic patients.

Laboratory diagnosis: the determination of cryoglobulins in clinical practice

To obtain cryoprecipitates, patients should be acclimatized to room temperature (20–25°C) for 15–30 min, and at least 15 ml of blood should be collected and immediately incubated at 37°C for 2 hours. The sample should then be centrifuged twice at 1500 rpm for 3 min at 37°C, and the serum cooled in a graduated tube at 4°C for 7 days before being centrifuged at 4°C for 15 min at 1700 rpm. The cryocrit is determined as the percentage of total serum volume.

To characterize the cryoglobulin, the cryoprecipitate should be resuspended in three volumes of icy saline and centrifuged three times at 3500 rpm for 10 min at 4°C (discarding the supernatant

Table 41.3 Results of immunophenotypic analysis of the liver lymphoid nodules of HCV positive MC-II, MC-III, and non-cryoglobulinemic chronic hepatitis (CH) on cryostat sections (modified from Monteverde *et al.* 1997)

	n	CD20	CD5	IgM	Bcl-2	Ki-67<3%
MC-II						
Minimal/mild activity	40	40 (100%)	40 (100%)	40 (100%)	40 (100%)	40 (100%)
Moderate-severe activity/cirrhosis	21	14 (67%)	14 (67%)	6 (28%)	15 (71%)	21 (100%)
MC-III						
Minimal/mild activity	11	11 (100%)	11 (100%)	0	8(73%)	11 (100%)
Moderate-severe activity cirrhosis	12	8 (67%)	8 (67%)	0	5(62%)	8 (100%)
CH						
Minimal/mild activity	22	18 (82%)	14 (64%)	0	12 (54%)	22 (100%)
Moderate-severe activity cirrhosis	22	18 (82%)	11 (50%)	0	8 (36%)	22 (100%)

Statistically significant differences were found between MC-II and the other two groups with regard to the IgMκ restriction. This was present both in earlier (minimal/mild activity) and later (moderate-severe activity/cirrhosis) stages of liver disease. *p* values for comparisons of patients with minimal/mild activity were: MC-II vs. MC-III, *p* <0.001; MC-II vs. CH, *p* <0.001. *p* values for comparisons of patients with moderate-severe activity/cirrhosis were: MC-II vs. MC-III, *p* = 0.05; MC-II vs. CH, *p* <0.05. Student's t-test was used for all comparisons.

after each washing). The cryoprecipitate should then be dissolved by incubation in three volumes of saline at 37°C for 1 hour (with periodic shaking).

Immunofixation is currently considered the technique of choice for typing cryoprecipitates. The samples are placed on thin-layer agarose gels which, after electrophoretic migration and the antiserum reaction, are washed three times at 37°C in a 10% NaCl solution before the plates are stained. A more sensitive technique is immunoblotting, which allows the typing of low-concentration (10–80 mg/l) cryoprecipitates.

Differential diagnosis

The differential diagnosis of MC includes diseases associated with leukocytoclastic vasculitis such as Henoch–Schönlein purpura, polyarteritis nodosa, and microscopic polyangiitis. The presence of a cryoprecipitate, HCV and RF positivity, low C4 levels, and a modest increase in transaminases support the diagnosis of cryoglobulinemic vasculitis. It should be remembered that major organ involvement may be present at the onset of MC.

Prognosis

The clinical course of MC is generally favorable. Monteverde *et al.* (1996) reported that more than 70% of the patients were alive ten or more years after the diagnosis, with causes of death that vary in different studies. The leading cause of death was renal impairment in the oldest series (Gorevic *et al.* 1980; Invernizzi *et al.* 1990), cardiovascular disorder and infections in one study (Tarantino *et al.* 1995), and progressive liver disease in another (Monteverde *et al.* 1996). A recent review of the causes of death of 57 patients at a mean age of 71.2 years found that the main cause was liver impairment, followed by cardiovascular disorders and renal insufficiency (Saccardo *et al.* unpublished data).

No prospective investigations have sought to define prognostic criteria. On the basis of retrospective study results, the signs and symptoms that are the main candidates for prognostic indices are:

1 severity and frequency of purpura relapses and the presence of cutaneous ulcers;

2 presence of MPGN;

3 severity and progression of liver disease.

Peripheral neuropathy impairs the patients' quality of life, but its role as a predictor of a poor outcome is unclear.

Treatment

MC has long been considered an immune disorder requiring immunosuppressive treatment, but the discovery of the role of HCV has radically changed therapeutic strategies. Incomplete knowledge of the immunopathological mechanisms involved, and the complexity of MC patients, still precludes a universally accepted treatment protocol. Therapeutic interventions used in cryoglobulinemic syndromes are shown in Table 41.4. Generally speaking, treatment should be aimed at the underlying cause in order to prevent the organ damage associated with MC progression and contain the exacerbations of the syndrome. Accordingly, the treatment of patients with HCV-associated MC is mainly focused on the etiology, namely antiviral drugs such as IFN and ribavirin, and when necessary on

Table 41.4 Therapeutic interventions used in cryoglobulinemic syndromes

Category	Therapy	Evidence
Supportive therapy	Avoid exposure to cold	A III
	Avoid prolonged standing	A III
	Avoid fatigue	B III
	Antihypertensive drugs as needed	A III
Etiological therapy	Interferon plus ribavirin (HCV-related MC)	A I
	Other etiological therapy if available (non HCV-related MC)	C II
Immunosuppressant or immunomodulating therapy	Cyclosporin	C II
	Cytotoxic agents	B II
	Anti-CD20 MoAbs	B II
	Glucocorticoids	A I
	Colchicine	C II
	Intravenous immunoglobulins	C II
Circulating immune complex reducing therapies	Plasmapheresis	B II
	Low-antigen content diet	B I

Categorization of evidence and recommendations according to Shekelle *et al.* 1999 (see Table 32.6 in Chapter 32 for definitions).

the pathogenetic features (rituximab or cyclophosphamide) or on symptom relief (glucocorticoids or plasmapheresis).

Etiological treatment

Interferon and antiviral drugs

Interferon (IFN) treatment for patients unresponsive to glucocorticoids and cytotoxic therapies was proposed in 1987 (Bonomo *et al.* 1987). Initially given because of its antiproliferative action on B lymphocytes, IFN is currently mainly used as an antiviral agent although it may also have an immunomodulatory effect in reducing circulating cryoglobulin levels.

A number of randomized studies have documented the short-term therapeutic efficacy of IFN in patients with HCV-related MC (Mazzaro *et al.* 1994; Misiani *et al.* 1994). The large majority of patients show complete remission of MC-associated symptoms and disappearance of HCV-RNA. However, the side effects of IFN should not be ignored: one multicenter, randomized controlled study (Pioltelli *et al.* 1995) did not find any difference between the efficacy of deflazacort and IFN, but the incidence of major toxic effects was high in the IFN arm (25%).

The combination of IFN and ribavirin used for the treatment of chronic hepatitis in HCV-infected individuals (Zuckerman *et al.* 2000) has also recently been adopted for HCV-positive MC. Over the last few years, treatment with subcutaneous PEGylated interferon-alpha 2b (1.0–1.5 mg/kg/week) plus oral ribavirin (800–1200 mg/day) has been found to lead to a complete clinical response in most patients with HCV-associated MC (Mazzaro *et al.* 2005; Cacoub *et al.* 2005).

Immunosuppressive treatment

Cytotoxic agents

Cytotoxic agents are believed to inhibit immunoglobulin production by effecting B lymphocytes. Cyclophosphamide (1–3 mg/kg/day given orally), chlorambucil, and azathioprine have been most frequently used, often in combination with glucocorticoids. Their use is limited in HCV-related MC because their immunosuppressive effects could theoretically favor complications or the progression of HCV disease.

The use of these drugs is not supported by controlled studies, and in combination with plasmapheresis, is currently restricted to particularly severe cases unresponsive to traditional therapies.

Anti-CD20 monoclonal antibody (rituximab)

The have been reports of favorable preliminary results using the anti-CD20 monoclonal antibody rituximab (Zaja et al. 2003; Sansonno et al. 2003). Rituximab may be a safe and effective alternative to standard immunosuppression when antiviral therapy is ineffective, contraindicated, or not tolerated (Kay and McCluskey 2005), but further investigations and follow-up studies are needed to evaluate its cost-efficacy profile and the duration of response.

Colchicine

Colchicine has been used to treat autoimmune disease and leukocytoclastic vasculitis (Plotnick et al. 1989). One uncontrolled, open-label trial involving MC patients has shown a dose of 1 mg/day can reduce the cryocrit and lead to a clinical improvement (Monti et al. 1995c).

Cyclosporin

An uncontrolled, open-label trial found that cyclosporin 2.5 mg/kg/day has favorable effects on purpura, neuropathy, cryocrit, and hepatic function, and may reduce bone marrow B lymphocyte infiltration in some cases of HCV-related type II MC unresponsive to standard therapy with IFN (Ballaré et al. 1995).

Symptomatic treatment

Glucocorticoids

Widely used in the past, glucocorticoids ameliorate arthralgia and purpura, but do not seem to affect the evolution of the disease. One randomized, prospective study has demonstrated the effectiveness of both deflazacort and prednisone in reducing cryocrit and controlling most of the symptoms of cryoglobulinemic syndrome in the short term (Vacca and Dammacco 1992). Medium-to-low doses of prednisone (0.1–0.3 mg/kg/day) are frequently used to control minor symptoms such as purpura, arthralgia, arthritis, and weakness, and higher doses (0.5–1.5 mg/kg/day) have been used to manage major complications such as renal disease, neuropathy, and ulcers. Intravenous high-dose pulses of methylprednisolone (1 g/day for 3 days), followed by prednisone at lower doses, have been successfully used in renal and vasculitic emergencies. Side-effects must always be considered, as well as a possible increase in the viral load of HCV-positive patients. No data are available concerning the effects of repeated glucocorticoid treatment on HCV disease progression.

Plasmapheresis

The main indications for plasmapheresis are hyperviscosity syndrome, rapidly progressive renal disease, or major sensorimotor neuropathy. In uncontrolled studies of small series of patients, plasmapheresis, alone or in combination with cytotoxic drugs or glucocorticoids, has proved to be effective in improving severe MC-related conditions (Ferri et al. 1986; Frankel et al. 1992; Geltner et al. 1981; Pietrogrande et al. 1999; Alric et al. 2004). The mechanism of action of plasmapheresis remains unknown, but it has been postulated that it rapidly reduces the levels of circulating immune complexes and inflammation mediators, modifies the quality of the immune complexes and their solubilisation, and restores reticuloendothelial system function (Tavoni et al. 1995).

Plasmapheresis techniques have improved considerably over the last 20 years (Siami and Siami 2001; Madore 2002). The commonly used apheretic procedures are non-selective plasma exchange, double filtration plasmapheresis (a selective procedure for removing large plasma molecules), and cryoapheresis, which selectively removes cryoglobulins. Immunosuppressive drugs (typically cyclophosphamide) are added with the aim of partially abolishing the postpheresis rebound of cryoglobulins and immune complexes.

Low-antigen content diet

In patients with cryoglobulinemic syndrome, the reticuloendothelial system must remove a large number of circulating immune complexes. A low-antigen content (LAC) diet could reduce the levels of high molecular weight exogenous substances crossing the mucosal barrier of the gut, and thus reduce the burden of a saturated reticuloendothelial system. This hypothesis has been tested in a short-term randomized cross-over study (Ferri et al. 1989) and a second similar trial (Bombardieri and Ferri 1992), but the improvement in cryoglobulinemic symptoms observed in these studies was not corroborated by another controlled, randomized study (Pioltelli et al. 1995).

Intravenous immunoglobulins

Preliminary studies indicate that a combination of high doses of intravenous immunoglobulins (IVIg) and plasmapheresis may have favorable effects on skin ulcers and cyoglobulinemic neuropathy (Pietrogrande et al. 1999). Other anecdotal reports have described the responsiveness of peripheral neuropathy associated with vasculitis, including MC (Levy et al. 2003; Russel and Weenig 2004), but the occurrence of adverse events suggests caution in the use of this treatment (Yebra et al. 2002).

Non-steroidal anti-inflammatory drugs

NSAIDs are used to treat arthralgias but, given the frequency of liver and kidney disease in cryoglobulinemic syndrome, they should be used with caution.

References

Agnello, V. (1997). The etiology and pathophysiology of mixed cryoglobulinemia secondary to hepatitis C virus infection. *Springer Seminars in Immunopathology*, **19**, 111–29.

Agnello, V. and Abel, G. (1997). Localization of hepatitis C virus in cutaneous vasculitic lesions in patients with type II cryoglobulinemia. *Arthritis and Rheumatism*, **40**, 2007–15.

Agnello, V., Chung, R. T. and Kaplan, L. M. (1992). A role for hepatitis C virus infection in type II cryoglobulinemia. *New England Journal of Medicine*, **327**, 1490–5.

Agnello, V. and De Rosa, F. G. (2004). Extrahepatic disease manifestations of HCV infection, some current issues. *Journal of Hepatology*, **40**, 341–52.

Agnello, V., Zhang, Q. X., Abel, G. and Knight, G. B.(1995). The association of hepatitis C virus infection with monoclonal rheumatoid factors bearing the WA cross-idiotype, implications for the etiopathogenesis and therapy of mixed cryoglobulinemia. *Clinical and Experimental Rheumatology*, 13 (Suppl. 13), S101–4.

Allain, J. P., Dong, Y., Vandamme, A. M., Moulton, V. and Salemi, M. (2000). Evolutionary rate and genetic drift of hepatitis C virus are not correlated with the host immune response: studies of infected donor-recipient clusters. *Journal of Virology*, 74, 2541–9.

Alric, L., Plaisier, E., Thebault, S., Peron, J. M., Rostaing, L., Pourrat, J., Ronco, P., Piette, J. C. and Cacoub, P. (2004). Influence of antiviral therapy in hepatitis C virus-associated cryoglobulinemic MPGN. *American Journal of Kidney Disease*, 43, 617–23.

Amoroso, A., Berrino, M., Canale, L., Cornaglia, M., Guarrera, S., Mazzola, G., Savoldi, S., Scolari, F., Sallberg, M., Clementi, M. and Gabrielli, A. (1998). Are HLA class II and immunoglobulin constant region genes involved in the pathogenesis of mixed cryoglobulinemia type II after hepatitis C virus infection? *Journal of Hepatology*, 29, 36–44.

Au, W. Y., Kwok, J. S., Chu, K. M. and Ma, E. S. (2005). Life-threatening cryoglobulinemia in HCV-negative Southern Chinese and a novel association with structural aortic abnormalities. *Annals of Hematology*, 84, 95–8.

Ballarè, M., Bobbio, F., Poggi, S., Bordin, G., Bertoncelli, M. C., Catania, E. and Monteverde, A. (1995). A pilot study on the effectiveness of cyclosporine in type II mixed cryoglobulinemia. *Clinical and Experimental Rheumatology*, 13 (Suppl. 13), S201–3.

Benetti, B., Invernizzi, F., Rizzuto, N., Bonazzi, M. L., Zanusso, G. L., Chinaglia, G. and Monaco, S. (1997). T-cell-mediated epineurial vasculitis and humoral-mediated microangiopathy in cryoglobulinemic neuropathy. *Journal of Neuroimmunology*, 73, 145–54.

Bombardieri, S. and Ferri, C. (1992). Low antigen content diet in the management of immunomediated diseases. *Israel Journal of Medical Sciences*, 28, 117–20.

Bombardieri, S., Paoletti, P., Ferri, C., Di Munno, O., Fornal, E. and Giuntini, C. (1979). Lung involvement in essential mixed cryoglobulinemia. *American Journal of Medicine*, 66, 748–56.

Bonomo, L., Casato, M., Afeltra, A. and Caccavo, D. (1987) Treatment of idiopathic mixed cryoglobulinemia with alpha interferon. *American Journal of Medicine*, 83, 726–30.

Booth, J. C., Kumar, U., Webster, D., Monjardino, J. and Thomas, H. C. (1998). Comparison of the rate of sequence variation in the hypervariable region of E2/NS1 region of hepatitis C virus in normal and hypogammaglobulinemic patients. *Hepatology*, 27, 223–7.

Boyer, O., Saadoun, D., Abriol, J., Dodille, M., Piette, J. C., Cacoub, P. and Klatzmann, D. (2004). CD4+CD25+ regulatory T-cell deficiency in patients with hepatitis C-mixed cryoglobulinemia vasculitis. *Blood*, 103, 3428–30.

Brandau, D. T., Trautman, P. A., Steadman, B. L., Lawson, E. Q. and Middaugh, C. R. (1986). The temperature-dependent stoichiometry of mixed cryoimmunoglobulins. *Journal of Biological Chemistry*, 26, 16385–91.

Brouet, J. C., Clauvel, J. P., Danon, F., Klein, M. and Seligmann, M. (1974). Biologic and clinical significance of cryoglobulins. A report of 86 cases. *American Journal of Medicine*, 57, 775–88.

Cacoub, P., Renou, C., Kerr, G., Hue, S., Rosenthal, E., Cohen, P., Kaplanski, G., Charlotte, F., Thibault, V., Ghillani, P., Piette, J. C. and Caillat-Zucman, S. (2001). Influence of HLA-DR phenotype on the risk of hepatitis C virus-associated mixed cryoglobulinemia. *Arthritis and Rheumatism*, 44, 2118–24.

Cacoub, P., Saadoun, D., Limal, N., Sene, D., Lidove, O. and Piette, J. C. (2005). PEGylated interferon alfa-2b and ribavirin treatment in patients with hepatitis C virus-related systemic vasculitis. *Arthritis and Rheumatism*, 52, 911–5.

Casato, M., Taliani, G., Pucillo, L. P., Goffredo, F., Lagana, B. and Bonomo, L. (1991). Cryoglobulinaemia and hepatitis C virus. *Lancet*, 337, 1047–8.

Casato, M., Lilli, D., Donato, G., Granata, M., Conti, V., Del Giudice, G., Rivanera, D., Scagnolari, C., Antonelli, G. and Fiorilli, M. (2003). Occult hepatitis C virus infection in type II mixed cryoglobulinemia. *Journal of viral hepatitus*, 10, 455–9.

Dammacco, F., Sansonno, D., Piccoli, C., Tucci, F. A. and Racanelli, V. (2001). The cryoglobulins, an overview. *European Journal of Clinical Investigation*, 31, 628–38.

Dienstag, J. L., Wands, J. R. and Isselbacher, K. J. (1977). Hepatitis B and essential mixed cryoglobulinemia. *New England Journal of Medicine*, 297, 946–7.

Disdier, P., Harle, J. R. and Weiller, P. J. (1991). Cryoglobulinaemia and hepatitis C infection. *Lancet*, 338, 1151–2.

Durand, J. M., Lefevre, P., Harle, J. R., Boucrat, J., Vitviski, L. and Soubeyrand, J. (1991). Cutaneous vasculitis and cryoglobulinaemia type II associated with hepatitis C virus infection. *Lancet*, 337, 499–500.

Fabris, M., Sacco, S., De Marchi, G. *et al.* (2005). B-lymphocyte stimulator (BlyS) in mixed cryoglobulinemic syndrome, pathological and clinical implications. (Abstract) *Arthritis and Rheumatism*, 52, S645.

Ferri, C., Moriconi, L., Gremignai, G., Migliorini, P., Paleologo, G., Fosella, P. V. and Bombardieri, S. (1986). Treatment of the renal involvement in mixed cryoglobulinemia with prolonged plasma exchange. *Nephrology*, 43, 246–53.

Ferri, C., Pietrogrande, M., Cecchetti, R., Tavoni, A., Cefalo, A., Buzzetti, G., Vitali, C. and Bombardieri, S. (1989). Low-antigen-content diet in the treatment of patients with mixed cryoglobulinemia. *American Journal of Medicine*, 87, 519–24.

Ferri, C., Mannini, L. and Bartoli, V. (1990). Blood viscosità and filtration abnormalities in MC patients. *Clinical and Experimental Rheumatology*, 8, 271–81.

Ferri, C., Greco, F., Longombardo, G., Palla, P., Marzo, E. and Moretti, A. (1991). Hepatitis C virus antibodies in mixed cryoglobulinemia. *Clinical and Experimental Rheumatology*, 9, 95–6.

Ferri, C., La Civita, L., Cirafisi, C., Siciliano, G., Longombardo, G., Bombardieri, S. and Rossi, B. (1992). Peripheral neuropathy in mixed cryoglobulinemia, clinical and electrophysiologic investigations. *Journal of Rheumatology*, 19, 889–95.

Ferri, C., Monti, M., La Civita, L., Longombardo, G., Greco, F., Pasero, G., Gentilizi, P., Bombardieri, S. and Zignego, A. L. (1993). Infection of peripheral blood mononuclear cells by hepatitis C virus in mixed cryoglobulinemia. *Blood*, 82, 3701–4.

Ferri, C., Caracciolo, F., Zignego, A. L., La Civita, L., Monti, M., Longombardo, G., Lombardini, F., Greco, F., Capochiani, E., Mazzoni, A., *et al.* (1994). Hepatitis C virus infection in patients with non-Hodgkin's lymphoma. *British Journal of Haematology*, 88, 392–4.

Ferri, C., Pilieri, S. and Zigniego, A. L. (2000). Hepatitis C virus B-cell disorders, and non-Hodgkin's lymphoma. In *Infectious causes of cancer* (Goedert, J.J., ed.), pp. 349–68. Humana Press, Totowa, New Jersey.

Florin-Christensen, A., Roux, M. E. and Arana, R. M. (1974). Cryoglobulins in acute and chronic liver diseases. *Clinical and Experimental Immunology*, 16, 599–605.

Frankel, A. H., Singer, D. R., Winearls, C. G., Evans, D. J., Rees, A. J. and Pusey, C. D. (1992). Type II essential mixed cryoglobulinaemia, presentation, treatment and outcome in 13 patients. *Quarterly Journal of Medicine*, 82, 101–24.

Gabrielli, A., Manzin, A., Candela, M., Caniglia, M. L., Paolucci, S., Danieli, M. G. and Clementi, M. (1994). Active hepatitis C virus infection in bone marrow and peripheral blood mononuclear cells from patients with mixed cryoglobulinaemia. *Clinical and Experimental Immunology*, 97, 87–93.

Galli, M. (1991). Cryoglobulinaemia and serological markers of hepatitis viruses. Lancet, 338, 758–9.

Galli, M. (1995). Viruses and cryoglobulinemia. *Clinical and Experimental Rheumatology*, 13 (Suppl. 13), S63–70.

Galli, M., Caredda, F., D'Arminio Monforte, A., Fiorenza, A. M., Messina, K. and Invernizzi, F. (1982). (Mixed cryoglobulinemias and liver diseases). *Minerva Medica*, **73**, 1159–60.

Galli, M., Invernizzi, F., Chemotti, M., Monti, G., Gasparro, M. G., Caredda, F., Negri, C. and Moroni, M. (1986). Cryoglobulins and infectious diseases. *La Ricerca in Clinica e Laboratorio*, **16**, 301–13.

Galli, M., Monti, G., Invernizzi, F., Monteverde, A., Bombardieri, S., Gabrielli, A., Migliaresi, S., Mussini, C., Ossi, E., Pietrogrande, M., *et al.* (1992a). Hepatitis B virus-related markers in secondary and in essential mixed cryoglobulinemias, a multicentric study of 596 cases. The Italian Group for theStudy of Cryoglobulinemias (GISC). *Annali Italiani di Medicina Interna*, **7**, 209–14.

Galli, M., Monti, G., Monteverde, A., Invernizzi, F., Pietrogrande, M., Di Girolamo, M., Mazzaro, C., Migliaresi, S., Mussini, C., Ossi, E., *et al.* (1992b). Hepatitis C virus and mixed cryoglubulinaemia. *Lancet*, **339**, 989.

Galli, M., Zehender, G., Monti, G., Ballare, M., Saccardo, F., Piconi, S., De Maddalena, C., Bertoncelli, M. C., Rinaldi, G., Invernizzi, F., *et al.* (1995). Hepatitis C virus RNA in the bone marrow of patients with mixed cryoglobulinemia and in subjects with non-cryoglobulinemic chronic hepatitis type C. *Journal of Infectious Diseases*, **171**, 672–5.

Geltner, D., Kohn, R. W., Gorevic, P. and Franklin, E. C. (1981). The effect of combination therapy (steroids, immunosuppressives, and plasmapheresis) on 5 mixed cryoglobulinemia patients with renal, neurologic, and vascular involvement. *Arthritis and Rheumatism*, **24**, 1121–7.

Gerotto, M., Dal Pero, F., Loffreda, S., Bianchi, F. B., Alberti, A. and Lenzi, M. (2001). A 385 insertion in the hypervariable region 1 of hepatitis C virus E2 envelope protein is found in some patients with mixed cryoglobulinemia type 2. *Blood*, **98**, 2657–63.

Gorevic, P. D., Kassab, H. J., Levo, Y., Kohn, R., Meltzer, M., Prose, P. and Franklin, E. C. (1980) Mixed cryoglobulinemia, clinical aspects and long-term follow-up of 40 patients. *American Journal of Medicine*, **69**, 287–308.

Hall, C. G. and Abraham, G. N. (1984). Reversible self-association of a human myeloma protein. Thermodynamics and relevance to viscosity effects and solubility. *Biochemistry*, **23**, 5123–9.

Hijikata, M., Shimizu, Y. K., Kato, H., Iwamoto, A., Shih, J. W., Alter, H. J., Purcell, R. H. and Yoshikura, H. (1993). Equilibrium centrifugation studies of hepatitis C virus, evidence for circulating immune complexes. *Journal of Virology*, **67**, 1953–8.

Invernizzi, F., Galli, M., Serino, G., Monti, G., Meroni, P. L., Granatieri, C. and Zanussi, C. (1983). Secondary and essential cryoglobulinemias. Frequency, nosological classification, and long-term follow-up. *Acta Haematologica*, **70**, 73–82.

Invernizzi, F., Monti, G. and Zanussi, C. (1990). The clinical spectrum of mixed cryoglobulinemic. In *Immunological aspects of malignant lymphomas and cryoglobulinemia* (Dammacco, F., ed.), pp. 221–34. Edi-Ermes, Milano.

Invernizzi, F., Pietrogrande, M. and Sagramoso, B. (1995). Classification of the cryoglobulinemic syndrome. *Clinical and Experimental Rheumatology*, **13** (Suppl. 13), S123–8.

Iori, G. P. and Buonanno, G. (1972). Chronic hepatitis and cirrhosis on the liver in cryoglobulinemic. *Gut*, **13**, 610–13.

Kaplanski, G., Marin, V., Maisonobe, T., Sbai, A., Farnarier, C., Ghillani, P., Thirion, X., Durand, J. M., Harle, J. R., Bongrand, P., Piette, J. C. and Cacoub, P. (2002). Increased soluble p55 and p75 tumour necrosis factor-alpha receptors in patients with hepatitis C-associated mixed cryoglobulinaemia. *Clinical and Experimental Immunology*, **127**, 123–30.

Kay, J. and McCluskey, R. T. (2005). Case records of the Massachusetts General Hospital. Case 31–2005. A 60-year-old man with skin lesions and renal insufficiency. *New England Journal of Medicine*, **353**, 1605–13.

Kayali, Z., Buckwold, V. E., Zimmerman, B. and Schmidt, W. N. (2002). Hepatitis C, cryoglobulinemia, and cirrhosis, a meta-analysis. *Hepatology*, **36**, 978–85.

Kipps, T. J., Tomhave, E., Chen, P. P. and Fox, R. I. (1989). Molecular characterization of a major autoantibody-associated cross-reactive idiotype in Sjogren's syndrome. *Journal of Immunology*, **142**, 4261–8.

Kuniyoshi, M., Nakamuta, M., Sakai, H., Enjoji, M., Kinukawa, N., Kotoh, K., Fukutomi, M., Yokota, M., Nishi, H., Iwamoto, H., Uike, N., Nishimura, J., Inaba, S., Maeda, Y., Nawata, H. and Muta, K. (2001). Prevalence of hepatitis B or C virus infections in patients with non-Hodgkin's lymphoma. *Journal of Gastroenterology and Hepatology*, **16**, 215–9.

Kunkel, II. G., Agnello, V., Joslin, F. G., Winchester, R. J. and Capra, J. D. (1973). Cross-idiotypic specificity among monoclonal IgM proteins with anti-gamma-globulin activity. *Journal of Experimental Medicine*, **137**, 331–42.

Kuroki, A., Kuroda, Y., Kikuchi, S., Lajaunias, F., Fulpius, T., Pastore, Y., Fossati-Jimack, L., Reininger, L., Toda, T., Nakata, M., Kojima, N., Mizuochi, T. and Izui, S. (2002). Level of galactosylation determines cryoglobulin activity of murine IgG3 monoclonal rheumatoid factor. *Blood*, **99**, 2922–8.

La Civita, L., Zignego, A. L., Monti, M., Longombardo, G., Pasero, G. and Ferri, C. (1995). Mixed cryoglobulinemia as a possible preneoplastic disorder. *Arthritis and Rheumatism*, **38**, 1859–60.

Lenzi, M., Frisoni, M., Mantovani, V., Ricci, P., Muratori, L., Francesconi, R., Cuccia, M., Ferri, S. and Bianchi, F. B. (1998). Haplotype HLA-B8-DR3 confers susceptibility to hepatitis C virus-related mixed cryoglobulinemia. *Blood*, **91**, 2062–6.

Lerner, A. B. and Watson, C. J. (1947). Studies on cryoglobulins. Unusual purpura associated with the presence of a high concentration of cryoglobulin (cold precipitate serum globulin). *American Journal of Medical Sciences*, **214**, 410–15.

Levo, Y. (1980). Nature of cryoglobulinaemia. *Lancet*, **1**, 1285–7.

Levo, Y, Gorevic, P. D., Kassab, H. J., Zucker-Franklin, D. and Franklin, E. C. (1977). Association between hepatitis B virus and essential mixed cryoglobulinemia. *New England Journal of Medicine*, **296**, 1501–4.

Levy, Y., Uziel, Y., Zandman, G. G., Amital, H., Sherer, Y., Langevitz, P., Goldman, B. and Shoenfeld, Y. (2003). Intravenous immunoglobulins in peripheral neuropathy associated with vasculitis. *Annals of the Rheumatic Diseases*, **62**, 1221–3.

Lospalluto, J., Dorward, B., Miller, W. Jr and Ziff, M. (1962). Cryoglobulinemia based on interaction between a gamma macroglobulin and 7S gamma globulin. *American Journal of Medicine*, **32**, 142–7.

Lunel, F., Musset, L., Cacoub, P., Frangeul, L., Leger, S. M., Huraux, J. M. *et al.* (1994). Mixed cryoglobulinemia and hepatitis C virus. *American Journal of Medicine*, **96**, 124–32.

Machida, K., Cheng, K. T. and Sung, V. M. (2004). Hepatitis C virus induces a mutator phenotype, enhanced mutations of immunoglobulins and protooncogenes. *Proceedings of the National Academy of Sciences USA*, **101**, 4262–7

Madi, N., Steiger, G., Estreicher, J. and Schifferli, J. A. (1991). Defective immune adherence and elimination of hepatitis B surface antigen/antibody complexes in patients with mixed essential cryoglobulinemia type II. *Journal of Immunology*, **147**, 495–502.

Madore, F. (2002). Plasmapheresis. Technical aspects and indications. *Critical Care Clinics*, **18**, 375–92.

Mageed, R. A., Carson, D. and Jefferis, R. (1988). Analysis of rheumatoid factor autoantibodies in patients with essential mixed cryoglobulinaemia and rheumatoid arthritis. *Scandinavian Journal of Rheumatology*, **75** (Suppl.), 172–8.

Matsuda, J., Tsukamoto, M., Gohchi, K., Saitoh, N. and Gotoh, M. (1994). Hepatitis C virus (HCV) RNA and human immunodeficiency virus (HIV) p24 antigen in the cryoglobulin of hemophiliacs with HIV and/or HCV infection. *Clinical Infectious Diseases*, **18**, 832–3.

Mazzaro, C., Pozzato, G., Moretti, M., Crovatto, M., Modolo, M. L., Mazzi, G. and Santini, G. (1994). Long-term effects of alpha-interferon therapy for type II mixed cryoglobulinemia. *Haematologica*, **79**, 342–9.

Mazzaro, C., Zagonel, V., Monfardini, S., Tulissi, P., Pussini, E., Fanni, M., Sorio, R., Bortolus, R., Crovatto, M., Santini, G., Tiribelli, C., Sasso, F., Masutti, R. and Pozzato, G. (1996). Hepatitis C virus and non-Hodgkin's lymphomas. *British Journal of Haematology*, **94**, 544–50.

Mazzaro, C., Zorat, F., Caizzi, M., Donada, C., Di Gennaro, G., Maso, L. D., Carniello, G., Virgolini, L., Tirelli, U. and Pozzato, G. (2005). Treatment with peg-interferon alfa-2b and ribavirin of hepatitis C virus-associated mixed cryoglobulinemia, a pilot study. *Journal of Hepatology*, **42**, 632–8.

Mcintosh, R. M., Koss, M. N. and Gocke, K. J. (1976). The nature and incidence of cryoproteins in hepatitis B antigen (HbsAg) positive patients. *Quarterly Journal of Medicine*, **45**, 23–38.

Mele, A., Pulsoni, A., Bianco, E., Musto, P., Szklo, A., Sanpaolo, M. G., Iannitto, E., De Renzo, A., Martino, B., Liso, V., Andrizzi, C., Pusterla, S., Dore, F., Maresca, M., Rapicetta, M., Marcucci, F., Mandelli, F. and Franceschi, S. (2003). Hepatitis C virus and B-cell non-Hodgkin lymphomas, an Italian multicenter case-control study. *Blood*, **102**, 996–9.

Meltzer, M. and Franklin, E. C. (1966). Cryoglobulinemia–a study of twenty-nine patients. I. IgG and IgM cryoglobulins and factors affecting cryoprecipitability. *American Journal of Medicine*, **40**, 828–36.

Meroni, P. L., Barcellini, W., DeBartolo, G., Invernizzi, F. and Zanussi, C. (1984). Abnormalities of in vitro immunoglobulin synthesis by peripheral blood lymphocytes from patients with essential mixed cryoglobulinemia. *Clinical Immunology and Immunopathology*, **33**, 245–57.

Meyers, C. M., Seeff, L. B., Stehman-Breen, C. O. and Hoofnagle, J. H. (2003). Hepatitis C and renal disease, an update. *American Journal of Kidney Diseases*, **42**, 631–57.

Migliaresi, S., Amendola, A., Di Iorio, G., Ambrosone, L., Ugolini, G., Sanges, G., *et al.* (1999). Autonomic dysfunction assessed by sympathetic skin response in patients with HCV-related mixed cryoglobulinemia. *Annals of Rheumatic Diseases*, **113**, (Abstract) 440.

Misiani, R., Bellavita, P., Fenili, D., Vicari, O., Marchesi, D., Sironi, P. L., Zilio, P., Vernocchi, A., Massazza, M., Vendramin, G., *et al.* (1994). Interferon alfa-2a therapy in cryoglobulinemia associated with hepatitis C virus. *New England Journal of Medicine*, **330**, 751–6.

Monga, G., Coppo, R., Piccoli, G. and Coda, R. (1986). Glomerular findings in mixed IgG-IgM cryoglobulinemic. Light, electron microscopi, immunofluorescence and histochemical correlation. *Virchows Archiv*, **20**, 185–96.

Montagnino, G. (1988). Reappraisal of the clinical expression of mixed cryoglobulinemia. *Springer Seminars in Immunopathology*, **10**, 1–19.

Monteverde, A., Ballare, M. and Pileri, S. (1997). Hepatic lymphoid aggregates in chronic hepatitis C and mixed cryoglobulinemia. *Springer Seminars in Immunopathology*, **19**, 99–110.

Monteverde, A., Invernizzi, F., Pilieri, S., Galli, M., Monti, G. and Ballarè, M. (1996). Le crioglobulinemie miste. In *Atti dei Congressi della Società Italiana di Medicina Interna*, 97° Congresso, Venezia, 15–19 ottobre, pp. 1–80. Luigi Pozzi Editore, Rome.

Monteverde, A., Rivano, M. T., Allegra, G. C., Monteverde, A. I., Zigrossi, P., Baglioni, P., Gobbi, M., Falini, B., Bordin, G. and Pileri, S. (1988). Essential mixed cryoglobulinemia, type II, a manifestation of a low-grade malignant lymphoma? Clinical-morphological study of 12 cases with special reference to immunohistochemical findings in liver frozen sections. *Acta Haematologica*, **79**, 20–5.

Monteverde, A., Sabattini, E., Poggi, S., Ballare, M., Bertoncelli, M. C., De Vivo, A., Briskomatis, A., Roncador, G., Falini, B. and Pileri, S. A. (1995). Bone marrow findings further support the hypothesis that essential mixed cryoglobulinemia type II is characterized by a monoclonal B-cell proliferation. *Leukemia and Lymphoma*, **20**, 119–24.

Monti, G., Galli, M., Invernizzi, F., Pioltelli, P., Saccardo, F., Monteverde, A., Pietrogrande, M., Renoldi, P., Bombardieri, S., Bordin, G., *et al.* (1995a). Cryoglobulinaemias, a multi-centre study of the early clinical and laboratory manifestations of primary and secondary disease. GISC. Italian Group for the Study of Cryoglobulinaemias. *Quarterly Journal of Medicine*, **88**, 115–26.

Monti, G., Saccardo, F., Pioltelli, P. and Rinaldi, G. (1995b). The natural history of cryoglobulinemia, symptoms at onset and during follow-up. A report by the Italian Group for the Study of Cryoglobulinemias (GISC). *Clinical and Experimental Rheumatology*, **13** (Suppl. 13), S129–33.

Monti, G., Saccardo, F., Rinaldi, G., Petrozzino, M. R., Gomitoni, A. and Invernizzi, F. (1995c). Colchicine in the treatment of mixed cryoglobulinemia. *Clinical and Experimental Rheumatology*, **13** (Suppl. 13), S197–9.

Monti, G., Pioltelli, P., Saccardo, F., Campanini, M., Candela, M., Cavallero, G., De Vita, S., Ferri, C., Mazzaro, C., Migliaresi, S., Ossi, E., Pietrogrande, M., Gabrielli, A., Galli, M. and Invernizzi, F. (2005). Incidence and characteristics of non-Hodgkin lymphomas in a multicenter casefile of patients with hepatitis C virus-related symptomatic mixed cryoglobulinemias. *Archives of Internal Medicine*, **165**, 101–5.

Musset, L., Diemert, M. C., Taibi, F., Thi Huong Du, L., Cacoub, P., Leger, J. M., Boissy, G., Gaillard, O. and Galli, J. (1992). Characterization of cryoglobulins by immunoblotting. *Clinical Chemistry*, **38**, 798–802.

Musset, L., Duarte, F., Gaillard, O., Du, L. T., Bilala, J., Galli, J. and Preud'homme, J. L. (1994). Immunochemical characterization of monoclonal IgG containing mixed cryoglobulins. *Clinical Immunology and Immunopathology*, **70**, 166–70.

Nakamura, M., Burastero, S. E., Notkins, A. L. and Casal, P. (1988). Human monoclonal rheumatoid factor-like antibodies from CD5 (Leu-1) + B cells are polyreactive. *Journal of Immunology*, **140**, 4180–6.

Newkirk, M. M. (2002). Rheumatoid factors, host resistance or autoimmunity? *Clinical Immunology*, **104**, 1–13.

Nityanand, S., Holm, G. and Lefvert, A. K. (1997). Immune complex mediated vasculitis in hepatitis B and C infections and the effect of antiviral therapy. *Clinical Immunology and Immunopathology*, **82**, 250–7.

Ogata, N., Alter, H. J., Miller, R. H. and Purcell, R. H. (1991). Nucleotide sequence and mutation rate of the H strain of hepatitis C virus. *Proceedings of the National Academy of Sciences USA*, **88**, 3392–6.

Okamoto, H., Kojima, M., Okada, S., Yoshizawa, H., Iizuka, H., Tanaka, T., Muchmore, E. E., Peterson, D. A., Ito, Y. and Mishiro, S. (1992). Genetic drift of hepatitis C virus during an 8.2-year infection in a chimpanzee: variability and stability. *Virology*, **190**, 894–9.

Pascual, M., Perrin, L., Giostra, E. and Schifferli, J. A. (1990). Hepatitis C virus in patients with cryoglobulinemia type II. *Journal of Infectious Diseases*, 162, 569–70.

Petermann, M. L. and Braunsteiner, H. (1954). A cryoglobulin of high sedimentation rate (macroglobulin) from human serum. *Archives of Biochemistry*, **53**, 491–500.

Pietrogrande, M., Marelli, F., Dilani, S., Pessina, I. and Invernizzi, F. (1999). Treatment of severe cryoglobulinemic sindrome with plasma exchange followed by high dose intravenous immunoglobulins, preliminary results. *Journal of Autoimmunity*, (Suppl), **12**, S-95.

Pileri, P., Uematsu, Y., Campagnoli, S., Galli, G., Falugi, F., Petracca, R., Weiner, A. J., Houghton, M., Rosa, D., Grandi, G. and Abrignani, S. (1998). Binding of hepatitis C virus to CD81. *Science*, **282**, 938–41.

Pioltelli, P., Gargantini, L., Cassi, E., Santoleri, L., Bellati, G., Magliano, E. M. and Morra, E. (2000). Hepatitis C virus in non-Hodgkin's lymphoma. A reappraisal after a prospective case-control study of 300 patients. Lombart Study Group of HCV-Lymphoma. *American Journal of Haematology*, **64**, 95–100.

Pioltelli, P., Maldifassi, P., Vacca, A., Mazzaro, C., Mussini, C., Migliaresi, S., Gabrielli, A., Pietrogrande, M., Monteverde, A. and Monti, G. (1995). GISC protocol experience in the treatment of essential mixed cryoglobulinaemia. *Clinical and Experimental Rheumatology*, **13** (Suppl. 13), S187–90.

Pioltelli, P., Zehender, G., Monti, G., Monteverde, A., Galli, M. (1996). HCV and non-Hodgking Lymphoma. *Lancet*, **347**, 624–5.

Plotnick, S., Huppert, A. S. and Kantor, G. (1989). Colchicine and leukocytoclastic vasculitis. *Arthritis and Rheumatism*, **32**, 1489–90.

Popp, J. W. Jr, Dienstag, J. L., Wands, J. R. and Bloch, K. J. (1980). Essential mixed cryoglobulinemia without evidence for hepatitis B virus infection. *Annals of Internal Medicine*, **92**, 379–83.

Radoux, V., Chen, P. P., Sorge, J. A. and Carson, D. A. (1986). A conserved human germline Vκ gene directly encodes rheumatoid factor light chains. *Journal of Experimental Medicine*, **164**, 2119–24.

Ramos-Casals, M., Brito-Zeron, P., Nardi, N., *et al.* (2005). Lifethreatening cryoglobulinemic vasculitis. Clinical presentation and outcome in a series of 560 patients with cryoglobulinemia. *Arthritis and Rheumatism*, **52** (Suppl.), S645–6.

Robinson, D. R. and Kirkham, S. E. (1984). A 33-year old woman with cutaneous vasculitis, arthralgia, and intermittent bloody diarrhea. *New England Journal of Medicine*, **311**, 904–11.

Roccatello, D., Morsica, G., Picciotto, G., Cesano, G., Ropolo, R., Bernardi, M. T., Cacace, G., Cavalli, G., Sena, L. M., Lazzarin, A., Piccoli, G. and Rifai, A. (1997). Impaired hepatosplenic elimination of circulating cryoglobulins in patients with essential mixed cryoglobulinaemia and hepatitis C virus (HCV) infection. *Clinical and Experimental Immunology*, **110**, 9–14.

Rosa, D., Saletti, G., De Gregorio, E., Zorat, F., Comar, C., D'Oro, U., Nuti, S., Houghton, M., Barnaba, V., Pozzato, G. and Abrignani, S. (2005). Activation of naïve B lymphocytes via CD81, a pathogenetic mechanism for hepatitis C virus-associated B lynphocite disorders. *PNAS*, **102**, 18544–9.

Russell, J. P. and Weenig, R. H. (2004). Primary cutaneous small vessel vasculitis. *Current Treatment Options in Cardiovascular Medicine*, **6**, 139–49.

Saadoun, D., Bieche, I., Maisonobe, T., Asselah, T., Laurendeau, I., Piette, J. C., Vidaud, M. and Cacoub, P. (2005). Involvement of chemokines and type 1 cytokines in the pathogenesis of hepatitis C virus-associated mixed cryoglobulinemia vasculitis neuropathy. *Arthritis and Rheumatism*, **52**, 2917–25.

Saccardo, F., Massaro, P., Monti, G., Angelopulos, N. and Galli, M. (1986). Causes of death in essential mixed cryoglobulinemia. *La Ricerca in Clinica e in Laboratorio*, **16**, 389–91.

Sansonno, D. and Dammacco, F. (2005). Hepatitis C virus, cryoglobulinaemia, and vasculitis, immune complex relations. *Lancet Infectious Diseases*, **5**, 227–36.

Sansonno, D., Cornacchiulo, V., Iacobelli, A. R., Di Stefano, R., Lospalluti, M. and Dammacco, F. (1995). Localization of hepatitis C virus antigens in liver and skin tissues of chronic hepatitis C virus-infected patients with mixed cryoglobulinemia. *Hepatology*, **21**, 305–12.

Sansonno, D., Iacobelli, A. R., Cornacchiulo, V., Iodice, G. and Dammacco, F. (1996a). Detection of hepatitis C virus (HCV) proteins by immunofluorescence and HCV RNA genomic sequences by non-isotopic in situ hybridization in bone marrow and peripheral blood mononuclear cells of chronically HCV-infected patients. *Clinical and Experimental Immunology*, **103**, 414–21.

Sansonno, D., Iacobelli, A. R., Cornacchiulo, V., Lauletta, G., Distasi, M. A., Gatti, P. and Dammacco, F. (1996b). Immunochemical and biomolecular studies of circulating immune complexes *European Journal of Clinical Investigation*, **26**, 465–75.

Sansonno, D., De Vita, S., Cornacchiulo, V., Carbone, A., Boiocchi, M. and Dammacco, F. (1996c). Detection and distribution of hepatitis C virus-related proteins in lymph nodes of patients with type II mixed cryoglobulinemia and neoplastic or non-neoplastic lymphoproliferation. *Blood*, **88**, 4638–45.

Sansonno, D., Gesualdo, L., Manno, C., Schena, F. P. and Dammacco, F. (1997). Hepatitis C virus-related proteins in kidney tissue from hepatitis C virus-infected patients with cryoglobulinemic membranoproliferative glomerulonephritis. *Hepatology*, **25**, 1237–44.

Sansonno, D., De Vita, S., Iacobelli, A. R., Cornacchiulo, V., Boiocchi, M. and Dammacco, F. (1998). Clonal analysis of intrahepatic B cells from HCV-infected patients with and without mixed cryoglobulinemia. *Journal of Immunology*, **160**, 3594–601.

Sansonno, D., De Re, V., Lauletta, G., Tucci, F. A., Boiocchi, M. and Dammacco, F. (2003a). Monoclonal antibody treatment of mixed cryoglobulinemia resistant to interferon alpha with an anti-CD20. *Blood*, **101**, 3818–26.

Sansonno, D., Lauletta, G., Nisi, L., Gatti, P., Pesola, F., Pansini, N. and Dammacco, F. (2003b) Non-enveloped HCV core protein as constitutive antigen of cold-precipitable immune complexes in type II mixed cryoglobulinaemia. *Clinical and Experimental Immunolonology*, **133**, 275–82.

Schifferli, J. A. (1996). Complement and immune complexes. *Research in Immunology*, **147**, 109–10.

Shalit, M., Wollner, S. and Levo, Y. (1982). Cryoglobulinemia in acute type-A hepatitis. *Clinical and Experimental Immunology*, **47**, 613–6.

Shekelle, P. G., Woolf, S. H., Eccles, M. and Grimshaw, J. (1999). Clinical guidelines: developing guidelines. *British Medical Journal*, **318**, 593–6.

Siami, G. A. and Siami, F. S. (2001). Current topics on cryofiltration technologies. *Therapeutic Apheresis*, **5**, 283–6.

Spertini, F., Gyotoku, Y., Shibata, T., Izui, S. and Lambert, P. H. (1988). Experimental model of murine cryoglobulinemia induced by monoclonal antibodies and modulation by anti-idiotypic antibodies. *Springer Seminars in Immunopathology*, **10**, 91–101.

Steinhardt, M. J. and Fisher, G. S. Case reports. (1954). Essential cryoglobulinemia. *American Journal of Medicine*, **65**, 848 58.

Stone, M. J. and Fedak, J. E. (1974). Studies on monoclonal antibodies. II. Immune complex (IgM-IgG) cryoglobulinemia, the mechanism of cryoprecipitation. *Journal of Immunology*, **113**, 1377–85.

Sutton, B., Corper, A., Bonagura, V. and Taussig, M. (2000). The structure and origin of rheumatoid factors. *Immunology Today*, **21**, 177–83.

Taillan, B., Garnier, G., Pesce, A., Ferrari, E., Fuzibet, J. G., Gratecos, N. and Dujardin, P. (1993). Cryoglobulinemia related to hepatitis C virus infection in patients with human immunodeficiency virus infection. *Clinical and Experimental Rheumatology*, **11**, 350.

Tarantino, A., Montagnino, G., Baldassarri, A., Barbiano di Belgioioso, G., Colasanti, A., Montoli, A., *et al.* (1986). Prognostic factors in essential mixed cryoglobulinemia nephropathy. In *Antiglobulins, cryoglobulins and glomerulonephritis* (Ponticelli, C., Minetti, L., D'Amico, G., eds), pp. 219–32. Martinus Nijoff, Dordrecht.

Tarantino, A., Campise, M., Banfi, G., Confalonieri, R., Bucci, A., Montoli, A., Colasanti, G., Damilano, I., D'Amico, G., Minetti, L., *et al.* (1995). Long-term predictors of survival in essential mixed cryoglobulinemic glomerulonephritis. *Kidney International*, **47**, 618–23.

Tavoni, A., Mosca, M., Ferri, C., Moriconi, L., La Civita, L., Lombardini, F. and Bombardieri, S. (1995). Guidelines for the management of essential mixed cryoglobulinemia. *Clinical and Experimental Rheumatology*, **13** (Suppl. 13), S191–5.

Tissot, J. D., Schifferli, J. A., Hochstrasser, D. F., Pasquali, C., Spertini, F., Clement, F., Frutiger, S., Paquet, N., Hughes, G. J. and Schneider, P. (1994). Two-dimensional polyacrylamide gel electrophoresis analysis of cryoglobulins and identification of an IgM-associated peptide. *Journal of Immunological Methods*, **173**, 63–75.

Tissot, J. D., Pietrogrande, M., Testoni, L. and Invernizzi, F. (1998). Clinical implications of the types of cryoglobulins determined by two-dimensional polyacrylamide gel electrophoresis. *Haematologica*, **83**, 693–700.

Toyoda, H., Fukuda, Y., Koyama, Y., Takamatsu, J., Saito, H. and Hayakawa, T. (1997). Effect of immunosuppression on composition of quasispecies population of hepatitis C virus in patients with Chronic hepatitis C coinfected with human immunodeficiency virus. *Journal of Hepatology*, **26**, 975–82.

Vacca, A. and Dalmacco, F. (1992). Deflazacort versus prednisone in the treatment of EMC, a controlled clinical study. *International Archives of Allergy and Immunology*, **99**, 306–13.

Wager, O., Rasanen, J. A. and Sihvonen, T. (1969). Immunological studies on mixed cryoglobulinemia. In *Human anti-human gammaglobulins* (Grubb, R. and Samuelsson, eds). pp. 161–71. Pergamon Press, Oxford, New York.

Walport, M. J., Peters, A. M., Elkon, K. B., Pusey, C. D., Lavender, J. P. and Hughes, G. R. (1985). The splenic extraction ratio of antibody-coated erythrocytes and its response to plasma exchange and pulse methylprednisolone. *Clinical and Experimental Immunology*, **60**, 465–73.

Wang, A. C. (1988). Molecular basis for cryoprecipitation. *Springer Seminars in Immunopathology*, **10**, 21–34.

Williams, R. C. Jr and Malone, C. C. (1994). Rheumatoid-factor-reactive sites on CH2 established by analysis of overlapping peptides of primary sequence. *Scandinavian Journal of Immunology*, **40**, 443–56.

Wintrobe, M. M. and Buell, M. V. (1933). Hyperproteinemia associated with multiple myeloma, with report of a case in which an extraordinary hyperproteinemia was associated with thrombosis of retinal veins and symptoms suggesting Raynaud's disease. *Bulletin of Johns Hopkins Hospital*, **52**, 156–72.

Yebra, M., Barrios, Y., Rincon, J., Sanjuan, I. and Diaz-Espada, F. (2002). Severe cutaneous vasculitis following intravenous infusion of gammaglobulin in a patient with type II mixed cryoglobulinemia. *Clinical and Experimental Rheumatology*, **20**, 225–7.

Zaja, F., De Vita, S., Mazzaro, C., Sacco, S., Damiani, D., De Marchi, G., Michelutti, A., Baccarani, M., Fanin, R. and Ferraccioli, G. (2003). Efficacy and safety of rituximab in type II mixed cryoglobulinemia. *Blood*, **101**, 3827–34.

Zehender, G., de Maddalena, C., Monti, G., Ballare, M., Saccardo, F., Piconi, S., Invernizzi, F., Monteverde, A. and Galli, M. (1995). HCV genotypes in bone marrow and peripheral blood mononuclear cells of patients with mixed cryoglobulinemia. *Clinical and Experimental Rheumatology*, **13** (Suppl. 13), S87–90.

Zehender, G., Meroni, L., De Maddalena, C., Varchetta, S., Monti, G. and Galli, M. (1997). Detection of hepatitis C virus RNA in CD19 peripheral blood mononuclear cells of chronically infected patients. *Journal of Infectious Diseases*, **176**, 1209–14.

Zehender, G., De Maddalena, C., Bernini, F., Ebranati, E., Monti, G., Pioltelli, P. and Galli, M. (2005). Compartimentalization of Hepatitis C virus quasispecies in blood mononuclear cells of patients with mixed cryoglobulinemic sindrome. *Journal of Virology*, **79**, 9145–56.

Zignego, A. L., Macchia, D., Monti, M., Thiers, V., Mazzetti, M., Foschi, M., Maggi, E., Romagnani, S., Gentilini, P. and Brechot, C. (1992). Infection of peripheral mononuclear blood cells by hepatitis C virus. *Journal of Hepatology*, **15**, 382–6.

Zignego, A. L., Ferri, C., Giannini, C., Monti, M., La Civita, L., Careccia, G., Longombardo, G., Lombardini, F., Bombardieri, S. and Gentilini, P. (1996). Hepatitis C virus genotype analysis in patients with type II mixed cryoglobulinemia. *Annals of Internal Medicine*, **124**, 31–4.

Zignego, A. L., Giannelli, F., Marrocchi, M. E., Giannini, C., Gentilini, P., Innocenti, F. and Ferri, C. (1997). Frequency of bcl-2 rearrangement in patients with mixed cryoglobulinemia and HCV-positive liver diseases. *Clinical and Experimental Rheumatology*, **15**, 711–2.

Zignego, A. L., Giannelli, F., Marrocchi, M. E., Mazzocca, A., Ferri, C., Giannini, C., Monti, M., Caini, P., Villa, G. L., Laffi, G. and Gentilini, P. (2000).T(14;18) translocation in chronic hepatitis C virus infection. *Hepatology*, **31**, 474–9.

Zinneman, H. H., Levi, D. and Seal, U. S. (1968). On the nature of cryoglobulins. *Journal of Immunology*, **100**, 594–603.

Zuckerman, E., Keren, D., Slobodin, G., Rosner, I., Rozenbaum, M., Toubi, E., Sabo, E., Tsykounov, I., Naschitz, J. E. and Yeshurun, D. (2000). Treatment of refractory, symptomatic, hepatitis C virus related mixed cryoglobulinemia with ribavirin and interferon-alpha. *Journal of Rheumatology*, **27**, 2172–8.

Zuckerman, E., Zuckerman, T., Sahar, D., Streichman, S., Attias, D., Sabo, E., Yeshurun, D. and Rowe, J. M. (2001). The effect of antiviral therapy on t(14;18) translocation and immunoglobulin gene rearrangement in patients with chronic hepatitis C virus infection. *Blood*, **97**, 1555–9.

CHAPTER 42

Miscellaneous forms of vasculitis

Gim Gee Teng, Sumapa Chaiamnuay, and W. Winn Chatham

For many patients presenting with clinical manifestations of vasculitis, the combination of historical features, physical findings, results of clinical laboratory tests, and histologic examination will identify a readily classifiable vasculitic syndrome, such as polyarteritis nodosa (PAN), or associated autoimmune disease, such as systemic lupus erythematosus (SLE). In some patients, an established associated infectious trigger such as hepatitis C virus or hepatitis B virus may be identified as the inciting factor. Less commonly, comprehensive evaluation will dictate consideration of either a rare disorder or one that, while not necessarily uncommon, has vasculitis as an uncommon feature. Recognition and appreciation of the unique clinical and histopathologic features of uncommon causes of vasculitis is important not only for optimal patient diagnosis and management but also for an understanding of the spectrum of vascular injury syndromes and their potential causes. These miscellaneous vasculitides are shown in Table 42.1.

Vasculitides induced by microbial pathogens

Infections have long been implicated as triggers of primary vasculitides although causality is yet to be affirmed in most syndromes. Nonetheless, certain infections are notorious mimickers of vasculitis (see Chapter 45). Inflammation of vessel walls due to direct or contiguous infection and septic embolism, as well as inflammation due to immune processes triggered by bacterial toxin or superantigen production, can compromise vascular integrity culminating in end organ damage. Many organisms with a propensity to involve blood vessels have been implicated in vascular inflammation (Table 42.1). Clinical manifestations overlap significantly with those of the primary vasculitides and range from non-specific constitutional symptoms, pyrexia, and a variety of skin lesions to infarction of major organs. A high index of suspicion for infection as a potential cause of vasculitis is prudent in that appropriate antimicrobial therapy can be directed at the underlying organism, and immunosuppressive therapy administered in the absence of antimicrobial therapy is likely to increase morbidity. This section considers pathogenesis of infection-related vasculitis, with focus on described viral and bacterial etiologies. Localized suppuration of vessel wall related to foreign material (catheter insertion, bypass grafts, etc.) or invasive procedures (angiography, vascular surgery, etc.) is beyond the scope of this text.

Endovascular bacterial infection

Bacterial endocarditis

Vascular injury simulating vasculitis of various sized intracranial vessels has been demonstrated on conventional angiography and on magnetic resonance angiography in patients with bacterial endocarditis and meningitis (Ferris *et al.* 1968; Abe *et al.* 2002; Jan *et al.* 2003); mycotic aneurysm, infarcts, and hemorrhage are dire consequences (Kastenbauer and Pfister 2003; Lee *et al.* 2005). In addition to directed antibiotic therapy, early adjunctive use of dexamethasone in selected patients may reduce vascular inflammation and neurological sequelae (McIntyre *et al.* 1997; de Gans and van de Beek, 2002).

Infectious aortitis

While Takayasu's arteritis (TA) and giant cell arteritis (GCA) are the most common types of vasculitis that cause aortitis, infective aortitis should be suspected in patients, often older men with atherosclerosis, presenting with prolonged fever, abdominal or back pain, palpable abdominal mass, and leukocytosis, with or without positive blood cultures. Infection may arise as a consequence of bacteremic seeding of a pre-existing aneurysm from distant endovascular foci of infection (such as infective endocarditis), invasive intravascular procedures, or bacteremia occurring in the setting of intravenous drug abuse. Extension from contiguous infection (Bronze *et al.* 1999) has been reported but occurs less commonly.

Whereas streptococci predominated in the preantibiotic era, enteric Gram-negative bacteria (especially salmonella) and *Staphylococcus aureus* have since become more frequent pathogens in infective aortitis (Foote *et al.* 2005). Mycotic aneurysm, aneurysm rupture, aortoduodenal fistula, and vertebral osteomyelitis are possible complications. In a clincopathologic study of 29 cases of surgical repair of infected aortic aneurysms, acute inflammation superimposed on severe chronic atherosclerosis was most prevalent, with approximately one-third of the cases exhibiting only chronic inflammatory changes, including lymphoplasmacytic inflammation, fibrosis, healed pseudoaneurysm, and chronic

Table 42.1 Miscellaneous forms of vasculitis

Vasculitides induced by microbial pathogens
  Viral
    Parvovirus B19
    Herpes viruses (varicella zoster virus, cytomegalovirus, Epstein–Barr virus)
    Hepatitis viruses (hepatitis B virus, hepatitis C virus)
    Retroviruses (human T lymphotrophic virus I, human immunodeficiency virus)
  Bacterial
    Staphylococci
    Streptococci
    Neisseria species
    Gram-negative enteric pathogens (Salmonella)
    Mycobacteria
  Spirochetes
  Fungal
    Aspergillus
    Coccidioides
    Candida
    Mucormycetes
  Parasites
  Cysticercosis
  Rickettsiae
  Mycoplasma
  Other infections

Vasculitis associated with immunodeficiency syndromes
  Wiskott–Aldrich syndrome
  X-linked lymphoproliferative disorder
  Purine nucleoside phosphorylase deficiency

Vasculitis associated with sarcoidosis

Cogan's syndrome

Degos' syndrome

Urticarial vasculitis

Erythema elevatum diutinum

Familial Mediterranean fever

Hyperimmunoglobulinemia D

Paraneoplastic vasculitis syndromes
  Myelodysplastic syndrome and myeloproliferative disorders
  Solid tumors

atherosclerotic changes without purulent inflammation. Acute inflammation tended to occur in patients with the shortest duration of symptoms and antibiotic therapy. Bacterial culture from the aneurysm wall was positive in less than half of surgical cases, although the frequency of negative blood or tissue cultures varies from 2% to 33% in other series (Miller *et al.* 2004).

The incidence of non-typhoid salmonellosis appears to be increasing in many countries (Centers for Disease Control 2003). Endovascular infections, most commonly of the abdominal aorta, are rare complications with insidious onset and typically a subacute course. The mean duration of symptoms in reported cases is 1 month (range 1 day to 6 months) (Soravia-Dunand *et al.* 1999), and prognosis is poor, as 40% of patients die of vessel rupture or sepsis before surgery (Lane *et al.* 1988). Moreover, rupture of non-aneurysmal infected aorta, cued by retroperitoneal collections, can occur (Cook and Christopoulous 1989). The most common isolates from patients

with endovascular infection are *Salmonella typhimurium* (serogroup B), *Salmonella enteritidis* (serogroup D1), and *Salmonella enterica* serotype Choleraesuis (*S. choleraesuis*; serogroup C1), in that order (Soravia-Dunand *et al.* 1999; Oskoui *et al.* 1993). Albeit extremely uncommon below the age of 50, risks factors should be sought in younger patients with salmonella bacteremia or arteritis, especially if recurrent. In a 20-year retrospective study of 373 cases of non-typhoid salmonellosis, SLE, liver cirrhosis, HIV infection, and solid organ cancers were shown to be independent risk factors for salmonella bacteremia but the only independent positive predictor of endovascular infection was atherosclerosis, contrary to the traditional belief that chronic immunosuppression such as immunodeficiency and malignancies may be at play (Hsu and Lin 2005).

Other categories of aortitis include syphilitic, tuberculous, tropical, and lepromatous (Umerah 2002), which are discussed below. In addition, the aorta and surrounding structures are affected in several syndromes falling under the label of chronic periaortitis, such as idiopathic retroperitoneal fibrosis (see Chapter 34), mediastinal fibrosis, and inflammatory aneurysm (see Figures 19.21, 19.22 and 19.23 in Chapter 19).

Computed tomography is the most useful imaging modality for evaluating suspected infectious aortitis. MRI should be considered for the evaluation of patients with contraindications for the use of iodinated contrast media. Optimal treatment with early excision of infected aorta and bypass grafting, in combination with prolonged antibiotic administration, have improved outcomes (Soravia-Dunand *et al.* 1999; Wang *et al.* 1996; Fernandez Guerrero *et al.* 2004).

Septic phlebitis

Lemierre's syndrome (postanginal sepsis) rarely complicates an oropharyngeal infection in adolescent and young adults, evolving as a septic thrombophlebitis of the internal jugular vein with subsequent septicemia and metastatic lesions to the lungs and other sites (Moreno *et al.* 1989). The usual etiologic agent is *Fusobacterium necrophorum*, which may not be uniquely anaerobic. An inflammatory prothrombotic state characterized by antiphospholipid antibodies and elevated factor VIII levels has been suggested as an attendant pathogenic mechanism in the syndrome (Goldenberg *et al.* 2005). Early diagnosis and aggressive antimicrobial therapies are usually curative while the role of anticoagulation is controversial (Chirinos *et al.* 2000).

Septic thrombophlebitis of intra-abdominal vessels (pyephlebitis), such as the portal vein, inferior mesenteric vein, and gonadal vein, historically results from perforated viscus, most commonly diverticultis, or abdominal sepsis from trauma or surgery (Saxena *et al.* 1996). Bacteremia (often polymicrobial) was present in most patients with *Bacteroides fragilis* being the most common blood isolate (Plemmons *et al.* 1995). Detection of thrombus and venous gas by computed tomography is diagnostic (Lee *et al.* 1996). Septic ovarian thrombosis must be sought in females with puerperal fever, pelvic pain, or post pelvic surgery, as potentially fatal complications such as sepsis, septic pulmonary thromboembolism, and thrombosis of the inferior vena cava and the renal veins can ensue (Hippach *et al.* 2000).

Rickettsial vasculitis

Rickettsiae are arthropod-borne (ticks), Gram-negative, obligate intracellular bacteria which primarily infect endothelial cells. They cause systemic, multiorgan diseases such as Rocky Mountain spotted fever (RMSF; caused by *Rickettsia rickettsii*), and bouton-neuse fever (caused by *Rickettsia conorii*), a sporadic syndrome which may remain persistent (Dumler and Walker 2005). RMSF can be fatal, even in young immunocompetent individuals, if not ade-quately treated with antibiotics early during the course of the illness.

When *R. rickettsii* is introduced into the skin, it spreads via lymphatics into the circulation, infecting and replicating in the cytoplasm of its target endothelial cells. Individual rickettsial organisms then traverse cell-to-cell, utilizing actin polymerization-based directional motility for intracellular movements and inter-cellular spread (Heinzen 2003). The outer membrane proteins (Omps), purported immunogens capable of eliciting protective immune responses in experimental animals (Walker 1989), facilitate attachment to the endothelial cell membrane. Attachment (mediated by OmpA) is then followed by "induced phagocytosis" of the patho-gen into the cytosol, and a myriad of host cell immune responses follow, including the expression of mediators with important physiological functions such as adhesion molecules, cytokines, chemokines, and regulatory components of the coagulation cascade (Eremeeva *et al.* 2000). Activation of NF-κB plays a crucial role by controlling the expression of several procoagulant and proinflam-matory genes (Shi *et al.* 1998) and by protecting the host cells from apoptosis (Clifton *et al.* 1998). Cell damage has been associated with rickettsial phospholipase A2 and protease activities and free-radical-induced injury (Walker 1989). The net effect is a lymphohistocytic response with widespread vasculitis, most importantly in the brain and lungs, causing increased vascular permeability, edema, hypo-tension, and multiorgan failure. Hyponatremia may be due to hypo-volemia from capillary leak or inappropriate antidiuretic hormone secretion (Mouallem *et al.* 1987). Interstitial pneumonia, myo carditis, perivascular glial nodules of the CNS, and similar vascular nodules in the skin, GI tract, pancreas, liver, skeletal muscles, and kidneys have been observed (Walker and Raoult 2000).

The non-specific presentation poses a diagnostic challenge, and often leads to delayed therapy. Symptoms usually commence 2–14 days after the tick-bite with fever, headache, myalgias, nausea with or without vomiting, and abdominal pain (Kirk *et al.* 1990). The characteristic rash appears after 3–5 days and evolves from macular to maculopapular to petechial, on the ankles and wrists and then spreads centrally and to the palms and soles. Absence of the typical rash ("viscerotropic" RMSF) frequently delays diagnosis and is more commonly associated with fatal outcomes (Hattwick *et al.* 1976). An eschar at the site of tick bite may be evident on careful history and physical examination (Walker *et al.* 1981). Meningoencephalitis and neurological involvement is generally ominous (Horney and Walker 1988). Non-cardiogenic pulmonary edema and adult respiratory distress may require mechanical venti-lation. Azotemia, skin necrosis, and thrombocytopenia (true dis-seminated intravascular coagulation is rare), retinal vasculitis, and multifocal rhabdomyolysis are other complications. In fulminant RMSF, death occurs within the first 5 days, and is more often observed with increasing age, male gender, and presence of glucose-6-phosphate dehydrogenase deficiency (Hattwick *et al.* 1976, Walker 1990).

It remains prudent to inquire about travel history and tick expo-sures in the appropriate epidemiologic setting as early clinical diag-nosis can be life saving with empirical therapy with a tetracycline class antibiotic (Kirkland *et al.* 1995). Serologic analysis confirms diagnosis restrospectively only when antibodies appear during convalescence and is not useful during initial management. Polymerase chain reaction (PCR) analysis is insensitive, and immu-nohistochemical analysis of skin-biopsy specimens for *R. rickettsii* antigen is not widely available.

Viral-induced vasculitides

Viruses are frequently considered to be causative agents in vasculitis due to the frequent occurrence of circulating immune complexes during acute viral infection and the tropism of some viruses for cells comprising the vasculature. The associations of hepatitis B and hepatitis C with polyarteritis nodosa (PAN) and cryoglobuli-nemia are well recognized and are discussed in detail elsewhere. Vasculitis induced by herpes viruses, including cytomegalovirus (CMV), varicella zoster virus (VZV), and Epstein–Barr virus (EBV), has been reported predominantly in the context of immuno-suppression, with most reports involving transplant recipients, patients on chemotherapy for cancer, or patients with immunodefi-ciency due to HIV infection. Evidence for infection with various other viruses, including parvovirus B19, in the clinical setting of vasculitis affecting small, medium, or large-caliber vessels, has been documented in various case reports. With the possible exception of PAN and cryoglobulinemia associated with hepatitis B and hepatitis C viruses, the true prevalence and pathogenic role of these viruses in systemic vasculitis syndromes is not established. Nonetheless, as the role of viruses in vasculitis becomes better understood, treat-ment regimens incorporating therapies targeting specific viruses are playing a greater role in the management of vasculitis.

Parvovirus B19

Infection with human parvovirus B19 has been documented in the clinical setting of leukocytoclastic vasculitis (Chapter 39) and Henoch–Schönlein purpura (HSP) (Chapter 40) using seroconver-sion data as well as PCR amplification of parvovirus DNA from blood samples (Ferguson *et al.* 1996; Veraldi *et al.* 1999). Its DNA has also been identified in dermal and glomerular capillary endo-thelial cells and surrounding the dermal inflammatory cells (Cioc *et al.* 2002). A higher prevalence of human parvovirus B19 non-structural (NS1) DNA, which encodes a cytotoxic protein, has been observed in skin tissues of patients with HSP and "hypersensitivity vasculitis" compared with normal controls (Ohtsuka and Yamazaki 2005). The NS1 has also been shown to upregulate human interleu-kin-6 gene expression (Moffat *et al.* 1996) and to induce apoptosis in cells of the erythroid lineage (Moffat *et al.* 1998).

Combined serologic and DNA amplification approaches have also been used to link parvovirus infection with some cases of Kawasaki's disease (KD), although other studies refute this finding (Holm *et al.* 1995; Nigro *et al.* 1994; Rowley *et al.* 1994). Serologic and DNA evidence of parvovirus infection has also been reported in association with WG and medium-sized vessel vasculitis charac-teristic of PAN (Finkel *et al.* 1994). The presence of parvovirus in such cases may alter expected response to therapy. In three of the reported cases, manifestations of vasculitis responded poorly to treatment with glucocorticoids and cytotoxic agents, only to resolve following courses of high-dose intravenous gamma globulin (IVIg) (Finkel *et al.* 1994). Parvovirus DNA has also been PCR amplified from temporal artery biopsy specimens of patients with GCA, sug-gesting a possible role for the virus in the development of large-vessel vasculitis (Gabriel *et al.* 1999), particularly in those patients with high viral load (Álvarez-Lafuente R *et al.* 2005); however, results of recent studies did not corroborate this observation (Salvarani *et al.* 2002; Rodriguez-Pla *et al.* 2004). Furthermore, a similar frequency of B19 DNA localization was found in arterial surgical specimens obtained from age-matched controls with atherosclerotic carotid or aortic disease (Salvarani *et al.* 2002).

Cytomegalovirus

While CMV commonly produces invasive disease affecting multiple organs in the immunocompromised host, it is also capable of infecting endothelial cells leading to a clinical presentation consistent with small to medium-sized vessel vasculitis (Golden *et al.* 1994). The lesions associated with CMV vasculitis are most common in the gut or the skin, but their appearance is frequently non-specific; neurologic deficits due to central or peripheral nervous system infarcts may also appear (Koeppen *et al.* 1981; Golden *et al.* 1994; Tatum *et al.* 1989). Biopsy of lesions to identify cytomegalic endothelia and macrophages with intranuclear inclusions is required to establish the diagnosis. Early recognition of CMV-induced vasculitis in immunosuppressed patients is critical, even after apparently adequate anti-CMV prophylaxis (Zandberg *et al.* 2005), as favorable outcomes require prompt institution of antiviral therapy (with ganciclovir or foscarnet) and a decrease in the immunosuppressive regimen (Golden *et al.* 1994).

In transplant recipients, CMV infection may be difficult to differentiate from allograft rejection. In studies of allograft biopsies, CMV infection is associated with a higher prevalence of subintimal arteriolar allograft inflammation, and it is postulated that infection with CMV may promote the development of atherosclerotic lesions in the allograft (Koskinen *et al.* 1994). A diagnostic and therapeutic challenge arises when CMV-induced vasculitis occurs in patients who are on immunosuppressive therapy for treatment of other vasculitides, including Wegener's granulomatosis (WG) (Sackier *et al.* 1991; Weiss *et al.* 1993). Manifestations of CMV infection in such patients may mimic recrudescence of the underlying vasculitis; appropriate cultures, PCR studies, and mucosal biopsy specimens to rule out CMV infection should be procured in previously stable patients who develop new lesions involving the skin, lungs, glomeruli, gut, or CNS.

It should be recognized that CMV-induced vasculitis involving small or medium-sized arteries has also been reported to occur in patients without known immunodeficiency. CMV-associated enteric vasculitis, alveolar hemorrhage, and classic PAN have been reported in otherwise healthy, immunocompetent individuals (Fernandes *et al.* 1999; Taniwaki *et al.* 1997; Magro *et al.* 2005). Pulmonary septal capillary injury without classic inclusion body cytopathic change, which is morphologically indistinguishable from small-vessel vasculitis involving the lungs, has been described. Therefore primary CMV infection should be suspected in a setting of clinical worsening despite traditional immunosuppression of purported autoimmune vasculitis (Magro *et al.* 2005). CMV DNA sequences and proteins have also been identified in inflammatory lesions of the aorta, suggesting the virus may play a role in the pathogenesis of aortitis (Tanaka *et al.* 1994). While necrotizing arteritis may require glucocorticoid treatment initially, appropriate antiviral therapy should be instituted concurrently and promptly in patients with CMV-associated vasculitis.

Varicella zoster virus

Varicella zoster virus (VZV) vasculopathy in the central nervous system (CNS) affects large and small cerebral vessels and can follow either primary infection or reactivation of the virus. Stroke syndromes due to large-vessel disease (called unifocal vasculopathy but also known as granulomatous angiitis) are well recognized complications that occur mainly in immunocompetent individuals, weeks to months after contralateral herpes zoster ophthalmicus (Gilden 2004). In a reported case, VZV DNA and antigens were identified in the affected arterial tissues of an elderly male with segmental granulomatous angiitis of the CNS, in the absence of cutaneous or ophthalmic zoster (Gilden *et al.* 1996).

In contrast, small-vessel disease (multifocal vasculopathy) usually afflicts the immunocompromised patients, such as those with organ transplant, cancer, or AIDS. Cutaneous or ophthalmic manifestations of herpes zoster are more frequently absent, and the clinical course relatively subacute and protracted. A similar angiitis of the CNS affecting medium and large-caliber vessels resulting in cerebral infarction with evidence of varicella zoster virus (VZV) in the cerebrospinal fluid has been reported among HIV patients (Picard *et al.* 1997). Vascular involvement in these cases was typically patchy and segmental rather than diffuse, with some lesions identifiable using magnetic resonance angiography (MRA) or digital subtraction angiography (DSA). These cases emphasize the need to analyze cerebrospinal fluid (CSF) by PCR for VZV DNA and presence of VZV-specific antibody in patients with primary angiitis of the CNS, particularly when there is evidence of segmental narrowing of larger vessels or infarction of white matter.

HTLV-1

Human T cell lymphotropic virus-1 (HTLV-1) is one of several retroviruses capable of directly or indirectly inducing vascular lesions. In addition to inducing T cell lymphomas, HTLV-1 has been identified as a causative factor in a number of non-malignant inflammatory lesions, most notably a myelopathy classically described as tropical spastic paraparesis. Vascular complications of HTLV-1 infection include inflammation of the uveal tract with anterior uveitis and retinal vasculitis (Hayasaka *et al.* 1991; Watanabe *et al.* 1997). HTLV-1 infection is diagnosed by the presence of elevated serum or CNS antibody titers to HTLV-1 in an appropriate clinical setting.

Human immunodeficiency virus

The vasculitis syndromes associated with human immunodeficiency virus (HIV) are heterogeneous with regard to their clinical presentation and histologic appearance. Vascular inflammation in HIV-infected patients may occur as a result of host responses to HIV, complications of opportunistic infection, or hypersensitivity to antimicrobial and antiviral drugs. Moreover, a state of immune activation is characteristically observed among patients infected with HIV, creating a favorable milieu for the development and perpetuation of vascular inflammation. These considerations emphasize the need to carefully consider both the role of opportunistic infection and the biology of HIV when formulating a diagnostic and treatment approach to HIV patients who present with signs of vasculopathy.

In reported case series of HIV-related vasculitis, small-caliber arterial vessels in dermal, muscular, and peripheral neural tissues are most commonly affected, with peripheral neuropathy a common presenting manifestation (Calabrese 1991; Gherardi *et al.* 1993). Like other viruses, HIV may induce vascular inflammation as a consequence of humoral immune responses to viral antigens with formation and deposition of immune complexes in the vasculature.

Circulating immune complexes in response to HIV or opportunistic infection are frequently detected in HIV-positive individuals (Gupta and Licorish 1984), and deposition of these complexes may trigger a necrotizing arteritis comparable to that in hepatitis C-associated cryoglobulinemia or hepatitis B-associated PAN. Peripheral neuropathy associated with HIV-related necrotizing arteritis has been reported to respond favorably to glucocorticoids (Libman *et al.* 1995; Massari *et al.* 1996); complete recovery of neurologic function without untoward effects has been reported when initial glucocorticoid therapy is followed by antiretroviral therapy concurrent with plasmapheresis (Cohen *et al.* 1993).

HIV antigens have been detected in the perivascular cells of inflamed muscular and neural vessels (Chad *et al.* 1990; Gherardi *et al.* 1993), and it has been suggested that vasculitis may occur as a consequence of T cell-mediated host responses to HIV replicating within vascular or perivascular cells (Gherardi *et al.* 1993). Concomitant opportunistic infection may be of particular relevance to the development of vascular inflammation through this mechanism, as perivascular macrophages constitute reservoirs for latent HIV, and macrophage activation by cytokines such as tumor necrosis factor can promote HIV replication (Fauci 1988; Hickey and Kimura 1988). Local cytokine release within the vasculature in response to either deposition of immune complexes or direct infection of intimal cells by opportunistic viruses may promote HIV replication within these perivascular macrophages, perpetuating immune activation.

T-cell responses to perivascular foci of HIV replication may account for angiocentric lymphoproliferative lesions reported in HIV-infected patients (Calabrese 1991; Anders *et al.* 1989; Katsetos *et al.* 1999). These lesions are characterized by perivascular accumulation and transmural infiltration of CD8+ T cells; monocytes and macrophages within the infiltrate are immunoreactive to the p24 HIV core protein (Katsetos *et al.* 1999). Although arterial necrosis is not observed, an occlusive vasculopathy may occur, resulting in CNS or visceral organ compromise (Calabrese 1991); the lesions may potentially evolve into malignant lymphoma (Anders *et al.* 1989). It should be recognized that these angiocentric lesions are immunologically and pathologically distinct from the diffuse infiltrative CD8 lymphocytosis syndrome involving salivary glands and other visceral organs, in which vasculitis has not been a described feature (Itescu *et al.* 1990).

The immunocompromised nature of late-stage HIV infection mandates that opportunistic infection be considered when lesions suggestive of vasculitis appear in visceral organs or the CNS. As noted above, CMV should be considered in the setting of cutaneous, pulmonary, enteric, renal, or CNS vasculitis. Arterial inflammation of the CNS merits consideration of VZV (Picard *et al.* 1997), despite a disproportionate number of primary angiitis of the CNS being reported (Calabrese 1991). *Toxoplasma gondii* and herpes simplex virus should also be included in the differential diagnosis of CNS vascular lesions (De Girolami *et al.* 1990; Huang and Chou 1988). Infiltration of pulmonary vessels by *Pneumocystis carinii* has been associated with necrotizing vasculitis in the pulmonary parenchyma (Liu *et al.* 1989).

Syndromes resembling Kawasaki's disease (KD) in adult HIV-positive patients present with a constellation of signs and symptoms very similar to non-HIV children, except gastrointestinal complaints are more common and cervical lymphadenopathy less pronounced (Johnson *et al.* 2001). Presence of IgA plasma cells and paucity of complement proteins within vasculitic lesions is a feature unique to pediatric KD and has been observed in coronary arteries of young HIV-infected males who died of acute myocardial infarction (without atherosclerosis) after a flu-like illness (Johnson *et al.* 2003).

Cutaneous leukocytoclastic vasculitis in HIV-infected patients, most commonly presenting as palpable purpura, also merits consideration of opportunistic infection with bacteria or viruses such as CMV, hepatitis B, hepatitis C, or EBV. Reactions to antiviral or antimicrobial drugs, most commonly sulfonamides, are observed frequently in HIV patients and should be considered a potential cause of cutaneous vasculitis (Battegay *et al.* 1989; Dover and Johnson 1991; Gordin *et al.* 1984). HSP with dermal vascular deposits of IgA has also been reported in patients with early as well as late-stage HIV infection (Gherardi *et al.* 1993). Microvascular inflammation may occur in the early, acute stage of HIV infection, but lesions in the exanthem are characterized by perivascular infiltrates of mononuclear cells without evidence of leukocytoclasis (Balslev *et al.* 1990; McMillan *et al.* 1989). Included in the spectrum of leukocytoclastic vasculitis associated-lesions that occurs in patients with HIV infection is erythema elevatum diutinum.

Epstein–Barr virus

By virtue of its tropism for, and transforming properties of, lymphoid cells, and its ability to trigger typical immune responses, EBV may be associated with an unusual variety of vascular and perivascular syndromes. EBV may infect cells comprising the vasculature, demonstrated by studies of patients with granulomatous angiitis involving medium-sized and large arteries, where EBV DNA sequences have been found in intimal and medial tissues (Ban *et al.* 1999; Murakami *et al.* 1998). Immune-complex mediated vasculitis involving smaller-caliber vessels and renal glomeruli has also been reported to occur during acute EBV infection (Lande *et al.* 1998).

A number of studies have demonstrated significant associations between infection with EBV and coronary artery aneurysms and other inflammatory lesions of the aorta reminiscent of KD. In several series of Japanese patients, a significantly greater prevalence of EBV DNA sequences has been demonstrated in circulating mononuclear cells of patients with KD and coronary artery aneurysms than among age-matched controls (Kikuta *et al.* 1991, 1992). Coronary artery aneurysms, similar to those observed in KD, have been reported among patients with acute or chronic EBV infection (Kanegane *et al.* 1994; Nakagawa *et al.* 1996). While not all patients with KD have evidence of EBV infection, the correlation between coronary artery aneurysms and systemic and local EBV infection in these patients is intriguing and worthy of continued investigation.

Transformation of EBV-infected B cell lymphocytes and NK cells may result in several vascular syndromes associated with angiocentric lymphoid proliferation. The majority of patients with lymphomatoid granulomatosis have evidence of EBV DNA sequences within the lymphoproliferative lesions. These EBV sequences are enriched in B cells and are not typically found in the large numbers of non-clonally related T cells (Guinee *et al.* 1994). These data have led to the hypothesis that vascular lesions in lymphomatoid granulomatosis (LG) constitute T cells responding to EBV-infected B cells in and around the vasculature. Such findings also serve to distinguish lymphomatoid granulomatosis from angiocentric T cell lymphomas, where there is evidence of clonal T-cell expansion (Guinee *et al.* 1994). Due to its propensity for multiorgan involvement, most frequently the lungs, and the histological features of angiitis, LG often mimics systemic vasculitis, most notably WG (Liebow *et al.* 1972). LG occurs most commonly in immunodeficiency states, such as AIDS, Wiskott–Aldrich syndrome, and post-transplantation immunodeficiency (Jaffe *et al.* 1997), but has been associated with autoimmune disorders including Sjögren's syndrome, rheumatoid arthritis (RA), and SLE (Beste *et al.* 2005). EBV transformation of NK cells resulting in multisystem vascular infiltration by clonally expanded, large, granular lymphocytes has also been reported (Gelb *et al.* 1994) further adding to the spectrum of EBV-associated vasculopathies.

Vasculitis associated with immunodeficiencies

Wiskott–Aldrich syndrome

Autoimmune manifestations, including vasculitis syndromes, are sometimes observed as a consequence of immune dysregulation in patients with genetic immunodeficiencies. The Wiskott–Aldrich syndrome (WAS) is an X-linked disorder manifested by thrombocytopenia, severe immunodeficiency, and eczema. The molecular basis of the disorder has been shown to reside in mutations of WASP, a protein mediating the transduction of signals from the cell membrane to the actin cytoskeleton in hematopoietic cells. Impairment of WASP-mediated signaling results in the disruption of a wide array of leukocyte functions, including maturation of thymocytes, neutrophil phagocytosis, T cell antigen receptor (TCR)-triggered proliferative responses and IL-2 production, and TCR-triggered apoptotic responses (Zhang *et al.* 1999).

A variety of vascular lesions has been reported in WAS patients, most commonly leukocytoclastic vasculitis and aortitis. Aortitis with aortic aneurysm and stenotic lesions of aortic branch vessels have been reported in children as well as adults (Lau *et al.* 1992; van Son *et al.* 1995). Aneurysmal dilatation of medium-caliber splanchnic and renal vessels with histologic evidence of necrotizing arteritis has also been reported, as has pulmonary vasculitis histologically indistinguishable from LG (Ilowite *et al.* 1986; McCluggage *et al.* 1999). It has been speculated that impaired host defense against viral pathogens known to engender vascular inflammation (see above) may account for some of the vasculitis complications observed in WAS (Ilowite *et al.* 1986).

X-linked lymphoproliferative disorder

EBV infection or reactivation within endothelial cells may precipitate a cytotoxic T lymphocyte (CTL)-mediated vasculitis in patients with X-linked lymphoproliferative (XLP) disease, an immunodeficiency characterized by fulminant EBV infection, lymphoproliferative disorder, and dysgammaglobulinemia (Dutz *et al.* 2001). The diagnosis can be confirmed by genetic analysis for mutated SH2D1A/DSHP/SLAM-associated protein (SAP). Mutations in the protein confer severe immune deficiency to EBV infection and EBV-transformed cells (Sharifi *et al.* 2004), perhaps via defective polarization of the lytic machinery of NK cells and cytotoxic T lymphocytes (Dupre *et al.* 2005).

Purine nucleoside phosphorylase deficiency

Cerebral vasculitis is a reported complication in patients with deficiency of purine nucleoside phosphorylase (PNP), a rare autosomal recessive condition accounting for approximately 5% of cases of severe combined immunodeficiency (Markert 1991). Deficiency of PNP results in accumulation of deoxyguanosine and deoxyinosine; the dGTP and dITP metabolites of these purines are highly toxic to developing T cells. Affected individuals experience frequent disseminated bacterial, fungal, and viral infections. It is conceivable that the cerebral vasculitis observed in the context of PNP deficiency may be due to infection with VZV.

Vasculitis associated with sarcoidosis

Sarcoidosis is a multisystem, inflammatory disease characterized by the presence of non-caseating granulomas in affected tissues. The cause of sarcoidosis has remained elusive, but recent work has implied a potential role for microbial pathogens (most notably cell wall-deficient L forms of mycobacteria) in triggering the granulomatous inflammation and other immune abnormalities seen in this disorder (Almenoff *et al.* 1996; Newman *et al.* 1997). Epithelioid cells surrounded by large numbers of CD4+ T lymphocytes exhibiting a Th1 phenotype characterize the immunopathology of sarcoid granulomas (Hunninghake and Crystal 1981). Although the prevalence of sarcoidosis is as high as 60/100,000 in Caucasians of northern European descent (Sartwell 1976) and 107/100,000 in African-American females (Rybicki *et al.* 1997), vasculitis occurs as a rare manifestation.

Consistent with the observation that sarcoidosis can affect almost any organ system, vascular complications may involve large, medium, or small-caliber vessels. Large-vessel granulomatous vasculitis in sarcoidosis involves the aortic arch and may be histologically indistinguishable from that of GCA or TA (Faye-Petersen *et al.* 1991; Marcussen and Lund 1989; Murai *et al.* 1986; Rose *et al.* 1990). GCA involving large vessels occurring in association with systemic non-necrotizing granulomatous disease has been reported most commonly in children but has also been reported in adults. Complications include aortic dissection, saccular aortic aneurysm, myocardial infarction, stroke, and limb ischemia (Faye-Petersen *et al.* 1991; Numata *et al.* 2005; Marcussen and Lund 1989; Murai *et al.* 1986). Although the prevalence of sarcoidosis among adult patients with GCA is unknown, the reported cases of large-vessel vasculitis in patients with granulomatous inflammation involving other organs emphasize the need to consider sarcoidosis in the differential diagnosis of large-vessel vasculitis. Moreover, the possibility of large-vessel involvement should be entertained in adult as well as pediatric patients with established sarcoidosis who present with syndromes consistent with visceral organ or limb ischemia.

Pulmonary vascular lesions in sarcoidosis are characterized by granulomatous angiitis involving veins or arteries. Published series of open lung and transbronchial biopsies of patients with established sarcoidosis indicate venous involvement in the vast majority of cases, combined venous and arterial involvement in one-fourth to one-third of patients, and isolated arterial involvement in 8–11% of biopsied patients (Rosen *et al.* 1977; Takemura *et al.* 1991). Necrotizing sarcoid granulomatosis (NSG) is a form of pulmonary vasculitis that may be a variant of nodular pulmonary sarcoidosis (Churg *et al.* 1979; Leavitt and Fauci 1986; Tauber *et al.* 1999). Histologically, these lesions are characterized by foci of confluent granulomas with variable amounts of tissue necrosis and hyalinization, and a granulomatous vasculitis that resembles the vascular lesions noted in open lung biopsies of patients with established sarcoidosis. Although the histologic appearance of granulomatous vasculitis associated with sarcoidosis may be similar to that seen in WG, the prognosis is much more favorable, with patients improving either without therapy or with a limited course of glucocorticoids (Churg *et al.* 1979; Tauber *et al.* 1999). Differentiating features include greater degrees of liquefactive necrosis, abundance of eosinophils, and paucity of perivascular lymphocytes and plasma cells in the WG lesions, and the absence of antineutrophil cytoplasmic antibodies and granulocytic vascular inflammation in patients with NSG (DeRemee 1994; Saldana *et al.* 1977; Popper *et al.* 2003).

Extrapulmonary complications of necrotizing or non-necrotizing granulomatous inflammation of small caliber arteries may include peripheral mononeuritis with foot drop, myelopathy, myositis, cutaneous ulcers, myositis, and digital gangrene (Diri *et al.* 1999; Gibson *et al.* 1994; Kwong *et al.* 1994; Petri *et al.* 1988; Prayson 1999; Takemura *et al.* 1997).

Circulating immune complexes may engender a leukocytoclastic vasculitis with various cutaneous manifestations, including erythema annulare centrifugum and palpable purpura (Aractingi *et al.* 1993; Branford *et al.* 1982; Cecchi and Giomi 1999; García-Porrua *et al.* 1998; Johnston and Kennedy 1984). These cutaneous complications occur most commonly in patients with early, acute disease, with erythema nodosum as an accompanying feature. Other reported manifestations of sarcoidosis attributed to inflammatory lesions of small vessels include posterior uveitis, retinitis (see Chapter 12), and cranial neuropathies (Babin *et al.* 1984; Caplan *et al.* 1983; Sivakumar and Chee 1998).

Manifestations of sarcoidosis due to vascular inflammation usually respond to limited courses of glucocorticoids. Acute pulmonary and neuromuscular complications can be successfully managed with the equivalent of 1.0 mg of prednisone per kg of body weight administered daily. Although the evidence is anecdotal, methotrexate (10–25 mg/week) has been used with success as a steroid-sparing agent, as has daily oral azathioprine (2 mg/kg) (Baughman and Lower 1977; Diri *et al.* 1999). Cyclophosphamide is not typically used for sarcoidosis, but may be required in the rare patient with extrapulmonary necrotizing vasculitis (Kwong *et al.* 1994).

Cogan's syndrome

Cogan's syndrome is a rare inflammatory disease consisting of interstitial keratitis, vestibular dysfunction, and sensorineural hearing loss. Although ocular and vestibuloauditory symptoms predominate, some patients develop features of systemic vasculitis, including aortitis and mesenteric arteritis. The disease occurs most frequently in young adults of either sex, but may develop in children or the elderly (Fidler and Jones 1989; Haynes *et al.* 1980; Shepherd 1994; Vollertsen *et al.* 1986).

The cause of Cogan's syndrome is unknown. Elevated antibody titers to *Chlamydia trachomatis* in some patients (Hammer *et al.* 1994; Haynes *et al.* 1980; Ljunstrom *et al.* 1997) and at least one instance of *Chlamydia psittaci* isolated from the conjunctiva of a patient with Cogan's syndrome (Darougar *et al.* 1978) have provoked interest in a possible role for chlamydia species in triggering the disease. Subsequent attempts to culture chlamydia from the eyes of other affected patients or identify chlamydial antigens in ocular tissues have been unsuccessful (St Clair and McCallum 1999). Similarities between the corneal and vascular findings seen in syphilis and those in Cogan's syndrome have prompted consideration of other spirochete species such as *Borrelia burgdorferi* as a causal link (Fox *et al.* 1990), but definitive evidence for infection with such organisms has not been established in patients with Cogan's syndrome.

The initial presentation of Cogan's syndrome may consist of ocular symptoms in the absence of vestibuloauditory symptoms or vice versa; however, the majority of patients develop symptoms referable to both organ systems within a year. Symptoms of the interstitial keratitis include blurred vision, photophobia, perilimbal erythema, and ocular pain. Subepithelial keratitis in the periphery of the anterior corneal stroma is an early finding on slit-lamp examination (Cobo and Haynes 1984). Deeper, granular corneal infiltrates are characteristic of more advanced lesions. Other less common ocular manifestations of Cogan's syndrome that may occur in the absence or presence of interstitial keratitis include conjunctivitis, episcleritis, anterior or posterior scleritis, and retinal vasculitis (Haynes *et al.* 1980; Shah *et al.* 1994; Vollertsen *et al.* 1986). Vestibular symptoms typically begin abruptly with vertigo, ataxia, nausea, or vomiting. Abnormal vestibular responses are seen on electronystagmometry and caloric testing. Hearing loss typically presents as poor speech discrimination, with audiometric testing revealing evidence of sensorineural hearing loss at middle and high frequencies. Changes in hearing often coincide with flares of disease activity, and permanent, severe hearing loss occurs frequently, in up to two-thirds of cases (Haynes *et al.* 1980; Vollertsen *et al.* 1986).

Histopathologic studies of corneal and vestibuloauditory organs from patients with early disease are limited. Corneal tissues from patients with interstitial keratitis are remarkable for infiltrates of plasma cells and lymphocytes into the deeper layers of the cornea, with variable degrees of scarring and neovascularization. Histologic sections of temporal bones obtained at autopsy have revealed infiltration of the spiral ligament with lymphocytes and plasma cells, demyelination and atrophy of the vestibular and cochlear nerves, and degeneration of the organ of Corti, cochlea, and vestibular apparatus (Fisher and Hellstrom 1961; Schuknecht and Nadol 1994). Evidence of vasculitis has not been seen; however, the shortest interval from disease onset to autopsy in cases reported to date has been 4 years.

Vasculitis involving the aorta, aortic arch vessels, or large muscular arteries occurs in approximately 10% of patients with Cogan's syndrome (Haynes *et al.* 1980; Vollertsen *et al.* 1986). Aortitis may produce thoracoabdominal aneurysm (Tseng *et al.* 1999), and involvement of the proximal ascending aorta as well as the valve cusps may result in aortic valve regurgitation necessitating valve replacement (Cochrane and Tatoulis 1991; Hammer *et al.* 1994; Livingston *et al.* 1992). Coronary arteries may be compromised due to arteritis or involvement of the coronary ostia in aortitis (Livingston *et al.* 1992; Vollertsen *et al.* 1986). Narrowing of the major branches of the aorta at their orifice similar to that observed in TA may result in upper extremity claudication (Cochrane and Tatoulis 1991; Raza *et al.* 1998). The histologic appearance of lesions in the aorta and large muscular arteries is similar to that observed in GCA, with lymphocytes, plasma cells, and neutrophils infiltrating the vessel wall, intimal proliferation, disruption of the internal elastic lamina, and multinucleate giant cells (Cochrane and Tatoulis 1991; Fisher and Hellstrom 1961; Gelfand *et al.* 1972; Haynes *et al.* 1980; Livingston *et al.* 1992).

Arteritis of medium-caliber vessels occurs in a smaller percentage of patients. Reported complications include limb ischemia, mesenteric insufficiency, renal artery rupture, and renal artery stenosis with hypertension (Allen *et al.* 1990; Bastug *et al.* 1997; Ho *et al.* 1999; Raza *et al.* 1998; Thomas 1992; Vella *et al.* 1997). Typical of arteritis affecting medium-caliber arteries, the walls of affected vessels are infiltrated with lymphocytes, plasma cells and, to a lesser extent, eosinophils and neutrophils (Fisher and Hellstrom 1961). Involvement of smaller caliber arteries as well as veins (Fisher and Hellstrom 1961) may account for the non-corneal ocular manifestations and other reported complications such as lacunar infarcts of the CNS, inflammatory arthritis, and pericarditis (Cheson *et al.* 1976; Karni *et al.* 1991; Pinals 1978).

The diagnosis of Cogan's syndrome rests on both ocular inflammation and evidence of vestibuloauditory dysfunction. Although evidence of vasculitis involving other organ systems is not required, Cogan's syndrome should be considered in any patient presenting with manifestations of systemic vasculitis accompanied by visual or vestibuloauditory symptoms. MRI may be useful in differentiating Cogan's syndrome from cerebellopontine angle tumors and other CNS disorders that could account for vestibuloauditory symptoms. In several patients with Cogan's syndrome, enhancement of vestibular and cochlear structures has been observed using gadolinium imaging (Majoor *et al.* 1993; St Clair and McCallum 1999). Obliteration of vestibular and labyrinth structures in some patients with well-established disease has been noted on MRI or CT scan (Casselman *et al.* 1994; Majoor *et al.* 1993).

Glucocorticoids constitute the mainstay of therapy for acute flares and recurrences of the ocular and vestibuloauditory manifestations. Keratitis and anterior uveitis are usually responsive to topical glucocorticoids, whereas posterior scleritis and retinitis require treatment with oral glucocorticoids (McCallum 1996; St Clair and McCallum 1999). Prompt and early treatment of vestibuloauditory manifestations with high-dose oral prednisone (1–2 mg/kg/day) is reported to improve outcomes and is recommended to prevent permanent hearing loss (Haynes *et al.* 1981). Azathioprine, methotrexate, cyclosporin, tacrolimus (FK506), or cyclophosphamide may be used as steroid-sparing agents or for steroid-resistant ocular inflammation or vestibuloauditory dysfunction (Allen *et al.* 1990; Reinte *et al.* 1996; Richardson 1994; Roat *et al.* 1991). For patients who develop permanent, severe bilateral hearing loss, cochlear implants have been shown to be a relatively safe and effective intervention for at least partial restoration of functional hearing (Degos 1966; Kohlmeier 1941).

Patients with aortitis respond favorably to oral glucocorticoids. Prescribed in a manner similar to that for the management of GCA or TA, initial treatment with prednisone (1 mg/kg/day) can be followed by slow tapering of the dose. Published experience of other immunosuppressive agents to manage aortitis or large-vessel vasculitis associated with Cogan's syndrome is limited to case reports. Concomitant therapy with daily cyclophosphamide, azathioprine, cyclosporin, or low-dose weekly methotrexate may be used to minimize the duration of high-dose glucocorticoid therapy (Allen *et al.* 1990; Raza *et al.* 1998; Tseng *et al.* 1999). Methotrexate has also been used to maintain remission of the vascular lesions following initial therapy with glucocorticoids and cyclophosphamide (Raza *et al.* 1998). Necrotizing vasculitis involving medium caliber vessels may be severe, if not life-threatening, and usually warrants the use of daily cyclophosphamide (2 mg/kg) concomitant with initiation of glucocorticoids.

Degos' syndrome

Initially described in independent case reports published in the early 1940s by Kohlmeier (1941) and Degos (1966), Degos' syndrome is a rare, occlusive vasculopathy of unknown etiology characterized by multiple cutaneous, mesenteric, and central nervous system infarcts. The disorder has been referred to by a number of eponyms including Kohlmeier–Degos disease, malignant atrophic papulosis, progressive arterial mesenteric vascular disease, or disseminated intestinal and cutaneous thromboangiitis. The skin lesions associated with Degos' syndrome are distinctive, typically appearing in crops of painless, minimally elevated papules less than 5 mm in diameter (Figure 42.1). Initially gray, pale yellow, or rose in color, the papules turn white and develop a depressed center, giving rise to the 'porcelain drop' lesions pathognomonic for the syndrome (Tzanck *et al.* 1948). Margins of the papules are initially erythematous or violaceous, later resolving into a filiform border. A detachable scale frequently develops over the top of the papule (Degos 1979). The cutaneous lesions, which are not pruritic and do not ulcerate, appear predominantly on the trunk and proximal extremities (Degos 1979).

Degos' syndrome has been reported to occur in young infants and in the elderly, but predominantly affects young and middle-aged adults (Cabre *et al.* 1974; Magrinat *et al.* 1989; Soter *et al.* 1982). Although the vast majority of reported cases involve Caucasians, the syndrome has also been reported in African-Americans, Asian Indians, and Japanese (Naylor *et al.* 1960; Ogawa *et al.* 1967; Premalatha *et al.* 1980). Clinical variants associated with the cutaneous appearance of Degos' lesions include a benign cutaneous type that affects only the skin, a systemic type wherein visceral manifestations occur months to years following the onset of the skin manifestations, and a hereditary type in which familial clustering has been observed (Kisch and Bruyzeel 1984; Newton and Black 1984).

In patients with the systemic variant of Degos' syndrome, the appearance of multiple dermal infarcts is the initial and dominant feature, but mesenteric and CNS infarcts are responsible for the fatal outcomes frequently seen in this variant. The initial symptoms of intestinal involvement are often non-specific. Hemorrhages and perforations complicated by peritonitis comprise the major serious intestinal complications of the vasculopathy. Typical findings at laparotomy and autopsy include white infarcts ranging from 0.5 to 3 cm on the bowel serosa, most commonly involving the small intestine (Degos 1979; Fruhwirth *et al.* 1997; Su *et al.* 1985). Other reported visceral complications include fibrous pericarditis, pulmonary infarcts, and pleural reactions (Degos 1979; Su *et al.* 1985). Neurological complications include: seizures; ptosis; diplopia; optic neuritis; loss of visual fields; stroke syndromes; and polyradiculoneuropathy (Degos 1979; Su *et al.* 1985; Subbiah *et al.* 1996). CNS infarcts and hemorrhages with intravascular thrombi, often in the absence of demonstrable vasculitis, are characteristic findings at autopsy (Subbiah *et al.* 1996).

It is important to note that cutaneous lesions that are grossly and histologically indistinguishable from Degos' lesions have also been demonstrated in patients with systemic lupus erythematosus (atrophie blanche), dermatomyositis, polymyositis, and systemic

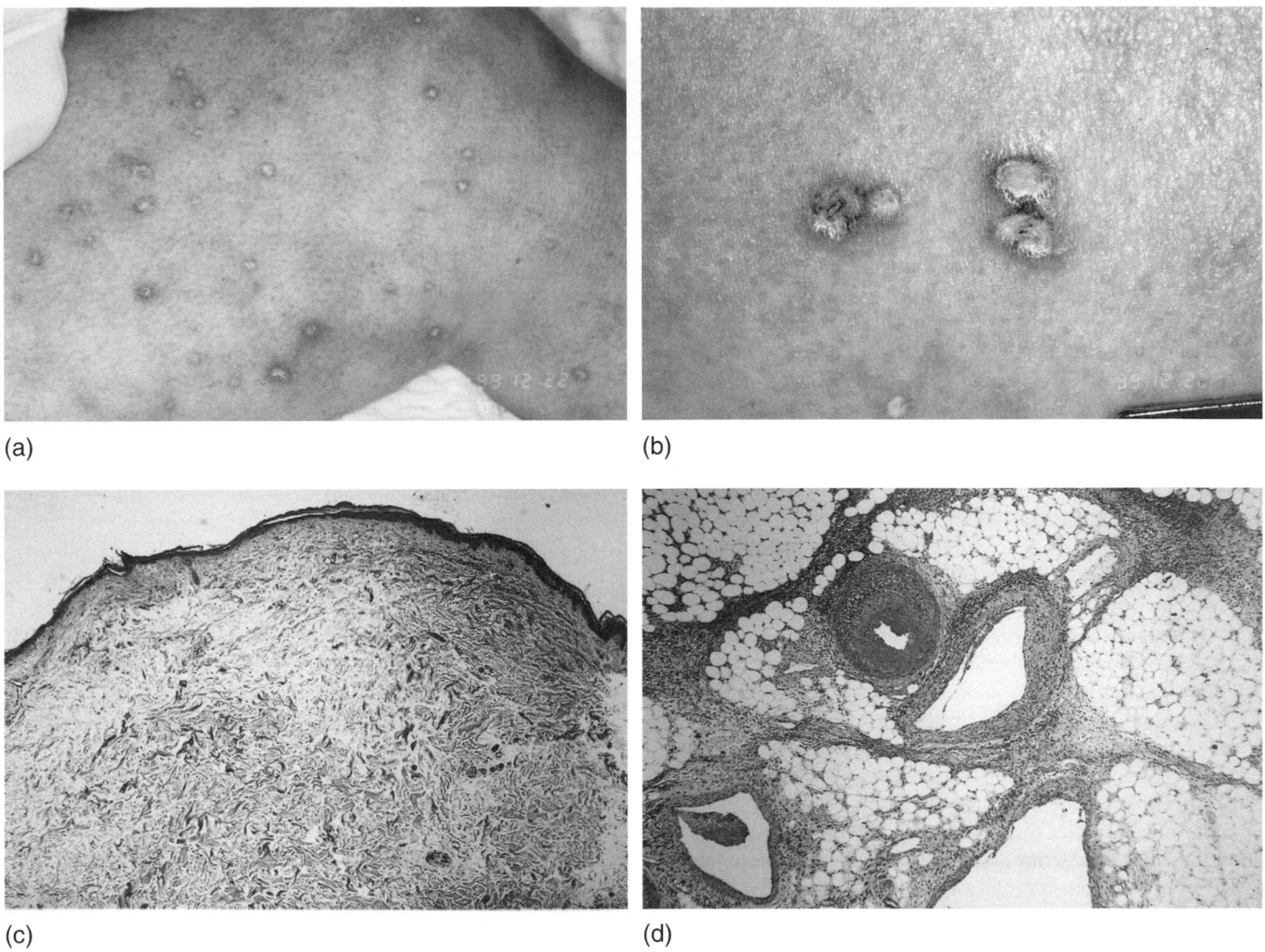

(a)

(b)

(c)

(d)

Figure 42.1 Cutaneous lesions of Degos' syndrome. (a) Skin lesions on the thigh of an affected individual.
(b) Close-up view of lesions demonstrating pale yellow papules with violaceous margins; lesion on the left has overlying scale.
(c) Photomicrograph of skin lesion demonstrating edematous, relatively acellular dermis. (d) Involved arteriole and vein
in subjacent pannicular tissue demonstrating perivascular lymphoid infiltrates, proliferation of endothelium, and arteriolar
thrombus. (Courtesy of Dr M. K. Abele.) (See Color Plate 120).

sclerosis (Black and Hudson 1976; Dubin and Stawiski 1974; Durie *et al.* 1969; Torok *et al.* 1993; Olmos and Laugier 1977; Sollberg 1987). Distinguishing features in the reported cases associated with SLE include the presence of other manifestations of lupus as well as granular basal membrane deposits of IgM, IgG, and C3 at the dermoepidermal junction (Black and Hudson 1976; Dubin and Stawiski 1974; Torok *et al.* 1993). Among these few reported cases associated with systemic autoimmune disease, the presence of Degos' lesions did not significantly impact on the course of the underlying disease (Black and Hudson 1976; Dubin and Stawiski 1974). The observation of Degos' lesions in other autoimmune disorders lends support to the contention that Degos' lesions may represent a common end point of a variety of vascular insults (High *et al.* 2004).

Histopathologic features of the cutaneous and visceral lesions of Degos' syndrome have engendered controversy with regard to whether the lesions arise primarily as a consequence of vascular inflammation, focal coagulation abnormalities, or abnormal

deposition of mucin (Magrinat *et al.* 1989). The characteristic histologic feature of the cutaneous lesion seen in Degos' syndrome is traditionally described as an "inverted cone of necrobiosis", with an atrophic hyperkeratotic epidermis at the base, a thrombosed dermal vessel at the apex, and accumulation of acid mucopolysaccharide or mucin in the edematous, acellular cone (Degos 1952; Soter *et al.* 1982; Su *et al.* 1985). Endothelial swelling and proliferation is seen in the affected dermal vessels, some of which contain platelet-fibrin thrombi within their lumens. A number of early histopathologic studies noted a paucity of vascular inflammation in Degos' lesions. With use of more refined techniques, infiltrates of lymphocytes and occasional monocytes can be demonstrated either within or around the walls of arterioles and venules in the majority of lesions (Soter *et al.* 1982; Su *et al.* 1985). There have been no reports of disruptions of the internal elastic lamina, infiltration by neutrophils, or leukocytoclasis.

The presence of thrombi in dermal and mesenteric vessels and the paucity of vascular inflammation observed by some investigators have prompted investigations to establish Degos' syndrome primarily as a coagulopathy (Daniel *et al.* 1982; Magrinat *et al.* 1989; Paramo *et al.* 1985). Levels of fibrinogen; antithrombin III; plasminogen; von Willibrand factor; protein C; activity of antithrombin III, plasminogen, and α2-antiplasmin; platelet aggregation times; activated partial thromboplastin times; and fibrin assembly kinetics are generally normal in patients with Degos' syndrome (Durie *et al.* 1969; Magrinat *et al.* 1989; Muller and Landry 1974; Sotrel *et al.* 1983). The failure to demonstrate evidence of a systemic coagulopathy has accordingly suggested that the platelet-fibrin thrombi observed in Degos' lesions form secondary to other factors related to the microvasculature. The concomitant occurrence of anticardiolipin antibodies and lupus anticoagulant with Degos' lesions has been reported, and Degos' lesions have been reported in lupus anticoagulant-positive patients with SLE (Englert *et al.* 1984; Stephansson *et al.* 1991). The overall prevalence of antiphospholipid antibodies among individuals with Degos' syndrome is not known.

Originally considered to be an epiphenomenon of the dermal injury and necrobiosis, the role of mucin accumulation in the evolution of Degos' lesions has been reconsidered (Magrinat *et al.* 1989). Mucin-related glycoproteins with thrombogenic potential are consistently found in early, as well as in established, Degos' lesions. It is conceivable that their accumulation in or around dermal vessels may promote formation of dermal thrombi (Kyung-Whan *et al.* 1980; Magrinat *et al.* 1989). Since activated T cells have been shown to induce mucin production by follicular keratinocytes (Reed 1981), mucin production in response to T-cell cytokines may constitute one of the mechanistic links between immunologic activation in and around the vasculature and the thrombosis with infarction observed in Degos' lesions.

Roles for immunologic mechanisms in triggering the endothelial abnormalities observed in Degos' syndrome have not been proven or excluded. Antibodies with specificity for arterial endothelium or other vessel wall components have been documented in the serum of patients with Degos' syndrome (Basset *et al.* 1969; Degos *et al.* 1967), but such antibodies lack disease specificity as they are found in patients with malignant hypertension or atherosclerosis, and are not uncommon in normal subjects (Cerilli *et al.* 1985; Gudbrandsson *et al.* 1981; Kristensen *et al.* 1984). The significance of these antibodies with regard to the evolution of the endothelial alterations in Degos' lesions remains undetermined. Antibody-mediated alterations of the vasculature otherwise appear to play a negligible role in Degos' syndrome, as deposits of immunoglobulin or complement have not been consistently demonstrated in lesions (with the exception of those associated with SLE) (Hall-Smith 1964; Muller and Landry 1974; Pallensen and Rasmussen 1979; Su *et al.* 1985).

The identification by electron microscopy of "virus-like" inclusions in the cytoplasm of affected endothelial cells has merited consideration of a viral etiology for Degos' syndrome (Bleehen 1977; Howard and Nishida 1969; Olmos and Laugier 1977); however, the observation of similar cytoplasmic inclusions in tumor cells, experimentally induced wounds, and in skin lesions of patients with SLE or dermatomyositis suggests that the inclusions in endothelial cells of Degos' lesions might be induced by factors other than viruses (Eady and Odland 1975; Olmos *et al.* 1979; Schaff *et al.* 1972; Uzman *et al.* 1971). The observation that recombinant alpha or beta interferons induce tubuloreticular structures such as those seen in Degos' lesions and other disorders has provided indirect evidence that interferon-secreting cells such as activated T lymphocytes might well be involved in the early events triggering modification of the endothelium (Rich 1981; Rich and Owens 1982).

Despite a postulated role for lymphocyte-mediated vascular inflammation and activated T cells in the pathogenesis of Degos' syndrome, the response to treatment with glucocorticoids and other immunosuppressive regimens has been uniformly disappointing (Englert *et al.* 1984; Hall-Smith 1969; Strole *et al.* 1967; Su *et al.* 1985; Subbiah *et al.* 1996). The ubiquitous appearance of luminal platelet-fibrin thrombi in Degos' lesions has prompted the use of antiplatelet agents and anticoagulants to avoid thrombotic complications. Several patients without known visceral complications improved during treatment with aspirin and dipyridamole (Su *et al.* 1985). In other cases with more systemic involvement, antiplatelet agents and plasma exchange were not helpful. Heparin appears to have been of benefit in some cases, but outcome data with regard to the use of chronic anticoagulation is not available.

Urticarial vasculitis

Chronic or recurrent urticaria is common, but only approximately 10% of patients with chronic urticarial lesions have associated vasculitis (Wisnieski 2000). Urticarial vasculitis (see Figure 10.3 in Chapter 10) may be a manifestation of SLE, Sjögren's syndrome, or mixed cryoglobulinemia. In patients with urticarial vasculitis, IgG antibodies reactive to the C1q subunit of the first component of complement, and markedly low serum levels of C1q, have traditionally been given a diagnosis of hypocomplementemic urticarial vasculitis (HUV) (Zeiss *et al.* 1980). In addition to low serum levels of C1q, patients with HUV may have modest to marked depletion of C4, C2, or C3. Levels of C1r, C1s, the fifth through ninth components of complement (C5–C9), as well as factor B and factor D are generally normal (Zeiss *et al.* 1980). Skin biopsy specimens of urticarial and purpuric lesions characteristically reveal leukocytoclastic vasculitis with granular deposition of C3, C1q, and immunoglobulin in the basement membrane zone (Davis *et al.* 1998; Sanchez *et al.* 1982).

Common extracutaneous clinical features observed in patients with HUV include angioedema, ocular inflammation, arthritis, and glomerulonephritis (Wisnieski *et al.* 1995; Zeiss *et al.* 1980). The arthritis is typically non-erosive and deforming, but may evolve into a Jaccoud's-like arthropathy with reversible subluxation of the metacarpophalangeal joints (Palazzo *et al.* 1993; Sturgess and Littlejohn 1988). Mesangial, and membranous, as well as membranoproliferative, lesions have been noted on renal biopsy (Fortson *et al.* 1986; Kobayashi *et al.* 1994; Wisnieski *et al.* 1995). A high prevalence of obstructive pulmonary disease, causing substantial morbidity and mortality, has been reported in HUV (Wisnieski *et al.* 1995). Although deaths from respiratory failure have been observed primarily in patients who smoke cigarettes, significant obstructive lung disease has also been reported in non-smokers with HUV (Eiser *et al.* 1997). Lung biopsies reveal severe emphysema with immunoglobulin deposition and thickening of blood vessel walls (Fortson *et al.* 1986). Less commonly reported clinical features include pericarditis, regurgitant valvular lesions, and vasculitis involving medium to large-caliber arteries (Babajanians *et al.* 1991; Palazzo *et al.* 1993; Sturgess and Littlejohn 1988).

Since the presence of antibodies to C1q and low levels of C1q, C2, C3, C4 are frequently observed in patients with SLE, and HUV may be a feature of SLE, it has been cogently argued that HUV represents a subset of SLE (Davis *et al.* 1998; Trendelenburg *et al.* 1999). In addition to the presence of antibodies to C1q and a continuous band of immunoreactants along the epidermal basement membrane, other immunologic features shared with SLE include a high prevalence of antiendothelial cell antibodies and shared anti-C1q IgG antibody binding properties (D'Cruz *et al.* 1995; Martensson *et al.* 1992; Nurnberg *et al.* 1995; Wisnieski and Jones 1992a, 1992b). In both HUV and SLE, the serum reactivity to C1q is primarily to either surface bound or complexed C1q rather than to native (fluid-phase) C1q. Moreover, with the possible exception of obstructive pulmonary disease, most of the extracutaneous features observed in patients with HUV are not uncommonly clinical features observed in patients with SLE. Since HUV may be a presenting feature of SLE (Trendelenburg *et al.* 1999), expectant observation for evolving SLE is prudent in any patient with HUV. Despite common clinical expression and immunologic features, differences in the epitope binding specificities of C1q-reactive IgG in HUV and SLE sera suggest there may be some differences in the pathogenetic mechanisms operative in SLE and HUV (Martensson *et al.* 1992).

HUV responds favorably to glucocorticoids, and many patients have an excellent response to dapsone (Eiser *et al.* 1997; Fortson *et al.* 1986; Nurnberg *et al.* 1995). Combinations of dapsone (100 mg/day) and pentoxifylline (300 mg TID) have been well tolerated and successful in resistant cases of HUV, as has hydroxychloroquine (Lopez *et al.* 1984; Nurnberg *et al.* 1995). Significant proteinuria, renal dysfunction, or other visceral manifestations should prompt consideration of, and assessment for, evolving SLE, with management directed toward its treatment as clinically indicated.

Erythema elevatum diutinum

Erythema elevatum diutinum (EED) is a rare, chronic, localized form of cutaneous leukocytoclastic vasculitis that is most frequently observed in systemically ill patients. EED has been reported most commonly in patients with HIV, celiac disease, and paraprotein gammopathies (Chow *et al.* 1996; Dronda *et al.* 1996; LeBoit and Cockerell 1993; Muratori *et al.* 1999; Soni *et al.* 1998; Suarez *et al.* 1998; Tasanen *et al.* 1997; Wilkinson *et al.* 1992). The lesions usually appear as bilateral symmetric plaques or nodules, often over extensor surfaces of joints (see Figure 10.2 in Chapter 10). Lesions may initially appear purpuric, later developing a pink or yellow hue. On visual inspection, EED lesions may be difficult to distinguish clinically from dermatofibroma, granuloma annulare, granuloma faciale, or dermatitis herpetiformis. In patients with HIV infection, the cutaneous appearance of the lesions may be similar to those of Kaposi's sarcoma or bacillary angiomatosis.

Biopsy of EED lesions reveals distinct histopathologic features consistent with an immune complex vasculitis. Early, acute lesions are characterized by dermal infiltrates of neutrophils and eosinophils with perivascular nuclear dust and fibrin within aggregates of spindled cells (LeBoit and Cockerell 1993; Sangueza *et al.* 1977). More established, chronic lesions are characterized by a dense fibrosis with proliferation of fibroblasts and myofibroblasts; lymphocytes, macrophages, and histiocytes containing cholesterol clefts and lipid droplets comprise the remainder of the dermal infiltrate (Kanitakis *et al.* 1993; Lee *et al.* 1989).

Dapsone has been reported to be effective in the treatment of EED, inducing regression of lesions in patients without known disease associations as well as in patients with HIV or gammopathies (Dronda *et al.* 1996; Katz *et al.* 1977; LeBoit and Cockerell 1993; Suarez *et al.* 1998). Dapsone may also be effective in EED associated with celiac disease but adherence to a gluten-free diet may be required for sustained remission (Rodriguez-Serna *et al.* 1993; Tasanen *et al.* 1997). Plasma exchange in conjunction with chlorambucil or cyclophosphamide has been successful in treating patients with EED lesions associated with exceedingly high levels of IgA (Chow *et al.* 1996). Fibrotic lesions may be less responsive to therapy.

Familial Mediterranean fever

Vasculitis is an important, but not readily appreciated, feature of familial Mediterranean fever (FMF), an autosomal recessive disease characterized by recurrent self-limited attacks of fever accompanied by peritonitis, pleuritis, and arthritis. The majority of FMF cases are attributable to mutations in the MEFV gene, presumed to be an important regulator of inflammation (The International FMF Consortium 1997; The French FMF Consortium 1997). Approximately 5–7% of individuals with FMF have been reported to experience attacks of Henoch–Schönlein purpura (HSP) (Ozdogan *et al.* 1997). A higher than expected percentage of FMF patients (~1%) experience PAN (Ozdogan *et al.* 1997; Tekin *et al.* 2000). Perirenal hematoma has been reported frequently in patients with FMF and PAN; its presence in a patient with FMF accordingly warrants careful evaluation for arteritis (Glikson *et al.* 1989). Vasculitis should also be considered in patients with FMF who experience protracted attacks of myalgia and fever, particularly in the presence of hypertension and thrombocytosis (Tekin *et al.* 1999). Unlike other acute manifestations of FMF, vasculitis in FMF responds favorably to glucocorticoids.

Hyperimmunoglobulinemia D

Among the patients with periodic fever syndromes, and distinct from those with familial Mediterranean fever or Still's disease, are those with significantly elevated levels of IgD who experience recurrent attacks of fever, arthritis, and cutaneous vasculitis. Levels of serum IgD in affected patients are consistently elevated, often exceeding 100 U/ml, and have been shown to correlate with percentages of circulating B cells expressing surface IgD (Kumano *et al.* 1997). Circulating immune complexes containing IgD have been observed in patients during and between attacks and IgD deposits have been identified by immunofluorescence in affected skin lesions (Boom *et al.* 1990).

In one of the largest reported case series from Western Europe, a familial association was observed (Drenth *et al.* 1994b). Attacks of arthritis, fever, and diarrhea with skin lesions and lymphadenopathy were the most common manifestations. The cutaneous lesions included tender erythematous nodules, urticarial-like plaques, and erythematous macules and papules (Drenth *et al.* 1994a). The arthritis was non-deforming, most commonly affecting the ankles and knees. The attacks frequently began in infancy, and in over half of the patients, immunizations were noted to precipitate attacks. In addition to marked elevations in IgD, significant elevations in serum IgA were observed in the majority of patients.

Elevated levels of IgD have been also been observed in patients with idiopathic retinitis as well as in patients with Behçet's syndrome and uveitis (Kumano *et al.* 1997). In this report, elevated IgD levels were not found in patients with uveitis associated with other disorders such as sarcoidosis. The mechanism(s) whereby enhanced production of IgD occurs in these patients remains unknown.

Vasculitis associated with malignancy

Malignancies may masquerade as vasculitis, such as occurs with angiocentric T-cell lymphomas, or they may trigger immune responses culminating in vascular inflammation, thus qualifying vasculitis as a true paraneoplastic syndrome. Although the latter syndromes are uncommon, it is important to recognize that in such cases the appearance of vasculitis not infrequently antedates the appearance of other manifestations of malignancy. The vast majority of paraneoplastic vasculitis syndromes involve small vessels with palpable purpura, urticaria, maculopapular lesions, erythema multiforme, arthralgias, and neuropathy as predominant manifestations; internal organ and muscle lesions occur with less frequency (Sanchez-Guerrero *et al.* 1990). The most common lesions reported in association with malignancy are leukocytoclastic vasculitis and polyarteritis nodosa (Kurzrock and Cohen 1995). Concomitant polyarthritis has been reported as migratory, non-deforming, non-erosive arthritis (Greer and Panush 1988). Although, in general, the presenting signs and symptoms of malignancy-associated vasculitis are similar to those observed in patients without malignancy, suspicion for malignancy should be heightened in older patients presenting with cutaneous vasculitis or vasculitic neuropathy without other identifiable cause, or in patients who have a suboptimal response to treatments which are usually effective for vasculitis (Bachmeyer *et al.* 2005; Hutson and Hoffman 2000).

The true prevalence of vasculitis in cancer patients remains unknown, but evidence of malignancy is reported in up to 5% of individuals presenting with vasculitis. In patients with malignancy and vasculitis, hematologic malignancies are most common and include hairy cell leukemia; Hodgkin's disease; non-Hodgkin's lymphoma; myelodysplastic syndrome; myeloproliferative disorders (especially chronic myelegenous leukemia); and multiple myeloma (Sanchez-Guerrero *et al.* 1990). Non-small cell lung cancer is most prevalent among the associated solid tumors (Kurzrock and Cohen 1993).

Vasculitis should be attributed to malignancy with great caution. Described criteria for mucocutaneous paraneoplastic syndromes are: (1) both conditions occur about the same time and (2) both conditions follow a parallel course (McLean 1986; Curth 1976). There is not a consistent temporal relationship between the occurrence of malignancy and vasculitis; the resolution of vasculitis after malignancies are successfully treated; and recurrence or persistence of vasculitis concurrent with the progression of malignancy. Since there are other causes of vasculitis in cancer patients, such as drug reactions, infections, or cryoglobulinemia, these conditions should be considered and appropriately addressed. In one review of hematologic malignancies and skin biopsy-confirmed vasculitis, 39% of 23 patients had vasculitis due to other identifiable causes (Bachmeyer *et al.* 2005).

The pathogenesis of malignancy-associated vasculitis is uncertain and may be multifactorial. Postulated mechanisms include: (1) direct effects of tumor cells (notably hairy cells) on vascular walls (Klima and Waddell 1984; Gabriel and Scott 1986); (2) tumor release or tumor-induced release of cytokines that promote destruction of vascular structures; and (3) formation of immune complexes of tumor associated antigen/ antibodies (Sanchez-Guerrero and Alarcon-Segovia 1990; Kurzrock and Cohen 1993).

Vasculitis associated with hematologic malignancy

Myeloproliferative and lymphoproliferative disorders account for up to two-thirds of all malignancy-associated vasculitis. Lymphoproliferative disorders, myelodysplastic syndrome, and multiple myeloma account for up to 90% of malignancy-associated leukocytoclastic vasculitis (Sanchez and Pascual 2004). Henoch–Schönlein purpura may be a presenting manifestation of myelodysplastic syndrome (Blanco *et al.* 1997b). As many as one-third of malignancies associated with Henoch–Schönlein purpura are myelodysplastic syndrome, non-Hodgkin's and Hodgkin's lymphoma, and multiple myeloma (Pertuiset *et al.* 2000). Patients with non-Hodgkin's lymphoma of B cell origin may present with vasculitis and tumor-derived circulating paraproteins and cryoglobulins (Farrell *et al.* 1999; Wooten and Jasin 1996) and may have skin and renal glomerular lesions. Several observations pertinent to vasculitis associated with hematologic malignancy other than paraprotein-secreting B cell lymphomas are noteworthy: (1) low complement levels are typically not present; (2) skin lesions typically stain negative for immunoglobulins and complement products; and (3) cutaneous vasculitis in myelodysplastic syndromes or chronic leukemia may antedate bone marrow disease but frequently diminishes with disease progression (Longley *et al.* 1986; Sanchez-Guerrero *et al.* 1990; Greer *et al.* 1988; Enright and Miller 1997).

The association of polyarteritis or cutaneous vasculitis with hairy cell leukemia (HCL) is well recognized, with arteritis most commonly developing following splenectomy or infections (Hasler *et al.* 1995; Elkon *et al.* 1979). Polyarteritis has also been described in patients with myelodysplastic syndrome and chronic monomyelocytic leukemia (Hamidou *et al.* 2001). Polyarteritis nodosa in association with malignancy resembles classic polyarteritis nodosa in terms of age of onset, male predominance, presence of visceral involvement, and elevation of sedimentation rate. Nevertheless, in one reported series there were some distinguishing features of polyarteritis in this population: (1) peripheral aneurysms (in radial, ulnar, brachial, temporal, occipital, dorsal pedal arteries) occurred in approximately half of patients with malignant-associated polyarteritis nodosa whereas it is rare in classic polyarteritis nodosa; and (2) rheumatoid factor, antinuclear antibody, hepatitis B surface antigen, circulating immune complexes, and decreased complement levels were observed to a lesser extent than might be expected in classic polyarteritis nodosa (Komadina and Houk 1989).

Granulomatous angiitis of the central nervous system (see Chapter 37) has been reported in a number of cases of Hodgkin's lymphoma, with favorable responses occurring following aggressive therapy directed toward both conditions (Rosen *et al.* 2000; Sheehy *et al.* 2003). Of questionable significance, GCA has been reported in one patient with lymphoma and hairy cell leukemia (Webster *et al.* 1986).

Vasculitis associated with solid tumors

The most common solid tumors associated with vasculitis are small-cell and non-small-cell lung carcinoma; prostate; breast; colon, and renal cell carcinoma. Vasculitis has also been reported in association with tumors of the nasopharynx, ovary, stomach, bile duct, small bowel, ovary, and endometrium (Blanco *et al.* 1997a; Hayem *et al.* 1997; Matsumuro *et al.* 1994; Mita *et al.* 1999; Miyachi *et al.* 1987; Oh *et al.* 1991; Pertuiset *et al.* 2000; Ponge *et al.* 1998; Stashower *et al.* 1999). Small-vessel vasculitis involving skin, muscle, and peripheral nerves, and HSP are the most common reported forms of solid tumor associated vasculitis (Pertuiset *et al.*2000; Kurzrock *et al.* 1994). Most cases (71%) occurred prior to and concurrent with the diagnosis or relapse of tumor (Kurzrock *et al.* 1994). Renal involvement with focal segmental glomerulonephritis has been reported in association with small-cell lung cancer, and retinitis is a rarely reported ocular manifestation (Ponge *et al.* 1998; Suzuki *et al.* 1996). Polyarteritis nodosa has been reported in association with solid tumors only rarely (Hayem *et al.* 1997).

It is noteworthy that approximately one-third of adult cases of HSP are associated with malignancy, most commonly occurring in older males with lung cancer and prostate cancer. Proteinuria and hematuria occurring in the context of biopsy-confirmed proliferative nephritis and necrotizing vasculitis affecting the kidney has been demonstrated in some patients with solid tumor-associated HSP (Kurzrock *et al.* 1994). Given that HSP is uncommon in adults, its occurrence in men older than 40 years of age should raise suspicion for malignancy (Pertuiset *et al.* 2000).

Malignancy-associated vasculitis targeting nerve or muscle is reported most often among patients with solid tumors, principally prostate and lung cancer (small cell and adenocarcinoma) (Kurzrock and Cohen 1993). In one series of biopsy-confirmed nerve-muscle vasculitis, malignancy was found in 14% of cases (Vincent *et al.* 1986). Patients may present with either symmetric polyneuropathy or mononeuropathy multiplex, with the lower extremities more frequently affected (Oh 1997). Cutaneous or other systemic organ involvement is often absent (Matsumuro *et al.* 1994), but erythrocyte sedimentation rate and protein in the cerebrospinal fluid are usually elevated (Oh 1997).

GCA has been described in patients with renal cell carcinoma, brain, lung, uterine cancer, and adenocarcinoma of unknown origin; however, the observed incidence of cancer in patients with giant cell arteritis does not appear to be different from that observed in an age-matched population (Kurzrock *et al.* 1994).

In a review of 200 patients with ANCA-associated vasculitis, coexisting malignancy was diagnosed within 6 months in 20 (10%). Patients with ANCA-associated vasculitis have an increased risk of cancer compared with aged-matched controls (relative risk 6.0, 95% confidence interval 3.7–9.4) (Pankhurst *et al.* 2004). Solid tumors were most common, notably colon cancer, breast cancer, and gynecologic cancer. In contrast, positive ANCA serology has been shown not to be predictive of malignancy (Pankhurst *et al.* 2004; Diez-Porres *et al.* 2005). Churg–Strauss vasculitis has been reported in a patient with metastatic melanoma (Cupps and Fauci 1982).

Treatment

The mainstay of treatment for malignancy-associated vasculitis is glucocorticoids. Prednisone is usually started at moderate to high doses (20 mg/day to 1 mg/kg/day) and the majority of patients have some response within 1 week. In most patients with vasculitis associated with myelodysplastic syndrome, responses to prednisone were favorable (Enright and Miller 1997; Enright *et al.* 1995; Longley *et al.* 1986); however, successful and sustained resolution of vasculitis usually requires treatment of the underlying malignancy (Kurzock and Cohen 1993; Kurzrock and Cohen 1995; Greer and Panush 1988). Polyarteritis associated with hairy cell leukemia responds favorably to glucocorticoids and cyclophosphamide, and success has been reported following treatment with interferon alone (Carpenter and West 1994). Immunosuppressive therapies, such as cyclophosphamide, have been used in the management of arteritis occurring in the context of other malignancies but such interventions should be used with caution since they could theoretically enhance tumor growth by suppression of tumor immunosurveillance. For patients in whom vasculitis emerges after initial successful treatment of malignancy, a thorough evaluation for evidence of recurrence should be completed before institution of immunosuppressive therapy.

References

Abe M., Takayama, Y. Yamashita, H., Noguchi, M., and Sagoh, T. (2002). Purulent meningitis with unusual diffusion-weighted MRI findings. *European Journal of Radiology*, **44**, 1–4.

Allen, N. B., Cox, C. C., Cobo, M., Kisslo, J., Jacobs, M. R., McCallum, R. M. and Haynes, B. F. (1990). Use of immunosuppressive agents in the treatment of severe ocular and vascular manifestations of Cogan's syndrome. *American Journal of Medicine*, **88**, 296–301.

Almenoff, P. L., Johnson, A., Lesser, M. and Mattman, L. H. (1996). Growth of acid fast L forms from the blood of patients with sarcoidosis. *Thorax*, **51**, 530–3.

Alvarez-Lafuente, R., Fernandez-Gutierrez, B. and Lamas, J. R. *et al.* (2005). Human parvovirus B19, varicella zoster virus, and human herpes virus 6 in temporal artery biopsy specimens of patients with giant cell arteritis: analysis with quantitative real time polymerase chain reaction. *Annals of the Rheumatic Diseases*, **64**, 780–2

Anders, K. H., Latta, H., Chang, B. S. *et al.* (1989). Lymphomatoid granulomatosis and malignant lymphoma of the central nervous system in the acquired immuno-deficiency syndrome. *Human Pathology*, **20**, 326–34.

Amene, P. C. (1985). Aortitis and mycotic aneurysms and probable tuberculous immunopathy. *West African Journal of Medicine*, **4**, 255.

Aractingi, S., Cadranel, J., Milleron, B., Saiag, P., Malepart, M. J. and Dubertret, L. (1993). Sarcoidosis associated with leucocytoclastic vasculitis. A case report and review of the literature. *Dermatology*, **187**, 50–3.

Babajanians, A., Chung-Park, M. and Wisnieski, J. J. (1991). Recurrent pericarditis and cardiac tamponade in a patient with hypocomplementemic urticarial vasculitis syndrome. *Journal of Rheumatology*, **18**, 752–5.

Babin, R., Liu, C. and Aschenbrener, C. (1984). Histopathology of neurosensory deafness in sarcoidosis. *Annals of Otology Rhinology and Laryngology*, **93**, 389–93.

Bachmeyer, C., Wetterwald, E., Aractingi, S. (2005). Cutaneous vasculitis in the course of hematologic malignancies. *Dermatology*, **210**, 8–14.

Balslev, E., Thomsen, H. K. and Weissman, K. (1990). Histopathology of acute human immunodeficiency virus exanthem. *Journal of Clinical Pathology*, **43**, 201–2.

Ban, S., Goto, Y., Kamada, K., Takahama, M., Watanabe, H., Iwahori, T. and Takeuchi, H. (1999). Systemic granulomatous arteritis associated with Epstein-Barr virus infection. *Virchows Archives*, **434**, 249–54.

Basset, A., Kurtz, D., Bergoend, H. *et al.* (1969). Paulose atrophiante maligne de Degos avec atteinte du systeme nerveux central et presence d'anticorps antiartere. *Bulletin de la Societe de Dermatologie et de Syphiligraphie*, **76**, 333–4.

Bastug, D. E., Dominic, A., Ortiz, O., DiBartolomeo, A. G., Kotzan, J. M. and Abraham, F. M. (1997). Popliteal artery thrombosis in a patient with Cogan syndrome: treatment with thrombolysis and percutaneous transluminal angioplasty. *Cardiovascular and Interventional Radiology*, **20**, 57–9.

Battegay, A. M., Opravil, M., Wuthrich, B. and Luthy, R.(1989). Rash with amoxacillin-clavulinate therapy in HIV-infected patients. *Lancet*, **2**, 1100.

Baughman, R. P. and Lower, E. E. (1977). Alternatives to corticosteroids in the treatment of sarcoidosis. *Sarcoidosis, Vasculitis, and Diffuse Lung Diseases*, **14**, 121–30.

Baughman, R. P. and Lower, E. E. (1999). A clinical approach to the use of methotrexate for sarcoidosis. *Thorax*, **54**, 742–6.

Beste, L. A., Ansari-Lari, A., Borowitz, M. and Flynn, J. A., (2005). Lymphadenopathy, cough, and fever in a 51-year-old woman with systemic lupus erythematosus: case report of lymphomatoid granulomatosis. *Arthritis and Rheumatism*, **53**, 621–4.

Black, M. M. and Hudson, P. M. (1976). Atrophie blanche lesions closely resembling malignant atrophic papulosis (Degos' disease) in systemic lupus erythematosus. *British Journal of Dermatology*, **95**, 649–52.

Blanco, R., González-Gay, M. A., Ibanez, D., Alba, C. and Perez de Llano, L. A. (1997a). Henoch-Schönlein purpura as a clinical presentation of small cell lung cancer. *Clinical and Experimental Rheumatology*, **15**, 545–7.

Blanco, R., González-Gay, M. A., Ibanez, D., Lopez-Viana, A., Ferran, C., Regueira, A. and Gonzalez-Vela, C. (1997b). Henoch-Schönlein purpura as clinical presentation of a myelodysplastic syndrome. *Clinical Rheumatology*, **16**, 626–8.

Bleehen, S. S. (1977). Intra-endothelial tubular aggregates in malignant atrophic papulosis (Degos' disease). *Clinical Experimental Dermatology*, **2**, 73–4.

Boom, B. W., Daha, M. R., Vermeer, B. J. and van der Meer, J. W. (1990). IgD immune complex vasculitis in a patient with hyperimmunoglobulinemia D and periodic fever. *Archives of Dermatology*, **126**, 1621–4.

Branford, W. A., Farr, P. M. and Porter, D. I. (1982). Annular vasculitis of the head and neck in a patient with sarcoidosis. *British Journal of Dermatology*, **106**, 713–6.

Bronze, M. S., Shirwany, A., Corbett, C. and Schaberg, D. R. (1999). Infectious aortitis: an uncommon manifestation of infection with Streptococcus pneumoniae. *American Journal of Medicine*, **107**, 627–30.

Cabre, J., Noguer-Debray, S., Bosch-Castane, J., *et al.* (1974). Papulose atrophiante maligne de Degos chez un nourrisson. *Bulletin de la Societe de Dermatologie et de Syphiligraphie*, **81**, 652–3.

Calabrese, L. H. (1991). Vasculitis and infection with the human immunodeficiency virus. *Rheumatic Diseases Clinic of North America*, **17**, 131–47.

Caplan, L., Corbett, J., Goodwin, J., Thomas, C., Shenker, D. and Schatz, N. (1983). Neuro-ophthalmologic signs in the angiitic form of neurosarcoidosis. *Neurology*, **33**, 1130–5.

Carpenter, M. T. and West, S. G. (1994). Polyarteritis nodosa in hairy cell leukemia: treatment with interferon-alpha. *Journal of Rheumatology*, **21**, 1150–2.

Casselman, J. W., Majoor, M. H.J. M. and Albers, F. W. (1994). MR of the inner ear in patients with Cogan's syndrome. *American Journal of Neuroradiology*, **15**, 131–8.

Cecchi, R. and Giomi, A. (1999). Annular vasculitis in association with sarcoidosis. *Journal of Dermatology*, **26**, 334–6.

Centers for Disease Control. (2003). Outbreaks of Salmonella serotype enteritidis infection associated with eating shell eggs-United States, 1999–2001. *Morbidity and Mortality Weekly Report*, **51**, 1149–52.

Cerilli, J., Brasile, L. and Karmady, A. (1985). Role of the vascular endothelial cell antigen system in the etiology of atherosclerosis. *Annals of Surgery*, **202**, 329–34.

Chad, D. A., Smith, T. W., Blumenfeld, A., Fairchild, P. G. and de Girolami, U. (1990). Human immunodeficiency virus (HIV)-associated myopathy: immunocytochemcal identification of an HIV antigen (gp41) in muscle macrophages. *Annals of Neurology*, **28**, 579–82.

Cheson, B. D., Bluming, A. Z. and Alroy, J. (1976). Cogan's syndrome: a systemic vasculitis. *American Journal of Medicine*, **60**, 549–55.

Chirinos, J. A., Lichtstein, D. M., Garcia, J. and Tamariz, L. J. (2002). The evolution of Lemierre syndrome: report of 2 cases and review of the literature. *Medicine* (Baltimore), **81**, 458–65

Chow, R. K., Benny, W. B., Coupe, R. L., Dodd, W. A. and Ongley, R. C. (1996). Erythema elevatum diutinum associated with IgA paraproteinemia successfully controlled with intermittent plasma exchange. *Archives of Dermatology*, **132**, 1360–4.

Churg, A., Carrington, C. B. and Gupta, R. (1979). Necrotizing sarcoid granulomatosis. *Chest*, **76**, 406–13.

Cioc, A, Sedmak D., Nuovo G., Dawood M., Smart G, and Magro C. (2002). Parvovirus B19 associated adult Henoch—Schönlein purpura. *Journal of Cutaneous Pathology*, **29**, 602–7.

Clifton, D. R., Goss, R. A., Sahni, S. K., van Antwerp D., Baggs, R. B., Marder, V. J., Silverman, D. J., and Sporn, L. A. (1998). NF-κB-dependent inhibition of apoptosis is essential for host cell survival during *Rickettsia rickettsii* infection. *Proceedings of the National Academy of Sciences USA*, **95**, 4646–51.

Cobo, M. and Haynes, B. F. (1984). Early corneal findings in Cogan's syndrome. *Ophthalmology*, **91**, 903–7.

Cochrane, A. D. and Tatoulis, J. (1991). Cogan's syndrome with aortitis, aortic regurgitation, and aortic arch vessel stenoses. *Annals of Thoracic Surgery*, **52**, 1166–7.

Cohen, P., Guillevin, L., Gayraud, M., Lhote, F., Jarrousse, B., Leon, A. and Gherardi, R. (1993). Successful treatment of HIV-related vasculitis with peripheral neuropathy with short-term steroids followed by the association of zidovudine and plasmapheresis. *Transfusion Science*, **14**, 383–9.

Cohen, P. S., O'Brien, T. F., Schoenbaum, S. C. and Medeiros, A. A. (1978). The risk of endothelial infection in adults with salmonella bacteraemia. *Annals of Internal Medicine*, **89**, 931–2.

Cook, A. M. and Christopoulos, D. (1989). Rupture of a non-aneuysmal salmonellainfected aorta. *Clinical Radiology*, **40**, 605–6.

Cupps, T.R. and Fauci, A.S. (1982). Neoplasm and systemic vasculitis: a case report. *Arthritis and Rheumatism*, **25**, 475–6.

Curth, H. (1976). *Skin lesions and internal carcinoma*. Philadelphia, PA, Saunders.

Daniel, F., Foix, C. and Gray, J. M. *et al.* (1982). Malignant atrophic papulosis with insufficiency of blood fibrinolysis. *Annals of Dermatology and Venereology*, **109**, 763–4.

Darougar, S., John, A. C., Viswalingam, M., Cornell, L. and Jones, B. R. (1978). Isolation of Chlamydia psittaci from a patient with interstitial keratitis and uveitis associated with otological and cardiovascular lesions. *British Journal of Ophthalmology*, **62**, 709–14.

Davis, M. D., Daoud, M. S., Kirby, B., Gibson, L. E. and Rogers, R. S. (1998). Clinicopathologic correlation of hypocomplementemic and normocomplementemic urticarial vasculitis. *Journal of the American Academy of Dermatology*, **38**, 899–905.

D'Cruz, D. P., Wisnieski, J. J., Asherson, R. A., Khamashta, M. A. and Hughes, G. R. (1995). Autoantibodies in systemic lupus erythematosus and urticarial vasculitis. *Journal of Rheumatology*, **22**, 1669–73.

De Gans, J. and van de Beek, D. (2002). Dexamethasone in adults with bacterial meningitis. *New England Journal of Medicine*, **347**, 1549–56.

De Girolami, U., Smith, T. W., Henin, D. and Hauw, J.-J. (1990). Neuropathology of the acquired immune deficiency syndrome. *Archives of Pathology and Laboratory Medicine*, **114**, 643–55.

Degos, R. (1952). Papulose atrophiante maligne (syndrome cuatneo-intestal mortel). *Annales de Dermatologie et de Syphiligraphie*, **79**, 410–17.

Degos, R. (1966). Malignant atrophic papulosis: A fatal cutaneo-intestinal syndrome. *British Journal of Dermatology*, **66**, 304–7.

Degos, R. (1979). Malignant atrophic papulosis. *British Journal of Dermatology*, **100**, 21–35.

Degos, R., Lortat-Jacob, E., Daniel, F., *et al.* (1967). Papulose atrophiante Maligne avec presence d'anticorps anti-artere. *Bulletin de la Societe de Dermatologie et de Syphiligraphie*, **74**, 715–17.

DeRemee, R. A. (1994). Sarcoidosis and Wegener's granulomatosis: a comparative analysis. *Sarcoidosis*, **11**, 7–18.

Diez-Porres, L., Rios-Blanco, J.J., Robles-Marhuenda, A., Gutierrez-Molina, M., Gil-Aguado, A. and Vazquez-Rodrigucz, J.J. (2005). ANCA-associated vasculitis as paraneoplastic syndrome with colon cancer: a case report. *Lupus*, **14**, 632–4.

Diri, E., Espinoza, C. G. and Espinoza, L. R. (1999). Spinal cord granulomatous vasculitis: an unusual clinical presentation of sarcoidosis. *Journal of Rheumatology*, **26**, 1408–10.

Dover, J. S. and Johnson, R. A. (1991). Cutaneous manifestations of human immunodeficiency virus infection: II. *Archives of Dermatology*, **127**, 1549–58.

Drenth, J. P., Boom, B. W., Toonstra, J. and Van der Meer, J. W. (1994a). Cutaneous manifestations and histologic findings in the hyperimmunoglobulinemia D syndrome. *Archives of Dermatology*, **130**, 59–65.

Drenth, J. P., Haagsma, C. J. and van der Meer, J. W. (1994b). Hyperimmunoglobulinemia D and periodic fever syndrome. The clinical spectrum in a series of 50 patients. *Medicine* (Baltimore), **73**, 133–44.

Dronda, F., Gonzalez-Lopez, A., Lecona, M. and Barros, C. (1996). Erythema elevatum diutinum in human immunodeficiency virus-infected patients – report of a case and review of the literature. *Clinical and Experimental Dermatology*, **21**, 222–5.

Dubin, H. V. and Stawiski, M. A. (1974). Systemic lupus erythematosus resembling malignant atrophic papulosis. *Archives of Internal Medicine*, **134**, 321–3.

Duffey, R. J. and Mammer, M. E. (1987). The ocular manifestations of Rocky Mountain spotted fever. *Annals of Ophthalmology*, **19**, 301–3, 306.

Dumler, J. S. and Walker, D. H. (2005). Rocky Mountain spotted fever–changing ecology and persisting virulence. *New England Journal of Medicine*, **353**, 551–3.

Dupre, L., Andolfi, G., Tangye, S. G., Clementi, R., Locatelli, F., Arico, M., Aiuti, A. and Roncarolo, M. G. (2005). SAP controls the cytolytic activity of CD8+ T cells against EBV-infected cells. *Blood*, **105**, 4383–9.

Durie, B. G.M., Stroud, J. D. and Kahn, J. K. (1969). Progressive systemic sclerosis with malignant atrophic papulosis. *Archives of Dermatology*, **100**, 575–81.

Dutz, J. P., Benoit, L., Wang, X., Demetrick, D. J., Junker, A., de Sa, D., and Tan, R. (2001). Lymphocytic vasculitis in X-linked lymphoproliferative disease. *Blood*, **97**, 95–100.

Eady, R. A. J. and Odland, G. F. (1975). Intraendothelial tubular aggregates in experimental wounds: Ultrastructural study. *British Journal of Dermatology*, **93**, 165–73.

Eiser, A. R., Singh, P. and Shanies, H. M. (1997). Sustained dapsone-induced remission of hypocomplementemic urticarial vasculitis – a case report. *Angiology*, **48**, 1019–22.

Elkon, K.B., Hughes, G.R., Catovsky, D., *et al.* (1979). Hairy-cell leukaemia with polyarteritis nodosa. *Lancet*, **2**, 280–2.

Englert, H. J., Hawkes, C. H., Bowy, M. L., *et al.* (1984). Degos' disease: Association with anticardiolipin antibodies and the lupus anticoagulant. *British Medical Journal*, **289**, 576.

Enright, H. and Miller, W. (1997). Autoimmune phenomena in patients with myelodysplastic syndromes. *Leukemia and Lymphoma*, **24**, 483–9.

Enright, H., Jacob, H. S., Vercellotti, G., Howe, R., Belzer, M. and Miller, W. (1995). Paraneoplastic autoimmune phenomena in patients with myelodysplastic syndromes: response to immunosuppressive therapy. *British Journal of Haematology*, **91**, 403–8.

Eremeeva, M. E., Dasch, G. A. and Silverman, D. J. (2000). Interaction of rickettsiae with eukaryotic cells: adhesion, entry, intracellular growth, and host cell responses. *Sub-cellular Biochemistry*, **33**, 479–516.

Farrell, A. M., Stern, S. C., El-Ghariani, K., Frankel, A., Woodrow, D., Muller, B. and Cream, J. J. (1999). Splenic lymphoma with villous lymphocytes presenting as leucocytoclastic vasculitis. *Clinical and Experimental Dermatology*, **24**, 19–22.

Fauci, A. S. (1988). The human immunodeficiency virus: infectivity and mechanism of pathogenesis. *Science*, **239**, 617–22.

Faye-Petersen, O., Frankel, S. R., Schulman, P. E., Raucher, H., Spiera, H. and Dische, M. R. (1991). Giant cell vasculitis with extravascular granulomas in an adolescent. *Pediatric Pathology*, **11**, 281–95.

Ferguson, P. J., Saulsbury, F. T., Dowell, S. F., Torok, T. J.,Erdman, D. D. and Anderson, L. J. (1996). Prevalence of human parvovirus B19 infection in children with Henoch-Schönlein purpura. *Arthritis and Rheumatism*, **39**, 880–1.

Fernandes, S. R., Bertolo, M. B., Rossi, C. L., Samara, A. M., Bonon, S. H., Durante, P. and Costa, S. C. (1999). Polyarteritis nodosa and cytomegalovirus: diagnosis by polymerase chain reaction. *Clinical Rheumatology*, **18**, 501–3.

Fernandez Guerrero, M. L., Aguado, J. M., Arribas, A., Lubreras, C. and de Gorgolas, M. (2004). The spectrum of cardiovascular infections due to Salmonella enterica: a review of clinical features and factors determining outcome. *Medicine* (Baltimore), **83**, 123–38.

Ferris, E. J., Rudikoff, J. C. and Shapiro, J. H. (1968). Cerebral angiography of bacterial infection. *Radiology*, **90**, 727–34.

Fidler, H. and Jones, N. S. (1989). Late onset Cogan's syndrome. *Journal of Laryngology*, **103**, 512–14.

Finkel, T. H., Torok, T. J., Ferguson, P. J., Durigon, E. L.,Zaki, S. R., Leung, D. Y., *et al.* (1994). Chronic parvovirus B19 infection and systemic narcotizing vasculitis: opportunistic infection or aetiological agent? *Lancet*, **343**, 1255–8.

Fisher, E. R. and Hellstrom, H. R. (1961). Cogna's syndrome and systemic vascular disease: analysis of pathologic features with reference to its relationship to thromboangiitis obliterans (Buerger). *Archives of Pathology*, **72**, 572–92.

Foote, E. A., Postier, R. G., Greenfield, R. A., and Bronze, M. S. (2005). Infectious Aortitis. *Current treatment options in cardiovascular disease*, **7**, 89–97.

Fortson, J. S., Zone, J. J., Hammond, M. E. and Groggel, G. C. (1986). Hypocomplementemic urticarial vasculitis syndrome responsive to dapsone. *Journal of the Academy of Dermatology*, **15**, 1137–42.

Fox, G. M., Heilskov, T. and Smith, J. L. (1990). Cogan's syndrome and seroreactivity of Lyme borreliosis. *Journal of Clinical Neuro-Ophthalmology*, **10**, 83–7.

Fruhwirth, J., Mischinger, H. J., Werkgartner, G., Beham, A. and Pfaffenthaller, E. C. (1997). Kohlmeier-Degos's disease with primary intestinal manifestation. *Scandinavian Journal of Gastroenterology*, **32**, 1066–70.

Gabriel, S. E., Conn, D. L., Phyliky, R. L., Pittelkow, M. R. and Scott, R. E. (1986). Vasculitis in hairy cell leukemia: review of literature and consideration of possible pathogenic mechanisms. *Journal of Rheumatology*, **13**, 1167–72.

Gabriel, S. E., Espy, M., Erdman, D. D., Bjornsson, J., Smith, T. F. and Hunder, G. G. (1999). The role of parvovirus B19 in the pathogenesis of giant cell arteritis: a preliminary evaluation. *Arthritis and Rheumatism*, **42**, 1255–8.

García-Porrua, C., González-Gay, M. A., García-Pais, M. J. and Blanco, R. (1998). Cutaneous vasculitis: an unusual presentation of sarcoidosis in adulthood. *Scandinavian Journal of Rheumatology*, **27**, 80–2.

Gelb, A. B., van de Rijn, M., Regula, D. P. Jr., Cornbleet, J. P.,Kamel, O. W., Horoupian, D. S., Cleary, M. L. and Warnke, R. A. (1994). Epstein-Barr virus-associated natural killer-large granular lymphocyte leukemia. *Human Pathology*, **25**, 953–60.

Gelfand, M. L., Kantor, T. and Gorstein, F. (1972). Cogan's syndrome with cardiovascular involvement: aortic insufficiency. *Bulletin of the New York Academy of Medicine*, **48**, 647–60.

Gherardi, R., Belec, L., Mhiri, C., Gray, F., Lescs, M.-C., Sobel, A., Guillevin, L. and Wechsler, J. (1993). The spectrum of vasculitis in human immunodeficiency virus-infected patients – A clinicopathologic evaluation. *Arthritis and Rheumatism*, **36**, 1164–74.

Gibson, L. E., el-Azhary, R. A., Smith, T. F. and Reda, A. M. (1994). The spectrum of cutaneous granulomatous vasculitis: histopathologic report of eight cases with clinical correlation. *Journal of Cutaneous Pathology*, **21**, 437–45.

Gilden, D. (2004). Varicella zoster virus and central nervous system syndromes. *Herpes*, **11** (Suppl. 2), 89A–94A.

Gilden, D. H., Kleinschmidt-DeMasters, B. K., Wellish, M., Hedley-Whyte, E. T., Rentier, B. and Mahalingam, R. (1996). Varicella zoster virus, a cause of waxing and waning vasculitis: the New England Journal of Medicine case 5–1995 revisited. *Neurology*, **47**, 1441–6.

Glikson, M., Galun, E., Schlesinger, M., Cohen, D., Haskell, L., Rubinow, A. and Eliakim, M. (1989). Polyarteritis nodosa and familial Mediterranean fever: a report of 2 cases and review of the literature. *Journal of Rheumatology*, **16**, 536–9.

Golden, M. P., Hammer, S. M., Wanke, C. A. and Albrecht, M. A. (1994). Cytomegalovirus vasculitis. Case reports and review of the literature. *Medicine* (Baltimore), **73**, 246–55.

Goldenberg, N. A., Knapp-Clevenger, R., Hays, T. and Manco-Johnson, M. J. (2005). Lemierre's and Lemierre's-like syndromes in children: survival and thromboembolic outcomes. *Pediatrics*, **116**, e543–8.

Goodless, D. R., Ramos-Caro, F. and Flowers, F. P. (1991). Reactional states in Hansen's disease: practical aspects of emergency management. *Southern Medical Journal*, **84**, 237–40.

Gordin, F. M., Simon, G. L., Wofsy, C. B. and Mills, J. (1984). Adverse reactions to trimethoprim-sulphamethoxazole in patients with acquired immunodeficiency syndrome. *Annals of Internal Medicine*, **100**, 495–9.

Greer, J. M., Longley, S., Edwards, N. L., Elfenbein, G. J. and Panush, R. S. (1988). Vasculitis associated with malignancy. Experience with 13 patients and literature review. *Medicine* (Baltimore), **67**, 220–30.

Gudbrandsson, T., Hansson, L., Herlitz, H. *et al.* (1981). Immunological changes in patients with previous malignant essential hypertension. *Lancet*, **1**, 406–8.

Guinee, D. Jr., Jaffe, E., Kingma, D., Fishback, N., Wallberg, K., Krishnan, J., Frizzera, G., Travis, W. and Koss, M. (1994). Pulmonary lymphomatoid granulomatosis. Evidence for a proliferation of Epstein-Barr virus infected B-lymphocytes with a prominent T-cell component and vasculitis. *American Journal of Surgical Pathology*, **18**, 753–64.

Gupta, S. and Licorish, K. (1984). Circulating immune complexes in AIDS. *New England Journal of Medicine*, **310**, 1530–31.

Hall-Smith, P. (1969). Malignant atrophic papulosis (Degos' disease): Two cases occurring in the same family. *British Journal of Dermatology*, **81**, 817–22.

Hall-Smith, S. P. (1964). Malignant atrophic papulosis (Degos' syndrome). *Proceedings of the Royal Society of Medicine*, **57**, 519–21.

Hamidou, M. A., Boumalassa, A., Larroche, C., El Kouri, D., Bletry, O. and Grolleau, J. Y. (2001). Systemic medium-sized vessel vasculitis associated with chronic myelomonocytic leukemia. *Seminars in Arthritis and Rheumatism*, **31**, 119–26.

Hammer, M., Witte, T., Mugge, A., Wollenhaupt, J., Laas, J., Laszig, R. and Zeidler, H. (1994). Complicated Cogan's syndrome with aortic insufficiency and coronary stenosis. *Journal of Rheumatology*, **21**, 552–5.

Hasler, P., Kistler, H. and Gerber, H. (1995). Vasculitides in hairy cell leukemia. *Seminars in Arthritis and Rheumatism*, **25**, 134–42.

Hattwick, M. A., O'Brien, R. J., and Hanson, B. F. (1976). Rocky Mountain spotted fever: epidemiology of an increasing problem. *Annals of Internal Medicine*, **84**, 732–9.

Hayasaka, S., Takatori, Y., Noda, S., Setogawa, T. and Hayashi, H. (1991). Retinal vasculitis in a mother and her son with human T-lymphotropic virus type 1 associated myelopathy. *British Journal of Ophthalmology*, **75**, 566–7.

Hayem, G., Gomez, M. J., Grossin, M., Meyer, O. and Kahn, M. F. (1997). Systemic vasculitis and epithelioma. A report of three cases with a literature review. *Revue du Rhumatisme*, (English), **64**, 816–24.

Haynes, B. F., Kaiser-Kupfer, M. I., Mason, P. and Fauci, A. S. (1980). Cogan syndrome: studies in thirteen patients, long-term follow-up, and a review of the literature. *Medicine* (Baltimore), **59**, 426–41.

Haynes, B. F., Pikus, A., Kaiser-Kupfer, M. and Fauci, A. S. (1981). Successful treatment of sudden hearing loss in Cogan's syndrome with corticosteroids. *Arthritis and Rheumatism*, **24**, 501–3.

Heinzen, R. A. (2003). Rickettsial actin-based motility: behavior and involvement of cytoskeletal regulators. *Annals of the New York Academy of Sciences*, **990**, 535–47.

Hickey, W. F. and Kimura, H. (1988). Perivascular microglia are bone marrow derived and present antigen in vivo. *Science*, **239**, 290–2.

High, W. A., Aranda J., Patel, S. B., Cockerel, C. J., Costner M. I. (2004). Is Degos' disease a clinical and histological end point rather than a specific disease? *Journal of the American Academy of Dermatology*, **50**, 895–9.

Hippach, M., Meyberg, R., Villena-Heinsen, C., Mink, D., Ertan, A. K., Schmidt, W. and Hippach, M. (2000). Postpartum ovarian vein thrombosis. *Clinical and Experimental Obstetrics and Gynecology*, **27**, 24–6.

Ho, A. C., Roat, M. I., Venbrux, A. and Hellmann, D. B. (1999). Cogan's syndrome with refractory abdominal aortitis and mesenteric vasculitis. *Journal of Rheumatology*, **26**, 1404–7.

Holm, J. M., Hansen, L. K. and Oxhoj, H. (1995). Kawasaki disease associated with parvovirus B19 infection. *European Journal of Pediatrics*, **154**, 633–4.

Horney, L. F. and Walker, D. H. (1988). Meningoencephalitis as a major manifestation of Rocky Mountain spotted fever. *Southern Medical Journal*, **81**, 915–8.

Howard, R. O. and Nishida, S. (1969). A case of Degos' disease with electron microscopic findings. *Transactions of the American Academy of Ophthalmology and Otolaryngology*, **73**, 1097–112.

Hsu, R. B. and Lin, F. Y. (2005). Risk factors for bacteraemia and endovascular infection due to non-typhoid salmonella: a reappraisal. *Quarterly Journal of Medicine*, **98**, 821–7

Huang, T. E. and Chou, S. M. (1988). Occlusive hypertrophic arteritis as the cause of discrete necrosis in CNS toxoplasmosis in the acquired immune deficiency syndrome. *Human Pathology*, **19**, 1210–14.

Hunninghake, G. W. and Crystal, R. G. (1981). Pulmonary sarcoidosis: a disorder manifest by excess helper T-lymphocyte activity at sites of disease activity. *New England Journal of Medicine*, **305**, 429–34.

Hutson, T. E. and Hoffman, G. S. (2000). Temporal concurrence of vasculitis and cancer: a report of 12 cases. *Arthritis Care Research*, **13**, 417–23.

Ilowite, N. T., Fligner, C. L., Ochs, H. D., Brichacek, B., Harada, S., Haas, J. E., Purtilo, D. T. and Wedgwood, R. J. (1986). Pulmonary angiitis with atypical lymphoreticular infiltrates in Wiskott-Aldrich syndrome: possible relationship of lymphomatoid granulomatosis and EBV infection. *Clinical Immunology and Immunopathology*, **41**, 479–84.

Issacson, C. (1961). Idiopathic aortitis in young Africans. *Journal of Pathology and Bacteriology*, **81**, 61.

Itescu, S., Brancato, L. J., Buxbaum, J., *et al.* (1990). A diffuse infiltrative CD8 lymphocytosis syndrome in human immunodeficiency virus (HIV) infection: A host immune response associated with HLA-DR5. *Annals of Internal Medicine*, **112**, 3.

Jaffe, E. S. and Wilson, W. H. (1997). Lymphomatoid granulomatosis: pathogenesis, pathology and clinical implications. *Cancer Surveys*, **30**, 233–48.

Jan W., Zimmerman, R. A., Bilaniuk, L. T., Hunter J. V., Simon, E. M., and Haselgrove, J. (2003). Diffusion-weighted imaging in acute bacterial meningitis in infancy. *Neuroradiology*, **45**, 634–9.

Joffe, N. (1965). Aortitis of obscure origin in the African. *Clinical Radiology*, **16**, 130–40.

Johnson, R. M., Little, J. R. and Storch, G. A. (2001). Kawasaki-like syndromes associated with human immunodeficiency virus infection. *Clinical Infectious Diseases*, **32**, 1628–34.

Johnson, R. M., Barbarini, G. and Barbaro, G. (2003). Kawasaki-like syndromes and other vasculitic syndromes in HIV-infected patients. *AIDS*, **17** (Suppl. 1), S77–82.

Johnston, C. and Kennedy, C. (1984). Cutaneous leucocytoclastic vasculitis associated with acute sarcoidosis. *Postgraduate Medical Journal*, **60**, 549–50.

Kanegane, H., Tsuji, T., Seki, H., Yachie, A., Yokoi, T., Miyawaki, T. and Taniguchi, N. (1994). Kawasaki disease with a concomitant primary Epstein-Barr virus infection. *Acta Paediatrica Japonica*, **36**, 713–6.

Kanitakis, J., Cozzani, E., Lyonnet, S. and Thivolet, J. (1993). Ultrastructural study of chronic lesions of erythema elevatum diutinum: 'extracellular cholesterosis' is a misnomer. *Journal of the American Academy of Dermatology*, **29**, 363–7.

Karni, A., Sadeh, M., Blatt, I. and Goldhammer, Y. (1991). Cogan's syndrome complicated by lacunar brain infarcts. *Journal of Neurology, Neurosurgery, and Psychiatry*, **54**, 169–71.

Kastenbauer, S. and Pfister, H. W. (2003). Pneumococcal meningitis in adults: spectrum of complications and prognostic factors in a series of 87 cases. *Brain*, **126**, 1015–25.

Katsetos, C. D., Fincke, J. E., Legido, A., Lischner, H. W., de Chadarevain, J. P., Kaye, E. M., Platsoucas, C. D. and Oleszak, E. L. (1999). Angiocentric CD3(+) T-cell infiltrates in human immunodeficiency virus type 1-associated central nervous system disease in children. *Clinical and Diagnostic Laboratory Immunology*, **6**, 105–114.

Katz, S. I., Gallin, J. I., Hertz, K. C., Fauci, A. S. and Lawley, T. J. (1977). Erythema elevatum diutinum: skin and systemic manifestations, immunologic studies, and successful treatment with dapsone. *Medicine* (Baltimore), **56**, 443–55.

Kikuta, H., Matsumoto, S. and Osato, T. (1991). Kawasaki disease and Epstein-Barr virus. *Acta Paediatrica Japonica*, **33**, 765–70.

Kikuta, H., Nakanishi, M., Ishikawa, N., Konno, M. and Matsumoto, S. (1992). Detection of Epstein-Barr virus sequences in patients with Kawasaki disease by means of the polymerase chain reaction. *Intervirology*, **33**, 1–5.

Kirk, J. L., Fine D. P., Sexton, D. J. and Munchmore, H. G. (1990). Rocky Mountain spotted fever. A clinical review based on 48 confirmed cases, 1943–1986. *Medicine* (Baltimore), **69**, 35–45.

Kirkland, K. B., Williamson, W. E. and Sexton, D. J. (1995). Therapeutic delay and mortality in cases of Rocky Mountain spotted fever. *Clinical Infectious Diseases*, **20**, 1118–21.

Kisch, L. S. and Bruyzeel, D. P. (1984). Six cases of malignant atrophic papulosis (Degos' disease) occurring in one family. *British Journal of Dermatology*, **111**, 469–71.

Klima, M. and Waddell, C.C. (1984). Hairy cell leukemia associated with focal vascular damage. *Human Pathology*, **15**, 657–9.

Kobayashi, S., Nagase, M., Hidaka, S., Arai, T., Ikegaya, N., Hishida, A. and Honda, N. (1994). Membranous nephropathy associated with hypocomplementemic urticarial vasculitis: report of two cases and a review of the literature. *Nephron*, **66**, 1–7.

Koeppen, A. H., Lansing, L. S., Peng, S. K. and Smith, R. S.(1981). Central nervous system vasculitis in cytomegalovirus infection. *Journal of Neurological Science*, **51**, 395–410.

Kohlmeier, W. (1941). Multiple Hautnekrosen beiThrombangiitis obliterans. *Archiv für Dermatologie und Syphilis*, **181**, 783–92.

Komadina, K. H. and Houk, R. W. (1989). Polyarteritis nodosa presenting as recurrent pneumonia following splenectomy for hairy-cell leukemia. *Seminars in Arthritis and Rheumatism*, **18**, 252–7.

Koskinen, P., Lemstrom, K., Bruggeman, C., Lautenschlager, I. and Hayry, P. (1994). Acute cytomegalovirus infection induces a subendothelial inflammation (endotheliitis) in the allograft vascular wall. A possible linkage with enhanced allograft arteriosclerosis. *American Journal of Pathology*, **144**, 41–50.

Kristensen, B. O., Andersen, P. L.M., Wiik, A. *et al.* (1984). Autoantibodies and vascular events in essential hypertension: A five-year longitudinal study. *Journal of Hypertension*, **2**, 19–24.

Kumano, Y., Nagato, T., Kurihara, K., Kikukawa, H., Goto, M., Kawano, Y., Ohnishi, Y. and Inomata, H. (1997). Hyperimmunoglobulinemia D in idiopathic retinal vasculitis. Graefes *Archives in Clinical and Experimental Ophthalmology*, **235**, 372–8.

Kurzrock, R. and Cohen, P. R. (1993). Vasculitis and cancer. *Clinical Dermatology*, **11**, 175–87.

Kurzrock, R., Cohen, P. R. and Markowitz, A. (1994). Clinical manifestations of vasculitis in patients with solid tumors. A case report and review of the literature. *Annals of Internal Medicine*, **154**, 334–40.

Kurzrock, R. and Cohen, P. R. (1995). Mucocutaneous paraneoplastic manifestations of hematologic malignancies. *American Journal of Medicine*, **99**, 207–16.

Kwong, T., Valderrama, E., Paley, C. and Ilowite, N. (1994). Systemic necrotizing vasculitis associated with childhood sarcoidosis. *Seminars in Arthritis and Rheumatism*, **23**, 388–95.

Kyung-Whan, M., Yorkey, F. and Sato, C. (1980). Mucin-producing adenoscarcinomas and nonbacterial thrombotic endocarditis: Pathogenetic role of tumor mucin. *Cancer*, **45**, 2375–82.

Lande, M. B., Mowry, J. A., Houghton, D. C., White, C. R. Jr. and Brozy, M. S. (1998). Immune complex disease associated with Epstein-Barr virus infectious mononucleosis. *Pediatric Nephrology*, **12**, 651–3.

Lane, G. P., Cochrane, A. D. and Fore, D. R. (1988). Salmonella mycotic abdominal-aortic aneurysm. *Medical Journal of Australia*, **149**, 95–7.

Lau, Y. L., Wong, S. N. and Lawton, W. M. (1992). Takayasu's arteritis associated with Wiskott-Aldrich syndrome. *Journal of Paediatrics and Child Health*, **28**, 407–9.

Leavitt, R. Y. and Fauci, A. S. (1986). Pulmonary vasculitis. *American Review of Respiratory Disease*, **134**, 149–66.

LeBoit, P. E. and Cockerell, C. J. (1993). Nodular lesions of erythema elevatum diutinum in patients infected with the human immunodeficiency virus. *Journal of the American Academy of Dermatology*, **28**, 919–22.

Lee, A. Y., Nakagawa, H., Nogita, T. and Ishibashi, Y. (1989). Erythema elevatum diutinum: an ultrastructural case study. *Journal of Cutaneous Pathology*, **16**, 211–7.

Lee, S. B., Jones L. K., and Giannini, C. (2005). Brainstem infarcts as an early manifestation of Streptococcus anginosus meningitis. *Neurocrit Care*, **3**, 157–60.

Lee, L., Kang, Y. S. and Astromoff, N. (1996). Septic thrombophlebitis of the inferior mesenteric vein associated with diverticulitis CT diagnosis. *Clinical Imaging*, **20**, 115–7.

Libman, B. S., Quismorio, F. P. Jr. and Stimmler, M. M. (1995). Polyarteritis nodosa-like vasculitis in human immunodeficiency virus infection. *Journal of Rheumatology*, **22**, 351–5.

Liebow, A. A., Carrington, C. R. and Friedman, P. J. (1972). Lymphomatoid granulomatosis. *Human Pathology*, **3**, 457–558.

Liu, Y. C., Tomashefski, J. F., Tomford, J. W. *et al.* (1989). Necrotizing pneumocystis carinii vasculitis associated with acquired immunodeficiency syndrome. *Archives of Pathology and Laboratory Medicine*, **113**, 494.

Liu, Y. Q. (1985). Radiology of aortoarteritis. *Radiologic Clinics of North America*, **23**, 671–88.

Livingston, J. Z., Casale, A. S., Hutchins, G. M. and Shapiro E. P. (1992). Coronary involvement in Cogan's syndrome. *American Heart Journal*, **123**, 528–30.

Ljunstrom, L., Franzen, C., Schlaug, M., Elowson, S. and Vidas, U. (1997). Reinfection with chlamydia pneumonia may induce isolated and systemic vasculitis in small and large vessels. *Scandinavian Journal of Infectious Diseases*, **104** (Suppl.), 37–40.

Longley, S., Caldwell, J. R. and Panush, R. S. (1986). Paraneoplastic vasculitis. Unique syndrome of cutaneous angiitis and arthritis associated with myeloproliferative disorders. *American Journal of Medicine*, **80**, 1027–30.

Lopez, L. R., Davis, K. C., Kohler, P. F. and Schocket, A. L.(1984). The hypocomplementemic urticarial-vasculitis syndrome: therapeutic response to hydroxychloroquine. *Journal of Allergy and Clinical Immunology*, **73**, 600–3.

McCallum, R. M. (1996). Cogan's syndrome. In *Current therapy of allergy, immunology, and rheumatology* (Lichtenstein, L. M. and Fauci, A. S., eds), 5th edn, pp. 255–60. Mosby, St Louis.

McCluggage, W. G., Armstrong, D. J., Maxwell, R. J., Ellis, P. K. and McCluskey, D. R. (1999). Systemic vasculitis and aneurysm formation in the Wiskott-Aldrich syndrome. *Journal of Clinical Pathology*, **52**, 390–2.

McIntyre, P. B., Berkey, C. S., King, S. M., Schaad, U. B., Kilpi, T. and Kanra, G. Y. (1997). Dexamethasone as adjunctive therapy in bacterial meningitis. A meta-analysis of randomized clinical trials since 1988. *Journal of the American Medical Association*, **278**, 925–31.

McLean, D. I. (1986). Cutaneous paraneoplastic syndromes. *Archives of Dermatology*, **86;122**, 765–7.

McMillan, A., Bishop, P. E., Aw, D. and Peutherer, J. F. (1989). Immunohistology of the skin rash associated with acute HIV infection. *AIDS*, **3**, 309–12.

Magrinat, G., Kerwin, K. S. and Gabriel, D. A. (1989). The clinical manifestations of Degos' syndrome. *Archives of Pathology and Laboratory Medicine*, **113**, 354–62.

Magro, C., Ali, N., Williams, J. D., Allen, J. N., and Ross, P. Jr (2005). Cytomegalovirus-associated pulmonary septal capillary injury sine inclusion body change: a distinctive cause of occult or macroscopic pulmonary hemorrhage in the immunocompetent host. *Applied Immunohistochemistry and Molecular Morphology*, **13**, 268–72.

Majoor, M. H. J. M., Albers, F. W. J. and Casselman, J. W. (1993). Clinical relevance of magnetic resonance imaging and computed tomography in Cogan's syndrome. *Acta Otolaryngologica*, (Stockholm), **113**, 625–31.

Marcussen, N. and Lund, C. (1989). Combined sarcoidosis and disseminated visceral giant cell vasculitis. *Pathology Research in Practice*, **184**, 325–30.

Markert, M. L. (1991). Purine nucleoside phosphorylase deficiency. *Immunodeficiency Review*, **3**, 45.

Martensson, U., Sjoholm, A. G., Sturfelt, G., Truedsson, L. and Laurell, A. B. (1992). Western blot analysis of human IgG reactive with the collagenous portion of C1q: evidence of distinct binding specificities. *Scandinavian Journal of Immunology*, **35**, 735–44.

Massari, M., Salvarani, C., Portioli, I., Ramazzotti, E., Gabbi, E. and Bonazzi, L. (1996). Polyarteritis nodosa and HIV infection: no evidence of a direct role of HIV. *Infection*, **24**, 159–61.

Matsumuro, K., Izumo, S., Umehara, F., Arisato, T., Maruyama, I., Yonezawa, S., Shirahama, H., Sato, E. and Osame, M. (1994). Paraneoplastic vasculitic neuropathy: immunohistochemical studies on a biopsied nerve and postmortem examination. *Journal of Internal Medicine*, **236**, 225–30.

Meehan, J. J., Bernard, H., Pastor, M. D., Anthony, V. and Torre, M. D. (1957). Dissecting aneurysm of aorta secondary to tuberculous aortitis. *Circulation*, **16**, 615–20.

Meyers, W. M. and Marty, A. M. (1991). Current concepts in the pathogenesis of leprosy. *Drugs*, **41**, 832–56.

Miller, D. V., Oderich, G. S., Aubry, M. C., Panneton, J. M., and Edwards, W. D. (2004). Surgical pathology of infected aneurysms of the descending thoracic and abdominal aorta: Clinicopathologic correlations in 29 cases (1976 to 1999). *Human Pathology*, **35**, 1112–20.

Mita, T., Nakanishi, Y., Ochiai, A., Shimoda, T., Kato, H., Yamaguchi, H. and Toda, G. (1999). Paraneoplastic vasculitis associated with esophageal carcinoma. *Pathology International*, **49**, 643–7.

Miyachi, H., Akizuki, M., Yamagata, H., Mimori, T., Yoshida, S. and Homma, M. (1987). Hypertrophic osteoarthropathy, cutaneous vasculitis, and mixed-type cryoglobulinemia in a patient with nasopharyngeal carcinoma. *Arthritis and Rheumatism*, **30**, 825–9.

Molbak, K. (2005). Human health consequences of antimicrobial drug-resistant Salmonella and other foodborne pathogens. *Clinical Infectious Diseases*, **41**, 1613–20.

Moffatt, S., Tanaka, N., Tada, K., Nose, M., Nakamura, M., Muraoka, O., Hirano, T. and Sugamura, K. (1996). A cytotoxic nonstructural protein, NS1, of human parvovirus B19 induces activation of interleukin-6 gene expression. *Journal of Virology*, **70**, 8485–91.

Moffatt, S., Yaegashi, N., Tada, K., and Sugamura, K. (1998). Human parvovirus B19 nonstructural protein induced apoptosis in erythroid lineage cells. *Journal of Virology*, **72**, 3018–24.

Moreno, S., Garcia Altozano, J., Pinilla, B., Lopez, J. C., de Quiros, B., Ortega, A., and Bouza, E. (1989). Lemierre's disease: postanginal bacteremia and pulmonary involvement caused by Fusobacterium necrophorum. *Review of Infectious Diseases*, **11**, 319–24.

Mouallem, M., Friedman, E., Pauzner, R., Schwartz, E., and Rubenstein, E. (1987). Rickettsiosis-associated hyponatremia. *Infection*, **15**, 315–6.

Muller, S. A. and Landry, M. (1974). Exchange autografts in malignant atrophic papulosis (Degos' disease). *Mayo Clinic Proceedings*, **49**, 884–8.

Murai, T., Imai, M., Inui, M., Watanabe, H. and Hosoda, Y. (1986). Generalized granulomatous arteritis with aortic dissection. *Zentralblatt fur Allgemeine Pathologie und Pathologische Anatomie*, **132**, 41–7.

Murakami, K., Ohsawa, M., Hu, S. X. Kanno, H., Aozasa, K. and Nose, M. (1998). Large-vessel arteritis associated with chronic active Epstein-Barr virus infection. *Arthritis and Rheumatism*, **41**, 369–73.

Muratori, S., Carrera, C., Gorani, A. and Alessi, E. (1999). Erythema elevatum diutinum and HIV infection: a report of five cases. *British Journal of Dermatology*, **141**, 335–8.

Nakagawa, A., Ito, M., Iwaki, T., Yatabe, Y., Asai, J. and Hayashi, K. (1996). Chronic active Epstein-Barr virus infection with giant coronary aneurysms. *American Journal of Clinical Pathology*, **105**, 733–6.

Naylor, D., Mullins, J. F. and Gilmore, J. F. (1960). Papulosis atrophicans maligna (Degos' syndrome): Report of the first United States case and review of the literature. *Archives of Dermatology*, **81**, 189–97.

Newman, L. S., Rose, C. S. and Maier, L. A. (1997). Medical progress: sarcoidosis. *New England Journal of Medicine*, **336**, 1224–34.

Newton, J. and Black, M. M. (1984). Familial malignant atrophic papulosis. *Clinical and Experimental Dermatology*, **9**, 298–9.

Nigro, G., Zerbini, M., Krzysztofiak, A., Gentilomi, G., Porcaro, M. A., Mango, T. and Musiani, M. (1994). Active or recent parvovirus B19 infection in children with Kawasaki disease. *Lancet*, **343**, 1260–1.

Numata, S., Kanda, K., Tanda, S., Inoue T., Doi, K., Sasaki S., Yaku, H. (2005). Sarcoidosis with double saccular abdomainl aortic aneurysm. *Journal of Vascular Surgery*, **41**, 1065.

Nurnberg, W., Grabbe, J. and Czarnetzki, B. M. (1995). Urticarial vasculitis syndrome effectively treated with dapsone and pentoxifylline. *Acta Dermato-Venereologica*, **75**, 54–6.

Ogawa, K., Ohmori, M., Kobayashi, S., *et al.* (1967). An autopsy case of papulose atrophiante maligne: The first case in Japan. *Acta Pathologica Japonica*, **17**, 457–63.

Oh, S. J. (1997). Paraneoplastic vasculitis of the peripheral nervous system. *Neurology Clinics*, **15**, 849–63.

Oh, S. J., Slaughter, R. and Harrell, L. (1991). Paraneoplastic vasculitic neuropathy: a treatable neuropathy. *Muscle and Nerve*, **14**, 152–6.

Ohtsuka, T. and Yamazaki, S. (2005). Prevalence of human parvovirus B19 component NS1 gene in patients with Henoch-Schonlein purpura and hypersensitivity vasculitis. *British Journal of Dermatology*, **152**, 1080–1.

Olmos, L. and Laugier, P. (1977). Ultrastructural study of a new case of Degos' disease, with a review of the literature. *Annals of Dermatology and Venereology*, **104**, 280–93.

Olmos, L., Hunziker, N. and Laugier, P. (1979). Microcylinders of endoplasmic reticulum in histiocytes in patients suffering from Degos' syndrome and dermatomyositis. *British Journal of Dermatology*, **100**, 137–45.

Oskoui, R., Davis, W. A. and Gomes, M. N. (1993). Salmonella aortitis. A report of a successfully treated case with a comprehensive review of the literature. *Archives of Internal Medicine*, **153**, 517–25.

Ozdogan, H., Arisoy, N., Kasapcapur, O., Sever, L., Caliskan, S., Tuzuner, N., Mat, C. and Yazici, H. (1997). Vasculitis in familial Mediterranean fever. *Journal of Rheumatology*, **24**, 323–7.

Palazzo, E., Bourgeois, P., Meyer, O., DeBandt, M., Kazatchkine, M. and Kahn, M. F. (1993). Hypocomplementemic urticarial vasculitis syndrome, Jaccoud's syndrome, valvulopathy: a new syndromic combination. *Journal of Rheumatology*, **20**, 1236–40.

Pallensen, R. M. and Rasmussen, N. R. (1979). Malignant atrophic papulosis (Degos' syndrome). *Acta Chirurgica Scandinavica*, **145**, 279–83.

Pankhurst, T., Savage, C. O., Gordon, C. and Harper, L. (2004). Malignancy is increased in ANCA-associated vasculitis. *Rheumatology* (Oxford), **43**, 1532–5.

Paramo, J. A., Rocha, E., Cuesta, B., *et al.* (1985). Fibrinolysis in Degos' disease. *Thrombosis and Haemostasis*, **54**, 730.

Pertuiset, E., Liote, F., Launay-Russ, E., Kemiche, F., Cerf-Payrastre, I. and Chesneau, A. M. (2000). Adult Henoch-Schönlcin purpura associated with malignancy. *Seminars in Arthritis and Rheumatism*, **29**, 360–7.

Petri, M., Barr, E., Cho, K. and Farmer, E. (1988). Overlap of granulomatous vasculitis and sarcoidosis: presentation with uveitis, eosinophilia, leg ulcers, sinusitis, and past foot drop. *Journal of Rheumatology*, **15**, 1171–3.

Pfaltzgraff, R. E. and Bryceson, A. (1985). Clinical leprosy. In *Leprosy* (Hastings, R. C., ed.), pp. 165–71. Churchill Livingstone, London.

Picard, O., Brunereau, L., Pelosse, B., Kerob, D., Cabane, J. and Imbert, J. C. (1997). Cerebral infarction associated with vasculitis due to varicella zoster virus in patients infected with the human immunodeficiency virus. *Biomedical Pharmacotherapy*, **51**, 449–54.

Pinals, R. S. (1978). Cogan's syndrome with arthritis and aortic insufficiency. *Journal of Rheumatology*, **5**, 294–8.

Plemmons, R. M., Dooley, D. P. and Longfield, R. N. (1995). Septic thrombophlebitis of the portal vein (pylephlebitis): diagnosis and management in the modern era. *Clinical Infectious Diseases*, **21**, 1114–20.

Podder, S. and Shepherd, R. C. (1994). Cogan's syndrome: a rare systemic vasculitis. *Archives of Diseases in Childhood*, **71**, 163–4.

Ponge, T., Boutoille, D., Moreau, A., Germaud, P., Dabouis, G., Baranger, T. and Barrier, J. (1998). Systemic vasculitis in a patient with small-cell neuroendocrine bronchial cancer. *European Respiratory Journal*, **12**, 1228–9.

Popper, H. H., Klemen, H., Colby, T. V. and Churg, A. (2003). Necrotizing sarcoid granulomatosis – is it different from nodular sarcoidosis? *Pneumonologie*, **57**, 268–71.

Prayson, R. A. (1999). Granulomatous myositis. Clinicopathologic study of 12 cases. *American Journal of Clinical Pathology*, **112**, 63–8.

Premalatha, S., Yesudian, P., Janaki, V. R., *et al.* (1980). Malignant atrophic papulosis (Degos' syndrome): First case report from India. *Clinical and Experimental Dermatology*, **5**, 370–71.

Raza, K., Karokis, D. and Kitas, G. D. (1998). Cogan's syndrome with Takayasu's arteritis. *British Journal of Rheumatology*, **37**, 369–72.

Reed, R. J. (1981). The T-lymphocyte, the mucinous epithelial interstitium, and immunostimulation. *American Journal of Dermatopathology*, **3**, 207–14.

Reinte, L., Taglione, E. and Berretini, S. (1996). Efficacy of methotrexate in Cogan's syndrome. *Journal of Rheumatology*, **23**, 1830–31.

Rich, S. A. (1981). Human lupus inclusions and interferon. *Science*, **213**, 772–5.

Rich, S. A. and Owens, T. R. (1982). Inducibility of human lupus inclusions by interferons. *Journal of Cellular Biochemistry*, S6, 279A.

Richardson, B. (1994). Methotrexate therapy for hearing loss in Cogan's syndrome. *Arthritis and Rheumatism*, **37**, 1559–61.

Roat, M. I., Thoft, R. A., Thomson, A. W., Jain, A., Funf, J. J. and Starzl, T. E. (1991). Treatment of Cogan's syndrome with FK506: a case report. *Transplantation Proceedings*, **23**, 3347.

Rodriguez-Pla, A., Bosch-Gil, J. A., Echevarria-Mayo, J. E., Rossello-Urgell, J., Solans-Laque, R., Huguet-Redecilla, P., Stone, J. H. and Vilardell-Tarres, M. (2004). No detection of parvovirus B19 or herpesvirus DNA in giant cell arteritis. *Journal of Clinical Virology*, **31**, 11–5.

Rodriguez-Serna, M., Fortea, J. M., Perez, A., Febrer, I., Ribes,C. and Aliaga, A. (1993). Erythema elevatum diutinum associated with celiac disease: response to a gluten-free diet. *Pediatric Dermatology*, **10**, 125–8.

Rose, A. G. and Sinclair-Smith, C. C. (1980). Takayasu's arteritis. A study of 16 autopsy cases. *Archives of Pathology Laboratory Medicine*, **104**, 231–7.

Rose, C. D., Eichenfield, A. H., Goldsmith, D. P. and Athreya,B. H. (1990). Early onset sarcoidosis with aortitis – juvenile systemic granulomatosis. *Journal of Rheumatology*, **17**, 102–6.

Rosen, C. L., DePalma, L. and Morita, A. (2000). Primary angiitis of the central nervous system as a first presentation in Hodgkin's disease: a case report and review of the literature. *Neurosurgery*, **46**, 1504–10.

Rosen, Y., Moon, S., Huang, C. T., Gourin, A. and Lyons, H. A. (1977). Granulomatous pulmonary angiitis in sarcoidosis. *Archives of Pathology and Laboratory Medicine*, **101**, 170–4.

Rowley, A. H., Wolinsky, S. M., Relman, D. A., Sambol, S. P., Sullivan, J., Terai, M. and Shulman, S. T. (1994). Search for highly conserved viral and bacterial nucleic acid sequences corresponding to an etiologic agent of Kawasaki disease. *Pediatric Research*, **36**, 567–71.

Rybicki, B. A., Major, M., Popovich, Jr. J. *et al.* (1997). Racial differences in sarcoidosis incidence: a 5-year study in a health maintenance organization. *American Journal of Epidemiology*, **145**, 234–41.

Sackier, J. M., Kelly, S. B., Clarke, D., Rees, A. J. and Wood, B. (1991). Small bowel haemorrhage due to cytomegalovirus vasculitis. *Gut*, **32**, 1419–20.

St Clair, E. W. and McCallum, R. M. (1999). Cogan's syndrome. *Current Opinion in Rheumatology*, **11**, 47–52.

Saldana, M. J., Patchefsky, A. S., Israel, H. I. and Atkinson, G. W. (1977). Pulmonary angiitis and granulomatosis. The relationship between histological features, organ involvement, and response to treatment. *Human Pathology*, **8**, 391–409.

Salvarani, C., Farnetti, E., Casal, B., Nicoli, D., Wenlan, L., Bajocchi, G., Macchioni, P., Lo Scocco, G., Grazia Catanoso, M., Boiardi, L. and Cantini, F. (2002). Detection of parvovirus B19 DNA by polymerase chain reaction in giant cell arteritis: a case-control study. *Arthritis and Rheumatism*, **46**, 3099–101.

Sanchez, N. B., Canedo, I. F., Garcia-Patos, P. E., de Unamuno Perez, P., Benito, A. V. and Pascual, A. M. (2004). Paraneoplastic vasculitis associated with multiple myeloma. *Journal of the European Academy of Dermatology and Venereology*, **18**, 731–5.

Sanchez, N. P., Winkelmann, R. K., Schroeter, A. L. and Dicken, C. H. (1982). The clinical and histopathologic spectrums of urticarial vasculitis: study of forty cases. *Journal of the American Academy of Dermatology*, **7**, 599–605.

Sanchez-Guerrero, J., Gutierrez-Urena, S., Vidaller, A., Reyes, E., Iglesias, A. and Alarcon-Segovia, D. (1990). Vasculitis as a paraneoplastic syndrome. Report of 11 cases and review of the literature. *Journal of Rheumatology*, **17**, 1458–62.

Sangueza, O. P., Pilcher, B. and Martin Sangueza, J. (1977). Erythema elevatum diutinum: a clinicopathological study of eight cases. *American Journal of Dermatopathology*, **19**, 214–22.

Sartwell, P. E. (1976). Racial differences in sarcoidosis. *Annals of the New York Academy of Sciences*, **278**, 368.

Saxena, R., Adolph, M., Ziegler, J. R., Murphy, W. and Rutecki, G. W. (1996). Pylephlebitis: a case report and review of outcome in the antibiotic era. *American Journal of Gastroenterology*, **91**, 1251–3.

Schaff, Z., Heine, U. and Dalton, A. J. (1972). Ultramorphological and ultracytochemical studies of tubuloreticular structures in lymphoid cells. *Cancer Research*, **32**, 2696.

Schuknecht, H. F. and Nadol, J. B. (1994). Temporal bone pathology in a case of Cogan's syndrome. *Laryngoscope*, **104**, 1135–42.

Sen, P. L., Kinare, S. G., Kulkarni, T. P. and Panulkar, G. B. (1962). Stenosing aortitis of unknown etiology. *Surgery*, **51**, 317–25.

Sharifi, R., Sinclair, J. C., Gilmour, K. C., Arkwright, P. D., Kinnon, C., Thrasher, A. J. and Gaspar, H. B. (2004). SAP mediates specific cytotoxic T-cell functions in X-linked lymphoproliferative disease. *Blood*, **103**, 3821–7.

Shah, P., Luqmani, R. A., Murray, P. I., Honan, W. P., Corridan, P. G. J. and Emery, P. (1994). Posterior scleritis: an unusual manifestation of Cogan's syndrome. *British Journal of Rheumatology*, **33**, 774–5.

Sharifi, R., Sinclair, J. C., Gilmour, K. C., Arkwright, P. D., Kinnon, C., Thrasher, A. J. and Gaspar, H. B. (2004). SAP mediates specific cytotoxic T-cell functions in X-linked lymphoproliferative disease. *Blood*, **103**, 3821–7.

Sheey, N., Sheehan, K, Brett, F., Kay, E., Grogan, L., and Delanty, N. (2003). Hodgkins disease presenting as granulomatous angiitis of the central nervous system. *Journal of Neurology*, **250**, 112–3.

Shi, R. J., Simpson-Haidaris, P. J., Lerner, N. B., Marder, V. J., Silverman, D. J. and Sporn, L. A. (1998). Transcriptional regulation of endothelial cell tissue factor expression during Rickettsia rickettsii infection: involvement of the transcription factor NF-κB. Infect. *Immunology*, **66**, 1070–5.

Singarayar, J. and Umerah, B. C. (1978). Tropical vasculitis. *Medical Journal of Zambia*, **12**, 74–6.

Sivakumar, M. and Chee, S. P. (1998). A case series of ocular disease as the primary manifestation in sarcoidosis. *Annals of the Academy of Medicine Singapore*, **27**, 560–6.

Soni, B. P., Wiiliford, P. M. and White, W. L. (1998). Erythematous nodules in a patient infected with the human immunodeficiency virus. Erythema elevatum diutinum (EED). *Archives of Dermatology*, **134**, 232–6.

Soravia-Dunand, V. A., Loo, V. G. and Salit, I. E. (1999). Aortitis due to Salmonella: report of 10 cases and comprehensive review of the literature. *Clinical Infectious Diseases*, **29**, 862–8.

Soter, N. A., Murphy, G. F. and Mihm, M. C. Jr (1982). Lymphocytes and necrosis of the cutaneous microvasculature in malignant atrophic papulosis: A refined light microscopy study. *Journal of American Academy of Dermatology*, **7**, 620–30.

Sotrel, A., Lacson, A. G. and Huff, K. R. (1983). Childhood Kohlmeier-Degos disease with atypical skin lesions. *Neurology*, **33**, 1146–51.

Stashower, M. E., Rennie, T. A., Turiansky, G. W. and Gilliland, W. R. (1999). Ovarian cancer presenting as leukocytoclastic vasculitis. *Journal of American Academy of Dermatology*, **40**, 287–9.

Stephansson, E. A., Niemi, K. M., Jouhikainen, T., Vaarala, O. and Palosuo, T. (1991). Lupus anticoagulant and the skin. A longterm follow-up study of SLE patients with special reference to histopathological findings. *Acta Dermato-Venereologica*, **71**, 416–22.

Strole, W. E. Jr., Clark, W. H. Jr. and Isselbacher, K. J. (1967). Progressive arterial occlusive disease (Kohlmeier-Degos): A frequently fatal cutaneo-systemic disorder. *New England Journal of Medicine*, **276**, 195–201.

Sturgess, A. S. and Littlejohn, G. O. (1988). Jaccoud's arthritis and panvasculitis in the hypocomplementemic urticarial vasculitis syndrome. *Journal of Rheumatology*, **15**, 858–61.

Su, W. P., Schroeter, A. L., Lee, D. A., Hsu, T. and Muller, S. A. (1985). Clinical and histologic findings in Degos' syndrome (malignant atrophic papulosis). *Cutis*, **35**, 131–8.

Suarez, J., Miguelez, M. and Villalba, R. (1998). Nodular erythema elevatum diutinum in an HIV-1 infected woman: response to dapsone and antiretroviral therapy. *British Journal of Dermatology*, **138**, 717–8.

Subbiah, P., Wijdicks, E., Muenter, M., Carter, J. and Connolly, S. (1996). Skin lesion with a fatal neurologic outcome (Degos' disease). *Neurology*, **46**, 636–40.

Suzuki, J. and Takaku, A. (1969). Cerebrovascular 'moya moya' disease showing abnormal net-like vessels in base of brain. *Archives of Neurology*, **20**, 288–99.

Suzuki, T., Obara, Y., Sato, Y., Saito, G., Ichiwata, T. and Uchiyama, T. (1996). Cancer-associated retinopathy with presumed vasculitis. *American Journal of Ophthalmology*, **122**, 125–7.

Takemura, T., Matsui, Y., Oritsu, M., Akiyama, O., Hiraga, Y., Omichi, M., Hirasawa, M., Saiki, S., Tamura, S. and Mochizuki, I. (1991). Pulmonary vascular involvement in sarcoidosis: granulomatous angiitis and microangiopathy in transbronchial lung biopsies. *Virchows Archives in Pathology Anatomy and Histopathology*, **418**, 361–8.

Takemura, T., Shishiba, T., Akiyama, O., Oritsu, M., Matsui, Y. and Eishi, Y. (1997). Vascular involvement in cutaneous sarcoidosis. *Pathology International*, **47**, 84–9.

Tanaka, S., Komori, K., Okadome, K., Sugimachi, K. and Mori, R. (1994). Detection of active cytomegalovirus infection in inflammatory aortic aneurysms with RNA polymerase chain. *Journal of Vascular Surgery*, **20**, 235–43.

Taniwaki, S., Kataoka, M., Tanaka, H., Mizuno, Y. and Hirose, M. (1997). Multiple ulcers of the ileum due to Cytomegalovirus infection in a patient who showed no evidence of an immunocompromised state. *Journal of Gastroenterology*, **32**, 548–52.

Tasanen, K., Raudasoja, R., Kallioinen, M. and Ranki, A.(1997). Erythema elevatum diutinum in association with coeliac disease. *British Journal of Dermatology*, **136**, 624–7.

Tatum, E. T., Sun, P. C. and Cohn, D. L. (1989). Cytomegalovirus vasculitis and colon perforation in a patient with the acquired immunodeficiency syndrome. *Pathology*, **21**, 235–8.

Tauber, E., Wojnarowski, C., Horcher, E., Dekan, G., and Frischer, T. (1999). Necrotizing sarcoid granulomatosis in a 14-yr-old female. *European Respiratory*, **13**, 703–5.

Tekin, M., Yalcinkaya, F., Tumer, N., Akar, N., Misirlioglu, M. and Cakar, N. (2000). Clinical, laboratory and molecular characteristics of children with familial Mediterranean fever-associated vasculitis. *Acta Paediatrica*, **89**, 177–82.

Tekin, M., Yalcinkaya, F., Tumer, N., Cakar, N., Kocak, H., Ozkaya, N. and Gencgonul, H. (1999). Familial Mediterranean fever – renal involvement by diseases other than amyloid. *Nephrology, Dialysis, Trasplantation*, **14**, 475–9.

The French FMF Consortium (1997). A candidate gene for familial Mediterranean fever. *Nature Genetics*, **17**, 25–31.

The International FMF Consortium. (1997). Ancient missense mutations in a new member of the RoRet gene family are likely to cause familial Mediterranean fever. *Cell*, **90**, 797–807.

Thomas, H. G. (1992). Case report: clinical and radiological features of Cogan's syndrome – non-syphilitic interstitial keratitis, audiovestibular symptoms and systemic manifestations. *Clinical Radiology*, **45**, 418–21.

Torok, L., Husz, S., Korom, I., Horvath, K. and Forizs, A. (1993). Systemic lupus erythematosus with pigmented skin. *Cutis*, **51**, 433–6.

Trendelenburg, M., Courvoisier, S., Spath, P. J., Moll, S., Mihatsch, M., Itin, P., and Schifferli, J. A. (1999). Hypocomplementemic urticarial vasculitis or systemic lupus erythematosus? *American Journal of Kidney Diseases*, **34**, 745–51.

Trottier, F., Dufour, M., Grondin, P., Bouchard, G., *et al.* (1994). Magnetic resource imaging in moya moya disease. *Canadian Association of Radiology Journal*, **45**, 137–9.

Tseng, J. F., Cambria, R. P., Aretz, H. T., and Brewster, B. C. (1999). Thoracoabdominal aortic aneurysm in Cogan's syndrome. *Journal of Vascular Surgery*, **30**, 565–8.

Tzanck, A., Civatte, A. and Sidi, E. (1948). Presentation de moulage: Ulerytheme porcelain en gouttes. *Bulletin de la Societe Francaise de Dermatologie et de Syphiligraphie*, **55**, 10–12.

Umerah B. C. (2002). Tropical aortitis (tropical vasculitis) and lepromatous vasculitis. In: *Vasculitis* (Ball G. V. and Bridges, S. L. Jr., eds), pp. 290–9. Oxford University Press, Oxford.

Umerah, B. C. (1980). Angiography of stroke in Central Africa. *American Journal of Roentgenology*, **134**, 963–5.

Uzman, B. G., Saito, H. and Kasac, M. (1971). Tubular arrays in the endoplasmic reticulum in human tumor cells. *Laboratory Investigation*, **24**, 492–8.

van Son, J. A., O'Marcaigh A. S., Edwards, W. D., Julsrud, P. R., and Danielson G. K. (1995). Successful resection of thoracic aortic aneurysms in Wiskott-Aldrich syndrome. *Annals of Thoracic Surgery*, **60**, 685–7.

Vella, J. P., O'Callaghan, J., Hickey, D., and Walshe, J. J. (1997). Renal artery stenosis complicating Cogan's syndrome. *Clinical Nephrology*, **47**, 407–8.

Veraldi, S., Mancuso, R., Rizzitelli, G., Gianotti, R., and Ferrante, P. (1999). Henoch-Schonlein syndrome associated with human Parvovirus B19 primary infection. *European Journal of Dermatology*, **9**, 232–3.

Vincent, D., Dubas, F., Hauw, J. J., *et al.* (1986). Nerve and muscle microvasculitis in peripheral neuropathy: a remote effect of cancer? *Journal of Neurology Neurosurgery and Psychiatry*, **49**, 1007–10.

Volini, F. I., Olfield, R. C., Thompson, J. R. and Kent, G. (1962). Tuberculosis of the aorta. *Journal of the American Medical Association*, **181**, 78–83.

Vollertsen, R. S., McDonald, T. J., Younge, B. R., Banks, P. M., Stanson, A. W. and Ilstrup, D. M. (1986). Cogan's syndrome: 18 cases and a review of the literature. *Mayo Clinic Proceedings*, **61**, 344–61.

Walker, D. H. (1989). Rocky Mountain spotted fever: A Disease in need of microbiological convern. *Clinical Microbiology Reviews*, **2**, 227.

Walker, D. H. (1990). The role of host factors in the severity of spotted fever and typhus rickettsioses. *Annals of the New York Academy of Sciences*, **590**, 10–9.

Walker, D. H., Gay, R. M., and Valdes-Dapena, M. (1981). The occurrence of eschars in Rocky Mountain spotted fever. *Journal of the American Academy of Dermatology*, **4**, 571–6.

Walker, D. H. and Raoult, D. (2000). *Rickettsia rickettsii* and other spotted fever group Rickettsiae (Rocky Mountain spotted fever and other spotted fevers). In *Bennett's Principles and Practice of Infectious Diseases* (Mandell, G. L., Bennett, J. E. and Dolin, R., eds), 5th edn, pp. 2037–8. Churchill Livingstone, Philadelphia, PA.

Wang, J. H., Liu, Y. C., Yen, M. Y., Chen, Y. S., Wann, S. R., and Cheng, D. L. (1996). Mycotic aneurysm due to non-typhi salmonella: report of 16 cases. *Clinical Infectious Diseases*, **23**, 743–7.

Watanabe, T., Mochizuki, M. and Yamaguchi, K. (1997). HTLV-1 uveitis (HU). *Leukemia*, **11** (Suppl. 3), 582–4.

Webster, E., Corman, L. C. and Braylan, R. C. (1986). Syndrome of temporal arteritis with perivascular infiltration by malignant cells in a patient with follicular small cleaved cell lymphoma. *Journal of Rheumatology*, **113**, 1163–6.

Weiss, D. J., Greenfield, J. W. Jr, O'Rourke, K. S., McCune, W. J. (1993). Systemic cytomegalovirus infection mimicking an exacerbation of Wegener's granulomatosis. *Journal of Rheumatology*, **20**, 155–7.

Wilkinson, S. M., English, J. S., Smith, N. P., Wilson-Jones, E. and Winkelmann, R. K. (1992). Erythema elevatum diutinum: a clinicopathological study. *Clinical and Experimental Dermatology*, **17**, 87–93.

Wisnieski, J. J. (2000). Urticarial vasculitis. *Current Opinion in Rheumatology*, **12**, 24–31.

Wisnieski, J. J. and Jones, S. M. (1992a). Comparison of autoantibodies to the collagen-like region of C1q in hypocomplementemic urticarial vasculitis syndrome and systemic lupus erythematosus. *Journal of Immunology*, **148**, 1396–403.

Wisnieski, J. J. and Jones, S. M. (1992b). IgG autoantibody to the collagen-like region of C1q in hypocomplementemic urticarial vasculitis syndrome, systemic lupus erythematosus, and 6 other musculoskeletal or rheumatic diseases. *Journal of Rheumatology*, **19**, 884–8.

Wisnieski, J. J., Baer, A. N., Christensen, J., Cupps, T. R., Flagg, D. N., Jones, J. V., Katzenstcin, P. L., McFadden, E. R., McMillen, J. J., Pick, M. A., *et al.* (1995). Hypocomplementemic urticarial vasculitis syndrome. Clinical and serologic findings in 18 patients. *Medicine* (Baltimore), **74**, 24–41.

Wooten, M. D. and Jasin, H. E. (1996). Vasculitis and lymphoproliferative diseases. *Seminars in Arthritis and Rheumatism*, **26**, 564–74.

Zandberg, M., de Maar, E. F., Hofker, H. S., Homan van der Heide, J. J., Rosati, S. and van Son, W. J. (2005). Initial cytomegalovirus prophylaxis with ganciclovir: no guarantee for prevention of late serious manifestations of CMV after solid organ transplantation. *Netherlands Journal of Medicine*, **63**, 408–12.

Zeiss, C. R., Burch, F. X., Marder, R. J., Furey, N. L., Schmid, F. R. and Gewurz, H. (1980). A hypocomplementemic vasculitic urticarial syndrome. Report of four new cases and definition of the disease. *American Journal of Medicine*, **68**, 867–75.

Zhang, J., Shehabeldin, A., da Cruz, L. A., Butler, J., Somani, A. K., McGavin, M., Kozieradzki, I., dos Santos, A. O., Nagy, A., Grinstein, S., Penninger, J. M. and Siminovitch, K. A. (1999). Antigen receptor-induced activation and cytoskeletal rearrangement are impaired in Wiskott-Aldrich syndrome protein-deficient lymphocytes. *Journal of Experimental Medicine*, **190**, 1329–42.

CHAPTER 43

Experimental therapies for vasculitis

Philip Seo and John H. Stone

Primary systemic vasculitis was not recognized as a clinical entity until 1866, when Adolf Kussmaul and Rudolf Maier described the case of a 27-year-old journeyman tailor who developed fever, myalgias, abdominal pain, and oliguria (Kussmaul and Maier 1866). On autopsy, they noted nodular inflammatory lesions of the medium- and small-sized arteries that today would be recognized as polyarteritis nodosa, the archetype for all forms of primary systemic vasculitis (Matteson 1999). In their famous description of this disorder, they wrote that he was "[o]ne of those patients for whom one can already give the prognosis before the diagnosis.... The first impression was one of a lost soul whose ... days were numbered...."

The prognosis for primary systemic vasculitis in the modern era is not nearly so grim. The use of cytotoxic agents for the treatment of these diseases has dramatically improved the immediate prognosis of patients with these diseases. The so-called Fauci–Wolff protocol (Fauci and Wolff 1973), which uses a prolonged course of cyclophosphamide and glucocorticoids for the treatment of Wegener's granulomatosis (WG) and microscopic polyangiitis (MPA), has provided a template that has been successfully applied to other forms of systemic vasculitis, resulting in a dramatic improvement in mortality.

This great success, unfortunately, highlights the shortcomings of current treatment strategies. A quick end has now been replaced by death by a thousand cuts, inflicted by the all too-common cycle of disease flare, control of inflammation through exposure to immunosuppressive agents, relapse upon tapering of these medications, and retreatment with the same potentially toxic therapies. Ironically, the treatments themselves frequently lead to the most serious consequences in terms of long-term morbidity and quality of life (Seo et al. 2005).

Renewed interest in the vasculitides has led to a groundswell of experience regarding the treatment of these complex diseases. Many of these new (but still unproven) therapies may be on the cusp of joining standard medications for the treatment of vasculitis. This chapter will explore some of the most promising experimental therapies that may eventually become part of a new standard of care for these diseases.

Antimetabolite agents

Immunity is dependent on rapidly dividing cells that require continual synthesis of DNA. These cells are particularly susceptible to antimetabolite agents that mimic the structure of natural substrates and thereby block nucleotide and nucleic acid synthesis. Azathioprine, for example, is metabolized to 6-mercaptopurine, which blocks de novo purine synthesis. Methotrexate, an analog of folate, blocks the synthesis of both purines and pyrimidines. The immunosuppressive properties of antimetabolites have long been recognized, and such drugs have been widely used in solid organ transplantation and the treatment of autoimmune diseases, including vasculitis.

In recent years, patients with the most severe forms of vasculitis have been treated with a two-step approach. First, the flare is quelled with the combination of high-dose glucocorticoids and a cytotoxic agent, such as cyclophosphamide. After remission is achieved, the cytotoxic agent is replaced by an antimetabolite, such as methotrexate or azathioprine. Although this strategy has become the standard of care, only recently has this approach been validated in randomized, controlled trials (Jayne et al. 2003; Wegener's Granulomatosis Etanercept Trial (WGET) Research Group 2005).

The use of antimetabolite agents has not been confined to remission-maintenance alone. Antimetabolites have been the medications of choice to treat forms of vasculitis that are not life threatening, due to their favorable toxicity profile. The "Non-Renal ANCA-associated vasculitis Alternatively treated with Methotrexate" (NORAM) trial is the first randomized clinical trial to examine this approach (De Groot et al. 2005). In this trial, 100 patients with early systemic WG or MPA were randomized to treatment with either oral cyclophosphamide or weekly methotrexate (in addition to standardized glucocorticoids in tapering doses). Approximately 90% of patients in both groups achieved remission in 6 months, further supporting the use of these agents as initial therapy in carefully selected patients with vasculitis.

Because these agents are generally well tolerated, there has been great interest in expanding their use for the treatment of systemic vasculitis. Much of that interest has focused on the development of mycophenolate mofetil as an alternative to methotrexate and azathioprine. There has also been recent experience with more aggressive use of older agents.

High-dose azathioprine

When used for the treatment of vasculitis, azathioprine is generally administered using a daily oral dose of 2 mg/kg of body weight. Whether this is the optimal dose and route, however, has never been established. High-dose, pulse intravenous azathioprine has previously been demonstrated to be efficacious and well-tolerated in patients with ulcerative colitis (Mahadevan et al. 2000), ankylosing spondylitis (Durez and Horsmas 2000), and refractory rheumatoid arthritis (Pickenpack et al. 2000; Matteson et al. 1999), raising the possibility that this treatment strategy may be effective for systemic vasculitis as well.

In 2004, Aries et al. reported their use of high-dose intravenous azathioprine for two patients with WG who had failed other forms of therapy (including infliximab and rituximab). Both patients were treated with monthly intravenous boluses of azathioprine (dosed at 17 mg/kg), supplemented by oral daily azathioprine both during pulse therapy, and afterward for remission maintenance. In both cases, clinical response was noted after the first two pulses of azathioprine, and continued improvement was noted throughout treatment.

In that same year, a second group reported their experience with a similar treatment protocol applied to four patients with WG, all of whom had been refractory to therapy with daily oral cyclophosphamide (with a mean cumulative dose of 29 g per patient) (Benenson et al. 2004). All four patients had received comparable doses of intravenous azathioprine, that is between 1200 mg and 1800 mg azathioprine per dose, and each patient received between two and six pulses, depending on clinical response. One patient entered a prolonged clinical remission after four intravenous pulses. A second patient remained in remission with the assistance of methotrexate and low-dose prednisone. The other two patients, however, failed to respond, with progression of pulmonary and ocular disease, respectively.

There are several possible explanations for why intravenous boluses of azathioprine might be more efficacious than standard oral dosing. Bioavailability of orally administered azathioprine is highly variable; moreover, the optimal dose–response relationship for azathioprine has never been thoroughly explored. Based on these data, it seems reasonable to conclude that the clinical efficacy of azathioprine may be limited by the imposition of arbitrary dosing strategies, and that the full potential of this drug for the treatment of vasculitis has not yet been realized.

Mycophenolate mofetil

In the 1960s, mycophenolate mofetil was identified as a promising new antibiotic (Ballio and Sermonti 1961). More recently, it was noted that mycophenolate mofetil also has immunosuppressive properties, based on its ability to inhibit the de novo synthesis of purines (Allison and Eugui 1991). In the modern era, it is most frequently used as an immunosuppressive agent for patients with solid organ transplants, particularly those involving the kidney.

Mycophenolate mofetil is rapidly metabolized to mycophenolic acid, which is chiefly responsible for its therapeutic effect. Free mycophenolic acid reversibly inhibits inosine monophosphate dehydrogenase, which is integral to the de novo synthesis of purines. Free mycophenolic acid preferentially binds the isoform expressed by lymphocytes; in theory, this preference should make this compound more lymphocyte-specific than azathioprine (Appel et al. 2005).

The most common reason for intolerance to this drug is mycophenolic acid glucuronide, an inactive metabolite that induces nausea in as many as 11% of all patients (Mok and Lai 2002). There is now an enteric-coated form of mycophenolic acid that may provide an option for patients who were previously intolerant of this drug (Salvadori et al. 2004). This may be particularly important for patients with severe renal dysfunction, who may be more likely to experience untoward effects due to impaired clearance of the metabolite (Haubitz and de Groot 2002).

Enthusiasm for the use of mycophenolate mofetil for the treatment of rheumatic diseases blossomed after the recent publication of studies indicating that it is non-inferior and potentially superior to cyclophosphamide for the treatment of diffuse proliferative lupus nephritis (Ginzler et al. 2005). Mycophenolate mofetil has been used for the treatment of several forms of vasculitis. Although definitive studies are forthcoming, current evidence provides clues as to the niche that this drug may occupy for the treatment of these challenging diseases.

Mycophenolate mofetil and Takayasu's arteritis

In 1999, Daina et al. published their experience using mycophenolate mofetil for the treatment of refractory Takayasu's arteritis. In this report, they described rapid resolution of both subjective and objective signs and symptoms of vasculitis after treatment with 1 g of mycophenolate mofetil taken twice daily (Daina et al. 1999). Since that time, however, many have been unable to replicate these results in clinical practice (Liang and Hoffman 2005). Moreover, no further reports documenting the successful use of mycophenolate mofetil for the treatment of Takayasu's arteritis have been published since.

Mycophenolate mofetil and Behçet's syndrome

Behçet's syndrome (BS) is a protean disorder that can lead to small, medium, and large-vessel vasculitis, in addition to the pathognomonic mucocutaneous ulcerations. Because the immunosuppressive effects of mycophenolate mofetil are similar to those of cyclosporine and azathioprine (both of which are known to be efficacious for the treatment of BS), it is logical to assume that mycophenolate mofetil might be effective for BS as well. In 2001, Adler et al. published their experience with a series of six patients who were treated with 2 to 3 g of mycophenolate mofetil daily in divided doses. Although these patients were enrolled as part of a much larger study, the trial was stopped after the sixth patient due to early evidence of futility (Adler et al. 2001). All patients were treated with mycophenolate mofetil and prednisolone 30 mg daily; as the prednisolone was withdrawn, all six patients experienced disease flares. This negative study highlights the extent to which the exact mechanism of immunosuppressive agents is poorly understood, and the importance of clinical trials to confirm the efficacy of ostensibly similar compounds.

Mycophenolate mofetil and ANCA-associated vasculitis

The greatest interest in mycophenolate mofetil has been generated by its potential use as a treatment for the ANCA-associated vasculitides, in particular WG and MPA. Because it is functionally similar to agents with known efficacy for the treatment of ANCA-associated vasculitis, it is tempting to assume that this agent would be equally efficacious for these diseases.

The first published report of the use of mycophenolate mofetil for the treatment of an ANCA-associated vasculitis appeared in 1999 (Waiser *et al.* 1999). Since that time, there have been two case series examining the potential use of this drug for the maintenance of cyclophosphamide-induced remission. The initial report was more sanguine; in 1999, Nowack *et al.* reported the successful use of mycophenolate mofetil for maintenance of remission in patients with ANCA-associated vasculitis, noting only one relapse among 11 patients followed for a median of 15 months (Nowak *et al.* 1999). More sobering is the experience reported by Langford *et al.* (2004) who noted a 42% relapse rate among 14 patients followed for a median of 18 months. The difference in outcome may have reflected differences in trial design, since the Nowak study allowed patients to remain on prednisone 5 mg daily as a maintenance dose, while the Langford study tapered patients completely off prednisone. This may highlight the importance of low-dose prednisone as an adjunctive remission maintenance agent, and the limitations of mycophenolate mofetil as monotherapy for vasculitis (Birck *et al.* 2005).

In 2005, Joy *et al.* reported their experience using mycophenolate mofetil for the induction of remission in patients with flares of ANCA-associated vasculitis. Twelve patients with vasculitis flares that were either non-life threatening or resistant to cyclophosphamide were treated with 1 g of mycophenolate mofetil twice daily. At 24 weeks, the average Birmingham Vasculitis Activity Score (BVAS) (see Chapter 23) fell from a mean of 9.1 to a mean of 2.8, with sustained effects at 52 weeks of follow-up (Joy *et al.* 2005). From the study design, it is not clear how important glucocorticoids were to maintaining remission, although this study gives further evidence that mycophenolate mofetil may be appropriate for the initial therapy of patients with these diseases.

The real answers likely lie in the results of the "International Mycophenolate mofetil Protocol to Reduce Outbreaks of Vasculitides" (IMPROVE) trial, which will compare mycophenolate mofetil to azathioprine for remission maintenance in ANCA-associated vasculitis (Little and Pusey 2005), and the ongoing Mayo Nephrology Clinical Group Trial of mycophenolate mofetil for the induction and maintenance of remission among patients with MPA.

Biologic agents

In retrospect, the first decade of the twenty-first century will be seen as having ushered in a new era in rheumatology therapeutics. This exciting time has seen the advent of biologic agents that target key components of the autoinflammatory response. This new era has been propelled by research in inflammatory arthritis and the discovery of the important role played by tumor necrosis factor (TNF) in rheumatoid arthritis and the spondyloarthropathies. With commercially-available TNF inhibitors, clinical improvement and even regression of erosive damage have become commonplace (Emery 2006).

Unfortunately, the resounding success of these agents for the treatment of inflammatory arthritis does not translate easily to other forms of autoimmune disease. Attempts to use these agents for systemic lupus erythematosus, scleroderma, and the inflammatory myopathies, for example, have not yielded a practical role for TNF blockade in the treatment of these diseases.

Despite some early failures, however, biologic agents still hold great promise for the treatment of the primary systemic vasculitides. Early work in this field focused on the use of TNF inhibitors; more recently, there has been significant work on the use of anti-CD20 monoclonal antibody therapy as a potential treatment for several forms of vasculitis.

TNF inhibitors and large-vessel vasculitis

Both Takayasu's arteritis and giant cell arteritis (GCA) are characterized by granulomatous vascular inflammation. Because TNF is vital to granuloma formation, TNF inhibition represents an approach worthy of thorough investigation. Moreover, there is evidence indicating that susceptibility to these diseases may be influenced by polymorphisms of the TNF gene (Mattey *et al.* 2000), making the use of TNF inhibitors even more tempting.

In 2004, Hoffman *et al.* reported the results of an open label trial examining the effect of anti-TNF therapy on patients with relapsing Takayasu's arteritis (Hoffman *et al.* 2004). Seven patients were treated with etanercept, and eight were treated with infliximab at varying doses. There was only one treatment failure; the remaining 14 patients all demonstrated clinical benefit, and 10 patients were successfully tapered off glucocorticoids. Of note, three of the patients initially treated with etanercept were switched to infliximab due to lack of availability of etanercept, but patients continued on etanercept therapy alone also demonstrated marked clinical response.

In 2005, Hoffman *et al.* reported the interim results of a double-blind, placebo-controlled trial of patients with active GCA, randomized to receive adjunctive therapy with infliximab (5 mg/kg intravenous every 8 weeks). This trial had enrolled 44 patients when it was stopped due to lack of clinical efficacy (Hoffman *et al.* 2005). Interim analysis demonstrated no significant difference in rate of relapse, cumulative glucocorticoid dose, and time to first relapse.

These disparate results are surprising, given the similarities in pathophysiology between these two diseases. Why this approach should succeed for one disease but not the other is not immediately clear. Regardless, this differential response to TNF inhibition provides a profound insight into the pathophysiology of these diseases, demonstrating how intrinsically different molecular pathways can lead to a clinically similar endpoint.

TNF inhibitors and ANCA-associated vasculitis

There is a considerable amount of indirect evidence supporting a role for TNF-α in the pathogenesis of ANCA-associated vasculitis. Polymorphisms of the TNF gene have been reported to influence the clinical course of patients with WG (Mascher *et al.* 1997). Moreover, TNF-α may be integral to priming the neutrophils that induce tissue damage (Kamesh *et al.* 2002). In one small study, patients with ANCA-associated vasculitis had detectable levels of serum TNF-α that normalized during disease remission (Jonasdottir *et al.* 2001). In an animal model of vasculitis, treatment with anti-TNF-α therapy prevents the onset of renal vasculitis (Karkar 2001). It therefore seems logical to assume that TNF-inhibitors would drastically influence the outcomes of these diseases. Data in this field primarily come from European case series that have focused on the use of infliximab, and a large American randomized clinical trial of etanercept as an adjunctive therapy for the treatment of WG.

Infliximab and ANCA-associated vasculitis

In 2002, Lamprecht *et al.* (2002b) reported their experience treating six patients with refractory WG with a combination of glucocorticoids, cyclophosphamide, and infliximab (5 mg/kg intravenous infusion every 6 weeks). Five patients experienced disease remission within 6 months. All patients demonstrated normalization of C-reactive protein levels, and ANCA titers became undetectable. One patient experienced a disease relapse after 12 months while receiving remission maintenance therapy with azathioprine. Two patients experienced untoward effects: one developed an infection that led the investigators to discontinue infliximab; the other developed a carcinoid tumor 12 months after disease remission was attained (Lamprecht *et al.* 2002a).

This report was rapidly followed by another, in which Bartolucci *et al.* described the use of infliximab in seven patients who were refractory to standard therapies (which consisted of glucocorticoids and at least one glucocorticoid-sparing agent). Patients were treated with a loading regimen, followed by maintenance infusions of infliximab dosed at 5 mg/kg every 8 weeks. All patients demonstrated some clinical benefit, with a decrease in the mean BVAS score from 9.1 to 1.3 at 6 months of follow-up, with no serious adverse events reported (Bartolucci *et al.* 2002).

In 2004, Booth *et al.* examined the effects of infliximab on 14 patients with ANCA-associated vasculitis, using response to acetylcholine stimulation as a surrogate marker for endothelial dysfunction (Booth *et al.* 2004a). In this study, infliximab infusion significantly improved responsiveness to acetylcholine as measured by forearm plethysmography, implying that TNF inhibition might improve the endothelium-dependent vasomotor response that was damaged by vasculitis.

In an open-label study conducted at the same time, 16 patients with acute flares of ANCA-associated vasculitis, and 16 patients with persistent "grumbling" disease were treated with 5 mg/kg of infliximab, administered at 0, 2, 6, and 10 weeks in addition to standard therapies (Booth *et al.* 2004b). Fourteen patients in each group achieved disease remission, with a decrease in BVAS from 12.3 to 0.3 at week 14 (P <0.001). This was accompanied by a significant decrease in serum C-reactive protein (CRP) levels. Despite this initial response, during a mean follow-up period of 16.8 months, one out of every five patients experienced disease flare while maintained on infliximab, and approximately one out of every five developed a severe infection, including pneumonia, urosepsis, abscess, and *Nocardia* endophthalmitis (Booth *et al.* 2004b).

Etanercept and ANCA-associated vasculitis

The Wegener's Granulomatosis Etanercept Trial (WGET) was a double-blinded trial of patients with active WG who were randomized to receive either etanercept or placebo, in addition to standard-of-care therapies (including cyclophosphamide or methotrexate, depending on disease severity). This trial, the largest of its kind to be conducted in the United States, enrolled 180 WG patients (128 of whom had severe disease). Patients who were randomized to the experimental arm received adjunctive therapy with etanercept 25 mg administered subcutaneously twice weekly. Patients in the WGET cohort were followed for a mean of 2.4 years after enrollment (Wegener's Granulomatosis Etanercept Trial (WGET) Study Group 2005).

This trial demonstrated no benefit of adding etanercept to standard therapies in terms of remission rate, frequency of sustained remission or low disease activity, time to sustained remission, or number of disease flares. In addition, six patients who had received etanercept had developed solid tumor malignancies, significantly more than would have been expected given the age and gender of the patients in the WGET cohort (Stone *et al.* 2005).

The reasons that this trial failed to demonstrate clinical benefit for adjunctive therapy with etanercept, which suppressed the enthusiasm engendered by early successes with infliximab, are not completely clear. Infliximab is a more efficient inhibitor of TNF than etanercept, and it seems possible that mechanistic differences may lead to differences in clinical response. Regardless, given the strongly negative results of the WGET trial and the potential association between TNF inhibitors and adverse events (including infection and malignancy), enthusiasm for continued investigations of TNF inhibition for ANCA-associated vasculitis is low.

B-cell targeted therapies

The first report linking a B-cell targeted therapy to vasculitis was published in 2001, in a case report documenting a possible causal link between rituximab and cutaneous vasculitis (Dereure *et al.* 2001). It is therefore ironic that rituximab, a chimeric monoclonal anti-CD 20 antibody that specifically targets the B-cell lineage, is the most promising of the new biologic agents for the treatment of systemic vasculitis. Rituximab has long been used as primary therapy for specific types of lymphoma, and more recently has found a niche for the treatment of autoimmune hematologic diseases, including antibody-mediated thrombocytopenia, chronic immune-mediated thrombocytopenia, and autoimmune hemolytic anemia. The resounding success of this drug in hematology and oncology has led to investigations in rheumatoid arthritis, systemic lupus erythematosus, and vasculitis (Gottenberg *et al.* 2005).

Fully humanized forms of anti-CD20 monoclonal antibodies and other antibodies targeting other molecules crucial to the B-cell lineage may rival rituximab in the next few years. Whether these new treatments will demonstrate clinical superiority (while maintaining the safety profile associated with the older drug) will need to be established in the near future.

Rituximab and cryoglobulinemia

In 2002, Arzoo *et al.* reported the successful use of rituximab to treat a 71-year-old woman who had developed glomerulonephritis, neuropathy, and cutaneous vasculitis due to mixed essential cryoglobulinemia not associated with hepatitis C infection (Arzoo *et al.* 2002). This report was followed by a larger case series of 15 patients with mixed cryoglobulinemia (due to hepatitis C in 12 cases) who had been refractory to other forms of therapy (Zaja *et al.* 2003). Patients were followed for 9 to 31 months after rituximab administration. All patients had evidence of clinical improvement accompanied by decreased levels of serum rheumatoid factor (thus corroborating the ability of rituximab to decrease the immune complex burden associated with a chronic infection). Additional case reports lend further credence to the hypothesis that rituximab is safe and efficacious for the treatment of hepatitis C-associated mixed cryoglobulinemia (Lamprecht *et al.* 2003; Roccatello *et al.* 2004).

Rituximab and ANCA-associated vasculitis

Specks *et al.* (2001) published a case report describing a patient with WG who was intolerant of cyclophosphamide, and had previously failed therapy with methotrexate, azathioprine, and mycophenolate mofetil. He was treated with rituximab using a standard lymphoma protocol of 4 infusions of 375 mg/m^2 at weekly intervals. After therapy, his ANCA titer was undetectable and he remained in clinical remission for 11 months (Specks *et al.* 2001). In 2005, Keogh *et al.* published their experience using rituximab to treat 11 patients with proteinase 3-ANCA-associated vasculitis who had either failed or were intolerant of cyclophosphamide. After treatment with rituximab (using a standard lymphoma protocol), all patients entered prolonged remissions that persisted as long as B-cell levels were undetectable (Keogh *et al.* 2005). Eriksson subsequently published his experience treating two patients with MPA and seven patients with WG with rituximab. All patients had previously failed therapy with cyclophosphamide, and were treated with weekly rituximab infusions for 2 to 4 weeks (depending on clinical response) in addition to mycophenolate mofetil, azathioprine, or a short course of cyclophosphamide. Six months after the initiation of therapy, all patients demonstrated clinical response, with an 89% remission rate (Eriksson 2005).

Rituximab-induced remission, while long-lasting, is likely not permanent (Omdal *et al.* 2005). Since disease flares seems to be restricted to patients who experience return of detectable circulating B-cells, routine retreatment with rituximab may provide an acceptable option to prolong the benefits of therapy (Keogh *et al.* 2006). The potential benefits of this treatment strategy (which would obviate cytotoxic drugs altogether) are enormous, and are being explored in randomized clinical trials both in North America and Europe.

Hematopoietic stem cell transplantation

Hematopoietic stem cell transplantation (with or without immunoablative therapy) is an appealing approach to the therapy of many serious inflammatory disorders because of its inherent logic (albeit unproven) and its theoretical potential for cure. Stem cell transplantation has been proposed as a potential therapy for rheumatoid arthritis, systemic lupus erythematosus, and scleroderma. Initial guidelines for the use of hematopoietic stem cell transplantation were established by the European League Against Rheumatism (EULAR) in 1995 (Marmont *et al.* 1995). Since that time, however, the potential of this therapy has not been realized in clinical practice, largely due to technical difficulties, including an unacceptably high mortality rate. Transplantation is also associated with significant upfront costs, although it has been argued that these costs are less than the cost of chronic treatment for a patient with a severe, relapsing autoimmune disease (Burt 1997). Although there is no direct evidence supporting the use of hematopoietic stem cell transplantation in patients with vasculitis, this continues to be a field of enormous interest for investigators, particularly to address the needs of patients with truly refractory forms of vasculitis.

Hematopoietic stem cell transplantation for the treatment of rheumatic diseases

In 1997, Nelson *et al.* published a retrospective review of patients who underwent allogeneic bone marrow transplantation at the Fred Hutchinson Cancer Research Center (and affiliated hospitals) between 1969 and 1989. They identified 13 patients who received a transplant from a living related donor, had at least 3 years of relapse-free survival, and had a pre-existing autoimmune disease, including systemic lupus erythematosus, rheumatoid arthritis, and vasculitis. After a median follow-up of 14 years after transplantation, none of these patients had recurrence of their autoimmune disease (Nelson *et al.* 1997).

There is virtually no published literature related to the use of hematopoietic stem cell transplantation for the treatment of vasculitis. From 1995 to 2004, however, more than 500 patients were reported to the European Group for Bone Marrow Transplantation (EMBT) registry as having received stem cell transplantation specifically for the treatment of autoimmune diseases, including rheumatoid arthritis, systemic lupus erythematosus, and systemic sclerosis (Burt *et al.* 2004). This combined experience has yielded a wealth of information, although the results are mixed, and await confirmation in randomized clinical trials (van Laar 2005).

By 2004, 76 patients in the United States and Europe had undergone autologous hematopoietic stem cell transplantation for severe, refractory rheumatoid arthritis (Snowden *et al.* 2004). One patient died as a result of a transplant-related complication. Of the remaining patients, three achieved complete remission, 33 patients (44%) achieved an ACR 70 response, and 13 patients (17%) achieved an ACR 50 response. Interestingly, 12 patients had no clinical response to transplant. As would be expected, the patients who did respond to transplantation had a significant overall decrease in tender joint count and HAQ score. After 12 months of follow-up, however, the majority of patients again required DMARD therapy, although approximately half of those patients had significantly milder disease than before the transplant.

A retrospective review of the EBMT registry during a similar period of time yielded 53 patients with systemic lupus erythematosus treated with autologous stem cell transplant for refractory disease (Jayne and Tyndall 2004). Remission was seen in 66% of patients at 6 months, but one-third of those patients relapsed after a median follow-up of 6 months. Seven patients (13%) died due to transplant-associated complications.

This experience was recently augmented by the publication of a single-center study of 50 patients with refractory systemic lupus erythematosus treated with hematopoietic stem cell transplantation (Burt *et al.* 2006). One patient died due to complications related to transplantation. For the remaining patients, the overall 5-year survival was 84%, with a 50% probability of a 5-year disease-free survival (defined as a prednisone dose of less than 10 mg/day and no additional immunosuppressive agents).

Based on these data, the use of autologous hematopoietic stem cell transplantation may be an appropriate option for patients with life-threatening, refractory forms of systemic vasculitis. It is difficult to project, however, the length of response that could be expected, since this may be disease-specific. For the majority of patients, it seems that this approach is likely to provide a reprieve, not absolution. Moreover, because of the speculative nature of these conclusions, and the high level of technical expertise required, stem cell transplantation should be offered only by highly experienced centers in the context of a clinical trial.

Other therapies
Acetylsalicylic acid

Aspirin is one of the oldest known treatments in Western medicine, but the mechanism of its anti-inflammatory properties is still being unraveled. To explore the effect of aspirin and other anti-inflammatory medications on giant cell arteritis, Weyand *et al.* developed a model of the disease that involved implanting inflamed temporal artery specimens into immunodeficient (SCID) mice. These mice were then treated with intraperitoneal injections of saline, acetylsalicylic acid, dexamethasone, or indomethacin for 3 weeks, after which the mice were sacrificed, and cytokine messenger RNA was quantified (Weyand *et al.* 2002). Using this model, acetylsalicylic acid (but not indomethacin) was found to be an effective inhibitor of cytokine transcription in temporal arteries, predominantly by suppressing interferon-γ transcripts. The anti-inflammatory properties of dexamethasone, in contrast, were attributed primarily to its inhibition of NF-κB-regulated cytokines (including IL-1 and IL-6). Because aspirin and dexamethasone exert anti-inflammatory effects through divergent pathways, using them in combination, in theory, might improve clinical outcomes for patients with giant cell arteritis.

This interpretation of Weyand's seminal work was recently supported by a retrospective chart review of 166 patients diagnosed with GCA in Jerusalem between 1980 and 2000 (Nesher *et al.* 2004). Temporal artery biopsy established the diagnosis in 92% of the patients; the others met American College of Rheumatology classification criteria for GCA (Hunder *et al.* 1990). Patients were divided into two groups, based on their use of prophylactic low-dose aspirin prior to the onset of vasculitis. There was no statistically significant difference in symptoms or laboratory data (including erythrocyte sedimentation rate, platelet count, and hemoglobin) between the two groups. The patients who were taking low-dose aspirin, however, were more likely to have risk factors for cerebrovascular disease but less likely to have an event. Of the 36 patients who had taken prophylactic aspirin, 14 (38.9%) had risk factors for cerebrovascular disease (such as hypertension, hypercholesterolemia, or diabetes) but only three (8%) had a cranial ischemic complication (such as a cerebrovascular accident, or visual loss due to anterior ischemic optic neuropathy). This differed significantly from the 139 patients who had not received prophylactic aspirin, 40 (29%) of whom had a cranial ischemic complication attributed to GCA, even though only 28 (20%) had risk factors for vascular disease.

This study cannot exclude the possibility that patients with GCA derive benefit from the cyclooxygenase inhibition of platelets (rather than the blockade of a secondary, glucocorticoid-resistant, inflammatory pathway). Given its low morbidity for patients without contraindications to salicylates, the adjunct use of aspirin in patients with GCA seems prudent. Whether patients with other forms of vasculitis may also benefit from the addition of aspirin is an important, but unanswered, question.

Pooled immunoglobulin

Intravenous immunoglobulin (IVIg) has been used for years for multiple forms of autoimmune illness, although its exact mechanism of action is not clear. Proposed mechanisms include nonspecific Fc receptor blockade, anti-idiotype antibodies, modulation of cytokine production, and B-cell inhibition. A particularly compelling model proposes that pooled immunoglobulin downregulates effector cells by inducing surface expression of an inhibitory Fc receptor (Samuelsson *et al.* 2001). Regardless of the exact mechanism, intravenous immunoglobulin has been used as a treatment for multiple rheumatic diseases, including inflammatory myopathy and vasculitis.

The use of pooled immunoglobulin for the treatment of Kawasaki's disease is now well-established as part of the standard of care, although its use in other forms of vasculitis remains unproven. Several case series seem to indicate that pooled immunoglobulin may have a role as a second-line agent for the treatment of refractory ANCA-associated vasculitis, although the benefits may be limited (Richter *et al.* 1995). In 2000, Jayne *et al.* conducted a placebo-controlled trial of 34 patients with refractory ANCA-associated vasculitis randomized to receive 5 days of intravenous immunoglobulin (at 0.4 g/kg/day) in addition to standard immunosuppressive therapies. A 50% reduction in BVAS was noted in 14 (82%) of patients treated with intravenous immunoglobulin, but only six (35%) of patients treated with placebo (P = 0.015). Despite an initial response, however, approximately 30% of patients treated with intravenous immunoglobulin experienced a disease flare within 3 months (Jayne *et al.* 2000).

The French Vasculitis Study Group conducted a subsequent open-label trial of 20 patients with ANCA-associated vasculitis who had previously failed other forms of therapy. Patients received monthly infusions of intravenous immunoglobulin (0.5 g/kg/day for 4 days) every month for 6 months; patients enrolled in this trial were allowed to remain on immunosuppressive therapy, but these medications could not be increased during this trial. At 9 months of follow-up, 12 patients (60%) were in complete remission (Martinez *et al.* 2005). Based on this experience, intravenous immunoglobulin may be a valuable adjunct therapy for the treatment of ANCA-associated vasculitis, although it may be only a temporizing measure that, in the long run, might be offset by the high costs associated with this treatment.

Plasma exchange

Plasma exchange has been used successfully as adjunctive therapy for the treatment of several autoantibody-driven diseases, including antiglomerular basement membrane disease (Stegmayr *et al.* 2004), and has long been advocated by the French Vasculitis Study Group as an important adjunct to immunosuppression for the treatment of several forms of vasculitis such as polyarteritis nodosa (Guillevin *et al.* 2005). More recently, plasma exchange has been used for the treatment of the ANCA-associated vasculitides (Frasca *et al.* 2003). Plasma exchange in these cases is predicated on the ideas that: (1) ANCA are either pathogenic or contribute substantially to disease pathophysiology; and (2) removal of ANCA through the process of plasma exchange will therefore affect the disease course favorably.

The European Union Vasculitis Study Group (EUVAS) has addressed this question with a recently completed trial designed to investigate whether plasma exchange is more effective than pulse methylprednisolone in leading to dialysis independence for patients presenting with severe renal dysfunction defined as serum creatinine level >500 μmol/liter (5.68 mg/dl) (de Groot and Jayne 2005). Patients randomized to receive plasma exchange underwent seven exchanges over 2 weeks; those who were randomized to pulse methylprednisolone received 1 g intravenously daily for 3 days. Patients in both groups received background treatment consisting of daily CYC (2.5 mg/kg/day) and prednisolone (60 mg/day).

The investigators randomized 137 patients to receive either plasma exchange or intravenous methylprednisolone. A total of 35 patients (26%) died during the trial. Among all patients enrolled, only 52% (71 of 137) had sufficient renal function to stay off hemodialysis 12 months after randomization (45% in the methylprednisolone group, 59% in the plasma exchange group; P = 0.125). Time to recovery of renal function was significantly faster among the patients who received plasma exchange, but the serum creatinine levels at the end of the trial were not significantly different between the two groups. Although plasma exchange may provide some limited benefit for patients with acute flares of ANCA-associated vasculitis, it is offset by the significant risk of mortality associated with the procedure, and the lack of long-term clinical benefit.

Conclusions

The abundance of new, experimental therapies for the treatment of vasculitis is an important measure of international interest in these diseases. In recent years, investigators have made great strides in applying completely novel therapies to the primary systemic vasculitides, and finding new uses for older ones. Throughout the development of these novel approaches, initial enthusiasm is frequently supplanted by more sober interpretations, and therefore, these early reports should be viewed warily. The early forays into experimental approaches to the treatment of systemic vasculitis highlight the need to test promising new therapies in randomized clinical trials.

Acknowledgment

Dr Seo is a Lowe Family Scholar in the Center for Innovative Medicine at Johns Hopkins Bayview Medical Center. Dr Stone is a Hugh and Renna Cosner Scholar in the Center for Innovative Medicine at Johns Hopkins Bayview Medical Center.

References

Adler, Y. D., Mansmann, U., Zouboulis, C. C. (2001). Mycophenolate mofetil is ineffective in the treatment of mucocutaneous Adamantiades-Behcet's disease. *Dermatology*, **203**, 322–4.

Allison, A. C. and Eugui, E. M. (1991). Immunosuppressive and long-acting anti-inflammatory activity of mycophenolic acid and derivative, RS-61443. *British Journal of Rheumatology*, **30**, 57–61.

Appel, G. B., Radhakrishnan, J. and Ginzler, E. M. (2005). Use of mycophenolate mofetil in autoimmune and renal diseases. *Transplantation*, **80**, S265–71.

Aries, P. M., Hellmich, B., Reinhold-Keller, E. and Gross, W. L. (2004). High-dose intravenous azathioprine pulse treatment in refractory Wegener's granulomatosis. *Rheumatology* (Oxford), **43**, 1307–8.

Arzoo, K., Sadeghi, S. and Liebman, H. A. (2002). Treatment of refractory antibody mediated autoimmune disorders with an anti-CD20 monoclonal antibody (rituximab). *Annals of the Rheumatic Diseases*, **61**, 922–4.

Ballio, A. and Sermonti, G. (1961). Action of mycophenolic acid on unstable diploids of Penicillium chrysogenum. *Nature*, **190**, 108–9.

Bartolucci, P., Ramanoelina, J., Cohen, P., *et al.* (2002). Efficacy of the anti-TNF-alpha antibody infliximab against refractory systemic vasculitides: an open pilot study on 10 patinets. *Rheumatology* (Oxford), **41**, 1126–32.

Benenson, E., Fries, J. W.U., Heilig, B., Pollok, M. and Rubbert, A. (2004). High-dose azathioprine pulse therapy as a new treatment option in patients with active Wegener's granulomatosis and lupus nephritis refractory or intolerant to cyclophosphamide. *Clinical Rheumatology*, **24**, 251–7.

Birck, R., Newman, M., Braun, C., *et al.* (2006). 15-Deoxyspergualin and cyclophosphamide, but not mycophenolate mofetil, prolong survival

and attenuate renal disease in a murine model of ANCA-associated crescentic nephritis. *Nephrology, Dialysis, Transplantation*, **21**, 58–63.

Booth, A., Harper, L., Hammad, T., *et al.* (2004b). Prospective study of TNF-α blockade with infliximab in anti-neutrophil cytoplasmic antibody-associated systemic vasculitis. *Journal of the American Society of Nephrology*, **15**, 717–21.

Booth, A. D., Jayne, D. R., Kharbanda, R. K., *et al.* (2004a). Infliximab improves endothelial dysfunction in systemic vasculitis: a model of vascular inflammation. *Circulation*, **109**, 1718–23.

Burt, R. K. (1997). Immune ablation and hematopoietic stem cell rescue for severe autoimmune diseases (SADS). *Cancer Treatment and Research*, **77**, 317–32.

Burt, R. K., Oyama, Y., Verda, L., *et al.* (2004). Induction of remission of severe and refractory rheumatoid arthritis by allogeneic mixed chimerism. *Arthritis and Rheumatism*, **50**, 2466–70.

Burt, R. K., Traynor, A., Statkute, L., *et al.* (2006). Nonmyeloablative hematopoietic stem cell transplantation for systemic lupus erythematosus. *Journal of the American Medical Association*, **295**, 527–35.

Daina, E., Schieppati, R. and Remuzzi, G. (1999). Mycophenolate mofetil for the treatment of Takayasu's arteritis: A report of three cases. *Annals of Internal Medicine*, **130**, 422–6.

De Groot, K. and Jayne, D. (2005). What is new in the therapy of ANCA-associated vasculitides? *Clinical Nephrology*, **64**, 480–4.

De Groot, K., Rasmussen, N., Bacon, P. A., *et al.* (2005). Randomized trial of cyclophosphamide versus methotrexate for induction of remission in early systemic antineutrophil cytoplasmic antibody-associated vasculitis. *Arthritis and Rheumatism*, **52**, 2461–9.

Dereure, O., Navarro, R., Rossi, J. F. and Guilhou, J. J. (2001). Rituximab-induced vasculitis. *Dermatology*, **203**, 83–4.

Durez, P. and Horsmas, Y. (2000). Dramatic response after an intravenous loading dose of azathioprine in one case of severe and refractory ankylosing spondylitis. *Rheumatology* (Oxford), **39**, 182–184.

Emery, P. (2006). Treatment of rheumatoid arthritis. *British Medical Journal*, **332**, 152–5.

Eriksson, P. (2005). Nine patients with anti-neutrophil cytoplasmic antibody-positive vasculitis successfully treated with rituximab. *Journal of Internal Medicine*, **257**, 540–8.

Fauci, A. S. and Wolff, S. M. (1973). Wegener's granulomatosis: studies in eighteen patients and a review of the literature. *Medicine* (Baltimore), **52**, 535–61.

Frasca, G. M., Soverini, M. L., Falaschini, A., Tampieri, E., Vangelista, A. and Stefoni, S. (2003). Plasma exchange treatment improves prognosis of antineutrophil cytoplasmic antibody-associated crescentic glomerulonephritis: a case-control study in 26 patietns from a single center. *Therapeutic Apheresis and Dialysis*, **7**, 540–6.

Ginzler, E. M., Dooley, M. A., Aranow, C., *et al.* (2005). Mycophenolate mofetil or intravenous cyclophosphamide for lupus nephritis. *New England Journal of Medicine*, **353**, 2219–28.

Gottenberg, J. E., Guillevin, L., Lambotte, O., *et al.* (2005). Tolerance and short term efficacy of rituximab in 43 patients with systemic autoimmune diseases. *Annals of the Rheumatic Diseases*, **64**, 913–20.

Guillevin, L., Mahr, A., Callard, P., *et al.* (2005). Hepatitis B virus-associated polyarteritis nodosa: clinical characteristics, outcome, and impact of treatment in 115 patients. *Medicine* (Baltimore), **84**, 313–22.

Haubitz, M. and de Groot, K. (2002). Tolerance of mycophenolate mofetil in end-stage renal disease patients with ANCA-associated vasculitis. *Clinical Nephrology*, **57**, 421–4.

Hoffman, G. S., Cid, M. C., Weyand, C. M., Stone, J. H., *et al.* (2005). Phase II study of the safety and efficacy of infliximab in giant cell arteritis (GCA): 22 week interim analysis (abstract). *Arthritis and Rheumatism*, **52**, S271.

Hoffman, G. S., Merkel, P. A., Brasington, R. D., Lenshow, D. J. and Liang, P. (2004). Anti-tumor necrosis factor therapy in patients with difficult to treat Takayasu arteritis. *Arthritis and Rheumatism*, **50**, 2296–304.

Hunder, G. G., Bloch, D. A., Michel, B. A., *et al.* (1990). The American College of Rheumatology 19990 criteria for the classification of giant cell arteritis. *Arthritis and Rheumatism*, **33**, 1122–8.

Jayne, D., Rasmussen, N., Andrassy, K., *et al.* (2003). A randomized trial of maintenance therapy for vasculitis associated with antineutrophil cytoplasmic autoantibodies. *New England Journal of Medicine*, **349**, 36–44.

Jayne, D. and Tyndall, A. (2004). Autologous stem cell transplantation for systemic lupus erythematosus. *Lupus*, **13**, 359–65.

Jayne, D. R., Chapel, H., Adu, D., *et al.* (2000). Intravenous immunoglobulin for ANCA-associated systemic vasculitis with persistent disease activity. *Quarterly Journal of Medicine*, **93**, 433–9.

Jonasdottir, O., Petersen, J. and Bendtzen, K. (2001). Tumor necrosis factor-α (TNF), lymphotoxin, and TNF receptor levels in serum from patients with Wegener's granulomatosis. *APMIS*, **109**, 781–6.

Joy, M. S., Hogan, S. L., Jennette, J. C., Falk, R. J. and Nachman, P. H. (2005). A pilot study using mycophenolate mofetil in relapsing or resistant ANCA small vessel vasculitis. *Nephrology, Dialysis, Transplantation*, **20**, 2725–32.

Kamesh, L., Harper, L. and Savage, C. O. (2002). ANCA-positive vasculitis. *Journal of the American Society of Nephrology*, **13**, 1953–60.

Karkar, A. M., Smith, J. and Pusey, C. D. (2001). Prevention and treatment of experimental crescentic glomerulonephritis by blocking tumor necrosis factor-α. *Nephrology, Dialysis, Transplantation*, **16**, 581–24.

Keogh, K. A., Wylam, M. E., Stone, J. H. and Specks, U. (2005). Induction of remission by B lymphocyte depletion in eleven patients with refractory antineutrophil cytoplasmic antibody-associated vasculitis. *Arthritis and Rheumatism*, **52**, 262–8.

Keogh, K. A., Ytterberg, S. R., Fervenza, F. C., Carlson, K. A., Schroeder, D. R. and Specks, U. (2006). Rituximab for refractory Wegener's granulomatosis: report of a prospective, open-label pilot trial. *American Journal of Respiratory and Critical Care Medicine*, **173**, 180–7.

Kussmaul, A. and Maier, R. (1866). Ueber eine bisher nicht beschriebenen Eigenthumliche arterienerkrankung (periarteritis nodosa), die mit Morbus Brightii und rapid fortschreitender allgemeiner muskellahmung Einhergeht. *Deutsches Archiv für Klinische Medizin*, **1**, 484–518.

Lamprecht, P., Arbach, O., Voswinkel, J., *et al.* (2002a). Induction of remission with infliximab in therapy-refractory Wegener's granulomatosis – Follow-up of six patients. *Deutsche Medizinische Wochenschrift*, **127**, 1876–80.

Lamprecht, P., Voswinkel, J., Lilienthal, T., *et al.* (2002b). Effectiveness of TNF-alpha blockade with infliximab in refractory Wegener's granulomatosis. *Rheumatology* (Oxford), **41**, 1303–7.

Lamprecht, P., Lerin-Lozano, C., Merz, H., *et al.* (2003). Rituximab induces remission in refractory HCV associated cryogloublinaemic vasculitis. *Annals of the Rheumatic Diseases*, **62**, 1230–3.

Langford, C. A., Talar-Williams, C. and Sneller, M. C. (2004). Mycophenolate mofetil for remission maintenance in the treatment of Wegener's granulomatosis. *Arthritis and Rheumatism*, **51**, 278–83.

Liang, P. and Hoffman, G. S. (2005). Advances in the medical and surgical treatment of Takayasu's arteritis. *Current Opinion in Rheumatology*, **17**, 16–24.

Little, M. A. and Pusey, C. D. (2005). Glomerulonephritis due to antineutrophil cytoplasm antibody-associated vasculitis: An update on approaches to management. *Nephrology*, **10**, 368–76.

Mahadevan, U., Tremaine, W. J., Johnson, T., *et al.* (2000). Intravenous azathioprine in severe ulcerative colitis: a pilot study. *American Journal of Gastroenterology*, **95**, 3463–8.

Marmont, A., Tyndall, A., Gratwohl, A. and Vischer, T. (1995). Haemopoietic precursor-cell transplants for autoimmune diseases. *Lancet*, **345**, 978.

Martinez, V., Cohen, P., Mouthon, L., Guillevin, L., French Vasculitis Study Group (2005). Intravenous immunoglobulins (IVIG) for relapses of ANCA-associated systemic vasculitides: final analysis of a prospective, open and multicenter trial (abstract). *Arthritis and Rheumatism*, **52**, S649.

Mascher, B., Schmitt, W., Csernok, E., Tatsis, E., Reil, A., Gross, W. L. and Seyfarth, M. (1997). Polymorphisms in the tumor necrosis factor genes in Wegener's granulomatosis. *Experimental and Clinical Immunogenetics*, **14**, 226–33.

Matteson, E. L. (1999). A history of early investigation in polyarteritis nodosa. *Arthritis Care and Research*, **12**, 294–302.

Matteson, E. L., Orces, C. H., Duddy, J., *et al.* (1999). Induction therapy with an intravenous loading dose of azathioprine for treatment of refractory, active rheumatoid arthritis. *Arthritis and Rheumatism*, **42**, 186–7.

Mattey, D. L., Hajeer, A. H., Dabadneh, A., *et al.* (2000). Association of giant cell arteritis and polymyalgia rheumatica with different tumor necrosis factory microsatellite polymorphisms. *Arthritis and Rheumatism*, **43**, 1749–55.

Mok, C. C. and Lai, K. N. (2002). Mycophenolate mofetil in lupus glomerulonephritis. *American Journal of Kidney Disease*, **40**, 447–57.

Nelson, J. T., Torrez, R., Louie, F. M., Choe, O. S., Storb, R. and Sullivan, K. M. (1997). Pre-existing autoimmune disease in patients with long-term survival after allogeneic bone marrow transplantation. *Journal of Rheumatology*, **48**, 23–9.

Nesher, G., Berkum, Y., Mates, M., Baras, M., Rubinow, A. and Sonnenblick, M. (2004). Low-dose aspirin and prevention of cranial ischemic complications in giant cell arteritis. *Arthritis and Rheumatism*, **50**, 1332–7.

Nowack, R., Gobel, U., Klooker, P., *et al.* (1999). Mycophenolate mofetil for maintenance therapy of Wegener's granulomatosis and MPA: a pilot study in 11 patients with renal involvement. *Journal of the American Society of Nephrology*, **10**, 1965–71.

Omdal, R., Wildhagen, K., Hansen, T., Gunnarsson, R. and Kristoffersen, G. (2005). Anti-CD20 therapy of treatment-resistant Wegener's granulomatosis: favourable but temporary response. *Scandinavian Journal of Rheumatology*, **34**, 229–32.

Pickenpack, A., Straub, R. H., Distler, O., *et al.* (2000). Safety and efficacy of an intravenous loading dose of azathioprine for the treatment of non-TPMT-deficient patients with rheumatic diseases. *Rheumatology* (Oxford), **39**, 1435–6.

Richter, C., Schnabel, A., Csernok, E., De Groot, K., Reinhold-Keller, E. and Gross, W. L. (1995). Treatment of anti-neturophil cytoplasmic antibody (ANCA)-associated systemic vasculitis with high-dose intravenous immunoglobulin. *Clinical and Experimental Immunology*, **101**, 2–7.

Roccatello, D., Baldovino, S., Rossi, D., *et al.* (2004). Long-term effects of anti-CD20 monoclonal antibody treatment of cryoglobulinaemic glomerulonephritis. *Nephrology, Dialysis, Transplantation*, **19**, 3054–61.

Salvadori, M., Holzer, H., De Mattos, A., *et al.* (2004). Enteric-coated mycophenolate sodium is therapeutically equivalent to mycophenolate mofetil in de novo renal transplant patients. *American Journal of Transplantation*, **4**, 231–6.

Samuelsson, A., Towers, T. L. and Ravetch, J. V. (2001). Anti-inflammatory activity of IVIG mediated through the inhibitory FC Receptor. *Science*, **291**, 484–5.

Seo, P., Min, Y. I., Holbrook, J. T., *et al.* (2005). Damage caused by Wegener's granulomatosis and its treatment: prospective data from the Wegener's Granulomatosis Etanercept Trial (WGET). *Arthritis and Rheumatism*, **52**, 2168–78.

Snowden, J. A., Passweg, J., Moore, J. J., *et al.* (2004). Autologous hemopoietic stem cell transplantation in severe rheumatoid arthritis: a report from the EBMT and ABMTR. *Journal of Rheumatology*, **31**, 482–8.

Specks, U., Fervenza, F. C., McDonald, T. J. and Hogan, M. C. (2001). Response of Wegener's granulomatosis to anti-CD20 chimeric monoclonal antibody therapy. *Arthritis and Rheumatism*, **44**, 2836–40.

Stegmayr, B., Ptak, J., Wikstrom, B., *et al.* (2005). World apheresis registry: report of 2004 data. *Therapeutic Apheresis and Dialysis*, **9**, A38.

Stone, J. H., Holbrook, J., Marriott, M., *et al.* (2005). Solid malignancies among Wegener's granulomatosis patients treated with etanercept: potential interaction with cyclophosphamide (abstract). *Arthritis and Rheumatism*, **52,** S272.

van Laar, J. M., Farge, D. and Tyndall, A. (2005). Autologous Stem cell Transplantation International Scleroderma (ASTIS) trial: hope on the horizon for patients with severe systemic sclerosis. *Annals of the Rheumatic Diseases*, **64,** 1515.

Waiser, J., Budde, K., Braasch, E. and Neumayer, H. H. (1999). Treatment of acute c-ANCA-positive vasculitis with mycophenolate mofetil. *American Journal of Kidney Diseases*, **34,** e9.

Wegener's Granulomatosis Etanercept Trial (WGET) Research Group (2005). Etanercept plus standard therapy for Wegener's granulomatosis. *New England Journal of Medicine*, **352,** 351–61.

Weyand, C. M., Kaiser, M., Yang, H., Younge, B. and Goronzy, J. J. (2002). Therapeutic effects of acetylsalicylic acid in giant cell arteritis. **46,** 457–66.

Zaja, F., De Vita, S., Mazzaro, C., *et al.* (2003). Efficacy and safety of rituximab in type II mixed cryoglobulinemia. *Blood*, **101,** 3827–34.

PART 6

Mimickers of vasculitis

CHAPTER 44

Antiphospholipid Syndrome

David P. D'Cruz, Munther A. Khamashta, and Graham R. V. Hughes

Introduction

It may seem a little curious to include a chapter on the antiphospholipid (Hughes) syndrome (APS) in a book on systemic vasculitis. However, this can be justified on several grounds. APS is one of the commonest causes of acquired thrombosis. It is characterized by a vasculopathy that involves the vessel wall, vascular endothelium, and procoagulant factors in the blood associated with the presence of antiphospholipid antibodies (aPL). In the early days of the description of this syndrome, it was often confused for vasculitis, especially when seen in the context of systemic lupus erythematosus (SLE), and patients received immunosuppression. It is now clear that this is a non-inflammatory vasculopathy. Nevertheless, it can sometimes be difficult to distinguish lesions seen in APS from those due to vasculitides such as polyarteritis nodosa. For example, Asherson et al. (1992) reported two patients with APS and skin lesions resembling vasculitis but who had microthrombosis at histology. Acalculous cholecystitis, an uncommon feature of vasculitis, has also been reported in APS (Dessailloud et al. 1998) and the angiographic appearance of APS may also rarely mimic vasculitis (Provenzale et al. 1998). Indeed, it is being increasing recognized that APS and systemic vasculitides can coexist, leading to diagnostic confusion and increased morbidity (Norden et al. 1995; Rocca et al. 1994; Rees et al. 2006).

The main clinical features of this syndrome are arterial and venous thrombosis, thrombocytopenia, and recurrent pregnancy loss; these have stood the test of time. However, the spectrum of clinical manifestations seen in APS continues to expand and virtually every branch of medicine has been influenced by this disorder.

APS: a brief history

The first test that detected an antibody against a phospholipid dates back to 1906 when Wasserman developed a serological test for syphilis. This involved a reaction between a lipid tissue antigen and an autoantibody in syphilitic sera. Subsequently, it was determined that an alcoholic extract of beef heart, the antigen in this test, contains a phospholipid, termed cardiolipin by Mary Pangborn in 1942. In 1952, Conley and Hartmann described the association between a circulating anticoagulant and SLE (Conley and Hartmann 1952). In the same year, Moore and Mohr recognized that biologically false-positive serological tests for syphilis could

occur, especially in lupus. Soon after, two reports (Beaumont 1954; Nillson and Laurell 1957) linked a circulating anticoagulant with recurrent fetal deaths, spontaneous abortions, and intrauterine growth retardation. Bowie et al. (1963) reported the paradoxical occurrence of thrombotic lesions in patients with a circulating anticoagulant. In 1972 the term "lupus" anticoagulant (LA) was introduced by Feinstein and Rapaport and in 1982, at the Heberden Round, Graham Hughes presented a patient with primary APS (PAPS). In 1983, the first solid-phase radioimmunoassay for the detection of anticardiolipin antibodies (aCL) was described (Harris et al. 1983). A few years later, Gharavi and colleagues developed an enzyme-linked immunosorbent assay (ELISA) while working in Hughes's laboratory (Gharavi et al. 1987). Between 1983 and 1990, numerous clinical associations were described including livedo reticularis; thrombosis in multiple sites; pulmonary hypertension; myelopathy; chorea; bowel infarction; dementia; and pregnancy-related complications. More recently, these observations have been extended to include stenotic lesions of the renal and celiac arteries, fractures, demyelinating syndromes, and involvement of the eyes and ears. In 1990, three groups (Takao Koike, Monica Galli, Steven Krilis and their colleagues) reported that in sera from patients with thrombosis, aCL bound to a plasma cofactor β_2-glycoprotein 1 (β_2GPI), a naturally occurring anticoagulant (McNeil et al. 1990; Galli et al. 1990; Matsuura et al. 1990). Several animal models were described during the 1990s and the link between accelerated atheroma and aPL has been elucidated, particularly by Vaarala (1997). In recognition of Graham Hughes's descriptions and major contributions to this field, the eponym "Hughes syndrome" was introduced in 1994.

Antiphospholipid antibodies: methods of detection

aPL are a heterogeneous group of immunoglobulins directed at phospholipid binding proteins. Anticardiolipin antibodies (aCL) may be detected routinely with phospholipid-dependent solid phase immunoassays (ELISAs). Prolongation of phospholipid-dependent coagulation tests with correction testing using a phospholipid source, such as washed platelets, detects the lupus anticoagulant (LA). The assays for aCL involve coating plastic plates with pure cardiolipin dissolved in ethanol, then blocking non-specific binding by incubation with fetal calf or adult bovine serum, and incubation with diluted patient test sera. Bound antibody is identified using radioactive or enzyme-labeled antihuman antibody. In 1990, three groups independently found that autoimmune aCL required a cofactor for binding to antigen (Galli *et al.* 1990; McNeil *et al.* 1990; Matsuura *et al.* 1990). The cofactor proved to be β_2GPI, a naturally occurring anticoagulant. β_2GPI is a 50-kD plasma protein that is a member of the complement control protein super family of molecules, possessing five characteristic domains that contain the cryptic epitopes for aCL binding (Reid *et al.* 1986). These epitopes are exposed when β_2GPI binds to negatively charged phospholipids such as cardiolipin or irradiated plastic plates (Matsuura *et al.* 1994). *In vitro*, β_2GPI binds to anionic phospholipids, DNA, and heparin, and has anticoagulant properties.

aCL found in infections such as HIV disease, unlike autoimmune-associated aCL, do not bind β_2GPI. This may explain the lack of thrombosis with infections. The presence of anti-β_2GPI antibodies may provide a higher positive predictive value for the development of thrombotic events compared to aCL (Amengual *et al.* 1996; Cabiedes *et al.* 1995; Teixido *et al.* 1997), although not all studies have confirmed this (Swadzba *et al.* 1997) and testing for anti-β_2GPI antibodies is neither universally available nor fully standardized.

The term "lupus anticoagulant" describes a common laboratory phenomenon in which plasma autoantibodies impair the function of anionic phospholipid in a variety of phospholipid-dependent *in vitro* coagulation tests. These include the activated partial thromboplastin time, the Russell viper venom clotting time, the kaolin clotting time, and the prothrombin time determined using dilute thromboplastin. The main problems come from the laboratory techniques that are necessary to detect the LA activity. These involve coagulation procedures that are subject to a variety of conditions. It is recommended that the presence of an LA be confirmed by a platelet neutralization test. To rule out coagulation factor deficiencies, the test should be performed with a mixture of patient and control plasmas (Brandt *et al.* 1995).

Growing evidence suggests that LA are not only directed against anionic phospholipids but against neoepitopes on plasma proteins, particularly β_2GPI and prothrombin (Edson *et al.* 1984; Fleck *et al.* 1988; Galli *et al.* 1992). LA may also be directed at oxidized low-density lipoprotein and other phospholipid-binding proteins such as protein C, protein S, and heparan sulfate.

Concordance rates for the presence of aCL and LA in a given patient have been estimated at between 60% and 70%. Some patients can be positive for only LA or aCL, but not both, and sera with both LA and aCL have been separated into fractions with only one reactivity each, suggesting that the antibodies are related but clearly differ in their binding to phospholipid (McNeil *et al.* 1989, 1991). For this reason, both tests should be requested when APS is suspected.

Other aPL have been identified including antibodies to phosphatidylserine, phosphatidylinositol, phosphatidic acid, phosphatidylcholine, phosphatidylethanolamine, sphingomyelin, or a mixture of these compounds. Other novel antigens that are undergoing clinical testing include antiprothrombin antibodies and antibodies to phosphatidylserine/ prothrombin complexes (Atsumi *et al.* 2000; Bertolaccini *et al.* 2005). At present, their detection adds little clinical information and is restricted to research centers.

Several studies have shown that LA has a greater positive predictive value for thrombosis than aCL. ELISAs can be very sensitive, detecting picograms of antibody in serum. In contrast, larger amounts of antibody are required to prolong coagulation assays. A positive result in an LA assay would suggest a higher titer of antibody than a positive result in an aCL assay, and the greater predictive value may be due to the lower sensitivity of these assays (Tincani *et al.* 1998). Thus LA may be more specific but less sensitive than aCL testing for APS, reinforcing the need to request both assays when suspecting this syndrome.

Demographics

APS has, perhaps misleadingly, been recognized largely as a disease of young women due to the association with SLE and pregnancy loss. The age of first thrombosis in APS has been shown to be predominately between 30 and 45 years (Piette and Cacoub 1998); however, the syndrome has been described in children and the elderly. There are problems with reporting bias, as young patients with thrombosis and pregnancy loss are more likely to be investigated, hence skewing the results. In fact, aPL are being increasingly recognized in a diverse number of conditions, and in older subjects. Among the latter, the prevalence may be as high as 7–12% (Fields *et al.* 1989; Schved *et al.* 1994) but the clinical significance is unclear. Racial differences have been noted, with IgA aCL more common in Afro-Caribbeans (Molina *et al.* 1997).

There have been several large studies of the prevalence of aPL in SLE patients. Perhaps the largest is the Euro-Lupus study which found a prevalence of 24% IgG aCL, 13% IgM aCL, and 15% LA in a cohort of 1000 patients with SLE (Cervera *et al.* 1993). The prevalence of aPL and definite APS may increase with longer follow-up, further pregnancies, and repeat testing for aPS. Thus Perez-Vazquez (1993) *et al.* showed that the prevalence of APS increased from 10% to 23% after 15–18 years in a large cohort of SLE patients. A further study of 1000 APS patients has detailed the clinical features of the disorder (Cervera *et al.* 2002). The Hopkins Lupus Cohort Study longitudinally studied aPL and showed that SLE patients positive for LA had a 50% chance of a venous thrombotic event within 10 years of diagnosis (Somers *et al.* 2002). In studies of patients with established APS, the risk of recurrent thrombotic events is substantially increased, especially if tight anticoagulation is not maintained (Khamashta *et al.* 1995).

Definition and classification of APS

An international consensus statement on classification criteria for definite APS was published after a workshop in 1998 (the so-called Sapporo criteria), which have recently been updated (Sydney criteria) (Table 44.1). Classification criteria are used to facilitate research studies and are not a substitute for diagnostic criteria. When considering a diagnosis of APS, it behooves the clinician to exclude other possible causes of thrombosis. It has to be said, however, that there are very few causes of arterial and venous events in combination with pregnancy morbidity that can occur in the same patient other than the APS.

Piette has urged clinicians to be aware of suspicious symptoms. Fever and weight loss are unusual in APS and suggest infection or malignancy. Splenomegaly is not a feature of APS unless complicated

Table 44.1 Classification criteria for antiphospholipid syndrome

Clinical criteria

1. Vascular thrombosis

   One or more clinical episodes of arterial, venous, or small vessel thrombosis, in any tissue or organ. Thrombosis must be confirmed by objective validated criteria, i.e. unequivocal findings of appropriate imaging studies or histopathology. For histopathologic confirmation, thrombosis should be present without significant evidence of inflammation in the vessel wall.

2. Pregnancy morbidity

   (a) One or more unexplained deaths of a morphologically normal fetus at or beyond the 10th week of gestation, with normal fetal morphology documented by ultrasound or by direct examination of the fetus, or

   (b) One or more premature births of a morphologically normal neonate at or before the 34th week of gestation because of (i) eclampsia or severe pre-eclampsia defined according to standard definitions or (ii) recognized features of severe placental insufficiency, or

   (c) Three or more unexplained consecutive spontaneous abortions before the 10th week of gestation, with maternal anatomic or hormonal abnormalities and paternal and maternal chromosomal causes excluded.

In studies of populations of patients who have more than one type of pregnancy morbidity, investigators are strongly encouraged to stratify groups of subjects according to (a), (b), or (c) above.

Laboratory criteria

1. **Lupus anticoagulant** present in plasma on two or more occasions at least 12 weeks apart, detected according to the guidelines of the International Society on Thrombosis and Hemostasis.

2. Anticardiolipin antibody of IgG and/or IgM isotype in serum or plasma, present in medium or high titer (i.e. >40 GPL or MPL or >99th percentile), on two or more occasions, at least 12 weeks apart, measured by a standard enzyme linked immunosorbent assay.

3. Anti-β2-glycoprotein 1 antibody of IgG and/or IgM isotype in serum or plasma (in titer >99th percentile), present on two or more occasions at least 12 weeks apart, measured by a standardized ELISA, according to recommended procedures.

Definite APS is considered to be present if at least one of the clinical and one of the laboratory criteria are met (Wilson *et al.* 1999, Miyakis *et al.* 2006).

Table 44.2 Indications for testing for antiphospholipid syndrome

Venous/arterial thrombosis before the age of 45 years
Thrombosis after trivial provocation
Association of arterial and venous thrombosis
Association of thrombosis and fetal loss
Recurrent thrombotic events
Family history
Thrombosis in an unusual site: retinal veins, portal, cerebral veins, renal veins, axillary veins
Coumarin-induced skin necrosis
Systemic lupus erythematosus
Recurrent superficial thrombophlebitis
Recurrent miscarriage
Fetal loss, especially stillbirth
Severe early pre-eclampsia

Indications for testing for aPL are shown in Table 44.2. Thrombosis may be spontaneous or it may occur in association with other recognized risk factors. These risk factors can be divided into primary (hereditary thrombophilias) and secondary (acquired) causes. The primary causes include protein C, S or antithrombin III deficiency, Factor V Leiden mutations, and homocystinuria, etc. The acquired causes are immobility, trauma, surgery, use of oral contraceptive pills, pregnancy, smoking, malignancy, diabetes, nephrotic syndrome, and vasculitis. There is some anecdotal evidence that thrombosis due to aPL may be more severe when occurring in association with the hereditary thrombophilias (Alarcón-Segovia *et al.* 1996; Ames *et al.* 1998; Brenner *et al.* 1996; Peddi and Kant 1995; Schutt *et al.* 1998).

The commonest site of venous thrombosis is the large veins of the lower limb; however, superficial thrombophlebitis, upper limb thrombosis, portal vein thrombosis, Budd–Chiari syndrome and cerebral venous thrombosis have all been reported.

Arterial thromboses, especially strokes in young patients, are a hallmark of this disorder. For example, Nencini *et al.* (1992) found 18% of young stroke patients (mean age 38 years) were positive for aPL (LA and aCL) whereas the Antiphospholipid Antibodies in Stroke Study Group (APASS 1993) found 9.7% of first stroke patients had a positive aCL. Acute occlusion of peripheral arteries is unusual, but it is clear that premature peripheral vascular disease may be a feature of APS.

In myocardial infarction, the prevalence of aCL is between 5% and 15% (Vaarala 1998). Although this does not necessarily imply causation, the high prevalence of both aPL and myocardial ischemia in SLE, combined with increasing evidence for a link between aPL and atherosclerosis, is suggestive.

Patients with persistent aPL may not experience thrombosis, though over time, patients with medium to high titer aPL have an increased risk of thrombosis (Shah *et al.* 1998). Many patients have recurrent pregnancy morbidity as the only manifestation of the disease. It is not clear whether these women are at increased risk of future thrombotic events. A recent, retrospective, case–control study of women with APS presenting with recurrent miscarriage showed no difference in the rate of thrombotic events compared to otherwise

by other conditions. Abnormal liver function tests, thrombocytosis, or leukocytosis are unusual (Piette 1998). HIV infection can be a great mimicker, reminiscent of syphilis in the centuries before effective treatment was available. Thrombosis associated with aPL in patients with HIV disease has occurred but is rare.

Clinical features of APS

Thrombosis

Arterial or venous thrombosis is one of the major features of the syndrome. aPL should be included in the work up of unexplained thrombosis, particularly in unusual sites or in young patients.

healthy women with recurrent miscarriage (Quenby *et al.* 2005). The various studies that have addressed the risk of thrombosis are summarized in Table 44.3. A major focus of research is identification of risk factors for thrombosis so that we can identify those patients who require more aggressive treatment. Although the data cited above suggests that 50% of patients with high titer aPL/LA may have a thrombotic event over 10 years, it is not possible to predict with any certainty which individual patients will go on to have an event. These studies also show that low-dose aspirin alone is not sufficient as primary prophylaxis against thrombosis. In order to address this, a prospective study of low-dose aspirin versus low-intensity anticoagulation with warfarin (target INR 1.5) is in progress to assess whether low-intensity warfarin may be an effective primary prevention strategy. At this stage, the best predictor

Table 44.3 Selected studies on thrombotic risk in APS

Study	Design	Patients	aPL type	Risk of thrombosis	Comments
Rosove, Brewer 1992	Retrospectve	Primary (51) and secondary APS (14) Course after first thrombosis	aCL, LA	53% recurrence rate, with mean follow-up 5.2 years	91% followed initial pattern of thrombosis Highest INR coincident with thrombosis: 2.6
Bongard *et al.* 1992	Retrospective	VTE (107) and suspected VTE (186)	aCL	No association	
Khamashta *et al.* 1995	Retrospective	SLE (85), PAPS (66), 10 years follow-up	LA, aCL	69% recurrence rate for thrombosis Significantly reduced rate of recurrent events in INR >3 group	20% had bleeding complications, all had INR >3
Horbach *et al.* 1996	Retrospective, multivariate analysis	SLE (175), PAPS (23) Controls (blood donors)	IgG, IgM aCL, LA	Odds ratio VTE: LA: 6.55*, IgM aCL>20 MPL units: 3.9* Arterial: LA: 9.77* aCL: NS	Higher titers of aCL in the thrombotic SLE groups No additional information from β_2-GPI
Ginsburg *et al.* 1992	Nested case control	American physicians	aCL	aCL>33GPL units Relative risk: VTE: 5.3* CVA: 1.35 NS	
Nencini *et al.* 1993	Case controlled	Young strokes (15–44 years), healthy volunteers	LA, aCL	18% young strokes positive for aPL, 2% healthy controls	Recurrence rate for stroke higher in the aPL-positive group
APASS 1993	Case controlled	Stroke (248) vs. non-stroke hospitalized (257)	IgM, IgG, IgA aCL	Odds ratio: 2.33*	Strength of association equivalent to hypertension
Ghirdello *et al.* 1994	Cross-sectional	SLE (107)	IgG aCL, LA	Thrombosis associated with LA, less extent aCL	
Ginsberg *et al.* 1995	Cross-sectional prospective cohort	VTE vs. no VTE	IgG aCL, LA	Odds ratio VTE LA: 9.4* aCL: 0.7 aCL >50GPL: 1.9 NS	
Vaarala *et al.* 1995 Helsinki Heart Study	Nested case control	Men with LDL cholesterol >5.2 mmol/l	IgG aCL	Cardiac end points (infarction, death) Highest quartile of aCL: Odds ratio: 2.0*	Risk independent of other risk factors aCL levels higher in smokers
Abu Shakra *et al.* 1995	Prospective cohort	SLE (390)	LA, aCL	LA: thrombosis, Odds ratio:7.96* aCL: Coombs, thrombocytopenia No association with thrombosis	No correlation with recurrent fetal loss
Simioni *et al.* 1996	Cross-sectional, case control	VTE(59) vs. no VTE (117)	LA	LA: Odds ratio for DVT: 10.7*	Prevalence of LA in idopathic VTE: 10.7%
Finazzi *et al.* 1996 Italian APS Registry	Prospective cohort	PAPS (165) Secondary APS:SLE (69)	IgG aCL, LA	IgG >40GPL units, relative risk for thrombosis: 3.66* LA: NS	With previous thrombotic history the relative risk rose to 4.9

Study	Design	Patients	aPL type	Risk of thrombosis	Comments
Schulman *et al.* 1998	Prospective cohort	VTE (897 first episode)	IgG aCL 6 months post-thrombosis	Risk ratio for recurrent VTE: 2.1*	No recurrence in group with INR 2.0–2.85 (follow-up 4 years) Of 20 recurrences in the aCL positive group, 14/20 had negative aCL at time of thrombosis
Kearon *et al.* 1999	Prospective	'Idiopathic VTE'	LA, aCL	Risk ratio for recurrence LA: 6.8* aCL: 2.3	
Wahl *et al.* 1997	Meta-analysis	SLE	LA, aCL	Odds ratio for VTE: LA: 6.32*, aCL: 2.17*	
Wahl *et al.* 1997	Meta-analysis	aPL-positive patients non-autoimmune disease or previous thrombosis	LA, aCL	Odds ratio for VTE: LA: 11.1* aCL: 1.64	Odds ratio increased to 3.21 for high titer aCL
Cervera *et al.* 2002	Prospective cohort 1000 patients	aPL-positive patients	LA, aCL	Primary APS: 53.1% APS with SLE: 36.2%	Largest series to date

* Significant result, NS, not significant; VTE, venous thromboembolism; CVA cerebrovascular accident; INR international normalized ratio.

appears to be previous thrombotic history, LA, and high titers of aCL.

Seronegative APS

Over the last few years it has become apparent that there are many patients with the typical clinical features of APS including pregnancy losses, thrombotic events, and livedo reticularis but who remain persistently negative for conventional testing for aPL: the so-called "seronegative APS" (Hughes and Khamashta 2003; Sangle et al. 2005a). A tiny minority of these patients may have anti-β2-glycoprotein 1 and/or antiprothrombin antibodies, but it may be that these patients have other explanations for their clinical features (Bertolaccini et al. 1998). Nevertheless, faced with a patient with recurrent thrombotic events, long-term anticoagulation is essential even if aPL remain negative.

Cutaneous disease

The most striking cutaneous lesion is that of livedo reticularis (Figure 44.1). "This is a cyanotic, mottled discolouration of the skin with a characteristic network pattern, which is accentuated by cold" (Rook *et al.* 1998). The mottling of livedo reticularis may correspond to watershed areas where the blood supply (larger arterioles) is relatively diminished; hence the discoloration is due to dilatation and stagnation of blood within capillaries and minute vessels. Livedo may be physiological (cutis marmorata), primary, or secondary to intravascular obstruction or vessel wall disease. Pathological livedo reticularis is usually extensive, occurring on the limbs, especially the forearms and knees, trunk, and buttocks and has a broken pattern. The list of pathological causes includes cardiac failure, oxalosis, thrombocythemia, cryoglobulins, cold agglutinins, and arteritis, including PAN. The changes are initially reversible if the underlying cause can be corrected, but after a time the vessels become permanently dilated. In APS, livedo reticularis is usually persistent and anticoagulation has no effect on its extent or severity. It is clear that livedo reticularis is a marker for poor prognosis and more severe disease in APS and as such is a powerful

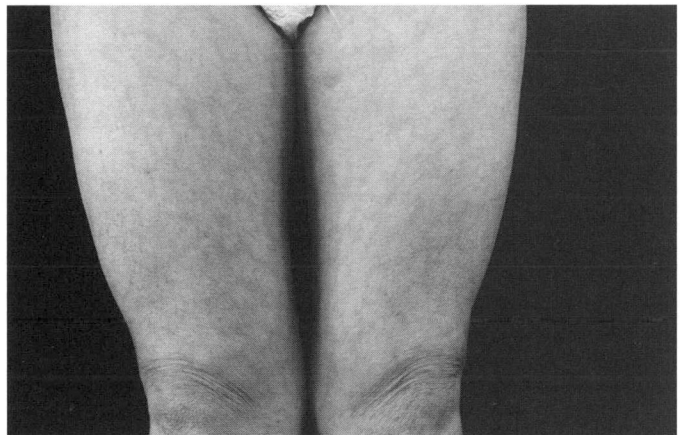

Figure 44.1 Livedo reticularis in a patient with systemic lupus erythematosus. (See Color Plate 121).

physical sign when this disorder is suspected (Toubi *et al.* 2005). Livedo reticularis may also be a useful sign in patients with seronegative APS (Sangle *et al.* 2005a).

Livedo can be seen with nodules (cutaneous polyarteritis nodosa), and with a segmental hyalinizing vasculitis, often with ulceration of the lower limbs, called livedoid vasculitis. This is also referred to as segmental hyalinizing vasculitis, or livedo reticularis with summer ulceration (Figure 44.2). The latter condition is a chronic disease with ulcers, which tend to heal with hyperpigmentation and atrophie blanche (Figure 44.3), affecting the feet and lower legs. The absence of a sufficient perivascular infiltrate is against vasculitis as a primary cause. It is not usually associated with aPL; however, Acland *et al.* (1999) have reported four patients in whom aPL were found. Successful treatment of resistant livedoid vasculitis in six patients with non-healing ulcers by tissue plasminogen activator (tPA) highlights that thrombosis may be a key factor in this condition (Klein and Pittelkow 1992).

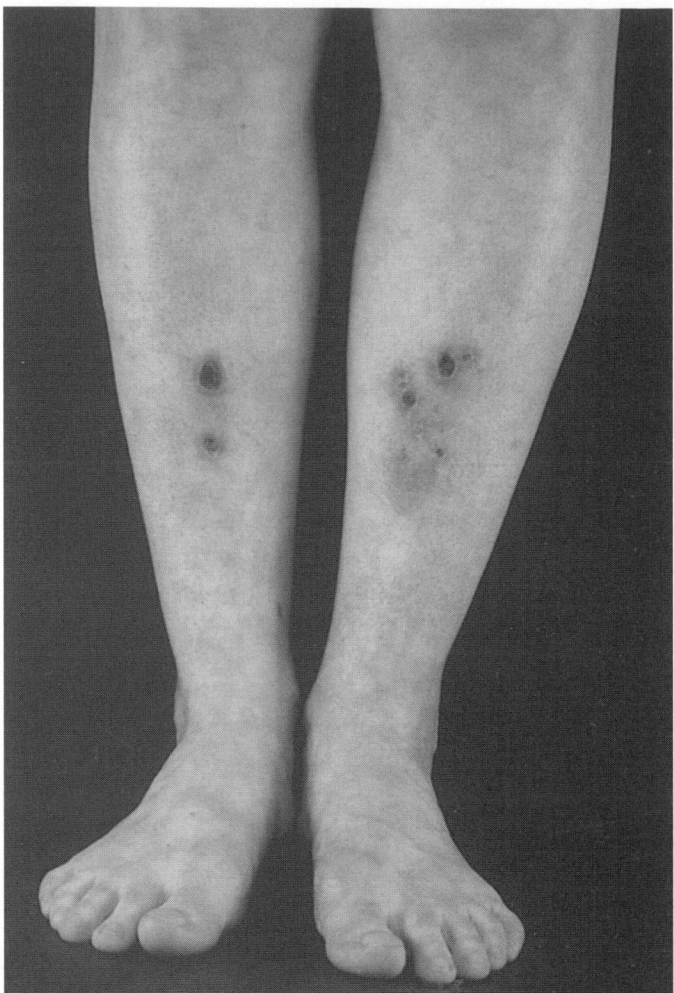

Figure 44.2 Livedo and leg ulceration in a patient with livedoid vasculitis.

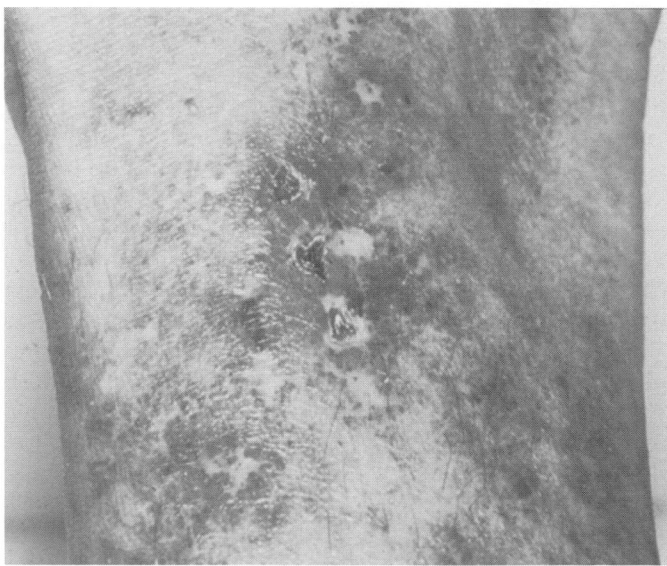

Figure 44.3 Livedo vasculitis. Characteristic lesions on the medial lower leg showing stellate shaped areas of necrosis and stellate white scars (atrophie blanche) surrounded by macular purpura and secondary hemosiderin pigmentation. (From Sams and Sams (2002) Cutaneous manifestations. In *Vasculitis*, Ball, G. V. and Bridges, S. L. Jr, eds. Oxford University Press) (See Color Plate 122).

Other reported cutaneous associations include anetoderma, ulcers, Degos' disease, splinter hemorrhages, superficial thrombophlebitis, distal cutaneous ischemia, and Sneddon's syndrome. However, closer examination of Sneddon's syndrome (strokes and livedo reticularis) reveals that many of these patients in fact have APS with the finding of aCL and antiprothrombin antibodies (Kalashnikova *et al.* 1990, 1999).

Neurological

There is a very broad spectrum of CNS involvement in APS, as shown in Table 44.4. Stroke is a hallmark of APS. The age of onset in APS, though, is several decades earlier than in the typical stroke population (Levine *et al.* 1995) and the ischemic events may occur in any territory (Coull *et al.* 1992).

In SLE patients, MRI abnormalities are common in both aPL positive and negative patients. Sailer *et al.* (1997) found that abnormalities greater than 8 mm in diameter were more likely to be aPL related than inflammatory (Figures 44.4 and 44.5). In many patients, these clinical and radiological signs may be mistaken for multiple sclerosis. Radiologically, it is almost impossible to distinguish large high-signal lesions on brain MRI due to APS from those due to multiple sclerosis (Cuadrado *et al.*). Anecdotally, some patients who apparently have multiple sclerosis but who are positive for aPL have benefited from anticoagulation, though this is often a difficult clinical decision (Ferreira *et al.* 2005).

Many patients complain of other problems such as migraine, poor memory, and cognitive impairment. Brain MRI is often helpful in these patients, revealing high-signal lesions. Electroencephalography (EEG) is also a useful test in these patients. Lampropoulos *et al.* (2005) showed that EEG abnormalities of bitemporal slow activity,

Table 44.4 Spectrum of CNS involvement in antiphospholipid syndrome (source: Brey and Escalante 1998)

Cerebrovascular ischemia
Stroke
Transient ischemic attack
Cerebral venous sinus thrombosis
Ocular ischemia
Dementia
Acute ischemic encephalopathy
with Sneddon's syndrome
without Sneddon's syndrome
Atypical migrainous-like events
Seizures
Chorea
Transverse myelopathy
Guillain–Barré syndrome
Diabetic peripheral neuropathy
Sensorineural hearing loss
sudden onset
progressive
Transient global amnesia
Psychiatric disorders
Orthostatic hypotension

AH

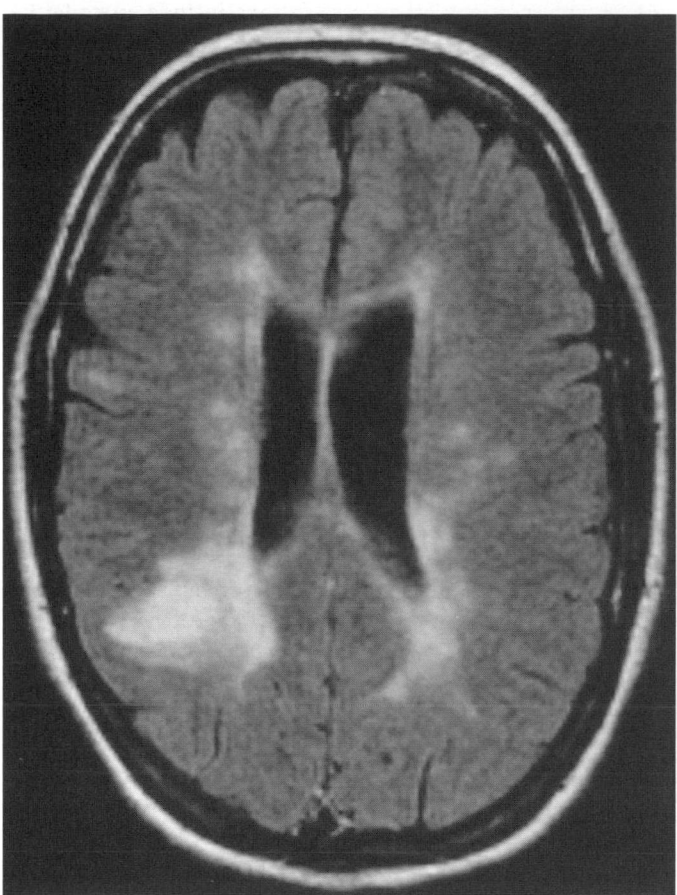

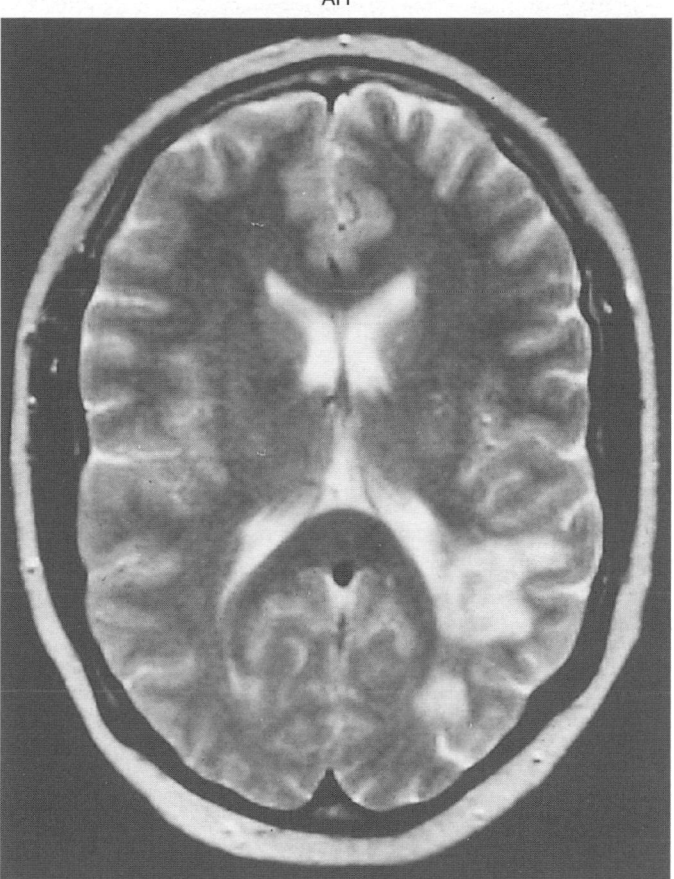

Figure 44.4 MRI of brain showing lesions indistinguishable radiologically from multiple sclerosis.

Figure 44.5 Large vessel disease with a parieto-occipital infarct.

suggesting cerebrovascular insufficiency, are common and correlate with the presence of aPL, even when the MRI is normal.

More severe associations include dementia (Gomez-Puerta *et al.* 2005b), psychosis, myelopathy, multiple sclerosis-like syndrome, chorea, sensorineural hearing loss, cerebral artery or vein occlusion, and retinal lesions. Although the pathological lesion is likely to be thrombotic (small or large-vessel ischemia), or embolic, there is some evidence for direct neurotoxicity (Furie *et al.* 1994).

Two controversial studies have examined the association between abnormal cognitive function and aPL. Hanly *et al.* (1999) prospectively studied cognitive function in SLE patients and found that psychomotor speed was reduced in patients who had persistently positive IgG aCL. Menon *et al.* (1999) found similar results in 45 SLE patients. Those patients with persistently elevated IgG aCL over a 2 to 3-year period performed poorer in tasks requiring speed of attention and concentration. No association was found with anti-DNA antibody or C3 levels.

The prevalence of aPL in migraine is debated. The largest case–control study failed to find an association in patients less than 60 years old for migraine with or without focal neurological deficits compared with controls (Tietjen *et al.* 1998).

Pregnancy

APS is frequently diagnosed following investigation for recurrent miscarriage, pregnancy morbidity being one of the major manifestations of the syndrome. In pregnancies that do not end in miscarriage or fetal loss, there is a high incidence of early-onset pre-eclampsia, intrauterine growth restriction, placental abruption, and premature delivery (Lima *et al.* 1996). Since the classification criteria for APS have been amended (Wilson *et al.* 1999; Miyakis *et al.* 2006), a patient with adverse pregnancy outcome may now be labeled as APS without a history of fetal loss. The prevalence of aPL in the general obstetric population is low (<2%), so universal screening is not warranted (Harris and Spinnato 1991); however, any woman with a history of three or more first trimester miscarriages should be tested for these antibodies. Rai *et al.* (1995) have reported that 15% of women with a history of three or more consecutive miscarriages have persistently positive aPL results. A recent study has reported that testing for aPL other than LA and aCL in women with recurrent miscarriage is of no clinical value (Branch *et al.* 1997). The risk of pregnancy loss is directly related to antibody titer, particularly IgG aCL, although many women with a history of recurrent loss have only IgM antibodies. Quantifying the risk is difficult, and the presence of aPL does not preclude successful pregnancy. The antibodies should be regarded as markers for a high-risk pregnancy. Once the diagnosis of APS is made and confirmed, serial aPL determinations are not useful. Previous poor obstetric history remains the most important predictor of future risk (Lima *et al.* 1996).

The mechanism of pregnancy loss in APS remains uncertain. It seems likely that progressive thrombosis of the microvasculature of the placenta, which leads to infarction (Figure 44.6) may cause

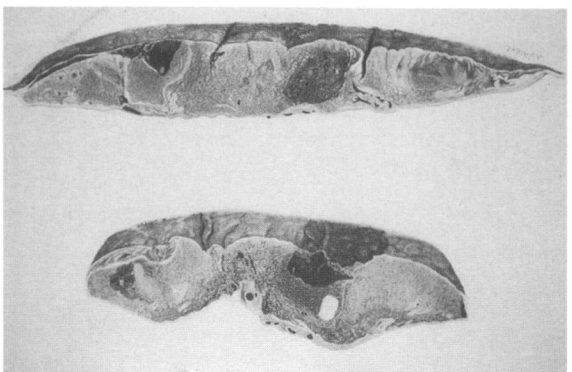

Figure 44.6 Placental infarcts.

placental insufficiency, which in turn leads to fetal growth restriction and fetal death in some patients. However, not all placentas examined have shown areas of thrombosis or infarction and it is, therefore, likely that other mechanisms are operative (Lockshin 1998). A variety of hypotheses have been proposed to explain how aPL might cause pregnancy loss, including: (1) inhibition of placental prostaglandins and thromboxane; (2) inhibition of placental gonadotrophin; (3) competition with Annexin V; (4) displacement of Annexin V; and (5) inhibition of trophoblast proliferation.

Recent landmark animal studies have suggested that complement, especially C5a, may have an important role in the pathogenesis of fetal loss (Girardi et al. 2004). Heparin may block the effects of complement and thus prevent fetal loss by an anti-inflammatory rather than antithrombotic mechanism. It is likely that these mechanisms pertain to the human situation but this remains to be seen.

Many investigators have found a statistically higher rate of aPL in women with infertility, though not all agree (Branch and Hatasaka 1998). Proof that aPL are associated with a specific type of infertility or influence pregnancy outcome with assisted reproductive technology is lacking.

Pulmonary

The commonest manifestation is pulmonary emboli and thromboembolic pulmonary hypertension. Gertner and Lie (1993) noted that other manifestations may be seen in primary APS including a syndrome resembling adult respiratory distress syndrome, alveolar hemorrhage, microvascular pulmonary thrombosis, transient/migratory infiltrates on chest radiography, and (pathologically) capillaritis.

Hematological

Thrombocytopenia has been found in up to 30% of primary APS, and is seen more frequently in SLE with aPL. Despite thrombocytopenia, some patients are still at risk of thrombosis. Coombs-positive hemolytic anemia may also occur.

Cardiac

Several cardiac lesions apart from coronary artery disease have been reported in association with aPL (Tenedios et al. 2006). Libman–Sacks endocarditis was first described in 1924 in patients with sterile lesions of the valvular and mural endocardium (Libman and Sacks 1924). The association between Libman–Sacks endocarditis and aPL was first noted in 1985 (D'Alton et al.) in a young woman with transient ischemic attacks, valvular disease, and LA. In 1989, other groups highlighted a probable role of aPLs in the pathogenesis of valvular lesions in patients with SLE (Chartash et al. 1989; Galve et al. 1989; Khamashta et al. 1989; Straaton et al. 1989). In the absence of SLE, Doppler echocardiogram has revealed a prevalence of valvular lesions in patients with APS of between 32% and 38% (Hojnik et al. 1996). In non-APS patients referred for valve replacement, aPL were found in 19 of 89 (21%) compared with 9% of controls (Bouillanne et al. 1996). The mitral valve is affected more commonly than the aortic valve and the lesions may be vegetations or valvular thickening (Khamashta et al. 1990). Functionally the valve may become regurgitant, but stenosis is rarely encountered. The hemodynamic significance is usually minor, although valve replacement has been required in some patients. The vegetations may be a source of thromboembolism. Infective endocarditis is uncommon, but a condition of pseudoendocarditis has been described in both SLE and primary APS, and is characterized by fever, murmurs, valve vegetations, splinter hemorrhages, increased aPL, and negative blood cultures.

It is likely that thrombosis on a damaged valve and healing with fibrosis are key players in the valve deformity. Whether aPL are instrumental in initial damage of the valves remains to be elucidated, but deposits of immunoglobulin (including aCL) and complement in diseased valves have been documented, suggesting a role in the development of valvular pathology.

Diastolic dysfunction has also been documented by a number of groups (Hasnie et al. 1995). Coudray et al. (1995) studied 18 patients with echocardiogram and found impairment of myocardial relaxation and filling dynamics of the left ventricle in PAPS compared with controls. They concluded that the abnormalities may be due to subclinical myocardial damage, possibly secondary to microvascular thrombosis. This is supported by the observation (Kaplan et al. 1992) that widespread cardiac dysfunction due to multiple arteriolar thrombi can occur in the absence of coronary artery disease.

Musculoskeletal

Avascular necrosis (AVN) of bone (also referred to as osteonecrosis) may be associated with aPL. Tektonidou et al. (2003) found MRI scanning to be a sensitive test with 20% of primary APS patients showing evidence of AVN. A previous group of 800 SLE patients were retrospectively reviewed and 37 were found to have developed AVN (4.6%); 27 (73%) were positive for aPL (Asherson et al. 1993). Given the aPL prevalence figures in SLE, the expected rate would have been 30–40%, suggesting that aPL may be a risk factor for AVN. However, Alarcón-Segovia et al. (1989) and Houssiau et al. (1998) failed to find any association between aPL and AVN in SLE patients. Although glucocorticoid treatment may influence the incidence of AVN in the SLE population, it has also been reported in primary APS patients who are glucocorticoid-naïve (Asherson et al. 1993; Nagasawa et al. 1989).

Spontaneous metatarsal fractures are another manifestation linked to aPL that have been described recently (Sangle et al. 2004). These patients presented with fractures that occurred either spontaneously or after trivial trauma and many had normal bone mineral density and were not taking glucocorticoids. How aPL cause these fractures remains unknown but speculatively it is possible that thrombosis of the blood supply to the bones may be an explanation.

Endocrine

Addison's disease due to adrenal thrombosis/ hemorrhage is a recognized clinical association of aPL. More recently, anterior pituitary failure has been reported in a patient with APS (Pandolfi *et al.* 1997).

Renal

Almost any part of the renal vasculature can be affected in the APS. Since the early descriptions of the disease, labile hypertension has been noted (Hughes *et al.* 1987). Amigo *et al.* (1992) found renal involvement in up to 25% of patients with primary APS. There are now several well-documented cases of renal artery thrombosis or stenosis occurring in primary or secondary APS (Asherson *et al.* 1991; Ostuni *et al.* 1990) (Figure 44.7). The exact etiology is unclear, as there are case reports of thrombosis and improvement with anticoagulation, while other lesions are probably atherosclerotic in nature. Godfrey *et al.* (2000) documented five cases of renal artery stenosis in APS patients, three of which developed in patients already on anticoagulation. A case–control study has confirmed these findings showing a significantly increased prevalence of renal artery stenosis in 26% of patients with aPL compared to 8% and 3% in control groups with hypertension or who were renal organ donors respectively. Furthermore, anticoagulation appeared to improve outcome in these patients (Sangle *et al.* 2005b). Renal cortical infarcts may occur due to occlusion of renal arteries secondary to thrombosis, stenosis, or embolism. Renal vein thrombosis has also been documented (Gluek *et al.* 1985; Morgan and Feneley 1994). Tektonidou *et al.* (2004) found a strong association between APS nephropathy, arterial thrombosis, and livedo reticularis.

Thrombotic microangiopathy occurs in primary or secondary APS (Bhandari *et al.* 1998). The microangiopathy can involve both the vascular tree and the glomerular tufts, and ischemic obsolescence of glomeruli may result, culminating in renal impairment or failure (Amigo *et al.* 1992). Renal impairment may also result from cortical renal ischemia due to occlusion of small renal vessels, which may give rise to foci of cortical necrosis. This may be multiple in the catastrophic APS.

It is not uncommon for patients with aPL to come to renal transplantation. This may be due to associated lupus nephritis or to the primary effect of aPL on the kidney. Loss of renal allograft may occur due to a thrombotic vascular lesion or to a recurrence of thrombotic microangiopathy (Vaidya *et al.* 1998). D'Cruz (2005) has reviewed the broad spectrum of renal complications of APS.

Gastrointestinal

Intestinal ischemia and perforations due to thrombosis are rare but well described, especially in the context of the catastrophic APS. Recently, there have been descriptions of mesenteric angina in aPL positive patients, some of whom had abdominal bruits. Investigation of these patients disclosed celiac (Figure 44.8) and mesenteric artery stenoses, further supporting the idea that a medium to large-vessel vasculopathy is a feature of the APS (Sangle *et al.* 2006).

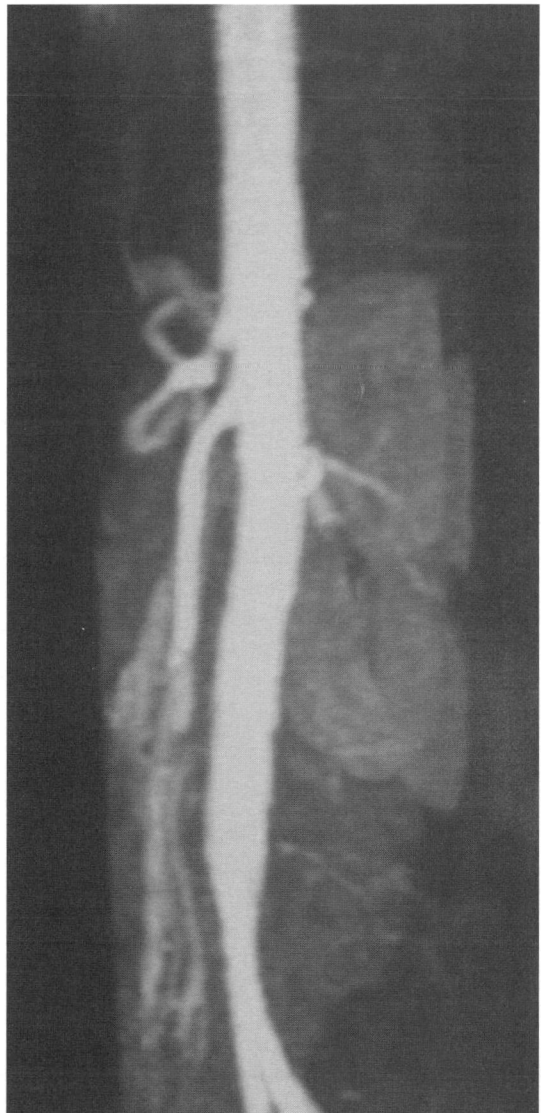

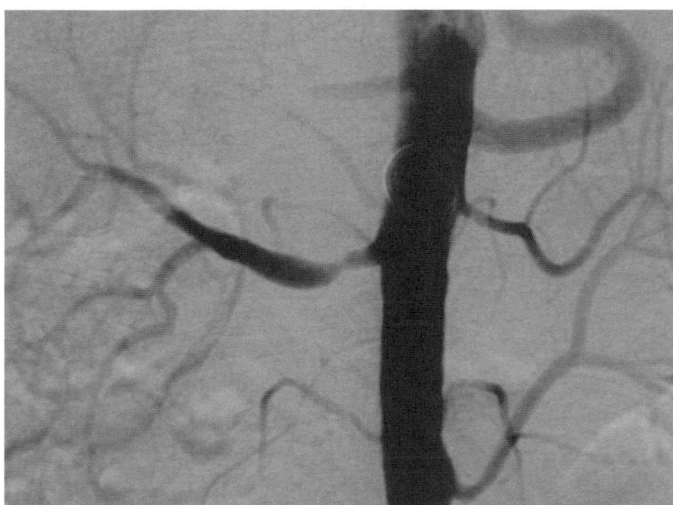

Fig. 44.7 Right renal artery stenosis in APS.

Fig. 44.8 Celiac artery stenosis in APS.

Catastrophic APS

The term catastrophic APS was first introduced by Asherson in 1992 to describe an accelerated form that results in multiorgan failure (Figure 44.9). The majority of the patients to date have suffered with primary APS and precipitating factors have been infections, operations, anticoagulant withdrawal, and drugs. Classification criteria for the catastrophic APS have been validated (Cervera *et al.* 2005).

Asherson (1998) initially reviewed 50 patients with catastrophic APS documented in the literature and this has recently been extended to 250 patients using registry data (Bucciarelli *et al.* 2006). Fatal outcome was seen in 44% with cerebral disease (mainly stroke), cerebral hemorrhage, and encephalopathy being the most common cause of death, followed by cardiac disease and infection. The most significant prognostic factor was the presence of SLE. Renal involvement, hypertension and pulmonary disease (ARDS in 50%, pulmonary emboli, pulmonary edema, and infrequently intra-alveolar hemorrhage) were also common.

Atherosclerosis

The etiology of atherosclerosis is multifactorial with traditional risk factors including hyperlipidemia, hypertension, smoking, diabetes, and family history. In recent years, the role of the immune system has begun to be appreciated. The role of aPL is also being unraveled. It is well recognized that SLE patients have accelerated atherosclerosis and the risk is increased in the setting of aPL. It is also known that aPL can bind and activate endothelial cells, increase monocyte adherence *in vitro*, and bind to oxidized LDL, perhaps resulting in increased uptake into vessel walls via Fc receptors (Del Papa *et al.* 1997). Hasunuma *et al.* (1997) showed that macrophages take up labeled oxidized LDL at an increased rate in the presence of aPL. Further evidence supporting a role for aPL in atherosclerosis comes from mouse models where immunization of LDL receptor-deficient mice with human β_2GPI led to acceleration of early atherosclerosis (George *et al.* 1998).

Recent studies using the ankle-brachial pressure index (ABI) have shown that an abnormal ABI (<1.0) occurs in 19% of APS

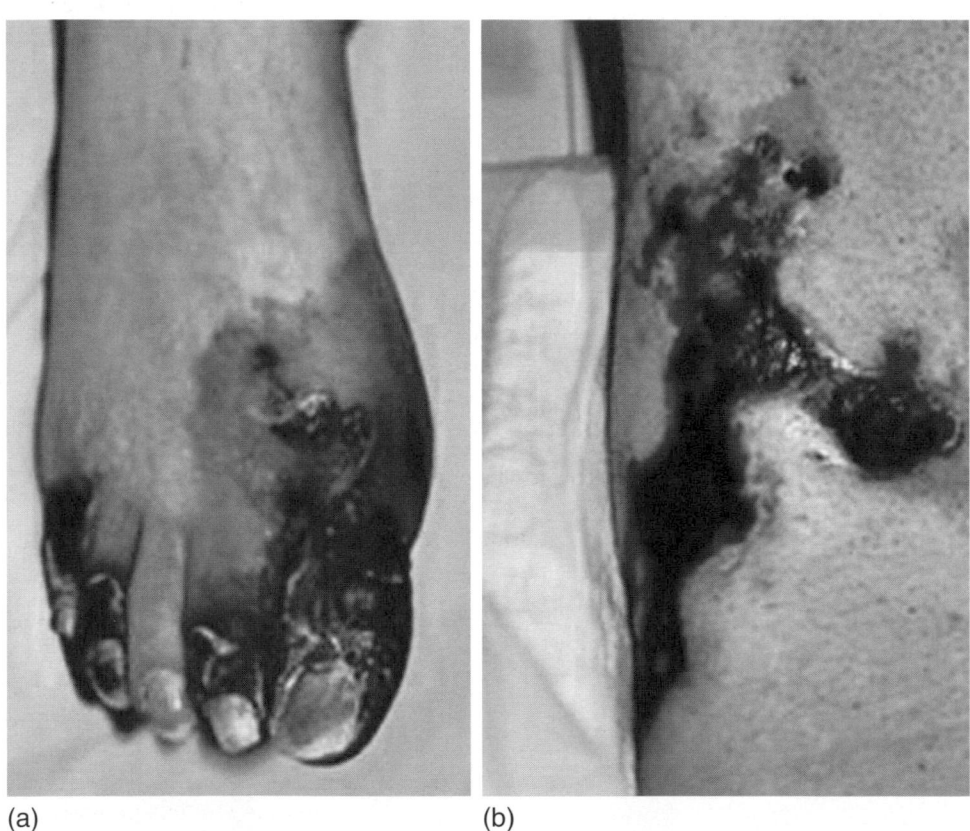

Fig. 44.9 (a and b) Catastrophic APS in a patient with severe skin necrosis and gangrene from widespread thrombosis. (See Color Plate 123).

(a)　　　　　　　　　　　　　　(b)

patients with a history of previous thrombotic events (Baron *et al.* 2005), and in APS patients with a previous history of pregnancy morbidity but without thrombotic events, an abnormal ABI was found in 23% of patients (Christodoulou *et al.* 2006). In both studies the prevalence of an abnormal ABI was significantly higher than in healthy controls. Furthermore, Medina *et al.* (2003) showed that patients with primary APS had significantly increased carotid artery intima–media thickness (IMT) compared to controls. These patients were also more likely to have reduced lumen diameter. Patients with increased IMT were more likely to have had arterial events such as strokes. The description of renal and celiac artery lesions further supports this idea, although the precise mechanisms remain elusive. Post-mortem histology in patients with SLE and aPL suggests that vascular intimal fibrous hyperplasia is a common finding (Sipek-Dolnicar *et al.* 2002).

Differences between primary and secondary APS

Vianna *et al.* (1994) found that primary APS and APS secondary to SLE had similar clinical features, but heart valve disease, autoimmune hemolytic anemia, lymphopenia, neutropenia, and low C4 levels were more common in patients with SLE. Anti-dsDNA antibodies or antibodies to extractable nuclear antigens (Sm and RNP) were not found in PAPS and their presence should suggest a secondary cause. The distinction between PAPS and APS due to SLE can sometimes be difficult. Features such as thrombocytopenia, anemia, renal, and CNS disease may be seen in both conditions. Piette *et al.* (1993) have been strong advocates of exclusion criteria for primary APS (Table 44.5). There does not appear to be any difference in rates of arterial or venous thrombosis, or fetal loss (Finazzi *et al.* 1996; Krnic-Barrie *et al.* 1997; Vianna *et al.* 1994). Shah *et al.* (1998) found IgM aCL more often in SLE than PAPS (22 of 42 patients, vs. 1 of 10 patients) but no difference in thrombotic rates.

The number of cases reported in the literature of patients with primary APS evolving into SLE is small. Silver *et al.* (1994) and Mujic *et al.* (1995) have reported the evolution in small numbers (7 of 71 and 3 of 80, respectively) but Asherson *et al.* (1989) and Vianna *et al.* (1994) did not find any such progression. The short

Table 44.5 Proposed exclusion criteria for primary APS (Piette *et al.* 1993)

Malar or discoid rash
Oral, pharyngeal, or nasal ulceration
Frank arthritis
Pleurisy/ pericarditis
Persistent proteinuria >0.5 g/day, due to biopsy proven immune complex related glomerulonephritis
Lymphopenia (<1000 cells/μl)
Antibodies to dsDNA (crithidia or radioimmunoassay), or ENA
ANA >1:320
Treatment with drugs known to produce aPL
Follow-up >5 years from the initial clinical manifestation.

period of follow-up may have been responsible for the latter result (5 and 2 years respectively), as several patients have developed the syndrome after 10 years. The presence of high titer ANA (>1:320) and lymphopenia may be predictive of subsequent SLE (Seisdedos *et al.* 1997). More recently, a large study of 128 patients confirmed the low rate of progression from primary APS to SLE: during the follow-up and after a median disease duration of 8 years, 11 (8%) patients developed SLE, and six (5%) developed lupus-like disease. A positive Coombs test increased the risk of developing SLE (Gomez-Puerta *et al.* 2005a).

Pathophysiology

Immunogenetics

A number of studies have examined HLA antigens in patients with primary and secondary APS. Most studies have involved small numbers of patients. In primary APS, an association has been noted with HLA-DR53, -DR4, -DQ7, and -DR7. In disease associated with SLE and aCL, HLA-DR7, -DR4, -DR53, or no association emerge (Granados *et al.* 1997; Schutt *et al.* 1998). Examination of alleles encoding complement components has found a variable association. There is geographical variation, with HLA-DR7 more common in Latins (Sebastiani *et al.* 1996).

The gene encoding β_2GPI (apolipoprotein H, or apoH) is located on chromosome 17 (Steinkasserer *et al.* 1992). A number of alleles, designated APOH*1, APOH*2, APOH*3, and APOH*4, have been identified and allele frequency varies among populations. The binding site of β_2GPI to anionic phospholipids resides in the fifth domain. Genetic mutations in the fifth domain of β_2GPI can affect aPL binding and the production of β_2GPI dependent aPL (Kamboh and Mehdi 1998).

Gharavi *et al.* (1999) have demonstrated that lysine-rich peptides from cytomegalovirus (CMV), adenovirus, and *Bacillus subtilis*, which have sequence homology for the phospholipid binding region of β_2GPI, can induce production of high levels of aPL and anti-β_2GPI antibodies when bound to bovine serum albumin in Freund's adjuvant. This may be a mechanism of production of infection-associated aPL, but the latter are not usually associated with thrombosis in humans, so this model may not explain the production of autoimmune aPL.

Mechanism of pathogenicity

The exact mechanism by which aPL leads to thrombosis is unknown. Mechanisms may be divided into those where antibodies interfere with hemostatic reactions of physiological anticoagulants or those that affect cell mediated events such as endothelial cells, monocytes, and platelets. The heterogeneity of the antibodies and the multiple proposed mechanisms may explain the clinical features, in particular why some individuals experience only pregnancy loss and others venous or arterial thrombosis.

At a simplistic level, the mechanism of thrombosis may be through binding of natural anticoagulants such as β_2GPI, protein C, protein S, or thrombomodulin, the primary activator of protein C (Oosting *et al.* 1993). However, under physiological conditions, β_2GPI is a weak anticoagulant and individuals who lack β_2GPI do not appear to suffer with thrombosis (Bancsi *et al.* 1992). Inhibition of the function of protein C has been documented and remains one of the major hypotheses for the mechanism of thrombosis.

Galli *et al.* (1998) have shown activated protein C resistance in patients with aPL; the effect was β_2GPI dependent, but antiprothrombin antibodies were not associated with the phenotype.

Various studies have shown that the sera or IgGs from patients with LA or aCL can induce tissue factor (a cell glycoprotein) expression in cultured endothelial cells and normal monocytes (Amengual *et al.* 1998; Cuadrado *et al.* 1997; Reverter *et al.* 1996; Tripplett 1995; Lopez-Pedrera *et al.* 2006). Tissue factor is not normally expressed by cells in contact with blood, but with inflammatory stimuli, tissue factor expression on monocytes and endothelial cells can be induced, which may then initiate normal and pathological coagulation.

β_2GPI can adhere to endothelial cells, offering suitable epitopes for circulating aPL, especially anti-β_2GPI, antibodies. Functional changes then occur to induce cell activation. This has been demonstrated *in vitro* by up-regulation of adhesion molecule expression and by production of proinflammatory cytokines rendering the endothelium prothrombotic (Del Papa *et al.* 1997; Simantov *et al.* 1995). Pierangeli *et al.* (1999) have demonstrated both *in vitro* and *in vivo* endothelial activation when affinity-purified aPL was presented to human umbilical vein endothelial cells, and in a mouse model of the microcirculation.

Analysis of monoclonal aPL has shown that arginine residues are critical in determining the binding of human monoclonal antiphospholipid antibodies to clinically relevant antigens (Giles *et al.* 2006).

Finally, a mechanism of action of LA through platelet activation has been postulated and demonstrated in primary APS by detection of activated platelets by flow cytometry (Emmi *et al.* 1997) as well as under flow conditions (Font *et al.* 2002).

It would seem likely that a two-hit hypothesis is necessary for thrombosis to occur. The prothrombotic state is present, but a second event may be necessary to trigger thrombosis. Various animal models exist but no model has been able to mimic all features of APS. In particular, venous thrombosis has been rarely produced without non-physiological stimuli. The pathogenesis of APS has been recently reviewed by Pierangeli *et al.* (2006).

A large number of conditions have been reported as causing aPL (Table 44.6). Thrombosis is unusual in most of these conditions except for SLE. In a prospective study, Merkel *et al.* (1996) found 16% of rheumatoid arthritis and SLE patients had either IgG or IgM aCL, compared with 4% of blood donors. Patients with scleroderma, myositis, undifferentiated connective tissue disease, and ANCA-associated vasculitis did not differ from the control blood donors in the prevalence of aPL. The manifestations of APS are not usually seen in infection- or drug-associated aCL, although occasional reports of the development of thrombosis in patients with AIDS and CMV infection have prompted recommendations to search for infections in patients developing APS (Soweid *et al.* 1995). Procainamide has been shown to produce β_2GPI-dependent antibodies that are potentially pathogenic (Merrill *et al.* 1997).

APS and systemic vasculitis

APS may complicate systemic vasculitis (Rees *et al.* 2006). aPL were found in 17% of 144 patients; nine patients had definite APS and a further four had clinical and serological features of APS but did not meet all the classification criteria. Previous studies showed that aPL may occur in the systemic vasculitides. Bleil *et al.* (1991) did not find significantly elevated levels in patients with Wegener's granulomatosis (WG) compared with controls, but there were significant associations with four patients with polyarteritis nodosa and 24 patients with polymyalgia rheumatica/ giant cell arteritis (GCA). Consistent with these findings, other authors have found significant associations with GCA (Duhaut *et al.* 1998; McHugh *et al.* 1990; Watts *et al.* 1990). Duhaut *et al.* (1998), in multivariate analyses, did not find any association with thrombosis. They postulated that aCL may be produced as a consequence of endothelial damage and not have a relationship to thrombosis. Thrombosis is a feature of Behçet's syndrome, however aPL have not been consistently found (Aydintug *et al.* 1993). Case reports have also described aPL in Takayasu's arteritis (Yokoi *et al.* 1996) and classical PAN (Dasgupta *et al.* 1997; Norden *et al.* 1995).

It is not clear if the aPL in these conditions are pathogenic and contribute to the clinical features, although it is postulated that a more severe clinical course may occur if both vasculitis and aPL are present at the same time (Norden *et al.* 1995). Given the recent description of a high rate of venous thromboses in Wegener's granulomatosis (Merkel *et al.* 2005) discussed elsewhere in this book, this finding may be highly relevant.

Treatment

General measures

Given the increased thrombotic risk of these patients and the possible association with atherosclerosis, vascular risk factors should be addressed. Lifestyle measures and management of risk factors, such as obesity, smoking, hypertension, diabetes, and hyperlipidemia, are important. The combined oral contraceptive pill and hormone replacement therapy should be avoided.

Table 44.6 Conditions associated with aPL

Autoimmune disorders
SLE/Sjögren's syndrome
Rheumatoid arthritis
Systemic vasculitis
Malignancy
Infection
Syphilis
Lyme disease
Human immunodeficiency virus
Hepatitis C
Cytomegalovirus
Mycoplasma
Drugs
Chlorpromazine
Quinine/ quinidine
Hydralazine
Procainamide
Phenytoin

Asymptomatic patients

Increasing numbers of asymptomatic or recurrent miscarriage patients are being detected due to improved awareness of the condition. A major dilemma is how these patients, who have not had a thrombotic event but remain persistently aPL positive, should be managed. There is no doubt that some of these patients will have a future event, but predicting those at high risk has proven difficult.

Many physicians recommend low-dose aspirin for management of those patients without previous thrombosis, particularly if titers of aPL are high; however, there is little objective evidence to support this. In SLE patients, there is some evidence supporting use of hydroxychloroquine, as it was protective against future thrombosis in the Hopkins Lupus Cohort (Petri 1997). It has also been used as a prophylactic agent to prevent DVT in patients undergoing orthopedic surgery.

Traveler's thrombosis has become topical and, in the absence of evidence, it seems reasonable to recommend simple measures such as support stockings, hydration, and exercises to APS patients undertaking long journeys by any transport mode. In very high risk aPL-positive patients, some clinicians recommend a single injection of heparin prior to commencing the journey, though this is clearly anecdotal. Other high-risk periods include the postoperative period, especially after abdominal, gynecological, and orthopedic surgery where heparin prophylaxis is important.

Thrombotic events

Arterial and venous events are treated in similar fashion, that is initially with unfractionated heparin or low molecular weight heparins, followed by oral anticoagulation with agents such as warfarin. When using unfractionated heparin, it is important to examine the baseline activated partial thromboplastin time (APTT) level, which may indicate the presence of LA. If there is concern that the APTT will not accurately reflect the degree of anticoagulation, other tests can be employed such as a factor Xa inhibition test. Alternatively, low molecular weight heparins such as tinzaparin or enoxaparin can be used. Similar problems may occur rarely with warfarin and the International Normalized Ratio (INR) level, but can be avoided by using chromogenic factor X levels and prothrombin-proconvertin times (Bartholomew and Kottke-Marchant 1998).

The current recommendation is that anticoagulation should be lifelong, given the risk of recurrent events; however, lifelong anticoagulation is not without hazard, with major bleeding occurring in up to 20–40% in some long-term studies of non-APS patients (Fihn et al. 1993; Landefeld and Goldman 1989). It is tempting not to recommend lifelong anticoagulation if the initial venous thrombosis is minor, particularly if there has been a clear-cut precipitating factor. In this situation, comorbid factors as well as titers of aPL should be considered and discussed with the patient. No such uncertainty should exist with arterial events, particularly cerebral, where lifelong anticoagulation is usually indicated.

The optimal intensity of anticoagulation has been debated. Khamashta et al. (1995) and Rosove and Brewer (1992) found no thrombosis in patients who maintained the INR greater than 3 and 2.9 respectively, and Schulman et al. (1998) found no recurrence in a group of patients with venous thromboembolic events who maintained their INR in the range of 2.0–2.85. In those patients that fail high-intensity warfarin, it has been our practice to add aspirin although little evidence, other than anecdotal, exists to support or discourage this approach. Recent randomized, controlled trials have suggested that lower INR levels may be sufficient in APS patients with only venous thrombotic events (reviewed in Lim et al. 2006).

Treatment of catastrophic APS has involved glucocorticoids, cyclophosphamide, plasmapheresis, intravenous gamma globulin, anticoagulation and, in the occasional patient, thrombolytic therapy. More than one modality has been tried in most patients. Although no clear approach has emerged, the most recent study of mortality suggests that anticoagulation, glucocorticoids, and plasma exchange may be useful treatments (Bucciarelli et al. 2006).

Thrombocytopenia is common in APS. Patients remain at risk of thrombosis despite this and warfarin should be continued unless the platelet count falls below 50×10^9/L. Anticoagulation may be continued even when the platelet count is below 50×10^9/L, but the intensity of anticoagulation may need to be reduced. In patients with severe thrombocytopenia, glucocorticoids and intravenous immunoglobulins are usually effective. Other agents such as danazol, dapsone, and even aspirin have been tried. There is some debate as to the effectiveness of splenectomy in APS patients. Hakim et al. (1998) and Galindo et al. (1999) have shown that splenectomy may allow successful long-term outcomes.

A frequent problem in the management of female patients is menorrhagia, particularly when INRs are maintained at high levels. In this situation, the "Mirena" coil, an intrauterine coil with a silastic capsule containing levonorgestrel, has been found to be helpful (Pisoni et al. 2006).

Pregnancy

The management of pregnancy in women with APS remains controversial. Antithrombotic treatment is preferred to glucocorticoids (which were once widely recommended). The current choice is aspirin or heparin, or both, and this has been reviewed in detail by Derksen et al. (2004). This area remains controversial, especially since Farquharson et al. (2002) showed in a randomized, controlled trial that high pregnancy success rates were achieved with low-dose aspirin and no advantage was gained by the addition of low molecular weight heparin. Women with APS and previous thromboembolism are at extremely high risk in pregnancy and the puerperium, and should be given antenatal thromboprophylaxis with subcutaneous heparin.

Warfarin exposure between 6 and 12 weeks of gestation can be associated with embryopathy, which is characterized by stippled epiphyses and nasal hypoplasia. Therefore, the change from warfarin to heparin should be achieved prior to 6 weeks' gestation. Heparin does not cross the placenta and is not known to cause any adverse fetal effects. Baglin et al. (2006) have published guidelines for the use of heparin, including the use of low molecular weight heparin in pregnancy. The risk of osteoporosis in the mother from long-term heparin use has probably been overestimated: a controlled study by Carlin et al. (2004) showed that bone loss is a feature of normal pregnancy and that low molecular weight heparin does not exacerbate this loss.

For patients who continue to have pregnancy losses despite heparin and low-dose aspirin treatment, intravenous immunoglobulin (IVIg) may be an option. IVIg is expensive and definitive proof of its efficacy is needed before endorsing its use as a first line therapy (Gordon and Kilby 1998).

Most authorities agree that one of the main reasons for the improving outcome of APS pregnancies is closer obstetric surveillance (Mascola and Repke 1997). Viable APS pregnancies have a high incidence of obstetric and fetal complications, including intrauterine growth restriction, prematurity and pre-eclampsia, hence, close monitoring including uterine artery Doppler scans and timely delivery may improve fetal outcome in these women.

Conclusions

The identification of APS and its pathophysiology have significantly advanced in the last 25 years, touching nearly all branches of medicine. In the field of systemic vasculitis, it is becoming clear that APS patients may also suffer the consequences of thrombosis, contributing to a poor prognosis. It would therefore be prudent to consider screening newly diagnosed systemic vasculitis patients for aPL.

References

Abu-Shakra, M., Gladman, D., Urowitz, M. and Farewell, V. (1995). Anticardiolipin antibodies in systemic lupus erythematosus: Clinical and Laboratory correlations. *American Journal of Medicine*, **99**, 624–8.

Acland, K., Darvay, A., Wakelin, S. and Russell Jones, R. (1999). Livedoid vasculitis: a manifestation of the antiphospholipid syndrome? *British Journal of Dermatology*, **140**, 131–5.

Alarcón-Segovia, D., Deleze, M., Oria, C., *et al.* (1989). Antiphospholipid antibodies and the antiphospholipid syndrome in systemic lupus erythematosus: A prospective study of 500 consecutive patients. *Medicine*, **68**, 353–65.

Alarcón-Segovia, D., Ruiz-Arguelles, G., Garces-Eisele, J., *et al.* (1996). Inherited activated protein C resistance in a patient with familial primary antiphospholipid syndrome. *Journal of Rheumatology*, **23**, 2162–5.

Amengual, O., Atsumi, T., Khamashta, M., Koike, T. and Hughes, G. (1996). Specificity of ELISA for antibody to β2-glycoprotein I in patients with antiphospholipid syndrome. *British Journal of Rheumatology*, **35**, 1239–43.

Amengual, O., Atsumi, T., Khamashta, M. and Hughes, G. (1998). The role of the tissue factor pathway in the hypercoaguable state in patients with the antiphospholipid syndrome. *Thrombosis and Haemostasis*, **79**, 276–81.

Ames, P., Tommasino, C., D'Andrea, G., Iannaccone, L., Brancaccio, V. and Margaglione, M. (1998). Thrombophilic genotypes in subjects with idiopathic antiphospholpid antibodies – Prevalence and significance. *Thrombosis and Haemostasis*, **79**, 46–9.

Amigo, M., Garcia-Torres, R., Robles, M., Bochiccio, T. and Reyes, P. (1992). Renal involvement in primary antiphospholipid syndrome. *Journal of Rheumatology*, **19**, 1181–5.

Antiphospholipid Antibodies in Stroke Study Group (APASS) (1993). Clinical, radiological, and pathological aspects of cerebrovascular disease associated with antiphospholipid antibodies. *Stroke*, **24** (Suppl. 1), 120–3.

Asherson, R. A. (1992). The catastrophic antiphospholipid syndrome. *Journal of Rheumatology*, **19**, 508–12.

Asherson, R. A. (1998). The catastrophic antiphospholipid syndrome. A review of the clinical features, possible pathogenesis and treatment. *Lupus*, **7** (Suppl. 2), S55–62.

Asherson, R., Khamashta, M., Ordi Ros, J., *et al.* (1989). The primary antiphospholipid syndrome: Major clinical and serological features. *Medicine*, **68**, 366–74.

Asherson R., Noble G. and Hughes G. (1991). Hypertension, renal artery stenosis and the 'primary' antiphospholipid syndrome. *Journal of Rheumatology*, **18**, 1413–5.

Asherson, R., Jacobelli, S., Rosenberg, H., Mckee, P. and Hughes G. (1992). Skin nodules and macules resembling vasculitis in the antiphospholipid syndrome: a report of two cases. *Clinical and Experimental Dermatology*, **17**, 266–9.

Asherson, R., Liote, F., Page, B., *et al.* (1993). Avascular necrosis of bone and antiphospholpid antibodies in systemic lupus erythematosus. *Journal of Rheumatology*, **20**, 284–8.

Atsumi, T., Ieko, M., Bertolaccini, M. L., Ichikawa, K., Tsutsumi, A., Matsuura, E. and Koike, T. (2000). Association of autoantibodies against the phosphatidylserine-prothrombin complex with manifestations of the antiphospholipid syndrome and with the presence of lupus anticoagulant. *Arthritis and Rheumatism*, **43**, 1982–93.

Aydintug, A., Tokgoz, G., D'Cruz, D., *et al.* (1993). Antibodies to endothelial cells in patients with Behcet's Disease. *Clinical Immunology and Immunopathology*, **67**, 157–62.

Baglin, T., Barrowcliffe, T. W., Cohen, A., Greaves, M,; British Committee for Standards in Haematology (2006). Guidelines on the use and monitoring of heparin. *British Journal of Haematology*, **133**, 19–34.

Bancsi, L., van der Linden, I. and Bertina, R. (1992). β₂-glyco-protein I deficiency and the risk of thrombosis. *Thrombosis and Haemostasis*, **67**, 649–53.

Baron, M. A., Khamashta, M. A., Hughes, G. R., D'Cruz, D. P. (2005). Prevalence of an abnormal ankle-brachial index in patients with primary antiphospholipid syndrome: preliminary data. *Annals of the Rheumatic Diseases*, **64**, 144–6.

Bartholomew, J. and Kottke-Marchant, K. (1998). Monitoring anticoagulant therapy in patients with the lupus anticoagulant. *Journal of Clinical Rheumatology*, **4**, 307–11.

Beaumont, J. (1954). Syndrome hemorrhagique acquis de a un anticoagulant. *Sang*, **25**, 1–5.

Bertolaccini, M. L., Atsumi, T., Koike, T., Hughes, G. R. and Khamashta, M. A. (2005). Antiprothrombin antibodies detected in two different assay systems. Prevalence and clinical significance in systemic lupus erythematosus. *Thrombosis and Haemostasis*, **93**, 289–97.

Bertolaccini, M. L., Roch, B., Amengual, O., Atsumi, T., Khamashta, M. A., Hughes, G. R. (1998). Multiple antiphospholipid tests do not increase the diagnostic yield in antiphospholipid syndrome. *British Journal of Rheumatology*, **37**, 1229–32.

Bhandari, S., Harnden, P., Brownjohn, A. and Turney, J. (1998). Association of anticardiolipin antibodies with intraglomeruli thrombi and renal dysfunction in lupus nephritis. *Quarterly Journal of Medicine*, **91**, 401–9.

Bleil, L., Manger, B., Winkler, T., *et al.* (1991). The role of antineutrophil cytoplasmic antibodies, anticardiolipin antibodies, von Willebrand factor antigen, and fibronectin for the diagnosis of systemic vasculitis. *Journal of Rheumatology*, **18**, 1199–206.

Bongard, O., Reber, G., Bounameaux, H. and de Moerloose, P. (1992). Anticardiolipin in acute venous thromboembolism. *Thrombosis and Haemostasis*, **67**, 724.

Bouillanne, O., Millaire, A., de Groote, P., *et al.* (1996). Prevalence and clinical significance of antiphospholipid antibodies in heart valve disease: a case control study. *American Heart Journal*, **132**, 790–5.

Bowie, E., Thompson, J., Pascuzzi, C. and Owen, C. (1963). Thrombosis in SLE despite circulating anticoagulants. *Journal of Laboratory and Clinical Medicine*, **62**, 416–30.

Branch, D., Silver, R., Pierangeli, S., Van Leeuwen, I. and Harris, E. (1997). Antiphospholipid antibodies other than lupus anticoagulant and anticardiolipin antibodies in women with recurrent pregnancy loss, fertile controls and antiphospholipid syndrome. *Obstetrics and Gynecology*, **89**, 549–55.

Brandt, J., Triplett, D., Alving, B. and Scharrer, I. (1995). Criteria for the diagnosis of lupus anticoagulants: an update. *Thrombosis and Haemostasis*, **74,** 1185–90.

Brenner, B., Vulfsons, S., Lanir, N. and Nahir, M. (1996). Coexistence of familial antiphospholipid syndrome and factor V Leiden: Impact on thrombotic diathesis. *British Journal of Haematology*, **94,** 166–7.

Brey, R. and Escalante, A. (1998). Neurological manifestations of antiphospholipid antibody syndrome. *Lupus*, **7** (Suppl. 2), S67–74.

Bucciarelli, S., Espinosa, G., Cervera, R., Erkan, D., Gomez-Puerta, J. A., Ramos-Casals, M., Font, J., Asherson, R. A.; European Forum on Antiphospholipid Antibodies (2006). Mortality in the catastrophic antiphospholipid syndrome: causes of death and prognostic factors in a series of 250 patients. *Arthritis and Rheumatism*, **54,** 2568–76.

Cabiedes, J., Cabral, A and Alarcon-Segovia, D. (1995). Manifestation of anti phospholipid syndrome in patients with the systemic lupus erythematosus associate more strongly with anti β_2-glycoprotein-1 than with antiphospholipid antibodies. *Journal of Rheumatology*, **22,** 381–5.

Carlin, A. J., Farquharson, R. G., Quenby, S. M., Topping, J. and Fraser, W. D. (2004). Prospective observational study of bone mineral density during pregnancy: low molecular weight heparin versus control. *Human Reproduction*, **19,** 1211–4.

Cervera, R., Khamashta, M. A., Font, J., Sebastiani, G. D., Gil, A., Lavilla, P., Domenech, I., Aydintug, A. O., Jedryka-Goral, A., de Ramon, E., *et al.* (1993). Systemic lupus erythematosus: clinical and immunologic patterns of disease expression in a cohort of 1,000 patients. The European Working Party on Systemic Lupus Erythematosus. *Medicine* (Baltimore), **72,** 113–24.

Cervera R, Piette JC, Font J, Khamashta MA, Shoenfeld Y, Camps MT, *et al.*; Euro-Phospholipid Project Group. (2002). Antiphospholipid syndrome: clinical and immunologic manifestations and patterns of disease expression in a cohort of 1,000 patients. *Arthritis and Rheumatism*, **46,** 1019–27.

Cervera, R., Font, J., Gomez-Puerta, J. A., Espinosa, G., Cucho, M., Bucciarelli, S., Ramos-Casals, M., Ingelmo, M., Piette, J. C., Shoenfeld, Y., Asherson, R. A.; Catastrophic Antiphospholipid Syndrome Registry Project Group (2005). Validation of the preliminary criteria for the classification of catastrophic antiphospholipid syndrome. *Annals of the Rheumatic Diseases*, **64,** 1205–9.

Chartash, E., Lans, D., Paget, S., Qamar, T. and Lockshin, M. (1989). Aortic insufficiency and mitral regurgitation in patients with systemic lupus erythematosus and the antiphospholipid syndrome. *American Journal of Medicine*, **86,** 407–12.

Christodoulou, C., Zain, M., Bertolaccini, M. L., Sangle, S., Khamashta, M. A., Hughes, G. R., D'Cruz, D. P. (2006). Prevalence of an abnormal ankle-brachial index in patients with antiphospholipid syndrome with pregnancy loss but without thrombosis: a controlled study. *Annals of the Rheumatic Diseases*, **65,** 683–4.

Conley, C. L. and Hartmann, R. C. (1952). A hemorrhagic disorder caused by circulating anticoagulant in patients with disseminated lupus erythematosus. *Journal of Clinical Investigation*, **31,** 621–2.

Coudray, N., de Zuttere, D., Bletry, O., *et al.* (1995). M Mode and doppler echocardiographic assessment of left ventricular diastolic function in primary antiphospholipid syndrome. *British Heart Journal*, **74,** 531–5.

Coull, B., Levine, S. and Brey, R. (1992). The role of antiphospholipid antibodies in stroke. *Neurology Clinics*, **10,** 125–43.

Cuadrado, M. J., Lopez-Pedrera, C., Khamashta, M., *et al.* (1997). Thrombosis in primary antiphospholipid syndrome: a pivotal role for monocyte tissue factor expression. *Arthritis and Rheumatism*, **40,** 834–41.

Cuadrado, M. J., Khamashta, M. A., Ballesteros, A., Godfrey, T., Simon, M. J., Hughes, G. R. (2000). Can neurologic manifestations of Hughes (antiphospholipid) syndrome be distinguished from multiple sclerosis? Analysis of 27 patients and review of the literature. *Medicine* (Baltimore), **79,** 57–68.

D'Alton, J., Preston, D., Bormanis, J., Green, M. and Kraag, G. (1985). Multiple transient ischaemic attacks, lupus anticoagulant and verrucous endocarditis. *Stroke*, **16,** 512–4.

D'Cruz, D. P. (2005). Renal manifestations of the antiphospholipid syndrome. *Lupus*, **14,** 45–8.

Dasgupta, B., Almond, M. and Tanqueray, A. (1997). Polyarteritis nodosa and the antiphospholipid syndrome. *British Journal of Rheumatology*, **36,** 1210–12

Del Papa, N., Guidali, L., Sala, A., *et al.* (1997). Endothelial cells as target for antiphospholpid antibodies: human polyclonal and monoclonal anti- β_2-glycoprotein 1 antibodies react in vitro with endothelial cells through adherent β_2-glycoprotein 1 and induce endothelial activation. *Arthritis and Rheumatism*, **40,** 551–61.

Derksen, R. H., Khamashta, M. A. and Branch, D. W. (2004). Management of the obstetric antiphospholipid syndrome. *Arthritis and Rheumatism*, **50,** 1028–39.

Dessailloud, R., Papo, T., Vaneecloo, S., Gamblin, C., Vanhille, P. and Piette, J. (1998). Acalculous ischaemic gallbladder necrosis in the catastrophic antiphospholipid syndrome. *Arthritis and Rheumatism*, **41,** 1318–20.

Duhaut, P., Berruyer, M., Pinede, L., *et al.* (1998). Anticardiolipin antibodies and giant cell arteritis: a prospective, multicenter case-control study. *Arthritis and Rheumatism*, **41,** 701–9.

Edson, J., Vogt, J. and Hasegawa, D. (1984). Abnormal prothrombin crossed-immunoelectrophoresis in patients with lupus inhibitors. *Blood*, **64,** 807–16.

Emmi, L., Bergamini, C., Spinelli, *et al.* (1997). Possible pathogenic role of activated platelets in the primary antiphospholipid syndrome involving the central nervous system. *Annals of the New York Academy of Science*, **823,** 188–200.

Farquharson, R. G., Quenby, S. and Greaves, M. (2002). Antiphospholipid syndrome in pregnancy: a randomized, controlled trial of treatment. *Obstetrics and Gynecology*, **100,** 408–13.

Ferreira, S., D'Cruz, D. P. and Hughes, G. R. (2005). Multiple sclerosis, neuropsychiatric lupus and antiphospholipid syndrome: where do we stand? *Rheumatology* (Oxford), **44,** 434–42.

Feinstein, D. and Rapaport, S. (1972). Acquired inhibitors of blood coagulation. *Progress in Haemostasis and Thrombosis*, **1,** 75–95.

Fields, R., Toubbeh, H., Searles R. and Bankhurst, A. (1989). The prevalence of anticardiolipin antibodies in a healthy elderly population and its association with antinuclear antibodies. *Journal of Rheumatology*, **16,** 623–5.

Fihn, S., McDonell, M., Martin, D., *et al.* (1993). Risk factors for complications of chronic anticoagulation: A multicentre study. *Annals of Internal Medicine*, **118,** 511–20.

Finazzi, G., Brancaccio, V., Moia, M., *et al.* (1996). Natural history and risk factors for thrombosis in 360 patients with antiphopsholipid antibodies. A four year prospective study from the Italian Registry. *American Journal of Medicine*, **100,** 530–6.

Fleck, R., Rapaport, S. and Rao, L. (1988). Antiprothrombin antibodies and the lupus anticoagulant. *Blood*, **72,** 512–9.

Font, J., Espinosa, G., Tassies, D., Pino, M., Khamashta, M. A., Gallart, T., Cervera, R., Escolar, G., Hughes, G. R., Ingelmo, M., Ordinas, A. and Reverter, J. C. (2002). Effects of beta2-glycoprotein I and monoclonal anticardiolipin antibodies in platelet interaction with subendothelium under flow conditions. *Arthritis and Rheumatism*, **46,** 3283–9.

Furie, R., Ishikawa, T., Dhawan, V. and Eidelberg, D. (1994). Alternating hemichorea in primary antiphospholipid syndrome: evidence for contralateral striatal metabolism. *Neurology*, **44,** 2197–9.

Galindo, M., Khamashta, M. and Hughes, G. (1999). Splenectomy for refractory thrombocytopenia in the antiphospholipid syndrome. *Rheumatology*, **38,** 848–53.

Galli, M., Confurius, P., Maassen, C., *et al.* (1990). Anticardiolipin antibodies directed not to cardiolipin but to a plasma protein cofactor. *Lancet*, **335,** 1544–7.

Galli, M., Comfurius, P., Barbui, T., Zwaal, R. and Bevers, E. (1992). Anticoagulant activity of β₂GPI is potentiated by a distinct group of anticardiolipin antibodies. *Thrombosis and Haemostasis*, **68**, 297–300.

Galli, M., Ruggeri, L. and Barbui, T. (1998). Differential effects of anti-β₂GP1 and antiprothrombin antibodies on the anticoagulant activity of activated protein C. *Blood*, **91**, 1999–2004.

Galve, E., Ordi, J., Candell-Riera, J., Permanyer-Miralda, G., Vilardell, M. and Soler-Soler, J. (1989). Valvular heart disease in systemic lupus erythematosus. *New England Journal of Medicine*, **320**, 740–1.

George, J., Afek, A., Gilburd, B., *et al.* (1998). Induction of early atherosclerosis in LDL receptor deficient mice by immunization with beta 2 glycoprotein 1. *Circulation*, **98**, 1108–15.

Gertner, E. and Lie, J. (1993). Pulmonary capillaritis, alveolar haemorrhage, and recurrent microvascular thrombosis in primary antiphospholipid syndrome. *Journal of Rheumatology*, **20**, 1224–8.

Gharavi, A. E., Harris, E. N., Asherson, R. A., and Hughes, G. R.V. (1987). Anticardiolipin antibody: isotype distribution and phospholipid specificity. *Annals of the Rheumatic Diseases*, **46**, 1–6.

Gharavi, E., Chaimovich, H., Cucurull, E., *et al.* (1999). Induction of antiphospholipid antibodies by immunisation with synthetic viral and bacterial peptides. *Lupus*, **8**, 449–55.

Ghirardello, A., Doria, A., Ruffati, A., *et al.* (1994). Antiphospholipid antibodies (aPL) in systemic lupus erythematosus. Are they specific tools for the diagnosis of aPL syndrome. *Annals of the Rheumatic Diseases*, **53**, 140–2.

Giles, I., Lambrianides, N., Pattni, N., Faulkes, D., Latchman, D., Chen, P., Pierangeli, S., Isenberg, D. and Rahman, A. (2006). Arginine residues are important in determining the binding of human monoclonal antiphospholipid antibodies to clinically relevant antigens. *Journal of Immunology*, **177**, 1729–36.

Ginsburg, K., Liang, M., Newcomer, L., *et al.* (1992). Anticardiolipin antibodies and the risk for ischaemic stroke and venous thrombosis. *Annals of Internal Medicine*, **117**, 997–1002.

Ginsberg, J., Wells, P., Brill-Edwards, P., *et al.* (1995). Antiphospholipid antibodies and venous thromboembolism. *Blood*, **86**, 3685–91.

Girardi, G., Redecha, P. and Salmon, J. E. (2004). Heparin prevents antiphospholipid antibody-induced fetal loss by inhibiting complement activation. *Nature Medicine*, **10**, 1222–6.

Gluek, H., Kant, K., Weiss, M., Pollak, V., Miller, M. and Coots, M. (1985). Thrombosis in systemic lupus erythematosus. Relation to the presence of circulating anticoagulants. *Archives of Internal Medicine*, **145**, 1389–95.

Godfrey, T., Abbs, I., Khamashta, M. and Hughes, G. (2000). Antiphospholipid syndrome and renal artery stenosis. *Quarterly Journal of Medicine*, **93**, 127–9.

Gomez-Puerta, J. A., Martin, H., Amigo, M. C., Aguirre, M. A., Camps, M. T., Cuadrado, M. J., Hughes, G. R. and Khamashta, M. A. (2005a). Long-term follow-up in 128 patients with primary antiphospholipid syndrome: do they develop lupus? *Medicine* (Baltimore), **84**, 225–30.

Gomez-Puerta, J. A., Cervera, R., Calvo, L. M., Gomez-Anson, B., Espinosa, G., Claver, G., Bucciarelli, S., Bove, A., Ramos-Casals, M., Ingelmo, M. and Font, J. (2005b). Dementia associated with the antiphospholipid syndrome: clinical and radiological characteristics of 30 patients. *Rheumatology* (Oxford), **44**, 95–9.

Gordon, C. and Kilby, M. D. (1998). Use of intravenous immunoglobulin therapy in pregnancy in systemic lupus erythematosus and antiphospholipid syndrome. *Lupus*, **7**, 429–33.

Granados, J., Vargas-Alarcon, G., Drenkard, C., *et al.* (1997). Relationship of anticardiolpin antibodies and antiphospholipid syndrome to HLA DR7 in Mexican patients with SLE. *Lupus*, **6**, 57–62.

Hakim, A., Machin, S. and Isenberg, D. (1998). Autoimmune thrombocytopenia in primary antiphospholipid syndrome and systemic lupus eyththematosus: The response to splenectomy. *Seminars in Arthritis and Rheumatism*, **28**, 20–25.

Hanly, J., Hong, C., Smith, S. and Fisk, J. (1999). A prospective analysis of cognitive function and anticardiolipin antibodies in systemic lupus erythematosus. *Arthritis and Rheumatism*, **42**, 728–34.

Harris, E. and Spinnato, J. (1991). Should anticardiolipin tests be performed in otherwise healthy pregnant women? *American Journal of Obstetrics and Gynecology*, **165**, 1272–7.

Harris, E., Gharavi, A., Boey, M., *et al.* (1983). Anticardiolipin antibodies: detection by radioimmunoassay and association with thrombosis in SLE. *Lancet*, **2**, 1211–14.

Hasnie, A., Stoddard, M., Gleason, C., *et al.* (1995). Diastolic dysfunction is a feature of the antiphospholipid syndrome. *American Heart Journal*, **129**, 1009–13.

Hasunuma, Y., Matsuura, E., Makita, Z., Katahira, T., Nishi, S. and Koike T. (1997). Involvement of β₂-glycoprotein 1 and anticardiolipin antibodies in oxidatively modified lowdensity lipoprotein uptake by macrophages. *Clinical and Experimental Immunology*, **107**, 569–73.

Hojnik, M., George, J., Ziporen, L. and Shoenfeld, Y. (1996). Heart valve involvement (Libman-Sacks endocarditis) in the antiphospholipid syndrome. *Circulation*, **93**, 1579–87.

Horbach, D., Oort, E., Donders, R., Derksen, R. and de Groot, P. (1996). Lupus anticoagulant is the strongest risk factor for both venous and arterial thrombosis in patients with systemic lupus erythematosus. *Thrombosis and Haemostasis*, **76**, 916–24.

Houssiau, F. A., N'Zeusseu Toukap, A., Depresseux, G., Maldague, B. E., Malghem, J., Devogelaer, J. P. and Vande Berg, B. C. (1998). Magnetic resonance imaging-detected avascular osteonecrosis in systemic lupus erythematosus: lack of correlation with antiphospholipid antibodies. *British Journal of Rheumatology*, **37**, 448–53.

Hughes, G., Hanis, E. and Gharavi, A. (1987). The anticardiolipin syndrome. *Journal of Rheumatology*, **13**, 486–9.

Hughes, G. R. and Khamashta, M. A. (2003). Seronegative antiphospholipid syndrome. *Annals of the Rheumatic Diseases*, **62**, 1127.

Kamboh, M. and Mehdi, H. (1998). Genetics of apolipoprotein H (2-glycoprotein 1) and anionic phospholipid binding. *Lupus*, **7** (Suppl. 2), S10–13.

Kalashnikova, L. A., Nasonov, E. L., Kushekbaeva, A. E. and Gracheva, L. A. (1990). Anticardiolipin antibodies in Sneddon's syndrome. *Neurology*, **40**, 464–7.

Kalashnikova, L. A., Korczyn, A. D., Shavit, S., Rebrova, O., Reshetnyak, T. and Chapman, J. (1999). Antibodies to prothrombin in patients with Sneddon's syndrome. *Neurology*, **53**, 223–5.

Kaplan, S., Chartash, E., Pizzarello, R. and Furies, R. (1992). Cardiac manifestations of the antiphospholipid syndrome. *American Heart Journal*, **124**, 1331–8.

Kearon, C., Gent, M., Hirsh, J., *et al.* (1999). A comparison of three months of anticoagulation with extended anticoagulation for a first episode of idiopathic venous thromboembolism. *New England Journal of Medicine*, **340**, 901–7.

Khamashta, M., Gil, A., Asherson, R., Vazquez, J. and Hughes, G. (1989). Antiphospholipid antibodies, valvular heart disease, and systemic lupus erythematosus (Letter). *American Journal of Medicine*, **86**, 633–4.

Khamashta, M., Cervera, R., Asherson, R., *et al.* (1990). Association of antibodies against phospholipids with heart valve disease in systemic lupus erythematosus. *Lancet*, **335**, 1541–2

Khamashta, M., Cuadrado, M., Mujic, F., *et al.* (1995). The management of thrombosis in the antiphospholipid-antibody syndrome. *New England Journal of Medicine*, **332**, 993–7.

Klein, K. and Pittelkow, M. (1992). Tissue plasminogen activator for treatment of livedoid vasculitis. *Mayo Clinic Proceedings*, **67**, 923–33.

Krnic-Barrie, S., O'Connor, C., Looney, S., Pierangeli, S. and Harris, N. (1997). A retrospective review of 61 patients with antiphospholipid syndrome. Analysis of factors influencing recurrent thrombosis. *Archives of Internal Medicine*, **157**, 2101–8.

Lampropoulos, C. E., Koutroumanidis, M., Reynolds, P. P., Manidakis, I., Hughes, G. R. and D'Cruz, D. P. (2005). Electroencephalography in the assessment of neuropsychiatric manifestations in antiphospholipid syndrome and systemic lupus erythematosus. *Arthritis and Rheumatism*, **52**, 841–6.

Landefeld, C. S. and Goldman L. (1989). Major bleeding in outpatients treated with warfarin: Incidence and prediction by factors known at the start of outpatient therapy. *American Journal of Medicine*, **87**, 144–52.

Levine, S., Brey, R., Sawaya, K., *et al.* (1995). Recurrent stroke and thrombo-occlusive events in the antiphospholipid syndrome. *Annals of Neurology*, **38**, 119–24.

Libman, E. and Sacks, B. (1924). A hitherto undescribed form of valvular and mural endocarditis. *Archives of Internal Medicine*, **33**, 701–37.

Lie, J. T. (1994). Vasculitis in the antiphospholipid syndrome: Culprit or consort? *Journal of Rheumatology*, **21**, 397–9.

Lim, W., Crowther, M. A. and Eikelboom, J. W. (2006). Management of antiphospholipid antibody syndrome: a systematic review. *Journal of the American Medical Association*, **295**, 1050–7.

Lockshin, M. (1998). Pregnancy loss and antiphospholipid antibodies. *Lupus*, **7** (Suppl. 2), S86–9.

Lopez-Pedrera, C., Buendia, P., Cuadrado, M. J., Siendones, E., Aguirre, M. A., Barbarroja, N., Montiel-Duarte, C., Torres, A., Khamashta, M. and Velasco, F. (2006). Antiphospholipid antibodies from patients with the antiphospholipid syndrome induce monocyte tissue factor expression through the simultaneous activation of NF-kappaB/Rel proteins via the p38 mitogen-activated protein kinase pathway, and of the MEK-1/ERK pathway. *Arthritis and Rheumatism*, **54**, 301–11.

McHugh, N., James, I. and Plant, G. (1990). Anticardilopin and antineutrophil antibodies in giant cell arteritis. *Journal of Rheumatology*, **17**, 916–22.

McNeil, H. P., Chesterman, C. N. and Krilis, S. A. (1989). Anticardiolipin and lupus anticoagulants comprise separate antibody subgroups with different phospholipid binding characteristics. *British Journal of Haematology*, **73**, 506–12.

McNeil, H., Simpson, R., Chesterman, C. and Krilis, S. (1990). Antiphospholipid antibodies are directed against a complexed antigen that includes a lipid binding inhibitor of coagulation: beta-2-glycoprotein 1. *Proceedings of the National Academy of Science, USA*, **87**, 4120–4.

McNeil, H. P., Chesterman, C. N. and Krilis, S. A. (1991). Immunology and clinical importance of antiphospholipid antibodies. *Advances in Immunology*, **49**, 193–280.

Mascola, M. A. and Repke, J. T. (1997). Obstetric management of the high-risk lupus pregnancy. *Rheumatic Disease Clinics of North America*, **23**, 119–32.

Matsuura, E., Igarasha, T., Fujimoto, M., Ichikawa, K. and Koike, T. (1990). Anticardiolipin cofactor(s) and differential diagnosis of autoimmune disease. *Lancet*, **336**, 117–8.

Medina, G., Casaos, D., Jara, L. J., Vera-Lastra, O., Fuentes, M., Barile, L. and Salas, M. (2003). Increased carotid artery intima-media thickness may be associated with stroke in primary antiphospholipid syndrome. *Annals of the Rheumatic Diseases*, **62**, 607–10.

Menon, S., Jameson-Shortall, E., Newman, S., Hall-Craggs, R., Chinn, R. and Isenberg, D. (1999). A longitudinal study of anticardiolipin antibody levels and cognitive functioning in sytemic lupus erythematosus. *Arthritis and Rheumatism*, **42**, 735–41.

Merkel, P., Chang, Y., Pierangeli, S., Convery, K., Harris, N. and Polisson, R. (1996). The prevalence and clinical association of anticardiolipin antibodies in a large inception cohort of patients with connective tissue diseases. *American Journal of Medicine*, **101**, 576–83.

Merkel, P. A. Lo, G. H. Holbrook, J. T., *et al.* (2005). Brief communication: high incidence of venous thrombotic events among patients with Wegener granulomatosis: the Wegener's Clinical Occurence of Thrombosis (WeCLOT) Study. *Annals of International Medicine*, **142**, 620–6.

Merrill, J., Shen, C., Gugnani, M., Lahita, R. and Mongey, A. (1997). High prevalence of antiphospholipid antibodies in patients taking procainamide. *Journal of Rheumatology*, **24**, 1083–8.

Miyakis, S., Lockshin, M. D., Atsumi, T., Branch, D. W., Brey, R. L., Cervera, R., *et al.* (2006). International consensus statement on an update of the classification criteria for definite antiphospholipid syndrome (APS). *Journal of Thromb Haemost*, **4**, 295–306.

Molina, J. F., Gutierrez-Urena, S., Molina, J., *et al.* (1997). Variability of anticardiolipin antibody isotype distribution in 3 geographic populations of patients with systemic lupus erythematosus. *Journal of Rheumatology*, **24**, 291–6.

Moore, J. and Mohr, C. (1952). Biologically false positive serological tests for syphilis. Type, incidence and cause. *Journal of the American Medical Association*, **150**, 467–73.

Morgan, R. and Feneley, C. (1994). Renal vein thrombosis caused by primary antiphospholipid syndrome. *British Journal of Urology*, **74**, 807–8.

Mujic, F., Cuadrado, M., Lloyd, M., *et al.* (1995). Primary antiphospholipid syndrome evolving into SLE. *Journal of Rheumatology*, **22**, 1589–92.

Nagasawa, K, Ishii, T., Mayumi, T., *et al.* (1989). Avascular necrosis of bone in systemic lupus erythematosus: Possible role of haemostatic abnormalities. *Annals of the Rheumatic Diseases*, **48**, 672–6.

Nencini, P., Baruffi, M., Abbate, R., Massai, G., Amaducci, L. and Inzitari, D. (1992). Lupus anticoagulant and anticardiolipin antibodies in young adults with cerebral ischaemia. *Stroke*, **23**, 189–93.

Nilison, I. and Laurell, A. (1957). Intrauterine death and circulating 'antithromboplastin'. *Acta Medica Scandinavica*, **197**, 153–9.

Norden, D., Ostrov, B., Shafritz, A. and Von Feldt, J. (1995). Vasculitis associated with antiphospholipid syndrome. *Seminars in Arthritis and Rheumatism*, **24**, 273–81.

Oosting, J., Derkson, R., Bobbink, I., Hackeng, T., Bouma, B. and de Groot, P. (1993). Antiphopsholipid antibodies directed against a combination of phospholipids with prothrombin, protein C, or protein S: an explanation for their pathogenic mechanism? *Blood*, **81**, 2618–25.

Ostuni, P., Lazzarin, P., Pengo, V., Ruffati, A., Schiavon, F. and Gambari, P. (1990). Renal artery thrombosis and hypertension in a 13-year-old girl with antiphospholipid syndrome. *Annals of the Rheumatic Diseases*, **49**, 184–7.

Pandolfi, C., Gianni, A., Fregoni, V., Nalli, G. and Faggi, L. (1997). Hypopituitarism and antiphospholipid syndrome. *Minerva Endocrinologica*, **22**, 103–5.

Pangborn, M. (1942). Isolation and purification of a serologically active phospholipid from beef heart. *Journal of Biological Chemistry*, **143**, 247–56.

Peddi, V. and Kant, K. (1995). Catastrophic secondary antiphospholipid syndrome with concomitant antithrombin III deficiency. *Journal of the American Society of Nephrology*, **5**, 1882–7.

Petri, M. (1997). Pathogenesis and treatment of APS. *Medical Clinics of North America*, **81**, 151–61.

Pierangeli, S., Colden-Stanfield, M., Liu, X., Barker, J., Anderson, G. and Harris, N. (1999). Antiphospholipid antibodies from antiphospholipid syndrome patients activate endothelial cell in vitro and in vivo. *Circulation*, **99**, 1997–2002.

Pierangeli, S. S., Chen, P. P. and Gonzalez, E. B. (2006). Antiphospholipid antibodies and the antiphospholipid syndrome: an update on treatment and pathogenic mechanisms. *Current Opinion in Hematology*, **13**, 366–75.

Piette, J. (1998). Criteria for the antiphosholipid syndrome. *Lupus*, **7** (Suppl. 2), S149–57.

Piette, J. and Cacoub, P. (1998). Antiphospholipid syndrome in the elderly: Caution. *Circulation*, **97**, 2195–6.

Piette, J., Weschler, B., Frances, C., Papo, T. and Godeau, P. (1993). Exclusion criteria for primary antiphospholipid syndrome. *Journal of Rheumatology*, **20**, 1802–4.

Pisoni, C. N., Cuadrado, M. J., Khamashta, M. A., Hunt, B. J. (2006). Treatment of menorrhagia associated with oral anticoagulation: efficacy and safety of the levonorgestrel releasing intrauterine device (Mirena coil). *Lupus*. **15**, 877–80.

Provenzale, J., Barboriak, D., Allen, N. and Ortel, T. (1998). Antiphospholipid antibodies: findings at arteriography. *American Journal of Neuroradiology*, **19**, 611–6.

Quenby, S., Farquharson, R. G., Dawood, F., Hughes, A. M. and Topping, J. (2005). Recurrent miscarriage and long-term thrombosis risk: a case-control study. *Human Reproduction*, **20**, 1729–32.

Rai, R. S., Regan, L., Clifford, K. *et al.* (1995). Antiphospholipid antibodies and β$_2$-Glycoprotein I in 500 women with recurrent miscarriage: results of a comprehensive screening approach. *Human Reproduction*, **10**, 2001–5.

Rees, J. D., Lanca, S., Marques, P. V., Gomez-Puerta, J. A., Moco, R., Oliveri, C., Khamashta, M. A., Hughes, G. R. and D'Cruz, D. P. (2006). Prevalence of the antiphospholipid syndrome in primary systemic vasculitis. *Annals of the Rheumatic Diseases*, **65**, 109–11.

Reid, K., Bentley, D. and Campbell, R. (1986). Complement system proteins which interact with C3b or C4b: A super-family of structurally related proteins. *Immunology Today*, **7**, 230–4.

Reverter, J., Tassies, D., Font, J., *et al.* (1996). Hypercoaguable state in patients with antiphospholipid syndrome is related to high induced tissue factor expression on monocytes and to low free protein S. *Arteriosclerosis, Thrombosis and Vascular Biology*, **16**, 1319–26.

Rocca, P., Siegel, L. and Cupps, T. (1994). The concomitant expression of vasculitis and coagulopathy: Synergy for marked tissue ischaemia. *Journal of Rheumatology*, **21**, 556–60.

Rook, A., Wilkinson, D. and Ebling, F. (1998). *Textbook of Dermatology* (Champion, R., Burton, J., Burns, D. and Breathnach, S., eds), Vol. 3, 6th edn, pp. 963. Blackwell Science, London.

Rosove, M. and Brewer, P. (1992). Antiphospholipid thrombosis: Clinical course after the first thrombotic event in 70 patients. *Annals of Internal Medicine*, **117**, 303–8.

Sailer, M., Burchert, W., Smid, H., *et al.* (1997). Positron emission tomography and magnetic resonance imaging for cerebral involvement in patients with SLE. *Journal of Neurology*, **244**, 186–93.

Sangle, S. R., D'Cruz, D. P., Jan, W., Karim, M. Y., Khamashta, M. A., Abbs, I. C. and Hughes, G. R. (2003). Renal artery stenosis in the antiphospholipid (Hughes) syndrome and hypertension. *Annals of the Rheumatic Diseases*, **62**, 999–1002.

Sangle, S., D'Cruz, D. P., Khamashta, M. A. and Hughes, G. R. (2004). Antiphospholipid antibodies, systemic lupus erythematosus, and non-traumatic metatarsal fractures. *Annals of the Rheumatic Diseases*, **63**, 1241–3.

Sangle, S., D'Cruz, D. P. and Hughes, G. R. (2005a). Livedo reticularis and pregnancy morbidity in patients negative for antiphospholipid antibodies. *Annals of the Rheumatic Diseases*, **64**, 147–8.

Sangle, S. R., D'Cruz, D. P., Abbs, I. C., Khamashta, M. A. and Hughes, G. R. (2005b). Renal artery stenosis in hypertensive patients with antiphospholipid (Hughes) syndrome: outcome following anticoagulation. *Rheumatology* (Oxford), **44**, 372–7.

Sangle, S. R., Jan, W., Lau, I. S., Bennett, A. N., Hughes, G. R. and D'Cruz, D. P. (2006). Coeliac artery stenosis and antiphospholipid (Hughes) syndrome/antiphospholipid anti-bodies. *Clinical and Experimental Rheumatology*, **24**, 349.

Schulman, S., Svenungsson, E., Granqvist, S. and the Duration of Anticoagulation Study Group. (1998). Anticardiolipin antibodies predict early recurrence of thromboembolism and death among patients with venous thromboembolism following anticoagulation therapy. *American Journal of Medicine*, **104**, 332–8.

Schutt, M., Kluter, H., Hagedorn-Greiwe, M., Fehm, H. and Wiedemann, G. (1998). Familial co-existence of primary antiphospholipid syndrome and Factor V Leiden. *Lupus*, **7**, 176–82.

Schved, J., Dupuy-Fons, C., Biron, C., Quere, I. and Janbon, C. (1994). A prospective epidemiological study on the occurrence of antiphospholipid antibody: The Montpellier Antiphospholipid (MAP) Study. *Haemostasis*, **24**, 175–82.

Sebastiani, G., Galeazzi, M., Morozzi, G. and Marcolongo, R. (1996). The immunogenetics of the antiphospholipid syndrome, anticardiolipin antibodies, and lupus anticoagulant. *Seminars in Arthritis and Rheumatism*, **25**, 414–20.

Seisdedos, L., Munos-Rodriguez, F., Cervera, R., Font, J. and Ingelmo, M. (1997). Primary antiphospholipid syndrome evolving into SLE. *Lupus*, **6**, 285–6.

Shah, N., Khamashta, M., Atsumi, T. and Hughes, G. (1998). Outcome of patients with anticardiolpin antibodies: a 10 year follow up of 52 patients. *Lupus*, **7**, 3–6.

Silver, R., Draper, M., Scoff, J., Lyon, J., Reading, J. and Branch, D. (1994). Clinical consequences of antiphospholipid antibodies. An historic cohort study. *Obstetrics and Gynaecology*, **83**, 372–7.

Simantov, R., LaSala, J., Lo, S., *et al.* (1995). Activation of cultured vascular endothelial cells by antiphospholipid antibodies. *Journal of Clinical Investigation*, **96**, 2211–19.

Simioni, P., Prandoni, P., Zanon, B., *et al.* (1996). Deep venous thrombosis and lupus anticoagulant. *Thrombosis and Haemostasis*, **76**, 187–9.

Sipek-Dolnicar, A., Hojnik, M., Bozic, B., *et al.* (2002). Clinical presentations and vascular histopathology in autopsied patients with systemic lupus erythematosus an anticardiolipin antibodies. *Clinical and Experimental Rheumatology*, **20**, 335–42.

Somers, E., Magder, L. S. and Petri, M. (2002). Antiphospholipid antibodies and incidence of venous thrombosis in a cohort of patients with systemic lupus erythematosus. *Journal of Rheumatology*, **29**, 2531–6.

Soweid, A., Hajjar, R., Hewan-Lowe, K. and Gonzalez, E. (1995). Skin necrosis indicating antiphospholipid syndrome in patients with AIDS. *Southern Medical Journal*, **88**, 786–8.

Steinkasserer, A., Cockburn, D., Black, D., Boyd, Y., Solomon, E. and Sim, R. (1992). Assignment of apolipoprotein H to human chromosome 17q23 qter; determination of the major expression site. *Cytogenetics and Cell Genetics*, **60**, 31–3.

Straaton, K., Chatham, W., Smith, S. and Koopman, W. (1989). Valvular heart disease in systemic lupus erythematosus. *New England Journal of Medicine*, **320**, 740.

Swadzba, J., De Clerk, L., Stevens, W., *et al.* (1997). Anticardiolipin, anti$_2$ glycoprotein1, antiprothrombin antibodies, and lupus anticoagulant in patients with systemic lupus erythematosus with a history of thrombosis. *Journal of Rheumatology*, **24**, 1710–15.

Teixido, M., Font, J., Reverter, J., *et al.* (1997). Anti-β2GP1 antibodies: a useful marker for the antiphospholipid syndrome. *British Journal of Rheumatology*, **36**, 113–6.

Tektonidou, M. G., Malagari, K., Vlachoyiannopoulos, P. G., Kelekis, D. A. and Moutsopoulos, H. M. (2003). Asymptomatic avascular necrosis in patients with primary antiphospholipid syndrome in the absence of corticosteroid use: a prospective study by magnetic resonance imaging. *Arthritis and Rheumatism*, **48**, 732–6.

Tektonidou, M. G., Sotsiou, F., Nakopoulou, L., Vlachoyiannopoulos, P. G. and Moutsopoulos, H. M. (2004). Antiphospholipid syndrome nephropathy in patients with systemic lupus erythematosus and antiphospholipid antibodies: prevalence, clinical associations, and long-term outcome. *Arthritis and Rheumatism*, **50**, 2569–79.

Tenedios, F., Erkan, D. and Lockshin, M. D. (2006). Cardiac manifestations in the antiphospholipid syndrome. *Rheumatic Disease Clinics of North America*, **32**, 491–507.

Tietjen, G., Day, M., Norris, L., *et al.* (1998). Role of anticardiolipin antibodies in young persons with migraine and transient focal neurological events. *Neurology*, **50**, 1433–40.

Tincani, A., Balestrieri, G., Spatola, L., Cinquini, M., Meroni, P. and Roubey, R. (1998). Anticardiolipin and anti-$\beta_2$glycoprotein 1 immunoassays in the diagnosis of antiphospholipid syndrome. *Clinical and Experimental Rheumatology*, **16**, 396–402.

Toubi, E., Krause, I., Fraser, A., Lev, S., Stojanovich, L., Rovensky, J., Blank, M. and Shoenfeld, Y. (2005). Livedo reticularis is a marker for predicting multi-system thrombosis in antiphospholipid syndrome. *Clinical and Experimental Rheumatology*, **23**, 499–504.

Tripplett, D. (1995). Protean clinical presentation of antiphospholipid - protein antibodies. *Thrombosis and Haemostasis*, **74**, 329–37.

Vaarala, O., Männttäri, M., Manninen, V., *et al.* (1995). Anti-cardiolipin antibodies and risk of myocardial infarction in a prospective cohort of middle aged men. *Circulation*, **91**, 23–7.

Vaarala, O. (1997). Atherosclerosis in SLE and Hughes' syndrome. *Lupus*, **6**, 489–90.

Vaarala, O. (1998). Antiphospholipid antibodies and myocardial infarction. *Lupus*, **7** (Suppl. 2), S132–4.

Vaidya, S., Wang, C., Gugliuzza, C. and Fish, J. (1998). Relative risk of post-transplant renal thrombosis in patients with antiphospholpid antibodies. *Clinical Transplantation*, **12**, 439–44.

Vianna, J., Khamashta, M., Ordi-Ros, J., *et al.* (1994). Comparison of the primary and secondary antiphospholipid syndrome: A European multicentre study of 114 patients. *American Journal of Medicine*, **96**, 3–9.

Wasserman, A., Neisser, A. and Bruck, C. (1906). Eine Serodiagnostiche reaktion bei Syphilis. *Deutsche Medizinische Wochenschrift*, **32**, 745–6.

Wahl, D., Guillemin, F., de Maistre, B., Perret, C., Lecompte, T. and Thibaut, G. (1997). Risk for venous thrombosis related to antiphospholipid antibodies in systemic lupus erythematosus- A meta analysis. *Lupus*, **6**, 467–73.

Wahl, D., Guillemin, F., de Maistre, B., Perret-Guillaume, C., Lecompte, T. and Thibaut, G. (1998). Meta-analysis of the risk of venous thrombosis in individuals with antiphospholipid antibodies without underlying autoimmune disease or previous thrombosis. *Lupus*, **7**, 15–22.

Watts, M., Greaves, M., Clearkin, L., *et al.* (1990). Antiphospholipid antibodies and ischaemic optic neuropathy. *Lancet*, **335**, 613–4.

Wilson, W., Gharavi, A., Koike, T., *et al.* (1999). International consensus statement on preliminary classification for definite antiphospholipid syndrome. Report of an International Workshop. *Arthritis and Rheumatism*, **42**, 1309–11.

Yokoi, K., Hosoi, E., Akaike, M., Shigekiyo, T. and Saito, S. (1996). Takayasu's arteritis associated with antiphospholipid antibodies. Report of two cases. *Angiology*, **47**, 315–9.

CHAPTER 45

Imitators of vasculitis

Sharon A. Chung and Kenneth E. Sack

Introduction

To most physicians, "vasculitis" connotes an immune-mediated disease. Yet, strictly speaking, the term simply means inflammation of the vessel wall, regardless of the cause. Confusion arises when non-inflammatory vascular damage produces the same signs and symptoms as those resulting from true vasculitis (Table 45.1). For these reasons, defining imitators of vasculitis becomes somewhat arbitrary. In this chapter, we describe conditions of both vascular and non-vascular etiology that foster the mistaken diagnosis of immune-mediated vasculitis and promote inappropriate use of immunosuppressive agents.

Mechanisms of vascular damage

The initial cause of vascular injury is often obscure because different stimuli can produce identical responses in the vessel wall. Non-immunologic causes of vascular injury include infection (Blanco 1999; Golden *et al.* 1994; Hogarth *et al.* 1999; Lie 1996; Pandey and LeRoy 1998; Somer and Finegold 1995; Walker and Mattern 1980), neoplasia (Bhawan *et al.* 1985; Fortin 1996; Harmon and Mark 1999; Fredericks 1991b; Kao *et al.* 1992; Lie 1992a; Otrakji *et al.* 1988; Petroff *et al.* 1989; Sheibani *et al.* 1986; Sienknecht 1995; Wick *et al.* 1986), ischemia, congenital or inherited abnormalities (Imahori *et al.* 1969; Olmsted and McGee 1977; Schievink 1997), and various forms of external (Martens 1996; Sijpkens *et al.* 1997; Nance 1997; Olivero 1997; Pineda *et al.* 1985; Shim 1998) and internal (Ryan and Wilkinson 1986) injury to the vessel wall.

Pitfalls of angiography

Irregularities in vessel walls, as well as segmental vascular occlusions and dilatations, are the commonly recognized angiographic manifestations of vasculitis (see Chapter 18). These same findings, however, occur in a host of other conditions (Table 45.2).

Pitfalls of histology

Histopathologic examination of vascular tissue does not always yield definitive information. A vessel damaged by any mechanism may accumulate immune complexes or fibrin; inflammation in neighboring tissues occasionally triggers an inflammatory response

Table 45.1 Non-inflammatory causes of vascular damage

Occlusive processes	Atheroembolic disease
	Thrombotic disorders
	Antiphospholipid antibody syndrome
	Thrombotic thrombocytopenic purpura
	Sickle cell anemia
	Thromboembolism
	Abnormal proteins
	Cryoglobulins
	Cryofibrinogens
	Paraproteins
Neoplasia	Cardiac myxoma
	Other neoplasms
External injury	Exposure to cold
	Radiation exposure
Internal injury	Hypertension, arterial dissection
Biochemical abnormalities	
Infection	(See Table 45.3)
Congenital or inherited abnormalities	Pseudoxanthoma elasticum
	Ehlers–Danlos syndrome
	Neurofibromatosis
	Fibromuscular dysplasia
Miscellaneous conditions	Drug effects
	Moyamoya disease
	Others (see Table 45.4)
	Non-vascular

in the vessel wall (Ryan and Wilkinson 1986). Furthermore, the microscopic findings are a function of the type of injury and the time between the original insult and the obtaining of tissue. Anoxia, for example, can damage vascular smooth muscle within 2 hours (Ryan and Wilkinson 1986). Conversely, radiation injury may cause

Table 45.2 Angiographic imitators of vasculitis

Imitator	Authors
Amyloidosis	Salvarani et al. 1994
Atheromatous emboli	Cappiello et al. 1989
Atrial myxoma	New et al. 1970; Thomas 1981
Cold exposure	Jacob et al. 1986
Drug abuse	Rumbaugh et al. 1971a; Sack 1997
Dye injection	
Ehlers–Danlos syndrome	Imahori et al. 1969; Miller and A.A.A.S 2005
Fibromuscular dysplasia	Meyers et al. 1974
Hypertension	Garner et al. 1990
Infection	Ferris et al. 1968; Marks and Kuskov 1995; Shimizu et al. 2004
Migraine	Masuzawa et al. 1983; Serdaru et al. 1984
Moyamoya	Provost et al. 1991; Ueki et al. 1994
Neurofibromatosis	Finley and Dabbs 1988; Tomsick et al. 1976
Neoplasia	Fredericks 1991b; Leeds and Rosenblatt 1972; Sack 1997
Pseudoxanthoma elasticum	Travers et al. 1979
Radiation exposure	McCready et al. 1983
Reperfusion of normal vessels	Sack 1997
Thrombotic thrombocytopenic purpura	Orbison 1952
Trauma	Savader et al. 1988; Suwanwela and Suwanwela 1972

atherosclerotic changes and periarterial fibrosis after a latency of 20 years (Lie 1992b). Associated illnesses and the site of the biopsy may also affect the histopathologic picture. Thus, acute arterial hypertension may cause fibrinoid changes in vessel walls, usually without cellular infiltration. In areas where stasis occurs, such as the lower leg, a mild degree of perivascular cellular infiltration and vascular hypertrophy are the rule (Ryan and Wilkinson 1986).

Representative syndromes

Occlusive processes

Atheroembolic disease

Clinical manifestations

The most frequent, visible manifestation of atheroembolic disease is purple discoloration of the toes, occasionally followed by ulceration and gangrene. In this situation, the peripheral pulses are usually normal, and the patient often has livedo reticularis symmetrically affecting the lower body (Anderson and Richards 1968; Falanga et al. 1986; Fisher et al. 1960; Kalter et al. 1985). Many cases of "blue toe" syndrome are probably caused by atheroemboli (Fisher et al. 1960; Moldveen-Geronimus and Merriam 1967; Nevelsteen et al. 1992; Hyman et al. 1987; O'Keeffe et al. 1992). Rarely, these emboli cause gangrene in the scrotum and penis or produce splinter hemorrhages in the nailbeds (Turakhia and Khan 1990).

Unexplained acute or progressive renal failure (Bradley 1995; Gupta et al. 1993; Hadjivassiliou 1998; Harrington et al. 1968; Lye et al. 1993; Jones and Iannaccone 1975; Mayo and Swartz 1996; Smith et al. 1981; Spring et al. 1998; Thadhani et al. 1995) or hypertension (Bradley 1995; Dahlberg et al. 1989; Handler 1956; Sack 1998) should also suggest atheroembolic disease. In most such cases the course is unrelentingly downhill (Dahlberg et al. 1989; Gupta et al. 1993; Lye et al. 1993), but occasionally, spontaneous resolution of the renal insufficiency occurs (Smith et al. 1981). Additional clinical conditions caused by atheroemboli include acute pancreatitis (Orvar and Johlin 1994; Probstein et al. 1957), amaurosis (Bradley 1995; Darsee 1979; Young et al. 1986), abdominal pain (with or without gastrointestinal bleeding) (Darsee 1979; Hendel et al. 1989; Moolenaar and Lamers 1996; Richards et al. 1965), angina pectoris (Cappiello et al. 1989), myocardial infarction (Darsee 1979), transient ischemic attacks (Cappiello et al. 1989; Stanton and Nickeleit 1996; Young et al. 1986), and other stroke syndromes (Cappiello et al. 1989; Meyer 1947; Sijpkens et al. 1997; Winter 1957; Young et al. 1986). Angioplasty does not increase the risk of embolization (Sanborn et al. 1982). Anticoagulation might predispose to atheroemboli by preventing the formation of a "protective" thrombus over an atheromatous plaque (Nevelsteen et al. 1992; Panum 1862; Moldveen-Geronimus and Merriam 1967; Teepe et al. 1986; Hyman et al. 1987). Thrombolytic therapy might also initiate the syndrome (Queen et al. 1990; Rivera-Manrique et al. 1998), but in many such reported cases the patient had received an anticoagulant (Gupta et al. 1993; Bhardwaj et al. 1989; Mendia et al. 1992; King and Carlson 1993). When there is no obvious triggering event, other signs and symptoms of atherosclerotic disease or an aortic aneurysm are usually present (Mayo and Swartz 1996; Stanton and Nickeleit 1996; Sack 1998; Cabili et al. 1993; Kalter et al. 1985; Smith et al. 1981; Fine et al. 1987; Jones and Iannaccone 1975; Karmody et al. 1976).

Atheromatous plaques dislodge and embolize in fragments or ulcerate and release cholesterol crystals or other components (Kennedy et al. 1989; Eliot et al. 1964). The emboli typically lodge in arteries 150–200 μm in diameter (Eliot et al. 1964). The affected vessels undergo successive pathologic changes (Leeds and Rosenblatt 1972; Hollenhorst 1961; Cross 1991; Retan and Miller 1966). Soon after the atheromatous material deposits in the arterial lumen, an acute inflammatory response occurs. Intimal hyperplasia and panarteritis follow rapidly, often accompanied by the appearance of foreign body giant cells. Intimal fibrosis ensues along with complete encasement of the cholesterol crystals by collagenous material. The vessel lumen, which initially contained slit-like passages (Figure 45.1), may eventually become completely occluded. Superimposed thrombosis is uncommon (Handler 1956; Retan and Miller 1966).

Laboratory evaluation

Crystalline cholesterol, as well as lipids from atheromata, can fix complement (Hammerschmidt et al. 1981; Cosio et al. 1985). This process not only causes hypocomplementemia but also results in the production of C5a (Hammerschmidt et al. 1981), a potent chemotactic factor for eosinophils and neutrophils (Cosio et al. 1985). Thus, eosinophilia and eosinophiluria are common concomitants of atheroembolic disease (Lye et al. 1993; Cosio et al. 1985; Cappiello et al. 1989; Kay et al. 1973; Kasinath and Lewis 1987; Ebert and McCluskey 1986; Fine et al. 1987; Wilson et al. 1991).

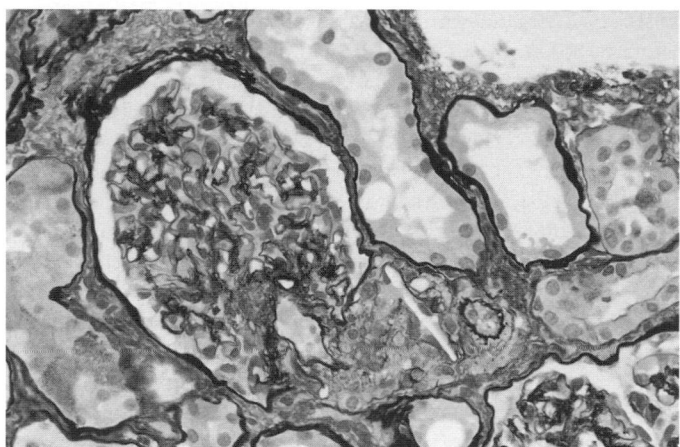

Figure 45.1 Atheromatous embolus lodged in an afferent renal arteriole. (See Color Plate 124).

Other laboratory abnormalities that commonly accompany atheroembolic disease are similar to those seen in immune-mediated conditions: markers of inflammation (anemia, leukocytosis, elevated erythrocyte sedimentation rate); azotemia; thrombocytopenia; hyperamylasemia; positive antinuclear antibody or rheumatoid factor; proteinuria; and granular or hyaline urinary casts (Sack 1998; Cappiello *et al.* 1989; Goldman *et al.* 1980; Young *et al.* 1986; Fine *et al.* 1987; Stanton and Nickeleit 1996; Ebert and McCluskey 1986; Wilson *et al.* 1991). Less common findings are elevated muscle enzymes, cryoglobulinemia, glycosuria, hematuria, pyuria, and urinary cellular casts (Sack 1997).

In the appropriate setting, biopsy of a skin lesion (Falanga *et al.* 1986) or the kidney (Gupta *et al.* 1993; Smith *et al.* 1981) yields the diagnosis. Occasionally, random biopsy of muscle (Anderson, 1965) or bone marrow (Pierce *et al.* 1978) is diagnostic. Usual methods for preparing histologic specimens dissolve cholesterol, leaving characteristic clefts (Figure 45.1). In cases where necrotizing angiitis is the dominant pathologic finding, these clefts may go unnoticed (Sijpkens *et al.* 1997; Anderson 1965; Anderson and Richards 1968; Rosansky 1982).

Treatment
Prognosis for recovery from atheroembolic disease is poor (Dahlberg *et al.* 1989; Gupta *et al.* 1993; Lye *et al.* 1993). The mortality is 70–90% in some series (Moolenaar and Lamers 1996; Hendel *et al.* 1989; Falanga *et al.* 1986; Fine *et al.* 1987), and the need for long-term dialysis is common (Lye *et al.* 1993). Survival probably relates to the cause and extent of the disease (Smith *et al.* 1981). Thus, a patient with limited emboli from a discrete source, such as an aneurysm or localized plaque, may do well upon removal of the offending lesion (Darsee 1979; Kazimer *et al.* 1966). Glucocorticoids can temporarily alleviate some of the disease manifestations but do not affect the outcome (Hendel *et al.* 1989). Use of low-molecular-weight dextran, antiplatelet drugs, or vasodilators does not alter the course substantially (Hendel *et al.* 1989; Kalter *et al.* 1985; Cappiello *et al.* 1989). Agents of potential benefit include pentoxifylline (Carr *et al.* 1994), lipid-lowering drugs (Woolfson and Lachmann 1998; Cabili *et al.* 1993; Cabili *et al.* 1993; Kawakami *et al.* 1990), and drugs with the ability to stabilize atherosclerotic plaques (Kullo *et al.* 1998). If anticoagulants precipitate the syndrome, the patient may improve after discontinuing them (Bruns *et al.* 1978).

Thrombotic disorders
Thrombosis in multiple vessels occasionally masquerades as vasculitis, and when inflammation and thrombosis occur together in a vessel, determining which came first is difficult (Jordan *et al.* 1987). The antiphospholipid antibody (APL) syndrome is the most common hypercoagulable state that simulates vasculitis (see Chapter 44). Of the many skin manifestations associated with APL syndrome, livedo reticularis, often accompanied by acrocyanosis, is the most characteristic (Alarcon-Segovia *et al.* 1997; Fisher *et al.* 1960; Ingram *et al.* 1987; Naldi *et al.* 1993; Sammaritano *et al.* 1990; Weinstein *et al.* 1987; Asherson 1992; Hughes 1993; Alegre *et al.* 1989; Bowles 1990; Smith *et al.* 1990; Stephens 1991), and is associated with arterial events (Frances *et al.* 2005). Other cutaneous manifestations include small, non-blanching, erythematous, or cyanotic areas on the hands and feet, as well as hemorrhages, ulcers, and gangrene (Asherson 1992; Hughes 1993; Alegre *et al.* 1989; Bowles 1990; Stephens 1991; Grob *et al.* 1991; Frances *et al.* 2005). Histopathologic examination of the skin occasionally shows inflammation of small vessels (Naldi *et al.* 1993; Grob and Bonerandi 1986; Goldberger *et al.* 1992), but thrombosis is likely the primary event (Dessailloud *et al.* 1998; Fessler 1997; Ingram *et al.* 1987; Bowles 1990; Smith *et al.* 1990; Stephens 1991; Lie 1994; Gertner and Lie 1994; Klein and Pittelkow 1992). The antibodies in this syndrome occasionally induce widespread thrombosis, causing ischemia in single (Dessailloud *et al.* 1998; Gertner 1999; Marie *et al.* 1997; Sneddon 1965) or multiple (Asherson *et al.* 1998) organs. In these instances, angiograms may demonstrate occlusions or narrowing of involved vessels (Roberts *et al.* 1994).

A pentad of microangiopathic hemolytic anemia, thrombocytopenic purpura, neurologic abnormalities, renal dysfunction, and fever is characteristic of thrombotic thrombocytopenic purpura (Fox *et al.* 1986; Jain *et al.* 1994). Histopathologic examination of tissues such as gingiva or kidney shows hyaline thrombi, microaneurysm formation, and endothelial cell proliferation in small arteries and arterioles (Orbison 1952; Fox *et al.* 1986; Jain *et al.* 1994). Similar changes occur when injury to vascular endothelium induces disseminated intravascular coagulation (Gilbert and Scalzi 1993).

Sickle cell anemia occasionally gives rise to vascular narrowing (Liebeskind *et al.* 1973; Calabrese *et al.* 1992). Thrombocythemia can cause digital gangrene and livedo reticularis without demonstrable arterial disease (Singh and Wetherley-Mein 1977).

Thromboembolism
Thromboembolism, by occluding multiple arterial beds, can create the clinical picture of vasculitis (Sprabery *et al.* 1994). The embolic material ordinarily comes from the heart (*in situ* thrombi, marantic valvular lesions) or a large artery (Halasz and Strauss 1998), but venous thrombi occasionally embolize paradoxically through a patent foramen ovale (Karl 1975). Rarely, the emboli consist of air, fat, or neoplastic tissue (Lee and Hodes 1967).

In addition to vasculitis, embolic disease is one of the many causes of "blue toe syndrome" (the sudden onset of discrete painful, blue or purple discolorations on the foot or toes). Other conditions associated with this phenomenon include *de novo* thrombi, various infections, cyanotic heart disease, hyperviscosity, calciphylaxis, and pheochromocytoma (Abdelmalek and Spittell 1995; Federman *et al.* 1994; Nevelsteen *et al.* 1992; O'Keeffe *et al.* 1992).

Abnormal proteins

Materials other than atheromatous or thrombotic debris can occlude vessels and simulate vasculitis. Temperature may play an important role in this process–cryoglobulins and cryofibrinogens precipitate in cold temperature and occlude blood vessels (Korst and Kratochvil 1955; Waxman and Dove 1969), causing cutaneous ulcerations and acral purpura (Selzer *et al.* 1972; Sack 1993; Stoane *et al.* 1966; Schwarz *et al.* 1972). Cryofibrinogens occur most commonly in patients with neoplasia or diabetes mellitus (Kirsner *et al.* 1993; Smith and Arkin 1972). The characteristic histopathologic feature is eosinophilic thrombi in dermal vessels associated with minimal signs of inflammation (Beightler *et al.* 1991; Burruss *et al.* 1994). Rarely, whole immunoglobulins or light chains can form occlusive crystals at cool temperatures giving rise to polyarthralgia, palpable purpura, necrotic cutaneous ulcers, nerve palsies, or combinations thereof (von Bonsdorff *et al.* 1938; Grossman *et al.* 1972; Dotten *et al.* 1976; Stone *et al.* 1989).

Non-cryoprecipitable paraproteins, such as those occurring in multiple myeloma, may cause an occlusive vasculopathy (Dornan *et al.* 1985). A similar vasculopathy also appears in a condition termed POEMS (polyneuropathy, organomegaly, endocrinopathy, M protein, and skin changes) (Lesprit 1996; Trentham *et al.* 1976; Bardwick *et al.* 1980; Viard *et al.* 1988; Manning *et al.* 1992; Soubrier *et al.* 1994). The cardinal feature of POEMS is severe, progressive sensorimotor polyneuropathy. Other common findings are plasma cell dyscrasia, in association with osteosclerotic bone lesions, production of an M protein, hepatosplenomegaly, lymphadenopathy, thickening and hyperpigmentation of the skin, and endocrine dysfunction (diabetes mellitus, hypothyroidism, adrenal insufficiency, amenorrhea, gynecomastia, or impotence).

Neoplasia

Cardiac myxoma

Clinical manifestations

Myxomas comprise over 50% of cardiac neoplasms. They usually are pedunculated and typically occur in the left atrium (Markel *et al.* 1987; Tazelaar *et al.* 1992), most often attached to the septum near the fossa ovalis (Reynen 1995; Markel *et al.* 1987; Greenwood 1968). Occasionally, these tumors appear in the right atrium, and about 5% involve the ventricles (Markel *et al.* 1987). Rarely, they attach to a cardiac valve or to the chordae tendinae (Markel *et al.* 1987). Cardiac myxomas usually affect patients between the ages of 30 and 60 years, are uncommon in blacks (Markel *et al.* 1987), and are sometimes familial (Siltanen *et al.* 1976; Liebler *et al.* 1976).

Myxomas characteristically cause systemic, obstructive, and embolic symptoms (Reynen 1995; Greenwood 1968; Markel *et al.* 1987; Goodwin 1963; Nasser *et al.* 1972; St. John Sutton *et al.* 1980). Some patients have fever, weight loss, arthralgias, myalgias, or Raynaud's phenomenon (Greenwood 1968; Reynen 1995; Thomas 1981; Wold and Lie 1980; Markel *et al.* 1987; Goodwin 1963; Nasser *et al.* 1972; St. John Sutton *et al.* 1980; MacGregor and Cullen 1959; Fitzpatrick *et al.* 1986; Cohen *et al.* 1963; Kaminsky *et al.* 1979; Boussen *et al.* 1991). In addition, a skin rash may appear that ranges from erythematous (or livedoid) macules or papules, to frank ulcerations or telangiectasias (Reynen 1995; Navarro *et al.* 1995; Gravallese 1995; Huston *et al.* 1978; Byrd *et al.* 1980; Bridges and Hector 1989). Clubbing may also occur (Reynen 1995; Greenwood 1968). Obstruction of the mitral valve can cause shortness of breath (which may improve on recumbency), fatigue, weakness, or syncope (Reynen 1995; Markel *et al.* 1987; Goodwin 1963; Nasser *et al.* 1972; St. John Sutton *et al.* 1980; MacGregor and Cullen 1959; Cohen *et al.* 1963; Harvey 1968; Symbas *et al.* 1971; Selzer *et al.* 1972; Peters *et al.* 1974). New-onset congestive heart failure, chest pain, and episodic pulmonary edema are the most common cardiac-related symptoms (Bulkley and Hutchins 1979). When shortness of breath improves in the supine position or when syncope occurs during reclining, atrial myxoma merits strong consideration (Markel *et al.* 1987).

One-quarter to one half of patients with atrial myxoma will have one or more embolic events (Greenwood 1968; Reynen 1995; Wold and Lie 1980; Bulkley and Hutchins 1979; Goodwin 1963; St. John Sutton *et al.* 1980), 50% of which affect the central nervous system (Schmidley 1993; Markel *et al.* 1987) causing focal abnormalities (New *et al.* 1970; Stoane *et al.* 1966; Schwarz *et al.* 1972; Yufe *et al.* 1976). Peripheral emboli may cause mononeuropathy multiplex, simulating vasculitis (Byrd *et al.* 1980). Right-sided myxomatous emboli often produce symptoms and signs of pulmonary thromboembolism, leading in some instances to pulmonary hypertension (Heath and Mackinnon 1964; Wold and Lie 1980; Markel *et al.* 1987; Goodwin 1963). The manifestations occasionally simulate those of constrictive pericarditis (Reynen 1995). Rarely, atrial myxomas occur in conjunction with spotty skin pigmentation and tumors of other organs – the so-called Carney complex (Carney *et al.* 1985; Edwards *et al.* 2003).

Clinical findings on cardiac examination may be normal (Bulkley and Hutchins 1979; Byrd *et al.* 1980). Some patients, however, have an accentuated first heart sound, an increased pulmonic component of the second heart sound, and a diastolic rumble suggesting mitral stenosis (Greenwood 1968; Markel *et al.* 1987; Goodwin 1963; St. John Sutton *et al.* 1980; Harvey 1968; Selzer *et al.* 1972). In those cases, however, atrial fibrillation and enlargement of the left atrium are unusual (Markel *et al.* 1987). A unique, but infrequent finding is a low-frequency tumor plop heard 0.08 to 0.15 seconds after the second heart sound; it is mistaken at times for an S3 or opening snap (Greenwood 1968; Markel *et al.* 1987; St. John Sutton *et al.* 1980; Harvey 1968). Rarely, a to-and-fro cardiac rub with a crunching quality may appear (Greenwood 1968). Right-sided myxomas can produce murmurs of tricuspid stenosis or regurgitation, jugular venous distension, hepatomegaly, edema, or ascites (Markel *et al.* 1987). Ventricular myxomas can cause signs of ventricular outflow obstruction (Markel *et al.* 1987; Wold and Lie 1980).

Pathogenesis

Cardiac myxomas are single (occasionally multiple), pedunculated, friable masses ranging in diameter from a few millimeters to greater than 10 cm (Wold and Lie 1980; Markel *et al.* 1987). Microscopic examination shows a paucicellular collection of polygonal and stellate cells in an amorphous mucopolysaccharide matrix with variable vascularity (Markel *et al.* 1987; Tazelaar *et al.* 1992). The cells contain few mitotic figures, but the fact that myxomas sometimes recur locally or in peripheral sites confirms their neoplastic nature (New *et al.* 1970; Heath and Mackinnon 1964; Price *et al.* 1970; Read *et al.* 1974). On immunohistochemical and ultrastructural study, myxoma cells may show endothelial, epithelial, smooth muscle, and fibroblastic features, suggesting a multipotential, mesenchymal cell origin (Reynen 1995; Landon *et al.* 1986; Goldman *et al.* 1987).

The location of these pedunculated tumors explains their ability to obstruct flow across the atrioventricular valve. The rarer sessile, relatively immobile, tumors cause valvular obstruction only when quite large (Markel *et al.* 1987). Atrial myxomas also may fragment and embolize to peripheral vascular beds or produce cytokines such as interleukin-6 (IL-6), a potent B-lymphocyte and hepatocyte-stimulating factor (Gravallese 1995; Reynen 1995; Hirano *et al.* 1987; Jourdan *et al.* 1990). A thrombus overlying the myxoma (Markel *et al.* 1987) or infection within the tumor (Revankar and Clark 1998; Rogers *et al.* 1978; Graham *et al.* 1976; Rajpal *et al.* 1979) can alter the clinical presentation.

Recent genetic studies of the Carney complex have disclosed a mutation of the R1α regulatory subunit of protein kinase A (Casey *et al.* 2000). A variant of the Carney complex occurs with trismus-pseudocamptodactyly syndrome, and is seen in association with a missense mutation in the perinatal myosin heavy-chain gene (Veugelers *et al.* 2004).

Laboratory evaluation

Echocardiography confirms a mass in virtually 100% of the cases (Markel *et al.* 1987; Rajpal *et al.* 1979). A two-dimensional echocardiogram shows not only its size, shape, and location, but also estimates its mobility (Markel *et al.* 1987; DePace *et al.* 1981; Alam and Sun 1991). Computed tomography (CT) and magnetic resonance imaging (MRI) can detect myxomas 0.5 cm or greater in diameter (Reynen 1995).

Embolic fragments of myxoma are sometimes detectable in tissue specimens (Greenwood 1968; Markel *et al.* 1987; Boussen *et al.* 1991), but occasionally one sees only "vasculitis" (Leonhardt and Kullenberg 1977). The angiographic findings of myxomatous emboli (vascular irregularities, dilatations, or aneurysms) (Thomas 1981; New *et al.* 1970; Markel *et al.* 1987; Boussen *et al.* 1991; Stoane *et al.* 1966; Schwarz *et al.* 1972; Leonhardt and Kullenberg 1977) may contribute to diagnostic confusion.

The common findings of anemia, leukocytosis, thrombocytopenia, hypocomplementemia, elevated ESR, acute phase reactants, and serum autoantibodies (Gravallese 1995; Reynen 1995; Greenwood 1968; Wold and Lie 1980; St. John Sutton *et al.* 1980; MacGregor and Cullen 1959; Byrd *et al.* 1980; Selzer *et al.* 1972; Goodwin 1968; Savige *et al.* 1988) likely result from the immune-stimulating properties of myxomas, for example the production of IL-6. For unclear reasons, polycythemia may accompany right atrial myxomas (Greenwood 1968; Wold and Lie 1980; Markel *et al.* 1987; St. John Sutton *et al.* 1980). An infected tumor may yield positive blood cultures and lead to an erroneous diagnosis of infective endocarditis (Revankar and Clark 1998; Rajpal *et al.* 1979).

Treatment

Improved methods of detection and better surgical techniques have increased survival substantially (Reynen 1995; Greenwood 1968; Markel *et al.* 1987; Bulkley and Hutchins 1979; Nasser *et al.* 1972; St. John Sutton *et al.* 1980; Peters *et al.* 1974; Richardson *et al.* 1979). Because the tumor is occasionally multicentric, direct visualization of all four cardiac chambers is important (Markel *et al.* 1987). Full thickness excision of the tumor at the base of its pedicle is usually curative. The operative mortality varies from 0 to 2.7%, and the recurrence rate varies from 0 to 14% (Reynen 1995; Markel *et al.* 1987; St. John Sutton *et al.* 1980; Peters *et al.* 1974; Richardson *et al.* 1979). Most recurrences are local and occur within the first or second year postoperatively. In some cases, however, the interval is longer (Desousa *et al.* 1978; Markel *et al.* 1987; St. John Sutton *et al.* 1980; Markel *et al.* 1986). Myxomas may also recur at extracardiac sites (Desousa *et al.* 1978; Markel *et al.* 1986), presumably from slow growth of the embolic tissue.

Other neoplasms

Neoplasms can injure blood vessels by: inducing immune-mediated inflammation (Fortin 1996; Hasler 1995; O'Donnell *et al.* 1980; Farcet *et al.* 1987; Tolosa-Vilella *et al.* 1990; Burnham 1972); occluding the vessel via embolization of tumor particles (Mertz and Conn 1992; Greenwood 1968; Markel *et al.* 1987; Boussen *et al.* 1991; Sheibani *et al.* 1986; Primka *et al.* 1993); inducing a hypercoagulable state (Taylor 1987; Mertz and Conn 1992; O'Keeffe *et al.* 1992; Nachman and Silverstein 1993; Fengler *et al.* 1990); producing an abnormal protein (Mertz and Conn 1992; Stone *et al.* 1989; Dornan *et al.* 1985; Kois *et al.* 1991); or by directly invading the vessel wall (Kanno 1987; Gabriel *et al.* 1986; Webster *et al.* 1986; Thomas *et al.* 1994; Leeds and Rosenblatt 1972; Liebeskind *et al.* 1973; Leeds *et al.* 1971; Lin and Siew 1971; Garces and Gosink 1972; Krieger *et al.* 1982). Furthermore, tumors sometimes invade the microscopic nerves supplying the vessel (O'Connor 1884) and in some instances the tumor involves major nerves *per se*, creating the picture of mononeuritis multiplex (Jones and Edgar 1995), thereby simulating vasculitis. Pheochromocytoma, perhaps by releasing catecholamines, can generate ischemic lesions and angiographic findings typical of vasculitis (Armstrong and Hayes 1961; McColl and Fraser 1995).

Angiotropic lymphomas and the related condition, lymphomatoid granulomatosis, can also imitate vasculitis (Glass 1993; Kleinschmidt-DeMasters 1992; Walker 1994; Roux 1995; Thomas *et al.* 1994; Anders *et al.* 1989; Lipford *et al.* 1988; Wu *et al.* 2005). Malignant angioendotheliomatosis, once considered a neoplasm of vascular endothelial cell origin (Petito *et al.* 1978; Braverman and Lerner 1961), is probably an angiotropic lymphoma (Fredericks 1991b; DiGiuseppe 1994; Sienknecht 1995; Bhawan *et al.* 1985; Sheibani *et al.* 1986; Kao *et al.* 1992; Otrakji *et al.* 1988; Petroff *et al.* 1989; Wick *et al.* 1986) with a predilection for vessels of the central nervous system (Lie 1992a; Kamesaki *et al.* 1990). Primary vascular sarcomas may obstruct vessels or embolize distally (Mason *et al.* 1982); occasionally they induce aneurysms (O'Donnell and O'Connell 1993).

External injury

The vascular narrowing seen on cerebral angiograms after severe head trauma could result from pathogenic mechanisms similar to those of the hypothenar hammer syndrome. In cases of head trauma, however, cerebral vasospasm consequent to intracranial hemorrhage may be an additional factor (Suwanwela and Suwanwela 1972). Trauma to the carotid artery can mimic cerebral vasculitis by causing dissection of the vessel wall (Nance 1997; Lanczik *et al.* 2003) or formation of a thrombus that embolizes distally (Thomas and Lowitt 1995). Likewise, if atlantoaxial subluxation causes injury to the vertebral arteries, multiple cerebellar infarctions may ensue (Shim 1998).

Exposure to cold

Prolonged exposure to non-freezing cold, particularly when the humidity is high, can cause the condition known as pernio, or chilblains (Herman *et al.* 1981; Jacob *et al.* 1986; Page and Shear 1988).

In the acute, self-limited form of this disorder, pruritic or painful purplish swellings appear on the extremities (or rarely the face) about 24 hours after the exposure. Tender blue nodules, and occasionally ulcerations, follow and persist for 10–14 days (Herman *et al.* 1981). Some patients acquire a chronic form of pernio in which the characteristic lesions recur during winter months. In such cases, the ulcerations are slow to heal and may leave scarring or postinflammatory pigmentation (Herman *et al.* 1981). Middle-aged women seem especially vulnerable (Herman *et al.* 1981; Jacob *et al.* 1986), perhaps because of hyper-reactivity of their arterial circulation to cold, or because of diminished temperature in the skin overlying a relatively thick layer of subcutaneous fat (Jacob *et al.* 1986; Page and Shear 1988). Other possible predisposing factors include systemic illness, nutritional deficiencies, neuromuscular dysfunction, and genetic traits (Millard and Rowell 1978; Herman *et al.* 1981; Thomas 1964; Kelly and Dowling 1985).

Histopathologic examination of cutaneous lesions demonstrates non-specific inflammation and edema in the papillary dermis along with perivascular mononuclear cell infiltration around dermal arterioles (Herman *et al.* 1981; Page and Shear 1988; Wall and Smith 1981). Proliferation of the vessel intima (Page and Shear 1988), deposition of fibrin, and a true lymphocytic vasculitis (Herman *et al.* 1981) are occasional findings. Angiography of an affected extremity may show vascular occlusions and aneurysms (Jacob *et al.* 1986).

Protection from cold is the *sine qua non* of treating pernio (Jacob *et al.* 1986; Page and Shear 1988). Additionally, a weight loss program could reduce the insulating layer of subcutaneous fat and thereby raise skin temperature (Page and Shear 1988). Use of calcium channel blockers is sometimes successful (Dowd *et al.* 1986) and glucocorticoid creams can decrease itching (Ganor 1983).

Polyvinyl chloride

Exposure to polyvinyl chloride tubing during hemodialysis can cause a necrotizing dermatitis. Histopathologic examination shows thrombosis of vessels in the corium, fibrin deposits in the walls of arterioles, and inflammatory infiltrates without leukocytoclasis. Precipitates of IgG and complement occur in small vessels, but serum levels of immunoglobulin and complement are normal. When polyurethane is substituted for polyvinyl chloride, the rash does not occur (Bommer *et al.* 1979).

Radiation

External radiation can injure vascular endothelial cells within hours (Fonkalsrud *et al.* 1977; Page and Shear 1988). There may be subsequent thickening and irregularity of the intima as well as focal fibrosis and necrosis of the media. Exposure to 3600 to 6800 rads (McCready *et al.* 1983) can cause rupture or occlusion of an artery within several weeks or after many years (Lie 1992b; McCready *et al.* 1983) (Figure 45.2).

Hypothenar hammer syndrome

The "hypothenar hammer syndrome" exemplifies how external trauma can affect a blood vessel (Masuzawa *et al.* 1983; Savader *et al.* 1988; Pineda *et al.* 1985; Laroche 1976; Vayssairat *et al.* 1987; Wernick and Smith 1989). The typical history is one of hitting or pushing a hard surface with the hypothenar aspect of the hand. This circumstance conjures up the picture of a blacksmith – the patient's hand is the "hammer", the hook of the hamate bone is the

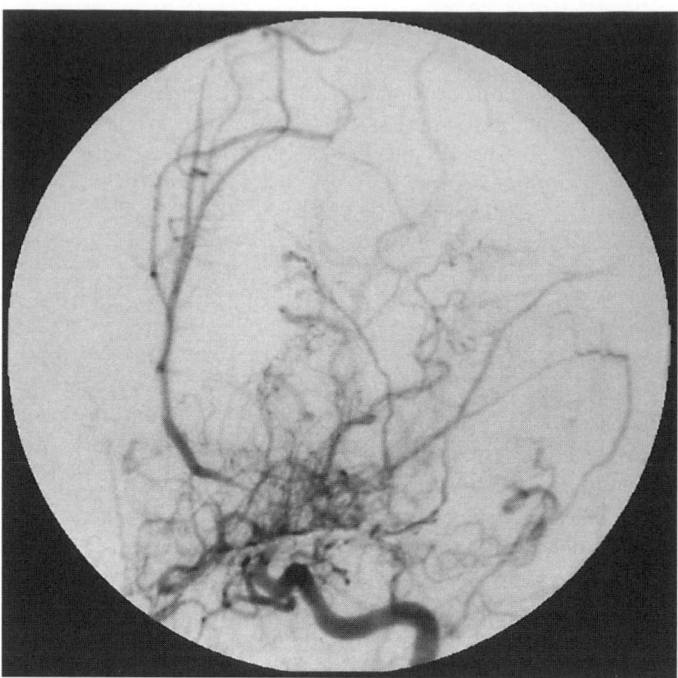

Figure 45.2 Radiation-induced vasculopathy – total occlusion of the middle cerebral artery and marked narrowing of the anterior cerebral artery in a young girl 3 years status post radiation therapy.

"anvil", and the unprotected superficial palmar branch of the ulnar artery is the "horseshoe". Intermittent lancinating pain ensues, followed by a dull ache over the hypothenar eminence. The subsequent ischemic symptoms often lead to a diagnosis of Raynaud's phenomenon, but careful questioning reveals that neither a triphasic color change nor involvement of the thumb occurs (Pineda *et al.* 1985). An angiogram will show an irregularity, an aneurysm, or an occlusion of the ulnar artery, sometimes in association with occlusion of the more distal arteries (Sack 1993; Savader *et al.* 1988; Pineda *et al.* 1985; Vayssairat *et al.* 1987) (see Figure 18.17 in Chapter 18). Histopathologic examination often demonstrates thrombosis on the intimal surface and fibrosis in the media of the affected vessels (Vayssairat *et al.* 1987). Trauma to the radial artery can cause a "thenar hammer syndrome", with digital cyanosis and splinter hemorrhages (White and Parke 2005).

Internal injury

Hypertension can be considered a form of internal vascular "trauma". Acute elevations of blood pressure may produce angiographic findings of vasoconstriction and dilatation of cerebral vessels (Garner *et al.* 1990). Segmental narrowing of these vessels may also occur in the postpartum period (Call *et al.* 1988; Bogousslavsky *et al.* 1989) as well as before, during, or after episodes of migraine (Masuzawa *et al.* 1983; Dukes and Vieth 1964; Ekbom and Greitz 1970; Serdaru *et al.* 1984; Call *et al.* 1988; Bogousslavsky *et al.* 1989). Dissections of extracranial and intracranial arteries, and occasionally of visceral arteries, may induce long foci of arterial narrowing on angiogram. This finding can prompt an erroneous diagnosis of arteritis (Caplan and Louis 1996). Obstruction of vasa vasorum by any mechanism can produce ischemic necrosis of an arterial wall. Mycotic aneurysms may form by such a process (Olmsted and McGee 1977).

Biochemical abnormalities

Amyloid

Amyloid angiopathy can appear as an isolated phenomenon in the central nervous system (Silbert 1995; Okazaki *et al.* 1989; Vanley *et al.* 1981; Gilbert and Vinters 1983; Mandybur 1986) or as part of systemic amyloidosis with an associated paraprotein (Breathnach and Wells 1980; Jennette *et al.* 1982). Its clinical features include progressive dementia, multiple cerebral infarctions, and signs suggesting temporal arteritis (Silbert 1995; Okazaki *et al.* 1989; Vanley *et al.* 1981; Gilbert and Vinters 1983; Mandybur 1986; Salvarani *et al.* 1994; Gertz *et al.* 1986; Rao and Allen 1993; Churchill *et al.* 2003). Moreover, when intracerebral hemorrhage accompanies dementia, amyloid cerebrovascular disease is a leading diagnostic consideration (Gilbert and Vinters 1983). Amyloid can also affect peripheral vessels and produce ischemic organ damage or purpura (Breathnach and Wells 1980; Jennette *et al.* 1982; Auethavekiat *et al.* 2004). Unexplained renal failure or hematuria, with or without proteinuria, sometimes heralds amyloidosis (Friman and Pettersson 1996). Angiography may show vascular narrowing or occlusion (Gertz *et al.* 1986; Auethavekiat *et al.* 2004). Histologic evaluation of affected vessels demonstrates infiltration with amyloid, accompanied at times by obliterative intimal changes, aneurysm formation, perivascular or transmural inflammatory infiltrates, and fibrinoid necrosis (Okazaki *et al.* 1989; Mandybur 1986; Breathnach and Wells 1980; Jennette *et al.* 1982).

α1-antitrypsin deficiency

α1-antitrypsin, the most abundant proteinase inhibitor in human plasma, plays a major role in protecting tissues (including blood vessels) from endogenous toxins (Cox 1994). A deficiency in this inhibitor reportedly increases the incidence of fibromuscular dysplasia (Schievink *et al.* 1994a), intracranial aneurysm (Schievink *et al.* 1994b), spontaneous dissection of cervical or peripheral arteries (Cattan *et al.* 1994), panniculitis (Schievink *et al.* 1994b), and vasculitis (Esnault *et al.* 1993). Some of these associations, however, remain unproven.

Calciphylaxis

In 1962, Selye showed that tissues could be rendered sensitive to calcification and termed this phenomenon calciphylaxis (Seyle 1962). In this model, vascular calcification did not occur, yet the calcific vasculopathy of renal failure has been termed calciphylaxis. Such arteriopathy typically occurs in patients with a high calcium phosphate product (Roe *et al.* 1994; Conn *et al.* 1973; Gipstein *et al.* 1976). Female gender and obesity may also be risk factors (Fine and Zacharias 2002; Janigan *et al.* 2000; Ahmed *et al.* 2001; Mazhar *et al.* 2001). Affected patients typically develop a livedo reticularis-like rash that becomes plaque-like, nodular, or bullous, and may progress to necrosis with ulceration. Infarction of major organs is rare (Adrogue *et al.* 1981). Parathyroidectomy (Blumberg and Weidmann 1977; Angelis *et al.* 1997) and hyperbaric oxygen (Vassa *et al.* 1994) may provide benefit, but the clinical course is often downhill (Roe *et al.* 1994).

Anderson–Fabry disease (angiokeratoma corporis diffusum)

Anderson-Fabry disease is unique among the sphingolipid storage diseases in that it is X-linked recessive and may cause symptoms in female carriers (Serdaru *et al.* 1984; Gupta *et al.* 2005; Rolfs *et al.* 2005). A deficiency in the lysosomal enzyme, α-galactosidase A,

results in widespread deposition of uncleaved glycosphingolipids, primarily trihexosylceramide (Anonymous 1990; Meschia *et al.* 2005). The characteristic skin manifestations are angiokeratomas (Figure 45.3), red-purple papules that blanch on pressure if not thrombosed. These lesions typically appear in a "bathing suit" distribution (genitalia, buttocks, and lower abdomen) during childhood or adolescence. Occasionally, they occur on the elbows, thighs, fingers, lips, and mucous membranes (Sack 1993; Serdaru *et al.* 1984; Anonymous 1990).

In adult men, virtually any organ system can be involved. As a consequence, the clinical findings vary considerably. A painful autonomic neuropathy frequently occurs early, manifesting as burning paresthesias, which may intensify with exertion or fever, and be accompanied by hypohidrosis (Desnick *et al.* 1989; Serdaru *et al.* 1984). Abnormalities of thermal sensation, especially cold sensitivity, are common, even in otherwise asymptomatic carriers (Morgan *et al.* 1990). A characteristic finding on slit-lamp examination of the cornea is a whorl-like lesion similar to that occasionally seen after use of phenothiazines, chloroquine, or indomethacin, which can be seen in asymptomatic carriers (Meschia *et al.* 2005). Additional ocular findings are cataracts, corneal opacities, and

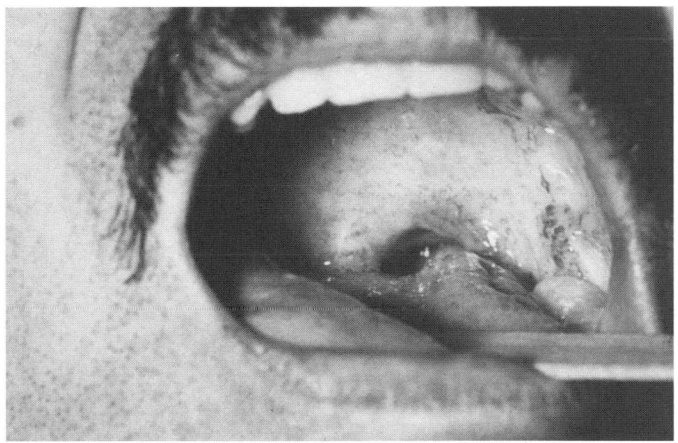

(a)

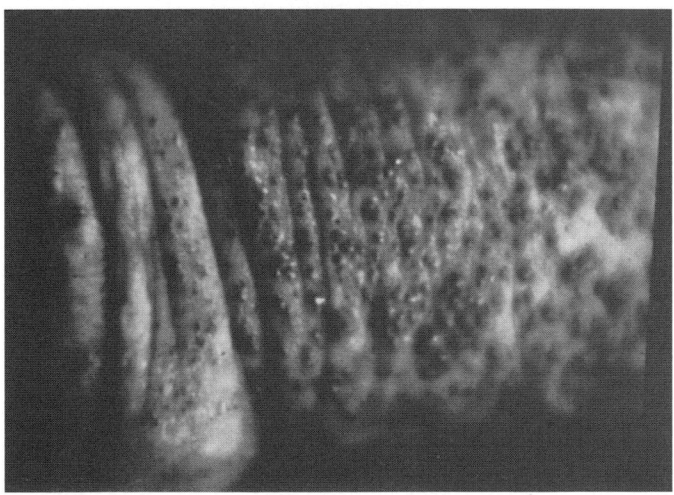

(b)

Figure 45.3 Angiokeratomas in the mouth (a) and on the penis (b) of a young man with Anderson–Fabry disease. (See Color Plate 125).

aneurysmal dilatations of conjunctival and retinal vessels (Klein 1986). Other manifestations of this disorder include: cerebrovascular occlusions (Serdaru *et al.* 1984); myocardial or cardiac valvular dysfunction (Nakao *et al.* 1995; Becker *et al.* 1975; Fisher *et al.* 1992); obstructive airway disease (Rosenberg *et al.* 1980); non-destructive arthropathy (Sheth and Bernhard 1979); ischemic necrosis of bone (Ross *et al.* 1993); bowel dysfunction (Rowe *et al.* 1974); vertigo; sensorineural hearing loss; and lymphadenopathy.

Affected men can be diagnosed by measuring α-galactosidase activity in plasma; affected women have low to normal levels of α-galactosidase activity and require genetic diagnosis (Meschia *et al.* 2005). Elevated serum levels of ceramide trihexoside help confirm the diagnosis (Serdaru *et al.* 1984). On biopsy, an angiokeratoma typically shows ectatic cutaneous capillaries protruding into a hyperkeratotic epidermis. Similar lesions, however, may appear in other inherited lysosomal disorders (Rodriguez-Serna *et al.* 1996; Kanzaki *et al.* 1993).

Treatment is largely symptomatic. Without dialysis, most patients succumb to renal failure by age 50 (Anonymous 1990). Renal transplantation, although occasionally of temporary benefit (Mosnier *et al.* 1991), does not appear to supply enough of the missing enzyme to stop progression of the disease. Enzyme replacement with human α-galactosidase A shows promise in reducing accumulated ceramide trihexose and in improving organ function and quality of life. The cost of such therapy, however, is prohibitive (Desnick *et al.* 2003; Schiffmann *et al.* 2001; Eng *et al.* 2001; Gahl 2001; Meschia *et al.* 2005).

Homocystinuria

Homocysteine can injure vascular endothelium, potentiate the oxidation of low-density lipoprotein cholesterol, and promote thrombosis (Stein and McBride 1998; Welch and Loscalzo 1998; Chambers *et al.* 1998; Clarke *et al.* 1991; Robinson *et al.* 1994). Patients who are homozygous for deficiency of cystathionine β-synthase have hyperhomocysteinemia (and homocystinuria) and are thereby susceptible to premature atherosclerosis and thromboembolism (Robinson *et al.* 1994). Heterozygote patients (approximately 1–2% of the population) have milder elevations of homocysteine levels but are also predisposed to occlusive vascular disease (Fassbender *et al.* 1999; Graham *et al.* 1997; Welch and Loscalzo 1998; Clarke *et al.* 1991; Boers *et al.* 1985; Selhub *et al.* 1995). Potential treatments include pyridoxine, folate, and vitamin B_{12} supplementation, as well as a diet low in methionine (Meschia *et al.* 2005). When low serum levels of folate accompany hyperhomocysteinemia, supplementation of this vitamin can decrease serum homocysteine levels and could conceivably ameliorate the associated vasculopathy (Stein and McBride 1998; Selhub *et al.* 1995; Stampfer and Malinow 1995). Patients with homocystinuria and a history of ischemic stroke should be placed on antiplatelet therapy (Meschia *et al.* 2005).

Hyperoxaluria

Hyperoxaluria is an autosomal recessive disorder that causes accumulation of oxalic acid, an endproduct of glycine metabolism (Baethge *et al.* 1988). Patients with this condition typically have a history of nephrocalcinosis, often beginning before age 5 (Kuiper 1996; Baethge *et al.* 1988; Blackburn *et al.* 1975). Renal failure may eventually ensue, after which calcium oxalate deposits in extrarenal tissues such as heart, skin, bone, joints, blood vessels, and eyes.

Oxalate crystals may also accumulate in the media of the vessel wall or physically occlude small vessels (Baethge *et al.* 1988; Blackburn *et al.* 1975). In addition, calcium oxalate activates complement and thus may trigger neutrophil-mediated injury of endothelial cells (Boogaerts *et al.* 1983). Thus, vascular complications are common (Kuiper 1996; Baethge *et al.* 1988; Blackburn *et al.* 1975), consisting of acrocyanosis, Raynaud's phenomenon, livedo reticularis, decreased pulses, and peripheral gangrene.

Finding an increased 24-hour urinary total oxalate excretion establishes the diagnosis of hyperoxaluria; biopsy of affected tissues reveals the vascular oxalate deposits (Kuiper 1996; Baethge *et al.* 1988). With the onset of renal failure, serum oxalate levels are difficult to interpret (Baethge *et al.* 1988). Consequently, distinguishing primary from secondary forms of oxalosis may require specific enzyme assays. Although oxalate is readily dialyzable, hemodialysis and peritoneal dialysis cannot keep up with its synthesis. Thus, most effective approaches for preserving renal function enhance oxalate solubility in the urine (phosphate, magnesium oxide, or citrate supplementation) or decrease its production (high doses of pyridoxine) (MacConnell and Ferro 1995; Milliner *et al.* 1994). Combined liver and renal transplantation offer the possibility of reversing the underlying metabolic defect (Bastani and Nahass 1999).

Infection

Direct infection of vessel walls, as well as infection-initiated immunologic or toxic processes, can compromise vascular integrity and simulate vasculitis (Sundy and Haynes 1995; Somer and Finegold 1995; Lie 1996; Mandel and Calabrese 1998). An array of organisms of various types may be the culprits (Table 45.3). The clinical manifestations range from non-specific systemic complaints and a variety of skin lesions to infarction of major organs. In addition, changes of "vasculitis" on cerebral angiograms may actually stem from: bacterial endocarditis (Leeds and Goldberg 1971); viral infection (Lie 1996; Victor and Green 1976); mycobacterial infection (Clarke *et al.* 2005); basilar meningitis secondary to bacteria, mycobacteria, fungi, or spirochetes (Ferris *et al.* 1968; Liebeskind *et al.* 1973; Leeds *et al.* 1971; Greitz 1964; Lehrer 1966; Wickbom and Davidson 1967; el Gammal 1969; Thomas and Hopkins 1972; Vatz *et al.* 1974; Tjia *et al.* 1985; Veenendaal-Hilbers *et al.* 1988; Wheat *et al.* 1990; Williams *et al.* 1992); or brain abscess. An example of Salmonella aortitis is shown in Figure 18.12 in Chapter 18.

Some infections cause cutaneous papules, nodules, and ulcers by non-vascular mechanisms. An example is the granulomatous panniculitis (erythema induratum) induced by *Mycobacterium tuberculosis* (Baselga 1997; Lebel and Lassonde 1986; Rademaker *et al.* 1989; Ollert *et al.* 1993). Infections with organisms such as *Strongyloides stercoralis* (Wachter *et al.* 1984; Reiman *et al.* 2002), trichinella (Frayha 1981), acanthamoeba (Murakawa 1995; Chandrasekar 1997; Slater *et al.* 1994), HIV (Roh and Gertner 1997; Lie 1996; Lipton and Ma 1996; Mandel and Calabrese 1998; Marks and Kuskov 1995; Simpson and Tagliati 1994), *Pythium insidiosum* (Prasertwitayakij *et al.* 2003), and rabies virus can also produce symptoms and signs identical to those of vasculitis. We have observed a patient with myalgias, scalp tenderness, jaw pain, and a markedly elevated ESR in whom the initial diagnosis of "giant cell arteritis" changed to orbital cellulitis when orbital swelling, proptosis, and gaze paralysis subsequently appeared.

Table 45.3 Infectious organisms, diseases, or syndromes associated with vasculitis

Organism, diseases, or syndrome	Reference(s)
Bacterial	
Neisseria gonorrhea	Mastrolonardo *et al.* 1994
Neisseria meningitides	Bitzer *et al.* 2003
Burkholderia pseudomallei (melioidosis)	Torrens *et al.* 1999
Fungal	Benedict 1992
Histoplasmosis	Rogers *et al.* 1978; Stone 1998
Aspergillus	Woods and Goldsmith 1990; Ledesma and Pearce 2000
Fusarium **species**	Nelson 1994
Sporotrichosis	Byrd 1998
Cryptococcus	Aberfeld and Gladstone 1967
Mycobacterial	
Mycobacterium tuberculosis	Baselga 1997; Blanco 1999; Clarke *et al.* 2005
Viral	
HIV/AIDS	Pumarola-Sune 1987; Gruber 1997; Calabrese 1991; Berger 1990; Mizusawa 1988; Marks and Kuskov 1995; Joshi 1987; Yankner 1986
Varicella-zoster virus	Morgello 1988; Erhard 1995; Linnemann and Alvira 1980; Gray 1994
Epstein–Barr virus	Murakami 1998
Rubella	Esterly and Oppenheimer 1967
Parvovirus B19	Finkel *et al.* 1994
Spirochetal/Rickettsial	
Neurosyphilis	Peters 1993
Borreliosis/ Lyme disease	Johnston *et al.* 1985; May and Jabbari 1990; Fontana 1996; Camponovo and Meier 1986
Rickettsia	Wenzel *et al.* 1986
Parasitic	
Chagas' disease (*Trypanosomiasis americana*)	Oddo 1992
Cysticercosis	Salgado 1997
Strongyloides	Wachter *et al.* 1984; Reiman *et al.* 2002
Visceral larva migrans	Kraus 1995
Toxoplasmosis	Huang and Chou 1988

Congenital and inherited abnormalities

Congenital weakness of an arterial wall may eventually lead to a saccular (Olmsted and McGee 1977) or dissecting (Schievink 1997) aneurysm. Inherited disorders of connective tissue, such as pseudoxanthoma elasticum (Nishida *et al.* 1990; Lebwohl *et al.* 1993; Travers *et al.* 1979) and Ehlers–Danlos syndrome

(Imahori *et al.* 1969), may cause premature vascular disease including aneurysms. Neurofibromatosis, a hamartomatous abnormality of neural crest tissue, can affect the intimal and adventitia of blood vessels, resulting in arterial stenoses or aneurysms (Tomsick *et al.* 1976; DiPrete *et al.* 1990; Finley and Dabbs 1988; Jones *et al.* 1998; Chan 1998; Meyers *et al.* 1974; Najafi 1966; den Butter *et al.* 1988) (see Figure 18.18 in Chapter 18). These abnormalities most commonly involve the renal arteries (DiPrete *et al.* 1990; Finley and Dabbs 1988), but other major vessels may be affected (Tomsick *et al.* 1976; DiPrete *et al.* 1990; Jones *et al.* 1998; Iwai *et al.* 1985; Rybka and Novick 1983; Stokes *et al.* 1996; Chan 1998; Malek *et al.* 1999).

Fibromuscular dysplasia can affect the intima, media, or adventita of vessels, causing stenosis, dilatation, or the formation of aneurysms (Slovut and Olin 2004). The renal arteries are the usual targets, but any artery can be involved (Slovut and Olin 2004). A recently described condition, segmental arterial mediolysis, may be a form of fibromuscular dysplasia (Slavin 1995) (see Figure 18.19 in Chapter 18).

Miscellaneous conditions
Drug effects

Ergot derivatives (Kapoor 1976; Henry *et al.* 1984) and sympathomimetic drugs (Fallis and Fisher 1985; Citron *et al.* 1970; Kalant and Kalant 1975; Matick *et al.* 1983; Lake *et al.* 1990; Sloan *et al.* 1991; Pearlson *et al.* 1993; Tapia and Schumacher 1993; Fredericks 1991a; Kaye and Fainstat 1987), particularly amphetamines and ephedrine (Calabrese and Mallek 1988), can induce vascular abnormalities. The cause of these abnormalities is likely multifactorial. Vasospasm plays a role, as evidenced by the transient segmental arterial constrictions visible on angiograms soon after exposure to the offending agent (Rumbaugh *et al.* 1971a; Kapoor 1976; Henry *et al.* 1984). In some instances, histopathologic studies show true vasculitic lesions (Citron *et al.* 1970; Tapia and Schumacher 1993), and angiograms occasionally show more permanent changes, for example aneurysms (Citron *et al.* 1970; Matick *et al.* 1983). Thus, vasoconstriction may be the initial event, followed by ischemia with resultant inflammation of the vessel wall (Fredericks 1991a; Rumbaugh *et al.* 1971b; Lake *et al.* 1990; Karch and Billingham 1988). Some drugs, on the other hand, can stimulate the release of toxic mediators or induce a coagulopathy (Rumbaugh *et al.* 1971a). Concomitant infection or emboli of drug contaminants occasionally play a role (Rumbaugh *et al.* 1971a; Citron *et al.* 1970) (see Figure 18.13).

Alpha-interferon, a protein with antiviral and antitumor activity, occasionally induces Raynaud's phenomenon or a thrombotic angiopathy (Schapira *et al.* 2002; Zuber *et al.* 2002). Likewise, recombinant human erythropoietin can induce a thrombotic vasculopathy (Gibson *et al.* 2005).

Tumor necrosis factor (TNF) inhibitors can induce vasculitic skin ulcerations, scleritis, mononeuritis (Jarrett *et al.* 2003), leukocytoclastic vasculitis, and proliferative lupus nephritis (Mor *et al.* 2005). These lesions resolve after withdrawal of the agent and treatment with glucocorticoids (Jarrett *et al.* 2003; Mor *et al.* 2005).

Cocaine use can cause a constellation of symptoms similar to Wegener's granulomatosis such as nasal septum destruction, ulcerated skin lesions, crescentic glomeruleronephritis, proteinuria, and positive antiproteinase 3 antibodies (Friedman and Wolfsthal 2005; Rowshani *et al.* 2004).

Female reproductive hormones may exert a toxic effect on the vasculature. Intimal proliferation reportedly occurs in the vessel walls of women who are pregnant, postpartum, or taking oral contraceptives (Irey and Norris 1973). Such changes might also be responsible for the "transient cerebrovascular disease of pregnancy" (Brick 1988).

Moyamoya disease

Moyamoya disease is an occlusive vasculopathy primarily affecting the arteries of the circle of Willis (Ueki *et al.* 1994; Suzuki and Takaku 1969; Takeuchi and Shimizu 1957). Although first recognized in Japan (Takeuchi and Shimizu 1957), it affects virtually all races (Ueki *et al.* 1994). The onset of disease has two peaks, one in the first and the other in the fourth decade of life (Ueki *et al.* 1994; Tzeng *et al.* 2005). Ischemic attacks characterize the childhood form, whereas cerebral hemorrhage predominates in adults. In the early stages, angiograms show stenoses of both carotid arteries at their suprasellar positions. As these arteries progressively narrow, a characteristic network of moyamoya ("hazy puff of smoke") vessels appears (Figure 45.4). These increase in prominence as major trunks of the anterior circle of Willis become occluded. With involvement of all the components (including the posterior cerebral arteries), the moyamoya vessels diminish in size and may completely disappear as collaterals develop from the extracranial circulation (Suzuki and Takaku 1969). Histopathologic examination of stenotic vessels shows fibrotic thickening. Dilated vessels have attenuation of the media and fragmentation of the elastic lamina (Yamashita *et al.* 1983).

Multiple factors may contribute to the pathogenesis of moyamoya disease (Hoshimaru *et al.* 1991; Yamamoto *et al.* 1998; Masuda *et al.* 1993; Tzeng *et al.* 2005). Case reports describe familial occurrences, an increased incidence in Down's syndrome (Ueki *et al.* 1994), and antibodies to Ro (SS-A) and La (SS-B) (Provost *et al.* 1991).

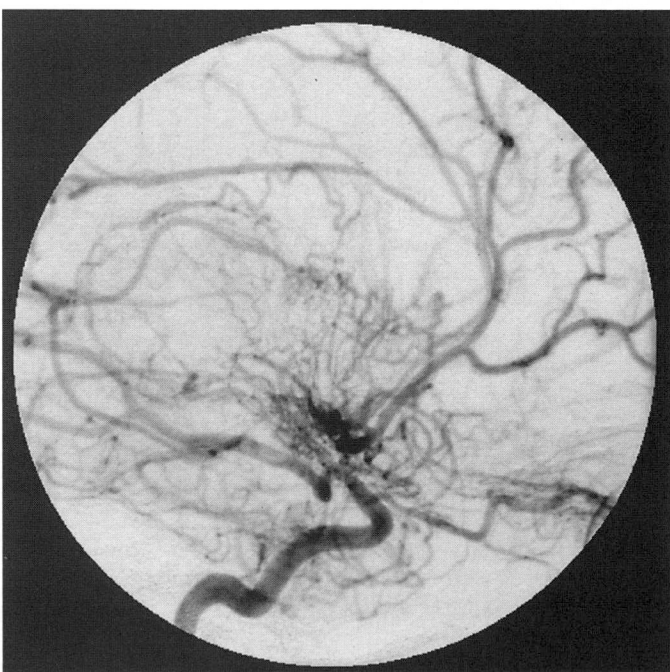

Figure 45.4 Moyamoya – total occlusion of the middle cerebral artery and marked narrowing of the anterior cerebral artery; prominent collateral moyamoya vessels.

This disease typically progresses and has a high mortality rate, especially in adults. Anastomotic surgical procedures may be beneficial (Kinugasa *et al.* 1993; Ueki *et al.* 1994).

A variety of other miscellaneous conditions may imitate vasculitis (Table 45.4).

Non-vascular diseases

Non-vascular diseases of almost any organ can simulate vasculitis (Rosenstein and Kramer 1994). For example, occult subacute thyroiditis can masquerade as giant cell arteritis, and antineutrophil cytoplasmic antibody can accompany inflammatory bowel disease (Stebbing *et al.* 1999) or infectious pulmonary processes (Byrd 1998). Keep in mind also that "imitators" may accompany

Table 45.4 Miscellaneous imitators of vasculitis

Imitator	Clinical features	Vasculitis simulated
Angiolymphoid hyperplasia with eosinophilia	Lymphadenopathy, erythematous papules	Polyarteritis nodosa
Anorexia nervosa	Livedo reticularis	Connective tissue disease
Atrophie blanche	Multifocal cutaneous infarctions of lower extremities	Cutaneous vasculitis
Brain abscess	Temporal headache	Giant cell arteritis
Cerebral autosomal dominant arteriopathy with subcortical infarcts and leukoencephalopathy (CADASIL)	Focal cerebral ischemia and progressive dementia	CNS vasculitis
Cerebral segmental vasoconstriction (reversible)	Headache, focal CNS ischemia	CNS vasculitis
Ear cerumen	Temporal headache	Giant cell arteritis
Glaucoma	Temporal headache	Giant cell arteritis
Gluten sensitivity	Ataxia	CNS vasculitis
Heparin-induced thrombotic thrombocytopenia	Skin necrosis, cerebral hemorrhage, GI bleeding, adrenal hemorrhage	Systemic vasculitis
Inflammatory bowel disease	CNS white matter lesions noted on MRI (without clinical findings)	CNS vasculitis
Mitochondrial myopathy, encephalopathy, lactic acidosis, and stroke-like episodes (MELAS)	Headache, CNS ischemia	CNS vasculitis
Non-bacterial thrombotic (marantic) endocarditis	Multiple organ infarctions	Polyarteritis nodosa
Orbital infection	Temporal headache	CNS vasculitis
Sickle cell anemia	Headache, CNS ischemia, segmental narrowing of cerebral vessels	CNS vasculitis
Small infarctions of the cochlear, retinal, and encephalic tissue (SICRET syndrome)	Focal CNS ischemia, visual and auditory disturbances	CNS vasculitis
Sphenoid pneumoceles	Episodic blindness	Giant cell arteritis

Table 45.5 Non-vascular cutaneous conditions that may simulate vasculitis

Familial leg ulcers
Infections
Insect bites (brown recluse spider)
Malignant neoplasm
Neutrophilic dermatosis (Sweet's syndrome, rheumatoid arthritis)
Panniculitis (erythema nodosum)
Polymorphic eruption of pregnancy
Pyoderma gangrenosum
Sarcoidosis
Scurvy

true vasculitis. Thus, pulmonary nodules or cavitary lesions in a patient with Wegener's granulomatosis or polyarteritis can just as easily result from infection as from vasculitis. And finally, non-vascular cutaneous conditions, such as those shown in Table 45.5, can simulate vasculitis.

References

Abdelmalek, M. F. and Spittell, P. C. (1995). 79-year-old woman with blue toes. *Mayo Clinic Proceedings*, **70**, 292–5.

Aberfeld, D. and Gladstone, J. (1967). Cryptococcal meningoencephalitis presenting with hemiplegia of sudden onset. *Journal of the American Medical Association*, **202**, 90–1.

Adrogue, H. J., Frazier, M. R., Zeluff, B. and Suki, W. N. (1981). Systemic calciphylaxis revisited. *American Journal of Nephrology*, **1**, 177–83.

Ahmed, S., O'Neill, K. D., Hood, A. F., Evan, A. P. and Moe, S. M. (2001). Calciphylaxis is associated with hyperphosphatemia and increased osteopontin expression by vascular smooth muscle cells. *American Journal of Kidney Diseases*, **37**, 1267–76.

Alam, M. and Sun, I. (1991). Transesophageal echocardiographic evaluation of left atrial mass lesions. *Journal of the American Society of Echocardiography*, **4**, 323–30.

Alarcon-Segovia, D., Mestanza, M., Cabiedes, J. and Cabral, A. R. (1997). The antiphospholipid/cofactor syndromes. II. A variant in patients with systemic lupus erythematosus with antibodies to beta 2-glycoprotein I but no antibodies detectable in standard antiphospholipid assays. *Journal of Rheumatology*, **24**, 1545–51.

Alegre, V. A., Gastineau, D. A. and Winkelmann, R. K. (1989). Skin lesions associated with circulating lupus anticoagulant. *British Journal of Dermatology*, **120**, 419–29.

Anders, K. H., Latta, H., Chang, B. S., Tomiyasu, U., Quddusi, A. S. and Vinters, H. V. (1989). Lymphomatoid granulomatosis and malignant lymphoma of the central nervous system in the acquired immunodeficiency syndrome. *Human Pathology*, **20**, 326–34.

Anderson, W. R. (1965). Necrotizing angiitis associated with embolization of cholesterol. Case report, with emphasis on the use of the muscle biopsy as a diagnostic aid. *American Journal of Clinical Pathology*, **43**, 65–71.

Anderson, W. R. and Richards, A. M. (1968). Evaluation of lower extremity muscle biopsies in the diagnosis of atheroembolism. *Archives of Pathology*, **86**, 535–41.

Angelis, M., Wong, L. L., Myers, S. A. and Wong, L. M. (1997). Calciphylaxis in patients on hemodialysis: a prevalence study. *Surgery*, **122**, 1083–9; discussion 1089–90.

Anonymous (1990). Anderson-Fabry disease [editorial]. *Lancet*, **336**, 24–5.

Armstrong, F. S. and Hayes, G. J. (1961). Segmental cerebral arterial constriction associated with pheochromocytoma. Report of a case with arteriograms. *Journal of Neurosurgery*, **18**, 843–6.

Asherson, R. A. (1992). The catastrophic antiphospholipid syndrome [editorial]. *Journal of Rheumatology*, **19**, 508–12.

Asherson, R. A., Cervera, R., Piette, J. C., *et al.* (1998). Catastrophic antiphospholipid syndrome. Clinical and laboratory features of 50 patients. *Medicine* (Baltimore), **77**, 195–207.

Auethavekiat, P., Murali, N. S. and Manek, N. J. (2004). Clinical images: Primary systemic amyloidosis masquerading as necrotizing vasculitis. *Arthritis and Rheumatism*, **50**, 3400.

Baethge, B. A., Sanusi, I. D., Landreneau, M. D., Rohr, M. S. and McDonald, J. C. (1988). Livedo reticularis and peripheral gangrene associated with primary hyperoxaluria. *Arthritis and Rheumatism*, **31**, 1199–203.

Bardwick, P. A., Zvaifler, N. J., Gill, G. N., Newman, D., Greenway, G. D. and Resnick, D. L. (1980). Plasma cell dyscrasia with polyneuropathy, organomegaly, endocrinopathy, M protein, and skin changes: the POEMS syndrome. Report on two cases and a review of the literature. *Medicine*, **59**, 311–22.

Baselga, E., Margall, N., Barnadas, M. A., Coll, P., deMoragas, J. M. (1997). Detection of Mycobacterium tuberculosis in lobular granulomatous panniculitis (erythema induratum-nodular vasculitis). *Archives of Dermatology*, **133**, 457–62.

Bastani, B. and Nahass, G. (1999). Images in clinical medicine. Type I primary hyperoxaluria. *New England Journal of Medicine*, **341**, 1979.

Becker, A. E., Schoorl, R., Balk, A. G. and van der Heide, R. M. (1975). Cardiac manifestations of Fabry's disease. Report of a case with mitral insufficiency and electrocardiographic evidence of myocardial infarction. *American Journal of Cardiology*, **36**, 829–35.

Beightler, E., Diven, D. G., Sanchez, R. L. and Solomon, A. R. (1991). Thrombotic vasculopathy associated with cryofibrinogenemia. *Journal of the American Academy of Dermatology*, **24**, 342–5.

Benedict, L., Kusne, S., Torre-Cisneros, J., Hunt, S. J. (1992). Primary cutaneous fungal infection after solid-organ transplantation: report of five cases and review. *Clinical Infectious Diseases*, **15**, 17–21.

Berger, J., Harris, J. O., Gregorios, J., Norenberg, M. (1990). Cerebrovascular disease in AIDS: a case-control study. *AIDS*, **4**, 239–44.

Bhardwaj, M., Goldweit, R., Erlebacher, J., Kashani, M., Levin, D. and Leber, G. (1989). Tissue plasminogen activator and cholesterol crystal embolization [letter]. *Annals of Internal Medicine*, **111**, 687–8.

Bhawan, J., Wolff, S. M., Ucci, A. A. and Bhan, A. K. (1985). Malignant lymphoma and malignant angioendotheliomatosis: one disease. *Cancer*, **55**, 570–6.

Bitzer, M., Armeanu, S., Krober, S. M., Horger, M. S. and Erley, C. M. (2003). A young woman with splenic infarction. *Lancet*, **362**, 1456.

Blackburn, W. E., McRoberts, J. W., Bhathena, D., Vazquez, M. and Luke, R. G. (1975). Severe vascular complications in oxalosis after bilateral nephrectomy. *Annals of Internal Medicine*, **82**, 44–6.

Blanco, F., Blas, M. S., Gonzalez, M. F. (1999). Histopathologic features of cerebral vasculitis associated with Mycobacterium tuberculosis. *Arthritis and Rheumatism*, **42**, 383.

Blumberg, A. and Weidmann, P. (1977). Successful treatment of ischaemic ulceration of the skin in azotaemic hyperparathyroidism with parathyroidectomy. *British Medical Journal*, **1**, 552–3.

Boers, G. H., Smals, A. G., Trijbels, F. J., *et al.* (1985). Heterozygosity for homocystinuria in premature peripheral and cerebral occlusive arterial disease [see comments]. *New England Journal of Medicine*, **313**, 709–15.

Bogousslavsky, J., Despland, P. A., Regli, F. and Dubuis, P. Y. (1989). Postpartum cerebral angiopathy: reversible vasoconstriction assessed by transcranial Doppler ultrasounds. *European Neurology*, **29**, 102–5.

Bommer, J., Ritz, E. and Andrassy, K. (1979). Necrotizing dermatitis resulting from hemodialysis with polyvinylchloride tubing. *Annals of Internal Medicine*, **91**, 869–70.

Boogaerts, M. A., Hammerschmidt, D. E., Roelant, C., Verwilghen, R. L. and Jacob, H. S. (1983). Mechanisms of vascular damage in gout and oxalosis: crystal induced, granulocyte mediated, endothelial injury. *Thrombosis and Haemostasis*, **50**, 576–80.

Boussen, K., Moalla, M., Blondeau, P., Ben Ayed, H. and Lie, J. T. (1991). Embolization of cardiac myxomas masquerading as polyarteritis nodosa. *Journal of Rheumatology*, **18**, 283–5.

Bowles, C. A. (1990). Vasculopathy associated with the antiphospholipid antibody syndrome. *Rheumatic Diseases Clinics of North America*, **16**, 471–90.

Bradley, M. (1995). Images in clinical medicine. Spontaneous atheroembolism. *New England Journal of Medicine*, **332**, 998.

Braverman, I. M. and Lerner, A. B. (1961). Diffuse malignant proliferation of vascular endolthelium. A possible new clinical and pathological entity. *Archives of Dermatology*, **84**, 22–30.

Breathnach, S. M. and Wells, G. C. (1980). Amyloid vascular disease: cord-like thickening of mucocutaneous arteries, intermittent claudication and angina in a case with underlying myelomatosis. *British Journal of Dermatology*, **102**, 591–5.

Brick, J. F. (1988). Vanishing cerebrovascular disease of pregnancy. *Neurology*, **38**, 804–6.

Bridges, B. F. and Hector, D. A. (1989). Possible association of cutaneous telangiectasia with cardiac myxoma. *American Journal of Medicine*, **87**, 483–5.

Bruns, F. J., Segel, D. P. and Adler, S. (1978). Control of cholesterol embolization by discontinuation of anticoagulant therapy. *American Journal of the Medical Sciences*, **275**, 105–8.

Bulkley, B. H. and Hutchins, G. M. (1979). Atrial myxomas: a fifty year review. *American Heart Journal*, **97**, 639–43.

Burnham, T. K. (1972). Antinuclear antibodies in patients with malignancies. *Lancet*, **2**, 436.

Burruss, J. B., Fabrae, V. C. and Callen, J. P. (1994). Painful acral purpuric nodules. *Arthritis and Rheumatism*, **37**, 1812–5.

Byrd, R., Hourany, J., Cooper, C. and Roy, T. M. (1998). False-positive antineutrophil cytoplasmic antibodies in a patient with cavitary pulmonary sporotrichosis. *American Journal of Medicine*, **104**, 101–3.

Byrd, W. E., Matthews, O. P. and Hunt, R. E. (1980). Left atrial myxoma presenting as a systemic vasculitis. *Arthritis and Rheumatism*, **23**, 240–3.

Cabili, S., Hochman, I. and Goor, Y. (1993). Reversal of gangrenous lesions in the blue toe syndrome with lovastatin–a case report. *Angiology*, **44**, 821–5.

Calabrese, L. H. (1991). Vasculitis and infection with the human immunodeficiency virus. *Rheumatic Diseases Clinics of North America*, **17**, 131–47.

Calabrese, L. H., Furlan, A. J., Gragg, L. A. and Ropos, T. J. (1992). Primary angiitis of the central nervous system: diagnostic criteria and clinical approach. *Cleveland Clinic Journal of Medicine*, **59**, 293–306.

Calabrese, L. H. and Mallek, J. A. (1988). Primary angiitis of the central nervous system. Report of 8 new cases, review of the literature, and proposal for diagnostic criteria. *Medicine*, **67**, 20–39.

Call, G. K., Fleming, M. C., Sealfon, S., Levine, H., Kistler, J. P. and Fisher, C. M. (1988). Reversible cerebral segmental vasoconstriction. *Stroke*, **19**, 1159–70.

Camponovo, F. and Meier, C. (1986). Neuropathy of vasculitic origin in a case of Garin-Boujadoux-Bannwarth syndrome with positive borrelia antibody response. *Journal of Neurology*, **233**, 69–72.

Caplan, D. and Louis, D. (1996). Case records of the Massacusetts General Hospital. *New England Journal of Medicine*, **335**, 952–9.

Cappiello, R. A., Espinoza, L. R., Adelman, H., Aguilar, J., Vasey, F. B. and Germain, B. F. (1989). Cholesterol embolism: a pseudovasculitic syndrome. *Seminars in Arthritis and Rheumatism*, **18**, 240–6.

Carney, J. A., Gordon, H., Carpenter, P. C., Shenoy, B. V. and Go, V. L. (1985). The complex of myxomas, spotty pigmentation, and endocrine overactivity. *Medicine*, **64**, 270–83.

Carr, M. E., Jr., Sanders, K. and Todd, W. M. (1994). Pain relief and clinical improvement temporally related to the use of pentoxifylline in a patient with documented cholesterol emboli–a case report. *Angiology*, **45**, 65–9.

Casey, M., Vaughan, C. J., He, J., *et al.* (2000). Mutations in the protein kinase A R1alpha regulatory subunit cause familial cardiac myxomas and Carney complex. *Journal of Clinical Investigation*, **106**, R31–8.

Cattan, S., Mariette, X., Labrousse, F. and Brouet, J. C. (1994). Iliac artery dissection in alpha 1-antitrypsin deficiency [letter; comment]. *Lancet*, **343**, 1371–2.

Chambers, J. C., McGregor, A., Jean-Marie, J. and Kooner, J. S. (1998). Acute hyperhomocysteinaemia and endothelial dysfunction. *Lancet*, **351**, 36–7.

Chan, R., Goodman, T. A., Aretz, T. H., Lie, J. T. (1998). Segmental mediolytic arteriopathy of the splenic and hepatic arteries mimicking systemic necrotizing vasculitis. *Arthritis and Rheumatism*, **41**, 935–8.

Chandrasekar, P., Nandi, P. S., Fairfax, M. R., Crane, L. R. (1997). Cutaneous infections due to Acanthamoeba in patients with acquired immunodeficiency syndrome. *Archives of Internal Medicine*, **157**, 569–72.

Churchill, C. H., Abril, A., Krishna, M., Callman, M. L. and Ginsburg, W. W. (2003). Jaw claudication in primary amyloidosis: unusual presentation of a rare disease. *Journal of Rheumatology*, **30**, 2283–6.

Citron, B. P., Halpern, M., McCarron, M., *et al.* (1970). Necrotizing angiitis associated with drug abuse. *New England Journal of Medicine*, **283**, 1003–11.

Clarke, P., Glick, S. and Reilly, B. M. (2005). Clinical problem-solving. On the threshold–a diagnosis of exclusion. *New England Journal of Medicine*, **352**, 919–24.

Clarke, R., Daly, L., Robinson, K., *et al.* (1991). Hyperhomocysteinemia: an independent risk factor for vascular disease [see comments]. *New England Journal of Medicine*, **324**, 1149–55.

Cohen, A. I., McIntosh, H. D. and Orgain, E. S. (1963). The mimetic nature of left atrial myxomas. Report of a case presenting as a severe systemic illness and simulating massive mitral insufficiency at cardiac catheterization. *American Journal of Cardiology*, **11**, 802–7.

Conn, J., Jr., Krumlovsky, F. A., Del Greco, F. and Simon, N. M. (1973). Calciphylaxis: etiology of progressive vascular calcification and gangrene? *Annals of Surgery*, **177**, 206–10.

Cosio, F. G., Zager, R. A. and Sharma, H. M. (1985). Atheroembolic renal disease causes hypocomplementaemia. *Lancet*, **2**, 118–21.

Cox, D. W. (1994). Alpha 1-antitrypsin: a guardian of vascular tissue [editorial; comment]. *Mayo Clinic Proceedings*, **69**, 1123–4.

Cross, S. S. (1991). How common is cholesterol embolism? *Journal of Clinical Pathology*, **44**, 859–61.

Dahlberg, P. J., Frecentese, D. F. and Cogbill, T. H. (1989). Cholesterol embolism: experience with 22 histologically proven cases. *Surgery*, **105**, 737–46.

Darsee, J. R. (1979). Cholesterol embolism: the great masquerader. *Southern Medical Journal*, **72**, 174–80.

den Butter, G., van Bockel, J. H. and Aarts, J. C. (1988). Arterial fibrodysplasia: rapid progression complicated by rupture of a visceral aneurysm into the gastrointestinal tract. *Journal of Vascular Surgery*, **7**, 449–53.

DePace, N. L., Soulen, R. L., Kotler, M. N. and Mintz, G. S. (1981). Two dimensional echocardiographic detection of intraatrial masses. *American Journal of Cardiology*, **48**, 954–60.

Desnick, R. J., Astrin, K. H. and Bishop, D. F. (1989). Fabry disease: molecular genetics of the inherited nephropathy. *Advances in Nephrology from the Necker Hospital*, **18**, 113–27.

Desnick, R. J., Brady, R., Barranger, J., *et al.* (2003). Fabry disease, an under-recognized multisystemic disorder: expert recommendations for diagnosis, management, and enzyme replacement therapy. *Annals of Internal Medicine*, **138**, 338–46.

Desousa, A. L., Muller, J., Campbell, R., Batnitzky, S. and Rankin, L. (1978). Atrial myxoma: a review of the neurological complications, metastases, and recurrences. *Journal of Neurology, Neurosurgery and Psychiatry*, **41**, 1119–24.

Dessailloud, R., Papo, T., Vaneecloo, S., Gamblin, C., Vanhille, P. and Piette, J. C. (1998). Acalculous ischemic gallbladder necrosis in the catastrophic antiphospholipid syndrome. *Arthritis and Rheumatism*, **41**, 1318–20.

DiGiuseppe, J., Nelson, WG, Seifter, EJ, Boitnott, JK, Mann, RB (1994). Intravascular lymphomatosis: a clinicopatgologic study of 10 casesand assessment of response to chemotherapy. *Journal of Clinical Oncology*, **12**, 2573–9.

DiPrete, D. A., Abuelo, J. G., Abuelo, D. N. and Cronan, J. J. (1990). Acute renal insufficiency due to renal infarctions in a patient with neurofibromatosis. *American Journal of Kidney Diseases*, **15**, 357–60.

Dornan, T. L., Blundell, J. W., Morgan, A. G., Burden, R. P., Reeves, W. G. and Cotton, R. E. (1985). Widespread crystallisation of paraprotein in myelomatosis. *Quarterly Journal of Medicine*, **57**, 659–67.

Dotten, D. A., Pruzanski, W., Olin, J. and Brown, T. C. (1976). Cryocrystalglobulinemia. *Canadian Medical Association Journal*, **114**, 909–12.

Dowd, P. M., Rustin, M. H. and Lanigan, S. (1986). Nifedipine in the treatment of chilblains. *British Medical Journal* (Clinical Research ed.), **293**, 923–4.

Dukes, H. T. and Vieth, R. G. (1964). Cerebral arteriography during migraine prodrome and headache. *Neurology*, **14**, 636–9.

Ebert, T. H. and McCluskey, R. T. (1986). Clinicopathological conference. *New England Journal of Medicine*, **315**, 308–15.

Edwards, R. J., Moss, T. and Sandeman, D. R. (2003). A syndrome lost in specialisation. *Lancet*, **362**, 1541.

Ekbom, K. and Greitz, T. (1970). Carotid angiography in cluster headache. *Acta Radiologica: Diagnosis*, **10**, 177–86.

el Gammal, T. (1969). Extra-ventricular communicating hydrocephalus: some observations on the midline ventricles. *American Journal of Roentgenology, Radium Therapy and Nuclear Medicine*, **106**, 308–28.

Eliot, R. S., Kanjuh, V. I. and Edwards, J. E. (1964). Atheromatous embolism. *Circulation*, **30**, 611–18.

Eng, C. M., Guffon, N., Wilcox, W. R., *et al.* (2001). Safety and efficacy of recombinant human alpha-galactosidase A–replacement therapy in Fabry's disease. *New England Journal of Medicine*, **345**, 9–16.

Erhard, H., Runger, T. M., Kreienkamp, M., Muller, J., Muller-Hermelink, H. K., *et al.* (1995). Atypical varicella-zoster virus infection in an immunocompromised patient: result of a virus-induced vasculitis. *Journal of the American Academy of Dermatology*, **32**, 908–11.

Esnault, V. L., Testa, A., Audrain, M., *et al.* (1993). Alpha 1-antitrypsin genetic polymorphism in ANCA-positive systemic vasculitis. *Kidney International*, **43**, 1329–32.

Esterly, J. and Oppenheimer, E. (1967). Vascular lesions in infants with congenital rubella. *Circulation*, **36**, 544–50.

Falanga, V., Fine, M. J. and Kapoor, W. N. (1986). The cutaneous manifestations of cholesterol crystal embolization. *Archives of Dermatology*, **122**, 1194–8.

Fallis, R. and Fisher, M. (1985). Cerebral vasculitis and hemmorrhage associated with phenylpropanolamine. *Neurology*, **35**, 405–7.

Farcet, J. P., Weschsler, J., Wirquin, V., Divine, M. and Reyes, F. (1987). Vasculitis in hairy-cell leukemia. *Archives of Internal Medicine*, **147**, 660–4.

Fassbender, K., Mielke, O., Bertsch, T., Nafe, B., Froschen, S. and Hennerici, M. (1999). Homocysteine in cerebral macroangiography and microangiopathy. *Lancet*, **353**, 1586–7.

Federman, D. G., Valdivia, M. and Kirsner, R. S. (1994). Syphilis presenting as the 'blue toe syndrome'. *Archives of Internal Medicine*, **154**, 1029–31.

Fengler, S. A., Berenberg, J. L. and Lee, Y. T. (1990). Disseminated coagulopathies and advanced malignancies. *American Surgeon*, **56**, 335–8.

Ferris, E. J., Rudikoff, J. C. and Shapiro, J. H. (1968). Cerebral angiography of bacterial infection. *Radiology*, **90**, 727–34.

Fessler, B. J. (1997). Thrombotic syndromes and autoimmune diseases. *Rheumatic Diseases Clinics of North America*, **23**, 461–79.

Fine, A. and Zacharias, J. (2002). Calciphylaxis is usually non-ulcerating: risk factors, outcome and therapy. *Kidney International*, **61**, 2210–7.

Fine, M. J., Kapoor, W. and Falanga, V. (1987). Cholesterol crystal embolization: a review of 221 cases in the English literature. *Angiology*, **38**, 769–84.

Finkel, T. H., Teoreok, T. J., Ferguson, P. J., *et al.* (1994). Chronic parvovirus B19 infection and systemic necrotising vasculitis, opportunistic infection or aetiological agent? [see comments]. *Lancet*, **343**, 1255–8.

Finley, J. L. and Dabbs, D. J. (1988). Renal vascular smooth muscle proliferation in neurofibromatosis. *Human Pathology*, **19**, 107–10.

Fisher, E. A., Desnick, R. J., Gordon, R. E., Eng, C. M., Griepp, R. and Goldman, M. E. (1992). Fabry disease: an unusual cause of severe coronary disease in a young man. Annals of *Internal Medicine*, **117**, 221–3.

Fisher, E. R., Hellstrom, H. R. and Myers, J. D. (1960). Disseminated atheromatous emboli. *American Journal of Medicine*, **29**, 176–80.

Fitzpatrick, A. P., Lanham, J. G. and Doyle, D. V. (1986). Cardiac tumours simulating collagen vascular disease. *British Heart Journal*, **55**, 592–5.

Fonkalsrud, E. W., Sanchez, M., Zerubavel, R. and Mahoney, A. (1977). Serial changes in arterial structure following radiation therapy. *Surgery, Gynecology and Obstetrics*, **145**, 395–400.

Fontana, P., Gabutti, L., Piffaretti, J. C. and Marone, C. (1996). Antibiotic treatment for giant cell arteritis? *Lancet*, **348**, 1630.

Fortin, P. (1996). Vasculitides associated with malignancy. *Current Opinion in Rheumatology*, **8**, 30–3.

Fox, D. A., Faix, J. D., Coblyn, J., Fraser, P., Smith, B. and Weinblatt, M. E. (1986). Thrombotic thrombocytopenic purpura and systemic lupus erythematosus. *Annals of the Rheumatic Diseases*, **45**, 319–22.

Frances, C., Niang, S., Laffitte, E., Pelletier, F., Costedoat, N. and Piette, J. C. (2005). Dermatologic manifestations of the antiphospholipid syndrome: two hundred consecutive cases. *Arthritis and Rheumatism*, **52**, 1785–93.

Frayha, R. A. (1981). Trichinosis-related polyarteritis nodosa. *American Journal of Medicine*, **71**, 307–12.

Fredericks, R., Lefkowitz, D. S., Challa, V. R. and Troost, B. T. (1991a). Cerebral vasculitis associated with cocaine abuse. *Stroke*, **22**, 1437–9.

Fredericks, R., Walker, F. O., Elster, A., Challa, V. (1991b). Angiotropic intravascular large-cell lymphoma (malignant angioendotheliomatosis): report of a case and review of the literature. *Surgical Neurology*, **35**, 218–23.

Friedman, D. R. and Wolfsthal, S. D. (2005). Cocaine-induced pseudovasculitis. *Mayo Clinic Proceedings*, **80**, 671–3.

Friman, C. and Pettersson, T. (1996). Amyloidosis. *Current Opinion in Rheumatology*, **8**, 62–71.

Gabriel, S. E., Conn, D. L., Phyliky, R. L., Pittelkow, M. R. and Scott, R. E. (1986). Vasculitis in hairy cell leukemia: review of literature and consideration of possible pathogenic mechanisms. *Journal of Rheumatology*, **13**, 1167–72.

Gahl, W. A. (2001). New therapies for Fabry's disease. *New England Journal of Medicine*, **345**, 55–7.

Ganor, S. (1983). Corticosteroid therapy for pernio [letter]. *Journal of the American Academy of Dermatology*, **8**, 136.

Garces, M. and Gosink, B. (1972). Aneurysm of the right iliac artery associated with fibrosarcoma. *Radiology*, **102**, 583–4.

Garner, B. F., Burns, P., Bunning, R. D. and Laureno, R. (1990). Acute blood pressure elevation can mimic arteriographic appearance of cerebral vasculitis–a postpartum case with relative hypertension. *Journal of Rheumatology*, **17**, 93–7.

Gertner, E. (1999). Diffuse alveolar hemorrhage in the antiphospholipid syndrome: spectrum of disease and treatment. *Journal of Rheumatology*, **26**, 805–7.

Gertner, E. and Lie, J. T. (1994). Systemic therapy with fibrinolytic agents and heparin for recalcitrant nonhealing cutaneous ulcer in the antiphospholipid syndrome. *Journal of Rheumatology*, **21**, 2159–61.

Gertz, M. A., Kyle, R. A., Griffing, W. L. and Hunder, G. G. (1986). Jaw claudication in primary systemic amyloidosis. *Medicine*, **65**, 173–9.

Gibson, A., Gardner, J. and O'Donnell, J. (2005). Erythropoietin and painful leg ulcers: thrombosis or vasculitis? *Arthritis and Rheumatism*, **53**, 792.

Gilbert, J. A., Jr. and Scalzi, R. P. (1993). Disseminated intravascular coagulation. *Emergency Medicine Clinics of North America*, **11**, 465–80.

Gilbert, J. J. and Vinters, H. V. (1983). Cerebral amyloid angiopathy: incidence and complications in the aging brain. I. Cerebral hemorrhage. *Stroke*, **14**, 915–23.

Gipstein, R. M., Coburn, J. W., Adams, D. A., *et al.* (1976). Calciphylaxis in man. A syndrome of tissue necrosis and vascular calcification in 11 patients with chronic renal failure. *Archives of Internal Medicine*, **136**, 1273–80.

Glass, J., Hochberg, F. H. and Miller, D. C. (1993). Intravascular lymphomatosis. *Cancer*, **71**, 3156–64.

Goldberger, E., Elder, R. C., Schwartz, R. A. and Phillips, P. E. (1992). Vasculitis in the antiphospholipid syndrome. A cause of ischemia responding to corticosteroids [see comments]. *Arthritis and Rheumatism*, **35**, 569–72.

Golden, M. P., Hammer, S. M., Wanke, C. A. and Albrecht, M. A. (1994). Cytomegalovirus vasculitis. Case reports and review of the literature. *Medicine*, **73**, 246–55.

Goldman, B. I., Frydman, C., Harpaz, N., Ryan, S. F. and Loiterman, D. (1987). Glandular cardiac myxomas. Histologic, immunohistochemical, and ultrastructural evidence of epithelial differentiation. *Cancer*, **59**, 1767–75.

Goldman, M., Goldman, A., Dereume, J. P., Heenen, M., Appelboom, T. and Bellens, R. (1980). Aortic atheromatosis presenting as a cutaneous vasculitis with antinuclear antibody [letter]. *Arthritis and Rheumatism*, **23**, 1407–8.

Goodwin, J. F. (1963). Diagnosis of left atrial myxoma. *Lancet*, **1**, 464–8.

Goodwin, J. F. (1968). The spectrum of cardiac tumors. *American Journal of Cardiology*, **21**, 307–14.

Graham, H. V., vonHartitzsch, B. and Medina, J. R. (1976). Infected atrial myxoma. *American Journal of Cardiology*, **38**, 658–61.

Graham, I. M., Daly, L. E., Refsum, H. M., *et al.* (1997). Plasma homocysteine as a risk factor for vascular disease. The European Concerted Action Project. *Journal of the American Medical Association*, **277**, 1775–81.

Gravallese, E., Waksmonski, C., Winters, G. L., Simms, R. W. (1995). Fever, arthralgias, skin lesions, and ischemic digits in a 59-year old man. Clinicopathologic conference. *Arthritis and Rheumatism*, **38**, 1161–8.

Gray, F., Belec, L., Lescs, M C., Chretien, F., Ciardi, A., Hassine, D., *et al.* (1994). Varicell-zoster virus infection of the central nervous system in the acquired immune deficiency syndrome. *Brain*, **117**, 987–99.

Greenwood, W. F. (1968). Profile of atrial myxoma. *American Journal of Cardiology*, **21**, 367–75.

Greitz, T. (1964). Angiography in tuberculous meningitis. *Acta Radiologica*, **2**, 369–78.

Grob, J. J. and Bonerandi, J. J. (1986). Cutaneous manifestations associated with the presence of the lupus anticoagulant. A report of two cases and a review of the literature. *Journal of the American Academy of Dermatology*, **15**, 211–19.

Grob, J. J., San Marco, M., Aillaud, M. F., *et al.* (1991). Unfading acral microlivedo. A discrete marker of thrombotic skin disease associated with antiphospholipid antibody syndrome [see comments]. *Journal of the American Academy of Dermatology*, **24**, 53–8.

Grossman, J., Abraham, G. N., Leddy, J. P. and Condemi, J. L. (1972). Crystalglobulinemia. *Annals of Internal Medicine*, **77**, 395–400.

Gruber, B., Schranz, J. A., Fuhrer, J. and Kane, P. B. (1997). Isolated pulmonary microangiitis mimicking pneumonia in a patient infected with human immunodeficiency virus. *Journal of Rheumatology*, **24**, 759–62.

Gupta, B. K., Spinowitz, B. S., Charytan, C. and Wahl, S. J. (1993). Cholesterol crystal embolization-associated renal failure after therapy with recombinant tissue-type plasminogen activator. *American Journal of Kidney Diseases*, **21**, 659–62.

Gupta, S., Ries, M., Kotsopoulos, S. and Schiffmann, R. (2005). The relationship of vascular glycolipid storage to clinical manifestations of Fabry disease: a cross-sectional study of a large cohort of clinically affected heterozygous women. *Medicine* (Baltimore), **84**, 261–8.

Hadjivassiliou, M., Grunewald, R. A., Chattopadhyay, A. K., Davies-Jones, G. A. B., Gibson, A., *et al.* (1998). Clinical, radiological, neurophysiological, and neuropathological characteristics of gluten ataxia. *Lancet*, **352**, 1582–5.

Halasz, C. L. and Strauss, E. B. (1998). Images in clinical medicine. Unilateral livedo reticularis. *New England Journal of Medicine*, **338**, 1127.

Hammerschmidt, D. E., Greenberg, C. S., Yamada, O., Craddock, P. R. and Jacob, H. S. (1981). Cholesterol and atheroma lipids activate complement and stimulate granulocytes. A possible mechanism for amplification of ischemic injury in atherosclerotic states. *Journal of Laboratory and Clinical Medicine*, **98**, 68–77.

Handler, F. P. (1956). Clinical and pathological significance of atheromatous embolization with emphasis on an etiology of renal hypertension. *American Journal of Medicine*, **20**, 366–73.

Harmon, D. C. and Mark, E. J. (1999). Case records of the Massachusetts General Hospital. *New England Journal of Medicine*, **340**, 1099–106.

Harrington, J. T., Sommers, S. C. and Kassirer, J. P. (1968). Atheromatous emboli with progressive renal failure. Renal arteriography as the probable inciting factor. *Annals of Internal Medicine*, **68**, 152–60.

Harvey, W. P. (1968). Clinical aspects of cardiac tumors. *American Journal of Cardiology*, **21**, 328–43.

Hasler, P., Kistler, H., Gerber, H. (1995). Vasculitides in hairy cell leukemia. *Seminars in Arthritis and Rheumatism*, **25**, 134–42.

Heath, D. and Mackinnon, J. (1964). Pulmonary hypertension due to myxoma of the right atrium. With special reference to the behavior of emboli of myxoma in the lung. *American Heart Journal*, **68**, 227–35.

Hendel, R. C., Cuenoud, H. F., Giansiracusa, D. F. and Alpert, J. S. (1989). Multiple cholesterol emboli syndrome. Bowel infarction after retrograde angiography. *Archives of Internal Medicine*, **149**, 2371–4.

Henry, P. Y., Larre, P., Aupy, M., Lafforgue, J. L. and Orgogozo, J. M. (1984). Reversible cerebral arteriopathy associated with the administration of ergot derivatives. *Cephalalgia*, **4**, 171–8.

Herman, E. W., Kezis, J. S. and Silvers, D. N. (1981). A distinctive variant of pernio. Clinical and histopathologic study of nine cases. *Archives of Dermatology*, **117**, 26–8.

Hirano, T., Taga, T., Yasukawa, K., *et al.* (1987). Human B-cell differentiation factor defined by an anti-peptide antibody and its possible role in autoantibody production. *Proceedings of the National Academy of Sciences of the USA*, **84**, 228–31.

Hogarth, M. B., Qureshi, T., Lloyd, J. and Rees, R. G. (1999). A blistering rash and swollen knees. *Lancet*, **353**, 978.

Hollenhorst, R. W. (1961). Significance of bright plaques in the retinal arterioles. *Journal of the American Medical Association*, **178**, 123–129.

Hoshimaru, M., Takahashi, J. A., Kikuchi, H., Nagata, I. and Hatanaka, M. (1991). Possible roles of basic fibroblast growth factor in the pathogenesis of moyamoya disease: an immunohistochemical study. *Journal of Neurosurgery*, **75**, 267–70.

Huang, T. and Chou, S. (1988). Occlusive hypertrophic arteritis as the cause of discrete necrosis in CNS toxoplasmosis in the acquired immunodeficiency syndrome. *Human Pathology*, **19**, 1210–14.

Hughes, G. R. (1993). The antiphospholipid syndrome: ten years on [see comments]. *Lancet*, **342**, 341–4.

Huston, K. A., Combs, J. J., Jr., Lie, J. T. and Giuliani, E. R. (1978). Left atrial myxoma simulating peripheral vasculitis. *Mayo Clinic Proceedings*, **53**, 752–6.

Hyman, B. T., Landas, S. K., Ashman, R. F., Schelper, R. L. and Robinson, R. A. (1987). Warfarin-related purple toes syndrome and cholesterol microembolization. *American Journal of Medicine*, **82**, 1233–7.

Imahori, S., Bannerman, R. M., Graf, C. J. and Brennan, J. C. (1969). Ehlers-Danlos syndrome with multiple arterial lesions. *American Journal of Medicine*, **47**, 967–77.

Ingram, S. B., Goodnight, S. H., Jr. and Bennett, R. M. (1987). An unusual syndrome of a devastating noninflammatory vasculopathy associated with anticardiolipin antibodies: report of two cases. *Arthritis and Rheumatism*, **30**, 1167–72.

Irey, N. S. and Norris, H. J. (1973). Intimal vascular lesions associated with female reproductive steroids. *Archives of Pathology*, **96**, 227–34.

Iwai, T., Konno, S., Hiejima, K., *et al.* (1985). Fibromuscular dysplasia in the extremities. *Journal of Cardiovascular Surgery*, **26**, 496–501.

Jacob, J. R., Weisman, M. H., Rosenblatt, S. I. and Bookstein, J. J. (1986). Chronic pernio. A historical perspective of cold-induced vascular disease. *Archives of Internal Medicine*, **146**, 1589–92.

Jain, R., Chartash, E., Susin, M. and Furie, R. (1994). Systemic lupus erythematosus complicated by thrombotic microangiopathy. *Seminars in Arthritis and Rheumatism*, **24**, 173–82.

Janigan, D. T., Hirsch, D. J., Klassen, G. A. and MacDonald, A. S. (2000). Calcified subcutaneous arterioles with infarcts of the subcutis and skin (calciphylaxis) in chronic renal failure. *American Journal of Kidney Diseases*, **35**, 588–97.

Jarrett, S. J., Cunnane, G., Conaghan, P. G., *et al.* (2003). Anti-tumor necrosis factor-alpha therapy-induced vasculitis: case series. *Journal of Rheumatology*, **30**, 2287–91.

Jennette, J. C., Sheps, D. S. and McNeill, D. D. (1982). Exclusively vascular systemic amyloidosis with visceral ischemia. *Archives of Pathology and Laboratory Medicine*, **106**, 323–7.

Johnston, Y. E., Duray, P. H., Steere, A. C., *et al.* (1985). Lyme arthritis. Spirochetes found in synovial microangiopathic lesions. *American Journal of Pathology*, **118**, 26–34.

Jones, D. B. and Iannaccone, P. M. (1975). Atheromatous emboli in renal biopsies. An ultrastructural study. *American Journal of Pathology*, **78**, 261–76.

Jones, H. and Edgar, M. (1995). Case records of the Massachusetts General Hospital. *New England Journal of Medicine*, **332**, 730–7.

Jones, H. J., Staud, R. and Williams, R. C., Jr. (1998). Rupture of a hepatic artery aneurysm and renal infarction: 2 complications of fibromuscular dysplasia that mimic vasculitis. *Journal of Rheumatology*, **25**, 2015–8.

Jordan, J. M., Allen, N. B. and Pizzo, S. V. (1987). Defective release of tissue plasminogen activator in systemic and cutaneous vasculitis. *American Journal of Medicine*, **82**, 397–400.

Joshi, V., Pawel, B., Connor, E., Sharer, L., Oleske, J. M., *et al.* (1987). Arteriopathy in children with acquired immune deficiency syndrome. *Pediatric Pathology*, **7**, 261–75.

Jourdan, M., Bataille, R., Seguin, J., Zhang, X. G., Chaptal, P. A. and Klein, B. (1990). Constitutive production of interleukin-6 and immunologic features in cardiac myxomas. *Arthritis and Rheumatism*, **33**, 398–402.

Kalant, H. and Kalant, O. J. (1975). Death in amphetamine users: causes and rates. *Canadian Medical Association Journal*, **112**, 299–304.

Kalter, D. C., Rudolph, A. and McGavran, M. (1985). Livedo reticularis due to multiple cholesterol emboli. *Journal of the American Academy of Dermatology*, **13**, 235–42.

Kamesaki, H., Matsui, Y., Ohno, Y., *et al.* (1990). Angiotropic lymphoma with histologic features of neoplastic angioendotheliomatosis presenting with predominant respiratory and hematologic manifestations. Report of a case and review of the literature [corrected] [published erratum appears in *American Journal of Clinical Pathology* (1992), **98**, 650] [see comments]. *American Journal of Clinical Pathology*, **94**, 768–72.

Kaminsky, M. E., Ehlers, K. H., Engle, M. A., Klein, A. A., Levin, A. R. and Subramanian, V. A. (1979). Atrial myxoma mimicking a collagen disorder. *Chest*, **75**, 93–5.

Kanno, J., Takemura, T. and Kasaga, T. (1987). Malignant endothelioma of the aorta. *Virchows Archiv A*, **412**, 183–8.

Kanzaki, T., Yokota, M., Irie, F., Hirabayashi, Y., Wang, A. M. and Desnick, R. J. (1993). Angiokeratoma corporis diffusum with glycopeptiduria due to deficient lysosomal alpha-N-acetylgalactosaminidase activity. Clinical, morphologic, and biochemical studies. *Archives of Dermatology*, **129**, 460–5.

Kao, N. L., Broy, S. and Tillawi, I. (1992). Malignant angioendotheliomatosis mimicking systemic necrotizing vasculitis. *Journal of Rheumatology*, **19**, 1133–5.

Kapoor, O. P. (1976). Iatrogenic ergot vasospastic angiitis. A case report. *Vascular Surgery*, **10**, 58–60.

Karch, S. B. and Billingham, M. E. (1988). The pathology and etiology of cocaine-induced heart disease. *Archives of Pathology and Laboratory Medicine*, **112**, 225–30.

Karl, M. (1975). Clinicopathologic conference. *American Journal of Medicine*, **59**, 837–43.

Karmody, A. M., Powers, S. R., Monaco, V. J. and Leather, R. P. (1976). Blue toe syndrome. An indication for limb salvage surgery. *Archives of Surgery*, **111**, 1263–8.

Kasinath, B. S. and Lewis, E. J. (1987). Eosinophilia as a clue to the diagnosis of atheroembolic renal disease [editorial]. *Archives of Internal Medicine*, **147**, 1384–5.

Kay, A. B., Shin, H. S. and Austen, K. F. (1973). Selective attraction of eosinophils and synergism between eosinophil chemotactic factor of anaphylaxis ECF-A and a fragment cleaved from the fifth component of complement C5a. *Immunology*, **24**, 969–76.

Kaye, B. R. and Fainstat, M. (1987). Cerebral vasculitis associated with cocaine abuse. *Journal of the American Medical Association*, **258**, 2104–6.

Kazimer, F. J., Sheps, S. G., Bernatz, P. E. and Sayre, G. P. (1966). Livedo reticularis and digital infarcts: a syndrome due to cholesterol emboli arising from atheromatous abdominal aortic aneurysms. *Vascular Disease*, **3**, 12–24.

Kelly, J. W. and Dowling, J. P. (1985). Pernio. A possible association with chronic myelomonocytic leukemia. *Archives of Dermatology*, **121**, 1048–52.

Kennedy, A., Cumberland, D. and Gaines, P. (1989). The pathology of cholesterol embolism arising as a complication of intra-aortic catheterization. *Histopathology*, **15**, 515–21.

King, A. J. and Carlson, J. A. (1993). Case records of the Massachusetts General Hospital. Weekly clinicopathological exercises. Case 38–1993. Renal failure and a painful toe in a 70-year-old man after an acute myocardial infarct. *New England Journal of Medicine*, **329**, 948–55.

Kinugasa, K., Mandai, S., Kamata, I., Sugiu, K. and Ohmoto, T. (1993). Surgical treatment of moyamoya disease: operative technique for encephalo-duro-arterio-myo-synangiosis, its follow-up, clinical results, and angiograms. *Neurosurgery*, **32**, 527–31.

Kirsner, R. S., Eaglstein, W. H., Katz, M. H., Kerdel, F. A. and Falanga, V. (1993). Stanozolol causes rapid pain relief and healing of cutaneous ulcers caused by cryofibrinogenemia. *Journal of the American Academy of Dermatology*, **28**, 71–4.

Klein, K. L. and Pittelkow, M. R. (1992). Tissue plasminogen activator for treatment of livedoid vasculitis [see comments]. *Mayo Clinic Proceedings*, **67**, 923–33.

Klein, P. (1986). Ocular manifestations of Fabry's disease. *Journal of the American Optometric Association*, **57**, 672–4.

Kleinschmidt-DeMasters, B., Filley, C. M. and Bitter, M. A. (1992). Central nervous system angiocentric, angiodestructive T-cell lymphoma (lymphomatoid granulomatosis). *Surgical Neurology*, **37**, 130–7.

Kois, J. M., Sexton, F. M. and Lookingbill, D. P. (1991). Cutaneous manifestations of multiple myeloma. *Archives of Dermatology*, **127**, 69–74.

Korst, D. R. and Kratochvil, C. H. (1955). Cryofibrinogen formation in a cse of lung neoplasm associated with thrombophlebitis migrans. *Blood*, **10**, 945–53.

Kraus, A., Valencia, X., Cabral, A. R., de la Vega, G. (1995). Visceral larva migrans mimicking rheumatic diseases. *Journal of Rheumatology*, **22**, 497–500.

Krieger, C., Robitaille, Y., Jothy, S. and Elleker, G. (1982). Intravascular malignant histiocytosis mimicking central nervous system vasculitis: an immunopathological diagnostic approach. *Annals of Neurology*, **12**, 489–92.

Kuiper, J. J. (1996). Initial manifestation of primary hyperoxaluria type I in adults– recognition, diagnosis, and management. *Western Journal of Medicine*, **164**, 42–53.

Kullo, I. J., Edwards, W. D. and Schwartz, R. S. (1998). Vulnerable plaque: pathobiology and clinical implications. *Annals of Internal Medicine*, **129**, 1050–60.

Lake, C. R., Gallant, S., Masson, E. and Miller, P. (1990). Adverse drug effects attributed to phenylpropanolamine: a review of 142 case reports. *American Journal of Medicine*, **89**, 195–208.

Lanczik, O., Szabo, K., Gass, A. and Hennerici, M. G. (2003). Tinnitus after cycling. *Lancet*, **362**, 292.

Landon, G., Ordaoanez, N. G. and Guarda, L. A. (1986). Cardiac myxomas. An immunohistochemical study using endothelial, histiocytic, and smooth-muscle cell markers. *Archives of Pathology and Laboratory Medicine*, **110**, 116–20.

Laroche, G. P. (1976). Traumatic vasospastic disease in chain-saw operators. *Canadian Medical Association Journal*, **115**, 1217–21.

Lebel, M. and Lassonde, M. (1986). Erythema induratum of Bazin. *Journal of the American Academy of Dermatology*, **14**, 738–42.

Lebwohl, M., Halperin, J. and Phelps, R. G. (1993). Brief report: occult pseudoxanthoma elasticum in patients with premature cardiovascular disease [see comments]. *New England Journal of Medicine*, **329**, 1237–9.

Ledesma, D. and Pearce, W. H. (2000). Images in clinical medicine. Septic (Aspergillus) embolus. *New England Journal of Medicine*, **342**, 1015.

Lee, K. F. and Hodes, P. J. (1967). Intracranial ischemic lesions. *Radiologic Clinics of North America*, **5**, 363–393.

Leeds, N. E. and Goldberg, H. I. (1971). Angiographic manifestations in cerebral inflammatory disease. *Radiology*, **98**, 595–604.

Leeds, N. E. and Rosenblatt, R. (1972). Arterial wall irregularities in intracranial neoplasms. The shaggy vessel brought into focus. *Radiology*, **103**, 121–4.

Leeds, N. E., Rosenblatt, R. and Zimmerman, H. M. (1971). Focal angiographic changes of cerebral lymphoma with pathologic correlation. A report of two cases. *Radiology*, **99**, 595–9.

Lehrer, H. (1966). The angiographic triad in tuberculous meningitis. A radiographic and clinicopathologic correlation. *Radiology*, **87**, 829–35.

Leonhardt, E. T. and Kullenberg, K. P. (1977). Bilateral atrial myxomas with multiple arterial aneurysms–a syndrome mimicking polyarteritis nodosa. *American Journal of Medicine*, **62**, 792–4.

Lesprit, P., Authier, F. J., Gherardi, R., Belec, L., Paris, D., *et al.* (1996). Acute arterial obliteration: a new feature of the POEMS syndrome? *Medicine*, **75**, 226–32.

Lie, J. (1996). Vasculitis associated with infectious agents. *Current Opinion in Rheumatology*, **8**, 26–9.

Lie, J. T. (1992a). Malignant angioendotheliomatosis intravascular lymphomatosis clinically simulating primary angiitis of the central nervous system [see comments]. *Arthritis and Rheumatism*, **35**, 831–4.

Lie, J. T. (1992b). Vasculitis simulators and vasculitis look-alikes. *Current Opinion in Rheumatology*, **4**, 47–55.

Lie, J. T. (1994). Vasculitis in the antiphospholipid syndrome: culprit or consort? [editorial] [see comments]. *Journal of Rheumatology*, **21**, 397–9.

Liebeskind, A., Cohen, S., Anderson, R., Schechter, M. M. and Zingesser, L. H. (1973). Unusual segmental cerebrovascular changes. *Radiology*, **106**, 119–22.

Liebler, G. A., Magovern, G. J., Park, S. B., Cushing, W. J., Begg, F. R. and Joyner, C. R. (1976). Familial myxomas in four siblings. *Journal of Thoracic and Cardiovascular Surgery*, **71**, 605–8.

Lin, J. P. and Siew, F. P. (1971). Glioblatoma multiforme presenting angiographically as intracranial atherosclerotic vascular disease. *Radiology*, **101**, 353–4.

Linnemann, C. and Alvira, M. (1980). Pathogenesis of Varicella-Zoster angiitis in the CNS. *Archives of Neurology*, **37**, 239–240.

Lipford, E. H., Jr., Margolick, J. B., Longo, D. L., Fauci, A. S. and Jaffe, E. S. (1988). Angiocentric immunoproliferative lesions: a clinicopathologic spectrum of post-thymic T-cell proliferations. *Blood*, **72**, 1674–81.

Lipton, S. and Ma, M. (1996). Case records of the Massachusetts General Hospital. *New England Journal of Medicine*, **335**, 1587–95.

Lye, W. C., Cheah, J. S. and Sinniah, R. (1993). Renal cholesterol embolic disease. Case report and review of the literature. *American Journal of Nephrology*, **13**, 489–93.

MacConnell, T. and Ferro, A. (1995). A sore eye and meningitis. *Lancet*, **346**, 1269.

MacGregor, G. A. and Cullen, R. A. (1959). The syndrome of fever, anemia, and high sedimentation rate with an atrial myxoma. *British Medical Journal*, **2**, 991–7.

Malek, A. M., Higashida, R. T., Phatouros, C. C. and Halbach, V. V. (1999). A strangled wife. *Lancet*, **353**, 1324.

Mandel, B. and Calabrese, L. (1998). Infections and systemic vasculitis. *Current Opinion in Rheumatology*, **10**, 51–7.

Mandybur, T. I. (1986). Cerebral amyloid angiopathy: the vascular pathology and complications. *Journal of Neuropathology and Experimental Neurology*, **45**, 79–90.

Manning, W. J., Goldberger, A. L., Drews, R. E., *et al.* (1992). POEMS syndrome with myocardial infarction: observations concerning pathogenesis and review of the literature. *Seminars in Arthritis and Rheumatism*, **22**, 151–61.

Marie, I., Levesque, H., Heron, F., Cailleux, N., Borg, J. Y. and Courtois, H. (1997). Acute adrenal failure secondary to bilateral infarction of the adrenal glands as the first manifestation of primary antiphospholipid antibody syndrome. *Annals of the Rheumatic Diseases*, **56**, 567–8.

Markel, M. L., Armstrong, W. F., Waller, B. F. and Mahomed, Y. (1986). Left atrial myxoma with multicentric recurrence and evidence of metastases. *American Heart Journal*, **111**, 409–13.

Markel, M. L., Waller, B. F. and Armstrong, W. F. (1987). Cardiac myxoma. A review. *Medicine*, **66**, 114–25.

Marks, C. and Kuskov, S. (1995). Pattern of arterial aneurysms in acquired immunodeficiency disease. *World Journal of Surgery*, **19**, 127–32.

Martens, P., Levine, J. A., Hunder, G. G. (1996). Splinter hemmorhages following arterial puncture. *Arthritis and Rheumatism*, **39**, 169–70.

Mason, M. S., Wheeler, J. R., Gregory, R. T. and Gayle, R. G. (1982). Primary tumors of the aorta: report of a case and review of the literature. *Oncology*, **39**, 167–72.

Mastrolonardo, M., Loconsole, F., Conte, A. and Rantuccio, F. (1994). Cutaneous vasculitis as the sole manifestation of disseminated gonococcal infection: case report. *Genitourinary Medicine*, **70**, 130–1.

Masuda, J., Ogata, J. and Yutani, C. (1993). Smooth muscle cell proliferation and localization of macrophages and T cells in the occlusive intracranial major arteries in moyamoya disease. *Stroke*, **24**, 1960–7.

Masuzawa, T., Shinoda, S., Furuse, M., Nakahara, N., Abe, F. and Sato, F. (1983). Cerebral angiographic changes on serial examination of a patient with migraine. *Neuroradiology*, **24**, 277–81.

Matick, H., Anderson, D. and Brumlik, J. (1983). Cerebral vasculitis associated with oral amphetamine overdose. *Archives of Neurology*, **40**, 253–4.

May, E. F. and Jabbari, B. (1990). Stroke in neuroborreliosis. *Stroke*, **21**, 1232–5.

Mayo, R. R. and Swartz, R. D. (1996). Redefining the incidence of clinically detectable atheroembolism. *American Journal of Medicine*, **100**, 524–9.

Mazhar, A. R., Johnson, R. J., Gillen, D., *et al.* (2001). Risk factors and mortality associated with calciphylaxis in end-stage renal disease. *Kidney International*, **60**, 324–32.

McColl, G. J. and Fraser, K. (1995). Pheochromocytoma and pseudovasculitis [letter]. *Journal of Rheumatology*, **22**, 1442–3.

McCready, R. A., Hyde, G. L., Bivins, B. A., Mattingly, S. S. and Griffen, W. O., Jr. (1983). Radiation-induced arterial injuries. *Surgery*, **93**, 306–12.

Mendia, R., D'Aloya, G., Cavaliere, G., *et al.* (1992). Does thrombolysis produce cholesterol embolisation? [letter]. *Lancet*, **339**, 562.

Mertz, L. E. and Conn, D. L. (1992). Vasculitis associated with malignancy. *Current Opinion in Rheumatology*, **4**, 39–46.

Meschia, J. F., Brott, T. G. and Brown, R. D., Jr. (2005). Genetics of cerebrovascular disorders. *Mayo Clinic Proceedings*, **80**, 122–32.

Meyer, W. W. (1947). Cholesterinkrystallemboli kleiner organarterien und ihre Folgen. *Virchows Archiv Pathological Anatomy*, **314**, 616–38.

Meyers, D. S., Grim, C. E. and Keitzer, W. F. (1974). Fibromuscular dysplasia of the renal artery with medial dissection. A case simulating polyarteritis nodosa. *American Journal of Medicine*, **56**, 412–6.

Millard, L. G. and Rowell, N. R. (1978). Chilblain lupus erythematosus Hutchinson. A clinical and laboratory study of 17 patients. *British Journal of Dermatology*, **98**, 497–506.

Miller, M. L., American College of Rheumatology Audiovisual Aids Subcommittee. (2005). Winners of the 2004 American College of Rheumatology Annual Slide Competition. *Arthritis and Rheumatism*, **52**, 679–80.

Milliner, D. S., Eickholt, J. T., Bergstralh, E. J., Wilson, D. M. and Smith, L. H. (1994). Results of long-term treatment with orthophosphate and pyridoxine in patients with primary hyperoxaluria. *New England Journal of Medicine*, **331**, 1553–8.

Mizusawa, H., Hirano, A., Llena, J. F., Shintaku, M. (1988). Cerebrovascular lesions in acquired immune deficiency syndrome (AIDS). *Acta Neuropathologica*, **76**, 451–7.

Moldveen-Geronimus, M. and Merriam, J. C., Jr. (1967). Cholesterol embolization. From pathological curiosity to clinical entity. *Circulation*, **35**, 946–53.

Moolenaar, W. and Lamers, C. B. (1996). Cholesterol crystal embolisation to the alimentary tract. *Gut*, **38**, 196–200.

Mor, A., Bingham, C., 3rd, Barisoni, L., Lydon, E. and Belmont, H. M. (2005). Proliferative lupus nephritis and leukocytoclastic vasculitis during treatment with etanercept. *Journal of Rheumatology*, **32**, 740–3.

Morgan, S. H., Rudge, P., Smith, S. J., *et al.* (1990). The neurological complications of Anderson-Fabry disease (alpha-galactosidase A deficiency)–investigation of symptomatic and presymptomatic patients. *Quarterly Journal of Medicine*, **75**, 491–507.

Morgello, S., Block, G. A., Price, R. W., Petito, C. K. (1988). Varicella-Zoster virus leukoencephalitis and cerebral vasculopathy. *Archives of Pathology and Laboratory Medicine*, **112**, 173–7.

Mosnier, J. F., Degott, C., Bedrossian, J., *et al.* (1991). Recurrence of Fabry's disease in a renal allograft eleven years after successful renal transplantation. *Transplantation*, **51**, 759–62.

Murakami, K., Oshawa, M., Hu, S. X., Kanno, H., Aozasa, K., *et al.* (1998). Large-vessel vasculitis associated with chronic active Epstein-Barr virus infection. *Arthritis and Rheumatism*, **41**, 369–73.

Murakawa, G., McCalmont, T., Altman, J., Telang, G. H., Hoffman, M. D., *et al.* (1995). Disseminated acanthamebiasis in patients with AIDS. *Archives of Dermatology*, **131**, 1291–6.

Nachman, R. L. and Silverstein, R. (1993). Hypercoagulable states [see comments]. *Annals of Internal Medicine*, **119**, 819–27.

Najafi, H. (1966). Fibromuscular hyperplasia of the external iliac arteries. An unusual cause of intermittent claudication. *Archives of Surgery*, **92**, 394–6.

Nakao, S., Takenaka, T., Maeda, M., *et al.* (1995). An atypical variant of Fabry's disease in men with left ventricular hypertrophy. *New England Journal of Medicine*, **333**, 288–93.

Naldi, L., Locati, F., Marchesi, L., *et al.* (1993). Cutaneous manifestations associated with antiphospholipid antibodies in patients with suspected primary antiphospholipid syndrome: a case-control study. *Annals of the Rheumatic Diseases*, **52**, 219–22.

Nance, J., Abbott, K., Morris, L., Couper, R. (1997). An unfortunate consequence of being tickled. *Lancet*, **349**, 1142.

Nasser, W. K., Davis, R. H., Dillon, J. C., *et al.* (1972). Atrial myxoma. I. Clinical and pathologic features in nine cases. *American Heart Journal*, **83**, 694–704.

Navarro, P. H., Bravo, F. P. and Beltran, G. G. (1995). Atrial myxoma with livedoid macules as its sole cutaneous manifestation. *Journal of the American Academy of Dermatology*, **32**, 881–3.

Nelson, P., Dignani, M. C., Anaissie, E. J. (1994). Taxonomy, biology, and clinical aspects of Fusarium species. *Clinical Microbiology Reviews*, **7**, 479–504.

Nevelsteen, A., Kutten, M., Lacroix, H. and Suy, R. (1992). Oral anticoagulant therapy: a precipitating factor in the pathogenesis of cholesterol embolization? *Acta Chirurgica Belgica*, **92**, 33–6.

New, P. F., Price, D. L. and Carter, B. (1970). Cerebral angiography in cardiac myxoma. Correlation of angiographic and histopathological findings. *Radiology*, **96**, 335–45.

Nishida, H., Endo, M., Koyanagi, H., Ichihara, T., Takao, A. and Maruyama, M. (1990). Coronary artery bypass in a 15-year-old girl with pseudoxanthoma elasticum. *Annals of Thoracic Surgery*, **49**, 483–5.

O'Connor, B. (1884). Symmetrical gangrene. *British Medical Journal*, **1**, 460.

Oddo, D., Casanova, M., Acuna, G., Ballesteros, J. and Morales, B. (1992). Acute Chagas' disease (*Trypanosomiasis americana*) in acquired immune deficiency syndrome: report of two cases. *Human Pathology*, **23**, 41–4.

O'Donnell, J. R., Keaveny, T. V. and O'Connell, L. G. (1980). Digital arteritis as a presenting feature of malignant disease. *Irish Journal of Medical Science*, **149**, 386–90.

O'Donnell, T. J. and O'Connell, J. X. (1993). Case records of the Massachusetts General Hospital. Weekly clinicopathological exercises. Case 26–1993. A 73-year-old man with an enlarging inguinal mass 10 years after treatment for prostate and colon cancers. *New England Journal of Medicine*, **329**, 43–8.

Okazaki, H., Reagan, T. J. and Campbell, R. J. (1989). Clinicopathologic studies of primary cerebral amyloid angiopathy. *Mayo Clinic Proceedings*, **54**, 22–31.

O'Keeffe, S. T., Woods, B. O., Breslin, D. J. and Tsapatsaris, N. P. (1992). Blue toe syndrome. Causes and management [see comments]. *Archives of Internal Medicine*, **152**, 2197–202.

Olivero, J. J. (1997). Case in point. *Hospital Practice*, **32**, 30.

Ollert, M. W., Thomas, P., Korting, H. C., Schraut, W. and Braun-Falco, O. (1993). Erythema induratum of Bazin. Evidence of T-lymphocyte hyperresponsiveness to purified protein derivative of tuberculin: report of two cases and treatment. *Archives of Dermatology*, **129**, 469–73.

Olmsted, W. W. and McGee, T. P. (1977). The pathogenesis of peripheral aneurysms of the central nervous system: a subject review from the AFIP. *Radiology*, **123**, 661–6.

Orbison, J. L. (1952). Morphology of thrombocytopenic purpura with demonstration of aneurysms. *American Journal of Pathology*, **28**, 129–43.

Orvar, K. and Johlin, F. C. (1994). Atheromatous embolization resulting in acute pancreatitis after cardiac catheterization and angiographic studies. *Archives of Internal Medicine*, **154**, 1755–61.

Otrakji, C. L., Voigt, W., Amador, A., Nadji, M. and Gregorios, J. B. (1988). Malignant angioendotheliomatosis–a true lymphoma: a case of intravascular malignant lymphomatosis studied by southern blot hybridization analysis. *Human Pathology*, **19**, 475–8.

Page, E. H. and Shear, N. H. (1988). Temperature-dependent skin disorders [see comments]. *Journal of the American Academy of Dermatology*, **18**, 1003–19.

Pandey, J. and LeRoy, E. (1998). Human cytomegalovirus and the vasculopathies of autoimmune diseases (especially scleroderma), allograft rejection, and coronary restenosis. *Arthritis and Rheumatism*, **41**, 10–15.

Panum, P. L. (1862). Experimentelle beitrage zur lehre von der embolie. *Virchows Archiv Pathologic Anatomy*, **25**, 308–31.

Pearlson, G. D., Jeffery, P. J., Harris, G. J., Ross, C. A., Fischman, M. W. and Camargo, E. E. (1993). Correlation of acute cocaine-induced changes in local cerebral blood flow with subjective effects. *American Journal of Psychiatry*, **150**, 495–7.

Peters, M., Gottschalk, D., Boit, R., Pohle, H. D. and Ruf, B. (1993). Meningovascular neurosyphilis in human immunodeficiency virus infection as a differential diagnosis of focal CNS lesions: a clinicopathological study. *Journal of Infection*, **27**, 57–62.

Peters, M. N., Hall, R. J., Cooley, D. A., Leachman, R. D. and Garcia, E. (1974). The clinical syndrome of atrial myxoma. *Journal of the American Medical Association*, **230**, 695–701.

Petito, C. K., Gottlieb, G. J., Dougherty, J. H. and Petito, F. A. (1978). Neoplastic angioendotheliosis: ultrastructural study and review of the literature. *Annals of Neurology*, **3**, 393–9.

Petroff, N., Koger, O. W., Fleming, M. G., *et al.* (1989). Malignant angioendotheliomatosis: an angiotropic lymphoma. *Journal of the American Academy of Dermatology*, **21**, 727–33.

Pineda, C. J., Weisman, M. H., Bookstein, J. J. and Saltzstein, S. L. (1985). Hypothenar hammer syndrome. Form of reversible Raynaud's phenomenon. *American Journal of Medicine*, **79**, 561–70.

Prasertwitayakij, N., Louthrenoo, W., Kasitanon, N., Thamprasert, K. and Vanittanakom, N. (2003). Human pythiosis, a rare cause of arteritis: case report and literature review. *Seminars in Arthritis and Rheumatism*, **33**, 204–14.

Price, D. L., Harris, J. L., New, P. F. and Cantu, R. C. (1970). Cardiac myxoma. A clinicopathologic and angiographic study. *Archives of Neurology*, **23**, 558–67.

Primka, E. J. D., King, C. and O'Keefe, E. J. (1993). Malignant melanoma of unknown origin presenting as a systemic vasculitis [letter]. *Archives of Dermatology*, **129**, 1205–7.

Probstein, J. G., Joshi, R. H. and Blumenthal, H. T. (1957). Atheromatous emboliztion: an etiology of acute pancreatitis. *Archives of Surgery*, **75**, 566–72.

Provost, T. T., Moses, H., Morris, E. L., *et al.* (1991). Cerebral vasculopathy associated with collateralization resembling moya moya phenomenon and with anti-Ro/SS-A and anti-La/SS-B antibodies. *Arthritis and Rheumatism*, **34**, 1052–5.

Pumarola-Sune, T., Navia, B. A., Cordon-Carlo, C., Cho, E. S., Price, R. W. (1987). HIV antigen in the brains of patients with the AIDS dementia complex. *Annals of Neurology*, **21**, 490–6.

Queen, M., Biem, H. J., Moe, G. W. and Sugar, L. (1990). Development of cholesterol embolization syndrome after intravenous streptokinase for acute myocardial infarction. *American Journal of Cardiology*, **65**, 1042–3.

Rademaker, M., Lowe, D. G. and Munro, D. D. (1989). Erythema induratum Bazin's disease. *Journal of the American Academy of Dermatology*, **21**, 740–5.

Rajpal, R. S., Leibsohn, J. A., Liekweg, W. G., *et al.* (1979). Infected left atrial myxoma with bacteremia simulating infective endocarditis. *Archives of Internal Medicine*, **139**, 1176–8.

Rao, J. K. and Allen, N. B. (1993). Primary systemic amyloidosis masquerading as giant cell arteritis. Case report and review of the literature. *Arthritis and Rheumatism*, **36**, 422–5.

Read, R. C., White, H. J., Murphy, M. L., Williams, D., Sun, C. N. and Flanagan, W. H. (1974). The malignant potentiality of left atrial myxoma. *Journal of Thoracic and Cardiovascular Surgery*, **68**, 857–68.

Reiman, S., Fisher, R., Dodds, C., Trinh, C., Laucirica, R. and Whigham, C. J. (2002). Mesenteric arteriographic findings in a patient with strongyloides stercoralis hyperinfection. *Journal of Vascular and Interventional Radiology*, **13**, 635–8.

Retan, J. W. and Miller, R. E. (1966). Microembolic complications of atherosclerosis. Literature review and report of a patient. *Archives of Internal Medicine*, **118**, 534–45.

Revankar, S. G. and Clark, R. A. (1998). Infected cardiac myxoma. Case report and literature review. *Medicine* (Baltimore), **77**, 337–44.

Reynen, K. (1995). Cardiac myxomas. *New England Journal of Medicine*, **333**, 1610–7.

Richards, A. M., Eliot, R. S., Kanjuh, V. I., Bloemendaal, R. D. and Edwards, J. E. (1965). Cholesterol embolism. A multiple-system disease masquerading as polyarteritis nodosa. *American Journal of Cardiology*, **15**, 696–707.

Richardson, J. V., Brandt, B. D., Doty, D. B. and Ehrenhaft, J. L. (1979). Surgical treatment of atrial myxomas: early and late results of 11 operations and review of the literature. *Annals of Thoracic Surgery*, **28**, 354–8.

Rivera-Manrique, E., Castro-Salomo, A., Azon-Masoliver, A. and Marin, L. M. (1998). Cholesterol embolism: a fatal complication after thrombolytic therapy for acute myocardial infarction. *Archives of Internal Medicine*, **158**, 1575.

Roberts, W. N., De Meo, J. H. and Breitbach, S. A. (1994). Well-imaged large vessel vasculitis attributed to anticardiolipin antibody. *Arthritis and Rheumatism*, **37**, 1254–7.

Robinson, K., Mayer, E. and Jacobsen, D. W. (1994). Homocysteine and coronary artery disease. *Cleveland Clinic Journal of Medicine*, **61**, 438–50.

Rodriguez-Serna, M., Botella-Estrada, R., Chabas, A., *et al.* (1996). Angiokeratoma corporis diffusum associated with beta-mannosidase deficiency. *Archives of Dermatology*, **132**, 1219–22.

Roe, S. M., Graham, L. D., Brock, W. B. and Barker, D. E. (1994). Calciphylaxis: early recognition and management. *American Surgeon*, **60**, 81–6.

Rogers, E. W., Weyman, A. E., Noble, R. J. and Bruins, S. C. (1978). Left atrial myxoma infected with *Histoplasma capsulatum*. *American Journal of Medicine*, **64**, 683–90.

Roh, S. and Gertner, E. (1997). Digital necrosis in acquired immune deficiency syndrome vasculopathy treated with recombinant tissue plasminogen activator. *Journal of Rheumatology*, **24**, 2258–61.

Rolfs, A., Bottcher, T., Zschiesche, M., *et al.* (2005). Prevalence of Fabry disease in patients with cryptogenic stroke: a prospective study. *Lancet*, **366**, 1794–6.

Rosansky, S. J. (1982). Multiple cholesterol emboli syndrome. *Southern Medical Journal*, **75**, 677–80.

Rosenberg, D. M., Ferrans, V. J., Fulmer, J. D., *et al.* (1980). Chronic airflow obstruction in Fabry's disease. *American Journal of Medicine*, **68**, 898–905.

Rosenstein, E. D. and Kramer, N. (1994). Occult subacute thyroiditis mimicking classic giant cell arteritis. *Arthritis and Rheumatism*, **37**, 1618–20.

Ross, G., Kuwamura, F. and Goral, A. (1993). Association of Fabry's disease with femoral head avascular necrosis. *Orthopedics*, **16**, 471–3.

Roux, S., Grossin, M., De Brandt, M., Palazzo, E., Vachon, F., *et al.* (1995). Angiotropic large cell lymphoma with mononeuritis multiplex mimicking systemic vasculitis. *Journal of Neurology, Neurosurgery and Psychiatry*, **58**, 363–6.

Rowe, J. W., Gilliam, J. I. and Warthin, T. A. (1974). Intestinal manifestations of Fabry's disease. *Annals of Internal Medicine*, **81**, 628–31.

Rowshani, A. T., Schot, L. J. and ten Berge, I. J. (2004). c-ANCA as a serological pitfall. *Lancet*, **363**, 782.

Rumbaugh, C. L., Bergeron, R. T., Fang, H. C. and McCormick, R. (1971a). Cerebral angiographic changes in the drug abuse patient. *Radiology*, **101**, 335–44.

Rumbaugh, C. L., Bergeron, R. T., Scanlan, R. L., *et al.* (1971b). Cerebral vascular changes secondary to amphetamine abuse in the experimental animal. *Radiology*, **101**, 345–51.

Ryan, T. J. and Wilkinson, D. S. (1986). Cutaneous vasculitis; angiitis. In *Textbook of dermatology* (Rook, A., Wilkinson, D. S., Ebling, F. J. G., Champion, R. H. and Burton, J. L., eds), pp. 1121–85. Blackwell Scientific.

Rybka, S. J. and Novick, A. C. (1983). Concomitant carotid, mesenteric and renal artery stenosis due to primary intimal fibroplasia. *Journal of Urology*, **129**, 798–800.

Sack, K. (1998). The difficulties of differentiating vasculitis from its mimics. *Cleveland Clinic Journal of Medicine*, **65**, 550–2.

Sack, K. E. (1993). When vasculitis is not vasculitis. *Hospital Practice Office Edition 28*, **94**, 97–100, 103.

Sack, K. E. (1997). Mimickers of vasculitis. In *Arthritis and allied conditions* (Koopman, W. J. ed.), 1525–46. Philadelphia, Lea and Febiger.

Salgado, P., Rojas, R. and Sotelo, J. (1997). Cysticercosis. Clinical classification based on imaging studies. *Archives of Internal Medicine*, **157**, 1991–7.

Salvarani, C., Gabriel, S. E., Gertz, M. A., Bjornsson, J., Li, C. Y. and Hunder, G. G. (1994). Primary systemic amyloidosis presenting as giant cell arteritis and polymyalgia rheumatica [see comments]. *Arthritis and Rheumatism*, **37**, 1621–6.

Sammaritano, L. R., Gharavi, A. E. and Lockshin, M. D. (1990). Antiphospholipid antibody syndrome: immunologic and clinical aspects. *Seminars in Arthritis and Rheumatism*, **20**, 81–96.

Sanborn, T. A., Faxon, D. P., Waugh, D., *et al.* (1982). Transluminal angioplasty in experimental atherosclerosis. Analysis for embolization using an in vivo perfusion system. *Circulation*, **66**, 917–22.

Savader, S. J., Savader, B. L. and Drewry, G. R. (1988). Hypothenar hammer syndrome with embolic occlusion of digital arteries. *Clinical Radiology*, **39**, 324–5.

Savige, J. A., Yeung, S. P., Davies, D. J., Ebeling, P. and Hunt, D. H. (1988). Anti-neutrophil cytoplasmic antibodies associated with atrial myxoma [letter]. *American Journal of Medicine*, **85**, 755–6.

Schapira, D., Nahir, A. M. and Hadad, N. (2002). Interferon-induced Raynaud's syndrome. *Seminars in Arthritis and Rheumatism*, **32**, 157–62.

Schievink, W. (1997). A surgeon with a nasty taste in his mouth. *Lancet*, **350**, 260.

Schievink, W. I., Bjeornsson, J., Parisi, J. E. and Prakash, U. B. (1994a). Arterial fibromuscular dysplasia associated with severe alpha 1-antitrypsin deficiency [see comments]. *Mayo Clinic Proceedings*, **69**, 1040–3.

Schievink, W. I., Prakash, U. B., Piepgras, D. G. and Mokri, B. (1994b). Alpha 1-antitrypsin deficiency in intracranial aneurysms and cervical artery dissection [see comments]. *Lancet*, **343**, 452–53.

Schiffmann, R., Kopp, J. B., Austin, H. A., 3rd, *et al.* (2001). Enzyme replacement therapy in Fabry disease: a randomized controlled trial. *Journal of the American Medical Association*, **285**, 2743–9.

Schmidley, J. W. (1993). Neurological presentations of atrial myxoma. *Heart Disease and Stroke*, **2**, 483–6.

Schwarz, G. A., Schwartzman, R. J. and Joyner, C. R. (1972). Atrial myxoma. Cause of embolic stroke. *Neurology*, **22**, 1112–21.

Selhub, J., Jacques, P. F., Bostom, A. G., *et al.* (1995). Association between plasma homocysteine concentrations and extracranial carotid-artery stenosis [see comments]. *New England Journal of Medicine*, **332**, 286–91.

Selzer, A., Sakai, F. J. and Popper, R. W. (1972). Protean clinical manifestations of primary tumors of the heart. *American Journal of Medicine*, **52**, 9–18.

Serdaru, M., Chiras, J., Cujas, M. and Lhermitte, F. (1984). Isolated benign cerebral vasculitis or migrainous vasospasm? *Journal of Neurology, Neurosurgery and Psychiatry*, **47**, 73–6.

Seyle, H. (1962). *Calciphylaxis*. Chicago, University of Chicago Press, pp. 1–16.

Sheibani, K., Battifora, H., Winberg, C. D., *et al.* (1986). Further evidence that malignant angioendotheliomatosis is an angiotropic large-cell lymphoma. *New England Journal of Medicine*, **314**, 943–8.

Sheth, K. J. and Bernhard, G. C. (1979). The arthropathy of Fabry disease. *Arthritis and Rheumatism*, **22**, 781–3.

Shim, S., Yoo, D. H., Lee, J. K., Koh, H. K., Lee, S. R., *et al.* (1998). Multiple cerebellar infarction due to vertebral artery obstruction and bulbar symptoms associated with verticle subluxation and atlanto-occipital subluxation in ankylosing spondylitis. *Journal of Rheumatology*, **25**, 2464–8.

Shimizu, J., Inatsu, A., Oshima, S. and Kubota, T. (2004). Unique angiopathy after herpes virus infection. *Journal of Rheumatology*, **31**, 925–30.

Sienknecht, C., Whetsell, W. O. and Pollock, P. (1995). Intravascular malignant lymphoma (malignant angioendotheliomatosis) mimicking primary angiitis of the central nervous system. *Journal of Rheumatology*, **22**, 1769–70.

Sijpkens, Y., Westendorp, R., van Kemenade, F., van Duinen, S. and Breedveld, F. (1997). Vasculitis due to cholesterol embolism. *American Journal of Medicine*, **102**, 302–3.

Silbert, P., Bartleson, J. D., Miller, G. M., Parisi, J. E., Goldman, M. S., *et al.* (1995). Cortical petechial hemorrhage, leukoencephalopathy, and subacute dementia associated with seizures due to cerebral amyloid angiopathy. *Mayo Clinic Proceedings*, **70**, 477–80.

Siltanen, P., Tuuteri, L., Norio, R., Tala, P., Ahrenberg, P. and Halonen, P. I. (1976). Atrial myxoma in a family. *American Journal of Cardiology*, **38**, 252–6.

Simpson, D. M. and Tagliati, M. (1994). Neurologic manifestations of HIV infection [published erratum appears in Ann Intern Med 1995 Feb 15;122 4,317] [see comments]. *Annals of Internal Medicine*, **121**, 769–85.

Singh, A. K. and Wetherley-Mein, G. (1977). Microvascular occlusive lesions in primary thrombocythaemia. *British Journal of Haematology*, **36**, 553–64.

Slater, C. A., Sickel, J. Z., Visvesvara, G. S., Pabico, R. C. and Gaspari, A. A. (1994). Brief report: successful treatment of disseminated acanthamoeba infection in an immunocompromised patient [see comments]. *New England Journal of Medicine*, **331**, 85–7.

Slavin, R., Saeki, K., Bhagavan, B., Maas, A. E. (1995). Segmental arterial mediolysis: a precursor to fibromuscular dysplasia? *Modern Pathology*, **8**, 287–94.

Sloan, M. A., Kittner, S. J., Rigamonti, D. and Price, T. R. (1991). Occurrence of stroke associated with use/abuse of drugs. *Neurology*, **41**, 1358–64.

Slovut, D. P. and Olin, J. W. (2004). Fibromuscular dysplasia. *New England Journal of Medicine*, **350**, 1862–71.

Smith, K. J., Skelton, H. G. D., James, W. D., *et al.* (1990). Cutaneous histopathologic findings in 'antiphospholipid syndrome'. Correlation with disease, including human immunodeficiency virus disease. *Archives of Dermatology*, **126**, 1176–83.

Smith, M. C., Ghose, M. K. and Henry, A. R. (1981). The clinical spectrum of renal cholesterol embolization. *American Journal of Medicine*, **71**, 174–80.

Smith, S. B. and Arkin, C. (1972). Cryofibrinogenemia: incidence, clinical correlations, and a review of the literature. *American Journal of Clinical Pathology*, **58**, 524–30.

Sneddon, I. B. (1965). Cerebro-vascular lesions and livedo reticularis. *British Journal of Dermatology*, **77**, 180–5.

Somer, T. and Finegold, S. (1995). Vasculitides associated with infections, immunization, and antimicrobial drugs. *Clinical Infectious Diseases*, **20**, 1010–36.

Soubrier, M. J., Dubost, J. J. and Sauvezie, B. J. (1994). POEMS syndrome: a study of 25 cases and a review of the literature. French Study Group on POEMS Syndrome. *American Journal of Medicine*, **97**, 543–53.

Sprabery, A. T., Newman, K. and Lohr, K. M. (1994). Aortic mural thrombus presenting as pseudovasculitis. *Chest*, **106**, 282–3.

Spring, M. W., Hartley, B., Scoble, J. E. and Viberti, G. C. (1998). A man with diabetes and unexplained renal failure. *Lancet*, **352**, 956.

St. John Sutton, M. G., Mercier, L. A., Giuliani, E. R. and Lie, J. T. (1980). Atrial myxomas: a review of clinical experience in 40 patients. *Mayo Clinic Proceedings*, **55**, 371–6.

Stampfer, M. J. and Malinow, M. R. (1995). Can lowering homocysteine levels reduce cardiovascular risk? [editorial; comment] [see comments]. *New England Journal of Medicine*, **332**, 328–9.

Stanton, R. C. and Nickeleit, V. (1996). Case records of the Massachusetts General Hospital. *New England Journal of Medicine*, **334**, 973–9.

Stebbing, J., Askin, F., Fishman, E. and Stone, J. (1999). Pulmonary manifestations of ulcerative colitis mimicking Wegener's granulomatosis. *Journal of Rheumatology*, **26**, 1617–21.

Stein, J. H. and McBride, P. E. (1998). Hyperhomocysteinemia and atherosclerotic vascular disease: pathophysiology, screening, and treatment. off. *Archives of Internal Medicine*, **158**, 1301–6.

Stephens, C. J. (1991). The antiphospholipid syndrome. Clinical correlations, cutaneous features, mechanism of thrombosis and treatment of patients with the lupus anticoagulant and anticardiolipin antibodies. *British Journal of Dermatology*, **125**, 199–210.

Stoane, L., Allen, J. H., Jr. and Collins, H. A. (1966). Radiologic observations in cerebral embolization from left heart myxomas. *Radiology*, **87**, 262–6.

Stokes, J. B., Bonsib, S. M. and McBride, J. W. (1996). Diffuse intimal fibromuscular dysplasia with multiorgan failure. *Archives of Internal Medicine*, **156**, 2611–4.

Stone, G. C., Wall, B. A., Oppliger, I. R., *et al.* (1989). A vasculopathy with deposition of lambda light chain crystals. *Annals of Internal Medicine*, **110**, 275–8.

Stone, J., Pomper, M. G., Hellmann, D. B. (1998). Histoplasmosis mimicking vasculitis of the central nervous system. *Journal of Rheumatology*, **25**, 1644–8.

Sundy, J. and Haynes, B. (1995). Pathogenic mechanisms of vessel damage in vasculitis syndromes. *Rheumatic Disease Clinics of North America*, **21**, 861–81.

Suwanwela, C. and Suwanwela, N. (1972). Intracranial arterial narrowing and spasm in acute head injury. *Journal of Neurosurgery*, **36**, 314–23.

Suzuki, J. and Takaku, A. (1969). Cerebrovascular moyamoya disease. Disease showing abnormal net-like vessels in base of brain. *Archives of Neurology*, **20**, 288–99.

Symbas, P. N., Abbott, O. A., Logan, W. D. and Hatcher, C. R., Jr. (1971). Atrial myxomas: special emphasis on unusual manifestations. *Chest*, **59**, 504–10.

Takeuchi, K. and Shimizu, K. (1957). Hypogenesis of bilateral internal carotid arteries. *No To Shinkei*, **9**, 37–43.

Tapia, J. and Schumacher, J. (1993). Case records of the Massachusetts General Hospital. New *England Journal of Medicine*, **329**, 117–24.

Taylor, L., Hauty, M. G., Edwards, J. M. and Porter, J. M. (1987). Digital ischemia as a manifestation of malignancy. *Annals of Surgery*, **206**, 62–8.

Tazelaar, H. D., Locke, T. J. and McGregor, C. G. (1992). Pathology of surgically excised primary cardiac tumors. *Mayo Clinic Proceedings*, **67**, 957–65.

Teepe, R. G., Broekmans, A. W., Vermeer, B. J., Nienhuis, A. M. and Loeliger, E. A. (1986). Recurrent coumarin-induced skin necrosis in a patient with an acquired functional protein C deficiency. *Archives of Dermatology*, **122**, 1408–12.

Thadhani, R. I., Camargo, C. A., Jr., Xavier, R. J., Fang, L. S. and Bazari, H. (1995). Atheroembolic renal failure after invasive procedures. Natural history based on 52 histologically proven cases. *Medicine* (Baltimore), **74**, 350–8.

Thomas, E. W. P. (1964). Chapping and chilblains. *Practioner*, **193**, 775–60.

Thomas, M. H. (1981). Myxoma masquerading as polyarteritis nodosa. *Journal of Rheumatology*, **8**, 133–7.

Thomas, P. and Lowitt, N. R. (1995). A traumatic experience. *New England Journal of Medicine*, **333**, 307–10.

Thomas, R., Vuitch, F. and Lakhanpal, S. (1994). Angiocentric T cell lymphoma masquerading as cutaneous vasculitis. *Journal of Rheumatology*, **21**, 760–2.

Thomas, V. H. and Hopkins, I. J. (1972). Arteriographic demonstration of vascular lesions in the study of neurologic deficit in advanced Haemophilus influenzae meningitis. *Developmental Medicine and Child Neurology*, **14**, 783–7.

Tjia, T. L., Yeow, Y. K. and Tan, C. B. (1985). Cryptococcal meningitis. *Journal of Neurology, Neurosurgery and Psychiatry*, **48**, 853–8.

Tolosa-Vilella, C., Ordi-Ros, J., Vilardell-Tarres, M., Selva-O'Callaghan, A. and Jordana-Comajuncosa, R. (1990). Raynaud's phenomenon and positive antinuclear antibodies in a malignancy [see comments]. *Annals of the Rheumatic Diseases*, **49**, 935–6.

Tomsick, T. A., Lukin, R. R., Chambers, A. A. and Benton, C. (1976). Neurofibromatosis and intracranial arterial occlusive disease. *Neuroradiology*, **11**, 229–34.

Torrens, J. K., McWhinney, P. H. and Tompkins, D. S. (1999). A deadly thorn: a case of imported melioidosis. *Lancet*, **353**, 1016.

Travers, R. L., Allison, D. J., Brettle, R. P. and Hughes, G. R. (1979). Polyarteritis nodosa: a clinical and angiographic analysis of 17 cases. *Seminars in Arthritis and Rheumatism*, **8**, 184–99.

Trentham, D. E., Masi, A. T. and Marker, H. W. (1976). Polyneuropathy and anasarca: evidence for a new connective-tissue syndrome and vasculopathic contribution. *Annals of Internal Medicine*, **84**, 271–4.

Turakhia, A. K. and Khan, M. A. (1990). Splinter hemorrhages as a possible clinical manifestation of cholesterol crystal embolization. *Journal of Rheumatology*, **17**, 1083–6.

Tzeng, D. Z., Fein, J., Boe, N. and Chan, A. (2005). A pregnant woman with headaches, seizures, and hypertension. *Lancet*, **365**, 2150.

Ueki, K., Meyer, F. B. and Mellinger, J. F. (1994). Moyamoya disease: the disorder and surgical treatment. *Mayo Clinic Proceedings*, **69**, 749–57.

Vanley, C. T., Aguilar, M. J., Kleinhenz, R. J. and Lagios, M. D. (1981). Cerebral amyloid angiopathy. *Human Pathology*, **12**, 609–16.

Vassa, N., Twardowski, Z. J. and Campbell, J. (1994). Hyperbaric oxygen therapy in calciphylaxis-induced skin necrosis in a peritoneal dialysis patient. *American Journal of Kidney Diseases*, **23**, 878–81.

Vatz, K. A., Scheibel, R. L., Keiffer, S. A. and Ansari, K. A. (1974). Neurosyphilis and diffuse cerebral angiopathy: a case report. *Neurology*, **24**, 472–6.

Vayssairat, M., Debure, C., Cormier, J. M., Bruneval, P., Laurian, C. and Juillet, Y. (1987). Hypothenar hammer syndrome: seventeen cases with long-term follow-up. *Journal of Vascular Surgery*, **5**, 838–43.

Veenendaal-Hilbers, J. A., Perquin, W. V., Hoogland, P. H. and Doornbos, L. (1988). Basal meningovasculitis and occlusion of the basilar artery in two cases of Borrelia burgdorferi infection. *Neurology*, **38**, 1317–9.

Veugelers, M., Bressan, M., McDermott, D. A., *et al.* (2004). Mutation of perinatal myosin heavy chain associated with a Carney complex variant. *New England Journal of Medicine*, **351**, 460–9.

Viard, J. P., Lesavre, P., Boitard, C., *et al.* (1988). POEMS syndrome presenting as systemic sclerosis. Clinical and pathologic study of a case with microangiopathic glomerular lesions. *American Journal of Medicine*, **84**, 524–8.

Victor, D. I. and Green, W. R. (1976). Temporal artery biopsy in herpes zoster ophthalmicus with delayed arteritis. *American Journal of Ophthalmology*, **82**, 628–30.

von Bonsdorff, B., Groth, H. and Packalen, T. (1938). On the presence of a high-molecular crystallizable protein in blood serum in myeloma. *Folia Haematol* (Leipz), **59**, 184–208.

Wachter, R. M., Burke, A. M. and MacGregor, R. R. (1984). Strongyloides stercoralis hyperinfection masquerading as cerebral vasculitis. *Archives of Neurology*, **41**, 1213–6.

Walker, D. H. and Mattern, W. D. (1980). Rickettsial vasculitis. *American Heart Journal*, **100**, 896–906.

Walker, U., Herbst, E. W., Ansorge, O. and Peter, H. H. (1994). Intravascular lymphoma simulating vasculitis. *Rheumatology International*, **14**, 131–3.

Wall, L. M. and Smith, N. P. (1981). Perniosis: a histopathological review. *Clinical and Experimental Dermatology*, **6**, 263–71.

Waxman, S. and Dove, J. T. (1969). Cryofibrinogenemia aggravated during hypothermia. *New England Journal of Medicine*, **281**, 1291–2.

Webster, E., Corman, L. C. and Braylan, R. C. (1986). Syndrome of temporal arteritis with perivascular infiltration by malignant cells in a patient with follicular small cleaved cell lymphoma. *Journal of Rheumatology*, **13**, 1163–6.

Weinstein, C., Miller, M. H., Axtens, R., Buchanan, R. and Littlejohn, G. O. (1987). Livedo reticularis associated with increased titers of anticardiolipin antibodies in systemic lupus erythematosus. *Archives of Dermatology*, **123**, 596–600.

Welch, G. N. and Loscalzo, J. (1998). Homocysteine and atherothrombosis. *New England Journal of Medicine*, **338**, 1042–50.

Wenzel, R. P., Hayden, F. G., Greoschel, D. H., *et al.* (1986). Acute febrile cerebrovasculitis: a syndrome of unknown, perhaps rickettsial, cause. *Annals of Internal Medicine*, **104**, 606–15.

Wernick, R. and Smith, D. L. (1989). Bilateral hypothenar hammer syndrome: an unusual and preventable cause of digital ischemia. *American Journal of Emergency Medicine*, **7**, 302–6.

Wheat, L. J., Batteiger, B. E. and Sathapatayavongs, B. (1990). Histoplasma capsulatum infections of the central nervous system. A clinical review. *Medicine*, **69**, 244–60.

White, W. B. and Parke, A. L. (2005). Acute pain in the tip of the index finger. *American Journal of Medicine*, **118**, 1223–4.

Wick, M. R., Mills, S. E., Scheithauer, B. W., Cooper, P. H., Davitz, M. A. and Parkinson, K. (1986). Reassessment of malignant angioendotheliomatosis. Evidence in favor of its reclassification as intravascular lymphomatosis. *American Journal of Surgical Pathology*, **10**, 112–23.

Wickbom, G. I. and Davidson, A. J. (1967). Angiographic findings in intracranial actinomycosis. A case report and consideration of pathogenesis. *Radiology*, **88**, 536–7.

Williams, P. L., Johnson, R., Pappagianis, D., *et al.* (1992). Vasculitic and encephalitic complications associated with Coccidioides immitis infection of the central nervous system in humans: report of 10 cases and review. *Clinical Infectious Diseases*, **14**, 673–82.

Wilson, D. M., Salazer, T. L. and Farkouh, M. E. (1991). Eosinophiluria in atheroembolic renal disease. *American Journal of Medicine*, **91**, 186–9.

Winter, W. J. (1957). Atheromatous emboli; a cause of cerebral infarction. *Archives of Pathology*, **64**, 137–42.

Wold, L. E. and Lie, J. T. (1980). Cardiac myxomas: a clinicopathologic profile. *American Journal of Pathology*, **101**, 219–40.

Woods, G. and Goldsmith, J. (1990). Aspergillus infection of the central nervous system in patients with acquired immunodeficiency syndrome. *Archives of Neurology*, **47**, 181–4.

Woolfson, R. G. and Lachmann, H. (1998). Improvement in renal cholesterol emboli syndrome after simvastatin. *Lancet*, **351**, 1331–2.

Wu, S. M., Min, Y., Ostrzega, N., Clements, P. J. and Wong, A. L. (2005). Lymphomatoid granulomatosis: a rare mimicker of vasculitis. *Journal of Rheumatology*, **32**, 2242–5.

Yamamoto, M., Aoyagi, M., Fukai, N., Matsushima, Y. and Yamamoto, K. (1998). Differences in cellular responses to mitogens in arterial smooth muscle cells derived from patients with moyamoya disease. *Stroke*, **29**, 1188–93.

Yamashita, M., Oka, K. and Tanaka, K. (1983). Histopathology of the brain vascular network in moyamoya disease. *Stroke*, **14**, 50–8.

Yankner, B., Skolnik, P. R., Shoukimas, G. M., Gabuzda, D. H., Sobel, R. A., *et al.* (1986). Cerebral granulomatous angiitis associated with isolation of human T-lymphotophic virus type III from the central nervous system. *Annals of Neurology*, **20**, 362–4.

Young, D. K., Burton, M. F. and Herman, J. H. (1986). Multiple cholesterol emboli syndrome simulating systemic necrotizing vasculitis. *Journal of Rheumatology*, **13**, 423–6.

Yufe, R., Karpati, G. and Carpenter, S. (1976). Cardiac myxoma: a diagnostic challenge for the neurologist. *Neurology*, **26**, 1060–5.

Zuber, J., Martinez, F., Droz, D., Oksenhendler, E. and Legendre, C. (2002). Alpha-interferon-associated thrombotic microangiopathy: a clinicopathologic study of 8 patients and review of the literature. *Medicine* (Baltimore), **81**, 321–31.

Index